Bone, Joints, and Soft Tissues—cont'd

Continued

Bone, Joints, and Soft Tissues—cont'd

PATHOLOGY	FIGURES	PATHOLOGY	FIGURES
Osteitis condensans illi	7-126, 17-65	Reticulohistiocytosis	19-5
Osteoblastoma	13-21, 17-48	Rheumatoid arthritis	9-2, 9-3, 9-4, 9-5, 9-6, 9-7,
Osteochondritis dissecans	8-11, 10-238, 10-239, 10-240,		9-8, 9-9, 9-10, 9-11, 9-12,
	10-241, 10-242, 10-243,		9-13, 9-16, 9-17, 9-18, 9-19,
	10-244, 11-1, 11-2, 11-3, 11-4		9-20, 9-24, 9-25, 9-149, 17-8,
Osteochondroma	10-120, 13-64, 13-65, 13-66,		17-22, 18-25, 19-6, 19-7, 19-8
	13-67, 13-72, 13-73, 17-51,	Rib fracture	10-22, 10-69, 10-70, 10-71,
	18-6, 18-7, 19-45, 20-5, 25-19,		10-72, 10-73, 10-74, 10-75,
	27-50		10-76
Osteogenesis imperfecta	8-33, 8-34, 19-1, 19-26	Rickets	14-35, 14-36, 14-37, 14-38,
Osteoid osteoma	13-17, 13-18, 13-19, 13-20, 18-55		14-40, 18-14, 18-61
Osteoma	13-15, 13-16, 16-13	Rotator cuff tendonopathy	10-114, 20-17, 20-18
Osteomalacia	14-33, 14-34	Sacroiliitis	9-12, 9-38, 9-39, 9-66, 17-66,
Osteopetrosis	8-35, 8-36, 8-37, 17-61,		17-67
	17-81, 17-82, 19-36, 20-1	Salter-Harris fracture	10-24, 10-25, 10-26, 10-27,
Osteopoikilosis	13-14		10-218
Osteoporosis	9-29, 10-13, 14-22, 14-23,	Sarcoidosis	19-19
	14-24, 14-25, 14-26, 14-27,	Scaphoid fracture	10-140, 10-142, 20-22, 20-138,
	19-24, 19-28, 15-25		20-139, 20-141
Osteosarcoma	13-23, 13-24, 13-25, 13-26,	Scaphoid subluxation	10-150, 10-152
	13-27, 13-28, 13-29, 18-42	Scapula fracture	10-101, 10-102, 10-103
Osteosclerosis	18-43, 19-35, 19-37, 19-41	Scheuermann's disease	8-39, 8-40, 8-41, 8-42, 17-79
Paget's disease	15-25, 15-26, 15-27, 15-28,	Schmorl's nodes	7-85, 7-81, 7-96, 7-97, 8-39,
	15-29, 15-30, 15-31, 15-32,		9-113, 9-114, 9-115, 17-80
	15-33, 15-34, 15-35, 15-36,	Scleroderma	9-31, 9-32, 9-33, 9-34, 18-2,
	15-37, 15-38, 15-39, 15-40,		19-50, 19-51
	15-41, 15-42, 15-43, 16-1,	Scoliosis	15-45, 15-46, 15-47, 15-48,
	16-26, 17-12, 17-42, 18-46,		15-49, 15-55, 15-56, 17-69
	19-32	Scurvy	14-41, 14-42, 14-43, 18-15,
Paracondylar process	7-10		18-62
Pars interarticularis fracture	10-80, 10-259	Sesamoid bone fracture	10-227, 10-228
Patella fracture	10-200, 20-38, 10-199	Shoulder impingement syndrome	10-114
Pectus excavatum	7-143, 7-144, 7-145	Sickle cell anemia	11-30, 11-31, 11-32, 17-3,
Pellegrini-stieda disease	19-47, 9-99		17-75, 17-85
Pelvic fracture	10-21, 10-173, 10-174,	Simple bone cyst	10-16, 13-159, 13-160, 13-161,
	10-175, 10-176, 10-177,		13-162, 13-163, 13-164,
	10-178, 10-179, 10-180		13-165, 13-166, 13-167,
Periosteal chondroma	18-52		13-168, 13-169, 18-23, 18-24
Phalanx dislocation	10-129, 10-168, 10-169	Sinusitis	16-17
Phalanx fracture	10-14, 10-26	Six lumbar vertebra	7-104
Pigmented villonodular synovitis	13-113, 13-114	Skull fracture	10-12
Plasmacytoma	13-30, 13-31, 13-32, 13-33	Slipped capital femoral epiphysis	10-246, 10-247
Platyspondylia	8-2, 8-22, 8-39	Spina bifida occulta	7-26, 7-34, 7-63, 7-98, 7-99,
Polydactyly	7-157		7-100, 7-101, 7-136
Ponticulus posticus	7-24, 7-25	Spondyloepiphyseal dysplasia	17-73
Posterior cruciate ligament tear	10-206	Spondylolisthesis	9-120, 10-248, 10-249, 10-250,
Protrusio acetabulum	8-33, 19-1, 19-2, 19-3, 19-4		10-251, 10-252, 10-253,
Pseudohypoparathyroidism	14-15, 14-16, 14-17		10-254, 10-255, 10-256,
Pseudopseudohypothyroidism	14-18		10-257, 10-258, 10-260,
Psoriatic arthritis	9-68, 9-70, 9-71, 9-72, 9-74,		10-261, 10-262, 10-263, 17-21
	9-75, 9-76, 9-78, 9-79,	Sprung pelvis	10-185
	9-80, 17-26, 19-10, 19-11	Sternal fracture	10-77
Pyknodysostosis	8-38, 16-11, 18-4, 19-37	Straight back syndrome	7-150
Radial fracture	10-125, 10-123, 10-128, 10-131	Stress fracture	10-18, 10-19, 10-20, 10-21,
Radiation necrosis	17-83, 17-84		10-22, 10-23
Red marrow Re-conversion	20-35	Sturge-Weber syndrome	16-15
Reiter's disease	9-60, 9-61, 9-62, 9-63, 9-64,	Stylohyoid ligament ossification	7-13, 7-14
	9-65, 9-66, 9-67, 19-12	Subchondral cysts	9-3, 9-8, 9-101, 9-148, 19-13,
Renal osteodystrophy	14-39		9-118, 9-119, 18-25

Bone, Joints, and Soft Tissues—cont'd

PATHOLOGY	FIGURES	PATHOLOGY	FIGURES
Subperiosteal hemorrhage	18-54	Transitional segments	7-108, 7-109, 7-110
Supracondylar process	10-118	Triquetrum fracture	10-147, 10-148
Swan-Neck deformity	9-6	Tumoral calcinosis	19-54, 19-55
Synovial osteochondromatosis	13-115, 13-116, 13-117, 13-118	Ulna fracture	10-131, 10-132, 10-122, 10-121,
Synovial sarcoma	13-119, 13-120		10-129
Syphilis	9-200, 9-201, 9-203, 12-1,	Uncinate process degeneration	9-128, 9-129, 9-130, 9-131,
	12-2, 18-57		9-178
Systemic lupus erythematosus	11-9, 19-9	Vacuum phenomena	9-109, 9-110, 9-111, 9-112,
Teardrop fracture	10-47, 10-48, 10-60, 10-92		9-117, 17-32, 9-103, 9-104
Tethered cord syndrome	20-12	Vertebral compression fracture	8-33, 10-15, 10-84, 10-85,
Thalassemia	11-33, 16-12, 19-25, 19-43		10-86, 10-87, 10-89, 10-90,
Tibia fracture	10-23, 10-201, 10-202,		17-20, 17-21
	10-218, 10-219, 20-39, 20-40	Wrist fibrocartilage tears	10-158
Torus fracture	10-11, 10-137, 10-145, 10-146,		
	10-144		

Chest

PATHOLOGY	FIGURES	PATHOLOGY	FIGURES
Adult respiratory distress syndrome	27-45	Pleural effusion	23-12, 23-13, 23-15, 23-16, 24-1
		Pneumonia	21-22, 24-1 through 24-12,
Asbestosis	26-3, 26-4, 26-5		24-14 through 24-17, 24-28,
Aspergillosis	24-14, 24-28		26-1
Atelectasis	22-2, 22-4, 22-7, 23-21, 24-27,	Pneumothorax	26-6, 26-7, 26-8, 26-9
	26-6, 27-3	Pulmonary abscess	24-2
Azygous fissure	21-15, 21-16	Pulmonary aneurysm	27-24
Bronchiectasis	22-8, 22-9, 27-1	Pulmonary arteriovenous malformation	23-9, 27-48
Bronchogenic carcinoma	25-1, 25-2, 25-3, 25-4, 25-7,	Pulmonary consolidation	24-1, 24-9, 24-12, 24-14, 24-17,
	25-8, 25-9, 25-10, 25-11,		24-18, 26-1, 27-13, 27-14
	25-12, 25-15, 25-16, 25-17,	Pulmonary edema	23-11, 23-19, 26-1, 27-46, 27-47
	25-25-29, 25-32, 25-37,	Pulmonary infarct	27-15
	27-2, 27-13, 27-19, 27-27,	Pulmonary nodules	25-13, 25-21, 25-22, 25-23,
	27-43, 27-49		25-24, 25-25, 25-28
Coarctation of aorta	23-8	Sarcoidosis	26-10, 26-11, 27-18, 27-21,
Congestive heart failure	23-10, 23-11, 23-21		27-22, 27-23
Cystic fibrosis	27-16	Septic emboli	27-28
Emphysema	22-12, 22-13, 22-14, 22-16, 27-5	Silicosis	26-5
Extrapleural sign	21-20	Substernal thyroid	25-45
Ganglioneuroma	27-41	Teratoma	25-44, 27-38
Granulomas	21-3, 21-4, 24-20, 24-23,24-24,	Thymoma	25-46
	24-25, 24-26, 25-26	Tracheal carcinoma	22-6
Hamartoma	25-33	Tuberculosis	12-3, 21-4, 24-18, 24-19, 24-21,
Hemothorax	26-6, 26-7, 26-8, 26-9		24-22, 24-23, 24-24, 24-26,
Histoplasmosis	24-20, 24-26		24-27, 24-28
Lipoma	27-35	Wegener's granulomatosis	27-29, 27-52
Lipomediastinum	27-36, 27-40		
Lymphoma	25-34, 25-35, 25-36, 27-20		
Mesothelioma	25-43		

Continued

Pathology Quick Reference—cont'd

Abdomen

PATHOLOGY	FIGURES	PATHOLOGY	FIGURES
Abscess	32-30	Horse-Shoe kidneys	32-59
Adrenal calcification	32-18	Hydatid cyst	31-10, 31-11, 31-12, 31-13
Adrenal carcinoma	32-45	Intraperitoneal gas	32-29
Adrenal cyst	32-15	Intrauterine device	32-70
Aortic aneurysm	17-49, 17-50, 17-15, 23-3, 23-5, 23-6, 23-7, 31-1, 31-2, 31-3, 31-4, 31-6, 31-7, 31-9, 32-9, 32-16, 32-49	Lithopedion	32-78
		Mesenteric cyst	32-51
		Mesenteric node calcification	32-23
		Nephroblastoma	29-2
Appendicolith	32-1	Nephrolithiasis	29-5, 29-6
Arterial calcification	32-65, 32-66, 32-67, 32-39, 32-10, 32-9	Ovarian carcinoma	29-10, 29-11
		Pancreatic calcification	32-3, 32-20
Ascites	32-35, 32-36	Pancreatic lithiasis	30-22, 30-23
Bladder calculi	29-1, 32-8	Phleboliths	32-4, 32-63
Bladder carcinoma	32-56	Pneumobilia	32-28
Chilaiditi syndrome	32-27	Pneumoperitoneum	32-26
Colon polyps	30-8, 30-9, 30-10	Prostate enlargement	32-52
Colon carcinoma	30-11	Prostatic calculi	32-5, 32-69
Crohn's disease	30-12, 30-13, 30-14, 30-15	Renal calcification	32-19
Cystadenoma	29-9, 32-54	Renal carcinoma	29-12, 29-13, 29-14, 29-15, 32-14, 32-46
Dermoid cyst	29-7, 29-8, 32-53		
Diverticulitis	30-10, 32-76	Renal cyst	32-46
Diverticulosis	30-16, 30-17, 30-18	Small bowel obstruction	32-31, 32-32
Endometrioma	32-55	Splenic calcification	32-10, 32-13, 32-17, 32-67
Foreign objects	32-72, 32-73, 32-74, 32-75	Splenomegaly	32-38, 32-39, 32-40, 32-44
Gallbladder calcification	30-1, 30-2, 30-6, 30-7, 32-2, 32-11, 32-62, 32-36	Staghorn calculus	29-5, 32-6
		Ulcerative colitis	30-26
Gallstones	30-3, 30-4, 30-5, 32-64	Ureteral stones	32-7
Gastric carcinoma	30-24, 32-43	Uterine leiomyoma	29-16, 29-17, 29-18, 29-19, 29-20, 29-21, 29-22, 32-21
Hepatic mass	32-42		
Hepatomegaly	32-37	Vas deferens calcification	32-12
Hiatal hernia	30-19, 30-20, 30-21	Volvulus	32-33, 32-34

Brain and Spinal Cord

PATHOLOGY	FIGURES	PATHOLOGY	FIGURES
Abscess	33-6, 33-7	Pituitary adenoma	33-16
Cerebral aneurysm	33-5	Syringomyelia	33-22, 33-23
Hematoma	33-2, 33-3	Tarlov cyst	33-24, 33-25
Hemorrhage	33-1	Tumors (primary)	33-10, 33-11, 33-12, 33-13, 33-14, 33-15, 33-16, 33-17, 33-18
Infarct	33-4		
Meningiomas	33-13		
Metastasis	33-19, 33-20, 33-21		
Multiple sclerosis	33-9		

CLINICAL IMAGING

With Skeletal, Chest, and Abdomen Pattern Differentials

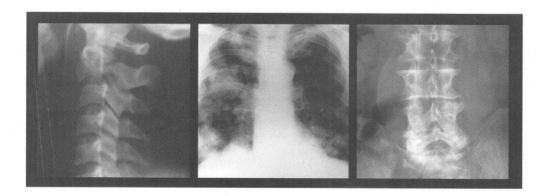

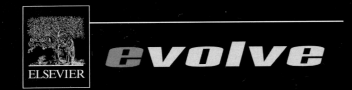

ELSEVIER

To access your Student Resources, visit the Web address below:

http://evolve.elsevier.com/Marchiori/clinicalimaging/

- **Student Image Bank**
  Based on the pathology quick reference listing in the front of the book,
  one good image for each pathology listed is provided

- **Review Questions and Answers**
  Self-tests provide extra resources for understanding the chapters.

- **Film Interpretation Checklists**
  Lateral Cervical Radiograph
  Anteroposterior Lower Cervical Radiograph
  Anteroposterior Open-Mouth Cervical Spine Radiograph
  Lateral Thoracic Radiograph
  Anteroposterior Thoracic Spine Radiograph
  Lateral Lumbar Radiograph
  Anteroposterior Lumbopelivc or Abdomen Radiograph
  Posteroanterior Chest Radiograph
  Lateral Chest Radiograph

- **Content Updates**
  New cases and information are provided on a regular basis.

- **WebLinks**
  Links to other interesting radiology sites are available.

CLINICAL IMAGING

With Skeletal, Chest, and Abdomen Pattern Differentials

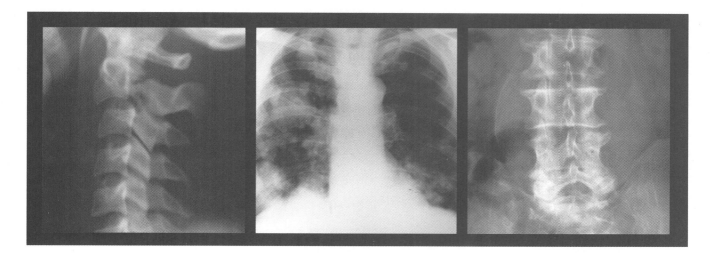

2nd edition

Dennis M. Marchiori, DC, MS, PhD (c), DACBR

Associate Professor
Department of Diagnosis and Radiology
Dean of Academic Affairs
Palmer College of Chiropractic
Davenport, Iowa

Illustrations by Mike Rekemeyer

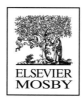

ELSEVIER
MOSBY

ELSEVIER
MOSBY

11830 Westline Industrial Drive
St. Louis, Missouri 63146

Notice

Chiropractic is an ever-changing field. Standard safety precautions must be followed, but as new research
and clinical experience broaden our knowledge, changes in treatment and drug therapy may become
necessary or appropriate. Readers are advised to check the most current product information provided by
the manufacturer of each drug to be administered to verify the recommended dose, the method and
duration of administration, and contraindications. It is the responsibility of the licensed prescriber,
relying on experience and knowledge of the patient, to determine dosages and the best treatment for each
individual patient. Neither the publisher nor the author assumes any liability for any injury and/or damage
to persons or property arising from this publication.

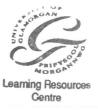

Publishing Director: Linda Duncan
Managing Editor: Christie Hart
Publishing Services Manager: Patricia Tannian
Project Manager: Sharon Corell
Senior Designer: Kathi Gosche

Printed in the United States of America

Last digit is the print number: 9   8   7   6   5   4   3   2   1

Contributors

Editor

Dennis M. Marchiori, DC, MS, PhD (c), DACBR
Associate Professor, Department of Diagnosis
   and Radiology
Dean of Academic Affairs
Palmer College of Chiropractic
Davenport, Iowa

Contributors

Tawnia L. Adams, DC, DACBR
Private Practitioner
Adams Radiology Consultants
Anchorage, Alaska

Richard Arkless, MD
President
Advanced Diagnostic Imaging Services
Seabeck, Washington
Instructor in Radiology
Western States Chiropractic College
Portland, Oregon

Linda Carlson, MS, RT
Coordinator of Radiography Instruction
Department of Diagnosis and Radiology
Palmer College of Chiropractic
Davenport, Iowa

Ray N. Conley, DC, DACBR
President, Regional MRI
President, Kansas State Board of Healing Arts
Overland Park, Kansas

Beverly L. Harger, DC, DACBR
Associate Professor and Chair
Department of Diagnostic Imaging
Western States Chiropractic College
Portland, Oregon

Lisa E. Hoffman, DC, DACBR
Assistant Professor
Department of Diagnostic Imaging
Western States Chiropractic College
Portland, Oregon

D. Robert Kuhn, DC, DACBR, ART
Professor and Chair
Clinical Science Division
Logan College of Chiropractic
St. Louis, Missouri

Tracey A. Littrell, DC
Assistant Professor
Department of Diagnosis and Radiology
Palmer College of Chiropractic
Davenport, Iowa

Gary A. Longmuir, DC, DACBR
Editor, Master of Applied Science Coordinating
Program Development Committee, Postgraduate Education
Southern California University of Health Sciences
Whittier, California

Ian D. McLean, DC, DACBR
Professor and Director, Clinical Radiology
Palmer Chiropractic Clinics
Palmer Chiropractic College
Davenport, Iowa

Timothy J. Mick, DC, DACBR, FICC
Associate Professor
Department of Radiology
Director, Radiological Consultation Service
Northwestern College of Chiropractic
Bloomington, Minnesota

Robert Percuoco, DC
Professor
Department of Diagnosis and Radiology
Palmer College of Chiropractic
Davenport, Iowa

Cynthia Peterson, RN, DC, DACBR, M.Med.Ed.
Professor and Chair
Department of Radiology
Canadian Memorial Chiropractic College
Toronto, Ontario, Canada

Gary D. Schultz, DC, DACBR
Vice President of Academic Affairs
Southern California University of Health Sciences
Whittier, California

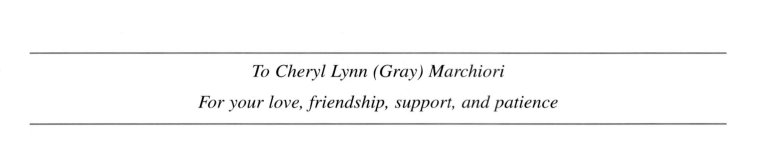

To Cheryl Lynn (Gray) Marchiori

For your love, friendship, support, and patience

Foreword to the First Edition

Although many excellent books deal with the several phases of radiology, this book takes a unique approach that is particularly valuable to students and nonradiologists.

Dr. Marchiori's Clinical Imaging is based on a gamut, or pattern, approach to radiology. The interpreter begins by using radiological signs to develop a differential list of possible diagnoses and then progresses to traditional discussions of the several diseases or conditions that are within that differential list. Until now, there has not been a book available that incorporates both pattern differentials and detailed traditional discussions of diseases in such a comprehensive format. This is the approach that I have tried to teach to students, particularly radiology residents, over the years. This book follows the approach to radiological interpretation that is usually used in clinical practice and is therefore valuable for students and helpful for practitioners who do not have the depth of radiological knowledge possessed by those whose primary practice is in radiological interpretation.

By enlisting the skills of contributors to cover areas in which they have particular expertise, Dr. Marchiori has produced a book that I feel will be welcomed by teachers, students, and many clinicians. The chapter outlines and quick-reference features make it easy to use. The approach to pattern recognition is simplified over that found in other books that deal with this subject. The disease chapters have sufficient depth to meet the needs of those in general clinical practice.

I congratulate Dr. Marchiori and his contributors on producing a book that will find its way into the libraries of many clinicians, chiropractic colleges, and students in training.

Joseph W. Howe, DC, DACBR, FACCR, FICC
Professor of Radiology;
Former Chairman, Radiology Department,
Los Angeles College of Chiropractic,
Whittier, California;
Former Chairman, Radiology Department,
National College of Chiropractic,
Lombard, Illinois

Advances in medical imaging have revolutionized diagnostic capabilities over the past 2 decades. The explosion in imaging technology has vastly improved diagnostic accuracy and thus benefited patient management. However, the negative aspect of this burgeoning technology has been the increasing cost of health care delivery. Even though medical imaging accounts for approximately only 4% of the total health care budget in the United States, rising costs and over-utilization of medical imaging concerns federal agencies, third-party payors, and politicians alike. Current medical practice and reimbursement schemes no longer permit all available tests to be performed on every patient. As radiologists, we have the responsibility to ensure that the different imaging methods are not indiscriminately used but selectively chosen according to their cost effectiveness and benefit for the patient's management.

Subspecialization leads to progress in medical imaging and provides expertise in the performance and interpretation of examinations in particular areas of radiology. However, when individuals need examinations in multiple areas, subspecialization requires many more radiologists than are needed. Under present financial constraints, subspecialization has become a luxury that is only affordable in a few major academic centers, even if it is recognized that radiology would be best served by individuals with expertise in a single area. With subspecialists participating in after-hours call, coverage within their department and consultation in areas outside their expertise become problematic. A subspecialty can be compared to a "feather in a cap" that is of little use without the cap.

A variety of excellent texts in all subspecialties dealing either with a specific imaging modality or a selective organ system is currently available. Texts in general radiology are fewer in number and tend to be either disease or pattern oriented. An imaging pattern is for a radiologist what a symptom is for a clinician. *From the Symptom to the Diagnosis* is a German text written by my former teacher, Walter Hadorn, Chairman of Internal Medicine at the University of Bern, Switzerland, that impressed me as a medical student by its practicality and usefulness. The book survived its author and is now in its eighth edition.

Correlation of an imaging pattern with clinical and laboratory findings was introduced by Fraser and Paré in 1970 with the original edition of their outstanding text entitled *Diagnosis of Diseases of the Chest*. These authors added a chapter to their text that comprised 17 tables of differential diagnosis with all the basic roentgenographic patterns of chest disease. Descriptions of specific imaging findings to be expected for a specific diagnosis as well as differential points aided the radiologist in arriving at a likely diagnosis and reasonable differential diagnosis. Using this concept, Martti Kormano and I introduced the first text covering the entire field of conventional radiology. This imaging pattern approach in tabular form has since been adopted by many authors, and we feel complimented by the old cliché, "Imitation is the sincerest form of flattery."

In his text, Dennis Marchiori has garnered contributions from an outstanding group of radiologists who represent the broad areas of subspecialization. The book is a successful attempt to combine the elements of a standard disease-oriented text with the pattern-oriented approach. Until Dennis Marchiori undertook this task, no publication fulfilled this need. The text provides a basic approach to both performance and interpretation of various imaging studies and can be recommended as an introductory text for the first year resident as well as reference book for general radiologists or subspecialists outside their area of expertise. Dennis Marchiori is to be congratulated on recognizing this need and carrying out the task of putting together such an outstanding text that combines the pattern with the more traditional disease-oriented approach.

Francis A. Burgener, MD
Professor of Radiology,
University of Rochester Medical Center,
Rochester, New York

As we enter the third century of clinical imaging, practitioners worldwide rely on noninvasive examinations of internal structures to diagnose disease and guide treatment. Popular tomographic methods, computer processing, and alternative forms of energy have not replaced the basic method used to depict Frau Roentgen's hand in 1895.

Recognition of anatomical silhouettes and tissues' characteristic patterns of x-ray absorption changed clinical practice forever. Simple x-ray photography remains by far the most important diagnostic technique for examination of the skeleton, chest, and abdomen.

Clinical Imaging: With Skeletal, Chest, and Abdomen Pattern Differentials builds its clinical teachings on the foundation of introductory chapters, efficiently covering the fundamentals of modern imaging technology. The strengths, weaknesses, pitfalls, and artifacts of clinical imaging are illustrated well.

This text usefully organizes the basic image patterns that must be recognized to accurately distinguish between diseased and normal anatomy. Basic principles of image interpretation are reduced into themes that can be applied over and over during academic training and in clinical practice.

The book is organized into four body regions that have distinctive clinical problems and imaging characteristics. Common, important, and diagnostic image findings are beautifully illustrated and summarized throughout this well-organized text.

This will be a most memorable introduction to practical clinical imaging for students and clinicians alike. Enjoy!

David D. Stark, MD, FACR
Professor and Chairman,
Department of Radiology,
University of Nebraska Medical Center,
Omaha, Nebraska

Preface

The goal of this book is to assist students and practitioners of the health sciences develop a better understanding of diagnostic imaging. In particular, the content of the book emphasizes plain film radiology, and to a lesser extent, magnetic resonance imaging. Currently, there are many excellent radiology books available, but the approach of this book is unique. The majority of currently available books employ a traditional approach. That is, diseases are presented individually within chapters devoted to broad categories (e.g., congenital, arthritides, tumor, trauma, etc.). However, a traditional design does not parallel strategies of diagnostic image interpretation.

Rather than publishing another exhaustive library of images and detailed descriptions, our efforts target the learner. We designed a textbook that will augment the connection between the findings on the image and the interpreter's need for clinical information. Interpreting radiographs, or other diagnostic images, begins with scanning the studies for abnormality. Once found, the abnormality is classified into broad patterns that suggest a list of differential diagnoses. Unfortunately, most traditional books do little to bridge the transition from image to differential diagnosis. It is a particularly serious deficit for nonradiologist interpreters, who are less familiar with the possible causes of a particular imaging presentation.

Our book is structured to help students and clinicians recognize patterns of abnormality and develop a list of related viable diagnostic possibilities. This is accomplished by allowing the reader to begin with the image presentation and progress to the responsible disease, rather than requiring the reader to begin with the disease and progress to the image presentation. Many currently available books that utilize a "pattern approach" leave out crucial detail about a particular disease. To avoid this limitation, we have combined the utility of a pattern approach with the detailed descriptions of disease entities found in more traditional designs. This provides an easy to use, comprehensive radiology resource for clinicians and students of the health sciences.

This book is divided into five parts: introduction, skeleton, chest, abdomen, and brain and spinal cord. A thumbnail along the right border of the book demarcates each section. The skeletal, chest, and abdomen parts are further subdivided into disease chapters and pattern chapters. Disease chapters follow a traditional design, presenting selected entities of a disease category (e.g., tumors, infections, trauma). Most disease entities are listed alphabetically and in a structured format of background, imaging findings, clinical comments, and key concepts, facilitating the reader's use of these chapters. The pattern chapters, found in the second portion of the skeletal, chest, and abdomen parts, consist of multiple tables of disease entries grouped by similarity of radiographic appearance, and for many of the chapters, subcategorize the entries as common or less common. The pattern or gamut approach of these chapters functions in two ways. First, it facilitates correlation between diseases of similar radiographic appearance. For instance, if the book is used as a textbook, readers will begin with the disease chapters and, after becoming familiar with the individual disease topics, will consult the pattern chapters as a capstone to their learning, to integrate similar appearances of individual diseases. Second, the pattern chapters will assist clinicians in developing a workable list of diseases that may be responsible for radiographic presentations they encounter. The list of differentials can be narrowed by reading the short comments that accompany each table entry. In addition, a page number accompanying most table entries in the pattern chapters refers the reader to a page in the disease chapters where more detailed descriptive information can be found. In particular, clinicians will find the clinical comments section of the disease chapters useful for patient management decisions. A glossary of radiological terms, figure tables, and mnemonics are also included within the book, and should prove to be a helpful learning aid to both students and clinicians.

This second edition is not merely an update of the content of the first edition, but rather an extensive rewrite. New to this edition are comprehensive chapters on the topics of normal anatomy and normal variants. Competence in these topics provides a foundation to image interpretation and, although the topics were covered in the first edition, we felt an expanded presentation was necessary. Also, we have provided a unique chapter on film interpretation and report writing, inclusive of checklists and identifying areas of the film that warrant particular attention during film interpretation. We feel this chapter will help novice and seasoned interpreters sharpen their skills and understand the process of image interpretation. Each chapter has been reworked, and the patient positioning, trauma, arthritides, and bone tumor chapters have been extensively reorganized and expanded. The last chapter on brain and spinal cord has been extensively expanded. Hundreds of new images and drawings have been added to illustrate the points made in the text.

In our preparation of the first, and now the second, edition we have resisted the tendency to become repetitious in our writing. Rather, every attempt was made to produce a concise, user-friendly resource for those in training, as well as those in clinical practice.

Dennis M. Marchiori

Acknowledgments to the First Edition

The completion of this project is due to the unselfish efforts of many individuals. My wife Cheryl is the first and foremost on the list of those I would like to acknowledge. Although she is not listed as a contributor, her involvement was certain and necessary. She assumed responsibility for nearly everything in our lives, allowing me to concentrate on this book. This task became especially arduous following the birth of our daughter Isabella, near the beginning of this three-year effort. Without the contributors, this book would not be worth reading; without Cheryl, there would not be a book.

I am especially fortunate to have been raised by very nurturing and loving parents, Phillip Valentino Marchiori and M. Judy (Bundy-Marchiori) Wymer. My late father was truly an inspiring man. He worked very hard to give his children opportunities that were not available to him. No one would be more proud of this book than my dad. We all miss him very much. Every child needs someone in their life who is irrationally devoted to them. I am lucky enough to be my mother's son and receive this kind of love.

There were few surprises on this project. Going into it, I thought it might be a lot of work. No surprise, it was. However, working with the contributors was surprising. All of the contributors were extremely enthusiastic and steadfast in their commitment. It was always a bit puzzling to me why many of them were so anxious to spend hundreds of hours working on their contributions for so little conventional reward. I have concluded they understand the importance of scholarship and are dedicated to their professions and to the topic of radiology. Each contributor has added an integral part to this book. Their contributions vary in size, but not in importance. I would also like to acknowledge their families and colleagues whose efforts and sacrifices are certainly nested within each contribution. The contributors' efforts have done more than produce a book; we have formed friendships and other collaborations that will extend into the future.

Ian McLean's writing is limited to the sections dealing with magnetic resonance imaging, but his influence is far greater. Ian introduced several of us on this project to the topic of radiology. Sometimes it is difficult to know where information gained from his teachings end, and our own thoughts begin.

Martha Sasser, Amy Christopher, Cathy Comer, and all of the staff at Mosby-Year Book, Inc. deserve special recognition. From my first phone conversation with Martha, to review of the last page proofs with Amy and Cathy, I found the entire experience to surpass any preconceived ideal I held going into the project.

Mike Daiuto is my research work-study, and with my wife, was the closest thing to staff we had on the book. He was particularly helpful in obtaining the citations for each chapter. His cheerful, easy manner was always appreciated. Mike Rekemeyer produced the line art illustrations. He turned the assignments around quickly and his rendition was always better than what I had envisioned. Jim Bandes photographed and developed a third of the half-tone illustrations; his dedication to detail is appreciated.

Most of the imaging studies in this book came from three sources. The first is Palmer Chiropractic Clinics. The second and third were personal libraries compiled by Joseph Howe and the combined efforts of Steven Brownstein and William Litterer. These individuals deserve tremendous recognition for compiling these collections which have assisted me and so many other students and authors over the past years.

Don Betz, Iftikar Bhatti, Robert (Bucky) Percuoco, Bill Meeker, and Clay McDonald provided the environment for this project to be conceived and completed. I admire each of these individuals for their strong commitment to educational excellence, faculty development, and our institution. As with most projects I am involved with, I found the advice and inspiration from my friend and colleague Chuck Henderson to be of particular value.

Palmer College has a proud tradition of excellence in chiropractic. The Palmers and other early fathers of the chiropractic profession underwent tremendous personal sacrifice to bring chiropractic to the world. It is in this proud tradition that we present this book. We hope this book helps students better serve their studies, teachers better serve their students, and practitioners better serve their patients.

Dennis M. Marchiori

Acknowledgments to the Second Edition

I begin acknowledgments of this second edition by reiterating my thanks to all those who contributed so importantly to the first edition. Their efforts are directly responsible for the first edition's tremendous success and have provided a firm foundation to accomplish the intended improvements of the second edition.

Talented academic people are always busy, with many available projects from which to choose. I am delighted and honored to have many of the contributors from our first edition dedicate the time, once again, to write for this book. I am equally pleased to incorporate the scholarly expertise of Linda Carlson, Ray Conley, Tracy Littrell, and Gary Longmuir into the project. Like the other contributors, each of these individuals has provided substantial effort to create an exceptional result. I also want to thank the contributors' families. Unfortunately, but very truly, the time and energy required to produce scholarship is nearly always diverted from family or leisure activities.

Efforts to revise the first edition began almost immediately after it was published. Many behind-the-scenes helpers provided tremendous support in advancing this second edition. I praise the following individuals for their undying contributions of time and talent. Organizing the case material was the first step in the revision process. Sean Mathers copied and organized much of the original case material and made it easier for me and the contributors to find the desired images. The need to update our pathology files to digital media presented an underestimated challenge. Heather Ganske provided the energy and expertise necessary to accomplish a large portion of this Herculean task. Laura Avitt also provided important assistance to this undertaking. The timeliness of their availability could not have been scripted better. Heather Wyant provided hundreds of hours of clerical work related to reference citations and the pathology table in the front of the book. Julie-Marthe Grenier gathered interesting case material from Palmer College's teaching clinics and provided detailed content reviews and suggestions for many of the chapters. Bryan Laneville spent countless hours writing on-line self-assessment questions that accompany the book chapters and provide an important learning resource for our readers. In addition to Sharon Corell and other Elsevier editors, the authors, and myself, the process of proofreading pages was accomplished by Drs. John Stites, Julie-Marthe Grenier, Tawnia Adams, Ian McLean, and Bob Rowell. The comments and attention to detail of all of these individuals is much appreciated. Vince De Bono is a friend and colleague who contributed immensely by writing the first edition's radiographic positioning chapter. His work influenced this second edition's chapter, written by Linda Carlson.

The images for the first edition were gathered from multiple sources. The greatest number of images were obtained from five collections: the first compiled by Dr. Joseph Howe, the second representing the combined collection of Drs. William Litterer and Steven Brownstein, the third constituting cases from the teaching clinics and radiology departments at Palmer College of Chiropractic, the fourth comprising cases provided by Dr. Ian D. Mclean, and the fifth including images from my personal collection. Dr. Joseph Howe is a living legend in the chiropractic profession. His professional work as the "teacher of the teachers" of radiology within the chiropractic profession is simply unparalleled. William Litterer and Steven Brownstein's shared film collection is immense, comprising more than 5 000 film cases and many times that number of slides and other media. These doctors' hard work and obvious dedication to radiology, chiropractic, and generosity to Palmer College have enabled me to bring their knowledge to thousands of students and practitioners. Who knows the ultimate magnitude of their work's impact on practitioners and the patients served? Dr. Litterer has passed away, and all will miss the delightfully engaging colleague and scholar of radiology. Dr. Steven Brownstein continues to practice radiology, collect cases, and teach, continuing the legacy Dr. Litterer established for both of them. Thank you, Dr. Brownstein, for all you have given to promote this book and its embedded goals.

I convey special thanks to Reed Phillips, Gary Schultz, and others at the Southern California College of Heath Sciences for their dedication to archiving case material and providing me access to their holdings, inclusive of the Joseph Howe teaching collection. Once the first edition was published, I was amazed at how many interesting cases were sent to me from various sources for possible inclusion in the second edition. Many of the cases do appear in this revision, and those contributions are recognized with credit lines accompanying the related images. Most notable is my appreciation to Gary Longmuir, who sent nearly 100 cases. Each of his cases was of special interest and excellent quality, and all but a few are included in this revision. Similarly, a brief query to my colleagues soliciting case material related to the chest prompted John Taylor to send 90 pounds of case material to Iowa. I remain overwhelmed by this generosity. Dr. Taylor's own book, *Skeletal Imaging,* is particularly known for its excellent collection of images, and I am thrilled to showcase other portions of his collection in my chapters. Good examples of pathology are not easily obtained. I thank the hundreds of doctors, students, and others who also provided images. Our readers will learn and grow from their contributions. I also acknowledge Bryan Hosler for supplying numerous hard-to-obtain images for the brain and spinal cord topics.

I am extremely fortunate that this text is an Elsevier title, providing me the opportunity to work with the highest caliber of professionals. Sharon Corell, Colin Odell, Kim Alvis, Kellie White, and everyone at Elsevier, especially my managing editor Christie Hart, were outstanding partners in this work. Christie exhibited the perfect balance of an uncompromising, assertive editor and a facilitating, encouraging friend. Working with her has been one of the most enjoyable aspects of this project. Her influence and ideas appear throughout this book and are greatly appreciated.

I would also like to thank my friends and co-workers Linda Carlson, Kevin Cunningham, Ian McLean, Pam Mullin, Robert "Bucky" Percuoco, Don Gran, and Dan Weinert for providing support and encouragement throughout the years of this project. Bucky Percuoco wrote an exceptional first chapter, which provides this book with firm initial footing; in addition, his good sense and intuition helped me navigate through many of the obstacles encountered during this project. Ian McLean is the behind-the- scenes Renaissance man of this project, acting as image archivist, author, and marketer. In addition to his outstanding contributions of Chapters 2 and 20, Ian provided extensive reviews and critiques of the contents and approach of the book. On the topic of radiology, for me and many others, he is our most valued counsel. I would also like to thank my graduate advisor, Al Henkin, for his always-valued advice related to this project and for specifically coordinating the schedule of my graduate work around this project. As always, my mother continues to be one of my strongest supporters, and although she does not entirely understand why this book was written or what function it might serve, she is absolutely positive that her son's book is the best one available … now and forever.

Lastly, and most reverently, I reserve the greatest outpouring of appreciation to my wife Cheryl for putting her aspirations on hold to advance mine. Her seemingly unending patience and understanding about this project and all the projects and diversions that have come before and during, and those likely to come after, underscore Cheryl's incredible importance to me as my amazing life partner. I am blessed with and completed by her love, support, and companionship. I thank our children Isabella, Sophia, Anthony, and Olivia for their patience during my time of absence. Perhaps an apology is more appropriate for the many times this book project deviated my valued attention from them. The sacrifices my family made so that readers could benefit from a more informed text hardly seemed worth it at times. Unfortunately, to accomplish such projects, it takes nearly exclusive focus and dedication. I've appreciated the fact that my family did not remind me too often over the last few years of my inverted sense of responsibility.

Dennis M. Marchiori

Contents

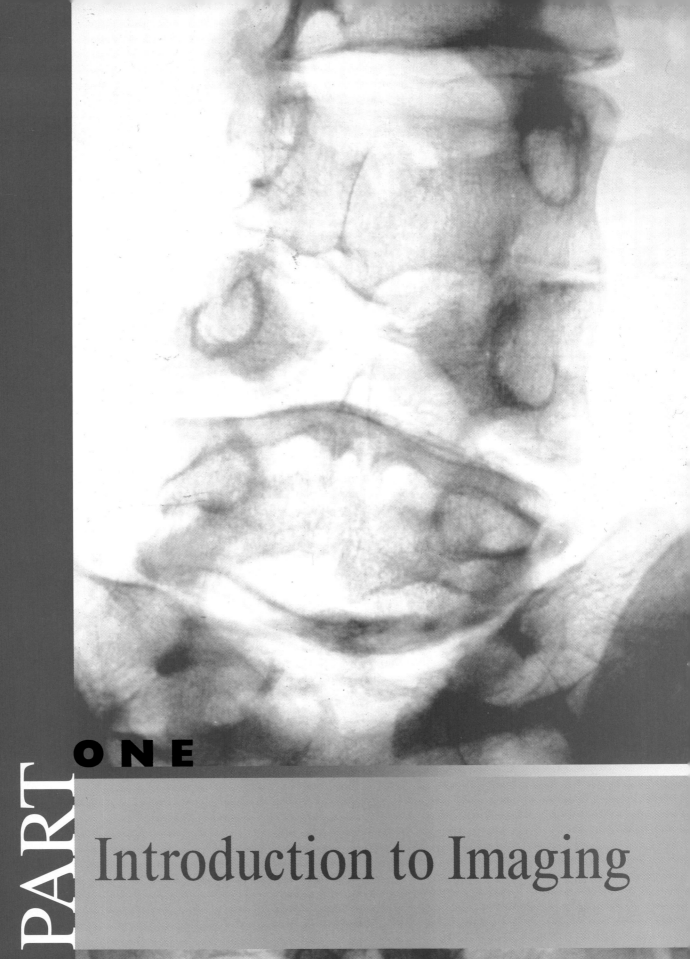

PART ONE

Introduction to Imaging

chapter 1

Plain Radiographic Imaging

ROBERT PERCUOCO

Concepts of Radiation

X-RAY DISCOVERY

X-rays were discovered by Wilhelm Konrad Roentgen on November 8, 1895, in Würzburg, Germany. As he activated a simple cathode ray tube, called *Crookes' tube,* he happened to observe visible light emanating from a nearby plate coated with a phosphorescent substance, barium platinocyanide. Light emission increased as he brought the plate closer to the tube. He found that the newly discovered ray passed through objects of various compositions. Roentgen named the strange phenomenon *x-light,* with *x* representing the unknown. The name *x-ray* was later adopted, although some called it a "roentgen ray" in honor of Roentgen.

PROPERTIES OF X-RAYS

Within months of Roentgen's discovery, he had uncovered nearly every property of x-rays known today. X-rays have the following properties:
• They are a type of electromagnetic radiation with neither mass nor charge that travel in straight lines at the speed of light.
• They travel in packets, or bundles, called *photons* or *quanta.*
• They produce chemical and biologic effects in matter because of their ionizing capability.
• They cause certain materials to fluoresce.
• They sensitize radiographic and photographic film.
• They cannot be detected by human senses.
• They produce secondary and scatter radiation.
• They obey the inverse square law, which describes changes in intensity over distance.
• They are absorbed by heavy, dense materials, such as lead and cement.
• They have a wave/particle dual nature.
• Because of their extremely short wavelengths, they penetrate materials that normally absorb or reflect light.
• They cannot be focused by a lens.
X-ray is a form of electromagnetic radiation that is produced when high-speed electrons in an electric circuit interact with a hard metal surface. The interaction takes place at the subatomic level and involves the electrical attributes of an atom.

ATOMIC STRUCTURE

In 1913 the German physicist Niels Bohr compared the atom with a miniature solar system. Current theories have evolved beyond the Bohr atom; however, Bohr's theory works well for illustrating and understanding atomic forces. Basically, Bohr described the atom as having a dense core, or *nucleus,* made up of neutrons and positively charged protons. Negatively charged electrons, spinning on their axes, orbit the nucleus at fixed distances called *quantum shells* or *energy levels.* Quantum shells are assigned the letters *K, L, M, N,* and so on, with *K* being the innermost shell (Fig. 1-1). Electrons occupying shells farther away from the nucleus have greater *potential energy* than those found closer to the nucleus.

In a neutral atom the number of protons in the nucleus, or *atomic number* (Z), is equal to the number of orbiting electrons. The maximum number of electrons occupying a given shell is determined by the formula $2n^2$, where *n* is the quantum shell number. The quantum shell number is obtained by counting the shells outward from the nucleus. The *K* shell ($n = 1$) can hold $2(1)^2$, or two, electrons; the *L* shell ($n = 2$) can hold $2(2)^2$, or eight, electrons; and so on. The outermost shell, or *valence shell,* never exceeds eight electrons at one time in a stable atom.

Positively charged nuclear protons exert an electrostatic attractive force that binds electrons to their orbit. Electron spin velocity counters the attractive force and keeps electrons at discrete distances from the nucleus. Electrons occupying shells closer to the nucleus are bound tighter. The amount of energy needed to remove an electron completely from its orbit is called *electron binding energy.* Electron binding energy is measured in *electron volts* (eV), the same units used to describe x-ray energy. A free electron is assumed to have zero binding energy; therefore a bound electron is in a negative energy state, because it takes positive energy to unbind or raise the binding energy to zero. Electrons occupying shells closer to the nucleus have greater binding energy than those found farther from the nucleus. The binding energy for any given electron increases as atomic number increases (Fig. 1-2).

3

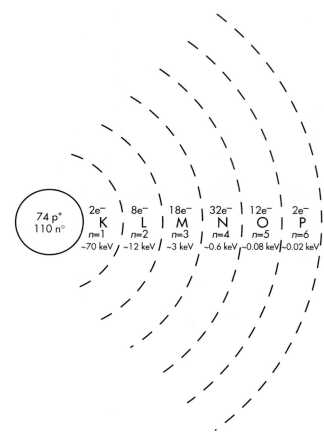

FIG. I-I   The closer an electron is to the nucleus, the stronger its attraction (binding energy) is to the nucleus.

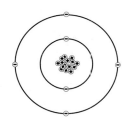

CARBON $\binom{12}{6}C$		
Shell	Number of electrons	Approximate binding energy (keV)
K	2	0.284
L	4	0.006

FIG. I-2   Atomic shell levels and estimated electron binding energies for carbon and tungsten. Inner shell electrons are more tightly bound than are the outer shell electrons.

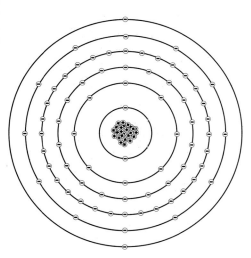

TUNGSTEN $\binom{184}{74}W$		
Shell	Number of electrons	Approximate binding energy (keV)
K	2	69.525
L	8	12.100
M	18	2.820
N	32	0.595
O	12	0.077
P	2	–

RADIATION

Energy is defined as the ability to do work. When energy is transmitted through space or matter, it is called *radiation*. Radiation takes on many forms, such as heat, light, and sound. Its energy often is described in the ability or inability to ionize matter. *Ionizing radiation* possesses sufficient energy to remove an orbital electron from a stable atom or molecule. X-rays, gamma rays, and alpha and beta particles are examples of ionizing radiation. *Nonionizing radiation* falls short of causing ionization; however, it may excite stable atoms by raising an orbital electron to a higher energy state. This type of radiation includes visible light, infrared rays, microwaves, and radio waves. Ionizing radiation is categorized as either *particle* or *electromagnetic* radiation.

Particle radiation. Particle radiation is made up of any subatomic particles, such as protons, neutrons, and high-speed electrons, capable of causing ionization. Alpha and beta particles are two of the more common types of particle radiation. They come from the nuclei of radioactive atoms through radioactive decay. Particle radiation has a mass component, may have a charge, and travels at varying speeds (slower than the speed of light).

Electromagnetic radiation. Electromagnetic radiation (EM) is an electric and magnetic disturbance traveling through space at the speed of light (2.998×10^8 m/s). It contains neither mass nor charge but travels in packets of radiant energy called *photons*, or *quanta*. Examples of EM radiation include radio waves and microwaves, as well as infrared, ultraviolet, gamma, and x-rays. Some sources of EM radiation include the cosmos (e.g., the sun and stars), radioactive elements, and manufactured devices. Electromagnetic radiation exhibits a dual *wave/particle nature*.

Electromagnetic radiation travels in a waveform at a constant speed. The wave characteristics of EM radiation are found in the relationship of *velocity to wavelength* (the straight line distance of a single cycle) and *frequency* (cycles per second, or hertz, Hz), expressed in the formula

$$c = \lambda v$$

where c = velocity, λ = wavelength, and v = frequency.

Because the velocity is constant, any increase in frequency results in a subsequent decrease in wavelength. Therefore wavelength and frequency are *inversely proportional*. All forms of EM radiation are grouped according to their wavelengths into an electromagnetic spectrum, seen in Figure 1-3.

The particle-like nature of EM radiation manifests in the interaction of ionizing photons with matter. The amount of energy *(E)* found in a photon is equal to its frequency *(v)* times Planck's constant *(h)*:

$$E = vh$$

Photon energy is *directly proportional* to photon frequency. Photon energy is measured in eV or keV (kilo electron volts). The energy range for diagnostic x-rays is 40 to 150 keV. Gamma rays, x-rays, and some ultraviolet rays possess sufficient energy (>10 keV) to cause ionizations.

The energy of EM radiation determines its usefulness for diagnostic imaging. Because of their extremely short wavelengths, gamma rays and x-rays are capable of penetrating large body parts. Gamma rays are used in radionuclide imaging. X-rays are used for plain film and computed tomography (CT) imaging. Visible light is applied to observe and interpret images. Magnetic resonance imaging (MRI) uses *radiofrequency* EM radiation as a transmission medium (see Fig. 1-3).

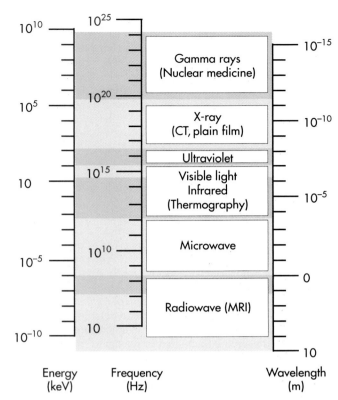

FIG. 1-3 The energy, frequency, and wavelength of the electromagnetic spectrum and their associated imaging modalities.

RADIATION UNITS OF MEASUREMENT

Four units used to measure radiation are the *roentgen* (R), *rad, rem,* and *curie*. The roentgen is a measurement of *radiation exposure,* or intensity, which creates 2.08×10^9 ion pairs in a cubic centimeter (cm³) of air. The SI system (Système Internationale d'Unités) is a modernized metric system based on meters-kilograms-seconds or centimeters-grams-seconds. The SI units are used more broadly in science and most countries of the world than are the British, or Customary, units of feet-pounds-seconds. The SI unit for radiation exposure is *coulombs/kilogram* (C/kg); 1 roentgen is equal to 2.58×10^{-4} C/kg. Radiation exposure emitted from x-ray machines is measured in roentgens or C/kg.

The *rad* is the unit that measures *absorbed dose*. It is a measure of energy (expressed in ergs) deposited into a mass of tissue (expressed in grams or kilograms) and is often related to the biologic effects of radiation. One rad is equal to 100 ergs in 1 gram of irradiated tissue. The SI unit for absorbed dose is the *gray* (Gy). One gray is equal to 100 rads. One rad is equal to 0.01 gray, or 1 *centigray* (cGy).

The unit that defines *absorbed dose equivalent* for humans is the *rem* (rad equivalent man). The rem is used exclusively for radiation protection reporting of occupational exposure. It is a measure of the biologic effectiveness of different types of radiation in humans. Compared with x-rays and gamma rays, radiation such as alpha and beta particles and fast neutrons produces different magnitudes of biologic effects, even at the same absorbed dose.

The National Council on Radiation Protection and Measurements (NCRP) is the governing body responsible for reporting guidelines for radiation protection and measurements. The most recent report, *NCRP No. 116: Limitations of Exposure to Ionizing Radiation,* which succeeds NCRP report No. 91, replaces the term *dose equivalent (H)* with the term *equivalent dose (H_{TR})*. The change goes beyond word semantics. Dose equivalent *(H)* is a measurement of absorbed dose at some certain location in tissue. Equivalent dose *(H_{TR})* is a measurement of an *average absorbed dose* in tissues and organs. Equivalent dose is the product of the average absorbed dose *(D_{TR})* of radiation *(R)* in a tissue *(T)* and a radiation weighting factor *(W_R):*

$$H_{TR} = W_R D_{TR}$$

The weighting factor replaces the previously used *quality factor* (QF) and accounts for the biologic effectiveness of specific types of radiation. The weighting factor for x-rays and gamma rays is 1; 1 rad of x-rays is equal to 1 rem. Alpha particles have a W_R of 20; 1 rad of alpha particles is equal to 20 rems. The SI unit for the rem is the *sievert* (Sv). A sievert is the product of the absorbed dose in grays and the radiation weighting factor. One Sv is equal to 100 rems, and 1 rem is equal to 10 mSv.

The *curie* (Ci) is a quantitative measure of *radioactive material.* It is defined as the amount of radioactive material in which 3.7×10^{10} atoms disintegrate every second. The radiation emitted from a curie of radioactive material is measured in roentgens, rads, and rems. The SI unit is the *becquerel* (Bq), defined as 1 disintegration per second. Millicurie (mCi) and microcurie (μCi) amounts are common in nuclear medicine procedures. The reporting units used in the radiologic sciences are listed in Table 1-1.

TABLE 1-1
Units of Measure in the Radiologic Sciences

Quantity	Customary unit	SI unit
Exposure	Roentgen (R)	Coulomb/ kilogram (C/kg)
Absorbed dose	Rad (rad)	Gray (Gy)
Dose equivalent	Rem (rem)	Sievert (Sv)
Activity	Curie (Ci)	Becquerel (Bq)

X-Ray Tube

Producing x-rays requires a source of electrons, a means to rapidly accelerate them, and a means to rapidly decelerate them. These factors are built into the x-ray apparatus. The three principal components of an x-ray machine are the *x-ray tube, generator,* and *control console.*

TUBE HOUSING

The *tube housing* is a grounded, lead-lined metal shelter that protects and supports the glass x-ray tube insert (Fig. 1-4). X-rays are emitted multidirectionally from the tube, but only those rays passing through an opening, or *port window,* in the housing expose the patient. All other rays are trapped in the housing wall, thereby decreasing unnecessary exposure to patients or x-ray personnel. Radiation emitted from the tube housing is called *primary radiation.*

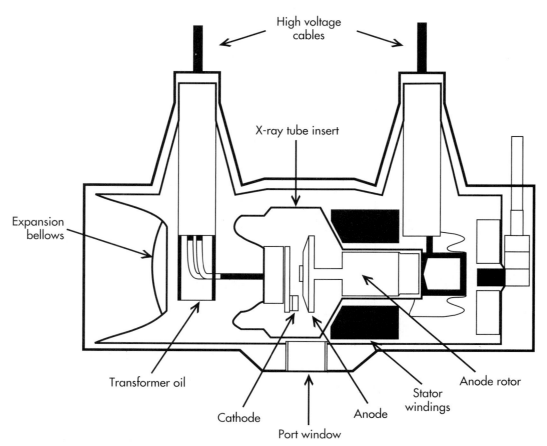

FIG. 1-4   A rotating anode x-ray tube within a housing assembly. (From Guebert G: Essentials of Diagnostic Imaging, St Louis, 1995, Mosby.)

Several high-voltage electrical cables connect through the back of the housing to the tube. The housing is factory packed with industrial grade oil to provide thermal and electrical insulation. Many modern x-ray machines have tube protection circuitry hooked into an expansion bellows inside the housing. As the oil expands with heating, the bellows trips a switch, which prohibits further exposure until the tube cools sufficiently. Industrial x-ray tubes may have a large heat exchanger that circulates and cools the oil.

GLASS ENVELOPE

X-rays are produced when high-speed electrons are rapidly decelerated in an x-ray tube. The x-ray tube is a device composed of two electrodes, *cathode* and *anode*, sealed in an evacuated borosilicate glass envelope. Electrons in an electric circuit, generated at the cathode, are accelerated toward and strike an anode target, which results mostly in heat energy and some x-ray energy. Approximately 1% of the kinetic energy of high-speed electrons produces x-rays.

Cathode. The cathode is the negative electrode and contains a *filament* embedded in a shallow depression called the *focusing cup*. Most diagnostic x-ray tubes are dual focus because they have two filaments: a large filament for exposures of high intensity and a small filament for exposures of low intensity.

The cathode *filament* supplies a controlled number of electrons to the anode. The filament is a thoriated tungsten wire drawn into a small, thin coil. Tungsten is used because its high atomic number (74) makes it electron rich. Current running through the filament heats it to white incandescence, which results in electrons being "boiled off" the tungsten by a process called *thermionic emission*. A cloud of electrons, or *space charge,* forms around the filament (Fig. 1-5). The space charge size is controlled by the amount of current running through the filament. Filament current is regulated

by the *mA (milliampere) selector* on the control console. The space charge generates *tube current* (mA), current between the cathode and anode. The tube current (mA) is directly proportional to radiation exposure or quantity of x-rays produced.

Electrons travel in only one direction in the tube, from cathode to anode. As the space charge builds, electrons repulse each other. This causes them to diverge, covering an unacceptable area on the anode. A *focusing cup* surrounding the filament carries a negative potential that tends to condense or "focus" the electron stream onto the anode target.

Anode. The anode is the positive electrode in the x-ray tube. The anode (1) produces x-rays, (2) conducts electricity, and (3) conducts heat away from the anode surface.

There are two types of anodes: *stationary* and *rotating*. Most diagnostic applications require the rotating type. The stationary anode is most applicable when a smaller electrical load is necessary for imaging (e.g., mammograph and dental radiograph).

A stationary anode consists of a copper shaft with a tungsten–rhenium target imbedded into a beveled surface (Fig. 1-6). Tungsten is used because of its high melting point (3410° C) and its high atomic number (74). The atomic number affects the ability of tungsten to produce x-rays in the diagnostic range. The beveled or angled surface affects the electron-loading capacity of the anode by providing more surface area for heat conduction. The angle on stationary anodes ranges from 30 to 45 degrees. The most common angle used on rotating anodes is 12 degrees with a useful range of 7 to 17 degrees.

A rotating anode allows significantly greater electron loading by providing a much larger surface area, or *focal track,* for heat conduction. The rotating anode consists of three component parts: (1) disc or target, (2) stem, and (3) rotor.

The disc is made of molybdenum and is covered with a tungsten–rhenium target material. An *electromagnetic induction motor* is used to rotate the anode disc an average of 3400 revolutions per minute (rpm) during the exposure, with high-speed anodes rotating at 10,000 rpm. Tube electron loading is directly proportional to anode rotation.

The stem connects the disc to the rotor and is made of copper for electrical conduction. The rotor is a shaftlike part composed of bars of copper around a soft iron core. The rotor is held in place in the tube by bearings that facilitate high-speed rotation. Outside of the evacuated glass tube and adjacent to the rotor is a series of pairs of electromagnets called a *stator.* Current running through the stator creates a magnetic field that crosses the rotor. The pairs of electromagnets are sequentially energized by multiphase current, creating a rotating magnetic field that turns the rotor (Fig. 1-7).

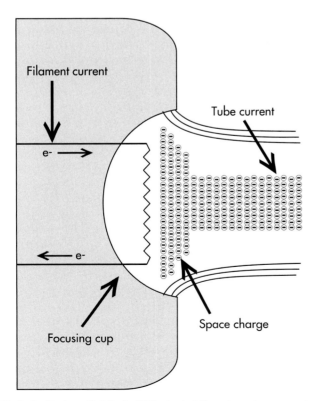

FIG. 1-5 Electrons that "boil off" the heated filament create a space charge surrounding the filament, which supplies the tube current.

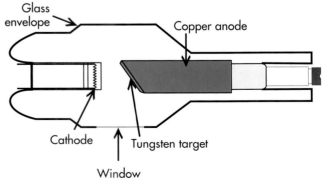

FIG. 1-6 Stationary anode x-ray tube.

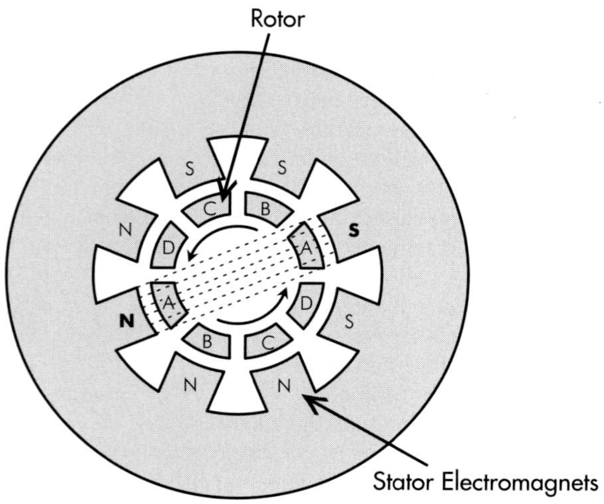

Rotor

Stator Electromagnets

FIG. 1-7   Anode rotation by electromagnetic induction. Stator electromagnets are activated in sequential pairs by multiphase current. Rotor windings move perpendicular to the magnetic lines of flux causing rotation.

Anode rotation is initiated by depressing the rotor or "prep" switch on the control console before activating the exposure. The filament circuit also is wired into the rotor switch so that filament current is boosted to preset levels at the time the rotor switch is depressed. Rotor speed and space charge are generated first in anticipation of the exposure. Depressing the exposure switch causes electrons to move from cathode to anode.

With many x-ray machines, the exposure switch alone activates all functions of the tube: rotation of the anode, creation of the space charge, and movement of electrons from cathode to anode. However, two-handed operation of the rotor and exposure switches allows the operator to control exactly when exposure occurs. Single-handed operation of the exposure switch alone is best when very fast exposure time (milliseconds) is used.

LINE-FOCUS PRINCIPLE

Electrons strike the surface of the anode at a target site called the *actual focal spot* (Fig. 1-8). An increase in either filament length or anode angle results in an increase in actual focal spot size. As the focal spot size is increased, the electrical loading capacity of the anode is increased, which safely allows exposures that require higher electrical loads. Although the entire target area emits x-rays, only those rays traveling in the direction of the patient are useful. The line-focus principle is used to reduce the effective area of the actual focal spot to that portion of the x-ray beam that is useful. The effective target area, or *effective focal spot,* is a measure of the width of the actual focal spot projected along the central ray and perpendicular to the plane of the x-ray port. As with the actual focal spot, the size of the effective focal spot is determined by the size of the filament and angle of the anode (see Fig. 1-8). Tube specifications typically are reported in effective focal spot size, which essentially is a measurement of the resolution afforded by a particular x-ray tube. In general, the smaller the effective focal spot size, the better the resolution. Effective focal spot sizes commonly used in diagnostic radiology range from 0.6 to 1 mm for small focus and 1.5 to 2 mm for large focus.

The anode angle on a rotating anode tube also determines maximum field coverage when the tube is placed at specified tube distances (Fig. 1-9). A standard angle of 12° is used for sectional imaging to cover 17 inches^2 at a 40-inch focal-spot-to-film distance. A 14° angle is needed to cover 36 inches^2 at a 72-inch focal-spot-to-film distance for scoliosis screening and other full-spine imaging needs.

Focal spot selection is linked to specific mA stations on the control console. For example, the small focal spot is coupled with mA stations below 200 mA on most diagnostic x-ray machines.

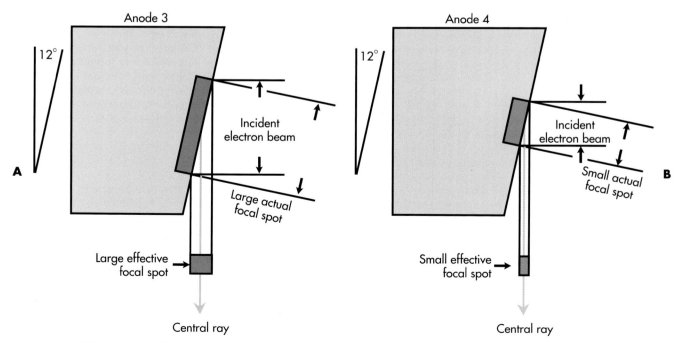

FIG. 1-8   **A** and **B,** As the filament size decreases, both actual and effective focal spots decrease in size.

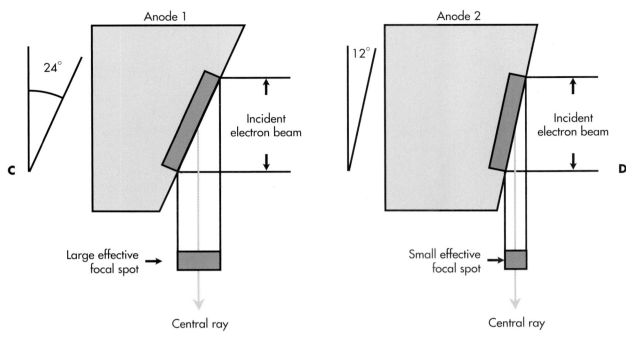

FIG. 1-8 cont'd The line-focus principle results in an effective focal spot that is smaller than the actual focal spot. **C** and **D,** As the anode angle decreases, both actual and effective focal spots decrease in size.

This limits the load on the anode and is best used with small body parts, such as the cervical spine and extremities. The large focal spot is coupled with the 200 mA and higher station to allow for greater electron loading of the anode. It is best used with large body parts, such as the lumbar spine. The small focus produces images with better detail than the large focus.

OFF-FOCUS RADIATION

Off-focus radiations results from rebounding electrons from the focal spot striking other areas of the anode, thereby producing a large low-intensity x-ray source. This extra-focal radiation increases patient dose and image blurring from shadowing, and decreases image contrast. Patient anatomy appearing outside of the exposure field (e.g., ears on a skull examination) is attributed to off-focus

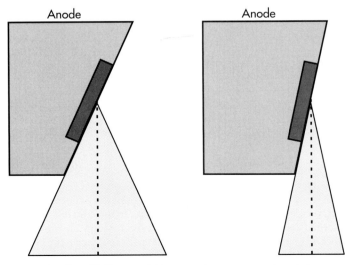

FIG. 1-9 **A** and **B,** Exposure field coverage increases as anode angle increases.

radiation. The upper fixed shutters of a *collimator* (beam-limiting device) help reduce the amount of off-focus radiation reaching the film.

HEEL EFFECT

X-ray intensity emanating from the tube is not uniform across the span of the beam. Exposure intensity is greater on the cathode side of the beam than the anode side. This is called the *anode heel effect.* Electrons penetrate the target at various depths, causing x-rays to be emitted with equal intensity in all directions. Those x-rays traveling into the substance of the anode are immediately absorbed. The angle at which x-rays emerge from the target surface toward the patient varies and causes some x-rays to be absorbed in the heel of the anode. The heel attenuates a portion of the x-ray beam and leaves less exposure (intensity) on the anode side of the beam (Fig. 1-10).

When body parts of different thicknesses are imaged, the heel effect can be used to advantage if the cathode portion of the beam is placed over the thickest part of the patient. The heel effect is less noticeable with smaller film sizes (8 × 10 inch) and longer tube distances (72-inch), because more of the central, uniform portion of the beam is used.

FILTRATION

Very-low-energy x-rays, or *soft rays,* add no diagnostic information to the image, because they are completely absorbed by the patient. To reduce patient dose from soft radiation, federal law requires a minimum of 2.5 mm equivalent of aluminum (equiv/Al) filtration for a beam greater than 70 kVp. Aluminum absorbs many of the low-energy photons while transmitting a large proportion of high-energy photons. The glass port window and oil within the tube housing provide inherent filtration of approximately 0.5 mm equiv/Al. The silver-coated mirror in the collimator is placed so that the x-ray beam must pass through it. It may supply another 1 mm equiv/Al of inherent filtration.

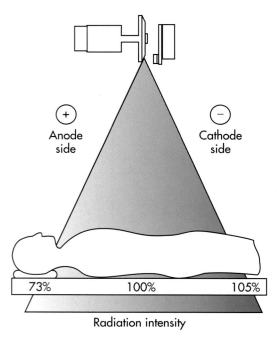

FIG. 1-10   Because of the anode heel effect, the x-ray exposure is more intense on the cathode side of the beam.

Another 2 mm of aluminum are *added* to most diagnostic x-ray machines to meet federal guidelines for total filtration. Inherent filtration plus added filtration equals *total filtration*. Compensating filters, used to offset variations in patient density, are not calculated into the total filtration needed to decrease the soft x-ray dose.

Generator (the Power to Generate X-Rays)

The electrical potential needed to accelerate electrons to high speed in the tube is provided by *single phase, three-phase,* and *constant potential (high-frequency)* generators. The scope of this chapter does not permit a detailed discussion on how these generators work; however, one must understand that the output waveform affects average x-ray energy, exposure time, and patient dose from soft radiation.

Alternating current (AC) is dispensed to the x-ray machine from an external source, but it is changed to direct current (DC) before it reaches the tube. AC manifests in electrons oscillating back and forth in a circuit and is graphically represented in Figure 1-11 by a sine wave. Each cycle of single-phase AC comprises a positive and negative pulsation. Running AC through the tube creates two problems: (1) it destroys the cathode when electrons reverse polarity during the negative pulsation, and (2) a secondary site for x-ray production is generated and negates any advantage of increased image detail produced by the line-focus principle.

AC is changed to DC through a process called *rectification*. For the purpose of this chapter, how rectification occurs is less important than why it occurs. Suppressing the negative pulsation of alternating current protects the tube and results in a type of pulsating DC called *half-wave rectification* (see Fig. 1-11). X-ray energy is produced at the peak of these pulsations (Fig. 1-12). Reversing the negative pulsation to a positive direction provides *full-wave rectification,* resulting in twice the number of pulsations per unit of time.

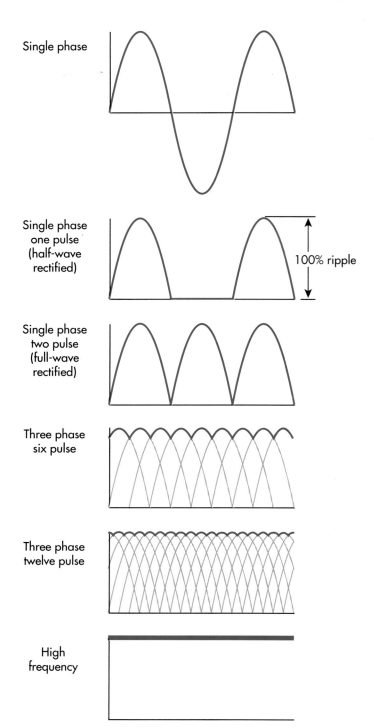

FIG. 1-11   Voltage waveforms from various types of x-ray generators. Single-phase generators produce 100% ripple, whereas high-frequency generators deliver a near-constant potential with less than 2% ripple.

This reduces the exposure time by half when compared with half-wave rectified circuits.

X-rays are produced when electrons strike the target at or near their peak potential, or *kilovolt peak* (kVp). In the case of full-wave rectified circuits, bursts of diagnostic *hard x-rays* are produced when the electrical potential reaches its peak with periods of lower energy (soft) or no x-rays produced between the peaks. The voltage drop from kVp is called *ripple* and represents the efficiency at

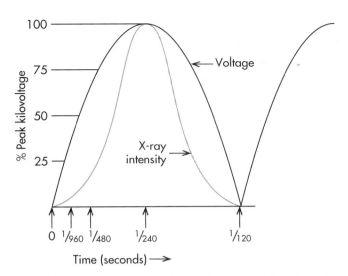

FIG. 1-12 After a slight lag, x-ray intensity increases rapidly as the voltage across the x-ray tube increases from zero to its peak value.

which x-rays are produced. The greater the ripple, the less efficient the x-ray production. A kVp of zero accompanies 100% ripple. A voltage potential that drops below peak kilovoltage produces x-ray photons with a wide spectrum of energies.

SINGLE-PHASE GENERATORS

Single-phase, full-wave rectified generators use a 220-volt, 100-amp, single-phase AC line source to produce two pulsations per cycle (120 pulsations per second), with 100% voltage ripple. With a constantly changing voltage potential, a spectrum of x-ray energies is produced with an average energy somewhere below peak kilovoltage. This pulsating beam results in an inefficient use of electricity, longer exposure time, and greater patient dose from lower-energy *soft x-rays* compared with more efficient generators that deliver a nonpulsating, constant electrical potential.

THREE-PHASE GENERATORS

A three-phase generator uses a three-phase AC line source for the purpose of creating more pulsations per unit time. This effectively reduces voltage ripple and increases efficiency of x-ray production. Three-phase power is best understood by imagining three single-phase line sources electrically intertwined to create greater incoming power. A *six-pulse generator* delivers six pulsations per cycle, which reduces voltage ripple to 13% of kVp (see Fig. 1-11). Changing the wiring configuration produces 12 pulses per cycle *(12-pulse generator)*, reducing voltage ripple to 3% of kVp. Using three-phase power results in greater photon output per unit of electrical input (mR/mAs) with higher average energy compared with single-phase units. Three-phase generators are expensive and rely on costly power line installations.

CONSTANT POTENTIAL GENERATORS

Medium- and high-frequency generators operate on either single-phase or three-phase power and virtually eliminate voltage ripple through rectification and smoothing circuits. Medium-frequency generators produce an electrical frequency in the 6- to 30-kHz range, and high-frequency generators produce an electrical frequency of approximately 100 kHz. Medium- and high-frequency generators allow more accurate control of tube voltages. Tube voltage regulates penetration of the x-ray beam. High-frequency generators deliver

the greatest mR/mAs output, the lowest soft radiation dosage to patients, the highest average (effective) x-ray energy, and the shortest exposure time.

TIMER CONTROL

Every x-ray exposure requires a certain predetermined tube current (mA) for a specific period of time. Both the timer and timer circuit are located on the control console and are electrically connected to the exposure switch.

Timers are described as mechanical, synchronous, or electronic. A simple mechanical timer is spring-loaded and unwinds at a set rate. Mechanical timers are used with single-phase, low-output x-ray generators such as those seen in dental offices. They are not very accurate and are limited to exposure times longer than ¼ second.

Synchronous timers operate from a synchronous motor running at 60 Hz. The time increments are in multiples of ¹/₆₀ second, such as ¹/₃₀, ¹/₂₀, and ¹/₁₀. The shortest exposure time is ¹/₁₂₀ second. Synchronous timers are not as accurate as electronic timers and cannot be used with serial exposures because they require a short recycling time.

An *electronic timer* is the most common timer in use today. It is accurate to less than 1 millisecond (msec) and to greater than 1 second. Electronic timers operate on sophisticated electronic circuitry by energizing a silicon-controlled rectifier (SCR), which activates the exposure. The combination of constant potential generators and very fast imaging systems (rare earth) require a timer accurate in milliseconds.

The product of mA and time, milliampere-seconds (mAs), determines the number of x-ray photons emitted and hence the relative darkness of the film. Patient part size and density govern how many mAs are needed to produce a diagnostic image. Calculating exposure by using units of mAs is common in a clinical setting. A *mAs timer* accurately provides the highest safe tube current with the shortest exposure time for a given mAs. Independent control of mA and time may not be possible with some *mAs* timers.

AUTOMATIC EXPOSURE CONTROL

Automatic exposure control (AEC), often called *phototiming,* terminates the exposure when a predetermined amount of film density (darkness) is reached by x-rays passing through the patient to the image receptor. The radiographer selects the appropriate beam penetration (kVp) and desired tube current (mA) for the part under examination. The phototiming device senses the exposure and, in response, creates an electronic signal that breaks the timer circuit.

Automatic exposure devices include the earlier photomultiplier tube and the more common ionization chamber. The photomultiplier tube converts a light signal from a fluorescent screen exposed to x-rays to an electronic signal that feeds back to terminate the exposure. The radiation-sensitive ionization chamber creates an electronic signal proportional to the number of ions produced by radiation exposure and feeds back to terminate the exposure.

The phototiming circuit usually has one, two, or three photocells of different shapes and positions in relation to the image receptor. From the control console, the operator may choose to use one or more photocells to determine exposure. When more than one photocell is used, the exposure is averaged between them. A manual backup timer is set to approximately 1.5 times the anticipated exposure to prevent tube overload and excessive patient dose. Setting the backup time too short may result in a risk of underexposure.

AEC decreases the need for repeat radiographs by adjusting for patient density and reducing human error in exposure calculation. However, positioning the body part under examination precisely over the photocell(s) is paramount to produce adequate exposure. Malposition results in overexposure or underexposure. Exposure area also affects the photosensor readings, especially considering scatter radiation production; therefore proper beam collimation is necessary to produce accurate exposure time. The calibration of the phototimer must be matched with the sensitivity of the image receptor (film/screen).

TUBE FAILURE

X-ray tubes can fail in a number of different ways. Most tube failure occurs as the result of thermal wear on the internal component parts. The wear usually develops over a period of time; however, an instantaneous load significantly above the tube rating can cause a tube to fail immediately. Common types of tube failure include worn rotor bearings, a cracked or pitted anode, gassing of the tube, and an open cathode filament.

To better prepare the tube to receive a high heat load, it is best to perform a *tube warm-up procedure.* Executing a couple of low-load exposures puts some heat into the anode and reduces the stress of an instantaneous large load on a cold anode. An example of a warm-up technique is an initial exposure of 50 kVp, 100 mA, at $1/30$ second, followed by a second exposure in which the mA is raised to 200. Other ways to maximize x-ray tube life include:
- Minimize filament boost (preparation) time.
- Limit rotor/start/stop operations.
- Use lower tube current (mA).
- Do not make a high mA exposure on a cold tube.
- Adhere to rating charts and anode heating and cooling curves.
- Limit operations to 80% of maximum single exposure ratings.
- Do not exceed the anode thermal capacity or dissipation rate of the target.

PRIMARY FACTORS CONTROLLING X-RAY EXPOSURE

Four primary exposure factors control the quantity and quality of x-ray films produced: peak kilovoltage, mA, time (seconds), and distance.
1. *Kilovoltage* (expressed in kVp) directly controls the speed of electrons traveling from cathode to anode. As electrons strike the target, their kinetic energy is transformed into x-ray and heat energy. X-ray *quality,* or *penetration power,* is directly proportional to kVp. Kilovoltage is the only controlling factor affecting x-ray beam energy (quality).
2. *Milliampere* (measured in mA) is a measure of tube current generated from the filament by thermionic emission. The number of electrons available to produce x-rays is directly proportional to milliampere. Changes in milliampere affect the *quantity* of x-rays produced. Milliampere output is linear in that as mA is doubled, exposure is doubled.
3. *Exposure time* is another factor controlling the number of x-rays *(quantity)* produced. Time is measured from milliseconds to seconds and is given the abbreviation *s.* Longer exposure time allows more electrons to be generated from the filament. Exposure time is also linear in that exposure is doubled as time is doubled.

   In clinical settings, exposure intensity (quantity) is commonly controlled by the product of milliamperes and time, or mAs. Ascribing mAs to a particular body part size is helpful in determining the total exposure needed to produce an acceptable image. Once the measurement of mAs is determined, any combination of milliampere and time to produce that same measurement of mAs yields a similar exposure. Kilovoltage is

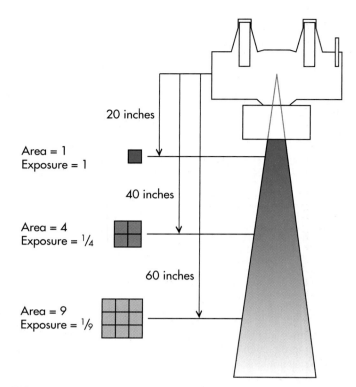

FIG. 1-13 Inverse square law. The intensity of the x-ray beam decreases with increasing distance from its source. The magnitude of intensity is inversely proportional to the square of the distance.

responsible for providing the penetration necessary to produce adequate subject contrast.
4. *Distance,* the fourth exposure parameter, is often expressed as *FFD* (focal-film distance), *SID* (source-to-image receptor distance), and *TFD* (tube-film distance). Distance affects the number of x-rays reaching the image receptor (film). As the x-ray tube is moved farther away from the film, the beam diverges and offers less x-ray photons per unit area. The number of x-ray photons striking the film is *inversely proportional* to the square of the distance. This is called the *inverse square law* and is expressed as

$$I = 1/d^2$$

where I = x-ray intensity and d = tube distance. If the distance is doubled, approximately $1/4$ of the number of x-rays reaches the film (Fig. 1-13).

Whereas x-ray beam intensity is inversely proportional to the square of the distance, tube load (mAs) is *directly proportional* to the square of the distance. An increase in distance mandates an increase in tube load expressed by the formula

$$\text{New mAs} = \text{Old mAs} \times (\text{FFD}_2/\text{FFD}_1)^2$$

where FFD_1 is the original distance, FFD_2 is the new distance, *old mAs* represents exposure (tube load) at the original distance, and *new mAs* represents exposure (tube load) at the new distance.

Control Console

Basic single-phase operating consoles (Fig. 1-14) provide selectors for *power (on/off), line-voltage compensation, peak kilovoltage, milliampere, time, focal spot, Bucky* (see Grids), *AEC, rotor,* and *exposure.*

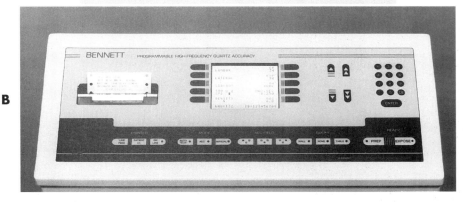

A

B

FIG. I-14 A and **B,** X-ray consoles. (From Guebert G: Essentials of Diagnostic Imaging, St Louis, 1995, Mosby.)

Control consoles have evolved with the use of computer technology. Manufacturers have reduced console size by replacing copper wiring, steel construction, and knob controls with microcircuitry. Menu-driven push-button controls, preprogrammed anatomic techniques, and AEC have dramatically reduced human error in the calculation and selection of exposure parameters.

Modern single-phase 300 mA/125 kVp x-ray machines may offer any or all of the following:

- Automatic line-voltage compensation (voltage fluctuation control)
- Kilovoltage selection by units of 1 kV, from 40 to 125 kVp
- Milliampere selection normally ranging from 25 to 300 mA and as high as 600 mA in 50- to 100-mA increments
- Automatic focal spot selection based on milliampere designation
- Electronic SCR timers with milliampere-seconds readout
- AEC with photocell selector and plus and minus density control
- Bucky selection
- Single- or double-switch operation of rotor control and exposure control
- Tube protection circuitry to safeguard against overload

X-Ray Production

X-rays are generated by two different yet simultaneous processes as high-speed electrons lose energy at the target. One reaction involves high-speed electrons interacting with the nucleus of tungsten target atoms to generate what is called *bremsstrahlung radiation.* The other involves collisions of high-speed electrons with inner shell electrons of target atoms to produce what is called *characteristic radiation.*

BREMSSTRAHLUNG RADIATION

Bremsstrahlung is the German word for *braking,* or slowing down. When a high-speed projectile electron from the cathode passes the nucleus of a tungsten atom in the target, the positively charged nucleus exerts an attractive force on the electron. A strong nuclear electric field inhibits penetration of the electron into the nucleus but causes the electron to decelerate and change direction (Fig. 1-15). This deceleration results in a loss of kinetic energy, which is converted into electromagnetic radiation (x-rays). The quality (or energy) of radiation released is contingent on the amount of deceleration and kinetic energy possessed by the incoming electron

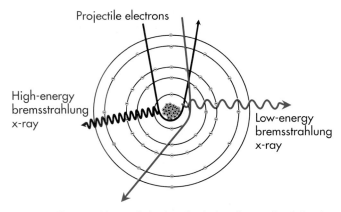

Projectile electrons

High-energy bremsstrahlung x-ray

Low-energy bremsstrahlung x-ray

FIG. I-15 Bremsstrahlung radiation is emitted when the speed and direction of a projectile electron is altered secondary to interaction with the target's nucleus.

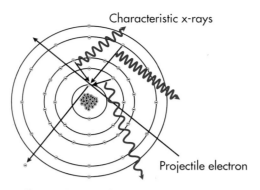

FIG. I-16 Characteristic radiation is emitted when an upper orbit electron fills the K-shell vacancy created by a projectile electron.

(measured in kVp). Deceleration is affected by the proximity in which electrons randomly approach the nucleus and size of the nucleus. Electrons directly striking the nucleus and giving up 100% of their kinetic energy generate the highest-energy x-rays.

Bremsstrahlung x-rays have a spectrum of energies, with an average energy somewhere below, but proportional to, the peak kilovolts used. Primary control of x-ray beam quality, or overall penetrating power, is a result of the effect of peak kilovolts on bremsstrahlung interactions. The quantity of bremsstrahlung x-rays is related more to milliampere-seconds (tube current) than peak kilovolts. Higher values of milliampere-seconds release more electrons to the target. Most of the x-rays produced in a diagnostic beam are of bremsstrahlung origin.

CHARACTERISTIC RADIATION

When a high-speed electron from the cathode interacts with a lower orbit (inner shell) electron in the tungsten target and the kinetic energy of the projectile electron exceeds the binding energy of the electron it interacts with, the orbital electron is ejected, leaving a vacancy in the inner shell (Fig. 1-16). Immediately, an upper orbit electron fills the vacancy, resulting in a release of a discrete amount of electromagnetic radiation (x-ray). The amount of energy released is equal to the difference in the binding energies of the orbital shells involved. For tungsten, atomic number 74, the following applies:

$$E_{Kshell} - E_{Lshell} = 69.5 \text{ keV} - 12.1 \text{ keV} = 57.4 \text{ keV x-ray}$$

A cascade effect causes all inner shell vacancies to be filled and lower energy photons to be released. The total amount of energy released equals the input energy necessary to remove the inner shell electron.

Binding energies are unique to each element. The radiation released is "characteristic" of the atom it is generated from, hence the name *characteristic radiation*. A *K*-characteristic x-ray of tungsten is 57.4 keV. A K-characteristic x-ray of molybdenum is 17.4 keV. It takes at least 70 keV (kVp) of input energy to release a *K*-shell electron in tungsten. Kilovoltage has no effect on the quality (energy) of characteristic radiation. However, the energy of characteristic x-rays increases as atomic number increases. Characteristic x-rays make up approximately 10% of the radiation emitted in the 80- to 100-kVp range. Figure 1-17 illustrates a filtered beam of bremsstrahlung and characteristic x-rays at 80 kVp.

Diagnostic X-Ray Interactions with Matter

One of three things can happen to a diagnostic x-ray as it encounters matter. It can (1) be totally absorbed, (2) be partially absorbed and scattered, or (3) pass through unaffected. The quality of the image produced is greatly affected by all three events.

PHOTOELECTRIC EFFECT

The *photoelectric effect* is a total absorption reaction in which x-ray photons interact with inner shell electrons of an absorbing medium to cause ionizations (Fig. 1-18). This is most likely to occur when the energy of the incident photon slightly exceeds the binding energy of an electron at the *K*- or *L*-shell level. The photon gives up all of its energy in overcoming the binding energy of an inner shell electron, and the photon ceases to exist. The *photoelectron* removed from the atom exits with kinetic energy equal to the energy of the incident photon minus the binding energy of the orbital electron. The empty shell is filled with an electron from an upper orbit, resulting in the release of characteristic radiation. The characteristic ray is called *secondary radiation* and is emitted randomly like scatter radiation. Most of these rays are reabsorbed in the body.

A photoelectric interaction is dependent on the atomic number of the absorbing medium and the energy of the x-ray. The tighter an electron is bound, the more likely it is to be involved in a photoelectric interaction. Also, the closer the x-ray energy is to the binding energy of an inner shell electron, the greater chance there is for a photoelectric effect. Absorption probability is inversely proportional to the cube of the x-ray photon energy (photoelectric adsorption = $1/E^3$) and it is directly proportional to the cube of the atomic number (Z), or Z^3.

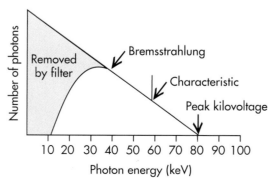

FIG. I-17 Photon energy spectrum typical for a machine operating at 80 kVp.

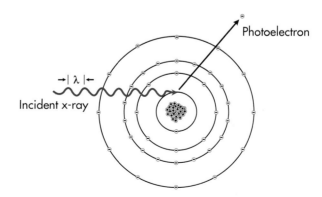

FIG. I-18 Photoelectric effect describes total absorption of the incident x-ray as it ejects an inner shell electron, known as a photoelectron. The empty shell is filled with an electron from an upper orbit, resulting in the release of characteristic radiation.

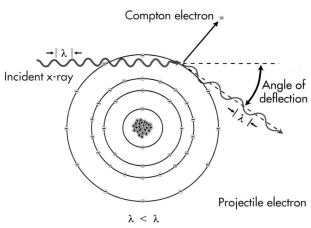

FIG. 1-19 Compton's effect describes the interaction between medium-energy x-rays and outer shell electrons. The interaction results in ionization of the target atom (with ejection of a Compton electron), deflection of the incident x-ray, and lower energy in the scattered x-ray.

The photoelectric effect is responsible for subject contrast seen on a radiograph. The x-ray beam is *attenuated,* or weakened, through absorption as it encounters tissues of different densities and atomic numbers. The resulting *differential absorption* produces subject contrast. With higher-energy x-rays (high peak kilovoltage), subject contrast is decreased as a result of an overall decrease in absorption.

COMPTON SCATTERING

Compton scattering is a partial absorption reaction that involves moderate-energy x-rays. As photon energy increases with a higher number of peak kilovolts, the x-ray gives up some of its energy as it strikes an outer shell electron in an absorbing medium (Fig. 1-19). The electron is ejected and the x-ray deflects from its original path. The photon energy loss results in a longer wavelength x-ray that is scattered. The angle of deflection is proportional to the energy loss. Radiation that scatters 180 degrees back in the direction of the tube is called backscatter. Scatter radiation delivers misinformation to the image receptor, which fogs the film and decreases image visibility. Scatter increases the overall darkness of the film, but not in a way that provides useful information.

The probability that an x-ray will undergo a Compton's interaction depends on the density of the absorbing medium and the energy of the x-ray. Water density tissues (e.g., muscle, blood, and solid organs) create the greatest amount of scatter radiation in the body. Tissues of greater density (e.g., bone) tend toward higher absorption of x-rays. Low-density tissues that contain air (e.g., lung and large bowel) allow greater penetration of x-rays. Higher-energy x-rays tend toward greater penetration, medium-energy x-rays tend toward partial absorption (scatter), and lower-energy x-rays tend toward total absorption.

CLASSICAL (RAYLEIGH) SCATTERING

Classical scattering involves very-low-energy x-rays (10 keV) and matter. An incoming, or incident, x-ray photon interacts with an atom, causing its electrons to vibrate at the same frequency as the photon (Fig. 1-20). The excited atom releases the excess energy in the form of a new photon. The new photon is randomly emitted as scatter and has a wavelength and energy equal to that of the incident photon. Rayleigh scattering accounts for less than 5% of scatter in the diagnostic range and does not significantly affect image quality.

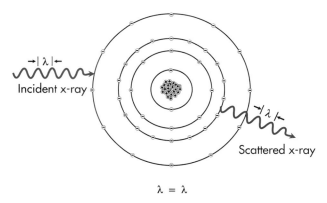

FIG. 1-20 Classical scattering describes an interaction between lower-energy x-rays and atoms. The wavelengths of the scatter rays are equal to those of the incident x-rays.

Scatter Radiation Control for Contrast Improvement

FACTORS CONTRIBUTING TO SCATTER RADIATION PRODUCTION

Beam energy, field size, patient size, and tissue type are the major contributors to scatter radiation production. As *beam energy* is increased, for example, from 70 to 90 kVp, fewer x-rays are completely absorbed. This leaves more photons to be scattered. The percentage of Compton interactions increases as peak kilovolts increases. As *field size* is increased, scatter production increases by expanding the area of tissue that interacts with primary radiation. As *patient size* increases, augmented by an increase in *soft tissue* water density, more scatter is produced.

METHODS OF SCATTER CONTROL

As mentioned, scatter radiation fogs a radiograph, thereby decreasing overall film contrast. Controlling scatter helps to increase contrast. Scatter may be regulated in the production phase or, once it is produced, by constraining it from reaching the film. Limiting peak kilovolts, minimizing beam size, and using patient recumbency, air-gap technique, and grids are all viable methods for controlling scatter.

Peak kilovolts limitation. Although the kilovoltage range for diagnostic x-rays is 40 to 150 kVp, scatter is best controlled by limiting peak kilovolts to 70 to 90 for the axial skeleton. The presentation of an obese patient may tempt the radiographer to drive the peak kilovolts higher; however, it is better to limit the peak kilovolts and increase the milliampere-seconds for scatter control.

Beam limitation. Limiting the exposure area is important to minimize patient dose and scatter radiation production. Field size is regulated by beam restrictors.

Aperture diaphragm. The simplest type of beam restrictor is an *aperture diaphragm.* An aperture diaphragm is a flat sheet of lead with an opening prescribed to cover a certain film size; it is attached to the tube housing at the port. The aperture diaphragm is used in situations in which film size and tube distance are constant, such as in dedicated head or chest radiography.

Cones and cylinders. *Cones* and *cylinders* are extension tubes attached to the tube housing to control beam size. Flared cones (Fig. 1-21) are designed to resemble a divergent x-ray beam, but they are often flared wider than the beam. The effectiveness is reduced to that of an aperture diaphragm. A cylinder provides true

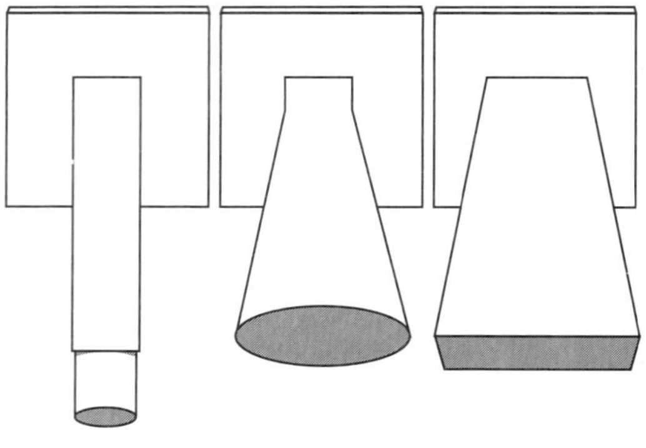

Adjustable   Circular   Rectangular
cylinder   flare   flare

FIG. 1-21   Cones and cylinders.

beam restriction as the field size is controlled by the constricted outer opening, which is farther away from the focal spot. Some cylinders are adjustable, which enhances versatility and effectiveness.

Collimators. A *collimator* is a variable-aperture beam-limiting device. It contains two sets of lead shutters, fixed upper shutters and adjustable lower shutters (Fig. 1-22). The upper shutters serve as an aperture diaphragm, controlling off-focus radiation. The lower shutters adjust in the vertical and horizontal directions to control the exposure area. A light field is projected through the lower shutter opening to help the radiographer estimate the exposure field. The light comes from a high-intensity lamp that reflects off a mirror strategically placed within the collimator. Collimators must be periodically checked to ensure that the light field and exposure field coincide.

To ensure patient protection, *positive beam limitation* (PBL) *collimators* are manufactured to make certain that the exposure field size never exceeds the film size. Distance and film size sensors regulate the function of the PBL collimator. If the distance sensor on the tube rail is not activated to indicate the tube distance, the collimator will not allow the exposure to initiate. Sensors in the Bucky tray convey film size to the collimator. If the film is improperly placed in the Bucky tray, the collimator reads an aberrant field size. If the Bucky tray is not pushed in such that the sensor in the end of the tray is connected back to the collimator, once again, the collimator blocks the exposure. *Semiautomatic PBL collimators* must be manually adjusted to film size to ensure exposure. *Fully automatic PBL collimators* possess a motorized mechanism in the collimator that automatically adjusts the lower shutters to the film size once the sensors are activated.

Manual collimators are less expensive and do not operate with a sensor system; therefore there is no check to ensure that the exposure field size does not exceed the film size.

Patient recumbency. When a patient is placed in a recumbent (lying down) position, soft tissue is more evenly distributed and the overall thickness of the patient is decreased, thereby reducing scatter production. The decreased patient thickness requires less peak kilovoltage for penetration, which also reduces scatter production. Measurement of the patient in the recumbent position is necessary to determine accurate exposure factors.

Air-gap technique. If the object-to-film (OFD) distance is increased to create an air space between the patient and film, some scatter traveling obliquely misses the film. Figure 1-23 shows the effect of an air-gap between the patient and film in reducing the scatter that reaches the film.

Compression devices. Different types of compression devices help decrease the thickness of tissue the x-ray beam must pass through. With a wider and flatter distribution of tissue, primary beam–tissue interactions decrease, resulting in less scatter.

FIG. 1-22   A collimator restricts the primary beam with fixed upper and adjustable lower shutters. An interposed mirror is used to reflect light through the opening created by the moveable shutters to yield a representation of the beam size during patient positioning.

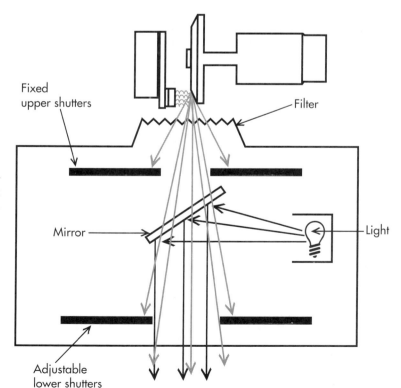

Fixed
upper shutters

Filter

Mirror

Light

Adjustable
lower shutters

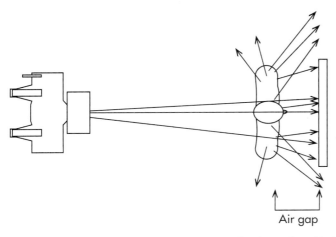

FIG. 1-23 Because scatter radiation travels in many directions, a 4- to 6-inch air-gap between the patient and the film reduces the amount of scatter that contacts the film.

Grids. A *grid* is a selective lead filter that increases film contrast by absorbing a large percentage of scatter radiation, tracking obliquely as it exits the patient. The grid is located behind the patient but in front of the film, so it absorbs scatter before it reaches the film.

Today's modern grid apparatus is derived from the combined inventions of medical radiologists Gustav Bucky and Hollis Potter in the early 1900s. Bucky designed a grid with lead lines spaced 2 cm apart, arranged in a cross-hatched pattern. Although the grid increased contrast, unsightly grid lines appeared on the film. Potter improved on the concept by reconfiguring the lines in a vertical direction only and laterally moving the grid during the exposure. Moving the grid caused the lead lines to blur and disappear from the film. Potter's invention is known as the *Potter-Bucky diaphragm,* or *Bucky.*

Grid design. Contemporary grids have thin lead strips configured in a linear or cross-hatched pattern with a *radiolucent interspacing* material between the strips (Fig. 1-24). Ideally the interspacing is designed to allow maximum penetration of the primary beam. Interspacing materials include cardboard, plastic, carbon fiber, and aluminum. Carbon fiber and aluminum are commercially available. Aluminum has a higher atomic number than carbon fiber. At higher peak kilovoltage, aluminum improves contrast by absorbing more lower-energy x-rays. However, at lower peak kilovoltage, aluminum absorbs more primary radiation than carbon fiber, which leads to higher patient dose. Carbon fiber grids are preferred in situations in which low peak kilovoltage techniques are employed (e.g., mammography), and their use can contribute to lower patient dose.

Linear grids are designed with parallel or focused lead strips. In a *parallel grid,* the lead strips and interspacing run parallel to one another (Fig. 1-25). A significant amount of cutoff of the primary beam at the periphery of the grid results when using a short tube

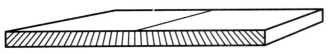

FIG. 1-24 Radiographic grid plate showing focused (*angled*) opaque lead lines with radiolucent interspacing.

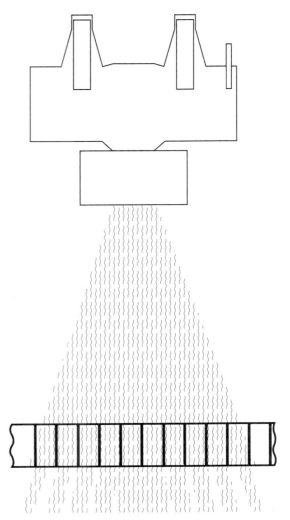

FIG. 1-25 A linear parallel grid is constructed with parallel grid lines. Primary beam cutoff occurs at the periphery of the image at a short source-to-image distance, because of a divergent x-ray beam.

distance (40 inches); therefore parallel grids are best used with a long distance (72 inches) in which more of the central, or perpendicular, part of the beam is used. Grid cutoff manifests as underexposure.

Focused grids are used more commonly than parallel grids for diagnostic imaging. In a *focused grid,* the lead strips and interspacing are angled toward the center of the grid to accommodate a divergent x-ray beam (Fig. 1-26). The intent is to reduce peripheral cutoff. The focus is determined by the angle of the divergent beam, which is governed by the distance between the grid and focal spot. If the lead lines were extended in space beyond the grid, they would converge at a focal point called the *grid radius.* When the x-ray tube is set at the grid radius distance, the grid is in optimum focus. The tube can be moved a short distance from the grid radius without significant peripheral cutoff. *Focal range* describes the distance plus or minus the grid radius in which the cutoff is not significant. Making exposures outside of the focal range results in noticeable cutoff. A focused grid must be accurately aligned to ensure that the center of the beam (central ray) is positioned in the middle of the grid. A misaligned grid results in peripheral cutoff to one side

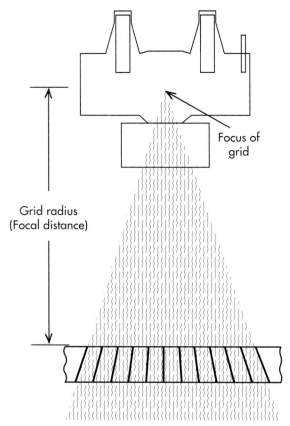

FIG. 1-26 A focused grid accommodates the divergence of the x-ray beam as long as the source-to-image distance (SID) is within the focal range. Primary beam cutoff occurs when the SID deviates from the focal range.

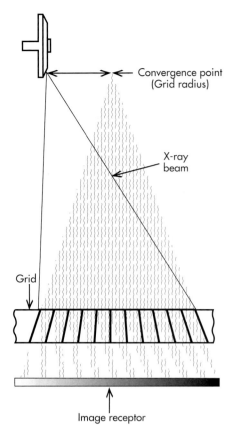

FIG. 1-27 An off-center grid produces grid cutoff, which manifests as a lighter density on one side of the film.

of the film and gives the appearance of underexposure (Figs. 1-27 and 1-28).

Grid ratio. Scatter cleanup is directly related to *grid ratio (GR)*. Grid ratio is described as the height of the lead strips *(h)* divided by the distance *(d)* between each lead strip, or

$$GR = h/d$$

The ratio measurement is taken from the edge of the grid in which the height of the lead strip is actually a measurement of the thickness of the grid plate (Fig. 1-29). Grid ratio can be increased by increasing the height of the lead or decreasing the space between the lines. Scatter radiation approaching at an angle that is not accommodated by the interspacing is trapped by the grid. Common grid ratios for diagnostic radiology include 6:1, 8:1, 10:1, and 12:1. Unfortunately, grids also absorb a significant amount of primary rays. To ensure sufficient primary ray transmission through the grid, exposure (milliampere-seconds) must be increased. Patient dose is three to five times higher when using a grid versus not using a grid.

Grid frequency. *Grid frequency* is a measure of the number of lead lines per inch (lines/inch) or per centimeter (lines/cm) (Fig. 1-30). Grids are manufactured with a frequency range between 60 and 200 lines/inch. For diagnostic imaging, frequencies between 85 and 103 lines/inch are most common. Fine line grids (103 lines/inch) are best used in a stationary mode in which the grid plate does not move during the exposure. The lines are thin and so close

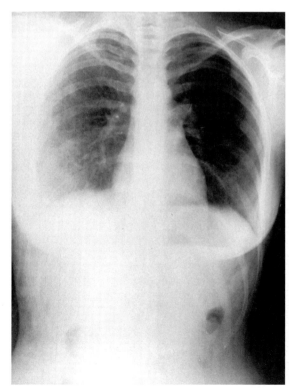

FIG. 1-28 Unequal density across the thorax secondary to misalignment of the grid and tube (grid cutoff).

together that they become virtually invisible. At higher frequencies (>103 lines/inch), the lead strips become too thin to be effective when using high peak kilovoltage techniques. Grids with 200 lines/inch can be used in mammography, because the peak kilovoltage range is 20 to 30 kVp. Lower-frequency grids (85 lines/inch) show lead lines on a film and should be used in a Potter-Bucky diaphragm. The diaphragm moves a linear grid in a reciprocating (back-and-forth) motion during exposure and blurs the lead lines. A cross-hatch grid requires an oscillating motion to blur all lines.

Application. Typically a grid is indicated if the body thickness measures greater than 10 cm or if greater than 70 kVp is necessary to penetrate the body part. Using grids may increase the contrast 1.5 to 3.5 times.

X-Ray Film

Of all image receptors used in diagnostic imaging, plain radiographic film is still the most common, although digital imaging is gaining in popularity. Film is photosensitive, which causes it to respond to wavelengths of light in the electromagnetic spectrum, particularly visible light and x-rays.

CONSTRUCTION

Radiographic film comprises two primary layers: a support layer (base) and a radiosensitive layer (emulsion) (Fig. 1-31). The *base* layer is made of polyester and is tinted with blue dye to reduce eyestrain for the interpreter. The base layer is unreactive to processing chemistry. The *emulsion* layer consists of a gelatinous matrix embedded with silver halide crystals, predominantly silver bromide. Silver halide is the photoactive ingredient in the emulsion. The gelatin provides a means for even distribution of silver halide crystals. It is water soluble, which allows easy penetration of processing chemistry to reach and act on the silver. The emulsion layer is attached to the base with a thin *adhesive* and is covered with a protective *supercoating*. For most diagnostic applications, radiographic film is coated with emulsion on both sides to increase film sensitivity and reduce patient dose.

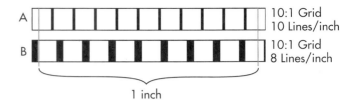

FIG. 1-30 Grid frequency is calculated by the number of grid lines per inch or centimeter. Grids A and B have the same grid ratio, but because B has thicker grid lines, it has a lower grid frequency.

FILM CHARACTERISTICS

Speed. Film speed, or sensitivity, is a measure of the response time of film to a minimal x-ray exposure. Film is blackened proportionally to exposure. A faster film requires less exposure time to sensitize. Film speed is governed by the thickness of the emulsion layer, size of the silver grains, emulsion coated on one or both sides of the film, and processing conditions.

Contrast. *Contrast* is the difference between adjacent exposure densities (darkness) on a film; it is described in gray scale from black to white. *Radiographic contrast* includes both subject contrast and detector contrast. *Subject contrast* is determined by attenuation of the beam by the patient, or subject, and is controlled by peak kilovoltage. *Detector contrast* refers to inherent film response characteristics in recording high and low contrast. Depending on clinical need, detector contrast varies. Compared with bone imaging, chest radiography often requires a film type with less contrast

Latitude. *Latitude* is the range of exposures over which the film responds with densities in the diagnostic range. *Latitude and contrast are inversely related.* Film with wide exposure latitude is low contrast. High-contrast film has narrow exposure latitude.

Spectral response. The *spectral response* of a film describes its sensitivity to different wavelengths (colors) of light. Screen film is manufactured to respond primarily to blue, green, and ultraviolet light. *Calcium tungstate* intensifying screens emit *blue* light; blue sensitive film is matched with these screens. *Rare earth* intensifying screens emit light in the *blue, green,* and *ultraviolet* ranges.

FILM TYPES

Direct-exposure film. Film that is exposed to only x-ray is called *direct-exposure,* or *nonscreen,* film. Direct-exposure film is used for *high-detail imaging.* In general, all x-ray film is much

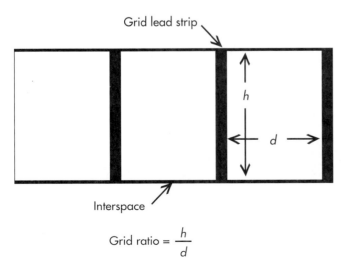

Grid lead strip

h

d

Interspace

$$\text{Grid ratio} = \frac{h}{d}$$

FIG. 1-29 Grid ratio is defined as the height of the lead strip (h) divided by the distance (d) between the lead strips (interspace).

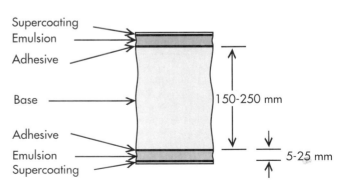

Supercoating
Emulsion
Adhesive

Base

Adhesive
Emulsion
Supercoating

150-250 mm

5-25 mm

FIG. 1-31 Cross section of x-ray film. The majority of the film is base. The emulsion contains the image.

more sensitive to visible light than to x-ray photons. It takes considerable exposure from x-ray alone to sensitize direct exposure film, limiting its use in general radiography. The emulsions are significantly thicker and contain more fine-grain silver than screen film. Limited medical applications include dental radiography (bite-wing), some mammography, imaging of occult (hidden) fractures of the small bones of the face and extremities, and localization of foreign objects. Its greatest application today is in industrial radiography, in which dose is not a concern.

Screen film. *Screen film* is the most common film type used in medical imaging. It is matched with intensifying screens that convert the energy of x-rays into visible light. Approximately 95% of exposure to screen film is by visible light. A double-emulsion film is routinely sandwiched between two intensifying screens. Screen film emulsions are considerably thinner than those on nonscreen film; however, when used in combination with intensifying screens, they are substantially faster. Resolution (detail) is diminished with screen film when compared with nonscreen film, but the dose-reduction benefit of screen film is an acceptable tradeoff. Screen film is commercially available in a wide variety of speeds, contrasts, spectral responses, and detail.

Single-emulsion film. Certain radiographic exams, such as mammography and extremity imaging, may use a single-emulsion, fine-grain film in conjunction with a single intensifying screen. The single emulsion/single screen combination offers better detail than a dual system and at a lower dose than a nonscreen film. Care should be taken to ensure that the emulsion side of a single-emulsion film is placed against the screen. Failure to do so results in some loss of speed.

Duplicating film. Radiographs often are duplicated for teaching files or for medico-legal reasons. The process involves a film duplicator that uses ultraviolet light. Regular x-ray film is a negative. *Duplicating film* is a single-emulsion positive film. Because duplicating film is exposed mostly in areas that are clearer on the original film and least exposed where the original film is darker, duplicating film reacts to exposure in an opposite manner to that of regular x-ray film. The silver crystals respond to light in an opposite fashion. More exposure time is needed to lighten a dark original. Less exposure time is needed to darken a light original.

STORAGE AND HANDLING

X-ray film is sensitive to light, x-rays, heat, moisture, pressure, fumes, and aging, all of which are capable of fogging the film or producing artifacts. Film should be stored in a cool, dry place (50° to 70° F, 30% to 50% relative humidity), safe from light and x-ray exposure. Film boxes should sit on end to decrease pressure sensitization. Stock should be rotated for use before the expiration date.

Intensifying Screens

An intensifying screen converts the energy of x-ray into visible light for the purpose of decreasing patient dose.

CONSTRUCTION

An intensifying screen consists of a protective coating, a phosphor layer, an undercoating layer, and a base layer (Fig. 1-32). The outer *protective coating* helps minimize abrasions of the sensitive phosphor layer. The *phosphor layer* is the photoactive layer of the screen. A *phosphor* is a phosphorescent substance that emits light when energized by x-rays (Fig. 1-33). Tiny phosphor crystals are evenly distributed in a polymer matrix. When energized, light is emitted

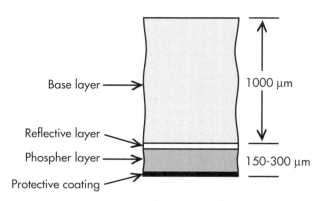

FIG. 1-32 Cross section of an intensifying screen.

isotropically (in all directions). The *undercoating layer* can be reflective or absorptive. Light traveling away from the film is reflected back to the film by a *reflective layer*. Screen speed is increased when a reflective layer is used. An absorptive undercoat decreases light flare from the screen, resulting in increased detail. The base, made of plastic or paper, is a support layer that is coated with an anticurl backing.

PHOSPHORS

Modern intensifying screens most frequently use blue-emitting calcium tungstate, or blue-green- or ultraviolet-emitting rare earth phosphors. Rare earth phosphors are named according to the family of elements from which they are formed. Lanthanum oxysulfide (green), lanthanum oxybromide (blue), and gadolinium oxysulfide (green) come from the lanthanide series of elements in the periodic table, otherwise known as the *rare earth elements*.

A suitable phosphor should have a high absorption capability. The peak kilovoltage used and the thickness and composition of the phosphor layer of the screen determine the *quantum detection efficiency* (QDE), or absorption capability of the screen. Phosphors also should have a high *conversion efficiency,* or ability to convert the energy of x-rays into visible light. Overall screen efficiency is the product of detection efficiency and conversion efficiency. Also, light emissions should cease at the instant an exposure is terminated. Persistence of luminance is called *screen lag,* or *afterglow,* and should be minimal.

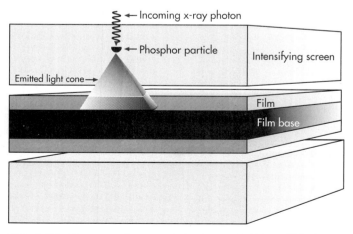

FIG. 1-33 The energy of an x-ray photon is converted into multiple photons of visible light by a phosphor crystal in the phosphor layer of an intensifying screen.

SCREEN SPEED

The amount of light emitted from an intensifying screen per unit of x-ray exposure defines *screen speed*. A faster screen emits more light per unit of x-ray exposure, thereby requiring less exposure, which results in lower patient dose. Manufacturers arbitrarily assign the number 100 to Par speed screens; the performance (speed) of all other screens is determined relative to the 100 Par speed screen. The term *relative speed* (RS) is used. Relative speed is determined by the type of phosphor used, the thickness of the phosphor layer, phosphor crystal size, the presence of a reflective layer, and the peak kilovoltage. Rare earth phosphors have a higher detection efficiency (QDE) and conversion efficiency than calcium tungstate phosphors, which makes rare earth phosphors faster. The increase in speed does not significantly diminish image detail. A 400-speed gadolinium oxysulfide screen produces an image with approximately the same resolution as a 200-speed calcium tungstate screen.

Screen speed varies across the useful peak kilovoltage range. With kilovoltage measurements below what is needed to ionize *K*-shell electrons in the phosphor, a noticeable decrease in light emission occurs because of a decrease in characteristic photon production. This is called the *K*-shell absorption edge phenomenon. The *K*-shell absorption edge varies for each phosphor. To compensate for the drop-off in light emissions, milliampere-seconds is increased. An increase in peak kilovoltage causes an increase in screen speed.

Speed is often referred to in respect to both film and screen, or film/screen speed. Matching film sensitivity to screen emission is the goal in maximizing speed, contrast, and resolution. Not all matches are perfect. Mixing and matching films with screens determines *working speed*. Working speed is one of the true indicators of how much exposure is needed; it is directly proportional to milliampere-seconds. Patient dose and image detail are *inversely related* to speed. Typical working speeds for calcium tungstate film/screens are 40 to 250; for rare earth, 40 to 1200. The slower speeds (40 to 80) are used in extremity radiography. Extremities are less radiosensitive than other organs of the body, so the increased dose is considered acceptable for the increase in detail. The most common working speed for rare earth imaging of the axial skeleton is 400.

Cassettes

Unexposed film must be housed in a light-tight holder to be handled in daylight conditions. The most common film holder is a *cassette*. Cassettes are designed specifically for screen film (Fig. 1-34). Two rigid surfaces are hinged together to support intensifying screens that are attached to the cassette with a compressive foam or felt. This ensures tight film-to-screen contact, which reduces blurring of the image. Some modern cassettes are made with biconcave surfaces to squeeze air out when closed. This helps maintain tight film-to-screen contact. The front cover is made of a radiolucent substance to minimize x-ray absorption by the cassette. *Bakelite* (e.g., lightweight) plastic and *carbon fiber* are the two substances most often used. Carbon fiber absorbs less radiation than the Bakelite, minimizing patient dose. The back cover is made of plastic or a lightweight metal, such as magnesium, with a thin foil of lead just inside the cover to absorb backscatter radiation.

Direct-exposure film is not used with intensifying screens; therefore it does not need an expensive film holder such as a cassette. Nonscreen film is placed in a cardboard holder or is individually wrapped in light-tight, moisture-proof paper.

The Latent Image

A physical change takes place when light and x-rays expose a film. The change is invisible to the naked eye. A *latent* (hidden) *image* is formed.

GURNEY-MOTT THEORY OF LATENT IMAGE FORMATION

The most accepted theory on latent image formation was proposed by Gurney and Mott in 1938. Silver halide crystals are manufactured in a lattice of silver, bromine, and iodine atoms. Ionic bonds couple positively charged silver (Ag^+) to negatively charged bromine and iodine (Br^- or I^-). The crystalline structure allows some migration of free silver ions and free electrons within the crystal. An impurity, called a *sensitivity speck,* is manufactured into the surface of many crystals and becomes an electrode for attracting free silver ions in the latent image process (Fig. 1-35).

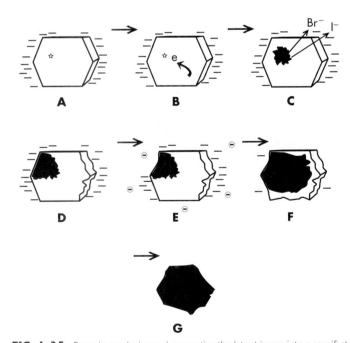

FIG. 1-35 Steps in producing and converting the latent image into a manifest image. **A,** Unexposed silver halide crystal. **B,** After irradiation of silver halide crystals, a minute number of electrons migrate to the sensitivity speck. **C,** Several silver ions are attracted to the sensitivity speck and neutralized to form atomic silver. **D,** The process is repeated many times, decreasing the amount of negative surface electrification and increasing the amount of atomic silver. **E** and **F,** The presence of reducing agents in the developer assists in further reducing the remaining silver ions to atomic silver. **G,** The process ends with the crystal completely converted to black atomic silver.

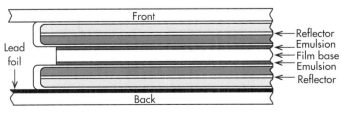

FIG. 1-34 Cross-section of a cassette, two intensifying screens, and radiographic film. A thin sheet of lead foil is mounted behind the second intensifying screen to absorb backscatter.

When light or x-rays interacts with the film, the input energy causes bromine or iodine to release an electron. The electron is free to wander and eventually may be trapped by the sensitivity speck. The more electrons that migrate to the sensitivity speck, the more electrically negative it becomes. The negatively charged speck attracts free silver ions, reducing them to atomic silver. A small mass of atomic silver begins to form at the sensitivity speck, invisible to the naked eye. Chemical development further reduces the silver in the latent image, causing the invisible image to become manifest.

Processing the Latent Image

DARKROOM ENVIRONMENT

The darkroom should be located as close to the exposure room as possible. The environment should be conducive to safe operations for both film and radiographer. The darkroom must be light-tight and safe from x-ray exposure. Common areas of light leaks include single-door thresholds and jambs and around drop ceilings. Using a double door or a light-tight revolving door may help remedy light leaks around the darkroom entrance. Contrary to popular belief, a darkroom does not have to be painted black. Rooms that are painted black typically require more intense safelighting to provide ample visibility. Safelight fog is directly related to safelight intensity. A light pastel color (preferably yellow) reflects low levels of light and helps minimize *postexposure fog*.

The darkroom should be properly ventilated to reduce the build-up of chemical fumes. Eye protection (goggles), rubber gloves, and aprons are basic protection apparel for darkroom workers. Chemical contact with skin must be minimized. A water source is needed for film processing and processor and darkroom maintenance.

Lighting. Two types of lighting are typically installed in a darkroom, *safelight* and *white light*. The white light is for general lighting when films are not being handled. White light is used when mixing chemicals, cleaning the automatic film processor, and for normal room maintenance. It is wise to strategically place the white light switch higher on the wall than a standard switch so that a conscious effort must be made to turn on the white light.

The safelight switch should be installed at a standard height. Safelighting is "relatively safe" for the film. Film sensitivity corresponds to a certain wavelength (color) of light. Safelight emissions are found at the other end of the visible light spectrum. A blue- or green-sensitive film is least sensitive to red light. Kodak's *GBX-2* red filter is commonly used with both green- and blue-sensitive film. Exposed film is many times more sensitive to light of any wavelength than unexposed film. Postexposure fog is directly proportional to safelight intensity. The type of filter, intensity of the bulb, number of safelights, distance between the safelight and film handling area, and handling time all affect the relative safeness of the light. Bulb wattage should not exceed 15 W; 7.5 W is preferred. The minimum distance between light and work area (and film processor) is 4 feet. By the inverse square law, light intensity is inversely proportional to the square of the distance; therefore as the distance between the safelight and film increases, postexposure fog decreases.

CHEMICAL PROCESSES

The latent image is made manifest by running the film through a series of chemical processes. The procedure may be done by hand or in an automatic film processor. The two main solutions are *developer* and *fixer*. Each solution is composed of several chemicals responsible for different functions in the chemical–film interaction.

The sequential steps in auto processing are as follows: *developing, fixing, washing,* and *drying*.

Developing. The critical phase in film processing is developing. Developer action is controlled by immersion *time*, solution *temperature*, and chemical concentration *(activity)*. The developer contains *reducing agents*, an *activator*, a *restrainer*, a *hardener*, and a *preservative*, all mixed in water.

A reducing agent readily gives up electrons to silver ions attracted to the sensitivity speck in the latent image. The reducing agents amplify the latent image more than a million times by completely reducing (neutralizing) exposed silver to black atomic silver. Figure 1-35 shows the interaction of the reducing agents with silver halides. Rapid process (RP) chemistry used in automatic film processing contains two reducing agents, hydroquinone and phenindone. *Hydroquinone* is slow acting and is responsible for the *heavy black densities*. *Phenindone* is fast acting, building *shades of gray* in the areas of lighter exposure on the film. Metol is used in manual processing chemistry in lieu of phenindone.

If a film is left in solution too long, or if the developer temperature is too high, unexposed silver ions are reduced, producing a *chemical fog* density, which leads to a darker film with decreased contrast. Oxidation (weakening) of the reducing agents through use or exposure to air, heat, light, or contaminants results in underdevelopment. A film developed in weakened developer appears light with low contrast. Increasing the milliampere-seconds to compensate for the lack of film density should be avoided because it results in a higher patient dose. To offset oxidation of reducing agents, a replenishment solution is periodically added to the developer. With automatic processing, replenishment is metered into the chemical tanks per inch of film travel at the time the film passes through the processor. Replenishment and changing chemicals monthly help control the symptoms of underprocessing resulting from weak developer, namely, low film density and contrast.

In addition to reducing agents, other agents affect the end result of development. A sodium carbonate *activator*, or accelerator, increases the permeability of the emulsion by causing the gelatin layer to swell. This allows the reducing agents to reach the silver halides within the emulsion. A potassium bromide (KBr) *restrainer* serves as an *antifogging agent*. It restrains the reducing agents from reducing unexposed silver. A glutaraldehyde *hardener* keeps the emulsion from *overswelling*, preventing scratches and abrasions in automatic processing. Glutaraldehyde helps maintain a uniform film thickness for easy travel through the roller transport system of an automatic processor. A sodium sulfite *preservative* minimizes *developer oxidation* caused by exposure to air.

Fixing. The fixer stops the developing process, removes undeveloped silver halides, and shrinks and hardens the emulsion. It contains an *acidifier, clearing agent, hardener, preservative,* and water as a solvent. Acetic acid acts as a stop bath in neutralizing the alkaline developer. Ammonium thiosulfate is the agent that clears the film of unexposed silver. The film takes on a milky white appearance if the unexposed silver is not completely removed. Aluminum chloride and potassium alum are hardeners that shrink and harden the emulsion. The preservative, sodium sulfite, ionizes the silver from the clearing agent so that it may remove more silver from the film. The buildup of silver ions in the fixer makes it environmentally unsafe. The silver must first be removed from the solution before the fixer can be discarded.

Washing. Water is used to wash developer and fixer from the film. Water should be of drinking quality. Relative hardness should be moderate, 40 to 150 ppm of calcium carbonate. Insufficient washing may result in brown, yellow, or green staining of the emulsion after several years. In an automatic processor, the environment may be conducive to algae growth in the wash water. Algae appear as black flecks on a radiograph. Adding 3 to 6 oz of liquid bleach to the wash tank at shutdown should eradicate the algae. If the problem persists, this procedure should be repeated two to three times per week. The tank should be thoroughly washed and the bleach eliminated before processing films. Draining the wash tank when the processor is shut down helps prevent algae growth.

Drying. Hot air forced over both sides of the film dries the film as it exits the processor. Air temperature varies from 110° F to 160° F, with 120° F being the average temperature. Films may emerge wet if the heater or blower is not functioning. Chemical-induced wetness may result from depleted hardener in the developer. Developer temperature also may affect film wetness. If the developer temperature exceeds 95° F, the emulsion may swell beyond the hardener's ability to control it.

TIME-TEMPERATURE METHOD

Film processing is based on *time* and *temperature*. *Optimum developer temperature is 68° F for manual processing.* Processing at this temperature provides latitude for human error. The higher the temperature, the greater the activity of the developer, and a compensatory decrease in developing time is needed. Strict adherence to manufacturers' time–temperature charts is necessary to produce consistent quality. Manual processing times range from 15 to 35 minutes before drying.

Automatic processing dictates no such single developer temperature at which all films are processed. Optimum temperature is determined by the manufacturer and is contingent on processing time, film, and chemistry. The temperature range is between 92° F and 96° F for a 90-second processor and lower for 2- and 3-minute processors. Automatic processing has distinct advantages over manual processing in reduced time and increased consistency of results. A film dropped into an auto processor emerges dry in 90 to 180 seconds and is ready for interpretation, analysis, or storage.

MANUAL PROCESSING APPARATUS AND PROCEDURE

Before the advent of automatic film processors in 1942, the time-consuming method of manually dipping films in chemical solutions predominated. Figure 1-36 shows a typical setup for manual processing. Equipment needs include the following:
1. Master tank filled with free-flowing water
2. In-line mixing valve to mix hot and cold water in the master tank; the circulating water is used to control chemical temperatures and to wash films
3. Two insert tanks with lids, one for developer and one for fixer
4. Thermometer to read chemical temperatures
5. Darkroom clock to monitor processing times
6. Separate stir paddles for developer and fixer
7. Time–temperature chart
8. Drying bin or area
9. Film hangers

Before a film is processed, chemicals must be stirred, developer temperature checked, clock set for the appropriate time, and the film placed on a hanger. Processing times are set according to film type, chemistry type, temperature, and concentration. Agitation may be necessary once a film is placed in the developer, depending on the type of chemistry. The film should not be taken out of solution before the development time has expired. The lid should be kept on the developer tank when the film is not being agitated. As the film is removed from the developer, chemicals running off the film should not be "dripped back" into the tank. This oxidized developer weakens the main volume of chemistry. At the end of development, the film is immersed in a rinse bath of water for approximately 15 seconds. The clock is reset for fixing time and the film, placed in the fixer, is agitated. Once the fixing time has expired, the film is removed and the excess fixer is allowed to drip back into the fixer tank. This ensures that ionic silver dripping off the film is retained in the fixer tank. The film is then placed in the wash water to remove fixer from the emulsion. Once the film is in the final

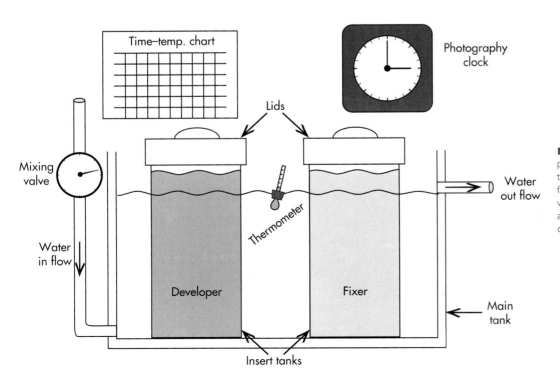

FIG. 1-36 Typical setup for manual processing. The developer and fixer tanks are seated into a larger tank filled with flowing water. The flowing water serves to maintain the temperature of the smaller tanks and also doubles as a wash.

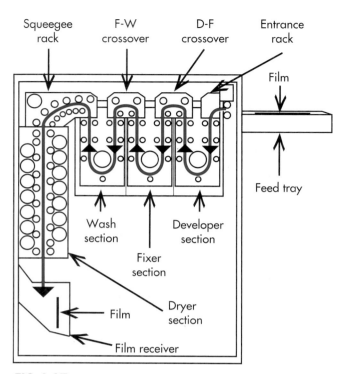

FIG. 1-37 Design and film path *(blue arrow)* of an automatic processor.

wash, the white light may be turned on for wet viewing. Finally the film is air-dried from 15 minutes to more than an hour, depending on the temperature and humidity of the drying area.

Replenishment should be added at the end of each day of film processing. Chemical manufacturers set mixing concentrations for replenishment and determine replenishment rates based on film size.

AUTOMATIC FILM PROCESSOR

The automatic processor is a collection of electrical and mechanical systems that control temperature, time, and chemical activity in a way that results in rapid processing of film (Fig. 1-37).

1. The auto processor has a *roller transport system* composed of rollers and deflector plates that transport film through the different tanks. A drive motor attached to a worm gear with a drive chain controls the feed rate.
2. Heaters regulated by thermostats make up the *temperature control system* for developer and dryer temperatures. Depending on the size of the developer tank, it takes between 15 and 30 minutes for developer temperatures to stabilize once the machine is turned on.
3. The *replenishment system* replenishes chemicals that are depleted through use, oxidation, or evaporation. Film sensors activate a pump to inject fresh chemicals from reservoirs outside the processor to regenerate volume and chemical activity.
4. The *circulation/filtration system* (composed of pumps, filters, and tubing) filters and circulates the water and chemicals to maintain uniform activity and stabilize temperatures.
5. Films are dried through a *dryer system,* which includes a blower, heater, and thermostat in addition to exhaust ducts.
6. The *electrical system* provides power to the other systems. Most processors are designed to partially shut down if a certain amount of time elapses between films being processed. When in "standby" mode, the drive motor and drying system (blower fan and heater) shut down to conserve energy. The developer heater

coil remains active at all times when the machine is on. This ensures a ready developer temperature anytime a film is to be processed. Placing a film in the processor activates all systems and takes the machine off standby.

Silver Recovery

Silver is a heavy metal that renders the fixer a hazardous waste, which causes damage to biologic systems. For this reason, silver must be recovered from spent fixer before it is discarded. Approximately 10% of the silver from a fresh film is recoverable, which also may generate a monetary return.

The fixer collecting system in the processor can be directly attached to a silver recovery unit. The unit has an outflow tube connected to a drain. Residual silver is recovered from fixing solutions through *metallic exchange, electrolysis* or *electroplating,* and *chemical precipitation.* Metallic replacement and electroplating can be performed in-house. Currently only commercial silver dealers use chemical precipitation.

A *metallic exchange unit* is a plastic bucket filled with steel wool or a steel screen. It has an inflow that accepts silver-laden fixer and outflow that passes silverless fixer to the drain. It is usually used in low-volume circumstances. No electricity is used. The iron in the steel gives up electrons to the silver, which causes silver to attach to the steel. Efficiency decreases with age based on total gallons of fixer treated or total silver exchanged. The useful life of a metallic exchange unit is approximately 6 months to 1 year.

An *electrolytic unit* uses an electric current passing between an anode and a cathode. The cathode offers electrons to ionic silver, converting it to atomic silver. The silver attaches to the cathode. Electrolytic units are designed for higher-volume circumstances. A properly sized electrolytic cell can recover 97% of the silver from the fixer.

Chemical precipitation requires the use of chemicals such as zinc chloride and sodium sulfite to precipitate metallic silver. The chemical reaction produces toxic chlorine gas and volatile hydrogen gas. The hazardous nature of the process requires a controlled environment not usually found in a radiology facility.

Silver also may be recovered from processed film through an industrial chemical process.

Image Quality

The goal of radiography is to maximize the amount of clearly defined anatomy on a film while maintaining a minimum dose to the patient. To realize this, the film must have adequate density (darkness and brightness), contrast (gray scale), and detail (clarity and resolution), with a minimum of distortion (aberrant size and shape). Film quality characteristics can be divided into *photographic properties* (image visibility), which include density, contrast, noise and fog factors, and *geometric properties* (structural sharpness), which include recorded detail and size and shape distortion.

PHOTOGRAPHIC PROPERTIES

Film density. *Film density* is described as the overall blackness seen on a finished radiograph. It results from the development of exposed silver halide crystals in the film emulsion. The greater the concentration of developed silver on a film, the less light is transmitted through the film, giving the appearance of a very dark area or image. From a photographic perspective, film may appear too dark, or *overexposed,* which demonstrates too much density;

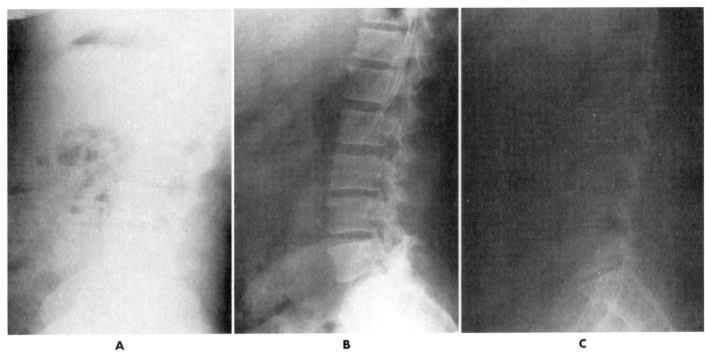

FIG. 1-38 A, Underexposed lateral lumbar film. **B,** An adequately exposed lateral lumbar film. **C,** Overexposed lateral lumbar film.

too light, or *underexposed,* which demonstrates too little density; or adequate exposure, which represents proper density (Fig. 1-38).

Film density is *inversely related* to patient density. The greater the patient density is, the lesser, or lighter, the film density will be. The body comprises tissues of different densities (expressed in *g/cm³*), which allow disparate amounts of x-ray radiation to penetrate. Radiographic contrast results from shades of these different film densities. Five observable radiographic densities result from x-ray interaction with patient density. They range from *radiolucent* (black) to *radiopaque* (white)—*air, fat, water, bone,* and *metal* (Fig. 1-39).

Film density is controlled by *milliampere-seconds,* because controlling milliampere-seconds regulates exposure. In a similar manner in which the brightness control knob on a black-and-white television controls overall darkness and lightness, milliampere-seconds controls the relative darkness of a radiograph. Individual film densities represented by tissues such as bone, muscle, and fat are affected more by peak kilovoltage than milliampere-seconds, because peak kilovoltage controls x-ray beam penetration. X-ray absorption is determined by beam penetration. Controlling factors and affecting factors for film density can be seen in Box 1-1.

Under normal conditions, affecting factors are standardized so that milliampere-seconds can be used to predictably control density. Milliampere-seconds is adjusted according to patient size and density. If affecting factors such as processing or peak kilovoltage become variable, then milliampere-seconds, and therefore film density, becomes less predictable.

The minimum change in milliampere-seconds necessary to cause a visible change in film density is 30%; however, repeating a radiograph only for a 30% change in milliampere-seconds is rarely clinically justified. Most commonly, films repeated for density require a doubling or halving of the milliampere-seconds. Within the useful range for film density, *density is doubled when milliampere-seconds is doubled and reduced to half when milliampere-seconds is halved.* Peak kilovoltage also has a direct effect on film density.

According to the *15% rule for peak kilovoltage,* a 15% increase in peak kilovoltage doubles film density. Conversely, a 15% decrease in peak kilovoltage reduces the density by half. Changes in peak kilovoltage affect density by altering the absorption-to-penetration ratio. Hence low-density tissues appear significantly darker than high-density tissues when peak kilovoltage is increased.

Film contrast. As discussed, *radiographic contrast* includes both subject and detector contrast. *Subject contrast* is determined by attenuation of the beam by the patient or subject and is controlled by peak kilovoltage. *Detector contrast* refers to inherent film response characteristics in recording high and low contrast. Subject contrast is variable.

Contrast is the difference between adjacent film densities and is described in gray scale from black to white (Fig. 1-40). A *high-contrast* radiograph demonstrates a *short gray scale,* or black and white, and is achieved with low peak kilovoltage. At lower peak kilovoltage, high-density tissues absorb more x-rays, which produce a very white appearance. Low-density tissues absorb little x-ray and appear very dark. A *low-contrast* radiograph portrays a *long gray scale,* or many shades of gray, and is achieved with high peak kilovoltage. High peak kilovoltage increases penetration to tissues of all densities, thereby decreasing the difference in blackening between tissues of various thicknesses and densities.

The primary controlling factor of contrast is *peak kilovoltage.* The kilovoltage selector works similarly to a contrast knob on a black-and-white television. An increase in peak kilovoltage with a subsequent decrease in milliampere-seconds decreases contrast. A decrease in peak kilovoltage with a compensatory increase in milliampere-seconds increases contrast. Milliampere-seconds alone plays no significant role in contrast because it has no effect on the absorption-to-penetration ratio. (Controlling factors and affecting factors for contrast can be found in Box 1-2.) Aberrant film processing and various fog factors can significantly compromise film contrast.

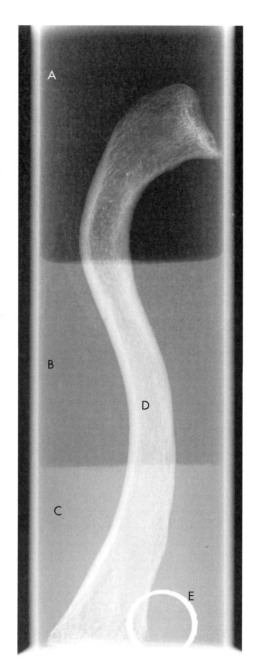

FIG. 1-39 Graduated cylinder representing the five different densities seen on a radiograph, from most radiolucent to most radiopaque: *A*, air; *B*, oil (fat); *C*, water; *D*, bone; and *E*, metal.

Visibility of detail. *Visibility of detail* is the visible perception of the structural details transferred to the film. Subject contrast, overall film density, fog, and noise factors all affect the visibility of detail. The term *noise* often is used to describe static found in audio systems. Video systems such as a television manifest noise as "snow." Radiographic "noise" is undesirable background information that is detected, but does not contribute to the quality of the image. Types of radiographic noise include *scatter radiation, film graininess, structural mottle,* and *quantum mottle.*

Image visibility relies greatly on film contrast. Low contrast caused from scatter radiation, safelight fog, and chemical fog decreases visibility of detail.

BOX 1-1
Film Density

Controlling factors
  Milliampere-seconds

Primary affecting factors
  Peak kilovoltage
  Film processing
  Film/intensifying screens
  Source-to-image distance
  Patient size, shape, and pathology

Secondary affecting factors
  Filtration
  Grid
  Beam limitation
  Fog
  Contrast media
  Anode heel effect

Film graininess results from the size and distribution of silver halide crystals in the emulsion. *Structural mottle* is the intensifying screen version of film graininess produced from large and widely distributed phosphor crystals in the screen. *Quantum mottle* results from the random interaction of x-ray photons with the image receptor and is the leading contributor to radiographic noise. With very fast imaging systems, a small amount of x-ray is needed to expose the film. The photons interact randomly with the phosphors

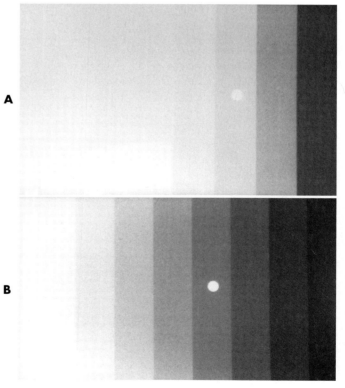

FIG. 1-40 Contrast describes the range of shades of gray in an image. **A** demonstrates higher contrast and a shorter scale of contrast than **B** because it progresses from white to dark with fewer shades of gray.

BOX 1-2
Film Contrast

Controlling factors
  Peak kilovoltage

Primary affecting factors
  Fog
  Grid
  Film processing
  Beam limitations
  Patient size, shape, and pathology
  Pulsations in waveform
  Contrast media
  Filtration

Secondary affecting factors
  Film/intensifying screens
  Compression devices
  Object-to-film distance

BOX 1-3
Film Detail

Factors affecting visibility of detail
  Density
  Contrast
  Noise
  Fog

Factors affecting recorded detail
  Motion
  Source-to-image distance
  Object-to-film distance
  Focal spot size
  Intensifying screen
  Object shape and density

Factors affecting distortion
  Object-to-film distance
  Source-to-image distance
  Patient thickness
  Central ray centering
  Object plane
  Film plane

---

in the intensifying screen, which produces a light output similar in effect to that of a low-resolution computer printer. A low-resolution printer prints fewer dots per inch (dpi) than a high-resolution printer, leaving a more mottled appearance. With faster imaging systems (>600), fewer numbers of x-ray photons are needed to produce the image (low dpi), thereby increasing quantum mottle and decreasing the visible quality of the image. All film/screen imaging systems inherently produce quantum mottle, with higher levels found in the faster systems.

Geometric Properties

Recorded detail. An image that appears "in-focus" with sharply defined structural borders and clarity of minute internal structures has good *recorded detail*. Various factors affecting geometric sharpness can be found in Box 1-3. X-rays do not emanate from a point source but rather from an area called a *focal spot*. Not all x-rays emitted from the focal spot hit a locus on an object at the same projectional angle (Fig. 1-41). The distinct core of the object is defined as the *umbra,* or area of geometric sharpness. The image may demonstrate an area of geometric unsharpness, or *penumbra,* adjacent to the umbral shadow. A large focal spot inherently produces a larger penumbra than a small focal spot.

Penumbra can be minimized by using a small focal spot, a long focal-film distance (FFD), and a short object-film distance (OFD). The penumbral effect contributing to geometric unsharpness may be calculated using the following formula:

Geometric unsharpness (penumbra) = (Focal spot size) × (OFD)/(FFD)

Other factors affecting image sharpness include motion unsharpness, intensifying screen unsharpness, and absorption unsharpness. *Motion unsharpness* most commonly results from patient movement during the exposure and compromises recorded detail (Fig. 1-42). A less common source of motion is vibration of the imaging equipment. Patients exhibit voluntary (gross movement) and involuntary motion (cardiac and respiratory motion). Radiographers have learned to control the effects of patient motion by using reliable immobilization techniques, short exposure time, and specific breathing instructions.

Intensifying screen unsharpness, also called *inherent unsharpness,* increases with larger phosphor crystals, thicker phosphor layers, use of a reflective layer, and poor contact between film and screen.

Variation in the absorption of the beam by the structural edges of an object may lead to *absorption unsharpness.* The shape and density of an object, in addition to the angle of incidence of the x-ray beam, may cause the edges to appear well defined or fuzzy. Absorption unsharpness gives the appearance of increased penumbra.

Distortion. *Distortion* is an exaggeration of the size or shape of an object because of unequal magnification of different parts of the object. *Shape distortion* occurs when any combination of film,

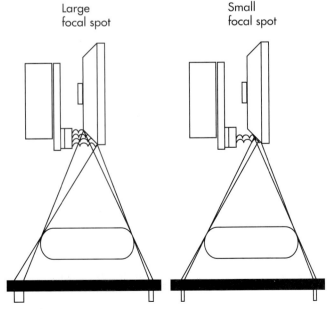

FIG. 1-41 A large focal spot produces a larger penumbra, resulting in less detail than a small focal spot.

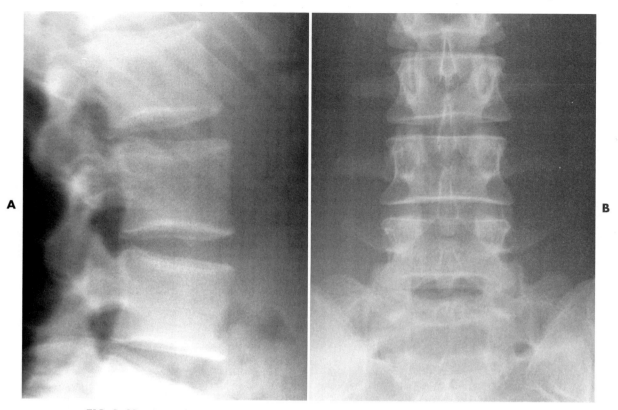

FIG. 1-42 A, Decreased detail caused by motion. **B,** No motion artifact, resulting in increased detail.

object, and central ray do not lie in the same plane (Fig. 1-43). Angulation of the film, object, or central ray (Fig. 1-44) causes an unequal elongation of the object, changing its shape. Off-centering of the object to the central ray also causes shape distortion. Simple *magnification,* in which the object size is increased, results in *size distortion.* Maintaining a short OFD and a long FFD minimizes magnification. Recorded detail is increased as size and shape distortion is reduced.

TROUBLESHOOTING IMAGE QUALITY

Common image problems seen in radiography include inadequate density, poor contrast, and loss of detail. A myriad of causes exists; however, some occur with greater frequency than others. Algorithms have been created to help troubleshoot the more common causes of poor image quality (see pages 32 to 34).

Technique

Radiography is an art form realized through the radiographer's ability to select proper exposure factors for a given examination. Although many influences exist, results are most predictable when many of the variables are standardized while varying a single factor. The two more common exposure theories in use today are *fixed peak kilovoltage/variable milliampere-seconds* and *variable peak kilovoltage/fixed milliampere-seconds techniques.*

FIXED PEAK KILOVOLTAGE/VARIABLE MILLIAMPERE-SECONDS TECHNIQUE

Peak kilovoltage affects many factors, such as contrast, density, patient dose, visibility of detail, penetration power, and scatter radiation production. These outcomes are more predictable when applying a fixed peak kilovoltage technique. In a fixed peak kilovoltage system, optimum kilovoltage is held constant for a

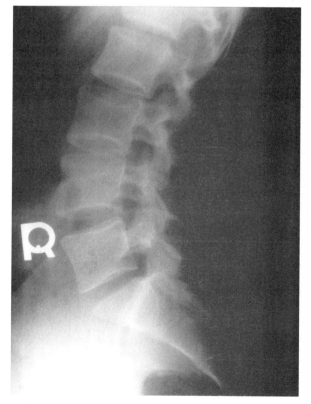

FIG. 1-43 Distortion of the lumbar spine with noted "hourglassing" effect. In this case, the convexity of the lumbar curve was not adjacent to the Bucky. Convention places the convexity of an aberrant spinal curvature against the Bucky to accommodate a divergent x-ray beam, thereby reducing projectional distortion.

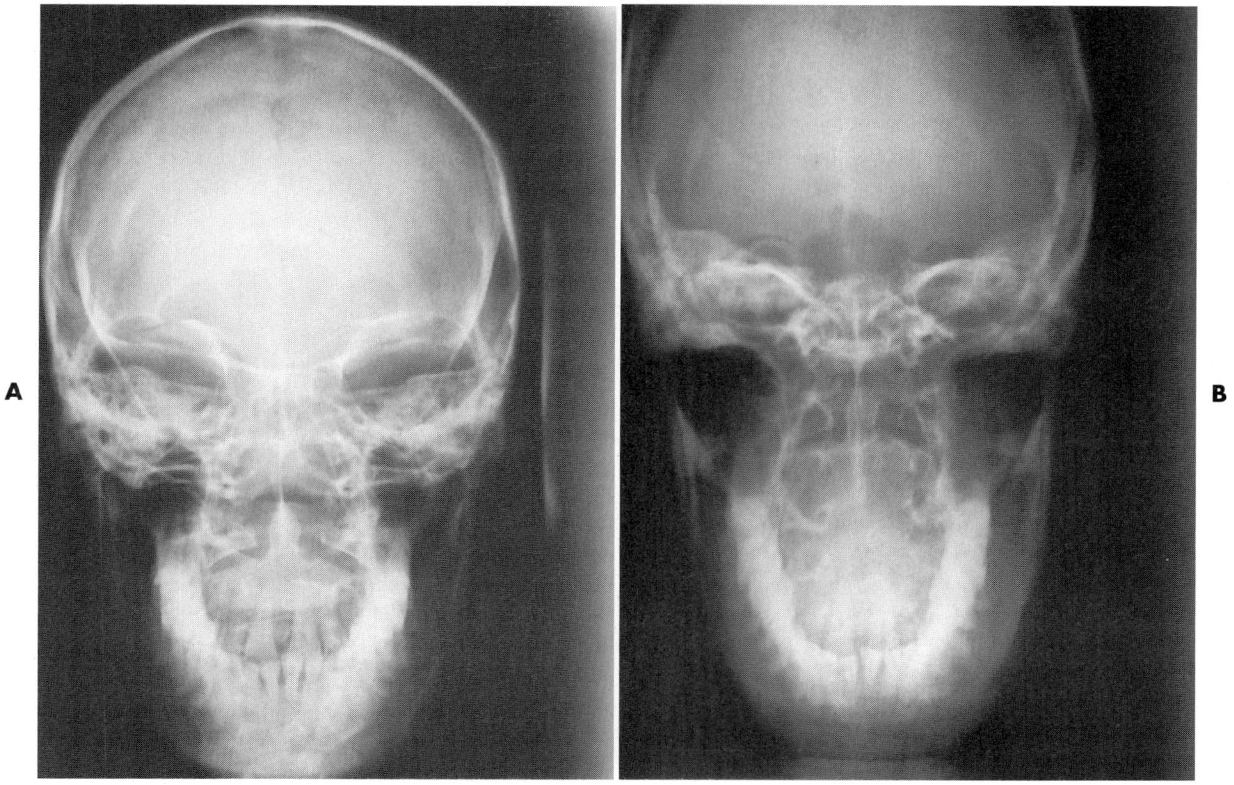

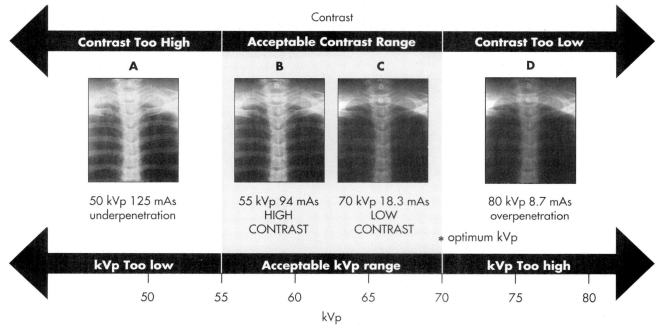

FIG. I-44 Distortion caused by tube tilt: **A,** which was taken with a 15° caudal tube tilt, is sharper and less distorted than **B,** which was taken with a 35° tube tilt.

Contrast

Contrast Too High	Acceptable Contrast Range		Contrast Too Low
A	**B**	**C**	**D**

50 kVp 125 mAs
underpenetration

55 kVp 94 mAs
HIGH
CONTRAST

70 kVp 18.3 mAs
LOW
CONTRAST

80 kVp 8.7 mAs
overpenetration

* optimum kVp

kVp Too low	Acceptable kVp range	kVp Too high

50   55   60   65   70   75   80

kVp

FIG. I-45 **A** through **D,** Optimum kVp. Although a range of acceptable peak kilovoltage exists per body part, optimum kVp is the highest peak kilovoltage that will produce acceptable contrast. Peak kilovoltages are shown within acceptable and unacceptable limits. The optimum peak kilovoltage for this body part is clearly marked.

TABLE 1-2

Suggested Optimum* Peak Kilovoltage (kVp) for Body Parts

Anatomy	Optimum kVp	
	Single phase	High frequency
Small extremity†	55-65	55-65
Large extremity‡	65-70	65-70
Lateral cervical spine	75	70
AP cervical spine	70	70
AP open mouth	75	70
Lateral thoracic spine	80	80
AP thoracic spine	75	70
Lateral lumbar spine	90	80
AP lumbar spine	80	75
AP pelvis	80	75
Abdomen	80	80
Ribs	70	70
Skull	80	75
Chest	110	110

*Pragmatic technique charts may list a small range of kVp settings accounting for extremes of body size.
†Small extremity: hand, wrist, forearm, elbow, foot, ankle.
‡Large extremity: upper arm, shoulder, knee, femur, hip.

given range of patient thickness, and milliampere-seconds is varied to attain the proper film density. *Optimum peak kilovoltage is the maximum kilovoltage that consistently produces an image with contrast within acceptable limits* (Fig. 1-45). Optimum peak kilovoltage provides greater penetration than what is minimally needed to penetrate the part. This ensures adequate penetration of a larger population of subjects without varying peak kilovoltage. With a fixed peak kilovoltage, milliampere-seconds changes with the patient measurement. The smallest increment of milliampere-seconds change on the technique chart is 30% because visible density changes cannot be detected below 30%. On average, milliampere-seconds doubles for every 5-cm increase in patient measurement.

Advantages of a fixed kilovoltage technique include lower patient dose, a wider exposure latitude (margin for exposure error), and longer gray scale. Those who prefer high-contrast films may negatively perceive the lower contrast. A disadvantage of optimum kilovoltage is an increase in scatter radiation production. Some subjectivity is involved in selecting optimum peak kilovoltage because of contrast preference of the radiologist. Table 1-2 lists suggested optimum peak kilovoltage for different body parts using single-phase and high-frequency generators.

VARIABLE PEAK KILOVOLTAGE/FIXED MILLIAMPERE-SECONDS TECHNIQUE

With variable peak kilovoltage technique, milliampere-seconds is fixed and peak kilovoltage varied, based on patient thickness. The size of the patient part determines the change in penetration of the beam. A range of kilovoltages from high to low can be used for any given body part. *Milliampere-second values are based primarily on film/screen speed, grid ratio, and body part size.* The quantity of radiation (mAs) remains constant from the smallest to the largest part.

Historically, with variable peak kilovoltage technique it is common practice to change peak kilovoltage by 2 for every 1 cm of patient tissue thickness. The following formula is applied:

Peak kilovoltage = 2 kVp × Part size + A base number

The base number varies, based on the minimum peak kilovoltage needed to penetrate the body part. For small extremities, the base number is 50; for cervical and thoracic spine and large extremities, 40; and for lumbar spine and pelvis, 30.

By design, lower peak kilovoltage is used in fixed peak kilovoltage techniques than in fixed peak kilovoltage systems. Advantages include high-contrast films and incremental changes in peak kilovoltage to compensate for variations in patient thickness. The disadvantages are higher patient dose, low exposure latitude, and variable contrast for the same body part as thickness changes.

TECHNIQUE APPLICATION

Multiple mechanisms exist to apply radiographic technique. *Automatic Exposure Control (AEC)* provides automated density control once peak kilovoltage is selected. Accuracy of exposure correlates to accuracy of positioning the anatomy over the photosensors and proper collimation. *Technique charts,* constructed based on fixed or variable peak kilovoltage, are customized to individual x-ray machines and imaging systems. Exposure accuracy is based on precise caliper measurements of the patient part. Charts are not easily transferable from one facility to another without some tinkering. The *SuperTech* technique calculator is a pocket-sized slide rule device with the versatility to provide accurate exposure information for many clinical situations. It can be applied easily to any x-ray setup. The newest innovation in technique application is the *anatomic preprogrammed technique.* The control console is outfitted with a software package that provides push-button selection of predetermined techniques based on anatomy and part thickness. All technique systems possess inherent error that must be monitored and eliminated. Fine tuning is essential to minimize repeat radiographs and patient dose.

Radiation Protection

Ionizing radiation exposures should be kept *As Low As Reasonably Achievable (ALARA).* ALARA is the overriding principle in radiation protection of patients and personnel.

PROTECTION OF THE PATIENT

The radiographer is responsible for understanding and applying safe radiologic procedures that minimize dose to patients. Unfortunately, many factors that contribute to producing a diagnostic image also increase patient dose. Such factors must be properly applied to minimize the dose while producing acceptable quality images. Recommendations to reduce patient dose are as follows:

1. *Technique.* Techniques that use high peak kilovoltage and low milliampere-seconds decrease patient dose. Proper attention ensures that the contrast is acceptable for the peak kilovoltage used.
2. *Grids.* Exposure must be increased when using a grid because both primary and scatter radiation are absorbed by the grid. Using the lowest acceptable grid ratio to improve contrast helps minimize dose.
3. *Beam restriction.* The exposure field size should be limited to the area of interest whenever possible and should never exceed the film size.
4. *Shielding.* To protect against genetic effects on the progeny of irradiated individuals, especially during child-bearing years, use of gonad shields is recommended whenever their use does not compromise diagnostic information. Collimation, properly applied, may minimize gonadal dose. Other radiosensitive organs such as eyes, thyroid, and female breasts should be shielded when appropriate.

5. *Filtration.* Inherent filtration plus added filtration help reduce soft radiation exposure to the patient. Compensating filters, such as wedge filters, help even out exposure to the film and at the same time reduce patient dose over the areas filtered.

6. *PA radiography.* Many radiosensitive organs (e.g., eyes, thyroid, breasts, and gonads) are located anteriorly in the patient. Projecting the beam through the patient posterior-to-anterior (PA) helps reduce organ exposure as the beam is attenuated in the patient.

7. *Image receptors.* The film/intensifying screen combination plays a pivotal role in reducing patient dose. Faster systems linearly reduce dose. A 400-speed system requires approximately one half the exposure of a 200-speed system. However, factors such as quantum mottle and film graininess must be considered when trying to balance patient dose with acceptable recorded detail.

8. *Repeat radiographs.* Common reasons for repeating radiographs include poor positioning of the patient, film, or tube; improper technique selection; inadequate film processing; artifacts; and patient motion. Patient dose increases any time a film is repeated. Many repeats could be avoided by effectively communicating with the patient initially and by being cognizant of the common errors that result in repeat films.

PROTECTION OF PERSONNEL

Laws entitle occupational radiation workers to a radiation-safe environment. A state inspector scrutinizes each facility for radiation safety annually or biannually. Basic principles of radiation protection for personnel include *time, distance,* and *shielding. Time* spent in the vicinity of x-ray exposure should be kept to a minimum. In accordance with the inverse square law, radiation exposure decreases significantly as *distance* is increased. Whenever possible, workers should maintain a safe distance from sources of ionizing radiation. Unfortunately, radiographers work very close to the x-ray machine, especially the fluoroscope, and fluoroscopic exposures run intermittently for minutes to an hour or more. In this case *shielding* is best applied. Shielding includes anything from a lead apron and gloves to a protective barrier placed between the source of radiation and the exposed individual.

For personal radiation protection, radiographers should follow these guidelines:
- Apply the rules of time, distance, and shielding.
- Maintain the smallest collimation field appropriate for the examination.
- Always wear a radiation monitoring device (e.g., film badge, thermoluminescent dosimeter [TLD], pocket dosimeter) to detect exposure.
- Avoid holding a patient during a radiographic examination. If using a restraining device is not possible and a patient must be held, no person should routinely hold patients.
- Ensure that anyone holding a patient is properly protected with a full lead apron and lead gloves.

Dose Limits. The federal government of the United States sets dose limits for radiation workers and the general public. The federal agency that enforces radiation safety laws and dose limits is the Nuclear Regulatory Commission (NRC). Dose limits are reported in the NCRP publications. NCRP Report No. 116, Limitation of Exposure to Ionizing Radiation (1993), provides the most up-to-date information on occupational and nonoccupational dose limits.[1] A summary of Report No. 116 can be found in Table 1-3. These dose limits *do not* pertain to patients receiving medical exposures for diagnostic or therapeutic purposes. The *annual effective dose limit* for

TABLE 1-3
Estimated Exposures*

Exposure	SI	Customary
Occupational exposures		
Effective dose limit		
Annual	50 mSv	5 rem
Cumulative	10 mSv × age	1 rem × age
Annual equivalent dose limits for tissues and organs		
Lens of eye	150 mSv	15 rem
Skin, hands, and feet	500 mSv	50 rem
Public exposures (annual)		
Effective dose limit		
Continuous or frequent exposure	1 mSv	0.1 rem
Infrequent exposure	5 mSv	0.5 rem
Equivalent dose limits for tissues and organs		
Lens of eye	15 mSv	1.5 rem
Skin, hands, and feet	50 mSv	5 rem
Education and training exposures (annual)		
Effective dose limit	1 mSv	0.1 rem
Equivalent dose limits for tissues and organs		
Lens of eye	15 mSv	1.5 rem
Skin, hands, and feet	50 mSv	5 rem
Embryo-fetus exposures (monthly)		
Effective dose limit	0.5 mSv	0.05 rem

*From National Council on Radiation Protection and Measurements: Report No. 116, Limitations of exposure to ionising radiation (supercedes NCRP report No. 91), Bethesda, Md, 1993, NCRP.

occupational exposures is *5 rem (50 mSv) per year.* The *cumulative effective dose limit* for occupational exposures is

$$1 \text{ rem} \times \text{Age of worker}$$

Dose limits are established primarily to minimize the risks of stochastic and nonstochastic radiation effects. A *stochastic radiation effect* is one in which the probability of occurrence, rather than severity, increases as the dose increases. No threshold dose exists below which risk is eliminated. Examples of stochastic effects are cancer and genetic effects.

A *nonstochastic radiation effect* is one that manifests with certainty after a certain dose and the severity increases as the dose increases. A threshold dose exists below which nonstochastic effects do not manifest. Examples include sterility changes, radiation burns, and cataract formation in the lens of the eye.

X-RAY AND PREGNANCY

Because of the radiosensitive nature of the embryo-fetus, especially in the first 14 weeks after conception, radiation exposure to the pregnant or potentially pregnant patient or worker should be significantly limited.

According to NCRP Report No. 54, Medical Radiation Exposure of Pregnant and Potentially Pregnant Women, the decision to x-ray a pregnant patient is relegated to the judgment of the physician.[2] When the protection of the patient's health requires a radiologic

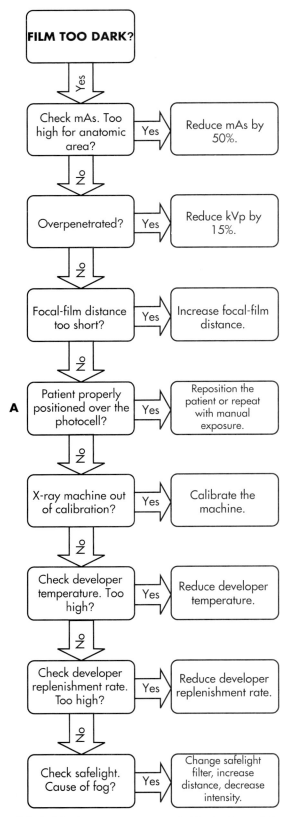

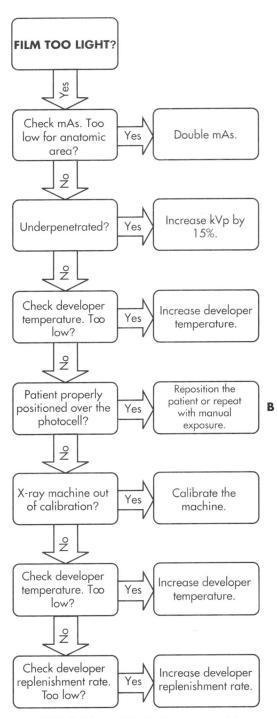

FIG. 1-46 Problem-solving charts. **A,** Film that is too dark.

FIG. 1-46 cont'd **B,** Film that is too light.

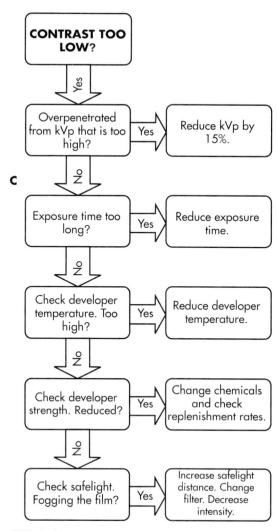

FIG. 1-46 cont'd **C,** Film with a contrast that is too low.

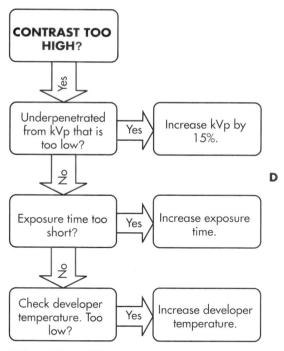

FIG. 1-46 cont'd **D,** Film with a contrast that is too high.

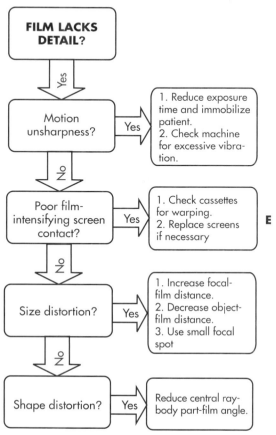

FIG. 1-46 cont'd **E,** Film that is fogged.

examination at a specific time, and adequate radiologic equipment and technique are used, in most cases, the potential benefits of the procedure outweigh the risks of the exposure. One in 1000 of all radiologic examinations (excluding fluoroscopy), performed properly, exposes the embryo-fetus to 1 rad or more of radiation. The NCRP Report No. 54 states that human embryo-fetus exposures below 5 rad are considered to be an acceptable risk when compared with the medical benefit of the radiologic examination to the patient.[2] Diagnostic procedures rarely result in a dose to the uterus as high as 5 rad. *The equivalent dose limit* (excluding medical exposure) *for the embryo should not exceed 0.05 rem (0.5 mSv) per month.*

Pregnant patients. Performing radiography on pregnant patients requires precisely collimated x-ray beams and properly positioned protective shields.

In the past, elective (nonemergent) radiologic procedures to the abdominal area of patients of child-bearing potential were recommended to be scheduled at a designated time to minimize exposure to an embryo in the early days of pregnancy. The *10-day rule* was applied to the 10-day period after the onset of menses, when the probability of pregnancy is low. The 10-day rule is now obsolete for medical procedures.

The pregnancy status of females of child-bearing potential should always be predetermined so that appropriate imaging decisions and radiation protection measures may be taken. When pregnancy is not known, it is common practice to solicit the date of the patient's last menses. If pregnancy is suspected, nonemergent exams may be rescheduled.

Pregnant workers. As stated, radiation exposure to the fetus of a pregnant worker must be limited. Pregnant workers should minimize or avoid rotations in fluoroscopy, portable radiography, and special procedures. Radiation protection practices such as time, distance, and shielding, should be reviewed and strictly enforced. Fetal dose may be monitored by having the worker wear a second personnel-monitoring device below a lead apron covering the abdomen. *The annual effective dose limit for the pregnant worker is reduced to the equivalent dose limit for the fetus, 0.05 rem per month, while the worker is pregnant.*

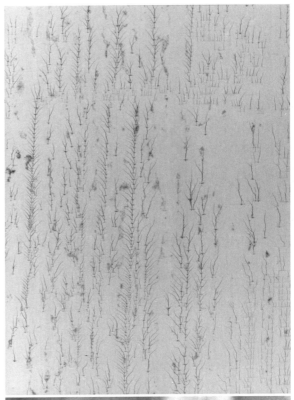

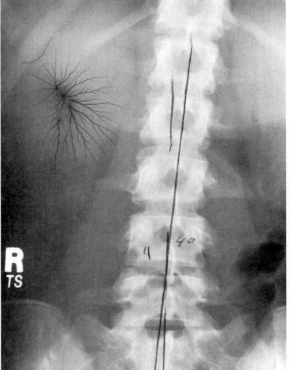

FIG. 1-47   **A–D,** Various static electricity markings.

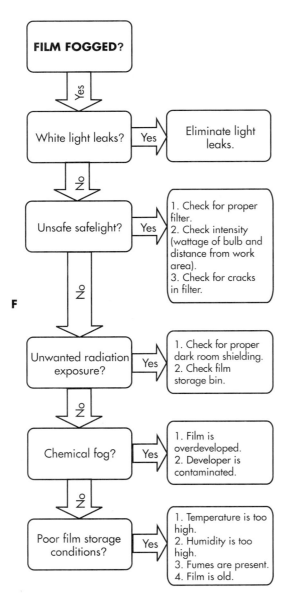

FILM FOGGED?

↓ Yes

White light leaks? → Yes → Eliminate light leaks.

↓ No

Unsafe safelight? → Yes →
1. Check for proper filter.
2. Check intensity (wattage of bulb and distance from work area).
3. Check for cracks in filter.

↓ No

Unwanted radiation exposure? → Yes →
1. Check for proper dark room shielding.
2. Check film storage bin.

↓ No

Chemical fog? → Yes →
1. Film is overdeveloped.
2. Developer is contaminated.

↓ No

Poor film storage conditions? → Yes →
1. Temperature is too high.
2. Humidity is too high.
3. Fumes are present.
4. Film is old.

F

FIG. 1-46 cont'd   **F,** Film that lacks detail.

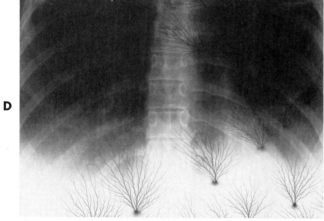

FIG. 1-47 cont'd (**D,** Courtesy Gary Longmuir, Phoenix, AZ.)

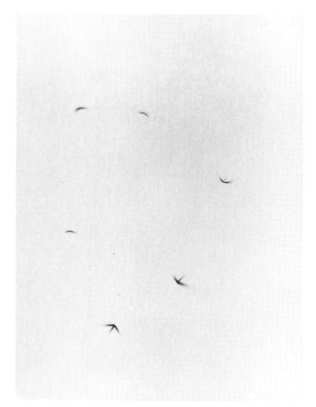

FIG. 1-48 Crescent artifacts that result from kinked film.

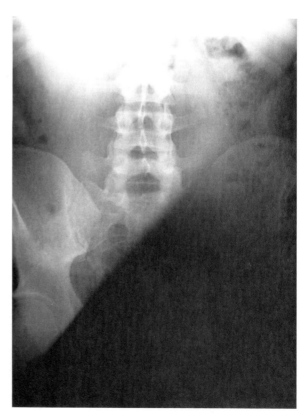

FIG. 1-49 Overexposed lower corner of the film secondary to light leak.

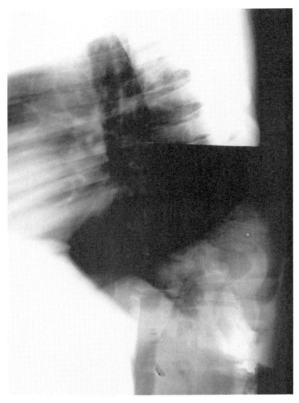

FIG. 1-50   Two films stuck together during processing.

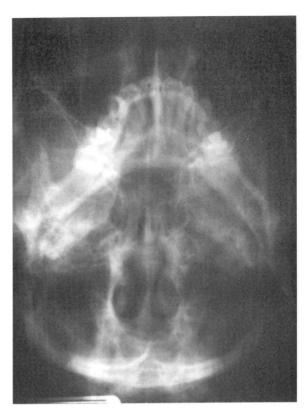

FIG. 1-51   Blurred, overexposed appearance caused by double exposure.

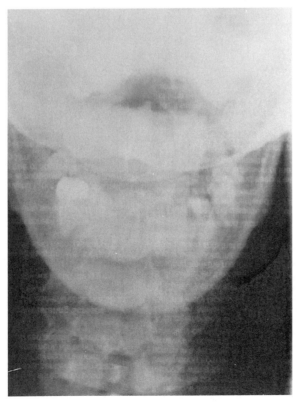

FIG. 1-52   Protective contact paper covering the intensifying screen of a new cassette was not removed before cassette use.

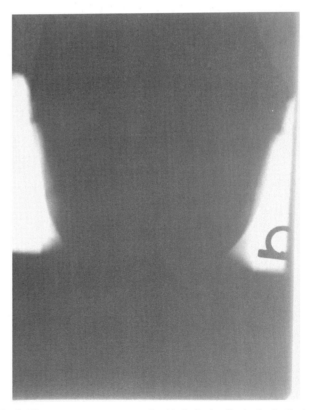

FIG. 1-53   Diagnostic exposure made with duplication film inadvertently placed in the cassette.

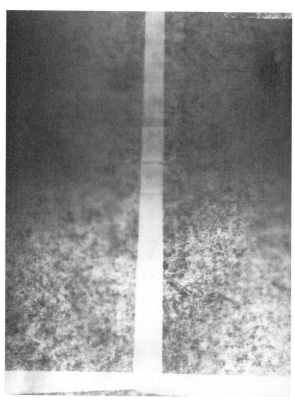

FIG. I-54 Exposed film was left in a paper film envelope in a lighted room while the radiographer went to lunch. After development, the light leaked through the paper envelope, creating this mottled appearance.

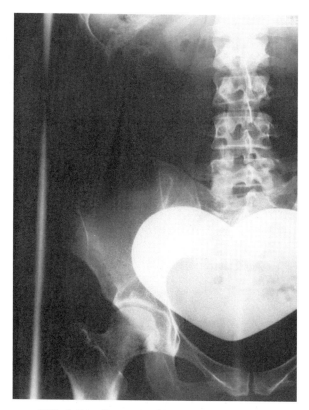

FIG. I-56 Cassette not fully pushed into the Bucky.

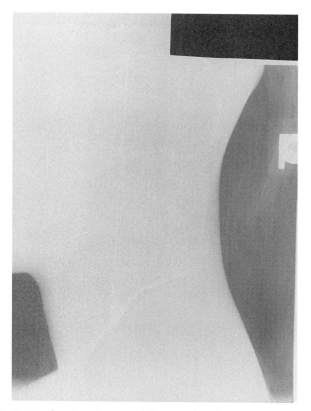

FIG. I-55 Grossly underexposed film caused by single-emulsion extremity film that was mistaken for spinal film.

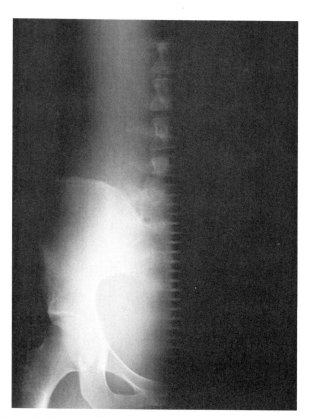

FIG. I-57 Darkroom light was turned on before the film had entirely entered the automatic processor.

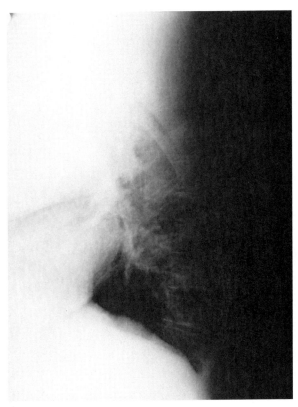

FIG. 1-58   Film fog resulting from a light leak.

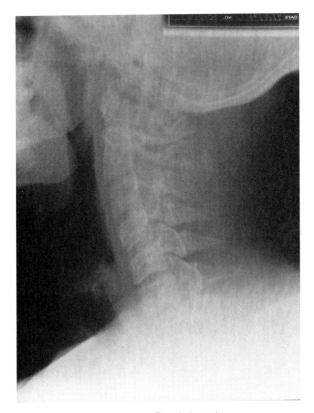

FIG. 1-60   Chemical streaks.

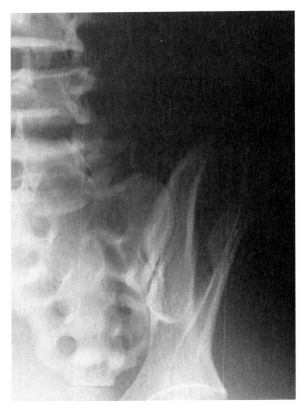

FIG. 1-59   Linear artifacts from processor's guide shoe.

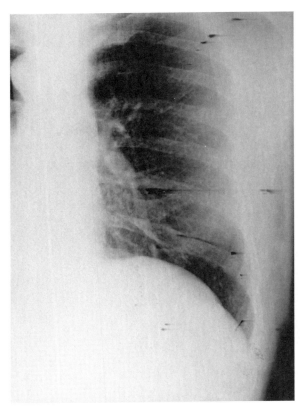

FIG. 1-61   Dark streaks from debris on rollers.

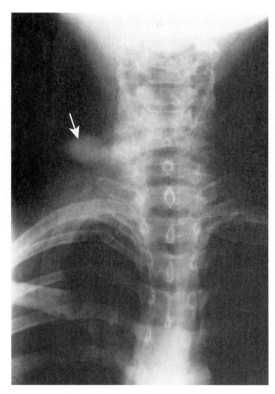

FIG. 1-62 Hair braid artifact *(arrow)*.

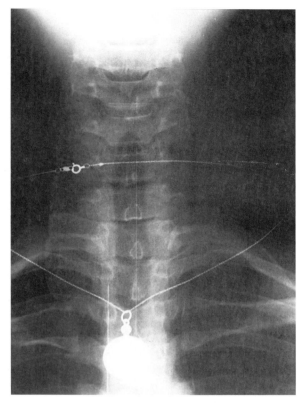

FIG. 1-64 Patient's necklace.

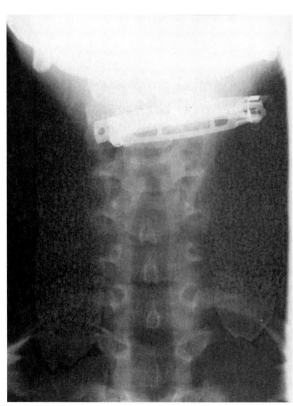

FIG. 1-63 Barrette artifact.

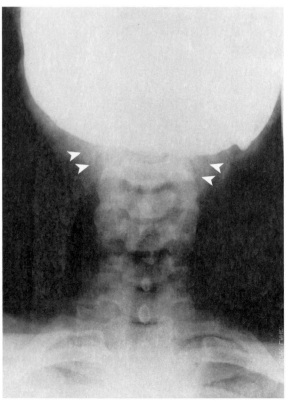

FIG. 1-65 Hair extensions artifact *(arrowheads)*.

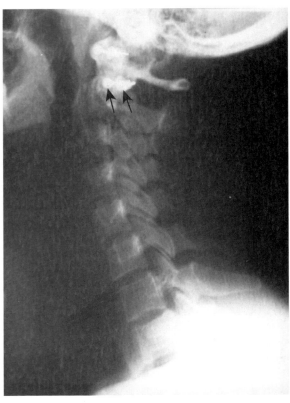

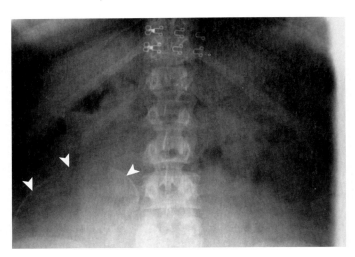

FIG. I-68 Bra clasp and infant's skull artifacts *(arrowheads)*.

FIG. I-66 Earring artifact *(arrows)*.

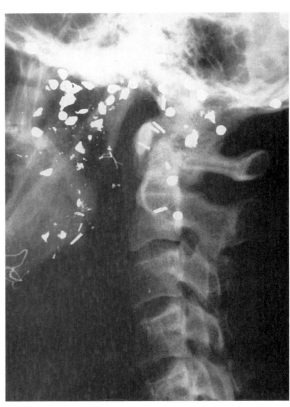

FIG. I-67 Gunshot to the face.

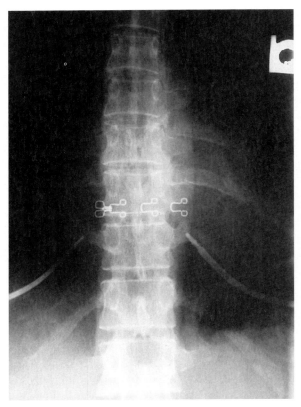

FIG. I-69 Bra clasp and underwire artifacts.

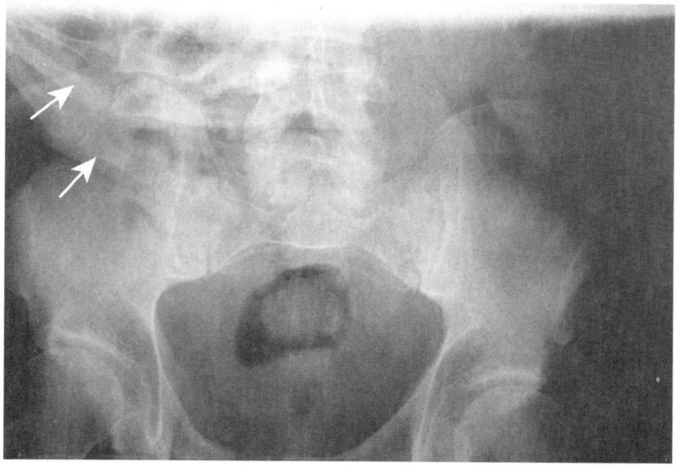

FIG. I-70 Hand artifact *(arrows)*.

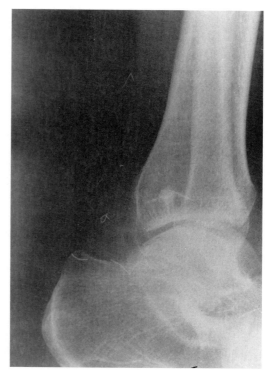

FIG. I-71 Acupuncture needle artifacts.

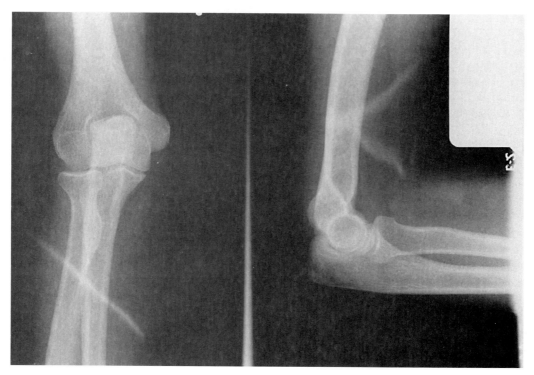

FIG. I-72 Clothing artifact.

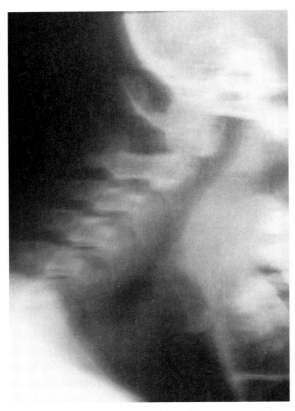

FIG. 1-73 Motion artifact causing a blurred appearance of the cervical anatomy.

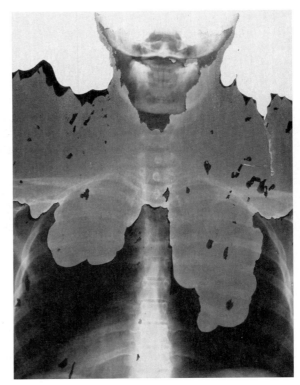

FIG. 1-74 Blotchy appearance of a film left in the fixer too long. (Courtesy Gary Longmuir, Phoenix, AZ.)

Problem Solving

The charts shown in Figure 1-46 are designed to assist radiographers in problem solving commonly encountered errors of image quality. Each radiograph warrants critical evaluation for density, contrast, and detail. If the radiograph is of diagnostic quality, close observation demonstrates areas that may be improved on for future studies. If the radiograph is not of diagnostic quality, the following charts assist the radiographer in determining which factors may be altered to improve the image.

Pictorial Summary

Figures 1-47 through 1-72 illustrate selected artifacts that are often encountered in clinical practice.

References

1. National Council on Radiation Protection and Measurements: Report No. 116, Limitations of exposure to ionizing radiation (supersedes NCRP Report No. 91), Bethesda, MD, 1993, NCRP.
2. National Council on Radiation Protection and Measurements: Report No. 54, Medical radiation exposure of pregnant and potentially pregnant women, Bethesda, MD, 1977, NCRP.

Suggested Readings

Burns EF: Radiographic imaging. A guide for producing quality radiographs, Philadelphia, 1992, WB Saunders.

Bushberg JT et al: The essential physics of medical imaging, Baltimore, 1994, Williams & Wilkins.
Bushong SC: Radiologic science for technologists: physics, biology, and protection, ed 7, St Louis, 2001, Mosby.
Carlton RR, Adler AM: Principles of radiographic imaging: an art and science, ed 2, Albany, 1996, Delmar Publishers.
Cullinan AM: Producing quality radiographs, Philadelphia, 1987, JB Lippincott.
Curry TS, Dowdey JE, Murry RC: Christensen's introduction to the physics of diagnostic radiology, ed 4, Philadelphia, 1990, Lea & Febiger.
Eastman Kodak Company: The fundamentals of radiography, ed 12, Rochester, 1980, Health Sciences Markets Division.
Grigg ERN: The trail of the invisible light: from x-Stahlen to radio(bio)logy, Springfield, IL, 1965, Charles C Thomas.
Lauer OG, Mayes JB, Thurston RR: Evaluating radiographic quality. The variables and their effects, Mankato, MN, 1990, Burnell.
Selman J: The fundamentals of x-ray and radium physics, ed 7, Springfield, IL, 1985, Charles C Thomas.
Sprawls P: Principles of radiography for technologists, Rockville, MD, 1987, Aspen.
Statkiewitcz-Sherer MA, Visconti PJ, Ritenour ER: Radiation protection in medical radiography, ed 4, St Louis, 2002, Mosby.
Tortorici M: Concepts in medical radiographic imaging, Philadelphia, 1992, WB Saunders.

chapter 2

Specialized Imaging

IAN D. McLEAN

Magnetic Resonance Imaging

HISTORY

Contemporary magnetic resonance imaging (MRI) developed from the nuclear magnetic resonance (NMR) technology that chemists use to evaluate the composition of laboratory samples. Laboratory use of NMR began in 1946, when Felix Bloch proposed that nuclei could behave as small magnets in the presence of a strong magnetic field.[1] Nearly three decades later, Raymond Damadien used this technology as an imaging tool when he produced a crude image of a rat tumor in 1974.[2] Damadien produced a successful image of a full body in July 3, 1977 with his MRI equipment, Indomitable, which is now housed in the Smithsonian.

MRI offers advantages over other diagnostic imaging modalities. In particular, MRI provides superior tissue contrast when compared with computed tomography (CT) and conventional radiography. The image contrast achieved in CT scanning is based on x-ray attenuation properties. Instead, MRI spatially analyzes the magnetic spin properties of tissue nuclei, principally hydrogen. Analysis of this information results in greater sensitivity to subtle differences among tissue types than is possible with imaging systems based on x-ray attenuation.

Notably MRI does not use ionizing radiation in the process of obtaining an image; therefore its use is not associated with the potential harmful effects of ionizing radiation. MRI uses high magnetic fields and radiofrequencies to analyze the magnetic spin properties of hydrogen nuclei. During the past century, the potential ill effects of magnetic or radiofrequency fields have been the focus of hundreds of papers. The specific concerns of past investigations have focused on changes in enzyme kinetics, nerve conductivity, effect on macromolecules and subcellular components, cardiac function, magnetohydrodynamic effects, membrane transportation, blood sedimentation, genetic effects, and other bioeffects. Reviews of this literature are available for the interested reader.[3-5] In general the parameters of MRI are without significant health risks, although the research is not conclusive enough to assume that MRI is absolutely safe.

EQUIPMENT

Principal components of the MRI scanner include a large homogeneous magnetic field, gradient magnetic coils, radiofrequency coils, and computer systems. On casual observation, the MRI scanner appears similar to a CT unit. Each is composed of a gantry, a couch for the patient, and a computer. The gantry of an MRI unit is longer than that of a CT scanner. The MRI gantry contains a large primary magnet to create a net magnetization of the hydrogen nuclei within the patient. Three principal types of magnets are used to generate the magnetic fields needed for MRI.[6]

1. *Superconducting magnets.* Superconducting magnets (Fig. 2-1) consist of primary magnetic coils supercooled by cryogens such as liquid helium or liquid nitrogen (Fig. 2-2). Supercooling the system dramatically decreases electrical resistance by allowing infinite conductivity. At infinite conductivity the primary magnet no longer requires a power supply, which means that the magnetic field can be interrupted only by ramping down the magnet by expelling (quenching) the cryogens. Further, the cryogens must be periodically replenished, which represents an ongoing financial cost. Superconducting magnet systems may be the most popular because they achieve good signal-to-noise ratio. They also tend to have a large peripheral (fringe) field, which can be a safety issue, especially for such medical devices as cardiac pacemakers.

2. *Permanent magnets.* Permanent magnets (Fig. 2-3) are constructed from individual bricks of ferromagnetic material. As a result, these scanners can be constructed with the popular open design (open MRI), which are less claustrophobic. Generally, these

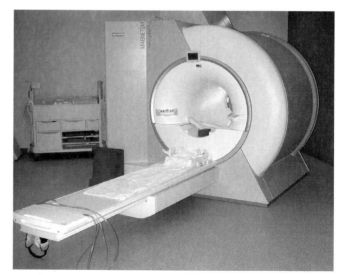

FIG. 2-1 Closed magnetic resonance imaging system using a supercooled magnet.

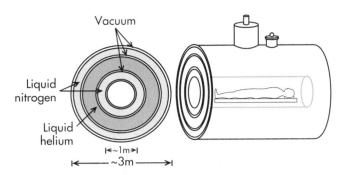

FIG. 2-2   Cross-section of a superconducting magnet.

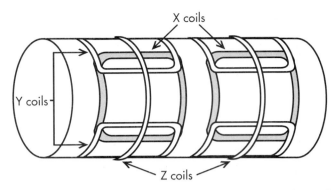

FIG. 2-4   The location of the three sets of gradient coils relative to the primary magnet. Gradient coils produce inhomogeneities of the magnet field that permit selection of slice thickness and pixel location within a slice.

systems are not able to obtain the high magnetic fields of super-conductive systems and present with field strength on the order of approximately 0.2 tesla (T) or less. Besides the lessened potential claustrophobia, other advantages include a minimal peripheral (fringe) magnetic field, minimal power consumption, and no need for relatively expensive cryogens.

3. *Resistive electromagnets.* This MRI system is based on the classical electromagnet in which large amounts of power are conducted through solenoidal loops of wire. These systems tend to have magnetic field strengths of 0.3 tesla or less. Although these systems may be of lower initial cost than superconducting magnets and of lower weight than permanent magnets, the power consumption is high. These scanners can be "turned off." Generally, however, these tend to be the least popular of the MRI designs.

MRI equipment with varying field strengths is widely available. Generally, low-field MRI is represented by equipment that has a magnetic field strength under 0.2 tesla. Midfield MRI is between 0.2 and 0.6 tesla. High-field MRI is 1 tesla and above. Considerable discussion can be found in the literature as to which magnet system (low-field versus high-field) is "better." High-field MRI equipment does allow for high-resolution images and improved

signal-to-noise ratio; however, advances in computer technology and imaging sequences have made mid- and low-field MRI very competitive, especially in musculoskeletal imaging. Further, high-field systems may be more prone to motion artifact and chemical shift artifact. Popular "open MRI" facilities generally are of the low-field variety because the open architecture of these systems is most compatible with permanent magnet designs (see Fig. 2-3).

Gradient magnetic coils are located within the gantry and allow "slicing" of the patient's anatomy along sagittal, coronal, or transverse planes (Fig. 2-4). These coils switch on and off very rapidly during the examination, which produces the characteristic, sometimes quite loud, tapping noise associated with an MRI scan.

Radiofrequency (RF) coils are placed on or near the area of the patient's anatomy being investigated. They are used to transmit and receive RF information pertaining to the location of the hydrogen nuclei. These RF coils or probes come in various designs adapted to most appropriately image the region of anatomy in question (Fig. 2-5).

IMAGE PRODUCTION

MR image production is based on the system's ability to spatially localize hydrogen atoms within body tissues. Within the body, the nuclei of hydrogen atoms are charged particles that generate small magnetic fields, similar to tiny bar magnets. Normally the hydrogen atoms are randomly oriented, their magnetic vectors cancel out, and no net magnetism of the tissue is produced. Hydrogen is particularly useful because it is plentiful, representing 80% of all atoms found in the body.

The MRI unit creates a strong magnetic field. Magnetic field strengths are measured in units of gauss (G) and T. One tesla is equal to 10,000 gauss. In comparison, the earth's magnetic field is approximately 0.5 gauss. Consequently, a 1.5-T MRI magnet is about 30,000 times the strength of the earth's magnetic field. The strength of electromagnets used to pick up cars in junkyards (1.5 to 2 T) generally is the same field strength of an MRI magnet.

When the patient is placed in the MRI scanner, each of the small magnetic fields of the patient's hydrogen atoms tends to orient with, or less often against, the stronger external magnetic field of the MRI unit. The hydrogen atoms are not statically polarized by the strong external magnetic force of the MRI unit; rather, they wobble like a child's top (Figs. 2-6 and 2-7).

Hydrogen wobbling is a phenomenon known as precession. In MRI, the rate of precession is intimately dependent on the element (in this case hydrogen) and the strength of the external

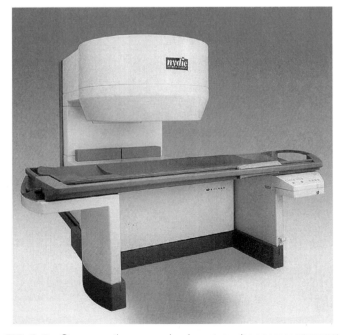

FIG. 2-3   Open magnetic resonance imaging system using a permanent magnet.

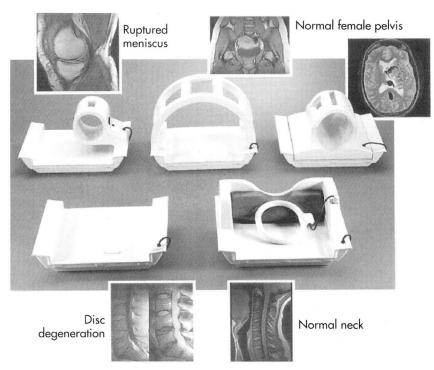

Ruptured meniscus

Normal female pelvis

AV malformation

Disc degeneration

Normal neck

FIG. 2-5 Radiofrequency coils are used to excite and localize the hydrogen nuclei magnetic fields. (Courtesy Picker International, Inc., Cleveland, OH.)

magnetic field created by the MRI. A linear relationship exists between the frequency of precession and the strength of an external magnetic field, known as the gyromagnetic ratio, and is measured in megahertz/tesla (MHz/T). For instance, when hydrogen is placed in a magnet of 1T, it assumes a characteristic precession frequency of 42.6 MHz. The relationship between the gyromagnetic ratio and magnetic field strength is described by the Larmor equation and forms the basis for MRI. The following is the Larmor equation:

Frequency of precession =
Gyromagnetic ratio × Strength of the external magnetic field

To obtain images, an RF identical to the Larmor frequency of precession is pulsed into the patient. For instance, if the hydrogen nuclei have precession frequency of 40 MHz, then these nuclei can be "excited" only by a 40-MHz radiofrequency pulse. This is the concept of resonance. A similar but more easily understood phenomenon occurs if an appropriately keyed tuning fork (e.g., D) is placed next to a guitar. The vibration from the tuning fork is propagated through air to cause selective vibration of just the D string of the six strings (Fig. 2-8).

With the pulses transmitted by the RF coils the hydrogen proton magnetic fields deviate from the plane of the main magnetic field and begin to precess with the same phase (see Figs. 2-6 and 2-7). When the RF pulse is turned off, the excited nuclei undergo longitudinal relaxation back to the equilibrium "parallel" plane of magnetism and transverse relaxation back to the equilibrium "out-of-phase" precession. During relaxation the accumulated energy is released in the form of RF, which is detected by the surface coil acting as an antenna system for the MRI equipment. The MRI signal received from the tissues is used to reconstruct an image;[7] therefore the dynamics of MRI can be summarized in four steps: resting, magnetism, excitation, and relaxation (Fig. 2-9).

IMAGING TECHNIQUES

As presented in the previous chapter, the production of a radiographic image is dependent on two principal controls that cover technique selection. These controls are kVp (peak kilovoltage) and mAs (milliampere-seconds). By carefully selecting kVp and mAs selections, radiographers can optimize the appearance of an image.

In MRI, image appearance is manipulated by controlling the timing of RF pulses sent into the patient (repetition time, TR) and the echo of the signal from the patient (echo time, TE). The most commonly used MRI technique is called a *spin-echo sequence*.

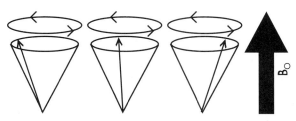

FIG. 2-6 When a patient is placed in the strong magnet field (B_o) of the magnetic resonance imaging unit, some of the patient's hydrogen atoms align themselves with the strong magnetic field as they precess or spin about a central axis. The individual spins of the hydrogen atoms are synchronized but are out of phase, until a radiofrequency pulse occurs.

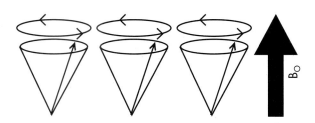

FIG. 2-7 After the application of a radiofrequency pulse identical to the Larmor frequency, the hydrogen atoms precess in phase.

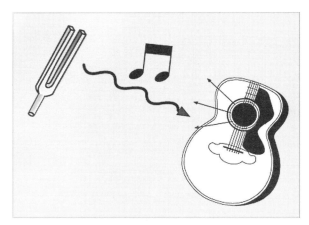

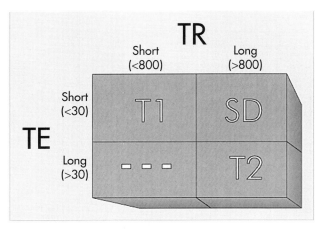

FIG. 2-8 Hydrogen nuclear resonance is the core phenomena of magnetic resonance imaging. The central idea is that a radiofrequency of the same energy wavelength as the magnetized hydrogen atoms will cause the hydrogen atoms to resonate. This is analogous to a tuning fork selectively vibrating a similarly tuned guitar string.

FIG. 2-10 Relationship of TR and TE to image weighting (T1-, T2-, and spin density). Hydrogens in fat yield high signal intensity (appear white) on T1-weighted images. Hydrogens in water yield high signal intensity (appear white) on T2-weighted images. The population of hydrogen in both fat and water yield high signal intensity (appear white) on spin-density images.

RF pulses are transmitted into the patient during this process. Typically the RF pulses are designed to "flip" or reorient the hydrogen magnetic field vectors to 90 or 180 degrees such that the associated emitted radiofrequencies can be detected by the antenna system within the RF coils.

As described, the RF pulses are discontinued after nuclear excitation and the hydrogen nuclei relax. RF is emitted from the tissue as they relax. This emitted MRI signal is received by the surface coil and used to reconstruct an image of the tissues being studied. The appearance of the image reflects the intensity of the emitted

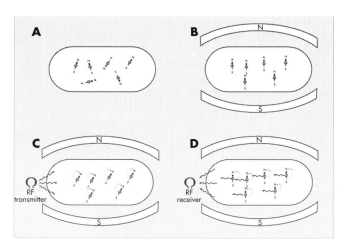

FIG. 2-9 Magnetic resonance imaging (MRI) phases. Because hydrogen atoms have a positive charge and move, they produce a tiny electrical current, and axiomatically associated magnetic currents, behaving as tiny bar magnets. In the resting state, **A,** the patient's hydrogen atoms (tiny bar magnets) are randomly oriented, so there is no net magnetism to the body. However, when the patient is placed in the strong magnetic field of the MRI unit, **B,** some (only about 7 per million) of the patient's freely moving hydrogen atoms align with (or less commonly against) the strong external polarity of the MRI unit. At this time, the addition of a prescribed radiofrequency, **C,** causes excitation of the aligned hydrogen atoms. As the hydrogen atoms absorb the applied radiofrequency pulse, they deflect from their parallel orientation. Once the applied radiofrequency pulse is turned off, **D,** the hydrogen atoms return to their equilibrium state, thereby emitting the radiofrequency energy they absorbed during excitation, **C.** The emitted signal, **D,** is collected and used to construct the MRI image.

signal from the examined body tissues. High signal intensity appears bright on the image; a low signal intensity appears dark.

Signal intensity is dependent on the population of hydrogen atoms and the environment in which the hydrogen are found. How hydrogen is "bound" also influences the MRI signal. Hydrogen that is tightly bound (e.g., within ligament) emanates minimal signal. Hydrogen that is loosely bound (e.g., within fluid) has the potential to exhibit a very bright signal with the appropriate MRI technique. The ability to evaluate hydrogen within varying by chemical and structural environments is accomplished by evaluating T1 and T2 relaxation times.

This is accomplished by manipulating the repetition of RF pulses (TR) and varying the collection time of the emitted signal (TE), which can dramatically influence which relaxation times are emphasized in the image. In other words, the resultant image can be based on the population of hydrogen (proton density) or emphasized to either the T1- or T2-weighted properties of the tissue (Figs. 2-10 and 2-11; Table 2-1).

For illustration purposes, a long TR is one that approximates 800 to 1000 milliseconds (msec) and a long TE exceeds 30 to 50 msec. Conversely, a short TR is often less than 800 msec and a short TE is often less than 30 msec. Alternative pulse sequences also are available and are used in certain clinical circumstances to enhance the delineation of pathologic processes. Among these are:
1. *Gradient echo.* A pulse sequence in which protons are "flipped" less than 90 degrees. As the flip angle tends toward 0 degrees the images create an increase in signal intensity from fluids, appearing with more T2-weighted emphasis. Because traditional spin-echo imaging requires a 90-degree pulse, these low flip angle sequences are considerably faster than conventional spin-echo sequences, especially when T2-weighted images are needed. Variations on the gradient echo sequences are also helpful in acquiring three-dimensional (3-D) data sets with subsequent multiplanar reformatting.
2. *STIR (short tau inversion recovery).* Pulse sequences used for fat suppression, in which a relatively short inversion time is used to null the fat signal while maintaining water and soft-tissue signal. These imaging sequences are particularly helpful in evaluating bone marrow pathology, including avascular necrosis (Fig. 2-12).

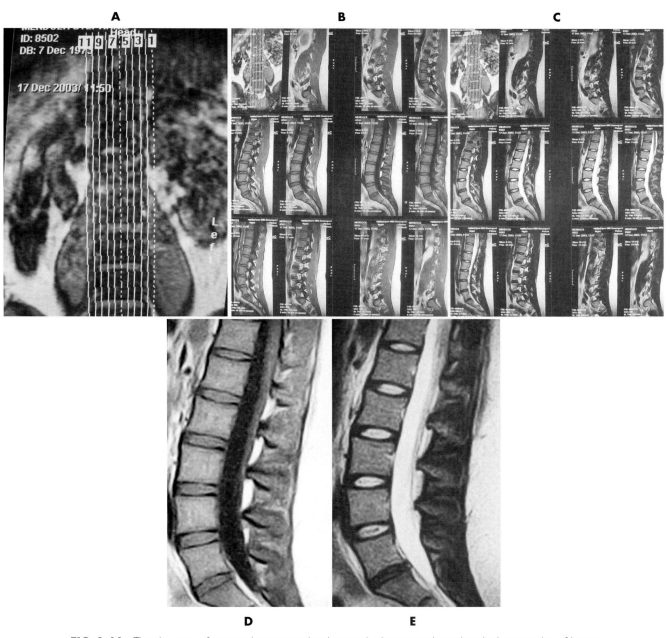

FIG. 2-11 The plan scans of a magnetic resonance imaging examination are used to orient the interpretation of images done in other plans. For instance, **A,** the coronal image, has vertical lines marked 1 to 11 denoting the 11 sagittal slices done in the sagittal plane. The sagittal images are displayed in groups, **B** and **C,** on 14 × 17 film where, **D,** individual T1-weighted spin density, or, **E,** T2-weighted images can be viewed. *Continued*

A typical lumbar spine MRI protocol begins with a coronal preliminary image, termed scout, localizer or plan scan (see Fig. 2-11). On this image, localizer lines are superimposed, corresponding to the subsequent sagittal T1- and T2-weighted sequences. The sagittal sequences usually extend from the left to the right neuroforamina or, depending on the MR equipment and the radiologist's preference. The direction of the sagittal slices always needs to be cross-checked before beginning interpretation. One of the middle sagittal sequences is used to "plan" the subsequent axial images. Axial images can be presented in two formats. One format is to have each slice parallel to each of the disc interspaces, most commonly for L3, L4, and L5, with the slices being angled to each disc plane line individually. The other format is to have a contiguous set of sequences extending from approximately L3 through S1. As depicted in the enclosed examples, the T1 sequences are noncontiguous, whereas the T2 sequences are contiguous. However, this is dependent on the inclination of the radiologist. The number of slices obtained is time dependent; therefore usually it is not common to evaluate the upper lumbar discs unless there is a probability of pathology specific to these regions. Similar protocols are used to evaluate other regions of the body, including the shoulder and knee.

FIG. 2-11 cont'd   Axial images can be accomplished with, **F,** contiguous slices or, **G,** slices angled to the disc plane. As with the sagittal images, the axial images, **H,** are printed on 14 × 17 film in groups so, **I,** each image can be interpreted.

TABLE 2-1
Signal Intensities of Various Tissues

Signal	T1-weighting	T2-weighting
Bright	Fat	Cerebrospinal fluid-water
	Yellow bone marrow	Cysts
	Subacute hemorrhage	Edema
	White matter of brain	Normal nucleus pulposus
		Tumor
Medium	Fluid	Dehydrated nucleus
	Intravenous pyelogram	pulposus
	Muscle	Fat
	Red bone marrow	Gray matter of brain
	Spinal cord	Muscle
	Tumor	Spleen
Dark	Air	Air
	Calcification	Calcification
	Cerebrospinal fluid	Cortical bone
	Cortical bone	Fast-moving blood
	Fast-moving blood	Fibrous tissue
	Fibrous tissue	Ligaments, tendons
	Ligaments, tendons	

PATIENT PREPARATION

The length of the total MRI examination can vary from 30 to 90 minutes, with an average examination taking 45 minutes. The length of the examination depends on the imaging sequences, which are gathered over 2- to 10-minute periods. Because of these prolonged examination times, it is critical that patients lie absolutely still for the duration of each imaging sequence. Referring physicians may find it beneficial to visit the MRI facility so that they can adequately explain the procedure to their patients. A well-informed patient is not likely to be overly anxious about the examination.

Patients should be asked to dress in comfortable clothing (e.g., a sweat suit) and without metal artifacts (e.g., jewelry, watches, and keys). These objects can result in suboptimal image quality because they can disturb the quality of the magnetic field. Credit cards should not be brought into the MRI facility because the large magnetic field erases the magnetic codes.

The patient is placed on the MRI table at the beginning of the examination. Surface coils, which transmit and receive radiofrequency data, are placed on the patient in the region to be examined at this juncture. Once this is accomplished the patient is glided into the MRI gantry. The technologists indicate to the patient when each of the examination sequences is to begin. The patient recognizes that the examination is ongoing by hearing a knocking noise

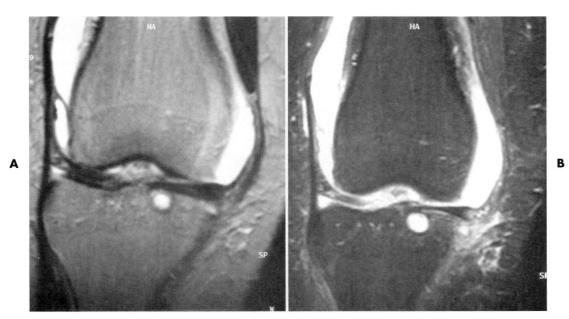

FIG. 2-12 **A** and **B,** Magnetic resonance imaging coronal T2-weighted and STIR (short tau inversion recovery) sequences. The patient demonstrated joint effusion and a subchondral cyst in the tibia.

coming from the MRI equipment. The typical rhythmic beating noise emanating from the MRI scanner comes from the gradient coils, which are intermittently energized to create cross-sectional images. Many MRI facilities also provide earphones with a choice of music. Noise suppression systems may be available as well.

Claustrophobia is the most common complication of an MRI examination; it is estimated to occur in up to 5% of patients. Although reassurance and positive interaction with the technologist works for most patients, a mild tranquilizer can be effective in alleviating high anxiety. Sometimes placing the patient within the scanner in a prone rather than supine position also reduces claustrophobia.

CONTRAINDICATIONS

A thorough history must be obtained from the patient before the MRI examination commences, with particular attention to a history of surgical intervention or industrial exposure to metals (Box 2-1). Generally, patients with pacemakers or other implanted electronic devices (including certain ear implants) cannot be examined. Many intracranial aneurysm clips are ferromagnetic, and torque or twist in a magnetic field; therefore MRI examinations are contraindicated in patients with vascular clips within the brain.

Some types of heart valves are affected also; however, this torque is usually less than the stress that normally occurs as a result of blood flow. Hence the presence of heart valves is not necessarily an absolute contraindication for an MRI examination. Orthopedic devices, although not usually contraindications to an MRI examination, can lead to considerable image degradation by causing significant alteration to the magnetic field homogeneity. In all circumstances, the presence of surgical devices should be made known to the MRI facility staff and radiologist. Especially in musculoskeletal MRI, patients should be encouraged to supply radiographs of the region to be examined, because correlation of the MRI examined with the x-rays can be extremely helpful to exclude metallic foreign bodies and aid in image interpretation.

Another potential hazard relating to MRI examination is ferromagnetic projectiles. This has received attention in the popular press by discussing circumstances in which ferromagnetic objects,

including oxygen tanks, have been attracted to the MRI magnet. These objects may be able to reach lethal speeds by the time they intercept the magnet. Reports include cleaning crews inadvertently entering the MRI suite with floor polishers that were dramatically wrested from the operator and pulled into the magnet bore. This represents an expensive situation in a high-field scanner.

MAGNETIC RESONANCE IMAGING CONTRAST AGENTS

MRI can obtain most anatomic information by relying on the inherent contrast of the body's tissues; however, under certain clinical circumstances an artificial contrast medium may be necessary. The first and most popular MRI contrast agent is gadopentetate dimeglumine (sold under the trade name Magnevist), a stable chelate made from the heavy metal gadolinium. Gadolinium is a paramagnetic

---

BOX 2-1

Selected Implants and Metal Artifacts That May Preclude or Interfere with a Magnetic Resonance Imaging Examination

Pacemakers
Implanted electromagnetic devices
Aneurysm clips (especially brain)
Vascular coils and filters
Heart valves
Porta-Cath device
Cochlear implants
Ocular implants
Surgical staples
Shrapnel
Contraceptive diaphragms or coils
Penile implants
Implanted insulin pumps
Bone or joint replacements
Tattoos or permanent eyeliner (contain metallic pigments)

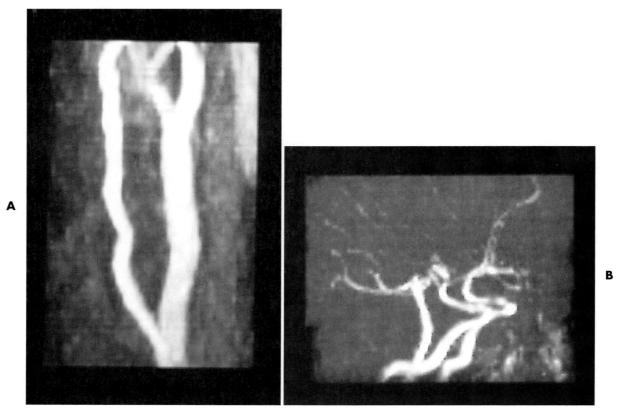

FIG. 2-13   A and **B**, Magnetic resonance angiography of the carotid and intracranial circulation.

substance that produces strong relaxation on the adjacent hydrogen nuclei;[8] therefore gadolinium acts as a T1-shortening agent that causes tissues containing this element to appear bright on T1-weighted images.

Gadolinium is not an iodinated contrast medium such as is used in CT examinations and angiography; subsequent adverse reactions are quite rare. Gadolinium chelates have been used safely as intravenous and intraarticular MRI contrast agents.[9] Gadolinium is especially useful in the detection of various central nervous system pathologies such as tumors and multiple sclerosis. Most commonly chiropractic patients with failed low back surgery require gadolinium to help differentiate recurrent disc herniation from scar formation.

MAGNETIC RESONANCE ANGIOGRAPHY

Magnetic resonance angiography (MRA) is a developing alternative to conventional angiography for the evaluation of vascular disease. This examination has the specific advantage of being totally noninvasive because no contrast medium is used. However, the spatial resolution of MRA is lower than routine angiographic examinations. Presently this examination is primarily used to study large vessels (Fig. 2-13).

Computed Tomography

BACKGROUND

CT is a diagnostic imaging procedure that constructs a cross-sectional image through the combination of x-ray physics and computer technology. Although early attempts to construct computed tomographic equipment occurred during the late 1950s, the first practical working model of a CT system was developed by

Godfrey Hounsfield in 1972.[10] Hounsfield, a computer engineer, worked at the Central Research Laboratory for Electric and Music Industry (EMI) in England, the company also notable for producing the works of the Beatles. Hounsfield won the Nobel Prize for Medicine and Physiology in 1979 for his work leading to the development of computed tomography. Hounsfield's original CT scan took hours to acquire a single slice of image data and more than 24 hours of computer time to reconstruct these data into a single image. By contrast, today's CT systems can acquire a single image in less than 1 second and reconstruct the image almost instantly.

IMAGE PRODUCTION

The CT scanner uses a radiographic tube contained within a gantry that emits a thin x-ray beam as it rotates about the patient (Figs. 2-14 and 2-15). An array of detectors on the opposite side of the tube intercepts those x-rays transmitted through the patient. The information from the attenuated x-ray beam is evaluated by a computer system that constructs the cross-sectional data directly in the axial plane line, with the ability to reformat the information into an indirect 3-D image. This overcomes a significant disadvantage of conventional x-ray in which three-dimensional (3-D) anatomy is superimposed on a two-dimensional (2-D) radiographic surface, representing a summation of superimposed densities.

In conventional radiography, information is displayed in analog form; it represents a "shadow" of anatomy created by differential absorption of the x-ray beam. Conversely, the images constructed by CT are digital. The x-ray beam is constantly attenuated by the incident anatomy as the x-ray tube rotates about the patient's body. The various resulting densities are attributed coefficients of attenuation, also called *CT numbers* or *Hounsfield units* (HU).

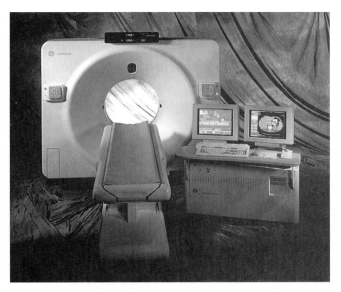

FIG. 2-14 Operator's console and spiral computed tomography imaging system. (From Bushong S: Radiologic science for technologists physics, biology, and protection, ed 7. St Louis, 2001, Mosby.)

BOX 2-2
Hounsfield Units for Various Tissues

−1000, air
−60, fat
0, water
+10, cerebrospinal fluid
+40, soft tissue/muscle
+400, bone/calcium
+2000, metallic surgical artifacts

The radiologist or radiologic technologist has the ability to alter the appearance of the images on the computer monitor (cathode-ray tube, CRT). Similar to a TV monitor, both the contrast (window width) and density (window level) can be manipulated to highlight the anatomy of interest. Typical abdominal window settings might be set at +40, which represents the central HU value with a range (width) of 400. This means that the CT image presents Hounsfield units between −160 and +240. All densities above +240 are white and below −160 are black. Once the desired gray scale is achieved, the images are printed to 14 × 17 inch film (Fig. 2-16). CT examinations of the spine usually are composed of both soft-tissue and bone window images for each axial slice, which demonstrate both osseous and soft-tissue anatomy (Fig. 2-17).

IMAGING TECHNIQUES

A typical CT examination technique of the lumbar spine uses axial slices parallel to the angle of each disc interspace, with each slice being approximately 3 to 5 mm thick. Thin slices are chosen to resolve small anatomy; however, with decreasing slice thickness less information is available from each voxel. A higher radiation dose is

The detector array is composed of x-ray–sensitive crystals or ionizing gas that produces electrical energy on stimulation by an x-ray photon. This information is gathered by the computer, and the anatomy within the examined slice is assigned gray scale values through a series of computer algorithms. The CT number for pure water is arbitrarily designated 0, air is approximately −1000, and dense bone is approximately +1000 (Box 2-2). In the language of computers, the various densities within a volume of tissue are called *voxels* (volume element). The CT image is ultimately displayed in pixels (picture element), which represent the various densities of the voxels.

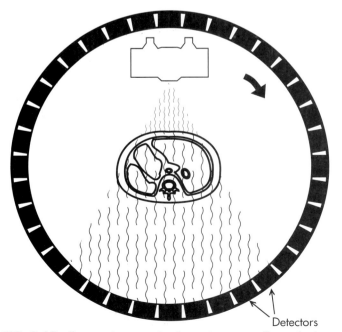

FIG. 2-15 Computed tomography does not use x-ray film as the image receptor system but relies on an array of detectors.

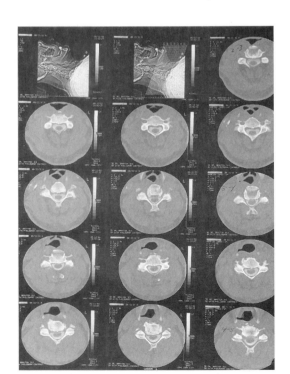

FIG. 2-16 Typical layout of computed tomography cervical spine images with the scout, or localizer, images in the upper left corner.

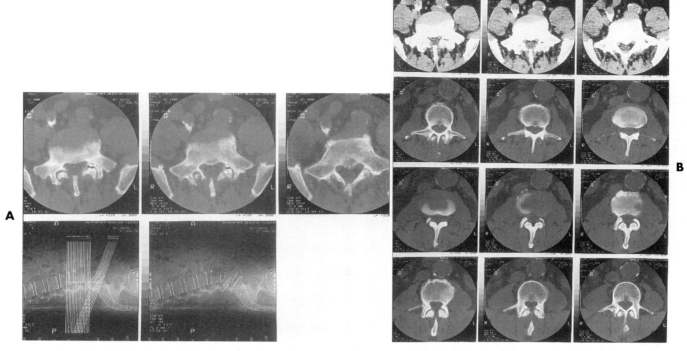

FIG. 2-17 **A,** The scout, or localizer, image allows accurate localization of the axial slices. **B,** Typical skeletal computed tomography examinations comprise two arrays of images; those that emphasize soft tissues (soft-tissue window) *(top row)* and those that emphasize the bone anatomy (bone window) *(bottom three rows)*.

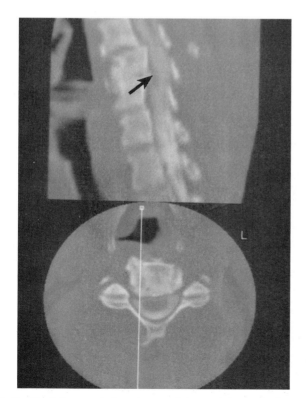

FIG. 2-18 Reformatted planar images of the cervical spine demonstrating hypertrophic spinal changes effacing the intrathecal contrast *(arrow)*.

necessary to acquire high-quality images to compensate for this. The gantry of the CT scanner also can be angled. This is particularly helpful in producing axial slices that conform to the disc plane line in examinations of the lumbar spine, which enhances the presentation of anatomy. Axial slices also can be obtained perpendicular to the tabletop. These contiguous axial slices then can be reformatted by the computer as sagittal or coronal images (Fig. 2-18). 3-D reformatted images are possible as well (Figs. 2-19 and 2-20).

The axial CT examination of the spine is preceded by digitized frontal or lateral scout views with appropriate numerical annotations, allowing for accurate localization of the subsequent axial slices. The scout images appear as a miniature radiograph on which the slice levels have been superimposed (see Fig. 2-17).

CLINICAL APPLICATION

CT renders high-resolution images that can be applied to most anatomic regions. Although MRI is often the procedure of choice to evaluate the brain, CT retains a prominent role in evaluating acute cerebral vascular lesions.

Spine and appendicular skeleton. CT, especially spiral CT, is the procedure of choice in the evaluation of spinal trauma. In particular CT should be performed as a primary evaluation technique in patients in whom there is strong clinical suspicion of cervical spine fracture. However, CT examination should be preceded by anteroposterior (AP) and lateral radiographs as a guideline for interpreting the CT study.[11,12]

CT is also helpful in evaluating appendicular skeleton trauma. In most cases CT mimics the findings of conventional radiography; however, precise localization of fracture fragments is obtained with reconstruction of the axial images into both coronal and sagittal planes. Although CT generally is able to depict all fractures, false-negative errors can occur when only axial imaging is employed.

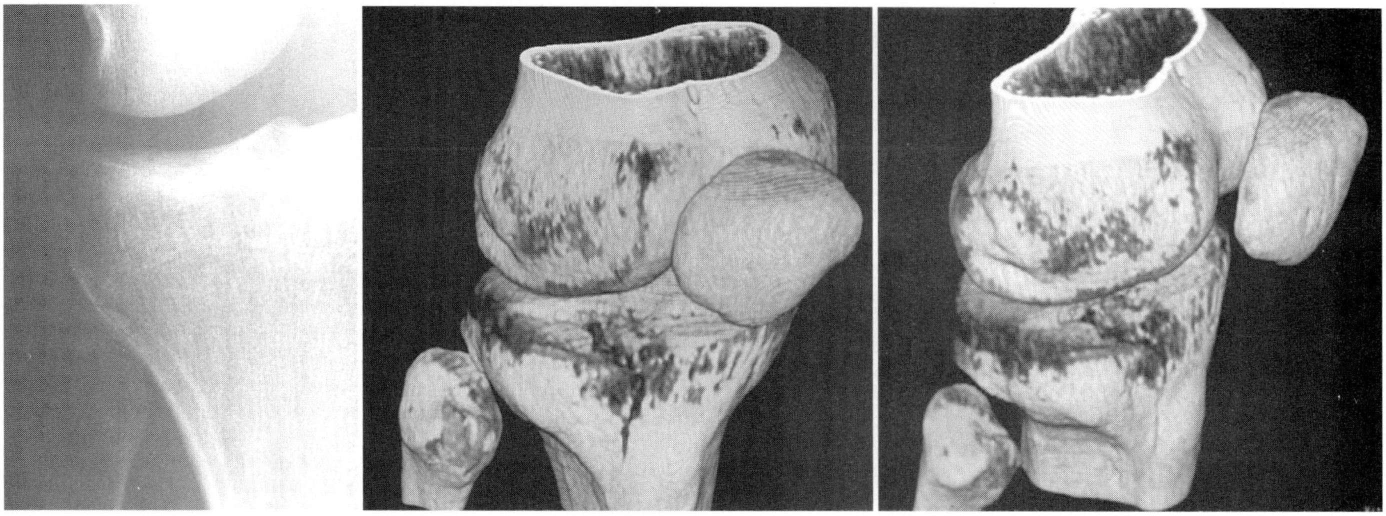

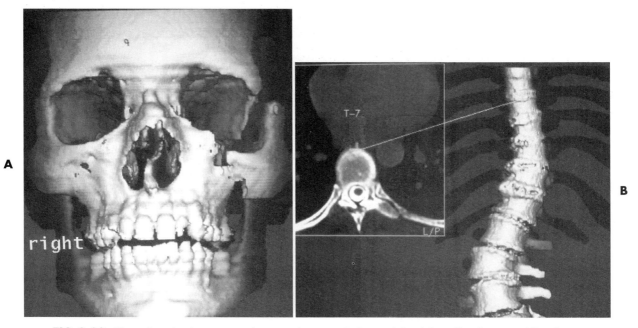

A	**B**	**C**

FIG. 2-19 A, Fracture of the lateral tibial plateau that is not clearly demonstrated on plain film. **B** and **C,** Imaging with reformatted computed tomography clarifies the location and extent of the injury.

If a fracture predominates in the axial plane (the same plane line as the slice), it may be unnoticed on the CT examination. Reconstructions of the axial data avoid this problem and yield additional information such as the morphology of possible defects of the articular surface (e.g., depression fractures).

CT may be useful in selected patients with spinal canal stenosis usually supplemented with contrast (CT myelography, CTM). CTM is most commonly performed in patients when there are contraindications for MRI, including implanted metal devices and claustrophobia. Multiplanar reformatted images and 3-D imaging techniques can be accomplished in selected patients as well.

Abdomen. CT is extremely helpful in evaluating the abdomen, including the major viscera. A common application is in

the evaluation of aortic aneurysm (Fig. 2-21), a lesion commonly discovered on conventional radiographs.

Chest. Solitary pulmonary nodules, a common incidental finding on both thoracic and chest radiographs, often require evaluation with CT, especially in patients clinically at risk for pulmonary malignancy. The advantages of CT over plain film include improved resolution of the pulmonary nodule margin characteristics. Benign lesions tend to have well-circumscribed smooth borders, whereas malignant nodules have irregular borders. CT allows more accurate detection and assessment of the calcification pattern within a pulmonary nodule than plain film. Calcification, which is more likely to be seen within a benign nodule, often allows differentiation from a malignant lesion; this can negate the

FIG. 2-20 Three-dimensional reconstructed computed tomography image of, **A,** a left maxillary fracture and, **B,** spine.

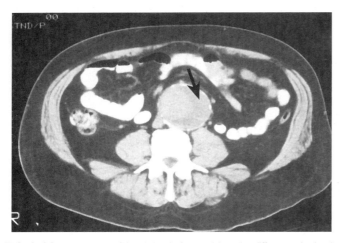

FIG. 2-21   Aneurysm of the abdominal aorta. Note the differences in density between the contrasted lumen of the vessel and the adjacent thrombus *(arrow)*.

need for a biopsy. However, if a biopsy is needed, it can be guided accurately by CT to ensure that the needle obtains tissue from the nodule.

Rapid image acquisition with helical CT has increased the application of this technology to evaluate pulmonary vascular abnormalities, including pulmonary embolism. Although pulmonary embolism is commonly evaluated with scintigraphy and digital subtraction pulmonary angiography, spiral CT is becoming a popular procedure because it is less invasive than pulmonary angiography and more specific than scintigraphy.

CONTRAST AGENTS

Like x-ray, CT images are dependent on inherent anatomic densities. Many soft-tissue CT examinations require the addition of contrast agents. CT contrast agents are applied to visualize specific tissues or organs. The majority of contrast agents used in CT are based on iodine. These agents can be delivered by various means, most commonly via oral ingestion, intravenous injection, or through the rectum. At times, contrast is injected directly into the subarachnoid space to produce a CT myelogram.

In the case of intravenous contrasts, once the contrast has entered the blood stream, it circulates to various organs. The x-ray beam of the CT scanner is attenuated by contrast within the organs, causing the organs to appear white on the CT image. In a short period of time, the kidneys and liver eliminate the contrast from the body. Intravascular contrast media can be applied to highlight blood vessels and vascular lesions. Cerebral pathologies that disrupt the blood–brain barrier are also contrasted with intravenous agents.

Side effects from iodinated contrast media are relatively minor; however, the radiologist and technologist should be informed if there is a history of allergies and reactions to previous iodine injections or shellfish. Because function of the kidneys and liver are directly related to the patient's ability to metabolize the contrast, patients older than 55 years usually are evaluated for basic renal function with blood urea nitrogen (BUN) or creatinine tests before the application of contrast.

COMPUTED TOMOGRAPHY MYELOGRAPHY

CTM describes a CT study made after the injection of contrast media into the subarachnoid space (Fig. 2-22). CTM provides excellent detail of the thecal sac, and in past literature has been shown to be

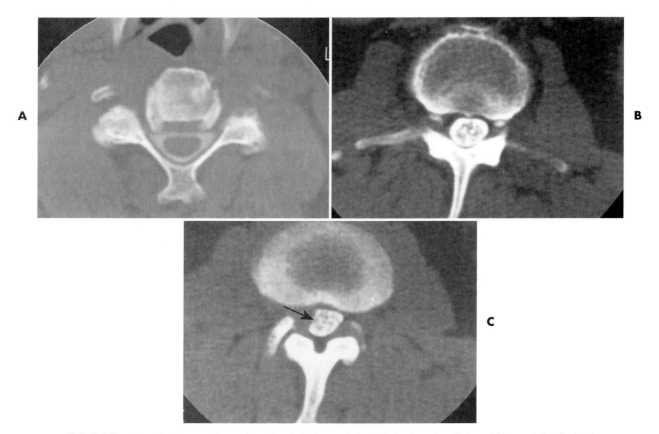

FIG. 2-22   Computed tomography myelography of, **A,** the cervical and, **B,** lumbar spine. **C,** An axial image at the disc level demonstrates effacement of the contrast-filled dural sac secondary to disc herniation *(arrow)*.

superior in the assessment of spondylosis and arachnoiditis of the cervical and thoracic spine when compared with MRI.[13] However, with the software and scanner improvements to high-resolution CT and MRI, CTM is less commonly considered as a routine examination procedure for the evaluation of spinal canal lesions. CTM may be helpful when MRI and CT do not provide the necessary information to resolve a clinical problem. CTM might also be a consideration in those patients not able to undergo an MRI study because of unavailability or claustrophobia. CTM is most helpful in the evaluation of arachnoiditis or fractures and malignancy that have effaced the spinal canal.

COMPUTED TOMOGRAPHY ARTHROGRAPHY

CT examination of a joint usually is done in conjunction with a contrast injection into the joint space. CT arthrography yields good anatomic detail but has become supplanted by MRI in many applications. Nevertheless CT arthrography remains helpful in cases of shoulder glenoid labrum tears.

COMPUTED TOMOGRAPHY DISCOGRAPHY

CT discography involves the application of CT to view the configuration of radiodense contrast that has been injected within the nucleus pulposus. It is a specific examination whose general application remains controversial.

PATIENT PREPARATION AND EXPERIENCE

The CT examination begins by placing the patient on the couch. The couch then slides into the gantry with the region of relevant anatomy positioned by laser cross-hairs. The scout image, essentially a digital radiograph, is taken before axial images are obtained. This digital image is used to spatially localize the subsequent cross-sectional slices. During the examination the patient typically is instructed to hold his or her breath and remain still for approximately 30 seconds. The technologist controls the examination from a workstation from which the patient can be observed. The patient may hear the tube rotating within the gantry and may feel the slight motion of the table as it moves through the gantry, activated by the computer for each slice sequence. Contrast may be administered during the examination. The most common side effect relating to the intravenous administration of an iodinated contrast media is a flushing sensation along with a metallic taste. On occasion, a skin reaction to the contrast develops; but this responds readily to treatment. More serious reactions include difficulty in breathing or swelling of the soft tissues of the airway. The patient must not eat for several hours before the examination if an oral contrast medium is used.

CONTRAINDICATIONS AND DISADVANTAGES

Contraindications to CT examinations are relatively few. As noted, some patients exhibit an allergic reaction to the contrast used in CT examinations. Additionally, the use of contrast media should be avoided in patients with renal insufficiency. Relative to other methods of imaging, CT imparts a higher radiation dose, ranging from 3 to 5 rads. To give some reference, a standard lumbar spine series imparts about 100 mrads. As a consequence, female pelvic examinations are best accomplished with relatively noninvasive technology such as ultrasonography. Pregnancy also represents a relative contraindication. CT examination of children has received recent attention, raising concerns about radiation dose, the need to optimize the technical settings for the patient's size, and the use of appropriate shielding.[14,15]

CT also has other drawbacks. CT images invariably are obtained in the axial or transverse plane. On occasion, this might result in suboptimal presentation of the anatomy in question. For instance, an odontoid fracture is oriented in the same plane line as an axial slice, which can make the lesion difficult to evaluate. In this circumstance, conventional radiography might better display this lesion. Alternatively, the axial images can be computer "reconstructed" in a coronal or sagittal plane line to enhance the axially oriented lesion.

Although CT produces high-quality images of viscera, they are dependent on inherent tissue densities to provide contrast. When pathologic tissue and adjacent anatomy are of similar density, contrast media may be needed for differentiation. Other imaging protocols might be preferred, principally MRI, which provides greater soft-tissue contrast. This is especially true if there is a history of contrast reaction.

SPIRAL/HELICAL AND MULTIDETECTOR COMPUTER TOMOGRAPHY

The x-ray tube within the gantry in a conventional CT unit is able to accomplish a 360-degree rotation about the patient; however, the tube must reverse for the second slice because of the attached high-voltage cables. Spiral CT describes the path of the x-ray beam during the scanning process made possible through the development of the "slip-ring" gantry, which replaces the high-voltage cables with a series of rotating electrical contacts. During the spiral CT examination, the couch on which the patient lies advances at a constant rate through the gantry while the x-ray tube forms a continuous spiral rotating path around the patient. The major advantage of spiral CT is that it can obtain entire anatomic regions in seconds. Contiguous volumetric data are obtained from which the computer formats images in 2-D plane lines (sagittal and coronal) along with 3-D reconstructions as needed. Multiplanar and 3-D imaging are particularly advantageous in assessing the spine with complex fractures.

Relatively recent innovations in spiral CT technology include multislice scanners that are able to collect at least 4 to 16 slices of data during each rotation at high speeds. This equipment has the ability to obtain multiple slices of data in as little as 500 msec, constructing 512 × 512 matrix images in a second. An entire chest examination can be accomplished in 5 to 10 seconds. This is of particular importance because it allows a complete examination of the thorax with a single breath hold.

Radionuclide Imaging

BACKGROUND

Radionuclide imaging is a relatively noninvasive technology that uses radiopharmaceuticals to evaluate pathophysiologic abnormalities of various organ systems. Imaging is dependent on certain substances concentrating selectively in different parts of the body. A radionuclide can be chemically tagged to these substances and consequently allow for evaluation of specific organ systems by imaging the radionuclide. The skeleton, lungs, liver, thyroid, and heart are common organ systems to be scanned with radionuclide imaging.

IMAGE PRODUCTION

Skeletal radionuclide imaging is performed with 99m technetium tagged to methylene diphosphonate (^{99m}Tc-MDP), a phosphate analog that is incorporated into the hydroxyapatite crystal of bone by the osteoblasts. Increased uptake of the radiopharmaceutical is seen in conditions that produce both an increased metabolic activity and blood supply, including tumors, infections, fractures, metabolic diseases, and joint diseases.[16] Radionuclide bone imaging is sensitive to early pathologic processes, but it is not as specific in defining anatomy as most other imaging systems. A major advantage of radionuclide imaging is that the entire skeleton can be imaged in a single examination.

Technetium is the most widely used radiopharmaceutical for bone scanning, because it is widely available, easily prepared, and it has a relatively short half-life (6 hours) with an acceptable whole-body radiation dose. The radiopharmaceutical is injected into a vein, where it is subsequently disseminated throughout the body. Images are most commonly obtained 2 to 3 hours after injection, which allows clearance of the isotope from the blood supply and incorporation into bone.

The imaging device in radionuclide scintigraphy is the gamma camera. After the injection of the radiopharmaceutical, the gamma-rays that are emitted from the patient's body are intercepted by a series of crystals within the gamma camera. The excited crystals emit the absorbed energy as a flash of light or scintillations (a process known as *scintigraphy*). These data are manipulated by the computer and the information is portrayed on the computer monitor. Ultimately the image is recorded (printed) on film by the technologist. The degree of film darkening reflects the degree of radionuclide activity. Images of both the whole body and specific collimated regions of interest are obtained.

Bone scans are often obtained in three phases (Fig. 2-23). The first phase, or *flow phase,* supplies a radionuclide angiogram,

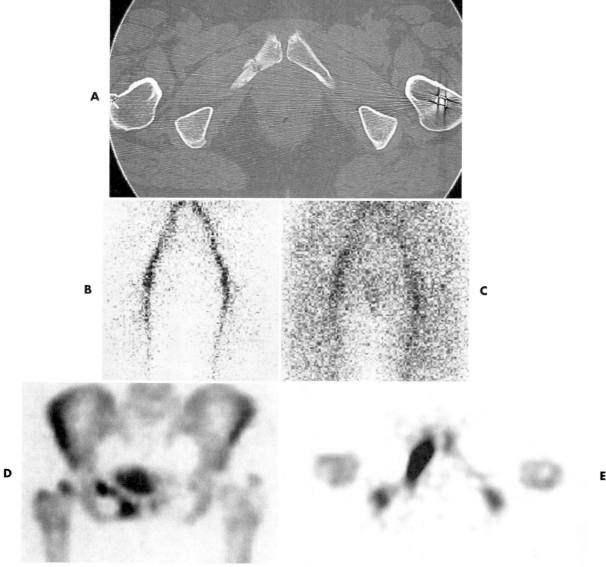

FIG. 2-23 Pubic fracture. **A,** The fracture is noted as a linear radiolucent defect noted on computed tomography. A three-phase bone scan is applied to demonstrate the region of the fracture. The first phase, known as the flow phase, occurs several seconds after injection of the radiotracer (**B,** at 4 seconds). After a few minutes, a blood pool image develops (**C,** at 52 seconds) as the radiotracer is further accumulated. The flow phase and blood flow phases of the bone scan demonstrate the perfusion of the examination area. Two to four hours after the radiotracer has been injected into the patient, the osteogenic component of the three-phase bone scan develops (**D,** at 3 hours). **E,** Additional information may be otained in other planes of the body by single proton emission computed tomography.

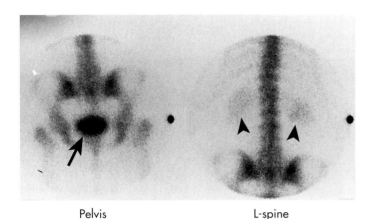

Pelvis   L-spine

FIG. 2-24 Normal radionuclide scintigraphy also demonstrating nonpathologic accumulation of the radioisotope within the bladder and kidney.

occurring within the first minute after the injection (Fig. 2-23, *B*). The second phase is noted as the *blood pool scan,* occurring 1 to 3 minutes after injection (Fig. 2-23, *C*). The third phase is the *static bone scan,* occurring 2 to 4 hours after injection (Fig. 2-23, *D*). With increased blood flow, the first and second phases demonstrate prominent collection. Collection of radionuclide in the third phase corresponds to osteogenic activity and blood flow.

Nonpathologic increased uptake is noted in the most metabolically active regions of the body (e.g., epiphyses, costochondral junctions, sacroiliac joints, and sternoclavicular joints). Increased uptake also is found in the kidneys secondary to the excretion of the radioisotope; therefore this affords the radiologist an opportunity to secondarily evaluate kidney anatomy and function (Fig. 2-24).

Single photon emission tomography (SPECT) imaging is an extension of simple planar radionuclide imaging. In a manner similar to CT, the SPECT scan can obtain data from multiple angles around the body. The computer reconstructs these data to present a tomographic or slice image of the area of interest. The images can be presented in coronal, sagittal, and axial projections that can provide enhanced spatial localization, superior to conventional radionuclide imaging. One common application of SPECT imaging is to examine for isolated defects of the pars interarticularis, as associated with spondylolisthesis.

PATIENT EXPERIENCE

Minimal patient preparation is necessary for this examination. No dietary changes are necessary before the examination. Depending on the imaging facility, after the injection of the radionuclide compound the patient is encouraged to ingest 500 to 1000 ml of fluid to promote renal excretion of the substance not taken up by bone.

Radionuclide examinations hold negligible risk for the patient. Pregnancy and breast-feeding represent the only relative contraindications for radionuclide imaging.

CLINICAL APPLICATION

The principal benefit of radionuclide scintigraphy is that it is able to detect physiologic abnormalities within a given tissue. In a bone scan, the uptake of the radionuclide within bone is dependent both on blood supply and bone metabolic activity. Any bone disease process that increases blood supply or osteoblastic activity will result in increased accumulation of the radiopharmaceutical. These focal regions of increased uptake are called *hot spots.* On occasion certain bone pathologies, such as infarction, create a focal decrease in radionuclide activity, representing a *cold spot.*

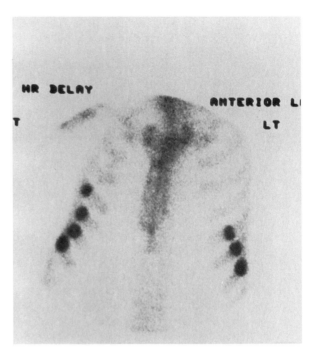

FIG. 2-25 Radionuclide scintigraphy revealing the typical linear distribution of "hot-spots" diagnostic of multiple rib fractures.

The most characteristic feature of an abnormal bone scan is asymmetric distribution of the radionuclide tracer (Fig. 2-25). Although MRI is also very sensitive to early physiologic osseous changes, a bone scan has two distinct advantages. Namely, a bone scan is less expensive and it has the ability to include the entire skeleton within the field of view.

The major disadvantage of radionuclide scintigraphy is that the findings generally are nonspecific. For example, on the basis of a bone scan, conditions such as Paget's disease cannot be readily differentiated from osseous metastasis. However, this may not be an impactful practical deficient. That is, a reasonably accurate differential diagnosis can be elucidated on the basis of the patient's clinical presentation and the pattern of the osseous radionuclide uptake. Generally, an abnormal radionuclide bone scan is followed by a more anatomy-specific imaging study, including x-ray, CT, or MRI in difficult cases.

Stress fractures. Radionuclide scintigraphy is a popular examination to evaluate stress fractures. Stress fractures occur in physically active people as a result of repetitive stress placed on normal bone. The repetitive stress eventually creates a collapse of the bony trabeculation and microfracture. On a bone scan, stress fractures are exhibited as focal regions of increased uptake of the radionuclide, often linear in presentation. Of particular clinical importance is the fact that bone scan changes often occur long before being evident on conventional radiographs, sometimes several weeks earlier. Therefore if a patient presents with clinical features of stress fracture but the radiographs are normal a bone scan can be applied as a more sensitive evaluation tool to exclude the existence of a stress fracture. As another example, radionuclide scintigraphy can reveal early defects in the pars interarticularis before the fracture is obvious on conventional radiographic studies, or before it becomes a completed lesion.

Reflex sympathetic dystrophy. Radionuclide scintigraphy can be useful in evaluating reflex sympathetic dystrophy (RSD). RSD is a poorly understood condition characterized by pain, swelling, vascular changes, and dystrophy of the distal extremities. The condition is often seen in conjunction with previous trauma and is possibly associated with an increased activity of the sympathetic nervous system. Radionuclide scintigraphy, principally the three-phase bone scan portion of the examination, can deliver characteristic, often diagnostic features of RSD. Acute RSD is characterized by increased blood pool activity along with delayed periarticular uptake about the involved extremity.[17]

Metastatic bone disease. A common use of a bone scan is to detect metastatic bone disease. A common scenario that might warrant a radionuclide bone scan is a patient with low back pain with a prior history of primary malignancy, especially of the breast or prostate. In contrast to radionuclide scintigraphy, conventional radiography is relatively insensitive in detecting metastatic bone disease. Approximately 30% of metastatic lesions evident on radionuclide scintigraphy are not noted on conventional radiographs. Approximately 50% trabecular bone destruction is necessary before being noted on x-ray. By contrast, only 2% of metastatic lesions noted on x-ray might be missed on radionuclide scintigraphy.[18]

Metastatic lesions that are most commonly associated with false-negative bone scans include anaplastic thyroid carcinoma and neuroblastoma. Multiple myeloma is also notorious for presenting a negative bone scan with radiographically evident bone destruction. Unfortunately, radionuclide bone imaging cannot always differentiate benign from malignant lesions. Definitive diagnosis often requires correlation with the clinical presentation and other diagnostic imaging studies. Ultimately biopsy might be needed.

In the spine, mild increased uptake also might be created by degenerative processes such as posterior facet arthrosis, but usually is easily differentiated from more serious pathology such as metastatic bone disease by the typical distribution of the hot spot in the region of the facet joints. Usually the degree of uptake is less intense with degeneration than with metastatic bone disease. Occult fractures, especially of the rib cage, are also well discriminated by radionuclide scintigraphy (see Fig. 2-25).

Paget's disease. Paget's disease is a relatively common radiographic finding. The condition is commonly polyostotic. Distribution of Paget's, disease is most efficiently evaluated with radionuclide scintigraphy. This should be accomplished, especially if there are multiple regions of bone pain, bone deformity, or significantly elevated alkaline phosphatase.

Infection. Radionuclide scintigraphy is very sensitive in detecting occult infections. However, specificity is reduced with consideration of other conditions that might mimic infection, including fracture, avascular necrosis, neuropathic arthropathy, and joint diseases. Technetium also can be used to label white blood cells, which have a potential to accumulate in areas are infection. In a similar fashion, these examinations also can be helpful in evaluating diabetic neuropathy, complicated by infection.

Pulmonary ventilation-perfusion (lung) scan. A lung scan is a radionuclide study performed to evaluate patients with potential pulmonary embolism. The examination is composed of two parts. For the ventilation component, the patient inhales a radioactive gas (xenon, technetium) with the distribution within the lungs being evaluated with the gamma camera. After this, an injection is made of a radiopharmaceutical tagged to macroaggregated albumin particles that are temporarily trapped within the pulmonary capillary bed. A normal lung scan is one in which there is symmetric distribution of the radiopharmaceutical on both the ventilation and perfusion study. With pulmonary embolism, cold spots are evident on the perfusion study, creating a mismatch with the ventilation component of the examination.

Dual Energy X-ray Absorptiometry (DEXA)

BACKGROUND

Bone mineral density measurement can be assessed by radiographs, quantitative computed tomography (QCT), single photon absorptiometry (SPA), dual photon absorptiometry (DPA), ultrasound, and dual energy x-ray absorptiometry (DEXA).[9] Of these methods, QCT is the most accurate, but because of associated radiation exposure and cost, DEXA is the most widely used method. DEXA is particularly helpful in evaluating patients at risk for osteoporosis, ideally before associated complications of bone fragility and fracture occur. Additionally, DEXA accurately functions as an effective follow-up method for monitoring response to treatment.[4]

IMAGE PRODUCTION

SPA employs a monoenergetic beam of radiation to measure the bone density of the peripheral skeleton, usually the calcaneous or distal radius. The bone density is a function of the beam's attenuation. With SPA, the bone density of clinically important areas, such as the lumbar spine or femoral neck, are extrapolated from the measured areas of the peripheral skeleton. However, the correlations between the bone density of the peripheral skeleton lumbar spine, for instance, are only moderate, leaving room for error in clinical evaluation and management. DPA uses radiation beams at two separate energy levels to measure the bone density of the hip and lumbar spine. DEXA is an advancement of the DPA technology, where the radionuclide source of radiation is exchanged for an x-ray tube, an advantage that leads to shorter examination times. Similarly to DPA, DEXA entails the use of two separate energy levels and depends on differential absorption of the tissue to create the measurement of bone density.

PATIENT EXPERIENCE

For a DEXA examination, the patient lies on the table and the x-ray source is directed over the region to be tested, principally the lumbar spine and proximal femora (Fig. 2-26). The examination takes approximate 10 to 20 minutes and delivers approximately $\frac{1}{10}$ the radiation dose of an average chest radiograph.

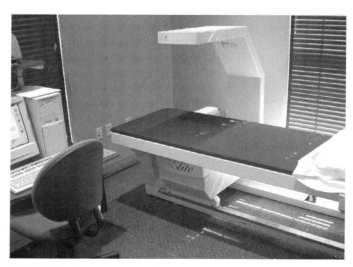

FIG. 2-26 Couch, scanner, and computer workstation of a dual energy x-ray absorptiometry unit.

CLINICAL APPLICATION

DEXA, or other measures of bone mineral density, are performed
to assess whether a patient has osteoporosis or osteopenia.
Osteoporosis is approximately four times more common in females
than in males and postmenopausal females are especially at high
risk. Genetics and aberrant health habits, inclusive of smoking and
alcoholism, contribute significantly to decreased bone material
density. Additionally, clinical disorders such as hyperparathyroidism, hyperthyroidism, and malabsorption are related to
decreased bone mineral density.

DEXA T-scores are used for diagnosis of osteopenia and osteoporosis. T-scores are calculated by subtracting the patient's bone
mineral density from a reference range of peak bone mineral density
in young women (or men), which is approximately of 35 years of
age. This value is then divided by the standard deviation of the reference sample to produce a T-score. According to the World Health
Organization (WHO), T-scores between +1.0 and −1.0 are considered
normal (Table 2-4). Osteopenia is defined as a T-score of between
−1.0 and −2.5. Osteoporosis is defined as a T-score of −2.5 or lower.
Severe osteoporosis is defined by a T-score lower than −2.5 and the
concurrent presence of one or more related fractures. There is a
strong correlation between low bone mineral density and prediction
of the occurrence of fractures.[6] Specifically, for every increase in
T-score the risk of fracture doubles. That is, at 1.0 the risk is 2×, at
−2.0 the risk is 4×, and at −3.0 the risk is 8 times that of the reference
population (T-score of 0) (Table 2-5). Clinical attention to prevent
further bone mineral loss begins when patients exibit T-scores below
−1 or −1.5, depending on other patient risk factors for fracture.

Z-scores are used to compare a patient's bone mineral density
to the bone density of persons of matched age, gender, and ethnicity. A Z-score of 0 indicates that half of the population has a
greater bone mineral density and half has less. If the Z-score was
"−1," 84% of the reference population would have greater bone
mineral density. A Z-score of −2.0 would indicate that the patient
is at the 2nd percentile and that 98% of the reference population
has a greater bone mineral density. Z-scores are useful to assess if

something unusual is contributing to the loss of bone mineral density.
Z-scores of less than −1.5 raise suspicion that something other than
age is accounting for the loss of bone mineral density, including
malnutrition, medicaions, and thyroid abnormalities.

When referring patient's for DEXA scans, it is important to
remember that the results of a DEXA scan do not necessarily translate
directly across all manufacturers and models of equipment. It is
best to schedule repeat evaluations at the same imaging center, on
the same equipment, to ensure the values are comparable.

Myelography

BACKGROUND

Myelography describes the introduction of contrast agents into the
subarachnoid space to aid the visualization of the spinal canal
anatomy. The procedure was first pioneered in the early 1900s with
the use of air.[22] Iodized poppy seed oil (Lipiodol) was the first positive contrast medium used.[23] However, widespread use proved
Lipiodol was a damaging agent, associated with high rates of
meningeal irritation and arachnoiditis complications. By the 1940s,
oil-based agents, namely, iophendylate (Myodil, Pantopaque), were
developed and became the standard in the United States for more than
30 years. Because the ionic, oil-based contrasts were also associated
with late meningeal pathology, development into safe alternatives
continued. After several iterations, relatively safe nonionic water-
based contrast agents such as metrizamide (Amipaque) were
generally available in the 1970s. Further improvement led to the
development of iohexol (Omnipaque) and iopamidol (Isovue) in the
1980s. These contrast agents are much safer than their predecessors.[24]

Patient selection is an important aspect of myelography. Patients
should be in good general health. Systemic conditions such as
alcoholism, diabetes, and cardiovascular disease may be contraindications to the examination. Additionally, patients should not exhibit
evidence of intracranial pressure (e.g., papilledema) or have bleeding
disorders. An allergy to contrast agents is an important consideration
before the examination.

Most patients experience minor discomfort during the examination. Headache remains the most common side effect of myelography and may be related to leakage of cerebrospinal fluid. Serious
side effects of myelography still occur, reflecting its invasive nature.
Serious but relatively rare complications include infections and
arterial bleeding; the latter usually associate with cervical puncture.

IMAGE PRODUCTION

Myelography is performed in the fluoroscopy suite of hospitals or
imaging centers. Nothing should be eaten during the 4 hours preceding the examination. The patient assumes a prone position on a
table that has the ability to tilt up or down. Under fluoroscopic
observation, the radiologist then inserts a needle (usually #22 or
#25 gauge) into the spinal canal and injects a radiopaque contrast
into the subarachnoid space. The needle is removed and the contrast is viewed by radiograph, fluoroscopy, or CT. Standard frontal,
lateral, and oblique projections are obtained. Abnormality is inferred
from alterations in the column of injected contrast into the subarachnoid space or its extensions. After the examination, the patient
rests with the torso slightly elevated for approximately 4 hours.
Fluids are encouraged.

CLINICAL APPLICATION

MRI is the primary imaging modality of the spine. MRI is considered to be the examination of choice in spinal infection, primary
and secondary malignant disease, and general lumbar disc disease.

Because MRI is less invasive and rapidly evolving, the use of myelography can be expected to decrease in the immediate future. Myelography will likely continue to be performed on those patients who cannot undergo an MRI examination, or for whom the resulting MRI images are of poor diagnostic accuracy or quality. Myelography combined with CT creates a valuable imaging tool for the spine, especially in areas of small anatomy such as lateral cervical disc herniations and cervical foraminal narrowing.

Myelography demonstrates the inner margins of the thecal sac, usually over a length of about three vertebrae. Myelography has several common applications in the cervical, thoracic, and lumbar regions, including the following.

Disc herniations. Disc herniations displace myelographic contrast media at the level of the disc interspace and also displace the dural sleeve around the corresponding nerve root. Diagnoses of disc bulge and disc herniation are possible. Accuracy of 97% has been recorded in distinguishing disc bulge from disc herniation. Ability to image disc herniations at the L5 level is decreased because of increased anterior epidural fat, which displays the myelographic contrast media within the subarachnoid space away from the offending disc lesion. The appearance of a disc herniation on a myelogram is marked by the following (Fig. 2-27):
- Sharp angular indentation on the lateral aspect of the thecal sac
- Narrowing of the disc space (a sign of disc degeneration)
- Enlargement of a nerve root secondary to edema
- Displacement of a nerve root secondary to nonfilling of a root sleeve

Arachnoiditis. Arachnoiditis is inflammation of the pia mater and arachnoid of the brain or spinal cord. It is a potential complication of myelography. Its presence is suggested by a blunted appearance of the nerve root sleeves.

Intradural-intramedullary lesions. An intradural-intramedullary lesion is a lesion within the spinal cord, including astrocytomas, ependymomas, and syringomyelia. Syringohydromyelia, representing cavitation within the spinal cord, is difficult if not impossible to differentiate from spinal cord intramedullary tumor and is consequently best evaluated with MRI. Characteristically, intradural-intramedullary lesions expand the spinal cord somewhat symmetrically with consequent effacement of the myelographic column.

Intradural-extramedullary lesions. Intradural-extramedullary pathologies are located within the subarachnoid space, external to the spinal cord. Common examples include meningiomas and neurofibromas. The characteristic findings of myelography are compression of the spinal cord with widening of the subarachnoid space at the site of the mass, with consequent widening of the overall thecal sac. The borders of the lesions may be sharply defined.

Extradural lesions. Extradural lesions are lateral to the thecal sac, the most common examples of which are disc herniations and degenerative spondylosis with osteophyte formation. The most common tumor type to create extradural myelographic effacement is spinal metastasis. The characteristic finding on myelography is displacement of the myelographic column away from the adjacent bone or disc interspace; displacement typically is asymmetric.

Discography

The procedure of directly injecting contrast agent into the center of the disc dates back to 1948 (Fig. 2-28).[25,26] The procedure has the ability to detail the structurally integrity of the outer nuclear envelope. In the healthy disc, contrast agent injected into the center of the nucleus does not transgress the outer nuclear envelope, appearing

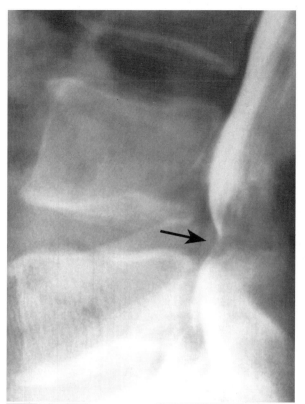
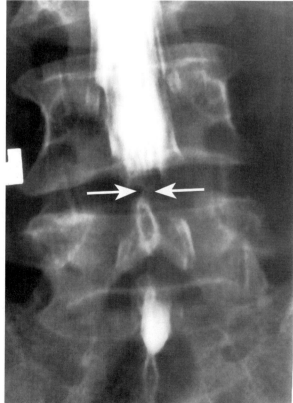

FIG. 2-27 Myelography of the lumbar spine showing an extradural defect consistent with disc herniation at the L4 level *(arrows)*.

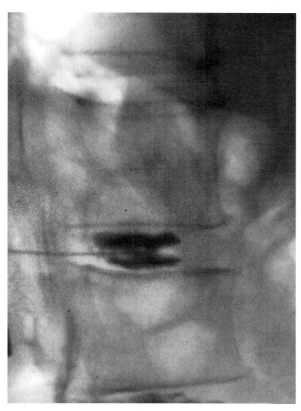

FIG. 2-28 Discography revealing normal disc structure with subtraction fluoroscopy.

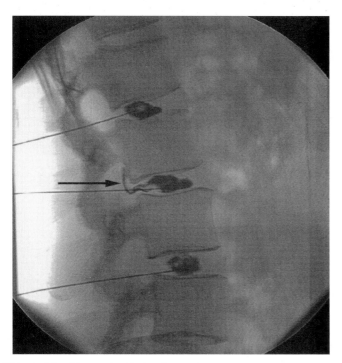

FIG. 2-29 Discography. Notice the needles placed in the center of the second, third, and fourth lumbar disc. When contrast is injected, the second and fourth discs appear of normal configuration, indicating healthy discs. However, the injected contrast migrates posteriorly in the third disc, a consistent finding of posterior disc rupture. (From Fenton DS, Czervionke LF: Image-guided spine intervention, Philadelphia, 2003, WB Saunders.)

oval, round, or as stacked ovals ("hamburger bun"). In the diseased disc, the injected contrast migrates through the nuclear envelope and moves through the annular tears and possibly the spinal canal or periphery of the disc (Fig. 2-29).

MRI and CT scans are regarded as the primary imaging modalities for the investigation of disc pathology. Discography is viewed as a follow-up to aid further evaluation in the complicated cases. Discography can be a provocative examination. For instance, the injection of contrast material into the center of the disc increases the intradiscal pressure and may replicate the patient's symptoms, thereby confirming a discogenic etiology to the patient's complaint. This may increase the diagnostic accuracy of whether the disc lesions are clinically important, or it may designate the symptomatic disc when multiple levels of herniation are present.

Digital X-Ray Imaging

A conventional radiographic image is an analog shadow produced as the x-ray beam traverses a patient's body, and the x-ray beam is differentially attenuated depending on the densities of the structures within the collimated beam. Digital radiography represents a relatively recent technology in which the x-ray beam is intercepted using detectors (rather than radiographic film) that convert the x-ray energy into digital data that can be computer stored, displayed, and manipulated (Fig. 2-30).

The benefits of digital x-ray imaging systems include potential reduction of x-ray dose, ability to enhance and manipulate the images with computer technology, ability to share images across computer platforms, digital archiving, and retrieval. Digital imaging also allows wider exposure latitude than radiographic film. Further, correction of overexposure and underexposure can occur within limits, which reduces patient reexaminations and unnecessary reexposure. In addition, consumable materials, including film

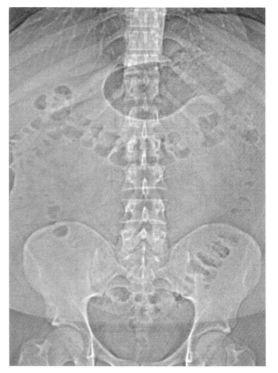

FIG. 2-30 Digital radiograph of the abdomen.

and chemicals, are no longer needed, which has a positive environmental impact.

Two major forms of digital imaging are available: direct capture radiography (DR) and computed radiography (CR). Both systems produce digital radiographs that can be transmitted, viewed, and stored in a computer-available format.

In analog x-ray imaging, the operator is necessary to expose a film-screen cassette that is then processed in a dark room environment. CR replaces the traditional film-cassette system with a photostimulable phosphor plate that is exposed to the x-ray beam. This plate absorbs the x-ray energy, essentially recording the image. After the exposure has occurred, the latent image stored on the phosphor plate is "read" by a laser scanner that traverses the imaging plate and stimulates a luminescence. The stimulated light emanating from the plate is converted into electrical energy and is sent as digital information to the computer. After completion of this process, the plate is erased with high-intensity light and then reused. This represents an "indirect" form of digital radiography.

DR directly transforms the x-ray energy into digital information without an intermediate scanning step through use of cesium iodide or charged couple devices. The images are produced immediately and are instantly accessible in this system. DR examinations have a more efficient image throughput because phosphor plate cassettes, which are an integral aspect of CR, are not necessary. Direct capture radiography is considerably more expensive than CR; however, these technologies are expected to eventually replace most film radiography applications.

Positron Emission Tomography

BACKGROUND

Positron emission tomography (PET) is a relatively noninvasive tomographic diagnostic imaging procedure for evaluating cellular and tissue metabolic activity through the detection of short-lived positron-emitting radiopharmaceuticals.

IMAGE PRODUCTION

In a process somewhat similar to radionuclide imaging, PET imaging involves the use of radioactive compounds. However, in contrast to radionuclide imaging, the compounds used in PET emit positrons through nuclear decay. An advantage of PET is that the atoms that have been "labeled" to become positron emitters also reside naturally in the body and include such elements as oxygen. Secondarily, the labeled compounds can be introduced in trace quantities such that they do not interfere with normally occurring metabolic activity. Radionuclides routinely produced for PET imaging studies include O-15 (2 min half-life), N-13 (10 min), C-11 (20 min), and F-18 (110 min). The most widely used radiotracer is F-18 2-fluoro-2-deoxy-D-glucose (FDG), commonly used to evaluate brain function and malignancy. This compound is similar to naturally occurring glucose with the addition of a radioactive fluorine atom (F-18).

A positron is an antimatter electron with identical mass but has a positive charge. In PET scanning, positrons are obtained from nuclear decay produced in a cyclotron by bombarding material with protons, which results in the ejection of a neutron from the nucleus. This new nucleus is unstable and eventually decays into a more stable form. The most prevalent PET scanning compound is formed when an isotope of oxygen (18-O) is bombarded, changing the atomic species to 18-F (fluorine). In this circumstance, one of the nuclear protons decays into a neutron and in the process emits

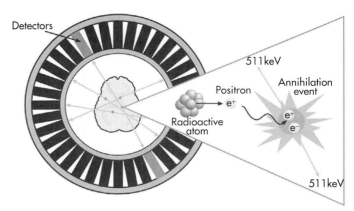

FIG. 2-31 When a nucleus decays by positron emission, a proton in the nucleus converts into a positron and a neutrino. Both are ejected from the nucleus, and the neutrino leaves without incident while the positron quickly interacts with a nearby electron as an annihilation event. The positron–electron annihilation event creates two 511 keV gamma rays (photons) that are emitted in opposite directions from the patient placed in the center of the gantry. Within the gantry photomultiplier-scintillator detectors record the locations of emitted gamma rays. This information is assessed by mathematical algorithms over many iterations (typically 10^7 to 10^8) and many different angles around the patient to map an image detailing where the radioactive substance has accumulated. The intensity detected at any point in the patient directly relates to the concentration of the radiotracer in the tissue.

both a neutrino and a positron. Ultimately the positron interacts with an electron, creating an annihilation episode. The annihilation produces two 511 keV gamma rays (photons) that travel off in opposite (180-degree) directions that are ultimately detected by the scanner (Fig. 2-31).

A small amount of the labeled compound is intravenously injected into the patient. After an appropriate amount of time the patient is scanned. This process measures and spatially localizes the radionuclide within the target tissue.

On casual review, the PET scanner appears similar to either a CT or MRI unit. Within the gantry, photomultiplier-scintillator detectors detect the gamma rays. A typical whole-body unit may contain 4096 crystals oriented into eight rings of 512 detectors per ring. The eight rings are used to collect eight direct slices of data. An additional seven slices are obtained by collecting photon interactions between adjacent direct planes for a total of 15 planes.

The scanner records the gamma rays being emitted, and the equipment computer uses the information and mathematical algorithms to map an image of the area where the radioactive substance has accumulated. The images can be displayed as cross-sectional, coronal, or sagittal sequences. 3-D images also can be constructed.

PATIENT EXPERIENCE

The patient is asked to fast for 6 hours and limit physical activity on the day previous to the examination to reduce muscular uptake. A blood glucose evaluation might be performed because high levels of glucose compete with the FDG, affecting the quality of the examination.

Other than the injection of the radiotracer, PET scanning is noninvasive. After the injection, it takes approximately 30 to 60 minutes for the compound to be absorbed by the tissue under study. During this time, the patient is asked to rest quietly in a partially darkened room and avoid significant movement or talking, which may alter the localization of the administered substance. Scanning begins after that time, which takes an additional 30 to 45 minutes. PET examinations can be performed in conjunction with stress testing in patients with potential cardiac disease.

After the examination the patient may be instructed to ingest fluids to flush the radioactive substance from the body, although the radiation dose is very low. Relative contraindications to PET examinations include patients who are pregnant or are breast-feeding.

CLINICAL APPLICATION

Positron emission tomography is most commonly used to evaluate cerebral and cardiac perfusion and tumors.

Oncology. Fluorodeoxyglucose (^{18}FDG) is particularly helpful in evaluating increased metabolic activity associated with tumors. Uptake of ^{18}FDG is high in malignancy because glucose use is higher than normal. As a result, PET imaging can discriminate between benign and malignant solitary pulmonary nodules with a greater than 90% sensitivity and specificity. Other malignancies that can be satisfactorily evaluated with PET scanning include colorectal cancer, lymphoma, melanoma, and breast tumors. As with any diagnostic imaging test, errors can occur.

False-positive findings can be seen in tumors that are benign but for various reasons might accentuate the accumulation of the radiotracer. Conversely, false-negative results might be seen in those tumors that, although malignant, have a lower metabolic activity. For instance, PET is rarely helpful in patients with prostate malignancy.

Cardiology. In patients with coronary artery disease, PET can evaluate decreased myocardial blood flow, which is representative of stenosed vessels. The examination is also usually accomplished as a component of a stress test.

Neurology. PET using ^{18}FDG can be used to localize brain lesions associated with epilepsy that might be amenable to surgical resection. PET is being used to define Alzheimer's disease, reducing diagnostic uncertainty.

IMAGE FUSION

Information from CT, MRI, SPECT, and PET can be superimposed (by computer) such that physiologic data from PET can be combined with anatomic data to assist in pathology interpretation. Common examples include combining PET and CT or MRI information. MRI and CT images also can be "fused"

TABLE 2-2
Appropriate Imaging Modalities Based on Pathology

Clinical presentation	MRI	CT	X-ray
Spine and spinal cord			
Disc herniation	Procedure of choice	Reasonably sensitive	Insensitive
Recurrent disc vs postoperative scar	Procedure of choice	Insensitive	Insensitive
Degenerative disc disease (DDD)	Very sensitive	Sensitive	Moderately sensitive
Radiculopathy	Procedure of choice	Reasonably sensitive	Adjunctive
Myelopathy	Procedure of choice	Insensitive	Adjunctive
Multiple sclerosis	Procedure of choice	Insensitive	Insensitive
Arnold Chiari malformation	Procedure of choice	Reasonably sensitive	Insensitive
Syringomyelia	Procedure of choice	Reasonably sensitive	Insensitive
Spinal metastasis, multiple myeloma	Very sensitive	Reasonably sensitive	Insensitive in early disease
Infections	Very sensitive	Reasonably sensitive	Insensitive in early disease
Cord tumors and "drop" metastases	Procedure of choice	Insensitive	Insensitive
Extremities (knee, shoulder, wrist, and ankle)			
Avascular necrosis	Procedure of choice	Insensitive	Insensitive in early disease
Cruciate ligament tears	Procedure of choice	Insensitive	Insensitive
Meniscal tears	Procedure of choice	Insensitive	Insensitive
Osteochondritis dessicans	Procedure of choice	Adjunctive	Insensitive in early disease
Posttrauma	Very sensitive	Sensitive	Procedure of choice
Chrondomalacia patella	Procedure of choice	Insensitive	Insensitive in early disease
Rotator cuff tear	Procedure of choice	Insensitive	Insensitive
Glenoid labrum tear	Sensitive	Sensitive	Insensitive
Tendonitis	Very sensitive	Insensitive	Insensitive
Joint effusions	Procedure of choice	Adjunctive	Insensitive
Cartilage degeneration (DJD)	Very sensitive	Adjunctive	Moderately sensitive
Infection, osteomyelitis	Very sensitive	Adjunctive	Insensitive in early disease
Tumor, multiple myeloma, metastasis	Very sensitive	Adjunctive	Insensitive in early disease
Brain			
Malignancy primary/metastasis	Procedure of choice	Adjunctive	Insensitive
Infections	Procedure of choice	Adjunctive	Insensitive
Chronic headaches	Procedure of choice	Adjunctive	Insensitive
Infarction	Procedure of choice	Adjunctive	Insensitive
Aneurysms	Very sensitive angiography	Procedure of choice	Insensitive
Hematoma, hemorrhage	Very sensitive angiography	Procedure of choice	Insensitive
Congenital anomalies	Procedure of choice	Sensitive	Insensitive
Pituitary lesions, tumor, empty sella	Procedure of choice	Adjunctive	Insensitive

such that the MRI component can show the soft-tissue aspects of a bone lesion to good advantage, whereas the CT component delineates the osseous aspects to better advantage. With fusion the radiologist has images that delineate the collective anatomic and physiologic components of a given pathology. Imaging equipment also is available in which CT is combined with PET into a single unit.

Table 2-2 presents common applications of MRI, CT, and plain film radiography for selected clinical pathologies.

References

1. Bloch F: The principle of nuclear induction, *Science* 118:425, 1953.
2. Kleinfield S: A machine called indomitable: the remarkable story of a scientist's inspiration, invention, and medical breakthrough, New York, 1985, Times Books.
3. Magin RL, Liburdy RP, Persson B: Biological effects and safety aspects of nuclear magnetic resonance imaging and spectroscopy, *Ann NY Acad Sci* 649:31, 1992.
4. Persson BRR, Stahlberg F: Health and safety of clinical NMR examinations, Boca Raton, FL, 1989, CRC Publishers.
5. Shellock FG, Kanal E: Magnetic resonance: bioeffects, safety, and patient management, Philadelphia, 1994, Lippincott-Raven.
6. Bushong SC: Magnetic resonance imaging, ed 3, St Louis, 2003, Mosby.
7. Armstrong P et al: Magnetic resonance imaging: basic principles of image production, *BMJ* 303:35, 1991.
8. Weinmann HJ et al: Characteristics of gadolinium-DPTA complex: a potential NMR contrast agent, *AJR Am J Roentgenol* 142:619, 1984.
9. Helgason JW, Vijay PC, Joseph SY: MR arthrography: a review of current technique and applications, *AJR Am J Roentgenol* 168:1473, 1997.
10. Friedland GW, Thurber BD: The birth of CT, *AJR Am J Roentgenol* 167:1365, 1996.
11. American College of Radiology: ACR practice guideline for general radiology, Reston, VA: American College of Radiology, 2001.
12. Daffner RH: Cervical radiography for trauma patients: a time effective technique? *AJR Am J Roentgenol* 175:1309, 2000.
13. Karnaze MG et al: Comparison of MR and CT myelography in imaging the cervical and thoracic spine, *AJR Am J Roentgenol* 150:397, 1988.
14. Pages J, Buls N, Osteaux M: CT doses in children: a multicentre study, *Br J Radiol* 76:803, 2003.
15. Paterson A, Frush DP, Donnelly LF: Helical CT of the body: are settings adjusted for pediatric patients? *AJR Am J Roentgenol* 176:297, 2001.
16. Hendler A, Hershkop M: When to use bone scintigraphy. It can reveal things other studies cannot, *Postgrad Med* 104:54, 1998.
17. Jimenez CE: Advantages of diagnostic nuclear medicine, *Phys Sportsmed* 27:13, 1999.
18. Katz DS, Math KR, Groskin SA: Radiology secrets, St Louis, 1998, Hanley & Belfus.
19. Deblinger L: Bone mineral density testing: who, when, how, *Patient Care* 1:62, 2001.
20. Bracker MD, Watts NB: How to get the most out of bone densitometry: results can help assess fracture risk and guide therapy. Symposium: second of four articles on osteoporosis, *Postgrad Med* 104:77, 1998.
21. Cummings SR, et al: Bone density at various sites for prediction of hip fractures. The study of osteoporotic fractures research group, *Lancet* 341:72, 1993.
22. Dandy WE: Roentgenography of the brain after injection of air into the spinal canal, *Ann Surg* 70:397, 1919.
23. Sicard JA, Forrestier JE: Methode general d'exploration radiologique par l'huile iodee (Lipiodol), *Bull Med Soc Med Hop Paris* 46:463, 1922.
24. MacPherson P et al: Iohexol versus Iopamidol for cervical mylography: a randomized double blind study, *Br J Radiol* 58:849, 1985.
25. Hirsch C: An attempt to diagnose level of disc lesion clinically by disc puncture, *Acta Orthop Scand* 18:132, 1948.
26. Lindblom K: Diagnostic puncture of intervertebral disks in sciatica, *Acta Orthop Scand* 17:231, 1948.

chapter 3

Radiographic Positioning

LINDA CARLSON

This chapter is designed as a quick reference guide to radiographic positioning and technique. Technical tips and supplemental views are provided to aid in obtaining optimal film quality using the most appropriate views. The routine study is highlighted in blue; this is the minimal number of views that must be performed in order to accomplish a complete evaluation of the area in question. For further information on the views included in this chapter, a textbook dedicated to radiographic positioning should be consulted. A list of recommended further reading is included at the end of this section.

RADIOGRAPHIC EQUIPMENT

The basic components of a radiography unit are a source of radiation (x-ray tube) and a receiving medium (x-ray film in the case of conventional plain film radiography). Figures 3-1 and 3-2 identify a stool, table, shields, side markers, and other accessories that are used for the radiographic setup.

RADIOGRAPHIC TECHNIQUE

The radiographic techniques listed in this chart were derived using the following parameters:
- 300/125 kVp single phase generator*
- 400-speed rare earth screens with matched film or
- Extremity detail screens with matched films†
- 10:1 stationary grids
- Automatic processor

The suggested technique is within a fixed kilovolt (kV) range per body part. In smaller patients the lower spectrum of the kV range is used; in larger patients the upper range of kV is used. In this system the milliampere-seconds (mAs) is variable and corrections in exposure factors require changing the mAs only. To correct the exposure factors in a film that is underexposed, the mAs must be changed by a minimum of 30% to note a detectable change or by 100% for a significant change. The reverse is true for films that are overexposed. When a fixed kV system is used, only one exposure factor, the mAs, needs to be changed to correct for errors. The techniques contained in the chart provide a starting point of adequate exposures for a radiographic system similar to the one listed in the preceding. Corrections for individual variations in machines are made by adjusting the mAs only because the chart was formulated using the fixed kV technique.

There may be instances when a change in penetration, or kVp, is necessary. When a film is critiqued, if the bony detail is too light so as to appear nonexistent, a 15% increase in kVp provides the

necessary penetration. An increase in mAs is required if the bony detail is present but the overall appearance of the film is too light.

PATIENT PREPARATION

Good patient education is essential and must include a thorough explanation of the study being performed and the patient's role during the examination. Protection methods and breathing instructions should be reviewed. Patients should be properly gowned and all artifacts should be removed before the radiographic examination begins (Fig. 3-3). Female patients of childbearing years should be assessed for possible pregnancy. If there is a possibility of pregnancy, the examination should be delayed, if possible, until it can be determined the patient is not pregnant, either by a negative human chorionic gonadotropin test or the start of menses. If possible, all radiographic examinations of the lumbar spine, abdomen, and pelvis should be scheduled during the first 10 days following the onset of menstruation because this is the least likely time for pregnancy to occur. Appropriate gonadal shielding should be used in both male and female patients whenever possible.

USING THE CHARTS

The following tables present commonly performed radiographic projections. The routine study is highlighted in blue. A routine study is the minimum number of views that must be performed to obtain a complete study of the area. Additional views are included in most sections and can be added to the basic study. Additional views are added to better demonstrate an area in question or to assess motion or stability. As reference, radiographic views are named by the body part being examined and either the direction the x-ray beam is passing through the body (anteroposterior, [AP]) or the portion of the body part touching the grid for oblique angles of the body (right posterior oblique [RPO]) (Fig. 3-4).

Each table explains the position setup, central ray placement, tube angulation, optimal film size, and focal film distance for each view. To conserve x-ray film and facilitate viewing, sometimes the film is divided so that multiple views of a body part are seen on a single film (Fig. 3-5). For each setup in the tables, there is a picture demonstrating the position and central ray placement and another to exhibit the anatomy demonstrated by the setup. The kV and mAs section lists the type of film screen combination used and whether the study is performed with the use of a grid or table top. If the use of a grid is listed, a fast film screen combination such as rare earth is suggested. If detailed or nongrid is listed, a slower speed film screen combination is suggested, such as those found in extremity cassettes or 100-speed cassettes. A suggested kV and mAs range is also provided for systems described in the previous section on technique. The "Additional Information" section describes other views that may be done to better demonstrate the desired anatomy. Technical tips are also included to aid in obtaining optimal studies.

---

*For high-frequency systems, lower the listed kV by 5 and decrease the mAs by half.

†100-Speed cassettes can be substituted for extremity detail screens. The same film used in 400-speed cassettes can be used in 100-speed cassettes as long as spectral matching remains the same.

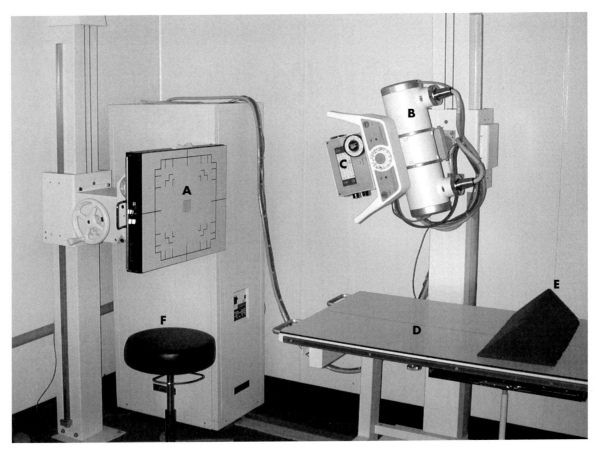

FIG. 3-1 Typical radiographic system and related equipment, including: *A*, grid cabinet (Bucky); *B*, x-ray tube; *C*, collimator; *D*, movable table; *E*, positioning sponge; and *F*, stool.

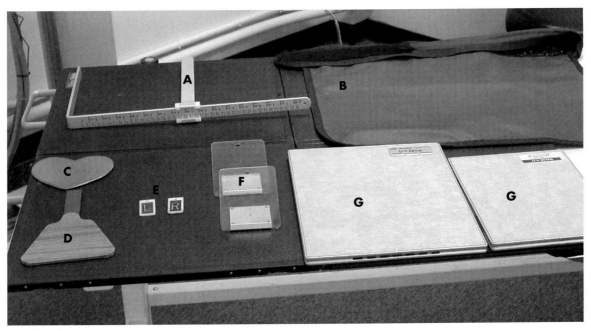

FIG. 3-2 Tools and accessories used for radiographic examinations, including: *A*, measuring calipers; *B*, lead apron; *C*, female gonad shield; *D*, male gonad shield; *E*, right and left side (Mitchell) markers; *F*, filters; and *G*, cassettes.

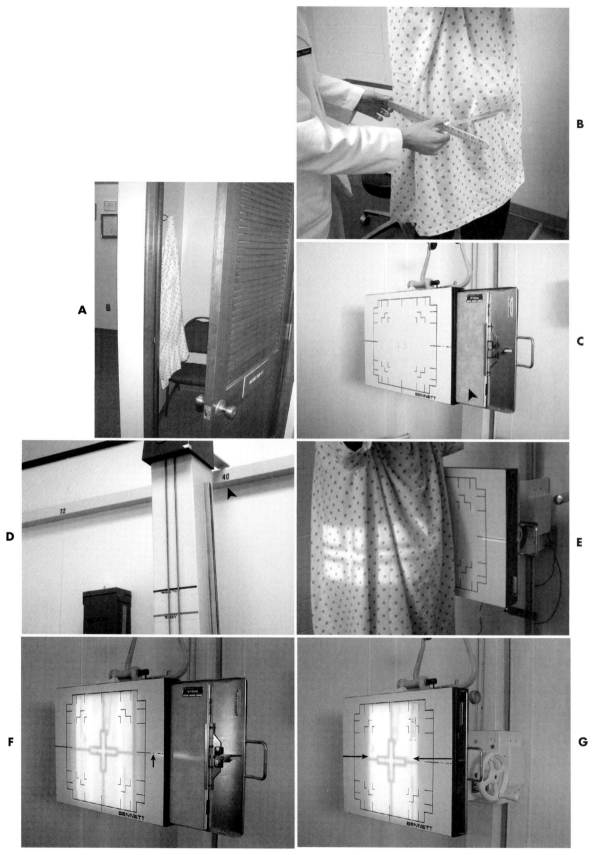

FIG. 3-3 The radiographic setup is done most proficiently by following a general sequence. The sequence begins with patient preparation, including, **A,** gowning; followed by, **B,** measurement technique selection; **C,** film selection and placement; **D,** choice of focal film distance; **E,** central ray placement; **F,** alignment of the center of the film and the central ray; **G,** collimation to film size.

Continued

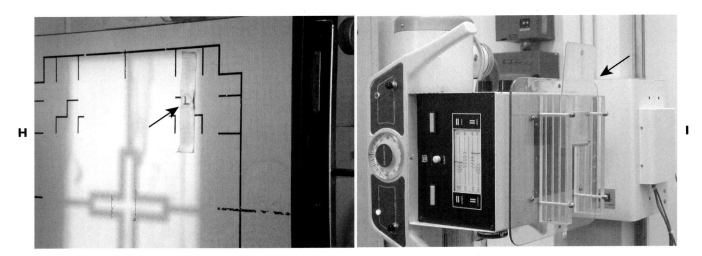

FIG. 3-3 cont'd   **H,** side marker placement; and sometimes, **I,** use of filter.

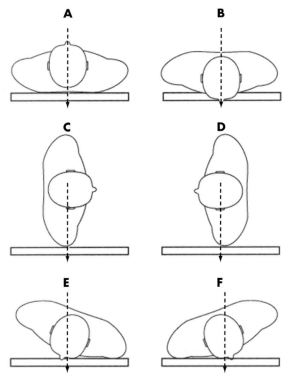

FIG. 3-4   Radiographic views. The term radiographic "projection" references the path of the central ray as it exits the x-ray tube and passes through the patient's body. For example, **A** denotes an anteroposterior (AP) projection and **B** a posteroanterior (PA) projection. In the extremities, lateral projections are similarly described by the direction of the central ray; hence, mediolateral and lateromedial projections are possible. However, when one deals with the head, neck, or body tunk, the lateral and oblique projections are further clarified by the specific "position" of the patient. Position denotes the placement of the patient's body, specifically the portion of the patient's anatomy that is in contact with the Bucky. For example, **C** indicates a lateral projection in a right lateral position and **D** indicates a lateral projection in a left lateral position. In **E,** the patient is in a left anterior oblique (LAO) position, and in **F** the patients is in a right anterior oblique (RAO) position, both corresponding to posteroanterior oblique projections.

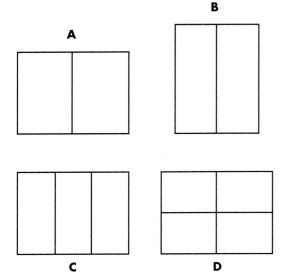

FIG. 3-5   **A** through **D,** For some small body parts (e.g., foot and wrist), the x-ray film may be divided to accommodate several projections.

TABLE 3-1
Skull: PA Caldwell, AP Towne, Lateral Skull

Position:	**PA Caldwell**
Patient Preparation:	Remove any artifacts in the desired field (e.g., earrings, dentures, hair appliances).
Measurement:	Place caliper base at the back of the skull. Slide the caliper arm until it rests lightly at the nasion.
Shielding:	Secure lead apron around patient.
Film Selection:	10 × 12
Film Placement:	Place vertical in Bucky.
ID Placement:	ID should be in lower corner of collimation field.
Patient Placement:	Place patient with nose and forehead against Bucky so that the orbitomeatal line is perpendicular to the film.
Technique Selection:	kVp 70 to 80; mAs 20 to 40
SID:	40″
Central Ray Placement:	Using a 15-degree caudal tube tilt, central ray enters the back of the skull so as to exit the nasion.
Collimation:	To film size.
Marker Placement:	Within the collimation field on either the right side or left side of patient's head.
Breathing Instructions:	Do not breathe. Do not move.
Anatomy Visualized:	Frontal bone, frontal and ethmoid sinuses, greater and lesser wing of the sphenoid, superior orbital fissure, foramen rotundum, orbital margins.
Additional Information:	The caudal tube angle may be increased to 30 degrees to optimally define the inferior orbital rim area.
	Petrous pyramids appear in the lower one third of the orbit as performed in the preceding. These are projected below the inferior orbital rim on the 30-degree angle.

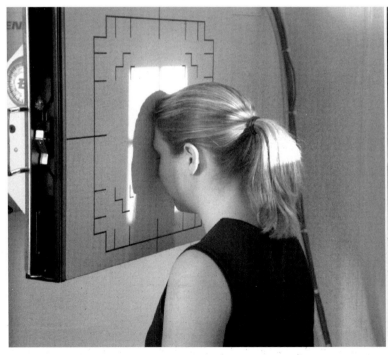 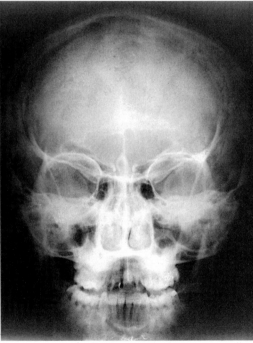

From Ballinger PW, Frank ED: Merril's atlas of radiographic positions and radiologic procedures, ed 10, St Louis, 2003, Mosby.

Continued

TABLE 3-1 cont'd
Skull: PA Caldwell, AP Towne, Lateral Skull

Position:	**AP Towne**
Patient Preparation:	Remove any artifacts in the desired field (e.g., earrings, dentures, hair appliances).
Measurement:	Place base bar of caliper on occiput. Slide moveable bar in toward the patient's head so as to touch the glabella.
Shielding:	Secure lead apron around patient.
Film Selection:	10 × 12
Film Placement:	Place vertically in Bucky.
ID Placement:	ID should be in lower corner of collimation field.
Patient Placement:	Place patient in AP position so back of head touches Bucky. Tuck the chin so the orbitomeatal line is perpendicular to the film.
Technique Selection:	kVp 70 to 80; mAs 30 to 60
SID:	40″
Central Ray Placement:	Central ray is angled 30 degrees caudally and enters 2″ above the glabella (superciliary arch).
Collimation:	To film size.
Marker Placement:	Within the collimation field on either the right side or left side of patient's head.
Breathing Instructions:	Do not breathe. Do not move.
Anatomy Visualized:	Occipital bone, petrous pyramids, foramen magnum with dorsum sellae and posterior clinoids projected through it.
Additional Information:	If the patient cannot tuck the chin sufficiently, adjust the head tilt so that the infraorbitomeatal line is perpendicular to the film and increase the tube tilt to approximately 37 degrees.

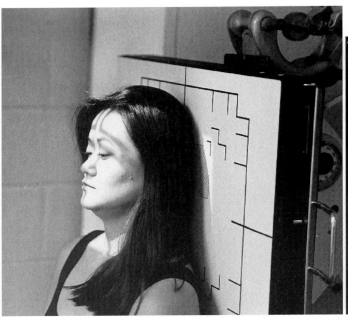
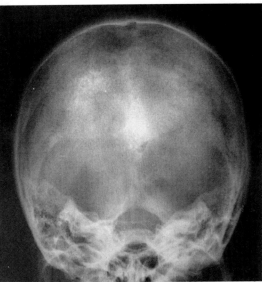

From Ballinger PW, Frank ED: Merril's atlas of radiographic positions and radiologic procedures, ed 10, St Louis, 2003, Mosby.

TABLE 3-1 cont'd
Skull: PA Caldwell, AP Towne, Lateral Skull

Position:	**Lateral Skull**
Patient Preparation:	Remove any artifacts in the desired field (e.g., earrings, dentures, hair appliances).
Measurement:	Place the base bar of the calipers on the temporal bone of one side of the head and move the slider bar toward the patient's head so as to touch the temporal bone on the other side of the head.
Shielding:	Secure lead apron around patient.
Film Selection:	10 × 12
Film Placement:	Place horizontally in Bucky.
ID Placement:	ID should be in lower corner of collimation field.
Patient Placement:	Place patient with side of head against Bucky. Oblique the patient's body for comfort. The interpupillary line is perpendicular to the film. The external occipital protuberance and the nasion should be equidistant from the film to prevent rotation.
Technique Selection:	kVp 70 to 80; mAs 20 to 40
SID:	40″
Central Ray Placement:	The central ray enters 1″ superior and anterior to the external auditory meatus.
Collimation:	To film size.
Marker Placement:	Within the collimation field denoting which side of the patient's head is touching the Bucky.
Breathing Instructions:	Do not breathe. Do not move.
Anatomy Visualized:	Lateral cranium closest to film, sella turcica, anterior and posterior clinoids, and ethmoid sinuses.
	AP, Anteroposterior; *ID,* identification; *PA,* posteroanterior; *SID,* source-to-image distance.

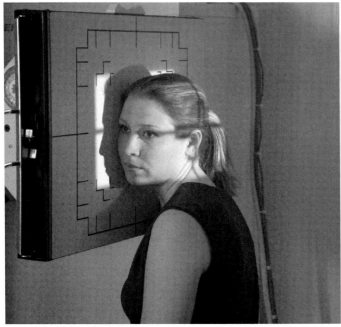
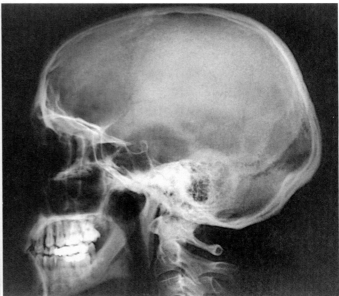

From Ballinger PW, Frank ED: Merril's atlas of radiographic positions and radiologic procedures, ed 10, St Louis, 2003, Mosby.

TABLE 3-2

Facial Bones: PA Waters, PA Caldwell, Lateral Facial Bones

Position:	**PA Waters**
Patient Preparation:	Remove any artifacts in the desired field (e.g., earrings, dentures, hair appliances).
Measurement:	Place base bar of calipers on back of skull and move slider bar toward patient's face until it touches between bottom lip and tip of chin.
Shielding:	Secure lead apron around patient.
Film Selection:	8 × 10
Film Placement:	Place vertically in Bucky so center of cassette is centered to the acanthion.
ID Placement:	ID should be in lower corner of collimation field.
Patient Placement:	Place patient in PA position with neck in slight extension so chin and nose rest against Bucky. The orbitomeatal line should form a 55-degree angle to the film.
Technique Selection:	kVp 70 to 80; mAs 20 to 40
SID:	40″
Central Ray Placement:	The central ray is directed perpendicular to the Bucky and is centered to the center of the cassette.
Collimation:	To film size.
Marker Placement:	Within the collimation field on either the right side or left side of patient's head.
Breathing Instructions:	Do not breathe. Do not move.
Anatomy Visualized:	Floor of the orbits, maxillary sinuses.
Additional Information:	Should be done in upright position to evaluate air fluid levels in the maxillary sinuses. Petrous ridges should be projected in the lower half of the maxillary sinuses below the inferior orbital rim. Good view for evaluation of possible "blowout" orbital fractures.

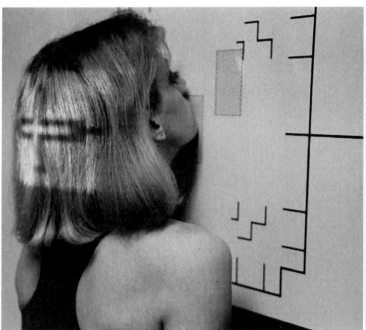
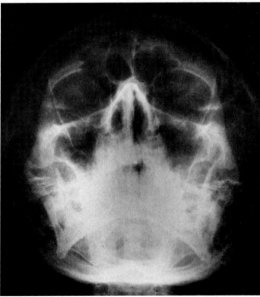

From Ballinger PW, Frank ED: Merril's atlas of radiographic positions and radiologic procedures, ed 10, St Louis, 2003, Mosby.

TABLE 3-2 cont'd
Facial Bones: PA Waters, PA Caldwell, Lateral Facial Bones

Position:	**PA Caldwell**
Patient Preparation:	Remove any artifacts in the desired field (e.g., earrings, dentures, hair appliances).
Measurement:	Place base bar of calipers against back of head. Move slider bar toward patient's face to rest on nasion.
Shielding:	Secure lead apron around patient.
Film Selection:	8 × 10
Film Placement:	Place vertically in Bucky with center of cassette aligned to the nasion.
ID Placement:	ID should be in lower corner of collimation field.
Patient Placement:	Place patient in the PA position against the Bucky so that the nose and forehead are against the Bucky and the orbitomeatal line is perpendicular to the cassette.
Technique Selection:	kVp 70 to 80; mAs 20 to 40
SID:	40″
Central Ray Placement:	The central ray is angled 15 degrees caudally and is centered to cassette.
Collimation:	To film size.
Marker Placement:	Within the collimation field on either the right side or left side of patient's head.
Breathing Instructions:	Do not breathe. Do not move.
Anatomy Visualized:	Orbital rim, maxillae, nasal septum, and zygomatic bones.
Additional Information:	For better definition of the inferior orbital rim area, increase the tube angle to 30 degrees.
	Petrous pyramids should be projected in the lower one third of the orbit with a 15-degree tube tilt and below the inferior orbital rim on the 30-degree tube tilt.

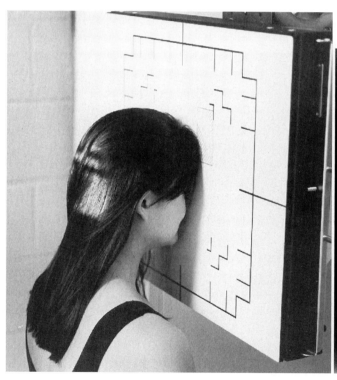
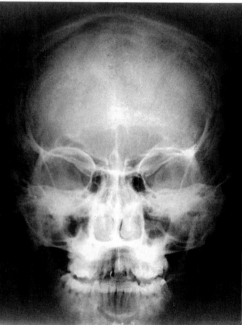

From Ballinger PW, Frank ED: Merril's atlas of radiographic positions and radiologic procedures, ed 10, St Louis, 2003, Mosby.

Continued

TABLE 3-2 cont'd

Facial Bones: PA Waters, PA Caldwell, Lateral Facial Bones

Position:	**Lateral Facial Bones**
Patient Preparation:	Remove any artifacts in the desired field (e.g., earrings, dentures, hair appliances).
Measurement:	Place the base bar of the calipers against the zygomatic arch. Move the slider bar of the calipers toward the patient's face so it rests on the opposite zygomatic arch.
Shielding:	Secure lead apron around patient.
Film Selection:	8 × 10
Film Placement:	Place vertically in Bucky.
ID Placement:	ID should be in lower corner of collimation field.
Patient Placement:	Place the patient in an anterior oblique position. Place the patient's head in a lateral position with the side of interest resting against the Bucky.
Technique Selection:	kVp 70 to 80; mAs 10 to 20
SID:	40″
Central Ray Placement:	The central ray enters ½″ posterior to the outer canthus.
Collimation:	To film size.
Marker Placement:	Within the collimation field denoting the side of the head that is closest to the Bucky.
Breathing Instructions:	Do not breathe. Do not move.
Anatomy Visualized:	Ethmoid, frontal, sphenoid, and maxillary sinuses in the lateral projection.
Additional Information:	This view should be performed with the patient in the upright position to evaluate air fluid levels in the sinuses.

ID, Identification; *PA*, posteroanterior; *RAO*, right anterior oblique; *SID*, source-to-image distance.

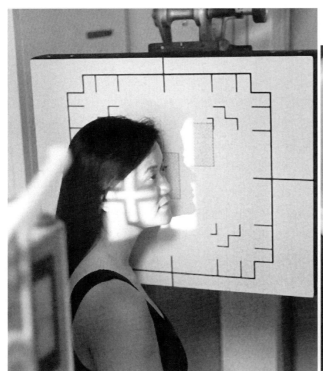

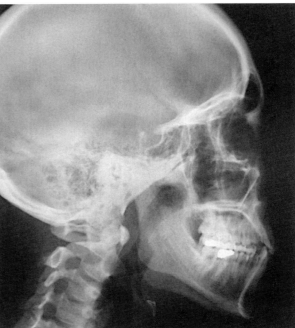

TABLE 3-3
Cervical Spine: Routine, Traumatic, and Palmer Upper Cervical

Routine: AP Open Mouth, AP Lower Cervical, Lateral Cervical

Position:	**AP Open Mouth**
Patient Preparation:	Remove any artifacts in the desired field (e.g., earrings, dentures, hair appliances).
Measurement:	Place base bar of calipers on back of head. Instruct patient to open mouth. Move slider bar in toward patient's face to corner of mouth (without touching patient's mouth).
Shielding:	Secure lead apron around patient.
Film Selection:	8 × 10
Film Placement:	Place vertically in Bucky.
ID Placement:	ID should be in lower corner of collimation field.
Patient Placement:	Place patient in the AP position with back of shoulders resting against Bucky. The plane of the upper occlusal plate and occiput with mouth open should be parallel to the floor.
Technique Selection:	kVp 70 to 80; mAs 10 to 15
SID:	40″
Central Ray Placement:	The central ray enters the midpoint of the open mouth.
Collimation:	Collimate just under the eyes vertically and to the mastoids horizontally.
Marker Placement:	Within the collimation field on either the right side or left side of patient's head.
Breathing Instructions:	Do not breathe. Do not move.
Anatomy Visualized:	Lateral masses, anterior and posterior arches of C1, odontoid process, pedicles, lamina, and spinous process of C2.
Additional Information:	Correct head placement is essential. If teeth superimpose odontoid, tip head back. If occiput superimposes odontoid, tip head forward. In extreme cases, the oblique odontoid or Fuchs view may be used.

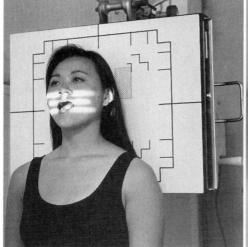 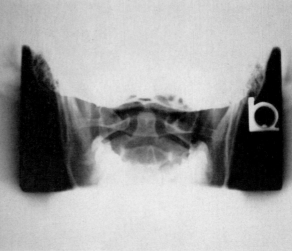

Continued

TABLE 3-3 cont'd
Cervical Spine: Routine, Traumatic, and Palmer Upper Cervical

Position:	**AP Lower Cervical**
Patient Preparation:	Remove any artifacts in the desired field (e.g., earrings, dentures, hair appliances).
Measurement:	Place the base bar of the calipers against the posterior aspect of the cervical spine at the level of C4.
	Move the slider bar toward the patient until it touches the anterior aspect of the cervical spine at C4.
Shielding:	Secure lead apron around patient.
Film Selection:	8 × 10
Film Placement:	Place vertically in Bucky.
ID Placement:	ID should be in upper corner of collimation field.
Patient Placement:	Place patient in the AP position with back of shoulders against the Bucky.
Technique Selection:	kVp 65 to 75; mAs 6 to 12
SID:	40″
Central Ray Placement:	The central ray should be angled 15 degrees cephalically so as to enter the area of C4 (thyroid cartilage).
Collimation:	To film size vertically. To mastoids horizontally.
Marker Placement:	Within the collimation field on either the right side or left side of patient's head.
Breathing Instructions:	Do not breathe. Do not move.
Anatomy Visualized:	Pedicles, lamina, transverse processes, vertebral bodies, and uncinate processes of C3 to C7. Lung apices are also visualized.
Additional Information:	If mandible obscures C3 and C4, elevate chin slightly or increase the angulation on the tube.
	If a lesion is suspected in visualized lung apices, a PA and lateral chest radiograph should be performed.

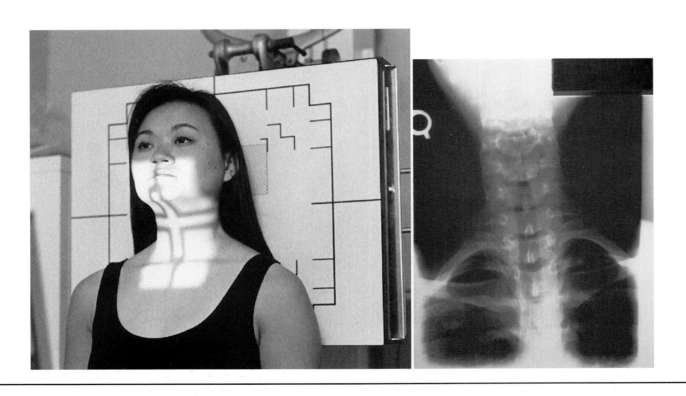

TABLE 3-3 cont'd
Cervical Spine: Routine, Traumatic, and Palmer Upper Cervical

Position:	**Lateral Cervical (Neutral Position)**
Patient Preparation:	Remove any artifacts in the desired field (e.g., earrings, dentures, hair appliances).
Measurement:	Place base bar of calipers on lateral side of patient's neck at C4 level. Move slider bar of calipers toward patient's neck so as to rest at the C4 level.
Shielding:	Secure lead apron around patient.
Film Selection:	8 × 10
Film Placement:	Place vertically in Bucky.
ID Placement:	ID should be in upper corner of collimation field.
Patient Placement:	Place patient (standing or seated) next to the Bucky in the lateral position.
Technique Selection:	kVp 70 to 80; mAs 15 to 30
SID:	72″
Central Ray Placement:	The central ray is directed horizontally to the C4-5 disc level.
Collimation:	To film size.
Marker Placement:	Within the collimation field on the side of the patient that is closest to the film.
Breathing Instructions:	Full exhalation, to drop shoulders.
Anatomy Visualized:	Vertebral bodies, intervertebral disc spaces, articular pillars, spinous processes, and anterior and posterior arch of atlas.
Additional Information:	This the most important view for the evaluation of cervical spine trauma. This film should be evaluated before continuing with the remainder of the cervical series in trauma cases. If C7 is poorly visualized, a swimmer's view may be used.

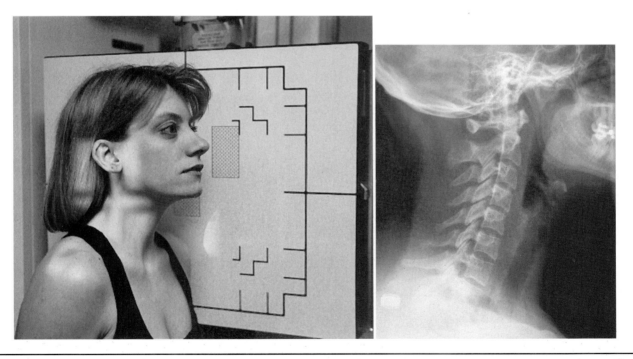

Continued

TABLE 3-3 cont'd
Cervical Spine: Routine, Traumatic, and Palmer Upper Cervical

Position:	Lateral Cervical (Flexion and Extension: for Trauma)
Patient Preparation:	Remove any artifacts in the desired field (e.g., earrings, dentures, hair appliances).
Measurement:	Same as Lateral Cervical (Neutral position).
Shielding:	Secure lead apron around patient.
Film Selection:	10 × 12
Film Placement:	Place vertically in Bucky.
ID Placement:	ID should be in upper corner of collimation field.
Patient Placement:	Same as Lateral Cervical (Neutral position). For *Flexion* view, ask patient to tuck chin into chest and roll head down so eyes rest on chest. For *Extension*, ask patient to roll head backward, looking toward the ceiling.
Technique Selection:	kVp 70 to 80; mAs 15 to 30
SID:	72″
Central Ray Placement:	Same as Lateral Cervical (Neutral position).
Collimation:	To film size.
Marker Placement:	Within the collimation field marking the side of the cervical spine that is closest to the film.
Breathing Instructions:	Full exhalation.
Anatomy Visualized:	These are additional views performed to demonstrate and evaluate excessive or diminished intersegmental mobility of the cervical spine.
Additional Information:	Flexion and Extension views should be performed only after the Lateral Cervical (Neutral position) view has been evaluated for a gross instability.

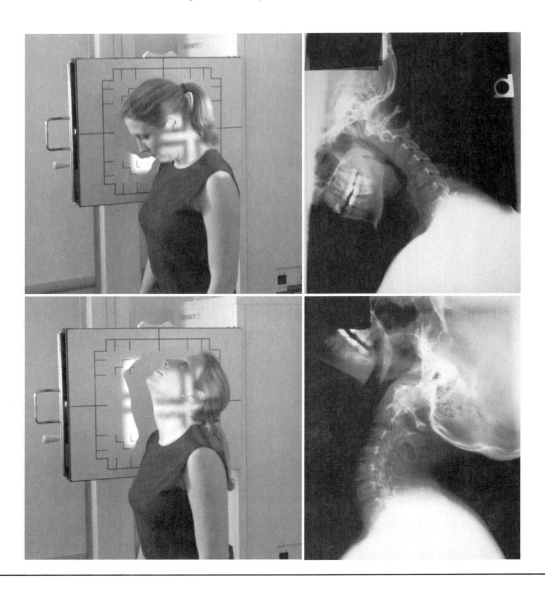

TABLE 3-3 cont'd
Cervical Spine: Routine, Traumatic, and Palmer Upper Cervical

Position:	**Cervical Oblique (for Trauma)**
Patient Preparation:	Remove any artifacts in the desired field (e.g., earrings, dentures, hair appliances).
Measurement:	Same as Lateral Cervical.
Shielding:	Secure lead apron around patient.
Film Selection:	8 × 10
Film Placement:	Place vertically in Bucky.
ID Placement:	ID should be in upper corner of collimation field.
Patient Placement:	The right and left oblique projections may be done in an anterior or posterior position. For anterior obliques (RAO and LAO), the anterior aspect of the patient's shoulder is placed against the Bucky and the body is angled 45 degrees with the grid. For posterior obliques (RPO and LPO), the posterior aspect of the patient's shoulder is placed against the Bucky and the body is angled 45 degrees with the grid. The anterior oblique position relates less radiation dose to the thyroid gland and better accommodates the diverging x-ray beam with the cervical lordosis.
Technique Selection:	kVp 70 to 80; mAs 15 to 30
SID:	72″
Central Ray Placement:	Angle tube 15 degrees cephalically for posterior obliques or 15 degrees caudally for anterior obliques at the level of C4.
Collimation:	To film size.
Marker Placement:	Within the collimation field on the side of the patient that is closest to the Bucky.
Breathing Instructions:	Full exhalation.
Anatomy Visualized:	Borders of the intervertebral foramen, pedicles, facet joints, uncinates and posterior vertebral bodies.
Additional Information:	Optimal view for visualization of bony foraminal effacement resulting from cervical spine spondylosis.
	Optimal view for evaluation of pedicles for possible fracture and relationship of superior and inferior facet joints for possible dislocation in trauma cases. The posterior cervical oblique positions (RPO and LPO) demonstrate the opposite side intervertebral foramen (e.g., RPO shows left foramen) and the anterior cervical oblique positions (RAO and LAO) demonstrate the same side intervertebral foramen (e.g., RAO shows right foramen). The anterior oblique position relates less radiation dose to the thyroid and the divergence of the x-ray beam better approximates the intervertebral disc angles, and therefore anterior obliques are typically preferred.

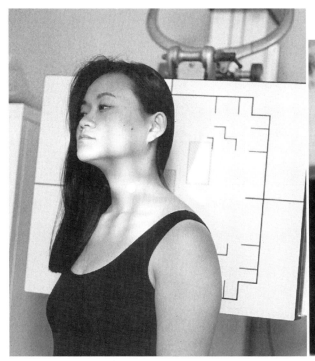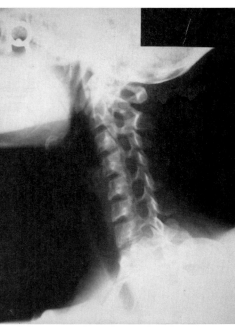

Continued

TABLE 3-3 cont'd
Cervical Spine: Routine, Traumatic, and Palmer Upper Cervical

Position:	**Oblique Odontoid (Kasabach method)**
Patient Preparation:	Remove any artifacts in the desired field (e.g., earrings, dentures, hair appliances).
Measurement:	Use recommended technique.
Shielding:	Secure lead apron around patient.
Film Selection:	8 × 10
Film Placement:	Place vertically in Bucky.
ID Placement:	ID should be in upper corner of collimation field.
Patient Placement:	AP with 45-degree rotation of the head.
Technique Selection:	kVp 75 to 85; mAs 15 to 25
SID:	40″
Central Ray Placement:	Central ray is angled 15 degrees caudally to enter midway between the outer canthus and the external auditory meatus.
Collimation:	To film size.
Marker Placement:	Within the collimation field on the side of the head that is touching the Bucky.
Breathing Instructions:	Do not breathe. Do not move.
Anatomy Visualized:	Demonstrates oblique view of odontoid process.
Additional Information:	This study is performed when the odontoid cannot be visualized on an AP open mouth view. In cases of trauma or in patients with decreased range of motion, the entire body can be rotated 45 degrees.

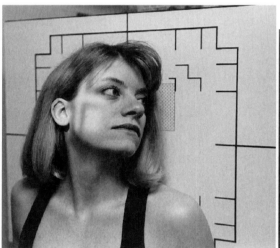 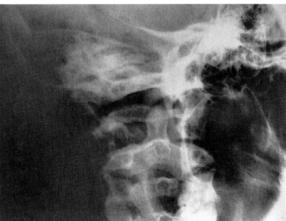

From Ballinger PW, Frank ED: Merril's atlas of radiographic positions and radiologic procedures, ed 10, St Louis, 2003, Mosby.

TABLE 3-3 cont'd
Cervical Spine: Routine, Traumatic, and Palmer Upper Cervical

Position:	**Fuchs (Nontrauma)**
Patient Preparation:	Remove any artifacts in the desired field (e.g., earrings, dentures, hair appliances).
Measurement:	Using the calipers, place the base bar under the chin. Move the slider bar so that it touches the patient at the vertex of the skull.
Shielding:	Secure lead apron around patient.
Film Selection:	8 × 10
Film Placement:	Place vertically in Bucky.
ID Placement:	ID can be either up or down because of collimation.
Patient Placement:	Patient is in the AP position with the neck extended so that the vertex of the skull touches the center of the Bucky.
Technique Selection:	kVp 70 to 80; mAs 10 to 15
SID:	40″
Central Ray Placement:	Central ray is angled 0-15 degrees (depending on the extent to which the patient can extend his or her neck) and enters 1″ below the chin.
Collimation:	To part size, approximately 5″ × 5″
Marker Placement:	Within the collimation field on either the right side or left side of patient's head.
Breathing Instructions:	Do not breathe. Do not move.
Anatomy Visualized:	AP projection of the odontoid process as it lies within the shadow of the foramen magnum.
Additional Information:	This view should not be performed on a trauma patient or a patient with limited range of motion. Use of linear tomography may be required to better visualize the odontoid in cases of suspected fractures. This is a supplemental view used when the dens cannot be visualized on the AP open mouth view.

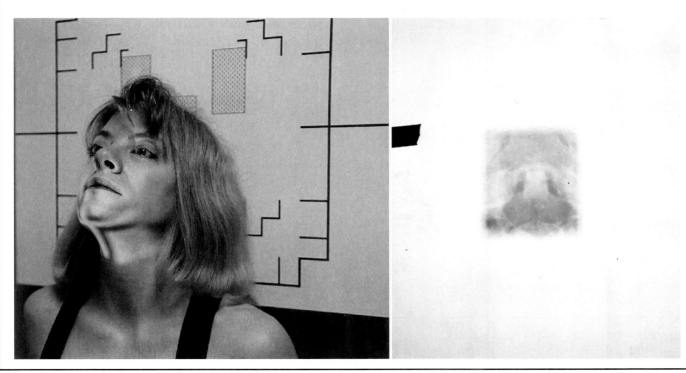

Continued

TABLE 3-3 cont'd
Cervical Spine: Routine, Traumatic, and Palmer Upper Cervical

Position:	**Pillar**
Patient Preparation:	Remove any artifacts in the desired field (e.g., earrings, dentures, hair appliances).
Measurement:	Same as AP Lower Cervical.
Shielding:	Secure lead apron around patient.
Film Selection:	8 × 10
Film Placement:	Place vertically in Bucky.
ID Placement:	ID should be in upper corner of collimation field.
Patient Placement:	Patient is in AP position with neck in full extension.
Technique Selection:	kVp 70 to 80; mAs 10 to 15
SID:	40″
Central Ray Placement:	Central ray is angled 35 degrees caudally and enters midline of the cervical spine, exiting at the C7 spinous process.
Collimation:	To film size.
Marker Placement:	Within the collimation field on either the right side or left side of patient's head.
Breathing Instructions:	Do not breathe. Do not move.
Anatomy Visualized:	Shape and height of the pillar.
Additional Information:	Computed tomography (CT) is the examination of choice to demonstrate pillar fractures, making this a view rarely performed.

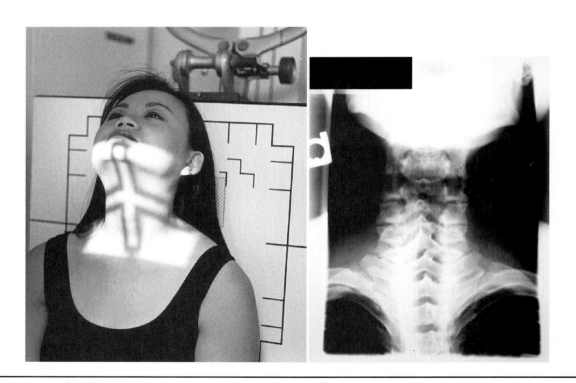

TABLE 3-3 cont'd
Cervical Spine: Routine, Traumatic, and Palmer Upper Cervical

Position:	**Vertebral Arch (AP Caudal Tilt)**
Patient Preparation:	Remove any artifacts in the desired field (e.g., earrings, dentures, hair appliances).
Measurement:	Same as AP Lower Cervical.
Shielding:	Secure lead apron around patient.
Film Selection:	8 × 10
Film Placement:	Place vertically in Bucky.
ID Placement:	ID should be in upper corner of collimation field.
Patient Placement:	Patient is in AP position with neck in full extension, head obliqued. Both obliques are performed for comparison.
Technique Selection:	kVp 70 to 80; mAs 10 to 15
SID:	40″
Central Ray Placement:	Central ray is angled 25 degrees caudally and enters midthyroid cartilage approximately 3″ below the external auditory meatus, exiting at the C7 spinous process.
Collimation:	To film size.
Marker Placement:	Within the collimation field denoting the side of the partient's head closest to the film.
Breathing Instructions:	Do not breathe. Do not move.
Anatomy Visualized:	Shape and continuity of the posterior arch of the vertebrae.
Additional Information:	Computed tomography (CT) is the examination of choice to demonstrate pillar fractures, making this a view rarely performed.

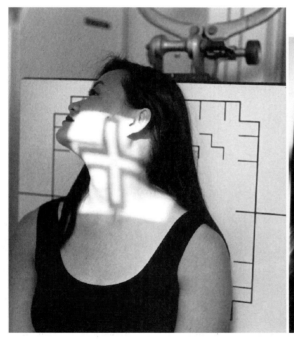 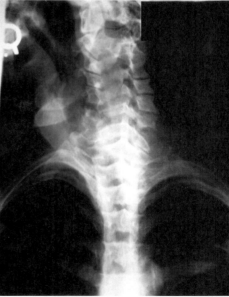

Continued

TABLE 3-3 cont'd
Cervical Spine: Routine, Traumatic, and Palmer Upper Cervical

Position:	**Nasium***
Patient Preparation:	Remove any artifacts in the desired field (e.g., earrings, dentures, hair appliances).
Measurement:	Using calipers, place base bar at the level of the occiput. Move the slider bar toward the patient's face until it rests on the glabella.
Shielding:	Secure lead apron around patient.
Film Selection:	8 × 10
Film Placement:	Place vertically in Bucky.
ID Placement:	ID should be in lower corner of collimation field.
Patient Placement:	Patient is seated in the AP position. Bucky is tilted so as to touch the patient's head and shoulders.
Technique Selection:	kVp 70 to 80; mAs 15 to 30
SID:	40″
Central Ray Placement:	Central ray is angled caudally so as to enter the glabella and exit the inferior tip of the mastoid process. The amount of angulation is determined by measurement obtained from the lateral cervical radiograph.
Collimation:	To film size.
Marker Placement:	Within the collimation field on either the right side or left side of patient's head.
Breathing Instructions:	Do not breathe. Do not move.
Anatomy Visualized:	Ocular orbits, lateral masses of C1, occipital condyles.
Additional Information:	Filtration is used to cover the eyes. Head clamps are used to ensure head is held in a neutral position. This view demonstrates atlas laterality.

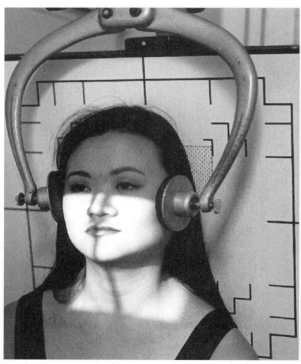
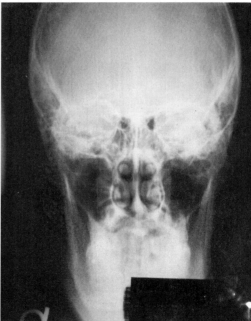

TABLE 3-3 cont'd
Cervical Spine: Routine, Traumatic, and Palmer Upper Cervical

Position:	**Base Posterior***
Patient Preparation:	Remove any artifacts in the desired field (e.g., earrings, dentures, hair appliances).
Measurement:	Using the calipers, place the base bar at the vertex of the skull. Move the slider bar toward the patient resting the bar 1″ below the chin.
Shielding:	Secure lead apron around patient.
Film Selection:	8 × 10
Film Placement:	Place vertically in Bucky. The Bucky is tilted 45 degrees with the top of the Bucky toward the tube.
ID Placement:	ID should be in lower corner of collimation field.
Patient Placement:	Patient is seated in the AP position with head in neutral position. The vertex of the skull is placed in the center of the Bucky.
Technique Selection:	kVp 75 to 85; mAs 20 to 30
SID:	40″
Central Ray Placement:	Central ray is angled cephalically entering 1″ below the chin, passing ½″ anterior to the external auditory meatus, and exiting the vertex of the skull.
Collimation:	To film size.
Marker Placement:	Within the collimation field on either the right side or left side of patient's head.
Breathing Instructions:	Do not breathe. Do not move.
Anatomy Visualized:	Atlas, axis, and nasal septum.
Additional Information:	Filter out the eyes. Head clamps may be used to hold head in neutral position. This view is used to demonstrate atlas rotation. The vertex may be used as an alternate view.

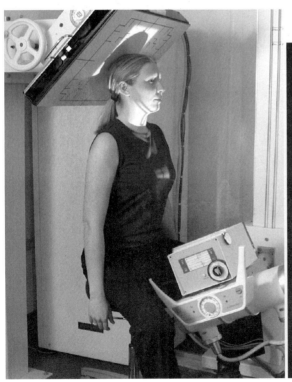
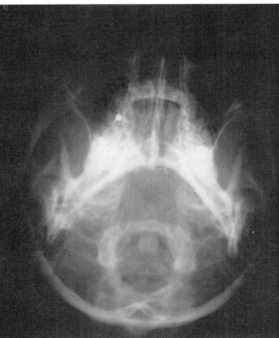

Continued

TABLE 3-3 cont'd

Cervical Spine: Routine, Traumatic, and Palmer Upper Cervical

Position:	**Palmer Open Mouth***
Patient Preparation:	Remove any artifacts in the desired field (e.g., earrings, dentures, hair appliances).
Measurement:	Using calipers, place the base bar against the occiput. Move the slider bar toward the patient's open mouth, stopping 1 cm short of touching the face.
Shielding:	Secure lead apron around patient.
Film Selection:	8 × 10
Film Placement:	Place vertically in Bucky. Bucky should be tilted to touch the back of the patient's head and shoulders.
ID Placement:	ID should be in upper corner of collimation field.
Patient Placement:	Patient is seated in AP position with mouth open.
Technique Selection:	kVp 70 to 80; mAs 10 to 15
SID:	40″
Central Ray Placement:	The central ray is angled to stimulate the direction of the line between the upper occlusal plate and the base of the occiput (0-5 degrees) and enters the corners of the mouth.
Collimation:	To film size.
Marker Placement:	Within the collimation field on either the right side or left side of patient's head.
Breathing Instructions:	Do not breathe. Do not move.
Anatomy Visualized:	Lateral masses, anterior and posterior arches of C1, odontoid process, pedicles, lamina and spinous process of C2, ocular orbits.
Additional Information:	Use filter to cover the ocular orbits. Head clamps may be used to hold head in neutral position. This view demonstrates axis listing.

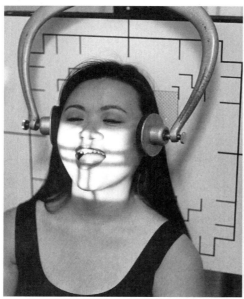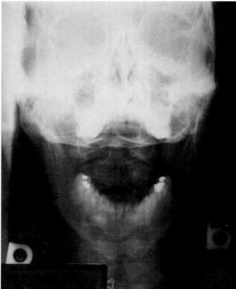

TABLE 3-3 cont'd

Cervical Spine: Routine, Traumatic, and Palmer Upper Cervical

Position:	**Palmer Lateral***
Patient Preparation:	Remove any artifacts in the desired field (e.g., earrings, dentures, hair appliances).
Measurement:	Using calipers, place base bar against one side of patient's neck. Move slider bar to rest comfortably on opposite side of neck.
Shielding:	Secure lead apron around patient.
Film Selection:	10 × 12
Film Placement:	Place vertically in Bucky.
ID Placement:	ID should be in upper corner of collimation field.
Patient Placement:	Patient is seated in a true lateral position with head in neutral position.
Technique Selection:	kVp 70 to 80; mAs 15 to 30
SID:	72″
Central Ray Placement:	Central ray is angled 90 degrees, perpendicular to film entering transverse process of C1.
Collimation:	To film size vertically. Horizontally, collimate to just behind the orbits.
Marker Placement:	Within the collimation field on the side of the body closest to the film.
Breathing Instructions:	Suspend respiration on exhalation to lower shoulders.
Anatomy Visualized:	Vertebral bodies, intervertebral disc spaces, articular pillars, spinous processes, and anterior and posterior arch of the atlas.
Additional Information:	This view demonstrates atlas superiority or inferiority. The measurements are also taken off of this view to determine the tube tilt for the nasium view.

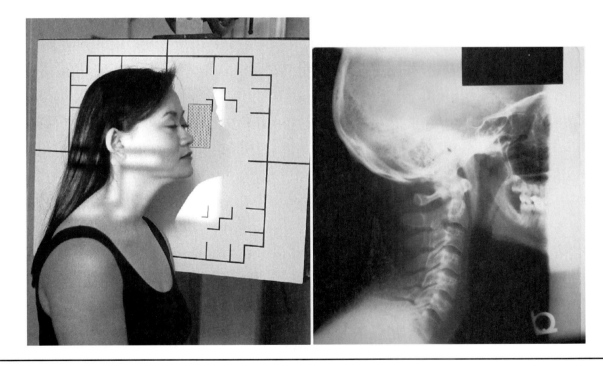

Continued

TABLE 3-3 cont'd

Cervical Spine: Routine, Traumatic, and Palmer Upper Cervical

Position:	**Vertex***
Patient Preparation:	Remove any artifacts in the desired field (e.g., earrings, dentures, hair appliances).
Measurement:	Same as Base Posterior.*
Shielding:	Secure lead apron around patient.
Film Selection:	8 × 10
Film Placement:	Place vertically in Bucky. The Bucky is tilted 45 degrees so the bottom of the Bucky is closest to the tube.
ID Placement:	ID should be in upper corner of collimation field.
Patient Placement:	Patient is seated facing the Bucky. With neck extended, the chin should rest in the center of the Bucky.
Technique Selection:	kVp 75 to 85; mAs 20 to 30
SID:	40″
Central Ray Placement:	The central ray enters the vertex of the skull, passes ½″ of the external auditory meatus, and exits 1″ below the chin.
Collimation:	To film size.
Marker Placement:	Within the collimation field on either the right side or left side of patient's head.
Breathing Instructions:	Do not breathe. Do not move.
Anatomy Visualized:	Atlas, axis, nasal septum.
Additional Information:	Filtration is used over the ocular orbits. Head clamps may be used to hold the head in a neutral position. This view demonstrates atlas rotation. It is used as an alternate to the base posterior view.

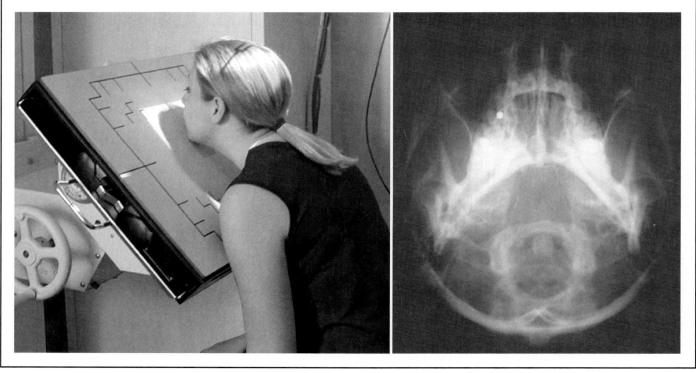

*Special view used for Palmer Upper Cervical technique analysis.
AP, Anteroposterior; *ID,* identification; *LAO,* left anterior oblique; *LPO,* left posterior oblique; *PA,* posteroanterior; *RAO,* right anterior oblique; *RPO,* right posterior oblique; *SID,* source-to-image distance.

TABLE 3-4
Thoracic Spine, Chest, Ribs, Sternum

Routine Thoracic Spine: AP and Lateral

Position:	**AP Thoracic Spine**
Patient Preparation:	Remove any artifacts in the desired field (e.g., clothing with hooks, snaps, zippers). Place patient in gown.
Measurement:	Using the calipers, place the base bar on the patient's spine. Rotate the caliper so that it is over the patient's shoulder. Then move the slider bar into the sternum of the patient.
Shielding:	Secure lead apron around patient.
Film Selection:	7 × 17 or 14 × 17
Film Placement:	Place vertically in Bucky. The top of the cassette should be 1″ to 1½″ above the vertebral prominence.
ID Placement:	ID should be in lower corner of collimation field.
Patient Placement:	The patient is standing in the AP position with back against the Bucky.
Technique Selection:	kVp 70 to 80; mAs 20 to 40
SID:	40″
Central Ray Placement:	Center to the center of the cassette, approximately 3″ to 4″ below the sternal notch.
Collimation:	To 7 × 17.
Marker Placement:	Within the collimation field on either the right side or left side of patient's spine.
Breathing Instructions:	Suspend on inspiration.
Anatomy Visualized:	Vertebral bodies, intervertebral disc spaces, pedicles, spinous and transverse processes, posterior ribs, and costovertebral joints. Paraspinal lines (pleural interface) can also be seen.
Additional Information:	For best results, the tube should be positioned so the anode is toward the patient's head and the cathode is down, taking advantage of the "heel effect." Wedge filtration should be used to achieve a more uniform density. The filter should be placed down to the midsternum.

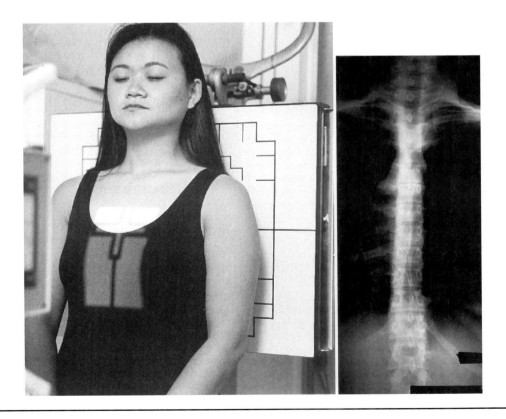

Continued

TABLE 3-4

Thoracic Spine, Chest, Ribs, Sternum

Position:	**Lateral Thoracic Spine**
Patient Preparation:	Remove any artifacts in the desired field (e.g., clothing with hooks, snaps, zippers). Place patient in gown.
Measurement:	Standing behind the patient, place base bar of calipers under left arm. Move slider bar so as to snugly rest under right arm.
Shielding:	Secure lead apron around patient.
Film Selection:	14 × 17
Film Placement:	Place vertically in Bucky. The top of the cassette should be 1½″ above the vertebral prominence.
ID Placement:	ID should be in upper corner of collimation field.
Patient Placement:	Patient is in lateral position (depending on direction of spinal curve) with arms raised and elbows flexed. Humeri should be parallel to floor.
Technique Selection:	kVp 75 to 85; mAs 40 to 60
SID:	40″
Central Ray Placement:	Central ray to center of previously placed cassette.
Collimation:	To film size vertically. To patient size horizontally.
Marker Placement:	Within the collimation field on the side of the patient that is closest to the Bucky.
Breathing Instructions:	Suspend on deep inspiration. OR use the breathing technique whereby the patient takes in a deep breath and blows out slowly, as if blowing through a straw.
Anatomy Visualized:	Thoracic vertebral bodies, intervertebral disc spaces, intervertebral foramen. Upper three to four vertebrae may not be visualized because of shoulder thickness.
Additional Information:	Use filtration from the bottom of the collimation field to the cross hairs of the central ray to provide a more uniform density of the entire thoracic spine.
	If using the breathing technique, use the longest exposure time with the smallest mA station that corresponds to the necessary mAs for each patient.

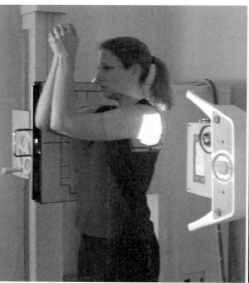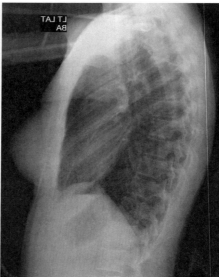

TABLE 3-4 cont'd

Thoracic Spine, Chest, Ribs, Sternum

Position:	**Swimmer's**
Patient Preparation:	Remove any artifacts in the desired field (e.g., clothing with hooks, snaps, zippers). Place patient in gown.
Measurement:	Same as Lateral Thoracic Spine.
Shielding:	Secure lead apron around patient.
Film Selection:	8 × 10 or 10 × 12
Film Placement:	Place vertically in Bucky.
ID Placement:	ID should be in lower corner of collimation field.
Patient Placement:	Patient can be seated or standing with arm closest to Bucky in full extension to pass alongside the ear. Shoulder nearest x-ray tube should be relaxed to its lowest point.
Technique Selection:	kVp 80 to 90; mAs 80 to 120
SID:	40″
Central Ray Placement:	The central ray enters the T1-T2 level along the midaxillary plane.
Collimation:	To film size.
Marker Placement:	Within the collimation field on either the right side or left side of patient depending on which lateral is performed.
Breathing Instructions:	Suspend on exhalation.
Anatomy Visualized:	Lower cervical and upper thoracic vertebral bodies and intervertebral disc spaces projected between the shoulders.
Additional Information:	A 5-degree caudal tube tilt may help to separate the shoulders and reduce superimposition of surrounding anatomy. This view may be used when C6-C7 cannot be visualized on the lateral cervical view.

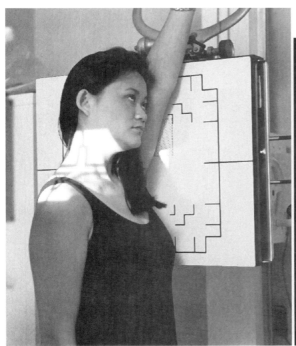
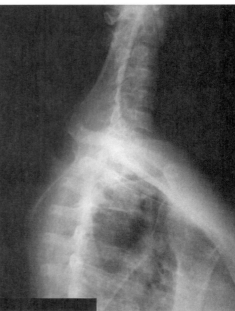

Continued

TABLE 3-4 cont'd
Thoracic Spine, Chest, Ribs, Sternum

Routine Chest: PA and Lateral

Position:	**PA Chest**
Patient Preparation:	Remove any artifacts in the desired field (e.g., clothing with hooks, snaps, zippers). Place patient in gown.
Measurement:	Same as AP Thoracic Spine.
Shielding:	Secure lead apron around patient.
Film Selection:	14 × 17
Film Placement:	Place either vertically or horizontally in Bucky depending on width of patient. The top of the cassette should be 1½" above the vertebral prominence.
ID Placement:	ID should be in upper corner of collimation field.
Patient Placement:	Patient is in PA position with chest against Bucky, head straight, chin slightly elevated, arms rolled forward.
Technique Selection:	kVp 110 to 120; mAs 1 to 4
SID:	72"
Central Ray Placement:	The central ray is centered to the previously placed cassette.
Collimation:	To film size.
Marker Placement:	Within the collimation field above the shoulder on either the right or left side.
Breathing Instructions:	Deep inhalation.
Anatomy Visualized:	Lungs, including apices, tracheal air shadow, heart, great vessels, and diaphragm. This view also demonstrates the costophrenic angles and bony thorax.
Additional Information:	The use of high kVp ensures an increased gray scale on the radiograph.
	Poor inspiratory efforts alter cardiothoracic ratio. One should be able to visualize the first four thoracic vertebral bodies and seven anterior ribs.
	In suspected apical lesions or middle lobe infiltrates, a lordotic view may be performed to better define these areas.
	If a pneumothorax is suspected, an additional view, a PA chest performed with full expiration accentuates the visceral–parietal pleural interspace.

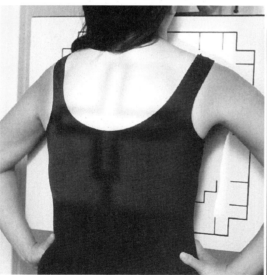
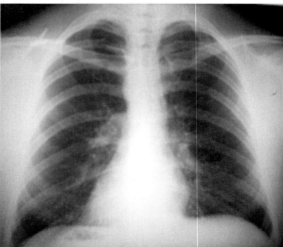

TABLE 3-4 cont'd

Thoracic Spine, Chest, Ribs, Sternum

Position:	**Lateral Chest**
Patient Preparation:	Remove any artifacts in the desired field (e.g., clothing with hooks, snaps, zippers). Place patient in gown.
Measurement:	Same as Lateral Thoracic Spine.
Shielding:	Secure lead apron around patient.
Film Selection:	14 × 17
Film Placement:	Place vertically in Bucky. Top of cassette should be 1½″ above vertebral prominence.
ID Placement:	ID should be in upper corner of collimation field.
Patient Placement:	Standing with left side against Bucky with both arms in full extension raised above head.
Technique Selection:	kVp 110 to 120; mAs 4 to 16
SID:	72″
Central Ray Placement:	Central ray is centered to center of cassette.
Collimation:	To film size.
Marker Placement:	Within the collimation field on the side of the patient closest to the film just below the ID blocker.
Breathing Instructions:	Deep inspiration.
Anatomy Visualized:	Lungs, trachea, heart, great vessels, diaphragm, posterior costophrenic angles, and bony thorax.
Additional Information:	The left lateral position is performed to reduce magnification of the heart shadow by having the heart closest to the film.

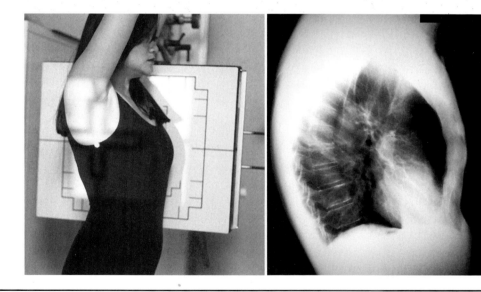

Continued

TABLE 3-4 cont'd

Thoracic Spine, Chest, Ribs, Sternum

Position:	**Apical Lordotic**
Patient Preparation:	Remove any artifacts in the desired field (e.g., clothing with hooks, snaps, zippers). Place patient in gown.
Measurement:	Same as PA Chest.
Shielding:	Secure lead apron around patient.
Film Selection:	14 × 17
Film Placement:	Place vertically in Bucky. Center to central ray.
ID Placement:	ID should be in lower corner of collimation field.
Patient Placement:	Patient is in AP position approximately 1′ from Bucky. Patient then leans back so back of shoulders comes in direct contact with Bucky.
Technique Selection:	kVp 110 to 120; mAs 1 to 4
SID:	72″
Central Ray Placement:	Central ray enters midsternum.
Collimation:	To film size.
Marker Placement:	Within the collimation field on either the right side or left side of patient.
Breathing Instructions:	Deep inspiration.
Anatomy Visualized:	This view demonstrates the apices of the lung free of superimposition of the clavicles. This view also demonstrates interlobar effusions, if present.
Additional Information:	This view may help to localize and define any lesions suspected to be posterior to the clavicle. This view also may demonstrate infiltrate in the right middle lobe.

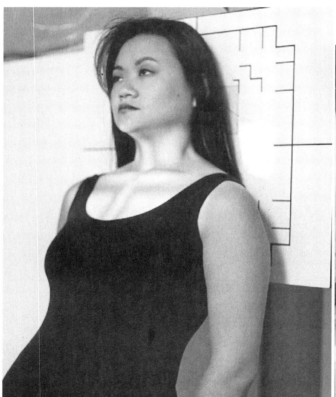 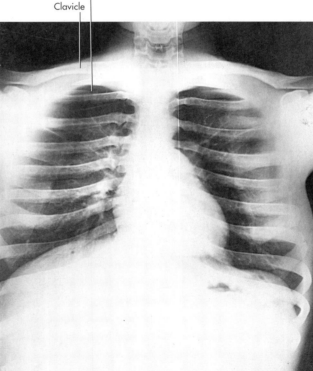

Lung apex
Clavicle

From Ballinger PW, Frank ED: Merril's atlas of radiographic positions and radiologic procedures, ed 10, St Louis, 2003, Mosby.

TABLE 3-4 cont'd

Thoracic Spine, Chest, Ribs, Sternum

Position:	**Lateral Decubitus**
Patient Preparation:	Remove any artifacts in the desired field (e.g., clothing with hooks, snaps, zippers, etc.). Place patient in gown.
Measurement:	Same as PA Chest.
Shielding:	Secure lead apron around patient.
Film Selection:	14 × 17
Film Placement:	Place horizontally in Bucky.
ID Placement:	ID should be in upper corner of collimation field.
Patient Placement:	Patient is lying on affected side (e.g., right side down for right lateral decubitus, left side down for left lateral decubitus). Arms are raised above head. Patient is placed on cart or table so the shoulders are 2″ to 3″ below top of film.
Technique Selection:	kVp 110 to 120; mAs 2 to 5
SID:	72″
Central Ray Placement:	To center of previously centered cassette.
Collimation:	To film size.
Marker Placement:	Within the collimation field on either the right side or left side of patient.
Breathing Instructions:	Deep inspiration.
Anatomy Visualized:	This view is performed when the patient cannot stand and pleural effusion is suspected. Because the side down is the dependent portion of the chest, small pleural effusions may be demonstrated *(arrows)*. This view helps delineate between small pleural effusions and scar tissue formation.
Additional Information:	Because pleural effusions less than 300 ccs usually cannot be seen clearly on routine PA chest radiography, decubitus films should be performed if pleural effusions are suspected.

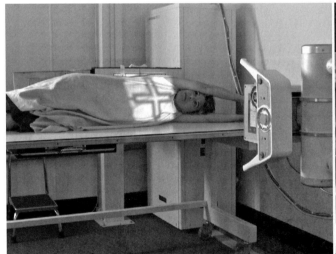 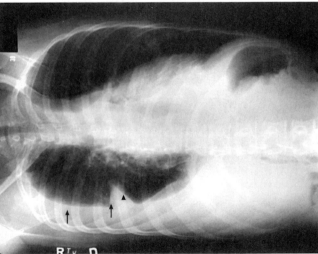

From Ballinger PW, Frank ED: Merril's atlas of radiographic positions and radiologic procedures, ed 10, St Louis, 2003, Mosby.

Continued

TABLE 3-4 cont'd
Thoracic Spine, Chest, Ribs, Sternum

Ribs: AP or PA Unilateral or Bilateral, Above or Below Diaphragm

Position:	**AP Bilateral Upper Ribs**
Patient Preparation:	Remove any artifacts in the desired field (e.g., clothing with hooks, snaps, zippers). Place patient in gown.
Measurement:	Same as AP Thoracic Spine.
Shielding:	Secure lead apron around patient.
Film Selection:	14 × 17
Film Placement:	Place transversely in Bucky. The top of the cassette should be 1½″ above the vertebral prominence.
ID Placement:	ID should be in lower corner of collimation field.
Patient Placement:	The patient is standing in the AP position.
Technique Selection:	kVp 65 to 75; mAs 20 to 40
SID:	40″
Central Ray Placement:	Central ray is centered to center of cassette.
Collimation:	To film size.
Marker Placement:	Within the collimation field on either the right side or left side of patient.
Breathing Instructions:	Suspend breathing on full inspiration.
Anatomy Visualized:	Ribs above the diaphragm, especially the posterior aspect of the ribs.
Additional Information:	The most common area of rib fracture is within the axillary margin of the rib, which is not clearly seen on this projection.
	Oblique views are required to visualize the axillary margin of the rib.
	A PA chest projection should be performed to rule out pneumothorax.

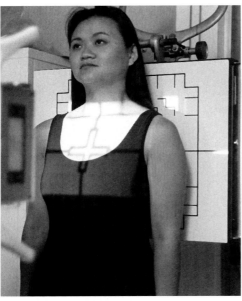
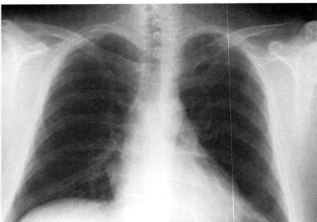

TABLE 3-4 cont'd
Thoracic Spine, Chest, Ribs, Sternum

Position:	**AP Bilateral Lower Ribs**
Patient Preparation:	Remove any artifacts in the desired field (e.g., clothing with hooks, snaps, zippers). Place patient in gown.
Measurement:	Measure AP through T12 area.
Shielding:	Secure lead apron around patient.
Film Selection:	14 × 17
Film Placement:	Place transversely in Bucky. The bottom of the cassette is 1″ below the top of the iliac crest.
ID Placement:	ID should be in upper corner of collimation field.
Patient Placement:	The patient is standing in the AP position.
Technique Selection:	kVp 70 to 80; mAs 30 to 60
SID:	40″
Central Ray Placement:	The central ray is directed to the center of the cassette.
Collimation:	To film size.
Marker Placement:	Within the collimation field on either the right side or left side of patient.
Breathing Instructions:	Suspend respiration on full exhalation.
Anatomy Visualized:	Ribs below the diaphragm.
Additional Information:	A computed tomography (CT) scan of the abdomen may be warranted to rule out damage to the internal organs, if a fracture of the lower ribs is suspected.

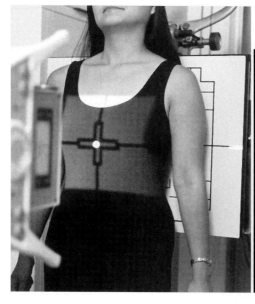 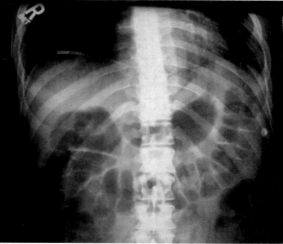

Continued

TABLE 3-4 cont'd
Thoracic Spine, Chest, Ribs, Sternum

Position:	**AP Ribs, Unilateral**
Patient Preparation:	Remove any artifacts in the desired field (e.g., clothing with hooks, snaps, zippers). Place patient in gown.
Measurement:	Same as AP Thoracic Spine.
Shielding:	Secure lead apron around patient.
Film Selection:	14 × 17
Film Placement:	Place vertically in Bucky. The top of the cassette should be 1½″ above the vertebral prominence for ribs above the diaphragm. If the lower ribs are of interest, the cassette should be placed so the bottom of the cassette is 1″ below the top of the iliac crest.
ID Placement:	ID should be in the corner of the collimation field opposite the area of interest.
Patient Placement:	The patient is standing with the midclavicular plane of the affected side centered to the center of the cassette.
Technique Selection:	kVp 65 to 75; mAs 20 to 40
SID:	40″
Central Ray Placement:	The central ray is directed to the center of the cassette.
Collimation:	To film size.
Marker Placement:	Within the collimation field on side of the patient that is closest to the Bucky.
Breathing Instructions:	For ribs above the diaphragm, suspend respiration on full inspiration. For ribs below the diaphragm, suspend respiration on full expiration.
Anatomy Visualized:	Ribs above or below the diaphragm. The view should include the area between the costovertebral joints to the axillary border of the ribs.
Additional Information:	This view is performed when patient presents with rib complaints on one side only.

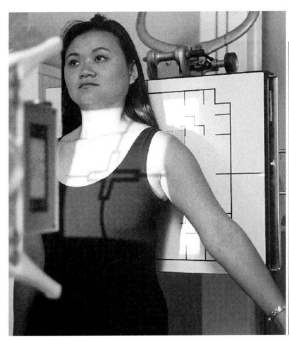
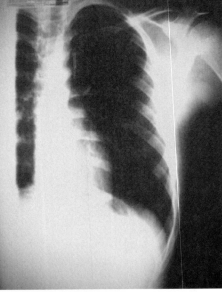

TABLE 3-4 cont'd
Thoracic Spine, Chest, Ribs, Sternum

Position:	**Oblique Ribs**
Patient Preparation:	Remove any artifacts in the desired field (e.g., clothing with hooks, snaps, zippers). Place patient in gown.
Measurement:	Same as AP Thoracic Spine.
Shielding:	Secure lead apron around patient.
Film Selection:	14 × 17
Film Placement:	Place vertically in Bucky. For ribs above the diaphragm, the cassette is placed 1½″ above the diaphragm. For ribs below the diaphragm, the bottom of the cassette is placed 1″ below the top of the iliac crest.
ID Placement:	ID should be in corner of collimation field opposite the area of interest.
Patient Placement:	The patient is standing in the AP position. Rotate the patient toward affected side 45 degrees. Right-sided rib injury requires an RPO; left-sided rib injury an LPO.
Technique Selection:	kVp 70 to 80; mAs 20 to 40
SID:	40″
Central Ray Placement:	The central ray is directed to the center of the cassette just lateral to the midsternal area.
Collimation:	To film size.
Marker Placement:	Within the collimation field on the side of the patient that is closest to the Bucky.
Breathing Instructions:	For ribs above the diaphragm, suspend respiration on full inhalation. For ribs below the diaphragm, suspend respiration on full exhalation.
Anatomy Visualized:	Axillary margin of ribs on the affected side.
Additional Information:	If oblique views cannot be performed with the patient in the posterior oblique position, anterior obliques may be done. The affected side is placed away from the film. An LAO is performed in right-sided injuries; an RAO is performed in left-sided injuries.

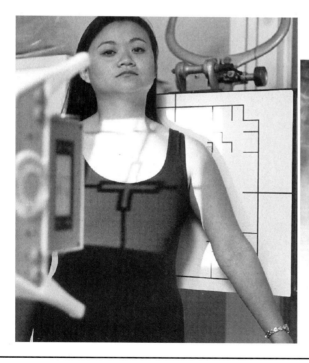
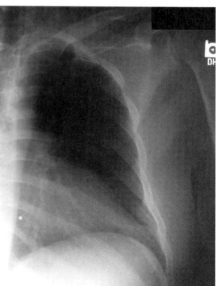

Continued

TABLE 3-4 cont'd
Thoracic Spine, Chest, Ribs, Sternum

Position:	**Costal Joints**
Patient Preparation:	Remove any artifacts in the desired field (e.g., clothing with hooks, snaps, zippers). Place patient in gown.
Measurement:	Same as AP Thoracic Spine.
Shielding:	Secure lead apron around patient.
Film Selection:	11 × 14 (a 14 × 17 can be used with appropriate collimation).
Film Placement:	Place vertically in Bucky. Center to central ray.
ID Placement:	ID should be in lower corner of collimation field.
Patient Placement:	Patient is standing in the AP position, centered to the Bucky.
Technique Selection:	kVp 70 to 80; mAs 20 to 40
SID:	40″
Central Ray Placement:	The central ray is angled 30 degrees cephalically so as to enter the lower aspect of the sternum, exiting at the level of T6.
Collimation:	To film size.
Marker Placement:	Within the collimation field on either the right or left side of patient.
Breathing Instructions:	Suspend respiration on full inspiration.
Anatomy Visualized:	Costovertebral and costotransverse joints of the upper to midthoracic spine.
Additional Information:	This view demonstrates changes to these joint spaces from entities such as rheumatoid arthritis and degenerative joint disease.

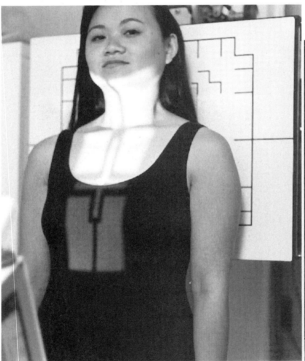 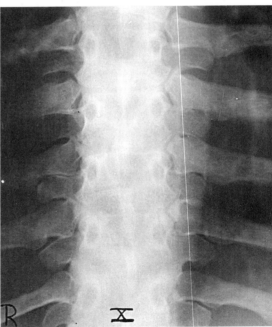

From Ballinger PW, Frank ED: *Merril's atlas of radiographic positions and radiologic procedures,* ed 10, St Louis, 2003, Mosby.

TABLE 3-4 cont'd

Thoracic Spine, Chest, Ribs, Sternum

Sternum: RAO and Lateral

Position:	**RAO Sternum**
Patient Preparation:	Remove any artifacts in the desired field (e.g., clothing with hooks, snaps, zippers). Place patient in gown.
Measurement:	AP through midline of sternum.
Shielding:	Secure lead apron around patient.
Film Selection:	10 × 12
Film Placement:	Place vertically in Bucky. Center to central ray.
ID Placement:	ID should be in lower corner of collimation field.
Patient Placement:	The patient is standing in the PA position, centered to the Bucky. Rotate the patient approximately 20 degrees so as to effect the RAO position.
Technique Selection:	kVp 75 to 85; mAs 30 to 40
SID:	40″
Central Ray Placement:	The central ray enters just left of the spine at the level of T6.
Collimation:	To film size.
Marker Placement:	Within the collimation field on the patient's right side.
Breathing Instructions:	Use the breathing technique whereby the patient takes even, shallow breaths, using a long exposure time.
Anatomy Visualized:	A slightly oblique PA projection of the sternum superimposed over the heart shadow.
Additional Information:	The RAO position is used so as to project the sternum over the heart shadow, which provides a homogenous background and increased visualization of the sternum.

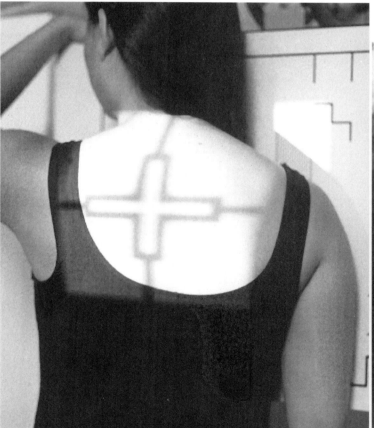 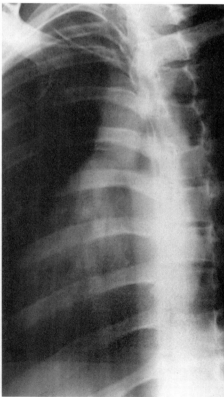

From Ballinger PW, Frank ED: Merril's atlas of radiographic positions and radiologic procedures, ed 10, St Louis, 2003, Mosby.

Continued

TABLE 3-4 cont'd
Thoracic Spine, Chest, Ribs, Sternum

Position:	**Lateral Sternum**
Patient Preparation:	Remove any artifacts in the desired field (e.g., clothing with hooks, snaps, zippers). Place patient in gown.
Measurement:	Measure laterally under the axilla.
Shielding:	Secure lead apron around patient.
Film Selection:	8 × 10
Film Placement:	Place vertically in Bucky.
ID Placement:	ID should be in corner of collimation field. The top of the cassette is placed 1″ above the suprasternal notch.
Patient Placement:	The patient is standing in a lateral position with hands clasped behind the back, forcing a slight forward thrust of the sternum.
Technique Selection:	kVp 75 to 85; mAs 40 to 60
SID:	40″
Central Ray Placement:	The central ray is directed to the center of the cassette at the level of the midsternum.
Collimation:	To film size.
Marker Placement:	Within the collimation field denoting either a right lateral or a left lateral.
Breathing Instructions:	Suspend respiration on full inspiration.
Anatomy Visualized:	The entire sternum is projected in the lateral position.
Additional Information:	If performing this view recumbent, raise the patient's arms above the head.
	In women, the breast should be moved out of the collimation field, if possible, and secured with a wrap so breast shadows do not obscure the lower aspects of the sternum.

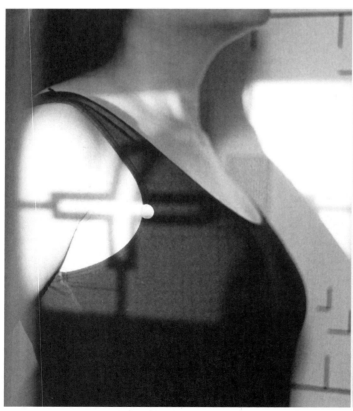 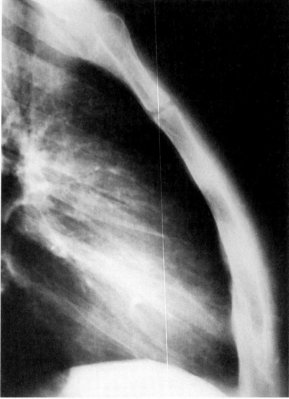

From Ballinger PW, Frank ED: Merril's atlas of radiographic positions and radiologic procedures, ed 10, St Louis, 2003, Mosby.

AP, Anteroposterior; *CT,* computed tomography; *ID,* identification; *LAO,* left anterior oblique; *LPO,* left posterior oblique; *PA,* posteroanterior; *RAO,* right anterior oblique; *RPO,* right posterior oblique; *SID,* source-to-image distance.

TABLE 3-5
Lumbar Spine

Routine Lumbar Spine: AP and Lateral

Position:	**AP Lumbar Spine**
Patient Preparation:	Remove any artifacts in the desired field (e.g., underwear, clothing with hooks, snaps, zippers). Place patient in gown.
Measurement:	Using the calipers, place the base bar on the patient's back. Move the slider bar toward the thickest part of the patient's abdomen.
Shielding:	Use appropriate gonadal shielding.
Film Selection:	14 × 17
Film Placement:	Place vertically in Bucky.
ID Placement:	ID should be in upper corner of collimation field.
Patient Placement:	The patient is standing in the AP position with the midsagittal plane in the center of the Bucky.
Technique Selection:	kVp 75 to 85; mAs 30 to 80
SID:	40″
Central Ray Placement:	The central ray is directed to a point 1″ below the iliac crest in females; 2″ below the crest in males so as to exit the disc interspace of L3-L4. Optimal positioning should include the ischial tuberosities on the film.
Collimation:	To film size.
Marker Placement:	Within the collimation field on either the right or left side of patient.
Breathing Instructions:	Suspend respiration on full exhalation.
Anatomy Visualized:	Lumbar vertebral bodies, intervertebral disc interspaces, lumbar spinous and transverse processes, lamina, pars interarticularis, SI joint, sacral ala, pelvis.
Additional Information:	In larger patients, recumbent radiography will provide better film quality. Compression also may be used to enhance film quality in upright radiography.

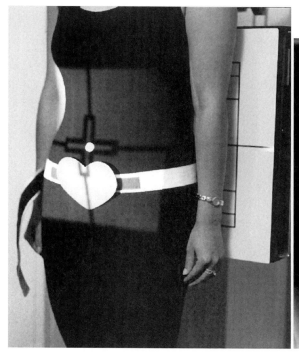
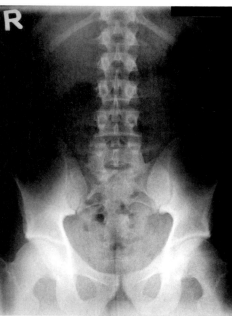

Continued

TABLE 3-5 cont'd
Lumbar Spine

Position:	**Lateral Lumbar Spine**
Patient Preparation:	Remove any artifacts in the desired field (e.g., underwear, clothing with hooks, snaps, zippers). Place patient in gown.
Measurement:	Using the calipers, place the base bar on one side of the patient. Move the slider bar toward the opposite side of the patient 1″ above the iliac crest.
Shielding:	Shielding is not necessary for this view.
Film Selection:	14 × 17
Film Placement:	Place vertically in Bucky.
ID Placement:	ID should be in upper corner of collimation field.
Patient Placement:	The patient is standing in the lateral position with the convexity of the lumbar curve next to the Bucky. The midaxillary plane is centered to the center of the cassette.
Technique Selection:	kVp 80 to 90; mAs 90 to 180
SID:	40″
Central Ray Placement:	The central ray is directed to a point 1″ above the iliac crest and halfway between the ASIS and PSIS.
Collimation:	To film size vertically. To patient size horizontally.
Marker Placement:	Within the collimation field on the side of the patient closest to the cassette.
Breathing Instructions:	Suspend respiration on full exhalation.
Anatomy Visualized:	Lumbar vertebral bodies, intervertebral disc interspaces, lumbar spinous processes, intervertebral foramina, sacrum, and coccyx in the lateral projection.
Additional Information:	This view may be performed with the patient in the lateral recumbent position for larger patients, providing improved radiographic quality.

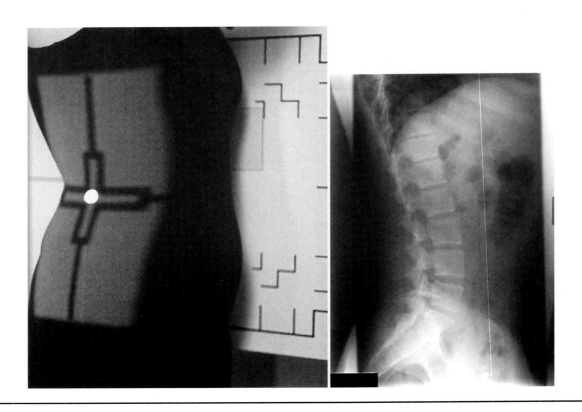

TABLE 3-5 cont'd
Lumbar Spine

Position:	L5-S1 Lateral Spot
Patient Preparation:	Remove any artifacts in the desired field (e.g., underwear, clothing with hooks, snaps, zippers). Place patient in gown.
Measurement:	Using the calipers, place the base bar 3″ below the iliac crest on one side of patient. Move the slider bar in so to rest on the opposite side of the patient, 3″ below the crest.
Shielding:	Shielding is unnecessary for this view.
Film Selection:	8 × 10
Film Placement:	Place vertically in Bucky.
ID Placement:	ID should be in upper corner of collimation field.
Patient Placement:	The patient is standing in the lateral position with the midaxillary plane centered to the center of the cassette. Arms are lifted and folded in front of the patient.
Technique Selection:	kVp 80 to 90; mAs 120 to 200
SID:	40″
Central Ray Placement:	The central ray enters 3″ below the iliac crest vertically and 1½ to 2″ anterior to the spinous of L5.
Collimation:	To film size.
Marker Placement:	Within the collimation field denoting the side of the patient closest to the Bucky.
Breathing Instructions:	Suspend respiration on full exhalation.
Anatomy Visualized:	L5-S1 disc interspace.
Additional Information:	A 5-degree caudal tube tilt may be used to better demonstrate the lumbosacral joint space. In larger patients, recumbent radiography improves film quality.

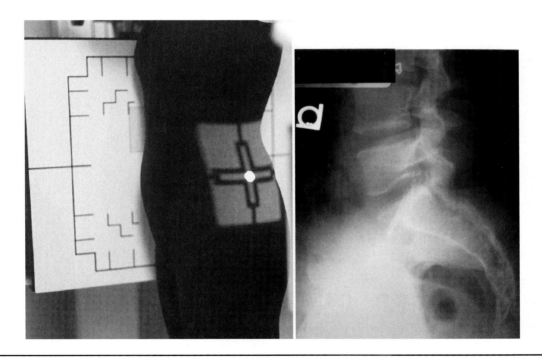

Continued

TABLE 3-5 cont'd
Lumbar Spine

Position:	**L5-S1 AP**
Patient Preparation:	Remove any artifacts in the desired field (e.g., underwear, clothing with hooks, snaps, zippers). Place patient in gown.
Measurement:	Same as AP Lumbopelvic.
Shielding:	Shielding is unnecessary for this view.
Film Selection:	8 × 10
Film Placement:	Place vertically in Bucky.
ID Placement:	ID should be in lower corner of collimation field.
Patient Placement:	The patient is standing in the AP position with the midsagittal plane centered to the center of the cassette.
Technique Selection:	kVp 75 to 85; mAs 30 to 80
SID:	40″
Central Ray Placement:	The central ray is angled 30 degrees cephalically to enter at the level of the ASIS to exit the L5 disc space.
Collimation:	To film size.
Marker Placement:	Within the collimation field on either the right side or left side of patient.
Breathing Instructions:	Suspend respiration on full exhalation.
Anatomy Visualized:	This projection opens up the L5-S1 interspace. This view also visualizes the SI joints.
Additional Information:	In females, the tube tilt should be increased to 35 degrees. This view demonstrates L5 transitional vertebra. This view better demonstrates the SI joints than the standard AP Lumbopelvic view.

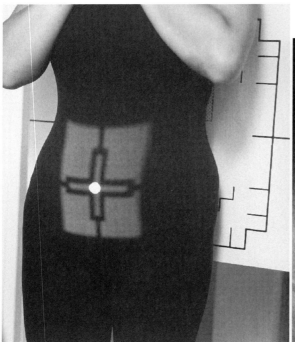
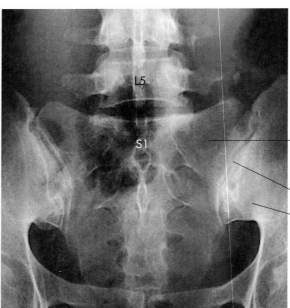

From Ballinger PW, Frank ED: Merril's atlas of radiographic positions and radiologic procedures, ed 10, St Louis, 2003, Mosby.

TABLE 3-5 cont'd
Lumbar Spine

Position:	**Oblique Lumbar Spine**
Patient Preparation:	Remove any artifacts in the desired field (e.g., underwear, clothing with hooks, snaps, zippers). Place patient in gown.
Measurement:	Same as AP Lumbopelvic.
Shielding:	Shielding is unnecessary for this view.
Film Selection:	10×12
Film Placement:	Place vertically in Bucky.
ID Placement:	ID should be in lower corner of collimation field.
Patient Placement:	The right and left lumbar oblique views may be done in an anterior or posterior patient position. The choice of performing either anterior or posterior oblique projections is influenced by two factors. The anterior oblique position better accommodates the diverging x-ray beam with the lordatic curvature of the lumbar spine. The posterior oblique position decreases the object-to-film (OFD) distance for an obese patient with a large abdomen. For anterior oblique positions (RAO and LAO), the anterior aspect of the patient's pelvis is placed against the grid and the body is angled 45 degrees with the grid. For posterior oblique positions (RPO and LPO), the posterior aspect of the patient's pelvis is placed against the grid and the body is angled 45 degrees with the grid.
Technique Selection:	kVp 75 to 85; mAs 30 to 80
SID:	40″
Central Ray Placement:	The central ray enters 1″ above the iliac crest and 1″ lateral to the spine on the side closest to the tube. For the LPO and RPO, the central ray is 1″ above the iliac crest with the vertical portion of the central ray positioned to the midpoint of the clavicle.
Collimation:	To film size.
Marker Placement:	Within the collimation field on the side of the patient that is closest to the Bucky.
Breathing Instructions:	Suspend respiration on full exhalation.
Anatomy Visualized:	Lumbar vertebral bodies and intervertebral disc interspaces, lumbar spinous and transverse processes, lamina, pars interarticularis, apophyseal joints. If properly positioned, the "Scotty dog" appearance formed by the pedicle, transverse process, superior and inferior articular facets, and pars interarticularis are visualized. The posterior oblique positions demonstrate the same side pars interarticulares (i.e., RPO shows right pars), and the anterior oblique positions demonstrate the opposite side pars interarticulares (i.e., RAO shows the left pars).
Additional Information:	Although posterior oblique positions can be performed, anterior oblique positions are preferred to minimize distortion. This view yields optimal visualization of the pars interarticularis when spondylolisthesis is suspected. For visualization of the apophyseal joints of the lower lumbar spine, a 30-degree rotation may be used.

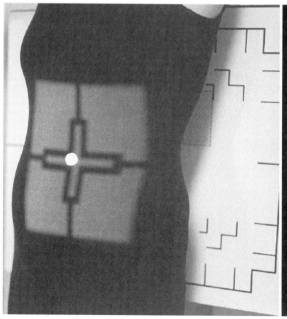 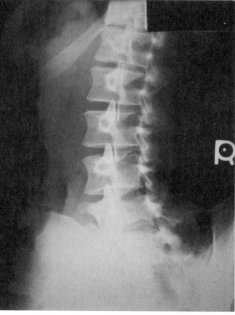

TABLE 3-5 cont'd
Lumbar Spine

Position:	**AP Sacrum**
Patient Preparation:	Remove any artifacts in the desired field (e.g., underwear, clothing with hooks, snaps, zippers). Place patient in gown.
Measurement:	Same as AP Lumbopelvic.
Shielding:	Shielding is unnecessary for this view.
Film Selection:	10 × 12
Film Placement:	Place vertically in Bucky.
ID Placement:	ID should be in lower corner of collimation field.
Patient Placement:	The patient is standing in the AP position with the midsagittal plane centered to the center of the Bucky.
Technique Selection:	kVp 75 to 85; mAs 30 to 80
SID:	40″
Central Ray Placement:	The central ray is angled 15 degrees cephalically to enter 2″ above the pubic symphysis.
Collimation:	To film size.
Marker Placement:	Within the collimation field on either the right or left side of patient.
Breathing Instructions:	Suspend respiration on full exhalation.
Anatomy Visualized:	True frontal projection of sacrum, SI joints, sacral ala, and sacral foramina.
Additional Information:	This view may be performed on larger patients in the recumbent position to improve film quality.
	Fecal material in rectosigmoid colon may obscure detail, so it may be helpful to radiograph patients immediately after evacuation.

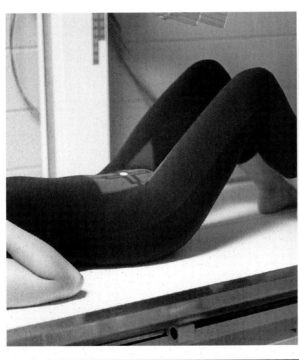
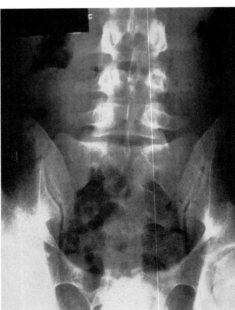

TABLE 3-5 cont'd
Lumbar Spine

Position:	**Lateral Sacrum**
Patient Preparation:	Remove any artifacts in the desired field (e.g., underwear, clothing with hooks, snaps, zippers). Place patient in gown.
Measurement:	Same as Lateral L5-S1.
Shielding:	Shielding is unnecessary for this view.
Film Selection:	10 × 12
Film Placement:	Place vertically in Bucky.
ID Placement:	ID should be in upper corner of collimation field.
Patient Placement:	Patient is standing in the lateral position with arms raised and folded in front of chest, or recumbant as depicted below.
Technique Selection:	kVp 75 to 85; mAs 90 to 180
SID:	40″
Central Ray Placement:	The central ray enters 3″ below the iliac crest vertically and midway between the ASIS and PSIS horizontally.
Collimation:	To film size.
Marker Placement:	Within the collimation field to denote the side of the patient closest to the Bucky.
Breathing Instructions:	Suspend respiration on full exhalation.
Anatomy Visualized:	Lateral projection of sacrum and coccyx.
Additional Information:	This view may be performed recumbent in larger patients.
	Bowel gas in the rectal vault may be helpful in this view because displacement of the rectal shadow is useful in evaluating trauma to the sacrum.

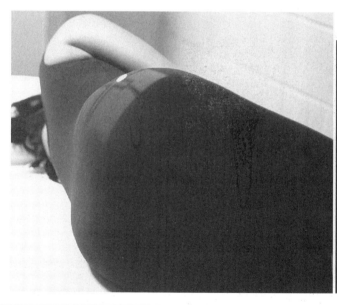 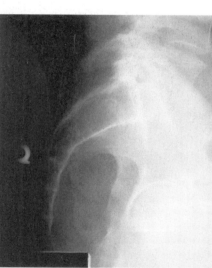

Continued

TABLE 3-5 cont'd
Lumbar Spine

Position:	SI Joints
Patient Preparation:	Remove any artifacts in the desired field (e.g., underwear, clothing with hooks, snaps, zippers). Place patient in gown.
Measurement:	Same as AP Lumbopelvic.
Shielding:	Shielding is unnecessary for this view.
Film Selection:	8 × 10
Film Placement:	Place vertically in Bucky.
ID Placement:	ID should be in lower corner of collimation field.
Patient Placement:	The patient is standing in the PA position with the unaffected side rotated 25 degrees away from the Bucky to perform an anterior oblique. In an RAO position the right SI joint is visualized; in LAO the left SI joint is visualized.
Technique Selection:	kVp 75 to 85; mAs 30 to 80
SID:	40″
Central Ray Placement:	The central ray enters the SI joint of the side closest to the Bucky at the level of the ASIS.
Collimation:	To film size.
Marker Placement:	Within the collimation field on the side of the patient closest to the Bucky.
Breathing Instructions:	Suspend respiration on full exhalation.
Anatomy Visualized:	Profile image of the SI joint nearest the film.
Additional Information:	Both obliques should be performed for comparison. Posterior obliques may be performed—the posterior oblique will demonstrate the SI joint that is farthest from the film.

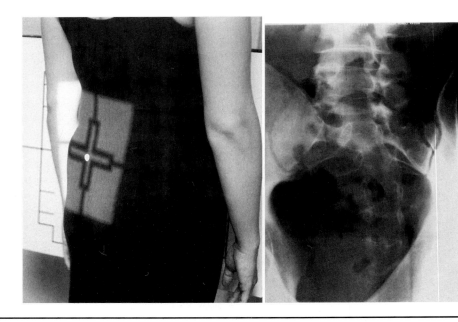

TABLE 3-5 cont'd
Lumbar Spine

Position:	**AP Coccyx**
Patient Preparation:	Remove any artifacts in the desired field (e.g., underwear, clothing with hooks, snaps, zippers). Place patient in gown.
Measurement:	Using calipers, place base bar at the top of the gluteal cleft. Move the slider bar to rest 2″ above pubic symphysis.
Shielding:	Shielding is unnecessary for this view.
Film Selection:	8 × 10
Film Placement:	Place vertically in Bucky.
ID Placement:	ID should be in upper corner of collimation field.
Patient Placement:	The patient is standing in the AP position with the midsagittal plane centered to the center of the Bucky.
Technique Selection:	kVp 70 to 80; mAs 30 to 50
SID:	40″
Central Ray Placement:	The central ray is angled 10 degrees caudally so as to enter midline 2″ above the pubic symphysis.
Collimation:	To part size.
Marker Placement:	Within the collimation field on either the right side or left side of patient.
Breathing Instructions:	Suspend respiration on full exhalation.
Anatomy Visualized:	True AP projection of the coccyx free of superimposition of the symphysis pubis.
Additional Information:	Fecal material in rectosigmoid colon may obscure the coccyx. For this reason, it may improve the quality of the radiograph to perform this view immediately following evacuation of the bowels.

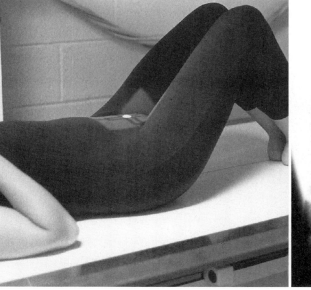
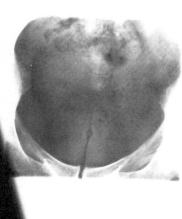

Continued

TABLE 3-5 cont'd
Lumbar Spine

Position:	**Lateral Coccyx**
Patient Preparation:	Remove any artifacts in the desired field (e.g., underwear, clothing with hooks, snaps, zippers). Place patient in gown.
Measurement:	Same as AP Coccyx.
Shielding:	Shielding is unnecessary for this view.
Film Selection:	8 × 10
Film Placement:	Place vertically in Bucky.
ID Placement:	ID should be in upper corner of collimation field.
Patient Placement:	The patient is best radiographed for this view in the recumbent position with the knees flexed.
Technique Selection:	kVp 70 to 80; mAs 30 to 50
SID:	40″
Central Ray Placement:	The central ray enters 2″ posterior to the greater trochanter.
Collimation:	To part size.
Marker Placement:	Within the collimation field to denote the side closest to the Bucky.
Breathing Instructions:	Suspend respiration on full exhalation.
Anatomy Visualized:	Lateral projection of the coccyx.
Additional Information:	A lead strip placed on the table behind the patient helps to absorb scatter radiation, thereby improving film quality.

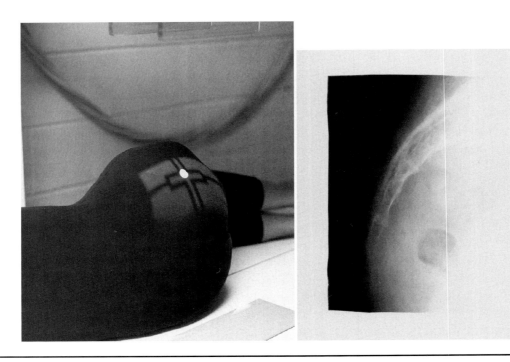

TABLE 3-5 cont'd
Lumbar Spine

Position:	**AP Full Spine**
Patient Preparation:	Remove any artifacts in the desired field (e.g., underwear, clothing with hooks, snaps, zippers). Place patient in gown.
Measurement:	Measure AP through the thickest portion of the patient.
Shielding:	Place appropriate gonadal shielding.
Film Selection:	14 × 36
Film Placement:	Place vertically in Bucky. The cassette should be centered so as to include C1 through the ischial tuberosities.
ID Placement:	ID should be in upper corner of collimation field.
Patient Placement:	The patient is standing in the AP position with the midsagittal plane centered to the center of the Bucky. The arms are at the patient's side and slightly abducted to remove them from the collimation field. The patient opens the mouth and the head is aligned to visualize C1 and C2.
Technique Selection:	kVp 80 to 90; mAs 50 to 100
SID:	72″
Central Ray Placement:	The central ray is centered to the cassette.
Collimation:	To film size vertically and to patient size horizontally.
Marker Placement:	Within the collimation field on either the right side or left side of patient.
Breathing Instructions:	Suspend respiration on full expiration.
Anatomy Visualized:	AP projection of the entire vertebral column, including the pelvis.
Additional Information:	Compensating filtration should be placed down to the midsternum to accommodate for different tissue densities.
	Large patients should be radiographed as sectional series for better visualization of the spine.
	This view is useful in scoliosis evaluation. It may be performed in the PA position to reduce breast and gonad dose.

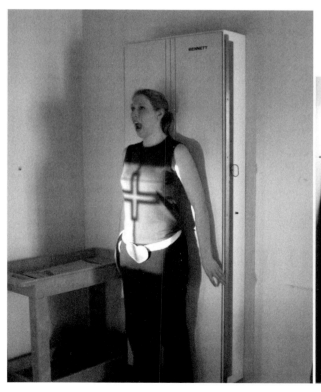
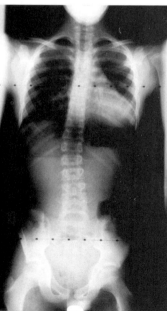

Continued

TABLE 3-5 cont'd
Lumbar Spine

Position: Lateral Full Spine

Because of technical limitations, which can result in suboptimal radiographic quality, this view is not recommended. Lateral sectional views should accompany the AP full spine for a complete study.

Routine Abdomen: AP and Upright

Position:	**AP Abdomen: Supine**
Patient Preparation:	Remove any artifacts in the desired field (e.g., clothing with hooks, snaps, zippers). Place patient in gown.
Shielding:	Do not use.
Film Selection:	14 × 17
Film Placement:	Place vertically in the table Bucky.
ID Placement:	ID blocker should be in the lower corner of the collimation field.
Patient Placement:	The patient is lying in the AP recumbent position centered to the midline of the table. The arms are placed by the patient's side.
Technique Selection:	kVp 70 to 80; mAs 40 to 60
SID:	40″
Central Ray Placement:	The central ray is directed perpendicular to the cassette at the level of the iliac crest.
Collimation:	To film size.
Marker Placement:	Within the collimation field, in a lower corner, denoting the patient's right or left side.
Breathing Instructions:	Suspend respiration on expiration.
Anatomy Visualized:	AP projection of the abdomen demonstrating size and shape of liver, spleen, and kidneys. Also demonstrates intraabdominal calcifications, bowel gas patterns, and evidence of tumor masses.
Additional Information:	Use of higher kVp results in a long scale of contrast necessary to delineate the various densities of the internal organs.

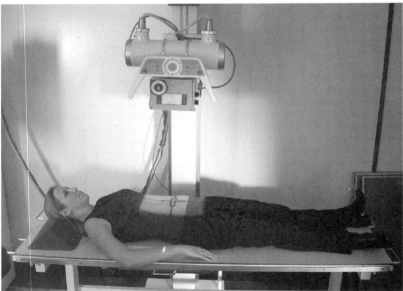

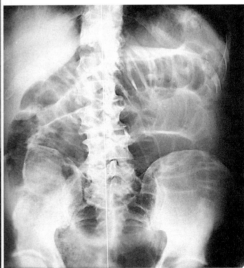

From Ballinger PW, Frank ED: Merril's atlas of radiographic positions and radiologic procedures, ed 10, St Louis, 2003, Mosby.

TABLE 3-5 cont'd
Lumbar Spine

Position:	**AP Abdomen: Upright**
Patient Preparation:	Remove any artifacts in the desired field (e.g., clothing with hooks, snaps, zippers). Place patient in gown.
Shielding:	None used.
Film Selection:	14 × 17
Film Placement:	Place vertically in the Bucky.
ID Placement:	ID should be in lower corner of collimation field.
Patient Placement:	The patient is standing in the AP position with back against Bucky and centered to midline of Bucky.
Technique Selection:	kVp 70 to 80; mAs 60 to 80
SID:	40″
Central Ray Placement:	The central ray is directed perpendicular to the film at a level of 2″ to 3″ above the crest to include the diaphragm.
Collimation:	To film size.
Marker Placement:	Within the collimation field denoting the patient's right or left side.
Breathing Instructions:	Suspend respiration on full expiration.
Anatomy Visualized:	AP projection of the abdomen demonstrating size and shape of liver, spleen, and kidneys. Also demonstrates intraabdominal calcifications, bowel gas patterns, and evidence of tumor masses. The upright also demonstrates intraperitoneal free air under the diaphragm, as well as air fluid levels within the bowel.
Additional Information:	The diaphragm must be included in upright abdomen for evaluation of free air. If intraperitoneal free air is suspected, lay the patient on the left side for 10 to 20 minutes to allow free air to rise into the area under the right hemidiaphragm where it is not superimposed by the gastric air bubble. This view is performed in addition to the supine abdomen, as its opposing perspective. A PA chest should be included to complete an abdominal series.

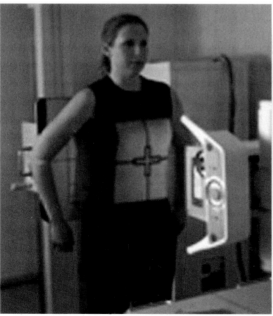
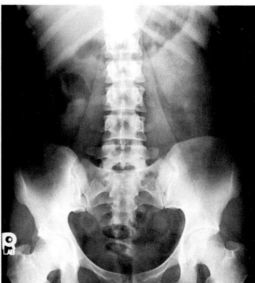

From Ballinger PW, Frank ED: Merril's atlas of radiographic positions and radiologic procedures, ed 10, St Louis, 2003, Mosby.

Continued

TABLE 3-5 cont'd
Lumbar Spine

Position:	Oblique Abdomen
Patient Preparation:	Remove any artifacts in the desired field (e.g., clothing with hooks, snaps, zippers). Place patient in gown.
Shielding:	None used.
Film Selection:	14 × 17
Film Placement:	Place vertically to the long axis of the patient in the Bucky.
ID Placement:	The ID should be in the corner of the collimation opposite the affected side.
Patient Placement:	The patient is lying recumbent on the table, obliquely rotated (approximately 30 degrees) so the affected side is touching the tabletop. The patient's hands can be placed over the chest to remove them from the desired area. Alternatively, the patient may be radiographed in the upright position, as depicted below.
Technique Selection:	kVp 70 to 80; mAs 40 to 60
SID:	40″
Central Ray Placement:	The central ray is perpendicular to the cassette at the level of the iliac crest.
Collimation:	To film size.
Marker Placement:	Within the collimation field denoting the affected side.
Breathing Instructions:	Suspend respiration on full expiration.
Anatomy Visualized:	Oblique projection of the abdomen, demonstrating a perpendicular renal shadow of the side closest to the film, whereas the renal shadow on the elevated side is projected in profile.
Additional Information:	The view is helpful in localizing intraabdominal radiopacities. By placing the affected side down, anteriorly located radiopacities, such as gallstones, are projected further away from the spine. The right posterior oblique position is the best position for this type of demonstration.
	Posterior radiopacities, such as kidney stones, are projected closer to the spine in the posterior oblique position.

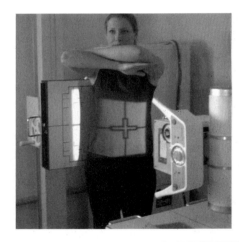

AP, Anteroposterior; *ASIS,* anterior superior iliac spine; *ID,* identification; *LAO,* left anterior oblique; *PA,* posteroanterior; *PSIS,* posterior superior iliac spine; *RAO,* right anterior oblique; *SI,* sacroiliac; *SID,* source-to-image distance.

TABLE 3-6
Upper Extremities

Routine Shoulder: Internal and External Rotation

Position:	**AP Shoulder Internal Rotation**
Patient Preparation:	Remove any artifacts in the desired field (e.g., clothing with hooks, snaps, zippers).
Shielding:	Secure lead apron around patient.
Film Selection:	10 × 12
Film Placement:	Place horizontally in Bucky. The top of the cassette is 1½″ above shoulder.
ID Placement:	ID should be in upper corner of collimation field.
Patient Placement:	The patient is standing in the AP position with back against Bucky, rotated slightly toward affected shoulder. The arm of the affected shoulder is internally rotated so that the epicondyles of the elbow are perpendicular to the plane of the film.
Technique Selection:	kVp 70 to 80; mAs 8 to 16
SID:	40″
Central Ray Placement:	The central ray enters the coracoid process.
Collimation:	To film size.
Marker Placement:	Within the collimation field denoting the affected shoulder.
Breathing Instructions:	Do not breathe. Do not move.
Anatomy Visualized:	Proximal humerus, scapula, humeral head in relation to the glenoid fossa. Internal rotation demonstrates the humerus in the true lateral position.
Additional Information:	This view demonstrates the subdeltoid bursa area.
	If the shoulder is too painful to be internally rotated, the affected side can be turned away from the film to obtain a similar view.

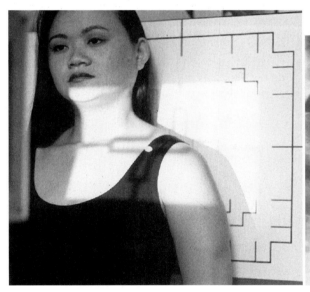 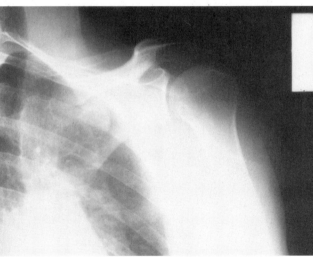

Continued

TABLE 3-6 cont'd
Upper Extremities

Position:	**AP Shoulder External Rotation**
Patient Preparation:	Remove any artifacts in the desired field (e.g., clothing with hooks, snaps, zippers).
Shielding:	Secure lead apron around patient.
Film Selection:	10 × 12
Film Placement:	Place horizontally in Bucky. The top of the cassette should be placed 1½″ above the top of the shoulder.
ID Placement:	ID should be in upper corner of collimation field.
Patient Placement:	The patient is standing in the AP position with back against Bucky, rotated slightly toward affected shoulder. The arm is rotated externally so that the epicondyles of the elbow are parallel to the plane of the film.
Technique Selection:	kVp 70 to 80; mAs 8 to 16
SID:	40″
Central Ray Placement:	The central ray enters the coracoid process.
Collimation:	To film size.
Marker Placement:	Within the collimation field denoting the affected shoulder.
Breathing Instructions:	Do not breathe. Do not move.
Anatomy Visualized:	Proximal humerus, scapula, humeral head in relation to glenoid fossa. External rotation demonstrates the proximal humerus in the true AP position.
Additional Information:	This view demonstrates calcified deposits in tendon insertions and the greater tuberosity of the proximal humerus in profile, which is the site of insertion of the supraspinatus tendon.

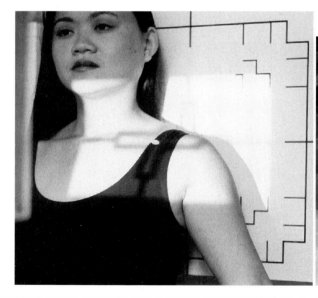 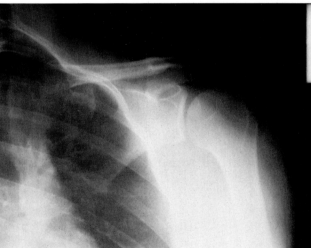

TABLE 3-6 cont'd
Upper Extremities

Position:	**AP Glenoid Fossa**
Patient Preparation:	Remove any artifacts in the desired field (e.g., clothing with hooks, snaps, zippers).
Shielding:	Secure lead apron around patient.
Film Selection:	10 × 12
Film Placement:	Place horizontally in Bucky with the top of the cassette 1½″ above the shoulder.
ID Placement:	ID should be in upper corner of collimation field.
Patient Placement:	The patient is standing in the AP position with back against Bucky. Rotate the patient 35 to 40 degrees toward affected side so that the scapula is parallel to the film. The arm is in the neutral position with hand slightly supinated.
Technique Selection:	kVp 70 to 80; mAs 8 to 16
SID:	40″
Central Ray Placement:	The central ray enters the glenohumeral joint space.
Collimation:	To film size.
Marker Placement:	Within the collimation field denoting the shoulder of interest.
Breathing Instructions:	Do not breathe. Do not move.
Anatomy Visualized:	Glenoid fossa in profile. The joint space between the humeral head and glenoid fossa is also demonstrated.
Additional Information:	The degree of patient rotation depends on how round-shouldered the patient is, and the angle increases as the degree of rounding increases.
	This view may be used in place of the standard AP placement for internal and external rotation.

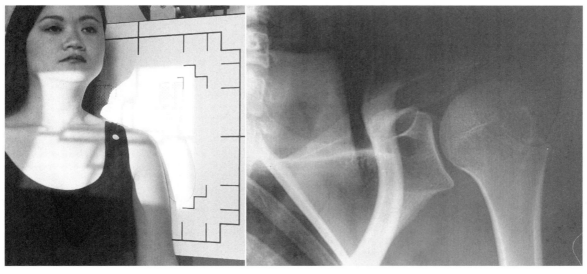

From Ballinger PW, Frank ED: Merril's atlas of radiographic positions and radiologic procedures, ed 10, St Louis, 2003, Mosby.

Continued

TABLE 3-6 cont'd
Upper Extremities

Position:	**AP Neutral Position**
Patient Preparation:	Remove any artifacts in the desired field (e.g., clothing with hooks, snaps, zippers).
Shielding:	Secure lead apron around patient.
Film Selection:	10 × 12
Film Placement:	Place horizontally in Bucky. The top of the cassette should be 1¹/2″ above the shoulder.
ID Placement:	ID should be in upper corner of collimation field.
Patient Placement:	The patient is standing in the AP position with back against Bucky. The arm is in the neutral position with no rotation.
Technique Selection:	kVp 70 to 80; mAs 8 to 16
SID:	40″
Central Ray Placement:	The central ray enters the coracoid process.
Collimation:	To film size.
Marker Placement:	Within the collimation field denoting the affected shoulder.
Breathing Instructions:	Do not breathe. Do not move.
Anatomy Visualized:	Proximal humerus, scapula, humeral head in relation to glenoid fossa, greater tuberle *(arrow)*.
Additional Information:	This view is used to detect fracture or dislocation within the shoulder girdle. In cases of suspected fracture or dislocation, DO NOT attempt to rotate the patient's arm.

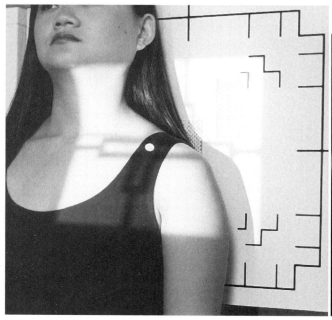
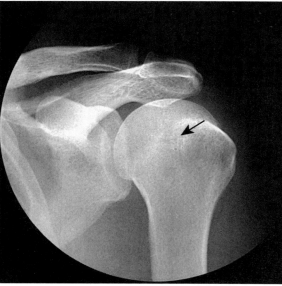

From Ballinger PW, Frank ED: Merril's atlas of radiographic positions and radiologic procedures, ed 10, St Louis, 2003, Mosby.

TABLE 3-6 cont'd
Upper Extremities

Position:	**Transthoracic Lateral**
Patient Preparation:	Remove any artifacts in the desired field (e.g., clothing with hooks, snaps, zippers).
Shielding:	Secure lead apron around patient.
Film Selection:	10 × 12
Film Placement:	Place vertically in Bucky with top of cassette placed 3″ above the top of the shoulder.
ID Placement:	ID should be in lower corner of collimation field.
Patient Placement:	The patient is standing with the affected side placed against the Bucky, opposite arm raised above head. The affected humerus is centered to the cassette.
Technique Selection:	kVp 75 to 85; mAs 40 to 60
SID:	40″
Central Ray Placement:	The central ray is angled 10 to 15 degrees cephalically and enters the opposite axilla so as to exit the surgical neck of the affected humerus.
Collimation:	To film size.
Marker Placement:	Within the collimation field denoting the affected humerus.
Breathing Instructions:	Do not breathe. Do not move.
Anatomy Visualized:	Upper half of the humerus in relation to the glenoid fossa projected through the thorax.
Additional Information:	The patient must be in a true lateral position to avoid superimposition of the thoracic spine. This view demonstrates anterior or posterior displacement of surgical neck fractures.

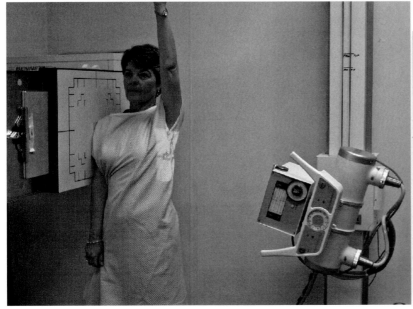
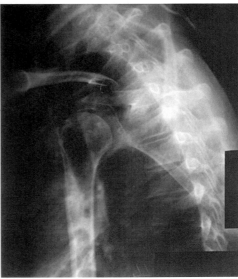

From Ballinger PW, Frank ED: Merril's atlas of radiographic positions and radiologic procedures, ed 10, St Louis, 2003, Mosby.

Continued

TABLE 3-6 cont'd
Upper Extremities

Routine Acromioclavicular Joints: Weighted and Unweighted

Position:	**Acromioclavicular Joints: Unweighted**
Patient Preparation:	Remove any artifacts in the desired field (e.g., clothing with hooks, snaps, zippers).
Shielding:	Secure lead apron around patient.
Film Selection:	8 × 10
Film Placement:	Place vertically in Bucky.
ID Placement:	ID should be in upper corner of field.
Patient Placement:	The patient is standing in the AP position with back against Bucky. Adjust the height of the cassette so that the AC joint is centered to the film.
Technique Selection:	kVp 60 to 70; mAs 6 to 12
SID:	40″
Central Ray Placement:	The central ray is angled 5 degrees cephalically so as to enter the AC joint.
Collimation:	To part size.
Marker Placement:	Within the collimation field.
Breathing Instructions:	Suspend respiration on full exhalation.
Anatomy Visualized:	Relationship of distal clavicle to the acromion process. Integrity of acromioclavicular joint.
Additional Information:	A tube tilt of 5 degrees may be used to elongate the AC joint in relation to the acromion.

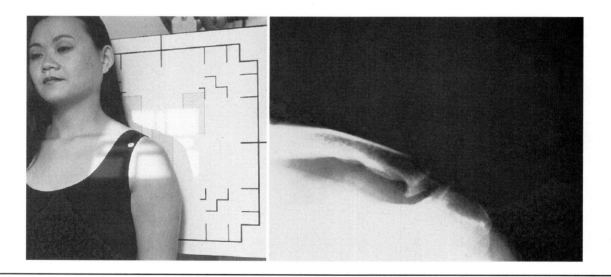

TABLE 3-6 cont'd
Upper Extremities

Position:	**Acromioclavicular Joints: Weighted**
Patient Preparation:	Remove any artifacts in the desired field (e.g., clothing with hooks, snaps, zippers).
Shielding:	Secure lead apron around patient.
Film Selection:	8 × 10
Film Placement:	Same as AC Joints, Unweighted.
ID Placement:	ID should be in corner of collimation field.
Patient Placement:	Same as for AC Joints, Unweighted.
Technique Selection:	kVp 60 to 70; mAs 6 to12
SID:	40″
Central Ray Placement:	Same as AC Joints, Unweighted.
Collimation:	To part size.
Marker Placement:	Within the collimation field.
Breathing Instructions:	Suspend respiration on full exhalation.
Anatomy Visualized:	Relationship of distal clavicle to the acromion process. Integrity of AC joint under stress.
Additional Information:	Instruct patient to hold a 5- to 10-lb. weight in each hand.
	The tube tilt may be increased to 5 degrees to elongate the AC joint in relation to the acromion.
	The inferior aspect of the acromion is compared with the distal clavicle in evaluating AC joint separation because the superior aspect of the clavicle normally is raised with respect to the acromion.

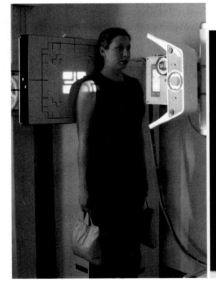
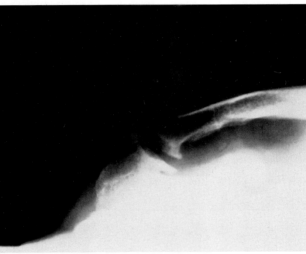

Continued

TABLE 3-6 cont'd
Upper Extremities

Position:	**PA Clavicle**
Patient Preparation:	Remove any artifacts in the desired field (e.g., clothing with hooks, snaps, zippers).
Shielding:	Secure lead apron around patient.
Film Selection:	10 × 12
Film Placement:	Place horizontally in Bucky.
ID Placement:	ID should be in corner of collimation field.
Patient Placement:	The patient is standing in the PA position with the clavicle of interest centered to the center of the cassette. The patient's head is turned away from the affected side.
Technique Selection:	kVp 60 to 70; mAs 8 to 16
SID:	40″
Central Ray Placement:	The central ray is directed midclavicle.
Collimation:	To film size horizontally. Collimate to approximately 4″ vertically.
Marker Placement:	Within the collimation field denoting the clavicle of interest.
Breathing Instructions:	Suspend respiration.
Anatomy Visualized:	Frontal projection of the clavicle and AC joint.
Additional Information:	Detail is increased when view is taken in the PA position because of decreased object–film distance.

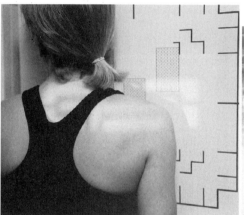 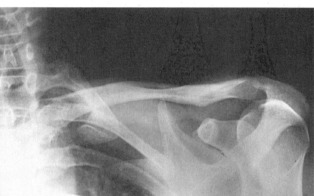

From Ballinger PW, Frank ED: Merril's atlas of radiographic positions and radiologic procedures, ed 10, St Louis, 2003, Mosby.

TABLE 3-6 cont'd
Upper Extremities

Routine Clavicle: PA and Axial

Position:	**AP Axial Clavicle**
Patient Preparation:	Remove any artifacts in the desired field (e.g., clothing with hooks, snaps, zippers).
Shielding:	Secure lead apron around patient.
Film Selection:	10 × 12
Film Placement:	Place horizontally in Bucky.
ID Placement:	ID should be in upper corner of collimation field.
Patient Placement:	The patient is standing in the AP position with back against Bucky and clavicle centered to center of cassette. Turn patient's head away from affected side.
Technique Selection:	kVp 60 to 70; mAs 8 to 16
SID:	40″
Central Ray Placement:	The central ray is angled 15 degrees cephalically so as to enter the subclavicular fossa at the midclavicle level.
Collimation:	To film size horizontally. To approximately 4″ vertically.
Marker Placement:	Within the collimation field denoting the affected clavicle.
Breathing Instructions:	Suspend on exhalation.
Anatomy Visualized:	Axial projection of the clavicle free of superimposition of underlying structures.
Additional Information:	Placing the patient in the lordotic position, one foot away from the Bucky, leaning backward so that the affected side is touching the Bucky further exaggerates the axial view, moving it even further away from underlying structures.

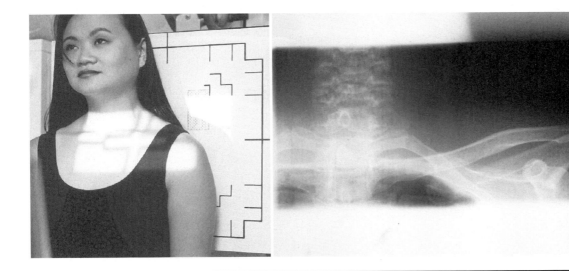

Continued

TABLE 3-6 cont'd
Upper Extremities

Routine Scapula: AP and Lateral

Position:	AP Scapula
Patient Preparation:	Remove any artifacts in the desired field (e.g., clothing with hooks, snaps, zippers).
Shielding:	Secure lead apron around patient.
Film Selection:	10 × 12
Film Placement:	Place vertically in Bucky.
ID Placement:	ID should be in upper corner of collimation field.
Patient Placement:	The patient is standing in the AP position with back against Bucky. The affected scapula is centered to the center of the Bucky with the arm abducted 90 degrees to draw the scapula laterally.
Technique Selection:	kVp 70 to 80; mAs 15 to 25
SID:	40″
Central Ray Placement:	The central ray is directed to enter 2″ below the coracoid, exiting midscapula.
Collimation:	To film size.
Marker Placement:	Within the collimation field denoting the affected scapula.
Breathing Instructions:	Do not breathe. Do not move.
Anatomy Visualized:	AP projection of the scapula with its lateral aspect free of superimposition of overlying structures.
Additional Information:	Do not rotate the patient toward the affected side because this superimposes the lateral border of the scapula over the bony thorax.
	The full scapula series (AP and Lateral) is performed in conjunction with the shoulder series when scapular fracture is suspected.

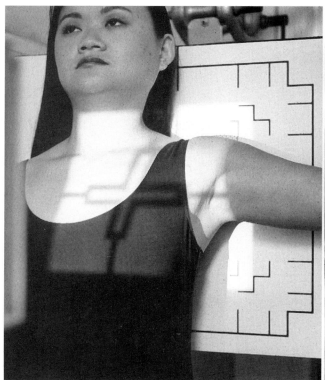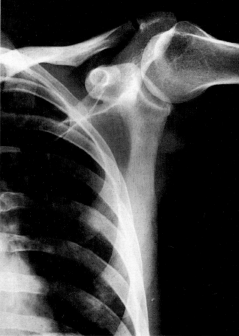

From Ballinger PW, Frank ED: Merril's atlas of radiographic positions and radiologic procedures, ed 10, St Louis, 2003, Mosby.

TABLE 3-6 cont'd
Upper Extremities

Position:	**Lateral Scapula**
Patient Preparation:	Remove any artifacts in the desired field (e.g., clothing with hooks, snaps, zippers).
Shielding:	Secure lead apron around patient.
Film Selection:	10 × 12
Film Placement:	Place vertically in Bucky with top of cassette approximately 2″ above the shoulder.
ID Placement:	ID should be in upper corner of collimation field.
Patient Placement:	The patient is standing in the anterior oblique position with the affected side against the Bucky. Instruct the patient to grasp the opposite shoulder with arm of affected side so that the scapula is in a true lateral position to the central ray.
Technique Selection:	kVp 70 to 80; mAs 20 to 40
SID:	40″
Central Ray Placement:	The central ray enters the midvertebral border of the scapula.
Collimation:	To film size.
Marker Placement:	Within the collimation field denoting the affected scapula.
Breathing Instructions:	Do not breathe. Do not move.
Anatomy Visualized:	Lateral view of the scapula free of superimposition of the ribcage.
Additional Information:	The patient is positioned at an approximately 60-degree oblique angle.
	This is the best view for demonstrating fractures within the body of the scapula.
	If possible, extend the patient's arm upward to rest on top of the head—this provides optimal view of the acromion and coracoid process.
	To better demonstrate the humeral head in relation to the glenoid fossa, align the patient's arm along the body so that the wing of the scapula superimposes it. This view can be used as an alternative to the transthoracic view in a traumatic shoulder series.

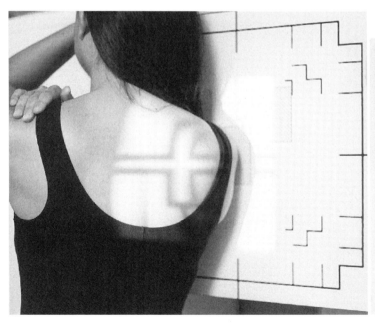
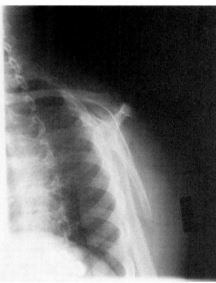

Continued

TABLE 3-6 cont'd
Upper Extremities

Routine Humerus: AP and Lateral

Position:	**AP Humerus**
Patient Preparation:	Remove any artifacts in the desired field (e.g., clothing with hooks, snaps, zippers).
Shielding:	Secure lead apron around patient.
Film Selection:	7 × 17 or collimated on a 14 × 17
Film Placement:	Place vertically in Bucky with the top of the cassette approximately 2″ above the shoulder or the bottom of the cassette 1″ below the elbow joint, depending on which joint is closest to the injury.
ID Placement:	ID should be in the upper corner of the collimation field if including the elbow joint as joint of interest or in the lower corner if the shoulder joint is the joint of interest.
Patient Placement:	The patient is standing in the AP position with back against the Bucky. Rotate the patient toward the affected side so that the humerus is in contact with the Bucky. Supinate the hand and slightly abduct arm.
Technique Selection:	kVp 60 to 70; mAs 5 to 10
SID:	40″
Central Ray Placement:	The central ray is directed to the midshaft of the humerus.
Collimation:	To film size.
Marker Placement:	Within the collimation field denoting the humerus of interest.
Breathing Instructions:	Do not breathe. Do not move.
Anatomy Visualized:	Frontal projection of the humerus.
Additional Information:	If the patient is in severe pain or fracture is suspected, do not supinate the hand. Perform the radiograph with the arm in the neutral position.

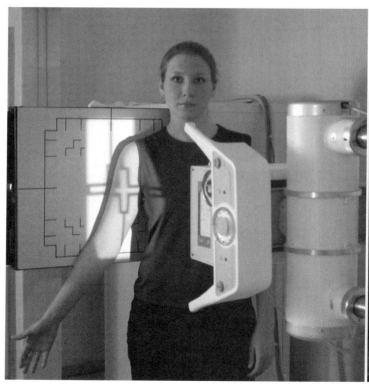
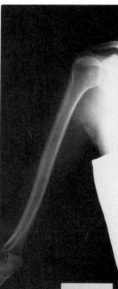

TABLE 3-6 cont'd
Upper Extremities

Position:	**Lateral Humerus**
Patient Preparation:	Remove any artifacts in the desired field (e.g., clothing with hooks, snaps, zippers).
Shielding:	Secure lead apron around patient.
Film Selection:	7 × 17 or collimated on 14 × 17
Film Placement:	Place vertically in Bucky.
ID Placement:	ID should be in corner of collimation field opposite the joint of interest.
Patient Placement:	The patient is standing in the AP position with back against the Bucky. The elbow is flexed and the forearm is adducted across the abdomen. The humerus is moved slightly lateral to avoid superimposition of the thorax. The hand is supinated so the palm points upward.
Technique Selection:	kVp 60 to 70; mAs 5 to 10
SID:	40″
Central Ray Placement:	The central ray is directed to the midshaft of the humerus.
Collimation:	To film size.
Marker Placement:	Within the collimation field denoting the humerus of interest.
Breathing Instructions:	Do not breathe. Do not move.
Anatomy Visualized:	Lateral projection of the humerus.
Additional Information:	The view can be obtained with the patient in the PA position to bring humerus closer to Bucky.
	If patient is experiencing severe pain, do not supinate hand, which rotates humerus into lateral position.

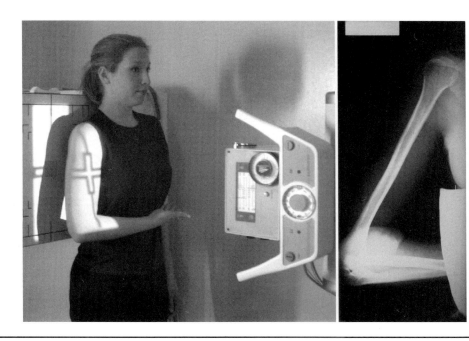

Continued

TABLE 3-6 cont'd
Upper Extremities

Position:	**Transthoracic Lateral**
Patient Preparation:	Remove any artifacts in the desired field (e.g., clothing with hooks, snaps, zippers).
Shielding:	Secure lead apron around patient.
Film Selection:	10 × 12
Film Placement:	Place vertically in Bucky with top of cassette placed 3″ above the top of the shoulder.
ID Placement:	ID should be in lower corner of collimation field.
Patient Placement:	The patient is standing with the affected side placed against the Bucky, opposite arm raised above head. The affected humerus is centered to the cassette.
Technique Selection:	kVp 75 to 85; mAs 40 to 60
SID:	40″
Central Ray Placement:	The central ray is angled 10 to 15 degrees cephalically and enters the opposite axilla so as to exit the surgical neck of the affected humerus.
Collimation:	To film size.
Marker Placement:	Within the collimation field denoting the affected humerus.
Breathing Instructions:	Do not breathe. Do not move.
Anatomy Visualized:	Upper half of the humerus in relation to the glenoid fossa projected through the thorax.
Additional Information:	The patient must be in a true lateral position to avoid superimposition of the thoracic spine. This view demonstrates anterior or posterior displacement of surgical neck fractures.

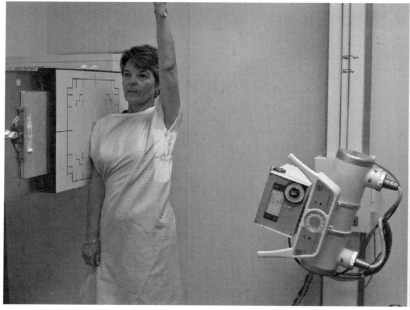

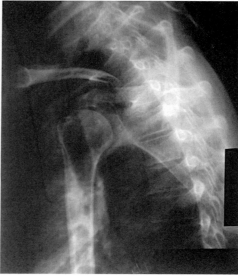

From Ballinger PW, Frank ED: Merril's atlas of radiographic positions and radiologic procedures, ed 10, St Louis, 2003, Mosby.

TABLE 3-6 cont'd
Upper Extremities

Routine Elbow: AP, Lateral, Internal, and External Oblique

Position:	AP Elbow
Patient Preparation:	Remove any artifacts in the desired field (e.g., clothing with hooks, snaps, zippers).
Shielding:	Secure lead apron around patient.
Film Selection:	10 × 12 placed horizontally and divided in half with AP elbow centered to half of cassette.
Film Placement:	Place cassette on tabletop.
ID Placement:	ID should be in corner of collimation field.
Patient Placement:	The patient is seated with affected elbow fully extended and hand supinated. The adjacent anatomy is lowered to the same plane as the tabletop.
Technique Selection:	kVp 55 to 65; mAs 15 to 30 (nongrid).
SID:	40″
Central Ray Placement:	The central ray is perpendicular to elbow joint and enters antecubital fossa.
Collimation:	To one half of film size.
Marker Placement:	Within the collimation field on one of the two elbow views.
Breathing Instructions:	Do not breathe. Do not move.
Anatomy Visualized:	AP projection of the elbow joint, proximal radius and ulna, distal humerus.
Additional Information:	Hand must be supinated to avoid superimposition of radius and ulna.
	If the patient can only partially extend elbow, two views must be taken: one with the forearm resting on the film and the second with the humerus resting on the film.

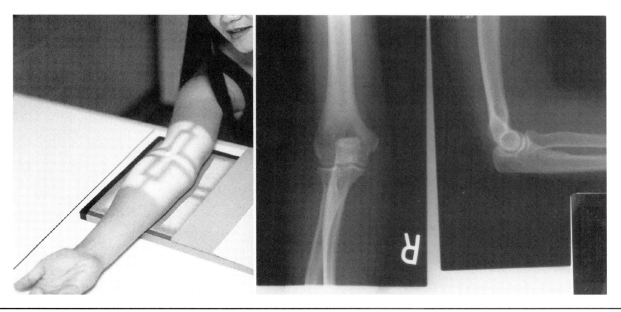

Continued

TABLE 3-6 cont'd
Upper Extremities

Position:	**Lateral Elbow**
Patient Preparation:	Remove any artifacts in the desired field (e.g., clothing with hooks, snaps, zippers).
Shielding:	Secure lead apron around patient.
Film Selection:	Use second half of 10 × 12 used for AP projection.
Film Placement:	Place film on tabletop.
ID Placement:	ID should be in corner of collimation field.
Patient Placement:	The patient is seated with the elbow flexed 90 degrees, forearm in true lateral position with thumb up. Drop shoulder to place adjacent anatomy in same plane as elbow joint.
Technique Selection:	kVp 55 to 65; mAs 15 to 30 (nongrid)
SID:	40″
Central Ray Placement:	The central ray enters elbow joint perpendicular to cassette.
Collimation:	To second half of film size used for AP.
Marker Placement:	Within the collimation field. If the marker was placed on the AP projection, none is needed for this view.
Breathing Instructions:	Do not breathe. Do not move.
Anatomy Visualized:	Lateral projection of elbow joint, proximal radius and ulna, distal humerus. Demonstrates olecranon process.
Additional Information:	This view demonstrates the elevation of the distal humeral fat pads. Elevation of distal humeral fat pads is indicative of intraarticular effusion, such as hemarthrosis from fracture, especially fracture of the radial head.

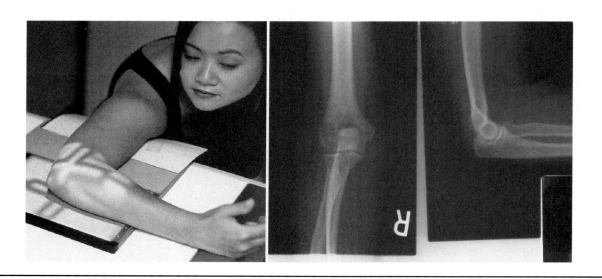

TABLE 3-6 cont'd

Upper Extremities

Position:	**External Oblique Elbow**
Patient Preparation:	Remove any artifacts in the desired field (e.g., clothing with hooks, snaps, zippers).
Shielding:	Secure lead apron around patient.
Film Selection:	10 × 12 divided horizontally into two sections.
Film Placement:	Place cassette on tabletop.
ID Placement:	ID should be in corner of collimation field.
Patient Placement:	The patient is seated with elbow in full extension and hand supinated. The humerus is lowered to the same plane as the elbow. Laterally rotate the entire arm so that the elbow joint is 45 degrees to the cassette.
Technique Selection:	kVp 55 to 65; mAs 15 to 30 (nongrid)
SID:	40″
Central Ray Placement:	The central ray enters perpendicular to the antecubital fossa.
Collimation:	To one half of film size.
Marker Placement:	Within the collimation field.
Breathing Instructions:	Do not breathe. Do not move.
Anatomy Visualized:	Oblique projection of the elbow joint, proximal radius and ulna, distal humerus. Best demonstrates the radial head, free of superimposition.
Additional Information:	This view demonstrates the coronoid process.
	If the patient is unable to laterally rotate the arm, leave in a true AP position and angle the tube 45 degrees to enter the medial aspect of the elbow and exit the elbow joint on the ulnar side.

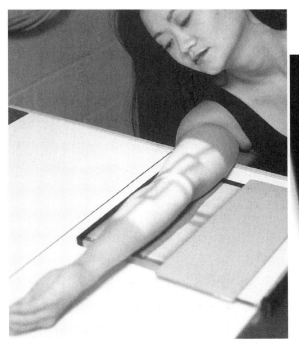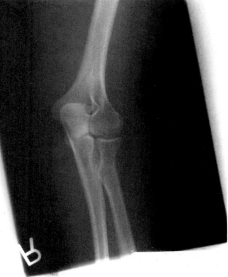

Continued

TABLE 3-6 cont'd
Upper Extremities

Position:	**Internal Oblique Elbow**
Patient Preparation:	Remove any artifacts in the desired field (e.g., clothing with hooks, snaps, zippers).
Shielding:	Secure lead apron around patient.
Film Selection:	10 × 12 divided in half—remaining side from External Oblique Elbow.
Film Placement:	Place horizontally on tabletop.
ID Placement:	ID should be in corner of collimation field.
Patient Placement:	The patient is seated with elbow in full extension, hand supinated. Lower the shoulder to the same plane as the elbow. Pronate the hand into a natural palm down position.
Technique Selection:	kVp 55 to 65; mAs 15 to 30 (nongrid)
SID:	40″
Central Ray Placement:	The central ray enters perpendicular to the antecubital fossa.
Collimation:	To one half film size.
Marker Placement:	Within the collimation field. If marked on External Oblique View, marker is not needed.
Breathing Instructions:	Do not breathe. Do not move.
Anatomy Visualized:	Oblique projection of the elbow joint, proximal radius and ulna, distal humerus. Demonstrates coronoid process free of superimposition of the radial head.
Additional Information:	This view demonstrates coronoid process.

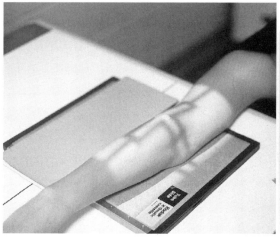
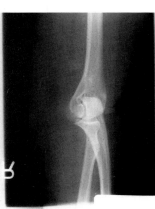

TABLE 3-6 cont'd
Upper Extremities

Position:	Axial Projection: Olecranon View
Patient Preparation:	Remove any artifacts in the desired field (e.g., clothing with hooks, snaps, zippers).
Shielding:	Secure lead apron around patient.
Film Selection:	8 × 10
Film Placement:	Place vertically on tabletop.
ID Placement:	ID should be in corner of collimation field.
Patient Placement:	The patient is seated with the elbow completely flexed (Jones position).
Technique Selection:	kVp 55 to 65; mAs 15 to 30 (nongrid)
SID:	40″
Central Ray Placement:	The central ray is perpendicular to the cassette entering approximately 2″ above tip of elbow.
Collimation:	To part size.
Marker Placement:	Within the collimation field denoting affected elbow.
Breathing Instructions:	Do not breathe. Do not move.
Anatomy Visualized:	Olecranon process superimposed distal humerus and proximal radius and ulna.
Additional Information:	If the distal humerus is the area of concern, center the central ray perpendicular to the film with no angle.
	If the distal forearm is the area of concern, angle the central ray to be perpendicular with the radius and ulna.

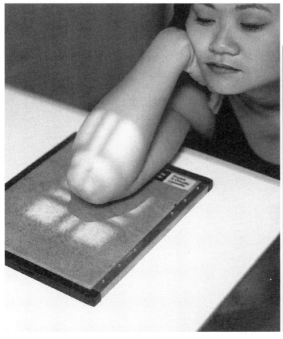
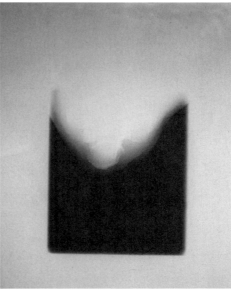

Continued

TABLE 3-6 cont'd
Upper Extremities

Routine Forearm: AP and Lateral

Position:	**AP Forearm**
Patient Preparation:	Remove any artifacts in the desired field (e.g., clothing with hooks, snaps, zippers).
Shielding:	Secure lead apron around patient.
Film Selection:	10 × 12 divided vertically.
Film Placement:	Place vertically on tabletop.
ID Placement:	ID should be in corner of collimation field opposite the joint closest to the injury.
Patient Placement:	The patient is seated with the elbow fully extended and hand supinated. The humerus is lowered to the same plane as the elbow and forearm. The forearm is placed so as to include both joints, if possible. The joint closest to injury must be included.
Technique Selection:	kVp 55 to 65; mAs 15 to 30 (nongrid)
SID:	40″
Central Ray Placement:	The central ray is directed perpendicular to the long axis of the forearm.
Collimation:	To one half of the film size vertically.
Marker Placement:	Within the collimation field on one of the two routine projections.
Breathing Instructions:	Do not breathe. Do not move.
Anatomy Visualized:	AP projection of the radius, ulna, and elbow joint.
Additional Information:	If the patient cannot hold hand in full supination, a sandbag may be placed in the hand to stabilize. The hand must be fully supinated to avoid the radius crossing over the ulna.

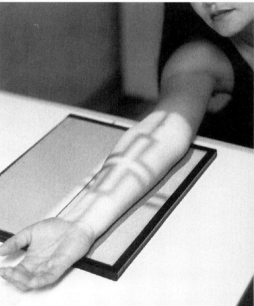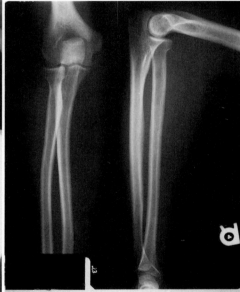

TABLE 3-6 cont'd
Upper Extremities

Position:	**Lateral Forearm**
Patient Preparation:	Remove any artifacts in the desired field (e.g., clothing with hooks, snaps, zippers).
Shielding:	Secure lead apron around patient.
Film Selection:	10 × 12 divided in half vertically.
Film Placement:	Place cassette on tabletop.
ID Placement:	ID should be in corner of collimation field opposite the joint closest to injury.
Patient Placement:	The patient is seated with the elbow flexed 90 degrees. The humerus must be lowered to the same plane as the elbow and forearm. The forearm and hand are in a true lateral position with the thumb pointing upward. The forearm is placed in the collimation field to include the joint closest to injury.
Technique Selection:	kVp 55 to 65; mAs 15 to 30 (nongrid)
SID:	40″
Central Ray Placement:	The central ray is directed perpendicular to the long axis of the forearm.
Collimation:	To one half of the film size vertically.
Marker Placement:	Within the collimation field on one of the two routine forearm projections.
Breathing Instructions:	Do not breathe. Do not move.
Anatomy Visualized:	This view demonstrates a lateral projection of the superimposed radius and ulna and elbow joint.

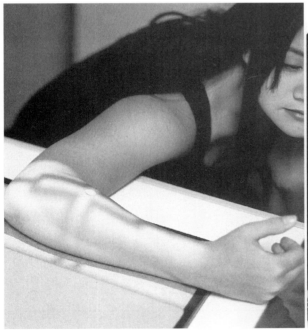 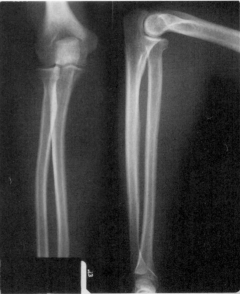

Continued

TABLE 3-6 cont'd

Upper Extremities

Routine Wrist: PA, Oblique, and Lateral

Position:	**PA Wrist**
Patient Preparation:	Remove any artifacts in the desired field (e.g., clothing with hooks, snaps, zippers).
Shielding:	Secure lead apron around patient.
Film Selection:	10 × 12 divided into thirds horizontally.
Film Placement:	Place horizontally on tabletop.
ID Placement:	ID should be in corner of collimation field in which the lateral wrist appears.
Patient Placement:	The patient is seated with the hand and forearm parallel to the long axis of the cassette. Partially flex fingers so that the wrist makes contact with the cassette. Place wrist in one third of the cassette.
Technique Selection:	kVp 55 to 60; mAs 12 to 24 (nongrid)
SID:	40″
Central Ray Placement:	The central ray is directed perpendicular to the wrist joint.
Collimation:	To one third of the cassette.
Marker Placement:	Within the collimation field in which the lateral wrist view appears.
Breathing Instructions:	Do not breathe. Do not move.
Anatomy Visualized:	PA projection of the carpals, distal radius and ulna, and the proximal metacarpals.
Additional Information:	If swelling makes midcarpal area difficult to locate, instruct the patient to slightly flex the wrist and place central ray perpendicular to the point of flexion.

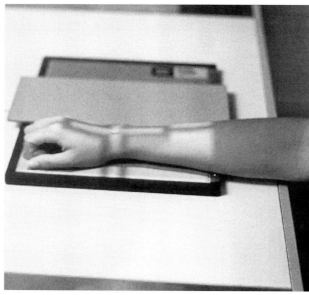

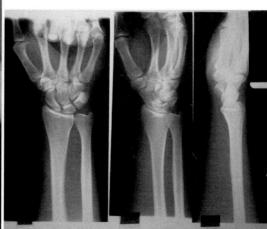

TABLE 3-6 cont'd
Upper Extremities

Position:	**Oblique Wrist**
Patient Preparation:	Remove any artifacts in the desired field (e.g., clothing with hooks, snaps, zippers).
Shielding:	Secure lead apron around patient.
Film Selection:	10 × 12 divided horizontally into thirds.
Film Placement:	Place oblique wrist in center third of cassette.
ID Placement:	ID should be in corner of collimation field in which the lateral wrist view appears.
Patient Placement:	The patient is seated with hand and forearm parallel to the long axis of the cassette. From the PA position, rotate the wrist laterally 45 degrees. The fingers may be slightly flexed for stability.
Technique Selection:	kVp 55 to 60; mAs 12 to 24 (nongrid)
SID:	40″
Central Ray Placement:	The central ray is directed perpendicular to the wrist joint.
Collimation:	To the center third of the cassette.
Marker Placement:	Within the collimation field in which the lateral wrist view appears.
Breathing Instructions:	Do not breathe. Do not move.
Anatomy Visualized:	This view provides better visualization of the carpals on the lateral aspect of the wrist. The scaphoid is projected free of superimposition.

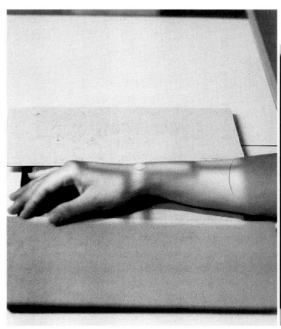
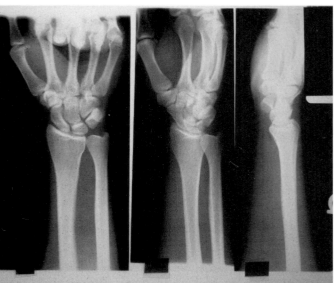

Continued

TABLE 3-6 cont'd
Upper Extremities

Position:	Lateral Wrist
Patient Preparation:	Remove any artifacts in the desired field (e.g., clothing with hooks, snaps, zippers).
Shielding:	Secure lead apron around patient.
Film Selection:	10 × 12 divided into thirds horizontally.
Film Placement:	Place horizontally on tabletop.
ID Placement:	ID should be in corner of collimation field in which this view appears.
Patient Placement:	The patient is seated with the forearm in the true lateral position with the fingers slightly flexed for stability.
Technique Selection:	kVp 55 to 60; mAs 12 to 24 (nongrid)
SID:	40″
Central Ray Placement:	The central ray is directed perpendicular to the wrist joint.
Collimation:	To one third of 10 × 12 placed horizontally.
Marker Placement:	Within the collimation field in which this view appears.
Breathing Instructions:	Do not breathe. Do not move.
Anatomy Visualized:	Lateral projection of the carpals, distal radius, ulna, and proximal metacarpals.
Additional Information:	The wrist must be placed in a true lateral position.

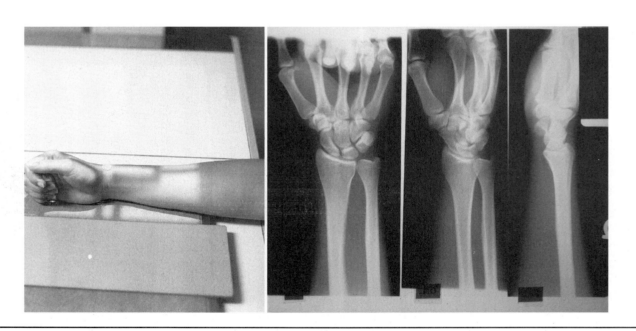

TABLE 3-6 cont'd
Upper Extremities

Position:	**Carpal Canal**
Patient Preparation:	Remove any artifacts in the desired field (e.g., clothing with hooks, snaps, zippers).
Shielding:	Secure lead apron around patient.
Film Selection:	8 × 10
Film Placement:	Place cassette on tabletop.
ID Placement:	ID should be in collimation field.
Patient Placement:	The patient is seated with the wrist in the PA position in the center of the cassette. The wrist is hyperextended, and this position is held stable by instructing the patient to pull back on a strap that has been placed around the fingers.
Technique Selection:	kVp 55 to 60; mAs 12 to 24 (nongrid)
SID:	40″
Central Ray Placement:	The central ray is angled 30 degrees cephalically to enter 1″ above the base of the fourth metacarpal.
Collimation:	To part size, approximately 5″ × 5″.
Marker Placement:	Within the collimation field.
Breathing Instructions:	Do not breathe. Do not move.
Anatomy Visualized:	Projection of the carpal canal, the palmar aspect of the greater and lesser multangulars, the tuberosity of the scaphoid, the capitate, the hook of the hamate, and the entire pisiform.
Additional Information:	This view demonstrates fractures of the pisiform and the hook of the hamate.
	If the patient is experiencing difficulty hyperextending the wrist, the central ray angulation can be increased to compensate.

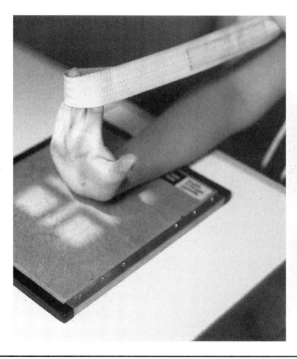
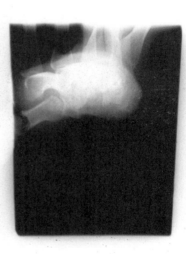

Continued

TABLE 3-6 cont'd
Upper Extremities

Position:	**Ulnar Flexion**
Patient Preparation:	Remove any artifacts in the desired field (e.g., clothing with hooks, snaps, zippers).
Shielding:	Secure lead apron around patient.
Film Selection:	8 × 10
Film Placement:	Place horizontally on the tabletop.
ID Placement:	ID should be placed so as not to superimpose required anatomy.
Patient Placement:	The patient is seated with the hand and forearm parallel to the long axis of the cassette. With the hand in the PA position, without moving the forearm, deviate (ulnar flex) the fingers as far as possible toward the radius without lifting the forearm.
Technique Selection:	kVp 55 to 60; mAs 12 to 24 (nongrid, detail).
SID:	40″
Central Ray Placement:	The central ray is angled 20 degrees to enter the web of the hand traveling parallel to the long axis of the forearm.
Collimation:	To part size.
Marker Placement:	Within the collimation field denoting either the patient's right or left.
Breathing Instructions:	Do not breathe. Do not move.
Anatomy Visualized:	This view demonstrates the scaphoid without the foreshortening that is present on the PA wrist position.

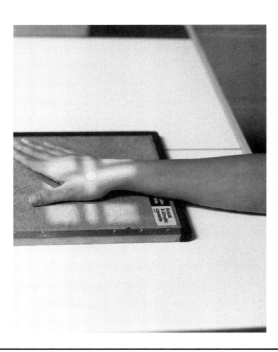

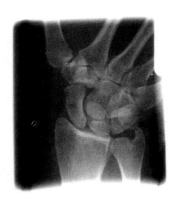

TABLE 3-6 cont'd
Upper Extremities

Routine Hand: PA and Lateral

Position:	**PA Hand**
Patient Preparation:	Remove any artifacts in the desired field (e.g., clothing with hooks, snaps, zippers).
Shielding:	Secure lead apron around patient.
Film Selection:	10 × 12 placed horizontally and divided in half.
Film Placement:	Place horizontally on the tabletop.
ID Placement:	ID should be in corner of collimation field in which the oblique view of the hand appears.
Patient Placement:	The patient is seated with the hand and forearm in the same plane, parallel to the long axis of the cassette. The hand is in pronation so that the palmar surface is in contact with the cassette.
Technique Selection:	kVp 55 to 60; mAs 12 to 24 (nongrid)
SID:	40″
Central Ray Placement:	The central ray is directed perpendicular to the third metacarpophalangeal joint.
Collimation:	To one half of the cassette.
Marker Placement:	Within the collimation field in which the oblique view of the hand appears.
Breathing Instructions:	Do not breathe. Do not move.
Anatomy Visualized:	PA projection of the carpals, metacarpals, and second to fifth phalanges; oblique projection of the first finger; demonstrates DIP, PIP, and MP joints.
Additional Information:	All fingers must be included in this view.

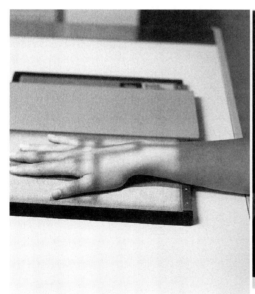
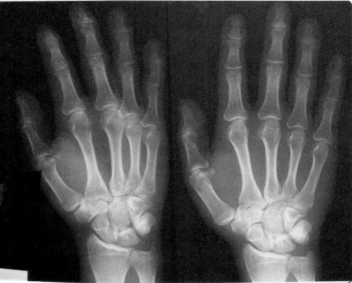

Continued

TABLE 3-6 cont'd
Upper Extremities

Position:	**Oblique Hand**
Patient Preparation:	Remove any artifacts in the desired field (e.g., clothing with hooks, snaps, zippers).
Shielding:	Secure lead apron around patient.
Film Selection:	10 × 12 divided in half.
Film Placement:	Place on tabletop.
ID Placement:	ID should be in corner of collimation field.
Patient Placement:	The patient is seated with the hand and forearm parallel to the long axis of the cassette. Place the hand in a lateral position and then guide the fingers toward the cassette so that each finger is in a 45-degree oblique position with the fingertips in contact with the cassette.
Technique Selection:	kVp 55 to 60; mAs 12 to 24 (nongrid)
SID:	40″
Central Ray Placement:	The central ray is directed perpendicular to the third metacarpophalangeal joint.
Collimation:	To one half of cassette.
Marker Placement:	Within the collimation field.
Breathing Instructions:	Do not breathe. Do not move.
Anatomy Visualized:	Oblique projection of the carpals, metacarpals, second to fifth phalanges; lateral projection of the first finger; DIP, PIP, and MP joints.
Additional Information:	A 45-degree wedge sponge can be used to further separate fingers on this view.

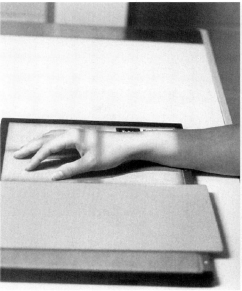
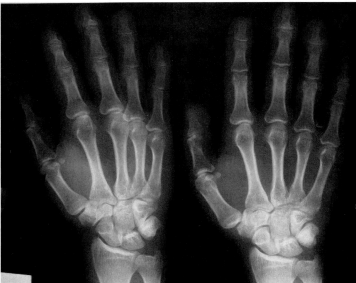

TABLE 3-6 cont'd
Upper Extremities

Position:	**Lateral Finger**
Patient Preparation:	Remove any artifacts in the desired field (e.g., clothing with hooks, snaps, zippers).
Shielding:	Secure lead apron around patient.
Film Selection:	8 × 10 or use a corner of the 10 × 12 used in the hand series.
Film Placement:	Place on tabletop.
ID Placement:	If performing a radiograph of the finger on an 8 × 10, the ID blocker can appear in either corner. If performing finger as part of the hand series on a 10 × 12, the ID should appear in the section in which the oblique hand appears.
Patient Placement:	Depending on area of injury, extend the affected finger and fold the remaining fingers inward. If the injury involves the second or third finger, place hand in lateral position with the radial side in contact with the cassette. If the injury involves the fourth to fifth finger, place the hand in the lateral position with the ulnar side in contact with the cassette.
Technique Selection:	kVp 50 to 55; mAs 6 to 12 (nongrid)
SID:	40″
Central Ray Placement:	The central ray is directed perpendicular to the finger of interest.
Collimation:	To part size.
Marker Placement:	Within the collimation field.
Breathing Instructions:	Do not breathe. Do not move.
Anatomy Visualized:	Lateral projection of affected phalanges.
Additional Information:	This view is done in conjunction with the hand series. Using a tongue depressor or tape to isolate the affected finger may provide a clearer view of the affected finger.
	Small avulsion fractures of phalanges can lead to permanent deformity and are best seen on lateral projections.

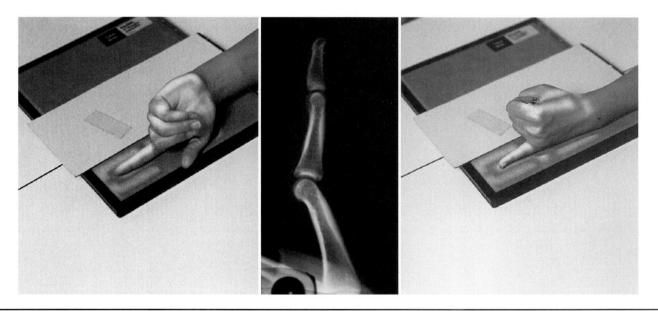

Continued

TABLE 3-6 cont'd
Upper Extremities

Position:	AP Thumb
Patient Preparation:	Remove any artifacts in the desired field (e.g., clothing with hooks, snaps, zippers).
Shielding:	Secure lead apron around patient.
Film Selection:	8 × 10 or corner of cassette on hand series.
Film Placement:	Place cassette on tabletop.
ID Placement:	ID should be in corner of cassette away from lateral thumb.
Patient Placement:	Internally rotate the hand until the posterior aspect of the thumb is in contact with the cassette. Instruct patient to hold fingers back with opposite hand.
Technique Selection:	kVp 50 to 55; mAs 6 to 12 (nongrid)
SID:	40″
Central Ray Placement:	The central ray is directed perpendicular to first MP joint.
Collimation:	To part size.
Marker Placement:	Within the collimation field.
Breathing Instructions:	Do not breathe. Do not move.
Anatomy Visualized:	AP projection of phalanges of first finger and MP and PIP joints.
Additional Information:	This view is performed in conjunction with hand series.
	On standard PA and oblique hand views, the thumb appears in an oblique and lateral position, respectively.

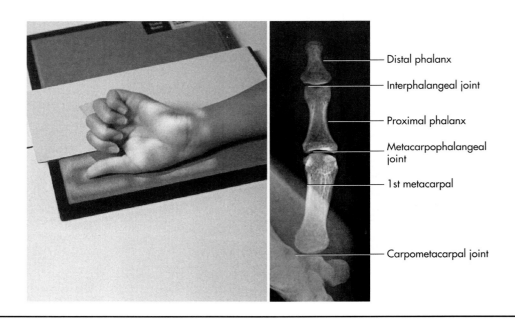

Labels (top to bottom): Distal phalanx, Interphalangeal joint, Proximal phalanx, Metacarpophalangeal joint, 1st metacarpal, Carpometacarpal joint

TABLE 3-6 cont'd
Upper Extremities

Position:	**Lateral Hand**
Patient Preparation:	Remove any artifacts in the desired field (e.g., clothing with hooks, snaps, zippers).
Shielding:	Secure lead apron around patient.
Film Selection:	8 × 10
Film Placement:	Place cassette on tabletop.
ID Placement:	ID should be placed away from anatomy.
Patient Placement:	The patient is seated with hand in true lateral position with fingers in full extension resting on ulnar aspect of hand.
Technique Selection:	kVp 55 to 60; mAs 12 to 24 (nongrid)
SID:	40″
Central Ray Placement:	The central ray is directed perpendicular to metacarpophalangeal joints.
Collimation:	To film size.
Marker Placement:	Within the collimation field.
Breathing Instructions:	Do not breathe. Do not move.
Anatomy Visualized:	Lateral projection of the hand in full extension.
Additional Information:	This view is performed for localization of foreign bodies within the soft tissue of the hand.

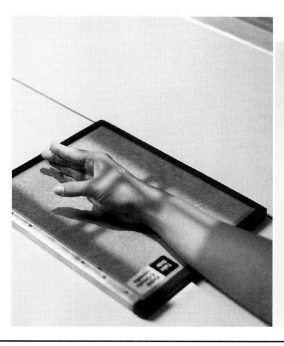
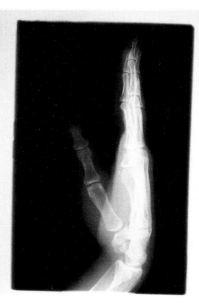

Continued

TABLE 3-6 cont'd
Upper Extremities

Position:	**Norgaard Method**
Patient Preparation:	Remove any artifacts in the desired field (e.g., clothing with hooks, snaps, zippers).
Shielding:	Secure lead apron around patient.
Film Selection:	10 × 12 placed horizontally.
Film Placement:	Place horizontally on tabletop.
ID Placement:	ID should be in upper corner of collimation field.
Patient Placement:	The patient is seated with both hands slightly supinated and placed in the center of the cassette.
Technique Selection:	kVp 55 to 60; mAs 12 to 24 (nongrid)
SID:	40″
Central Ray Placement:	The central ray is directed perpendicular to the center of the cassette.
Collimation:	To film size.
Marker Placement:	Within the collimation field denoting either left hand or right hand.
Breathing Instructions:	Do not breathe. Do not move.
Anatomy Visualized:	This view demonstrates the hands in a 45-degree oblique position.
Additional Information:	This view is useful in detecting early radiologic changes associated with rheumatoid arthritis. It demonstrates the medial aspect of the metatarsal heads, one of the first areas affected. This view also demonstrates the pisiform, another sight of early erosions in rheumatoid arthritis.

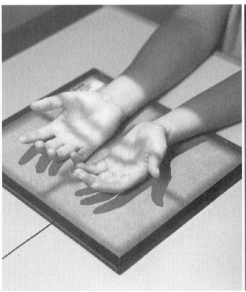 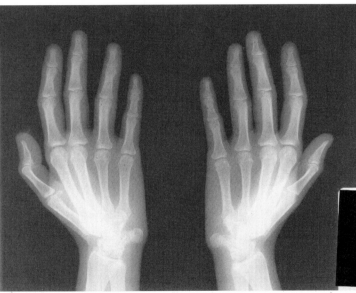

AC, Acromioclavicular; *AP,* anteroposterior; *DIP,* distal interphalangeal joint; *ID,* identification; *MP,* metacarpophalangeal; *PA,* posteroanterior; *PIP,* proximal interphalangeal joint; *SID,* source-to-image distance.

TABLE 3-7

Lower Extremities

Position:	**AP Pelvis**
Patient Preparation:	Remove any artifacts in the desired field (e.g., clothing with hooks, snaps, zippers).
Shielding:	Do not shield for this view.
Film Selection:	14 × 17
Film Placement:	Place in Bucky in the horizontal position. The top of the cassette is placed 1″ above the iliac crest.
ID Placement:	ID should be in lower corner of collimation field.
Patient Placement:	The patient is either standing or lying recumbent centered to the table or Bucky. Internally rotate the patient's legs 15 degrees or to patient's tolerance to visualize the surgical neck of the femur and place the greater trochanter in profile.
Technique Selection:	kVp 75 to 85; mAs 30 to 80
SID:	40″
Central Ray Placement:	The central ray is directed perpendicular to the center of the cassette.
Collimation:	To film size in the horizontal direction.
Marker Placement:	Within the collimation field denoting the patient's left or right side.
Breathing Instructions:	Suspend respiration.
Anatomy Visualized:	AP projection of the pelvis and femoral head, neck, trochanter, and proximal one third of the femoral shaft.
Additional Information:	A gonadal shield should be used, if possible.
	If fracture of the femoral neck is suspected, internal rotation of the legs should be avoided.

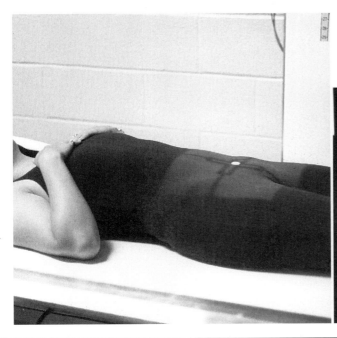
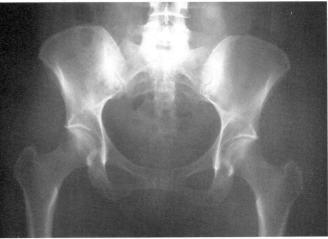

Continued

TABLE 3-7 cont'd
Lower Extremities

Routine Hip: AP and Frogleg Lateral

Position:	**AP Hip**
Patient Preparation:	Remove any artifacts in the desired field (e.g., clothing with hooks, snaps, zippers).
Shielding:	Use gonadal shielding, if possible.
Film Selection:	10 × 12
Film Placement:	Place vertically in Bucky.
ID Placement:	ID should be in upper corner of collimation field.
Patient Placement:	The patient is either standing in the AP position or lying recumbent on the table. Center the femoral head of the affected hip to the center of the cassette. Rotate the leg of the affected hip 15 degrees internally or to patient's tolerance.
Technique Selection:	kVp 75 to 80; mAs 20 to 50
SID:	40″
Central Ray Placement:	The central ray is directed perpendicular to the joint space.
Collimation:	To film size.
Marker Placement:	Within the collimation field denoting the patient's right or left hip.
Breathing Instructions:	Do not breathe. Do not move.
Anatomy Visualized:	Femoral head, neck, greater trochanter, and acetabulum.
Additional Information:	Do not attempt internal rotation of affected hip, if fracture is suspected.
	The AP pelvis is included in the initial examination of a patient with suspected hip pathology.

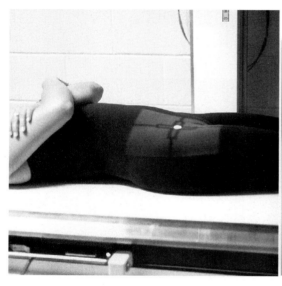
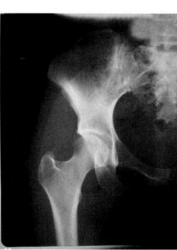

TABLE 3-7 cont'd

Lower Extremities

Position:	**Frogleg Lateral Hip**
Patient Preparation:	Remove any artifacts in the desired field (e.g., clothing with hooks, snaps, zippers).
Shielding:	Use gonadal shielding, if possible.
Film Selection:	10 × 12
Film Placement:	Place vertically in Bucky.
ID Placement:	ID should be in upper corner of collimation field.
Patient Placement:	Patient is either standing in the AP position or lying recumbent with back against Bucky. Instruct the patient to flex knee and draw up thigh so as to rest bottom of foot against inside of opposite thigh. Rotate the patient slightly toward the affected hip so that affected femoral shaft is parallel to Bucky.
Technique Selection:	kVp 75 to 80; mAs 20 to 50
SID:	40"
Central Ray Placement:	The central ray is directed perpendicular to the hip joint.
Collimation:	To film size.
Marker Placement:	Within the collimation field denoting patient's right or left hip.
Breathing Instructions:	Do not breathe. Do not move.
Anatomy Visualized:	Lateral view of femoral head, neck and greater trochanter, and acetabulum.
Additional Information:	This view is best accomplished with the patient in the recumbent position. If attempted in the upright position, provide a chair for the patient to grasp for stability.
	This view should not be attempted when fracture is suspected.
	The use of a 20-degree cephalic tube tilt better demonstrates the femoral neck.

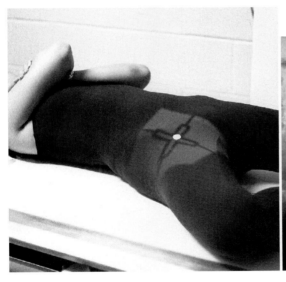 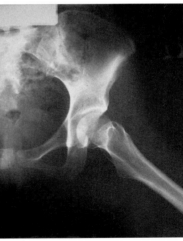

Continued

TABLE 3-7 cont'd
Lower Extremities

Routine Femur: AP and Lateral

Position:	**AP Femur**
Patient Preparation:	Remove any artifacts in the desired field (e.g., clothing with hooks, snaps, zippers).
Shielding:	Use gonadal shielding, if possible.
Film Selection:	7 × 17 or 14 × 17 collimated.
Film Placement:	Place vertically in Bucky.
ID Placement:	ID should be in corner of collimation field nearest the hip.
Patient Placement:	The patient is in the supine position on the radiographic table with leg in full extension, foot at 90-degree angle to lower leg. Internally rotate the femur so that femoral epicondyles are parallel to the table.
Technique Selection:	kVp 75 to 85; mAs 20 to 40
SID:	40″
Central Ray Placement:	The central ray is directed perpendicular to the center of the cassette.
Collimation:	To 7 × 17 collimation field.
Marker Placement:	Within the collimation field denoting patient's right or left femur.
Breathing Instructions:	Do not breathe. Do not move.
Anatomy Visualized:	AP projection of the femur including the knee or hip joint.
Additional Information:	If the injury is located in the upper one third of the femur, a hip series (AP and frog-leg lateral) should be included.
	Internal rotation of the femur goes to patient's tolerance.

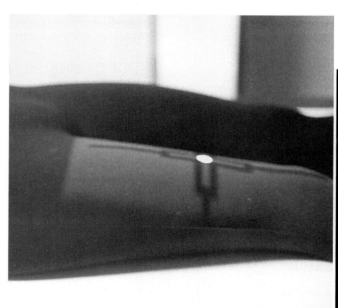

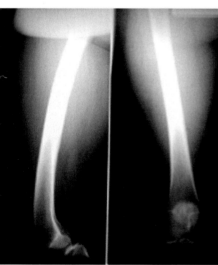

TABLE 3-7 cont'd
Lower Extremities

Position:	Lateral Femur
Patient Preparation:	Remove any artifacts in the desired field (e.g., clothing with hooks, snaps, zippers).
Shielding:	Use gonadal shielding, if possible.
Film Selection:	7 × 17 or 14 × 17 collimated.
Film Placement:	Place vertically in Bucky so as to include the knee joint.
ID Placement:	ID should be in corner of collimation field closest to the hip.
Patient Placement:	The patient is lying recumbent on the table on the affected side. The opposite leg is drawn up and is crossed over the affected leg. The shaft of the affected femur is placed parallel to the center of the table. Flex the knee 20 to 30 degrees so that epicondyles are perpendicular to the table.
Technique Selection:	kVp 75 to 80; mAs 20 to 40
SID:	40″
Central Ray Placement:	The central ray is directed perpendicular to the center of the cassette.
Collimation:	To 7 × 17 collimation field.
Marker Placement:	Within the collimation field denoting the patient's affected extremity.
Breathing Instructions:	Do not breathe. Do not move.
Anatomy Visualized:	Lateral view of the femur to include the knee joint.

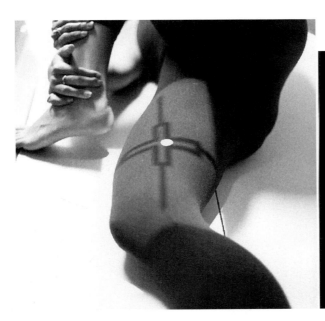
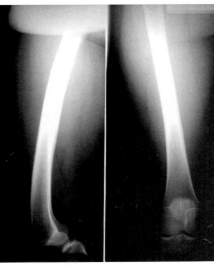

Continued

TABLE 3-7 cont'd
Lower Extremities

Routine Knee: AP, Lateral, and Open Joint

Position:	**AP Knee**
Patient Preparation:	Remove any artifacts in the desired field (e.g., clothing with hooks, snaps, zippers).
Shielding:	Use gonadal shielding, if possible.
Film Selection:	8 × 10
Film Placement:	Place vertically on tabletop.
ID Placement:	ID should be in lower corner of collimation field.
Patient Placement:	The patient is seated on radiographic table with knee in full extension, foot forming 90-degree angle with lower leg, leg internally rotated 5 degrees.
Technique Selection:	kVp 60 to 65; mAs 20 to 40 (nongrid)
SID:	40″
Central Ray Placement:	The central ray is angled 5 degrees cephalic entering ½″ below the apex of the patella.
Collimation:	To film size.
Marker Placement:	Within the collimation field denoting the affected extremity.
Breathing Instructions:	Do not breathe. Do not move.
Anatomy Visualized:	AP projection of the knee.
Additional Information:	If the knee measures greater than 14 cm, the view should be performed using the Bucky.

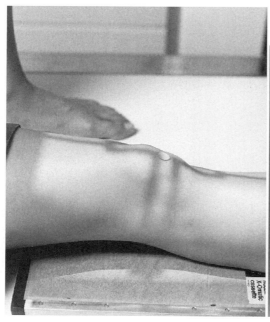 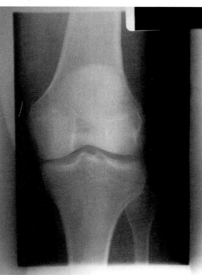

TABLE 3-7 cont'd

Lower Extremities

Position: Lateral Knee

Patient Preparation:	Remove any artifacts in the desired field (e.g., clothing with hooks, snaps, zippers).
Shielding:	Use gonadal shielding, if possible.
Film Selection:	8 × 10
Film Placement:	Place vertically on tabletop.
ID Placement:	ID should be in upper corner of collimation field.
Patient Placement:	The patient is in the lateral recumbent position on the radiographic table with the affected knee in contact with the table. The femur of the affected side is centered to the center of the table. Flex the knee 20 to 30 degrees so that femoral epicondyles are perpendicular to the table.
Technique Selection:	kVp 60 to 65; mAs 20 to 40 (nongrid)
SID:	40″
Central Ray Placement:	The central ray is directed 5 degrees cephalic entering 1″ distal to the medial epicondyle.
Collimation:	To film size.
Marker Placement:	Within the collimation field denoting the affected extremity.
Breathing Instructions:	Do not breathe. Do not move.
Anatomy Visualized:	Lateral projection of the knee joint, including the distal end of the femur, proximal end of the tibia and fibula, patella, and patellofemoral joint.
Additional Information:	Flexion of the knee should not exceed 30 degrees because further flexion tightens muscles and tendons, causing the patella to be drawn into the intercondylar sulcus. This may obscure diagnostic information, such as fat pad displacement resulting from effusion.

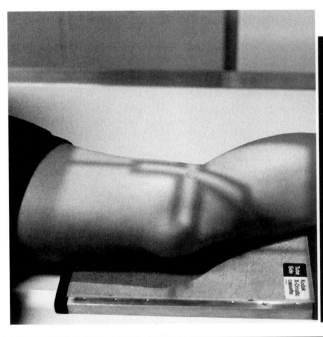
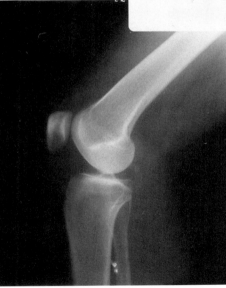

Continued

TABLE 3-7 cont'd
Lower Extremities

Position:	**Open Joint (Homblad method)**
Patient Preparation:	Remove any artifacts in the desired field (e.g., clothing with hooks, snaps, zippers).
Shielding:	Use gonadal shielding, if possible.
Film Selection:	8 × 10
Film Placement:	Place vertically on the tabletop.
ID Placement:	ID should be in upper corner of collimation field.
Patient Placement:	The patient is on the radiographic table on hands and knees, with affected leg slightly extended. The joint space is centered to the center of the cassette. The femur forms a 20-degree angle with the central ray.
Technique Selection:	kVp 65 to 70; mAs 20 to 40 (nongrid)
SID:	40″
Central Ray Placement:	The central ray is directed perpendicular to the popliteal fossa.
Collimation:	To film size.
Marker Placement:	Within the collimation field denoting the affected extremity.
Breathing Instructions:	Do not breathe. Do not move.
Anatomy Visualized:	Intercondylar fossa, medial and lateral intercondylar tubercles of the intercondylar eminence in profile.
Additional Information:	A variation to the mentioned positioning method is to have the patient standing with the affected knee flexed and placed on a stool, using a chair for support.
	This view is helpful in the evaluation for radiopaque loose bodies with the knee joint. It is also useful in evaluation of femoral condyles in entities such as osteochondritis dissecans.

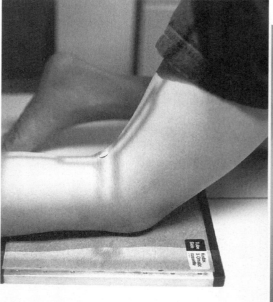
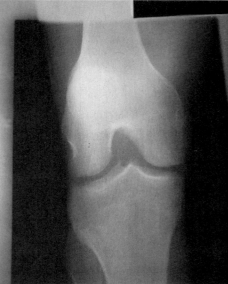

TABLE 3-7 cont'd

Lower Extremities

Position:	**Open Joint (Camp-Coventry Method)**
Patient Preparation:	Remove any artifacts in the desired field (e.g., clothing with hooks, snaps, zippers).
Shielding:	Use gonadal shielding, if possible.
Film Selection:	8 × 10
Film Placement:	Place vertically on the tabletop.
ID Placement:	ID should be in lower corner of collimation field.
Patient Placement:	The patient is in the prone position on the radiographic table with the knee flexed to a 40- to 45-degree angle resting the foot on support. The knee joint is centered to the middle of the cassette.
Technique Selection:	kVp 65 to 70; mAs 20 to 40 (nongrid)
SID:	40″
Central Ray Placement:	The central ray is angled caudally 40 to 45 degrees entering the popliteal fossa.
Collimation:	To film size.
Marker Placement:	Within the collimation field denoting the affected extremity.
Breathing Instructions:	Do not breathe. Do not move.
Anatomy Visualized:	Intercondylar fossa, medial and lateral intercondylar tubercles of the intercondylar eminence in profile.
Additional Information:	This view is an alternate to the Homblad method. It is used when the patient cannot bear weight on the affected knee.

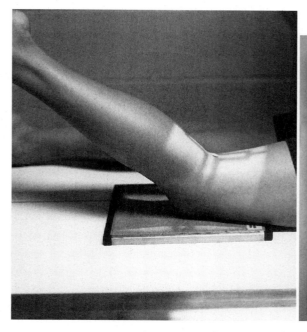 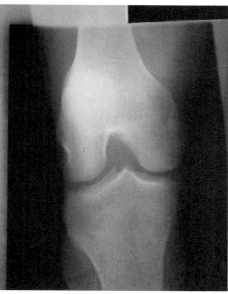

Continued

TABLE 3-7 cont'd

Lower Extremities

Position:	**Bilateral AP Weight Bearing**
Patient Preparation:	Remove any artifacts in the desired field (e.g., clothing with hooks, snaps, zippers).
Shielding:	Use gonadal shielding, if possible.
Film Selection:	14 × 17
Film Placement:	Place vertically in Bucky.
ID Placement:	ID should be in upper corner of collimation field.
Patient Placement:	The patient is standing in the AP position with knees centered to the Bucky. The toes point straight ahead, knees fully extended with weight equally distributed.
Technique Selection:	kVp 60 to 70; mAs 10 to 20
SID:	40"
Central Ray Placement:	The central ray is directed perpendicular to center of cassette midway between the knees at the level of the apices of the patellae.
Collimation:	To film size.
Marker Placement:	Within the collimation field denoting the patient's right or left side.
Breathing Instructions:	Do not breathe. Do not move.
Anatomy Visualized:	Evaluates joint spaces of both knees. Also useful in evaluation of varus and valgus deformities of the knee joint.
Additional Information:	This view is useful in evaluation of the arthritic knee. Weight-bearing studies reveal joint space narrowing that is not apparent on non–weight-bearing studies.

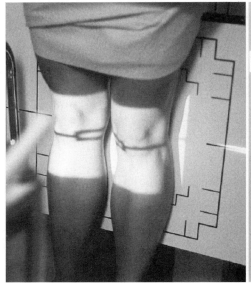
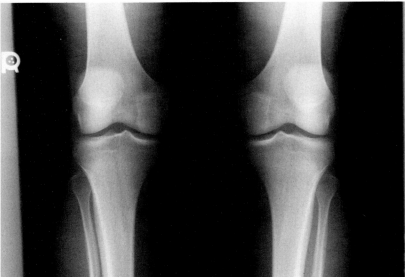

TABLE 3-7 cont'd

Lower Extremities

Position:	**Axial Patella (Settegast Method)**
Patient Preparation:	Remove any artifacts in the desired field (e.g., clothing with hooks, snaps, zippers).
Shielding:	Use gonadal shielding, if possible.
Film Selection:	8 × 10
Film Placement:	Place vertically on tabletop.
ID Placement:	ID should be in upper corner of collimation field.
Patient Placement:	The patient is in the prone position on the radiographic table. The knee is flexed to the patient's tolerance. The patella is centered to the middle of the cassette.
Technique Selection:	kVp 65 to 70; mAs 20 to 40 (nongrid)
SID:	40″
Central Ray Placement:	The central ray is angled 10 to 20 degrees cephalic to enter the patellofemoral joint.
Collimation:	To part size.
Marker Placement:	Within the collimation field denoting the affected extremity.
Breathing Instructions:	Do not breathe. Do not move.
Anatomy Visualized:	Axial view of the patella and patellofemoral joint, including the intercondylar sulcus in profile. Demonstrates vertical patella fractures.
Additional Information:	Extreme flexion of the knee should not be attempted until fractures of the patella have been ruled out.
	The degree of tube tilt is dependent on the degree of flexion present. Increase the tube tilt as the degree of knee flexion decreases.
	Quadriceps femoris is contracted in this view, pulling the patella into the intercondylar sulcus, making evaluation of patellar subluxation difficult. Suspected patellar subluxation warrants use of Merchant view.

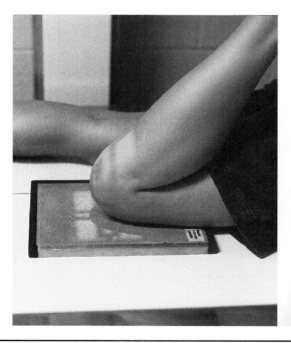
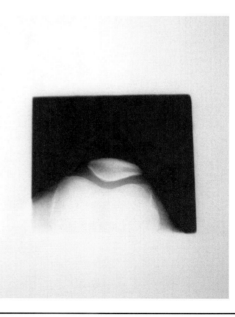

Continued

TABLE 3-7 cont'd
Lower Extremities

Position:	**Merchant View**
Patient Preparation:	Remove any artifacts in the desired field (e.g., clothing with hooks, snaps, zippers).
Shielding:	Use gonadal shielding, if possible.
Film Selection:	14 × 17
Film Placement:	Place cassette in Merchant holder.
ID Placement:	ID should be in upper corner of collimation field.
Patient Placement:	The patient is supine on the radiographic table with knees flexed 45 degrees over the edge of the table and resting on the Merchant board support. The knees are placed together and the legs are secured below the knee.
Technique Selection:	kVp 60 to 65; mAs 5 to 10 (nongrid)
SID:	40″
Central Ray Placement:	The central ray is angled 30 degrees caudal and enters midway between the patellae.
Collimation:	To film size.
Marker Placement:	Within the collimation field denoting either the left or right knee.
Breathing Instructions:	Do not breathe. Do not move.
Anatomy Visualized:	Bilateral axial projection of the patellae. Patellofemoral joint space without distortion of quadriceps femoris contraction.
Additional Information:	The quadriceps femoris muscles must be relaxed to aid in accurate diagnosis of patellar subluxation.

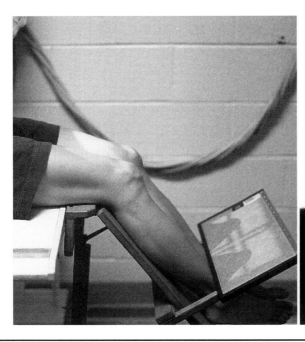
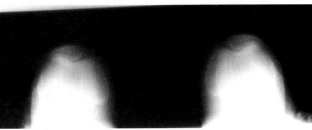

TABLE 3-7 cont'd
Lower Extremities

Position:	**PA Patella**
Patient Preparation:	Remove any artifacts in the desired field (e.g., clothing with hooks, snaps, zippers).
Shielding:	Use gonadal shielding, if possible.
Film Selection:	8 × 10
Film Placement:	Place vertically on tabletop.
ID Placement:	ID should be in upper corner of collimation field.
Patient Placement:	The patient is in the prone position on the radiographic table. Center the patella to the middle of the cassette.
Technique Selection:	kVp 64 to 68; mAs 20 to 40 (nongrid)
SID:	40″
Central Ray Placement:	The central ray is directed perpendicular to the popliteal fossa, passing through the patella.
Collimation:	To part size.
Marker Placement:	Within the collimation field denoting the affected extremity.
Breathing Instructions:	Do not breathe. Do not move.
Anatomy Visualized:	PA projection of the knee with improved demonstration of the patella than in the AP knee view.
Additional Information:	If suspected fraction of the patella is present, do not place patella directly on cassette. Place support under the femur to elevate patella slightly, decreasing pressure on the patella.

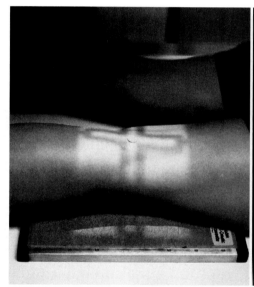 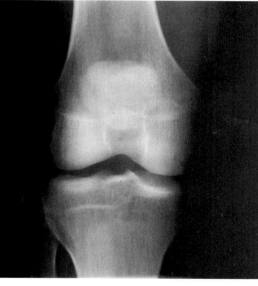

Continued

TABLE 3-7 cont'd
Lower Extremities

Position:	**Lateral Patella**
Patient Preparation:	Remove any artifacts in the desired field (e.g., clothing with hooks, snaps, zippers).
Shielding:	Place lead apron over patient's pelvic area.
Film Selection:	8 × 10
Film Placement:	Place vertically on tabletop.
ID Placement:	ID should be in lower corner of collimation field.
Patient Placement:	The patient is in the lateral recumbent position with affected patella in contact with the cassette. Center the patella to the midline of the cassette with knee flexed 20 to 30 degrees so that the femoral epicondyles are perpendicular to the cassette.
Technique Selection:	kVp 56 to 62; mAs 20 to 40 (nongrid)
SID:	40″
Central Ray Placement:	The central ray is directed perpendicular to the film entering the patellofemoral joint space.
Collimation:	To part size.
Marker Placement:	Within the collimation field denoting the affected extremity.
Breathing Instructions:	Do not breathe. Do not move.
Anatomy Visualized:	Lateral projection of the patella and patellofemoral joint space.
Additional Information:	If there is a suspected fracture of the patella, decrease knee flexion to 5 to 10 degrees to avoid fracture fragment displacement.

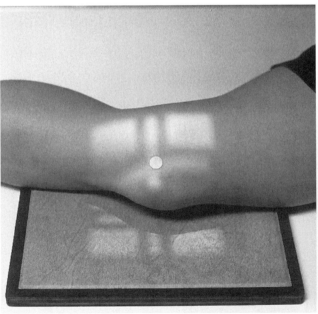
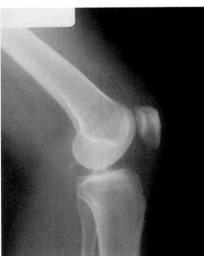

TABLE 3-7 cont'd
Lower Extremities

Routine Lower Leg: AP and Lateral

Position:	**AP Leg**
Patient Preparation:	Remove any artifacts in the desired field (e.g., clothing with hooks, snaps, zippers).
Shielding:	Place apron over pelvic area.
Film Selection:	7 × 17 or one half of 14 × 17.
Film Placement:	Place vertically on tabletop.
ID Placement:	ID should be in corner away from the joint of interest.
Patient Placement:	The patient is in the supine position on the table with leg in full extension, foot forming 90-degree angle with lower leg, leg rotated internally 5 degrees.
	The joint closest to injury must be included. The long axis of the lower leg is centered to the cassette.
Technique Selection:	kVp 60 to 65; mAs 3 to 5 (nongrid)
SID:	40″
Central Ray Placement:	The central ray is directed perpendicular to the midshaft of the tibia.
Collimation:	To film size.
Marker Placement:	Within the collimation field denoting the affected extremity.
Breathing Instructions:	Do not breathe. Do not move.
Anatomy Visualized:	AP projection of the tibia and fibula.
Additional Information:	If possible, both joints should be included. If not, the joint closest to the injury must be included.
	A sandbag may be placed against the foot to stabilize the leg.
	If a fracture of the distal leg is discovered, it is important o include the proximal tibiofibular joint because it is common to have an accompanying fracture at this site as well.

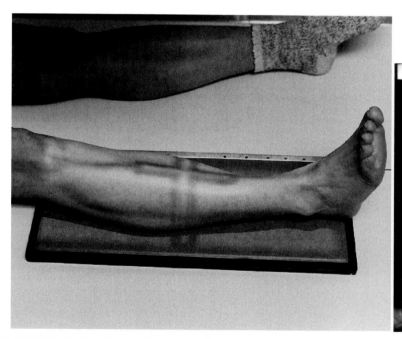

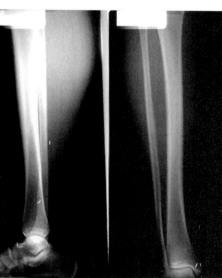

Continued

TABLE 3-7 cont'd
Lower Extremities

Position:	**Lateral Lower Leg**
Patient Preparation:	Remove any artifacts in the desired field (e.g., clothing with hooks, snaps, zippers).
Shielding:	Place apron over pelvic area.
Film Selection:	7 × 17 or one half of 14 × 17.
Film Placement:	Place vertically on tabletop.
ID Placement:	ID should be in corner of cassette that is away from the joint of interest.
Patient Placement:	The patient is in the lateral recumbent position on the table with the affected leg closest to the cassette. The long axis of the lower leg is centered to the long axis of the cassette. The foot forms a 90-degree angle with the lower leg.
Technique Selection:	kVp 60 to 65; mAs 3 to 5 (nongrid)
SID:	40″
Central Ray Placement:	The central ray is perpendicular to the midshaft of the tibia.
Collimation:	To film size.
Marker Placement:	Within the collimation field denoting the affected extremity.
Breathing Instructions:	Do not breathe. Do not move.
Anatomy Visualized:	Lateral projection of the tibia and fibula.

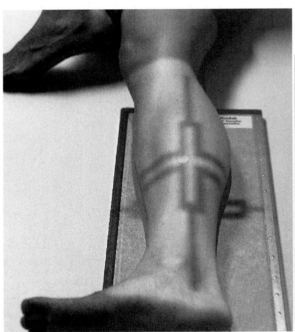 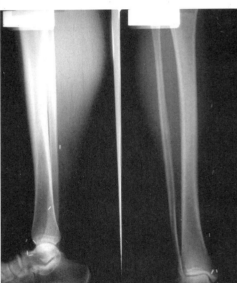

TABLE 3-7 cont'd
Lower Extremities

Routine Ankle: AP, Oblique, and Lateral

Position:	**AP Ankle**
Patient Preparation:	Remove any artifacts in the desired field (e.g., clothing with hooks, snaps, zippers).
Shielding:	Place apron over pelvic area.
Film Selection:	10 × 12
Film Placement:	Place horizontally on tabletop.
ID Placement:	ID should be in lower corner of cassette.
Patient Placement:	The patient is supine on table with leg in full extension, foot forming 90-degree angle with lower leg, leg rotated internally 5 degrees. Center the ankle joint to the center of one half of the 10 × 12 cassette.
Technique Selection:	kVp 65 to 70; mAs 15 to 30 (nongrid)
SID:	40″
Central Ray Placement:	The central ray is perpendicular to the cassette entering the ankle joint.
Collimation:	To one half film size.
Marker Placement:	Within the collimation field denoting the affected extremity.
Breathing Instructions:	Do not breathe. Do not move.
Anatomy Visualized:	AP projection of the ankle joint, including the distal tibia and fibula and proximal talus.
Additional Information:	The lateral portion of the ankle mortise does not appear open on a true AP ankle because the malleoli are not equidistant from the film in this position. If the lateral portion of the mortise joint appears open on this view, it is indicative of a spread of the ankle mortise resultant of ruptured ligaments.

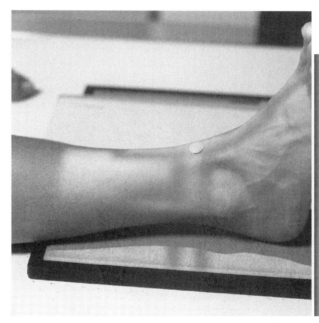
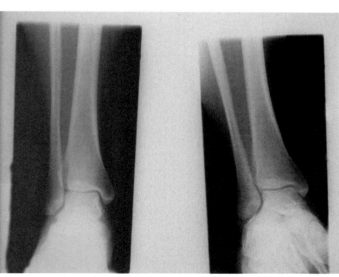

Continued

PART ONE

TABLE 3-7 cont'd
Lower Extremities

Position:	Oblique Ankle (Mortise View)
Patient Preparation:	Remove any artifacts in the desired field (e.g., clothing with hooks, snaps, zippers).
Shielding:	Place apron over pelvic area.
Film Selection:	10 × 12
Film Placement:	Place horizontally on tabletop.
ID Placement:	ID should be in upper corner of cassette.
Patient Placement:	The patient is supine on the table with leg fully extended. Internally rotate the leg 15 to 20 degrees so that intermalleolar plane is parallel to the cassette. Dorsiflex the foot. Center the ankle joint to the second half of the 10 × 12 used for the AP ankle.
Technique Selection:	kVp 65 to 70; mAs 15 to 30 (nongrid)
SID:	40″
Central Ray Placement:	The central ray is perpendicular to the cassette entering the ankle joint.
Collimation:	To one half of the film size.
Marker Placement:	Within the collimation field denoting the affected extremity.
Breathing Instructions:	Do not breathe. Do not move.
Anatomy Visualized:	Ankle mortise without superimposition of the lateral malleolus on the talus.
Additional Information:	In cases of suspected ligament ruptures or instability, a stress view may be accomplished.

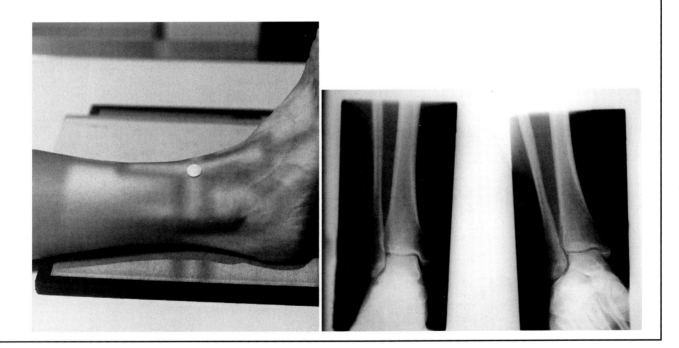

TABLE 3-7 cont'd
Lower Extremities

Position:	**Lateral Ankle**
Patient Preparation:	Remove any artifacts in the desired field (e.g., clothing with hooks, snaps, zippers).
Shielding:	Place apron over pelvic area.
Film Selection:	8 × 10
Film Placement:	Place vertically on tabletop.
ID Placement:	ID should be in upper corner of collimation field.
Patient Placement:	The patient is in the lateral recumbent position on the table with the affected ankle closest to the cassette. Center the affected ankle to the midline of the cassette in a true lateral position with foot in dorsiflexion.
Technique Selection:	kVp 65 to 70; mAs 15 to 30 (nongrid)
SID:	40″
Central Ray Placement:	The central ray is perpendicular to the cassette entering the medial side of the ankle joint.
Collimation:	To film size.
Marker Placement:	Within the collimation field denoting the affected extremity.
Breathing Instructions:	Do not breathe. Do not move.
Anatomy Visualized:	Lateral projection of the ankle joint to include the distal tibia and fibula, proximal talus, calcaneus, and the base of the fifth metatarsal.
Additional Information:	The base of the fifth metatarsal should be included on this view because this is a common area of fracture in ankle inversion injuries.

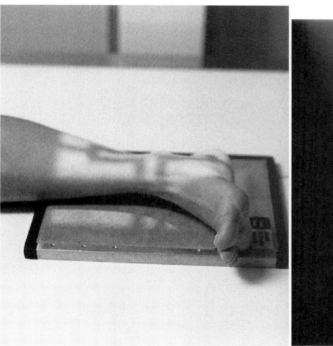 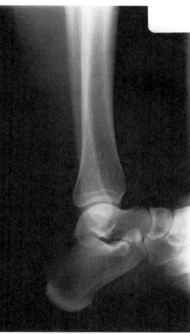

Continued

TABLE 3-7 cont'd
Lower Extremities

Position:	**AP Ankle Inversion Stress**
Patient Preparation:	Remove any artifacts in the desired field (e.g., clothing with hooks, snaps, zippers).
Shielding:	Place apron over pelvic area.
Film Selection:	10 × 12
Film Placement:	Place vertically on tabletop.
ID Placement:	ID should be in upper corner of cassette.
Patient Placement:	The patient is supine of the table with leg in full extension. Center the ankle joint to the center of the cassette. With the doctor wearing lead gloves, the lower leg is stabilized and with the opposite hand, inversion stress is applied to the ankle.
Technique Selection:	kVp 65 to 70; mAs 15 to 30 (nongrid)
SID:	40″
Central Ray Placement:	The central ray is perpendicular to the cassette entering the ankle joint.
Collimation:	To film size.
Marker Placement:	Within the collimation field denoting the affected extremity.
Breathing Instructions:	Do not breathe. Do not move.
Anatomy Visualized:	Ankle joint for evaluation of joint separation as a result of ligament rupture or tear.
Additional Information:	Stress should only be applied by a physician because further damage to ligaments may occur if too great a stress is applied.

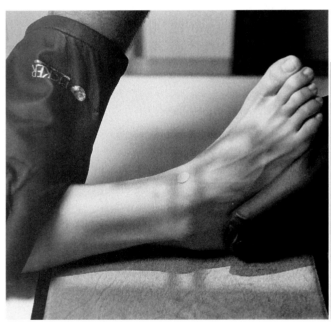
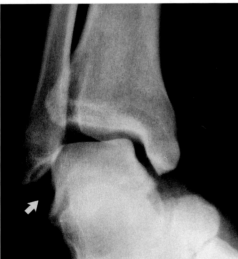

From Ballinger PW, Frank ED: Merril's atlas of radiographic positions and radiologic procedures, ed 10, St Louis, 2003, Mosby.

TABLE 3-7 cont'd

Lower Extremities

Routine Foot: AP, Oblique, and Lateral

Position:	**AP Foot**
Patient Preparation:	Remove any artifacts in the desired field (e.g., clothing with hooks, snaps, zippers).
Shielding:	Place apron over pelvic area.
Film Selection:	10 × 12
Film Placement:	Place vertically on tabletop.
ID Placement:	ID should be in corner of cassette closest to calcaneus.
Patient Placement:	The patient is supine on the table with the knee flexed and the plantar surface of the affected foot flat on one half of the cassette. The foot should be placed to include the toes.
Technique Selection:	kVp 60 to 65; mAs 15 to 30 (nongrid)
SID:	40″
Central Ray Placement:	The central ray is directed perpendicular to the long axis of the metatarsals (5 to 20 degrees) entering the base of the third metatarsal.
Collimation:	To half of the film size.
Marker Placement:	Within the collimation field denoting the affected extremity.
Breathing Instructions:	Do not breathe. Do not move.
Anatomy Visualized:	AP projection of the tarsals anterior to the talus, metatarsals, and phalanges.
Additional Information:	The pes planus or pes cavus of the foot determines the degree of tube tilt. A filter may be used to increase the radiographic quality of the phalanges. It is placed so that it covers the phalanges from the tips to the first metatarsophalangeal joint.

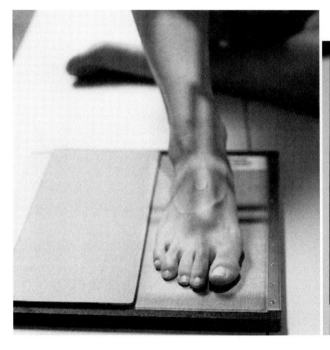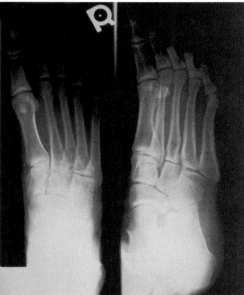

Continued

TABLE 3-7 cont'd
Lower Extremities

Position:	**Medial Oblique Foot**
Patient Preparation:	Remove any artifacts in the desired field (e.g., clothing with hooks, snaps, zippers).
Shielding:	Place apron over pelvic area.
Film Selection:	10 × 12
Film Placement:	Place vertically on tabletop.
ID Placement:	ID should be in corner of cassette nearest the calcaneus.
Patient Placement:	The patient is supine on the table with the knee flexed and the plantar surface of the affected foot flat on the cassette. Internally rotate the foot until the plantar surface forms a 30-degree angle to the cassette. The foot is centered to the center of the second half of the cassette used with the AP Ankle view. The toes must be included in this view.
Technique Selection:	kVp 60 to 65; mAs 15 to 30 (nongrid)
SID:	40″
Central Ray Placement:	The central ray is perpendicular to the long axis of the metatarsals (5 to 20 degrees) entering the base of the third metatarsal.
Collimation:	To one half of the film size.
Marker Placement:	Within the collimation field denoting the affected extremity.
Breathing Instructions:	Do not breathe. Do not move.
Anatomy Visualized:	Joint spaces of the cuboid articulations, joint space between the navicular and the talus, and oblique projection of the metatarsals and phalanges to include the tuberosity of the base of the fifth metatarsal. The sinus tarsus is well demonstrated on this view.
Additional Information:	Increasing the obliquity of the foot to 45 degrees may better demonstrate separation at the bases of the second to fifth metatarsals and in individual tarsals.
	A filter may be used to increase the radiographic quality of the phalanges. It is placed so that it covers the phalanges from the tips to the first joint.

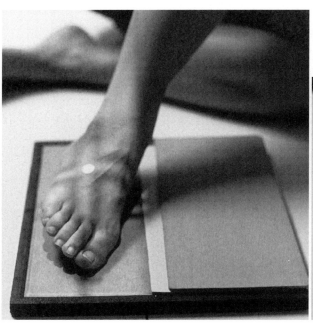
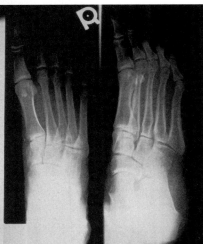

TABLE 3-7 cont'd

Lower Extremities

Position:	**Lateral Foot**
Patient Preparation:	Remove any artifacts in the desired field (e.g., clothing with hooks, snaps, zippers).
Shielding:	Place apron over pelvic area.
Film Selection:	8 × 10
Film Placement:	Place on tabletop.
ID Placement:	ID should be in corner of cassette opposite toes and calcaneus.
Patient Placement:	The patient is in the lateral recumbent position on table with affected side closest to cassette. Center the foot to the midline of the film in the true lateral position with the foot in dorsiflexion. The lower leg should be in the same plane as the foot.
Technique Selection:	kVp 60 to 65; mAs 15 to 30 (nongrid)
SID:	40″
Central Ray Placement:	The central ray is perpendicular to the cassette entering the first cuneiform.
Collimation:	To part size.
Marker Placement:	Within the collimation field denoting the affected extremity.
Breathing Instructions:	Do not breathe. Do not move.
Anatomy Visualized:	Lateral projection of the foot, ankle joint, and distal tibia and fibula.
Additional Information:	The cassette may be angled to accommodate the size of the foot, or a 10 × 12 cassette may be substituted.

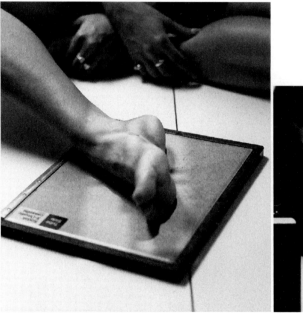
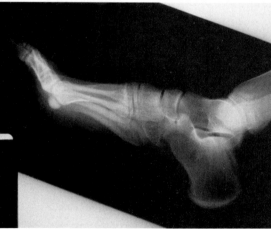

Continued

TABLE 3-7 cont'd
Lower Extremities

Routine Calcaneus: Axial and Lateral

Position:	**Axial Calcaneus**
Patient Preparation:	Remove any artifacts in the desired field (e.g., clothing with hooks, snaps, zippers).
Shielding:	Place apron over pelvic area.
Film Selection:	8 × 10
Film Placement:	Place horizontally on tabletop.
ID Placement:	ID should be in the corner of the cassette containing this view.
Patient Placement:	The patient is supine on the table with the leg in full extension. The foot is dorsiflexed as far as the patient is able to flex. The patient may loop a strap around the toes to assist in dorsiflexion. Center the calcaneus to the center of one half of the cassette.
Technique Selection:	kVp 65 to 70; mAs 15 to 30 (nongrid)
SID:	40″
Central Ray Placement:	The central ray is angled 35 to 45 degrees cephalically, entering the level of the talocalcaneal joint.
Collimation:	To one half of the film size.
Marker Placement:	Within the collimation field denoting the affected extremity.
Breathing Instructions:	Do not breathe. Do not move.
Anatomy Visualized:	Axial projection of the calcaneus from the tuberosity to the talocalcaneal joint. The sustentaculum tali appear in profile.
Additional Information:	It is important to avoid rotation of the ankle. The base of the first or the fifth metatarsals should not be visible on either side.

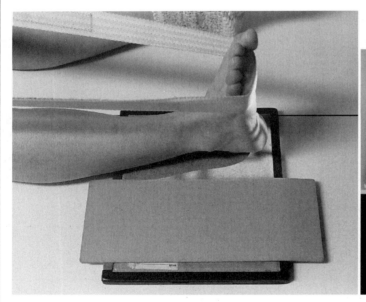
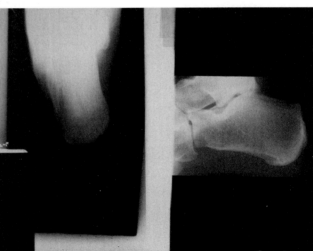

TABLE 3-7 cont'd

Lower Extremities

Position:	**Lateral Calcaneus**
Patient Preparation:	Remove any artifacts in the desired field (e.g., clothing with hooks, snaps, zippers).
Shielding:	Place apron over pelvic area.
Film Selection:	8 × 10
Film Placement:	Place horizontally on tabletop.
ID Placement:	ID should appear on one half of film containing axial calcaneus.
Patient Placement:	The patient is in the lateral recumbent position with the affected calcaneus centered to one half of the cassette. The leg is in full extension with the foot forming a 90-degree angle with the lower leg.
Technique Selection:	kVp 65 to 70; mAs 15 to 30 (nongrid)
SID:	40″
Central Ray Placement:	The central ray is directed perpendicularly entering 1″ below the medial malleolus.
Collimation:	To one half of the film size.
Marker Placement:	Within the collimation field denoting the affected extremity.
Breathing Instructions:	Do not breathe. Do not move.
Anatomy Visualized:	This view demonstrates the lateral projection of the calcaneus to include the calcaneocuboid and talonavicular joint spaces.
Additional Information:	The axial calcaneus is placed on the other side of the film.

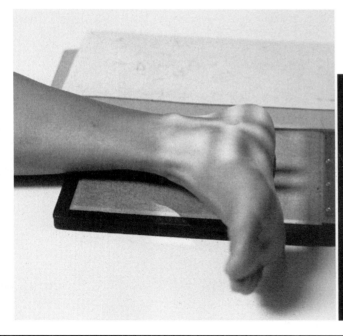
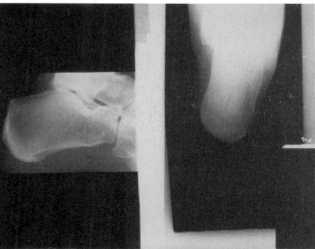

AP, Anteroposterior; *ID,* identification; *PA,* posteroanterior; *SID,* source-to-image distance.

chapter 4

Roentgenometrics

DENNIS M. MARCHIORI

Roentgenometrics play an important role in film interpretation by allowing quantification of observed structural and biomechanical alterations. The importance of roentgenometrics in cases of scoliosis, spinal instability, and so on cannot be overstated. Because many sources of measurement error and anatomic variation exist, results should be interpreted in light of clinical data. The reliability, validity, and clinical usefulness of each measure should be considered. However, when carefully used, roentgenometrics provide a useful tool for image interpretation.

The measures listed in Tables 4-1 through 4-4 are stratified by anatomic location.

TABLE 4-1
Skull Measures

Description	Significance
Basilar angle On the lateral skull or cervical projection, two lines are drawn. The first connects the frontal–nasal junction (nasion) to the center of the sella turcica. The second connects the anterior margin of the foramen magnum (basion) with the center of the sella turcica. The angle of intersection $(x°)$ should not exceed 152 degrees, with a minimum value of 137 degrees (Fig. 4-1).	Abnormally high angle measurements indicate an elevation of the skull base in relation to the anterior portion of the skull. This occurs with basilar invagination/impression secondary to congenital bone deformity or acquired bone softening disease (e.g., Paget's disease, fibrous dysplasia).
Chamberlain's line On the lateral skull or cervical projection a line is drawn from the posterior aspect of the hard palate to the posterior aspect of the foramen magnum (opisthion). The tip of the odontoid should not extend more than 7 mm above the line (x) (Fig. 4-2).	Elevation of the odontoid tip suggests basilar invagination/ impression or upward deformity of the skull base. This may occur secondary to congenital or acquired bone softening disorders (e.g., Paget's disease, fibrous dysplasia).
Digastric line On the frontal skull or cervical projection a line is drawn connecting the right and left digastric grooves (just medial to the mastoid processes). The tip of the odontoid should not project above this line (Fig. 4-3).	Elevation of the odontoid tip suggests basilar impression or upward deformity of the skull base. This may occur secondary to congenital or acquired bone softening disorders (e.g., Paget's disease, fibrous dysplasia).
McGregor's line On the lateral skull or cervical projection a line is drawn from the posterior aspect of the hard palate to the inferior surface of the occiput. The tip of the odontoid should be below the line (x) and is always abnormal if it extends more than 8 mm above the line in men and 10 mm in women (Fig. 4-4).	Elevation of the odontoid tip suggests basilar impression or upward deformity of the skull base. This may occur secondary to congenital or acquired bone softening disorders (e.g., Paget's disease, fibrous dysplasia). McGregor's method is considered the best method to assess for basilar impression.
McRae's line On the lateral skull or cervical projection a line is drawn between the anterior (basion) and posterior (opisthion) margin of the foramen magnum. The posterior portion of the occiput should be below this line. In addition, a vertical line extended from the tip of the odontoid process should intersect in the anterior fourth of the foramen magnum line (Fig. 4-5).	If the posterior occiput is convex upward or extends above the foramen magnum line, an upward deformity of the skull surrounding the foramen magnum is present. This occurs with basilar impression secondary to congenital or acquired bone softening disorders (e.g., Paget's disease, fibrous dysplasia). If the tip of the odontoid is found posterior to the anterior fourth of the foramen magnum line, fracture or dislocation is suspected.

Continued

175

TABLE 4-1 cont'd
Skull Measures

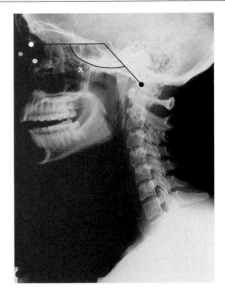

FIG. 4-1

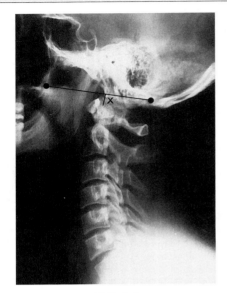

FIG. 4-2

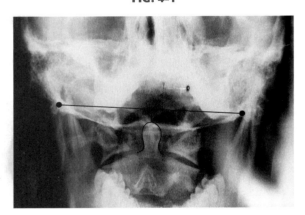

FIG. 4-3

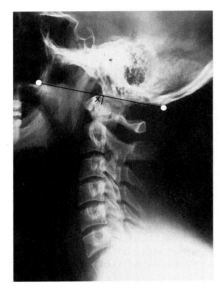

FIG. 4-4

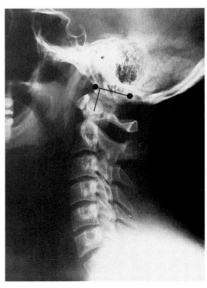

FIG. 4-5

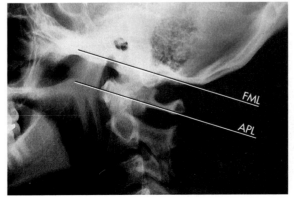

FIG. 4-6

TABLE 4-1 cont'd

Skull Measures

Description	Significance
Occipitoatlantal alignment On the lateral skull or cervical projection, two lines are constructed: a foramen magnum line (FML) is drawn along the inferior margin of the occiput, and an atlas plane line (APL) is drawn through the center of the anterior tubercle and the narrowest portion of the posterior arch of atlas. The FML and APL should be parallel (Fig. 4-6).	Divergence of the FML and APL anteriorly suggests anterior-superior malposition of the occiput. Divergence of the lines posteriorly suggests posterior-superior malposition of the occiput.
On the frontal open-mouth cervical projection, two lines are constructed: a transverse condylar line (TCL) is drawn connecting the grooves on the medial aspect of the mastoid processes bilaterally, and a transverse atlas line (TAL) is drawn connecting the lower junctions of the transverse processes and the lateral masses. The TCL and TAL should be parallel (Fig. 4-7).	Divergence of the TCL and TAL to the right suggests right occiput laterality. Divergence of the TCL and TAL to the left suggests left occiput laterality.
On the frontal open-mouth cervical projection, atlas rotational malposition is suggested by asymmetry in the width of the lateral masses. Occiput rotation is assumed to occur opposite atlas rotation.	The lateral mass with the wider measure is the side with anterior rotation of the atlas and posterior rotation of the occiput. Often the medial margin of the anteriorly rotated lateral mass appears more radiopaque.
Sella turcica size In the lateral skull projection (40 inches focal film distance [FFD]), the greatest horizontal dimension of the sella turcica should not exceed 16 mm, and the depth should not exceed 12 mm (Fig. 4-8).	An enlarged sella turcica may represent a normal variant or suggest the presence of a space-occupying lesion or condition (e.g., pituitary tumor, carotid aneurysm, and empty sella syndrome)

TABLE 4-2

Spine Measures

Description	Significance
Atlantoaxial "overhang" sign On the anteroposterior open-mouth projection the lateral margin of the lateral masses of atlas should not appear more lateral than the superior articular processes of the axis (Fig. 4-9).	Lateral displacement suggests fracture (atlas or odontoid process) or dislocation. A mild degree of "overhanging" of the atlas may be a normal variant in children.
Atlantodental interval (ADI) On the lateral cervical projection the distance (x) between the posterior surface of the anterior tubercle of the atlas and the anterior surface of the odontoid process of the axis should not exceed 3 mm in adults and 5 mm in children. The flexion lateral projection places the most stress on the atlantoaxial joint and would be most likely to reveal an abnormality. The ADI may appear V-shaped. In such cases the smallest portion of the joint space should be measured to limit false-positives (Fig. 4-10).	An enlarged atlantodental interval may result from congenital absence or weakness of the transverse atlantal ligament (e.g., Down syndrome, Morquio's syndrome, Larsen syndrome), trauma, infection, or an inflammatory arthritide (e.g., rheumatoid arthritis, ankylosing spondylitis).
Atlas alignment On the lateral cervical projection, two lines are constructed. An atlas plane line (APL) is drawn through the anterior tubercle and the narrowest portion of the posterior arch. Next an odontoid line (OL) is drawn to bisect the odontoid process. It is thought a line drawn perpendicular to the odontoid line (odontoid perpendicular line [OPL]) should be parallel to the APL (Fig. 4-11).	Anterior divergence of the lines suggests an anterior-superior malposition of the atlas in relation to the axis. Anterior convergence of the lines suggests an anterior-inferior malposition of the atlas.

Continued

TABLE 4-2 cont'd
Spine Measures

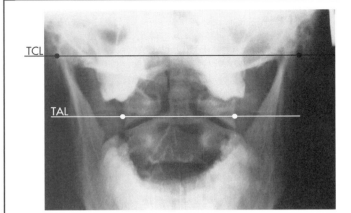

FIG. 4-7

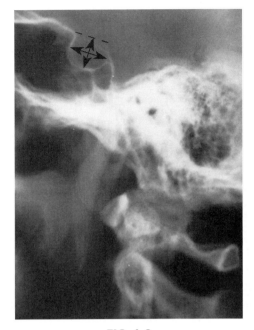

FIG. 4-8

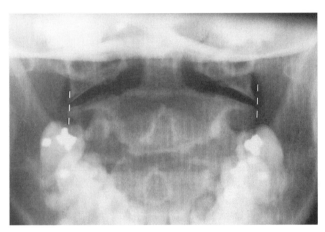

FIG. 4-9

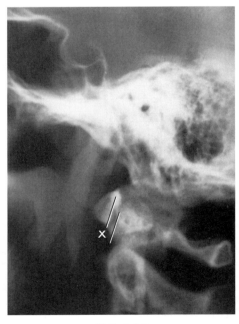

FIG. 4-10

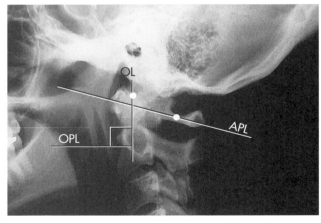

FIG. 4-11

TABLE 4-2 cont'd

Spine Measures

Description	Significance
Atlas alignment cont'd On the frontal open-mouth cervical projection, two lines are constructed: a transverse atlas line (TAL) is drawn connecting the lower junction of the transverse processes and the lateral masses, and an axis plane line (AxPL) is drawn between the lamina–pedicle junctions bilaterally. The TAL and AxPL should be parallel (Fig. 4-12).	Right atlas lateral malposition is suggested if the TAL and AxPL diverge to the right. Left atlas lateral malposition is suggested if the TAL and AxPL diverge to the left.
On the frontal open-mouth cervical projection, atlas rotational malposition is suggested by asymmetry in the width of the lateral masses (Fig. 4-13).	The lateral mass with the wider measure is the side with anterior rotation. Often the medial margin of the anteriorly rotated lateral mass appears more radiopaque.
Cervical gravity line In the lateral cervical projection, a vertical line drawn from the tip of the odontoid should intersect the seventh cervical vertebral body (Fig. 4-14).	An anterior weight-bearing posture is noted if the line is found anterior to C7 (as shown in figure), and a posterior weight-bearing posture is noted if the line is behind C7.
Cervical Jackson's stress lines On the lateral cervical flexion and extension projections, lines are drawn along the posterior aspect of C2 and C7. The posterior body lines should intersect the C5-C6 intervertebral disc space on the flexion film and C4-C5 intervertebral disc space on the extension film (Figs. 4-15 and 4-16).	The intersection of the lines is postulated to occur at the levels of greatest stress. Degeneration, muscle spasm, aberrant intersegmental mechanics, and other conditions may alter the levels of intersection.
Cervical lordosis *Harrison posterior tangent methods* On the lateral cervical projection, lines are drawn along the posterior body of C2 and a second line is drawn along the posterior body of C7. The superior or inferior angle of intersection $(x°)$ is measured as the cervical lordosis. Another application of the posterior tangent lines employs a comparison of lines of adjacent segments, yielding a measure of relative rotational angles. Normative values for such are found in the related literature (Fig. 4-17).	The average value of the cervical curvature from C2 to C7 using these methods is 34 degrees with a standard deviation of 9 degrees as reported by Harrison and others (1996). This method can be extended to the thoracic or lumbar regions.
Visual assessment On the lateral cervical projection a subjective appraisal of the cervical curve is made. Well-maintained anterior convexity is lordosis, exaggerated anterior convexity is hyperlordosis, slight anterior convexity is hypolordosis, lack of curvature is alordotic, and posterior convexity is kyphosis.	Altered cervical lordosis may be caused by factors such as trauma, degeneration, muscle spasm, and aberrant intersegmental mechanics.
Depth method On the lateral cervical projection a line is drawn from the tip of the odontoid process to the posterior surface of C7. A horizontal measure is taken from the vertical line to the posterior surface of the C4 body $(x°)$. The average depth is 12 mm. (Fig. 4-18)	Negative values indicate kyphosis, and large values indicate hyperlordosis. The depth method provides a more accurate assessment of cervical lordosis than the angle method. Lower measurements may result from factors such as trauma, degeneration, muscle spasm, and aberrant intersegmental mechanics.
Angle of curve On the lateral cervical projection a line is drawn connecting the anterior and posterior tubercles of the atlas, and a second line is drawn along the inferior endplate of C7. Perpendicular lines are drawn from the atlas and C7 lines, and their angle of intersection is recorded as the cervical lordosis $(x°)$. The average value is 40 degrees, although a variety of average values has been reported in the literature (Fig. 4-18).	Negative values indicate kyphosis, and large values indicate hyperlordosis. This method of measuring cervical lordosis is more common but less accurate than the depth method. Because the measurements depend only on C1 and C7, a kyphotic curve with compensatory extension of C1 has the false measurement of a lordotic curve. Reduced cervical curvature may be caused by factors such as trauma, degeneration, muscle spasm, and aberrant intersegmental mechanics.

Continued

TABLE 4-2 cont'd
Spine Measures

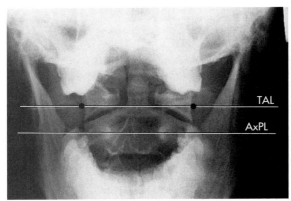

FIG. 4-12

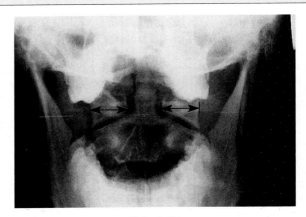

FIG. 4-13

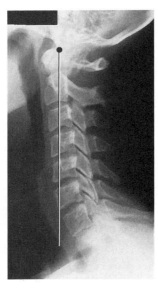

FIG. 4-14

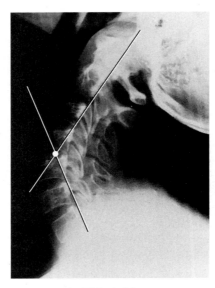

FIG. 4-15

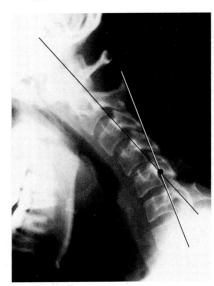

FIG. 4-16

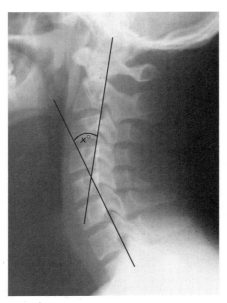

FIG. 4-17

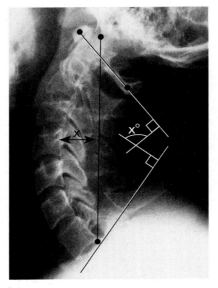

FIG. 4-18

TABLE 4-2 cont'd

Spine Measures

Description	Significance
Harrison modified Risser-Ferguson method (cervical spine) On the anteroposterior (AP) cervical radiograph, the narrow waists of the articular pillars are used to find the center of the vertebrae. Second, the spinous–lamina junctions are identified. The centrad for each vertebra is found by bisecting these two points on the segment. Next best-fit lines are constructed from C2 to the lowest visible thoracic vertebra. The angle of intersection of the best-fit line of the upper cervical vertebrae and the best-fit line of the lower cervical and upper thoracic vertebrae is measured as the cervical dorsal (CD) angle. In addition, the angle created by the best-fit line of the lower cervical and upper thoracic vertebrae and a true vertical line create a lateral flexion angle termed R_z^{T1-T4}. These lines and angles have been studied for reliability, yielding intraclass correlations in the good-to-excellent range with low mean absolute value of observer differences (see Harrison, 2002) (Fig. 4-19).	The Harrison modified Riser-Ferguson method for measurement of the AP cervical regions is based on the location of the two-dimensional center of mass of each vertebra. The resultant CD angle provides information of spinal distortion in a sagittal plane. The benefit of this method is that it accounts for both axial rotation and lateral bending displacements of vertebra. It can be applied to the cervical, thoracic, or lumbar region. The R_z^{T1-T4} angle is a measurement of lateral bending of the upper dorsal region.
Cervical prevertebral soft tissues On the lateral cervical projection the distance between the anterior aspect of C2 and the pharyngeal air shadow should not exceed 5 mm, and the distance between C6 and the tracheal air shadow should not exceed 20 mm (Fig. 4-20).	Posttraumatic hematoma, tumor, abscess, or other space-occupying lesion of the prevertebral space may distend these measures beyond their normal values.
Cervical spinal canal On the lateral cervical projection the horizontal width of the spinal canal between the posterior surface of the vertebral body (or odontoid) and the spinolaminar line should be at least 16 mm at C1, 14 mm at C2, 13 mm at C3, and 12 mm at C4-C7. (These measurements are for adults.) (Fig. 4-21.)	Sagittal canal widths less than these values indicate spinal canal stenosis. Spinal stenosis is more accurately assessed on the axial images provided by magnetic resonance imaging (MRI) or computed tomography (CT).
Cervical spinolaminar line On the lateral cervical projection a curvilinear line is drawn along the spinous process and lamina junctions. The curve should have a smooth contour without segmental disruption (Fig. 4-22).	Disruption is caused by segmental anterolisthesis or retrolisthesis. Disruptions at multiple consecutive levels may be caused by normal flexion and extension patterns. Care should be taken not to interpret this as abnormal.
Cervical, thoracic, and lumbar endplate lines On the lateral cervical projection, lines are drawn along the inferior endplate of the C2-T1 vertebrae and extended posteriorly to the cervical spine. The cervical endplate lines should all intersect at a common point located posterior to the spine (Fig. 4-23).	Lack of convergence suggests alterations in the normal lordotic cervical spine curve or intersegmental malpositions. Lines that cross closely to the spine suggest extension malposition of the superior segment. Lines that diverge sharply suggest flexion malposition of the superior segment.
On the frontal cervical, thoracic, and lumbar projections, lines are drawn to approximate the inferior vertebral endplates. The lines at adjacent levels should be parallel (Fig. 4-24).	Divergence of the endplate lines drawn on the frontal projection suggests lateral flexion malposition opposite the side of divergence.
Cervical, thoracic, and lumbar vertebral rotation *Body width method* On the frontal cervical, thoracic, and lumbar projections, the distance from the lateral margins of the vertebral bodies to the origin of the spinous process (*a* and *b*) should be equal bilaterally (Fig. 4-25).	If the distances from the base of the spinous process to the lateral margins of the vertebra are not equal, vertebral rotation is suggested, with spinous process deviation to the side of the smaller distance. A better analysis of vertebral rotation would probably incorporate the rotation of the vertebra above and below the segment in question. For instance, if a vertebra demonstrates 5 mm rotation to the right, and the segment below demonstrates 7 mm rotation to the right, the first segment demonstrates 2 mm of relative rotation to the left. Analysis of relative rotation attempts to limit spurious measurements of vertebral rotation caused by errors in patient positioning.

Continued

TABLE 4-2 cont'd
Spine Measures

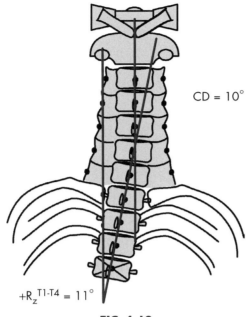

$CD = 10°$

$+R_z^{T1\text{-}T4} = 11°$

FIG. 4-19

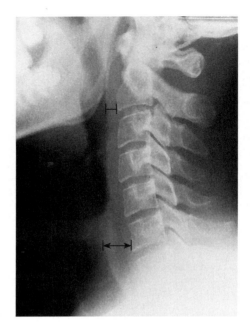

FIG. 4-20

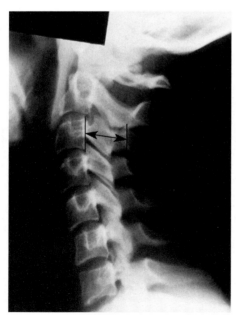

FIG. 4-21

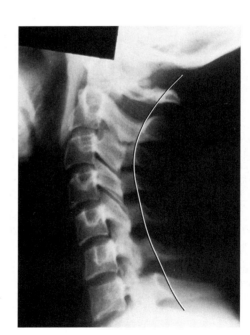

FIG. 4-22

TABLE 4-2 cont'd
Spine Measures

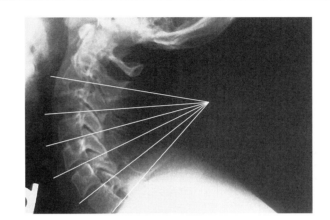

FIG. 4-23

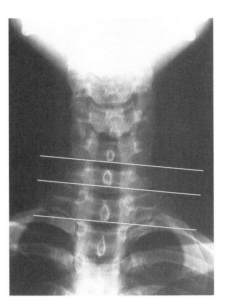

FIG. 4-24

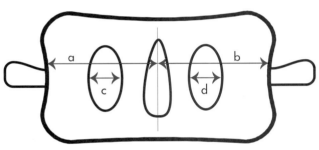

FIG. 4-25

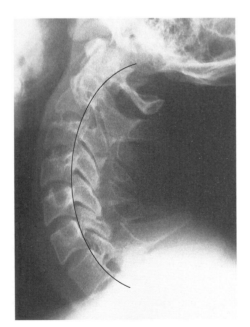

FIG. 4-26

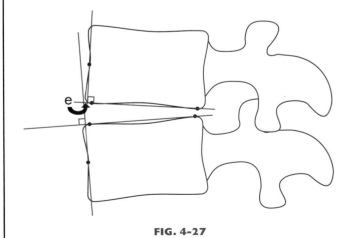

FIG. 4-27

Continued

TABLE 4-2 cont'd
Spine Measures

Description	Significance
Pedicle method On the frontal cervical, thoracic, and lumbar projections the appearance of the pedicle shadows may suggest vertebral rotation. It is expected that the pedicle shadows demonstrate bilateral symmetry (*c* and *d*).	If the width of a pedicle shadow appears narrower than the contralateral pedicle shadow, it suggests (1) segmental rotation with the spinous process deviated to the side of the narrower pedicle shadow, and (2) posterior vertebral body rotation to the side of the wider pedicle shadow.
Cervical, thoracic, and lumbar vertebral sagittal alignment *George's line* On the lateral cervical, thoracic, and lumbar projections, a curvilinear line is drawn along the posterior surfaces of the vertebral bodies. The curve should maintain a smooth contour throughout the spinal region without segmental disruption (Fig. 4-26).	Disruption is caused by segmental anterolisthesis or retrolisthesis. Disruptions at multiple consecutive levels may be caused by normal flexion and extension patterns. Care should be taken not to interpret this as abnormal. However, the adjacent posterior body lines should not demonstrate more than 3.5 mm of net relative translation in a comparison of the flexion and extension radiographs.
Barge's "e" space On the lateral lumbar projection, lines are drawn along the superior and inferior vertebral endplates of each segment. Lines perpendicular to each endplate line are then drawn and extended across the intervertebral disc space. The distance between the perpendicular lines at the inferior endplate of each lumbar segment is measured as the "e" space. The space should not exceed 3 mm (Fig. 4-27).	A larger Barge's "e" space suggests retrolisthesis of the segment above. Negative values indicate anterolisthesis. A more complete assessment would include the "e" space measurements at adjacent levels to determine relative retrolisthesis or anterolisthesis, thereby reducing spurious measurements that are caused by patient posture.
Visual method Segmental retrolisthesis may be indicated by the presence of the following: • Intervertebral disc degeneration (osteophytes, eburnation, reduced disc space, Schmorl's nodes, endplate irregularity) • The lowest segment of a "stack" of three or more vertebrae that do not contribute to a sagittal curvature may be posterior • The lowest involved segment of three or more consecutive segments that appear to be flexed or extended during neutral patient posture may be posterior • Segmental rotation in a coronal plane that produces an hourglass appearance • Narrowed sagittal diameter of the intervertebral foramen • Visual disparity of segmental alignment when comparing the margins of adjacent vertebrae	Retrolisthesis of L5 is often seen as a normal variant, accompanying short pedicles.
Cervical toggle analysis *Atlas tilt* On the lateral cervical projection, three lines are constructed: An occipital condyle line (OCL) is drawn along the base of the occipital condyles, an atlas plane line (APL) is drawn through the center of the anterior tubercle and the narrowest portion of the posterior arch of the atlas, and a listing line (LL) is drawn parallel to the occipital condyle line and through the narrowest portion of the posterior arch of the atlas. The atlas plane line should be 4 degrees above the listing line (Fig. 4-28).	If the APL is more than 4 degrees above the listing line, a superior malposition of the atlas is suspected; if the measure is less than 4 degrees, an inferior malposition of atlas is suspected. (*Note:* The malposition of the atlas is described with four letters. The first letter is always "A," the second indicates superior [S] or inferior [I] malposition, the third letter designates to right [R] or left [L] laterality, and the fourth letter designates whether the lateral malposition is anteriorly [A] or posteriorly [P] rotated.)

TABLE 4-2 cont'd

Spine Measures

Description	Significance
Atlas laterality On a frontal cervical projection taken horizontal to the atlas (nasium projection), four lines are constructed: A horizontal ocular orbit line (OOL) is drawn through similar matched points of the orbits, a superior basic line (SBL) is drawn parallel to the OOL through the tip of the most superior occipital condyle, an inferior basic line (IBL) is drawn through the inferior tips of the lateral masses, and a vertical median line (VML) is drawn perpendicular to the OOL and through the center of the foramen magnum. The distances between the inferior lateral tip of each lateral mass and the VML should be equal (Fig. 4-29).	The atlas is lateral toward the side of the greater measurement when the distances between the lateral inferior tip of each lateral mass and the VML are not equal. In addition, the SBL and IBL lines are thought to converge to the side of atlas laterality 70% of the time.
Atlas rotation On a cervical film whose projection is directed vertical to the atlas (base posterior), two lines are constructed: A transverse atlas line (TAL) is drawn through the transverse foramen bilaterally, and a perpendicular skull line (PSL) is drawn through points representing the centers of the nasal septum and the basal process of the occiput. The angle of intersection of the two lines should be approximately 90 degrees (Fig. 4-30).	The atlas is rotated posteriorly on the side of the larger angle created by the intersection of the PSL and TAL. In addition, 70% of the time the atlas is posteriorly rotated to the side of the diverging superior basic line (SBL) and inferior basic line (IBL) on the frontal open-mouth projection.
Axis malpositions On the frontal open-mouth projection, four lines are constructed: An ocular orbit line (OOL) is drawn through a set of similar points of the orbit (see *Atlas Laterality*), a superior basic line (SBL) is drawn bilaterally through the jugular processes, the inferior basic line (IBL) is drawn through the lateral inferior tip of both lateral masses, and a vertical median line (VML) is drawn perpendicular to the OOL through the center of the foramen magnum. The VML should approximate the center of the odontoid process base (Fig. 4-31).	If the VML does not bisect the odontoid, the axis is laterally malpositioned to the side opposite the VML. In addition, the center of the odontoid process base is compared with the center of the spinous process to assess for possible spinous deviation. The direction and magnitude of spinous process lateral malposition may be different from the lateral malposition of the axis body (e.g., the body of the axis may be exhibit right laterality with left spinous deviation).
Cobb's method for scoliosis On the frontal cervical, thoracic, or lumbar projection, lines are drawn along the superior endplate of the upper and inferior endplate of the lower vertebrae involved in the curvature. The end vertebrae chosen for measurement are the ones that tilt the most severely toward the scoliosis concavity. Perpendicular lines are constructed from the endplate lines, and the superior angle at their intersection *(x°)* is measured (Fig. 4-32).	This is the preferred method of quantifying the degree of scoliosis.
Coupled spinal motion sign Spinal motion is not pure and occurs in directions other than the primary direction of movement. For example, on frontal cervical, thoracic, or lumbar lateral bending projections, the lateral tilting of each vertebra is accompanied by concurrent vertebral rotation. In the cervical and upper thoracic region the spinous processes rotate to the convexity of the curve. In the lumbar and lower thoracic region the spinous processes rotate to the concavity of the curve. The amount of coupled motion may be small and therefore radiographically imperceptible (Fig. 4-33).	Alteration of the normal coupled motion occurs with aberrant intersegmental mechanics, muscle spasm, and vertebral fusion.

Continued

TABLE 4-2 cont'd
Spine Measures

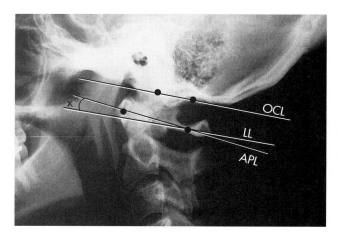

FIG. 4-28

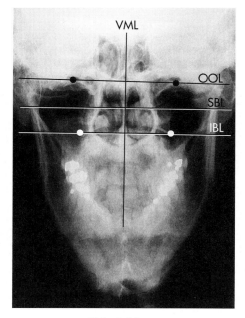

FIG. 4-29

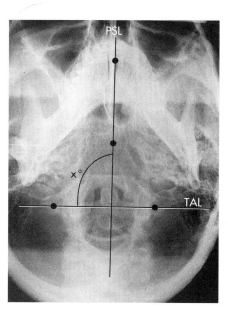

FIG. 4-30

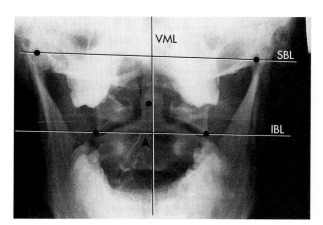

FIG. 4-31

TABLE 4-2 cont'd
Spine Measures

Description	Significance
Interpedicular distance On the frontal cervical, thoracic, or lumbar projections, the width *(x)* between opposing paired pedicles is typically 30 mm in the cervical spine, 20 mm in the thoracic spine, and 25 mm (L1-L3) to 30 mm (L4-L5) in the lumbar spine (Fig. 4-34).	Narrowed interpedicular distance results from congenital maldevelopment (e.g., achondroplasia) and is an indicator of spinal stenosis. Enlargement of the interpedicular distance occurs secondary to expanding canal lesions (e.g., tumor).
Thoracic cage dimension On the lateral chest radiograph the distance *(x)* between the posterior surface of the sternum and the anterior margin of T8 should be at least 9 cm in females and 11 cm in males (Fig. 4-35).	Narrowed anteroposterior dimension of the thoracic cage may result in cardiac compression.
Thoracic spine kyphosis On the lateral thoracic projection, lines are drawn along the superior endplate of T1 and the inferior endplate of T12. Vertical perpendicular lines are extended from these endplate lines, and the angle of intersection *(x°)* is measured, with values averaging near 30 degrees. The upper limit of normal is 56 degrees in women and 66 degrees in men (Fig. 4-36).	Measures of thoracic kyphosis are largely age dependent. Younger patients demonstrate less kyphosis, and older individuals demonstrate greater kyphosis.
Harrison posterior tangent method (thoracic spine) On the lateral thoracic projection, lines are drawn along the posterior body of T3 and a second line is drawn along the posterior body of T10. The superior or inferior angle of intersection *(x°)* is measured as the thoracic kyphosis (Fig. 4-37).	The value of the thoracic kyphosis from T3 to T10 using the methods described averages 37.4 degrees with a standard deviation of 11.1 degrees as reported by Harrison and others (2003).
Lumbar intervertebral disc angles On the lateral projection, lines are drawn along the superior and inferior vertebral endplates. The lines corresponding to each disc level intersect posterior to the lumbar spine. The disc angles *(x°)* increase with descending lumbar levels: L1—8 degrees, L2—10 degrees, L3—12 degrees, L4—14 degrees, and L5—14 degrees (Fig. 4-38).	Alterations of the lumbar disc angles occur with postural changes, aberrant intersegmental mechanics, muscular imbalances, and intervertebral disc pathology (e.g., herniations).
Lumbar intervertebral disc height ***Visual assessment*** On the lateral projection a subjective appraisal is made of the disc height compared with the adjacent levels and past experience.	Narrowing of the intervertebral disc space usually indicates degeneration. If narrowing occurs at the L5 level without concurrent findings of degeneration, underdevelopment is most probable. More aggressive pathology (e.g., infection) or surgery may narrow the disc space.
Ratio method On the lateral projection the anterior *(a)* and posterior *(b)* heights of the intervertebral disc space are averaged and divided by the horizontal width *(c)* of the middle portion of the disc. Therefore the disc height is expressed as a ratio of the disc width and height, which offers a method to control for differing patient sizes. In the lumbar spine, normal disc ratios increase with descending lumbar levels: L1—0.17, L2—0.18, L3—0.20, L4—0.25, and L5—0.28 (Fig. 4-39).	Narrowing of the intervertebral disc space usually indicates degeneration. If narrowing occurs at the L5 level without concurrent findings of degeneration, underdevelopment is most probable. More aggressive pathology (e.g., infection) or surgery may narrow the disc space.

Continued

TABLE 4-2 cont'd
Spine Measures

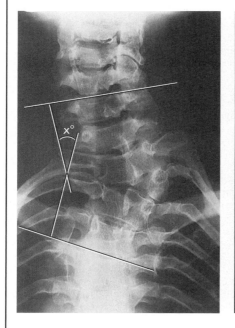

FIG. 4-32

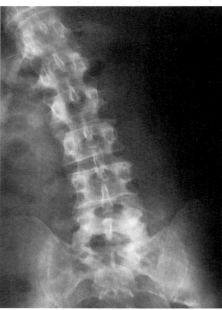

FIG. 4-33

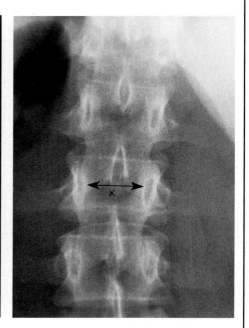

FIG. 4-34

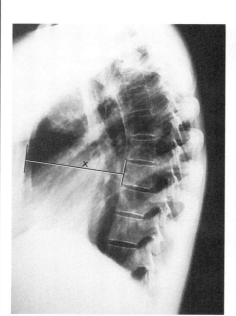

FIG. 4-35

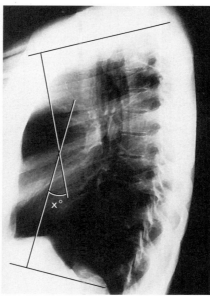

FIG. 4-36

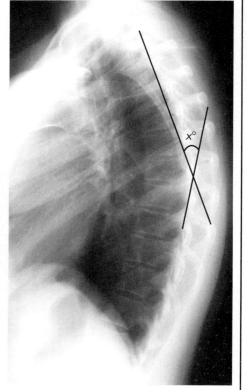

FIG. 4-37

TABLE 4-2 cont'd
Spine Measures

Description	Significance

Lumbar facet (Hadley's "S") curve
On the lateral or oblique lumbar projection, it should be possible to construct a smooth curve along the inferior margin of a transverse process that extends along the lateral margin of the inferior articular process, across the facet joint, and along the lateral margin of the superior articular process of the segment below (Fig. 4-40).

Alterations in the smooth progression of the curve suggest facet arthrosis or malposition.

Lumbar gravity line
On the lateral lumbar projection a vertical line is drawn from the center of the L3 vertebral body inferiorly. Normally the vertical line will pass through the anterior third of the sacral base (Fig. 4-41).

If the line falls more than 1 to 2 cm anterior to the sacrum, it suggests anterior weight-bearing with increased shear stress on the lower lumbar discs and facet joints (see figure). Posterior weight-bearing may lead to more weight distribution on the facet joints.

Lumbar instability (Van Akkerveeken's) lines
On the neutral or extension lateral lumbar projection, lines are drawn along the superior and inferior vertebral endplates adjacent to the same disc space. The distance between the posterior margin of each vertebra and the intersection of the two lines is measured (*a* and *b*). The presence of an abnormality is suggested if the measurements differ by more than 3 mm (Fig. 4-42).

Ligamentous injury to the disc or other spinal ligaments may result in increased translation and abnormal measurements. The extension radiograph is more likely to demonstrate an abnormality.

Lumbar spine lordosis
On the lateral lumbar projection, lines are drawn along the superior endplate of L1 and the base of sacrum. Vertical perpendicular lines are drawn from the endplate and sacral lines, and the angle of intersection *(x°)* averages 50 to 60 degrees (Fig. 4-43).

Wide variations in lordosis measurements have been noted. Alterations have been related to low back pain, disc herniations, altered posture, and other findings.

Harrison posterior tangent method (lumbar spine)
On the lateral lumbar projection, lines are drawn along the posterior body of L1 and a second line is drawn along the posterior body of L5. The superior or inferior angle of intersection *(x°)* is measured as the lumbar lordosis (Fig. 4-44).

The value of the lumbar lordosis from L1 to L5 using the methods described averages 39.7 degrees with a standard deviation of 9.1 degrees as reported by Janik and others (1998).

Lumbar spinal canal
Eisenstein's method
On the lateral lumbar projection a line is drawn connecting the tips of the superior and inferior articular processes of the same segment. The canal width *(x)* is expressed as the distance from the posterior body margin to the middle portion of the facet line. The canal dimension should not fall below 15 mm (although some use 14 mm or 12 mm as the cutoff) (Fig. 4-45).

Smaller measurements may indicate spinal stenosis. However, spinal stenosis is more accurately assessed on axial MRI and CT images, which provide additional information regarding canal shape.

Ratio method
On the frontal lumbar projection the interpedicular distance is multiplied by sagittal width obtained using Eisenstein's method as described on the lateral lumbar projection. Next, on the frontal lumbar projection the coronal width of the vertebrae is multiplied by the sagittal width of the vertebrae obtained from the lateral lumbar projection. The product of the two canal measures is divided by the product of the two vertebral measures, expressing the canal size as a ratio of the vertebral body. In the lumbar spine, the canal ratio should not fall below 1:3.

Smaller measurements may indicate spinal stenosis. However, spinal stenosis is much more accurately assessed on axial MRI and CT images, which provide additional information regarding canal shape.

Continued

TABLE 4-2 cont'd
Spine Measures

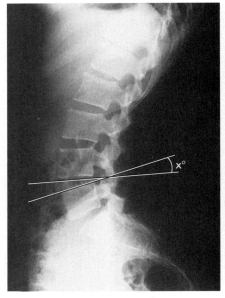

FIG. 4-38

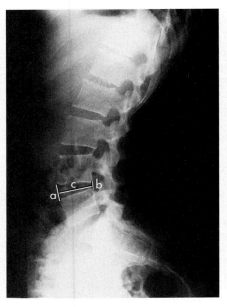

FIG. 4-39

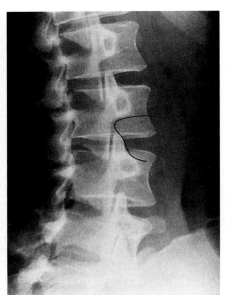

FIG. 4-40

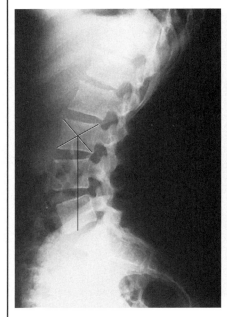

FIG. 4-41

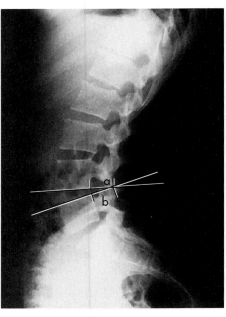

FIG. 4-42

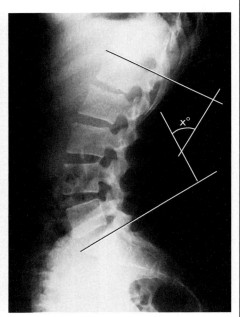

FIG. 4-43

TABLE 4-2 cont'd

Spine Measures

Description	Significance
Meyerding's grading for spondylolisthesis On the lateral lumbar projection the sacral base is divided into four quadrants. A line drawn along the posterior surface of the L5 vertebra should not intersect the sacral base (Fig. 4-46).	If L5 spondylolisthesis is present, the posterior body line intersects the sacral base. The sacral base quadrant that is intersected is used to qualify the amount of anterior displacement into Grades I to IV. (The figure shows a Grade I spondylolisthesis.) The method can be used at other spinal levels by dividing the segment below the spondylolisthesis into quadrants.
Risser-Ferguson method for scoliosis On the frontal, cervical, thoracic, or lumbar projection, lines are drawn from the center of the upper vertebra to the center of the vertebra at the apex of the lateral curvature (apical vertebra) and from the center of the lower vertebra to the center of the apical vertebra. The inferior angle *(x°)* at the intersection of these lines is measured. The apical vertebra is the one that is the most laterally deviated. The end vertebrae are most severely tilted to the concavity of the curve (Fig. 4-47).	This method is not used as often as Cobb's method to quantify scoliosis.
Harrison modified Risser-Ferguson method for measurement of AP lumbar views On the frontal lumbar film, the narrow-waisted lateral margins of the vertebral bodies are used to find the middle of the vertebrae. Next, the spinous–lamina junction is identified and the center of mass of the vertebra is established as the point halfway between the middle point of the vertebra and the spinous–lamina junction. Best-fit lines connect these two-dimensional centers of mass from T12 to L5. The upper best-fit line, connecting T11-L2, is drawn to cross the lower lumbar (L3-5) best-fit line. The angle measured is termed the lumbodorsal (LD) angle. The lower lumbar best-fit line is extended to the top of the sacral base line. This lower lumbar to sacral line creates a second angle known as the (coronal) lumbosacral (LS) angle. A third line is the sacral base angle to horizontal termed the HB angle (Fig. 4-48).	The Harrison modified Risser-Ferguson method for measurement of the AP lumbar regions is based on the location of the two-dimensional center of mass of each vertebra. The resultant LD angle provides information of spinal and sacral distortion in a sagittal plane. The benefit of this method is that it accounts for both axial rotation and lateral bending displacements of vertebrae. This method can be applied to the cervical, thoracic, or lumbar regions. The LS angle is a measure of lower lumbar lateral bending. The HB angle is a measure of lateral sacral tilt.
These AP lumbar lines and angles have been studied for reliability and have intraclass correlations in the good to excellent range with low mean absolute value of observer differences (see Harrison, 2002).	
Sacral angle *Barge's angle (a°)* On the lateral weight-bearing lumbar projection a line is drawn along the sacral base. The inferior angle of intersection between the sacral base line and a vertical line drawn parallel to the vertical edge of the film average 53 degrees, with a standard deviation of 4 degrees (Fig. 4-49).	Smaller Barge's angles and larger Ferguson's angles are associated with increased compressive forces at the facets or transverse shearing forces at the disc. Larger Barge's angles and smaller Ferguson's angles are associated with increased axial loading of the disc of increased axial shearing forces at the facets.
Ferguson's angle (b°) On the lateral lumbar projection a line is drawn along the sacral base. The inferior angle of intersection between the sacral base line and a horizontal line drawn parallel to the horizontal edge of the film average 41 degrees, with a standard deviation of 2 degrees and average values of 27 to 56 degrees.	
Ulmann's line On the lateral lumbar projection a line is drawn along the sacral base. A second line is drawn perpendicular to the sacral base line just anterior to the sacrum. Normally the L5 vertebra is found posterior to the perpendicular line (Fig. 4-50).	If the L5 vertebra crosses the perpendicular line, spondylolisthesis may be present. Ulmann's line is less sensitive to spondylolisthesis than George's posterior body line.

Continued

TABLE 4-2 cont'd
Spine Measures

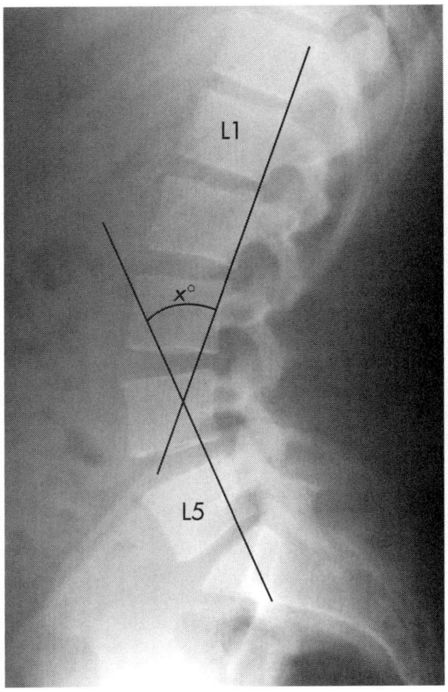

FIG. 4-44

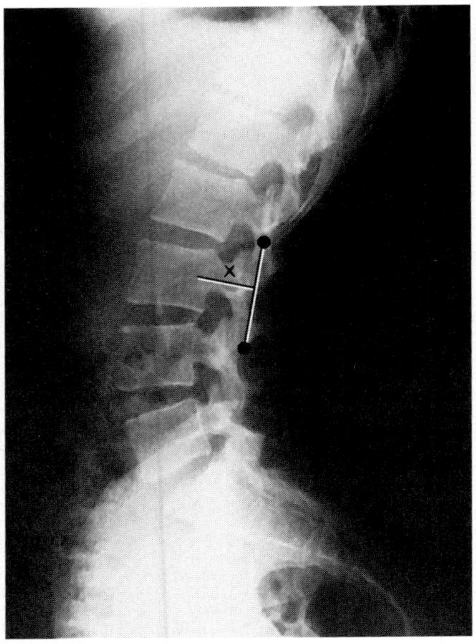

FIG. 4-45

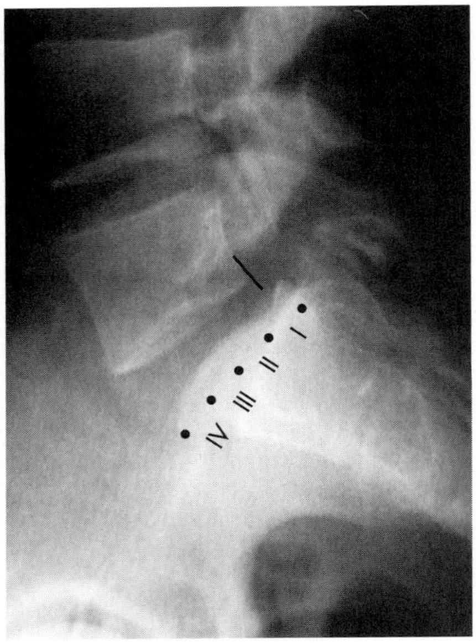

FIG. 4-46

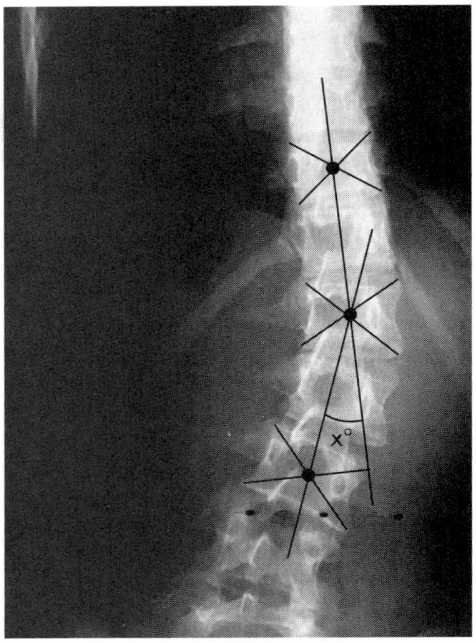

FIG. 4-47

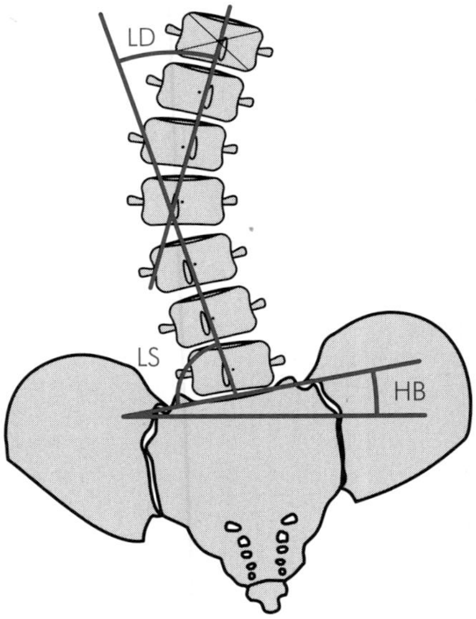

FIG. 4-48

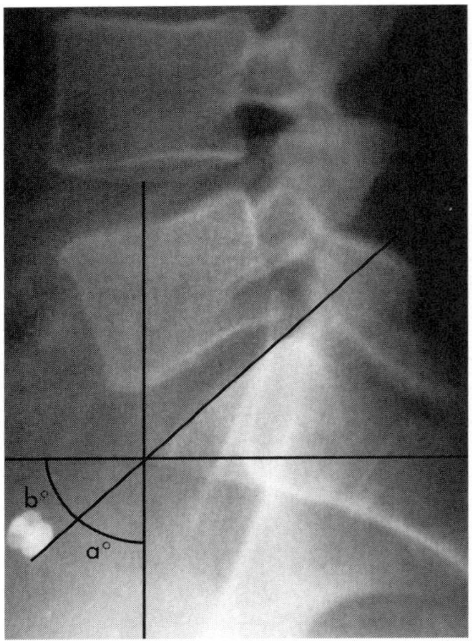

FIG. 4-49

TABLE 4-2 cont'd
Spine Measures

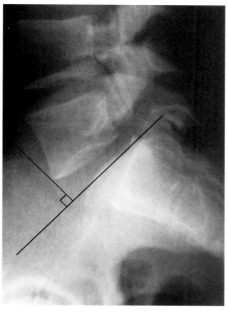

FIG. 4-50

TABLE 4-3
Upper Extremity Measures

Description	Significance
Acromioclavicular joint space On the anteroposterior shoulder or acromioclavicular projection, the space *(x)* between the distal clavicle and proximal acromion process averages 3 mm (Fig. 4-51).	An enlarged space suggests fracture, traumatic ligament tears, or bone resorption (e.g., due to hyperparathyroidism). A narrowed space is associated with degeneration.
Acromiohumeral joint space On the anteroposterior shoulder projection, the distance *(x)* from the inferior surface of the acromion to the humeral head averages 10 mm (Fig. 4-52).	A narrowed space is indicative of superior shoulder displacement, which is often secondary to shoulder impingement syndrome with rotator cuff tendinopathy. An enlarged space is associated with dislocation, joint effusion, and paralysis.
Glenohumeral joint space On the anteroposterior shoulder projection, the distance *(x)* from the glenoid to the humeral head averages 5 mm (Fig. 4-53).	An enlarged glenohumeral space is suggestive of joint effusion, acromegaly, and posterior humeral dislocation. A narrowed space is often secondary to degeneration and rheumatoid arthritis.
Anterior humeral line On the lateral elbow projection a line drawn along the anterior surface of the humerus should intersect the middle third of the lateral condylar ossific center (Fig. 4-54).	If the line passes anterior or posterior to the middle third of the lateral condyle, a fracture may be present.

Continued

TABLE 4-3 cont'd
Upper Extremity Measures

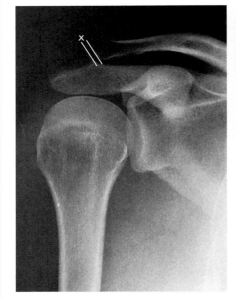

FIG. 4-51

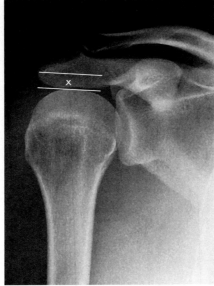

FIG. 4-52

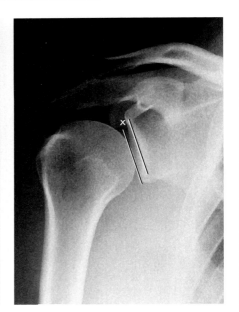

FIG. 4-53

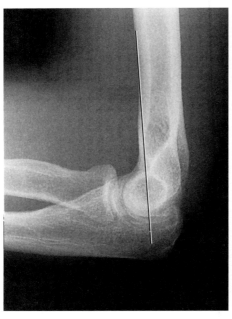

FIG. 4-54

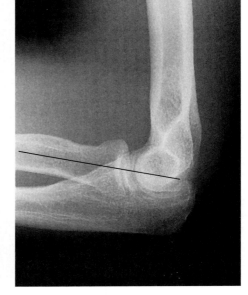

FIG. 4-55

TABLE 4-3 cont'd

Upper Extremity Measures

Description	Significance
Radiocarpal line On the lateral elbow projection a line is drawn through the center of the radius to approximate its long axis. The line should pass through the elbow joint to intersect the center of the capitellum (Fig. 4-55).	Assessment assists in determining the presence of fracture or dislocation.
Capitolunate sign On the lateral wrist projection, lines are drawn to approximate the long axes of the lunate and capitate. Their angle of intersection $(x°)$ should be less than 20 degrees (Fig. 4-56).	Carpal instability is suggested if the angle exceeds 20 degrees.
Metacarpal sign On the posteroanterior hand projection, an oblique line drawn along the distal articular surfaces of the fourth and fifth metacarpals should also intersect the distal articular surface of the third metacarpal (Fig. 4-57).	If the oblique line intersects the third metacarpal at a more proximal point than the distal articular surface, the fourth metacarpal may be abnormally short. This finding is often seen in gonadal dysgenesis (Turner's syndrome) or metacarpal fracture.
Radiolunate angle (lunate tilt) On the lateral wrist projection, lines drawn to approximate the long axes of the radius and lunate should be parallel (Fig. 4-58).	If the lunate is flexed more than 15 degrees, volar intercalated segment instability (VISI) is suggested. If the angle is greater than 10 degrees in extension, dorsal intercalated segment instability (DISI) is suggested. Occasionally VISI and usually DISI occur with scapholunate dissociation; VISI is also related to triquetrolunate dissociation.
Radioulnar variance On the anteroposterior wrist projection, the distal ulnar articular surface should align with the inner portion of the distal radial articular surface (Fig. 4-59).	A short ulna (e.g., negative ulnar variance) is associated with avascular necrosis of the lunate (Kienböck disease) and greater carpal stress distribution to the radius. A long ulna (e.g., positive ulnar variance) is associated with greater carpal stress distribution to the ulna. Differences of less than 5 mm are probably not significant.
Scapholunate angle (scaphoid tilt) On the lateral wrist projection, lines are drawn to approximate the long axes of the scaphoid and lunate. Their angle of intersection $(x°)$ averages 47 degrees with variance between 62 and 32 degrees (Fig. 4-60).	If the angle is greater than 80° and the lunate is also extended (dorsiflexed), DISI is suggested.

Continued

TABLE 4-3 cont'd
Upper Extremity Measures

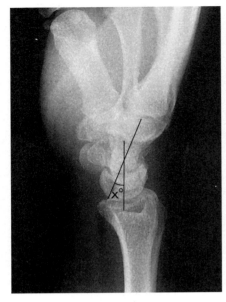

FIG. 4-56

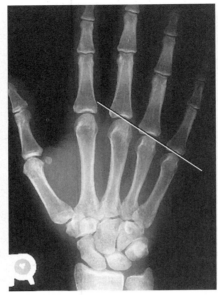

FIG. 4-57

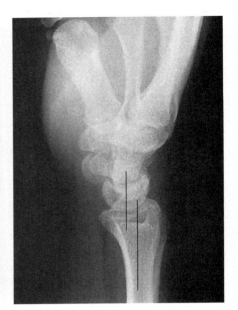

FIG. 4-58

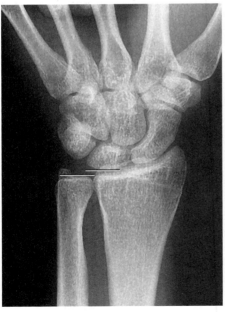

FIG. 4-59

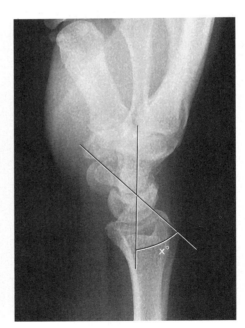

FIG. 4-60

TABLE 4-4
Lower Extremity Measures

Description	Significance
Acetabular (Wiberg's) center-edge angle On the anteroposterior pelvic or hip projection, a vertical line is drawn from the center of the femoral head superiorly through the acetabulum. A second line is drawn from the lateral aspect of the acetabulum to the center of the femoral head. The angle *(x°)* formed by the two lines is normally between 20 and 35 degrees (Fig. 4-61).	The angle serves as a width measure of the amount of coverage the acetabular roof provides. A shallow angle (e.g., less than 20 degrees) may be caused by acetabular dysplasia and is associated with hip dislocation and hip degeneration.
Acetabular index On the anteroposterior pelvic projection, a horizontal line *(a)* is drawn through the right and left triradiate cartilage (Y-Y or Hilgenreiner's line). Another line is drawn along each of the acetabuli *(b)* to intersect the horizontal triradiate cartilage line. The angles of intersection *(x°)* should not exceed standards based on age: at birth—less than 36 degrees in females, less than 30 degrees in males; 6 months—less than 28 degrees in females, less than 25 degrees in males; 1 year—less than 25 degrees in females, 24 degrees in males; 7 years—less than 19 degrees in females, less than 18 degrees in males (Fig. 4-62).	An enlarged angle is associated with acetabular dysplasia and possible lateral congenital dislocation of the hip. A shallow angle is seen in patients with Down syndrome.
Acetabular protrusion (Köhler's) line On the anteroposterior pelvic projection, a nearly vertical line is drawn from the outer border of the obturator foramen superiorly to the lateral cortical margin of the pelvic inlet. The floor of the acetabulum should not extend medially to this line (Fig. 4-63).	If the floor of the acetabulum extends medially to Köhler's line, protrusio acetabuli is present. Protrusio acetabuli is secondary to rheumatoid or degenerative arthritis, Paget's disease, osteogenesis imperfecta, and idiopathic or other bone-softening disorders.
Femoral neck angle On the anteroposterior pelvic or hip projection, a nearly vertical line is drawn approximating the femoral shaft *(a)*. A second line is drawn through the center of the femoral neck *(b)*. The angle of intersection *(x°)* is normally 124 degrees and should not be less than 110 degrees or more than 130 degrees (Fig. 4-64).	An angle of less than 110 degrees is termed *coxa vara*. A measure greater than 130 degrees is termed *coxa valga*.
Hip joint space On the anteroposterior pelvic or hip projection, the hip joint between the cortex of the femoral head and the acetabulum should not exceed 6 mm superiorly *(s)*, 7 mm axially *(a)*, or 13 mm medially *(m)* (Fig. 4-65).	A wider hip joint distance is associated with hip joint effusion. The superior joint space is usually narrowed by degeneration. The axial space is more commonly affected by an inflammatory arthritide (e.g., rheumatoid arthritis). The medial joint space is narrowed by degeneration and an inflammatory arthritide.
Iliofemoral line On the anteroposterior pelvic or hip projection, it should be possible to draw a smooth curve along the outer surface of the lower ilium that extends inferiorly along the femoral neck. The line should be bilaterally symmetric (Fig. 4-66).	Disruption of the smooth line is associated with hip dislocation, femoral neck fracture, and slipped capital femoral epiphysis.
Klein's (femoral epiphysis) line On the anteroposterior pelvic, anteroposterior hip, or frogleg hip projection, a line drawn along the outer border of the femoral neck should intersect the femoral capital epiphysis (Fig. 4-67).	Slipped capital femoral epiphysis is suspected if the femoral capital epiphysis is found medial to the femoral neck line or if the line transects less of the epiphysis than is found on the contralateral side.

Continued

TABLE 4-4 cont'd
Lower Extremity Measures

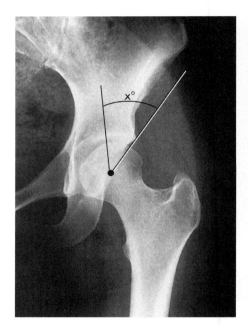

FIG. 4-61

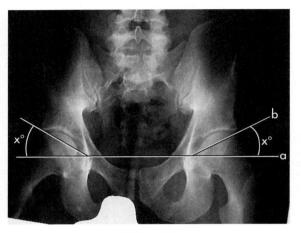

FIG. 4-62

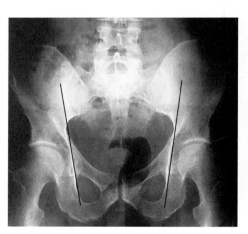

FIG. 4-63

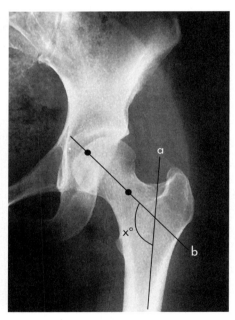

FIG. 4-64

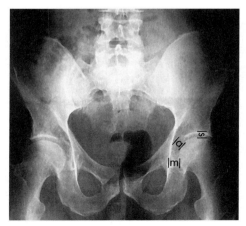

FIG. 4-65

TABLE 4-4 cont'd
Lower Extremity Measures

Description	Significance
Shenton's hip line On the anteroposterior pelvic or hip projection, it should be possible to draw a smooth curve along the medial and superior surface of the obturator foramen to the medial aspect of the femoral neck (Fig. 4-68).	Disruption of the smooth line is associated with hip dislocation, femoral neck fracture, and slipped capital femoral epiphysis.
Skinner's (femoral angle) line On the anteroposterior pelvic or hip projection, a nearly vertical line is drawn approximating the femoral shaft. A second line is drawn perpendicular to the first line at the level of proximal tip of the greater trochanter. The fovea capitis should be found at the level of or above the perpendicular line (Fig. 4-69).	If the fovea capitis is found below the perpendicular line, fracture or bone-softening conditions causing coxa vara are suspected.
Teardrop distance On the anteroposterior pelvic projection, the distance between the most medial portion of the femoral head and the most lateral portion of the teardrop at the inner acetabulum should not exceed 11 mm or differ from the contralateral side by more than 2 mm (which is Waldenström's sign) (Fig. 4-70).	A wider teardrop distance is associated with hip joint effusion.
Pelvis *Iliac angle* On the anteroposterior pelvic projection, a horizontal line is drawn through the right and left triradiate cartilage. Two additional lines are drawn, one along the lateral margin of each ilium. The sum of the right and left angles *(x°)* of intersection (the iliac index) should not be less than 60 degrees in a newborn (Fig. 4-71).	A sum (iliac index) of less than 60 degrees is indicative of Down syndrome. A sum between 60 and 68 degrees is suggestive of Down syndrome.
Pelvic misalignment *Innominate rotation* On the weightbearing frontal pelvic projection, a femoral head line (FHL) is drawn along the superior margins of the femoral heads bilaterally. A perpendicular line from the FHL is constructed to intersect the second sacral tubercle and should pass through the center of the pubic symphysis when extended inferiorly (Fig. 4-72).	If the perpendicular line intersects the pubic bone instead of the symphysis, the innominate is externally rotated on the side the line crosses through. The innominate on the opposite side is internally rotated. Rotation can be double-checked by measuring the width of the ilium *(a)* and the obturator foramen *(b)* External rotation of the innominate, using the posterior superior iliac spine (PSIS) as a reference point, is accompanied by a narrower ilium width and a wider obturator foramen on the ipsilateral side. Internal rotation is associated with a wider ilium and narrower obturator width ipsilaterally.
Innominate flexion-extension On the weight-bearing frontal pelvic projection, the distance from the top of the iliac crest to the inferior margin of the ischial tuberosity should be bilaterally similar.	The vertical measurement of the innominate is larger on the flexed side (the PSIS has moved posterior and inferior) and smaller on the extended side (the PSIS has moved anterior and superior).
Sacrum rotation On the weight-bearing frontal pelvic projection, the distances from the lateral margins of the sacrum to the second sacral tubercle (*c* and *d*) are measured parallel to the FHL and should be similar.	The sacrum is rotated posteriorly on the wider side and anteriorly on the narrower side.
Leg length inequality On the frontal weight-bearing pelvic projection, a line is drawn parallel to the lower margin of the film to the superior margin of the highest femoral head. The line should approximate both femoral heads if the legs are of equal length.	If the line constructed parallel to the bottom of the film does not approximate the femoral heads bilaterally, the line is drawn to the higher femoral head, and the distance from the line to the lower femoral head estimates the measured leg length deficiency. The clinical interpretation of a measured deficiency is dependent on accompanying pelvic misalignment.

Continued

TABLE 4-4 cont'd
Lower Extremity Measures

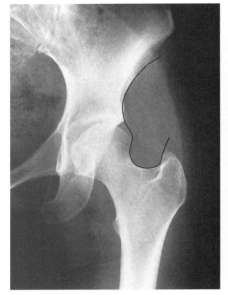

FIG. 4-66

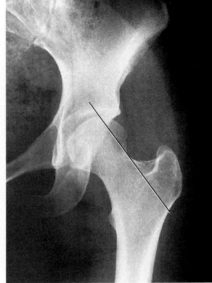

FIG. 4-67

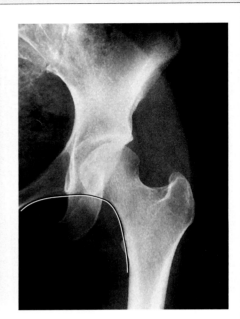

FIG. 4-68

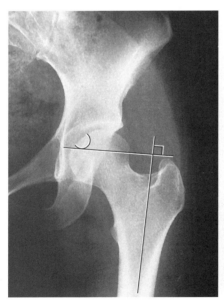

FIG. 4-69

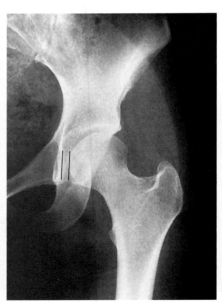

FIG. 4-70

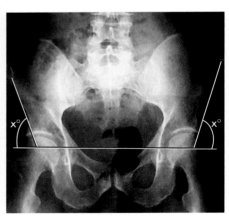

FIG. 4-71

TABLE 4-4 cont'd
Lower Extremity Measures

Description	Significance
Leg length inequality cont'd	It is believed that a flexed (PI) or externally rotated (EX) innominate decreases the leg length discrepancy when the innominate misalignment is corrected on the ipsilateral side of the short leg. In other words, correction of a flexed or externally rotated innominate raises the ipsilateral femoral head. Conversely, an extended (AS) or internally (IN) rotated innominate increases the leg length discrepancy when corrected on the ipsilateral side of the short leg. The opposite is noted if the short leg is on the contralateral side of the innominate misalignment. It has been estimated that the magnitude of leg length change is anticipated to be 40% of the measured misalignment of the innominate. Consideration of the pelvic misalignment allows an estimation of the actual leg length deficiency.
Presacral space On the lateral sacral projection the space *(x)* between the anterior sacral cortex and the posterior margin of the rectal gas should not exceed 2 cm in adults and 5 mm in children (Fig. 4-73).	An enlarged presacral space is associated with expansile lesion of the sacrum, soft tissue masses associated with abnormality of the sacrum, sacral trauma, or abnormalities of the bowel.
Symphysis pubis On the anteroposterior pelvic projection the pubic symphysis *(x)* should not exceed 6 mm in females and 7 mm in males (Fig. 4-74).	A widened space occurs with cleidocranial dysostosis, trauma, hyperparathyroidism, bladder exstrophy, and secondary to an inflammatory arthritide.
Lateral patellofemoral angle On a tangential or Merchant's knee projection, a line is drawn along the femoral condyles. A second line is drawn along the lateral margin of the patella. The angle of intersection *(x°)* of these two lines usually opens laterally (Fig. 4-75).	If the lines are parallel or their angle opens medially, recurrent patellar subluxation is likely.
Patellar displacement (Insall ratio) On the lateral knee projection a ratio of the greatest height of the patella *(a)* to the distance from the inferior pole of the patella to the tibial tubercle *(b)* should be 1:1; a 20% variation is often seen (Fig. 4-76).	A high patella (1:1.2, patella alta) may be the result of trauma or chondromalacia patella. A low patella (1:0.8, patella baja) is seen in patients with achondroplasia, polio, or juvenile rheumatoid arthritis.
Patellar sulcus On a tangential or Merchant's knee projection, a sulcus angle *(x°)* is formed by drawing a line from the highest portion of the medial femoral condyle to the lowest portion of the intercondylar notch; the line is also drawn for the lateral femoral condyle. The intersection of these lines forms the sulcus angle. The angle ranges from 126 to 150 degrees, with the average being 138 degrees (Fig. 4-77).	Larger sulcus angles are associated with subluxation or dislocation of the patella.
Boehler's angle On the lateral foot or calcaneus projection, an angle *(x°)* formed along the superior margin of the calcaneus is normally between 30 and 35 degrees; a measurement of less than 28 degrees is abnormal (Fig. 4-78).	The angle is decreased or increased by calcaneal dysplasia or fracture.
First metatarsal angle On the anteroposterior foot projection, lines drawn to approximate the long axes of the first metatarsal and proximal first phalanx should form an angle *(x°)* of less than 15 degrees (Fig. 4-79).	An increased angle indicates a hallux valgus deformity.

Continued

TABLE 4-4 cont'd
Lower Extremity Measures

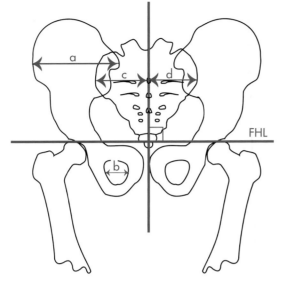

FIG. 4-72

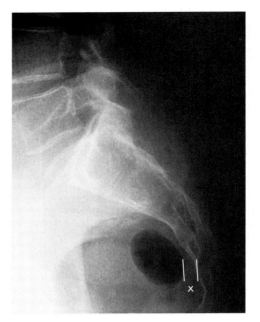

FIG. 4-73

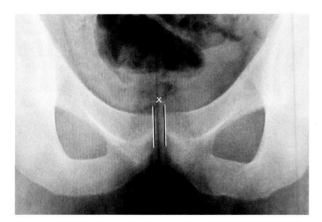

FIG. 4-74

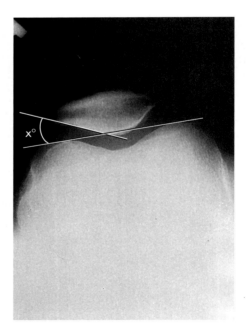

FIG. 4-75

TABLE 4-4 cont'd
Lower Extremity Measures

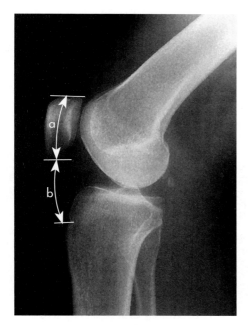

FIG. 4-76

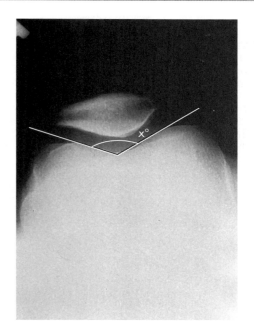

FIG. 4-77

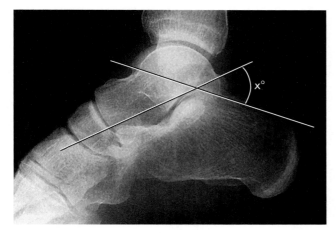

FIG. 4-78

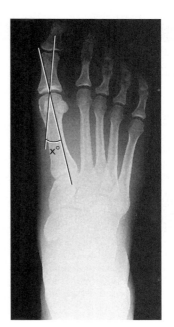

FIG. 4-79

Continued

TABLE 4-4 cont'd
Lower Extremity Measures

Description	Significance
Heel pad measurement On the non–weight-bearing lateral foot or calcaneus projection, the soft tissue of the heel inferior to the calcaneus should not exceed 23 mm in females and 25 mm in males (Fig. 4-80).	Increased heel pad thickness is associated with acromegaly, obesity, and edema.
Meary's angle On the lateral foot projection, lines drawn to approximate the longitudinal axis of the first metatarsal and talus should be parallel (Fig. 4-81).	If the lines are not parallel and form an angle that is greater than 0 degrees, forefoot cavus deformity is indicated.

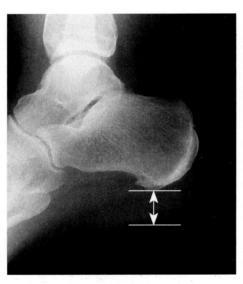

FIG. 4-80

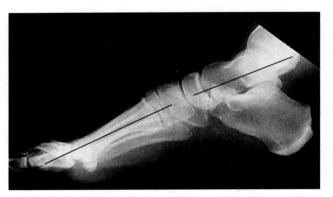

FIG. 4-81

Suggested Readings

Armbruster JG et al: The adult hip: an anatomic study. I. The bony landmarks, *Radiology* 128:1, 1978.

Barge FH: Chiropractic technique: tortipelvis, the slipped disc syndromes: its causes and correction, ed 4, Davenport, IA, 1986, Bawden Bros.

Brant WE, Helms CA: Fundamentals of diagnostic radiology, Baltimore, 1994, Williams & Wilkins.

Eyring EJ, Bjornson DR, Peterson CA: Early diagnostic and prognostic signs in Legg-Calvé-Perthes disease, *AJR Am J Roentgenol* 93:392, 1965.

Hak DJ, Gautsch TL: A review of radiographic line and angles used in orthopedics, *Am J Orthop* 24:590, 1995.

Harrison DD et al: Comparisons of lordotic cervical spine curvatures to a theoretical ideal model of the static sagittal cervical spine, *Spine* 21(2):667–675, 1996.

Harrison DE et al: Further reliability analysis of the Harrison radiographic line drawing methods: crossed ICCs for lateral posterior tangents and AP modified Risser-Ferguson, *J Man Physiol Ther* 25(2):93–98, 2002.

Harrison DD et al: Do alterations in vertebral and disc dimensions affect an elliptical model of the thoracic kyphosis? *Spine* 463–469, 2003.

Hellems HK, Keats TE: Measurement of the normal lumbosacral angle, *AJR Am J Roentgenol* 113(4):642, 1971.

Hubbard MJ: The measurement and progression of protrusio acetabuli, *AJR Am J Roentgenol* 106(3):506, 1969.

Insall J, Salvati E: Patella position in the normal knee joint, *Radiology* 101(1):101, 1971.

Janik TJ et al: Can the sagittal lumbar curvature be closely approximated by an ellipse? *J Orthop Res* 16(6):766–770, 1998.

Keats TE: Atlas of roentgenographic measurement, ed 7, St Louis, 2001, Mosby.

Marchiori DM et al: A comparison of radiographic findings of degeneration to corresponding MRI signal intensities in the lumbar spine, *J Man Physiol Ther* 17(4):238, 1994.

Meyerding HW: Spondylolisthesis, *Surg Gynecol Obstet* 54:371, 1932.

Nelson SW: Some important diagnostic and technical fundamentals in the radiology of trauma with particular emphasis on skeletal trauma, *Radiol Clin North Am* 4(2):241, 1966.

Petersson CJ, Redlund-Johnell I: Joint space in normal gleno-humeral radiographs, *Acta Orthop Scand* 54(2):274, 1983.

Plaugher GP: Textbook of clinical chiropractic: a specific biomechanical approach, Baltimore, 1993, Williams & Wilkins.

Rigler LG, O'Laughlin BJ, Tucker RC: Significance of unilateral enlargement of hilus shadow in early diagnosis of carcinoma of the lung with observations on method of mensuration, *Radiology* 59:683, 1952.

Tuck AM, Peterson CK: Accuracy and reliability of chiropractors and AECC students at visually estimating the lumbar lordosis from radiographs, *J Chiro Tech* 10:19, 1998.

chapter 5

Film Interpretation
and Report Writing

Film Interpretation
DENNIS M. MARCHIORI

Report Writing
CYNTHIA PETERSON

Focus on Radiographs

Since its inception, diagnostic imaging has played a fundamental role in patient evaluation. Diagnostic imaging began more than 100 years previously with plain film radiography, and has progressing to advanced modalities, such as digital radiography, magnetic resonance imaging (MRI), computed tomography (CT), and positron emission tomography (PET). Diagnostic imaging remains an essential tool to recognize, define, identify, and exclude many of the common and not so common pathologies encountered in a health care setting.

For most clinical assessments, the historically dominant modality of plain film radiography continues to be the first step, with more sophisticated specialized imaging systems such as MRI and CT often applied as follow-ups to negative, equivocal, or ambiguous results of the plain film study, or for clinical questions for which plain films are known to be insensitive. Plain film radiology is widely available, relatively inexpensive, and rapidly obtained, predicting it will likely remain as the most common imaging method into the near future.

Plain film radiology represents a common denominator to many health professions. Dentists, podiatrists, chiropractors, medical physicians, and many practitioners in allied heath professions routinely rely on information obtained from plain film radiographs to manage their patients. With this in mind, the present chapter is focused on the interpretation and reporting of plain film radiographs. However, with little modification, the concepts presented here and targeted to plain film radiology equally relate to other more specialized imaging modalities. Therefore the goal of this chapter is to provide the reader with an understanding of issues related to when radiographs should be taken, methods to successfully search radiographs for abnormal findings, the ability to categorize these findings by appearance and location into common patterns, and steps to summarize and report on these findings successfully.

Common Uses of Radiographs

In 2000 an estimated $1.3 trillion was spent on personal health care in the United States.[36] Heath care expenditure was 13.1% of the gross domestic product in 2000, representing a per capita expenditure of $4377.[36] Of the most current data available, in 1990, an estimated 3.5% of these expenditures were for radiologic services,[139,140] much of it directed to nonradiologists.

Diagnostic imaging is common to clinical practice. More than 80% of chiropractors use radiographs as part of their clinical protocol and have the necessary equipment to produce radiographs in their offices.[4] Although national data are not available, a survey of Minnesota medical physicians found that approximately 87% had onsite radiology equipment.[61]

Developing film interpretation skills is of obvious interest to radiologists, but developing these skills is also important to nonradiologist medical physicians, chiropractors, and other health care providers who often take and interpret radiographs as part of patient evaluation and management. For instance, most chiropractors do not regularly consult with radiologists to assist their interpretations.[63] In fact, fewer than 20% of hospitals have full-time onsite coverage by a board-certified radiologist.[101] During these off hours, the initial interpretation and related decisions are often done by nonradiologist clinicians, most to be overread by radiologists later. Moreover, of the radiologic services done in a private medical practice setting, 57%[139,140] to 70%[90,132] are performed and interpreted by nonradiologists.

Questions arise related to the appropriateness of training of nonradiologists to interpret imaging and under what circumstance it is best to consult with a radiologist. The American College of Radiology (ACR) recommends that radiographs be interpreted by certified radiologists or physicians who have documented training in an approved residency, including radiographic training on all body areas. This indicates the basic need for formal training, but does not limit interpretations to radiologists.[5] Literature within the chiropractic profession advocates for greater use of chiropractors who are certified with advanced training in radiology (Diplomates of the American College of Radiology [DACBR]) as a method of limiting liability and enhancing accuracy of image interpretation.[51]

Taylor[145] found that the degree of training positively influences the ability of medical and chiropractic clinicians and students to correctly identify selected bone and joint pathology. As one might expect, the concordance between the radiographic interpretation of radiologists and nonradiologists is best for extremity bone radiographs (approximately 95%) and lower for more complex studies, such as chest radiographs (generally ranging from 40% to 90%).*

Criteria for Ordering Radiographs

The most effective application of diagnostic imaging for many common clinical presentations is widely debated. The multifaceted and unique clinical presentations of most patients make the formation of common criteria for ordering diagnostic imaging problematic at best. Everyone agrees that all radiographic examinations should follow clear historical and clinical indications because of the examination costs and potentially hazardous effect of ionizing radiation.[96] Unfortunately, there is no general agreement on exactly what these historical and clinical indications should be to satisfy the competing needs of gaining information while limiting cost and radiation exposure.

To date, diverse opinions exist about what constitutes accepted clinical criteria for ordering radiographs for patients with musculoskeletal complaints. Although the literature documents many attempts to develop criteria for ordering radiographs for patients with complaints of the spine,† no system has been generally accepted. As a matter of observation, the use rates of plain film radiographs vary widely. Developing and embedding guidelines seem easier tasks for a narrow-scope presentation of something such as ankle[112,134] or knee trauma,[135,136] but are less successful for case presentations of increasing complexity and ambiguity (e.g., back pain) and applied management (e.g., pharmaceuticals versus manual adjustments or manipulation of the spine).

Opinions vary widely about the use of radiographs in the evaluation of patients experiencing back pain. Multiple questions cloud the issue. Should radiographs be taken of patients who are experiencing acute but not chronic back pain? What are the appropriate film-ordering criteria that maximize clinical information yet minimize patient cost and radiation exposure?

Despite the fact that these topics have garnered considerable attention over the past decade, evidence-based guidelines for the use of plain film radiology (or CT and MRI) are not widely used in the clinical setting.[52] In 1987 the Quebec Task Force, and later the United States' Agency for Health Care Policy and Research (AHCPR), developed guidelines for the use of plain film imaging related to patient presentation of acute low back pain. Similar efforts occurred in other countries.[27,36,122] The premise is that guidelines effectively influence practitioners' use of plain films, as has been shown to occur in some instances.[42,78] However, guidelines prove less effective as the population and clinical problems become less homogeneous and more complex.

Factors affecting whether radiographs are taken include clinical data, patient expectations, and clinicians' attempts to reassure patients or themselves.[91,104,157] Also the type of practitioner is very important: The use of radiographs for low back complaints varies from 2% to 48%, depending on the type of practitioner.[52] Chiropractors—who employ a manual approach to patient care—and orthopedic specialists demonstrate increased use of plain film radiographs compared with medical physicians in family practice who manage patients with acute low back pain.[32] This observation may result in part from a bias toward searching for a musculoskeletal derangement as the cause of the patient's complaint; however, it probably also reflects varying therapeutic approaches to patients' complaints and the need for structural information related to the delivery of care and patient management.

In chiropractic practice, radiographs generally are considered a standard first-step imaging protocol when evaluating degenerative and inflammatory joint disease, fractures, infections, and neoplasms.[57] The hands-on management approach of chiropractors warrants attention to biomechanical influences and potential structural contraindications to intended interventions (Fig. 5-1). Nonchiropractic clinicians, whose management of low back pain centers on exercise, patient education, pharmaceuticals, and other clinician-passive therapies, have less use for the biomechanical or structural information obtained from radiographs. Therefore these practitioners can easily adopt a more conservative approach to taking radiographs for musculoskeletal spine complaints than can chiropractors or other practitioners, who apply manual intervention.

Many radiographs taken in a chiropractic setting are interpreted as normal for serious bone pathology,[82] but they may relate biomechanical or structural information that allows the chiropractor to be more successful with technical aspects of formulating and applying the patient's management plan. However, more research into the reliability, validity, and clinical usefulness of biomechanical and structural information gleaned from radiographs is necessary. Also evidence is needed to clearly justify the added costs, define criteria of patient selection, and facilitate advancements in care delivery.

All clinicians, regardless of therapeutic approach, are concerned with serious pathology masking as routine low back pain. Clinical red flags that suggest the presence of serious pathology have been developed and are helpful to direct patient selection (Box 5-1). In the absence of these red flags, significant spinal pathology is estimated in only 1 of 2500 patients.[152] Deyo and Diehl[43] evaluated 1975 walk-in patients at a public hospital to estimate the prevalence of cancer as an underlying cause of the patient's back pain. Using a developed algorithm that generally reflects the questions listed in Box 5-1, only 22% of these patients would have received x-rays; this proportion includes all those who were later found to have cancer.

It should not be assumed that instituting guidelines, such as those listed in Box 5-1, will lead to less use. For example, Canadian researchers found that if the guidelines listed in Box 5-1 had been applied to their study population of 963 patients in a private medical family practice setting, 44% would have undergone radiography, increasing actual use by 238%. Considering patient follow-up, these researchers concluded that the sensitivity of the guidelines to detect fractures and tumors was higher than the physicians' use patterns, but their specificity and positive predictive values were low.[138]

Parallel and similarly controversial issues surround the application of specialized imaging. (e.g., whether MRI should be ordered for a patient in whom a disc herniation is clinically suspected yet

---

*References 19, 60, 72, 81, 83, 137.
†References 1, 41, 42, 44, 46, 98, 111, 119, 127, 133, 149.

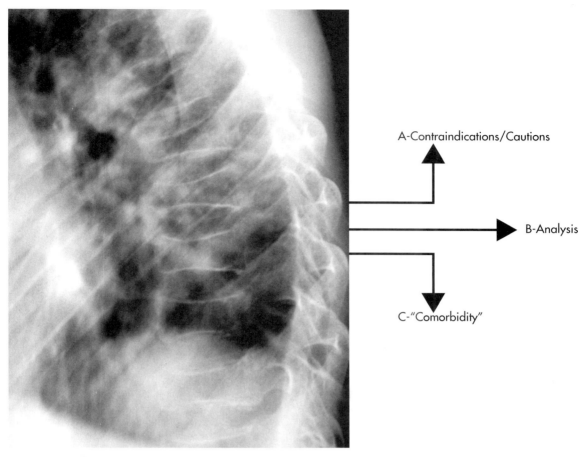

A-Contraindications/Cautions

B-Analysis

C-"Comorbidity"

FIG. 5-1 Three streams of information from the radiograph. In the context of delivering chiropractic care (or other manual approaches to patient care), radiographs provide three types of information: (a) information related to possible structural contraindications or cautions to delivering a corrective force into the demonstrated anatomy; (b) information that may influence the direction or technical approach to delivering a corrective force; and (c) information related to diseases, conditions, or findings that are seen in addition to the chiropractic subluxation, osteopathic lesion, or primary reasons the radiographs were taken. For instance, this radiograph demonstrates osteopenia that will influence the delivery of the chiropractic adjustment *(stream A)*. There may be biomechanical or degenerative features that will cause the chiropractor to adjust one segment over another, thereby influencing the technical approach to the patient *(stream B)*. Last, the compression fractures may result from an underlying aggressive pathology such as metastasis that would be of great concern to the clinician, beyond the issue related to the chiropractic subluxation or the initial concerns of the clinician *(stream C)*.

BOX 5-1

Clinical Red Flags of Serious Spinal Pathology (e.g., Infection, Tumor, or Fracture)

Unexplained weight loss
Personal history of cancer
Unexplained fever
Age more than 50 years
Intravenous drug use
Prolonged corticosteroid use
Severe, unremitting pain at night
Trauma sufficient to cause fracture or injury
Pain that worsens when the patient is lying down
Features of cauda equina syndrome
Urinary retention
Bilateral neurologic signs or symptoms
Saddle anesthesia

From Deyo RA, Diehl AK: Lumbar spine films in primary care: current use and effects of selective ordering criteria, *J Gen Intern Med* 1:20, 1986.

neurologic findings are limited). This is especially true when the literature suggests that approximately 25% of normal adults demonstrate acquired spinal stenosis and 33% have a disc herniation,[44] two key MRI findings.

In the absence of clear guidelines, clinicians must adhere to a logical rule for the use of all diagnostic procedures: If the patient's diagnosis or management is likely to significantly change from information routinely provided by the diagnostic procedure in question, then the study should be performed; if the necessary information is not routinely provided by the procedure or knowing the information obtained will not change the patient's management, then the procedure should not be performed.

Image Interpretation

EQUIPMENT AND RESOURCES

Before the skills and knowledge of the interpreter can be brought to task, the images should be clearly displayed and reference material should be close at hand. This is a digital age, but clearly the

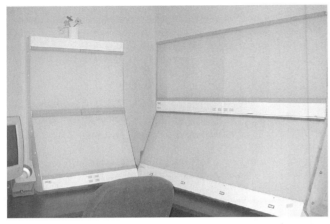

FIG. 5-2   View box station. View boxes are arranged in various formats to construct a viewing station. This picture exhibits a simple four over four bank on the right and a two over two bank to the left of it.

revolution has not permeated all segments of the population evenly. Although many clinics have moved to filmless methods for acquiring and displaying images, not all are so advanced. Much radiology, particularly plain film, is still accomplished traditionally; this produces radiographs that should be viewed on illuminated light boxes. These view boxes generally are available in two sizes, the standard 14 × 17 inch view box, and a larger 14 × 36 inch view box that accommodates a full spine radiograph, the type often used to assess scoliosis. Standard 14 × 17 inch view boxes are combined in various configurations to create a viewing station (Fig. 5-2).

High-volume centers may invest in a viewing system with rotating panels or belts that pass the films in front of a stationary bank of lights, because placing the films on and off the view box can consume a considerable amount of time. This system allows many cases to be stored and viewed quickly, without the need to shuffle through the films of each case as they are put on and off the view box.

A "hot" or "bright" light is another important tool necessary for film interpretation (Fig. 5-3). The hot light produces a controllable high-intensity beam of light that helps the interpreter view the

overexposed (dark or radiolucent) areas of the film. The intensity of the light can be controlled with a pedal that allows the interpreter to match the brightness of the light to the darkness of the radiograph. Even radiographs that are executed under the highest technical standard have regions of overexposed anatomy. Some of the more common and significant pathologies often hide in the overexposed areas of the film, making it difficult to recognize them when viewing the films only on a view box. Therefore a hot light is an essential tool to a thorough film interpretation.

It has been said that "a radiologist with a ruler is a radiologist in trouble."[97] Although the sentiment underscores the importance of clinical intuition, observation, and training, the reality is that handy access to rulers, protractors, or other measuring devices allows more accurate quantification of structural abnormalities. For instance, the degree of spondylolisthesis is related to the likelihood of its further progression, the rate of growth of a pulmonary nodule is predictive of its malignant potential, the degree of scoliosis is central to the management of the case, and so on.

Reference texts should be close at hand. The usefulness of some radiology books transcend the typical, such as Keats' *Atlas of Normal Roentgen Variants That May Simulate Disease.*[76] A recent edition of Keats' atlas should be close to the reading area. As the title describes, this book is a regional atlas of abnormal film findings that are normal variants of anatomy. This book is comprehensive and includes both subtle and grossly abnormal cases. Recognizing that an abnormal finding is a normal variant saves time and examination costs related to erroneous additional evaluation. For example, view the case exhibited in Figure 5-4 of a 12-year-old with a history of trauma. The calcaneus clearly looks fractured, but the radiolucent defect actually represents an unfused secondary growth at the center of the calcaneal tuberosity. A similar case is noted in the third edition of Keats' book.[76] Recognizing that this is a normal

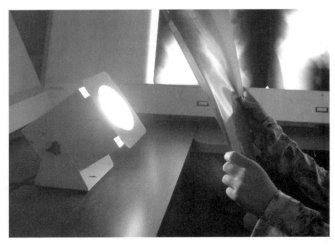

FIG. 5-3   Hot light. The hot light (also known as a *bright light*) is an essential tool to film interpretation. By using a hot light, the interpreter is able to view the overexposed regions of the film. Some of the most serious pathologies (e.g., lung nodules, aneurysms) are common to the overexposed regions of a radiograph and are more easily seen with the aid of a hot light.

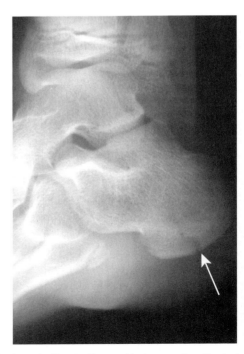

FIG. 5-4   Lateral ankle of a 12-year-old who recently suffered a trauma to the calcaneus. The radiolucent line appearing as a fracture *(arrow)* actually represents a normal appearance of the secondary growth centers. This case demonstrates how closely some normal findings and variants of normal may simulate a disease state. (Courtesy C. Robert Tatum, Davenport, IA.)

variant and not a fracture ensures that time and expense are not wasted.

ERRORS IN FILM INTERPRETATION

Interpreter error may arise from a failure to see, recognize, or understand the significance of a lesion. Although errors rates of 20% to 30% have been reported,[55] the more contemporary literature indicates that approximately 1% to 3% of plain film interpretations done by nonradiologists contain important errors.* Most of these studies are done by emergency department personnel.

Seltzer[128] estimates that 8% of interpretations by medical radiology residents contain potentially clinically important errors, which suggests that misinterpretation is increased in interpreters with fewer qualifications. Complex studies (e.g., CT)[2] and studies on pediatric patients[129] also increase misinterpretation. Fractures are the most often-missed lesions.[30,118,155] Training is associated with more accurate interpretation,[145] but radiologists are not immune to misinterpretations, as studied with various methods and imaging modalities.[65-69,93,116] Most studies focus on false-negative readings; however, false-positive readings occur among radiologists[30] and nonradiologists[153] alike. False-positives promote continued patient evaluation, adding to the cost, which is estimated to average $85 per false-positive reading.[153] Unnecessary examinations also result in increased risk of complications associated with imaging.

Alleged diagnostic errors account for the majority of legal cases related to radiology departments.[20] However, not every missed lesion constitutes evidence of negligence. Statistics pointing to related rates of missed lesions, limitations of normal human visual perception, image quality, and many other factors influence image interpretation, and may be mitigating factors for image misinterpretation.[20-24,130] The conceptual difference between errors in interpretation and those arising from perceptual variations is well described by Robinson.[117] The former assumes the diagnosis is known and generally agreed upon as a lesion; the latter does not (Fig. 5-5).

The goal of film interpretation is to eliminate as many misinterpretations as possible. There is a substantial literature addressing the topic of radiologic interpretation (see Table 5-1). The literature and conventional wisdom indicate that although it is impossible to eliminate human error, and therefore mistakes of radiologic interpretation, then attention to common principles should prove beneficial (Box 5-2).

For example, after careful review of the anteroposterior (AP) and lateral projections of the 56-year-old woman shown in Figure 5-6, it is apparent that the x-ray quality could be better. The patient is a large woman, and the typical problems of this circumstance are exhibited on these radiographs, such as the general "gray" appearance of the images related to excessive beam scatter. The anatomy of the lateral projection appears more radiodense in the lower portion of the lumbar spine and sacrum because the patient is wider at her hips than waist. Also, the overlying osseous shadows of the ilia add radiodensity. A skin fold creates a radiolucent transverse band at the level of the L3 disc space on the lateral projection. A degenerative spondylolisthesis is noted at L4 on L5. Multiple metallic clips are noted incidentally on the anteroposterior (AP) projection positioned along the periphery of the pelvis. The clips are related to a surgical procedure the patient underwent months earlier to remove a uterine carcinoma. Unfortunately, the surgical removal was not curative, and pulmonary metastasis is evidenced by the large mass appearing immediately superior to the apex of the

*References 30, 50, 58, 79, 113, 118, 148, 153, 155.

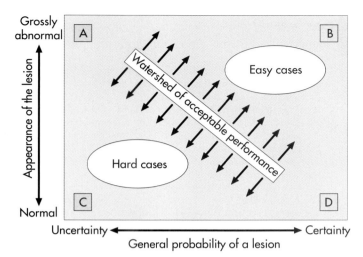

FIG. 5-5 Errors in image interpretation. This figure depicts a relationship between the imaging appearance of a lesion (size, shape, etc.) and the probability that the apparent lesion truly is one. *(A)* At times, their may be an uncertain or mixed interpretation of a grossly abnormal feature (e.g., importance of a lumbosacral transitional segmentation or spondylolisthesis). *(B)* Easy cases to interpret are defined as those that appear clearly abnormal on imaging and have a high degree of certainty that they are real lesions. Misinterpreting such a case is a clear error. *(C)* In contrast, difficult cases are those that present with only mild departures from the appearance of normal anatomy and are associated with doubtful conclusions on whether a true lesion is present. Misinterpreting this case may reflect a genuine difference of opinion among experts, representing variation in opinion more than direct error. *(D)* Last, only a small deviation from normal anatomy may correlates to a certain lesion. For example, a small corner fracture of the phalanx appears subtle, but has a certain interpretation as a lesion. The watershed of acceptable performance represents the line between clear-cut error and the inevitable difference in opinion existing between and among professionals. (From Robinson PJ: Radiology's Achilles' heel: error and variation in the interpretation of the Roentgen image, *Br J Radiol* 70:1085, 1997.)

diaphragm adjacent to the gastric air bubble, as seen on the lateral projection (Fig. 5-6, *A*). The presentation of the lung mass at the periphery of the film could cause it to be missed during initial review of the radiograph. Lesions appearing on the periphery of the film are not as evident as those appearing in the center. Remembering to give equal attention to the periphery of the image and adhering to the other principles of film interpretation (many listed in Box 5-2) reduces the rate of missed lesions.

Perceptual variations are more likely to occur when the lesion is subtle and its clinical interpretation is unknown or undecided. There are also limitations in the visual process. Two such limitations (ambiguous images and Mach bands) are discussed in the following.

Ambiguous image. When it comes to plain film radiography, our visual systems are constrained by interpreting two-dimensional representations of three-dimensional anatomy. The mental image formed may represent assumptions made of the depth of every point in the image. These assumptions may change over time, yielding dramatically different anatomic interpretations. This phenomenon can be self-demonstrated by viewing ambiguous images (Figs. 5-7 and 5-8). Ambiguous images cause perceptional vacillation, although the optical input remains constant. Fluctuations in perception are thought to reflect ambiguous information about the nature of an object at a given location in visual space. The brain reacts to uncertainty by fluctuating between different neural states

BOX 5-2
Suggestions to Reduce Radiologic Interpretation Errors

1. *Become familiar with the patient data.* The age, gender, and ethnicity of the patient may offer potent predictors of what disease process is represented on the radiographs. For instance, a 2-cm solitary radiodense defect of the L4 vertebral body is likely a bone island in a patient under 30 years of age. By contrast, a metastatic deposit needs to be excluded in a patient more than 40 years of age. Patient demographics directly influence clinical decision making.

2. *Become familiar with the clinical context of the study.* The clinical rationale for the study should be known before a patient's images are viewed. The interpreter should have a good idea of what he or she will encounter before the films come out of the processor. For example, are the films done to evaluate the patient for a clinically suspected rib fracture? Knowing the clinical context is essential to a thorough interpretation.

3. *Assess technical factors, image quality, and artifacts.* The images should be of sufficient quality and the correct area of clinical interest. Film interpretation is directly and negatively influenced by poor technical factors, such as improper patient positioning, patient motion, and many others problems that are more fully discussed in Chapter 1. Faint shadows of pathology may not be visible if the images are underexposed or overexposed. Patient motion is probably the most common technical defect that degrades image interpretation. Also, all of the clinically relevant anatomy must be visible to the degree expected. Images taken when the patient is recumbent may cause some of the anatomy to appear quite different. A case in point is the difference in size of the heart shadow on recumbent and upright films, or inspiration versus expiration patient instructions on upright films. Clothing and other artifacts can form ambiguous presentations on radiographs.

4. *Search the images using an intentional, thorough visual path.* Image interpretation has a greater chance of being successful if steps are taken to view the entire image in a complete manner. One popular approach to film interpretation involves a review of the alignments (A) of structures, bone (B) elements, cartilage (C) or joint spaces, and soft tissues (S). This is known as the "ABCS" approach to film interpretation and the method ensures that all of the anatomy is viewed completely. However, the interpreter should not be a slave to the ABCS sequence of film interpretation. For some, the ABCS approach may be more naturally applied as a BCAS or CABS sequence. The important point is that all of the anatomy is viewed; the order is less critical.

   When an abnormal finding is discovered, a free search path is invoked to follow the features of the disease. Once all of the related findings have been observed, the interpreter returns to a fixed sequence to ensure that all of the anatomy has been viewed. The search path never should be haphazard. It needs to intentionally follow the predetermined path of the anatomy (e.g., alignments, bone, cartilage, soft tissue) or trail of pathologic findings (e.g., observed fracture line, associated angulation, soft-tissue distension).

5. *Patients are entitled to more than one problem.* As mentioned, the radiographs should be searched completely for defects in the alignment, bones, cartilage joint spaces, and soft tissues. It is especially important to be vigilant to a complete search pattern after a lesion is uncovered. For instance, at times the interpreter may become so preoccupied with the first abnormality detected that a second or third lesion may be overlooked. This is a well-established phenomenon known as a "satisfaction of search error."[7,16] By definition, satisfaction of search errors represent omissions of underreading images. The satisfaction of search phenomenon is more likely to manifest when the first lesion is generally more attention-grabbing than the subsequent, more subtle lesion.[124]

   Although the causes of satisfaction of search errors are not explicitly defined, these errors may be reduced if interpreters are aware of the tendency to miss subsequent lesions, and hopefully develop a tendency to closely look for a second lesion whenever a first lesion is found, a third when a second is found, and so on until the anatomy is viewed completely. A complete search pattern is the only defense to avoid this well-known pitfall of image interpretation.

6. *Compare what is seen with the "mind's eye of normal."* After a review of the patient's demographics, the rationale for examination, and technical issues related to the image, image interpretation next begins with a thorough search of the displayed anatomy for any deviations from normal. This step is the most crucial of the film interpretation process. Image interpretation requires an excellent knowledge of normal anatomy. Abnormality quickly catches the eye when normal is understood.[87]

7. *Common things are commonly seen (or, rare things are rarely seen).* This concept underscores the importance of trying to explain the cause of abnormal findings by starting with the common pathologies and working to the less common differentials. For instance, a fragmented, radiodense, small proximal epiphysis appearing on hip radiographs of a 6-year-old boy could signify hypothyroidism, but there is a better chance that it represents traumatically induced avascular necrosis.

8. *Be proactive, not reactive.* Excluding common pathologic presentations should be proactively attempted; that is, pathologies that are common to some radiographs should be routinely investigated. For example, when an anteroposterior (AP) open-mouth projection is viewed, an odontoid fracture should specifically be looked for. Signs of an aneurysm of the abdominal aorta on a lateral lumbar projection, a femoral neck fracture on an AP view of the pelvis, and so on should be checked. Features of the pathology should not simply be reacted to; common pathologic presentations should be proactively eliminated, especially those suggested clinically.

9. *There is no substitute for experience.* Critically interpreting large numbers of radiographs will help interpreters develop a strong sense of normal anatomy, and allow subtle abnormal shadows to be more apparent.

10. *Consult with someone on difficult or ambiguous cases.* The social literature says that two minds are better than one. A group decision generally is more accurate than an individual conclusion. Keeping with this theme, when ambiguous findings are recognized or intuitively suspected, it may be helpful to obtain a second opinion to resolve any controversy and arrive at a valid film interpretation. Interestingly, research suggests that when asking another interpreter to view the film, it is better to blind the second interpreter to the suspicious areas of the film found by the first examiner. Swenson and Theodore[142] found that second interpreters of chest films were more accurate if they read the films using a "free search pattern," unencumbered and independent of the exact prior concerns of the first interpreter. The theory that supports this assertion is described as "superiority of search." The theory holds that when interpreters review standard radiographic views (e.g., posteroanterior (PA) chest film), they go through a process of skilled perceptual filtering that allows them to recognize abnormal findings. Diagnostic radiology is a visual interpretation reliant on knowledge and visual acuity. It is dependent on the ability to sort information to arrive at clinically meaningful conclusions.

Moreover, if the search pattern used by the radiologist is interrupted (in this case, by being tipped off to what to look at), the perceptual mechanisms are bypassed, resulting in a less accurate interpretation.[142] There is empiric evidence that second opinions are helpful to the interpretation of chest radiographs,[67,159] barium enemas,[103] and mammography.[6,25,29]

11. *Search for links between findings and various views*. Cognitively linking related findings together should be attempted in hopes of developing a perceptional flow to the image interpretation. Triangulation between the available views of the region (e.g., PA and lateral chest or AP, AP open-mouth, lateral cervical spine) should be used. Some interpreters embrace the concept that related anatomy should be reviewed together. For instance, when viewing a PA chest film it makes more sense to view all of the ribs separate from viewing the pulmonary tissues, as opposed to viewing the first rib and estimated pulmonary tissues concurrently.

12. *Eliminate extraneous light*. The ambient room light should be low, and view boxes that are not displaying images should be turned off.

13. *Compare current findings with those on past radiographs*. Past imaging studies are very useful to aid in the interpretation of current radiographs.[12,156] Berbaum found that normal comparison images were especially helpful for those interpreters who were in the earlier stage of training.[12] This is believed to be related to the perceptual operation in which single perceptions from the old and new film combine to form a common, third, unique perception. Comparison with past radiographs also helps to document the progression of a lesion. The stability of a lesion over time is a key predictor of its aggressiveness. For example, a 1-cm lung nodule not seen on radiographs 6 months previously likely indicates a malignant etiology of the nodule. If the nodule was on an early film and of consistent size on the past images, an etiology of granulomatous infection is likely to explain the nodule. However, caution is necessary. At times the progression of a pathology may be so subtle as to be missed when very recent past radiographs are viewed. Use of multiple comparisons, including old past images, is best to avoid this pitfall.

14. *The problem is perception*. Image interpretation is a function of perception more than visual acuity. The question is not what can be seen, but identifying what is seen. Interpreters tend to overlay personal bias onto the process of image interpretation. It takes discipline to focus on the objective interpretation of the demonstrated anatomy. Perception is made better by experience and continually correlating what is seen to what is actually present. This is learned best by iterations of comparing one's interpretation with that of someone more proficient.

15. *Is the abnormal finding real?* When abnormal shadows are seen on the image, it should first be considered that they may represent nothing more than a presentation of normal anatomy, artifact, or confluence of overlying shadows. It is common for superimposed structures to form a resultant shape. For instance, the pulmonary arteries coursing in multiple directions across the lung may combine to give the appearance of a circular, cystic

pulmonary defect. The resulting "virtual image" is termed a subjective image. It is not real; rather, it is an illusion conjured in the mind of the interpreter.

16. *Give special attention to the problem areas of the radiograph*. Some areas on the film are more likely to contain pathology than others. For instance, attention must be paid to interpret the lung apices on the AP lower cervical radiograph; the atlantodental interval and sella turcica are important areas that are often neglected on the lateral radiograph. Problem areas for various projections are listed in Figures 5-12 to 5-20. Generally, special attention should be given to the overexposed, radiolucent areas of all projections as common sites for pathology.

17. *Be organized*. Successful film interpretation requires some attention to detail. The patient's images should be accompanied by a correlating history and pertinent clinical data, inclusive of any past imaging studies that may assist the interpretation. Resources (e.g., books, rulers, protractors, voice recorders, alcohol to erase pencil lines, dry erase markers for annotating abnormal findings) should be close at hand. Part of being organized involves consistency in how the images are assembled on the view boxes. For instance, many interpreters feel compelled to place the lateral radiographs on the view box so the patients are facing to the interpreter's reading left, or view the films in a consistent sequence: lateral . . . AP . . . oblique, etc.

18. *Attention to environment*. The film reading environment should be quiet and free of distractions. Maintaining low ambient room light and turning off view boxes without films are both empirically associated with successful image interpretation.

19. *What is the clinical impact?* The purpose of diagnostic imaging is to gather data to assist clinical decision making. Therefore all abnormal findings should be interpreted in light of their clinical significance with appropriate follow-up imaging or procedures formulated into the report generated from the images.

20. *Do not ignore intuition*. The largest portion of the variation in film interpretation is unexplained. Sometimes the only predictor of an abnormality is that lingering sense that something is being missed. This feeling often drives extra attention that may eventually reveal a subtle defect. Perhaps the eyes are seeing something that the brain cannot immediately comprehend.

21. *Resist overinterpreting the study*. No matter how closely they are scrutinized, plain film radiographs do not reliably detail a disc lesion, ependymoma, hydrosyringomyelia, or a host of other defects. The clinical utility of the imaging modality must always be matched to the clinical question, and the modality's limitations must be considered. The temptation must be resisted to assume that the patient's problem is illustrated on the imaging study being reviewed. Also, a link must not be assumed between the patient's clinical problem and radiographic abnormalities that happen to be present. The early literature is replete with assumptive correlations that could not be supported when investigated in greater depth.

22. *Confirm findings with other views or studies*. If findings are equivocal, further views, contrast, specialized imaging, and so on should be used to increase the certainty about something found.

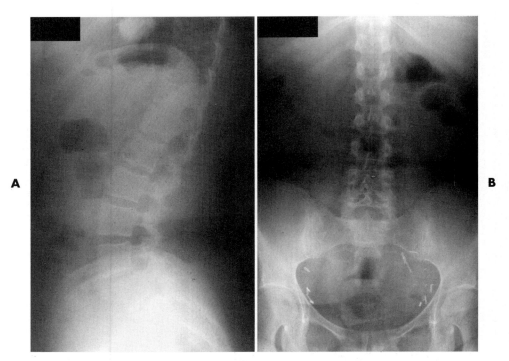

FIG. 5-6 **A,** Lateral and, **B,** anteroposterior projection of the lumbopelvic skeleton (see text for description of the findings).

over time.[8,80] Ambiguous images and other pitfalls of image perception and interpretation are possible. Generally, the film interpreter is cautioned not to assume that perception is reality.

Mach bands. A Mach band illusion is another common source of radiographic misinterpretation (Fig. 5-9). The human visual system may accentuate an abrupt change in brightness of an image so that regions of constant brightness appear to have varying brightness. This appearance is an illusion caused by the brain trying to enhance the contrast between slightly different hues of color (or gray scale). For example, in an AP open-mouth projection of the upper cervical spine, there may appear to be a transverse

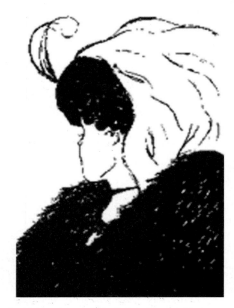

FIG. 5-8 Ambiguous image. A classical ambiguous image was developed by E.G. Boring, and inspired by earlier renditions of the image that appeared on postcards and advertisements. The image depicts a young woman from the perspective of looking over her left shoulder as she wears a large boa and hat with a posteriorly directed feather. If you look at the image long enough, instead of a young woman, you will see an old woman from her left anterior perspective. The jaw line of the young woman becomes the lower margin of the nose of the old woman, the young woman's ear becomes the old woman's left eye, and the young woman's necklace becomes the old woman's month, partially open. Ambiguous images arise from difficulties in interpreting three-dimensional structures from two dimensional imaging modalities. The film interpreter is cautioned to consider the impact of ambiguous images on their perceptions during image interpretation. (From Boring EG: A new ambiguous figure, *Amer J Psychol* 42: 444, 1930.)

FIG. 5-7 Ambiguous image. An ambiguous image has the potential for more than one interpretation. For example, notice that the white cup can also be interpreted as the profile of two dark gray opposing faces.

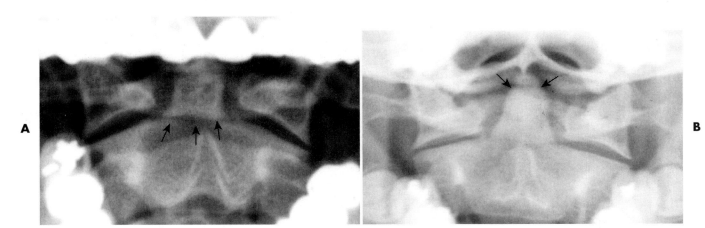

FIG. 5-9 Mach bands. The human visual system may accentuate an abrupt change in brightness of an image so that selected regions of constant brightness appear to have varying brightness. **A,** For example, the gradient above has three even steps, but there is a perception of a brighter strip immediately before each gradient change and darker strip immediately after the gradient change. This phenomenon can be graphically represented by the solid black line indicating the three steps in brightness that occur between each of the four shades of gray scale. The human visual system will accentuate the actual (black line) change in brightness to give the illusion of darker stripes parallel to and just before the gradient change and brighter line running parallel to and immediately after the gradient change. This perceived gradient change is depicted by the dashed blue line. **B,** Another example is this circular gradient change. Notice how there appears to be a white halo around the black (center) to white (periphery) gradient. In this example, the white halo is a mach band.

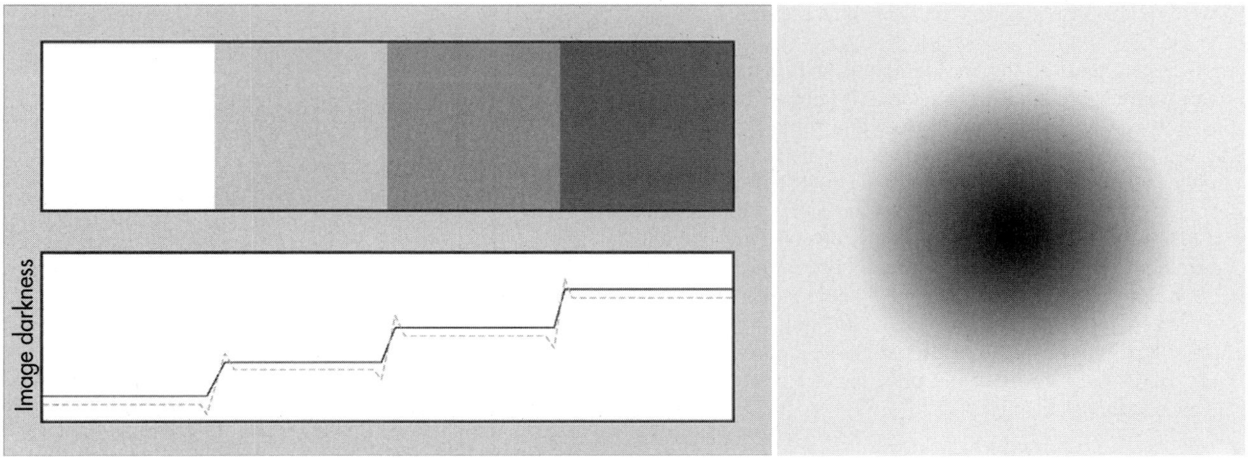

fracture of the odontoid process immediately adjacent to the overlapping anterior arch of the atlas. This illusion is caused by a perceived change in the radiodensity of the odontoid process (Fig. 5-10). A band of perceived (but not real) contrast enhancement is termed a *Mach band*.[49] A Mach band appears as a thin bright band on the lighter side and a thin dark band on the darker side of the gray scale, or color, gradient. Verification of a Mach band can be performed by a densitometer; the meter will not fluctuate across the perceived contrast enhancement.

APPEARANCE OF THE RADIOGRAPH

A typical family photograph is a positive image. Everything that is white appears white; everything that is black appears black; and

so on. A radiograph is a negative image. In reference to subject density, dense structures (a function of mass and volume), such as metal and bone, appear whiter than do less dense structures, such as fat or water. In this sense, the radiograph is a shadow of anatomy. Dense structures impede more of the x-ray beam from striking the radiographic film; therefore after chemical development, the area appears white (or light gray) when the radiograph is back-lighted on a view box. Less dense anatomy appears dark gray or black on the film. The term *radiopaque* describes dense structures that block most of the x-ray beam and consequently appear white on the radiograph. The term *radiolucent* describes less dense structures that block little of the x-ray beam and consequently appear dark gray or black on the radiograph. In distinction to subject density, film

FIG. 5-10 Mach bands across the odontoid process. **A,** Notice the radiolucent line across the base of the odontoid process (arrows). The radiolucent line is not real, but rather is caused by the overlapping posterior arch of the atlas above. The overlapping posterior arch changes the density gradient of the image and promotes the interpretation of a radiolucent line adjacent to the radiodense shadow. The odontoid is not really fractured. **B,** The overlapping inferior margin of the skull causes the appearance of a separated tip of the odontoid process (arrows). As in **A,** the odontoid is not really fractured. At times, it is difficult to separate a Mach band from a true fracture. When in doubt, the projection could be retaken with a slightly different head tilt. On the repeat radiograph, the Mach band should move; the fracture will not.

density describes the film's ability to stop light passing through the film.

The final appearance of the radiograph is a function of the summation of many superimposed structures. It may be that several superimposed structures of medium to low density appear on the radiograph as a lighter gray shadow than a single dense object. An x-ray beam that traverses a thin bone may appear more radiolucent (sometimes termed less dense) than when the same x-ray beam traverses a medium-sized organ (e.g., water density). In general, five radiographic densities are listed—metal, bone, water, fat, and air—from most radiolucent (black) to most radiopaque or radiodense (white) (Fig. 5-11). Of course, metal does not occur in the body naturally but may be present after surgery, dental work, or foreign body intrusion; or reflect the presence of overlying artifacts (e.g., necklaces or earrings).

BOX 5-3
Steps in Radiographic Interpretation

1. Understand the clinical rationale for the study.
2. Search the images for abnormal findings.
3. List and define any abnormal findings.
4. Summarize any abnormal findings by either concluding on an obvious diagnosis (an Aunt Minnie) or attempting to identify a general pattern or gamut described by the abnormal findings. Selected radiologic patterns of abnormality are listed in Box 5-13.
5. Integrate the radiologic findings and list of possible diseases that may explain these findings with pertinent data obtained from the history, clinical examination, laboratory testing, and further or past diagnostic imaging. The goal is to follow a systematic, rational process that narrows the list of radiologic and clinical considerations to identify a definitive diagnosis that will assist in successful patient management.

BOX 5-4
Interpretation Checklist for a Lateral Cervical Radiograph

Patient information
- Review and verify the date of examination and patient information.

Image quality
- Evaluate photographic properties: density, contrast, and noise factors (quantum mottle, fog, etc.).
- Evaluate geometric factors: size, shape, detail, and distortion.

Patient positioning and technical defects
- Are there signs of positioning errors, motion artifact, static marks, or other technical defects?
- Are the films done recumbent or upright?

Field of view
- Does the vertical field of view extend from the base of the occiput to below the C7 vertebra?
- Does the horizontal field of view include angles of the mandible to the C7 spinous process?

Common artifacts
- Are there stems of eyeglasses, earrings, necklaces, clothing, and so on?

Common foreign bodies
- Are there any dental fillings?

Alignment
- Is the cervical lordosis maintained?
- Is the tip of the odontoid vertically centered over the C7 body?
- Are the articular pillars offset, suggesting facet dislocation, or do they closely overlap as usual?
- Are the posterior borders of the rami of the mandible generally overlapped? (Projectional distortion causes them not to be directly overlapped.)
- Are the seven vertical lines maintained?
  - Line 1: along posterior tips of spinous processes
  - Line 2: along spinal laminal lines
  - Line 3: along posterior margins of posterior joints
  - Line 4: along anterior margins of posterior joints
  - Line 5: along posterior margins of bodies C2 to C7 (George's line)

Line 6: along anterior margins of bodies C2 to C7
Line 7: along posterior margin of pharynx and tracheal air shadows

Bones
- Are radiodensity, size, shape, and configuration of each vertebra normal?
  - Vertebral body
  - Transverse process
  - Pedicle
  - Lamina
  - Spinal laminar junction line
  - Spinous process
  - Odontoid process of C2
- Do the mandible, maxilla, and teeth appear normal?
- Are the radiodensity, size, shape, and configuration of the base of the skull normal?
- Is the sella turcica normal?
- Is the spinal canal maintained?

Joint spaces
- Is the atlantodental interval increased (>3 mm in adults or 5 mm in children)?
- Are the intervertebral disc spaces well maintained?
- Are cervical disc spaces wedged to the anterior?
- Are the posterior joint surfaces parallel with visible joint spaces from C3 to C7?
- Is the intervertebral foramen maintained?
- Is the space between the occiput and the atlas, and the interspinous spaces from C2 to C7 maintained?

Soft tissue
- Is the retropharyngeal space less than 5 mm at C2 and the retrotracheal space less than 20 mm at C6? (An in situ nasogastric tube will invalidate these measures.)
- Do the paranasal sinuses appear radiolucent?
- Is there physiologic calcification of the laryngeal cartilages?

Problem areas
- Atlantodental interval, sella turcica, C7 spinous process, and so on (Fig. 5-12)

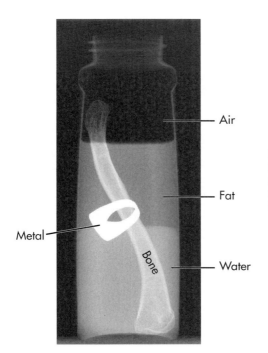

FIG. 5-11 Five radiographic densities. This is the radiograph of a baby's bottle in which the lower third of the bottle is filled with water, the middle third is filled with with oil (fat), and the upper third is left open to air. A clavicle and ring are inserted into the beaker. The constituents resemble each of the five radiographic densities of air, oil, water, bone, and metal, listed from black (radiolucent) to white (radiodense).

Air

Fat

Metal

Bone

Water

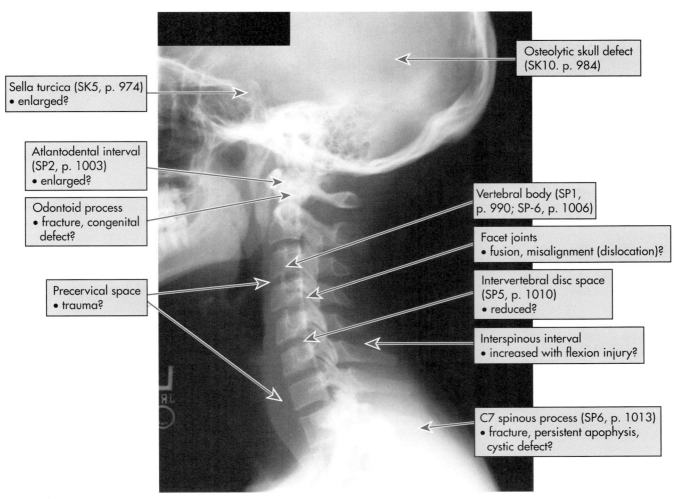

Osteolytic skull defect (SK10. p. 984)

Sella turcica (SK5, p. 974)
• enlarged?

Atlantodental interval (SP2, p. 1003)
• enlarged?

Odontoid process
• fracture, congenital defect?

Vertebral body (SP1, p. 990; SP-6, p. 1006)

Facet joints
• fusion, misalignment (dislocation)?

Precervical space
• trauma?

Intervertebral disc space (SP5, p. 1010)
• reduced?

Interspinous interval
• increased with flexion injury?

C7 spinous process (SP6, p. 1013)
• fracture, persistent apophysis, cystic defect?

FIG. 5-12 Lateral cervical radiograph: *key problem areas.*

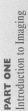

PART ONE Introduction to Imaging

BOX 5-5

Interpretation Checklist for an Anteroposterior Lower Cervical Radiograph

Patient information
- Review and verify the date of examination and patient information.

Image quality
- Evaluate photographic properties: density, contrast, and noise factors (quantum mottle, fog, etc.).
- Evaluate geometric factors: size, shape, detail, and distortion.

Patient positioning and technical defects
- Are there signs of positioning errors, motion artifact, static marks, or other technical defects?
- Are the films done recumbent or upright?

Field of view
- Does the vertical field of view extend from the angles of the mandible to the apices of the lung?
- Does the horizontal field of view include several centimeters of soft tissue on either side of the spine?

Common artifacts
- Are there eyeglasses, necklaces, hairpins, hair braids, clothing, and so on?

Common foreign bodies
- Are there any dental fillings, surgical staples from carotid enterectomy, and so on?

Alignment
- Is there a right or left cervical list or head tilt?
- Is there a right or left lateral curvature?
- Are the spinous processes generally aligned vertically?
- Is there a right or left laterolisthesis of any vertebrae?

Bones
- Are the radiodensity, size, shape, and configuration of each vertebra normal?
  - Vertebral body
  - Uncinate processes
  - Transverse processes
  - Pedicles
  - Laminae
  - Articular pillars
  - Spinous processes
  - Odontoid process of C2
- Are the radiodensity, size, shape, and configuration of the ribs normal?
- Are the radiodensity, size, shape, and configuration of the clavicle normal?
- Are the mastoid processes normal?
- Is the superior margin of the sternum normal?

Joint spaces
- Are the intervertebral disc spaces well maintained?
- Are the uncinate joint spaces well maintained?
- Are the costotransverse joints normal?

Soft tissue
- Is the piriform sinus, rima glottis, and tracheal air shadow midline?
- Does the paranasal sinus appear radiolucent?
- Are the apices of the lung clear of mass, infiltrate, or other defect?
- Is the aortic knob of normal configuration?
- Is there carotid artery calcification?
- Are the paraspinal tissues clear of mass or defect?

Problem areas
- Lung apices, uncinate processes, upper ribs, and so on (Fig. 5-13)

VISUAL SEARCH

Image interpretation involves gathering visual information to produce specific perceptions. The attitudes, beliefs, biases, and expectations of the examiner influence both what is observed during visual assessment and what is concluded from those observations. Although film interpretation is truly an art, generally accepted sequential steps define the process of image interpretation (Box 5-3). The first step is for the interpreter to become familiar with the study's clinical rationale. Is a fracture suspected? Does the 65-year-old patient with unrelenting low back pain have a history of night pain, unexplained weight loss, or past malignancy? Next the images should be viewed completely with a thorough visual search path. A complete search path is used to ensure that all of the anatomy has been observed. The best search path is a unique one developed by the interpreter over time, which compensates for the interpreter's inherent weaknesses in observation. For instance, if an interpreter has difficulty remembering to look at the sella turcica on a lateral radiograph of the cervical spine, the search path should be altered to emphasize that region; this will compensate for the interpreter's inherent tendency to underinterpret that portion of the film.

ABCS of film interpretation. The ABCS of film interpretation describes a commonly taught generic search path for film

interpretation. "ABCS" is a learning aid to prompt the interpreter to review all of the imaged anatomy by concentrating on four components in a fixed sequence: alignment, bone, cartilage (joint spaces), and soft tissue separately. By deconstructing the search path into manageable components (e.g., alignment and bone), the interpreter is less likely to omit aspects of the anatomy from the search path. Instead of following the ABCS format in direct sequence, some interpreters prefer to inspect the areas in other sequences, such as BCAS (bone, cartilage, alignment, and soft tissue) or ACBS (alignment, cartilage, alignment, and soft tissue).

Alternatively, some interpreters like to employ a "free" search pattern that allows interpreters' gaze to scan the anatomy in any sequence that grabs their visual attention. Regardless of the method (fixed or free), the search path must be comprehensive for reasons of accuracy, and concise for reasons of practicality.

Use of checklists in film interpretation. Some interpreters, especially beginners, are helped by consulting checklists of structures to assist in film interpretation. In a general sense, the ABCS approach to film interpretation is a brief checklist, reminding and sequencing the visual path of the interpreter through the presenting alignment, bone, cartilage (joint space) and soft tissues. All of the visualized anatomy needs to be closely scrutinized for possible defects.

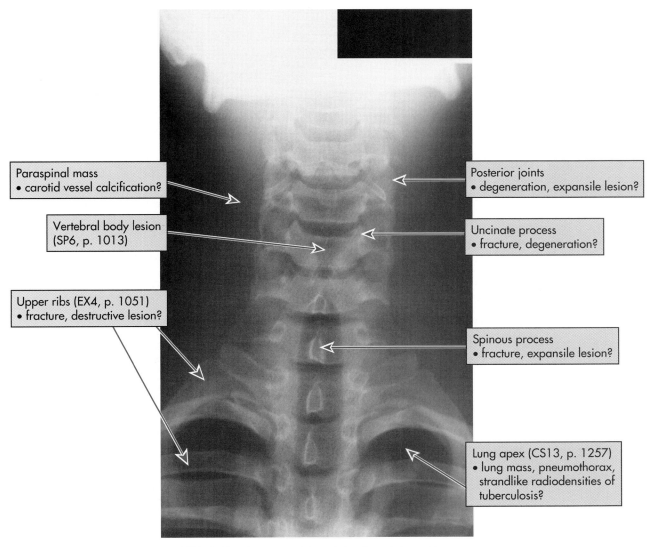

Paraspinal mass
• carotid vessel calcification?

Vertebral body lesion
(SP6, p. 1013)

Upper ribs (EX4, p. 1051)
• fracture, destructive lesion?

Posterior joints
• degeneration, expansile lesion?

Uncinate process
• fracture, degeneration?

Spinous process
• fracture, expansile lesion?

Lung apex (CS13, p. 1257)
• lung mass, pneumothorax,
strandlike radiodensities of
tuberculosis?

FIG. 5-13   Anteroposterior cervical radiograph: *key problem areas.*

Boxes 5-4 to 5-12 present developed checklists to ensure a comprehensive review of selected radiographic projections. Developing a truly all-inclusive checklist for each radiographic projection listed is not feasible. Instead the checklists enumerate the major technical considerations and anatomy (ABCS approach discussed in the preceding), and list problem areas that require extra attention.

Common problem areas of film interpretation. An effective search path is complete, scanning all of the visible anatomy. However, some anatomic regions deserve a second or extended look because they are common sites of pathology. Figures 5-12 through 5-20 accompanying Boxes 5-4 to 5-12 present selected radiographic projections with annotations corresponding to areas of the film that warrant special attention because they have a tendency to exhibit common or serious pathology.

IDENTIFY, DEFINE, AND SUMMARIZE ABNORMAL FINDINGS

The goal remains the same whether the interpreter chooses to rely on a checklist and resulting fixed visual path of inspection or employ a free visual path to evaluate the image. The goal is to identify, define, and summarize any and all deviations of normal anatomy.

In his text, *Medical Imaging,* Peter Scally[126] likens the process of identifying deviations of normal anatomy to the visual quizzes found in the comics section of most newspapers, in which the reader is instructed to spot differences between two frames of subtly different scenes. The difference, Dr. Scally points out, is that when it comes to interpreting radiographs, nobody is there to tell the interpreter how many differences are present. Following this analogy, one should develop a strong mental image of normal findings so that when abnormal findings present they will quickly attract attention.

A good portion of the problem is solved once the film has been searched and all of the abnormalities have been recognized. Then the interpreter must define and succinctly summarize the findings, allowing clinical attention to be directed most effectively. Ultimately the importance of an abnormality is judged in the context of its clinical impact.

BOX 5-6

Interpretation Checklist for an Anteroposterior Open-Mouth Cervical Spine Radiograph

Patient information
- Review and verify the date of examination and patient information.

Image quality
- Evaluate photographic properties: density, contrast, and noise factors (quantum mottle, fog, etc.).
- Evaluate geometric factors: size, shape, detail, and distortion.

Patient positioning and technical defects
- Are there signs of positioning errors, motion artifact, static marks, or other technical defects?
- Are the films done recumbent or upright?

Field of view
- Does the vertical field of view extend from above the tip of the odontoid to below the C2 spinous process?
- Does the horizontal field of view extend laterally to the tips of the transverse processes of the atlas?

Common artifacts
- Are there artifacts such as tongue jewelry, hairpins, and so on?

Common foreign bodies
- Are there any dental fillings, and so on?

Alignment
- Are the widths of the lateral masses bilaterally comparable?
- Are the paraodontoid spaces symmetric?
- Does the lateral mass extend laterally beyond the margin of the superior articular processes of C2?
- Is the center of the C2 spinous process vertically aligned with the center of the odontoid process?

Bones
- Are the radiodensity, size, shape, and configuration of the atlas normal?
  - Lateral masses
  - Transverse processes
  - Transverse foramen
  - Anterior arch
  - Posterior arch
- Are the radiodensity, size, shape, and configuration of the C2 segment normal?
  - Odontoid process
  - Body
  - Pedicles
  - Superior articular processes
  - Spinous process
- Are the radiodensity, size, shape, and configuration of the base of the occiput normal?
- Are the occipital condyles normal?
- Are the rami of the mandible normal?

Joint spaces
- Is the occipitoatlantal joint space maintained?
- Are the atlantoaxial joints maintained?
- Is the C2-C3 disc space maintained?

Soft tissue
- Is there ossification of the stylohyoid ligaments?

Problem areas
- Odontoid process, alignment of the lateral mass, and so on (Fig. 5-14)

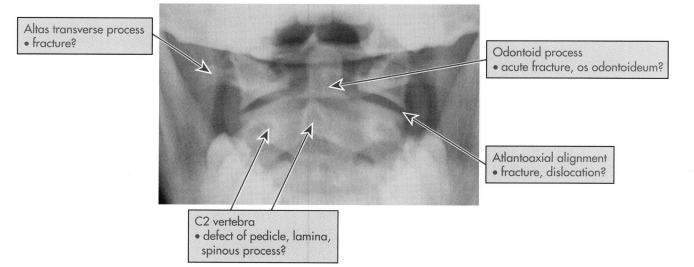

Altas transverse process
• fracture?

Odontoid process
• acute fracture, os odontoideum?

Atlantoaxial alignment
• fracture, dislocation?

C2 vertebra
• defect of pedicle, lamina, spinous process?

FIG. 5-14   Anteroposterior open mouth cervical radiograph: *key problem areas.*

BOX 5-7
Interpretation Checklist for a Lateral Thoracic Radiograph

Patient information
- Review and verify the date of examination and patient information.

Image quality
- Evaluate photographic properties: density, contrast, and noise factors (quantum mottle, fog, etc.).
- Evaluate geometric factors: size, shape, detail, and distortion.

Patient positioning and technical defects
- Are there signs of positioning errors, motion artifact, static marks, or other technical defects?
- Are the films done recumbent or upright?

Field of view
- Does the vertical field of view extend from above T1 to below T12?
- Does the horizontal field of view extend from near the sternum to include the posterior angles of the ribs?

Common artifacts
- Are there necklaces, hair braids, clothing, and so on?

Common foreign bodies
- Are there any sternal wires, pacemaker, valve prosthesis, and so on?

Alignment
- Is the thoracic kyphosis maintained?
- Is there any vertebral retrolisthesis or spondylolisthesis?
- Are the spinous processes generally aligned vertically?

Bones
- Are the radiodensity, size, shape, and configuration of each vertebra normal?
  - Vertebral body
  - Pedicles
  - Spinous process
- Are the radiodensity, size, shape, and configuration of each rib normal?
- Is the spinal canal maintained?

Joint spaces
- Are the intervertebral disc spaces maintained?
- Is the intervertebral foramen of normal size?

Soft tissue
- Is the tracheal air shadow centrally located?
- Is the heart shadow generally of normal size and configuration?
- Are the lung tissues clear of mass, infiltrate, or other defect?
- Are the ascending, transverse, and descending segments of the aorta normal?
- Are the aortic-pulmonary window and hila defined and clear?
- Is the diaphragm of normal position?
- Is the gastric air bubble of normal size and location below the diaphragm?

Problem areas
- Vertebral stature, lung tissue, hila, and so on (Fig. 5-15)

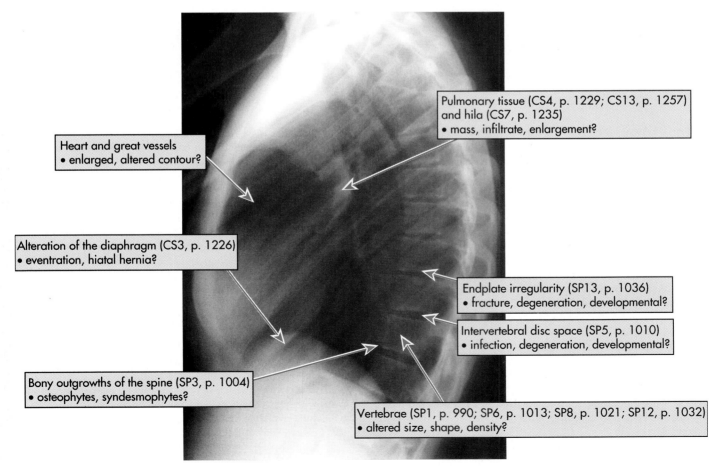

Heart and great vessels
• enlarged, altered contour?

Pulmonary tissue (CS4, p. 1229; CS13, p. 1257) and hila (CS7, p. 1235)
• mass, infiltrate, enlargement?

Alteration of the diaphragm (CS3, p. 1226)
• eventration, hiatal hernia?

Endplate irregularity (SP13, p. 1036)
• fracture, degeneration, developmental?

Intervertebral disc space (SP5, p. 1010)
• infection, degeneration, developmental?

Bony outgrowths of the spine (SP3, p. 1004)
• osteophytes, syndesmophytes?

Vertebrae (SP1, p. 990; SP6, p. 1013; SP8, p. 1021; SP12, p. 1032)
• altered size, shape, density?

FIG. 5-15 Lateral thoracic radiograph: *key problem areas.*

BOX 5-8
Interpretation Checklist for an Anteroposterior Thoracic Spine Radiograph

Patient information
- Review and verify the date of examination and patient information.

Image quality
- Evaluate photographic properties: density, contrast, and noise factors (quantum mottle, fog, etc.).
- Evaluate geometric factors: size, shape, detail, and distortion.

Patient positioning and technical defects
- Are there signs of positioning errors, motion artifact, static marks, or other technical defects?
- Are the films done recumbent or upright?

Field of view
- Does the vertical field of view extend from above T1 to below T12?
- Does the horizontal field of view include about 7 cm of soft tissue on either side of the spine?

Common artifacts
- Are there necklaces, hair braids, clothing, and so on?

Common foreign bodies
- Are there sternal wires, pacemaker, valve prosthesis, and so on?

Alignment
- Is there a right or left lateral curvature?
- Are the spinous processes generally aligned vertically?
- Are there any right or left vertebral translations?

Bones
- Are the radiodensity, size, shape, and configuration of each vertebra normal?

- Vertebral body
- Transverse processes
- Pedicles
- Laminae
- Articular processes
- Spinous process
- Are the radiodensity, size, shape, and configuration of the ribs normal?
- Are the radiodensity, size, shape, and configuration of the medial segments of the clavicles normal?
- Are radiodensity, size, shape, and configuration of the sternum normal?

Joint spaces
- Are the intervertebral disc spaces well maintained?
- Are the costotransverse joints normal?
- Are the costovertebral joints normal?

Soft tissue
- Is the tracheal air shadow midline?
- Is the heart shadow generally of normal size and configuration?
- Are the hila of normal size and configuration?
- Is the mediastinum midline and of expected size?
- Are the lung tissues clear of mass, infiltrate, or other defect?
- Are the ascending, transverse, and descending segments of the aorta normal?
- Is the diaphragm of normal position?
- Is the gastric air bubble of normal size and location?

Problem areas
- Hila, lung tissue, pedicle, ribs, and so on (Fig. 5-16)

The "Aunt Minnie" phenomenon. Sometimes (and increasingly with experience) the radiographic appearance is familiar to the interpreter as a characteristic expression of a known disease process. For instance, the appearance of a nearly symmetrically enlarged vertebral body with especially thickened cortices is a characteristic feature ("picture frame" vertebra) of Paget's disease. The simultaneous appearance of an enlarged vertebra with a thickened cortex is a unique feature of Paget's disease. After seeing this appearance once, the interpreter is sure to recognize it again.

In radiology, the phenomenon of correctly identifying a disease process by its unique radiologic presentation is termed an *Aunt Minnie*. Perhaps the majority of the diseases recognized by radiologists occur though the Aunt Minnie mechanism. Over time, a veteran radiologist memorizes the visual data of classic disease presentations and the Aunt Minnie mechanism becomes highly functional. It has been said that a radiologist's ability is dependent on skills of observation and memory; the latter endorses the Aunt Minnie mechanism. As defined on the website that carries her name, "Aunt Minnie" probably was coined by the famous radiologist Ben Felson, who applied the term to describe "a case with radiologic findings so specific and compelling that no realistic differential diagnosis exists."[35]

However, invoking the Aunt Minnie mechanism to summarize abnormal imaging findings assumes that the interpreter has a good knowledge of pathologic presentations and that the presentation is somewhat characteristic of the disease represented. It often turns out that this is too much to assume. For many interpreters, especially nonradiologist clinicians, a rational approach must be used to summarize abnormalities seen on imaging studies when a classic or characteristic presentation is not represented. Also, jumping to a definitive diagnosis by the Aunt Minnie process can result in a shortened interpretive process and diagnostic error.

The anatomic (pattern or gamut) approach. Once the radiograph has been reviewed, a rational method better defines abnormal radiologic findings and identifies disease processes. This method begins by categorizing the abnormal imaging findings into one or more succinct patterns of abnormality (Box 5-13). The patterns are based on the aberrant anatomy involved (e.g., enlarged vertebrae with thick cortex). An accurate summary of the radiographic findings is dependent on the interpreter's knowledge, experience, visual acuity, and so on.

The summarizing process can be thought of as a funnel (Fig. 5-21). The radiologic findings enter the broad end of the funnel. Consistent with the visual image of a funnel, the consideration of possible diseases needs to be broad: the broader the consideration, the less the chance of missing the correct explanation. However, the broader the list of differentials, the less practical it is to formulate a meaningful patient management plan. Therefore like the image of a funnel, the interpreter begins to eliminate the less likely differentials to develop a terse, more workable differential list of

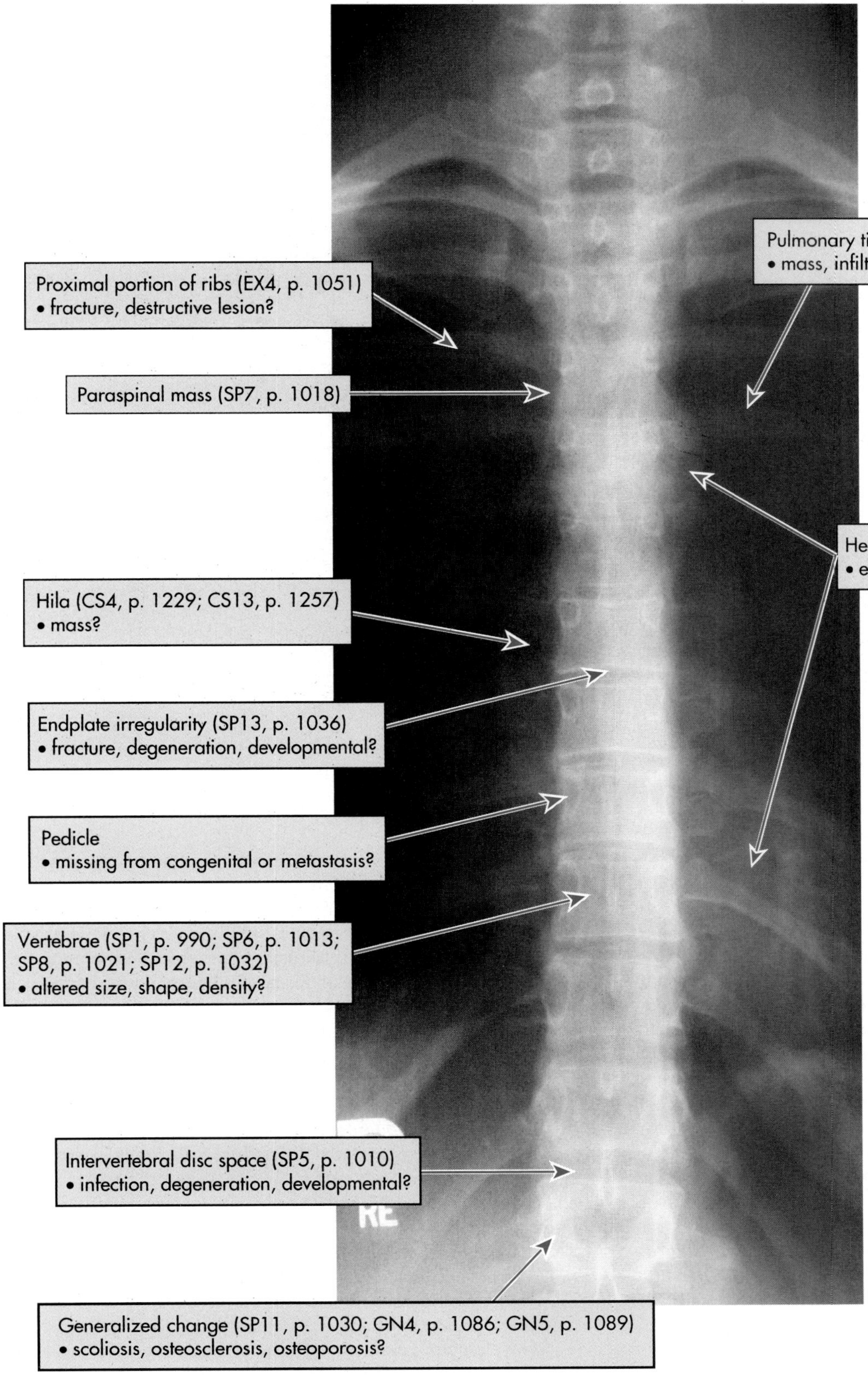

Proximal portion of ribs (EX4, p. 1051)
• fracture, destructive lesion?

Paraspinal mass (SP7, p. 1018)

Pulmonary tissue (CS4, p. 1229; CS13, p. 1257)
• mass, infiltrate?

Heart and great vessels
• enlarged, altered contour?

Hila (CS4, p. 1229; CS13, p. 1257)
• mass?

Endplate irregularity (SP13, p. 1036)
• fracture, degeneration, developmental?

Pedicle
• missing from congenital or metastasis?

Vertebrae (SP1, p. 990; SP6, p. 1013; SP8, p. 1021; SP12, p. 1032)
• altered size, shape, density?

Intervertebral disc space (SP5, p. 1010)
• infection, degeneration, developmental?

Generalized change (SP11, p. 1030; GN4, p. 1086; GN5, p. 1089)
• scoliosis, osteosclerosis, osteoporosis?

FIG. 5-16 Anteroposterior thoracic radiograph: *key problem areas.*

BOX 5-9
Interpretation Checklist for a Lateral Lumbar Radiograph

Patient information
- Review and verify the date of examination and patient information.
- Review image quality.
- Evaluate photographic properties: density, contrast, and noise factors (quantum mottle, fog, etc.).
- Evaluate geometric factors: size, shape, detail, and distortion.

Patient positioning and technical defects
- Are there signs of positioning errors, motion artifact, static marks, or other technical defects?
- Are the films done recumbent or upright?

Field of view
- Does the vertical field of view extend from above L1 to below the coccyx?
- Does the horizontal field of view extend from about 15 cm anterior to the lumbar spine to about 5 cm behind the lumbar spine bilaterally?

Common artifacts
- Are there any pieces of umbilical jewelry, clothing, and so on?

Common foreign bodies
- Are there any surgical staples, and so on?

Alignment
- Is the lumbar lordosis maintained?
- Are there any anterior or posterior vertebral translations?
- Is the coccyx deviated sharply anterior?
- Is the sacrum angle increased?

Bones
- Are the radiodensity, size, shape, and configuration of each vertebra normal?
  - Vertebral body
  - Spinous process
  - Superior and inferior articular processes
  - Pars interarticularis
  - Laminae
- Are the radiodensity, size, shape, and configuration of the sacrum and coccyx normal?
- Are the radiodensity, size, shape, and configuration of the ilia normal?
- Are the radiodensity, size, shape, and configuration of the lower ribs normal?

Joint spaces
- Are the intervertebral disc spaces maintained?

Soft tissue
- Is the gastric air bubble displaced superior to the diaphragm?
- Is the colon of normal size, shape, and placement without dilation or air-fluid levels?
- Are there any calculi or other radiodense shadows in the abdomen or pelvis?
- Is the posterior costophrenic angle sharply defined?

Problem areas
- Aneurysm, spondylolisthesis, and so on (Fig. 5-17)

---

possible diseases, and a corresponding patient management plan. The larger differential list is narrowed by clinical information related to the patient's complaint, patient demographics, past imaging studies, and further imaging or laboratory testing.

This book embraces a pattern or gamut approach to summarizing abnormalities seen on imaging studies. The identified pattern (e.g., radiodense vertebrae, cystic lesion of bone, solitary pulmonary nodule) allows the film interpreter to develop a workable differential list of possible explanations for the abnormal features noted during the search of the images. As the interpreter gains experience, a workable differential list becomes second nature. For example, the pattern of a pathologic compression fracture warrants further investigation to exclude advanced osteoporosis, metastatic bone disease, and multiple myeloma. This short differential list is used so commonly in clinical practice that it becomes rote. Alternatively, the radiographic feature may be so simple that further differential considerations are not needed. For instance, the sole finding of an oblique radiolucent line traversing the shaft of the fifth metatarsal does not warrant the development of an extensive differential list. It is simply a fracture . . . an Aunt Minnie.

Developing differential lists is integral to film interpretation. The list of possible diseases is certainly longer than the list of radiographic expressions of abnormality. In short, many diseases manifest similarly on imaging studies. The limited number of expressions demands broad consideration of possible etiologies when a "general" abnormal feature appears. This is an especially difficult task when dealing with something not often encountered

in general clinical practice; for example, the finding of radiodense metaphyseal bands. Textbooks or similar resources should be consulted in such instances to help build a functional differential list of possibilities.

This book is formatted to facilitate a "pattern-based" approach to film interpretation. Sections of this book address common radiologic patterns of abnormality in bone, chest, and abdomen imaging. In addition, diseases commonly present on MRI scans are tabulated by body region (see Chapter 20). The differential list of diagnoses listed for the common patterns of abnormalities can be used to suggest further differential possibilities. The patient's clinical data, including results of additional imaging and laboratory studies, then can be consulted to narrow the differential list to a few possibilities or a single diagnosis.

Chapters 16 to 20, 27, and 32 list many imaging patterns divided into chapters on skull, spine, extremity, MRI, chest, and abdomen. The reader is encouraged to use these chapters to generate a functional list of differential possibilities for abnormal imaging findings. Moreover, the mnemonics inside the back cover of the text may be helpful to this end.

Many famous volumes and articles have been written about the pattern-approach theme. One traditional favorite is *Reeder and Felson's Gamuts in Radiology*,[115] a long-time standard radiology reference book. Burgener and Kormona's *Differential Diagnosis in Conventional Radiology* is a phenomenal treatise on the pattern-approach theme.[31] Eisenberg's *Clinical Imaging: an Atlas of Differential Diagnosis,* also written with a pattern-approach theme,

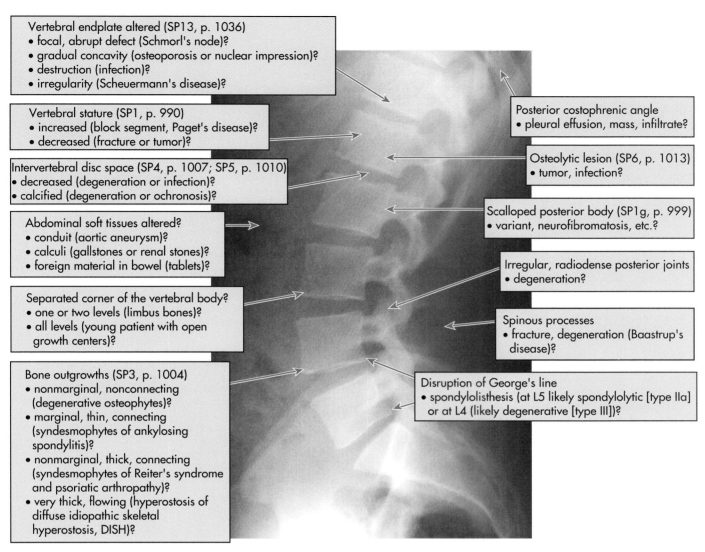

Vertebral endplate altered (SP13, p. 1036)
- focal, abrupt defect (Schmorl's node)?
- gradual concavity (osteoporosis or nuclear impression)?
- destruction (infection)?
- irregularity (Scheuermann's disease)?

Vertebral stature (SP1, p. 990)
- increased (block segment, Paget's disease)?
- decreased (fracture or tumor)?

Intervertebral disc space (SP4, p. 1007; SP5, p. 1010)
- decreased (degeneration or infection)?
- calcified (degeneration or ochronosis)?

Abdominal soft tissues altered?
- conduit (aortic aneurysm)?
- calculi (gallstones or renal stones)?
- foreign material in bowel (tablets)?

Separated corner of the vertebral body?
- one or two levels (limbus bones)?
- all levels (young patient with open growth centers)?

Bone outgrowths (SP3, p. 1004)
- nonmarginal, nonconnecting (degenerative osteophytes)?
- marginal, thin, connecting (syndesmophytes of ankylosing spondylitis)?
- nonmarginal, thick, connecting (syndesmophytes of Reiter's syndrome and psoriatic arthropathy)?
- very thick, flowing (hyperostosis of diffuse idiopathic skeletal hyperostosis, DISH)?

Posterior costophrenic angle
- pleural effusion, mass, infiltrate?

Osteolytic lesion (SP6, p. 1013)
- tumor, infection?

Scalloped posterior body (SP1g, p. 999)
- variant, neurofibromatosis, etc.?

Irregular, radiodense posterior joints
- degeneration?

Spinous processes
- fracture, degeneration (Baastrup's disease)?

Disruption of George's line
- spondylolisthesis (at L5 likely spondylolytic [type IIa] or at L4 (likely degenerative [type III])?

FIG. 5-17 Lateral lumbar radiograph: *key problem areas.*

is very well done.[48] Last, the excellent recent text authored by Taylor and Resnick, *Skeletal Imaging: Atlas of the Spine and Extremities,* is organized by a regional theme, allowing the reader to easily broaden the list of diagnostic entities that may be responsible for given radiologic findings.[146]

Use of mnemonics and disease categories. Mnemonics are a commonly used learning aid to remember long lists of diseases associated with radiologic expression. For example, the differential considerations of a presenting cystic bone lesion are summarized by the mnemonic FEGNOMASHIC, defined by *f*ibrous dysplasia, *e*nchondroma, *g*iant cell tumor, *n*onossifying fibroma, *o*steoblastoma, *m*ultiple myeloma/metastatic disease, *a*neurysmal bone cyst, *s*imple bone cyst, *h*yperparathyroidism/hemophilic pseudotumor, *i*nfection, and *c*hondroma, and listed with many others inside the back cover of this book. There are hundreds of mnemonics, limited only by the imagination of their creators.

Mnemonics are useful to derive a differential list. They function as prompts to expand the interpreter's consideration of differential causes for a specific radiologic presentation. Typically mnemonics are very specific; however, a few exceptions are worth noting. CAT BITES (defining *c*ongenital, *a*rthritide, *t*rauma, *b*lood, infection, *t*rauma, *e*ndocrine, and *s*oft tissue) serves as a universal mnemonic, providing a comprehensive list of disease categories.[73] Another universal mnemonic is described by VINDICATE (defining *v*ascular, *i*nflammatory, *n*eoplastic, *d*egenerative/drugs, *c*ongenital, *a*llergic/autoimmune, *t*raumatic, and *e*ndocrine/metabolic).[40] A short version is expressed by MINT (defining *m*alformations, *i*nflammation/intoxication, *n*eoplasms, and *t*rauma).[40]

Regardless of the exact approach used to view and summarize radiologic data, the interpreter must view all findings in light of their clinical impact. Diagnostic imaging is a wonderfully valuable aid to assist clinical diagnosis and patient management. One is cautioned not to manage patients from their imaging studies, or limit the investigation of the patient's problem to only that data obtained from diagnostic imaging. What appears as a puzzling presentation on an imaging study may be easily clarified by laboratory studies, use of more advanced imaging procedures, further physical examination, comparison with past imaging studies, or further elaborating the patient's history.

BOX 5-10
Interpretation Checklist for an Anteroposterior Lumbopelvic or Abdomen Radiograph

Patient information
- Review and verify the date of examination and patient information.

Image quality
- Evaluate photographic properties: density, contrast, and noise factors (quantum mottle, fog, etc.).
- Evaluate geometric factors: size, shape, detail, and distortion.

Patient positioning and technical defects
- Are there signs of positioning errors, motion artifact, static marks, or other technical defects?
- Are the films done recumbent or upright?

Field of view
- Does the vertical field of view extend from above L1 to below the ischial tuberosities?
- Does the horizontal field of view include the iliofemoral joints bilaterally?

Common artifacts
- Is there any umbilical jewelry, clothing, and so on?

Common foreign bodies
- Are there any surgical staples, hip prostheses, and so on?

Alignment
- Is there pelvic unleveling?
- Are there any lateral lumbar curvatures?
- Are there any anterior or posterior vertebral translations?
- Are the spinous processes generally aligned vertically?

Bones
- Are the radiodensity, size, shape, and configuration of each vertebra normal?
  - Vertebral body
  - Pedicles
  - Spinous process
    - Transverse processes
    - Superior and inferior articular processes
    - Pars interarticularis
    - Laminae
- Are the radiodensity, size, shape, and configuration of the sacrum normal?
  - Transverse sacral ridges
  - Sacral foramen
- Are the radiodensity, size, shape, and configuration of the ilia normal?
- Are the radiodensity, size, shape, and configuration of the proximal femora normal?
- Are the radiodensity, size, shape, and configuration of the lower ribs normal?

Joint spaces
- Are the intervertebral disc spaces maintained?
- Are the sacroiliac joints maintained?
- Are the iliofemoral joints maintained?
- Is the symphysis pubis maintained?

Soft tissue
- Is the liver of normal size, shape, and location?
- Is the spleen of normal size, shape, and location?
- Are the kidneys of normal size, shape, and location?
- Is the bladder of normal size, shape, and location?
- Are the small intestine and ascending, transverse, and descending colon of normal size, shape, and placement without dilation or air-fluid levels?
- Are the psoas muscles of normal size, shape, and location?
- Are the gluteal and adductor fascial planes about the hips normal?
- Are there any calculi or other radiodense shadows in the abdomen or pelvis?

Problem areas
- Pedicles, femoral neck, vertebrae, and so on (Fig. 5-18)

Report Writing

The radiology report is an integral component of the patient's medicolegal record. As such, care must be given to ensure that the information contained in this report is as accurate as possible while still being concise. Many practitioners consider the task of writing the radiologic report to be unnecessarily time consuming and onerous. As a result, they either write a brief summary of their impressions or make no written record whatsoever.[92,120] Failing to report on the patient's radiographs in writing is analogous to performing a physical examination without making any written entries into the patient's file.[125] The medicolegal implications are obvious.

The radiographs should confirm or exclude a clinical suspicion. Thus an important component of the report should be the attempt to link the radiologic signs with the history and physical examination findings.[107] Radiologic reports also offer the opportunity to monitor radiographic quality to act as a form of ongoing audit.[125] They can help the practitioner maintain and improve standards of radiographic quality while keeping radiation dosages to a minimum. Other important benefits of radiologic reports include the fact that they provide (a) a standard of comparison with previous or later examinations, (b) a permanent record if radiographs are lost or not immediately available, and (c) a way to expedite the treatment regimen by providing a resume of important indications and contraindications for therapy.

As with all components of the medical record, the radiologic report is a reflection of the abilities and professionalism of the practitioner. It also serves to facilitate interprofessional and intraprofessional communication. Unfortunately, the format and terminology of radiologic reports are not standardized, with the literature clearly pointing out their wide variation in length and style.[53,54,95,102]

PITFALLS IN RADIOLOGIC INTERPRETATION
Before embarking directly on the task of writing the radiologic report, several areas of caution must be addressed. Up to 20% of statements in radiology reports by medical radiologists or radiology residents have been found to be erroneous, with a small percentage of these statements having life-threatening consequences.[71,116,141] Not surprisingly, the error rate is higher among less experienced radiology residents.[38,47,116] Nonradiologist practitioners should keep these concepts in mind when interpreting their own radiographs. In contrast, chiropractic and medical radiologists were shown to

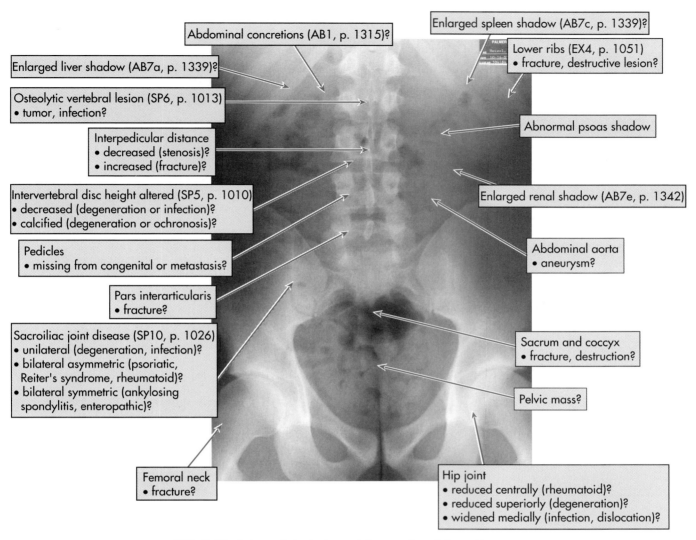

Enlarged spleen shadow (AB7c, p. 1339)?

Lower ribs (EX4, p. 1051)
• fracture, destructive lesion?

Abdominal concretions (AB1, p. 1315)?

Enlarged liver shadow (AB7a, p. 1339)?

Osteolytic vertebral lesion (SP6, p. 1013)
• tumor, infection?

Abnormal psoas shadow

Interpedicular distance
• decreased (stenosis)?
• increased (fracture)?

Intervertebral disc height altered (SP5, p. 1010)
• decreased (degeneration or infection)?
• calcified (degeneration or ochronosis)?

Enlarged renal shadow (AB7e, p. 1342)

Pedicles
• missing from congenital or metastasis?

Abdominal aorta
• aneurysm?

Pars interarticularis
• fracture?

Sacroiliac joint disease (SP10, p. 1026)
• unilateral (degeneration, infection)?
• bilateral asymmetric (psoriatic, Reiter's syndrome, rheumatoid)?
• bilateral symmetric (ankylosing spondylitis, enteropathic)?

Sacrum and coccyx
• fracture, destruction?

Pelvic mass?

Femoral neck
• fracture?

Hip joint
• reduced centrally (rheumatoid)?
• reduced superiorly (degeneration)?
• widened medially (infection, dislocation)?

FIG. 5-18 Anteroposterior lumbar or abdomen radiograph: *key problem areas.*

demonstrate significantly superior radiologic interpretative abilities as compared with nonradiologist practitioners, including chiropractors, in the evaluation of skeletal radiographs.[145] Although the debate about who should carry out radiologic reporting continues, the fact remains that many private practitioners choose to report on the majority of cases within their own practices.

Because all nonradiologist practitioners may be held legally responsible for failing to properly interpret radiographs,[70] increasing numbers are choosing to use the facilities of either chiropractic or medical radiologists for radiographic diagnosis and reporting. Although the use of these specialists should increase diagnostic accuracy and decrease the potential for litigation, no human being is infallible, and all practitioners should double-check all radiographs and reports themselves.

Radiographs must be evaluated in the proper environment. Radiographs should never be read for the first time in front of a patient or member of a patient's family. If a serious pathology is found, the clinician may inadvertently say something that is inappropriate and cannot easily be retracted. Similarly, significant pathology may be missed at first and discovered later when sufficient time is allocated for the interpretation. Radiographs cannot be read quickly. A quiet, dark room that is free of distractions is necessary. The patient's file, containing the history and physical examination information, should be readily available for correlation with the radiographic findings. The identification labels and film dates should be carefully checked to ensure they are correct. Comparison of current radiographs with old films is extremely valuable when these records are available.

Errors in radiologic diagnosis can be caused by several factors. These errors are commonly classified as either errors of observation or errors of interpretation. Another way of classifying these radiologic errors is false-positive or false-negative. A false-negative error occurs when a significant abnormal finding is not detected or is detected but interpreted as normal. False-positive errors are those in which a significant abnormality is "found" in a radiographic region that is actually normal.[116] Faulty and incomplete search patterns are responsible for many of the errors in radiologic diagnosis.[109] Observational errors also can be related to a lack of didactic knowledge, particularly in relationship to issues of image ambiguity. Errors of interpretation reflect lack of knowledge of the significance of abnormal radiographic signs, or the inability to link the signs with key clinical information.[109]

BOX 5-11

Interpretation Checklist for a Posteroanterior Chest Radiograph

Patient information
- Review and verify the date of examination and patient information.

Image quality
- Evaluate photographic properties: density, contrast, and noise factors (quantum mottle, fog, etc.).
- Evaluate geometric factors: size, shape, detail, and distortion.

Patient positioning and technical defects
- Are there signs of motion artifact, static marks, or other technical defects?
- Are there signs of positional error in rotation? (Are the medial ends of the clavicles equidistant from the T3 or T4 spinous process?)
- Are there 10 posterior (or 7 anterior) rib portions above the right hemidiaphragm consistent with a proper respiratory result?

Field of view
- Does the vertical field of view include the lung apices to the lateral costophrenic angles?
- Does the horizontal field of view include the lateral margins of the body wall?

Common artifacts
- Are there necklaces, clothing, tubes, lines, and so on?
- Identify common foreign bodies.
- Are there any surgical staples, sternal wires, and so on?

Alignment
- Are there any lateral thoracic curvatures?

Bones
- Are the radiodensity, size, shape, and configuration of the first four or so visible vertebrae normal?
- Are the radiodensity, size, shape, and configuration of the shoulder girdle (scapula, clavicle, proximal humerus) normal?
- Are the radiodensity, size, shape, and configuration of the ribs and sternum normal?
- Does the body wall exhibit a normal bell shape?

Joint spaces
- Are the intervertebral disc spaces maintained?
- Are the acromioclavicular joint spaces maintained?

Soft tissue
- Is the heart of normal width (<0.5 of thorax), shape, location, and silhouette?
- Is the mediastinum of normal width (<0.25 of thorax), size, shape, location, and silhouette?
- Is the diaphragm of normal size, shape, location, and silhouette?
  - Is the right side slightly higher than the left (not >4 cm)?
- Are the pleura and fissures of normal size, shape, and location?
- Are the trachea and bronchi of normal size, shape, and location?
- Are the hila of normal size, shape, and location (right slightly lower than left)?
- Is the pulmonary vasculature of normal size, shape, and location?
- Are the ascending, arch, and descending aorta of normal size, shape, and location?
- Is the lung parenchyma (e.g., lung field) clear of nodule, mass, and infiltrate?
- Is the gastric air bubble of normal size, shape, and location?

Problem areas
- Area behind the heart, hila, lung parenchyma, chest wall, and so on (Fig. 5-19)

Practitioners who are aware of the potential pitfalls in radiologic interpretation and their own abilities in radiologic interpretation, and who are determined to provide the best diagnostic service to the patient, are in a good position to determine which cases they should interpret themselves and which may benefit from a second opinion. Although digital media for radiographic images are not universally available at a reasonable cost, timely radiology reports are generated on films mailed to radiologists (medical and chiropractic), with reports being quickly faxed or e-mailed to the ordering clinician.

GENERATING THE RADIOLOGY REPORT

General. Many radiologists and practitioners dictate the radiology report, which then is typed by a transcriptionist.[26] Although this method is quick and efficient for the clinician, it requires the services of a typist and careful proofreading. Computer macros—parts of reports and common phrases that are preprogrammed into the computer—can decrease transcription time, although a typist is still needed.[26]

The need for a transcriptionist can be eliminated by using automated radiology reporting systems with software that presents radiologic findings and anatomic terms in graphic form and allows the desired terms to be selected using a track ball or touch-sensitive screen.[26] However, these systems do require more of the clinician's time than simply dictating the report. Another drawback of the automated reporting system is that the clinician must frequently look away from the radiographs to the computer screen, which could increase the error rate in interpretation.

Standard or "canned" radiology reports have been available to the medical profession for many years.[9] These are very economical and can be created easily on the computer for normal studies. However, standard reports for abnormal studies are not currently practical. Voice recognition by computers is the current preferred method of reporting by many radiologists.[9]

The radiologist simply dictates directly into the computer, and a report is generated without additional typing. "Dragon Naturally Speaking" is a very popular voice recognition system for radiology and medical reporting. This eliminates transcription and allows immediate proofreading and signing of the report. Preliminary studies have demonstrated that the accuracy of the speech recognition system for chest radiologic reports is between 96% and 99%.[9]

At the opposite extreme a few practitioners may still prefer to hand write their radiology reports. Regardless of the way in which the radiology report is generated, it should always contain the following components:[38,95,102,147,160]

1. Heading (preliminary information)
2. Clinical information (brief)
3. Findings
4. Conclusions
5. Recommendations (optional)
6. Signature

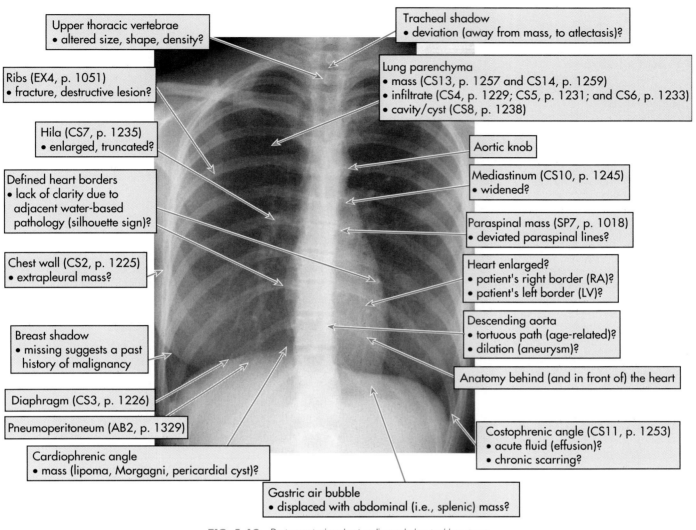

Upper thoracic vertebrae
• altered size, shape, density?

Ribs (EX4, p. 1051)
• fracture, destructive lesion?

Hila (CS7, p. 1235)
• enlarged, truncated?

Defined heart borders
• lack of clarity due to adjacent water-based pathology (silhouette sign)?

Chest wall (CS2, p. 1225)
• extrapleural mass?

Breast shadow
• missing suggests a past history of malignancy

Diaphragm (CS3, p. 1226)

Pneumoperitoneum (AB2, p. 1329)

Cardiophrenic angle
• mass (lipoma, Morgagni, pericardial cyst)?

Tracheal shadow
• deviation (away from mass, to atlectasis)?

Lung parenchyma
• mass (CS13, p. 1257 and CS14, p. 1259)
• infiltrate (CS4, p. 1229; CS5, p. 1231; and CS6, p. 1233)
• cavity/cyst (CS8, p. 1238)

Aortic knob

Mediastinum (CS10, p. 1245)
• widened?

Paraspinal mass (SP7, p. 1018)
• deviated paraspinal lines?

Heart enlarged?
• patient's right border (RA)?
• patient's left border (LV)?

Descending aorta
• tortuous path (age-related)?
• dilation (aneurysm)?

Anatomy behind (and in front of) the heart

Costophrenic angle (CS11, p. 1253)
• acute fluid (effusion)?
• chronic scarring?

Gastric air bubble
• displaced with abdominal (i.e., splenic) mass?

FIG. 5-19 Posteroanterior chest radiograph: *key problem areas.*

Heading. The radiology report should be written on the clinician's stationery and should include the name and address of the individual or clinic. Additional information contained in the heading should include the following:[63,110,147]

1. Date of the actual report
2. Patient information
   a. Name
   b. Date of birth (or age)
   c. Gender
   d. Date the radiographs were taken
   e. X-ray number (if available)
   f. Physician (if other than the person writing the report)
3. Radiographic information
   a. Part imaged
   b. Views obtained

Note: It may be advantageous to write separate reports for each region that has been imaged to improve the clarity and reduce potential reading and reporting errors. For example, if radiographs are taken of both the cervical and lumbar regions, two separate reports may be written rather than one that combines all of the information. Including the technical parameters into the heading of the report is optional.

Variation for computed tomography reports. Special imaging procedures should come complete with the radiologist's report to the practitioner ordering the study. It should be rare for a nonradiologist practitioner to be required to report on these images without a second opinion. However, the following information may prove useful in the interpretation of CT scan reports or for cases in which the clinician does not have access to the original report.

1. Part imaged: Note the exact area imaged by referring to the longitudinal "scout" view (e.g., L3 to S1 contiguous slices).
2. Views obtained: Record the imaging plane (e.g., axial) and whether there was gantry angulation to the slices. It also may be useful to note the thickness of the slices; include reformatted coronal and sagittal images if applicable. Also state which windows are included. Both bone and soft-tissue windows should be provided. The use of intrathecal or intravenous contrast agents also must be mentioned (e.g., "with myelogram").

The following is a summary of information that should be included in the heading of a CT report:

1. Levels imaged
2. Contiguous or interrupted slices
3. Slice thickness*
4. Plane of imaging

BOX 5-12
Interpretation Checklist for a Lateral Chest Radiograph

Patient information
- Review and verify the date of examination and patient information.

Image quality
- Evaluate photographic properties: density, contrast, and noise factors (quantum mottle, fog, etc.).
- Evaluate geometric factors: size, shape, detail, and distortion.

Patient positioning and technical defects
- Are there signs of positioning errors, motion artifact, static marks, or other technical defects?
- Are the arms obstructing the retrosternal space?

Field of view
- Does the vertical field of view extend from T1 to below the posterior costophrenic angle?
- Does the horizontal field of view extend from the sternum to include the posterior angles of the ribs?

Common artifacts
- Are there necklaces, hair braids, clothing, and so on?

Common foreign bodies
- Are there any sternal wires, pacemaker, valve prosthesis, and so on?

Alignment
- Is the thoracic kyphosis maintained?
- Is there any vertebral retrolisthesis or spondylolisthesis?
- Are the spinous processes generally aligned vertically?

Bones
- Are the radiodensity, size, shape, and configuration of each vertebra normal?
  - Vertebral body
  - Pedicles
  - Spinous process
- Are the radiodensity, size, shape, and configuration of each rib normal?
- Is the spinal canal maintained?

Joint spaces
- Are the intervertebral disc spaces maintained?
- Is the intervertebral foramen of normal size?

Soft tissue
- Is the tracheal air shadow centrally located?
- Is the heart shadow generally of normal size and configuration?
- Are the lung tissues clear of mass, infiltrate, or other defect?
- Are the ascending, transverse, and descending segments of the aorta normal?
- Are the aortic-pulmonary window and hila defined and clear?
- Is the diaphragm of normal position?
- Is the gastric air bubble of normal size and location below the diaphragm?
- Are the anterior and posterior costophrenic angles sharply defined?
- Are the retrosternal and retrocardiac spaces clear of mass or infiltrate?

Problem areas
- Vertebrae, hiatal hernia, hila, arch of aorta, and so on (Fig. 5-20)

---

5. Angulation of the gantry
6. Reformatting*
7. Windows provided
8. Use of contrast agent*

Variation for magnetic resonance imaging reports. As with CT scanning the clinician should not be expected to provide original reports on MRI scans. The following information is unique to the heading of these reports and may help the practitioner understand some of the differences between CT and MRI.

1. Area imaged: MRI has the advantage over CT scanning of being able to image an entire region (e.g., the entire cervical or lumbar spine at the very least).
2. Imaging planes: Most scans provide at least the sagittal plane, with axial images of areas of interest. Coronal scans also can be included. These imaging planes are not reformatted (reconstructed) images as they are in CT scans, so these terms should not be used. As a result, the detail of MRI images of the sagittal and coronal planes is superior to CT reformatted images.
3. Imaging sequences: T1- and T2-weighted spin-echo pulse sequences are commonly used. However, each imaging center has its own parameters, which may include gradient-echo pulse sequences and fat suppression imaging. Do not use the terms *bone* or *soft-tissue windows* in the description of MRI images.

Clinical information. Although some authors do not include the clinical information within the radiology report, it has been proved that practitioners who can easily link clinical information with radiographic findings are significantly more accurate in their radiologic diagnoses.[102,107,147] Providing a brief summary of the relevant features in the patient history, physical examination, and laboratory analysis may help the clinician focus attention on certain areas of the radiograph (while still considering others) or interpret the radiologic signs more precisely.

The following information should be included in the radiologic report after *Heading:*

1. Location, duration, onset, and type of symptoms
2. History of traumatic injury and exact dates received
3. Positive orthopedic or neurologic tests
4. Abnormal laboratory studies
5. Any other abnormal physical examination findings that may be related to the area imaged

Skeletal radiology reports

Findings. The *Findings* section is the body of the report and contains the relevant abnormal (and occasionally normal) radiographic signs. It is written in narrative form using professional terminology, complete sentences, and proper grammar. This is the portion of the report in which the clinician should describe abnormalities, not state diagnoses.[147] However, occasional exceptions to this rule exist, especially in cases involving fractures and dislocations. A tumor or other destructive lesion should be described in

---

*Optional considerations.

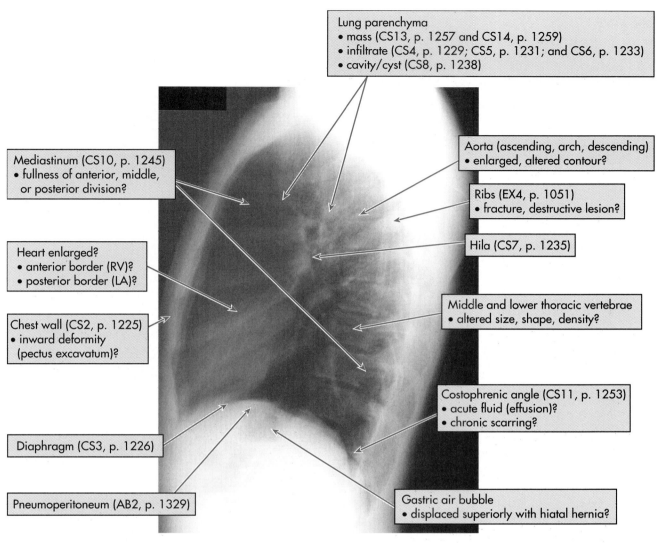

Lung parenchyma
• mass (CS13, p. 1257 and CS14, p. 1259)
• infiltrate (CS4, p. 1229; CS5, p. 1231; and CS6, p. 1233)
• cavity/cyst (CS8, p. 1238)

Aorta (ascending, arch, descending)
• enlarged, altered contour?

Mediastinum (CS10, p. 1245)
• fullness of anterior, middle, or posterior division?

Ribs (EX4, p. 1051)
• fracture, destructive lesion?

Hila (CS7, p. 1235)

Heart enlarged?
• anterior border (RV)?
• posterior border (LA)?

Middle and lower thoracic vertebrae
• altered size, shape, density?

Chest wall (CS2, p. 1225)
• inward deformity (pectus excavatum)?

Costophrenic angle (CS11, p. 1253)
• acute fluid (effusion)?
• chronic scarring?

Diaphragm (CS3, p. 1226)

Pneumoperitoneum (AB2, p. 1329)

Gastric air bubble
• displaced superiorly with hiatal hernia?

FIG. 5-20 Lateral chest radiograph: *key problem areas.*

Findings and diagnosed under *Conclusions.* The erosions or osteophytes associated with an arthritic condition should be described in *Findings* and the specific diagnosis included in *Conclusions.* *Findings* is the most controversial section of the report in the literature. The choice of terminology often has been determined by personal preference,[102] and subjectivity is the order of the day. In the *Handbook of Radiologic Dictation,* it is recommended that this section of the report be kept short (but complete) and simple with minimal use of pompous terms.[106]

It may be appropriate to occasionally comment on normal radiographic appearances if some peculiarity of positioning or superimposition could lead to misinterpretation of the normal appearance as pathologic. It is also important to indicate the level of certainty about the presence or absence of abnormal radiologic signs;[147] however, clinicians should not purposely and unnecessarily make noncommittal statements about the findings. If the findings are "equivocal," it should not be the result of insufficient knowledge or experience on the part of the interpreter.

Several authors recommend dividing *Findings* into paragraphs.[106,147,160] These paragraphs may reflect the organization of the various findings into related categories. One commonly used method of organizing reports for skeletal radiology is the ABCS approach:

A = Alignment
B = Bone
C = Cartilage
S = Soft tissues

The ABCS format is discussed in depth earlier in this chapter. Interpreters who employ a flexible search pattern may be more successful than those rigidly following an ABCS sequence of film interpretation.[110] However, even though a rigid ABCS format may be inadequate at times as a search pattern approach for evaluating the radiographs, it can work very well in most situations as a guide for actually writing an organized report.

Clinicians should feel free to be flexible about the order in which the various radiologic findings are organized in the report. It may be more appropriate to record the findings of a patient with a large abdominal aortic aneurysm who also has signs of diffuse idiopathic skeletal hyperostosis (DISH) in the order SBCA (a resequencing of ABCS). This organizes the radiologic findings by priority or severity. In addition, segregating the findings strictly into the ABCS categories not only may be burdensome but also confusing.

BOX 5-13
Radiologic Patterns of Abnormalities Listed in Chapters 16, 17, 18, 19, 27, and 32

Radiologic patterns of the skull (Chapter 16)
SK1. Basilar invagination (p. 968)
SK2. Button sequestration (p. 969)
SK3. Cystic lesions of the mandible (p. 970)
SK4. Diffuse demineralization (p. 973)
SK5. Enlargement or destruction of the sella turcica (p. 974)
SK6. Increased radiodensity of the calvarium (p. 976)
SK7. Intracranial calcification (p. 979)
SK8. Mass in the paranasal sinuses (p. 981)
SK9. Multiple wormian bones (p. 983)
SK10. Osteolytic defects of the skull (p. 984)
SK11. Radiodense mandible lesions (p. 987)

Radiologic patterns of the spine (Chapter 17)
SP1. Altered vertebral shape
    SP1a. Beaked or hooked vertebrae (p. 990)
    SP1b. Biconcave vertebrae (p. 991)
    SP1c. Blocked vertebrae (p. 993)
    SP1d. Wide enlarged vertebrae (p. 995)
    SP1e. Tall enlarged vertebrae (p. 997)
    SP1f. Anterior scalloped vertebrae (p. 998)
    SP1g. Posterior scalloped vertebrae (p. 999)
    SP1h. Square vertebrae (p. 1000)
    SP1i. Wedged vertebrae (p. 1001)
SP2. Atlantoaxial subluxation (p. 1003)
SP3. Bony outgrowths of the spine (p. 1004)
SP4. Calcification of the intervertebral discs (p. 1007)
SP5. Narrow intervertebral disc height (p. 1010)
SP6. Osteolytic lesions of the spine (p. 1013)
SP7. Paraspinal mass (p. 1018)
SP8. Radiodense "ivory" vertebrae (p. 1021)
SP9. Radiodense vertebral stripes (p. 1024)
SP10. Sacroiliac joint disease (p. 1026)
SP11. Scoliosis (p. 1030)
SP12. Vertebral collapse (p. 1032)
SP13. Vertebral endplate alterations (p. 1036)

Radiologic patterns of the extremities (Chapter 18)
EX1. Acroosteolysis (p. 1042)
EX2. Calcified intraarticular loose bodies (p. 1045)
EX3. Change in size and shape of epiphyses (p. 1046)
EX4. Cystic lesions of extremities and ribs (p. 1051)
EX5. Aggressive osteolytic lesions of extremities and ribs (p. 1057)
EX6. Osteosclerotic bone lesions (p. 1062)
EX7. Periosteal reactions
    EX7a. Localized periosteal reactions (p. 1064)
    EX7b. Generalized periosteal reactions (p. 1067)
EX8. Radiodense metaphyseal bands (p. 1070)
EX9. Radiolucent metaphyseal bands (p. 1072)

Radiologic patterns of the general skeleton (Chapter 19)
GN1. Acetabular protrusion (p. 1074)
GN2. Arthritides (p. 1076)
GN3. Dwarfism (p. 1084)
GN4. Generalized osteoporosis (p. 1086)
GN5. Generalized osteosclerosis (p. 1089)
GN6. Polyostotic bone lesions (p. 1094)
GN7. Soft-tissue calcification and ossification
    GN7a. Calcification (p. 1099)
    GN7b. Ossification (p. 1106)

Radiologic patterns of the chest (Chapter 27)
CS1. Atelectasis (p. 1222)
CS2. Chest wall pleural-based lesions (p. 1225)
CS3. Diaphragmatic abnormalities
    CS3a. Depressed diaphragm (p. 1226)
    CS3b. Elevated diaphragm (p. 1227)
CS4. Diffuse alveolar (air space) disease (p. 1229)
CS5. Localized alveolar (air space) disease (p. 1231)
CS6. Diffuse interstitial disease (p. 1233)
CS7. Enlarged hilum (p. 1235)
CS8. Focal radiolucent lesions
    CS8a. Cavities (p. 1238)
    CS8b. Cysts (p. 1241)
CS9. Intrathoracic calcifications
    CS9a. Cardiovascular calcifications (p. 1242)
    CS9b. Hilar/mediastinal calcifications (p. 1243)
    CS9c. Lung parenchymal calcifications (p. 1244)
    CS9d. Pleural calcifications (p. 1244)
CS10. Mediastinal lesions
    CS10a. Anterior mediastinum (p. 1245)
    CS10b. Middle mediastinum (p. 1249)
    CS10c. Posterior mediastinum (p. 1251)
CS11. Pleural effusion (p. 1253)
CS12. Pulmonary edema (p. 1254)
CS13. Solitary pulmonary nodule and mass (p. 1257)
CS14. Multiple nodules and masses (p. 1259)

Radiologic patterns of the abdomen (Chapter 32)
AB1. Abdominal calcifications
    AB1a. Concretions (p. 1315)
    AB1b. Conduit wall calcification (p. 1319)
    AB1c. Cystic calcification (p. 1322)
    AB1d. Solid mass calcification (p. 1325)
AB2. Pneumoperitoneum
    AB2a. Most common causes of pneumoperitoneum (p. 1329)
    AB2b. Plain film technique for detection of pneumoperitoneum (p. 1329)
    AB2c. Signs of pneumoperitoneum on suspine abdominal films (p. 1330)
    AB2d. Pseudopneumoperitoneum (p. 1331)
AB3. Abnormal localized intraperitoneal gas collections (p. 1332)
AB4. Pneumoretroperitoneum (p. 1334)
AB5. Abnormal bowel gas resulting from obstruction (p. 1335)
AB6. Ascites (p. 1337)
AB7. Enlarged organ shadows
    AB7a. Hepatomegaly (p. 1339)
    AB7b. Gallbladder enlargement (p. 1340)
    AB7c. Spleen enlargement (p. 1340)
    AB7d. Gastric distention (p. 1342)
    AB7e. Right kidney enlargement (p. 1342)
    AB7f. Left kidney enlargement (p. 1343)
    AB7g. Adrenal enlargement (p. 1343)
AB8. Abdominal masses
    AB8a. True abdominal masses (p. 1344)
    AB8b. Pseudomasses (p. 1353)
AB9. Diseases of the gallbladder (p. 1354)
AB10. Vascular calcifications (p. 1357)
AB11. Miscellaneous radiopacities and abdomen artifacts (p. 1359)

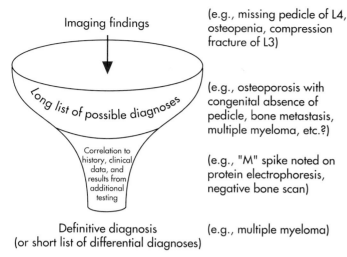

Imaging findings

(e.g., missing pedicle of L4, osteopenia, compression fracture of L3)

Long list of possible diagnoses

(e.g., osteoporosis with congenital absence of pedicle, bone metastasis, multiple myeloma, etc.?)

Correlation to history, clinical data, and results from additional testing

(e.g., "M" spike noted on protein electrophoresis, negative bone scan)

Definitive diagnosis (or short list of differential diagnoses)

(e.g., multiple myeloma)

FIG. 5-21 The mental process of radiologic interpretation reflects the function of a funnel, beginning with a broad array of imaging findings and leading to a narrow list of explanations for the findings. The narrowing or elimination process is augmented by correlating further imaging, laboratory, historic, and clinical data. At times, imaging findings are pathognomonic for a specific condition (an "Aunt Minnie"), but more often the imaging findings are best summarized by a "pattern" of abnormality. The pattern of abnormality leads to a list of differential diagnoses that are known to cause the observed appearance. The list of differential possibilities is narrowed, if possible, to a definitive diagnosis or group of related possibilities that can be used to formulate the patient's management plan.

Arthritic conditions usually present with both cartilaginous and bony abnormalities at the very least. Organizing together the various findings that relate to a particular condition may make more sense than separating them. For example, consider the following two excerpts from reports on the same set of lumbopelvic radiographs:

Version 1. Erosions and sclerosis of both sacroiliac joints are noted with a marginal syndesmophyte at the adjacent left lateral body margins between L1-L2. Moderate narrowing of the L5-S1 disc space is present with an approximate 10% anterolisthesis of L5 and hypertrophy of the L5-S1 facet articulations.

Version 2. An approximate 10% anterolisthesis of L5 is noted. *(Alignment)*

There is hypertrophy of the L5-S1 facet articulations. *(Bone)*

Erosions and sclerosis of both sacroiliac joints are noted. Moderate narrowing of the L5-S1 disc space is present. *(Cartilage)*

There is a marginal syndesmophyte at the adjacent left lateral body margins between L1 and L2. *(Soft tissues)*

Both versions are technically correct and acceptable. Version 2 most likely is easier for a student beginning the process of radiology report writing to record. Its rote format can be followed, ensuring that no important radiologic signs are missed. However, advanced students and practicing clinicians should recognize that version 1 logically organizes the related abnormal findings together. It is also clear from the way in which the report is written that the practitioner is aware these findings are related, which shows that the practitioner is thinking like an expert diagnostician.[109] Paragraphs can still be used with version 1; the current example has them organized according to pathologic processes rather than ABCS.

For the sake of simplicity, this book uses the ABCS approach to the way various findings should be written into the body of a report. Modifications can be made at the clinician's discretion.

Alignment. Roentgenometric lines, angles, and various measurements should be included in the report when appropriate. Include a normal or an abnormal measurement if it helps substantiate or refute a clinical suspicion based on the history and examination.[63,110] As a general rule of thumb, also include a measurement if it falls significantly outside the accepted normal range. This section should include information such as alterations of spinal curves, olisthesis, apparent leg length discrepancies, joint misalignments resulting from arthritic conditions, and the alignment of fracture fragments.[147] Marked static vertebral malpositions also may be mentioned in this section. However, the recognition of these malpositions does not necessarily confirm a clinically significant finding. They must be correlated to the patient's symptoms and other examination results.

It is critical to know that visual estimation of spinal curves should be avoided. Actual measurements help prevent this part of the report from being discredited at a later date. The interexaminer and intraexaminer reliability of chiropractors and students visually estimating cervical and lumbar lordosis has proved to be poor.[11,150] Furthermore, the validity (e.g., accuracy) of visually estimating these curves is equally inadequate.[11,150] Boxes 5-14 to 5-16 include guidelines for incorporating various spinal measurements into the radiologic report.[63,110]

If no abnormalities are detected, a negative statement attesting to this fact should be included under the heading *Alignment* (e.g., "Alignment of the visualized osseous structures is within normal limits.") Another way of saying the same thing is, "There are no abnormalities in alignment detected." Including a negative statement about a particular component in the radiology report indicates that the clinician actually evaluated this aspect of the films.

Bone. Descriptions of any congenital or acquired osseous abnormalities are included under the heading *Bone* in the report. In general, no conclusions should be made in this section of the report. The exception to this rule occurs in the event of a patient with a fracture. It is much clearer to state that, "There is an oblique fracture through the distal one third of the shaft of the left radius" than, "There is an oblique lucent line that disrupts the cortices of the distal one third of the left radius." Similarly, if the finding is a simple normal variant or trivial finding, it is not necessary to provide an elaborate generic description and then follow up with listings in the *Conclusions* section.

Concise descriptions using appropriate radiologic terminology are written to describe any abnormalities in the size, shape, density, or number of bones or cortical disruption or osseous destruction.[147] Advanced students and practitioners should report on more serious bone abnormalities first, before including less significant abnormalities.[63,110]

If no abnormalities are noted under the heading *Bone,* a negative statement about this should be included to confirm that the practitioner thoroughly evaluated this area in case future medicolegal questions arise. Because the radiographs should confirm or rule out a clinical suspicion, negative statements can be targeted specifically to the clinical concerns. For example, the statement, "No evidence of osseous destruction or focal sclerotic or lytic lesions is detected" could be included in the report for a patient being evaluated for possible metastatic bone disease. "No evidence of recent fracture or dislocation is evident" can be stated in the report on a patient with a history of recent trauma. A generic negative statement may read, "The osseous structures appear normal."

Cartilage. Articular cartilage is not normally visible on a radiograph. Instead the clinician evaluates the joint spaces and pathophysiologic impact of the joint disease on the adjacent osseous structures. Abnormalities in joint space width, symmetry, subchondral bone, fusion, and joint congruity are described in this section.[147]

BOX 5-14
Guidelines for Cervical Spine Roentgenometrics

Lordosis
- Assess patient positioning by evaluating Chamberlain's line. A horizontal Chamberlain's line indicates a neutral lateral position. Poor patient positioning gives false impressions of hyperlordosis or hypolordosis.
- Evaluate the architecture of the articular pillars on the lateral view. Hyperplasia causes a local loss of lordosis because of a structural alteration.[75,77]
- There are at least nine different roentgenometric methods of evaluating cervical lordosis. They do not all appear to have concurrent validity.[11,77]
- The angle of cervical lordosis is commonly measured using the atlas plane line and the inferior end plate of C7; normal is 35 to 45 degrees.[160] This method seems to be overly influenced by the tilt of the atlas; the depth method probably is a better alternative (see Chapter 14).

Chamberlain's line
- Assess this line to evaluate patient positioning.

McGregor's line
- This is an important line to evaluate for basilar invagination/impression.
- Only mention results if they are positive.

Atlantodental interval
- Give particular attention to all patients with inflammatory arthropathy, who have suffered a traumatic injury, or who have Down syndrome.
- Normal is greater than 3 mm in adults and greater than 5 mm in children.[160]

Sella turcica size
- Mention the size only if the sella turcica is enlarged (e.g., >12 × 16 mm).
- Enlargement may be associated with increased intracranial pressure.

George's line
- Evaluation is used to assess for the presence of anterolisthesis, retrolisthesis, or instability.

Posterior spinal (spinolaminar) line
- Evaluation is used to assess for anterolisthesis, retrolisthesis, or instability.

Prevertebral soft tissues
- Retropharyngeal is less than 5 mm. Retrotracheal is greater than 20 mm.
- Tissues may become enlarged because of trauma, infection, or tumor.

Flexion and extension studies
- Template flexion/extension studies are used to assess for the following:
  Relative anterolisthesis/retrolisthesis greater than 3.5 mm from flexion to extension
  Hypomobility/hypermobility
  Evidence of instability
  Aberrant motion at levels other than C0/C1

The practitioner must evaluate the apophyseal, uncovertebral, costotransverse, and costovertebral joints, as well as the disc spaces on spinal radiographs. It is too easy for the clinician to evaluate the obvious disc spaces while ignoring or missing significant abnormalities in the synovial spinal joints.

As stated for the other components of the radiologic report, if all joint spaces visualized are normal, a statement to that effect needs to be included (e.g., "The visualized joint or disc spaces are within normal limits.")

Soft tissues. This is a very important section in the skeletal radiologic report because it is a commonly overlooked area by clinicians who are concerned primarily with skeletal structures. Clinicians must be aware of this potentially dangerous omission and discipline themselves to always evaluate these structures. Success in correctly identifying abnormalities within the soft tissues depends on a thorough knowledge of structures expected to be seen in the region and their normal radiologic appearance. Organ enlargement or displacement, displacement of normal structures (e.g., the trachea), abnormal accumulations of gas, abnormal soft-tissue calcifications, prevertebral or paraspinal soft-tissue swelling, foreign bodies (including surgical clips and sutures), masses, and displacement or blurring of fat or fascial planes are the soft-tissue abnormalities that should be described in this section. Diagnostic conclusions should not be included.

If no abnormalities are observed within the visualized soft tissues, a negative statement is included as proof that these structures were thoroughly evaluated. This negative statement can be targeted specifically to a clinical suspicion or can be generic. Examples could include, "No abnormalities are detected within the visualized soft tissues," "The visualized soft tissues are within normal limits," or, "The splenic shadow does not project below the twelfth rib with no displacement of the gastric air bubble. The remainder of the soft tissues are unremarkable."

Conclusion. Although some authors recommend the use of the term *Impressions* for this section of the report, it may be

---

BOX 5-15
Guidelines for Thoracic Spine Roentgenometrics

Scoliosis evaluation
- Six components of each abnormal curvature must be mentioned:
  1. Configuration of curve (S or C)
  2. Direction of curve (right or left)
  3. Area of involvement (e.g., lumbar, thoracolumbar)
  4. Apex (apices)
  5. Cobb or Risser's Ferguson angle if greater than 10 degrees
  6. Axial rotation of the apical segment

Kyphosis evaluation
- The method of measurement is similar to Cobb's method for scoliosis evaluation.
- The superior end plate of T1 usually is difficult to see.
- The upper limit of normal is 56 degrees in females and 66 degrees in males.[160]

PART ONE
Introduction to Imaging

BOX 5-16
Guidelines for Lumbar Spine Roentgenometrics

Lordosis evaluation
- Several different roentgenographic methods using different anatomic landmarks have been used.[158]
- The full significance of hyperlordosis/hypolordosis has not been determined.
- A common procedure is to use the superior end plate of L1 and superior end plate of S1; average is 50 to 60 degrees. Because L1 is commonly wedge shaped, this is probably not appropriate. The inferior end plate of L1 may be preferred.[151]

Sacral base (Ferguson) angle
- This is the most researched angle of the lumbopelvic region.
- The normal range is 27 to 56 degrees (standard deviation = 2). The mean is 41 degrees in the upright position.
- Persons with spondylolytic spondylolisthesis have a statically significantly higher sacral base angle.[121]
- Increased angles may be associated with increased compressive forces at the facets or transverse shearing forces at the disc.[160]
- Decreased angles may be associated with increased axial loading of the disc or increased axial shearing forces at the facets.

Lumbosacral disc angle
- The normal range is 10 to 20 degrees.
- Larger angles may be associated with facet syndrome.
- Smaller angles may be associated with acute disc injuries and transitional segments.

Gravitational line from L3
- The line normally intersects the anterior one third of the sacral base. It also may fall anterior to the sacral base a distance equal to one third of the sacral base sagittal diameter and still be normal.

- The posterior line may be associated with increased axial forces to the facet joints.
- The anterior line may be associated with increased transverse forces to the facet joints and anterior compressive forces to the disc.

Anterolisthesis
- Evaluate the extent of anterior slippage using either the Meyerding classification system or preferably the percentile measurement.
- State whether pars defects can be observed.

Retrolisthesis/lateral listheses
- Evaluate the severity of slippage using percentile measurement.

Sagittal canal diameter
- A value of less than 15 mm may indicate spinal stenosis (according to Eisenstein's method).
- The measurement should be given serious consideration if associated findings such as hypertrophy of the facets or posterior vertebral body osteophytes are detected.

Flexion and extension studies
- Relative displacement of greater than 3.5 mm from full flexion to full extension may indicate instability.
- Up to 5 mm translation may be normal at L3-4 and L4-5.[144]
- Up to 4 mm translation may be normal at L5-S1.[144]
- There is a large range of variation in normal.
- Greater than 25 to 26 degrees of angular motion at L5-S1 is abnormal.[144]
- If one motion segment translates significantly more than the adjacent segments, it is probably abnormal.

---

inappropriate because it "... suggests knowledge is vague, subjective, and unreliable."[102] The suggested words to use are *Conclusions, Diagnosis, Judgment, Interpretation,* or *Reading.*[102]

The section of the report called *Conclusions* is a point-by-point summation of *Findings* (and includes all of the ABCS components). Complete sentences are not necessary in this section, and it is expected that diagnostic terminology will be used. This section is the appropriate portion of the report in which to label the condition or conditions (e.g., lytic metastatic disease, rheumatoid arthritis, new compression fracture). The diagnoses should be listed in the order of severity, starting with the most serious condition. For example, "metastatic disease" would be listed before "osteoarthritis." If the entire radiographic series reveals no abnormalities, *Conclusions* may simply read "Radiographically negative (cervical, thoracic, lumbar, etc.) series."

Recommendations. The *Recommendations* section is optional and only should be included if specific follow-up procedures are indicated.[147] Additional plain radiographs (e.g., "spot" or supplementary views), special imaging procedures, laboratory evaluations, and referrals to other health care providers are examples of appropriate recommendations. If recommendations are included, they must be specific and appropriate for the conditions diagnosed or suspected from the original radiographs. It is not acceptable to simply state, "Further laboratory tests are indicated" without explaining exactly which laboratory procedures are needed.

Recommendations about improvement of quality of the original radiographs also can be included in this section. Comments referring to improved patient positioning or altered technical factors for repeat radiographs can be mentioned.

Signature. All reports must be signed by the author and include credentials. Box 5-17 summarizes the sections in the skeletal radiology report.

Chest radiology reports. Controversy exists within the medical profession about the quantity of detail desired in chest x-ray reports.[95] Because of the work load of medical radiologists, a common chest x-ray report simply states that the examination is normal (if that is true), with no other remarks. However, for patients with specific chest complaints, referring physicians are not satisfied with these one-line reports; they prefer detailed reports targeting the specific symptoms.[95] Unfortunately, physicians cannot agree on how much detail should be included or the format of the reports. For those in chiropractic practice, it is better to err on the side of caution and include comments on all aspects of the chest radiograph.

The ABCS format is not applied to chest radiology reports in the same way that it is applied to skeletal reports. The purpose of taking chest radiographs is to evaluate the various soft-tissue structures rather than the osseous components. Therefore it is necessary to include much more detail about these soft tissues in the body of the report. The *Heading* and *Clinical Information* for a chest x-ray

---

BOX 5-17

Template for Writing a Skeletal Radiology Report

Heading
Practitioner and clinic information
Patient information
X-ray details

Clinical information
Relevant history
Pertinent examination findings
Abnormal laboratory studies

Findings (body of report)
ABCS format in appropriate order
Starts with most serious pathology first

Alignment	*or*	Bone	*or*	Soft tissues
Bone		Cartilage		Alignment
Cartilage		Alignment		Bone
Soft tissues		Soft tissues		Cartilage

Conclusions
Diagnosis or differential diagnosis

Recommendations*
Follow-up plain radiographs
Special imaging procedures
Specific laboratory tests
Technical comments

Signature

*Optional.

BOX 5-18

Template for Writing a Chest Radiology Report

Heading
Practitioner and clinic information
Patient information
X-ray details

Clinical information
Relevant history
Pertinent examination findings
Abnormal laboratory studies

Findings (body of report)
Emphasis on *soft tissues*
Starts with most serious pathology first

   Soft tissues
   Heart and mediastinum
   Lung parenchyma
   Pleura and costophrenic angles
   Soft tissues of chest wall

   Bone

   Cartilage

   Alignment*

Conclusions
Diagnosis or differential diagnosis

Recommendations*
Follow-up plain radiographs
Special imaging procedures
Specific laboratory tests
Technical comments

Signature

*Optional.

---

report follow the same format as the one included previously for skeletal radiographs. Box 5-18 contains a suggested template for writing chest x-ray reports.

Findings. The body of the chest x-ray report can use the ABCS format, but the section *Soft Tissues* is significantly expanded and usually starts the report. The soft tissues expected to be evaluated on these radiographs include the following:

- Heart and mediastinum
- Lung parenchyma
- Pleura and costophrenic angles
- Infradiaphragmatic (abdominal) soft tissues
- Soft tissues of the chest wall

Once comments have been included for each of the soft-tissue areas, the skeletal structures should be examined. Because chest radiographs are primarily taken to assess the heart, mediastinum, lungs, and pleura, clinicians may forget to evaluate the osseous structures, missing significant abnormal pathologic processes. Thus there is no substitute for a thorough search pattern. Being forced to write an x-ray report may help the clinician to thoroughly evaluate all aspects of each film.

If no abnormalities are detected in each of the components of the soft-tissue analysis, negative statements attesting to these facts should be included within the body of the report. An example of a normal chest report follows:

> The posteroanterior (PA) projection demonstrates a full inspiration with no signs of pathology in the heart or mediastinum. The lung parenchymas are symmetric in density with normal pulmonary markings and no masses evident. There is no pleural thickening and the costophrenic angles are sharp. No abnormalities are

detected in the visualized infradiaphragmatic structures or soft tissues of the chest wall. The thoracic cage is symmetric with no evidence of pathology in the ribs or other visualized osseous structures.

This example may seem lengthy for a normal chest report. However, by using computer macros or voice-activated dictation, the generation of such a report takes only a few seconds. In addition, the report indicates that the person evaluating the radiographs was thorough in assessing all aspects of the films.

Abdomen radiology reports. The chiropractor rarely should be called upon to write radiology reports on plain films of the abdomen. These radiographs initially should be taken in the recumbent position with technical factors chosen to enhance visualization of the abdominal soft tissues rather than the osseous structures. The plain abdominal radiograph often is used as a "scout" (preliminary search) film preceding various contrast studies. However, plain radiographs of the abdomen may be used alone to identify abnormalities in gas patterns, evaluation of the size and location of certain organs, the presence or absence of foreign bodies, and the identification of abnormal calcifications.

While the radiology report for abdominal films is being written, it should be remembered which anatomic structures can and cannot normally be visualized (Box 5-19).

Box 5-20 offers a template for the creation of plain film abdominal radiology reports. Although abdominal radiology reports emphasize the soft-tissue component of the anatomy, it is imperative that the clinician evaluate the entire radiograph, including the osseous and cartilaginous structures. Alignment also should be considered, even though these radiographs usually are taken in the recumbent position.

Spine computed tomography and magnetic resonance imaging reports. No consensus exists about the proper length or content of special imaging reports. As mentioned, general practice chiropractors should not be expected to report on special imaging procedures. However, they frequently must interpret the radiologist's report and explain abnormalities seen on special imaging procedures to the patient.

Both CT and MRI reports on the spine should contain information about the presence or absence of disc herniation. If herniation is detected, its exact location, size, and type should be mentioned using standard, universally accepted terminology. Displacement or obliteration of the spinal cord, thecal sac, or nerve roots also must be stated. Information confirming no visible encroachment onto these structures should be included. Stenosis of the central spinal canal, lateral recess, or intervertebral foramina should be mentioned, as well as an identification of the anatomic structures responsible for the stenosis and its severity.

Reports for both CT and MRI scans should address the clinical concern (as should all other radiology reports). If a tumor or infectious disease is suspected because of the history or examination findings, the special imaging procedure should confirm or rule out the clinical suspicion, with appropriate statements appearing in the body of the report.

Abnormalities of signal intensity, their specific anatomic location and imaging sequence, and the significance of these alterations also must be mentioned in MRI reports. For example, decreased signal intensity of intervertebral discs is seen with dehydration of the disc, which is associated with degenerative disc disease. This same finding is not seen on CT scans.

The radiology report should reflect the purpose of the abdominal study that was performed. If a plain abdominal radiograph is taken because a patient has the signs and symptoms of a kidney stone, the first statement within the body of the report should reflect this concern and comment on the presence or absence of a calcific density in the region of the kidney or ureter. If the clinician palpates a pulsating abdominal mass, the radiologic report must address this finding by noting whether a dilated, calcified abdominal aorta or iliac artery is present.

As in the chest radiology report, the ABCS format does not strictly apply to abdominal reports. The *Soft Tissues* section is emphasized and expanded, including appropriate negative statements added for the various organs and anatomic structures normally visualized. Although this process may seem unusually lengthy and cumbersome, computer macros or voice-activated dictation allow these reports to be completed in minimal time while enhancing thorough scrutiny of the radiographs and professional competence.

*Optional.

Summary

The quality and thoroughness of the radiology report is a reflection of the professionalism and competence of the clinician. As an important component of the medicolegal record, information contained in these reports is vital to the current and ongoing care of the patient, facilitates interprofessional and intraprofessional communication, and may help protect the patient and clinician in litigious circumstances. Each report should be tailored to the individual patient and clinical suspicions. However, because of the development of voice-activated dictation systems with instant report generation, as well as computer macros, individualized reports are no longer extraordinarily time-consuming tasks.

Sample Radiology Reports

The following case studies provide examples of written radiology, CT, and MRI reports.

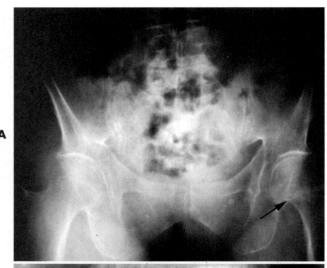

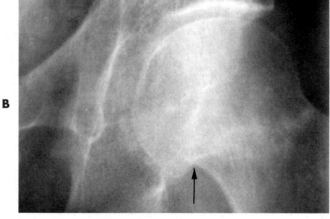

FIG. 5-22 **A** and **B,** Recent impaction fracture of the left femoral neck *(arrow).*

CASE STUDY I

Report date: December 2, 1992

Clinician:	Dr. Marc Adams
Patient:	Mrs. I. Stepson
Age/sex:	61/F
X-ray number:	A4291
Imaging date:	12/02/97
Part:	Pelvis
Views:	Recumbent AP

CLINICAL INFORMATION

Fell 2 weeks previously and has had left hip pain since the fall. Was diagnosed with degenerative joint disease (DJD) by a general practitioner (GP) and an orthopedist. Has had no previous radiographs. Has been on corticosteroids for the past 2 years because of asthma.

FINDINGS

A sclerotic line is noted traversing the neck of the left femur with disruption of the cortex medially at the junction of the femoral head and neck (Fig. 5-22). The remainder of the cortices are intact. The bone density reveals a marked generalized osteopenia.

No abnormalities are detected in the hip joints, sacroiliac articulations, or symphysis pubis.

There is a slight right lateral olisthesis of L3.

Several amorphous calcific densities are noted in the vicinity of the midsacrum (most likely superimposed over the sacrum). The remainder of the visualized soft tissues are unremarkable.

CONCLUSIONS

1. Recent impaction fracture of the left femoral neck
2. Marked osteoporosis, most likely resulting from a combination of age, gender, and long-term use of corticosteroids
3. Mild degenerative right lateral olisthesis of L3
4. Sclerotic densities in the region of the sacrum, most likely calcified lymph nodes from an old healed infectious process

RECOMMENDATIONS

1. The patient should receive an immediate orthopedic referral for consideration of surgical pinning.
2. Long-term monitoring is needed to detect possible development of avascular necrosis of the femoral head, conducted most effectively with MRI.

Cynthia Peterson, RN, DC, DACBR, MMedEd

CASE STUDY 2

Report date: July 27, 1997

Clinician:	Dr. Denise Marcos Adams
Patient:	Mr. D. Smith
Age/sex:	62/M
X-ray number:	B9393
Imaging date:	7/26/97
Part:	Cervical spine
Views:	Upright AP and lateral

CLINICAL INFORMATION

Long history of progressive neck pain and stiffness

FINDINGS

Thick, flowing hyperostosis is noted along the adjacent anterior body margins of C3-C7. Thin, nonmarginal syndesmophytes are visualized at the adjacent anterior body margins of C2-C3. There is a thick longitudinal osseous band extending from the posterior odontoid process to the posterior inferior body margin of C3 (Fig. 5-23), with apparent fusion to the posterior aspect of C3 and separation from the body of C2 and the dens. This osseous band occupies approximately 32% of the sagittal diameter of the spinal canal at the C3 level. Mild to moderate hypertrophy and sclerosis of the facet articulations is present bilaterally at the C3-C7 levels.

The visualized disc spaces are well preserved. The uncovertebral joints are difficult to evaluate because of underpenetration of the AP radiograph.

Calcific densities are present at the tips of the spinous processes of C6, C7, and T1.

No abnormalities of alignment are detected.

CONCLUSIONS

1. DISH with ossification of the posterior longitudinal ligament (OPLL). Significant encroachment into the spinal canal. Calcific densities at the tips of the spinous processes: common with DISH; represent calcification or ossification of the supraspinous ligament.
2. Mild to moderate facet arthrosis of C3-C7.

RECOMMENDATIONS

1. If any neurologic deficits are detected, CT or MRI of the cervical spine is indicated to evaluate the severity of canal stenosis caused by the OPLL.
2. Test for the possibility of diabetes mellitus, which has been associated with DISH.

Cynthia Peterson, RN, DC, DACBR, MMedEd

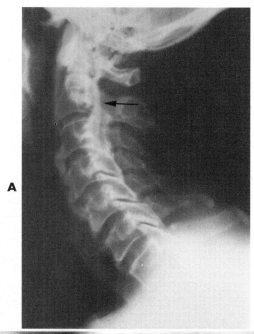

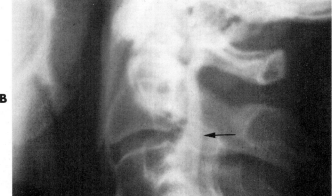

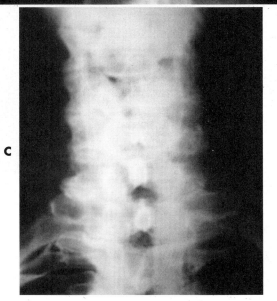

FIG. 5-23 A to **C,** Diffuse idiopathic skeletal hyperostosis with ossification of the posterior longitudinal ligament *(arrow).*

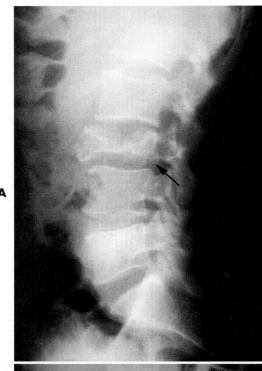

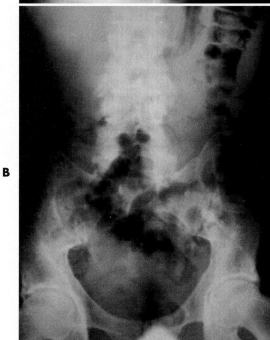

FIG. 5-24   **A** and **B,** Malignant pathologic fracture of L3. *Arrows* point to the osseous fragment at the posterior inferior corner of L3 and the medial displacement of the colon.

CASE STUDY 3

Report date: April 12, 1996

Clinician:	Dr. Prospero Antonuccio
Patient:	Mr. M. Melvin
Age/sex:	43/M
Imaging date:	4/12/96
X-ray number:	B8050
Part:	Lumbar spine
Views:	Recumbent AP and lateral

CLINICAL INFORMATION

Eight months of increasing low back pain. "Electric" type of pain radiating into both posterior legs. Numbness in groin, testicles, and penis. Difficulty urinating. Atrophy of quadriceps, hamstrings, and calf muscles. Has been treated by a physical therapist with no improvement.

FINDINGS

There is lytic destruction of the vertebral body of L3 with pathologic collapse and sagittal elongation (Fig. 5-24). A separate osseous fragment is noted at the posterior inferior body of L3. No other lytic lesions are detected.

Marked medial displacement of the descending colon is evident because of the presence of a large soft-tissue mass within the lateral aspect of the left side of the abdomen. A marked quantity of gas and fecal material is noted within the large bowel. A small, round osseous dense region is present adjacent to the superolateral margin of the right acetabulum.

The visualized disc spaces, hips, and sacroiliac joints are within normal limits.

No significant abnormalities of alignment are noted.

CONCLUSIONS

1. Malignant tumor of L3 with abdominal mass, which may represent a primary abdominal malignancy with metastatic spread to L3. However, also may be lymphoma, considering the patient's age and the radiographic findings. Malignant destruction of L3 is likely responsible for the patient's clinical presentation of cauda equina syndrome.
2. Os acetabulum right hip.

RECOMMENDATION

The patient should receive immediate referrals for an abdominal CT, a spinal MRI, and a biopsy.

Cynthia Peterson, RN, DC, DACBR, MMedEd

CASE STUDY 4

Report date: January 30, 1998

Clinician:	Dr. Doug Smith
Patient:	Mr. R. Hinley
Age/sex:	40/M
Imaging date:	1/12/98
Part:	Lumbar spine
Views:	Upright AP and lateral

CLINICAL INFORMATION

Long history of low back pain with recent severe, colicky left flank pain.

FINDINGS

There is a small, oval calcific density in the left upper quadrant, lateral to the L2-L3 disc space (Fig. 5-25). This is also suggested on the lateral view superimposed over the L2-L3 disc space. No other abnormalities are noted within the visualized soft tissues.

The lower two thirds of both sacroiliac joints are sclerotic with joint space narrowing and ill-defined subchondral bone. The remainder of the osseous and cartilaginous structures are within normal limits.

No significant abnormalities of alignment are detected.

CONCLUSIONS

1. Kidney stone on the left (nephrolithiasis).
2. Bilateral sacroiliitis. Differential diagnosis includes: ankylosing spondylitis, enteropathic spondylitis, Reiter's syndrome, and psoriatic arthritis. Clinical correlation is indicated.

RECOMMENDATIONS

1. The patient should receive a referral to a urologist for management of the kidney stone.
2. A spot angled (oblique) lumbosacral radiograph should be obtained to better visualize the sacroiliac joints.
3. Erythrocyte sedimentation rate (ESR) and HLA-B27 lab tests may be useful.

Cynthia Peterson, RN, DC, DACBR, MMedEd

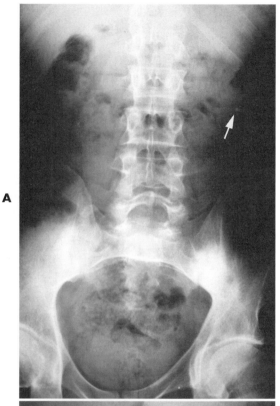

A

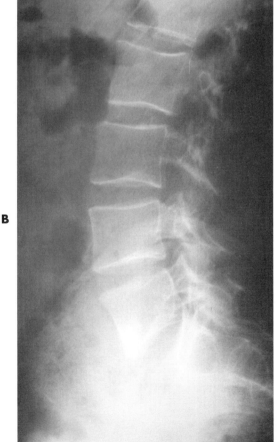

B

FIG. 5-25 **A** and **B,** Bilateral sacroiliitis with kidney calculus *(arrow).*

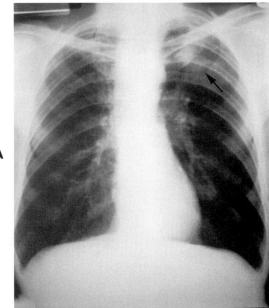

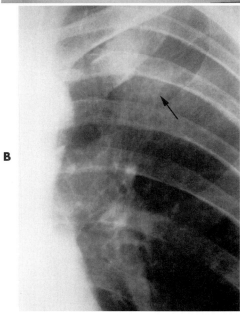

FIG. 5-26   **A** and **B,** Chronic obstructive airway disease with enlarged left hilus and mass in the left upper lung field *(arrow).*

CASE STUDY 5

Report date: March 10, 1998

Clinician:	Dr. Nancy Dafner
Patient:	Mr. Anthony Charminster
Age/sex:	62/M
Imaging date:	3/9/98
Part:	Chest
Views:	Upright PA

CLINICAL INFORMATION

Increasing dyspnea and long history of cigarette smoking.

FINDINGS

An ill-defined area of partial consolidation measuring approximately 2 × 3 cm barely appears in the left upper lung field between the posterior aspects of the fifth and sixth ribs, partially superimposed over the fifth rib (Fig. 5-26). The left hilar region appears enlarged.

The hemidiaphragms are low and flat bilaterally, at the level of the twelfth ribs. The lung fields appear hyperlucent.

The heart and mediastinal structures other than the left hilus appear to be within normal limits.

The costophrenic angles are sharp, and there is no pleural thickening.

No abnormalities are detected in the infradiaphragmatic or chest wall soft tissues.

The visualized osseous and articular structures are unremarkable. The thoracic cage is symmetric.

CONCLUSIONS

1. Left upper lobe infiltrate combined with prominent left hilus: must be considered malignant until proved otherwise. The most likely diagnosis (because of patient's long smoking history) is bronchogenic carcinoma with possible metastatic spread. Primary neoplasm: may be hilar with peripheral spread to the lung parenchyma or parenchymal infiltrate may represent primary lesion with spread to mediastinum.
2. Chronic obstructive pulmonary disease.

RECOMMENDATION

The patient should receive an immediate referral for CT of the chest, a cytology examination of sputum, a possible bronchoscopy, and a biopsy.

Cynthia Peterson, RN, DC, DACBR, MMedEd

CASE STUDY 6

Report date: April 9, 1997

Clinician:	Dr. Abraham Weir
Patient:	Mrs. J. Van der Veer
Age/sex:	44/F
Imaging date:	3/14/97
Part:	Lumbar spine
Procedure:	CT scan of L3-S1 intervertebral discs; angled gantry; soft-tissue window only

CLINICAL INFORMATION

Signs and symptoms of right-sided radiculopathy into the lateral aspect of the foot.

FINDINGS

There is a very large right posterolateral disc protrusion at the L5-S1 level that is best seen on slices 16 and 17 (Fig. 5-27). This encroaches posteriorly on approximately 65% of the sagittal canal diameter with displacement of the thecal sac without visualization of the right S1 nerve root.

Accurate assessment of the lateral recesses and osseous structures cannot be achieved without the corresponding "bone" windows.

No other abnormalities are detected.

CONCLUSION

Large right posterolateral disc herniation at L5-S1 affecting the right S1 nerve root and thecal sac, which correlates with the patient's clinical complaints.

RECOMMENDATION

If further imaging evaluation is warranted, an MRI would best demonstrate the lesion and its impact on the contents of the spinal canal. Additionally, an orthopedic evaluation may be warranted, especially if conservative management does not resolve the patient's clinical complaint.

Cynthia Peterson, RN, DC, DACBR, MMedEd

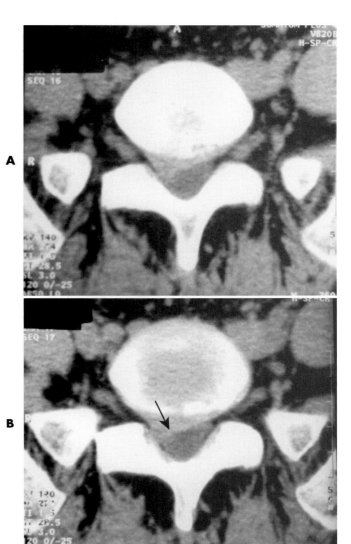

FIG. 5-27 **A** and **B,** Right posterior disc herniation at L5-S1 *(arrow).*

CASE STUDY 7

Report date: April 12, 1997

Clinician:	Dr. Michelle Hansell
Patient:	Miss J. Adams
Age/sex:	35/F
Imaging date:	4/9/97
Part:	Lumbar spine
Procedure:	T1- and T2-weighted sagittal scans, T1-weighted axial scans.

CLINICAL INFORMATION

Acute onset of severe low back and leg pain with neurologic deficits after lifting heavy glider wing

FINDINGS

A large left posterocentral intervertebral disc extrusion is noted at the L5-S1 level with inferior migration of the large discal fragment posterior to the body of S1 suggesting sequestration (Fig. 5-28). The discal fragment extends posteriorly approximately 75% of the sagittal canal diameter. Marked posterior and right displacement of the thecal sac is present at this level. The left S1 nerve root is still faintly visualized.

Slight decreased signal intensity of the L4-5 and L5-S1 discs is noted.

S1 appears to be somewhat transitional, with a remnant S1-2 disc.

No other abnormalities are detected.

CONCLUSIONS

1. Huge left posterocentral disc herniation with inferior migration of the sequestered fragment. Encroachment on approximately 75% of the sagittal canal diameter.
2. Decreased signal intensity at the L4-5 and L5-S1 levels that is consistent with early degenerative disc disease.

RECOMMENDATION

Neurosurgical consultation should be considered.

Cynthia Peterson, RN, DC, DACBR, MMedEd

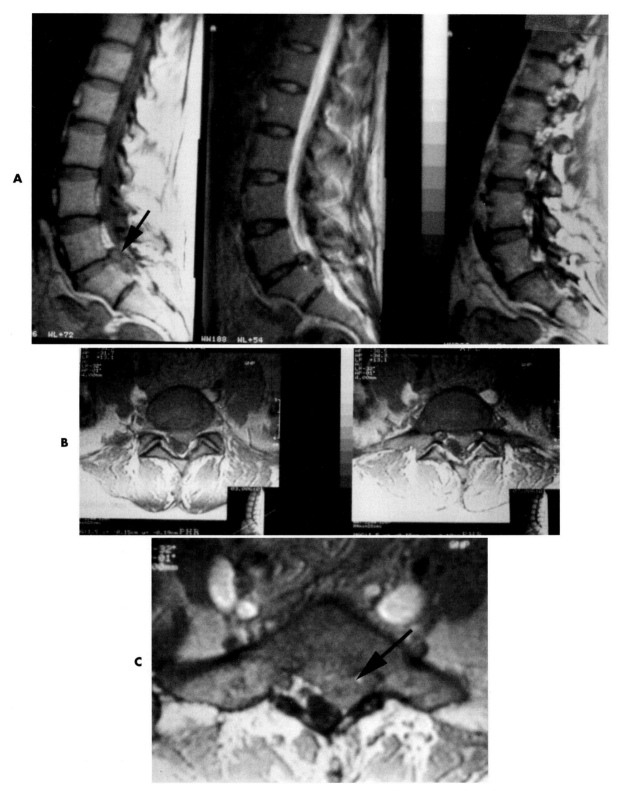

FIG. 5-28 **A** to **C,** Huge posterocentral disc herniation with sequestration *(arrows).*

TABLE 5-1

Annotated Bibliography of Selected Articles Addressing Radiologic Image Interpretation

Topic	Article	Summary
Ambient light	Alter AJ et al[3]	Employing low ambient room light, illuminating only films being viewed, and masking the radiograph around areas of interest improves visual performance; however, is cumbersome to implement completely in a clinical setting.
Appearance of the lesion	Krupinski EA et al[85]	This study found that physical features of pulmonary nodules do not attract attention as measured by "first hit" fixation of the interpreter's gaze; however, certain features do tend to hold the attention once the nodule has been fixated. The combination of all features influences whether or not it is detected.
Experience	Herman PG et al[66]	After having several interpreters view a series of chest radiographs, the authors found that, "Once an individual's radiology education has progressed beyond a fundamental level, individual reader characteristics overshadow experience (and training) in the accuracy of chest film interpretation."
Experience	Nodine CF et al[100]	Differences in resident performance resulted primarily from lack of perceptual-learning experience during mammography training, which limited object recognition skills and made it difficult to determine differences between malignant lesions, benign lesions, and normal image perturbations. A proposed solution is systematic mentor-guided training that links image perception to feedback about the reasons underlying decision making.
Experience	Qu G, Huda W, Belden CJ[114]	Trained observers are superior to untrained observers when assessing characteristics of phantom images.
Experience	Krupinski EA, Weinstein RS, Rozek LS[86]	There is a positive correlation between years of clinical experience and ability to successfully interpret radiographic images.
Experience	Nodine CF, Krupinski EA[99]	Performance on two visual search and detection tasks indicate that radiologists do not possess superior visual skills compared with lay people. Radiology expertise is more likely to be a combination of specific visual and cognitive skills derived from medical training and experience in detecting and determining the diagnostic importance of radiographic findings.
Experience	Rhea JT, Potsaid MS, DeLuca SA[116]	Experienced interpreters exhibited lower rates of false-positive and false-negative readings.
Experience	Sowden PT, Rose D, Davies IR[131]	Performance of a wide range of simple visual tasks improves with practice. This learning may be a specific function of the eye.
Experience	Taylor JAM et al[145]	This study demonstrated a significant association between the interpreters (both medical and chiropractic) training and their ability to recognize abnormal radiographs of the lumbosacral spine and pelvis.
Eye dwell time and axis of gaze	Carmody DP, Nodine CF, Kundel HL[34]	"Our findings indicate that a dwell time of 300 ms was sufficient to detect 85% of the nodules when they were viewed directly. Detection accuracy was reduced by one-half when the tumor was located 5 degrees from the axis of gaze."
Eye gaze durations, scan paths, and detection times	Krupinski EA[84]	Readers with more experience tended to detect lesions earlier in the search than did readers with less experience, but those with less experience tended to spend more time overall searching the images and cover more image area than did those with more experience.
Confidence level	Mayhue FE et al[94]	Prospective interpretations of nearly 1900 emergency room radiographs were performed by multiple interpreters. The concordance of agreement varied by level of confidence, but not training level among the interpreters.
Influence of patient history	Berbaum KS et al[15]	This study tested whether accompanying patient clinical information would improve perception or simply decision making. The report found that the interpreter's detection of pathology was significantly better with history provided before film inspection. Detection did not differ for history provided after inspection and inspection without history. The authors concluded, "clinical history affected perception in interpreting radiographs, not simply decision making."
Influence of patient history	Berbaum KS, Franken EA, el-Khoury GY[17]	A brief patient history may provide localization clues that improve the ability of interpreters to detect fractures and other features of trauma. When localization clues are withheld or unavailable, radiologists and nonradiologists alike are less successful in finding trauma lesions; although the accuracy of the radiologists suffers less.

TABLE 5-1 cont'd
Annotated Bibliography of Selected Articles Addressing Radiologic Image Interpretation

Topic	Article	Summary
Influence of patient history	Good BC et al[56]	Researchers found that knowledge of clinical history does not affect the accuracy of radiologists' interpretations of chest films for the detection of pathologies such as interstitial disease, nodules, and pneumothoraces.
Miss rates	Robinson PJ[117]	This is a literature review of strategies for reducing error in radiograph interpretation. Methods include: attention to viewing conditions, training of observers, availability of previous films and relevant clinical data, dual or multiple reporting, standardization of terminology and report format, and assistance from computers.
Miss rates	Herman PG et al[65]	These authors found that 41% of chest radiograph reports contained potentially significant errors and 56% showed indeterminate disagreement. In addition, 78% of all errors were false-negatives and 22% were false-positives.
Perception of the image	Kundel HL, Nodine CF[89]	These authors advocate that image perception begins with characterization of the scene integrating data from the retina and memory to form a visual concept. This theory holds that it may be necessary to have seen radiologic abnormalities in the past to be able to form an appropriate visual concept for a current abnormality.
Prior studies	Berbaum KS, Smith WL[18]	"Old reports add value to current interpretation by providing a form of 'second reading' and providing clinical history. Two years is sufficient old report access in 85% of situations."
Satisfaction of search errors	Berbaum KS et al[16]	This defines the satisfaction of search phenomenon in diagnostic radiology and the development of statistical methods to measure observer performance.
Satisfaction of search errors	Ashman CJ, Yu JS, Wolfman D[7]	The satisfaction of search phenomena describes a situation in which the detection of one radiographic abnormality interferes with the detection of others. Satisfaction of search defects of film interpretation is operative in the interpretation of radiographs of the musculoskeletal system.
Satisfaction of search errors	Berbaum KS et al[14]	It appears that satisfaction of search errors originate from recognition failures more than poor decision making.
Satisfaction of search errors	Berbaum KS et al[13]	An appropriate history appears to reduce satisfaction of search errors. It is believed that detailed histories direct the interpreter's perceptual resources to the prompted abnormalities, reducing the satisfaction of search error.
Search path	Kundel HL, Nodine CF[88]	This experiment quickly flashed the image as a means of negating the ability for observers to visually scan the image, resulting in an overall true-positive rate of 70%. As anticipated, the rate improved to 97% with the addition of a free search of the images. These data support the fact that visual search begins with a global response of the interpreter to the image to establish content and detect gross deviations from normal.
Search path	Beard DV et al[10]	Radiologists' film interpretation has a typical sequence. Films are mounted in order; radiologists generally start a sequential scan through the entire examination; this is followed by a detailed viewing of two to four clusters of three to six images; and last the findings are dictated or otherwise recorded.
Search path	Hu CH et al[74]	More systematic scanning patterns were observed for experienced than inexperienced observers.
Search path	Carmody DP, Kundel HL, Toto LC[33]	Although radiologists are formally trained to search radiographs using a systematic and directive search path with comparison of bilateral features, only 4% of visual activity was accomplished with bilateral comparison when observed. Most radiologists used a flexible search path.
Search path	Swensson RG, Hessel SJ, Herman PG[143]	Data collected on readings of chest radiographs found that "radiologists could distinguish between normal and abnormal radiographs better when searching the chest films for any abnormal findings than when explicitly evaluating" the radiographs for specific features to which their attention is directed. The authors theorize that "the recognition of abnormal findings may have been augmented by perceptual mechanisms that functioned only during the process of visual search."
Search path	Peterson C[107]	The authors found that chiropractic students who employed a flexible but complete search pattern when interpreting radiographs performed significantly better than their peers using any other search pattern approach.
Second opinions	Swensson RG, Theodore GH[142]	This study involved multiple interpretations of chest radiographs and found that second opinions are more accurate if the second interpreter is not aware of the concerns or findings of the first interpreter.

References

1. AHCPR Low Back Pain Guidelines Panel: Acute Low Back Pain Problems in Adults, Clinical Practice Guideline No. 14. Washington, DC: Department of Health and Human Services, Public Health Service, Agency for Health Care Policy and Research; 1995, AHCPR publication no. 95-0644.
2. Alfaro D et al: Accuracy of interpretation of cranial computed tomography scans in an emergency medicine residency program, *Ann Emerg Med* 25:169, 1995.
3. Alter AJ et al: The influence of ambient and view box light upon visual detection of low-contrast targets in a radiograph, *Invest Radiol* 17:402, 1992.
4. American Chiropractic Association: Statistics on chiropractic offices and equipment, *J Am Chiropract Assoc* 24:56, 1987.
5. American College of Radiology: ACR practice guideline for general radiology, Reston, VA, 2001, American College of Radiology.
6. Anderson EDC et al: The efficacy of double reading mammograms in breast screening, *Clin Radiol* 49:248, 1994.
7. Ashman CJ, Yu JS, Wolfman D: Satisfaction of search in osteoradiology, *AJR Am J Roentgenol* 175:541, 2000.
8. Attneave F: Multistability in perception, *Sci Am* 225:63, 1971.
9. Bauman RA: Reporting and communications, *Radiol Clin North Am* 34:597, 1996.
10. Beard DV et al: A study of radiologists viewing multiple computed tomography examinations using an eye tracking device, *J Digit Imag* 3:230, 1990.
11. Beck C: Accuracy and reliability of chiropractors and AECC students at visually estimating the cervical lordosis from radiographs, unpublished student project, Bournemouth, England, 1997, Anglo-European College of Chiropractic.
12. Berbaum K, Franken EA, Smith WL: The effect of comparison films upon resident interpretation of pediatric chest radiographs, *Invest Radiol* 20:124, 1985.
13. Berbaum KS et al: The influence of clinical history on visual search with single and multiple abnormalities, *Invest Radiol* 28:191, 1993.
14. Berbaum KS et al: Role of faulty decision making in the satisfaction of search effect in chest radiography, *Acad Radiol* 7:1098, 2000.
15. Berbaum KS et al: Influence of clinical history on perception of abnormalities in pediatric radiographs, *Acad Radiol* 1:217, 1994.
16. Berbaum KS et al: Satisfaction of search in diagnostic radiology, *Invest Radiol* 25:133, 1990.
17. Berbaum KS, Franken EA Jr, el-Khoury GY: Impact of clinical history on radiographic detection of fractures: a comparison of radiologists and orthopedists. *AJR Am J Roentgenol* 153:1221, 1989.
18. Berbaum KS, Smith WL: Use of reports of previous radiologic studies, *Acad Radiol* 5:111, 1998.
19. Bergus GR et al: Radiologic interpretation by family physicians in an office practice setting, *J Fam Pract* 41:352, 1995.
20. Berlin L, Berlin JW: Malpractice and radiologists in Cook County, IL: trends in 20 years of litigation, *AJR Am J Roentgenol* 165:781, 1995.
21. Berlin L, Hendrix RW: Perceptual errors and negligence, *AJR Am J Roentgenol* 170:863, 1998.
22. Berlin L: Malpractice issues in radiology. Perceptual errors, *AJR Am J Roentgenol* 167:587, 1996.
23. Berlin L: Malpractice issues in radiology. Errors in judgment, *AJR Am J Roentgenol* 166:1259, 1996.
24. Berlin L: Malpractice issues in radiology. Processing ordinary knowledge, *AJR Am J Roentgenol* 166:1027, 1996.
25. Bird RE: Professional quality assurance for mammography screening programmes, *Radiology* 177:587, 1990.
26. Bluemke DA, Eng J: An automated radiology reporting system that uses hypercard, *AJR Am J Roentgenol* 160:185, 1993.
27. Bogduk N: Evidence based clinical guidelines for the management of acute low back pain, NHMRC, November, 1999.
28. Boring EG: A new ambiguous figure, *Am J Psychol* 42:444, 1930.
29. Brenner RJ: Medicolegal aspects of breast imaging: variable standards of care relating to different types of practice, *AJR Am J Roentgenol* 156:719, 1991.
30. Brunswick JE et al: Radiographic interpretation in the emergency department, *Am J Emerg Med* 14:346, 1996.
31. Burgener FA, Kormano M: Differential diagnosis in conventional radiology, ed 2, New York, 1991, Thieme Medical Publishers.
32. Carey TS, Garrett J: Patterns of ordering diagnostic tests for patients with acute low back pain, The North Carolina Back Pain Project, *Ann Intern Med* 125:807, 1996.
33. Carmody DP, Kundel HL, Toto LC: Comparison scans while reading chest images. Taught, but not practiced, *Invest Radiol* 19:462, 1984.
34. Carmody DP, Nodine CF, Kundel HL: An analysis of perceptual and cognitive factors in radiographic interpretation, *Perception* 9:339, 1980.
35. Casey B: About Aunt Minnie, *http://www.auntminnie.com*.
36. Centers for Medicare and Medicaid Services (CMMS), National Health Statistics Group, Office of the Actuary: National health expenditures, 2000, *http://cms.hhs.gov*.
37. Cherkin DC et al: Physician variation in diagnostic testing for low back pain. Who you see is what you get, *Arthritis Rheum* 37:15, 1994.
38. Christensen E et al: The effect of search time on perception, *Diag Radiol* 138:361, 1981.
39. Clinical Standards Advisory Group (CSAG): Report on back pain, HMSO, 1994.
40. Collins RD: Differential diagnosis in primary care, ed 2, Philadelphia, 1987, JB Lippincott.
41. Deyo RA, Bigos SJ, Maravilla KR: Diagnostic imaging procedures for the lumbar spine, *Ann Intern Med* 111:865, 1989.
42. Deyo RA, Diehl AK, Rosenthal M: Reducing roentgenography use: can patient expectations be altered? *Arch Int Med* 147:141, 1987.
43. Deyo RA, Diehl AK: Cancer as a cause of back pain: frequency, clinical presentation, and diagnostic strategies, *J Gen Intern Med* 3:230, 1988.
44. Deyo RA, Diehl AK: Lumbar spine films in primary care: current use and effects of selective ordering criteria, *J Gen Intern Med* 1:20, 1986.
45. Deyo RA, Phillips WR: Low back pain. A primary care challenge, *Spine* 21:2826, 1996.
46. Deyo RA, Rainville J, Kent D: What can the history and physical examination tell us about low back pain? *JAMA* 268:760, 1992.
47. Doubilet P, Herman P: Interpretation of radiographs: effect of clinical history, *AJR Am J Roentgenol* 137:1055, 1981.
48. Eisenberg RL: Clinical imaging: an atlas of differential diagnosis, ed 2, Gaithersburg, MD, 2002, Aspen Publishers.
49. Fishler M, Firschein O: Intelligence, the eye, the brain and the computer, Boston, 1988, Addison Wesley.
50. Fleisher G, Ludwig S, McSorley M: Interpretation of pediatric x-ray films by emergency department pediatricians, *Ann Emerg Med* 12:153, 1983.
51. Foreman SM, Stahl MJ: Medical-legal issues in chiropractic, Baltimore, 1990, Williams & Wilkins.
52. Freeborn DK et al: Primary care physicians' use of lumbar spine imaging tests: effects of guidelines and practice pattern feedback, *J Gen Intern Med* 12:619, 1997.
53. Friedman C et al: A general natural-language text processor for clinical radiology, *J Am Med Inform Assoc* 1:161, 1994.
54. Friedman C, Cimino JJ, Johnson SB: A schema for representing medical language applied to clinical radiology, *J Am Med Inform Assoc* 1:233, 1994.
55. Garland LH: Studies on the accuracy of diagnostic procedures, *AJR Am J Roentgenol* 32:25, 1959.
56. Good BC et al: Does knowledge of the clinical history affect the accuracy of chest radiograph interpretation? *AJR Am J Roentgenol* 154:709, 1990.
57. Guidelines for Chiropractic Quality Assurance and Practice Parameters, Proceedings of the Mercy Center Consensus Conference, Baltimore, January 25–30, 1992, Aspen Publishers.

58. Gratton MC, Salomone JA, Watson WA: Clinically significant radiograph misinterpretations at an emergency medicine residency program, *Ann Emerg Med* 19:497, 1990.

59. Halpin SFS, Yeoman L, Dundas DD: Radiographic examination of the lumbar spine in a community hospital: an audit of current practice, *BMJ* 303:813, 1991.

60. Halvorsen JG et al: The interpretation of office radiographs by family physicians, *J Fam Pract* 28:426, 1989.

61. Halvorsen JG, Kunian A: Radiology in family practice: experience in community practice, *Fam Med* 20:112, 1988.

62. Harger BL et al: Chiropractic radiologists: a survey of chiropractors' attitudes and patterns of use, *J Man Physiol Ther* 20:311, 1998.

63. Harger BL, Taylor JAM, Peterson CK: Radiology report writing guidelines, class notes, Portland, OR, 1997, Western States Chiropractic College.

64. Health Care Financing Administration, Office of Actuary, National Health Statistics Group: National health expenditures aggregates, per capita, percent distribution, and annual percent change by source of funds: calendar years 1960–1997.

65. Herman PG et al: Disagreements in chest roentgen interpretation, *Chest* 68:278, 1975.

66. Herman PG, Hessel SJ: Accuracy and its relationship to experience in the interpretation of chest radiographs, *Invest Radiol* 10:62, 1975.

67. Hessel SJ, Herman PG, Swensson RG: Improving performance by multiple interpretations of chest radiographs: effectiveness and cost, *Radiology* 127:589, 1978.

68. Hillman BJ et al: Improving diagnostic accuracy: a comparison of interactive and Delphi consultations, *Invest Radiol* 12:112, 1977.

69. Hillman BJ et al: The value of consultation among radiologists, *AJR Am J Roentgenol* 127:807, 1976.

70. Hirtle RL: Chiropractic malpractice, *ACA J Chiropract* 24:35, 1987.

71. Holman BL et al: Medical impact of unedited preliminary radiology reports, *Radiology* 191:519, 1994.

72. Hopper KD et al: Diagnostic radiology peer review: a method inclusive of all interpreters of radiographic examinations regardless of speciality, *Radiology* 180:557, 1991.

73. Howe JW: A suggested approach to radiographic interpretation and reporting, ACA, Council Roentgenol Roentgen Brief, 1982.

74. Hu CH et al: Searching for bone fractures: a comparison with pulmonary nodule search, *Acad Radiol* 1:25, 1994.

75. Isdahl M: Inter- and intra-examiner reliability in determining hyperplastic articular pillars on lateral cervical radiographs, chiropractic student project, Bournemouth, England, 1997, Anglo-European College of Chiropractic.

76. Keats TE: Atlas of normal roentgen variants that may simulate disease, St Louis, 2001, Mosby.

77. Kirk R: Effect of hyperplastic articular pillars on cervical lordosis, chiropractic student project, Bournemouth, England, 1997, Anglo-European College of Chiropractic.

78. Klein BJ et al: Bridging the gap between science and practice in managing low back pain. A comprehensive spine care system in a health maintenance organization setting, *Spine* 25:47, 2000.

79. Klein EJ et al: Discordant radiograph interpretation between emergency physicians and radiologists in a pediatric emergency department, *Pediatr Emerg Care* 15:245, 1999.

80. Kleinschmidt A et al: Human brain activity during spontaneously reversing perception of ambiguous figures, *Proc R Soc Lond B* 265, 2427, 1998.

81. Knollmann BC et al: Assessment of joint review of radiologic studies by a primary care physician and a radiologist, *J Gen Intern Med* 11:608, 1996.

82. Kovach SG et al: Prevalence of diagnosis on the basis of radiographic evaluation of chiropractic cases, *J Man Physiol Ther* 6:197, 1983.

83. Kruitzky L, Haddy RI, Curry RW: Interpretation of chest roentgenograms by primary care physicians, *South Med J* 80:1347, 1987.

84. Krupinski EA: Visual scanning patterns of radiologists searching mammograms, *Acad Radiol* 3:137, 1996.

85. Krupinski EA et al: Searching for nodules: what features attract attention and influence detection? *Acad Radiol* 10:861, 2003.

86. Krupinski EA et al: Experience-related differences in diagnosis from medical images displayed on monitors, *Telemed J* 2:101, 1996.

87. Kundel HL, La Follette PS: Visual search patterns and experience with radiological images, *Radiology* 103:523, 1972.

88. Kundel HL, Nodine CF: Interpreting chest radiographs without visual search, *Radiology* 116:527, 1975.

89. Kundel HL, Nodine CF: A visual concept shapes image perception, *Radiology* 146:363, 1983.

90. Levin DC, Merrill C: The practice of radiology by nonradiologists: cost, quality and utilization issues, *AJR Am J Roentgenol* 162:513, 1994.

91. Little P et al: Why do GPs perform investigations? The medical and social agendas in arranging back x-rays, *Fam Pract* 15:264, 1998.

92. Mackintosh CE: Radiology: is reporting important? *Br J Hosp Med* 24:259, 1980.

93. Markus JB et al: Double-contrast barium enema studies: effect of multiple reading on perception error, *Radiology* 175:155, 1990.

94. Mayhue FE et al: Accuracy of interpretations of emergency department radiographs: effect of confidence levels, *Ann Emerg Med* 18:826, 1989.

95. McLoughlin RF et al: Radiology reports: how much descriptive detail is enough? *AJR Am J Roentgenol* 165:803, 1995.

96. McNeil BJ: Use of medical radiographs: extent of variation and associated active bone marrow doses, *Radiology* 156:51, 1985.

97. Miller G: A radiologist with a ruler..., *AJNR* 24:556, 2003.

98. Nicholson DA, Driscoll P: ABC of emergency radiology, London, 1995, BMJ Publishing.

99. Nodine CF, Krupinski EA: Perceptual skill, radiology expertise, and visual test performance with NINA and WALDO, *Acad Radiol* 5:603, 1998.

100. Nodine CF et al: How experience and training influence mammography expertise, *Acad Radiol* 6:575, 1999.

101. O'Leary MR et al: Physician assessments of practice patterns in emergency department radiograph interpretation, *Ann Emerg Med* 17:1019, 1988.

102. Orrison WW et al: The language of certainty: proper terminology for the ending of the radiologic report, *AJR Am J Roentgenol* 145:1093, 1985.

103. Ott DJ, Gelfand DW, Ramquist NA: Causes of error in gastrointestinal radiology: II Barium enema examination, *Gastrointest Radiol* 5:99, 1980.

104. Owen JP et al: Survey of general practitioners' opinions on the role of radiology in patients with low back pain, *Br J Gen Pract* 40:98, 1990.

105. Paakkala T: Training of general practitioners in interpreting chest radiographs, *Med Educ* 22:449, 1998.

106. Paris A: Handbook of radiologic dictation, Cincinnati, 1995, MRI-EFI Publications.

107. Peterson CK: Factors associated with success or failure in radiological interpretation: diagnostic thinking approaches, *Med Educ* 33:251, 1999.

108. Peterson CK, Haas M, Harger BL: A radiographic study of sacral base, sacrovertebral and lumbosacral disc angles in persons with and without defects in the pars interarticularis, *J Man Physiol Ther* 13:491, 1990.

109. Peterson CK: Factors associated with success or failure in diagnostic radiology, master's thesis, Scotland, 1996, University of Dundee Centre for Medical Education.

110. Peterson CK: Outline for radiological report, class notes, Bournemouth, England, 1997, Anglo-European College of Chiropractic.

111. Phillips RB: Plain film radiology in chiropractic, *J Man Physiol Ther* 15:47, 1992.

112. Pigman EC et al: Evaluation of the Ottawa clinical decision rules for the use of radiography in acute ankle and midfoot injuries in the emergency department: an independent site assessment, *Ann Emerg Med* 24:41, 1994.

113. Preston CA et al: Reduction of "call-backs" to the emergency department due to discrepancies in the plain radiograph interpretation, *Am J Emerg Med* 16:160, 1998.

114. Qu G, Huda W, Belden CJ: Comparison of trained and untrained observers using subjective and objective measures of imaging performance, *Acad Radiol* 3:31, 1996.

115. Reeder MM, Bradley WG: Reeder and Felson's gamuts in radiology, ed 3, New York, 1993, Springer-Verlag.

116. Rhea JT, Potsaid MS, DeLuca SA: Errors of interpretation as elicited by a quality audit of an emergency radiology facility, *Radiology* 132:277, 1979.

117. Robinson PJ: Radiology's Achilles' heel: error and variation in the interpretation of the Roentgen image, *Br J Radiol* 70:1085, 1997.

118. Robinson PJ et al: Variation between experienced observers in the interpretation of accident and emergency radiographs, *Br J Radiol* 72:323, 1999.

119. Rockey PH et al: The usefulness of x-ray examinations in the evaluation of patients with back pain, *J Fam Pract* 7:455, 1978.

120. Rose JF, Gallivan S: Plain film reporting in the UK, *Clin Radiol* 44:192, 1991.

121. Rosok G, Peterson CK: Comparison of the sacral base angle in females with and without spondylolysis, *J Man Physiol Ther* 16:447, 1993.

122. Royal College of General Practitioners (RCGP): Clinical guidelines for the management of acute low back pain, London, 1996, Royal College of General Practitioners.

123. Royal College of Radiologists: Statement on reporting in departments of clinical radiology, London, 1995, RCR.

124. Samuel S et al: Mechanism of satisfaction of search: eye position recordings in the reading of chest radiographs, *Radiology* 194:895, 1995.

125. Saxton HM: Should radiologists report on every film? *Clin Radiol* 45:1, 1992.

126. Scally P: Medical imaging, Oxford, UK, 1999, Oxford University Press.

127. Scavone JG, Latshaw RF, Rohrer GV: Use of lumbar spine films: statistical evaluation at a university hospital, *JAMA* 246:1105, 1981.

128. Seltzer SE et al: Resident film interpretations and staff review, *AJR Am J Roentgenol* 137:129, 1980.

129. Simon HK et al: Pediatric emergency physician interpretation of plain radiographs: is routine review by a radiologist necessary and cost-effective? *Ann Emerg Med* 27:295, 1996.

130. Smith MJ: Error and variation in diagnostic radiology. Springfield, IL, 1967, Charles C Thomas.

131. Sowden PT, Rose D, Davies IR: Perceptual learning of luminance contrast detection: specific for spatial frequency and retinal location but not orientation, *Vision Res* 42:1249, 2002.

132. Spettell CM et al: Practice patterns of radiologists and nonradiologists: national Medicare data on the performance of chest and skeletal radiography and abdominal and pelvic sonography, *AJR Am J Roentgenol* 171:3, 1998.

133. Spitzer WO: Scientific approach to the assessment and management of activity related spinal disorders, a monograph for clinicians: report of the Quebec Task Force on Spinal Disorders, *Spine* 12:S1, 1987.

134. Stiell IG et al: A study to develop clinical decision rules for the use of radiography in acute ankle injuries, *Ann Emerg Med* 21:384, 1992.

135. Stiell IG et al: Derivation of a decision rule for the use of radiography in acute knee injuries, *Ann Emerg Med* 26:405, 1995.

136. Stiell IG et al: Implementation of the Ottawa Knee Rule for the use of radiography in acute knee injuries, *JAMA*, 278:2075, 1997.

137. Strasser RP, Bass MJ, Brennan M: The effect of an on-site radiology facility on radiologic utilization in family practice, *J Fam Pract* 24:619, 1987.

138. Suarez-Almazor ME et al: Use of lumbar radiographs for the early diagnosis of low back pain. Proposed guidelines would increase utilization, *JAMA* 277:1782, 1997.

139. Sunshine JH, Bansal S, Evens RG: Radiology performed by non-radiologists in the United States: Who does what? *AJR Am J Roentgenol* 161:419, 1993.

140. Sunshine JH, Mabry MR, Bansal S: The volume and cost of radiologic services in the United States in 1990, *AJR Am J Roentgenol* 161:419, 1993.

141. Swensson RG, Hessel S, Herman R: Omissions in radiology: faulty search or stringent reporting criteria? *Radiology* 123:563, 1977.

142. Swensson RG, Theodore GH: Search and nonsearch protocols for radiographic consultation, *Radiology* 177:851, 1990.

143. Swensson RG, Hessel SJ, Herman PG: Radiographic interpretation with and without search: visual search aids the recognition of chest pathology, *Invest Radiol* 17:145, 1982.

144. Tallroth K, Alaranta H, Soukka A: Lumbar mobility in asymptomatic individuals, *J Spinal Disord* 5:481, 1992.

145. Taylor JAM et al: Interpretation of abnormal lumbosacral spine radiographs: a test comparing students, clinicians, radiology residents and radiologists in medicine and chiropractic, *Spine* 20:1147, 1995.

146. Taylor JAM, Resnick D: Skeletal imaging: atlas of the spine and extremities, Philadelphia, 2000, WB Saunders.

147. Taylor JAM: Writing radiology reports in chiropractic, *J Can Chiropract Assoc* 34:30, 1990.

148. Thomas HG et al: Value of radiograph audit in an accident service department, *Injury* 23:47, 1992.

149. Touquet R, Driscoll P, Nicholson D: Teaching in accident and emergency medicine: 10 commandments of accident and emergency radiology, *BMJ* 310:642, 1995.

150. Tuck AM, Peterson CK: Accuracy and reliability of chiropractors and AECC students at visually estimating the lumbar lordosis from radiographs, *J Chiropract Tech* 10:19, 1998.

151. Vix VA, Ryu CY: The adult symphysis pubis: normal and abnormal, *AJR Am J Roentgenol* 112:517, 1971.

152. Waddell G: The back pain revolution, ed 2, Edinburgh, 2004, Churchill Livingstone.

153. Walsh-Kelly CM, Hennes HM, Melzer-Lange MD: False-positive preliminary radiograph interpretations in a pediatric emergency department: clinical and economic impact, *Am J Emerg Med* 15:354, 1997.

154. Walsh-Kelly CM et al: Clinical impact of radiograph misinterpretation in a pediatric ED and the effect of physician training level, *Am J Emerg Med* 13:262, 1995.

155. Warren JS et al: Correlation of emergency department radiographs: results of a quality assurance review in an urban community hospital setting, *J Am Board Fam Pract* 6:255, 1993.

156. White K, Berbaum K, Smith WL: The role of previous radiographs and reports in the interpretation of current radiographs, *Invest Radiol* 29:263, 1994.

157. Wilson IB et al: Patients' role in the use of radiology testing for common office practice complaints, *Arch Int Med* 161:256, 2001.

158. Worrill NA, Peterson CK: Effect of anterior wedging of L1 on the measurement of lumbar lordosis: comparison of two roentgenological methods, *J Man Physiol Ther* 20:459, 1997.

159. Yerushalmy J, Harkness JT, Kennedy BR: The role of dual reading in mass radiography. *Am Rev Tuberculosis* 61:443, 1950.

160. Yochum TR, Rowe LJ: Essentials of skeletal radiology, ed 2, Baltimore, 1996, Williams & Wilkins.

chapter 6

Normal Anatomy

TRACEY A. LITTRELL

Embryology
Bone
Joints
Anatomic Figures

Embryology

The fertilized ovum migrates down the uterine tube and implants itself on the uterine mucosa. Implantation is followed by a period of rapid mitosis, passing through morula, blastocyst, and two-layer (endoderm and ectoderm) embryonic disc stages. A portion of the ectoderm extends ventrally, proliferates, and gives rise to the mesoderm, which separates the endoderm and ectoderm.

The neural plate of the ectoderm involutes to form the neural tube (future spinal cord). A rod of cells, known as the *notochord,* is situated between the developing gut and neural tube. The notochord guides the development of the spine.

The dorsal portion of the mesoderm located on either side of the notochord begins to condense and segment into 42 to 44 pairs of somites (four occipital, eight cervical, twelve thoracic, five lumbar, five sacral, and eight to ten coccygeal). Within each somite, cells exist that form the sclerotomal tissues (bone and dense connective tissues). These cells are guided by the notochord to form the vertebrae and ribs with further lateral migration to form the limb buds and extremities. The sclerotomal cells forming the vertebral bodies develop intervertebral fissures filled with mesenchyme that become the intervertebral disc. The notochordal elements within the disc become the nucleus pulposus. The somite also gives rise to myotomal (muscles) and dermatomal (dermis) structures.

Bone

BONE DEVELOPMENT

Bone functions to protect and support the body. Bone is a connective tissue and is composed of fibers, cells, and noncellular matrix material (ground substance). Bone is truly a remarkable substance that offers high tensile and compressive strength while maintaining some degree of elasticity. Bone is a relatively lightweight and resilient tissue. Contrary to popular belief, bone is not dead; it is highly dynamic and metabolically active. Bone provides a storehouse of calcium, phosphorus, and other minerals. It is constantly remodeling; atrophy occurs in areas of understress and hypertrophy in areas of overstress.

BONE COMPOSITION

Like any connective tissue, bone is composed of cells and matrix. The matrix is composed of fibers, inorganic salts, and ground substance. The fibers are mostly collagen; elastic fibers are minimal.

Collagen fibers are present to a greater degree than in other tissues, giving bone strength and resiliency. Organic salts give bone hardness and rigidity. Organic salts are present in crystal as hydroxyapatite crystals, a form of calcium phosphate. The ground substance consists of glycosaminoglycans (GAGs), namely, chondroitin sulfate, keratan sulfate, and hyaluronic acid.

BONE FORMATION

The cellular constituents and chemical reactions are the same for all bones formed in the body. Bone always forms by replacing some other preexisting material. The histogenesis of bone is dichotomized into bones that form in preexisting cartilage and bones that form from preexisting embryonic mesenchyme. The two types of bone production are not mutually exclusive. Both processes often occur within the same bone. For instance, the femoral bone is lengthened by enchondral bone formation at its metaphyses, but increased width of the bone occurs from intermembranous bone in the periosteum.

Enchondral ossification. Enchondral bone formation represents bones formed in a hyaline cartilage template. This is the most common method by which bones form. Examples include the femur, tibia, vertebrae, and metacarpals. The process begins in centers of ossification located in the embryonic skeleton and continues into the late teen years. Lengthening of the bone occurs in the epiphyseal growth plate. Cells on the metaphyseal side ossify (zone of provisional calcification), and cells on the epiphyseal side multiply (zone of proliferation).

Intermembranous ossification. Intermembranous bone formation occurs when embryonic mesenchyme condenses into highly vascular connective tissue, which produces a thin layer of matrix and collagen. Peripheral connective tissue cells differentiate into osteoblasts, which produce additional matrix and collagen. Calcification of the matrix occurs, trapping the osteoblasts within the newly formed bone, thereby converting them to osteocytes. Examples include the mandible and bones of the cranium.

BONE STRUCTURE

Macroscopic structure. Inspection of a longitudinal section of a long bone reveals two different types of bone structure: compact (substantia compacta) and spongy (substantia spongiosa), or cancellous, bone. Compact bone is found at the outer border of a bone; cancellous bone is the latticelike network within a bone. Both compact and cancellous bone are lamellar. Woven bone represents immature bone, which is replaced with lamellar bone over time.

TABLE 6-1
Classification of Joints by Function and Structure

Classification	Description	Examples
Function		
Synarthrosis	Fixed joints, no motion	Skull sutures
Amphiarthrosis	Deformable joints, slight motion	Intervertebral disc
Diarthrosis	Free joints, wide range of motion	Knee
Structure		
Fibrous	Apposing elements are connected by fibrous tissue; no joint cavity	Skull sutures, teeth
Cartilaginous	Apposing elements are connected by hyaline cartilage (synchondrosis) or fibrocarcartilage (symphysis); no joint space	Costochondral, intervertebral disc
Synovial	Apposing elements are separated by a joint space, surrounded by a fibrous joint capsule, may contain articular disc or meniscus, and are lined by a synovial membrane	Knee, ankle, elbow

A typical long bone is divided into a diaphysis (shaft), metaphysis, and epiphysis. The diaphysis is the central portion or shaft of the long bone, with a hollow inner medullary cavity (marrow cavity) encased by a thick, compact bony cortex. The ends of a long bone are capped by epiphyses, representing secondary centers of ossification.

In the immature skeleton, epiphyses are separated from the shaft of the long bone by a thin, cartilaginous epiphyseal plate. Cartilaginous epiphyseal plates are attached to the bony diaphysis by a transitional region, known as the *metaphysis*. The epiphysis and portions of the metaphysis contain a lattice of small bone spicules known as *trabeculae*.

In the adult, once the cartilaginous plates ossify, the medullary cavity of the diaphysis is continuous with the intertrabecular spaces of the metaphysis and epiphysis. At each end of the bone, a thin layer of articular cartilage covers the thin cortex of the epiphyses.

The periosteum represents a specialized connective tissue that covers the bone. It is composed of two layers: an inner layer that has the ability to form bone through intramembranous ossification, and an outer fibrous layer that anchors into the compact bone by Sharpey's fibers. Periosteum does not cover the ends of the bone in which articular cartilage exists, nor does it extend under joint capsules. The femoral neck and talus are examples of bone structures that lack periosteum. Fractures in these areas heal more precariously because of the absence of the osteogenic capabilities of the inner layer of the periosteum. Periosteum is also absent on bones formed within tendons (e.g., sesamoids, patella) and at ligament and tendon insertions.

The medullary cavity and interspaces of the cancellous bone are lined with endosteum. Endosteum lacks the tough fibrous nature of the periosteum, but, similar to the periosteum, it possesses osteogenic properties.

In the flat bones of the skull, the cortex forms two thick layers of bone (inner and outer table), which sandwich an interposed layer of spongy bone (diploë). The periosteum is known as *pericranium,* and the inner surface of the bone is lined by dura mater.

Microscopic structure

Compact bone. The basic anatomic unit of compact bone is the *osteon.* An osteon consists of 4 to 20 lamellae surrounding a central osteonal canal. Osteocytes are located within lacunae found between adjacent lamellae. Adjacent osteocytes communicate through tiny canals extending radially from the lacunae, known as *canaliculi.* Blood vessels are found in the osteonal canals

with radial branches extending through lateral canals to reach the periphery of the osteon. Between each osteon are partially resorbed or restructured osteons known as *interstitial systems.*

Cancellous bone. Cancellous bone does not form an orderly osteon, as in compact bone. Cancellous bone is found in sheets or layers. Osteocytes are found in lacunae orderly aligned in rows. Osteocytes are nourished by nutrient diffusion through canaliculi. An osteonal system is not needed because of the proximity of the rich blood supply in the bone marrow.

Cells. Osteoblasts form bone; they produce the matrix and collagen fibers. Once the bone is formed, osteoblasts become trapped and are known as *osteocytes. Osteoclasts* are large multinucleated cells responsible for the breakdown of bone by secreting osteolytic enzymes.

Joints

Joints, or articulations, represent connections between adjacent skeletal structures. The connections are maintained by connective tissues. The movement of the joint is largely dependent upon its structure and the nature of surrounding connective tissues. Joints are classified by either their degree of motion or the type of intervening connective tissue (Table 6-1).

Anatomic Figures

Figures 6-1 through 6-149 present normal anatomy of the brain, spine, thorax, and extremities. Plain film radiography and advanced imaging with magnetic resonance imaging and computed tomography are used. The images are presented in anatomic position, with the reader viewing the anterior aspect of the patient in face-to-face orientation.

Suggested Readings

Ballinger PW: Merrill's atlas of radiographic positioning, ed 8, St Louis, 1995, Mosby.

Haaga JR: CT and magnetic resonance imaging of the whole body, ed 4, vol 1, St Louis, 2003, Mosby.

Kelley LL: Sectional anatomy for the imaging professionals, St Louis, 1997, Mosby.

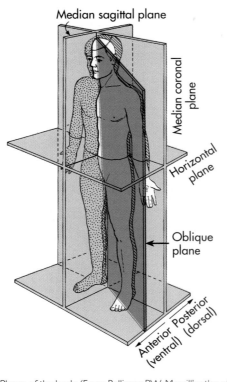

FIG. 6-1 Planes of the body. (From Ballinger PW: Merrill's atlas of radiographic positioning and radiologic procedures, ed 8, St Louis, 1995, Mosby.)

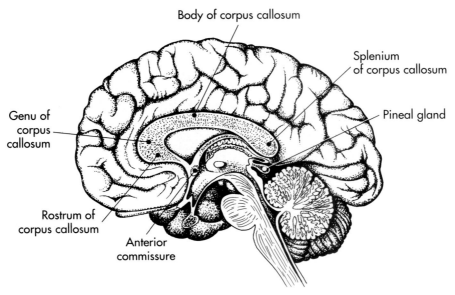

FIG. 6-2 Sagittal view of cerebral cortex. (From Kelley LL: Sectional anatomy for imaging professionals, St Louis, 1997, Mosby.)

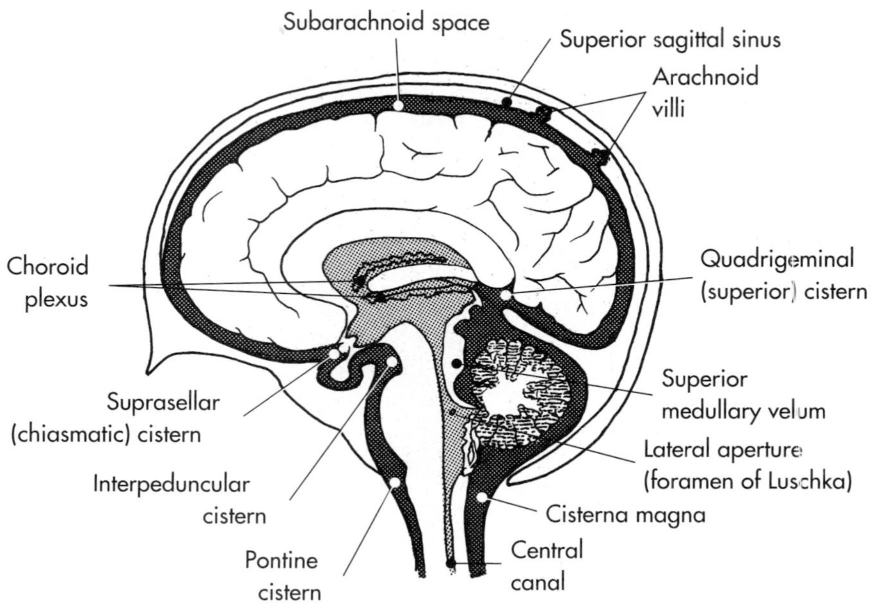

Subarachnoid space

Superior sagittal sinus

Arachnoid villi

Choroid plexus

Quadrigeminal (superior) cistern

Suprasellar (chiasmatic) cistern

Superior medullary velum

Interpeduncular cistern

Lateral aperture (foramen of Luschka)

Cisterna magna

Pontine cistern

Central canal

FIG. 6-3   Sagittal view of choroid plexus and cisterns of ventricular system. (From Kelley LL: Sectional anatomy for imaging professionals, St Louis, 1997, Mosby.)

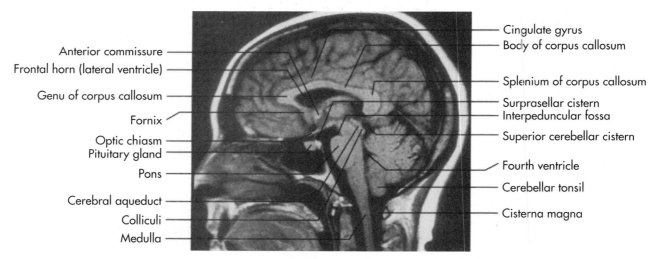

Anterior commissure

Frontal horn (lateral ventricle)

Genu of corpus callosum

Fornix

Optic chiasm

Pituitary gland

Pons

Cerebral aqueduct

Colliculi

Medulla

Cingulate gyrus

Body of corpus callosum

Splenium of corpus callosum

Surprasellar cistern

Interpeduncular fossa

Superior cerebellar cistern

Fourth ventricle

Cerebellar tonsil

Cisterna magna

FIG. 6-4   Sagittal T1-weighted magnetic resonance imaging scan at the midsagittal level. (From Haaga JR: CT and MRI of the whole body, ed 4, vol 1, St Louis, 2003, Mosby.)

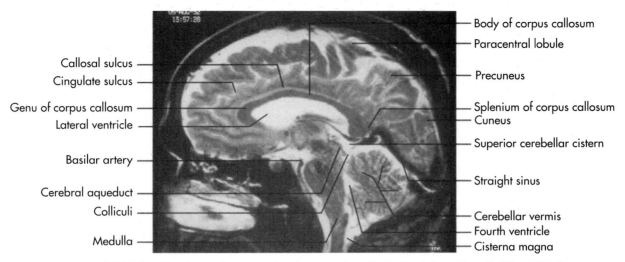

Callosal sulcus

Cingulate sulcus

Genu of corpus callosum

Lateral ventricle

Basilar artery

Cerebral aqueduct

Colliculi

Medulla

Body of corpus callosum

Paracentral lobule

Precuneus

Splenium of corpus callosum

Cuneus

Superior cerebellar cistern

Straight sinus

Cerebellar vermis

Fourth ventricle

Cisterna magna

FIG. 6-5 Sagittal T2-weighted magnetic resonance imaging scan at the midsagittal level. (From Haaga JR: CT and MRI of the whole body, ed 4, vol 1, St Louis, 2003, Mosby.)

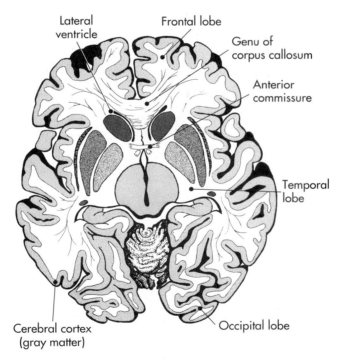

Lateral ventricle

Frontal lobe

Genu of corpus callosum

Anterior commissure

Temporal lobe

Cerebral cortex (gray matter)

Occipital lobe

FIG. 6-6 Axial view of cerebral cortex and corpus callosum. (From Kelley LL: Sectional anatomy for imaging professionals, St Louis, 1997, Mosby.)

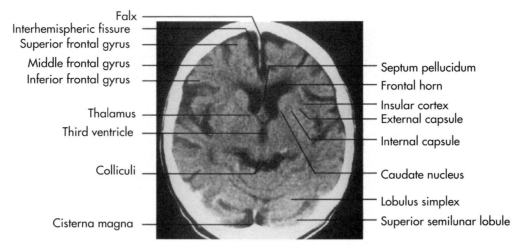

Falx
Interhemispheric fissure
Superior frontal gyrus
Middle frontal gyrus
Inferior frontal gyrus
Thalamus
Third ventricle
Colliculi
Cisterna magna

Septum pellucidum
Frontal horn
Insular cortex
External capsule
Internal capsule
Caudate nucleus
Lobulus simplex
Superior semilunar lobule

FIG. 6-7   Enhanced axial computed tomography scan at the third ventricular level. (From Haaga JR: CT and MRI of the whole body, ed 4, vol 1, St Louis, 2003, Mosby.)

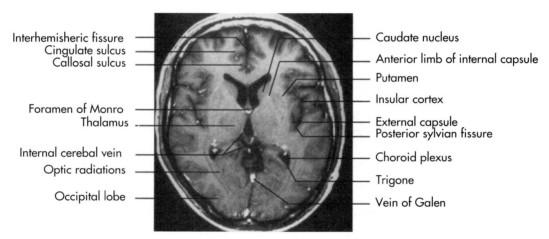

Interhemisheric fissure
Cingulate sulcus
Callosal sulcus
Foramen of Monro
Thalamus
Internal cerebal vein
Optic radiations
Occipital lobe

Caudate nucleus
Anterior limb of internal capsule
Putamen
Insular cortex
External capsule
Posterior sylvian fissure
Choroid plexus
Trigone
Vein of Galen

FIG. 6-8   Axial T1-weighted magnetic resonance imaging scan at the third ventricular level. (From Haaga JR: CT and MRI of the whole body, ed 4, vol 1, St Louis, 2003, Mosby.)

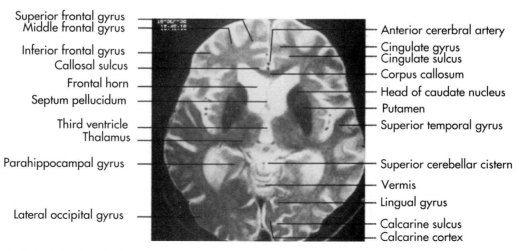

Superior frontal gyrus
Middle frontal gyrus
Inferior frontal gyrus
Callosal sulcus
Frontal horn
Septum pellucidum
Third ventricle
Thalamus
Parahippocampal gyrus
Lateral occipital gyrus

Anterior cererbral artery
Cingulate gyrus
Cingulate sulcus
Corpus callosum
Head of caudate nucleus
Putamen
Superior temporal gyrus
Superior cerebellar cistern
Vermis
Lingual gyrus
Calcarine sulcus
Calcarine cortex

FIG. 6-9   Axial T2-weighted magnetic resonance imaging scan at the third ventricular level. (From Haaga JR: CT and MRI of the whole body, ed 4, vol 1, St Louis, 2003, Mosby.)

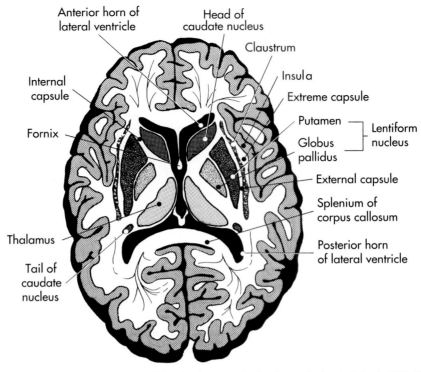

FIG. 6-10 Axial view of basal ganglia. (From Kelley LL: Sectional anatomy for imaging professionals, St Louis, 1997, Mosby.)

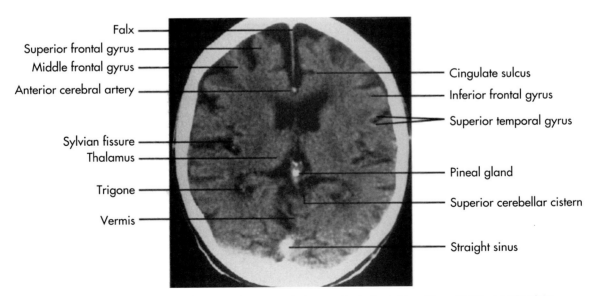

FIG. 6-11 Enhanced axial computed tomography scan at the low ventricular level. (From Haaga JR: CT and MRI of the whole body, ed 4, vol 1, St Louis, 2003, Mosby.)

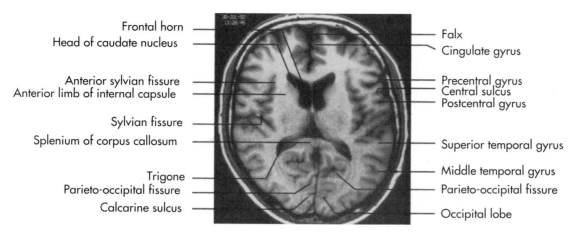

Frontal horn
Head of caudate nucleus

Anterior sylvian fissure
Anterior limb of internal capsule

Sylvian fissure
Splenium of corpus callosum

Trigone
Parieto-occipital fissure
Calcarine sulcus

Falx
Cingulate gyrus

Precentral gyrus
Central sulcus
Postcentral gyrus

Superior temporal gyrus

Middle temporal gyrus
Parieto-occipital fissure

Occipital lobe

FIG. 6-12 Axial T1-weighted magnetic resonance imaging scan at the low ventricular level, slightly above the computed tomography scan level. (From Haaga JR: CT and MRI of the whole body, ed 4, vol 1, St Louis, 2003, Mosby.)

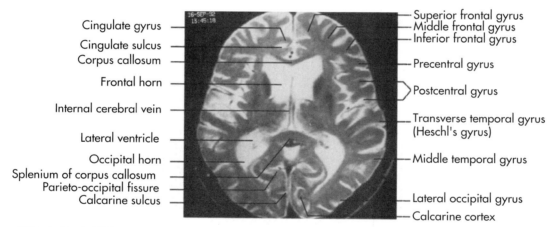

Cingulate gyrus

Cingulate sulcus
Corpus callosum

Frontal horn

Internal cerebral vein

Lateral ventricle

Occipital horn
Splenium of corpus callosum
Parieto-occipital fissure
Calcarine sulcus

Superior frontal gyrus
Middle frontal gyrus
Inferior frontal gyrus

Precentral gyrus

Postcentral gyrus

Transverse temporal gyrus
(Heschl's gyrus)

Middle temporal gyrus

Lateral occipital gyrus
Calcarine cortex

FIG. 6-13 Axial T2-weighted magnetic resonance imaging scan at the low ventricular level, slightly above the computed tomography scan level. (From Haaga JR: CT and MRI of the whole body, ed 4, vol 1, St Louis, 2003, Mosby.)

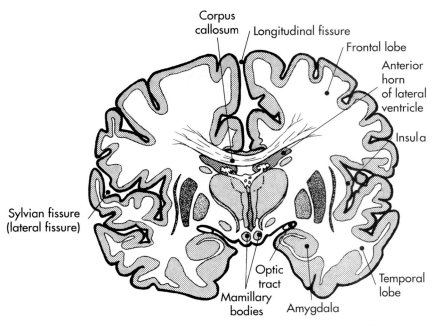

FIG. 6-14 Coronal view of cerebral lobes and insula. (From Kelley LL: Sectional anatomy for imaging professionals, St Louis, 1997, Mosby.)

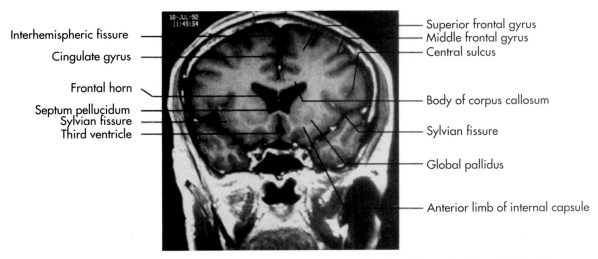

FIG. 6-15 Coronal T1-weighted magnetic resonance imaging scan at the level of the frontal horns. (From Haaga JR: CT and MRI of the whole body, ed 4, vol 1, St Louis, 2003, Mosby.)

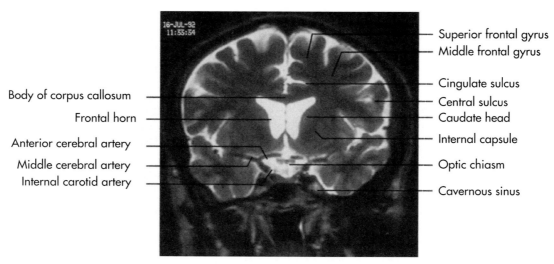

Superior frontal gyrus
Middle frontal gyrus
Cingulate sulcus
Central sulcus
Caudate head
Internal capsule
Optic chiasm
Cavernous sinus

Body of corpus callosum
Frontal horn
Anterior cerebral artery
Middle cerebral artery
Internal carotid artery

FIG. 6-16 Coronal T2-weighted magnetic resonance imaging scan at the level of the frontal horns. (From Haaga JR: CT and MRI of the whole body, ed 4, vol 1, St Louis, 2003, Mosby.)

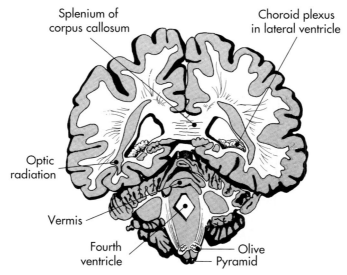

Splenium of
corpus callosum

Choroid plexus
in lateral ventricle

Optic
radiation

Vermis

Fourth
ventricle

Olive
Pyramid

FIG. 6-17 Coronal view of medulla oblongata. (From Kelley LL: Sectional anatomy for imaging professionals, St Louis, 1997, Mosby.)

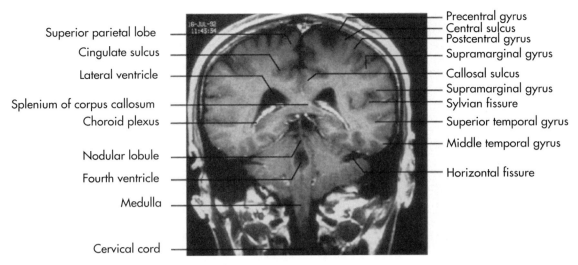

FIG. 6-18 Coronal T1-weighted magnetic resonance imaging scan at the mid-to-posterior ventricular level. (From Haaga JR: CT and MRI of the whole body, ed 4, vol 1, St Louis, 2003, Mosby.)

Labels (left side, top to bottom): Superior parietal lobe; Cingulate sulcus; Lateral ventricle; Splenium of corpus callosum; Choroid plexus; Nodular lobule; Fourth ventricle; Medulla; Cervical cord

Labels (right side, top to bottom): Precentral gyrus; Central sulcus; Postcentral gyrus; Supramarginal gyrus; Callosal sulcus; Supramarginal gyrus; Sylvian fissure; Superior temporal gyrus; Middle temporal gyrus; Horizontal fissure

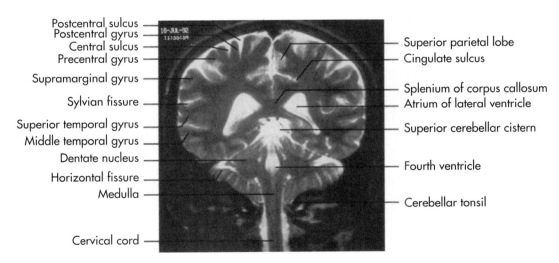

FIG. 6-19 Coronal T2-weighted magnetic resonance imaging scan at the mid-to-posterior ventricular level. (From Haaga JR: CT and MRI of the whole body, ed 4, vol 1, St Louis, 2003, Mosby.)

Labels (left side, top to bottom): Postcentral sulcus; Postcentral gyrus; Central sulcus; Precentral gyrus; Supramarginal gyrus; Sylvian fissure; Superior temporal gyrus; Middle temporal gyrus; Dentate nucleus; Horizontal fissure; Medulla; Cervical cord

Labels (right side, top to bottom): Superior parietal lobe; Cingulate sulcus; Splenium of corpus callosum; Atrium of lateral ventricle; Superior cerebellar cistern; Fourth ventricle; Cerebellar tonsil

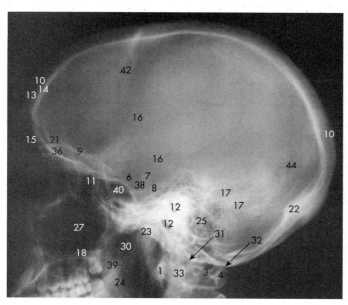

FIG. 6-20   Lateral skull radiograph. (See Key for Figures 6-20 through 6-22.)

KEY FOR FIGURES 6-20 THROUGH 6-22

1. Atlas/C1 anterior tubercle
2. Atlas/C1 lateral mass
3. Atlas/C1 posterior arch
4. Atlas/C1 posterior tubercle
5. Axis/C2 vertebral body
6. Clinoid process, anterior
7. Clinoid process, posterior
8. Clivus
9. Crista galli
10. Ciploic space
11. Ethmoid sinus
12. External/internal acoustic meatus
13. Frontal bone, external lamina
14. Frontal bone, internal lamina
15. Frontal sinus
16. Groove for middle meningeal vessels
17. Groove for sigmoid sinus
18. Hard palate
19. Inferior nasal concha
20. Innominate line
21. Internal frontal crest
22. Internal occipital protuberance
23. Mandible, condylar process
24. Mandible, ramus
25. Mastoid air cells
26. Mastoid process
27. Maxillary sinus
28. Nasal septum
29. Nasal spine
30. Nasopharynx
31. Occipital bone, basion
32. Occipital bone, opisthion
33. Odontoid process/dens
34. Orbit, lateral margin
35. Orbit, medial margin
36. Orbit, superior margin
37. Petrous ridge
38. Sella turcica/hypophyseal fossa
39. Soft palate
40. Sphenoid sinus
41. Superior orbital fissure
42. Suture, coronal
43. Suture, frontozygomatic
44. Suture, lambdoidal
45. Suture, sagittal
46. Zygomatic arch
       Dotted line, foramen magnum

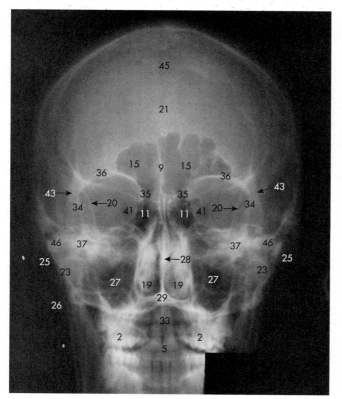

FIG. 6-21   Posteroanterior skull radiograph. (See Key for Figures 6-20 through 6-22.)

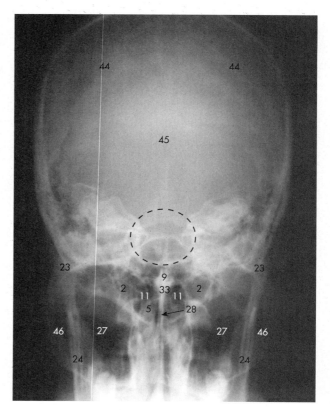

FIG. 6-22   Anteroposterior Towne skull radiograph. (See Key for Figures 6-20 through 6-22.)

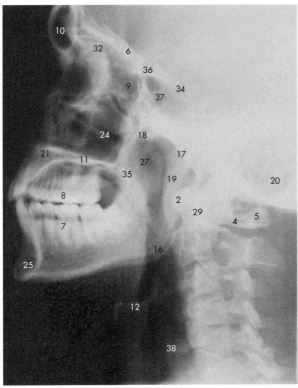

FIG. 6-23 Lateral sinus radiograph. (See Key for Figures 6-23 through 6-25.)

KEY FOR FIGURES 6-23 THROUGH 6-25

1. Atlas/C1 anterior arch
2. Atlas/C1 anterior tubercle
3. Atlas/C1 lateral mass
4. Atlas/C1 posterior arch
5. Atlas/C1 posterior tubercle
6. Crista galli
7. Dental arch, inferior
8. Dental arch, superior
9. Ethmoid sinuses
10. Frontal sinus
11. Hard palate;
12. Hyoid bone
13. Inferior nasal concha
14. Innominate line
15. Internal occipital protuberance
16. Mandible, angle
17. Mandible, condylar process
18. Mandible, coronoid process
19. Mandible, ramus
20. Mastoid air cells

21. Maxilla, alveolar process
22. Maxilla, frontal process
23. Maxilla, zygomatic process
24. Maxillary sinus
25. Mental protuberance
26. Nasal septum
27. Nasopharynx
28. Occipital bone, jugular process
29. Odontoid process/dens
30. Orbit, lateral margin
31. Orbit, medial margin
32. Orbit, superior margin
33. Petrous ridge
34. Sella turcica/ hypophyseal fossa
35. Soft palate
36. Sphenoid plane
37. Sphenoid sinus
38. Thyroid cartilage
39. Zygomatic arch

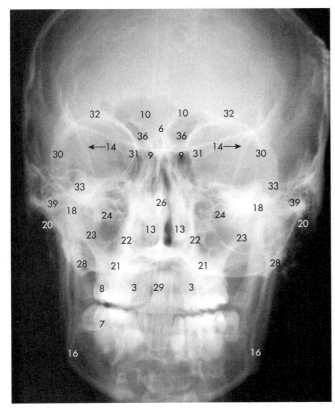

FIG. 6-24 Posteroanterior sinus radiograph. (See Key for Figures 6-23 through 6-25.)

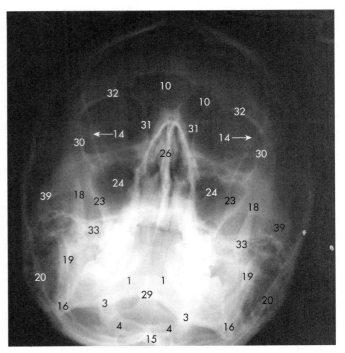

FIG. 6-25 Posteroanterior Waters radiograph. (See Key for Figures 6-23 through 6-25.)

KEY FOR FIGURES 6-26 THROUGH 6-31

1. Articular process, inferior
2. Articular process, superior
3. Atlantodental interval (ADI)
4. Atlas/C1 and axis/C2 articulation
5. Atlas/C1 anterior arch
6. Atlas/C1 anterior tubercle
7. Atlas/C1 lateral mass
8. Atlas/C1 posterior arch
9. Atlas/C1 posterior tubercle
10. Atlas/C1 transverse process
11. Clavicle
12. Clinoid process, anterior
13. Clinoid process, posterior
14. Clivus
15. Costotransverse articulation
16. Cribriform plate
17. Crista galli
18. Dental amalgam
19. Dental arch, inferior
20. Dental arch, superior
21. Diploic space
22. Ethmoid air cells
23. External/internal acoustic meatus
24. External occipital protuberance
25. Frontal sinus
26. Hard palate
27. Hyoid bone
28. Inferior nasal concha
29. Innominate line
30. Internal occipital protuberance
31. Intervertebral disc space, C2
32. Intervertebral disc space, C6
33. Lambdoidal suture
34. Lamina
35. Laryngopharynx
36. Mandible, angle
37. Mandible, body
38. Mandible, condylar process
39. Mandible, coronoid process
40. Mandible, foramen
41. Mandible, ramus
42. Manubrium
43. Mastoid air cells
44. Mastoid process
45. Maxillary sinus
46. Nasal septum
47. Nasopharynx
48. Occipital bone, external lamina
49. Occipital bone, internal lamina
50. Occipital condyle
51. Odontoid process/dens
52. Orbit, lateral margin
53. Orbit, medial margin
54. Orbit, superior margin
55. Oropharynx
56. Pedicle
57. Petrous ridge
58. Sella turcica/hypophyseal fossa
59. Sphenoid sinus
60. Spinolaminar line
61. Spinous process
62. T1 rib
63. T1 rib, tubercle
64. T2 rib, posterior aspect
65. T3 rib, posterior aspect
66. T4 rib, posterior aspect
67. Thyroid cartilage
68. Tracheal walls
69. Transverse process
70. Transverse process foramen
71. Uncinate process/Luschka joint
72. Uvula
73. Vertebral endplate, inferior
74. Vertebral endplate, superior
75. Zygomatic arch
    Dotted lines, piriform sinuses/pharyngeal sinuses

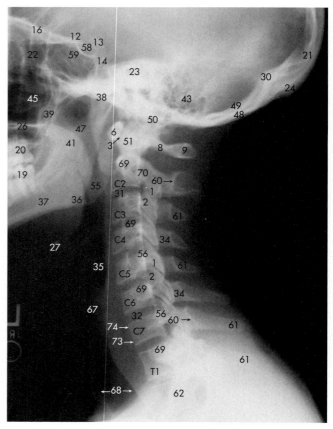

FIG. 6-26   Lateral cervical radiograph. (See Key for Figures 6-26 through 6-31.)

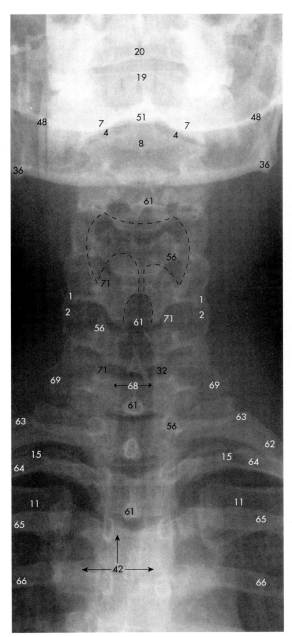

FIG. 6-27 Anteroposterior cervical radiograph. (See Key for Figures 6-26 through 6-31.)

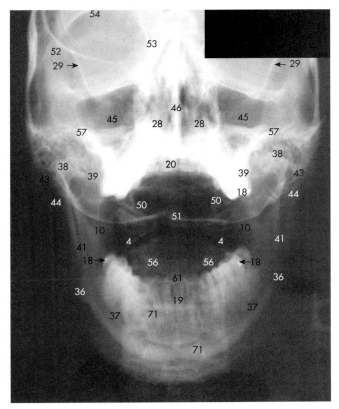

FIG. 6-28 Anteroposterior open-mouth radiograph. (See Key for Figures 6-26 through 6-31.)

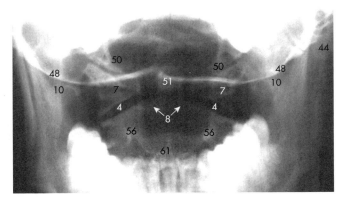

FIG. 6-29 Anteroposterior open-mouth close-up. (See Key for Figures 6-26 through 6-31.)

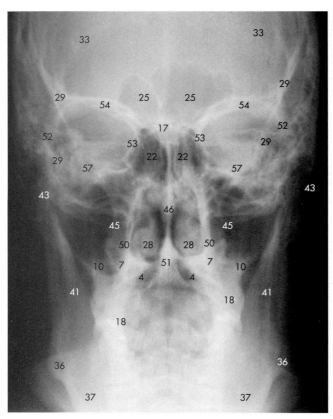

FIG. 6-30   Nasium radiograph. (See Key for Figures 6-26 through 6-31.)

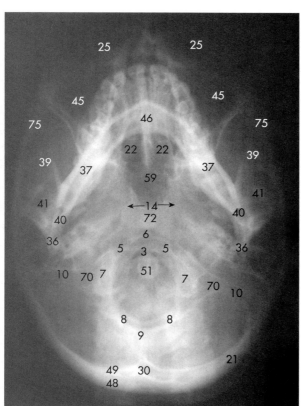

FIG. 6-31   Base posterior radiograph. (See Key for Figures 6-26 through 6-31.)

KEY FOR FIGURES 6-32 THROUGH 6-34

1. Articular process, inferior
2. Articular process, inferior, left
3. Articular process, inferior, right
4. Articular process, superior
5. Articular process, superior, left
6. Articular process, superior, right
7. Atlas/C1 anterior tubercle
8. Atlas/C1 posterior arch
9. Atlas/C1 posterior tubercle
10. Clavicle
11. Clinoid process, anterior
12. Clinoid process, posterior
13. Clivus
14. Dental arch, inferior
15. Dental arch, superior
16. Diploic space
17. External occipital protuberance
18. External/internal acoustic meatus
19. Hard palate
20. Hyoid bone
21. Internal occipital protuberance
22. Intervertebral disc space, C3
23. Intervertebral disc space, C5
24. Intervertebral foramen, left
25. Intervertebral foramen, right
26. Lambdoidal suture
27. Lamina, left
28. Lamina, right
29. Laryngopharynx
30. Mandible, angle
31. Mandible, body
32. Mandible, condylar process
33. Mandible, ramus
34. Mastoid air cells
35. Mental protuberance
36. Nasopharynx
37. Occipital bone, external lamina
38. Occipital bone, internal lamina
39. Occipital condyle
40. Odontoid process/dens
41. Oropharynx
42. Pedicle, left
43. Pedicle, right
44. Pinna of the ear
45. Ponticle/ponticulus posticus
46. Sella turcica/hypophyseal fossa
47. Sphenoid sinus
48. Spinolaminar line
49. Spinous process
50. Thyroid cartilage
51. Tracheal walls
52. Transverse process, C3
53. Transverse process, C5
54. Vertebral endplate, inferior
55. Vertebral endplate, superior

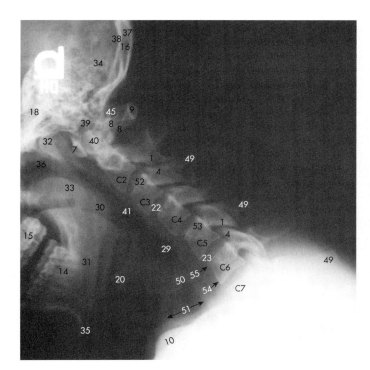

FIG. 6-32 Cervical flexion radiograph. (See Key for Figures 6-32 through 6-34.)

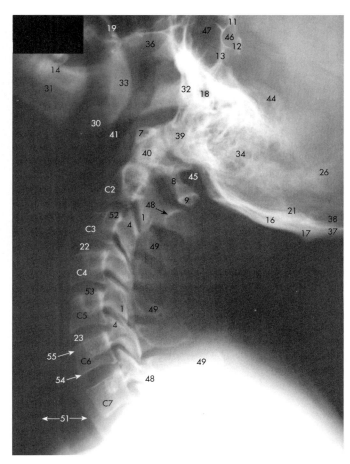

FIG. 6-33 Cervical extension radiograph. (See Key for Figures 6-32 through 6-34.)

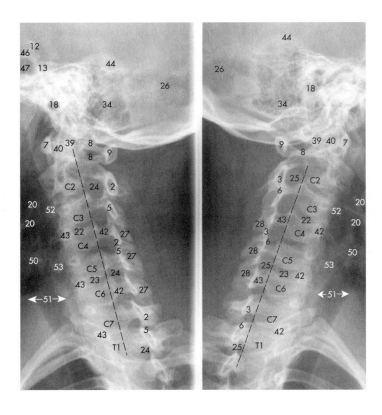

FIG. 6-34 Right and left posterior oblique cervical radiographs. (See Key for Figures 6-32 through 6-34.)

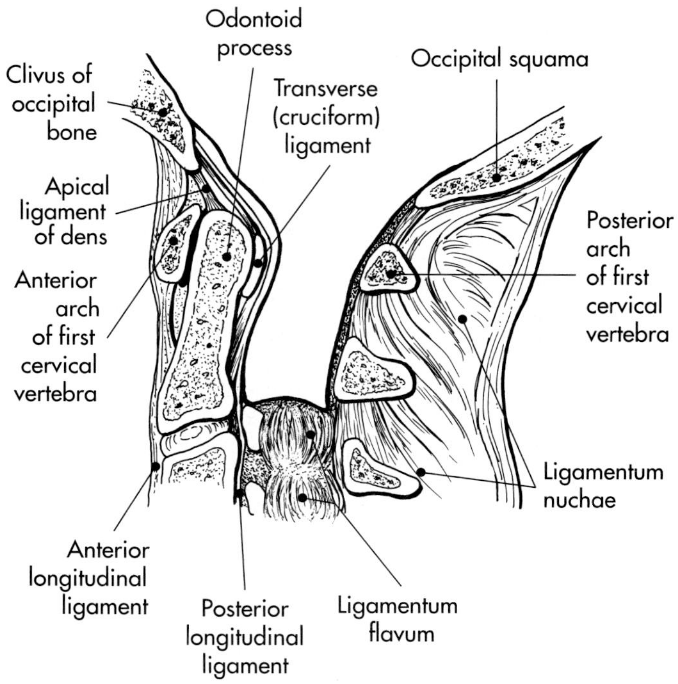

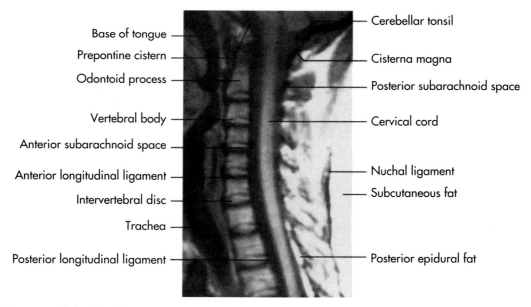

Clivus of occipital bone

Apical ligament of dens

Anterior arch of first cervical vertebra

Odontoid process

Transverse (cruciform) ligament

Occipital squama

Posterior arch of first cervical vertebra

Ligamentum nuchae

Anterior longitudinal ligament

Posterior longitudinal ligament

Ligamentum flavum

FIG. 6-35   Median section of cervical spine demonstrating spinal ligaments. (From Kelley LL: Sectional anatomy for imaging professionals, St Louis, 1997, Mosby.)

Base of tongue

Prepontine cistern

Odontoid process

Vertebral body

Anterior subarachnoid space

Anterior longitudinal ligament

Intervertebral disc

Trachea

Posterior longitudinal ligament

Cerebellar tonsil

Cisterna magna

Posterior subarachnoid space

Cervical cord

Nuchal ligament

Subcutaneous fat

Posterior epidural fat

FIG. 6-36   Sagittal T1-weighted magnetic resonance imaging of cervical spine. (From Haaga JR: CT and MRI of the whole body, ed 4, vol 1, St Louis, 2003, Mosby.)

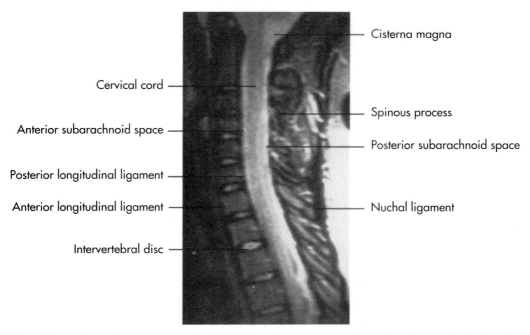

Cisterna magna

Cervical cord

Anterior subarachnoid space

Spinous process

Posterior subarachnoid space

Posterior longitudinal ligament

Anterior longitudinal ligament

Nuchal ligament

Intervertebral disc

FIG. 6-37 Sagittal gradient echo study of cervical spine showing increased signal intensity of cerebrospinal fluid, similar to that in a T2-weighted study. (From Haaga JR: CT and MRI of the whole body, ed 4, vol 1, St Louis, 2003, Mosby.)

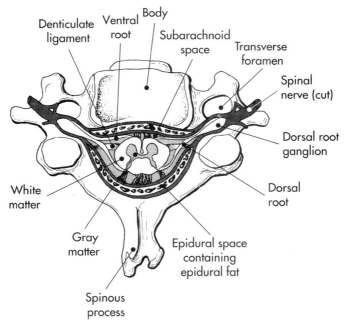

Denticulate ligament

Ventral root

Body

Subarachnoid space

Transverse foramen

Spinal nerve (cut)

Dorsal root ganglion

Dorsal root

White matter

Gray matter

Epidural space containing epidural fat

Spinous process

FIG. 6-38 Axial section of spinal cord. (From Kelley LL: Sectional anatomy for imaging professionals, St Louis, 1997, Mosby.)

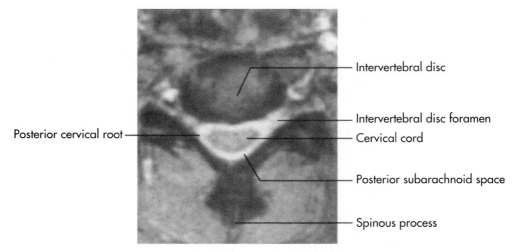

Intervertebral disc

Intervertebral disc foramen

Cervical cord

Posterior cervical root

Posterior subarachnoid space

Spinous process

FIG. 6-39 Axial gradient echo magnetic resonance imaging scan through the intervertebral foramen in the midcervical region. (From Haaga JR: CT and MRI of the whole body, ed 4, vol 1, St Louis, 2003, Mosby.)

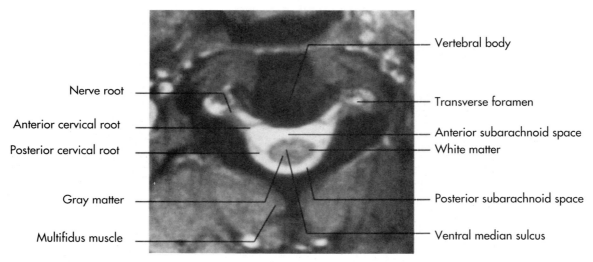

Vertebral body

Nerve root

Anterior cervical root

Posterior cervical root

Transverse foramen

Anterior subarachnoid space

White matter

Gray matter

Multifidus muscle

Posterior subarachnoid space

Ventral median sulcus

FIG. 6-40 Axial gradient echo magnetic resonance imaging scan in the midcervical region, just caudal to the image shown in Figure 6-39. (From Haaga JR: CT and MRI of the whole body, ed 4, vol 1, St Louis, 2003, Mosby.)

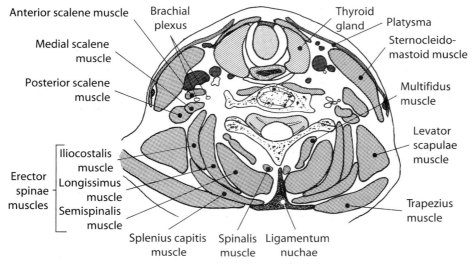

Anterior scalene muscle

Brachial plexus

Thyroid gland

Platysma

Sternocleido-mastoid muscle

Medial scalene muscle

Posterior scalene muscle

Multifidus muscle

Levator scapulae muscle

Erector spinae muscles

Iliocostalis muscle

Longissimus muscle

Semispinalis muscle

Trapezius muscle

Splenius capitis muscle

Spinalis muscle

Ligamentum nuchae

FIG. 6-41 Axial section of cervical vertebra with musculature. (From Kelley LL: Sectional anatomy for imaging professionals, St Louis, 1997, Mosby.)

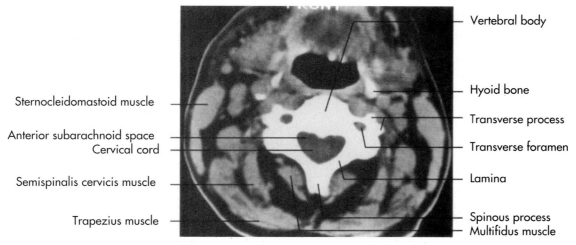

FIG. 6-42 Axial computed tomography scan through a cervical vertebral body. (From Haaga JR: CT and MRI of the whole body, ed 4, vol 1, St Louis, 2003, Mosby.)

Sternocleidomastoid muscle

Anterior subarachnoid space
Cervical cord

Semispinalis cervicis muscle

Trapezius muscle

Vertebral body

Hyoid bone

Transverse process

Transverse foramen

Lamina

Spinous process
Multifidus muscle

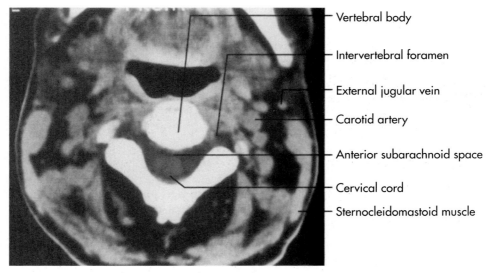

FIG. 6-43 Axial computed tomography scan through the intervertebral foramen in the midcervical region. (From Haaga JR: CT and MRI of the whole body, ed 4, vol 1, St Louis, 2003, Mosby.)

Vertebral body

Intervertebral foramen

External jugular vein

Carotid artery

Anterior subarachnoid space

Cervical cord

Sternocleidomastoid muscle

KEY FOR FIGURES 6-44 THROUGH 6-46

1. Aorta, descending thoracic portion
2. Aortic arch/aortic knob
3. Articular process, inferior
4. Articular process, superior
5. Bronchovascular markings
6. Bronchus, left
7. Bronchus, right
8. Cardiac shadow
9. Clavicle
10. Clavicle, nearest to film
11. Diaphragm, left
12. Diaphragm, posterior sulcus, left
13. Diaphragm, posterior sulcus, right
14. Diaphragm, right
15. Gastric air bubble/magenblase
16. Humerus, diaphysis, nearest to film
17. Humerus, head, nearest to film
18. Intervertebral disc space
19. Lamina
20. Manubrium
21. Pedicle
22. Rib, T1
23. Rib, T2, posterior aspect
24. Rib, T3, posterior aspect
25. Rib, T4, posterior aspect
26. Rib, T5, posterior aspect
27. Rib, T6, posterior aspect
28. Rib, T7, posterior aspect

29. Rib, T8, posterior aspect
30. Rib, T9, posterior aspect
31. Rib, T10, posterior aspect
32. Rib, T11, posterior aspect
33. Rib, T12, posterior aspect
34. Scapula, acromion
35. Scapula, body
36. Scapula, inferior angle
37. Soft tissue of the arm
38. Spinous process, C3
39. Spinous process, C5
40. Spinous process, C7
41. Spinous process, T1
42. Spinous process, T2
43. Spinous process, T3
44. Spinous process, T4
45. Spinous process, T5
46. Spinous process, T6
47. Spinous process, T7
48. Spinous process, T8
49. Spinous process, T9
50. Spinous process, T10
51. Spinous process, T11
52. Spinous process, T12
53. Spinous process, L1
54. Spinous process, L2
55. Sternum
56. Tracheal walls
57. Transverse process
58. Vertebral body, inferior endplate
59. Vertebral body, superior endplate

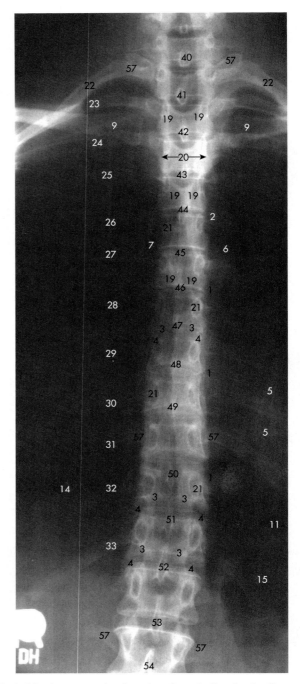

FIG. 6-45 Anteroposterior thoracic radiograph. (See Key for Figures 6-44 through 6-46.)

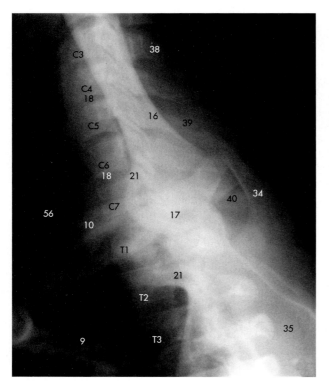

FIG. 6-44 Swimmer's projection of the lower cervical and upper thoracic spine. (See Key for Figures 6-44 through 6-46.)

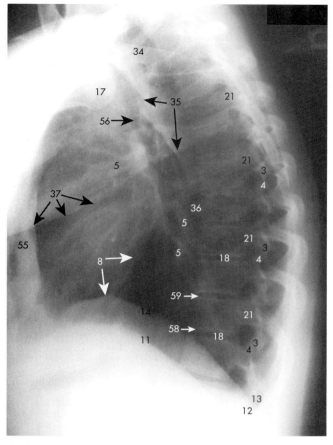

FIG. 6-46 Lateral thoracic radiograph. (See Key for Figures 6-44 through 6-46.)

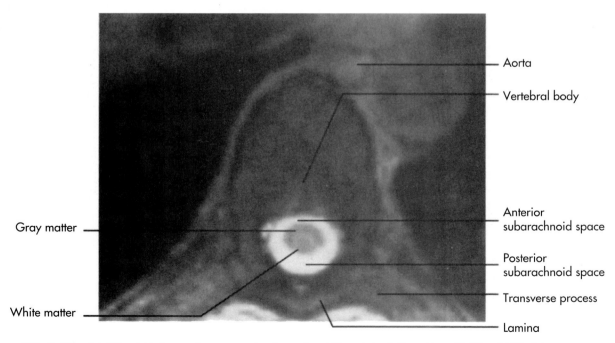

FIG. 6-47 Axial T2-weighted magnetic resonance imaging at the midthoracic level. (From Haaga JR: CT and MRI of the whole body, ed 4, vol 1, St Louis, 2003, Mosby.)

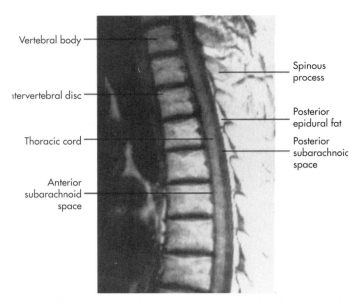

FIG. 6-48 Sagittal T1-weighted magnetic resonance imaging study of the thoracic spine. (From Haaga JR: CT and MRI of the whole body, ed 4, vol 1, St Louis, 2003, Mosby.)

Vertebral body

Intervertebral disc

Thoracic cord

Anterior subarachnoid space

Spinous process

Posterior epidural fat

Posterior subarachnoid space

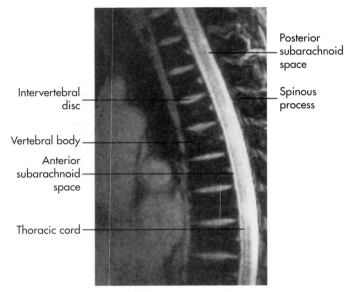

FIG. 6-49 Sagittal T2-weighted magnetic resonance imaging study of the thoracic spine. (From Haaga JR: CT and MRI of the whole body, ed 4, vol 1, St Louis, 2003, Mosby.)

Posterior subarachnoid space

Spinous process

Intervertebral disc

Vertebral body

Anterior subarachnoid space

Thoracic cord

KEY FOR FIGURES 6-50 THROUGH 6-56

1. Aortic knob/aortic arch
2. Aortopulmonary windo
3. Ascending aorta
4. Bronchus intermedius
5. Clavicle
6. Costophrenic sulcus
7. Descending aorta
8. Diaphragm
9. Left atrium
10. Left innominate vein
11. Left lower lobe
12. Left lower lobe bronchus
13. Left main stem bronchus
14. Left major fissure (oblique)
15. Left pulmonary artery
16. Left upper lobe
17. Left upper lobe bronchus orifice
18. Left ventricle
19. Lingula
20. Minor fissure (horizontal)
21. Posterior wall of bronchus intermedius
22. Retrosternal clear space
23. Rib, T1
24. Rib, T2, anterior aspect
25. Rib, T3, anterior aspect
26. Rib, T4, anterior aspect
27. Rib, T5, anterior aspect
28. Rib, T6, anterior aspect
29. Rib, T7, anterior aspect
30. Right atrium
31. Right innominate vein
32. Right lower lobe
33. Right main stem bronchus
34. Right major fissure (oblique)
35. Right middle lobe
36. Right pulmonary artery
37. Right upper lobe
38. Right upper lobe bronchus orifice
39. Right ventricle
40. Scapula, lateral border
41. Scapula, medial border
42. Scapula, superior angle
43. Superior vena cava
44. Trachea
45. Transverse process, T1
46. Transverse process, T2

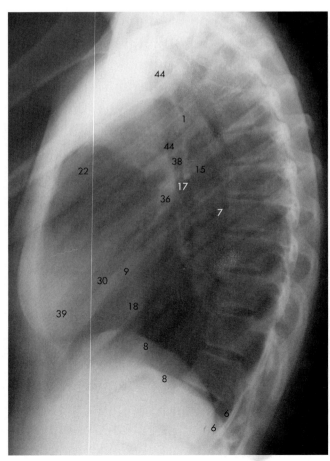

FIG. 6-50 Lateral chest radiograph. (See Key for Figures 6-50 through 6-56.)

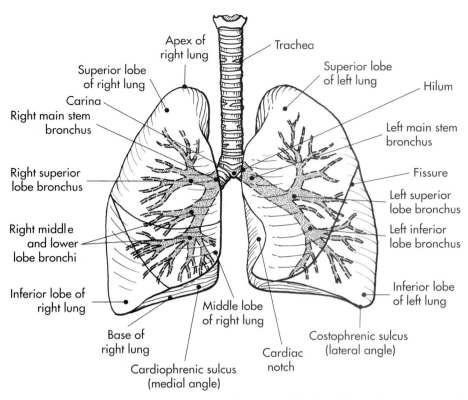

FIG. 6-51 Anterior view of the lungs. (See Key for Figures 6-50 through 6-56.) (From Kelley LL: Sectional anatomy for imaging professionals, St. Louis, 1997, Mosby.)

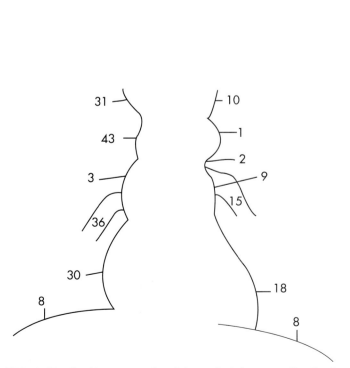

FIG. 6-52 Graphic representation of the mediastinal contours. (See Key for Figures 6-50 through 6-56.)

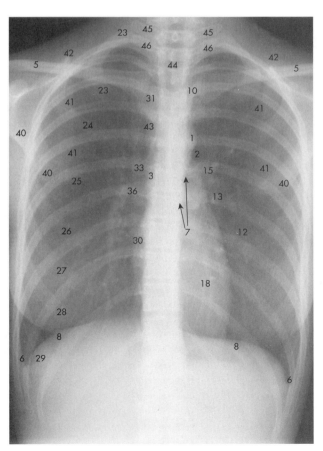

FIG. 6-53 Posterior chest radiograph. (See Key for Figures 6-50 through 6-56.)

KEY FOR FIGURES 6-50 THROUGH 6-56

1. Aortic knob/aortic arch
2. Aortopulmonary window
3. Ascending aorta
4. Bronchus intermedius
5. Clavicle
6. Costophrenic sulcus
7. Descending aorta
8. Diaphragm
9. Left atrium
10. Left innominate vein
11. Left lower lobe
12. Left lower lobe bronchus
13. Left main stem bronchus
14. Left major fissure (oblique)
15. Left pulmonary artery
16. Left upper lobe
17. Left upper lobe bronchus orifice
18. Left ventricle
19. Lingula
20. Minor fissure (horizontal)
21. Posterior wall of bronchus intermedius;
22. Retrosternal clear space
23. Rib, T1
24. Rib, T2, anterior aspect
25. Rib, T3, anterior aspect
26. Rib, T4, anterior aspect
27. Rib, T5, anterior aspect
28. Rib, T6, anterior aspect
29. Rib, T7, anterior aspect
30. Right atrium
31. Right innominate vein
32. Right lower lobe
33. Right main stem bronchus
34. Right major fissure (oblique)
35. Right middle lobe
36. Right pulmonary artery
37. Right upper lobe
38. Right upper lobe bronchus orifice
39. Right ventricle
40. Scapula, lateral border
41. Scapula, medial border
42. Scapula, superior angle
43. Superior vena cava
44. Trachea
45. Transverse process, T1
46. Transverse process, T2

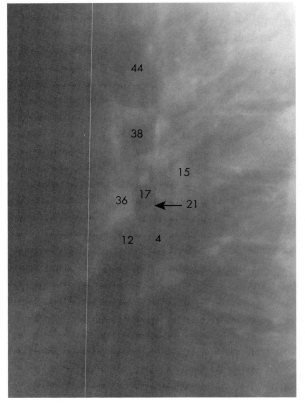

FIG. 6-54   Close-up of the hilar structures as seen on the lateral chest radiograph. (See Key for Figures 6-50 through 6-56.)

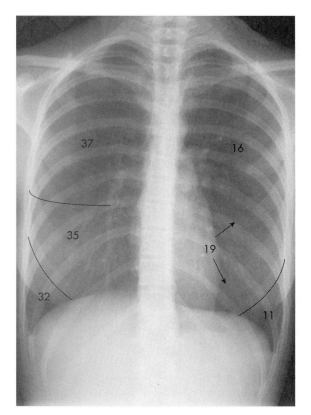

FIG. 6-55   Pleural fissures as seen on the lateral chest radiograph. (See Key for Figures 6-50 through 6-56.)

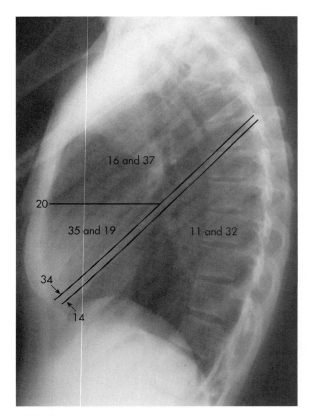

FIG. 6-56   Pleural fissures as seen on the posteroanterior chest radiograph. (See Key for Figures 6-50 through 6-56.)

KEY FOR FIGURES 6-57 THROUGH 6-67

a	Aorta	ma	Manubrium
ar	Aortic arch	mbr	Main stem bronchi
asa	Ascending aorta	ob	Oblique fissure of left lung
Az	Azygous vein		
brA	Brachiocephalic artery	pul	Pulmonary trunk
		ra	Right atrium
ca	Carina	rbrA	Right brachiocephalic artery
cl	Clavicle		
da	Descending aorta	rbrV	Right brachiocephalic vein
es	Esophagus		
h	Heart	rCA	Right coronary artery
la	Left atrium	rib	First rib
lbrV	Left brachiocephalic vein	rPA	Right pulmonary artery
		rPV	Right pulmonary vein
lCA	Left coronary artery	rv	Right ventricle
lCCA	Left common carotid artery	sbr	Secondary bronchi
		SCjt	Sternoclavicular joint
lPA	Left pulmonary artery	SVC	Superior vena cava
		tbr	Tertiary bronchi
lPV	Left pulmonary vein	tha	Thoracic aperture
lSA	Left subclavian artery	tr	Trachea
lv	Left ventricle		

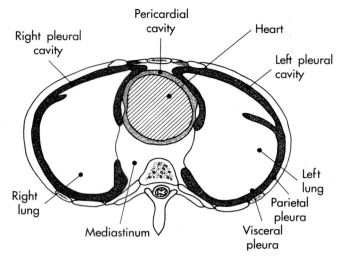

FIG. 6-57 Axial cross-section of the pleural cavity. (See Key for Figures 6-57 through 6-67.) (From Kelley LL: Sectional anatomy for imaging professionals, St. Louis, 1997, Mosby.)

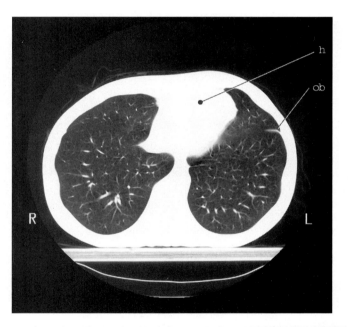

FIG. 6-58 Axial computed tomography scan of the lungs with fissures. (See Key for Figures 6-57 through 6-67.) (From Kelley LL: Sectional anatomy for imaging professionals, St Louis, 1997, Mosby.)

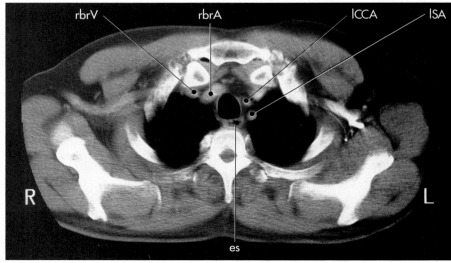

FIG. 6-59 Axial computed tomography scan of chest with aortic branches and superior vena cava tributaries. (See Key for Figures 6-57 through 6-67.) (From Kelley LL: Sectional anatomy for imaging professionals, St Louis, 1997, Mosby.)

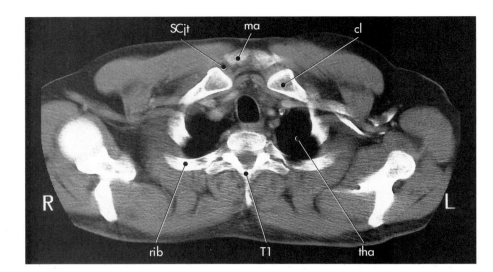

FIG. 6-60   Axial computed tomography scan of the thoracic inlet. (See Key for Figures 6-57 through 6-67.) (From Kelley LL: Sectional anatomy for imaging professionals, St Louis, 1997, Mosby.)

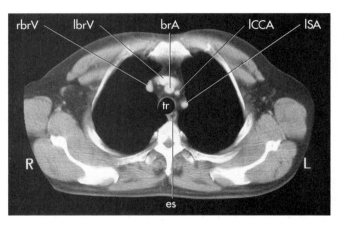

FIG. 6-61   Axial computed tomography scan of the chest with aortic arch branches and brachiocephalic veins. (See Key for Figures 6-57 through 6-67.) (From Kelley LL: Sectional anatomy for imaging professionals, St Louis, 1997, Mosby.)

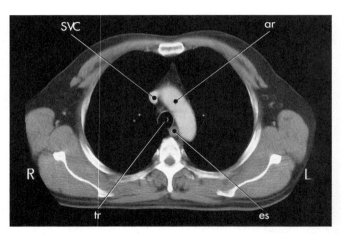

FIG. 6-62   Axial computed tomography scan of the chest with aortic arch. (See Key for Figures 6-57 through 6-67.) (From Kelley LL: Sectional anatomy for imaging professionals, St Louis, 1997, Mosby.)

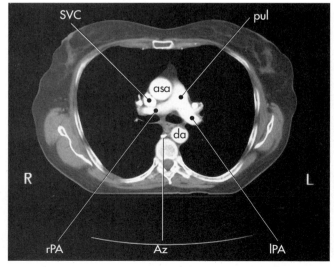

FIG. 6-63   Axial computed tomography scan of the chest with pulmonary trunk. (See Key for Figures 6-57 through 6-67.) (From Kelley LL: Sectional anatomy for imaging professionals, St Louis, 1997, Mosby.)

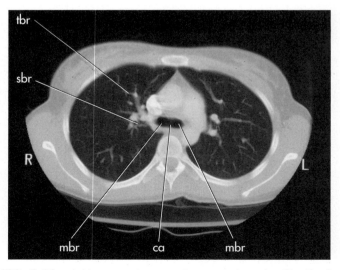

FIG. 6-64   Axial computed tomography scan at the carina. (See Key for Figures 6-57 through 6-67.) (From Kelley LL: Sectional anatomy for imaging professionals, St Louis, 1997, Mosby.)

KEY FOR FIGURES 6-57 THROUGH 6-67

a	Aorta	ma	Manubrium
ar	Aortic arch	mbr	Main stem bronchi
asa	Ascending aorta	ob	Oblique fissure of left
Az	Azygous vein		lung
brA	Brachiocephalic	pul	Pulmonary trunk
	artery	ra	Right atrium
ca	Carina	rbrA	Right brachiocephalic
cl	Clavicle		artery
da	Descending aorta	rbrV	Right brachiocephalic
es	Esophagus		vein
h	Heart	rCA	Right coronary artery
la	Left atrium	rib	First rib
lbrV	Left brachiocephalic	rPA	Right pulmonary
	vein		artery
lCA	Left coronary artery	rPV	Right pulmonary vein
lCCA	Left common carotid	rv	Right ventricle
	artery	sbr	Secondary bronchi
lPA	Left pulmonary	SCjt	Sternoclavicular joint
	artery	SVC	Superior vena cava
lPV	Left pulmonary vein	tbr	Tertiary bronchi
lSA	Left subclavian artery	tha	Thoracic aperture
lv	Left ventricle	tr	Trachea

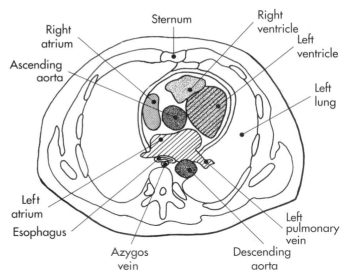

FIG. 6-65 Axial view of the heart with four chambers. (From Kelley LL: Sectional anatomy for imaging professionals, St Louis, 1997, Mosby.)

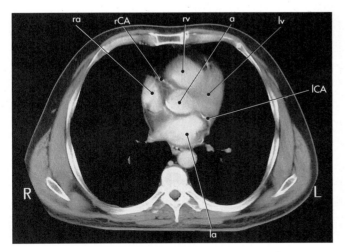

FIG. 6-66 Axial computed tomography scan of the heart with left and right coronary arteries. (See Key for Figures 6-57 through 6-67.) (From Kelley LL: Sectional anatomy for imaging professionals, St Louis, 1997, Mosby.)

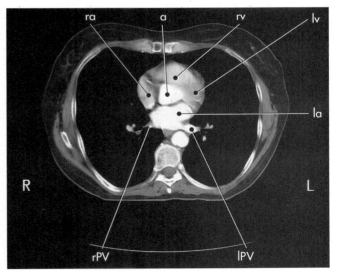

FIG. 6-67 Axial computed tomography scan of the chest with pulmonary veins. (See Key for Figures 6-57 through 6-67.) (From Kelley LL: Sectional anatomy for imaging professionals, St Louis, 1997, Mosby.)

KEY FOR FIGURES 6-68 THROUGH 6-77

1. Acetabular fossa
2. Acetabular fossa, inferior (Köhler's teardrop)
3. Acetabular rim, superior aspect
4. Anterior inferior iliac spine (AIIS)
5. Anterior superior iliac spine (ASIS)
6. Articular process, inferior, left
7. Articular process, inferior, right
8. Articular process, superior, left
9. Articular process, superior, right
10. Articular process, inferior
11. Articular process, superior
12. Coccyx
13. Diaphragm
14. Exostosis of obturator ("pubic ears")
15. Fascial plane line, gluteus medius
16. Fascial plane line, iliopsoas
17. Fascial plane line, obturator internus
18. Femur, fovea capitis
19. Femur, greater trochanter
20. Femur, head
21. Femur, lesser trochanter
22. Femur, neck
23. Gas in the ascending colon
24. Gas in the descending colon
25. Gastric air bubble/magenblase
26. Gluteal fold
27. Iliac crest
28. Iliac crest, left
29. Iliac crest, right
30. Iliac fossa
31. Iliopectineal line/arcuate line
32. Intertrochanteric line
33. Intervertebral disc space
34. Intervertebral foramen
35. Ischial spine
36. Ischial tuberosity
37. Ischium
38. Lamina, left
39. Lamina, right
40. Liver, inferior margin
41. Obturator foramen
42. Pars interarticularis, left
43. Pars interarticularis, right
44. Pedicle, left
45. Pedicle, right
46. Posterior inferior iliac spine (PIIS)
47. Posterior superior iliac spine (PSIS)
48. Psoas muscle shadow
49. Pubic ramus, inferior
50. Pubic ramus, superior
51. Pubic symphysis
52. Renal shadow
53. Sacral ala
54. Sacral foramen
55. Sacral hiatus/notch
56. Sacral promontory
57. Sacroiliac articulation
58. Sciatic notch, greater
59. Spinous process, T12
60. Spinous process, L1
61. Spinous process, L2
62. Spinous process, L3
63. Spinous process, L4
64. Spinous process, L5
65. T11 rib
66. T12 rib
67. Transverse process/costal process, left
68. Transverse process/ costal process, right
69. Urinary bladder

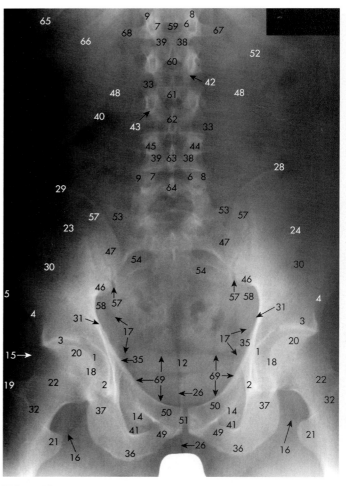

FIG. 6-68   Anteroposterior lumbopelvic radiograph. (See Key for Figures 6-68 through 6-71.)

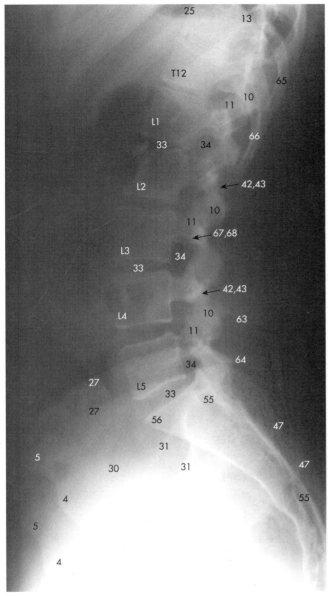

FIG. 6-69 Lateral lumbopelvic radiograph. (See Key for Figures 6-68 through 6-71.)

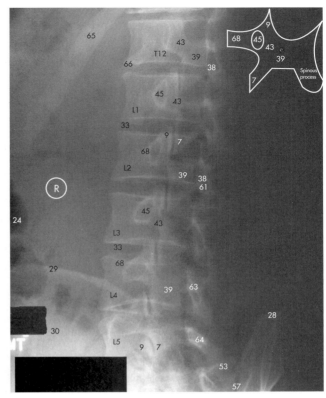

FIG. 6-70 Right posterior oblique lumbar radiograph. (See Key for Figures 6-68 through 6-71.)

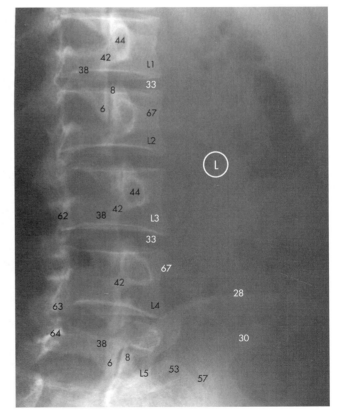

FIG. 6-71 Left posterior oblique lumbar radiograph. (See Key for Figures 6-68 through 6-71.)

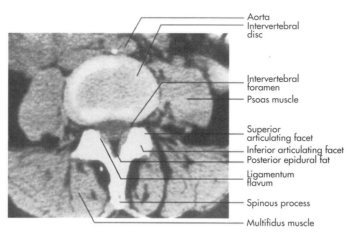

Aorta
Intervertebral disc

Intervertebral foramen
Psoas muscle

Superior articulating facet
Inferior articulating facet
Posterior epidural fat
Ligamentum flavum
Spinous process
Multifidus muscle

FIG. 6-72   Axial computed tomography scan through the intervertebral disc in the midlumbar region in a narrow window setting. (From Haaga JR: CT and MRI of the whole body, ed 4, vol I, St Louis, 2003, Mosby.)

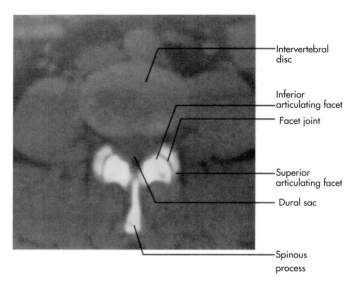

Intervertebral disc

Inferior articulating facet
Facet joint

Superior articulating facet

Dural sac

Spinous process

FIG. 6-73   Axial computed tomography scan through the intervertebral disc in a wide window setting. (From Haaga JR: CT and MRI of the whole body, ed 4, vol I, St Louis, 2003, Mosby.)

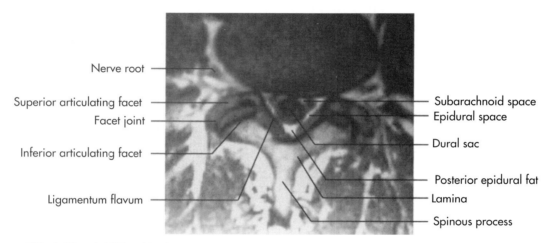

Nerve root

Superior articulating facet
Facet joint

Inferior articulating facet

Ligamentum flavum

Subarachnoid space
Epidural space

Dural sac

Posterior epidural fat

Lamina

Spinous process

FIG. 6-74   Axial T1-weighted magnetic resonance imaging through the facet joints. (From Haaga JR: CT and MRI of the whole body, ed 4, vol I, St Louis, 2003, Mosby.)

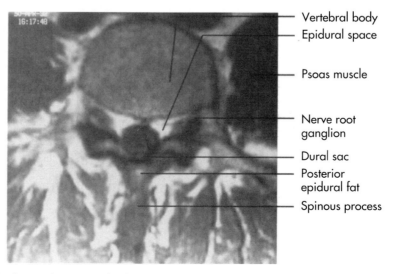

Vertebral body
Epidural space

Psoas muscle

Nerve root ganglion

Dural sac
Posterior epidural fat

Spinous process

FIG. 6-75   Axial T1-weighted magnetic resonance imaging through the midportion of the vertebral body in the lumbar region. (From Haaga JR: CT and MRI of the whole body, ed 4, vol I, St Louis, 2003, Mosby.)

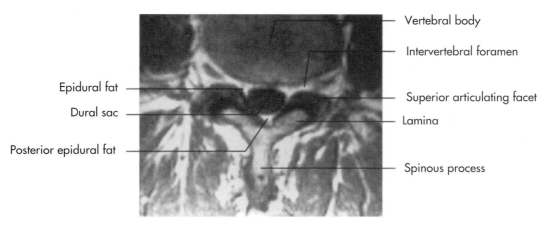

FIG. 6-76 Axial T1-weighted magnetic resonance imaging of fat in the epidural space. (From Haaga JR: CT and MRI of the whole body, ed 4, vol 1, St Louis, 2003, Mosby.)

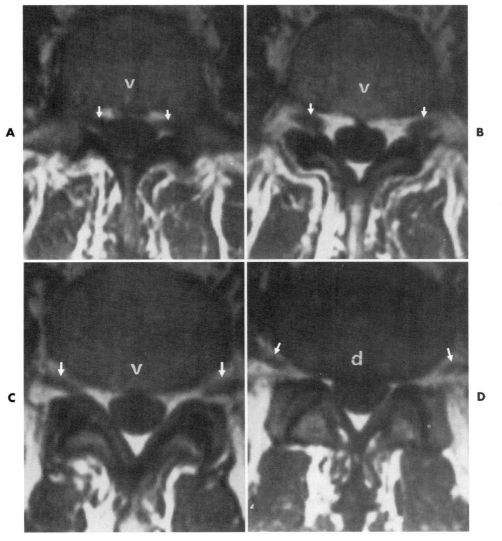

FIG. 6-77 Axial T1-weighted magnetic resonance imaging depicts the path of lumbar nerve roots through the canal; *d*, disc; *v*, vertebral body. **A,** At the midbody level, the preexisting roots *(arrows)* are positioned in the lateral recesses. **B** and **C,** Just inferior to **A** at the superior aspect of the discovertebral junction, the roots lie within the foramina *(arrows)*. **D,** At the inferior aspect of the discovertebral junction, the roots have already exited the foramina *(arrows)*. (From Haaga JR: CT and MRI of the whole body, ed 4, vol 1, St Louis, 2003, Mosby.)

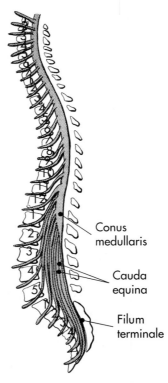

FIG. 6-78 Sagittal section of conus medullaris, cauda equina, and filum terminale. (From Kelley LL: Sectional anatomy for imaging professionals, St Louis, 1997, Mosby.)

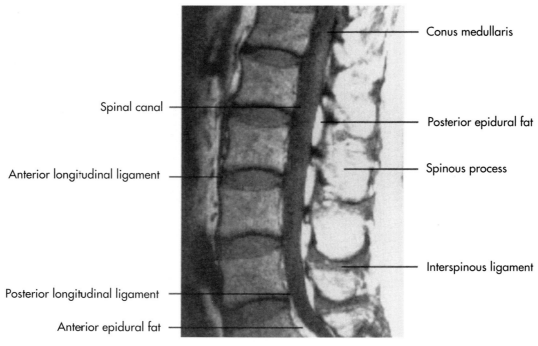

FIG. 6-79 Sagittal T1-weighted magnetic resonance imaging study of the lumbar spine in midline. (From Haaga JR: CT and MRI of the whole body, ed 4, vol 1, St Louis, 2003, Mosby.)

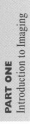

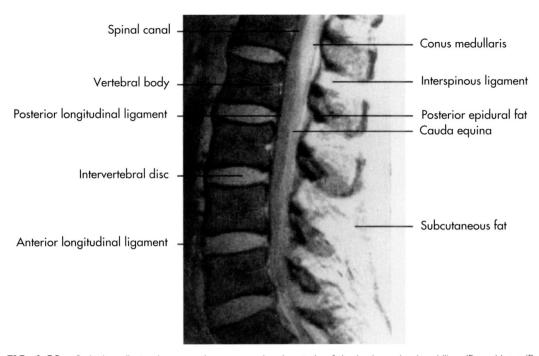

Spinal canal

Vertebral body

Posterior longitudinal ligament

Intervertebral disc

Anterior longitudinal ligament

Conus medullaris

Interspinous ligament

Posterior epidural fat
Cauda equina

Subcutaneous fat

FIG. 6-80 Sagittal gradient echo magnetic resonance imaging study of the lumbar spine in midline. (From Haaga JR: CT and MRI of the whole body, ed 4, vol 1, St Louis, 2003, Mosby.)

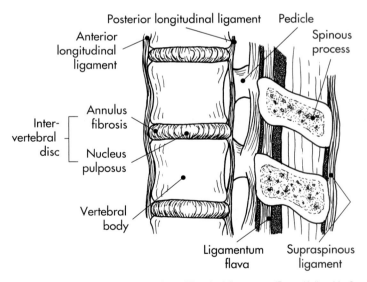

Posterior longitudinal ligament   Pedicle

Anterior longitudinal ligament

Spinous process

Inter-vertebral disc

Annulus fibrosis

Nucleus pulposus

Vertebral body

Ligamentum flava

Supraspinous ligament

FIG. 6-81 Sagittal section of the lumbar spine with spinal ligaments. (From Kelley LL: Sectional anatomy for imaging professionals, St Louis, 1997, Mosby.)

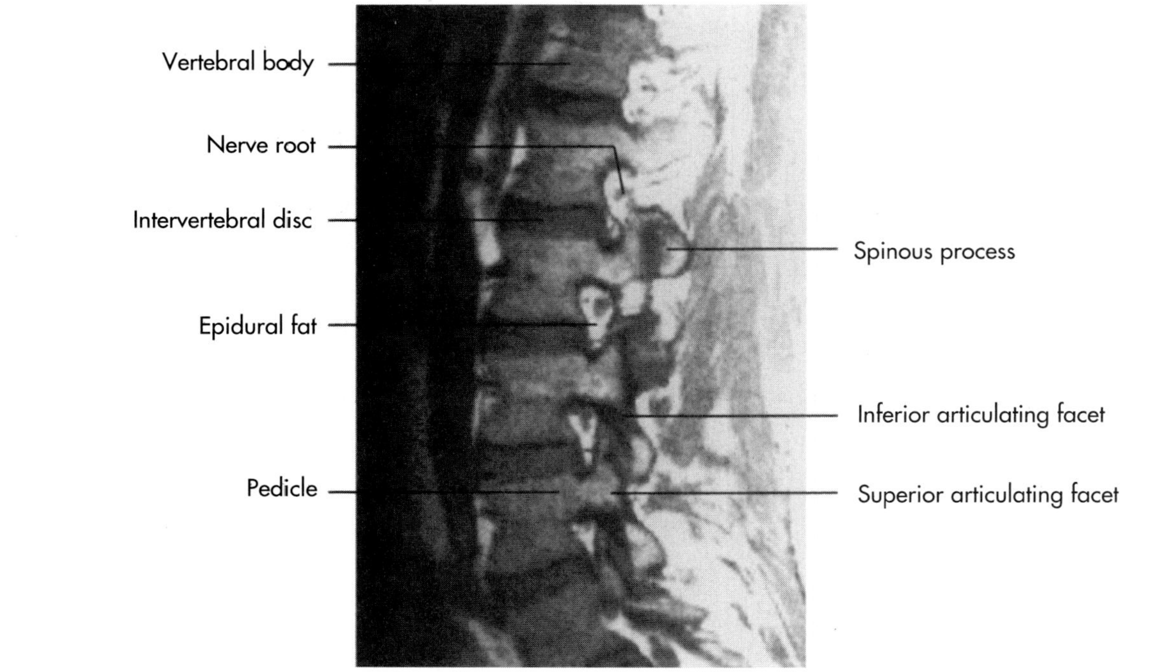

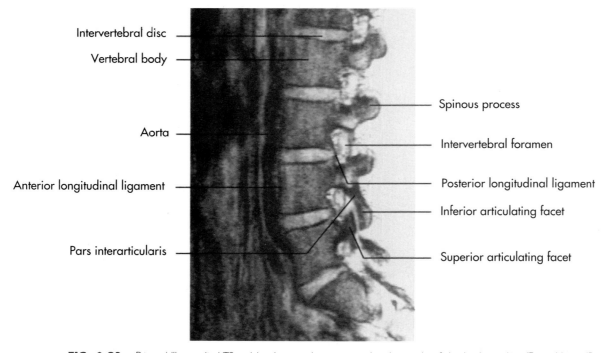

Vertebral body

Nerve root

Intervertebral disc

Epidural fat

Pedicle

Spinous process

Inferior articulating facet

Superior articulating facet

FIG. 6-82   Para-midline sagittal T1-weighted magnetic resonance imaging study of the lumbar spine. (From Haaga JR: CT and MRI of the whole body, ed 4, vol 1, St Louis, 2003, Mosby.)

Intervertebral disc
Vertebral body

Aorta

Anterior longitudinal ligament

Pars interarticularis

Spinous process

Intervertebral foramen

Posterior longitudinal ligament

Inferior articulating facet

Superior articulating facet

FIG. 6-83   Para-midline sagittal T2-weighted magnetic resonance imaging study of the lumbar spine. (From Haaga JR: CT and MRI of the whole body, ed 4, vol 1, St Louis, 2003, Mosby.)

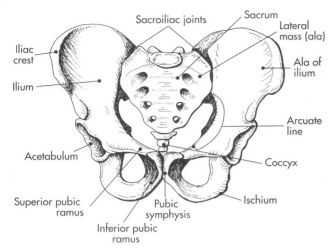

FIG. 6-84 Anterior view of the pelvis. (From Kelley LL: Sectional anatomy for imaging professionals, St Louis, 1997, Mosby.)

KEY FOR FIGURE 6-85

1. Acetabular fossa
2. Acetabular fossa, inferior aspect (Köhler's teardrop)
3. Acetabular rim, superior aspect
4. Anterior inferior iliac spine (AIIS)
5. Anterior superior iliac spine (ASIS)
6. Articular facet, inferior
7. Articular facet, superior
8. Fascial plane line, gluteus medius
9. Fascial plane line, iliopsoas
10. Fascial plane line, obturator internus
11. Femur, fovea capitis
12. Femur, greater trochanter
13. Femur, head
14. Femur, lesser trochanter
15. Femur, neck
16. Gas in the ascending colon
17. Gas in the descending colon
18. Gluteal fold
19. Gonadal shield
20. Iliac crest
21. Iliac fossa
22. Intertrochanteric line
23. Intervertebral disc space
24. Ischial spine
25. Ischial tuberosity
26. Ischium
27. Lamina
28. Obturator foramen
29. Pedicle
30. Pubic ramus, inferior
31. Pubic ramus, superior
32. Pubic symphysis
33. Spinous process, L3
34. Spinous process, L4
35. Spinous process, L5
36. Transverse process/costal process

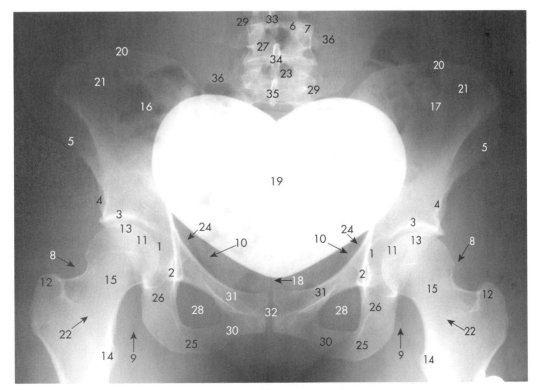

FIG. 6-85 Anteroposterior pelvic radiograph. (See Key for Figure 6-85.)

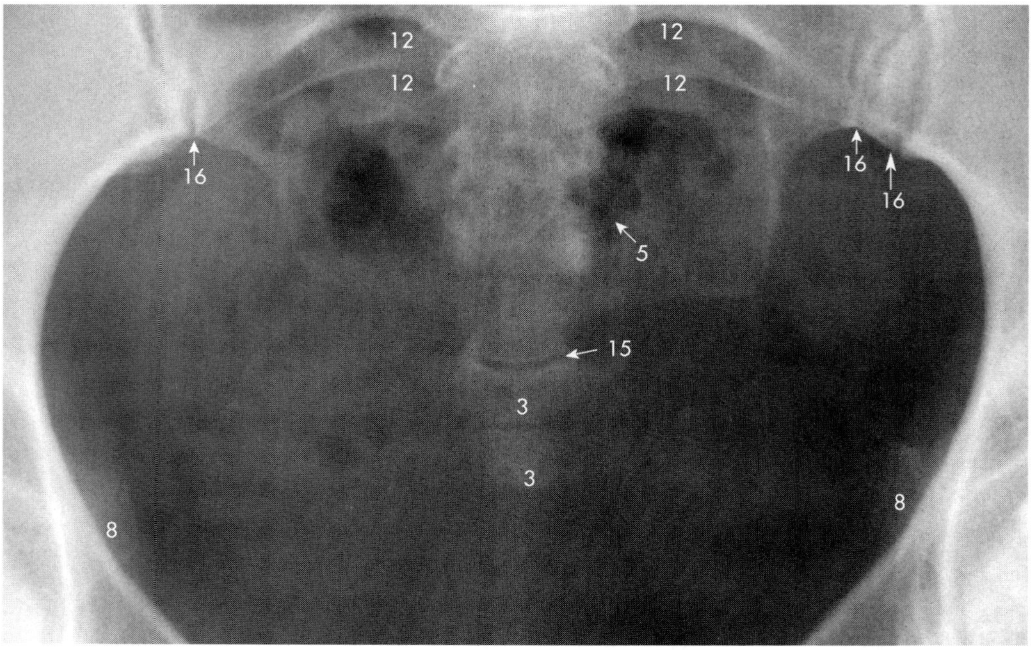

FIG. 6-86 Anteroposterior sacrum and coccyx radiograph. (See Key for Figures 6-86 through 6-87.)

KEY FOR FIGURES 6-86 THROUGH 6-87

1. Acetabular fossa
2. Acetabular rim
3. Coccyx segment
4. Femoral head
5. Gas in the sigmoid colon
6. Iliac crest
7. Iliopectineal line
8. Ischial spine
9. Ischium
10. Posterior superior iliac spine (PSIS)
11. Sacral canal
12. Sacral foramen
13. Sacral horn
14. Sacral promontory
15. Sacrococcygeal joint
16. Sacroiliac articulation
17. Sciatic notch, greater
18. Sciatic notch, lesser

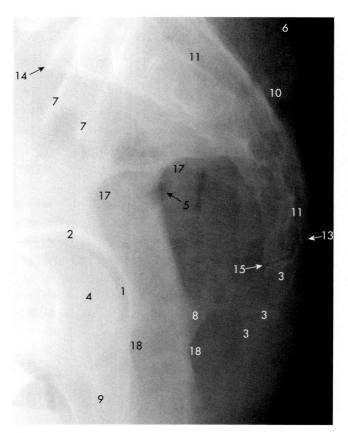

FIG. 6-87 Lateral sacrum and coccyx radiograph. (See Key for Figures 6-86 through 6-87.)

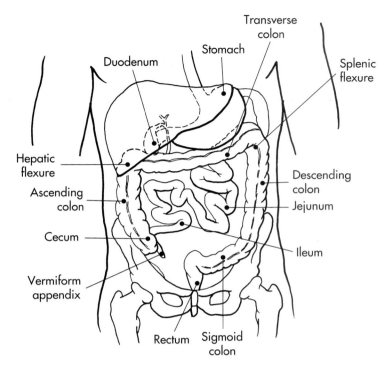

FIG. 6-88   Anterior view of the intestines. (From Kelley LL: Sectional anatomy for imaging professionals, St Louis, 1997, Mosby.)

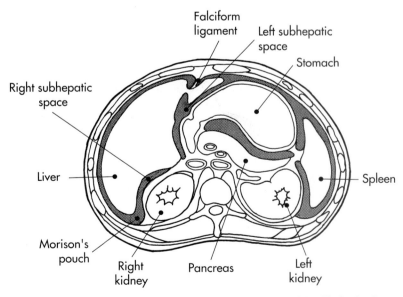

FIG. 6-89   Axial view of the subhepatic spaces and Morison's pouch. (From Kelley LL: Sectional anatomy for imaging professionals, St Louis, 1997, Mosby.)

KEY FOR FIGURES 6-90 THROUGH 6-95

1. Cecum
2. Gas in ascending colon
3. Gas in descending colon
4. Gas in hepatic flexure
5. Gas in sigmoid colon
6. Gas in splenic flexure
7. Gluteal fold
8. Kidney, left
9. Kidney, right
10. Liver, inferior margin
11. Psoas muscle shadow
12. Urinary bladder

A	Aorta
asc	Ascending colon
b	Body of pancreas
CBD	Common bile duct
desc	Descending colon
IMV	Inferior mesenteric vein

IVC	Inferior vena cava
li	Liver
LRA	Left renal artery
LRV	Left renal vein
n	Neck of pancreas
p	Peritoneum
pa	Pancreas
PD	Pancreatic duct
RRA	Right renal artery
SMA	Superior mesenteric artery
smb	Small bowel
SMV	Superior mesenteric vein
sp	Spleen
st	Stomach
t	Tail of pancreas
tra	Transverse colon

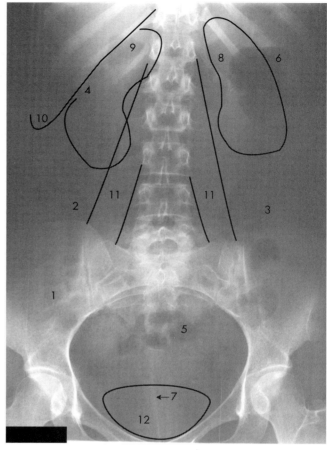

FIG. 6-90　Recumbent abdomen/kidney, ureter, and bladder radiograph. (See Key for Figures 6-90 through 6-95.)

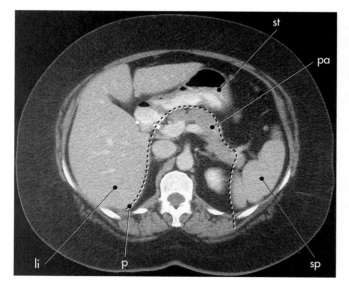

FIG. 6-91　Axial computed tomography scan of peritoneal and retroperitoneal structures, separated by dotted lines. (See Key for Figures 6-90 through 6-95.) (From Kelley LL: Sectional anatomy for imaging professionals, St Louis, 1997, Mosby.)

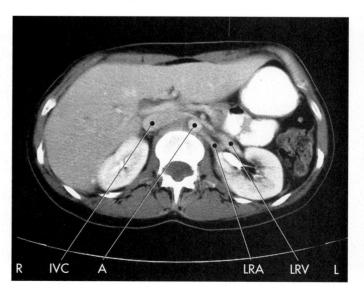

FIG. 6-92　Axial computed tomography scan with renal arteries and veins. (See Key for Figures 6-90 through 6-95.) (From Kelley LL: Sectional anatomy for imaging professionals, St Louis, 1997, Mosby.)

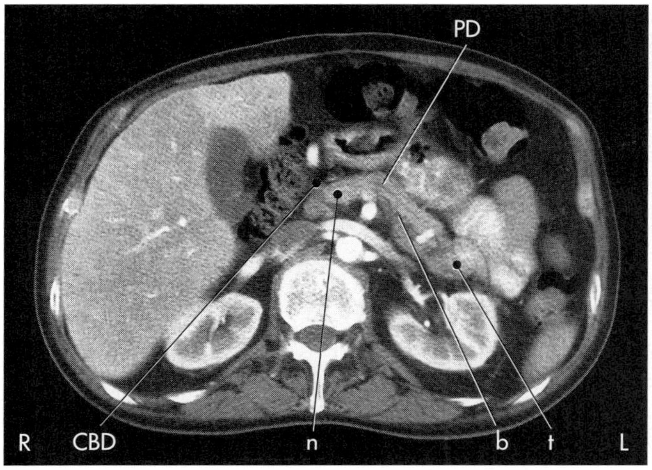

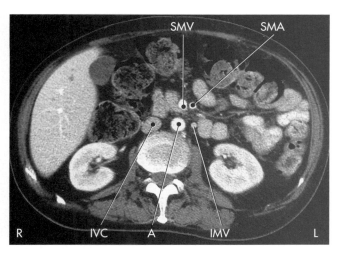

FIG. 6-93 Axial computed tomography scan of pancreas and pancreatic duct. (See Key for Figures 6-90 through 6-95.) (From Kelley LL: Sectional anatomy for imaging professionals, St Louis, 1997, Mosby.)

FIG. 6-94 Axial computed tomography scan with superior mesenteric veins. (See Key for Figures 6-90 through 6-95.) (From Kelley LL: Sectional anatomy for imaging professionals, St Louis, 1997, Mosby.)

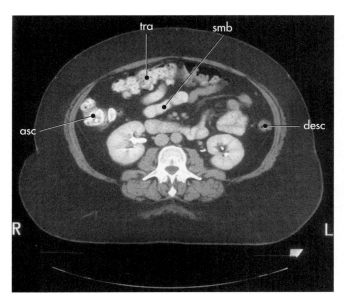

FIG. 6-95 Axial computed tomography scan with transverse colon. (See Key for Figures 6-90 through 6-95.) (From Kelley LL: Sectional anatomy for imaging professionals, St Louis, 1997, Mosby.)

KEY FOR FIGURES 6-96 THROUGH 6-102

1. Acromioclavicular articulation
2. Clavicle
3. Clavicle, conoid tubercle
4. Filter marker
5. Humerus, anatomic neck
6. Humerus, diaphysis
7. Humerus, greater tuberosity
8. Humerus, head
9. Humerus, lesser tuberosity
10. Humerus, surgical neck
11. Manubrium
12. Scapula, acromion process
13. Scapula, coracoid process
14. Scapula, glenoid fossa
15. Scapula, lateral border
16. Scapula, medial border
17. Scapula, spine
18. Scapula, superior angle
19. T1 rib
20. T2 rib, lateral aspect
21. T3 rib, lateral aspect
22. T4 rib, lateral aspect

ac	Acromion process
bi	Biceps tendon
ghl	Glenohumeral ligament
gl	Glenoid
grt	Greater tuberosity
inf	Infraspinatus
la	Labrum
sup	Supraspinatus
tr	Trapezius

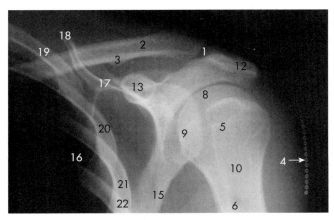

FIG. 6-96 Anteroposterior internal rotation shoulder radiograph. (See Key for Figures 6-96 through 6-102.)

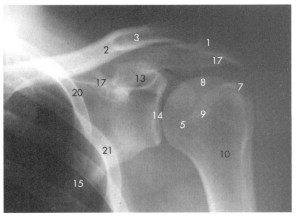

FIG. 6-97 Anteroposterior external rotation shoulder radiograph. (See Key for Figures 6-96 through 6-102.)

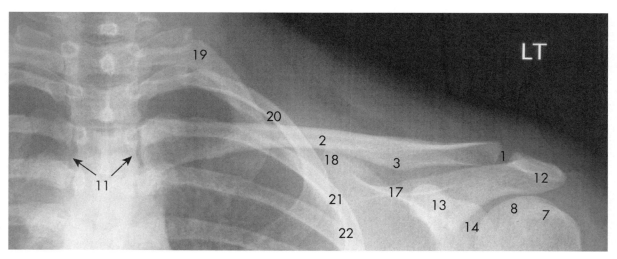

FIG. 6-98   Acromioclavicular radiograph. (See Key for Figures 6-96 through 6-102.)

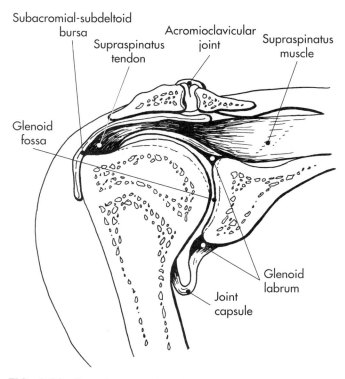

FIG. 6-99   Coronal cross section of the shoulder with glenoid labrum. (See Key for Figures 6-96 through 6-102.) (From Kelley LL: Sectional anatomy for imaging professionals, St Louis, 1997, Mosby.)

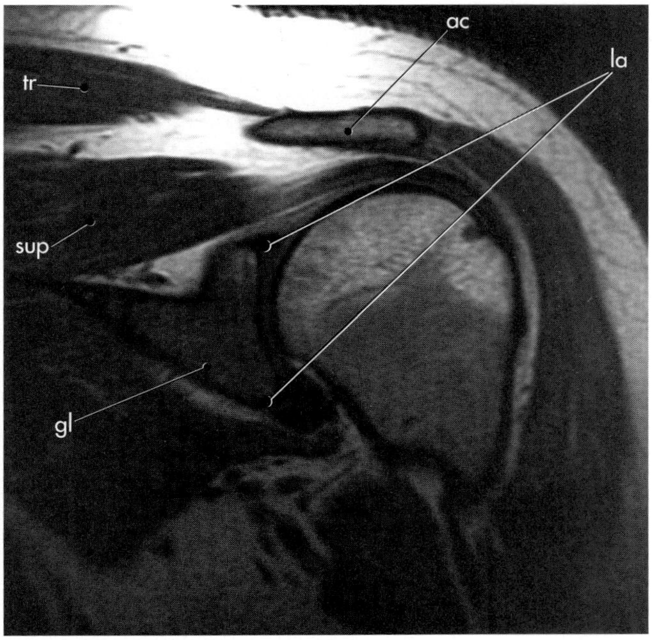

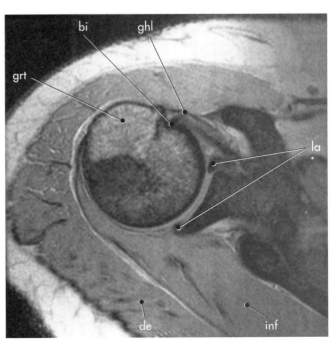

FIG. 6-100 Coronal oblique magnetic resonance imaging scan of the shoulder with glenoid labrum. (See Key for Figures 6-96 through 6-102.) (From Kelley LL: Sectional anatomy for imaging professionals, St Louis, 1997, Mosby.)

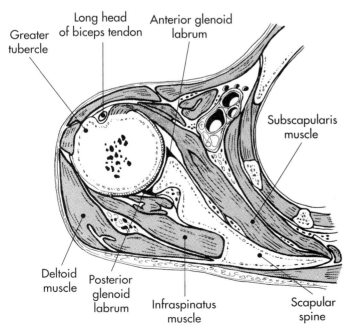

FIG. 6-101 Axial view of the shoulder muscles. (See Key for Figures 6-96 through 6-102.) (From Kelley LL: Sectional anatomy for imaging professionals, St Louis, 1997, Mosby.)

FIG. 6-102 Axial magnetic resonance imaging scan of the shoulder muscles at the midjoint. (See Key for Figures 6-96 through 6-102.) (From Kelley LL: Sectional anatomy for imaging professionals, St Louis, 1997, Mosby.)

KEY FOR FIGURES 6-103 THROUGH 6-106

1. Anterior humeral fat pad
2. Humerus, capitulum
3. Humerus, coronoid fossa
4. Humerus, diaphysis
5. Humerus, lateral epicondyle
6. Humerus, medial epicondyle
7. Humerus, olecranon fossa
8. Humerus, superimposed medial and lateral condyles
9. Humerus, trochlea
10. Proximal radioulnar joint
11. Radius, diaphysis
12. Radius, head
13. Radius, neck
14. Radius, tuberosity
15. Supinator fat line
16. Trochlear notch/semilunar notch
17. Ulna, coronoid process
18. Ulna, diaphysis
19. Ulna, olecranon

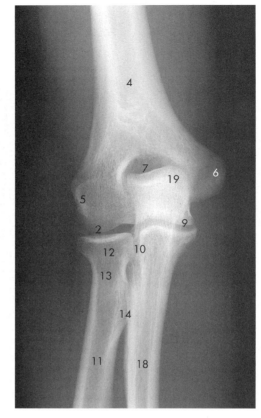

FIG. 6-103   Anteroposterior elbow radiograph. (See Key for Figures 6-103 through 6-106.)

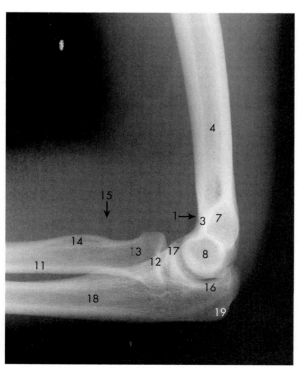

FIG. 6-104   Lateral elbow radiograph. (See Key for Figures 6-103 through 6-106.)

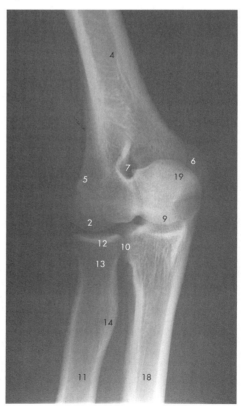

FIG. 6-105   External oblique elbow radiograph. (See Key for Figures 6-103 through 6-106.)

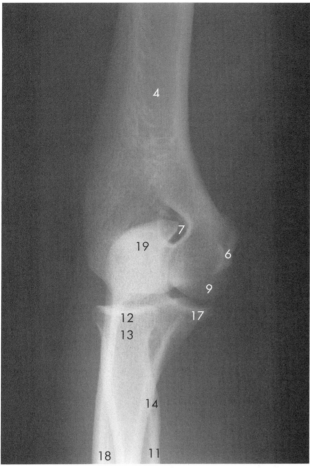

FIG. 6-106 Internal oblique elbow radiograph. (See Key for Figures 6-103 through 6-106.)

KEY FOR FIGURES 6-107 THROUGH 6-110

1. Carpal, scaphoid
2. Carpal, lunate
3. Carpal, triquetrum
4. Carpal, pisiform
5. Carpal, trapezium
6. Carpal, trapezoid
7. Carpal, capitate
8. Carpal, hamate
9. Carpal, hamate, hook of the hamate
10. Interphalangeal articulation
11. Interphalangeal articulation, distal
12. Interphalangeal articulation, proximal
13. Metacarpal, base
14. Metacarpal, diaphysis of first metacarpal
15. Metacarpal, diaphysis of second metacarpal
16. Metacarpal, diaphysis of third metacarpal
17. Metacarpal, diaphysis of fourth metacarpal
18. Metacarpal, diaphysis of fifth metacarpal
19. Metacarpal, head
20. Metacarpophalangeal articulation
21. Phalanx, distal
22. Phalanx, intermediate
23. Phalanx, proximal
24. Phalanx, diaphysis
25. Phalanx, base
26. Phalanx, head
27. Radius
28. Radius, styloid process
29. Sesamoid bone
30. Ulna
31. Ulna, styloid process
32. Ulnar notch/distal radioulnar joint
33. Ungual tuft/acral tuft

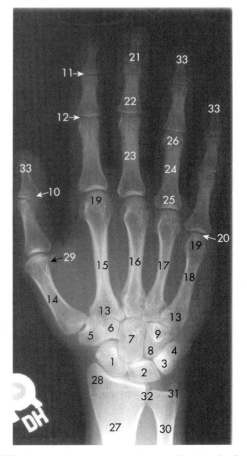

FIG. 6-107 Posteroanterior hand radiograph. (See Key for Figures 6-107 through 6-110.)

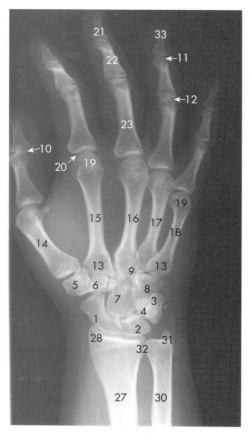

FIG. 6-108 Oblique hand radiograph. (See Key for Figures 6-107 through 6-110.)

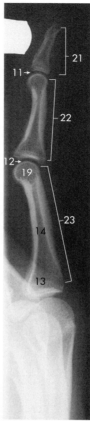

FIG. 6-109 Lateral finger radiograph. (See Key for Figures 6-107 through 6-110.)

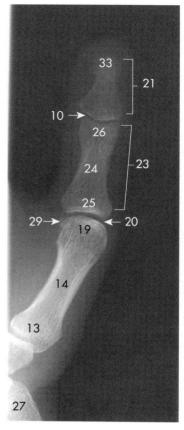

FIG. 6-110 Anteroposterior thumb radiograph. (See Key for Figures 6-107 through 6-110.)

KEY FOR FIGURES 6-111 THROUGH 6-117

1. Carpal, scaphoid
2. Carpal, lunate
3. Carpal, triquetrum
4. Carpal, pisiform
5. Carpal, trapezium
6. Carpal, trapezoid
7. Carpal, capitate
8. Carpal, hamate
9. Carpal, hamate, hook of the hamate
10. Interphalangeal articulation
11. Metacarpal, base
12. Metacarpal, diaphysis of first metacarpal
13. Metacarpal, diaphysis of second metacarpal
14. Metacarpal, diaphysis of third metacarpal
15. Metacarpal, diaphysis of fourth metacarpal
16. Metacarpal, diaphysis of fifth metacarpal
17. Metacarpal, head
18. Phalanx, distal
19. Phalanx, intermediate
20. Phalanx, proximal
21. Radius
22. Radius, styloid process
23. Sesamoid bone
24. Ulna
25. Ulna, styloid process
26. Ulnar notch/distal radioulnar joint

1st First metacarpal
c   Capitate
ex Extensor tendons
fl Flexor tendons
flr Flexor retinaculum
h   Hamate
mn Median nerve
td Trapezoid
tm Trapezium
ua Ulnar artery

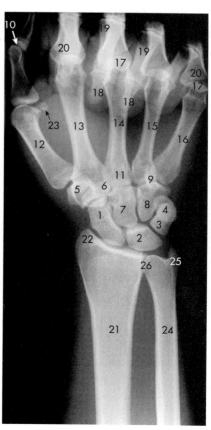

FIG. 6-111 Posteroanterior wrist radiograph. (See Key for Figures 6-111 through 6-117.)

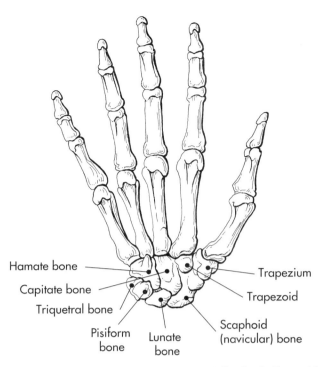

FIG. 6-112 Posterior view of the wrist and hand. (See Key for Figures 6-111 through 6-117.) (From Kelley LL: Sectional anatomy for imaging professionals, St Louis, 1997, Mosby.)

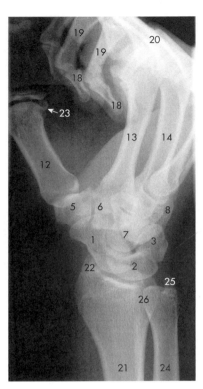

FIG. 6-113 Oblique wrist radiograph. (See Key for Figures 6-111 through 6-117.)

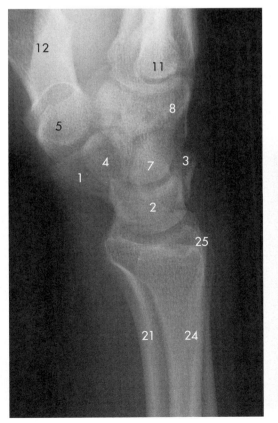

FIG. 6-114 Lateral wrist radiograph. (See Key for Figures 6-111 through 6-117.)

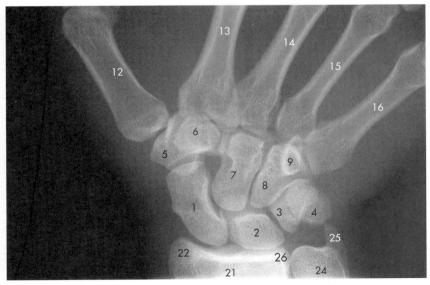

FIG. 6-115 Ulnar deviation wrist radiograph. (See Key for Figures 6-111 through 6-117.)

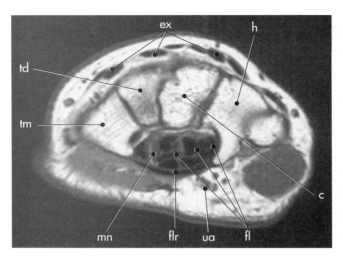

FIG. 6-116 Axial magnetic resonance imaging scan with neurovasculature of the wrist. (See Key for Figures 6-111 through 6-117.) (From Kelley LL: Sectional anatomy for imaging professionals, St Louis, 1997, Mosby.)

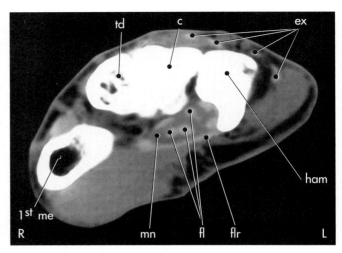

FIG. 6-117 Axial computed tomography scan of the wrist with flexor and extensor tendons and median nerve. (See Key for Figures 6-111 through 6-117.) (From Kelley LL: Sectional anatomy for imaging professionals, St Louis, 1997, Mosby.)

KEY FOR FIGURES 6-118 THROUGH 6-123

1. Acetabular fossa
2. Acetabular fossa, anterior margin
3. Acetabular fossa, inferior margin (Köhler's teardrop)
4. Acetabular rim
5. Anterior inferior iliac spine (AIIS)
6. Anterior superior iliac spine (ASIS)
7. Bowel gas and fecal material
8. Coccyx
9. Fascial plane line, gluteus medius
10. Fascial plane line, iliopsoas
11. Fascial plane line, obturator internus
12. Femur, diaphysis
13. Femur, fovea capitis
14. Femur, greater trochanter
15. Femur, head
16. Femur, intertrochanteric crest
17. Femur, lesser trochanter
18. Femur, neck
19. Greater sciatic notch
20. Iliac fossa
21. Iliopectineal line/arcuate line

22. Ischial spine
23. Ischial tuberosity
24. Ischium
25. Obturator foramen
26. Penis shadow
27. Pubic ramus, inferior
28. Pubic ramus, superior
29. Pubic symphysis
30. Sacral foramen
31. Sacroiliac articulation

ace	Acetabulum
acol	Anterior column
af	Acetabular fossa
fh	Femoral head
fov	Fovea capitis
gmax	Gluteus maximus
gmed	Gluteus medius
gmin	Gluteus minimus
ilig	Iliofemoral ligament
ilps	Iliopsoas
la	Labrum
obi	Obturator internus
pcol	Posterior column
quad	Quadratus femoris
sar	Sartorius
sGem	Superior gemellus
tere	Ligamentum teres
TFL	Tensor fascia latae
tlig	Transverse ligament

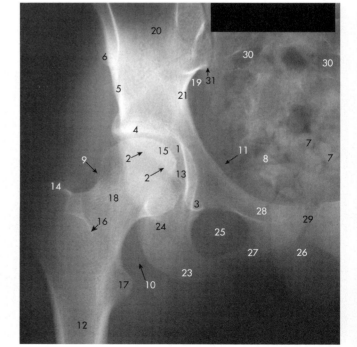

FIG. 6-118 Anteroposterior iliofemoral radiograph. (See Key for Figures 6-118 through 6-123.)

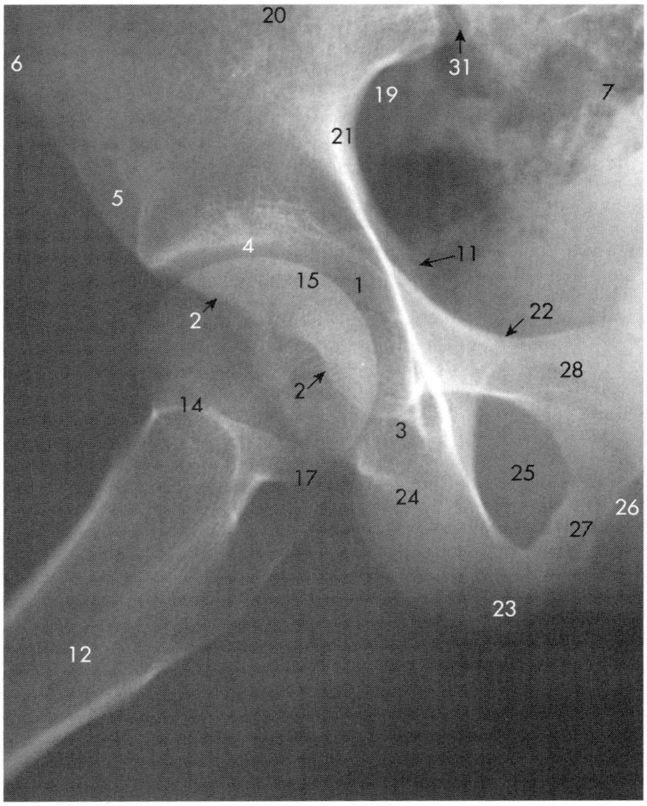

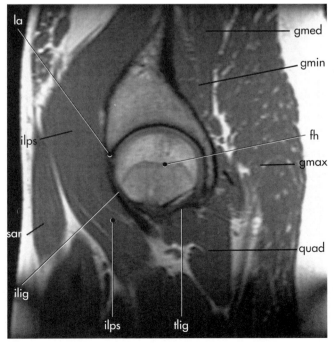

FIG. 6-119 Frog-leg iliofemoral radiograph. (See Key for Figures 6-118 through 6-123.)

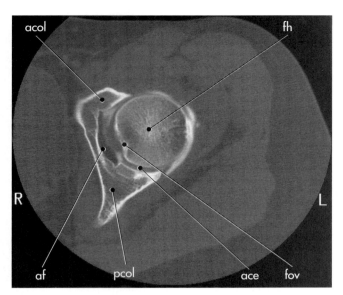

FIG. 6-120 Axial computed tomography scan of the hip joint. (See Key for Figures 6-118 through 6-123.) (From Kelley LL: Sectional anatomy for imaging professionals, St Louis, 1997, Mosby.)

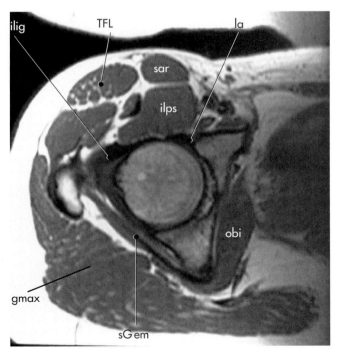

FIG. 6-121 Sagittal magnetic resonance imaging scan of the hip with iliofemoral ligaments. (See Key for Figures 6-118 through 6-123.) (From Kelley LL: Sectional anatomy for imaging professionals, St Louis, 1997, Mosby.)

FIG. 6-122 Axial magnetic resonance imaging scan of the hip with iliofemoral ligaments. (See Key for Figures 6-118 through 6-123.) (From Kelley LL: Sectional anatomy for imaging professionals, St Louis, 1997, Mosby.)

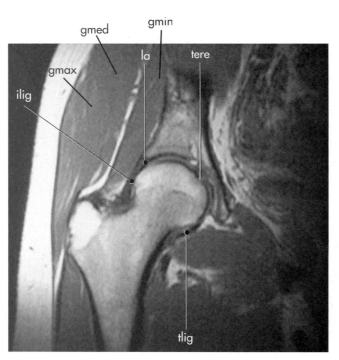

FIG. 6-123 Coronal magnetic resonance imaging scan of the hip with iliofemoral ligaments. (See Key for Figures 6-118 through 6-123.) (From Kelley LL: Sectional anatomy for imaging professionals, St Louis, 1997, Mosby.)

KEY FOR FIGURES 6-124 THROUGH 6-134

1. Fabella (sesamoid bone)
2. Femur, adductor tubercle
3. Femur, diaphysis
4. Femur, lateral condyle
5. Femur, lateral epicondyle
6. Femur, medial condyle
7. Femur, medial epicondyle
8. Femur, superimposed medial and lateral condyles
9. Fibula, apex of the head
10. Fibula, diaphysis
11. Fibula, head
12. Growth line/physis line
13. Infrapatellar fat pad
14. Intercondylar eminence
15. Intercondylar eminence, lateral
16. Intercondylar eminence, medial
17. Patella
18. Patella, articular surface
19. Patella, inferior pole
20. Patella, lateral articular facet
21. Patella, medial articular facet
22. Patella, superior pole
23. Popliteal groove
24. Suprapatellar bursa
25. Tibia, diaphysis
26. Tibia, lateral condyle
27. Tibia, medial condyle
28. Tibia, tuberosity

ACL	Anterior cruciate ligament
gas	Gastrocnemius muscle
lcol	Lateral collateral ligament
lmen	Lateral meniscus
lmenp	Lateral meniscus, posterior horn
mcol	Medial collateral ligament
mmen	Medial meniscus
pl	Patellar ligament
pop	Popliteus muscle
PCL	Posterior cruciate ligament
qten	Quadriceps tendon
slmena	Lateral meniscus, anterior horn
sol	Soleus muscle

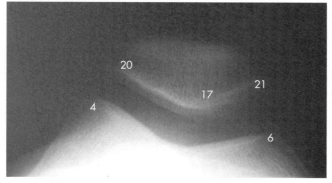

FIG. 6-124   Axial patella (Settegast method). (See Key for Figures 6-124 through 6-134.)

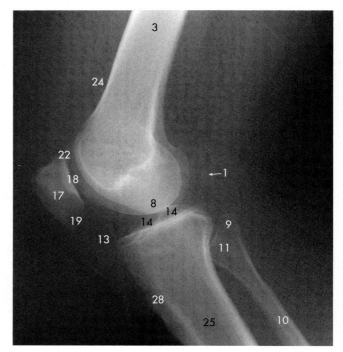

FIG. 6-125   Lateral knee radiograph. (See Key for Figures 6-124 through 6-134.)

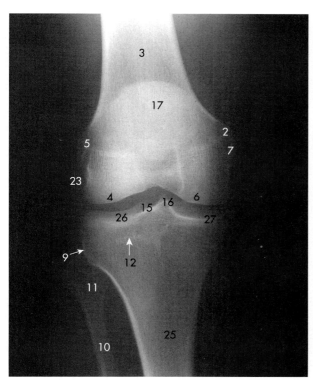

FIG. 6-126 Anteroposterior knee radiograph. (See Key for Figures 6-124 through 6-134.)

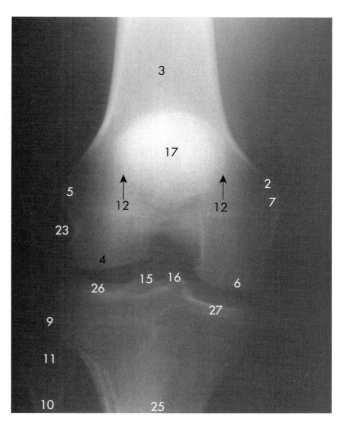

FIG. 6-127 Open joint knee radiograph. (See Key for Figures 6-124 through 6-134.)

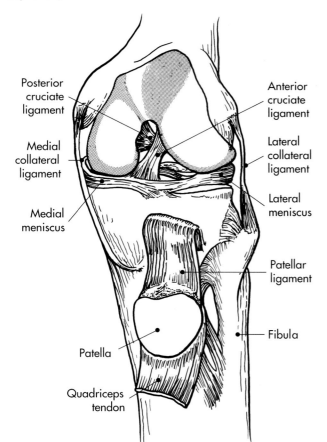

Posterior cruciate ligament

Anterior cruciate ligament

Medial collateral ligament

Lateral collateral ligament

Medial meniscus

Lateral meniscus

Patellar ligament

Fibula

Patella

Quadriceps tendon

FIG. 6-128 Anterior view of the meniscus and ligaments of the knee. (See Key for Figures 6-124 through 6-134.) (From Kelley LL: Sectional anatomy for imaging professionals, St Louis, 1997, Mosby.)

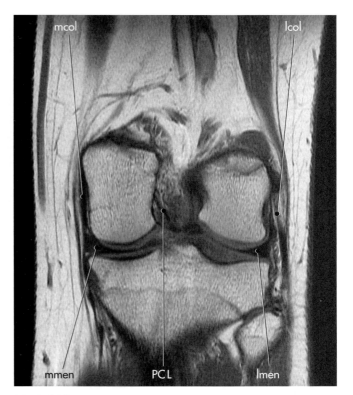

mcol

lcol

mmen

PCL

lmen

FIG. 6-129 Coronal magnetic resonance imaging scan of the knee with meniscus and ligaments. (See Key for Figures 6-124 through 6-134.) (From Kelley LL: Sectional anatomy for imaging professionals, St Louis, 1997, Mosby.)

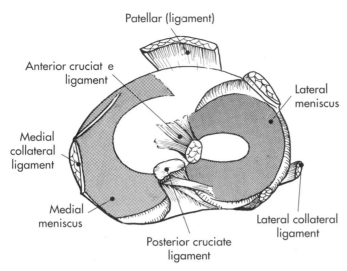

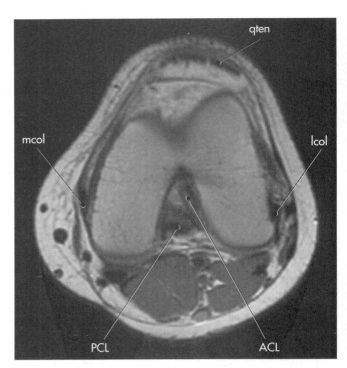

FIG. 6-130   Axial view of the meniscus and ligaments of the knee. (See Key for Figures 6-124 through 6-134.) (From Kelley LL: Sectional anatomy for imaging professionals, St Louis, 1997, Mosby.)

FIG. 6-131   Axial magnetic resonance imaging scan of the knee with cruciate and collateral ligaments. (See Key for Figures 6-124 through 6-134.) (From Kelley LL: Sectional anatomy for imaging professionals, St Louis, 1997, Mosby.)

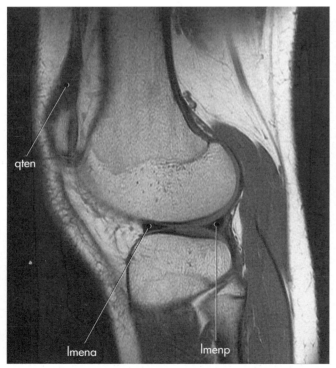

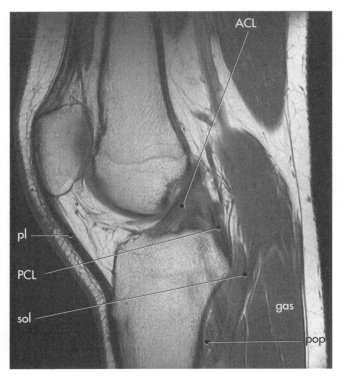

FIG. 6-132   Sagittal magnetic resonance imaging scan of the knee with meniscus and ligaments. (See Key for Figures 6-124 through 6-134.) (From Kelley LL: Sectional anatomy for imaging professionals, St Louis, 1997, Mosby.)

FIG. 6-133   Sagittal magnetic resonance imaging scan of the knee with anterior cruciate ligament. (See Key for Figures 6-124 through 6-134.) (From Kelley LL: Sectional anatomy for imaging professionals, St Louis, 1997, Mosby.)

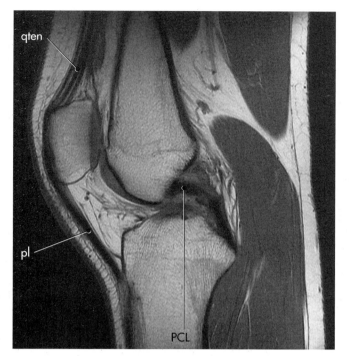

FIG. 6-134 Sagittal magnetic resonance imaging scan of the knee with posterior cruciate ligament. (See Key for Figures 6-124 through 6-134.) (From Kelley LL: Sectional anatomy for imaging professionals, St Louis, 1997, Mosby.)

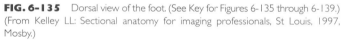

FIG. 6-135 Dorsal view of the foot. (See Key for Figures 6-135 through 6-139.) (From Kelley LL: Sectional anatomy for imaging professionals, St Louis, 1997, Mosby.)

KEY FOR FIGURES 6-136 THROUGH 6-139

1. Calcaneocuboid joint
2. Calcaneus
3. Calcaneus, anterior tubercle
4. Calcaneus, insertion of the Achilles' tendon
5. Calcaneus, insertion of the plantar aponeurosis
6. Calcaneus, middle tubercle
7. Calcaneus, posterior tubercle
8. Cuboid
9. Cuneiform, intermediate
10. Cuneiform, lateral
11. Cuneiform, medial
12. Fibula, diaphysis
13. Fibula, lateral malleolus
14. Interphalangeal articulation
15. Interphalangeal articulation, distal
16. Interphalangeal articulation, proximal
17. Metatarsal, base
18. Metatarsal, head
19. Metatarsal, diaphysis of the first metatarsal
20. Metatarsal, diaphysis of the second metatarsal
21. Metatarsal, diaphysis of the third metatarsal
22. Metatarsal, diaphysis of the fourth metatarsal
23. Metatarsal, diaphysis of the fifth metatarsal
24. Navicular
25. Os peroneum (accessory ossicle)
26. Phalanx, distal
27. Phalanx, intermediate
28. Phalanx, proximal
29. Phalanx, variant of two phalanges of fifth digit
30. Sesamoid bone
31. Talonavicular joint
32. Ttalus, dome/trochlea
33. Talus, head
34. Talus, neck
35. Talus, posterior process
36. Tarsal sinus
37. Tibia, diaphysis
38. Tibia, medial malleolus
39. Tuberosity of the fifth metatarsal

  C   Calcaneus
  cu Cuboid
  n   Navicular
  i   Sustentaculum tali
  I   Medial cuneiform
  III Lateral cuneiform

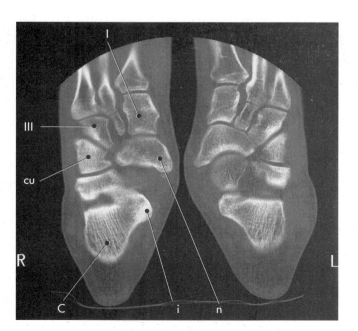

FIG. 6-136 Axial computed tomography scan of the ankle with tarsal bones. (See Key for Figures 6-136 through 6-139.) (From Kelley LL: Sectional anatomy for imaging professionals, St Louis, 1997, Mosby.)

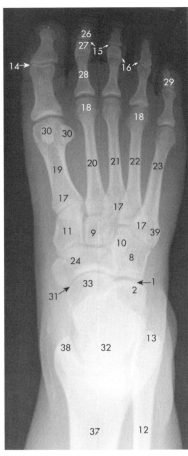

FIG. 6-137 Anteroposterior (dorsoplantar) foot radiograph. (See Key for Figures 6-136 through 6-139.)

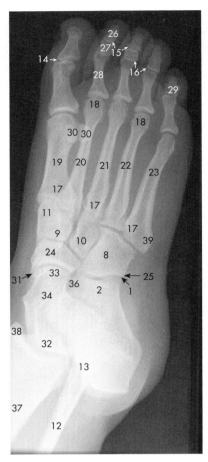

FIG. 6-138 Oblique foot radiograph. (See Key for Figures 6-136 through 6-139.)

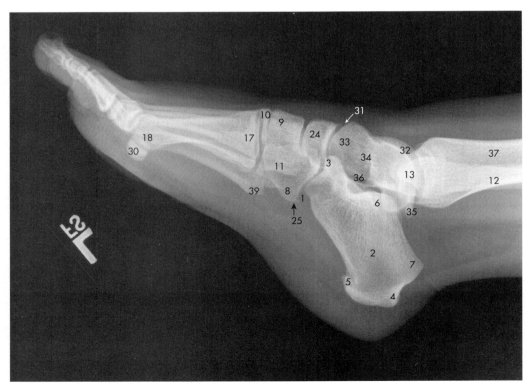

FIG. 6-139 Lateral foot radiograph. (See Key for Figures 6-136 through 6-139.)

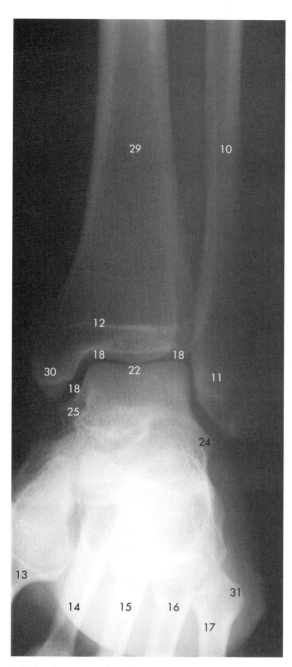

FIG. 6-140 Anteroposterior ankle radiograph. (See Key for Figures 6-140 through 6-149.)

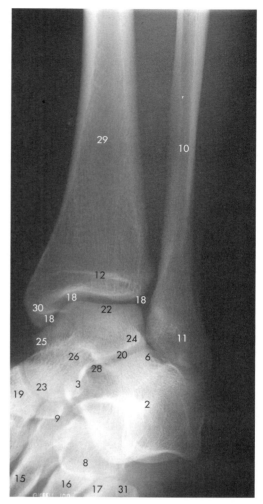

FIG. 6-141 Oblique ankle radiograph. (See Key for Figures 6-140 through 6-149.)

KEY FOR FIGURES 6-140 THROUGH 6-149

1. Calcaneocuboid joint
2. Calcaneus
3. Calcaneus, anterior tubercle
4. Calcaneus, insertion of the Achilles' tendon
5. Calcaneus, insertion of the plantar aponeurosis
6. Calcaneus, middle tubercle
7. Calcaneus, posterior tubercle
8. Cuboid
9. Cuneiform, overlapping lateral, intermediate, and medial
10. Fibula, diaphysis
11. Fibula, lateral malleolus
12. Growth line/physis line
13. Metatarsal, first
14. Metatarsal, second
15. Metatarsal, third
16. Metatarsal, fourth
17. Metatarsal, fifth
18. Mortise joint/talocrural joint
19. Navicular
20. Subtalar joint
21. Talonavicular joint
22. Talus, dome/trochlea
23. Talus, head
24. Talus, lateral process
25. Talus, medial process
26. Talus, neck
27. Talus, posterior process
28. Tarsal sinus
29. Tibia, diaphysis
30. Tibia, medial malleolus
31. Tuberosity of the fifth metatarsal

KEY FOR FIGURES 6-140 THROUGH 6-149

1. Calcaneocuboid joint;
2. Calcaneus
3. Calcaneus, anterior tubercle
4. Calcaneus, insertion of the Achilles' tendon
5. Calcaneus, insertion of the plantar aponeurosis
6. Calcaneus, middle tubercle
7. Calcaneus, posterior tubercle
8. Cuboid
9. Cuneiform, overlapping lateral, intermediate, and medial
10. Fibula, diaphysis
11. Fibula, lateral malleolus
12. Growth line/physis line
13. Metatarsal, firs
14. Metatarsal, second
15. Metatarsal, third
16. Metatarsal, fourth
17. Metatarsal, fifth
18. Mortise joint/talocrural joint
19. Navicular
20. Subtalar joint
21. Talonavicular joint
22. Talus, dome/trochlea
23. Talus, head
24. Talus, lateral process
25. Talus, medial process
26. Talus, neck
27. Talus, posterior process
28. Tarsal sinus
29. Tibia, diaphysis
30. Tibia, medial malleolus
31. Tuberosity of the fifth metatarsal

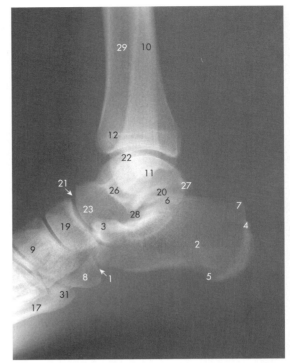

FIG. 6-142   Lateral ankle radiograph. (See Key for Figures 6-140 through 6-149.)

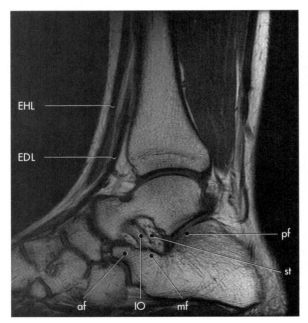

FIG. 6-143   Sagittal magnetic resonance imaging scan of the ankle. (See Key for Figures 6-140 through 6-149.)(From Kelley LL: Sectional anatomy for imaging professionals, St Louis, 1997, Mosby.)

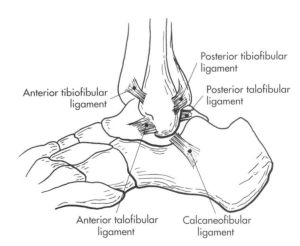

FIG. 6-144   Lateral ligaments of the ankle. (See Key for Figures 6-140 through 6-149.) (From Kelley LL: Sectional anatomy for imaging professionals, St Louis, 1997, Mosby.)

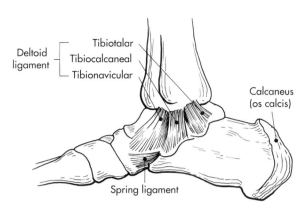

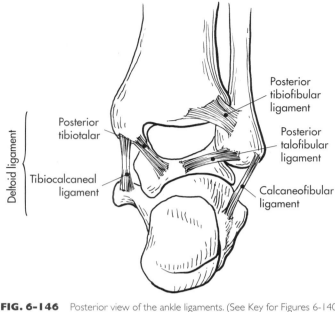

FIG. 6-145 Medial view of the ankle with deltoid ligaments. (See Key for Figures 6-140 through 6-149.) (From Kelley LL: Sectional anatomy for imaging professionals, St Louis, 1997, Mosby.)

FIG. 6-146 Posterior view of the ankle ligaments. (See Key for Figures 6-140 through 6-149.) (From Kelley LL: Sectional anatomy for imaging professionals, St Louis, 1997, Mosby.)

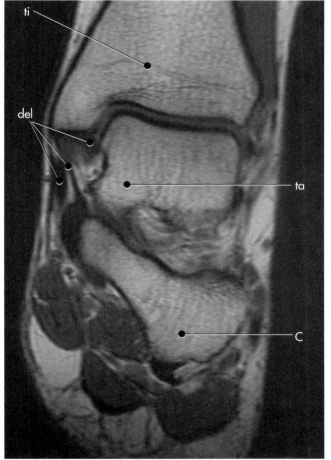

FIG. 6-147 Coronal magnetic resonance imaging scan of the ankle with deltoid ligaments. (See Key for Figures 6-140 through 6-149.) (From Kelley LL: Sectional anatomy for imaging professionals, St Louis, 1997, Mosby.)

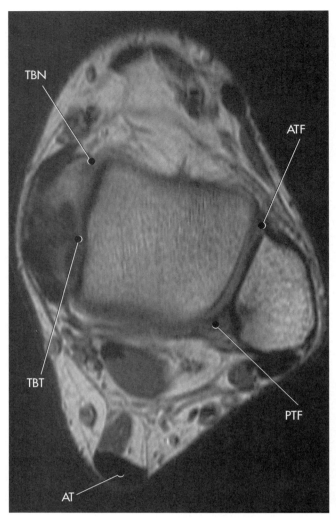

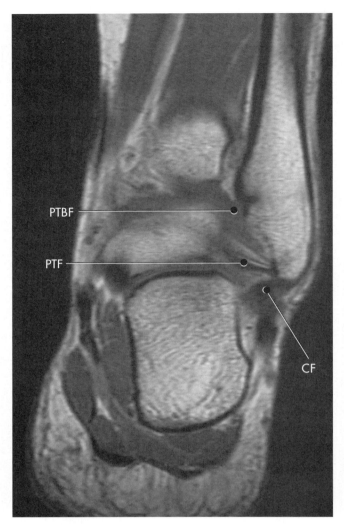

FIG. 6-148 Axial magnetic resonance imaging scan of the ankle with ligaments. (See Key for Figures 6-140 through 6-149.) (From Kelley LL: Sectional anatomy for imaging professionals, St Louis, 1997, Mosby.)

FIG. 6-149 Coronal magnetic resonance imaging scan of the ankle with lateral ligaments. (See Key for Figures 6-140 through 6-149.) (From Kelley LL: Sectional anatomy for imaging professionals, St Louis, 1997, Mosby.)

chapter *7*

Normal Variants

DENNIS M. MARCHIORI

Skeletal variants, anomalies, and defects are commonly encountered findings of plain film interpretation. A general understanding of their presentation is important because many appear to be similar to more aggressive pathologic disease states and traumas. Therefore successfully identifying a normal variant saves time, effort, and expense.

Tables 7-1 through 7-7 list selected variants, anomalies, and other defects by region. The selected entries are by no means exhaustive. Interested readers are referred to the extensive volumes by others (Keats TE: Atlas of normal variants that may simulate disease, St Louis, 2001, Mosby; Schmidt H et al: Kohler/Zimmer borderlands of the normal and early pathologic in skeletal pathology, New York, 1993, Thieme Medical Publishers).

TABLE 7-1
Skeletal Variants, Anomalies, and Defects of the Skull

Variant/Artifact	Comments
Artifacts (Figs. 7-1 and 7-2)	Common artifacts visualized are hearing aids, hairpins, dental fillings, etc.
Arnold-Chiari malformation	Arnold-Chiari malformation describes the presence of a myelomeningocele with varying degrees of caudal displacement of the cerebellar tonsils and hindbrain. It is discussed more fully in Chapter 33.
Basilar invagination (Fig. 7-3)	Basilar invagination describes a cephalic deformity of the margins of the foramen magnum with resulting deformity of the condyles and skull base (basilar impression). Although some authors separate the upward displacement of the foramen magnum (basilar invagination) from the resulting deformity of the skull base (basilar impression), most sources use the terms as synonyms. The presentation is either primary (congenital syndromes such as Klippel-Feil syndrome and Arnold-Chiari malformation) or acquired (bone softening pathologies such as osteomalacia, fibrous dysplasia, or Paget's disease). Primary basilar impression is also known as Bull-Nixon syndrome. The deformity is identified on the lateral projection by constructing lines from the posterior extreme of the hard palate to either the posterior margin of the foramen magnum (Chamberlain's line) or lower margin of the base of the occiput (McGregor's line), and examining the distance between the constructed line and the tip of the odontoid process. (See Chapter 4 for more detail on construction of these roentgenometrics.) In contrast to describing the relationship of the odontoid to the skull base, as is done for basilar invagination, the term *platybasia* (meaning "flat base") describes the morphology of the skull base without using the odontoid as a reference point. Platybasia is assessed by constructing approximations of the hard palate and clivus. If the resulting angle (Martin's basilar angle, see Chapter 4) is greater than 152 degrees, platybasia is present. Basilar impression increases the risk of neurologic damage and circulatory embarrassment.
Cerebral falx calcification	A calcified cerebral falx appears as a single sheet of calcification extending from the frontal bone. It is related to infection, trauma, and normal aging. A multiple layer (lamellar) appearance of calcification is seen in Gorlin syndrome.

Continued

PART ONE Introduction to Imaging

TABLE 7-I cont'd
Skeletal Variants, Anomalies, and Defects of the Skull

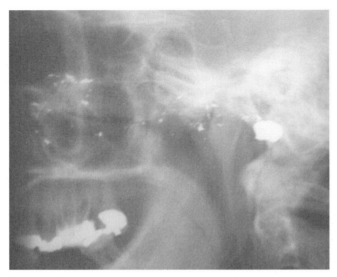

FIG. 7-1 A bullet and related trail of lead fragments is noted in this ambulatory patient who presented to a chiropractor's office.

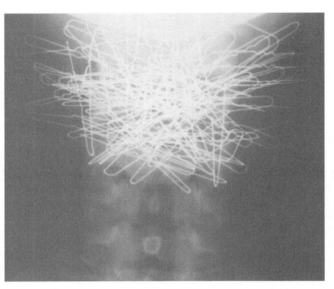

FIG. 7-2 Multiple hair pins obstructing the view of the lower skull. (Courtesy Robert C. Tatum, Davenport, IA.)

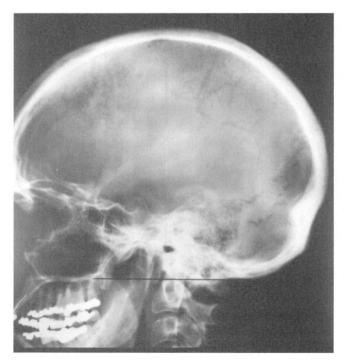

FIG. 7-3 Complete bony assimilation of C1 to occiput (occipitalization) and congenital basilar impression. This is diagnosed by observing the tip of the dens significantly above McGregor's line (in this case >15 mm). This may be associated with Chiari type 1 malformation, and magnetic resonance imaging often is indicated. (Courtesy Tim Mick, Bloomington, MN.)

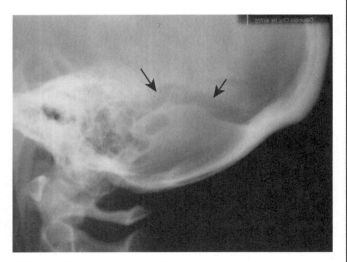

FIG. 7-4 The lateral view of the skull exhibits a radiolucent band representing the dural venous sinus *(arrows)*. (Courtesy Jamie and Lori Kirgis, Columbia City, IN.)

TABLE 7-1 cont'd
Skeletal Variants, Anomalies, and Defects of the Skull

Variant/Artifact	Comments
Choroid plexus calcification	Calcification of the choroid plexus is one of the most common normal intracranial calcifications, nearly always occurring in the lateral ventricles. It is noted as a stippled pattern of calcification located immediately superior to the orbits on a frontal projection and slightly superior and posterior to the pinna of the ear on the lateral film. Usually beginning during the third decade it should be differentiated from the punctuate cortical and linear basal ganglia calcifications that are associated with toxoplasmosis.
Dermoid	Dermoids are small (<1 cm), midline, well-marginated, radiolucent defects of the skull representing a congenital inclusion of ectoderm, mesoderm, and endoderm.
Digital impressions	Digital impressions are shallow, broad grooves on the inner table of the skull corresponding to the adjacent cerebral gyri. They are most conspicuous between 4 and 8 years of age, typically in the parietal bone of children and squamous portion of the temporal bone in adults. Craniosynostosis may cause accentuation of the local digital impressions. In children older than 1 year, an absence of digital impression suggests underdevelopment of the cerebrum.[97]
Doughnut lesion	A doughnut lesion describes a small (<1 cm) radiolucent defect with well-defined surrounding sclerosis and often a central calcification. They are normal variants of little clinical significance and are differentiated from the more clinically relevant button sequestrations by the absence of reported pain and disability.
Dural venous sinus (Fig. 7-4)	A radiolucent defect may be seen in the skull corresponding to the dural venous sinus.
Emissary veins	Emissary veins are normal conduits connecting dural venous sinuses to extracranial venous pathways. Their foramina may appear on radiographs of the skull as unilateral or bilateral radiolucent defects, typically in the frontal, parietal, and occipital bones. Their enlargement suggests elevated intracranial pressure or possibly dural arteriovenous malformation.
Empty sella syndrome (see Fig. 16-8 in Chapter 16)	Empty sella syndrome describes a small, flattened, or absent pituitary gland within a usually enlarged sella turcica. It is caused by a congenital (primary) or acquired (secondary to trauma, surgery, radiation, etc.) defect of the diaphragm sellae that allows an intrasellar extension of the suprasellar arachnoid space. Pulsations of the cerebrospinal fluid are thought to cause enlargement of the sella turcica and compression of the pituitary gland. Secondary empty sella syndrome is common among women who are overweight or have high blood pressure. Symptom expression is highly variable and may include headache, galactorrhea, hyperprolactinemia, dysmenorrhea, visual disturbance, and runny nose. Usually the pituitary function is normal. Primary empty sella syndrome typically is an incidental finding on radiologic imaging of the brain. Patients are usually without symptoms, and pituitary function usually is normal. Rarely, primary empty sella syndrome presents with abnormal facial features, short stature, highly arched palate, and osteosclerosis. Plain film findings demonstrate an enlarged sella turcica (width >16 mm, or depth >12 mm). Computed tomography (CT) and magnetic resonance imaging additionally demonstrate a small or absent pituitary gland.
Encephalocele	An encephalocele is the extension of intracranial tissue through a cranial defect. Usually the defect is congenital. Encephaloceles are most common in the occiput, and may be supratentorial or infratentorial. Ultrasound is used for antenatal evaluation. Magnetic resonance imaging details the type and extent of the lesion. Encephaloceles may be associated with Meckel-Gruber syndrome, microcephaly, cystic dysplastic kidneys, and polydactyly
Frontal sinus hypoplasia (Fig. 7-5)	The frontal sinuses commonly lack symmetry (hypoplasia), or are completely missing on one or both sides (aplasia). Rarely, hypoplasia of the frontal sinuses presents with sinusitis, bronchiectasis, and situs inversus; together this latter triad is known as Kartagener (dyskinetic cilia) syndrome.
Habenular calcification	Habenular calcification appears as a characteristic C-shaped or comma-shaped radiodensity sometimes noted on plain film and commonly noted on CT scans. It is of no clinical significance and is differentiated from pineal gland calcification by its smaller size and C-shaped configuration.

TABLE 7-1 cont'd
Skeletal Variants, Anomalies, and Defects of the Skull

Variant/Artifact	Comments
Hyperostosis frontalis interna (enostosis crani) (Fig. 7-6)	Hyperostosis frontalis interna is an idiopathic thickening of the internal table of the frontal bone. It progresses slowly over time in a bilateral fashion, but spares the midline. The condition is most common in women more than 40 years of age. It is not uncommon for the condition to spread to proximate regions of adjacent bones. If other bones are extensively involved, the term *hyperostosis interna generalisata* is used. Morgagni's-Stewart-Morel syndrome describes the combined presentation of hyperostosis frontalis interna, obesity, and hirsutism and virilism.
Lacunar skull	Lacunar skull (Lückenschädel, craniolacunia) describes an appearance of multiple radiolucent areas of calvarial thinning seen in newborns and infants. The appearance may be seen in association with meningoceles, encephalocele, or Arnold-Chiari malformations. The appearance may lessen or completely resolve within a few years. It is not analogous to the normal cortical sulcal impressions (digital impressions; see the preceding) that are a feature of young children. Also, lacunar skull is in contrast to the "beaten silver" appearance seen with increased intracranial pressure.
Lenticular calcification (Fig. 7-7)	The lens of the eye may calcify as a consequence of injury, inflammation, or old age. It appears as a ring or semicircular shadow in the orbit.[53] Calcifications larger than 1 cm may represent vitreous calcifications.[94]
Metopic suture	The two halves of the frontal bone fuse by 3 years of age. Less than 5% to 10% of individuals may demonstrate a persistent frontal (or metopic) suture. Trigonocephaly refers to premature closure of the frontal suture resulting in a triangular forehead with pinching of the temples laterally.
Occipital vertebra (Fig. 7-8)	Uncommonly, a portion of the caudal occipital somite or cephalic cervical somite detaches, forming a separate ossicle positioned between the occiput and atlas. If the ossicle is located anteriorly between the anterior tubercle of atlas and the occiput, it is termed a proatlas ossicle. These ossicles usually are of no clinical significance
Occipitalization of atlas (Fig. 7-9)	Also known as *assimilation of atlas* or *occipitocervical synostosis,* this anomaly arises from a defect of formation of the most caudal occipital somite resulting in partial or complete fusion of the atlas to the base of the occiput. Occipitalization is the most cephalic example of congenital blocked segmentation. The radiographic features are marked by decreased space between the atlas and the occiput. On sagittal plane flexion and extension radiographs, an occipitalized atlas demonstrates a consistent atlantooccipital space, instead of the typical enlargement of the atlantooccipital space during cervical flexion and narrowing of the same space during cervical extension. Magnetic resonance imaging provides an assessment for the extent of neurologic involvement. When presenting as an isolated phenomenon, occipitalization of atlas generally is viewed as clinically insignificant, although accompanying defects of the transverse atlantal ligament may make stress radiography prudent, especially if congenital blocks of other cervical vertebrae are found. Occipitalization has been associated with limited range of motion, vertigo, unsteady gait, paresthesias, more severe neurologic finding, and even death.[100,101] Also, occipitalization of atlas may present in association with Klippel-Feil syndrome, platybasia, Goldenhar syndrome, and Sturge-Weber syndrome.
Pacchionian granulations	Pacchionian granulations are multiple, nearly circular, smooth, radiolucent, usually symmetric, parasagittal erosions of the inner table of the skull. They are common in the frontal bone and generally of no clinical significance.
Paracondylar processes (Fig. 7-10)	A paracondylar process originates from or adjacent to the occipital condyle and extends inferiorly to or near the transverse process of the atlas. It is of little clinical significance, unless significance synostosis between the atlas and occiput exist that limits range of motion across the occipitoatlantal joint.[49,64] It is differentiated from an epitransverse process that arises in the opposite direction, from the transverse process of the atlas and extends superiorly to the occiput.
Parietal foramina	Parietal foramina are variants presenting as well-marginated, symmetric, parasagittal, radiolucent defects, representing passageways for emissary veins.

TABLE 7-1 cont'd

Skeletal Variants, Anomalies, and Defects of the Skull

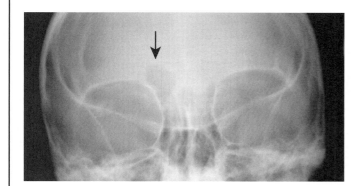

FIG. 7-5 The reading left frontal sinus is small (hypoplasia) *(arrow)* and the right side is missing (aplasia). (Courtesy Maureen Work, Ottawa, IL.)

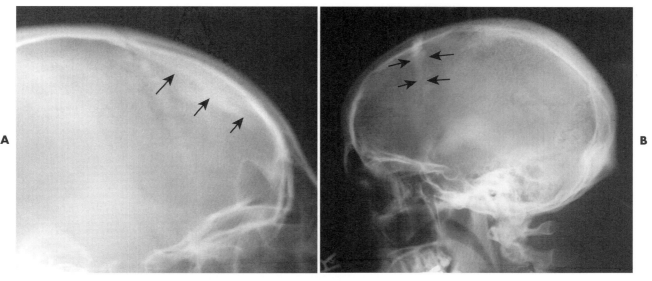

FIG. 7-6 A, The inner table of the frontal bone is thickened *(arrows)* representing a mild expression of hyperostosis frontalis interna. **B,** Similar changes are noted along the margins of the sutures in a different case *(arrows)*. (**A,** Courtesy Steven P. Brownstein, MD, Springfield, NJ; **B,** Courtesy Gary Longmuir, Phoenix, AZ.)

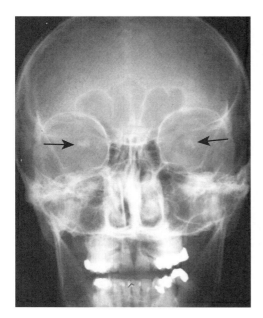

FIG. 7-7 Bilateral small foci of calcification are noted in the lens of the eyes of this 63-year-old man *(arrows)*. (Courtesy Steven P. Brownstein, MD, Springfield, NJ.)

TABLE 7-1 cont'd
Skeletal Variants, Anomalies, and Defects of the Skull

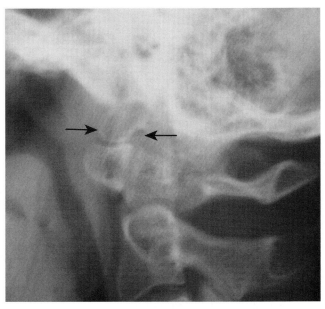

FIG. 7-8   There is a smooth bone projection extending inferiorly from the occiput, similar to a proatlas ossicle, except that it is not separated *(arrows)*. Additionally, a partially formed posterior ponticle is noted along the superior margin of the atlas. (Courtesy Ian D McLean, LeClaire, IA.)

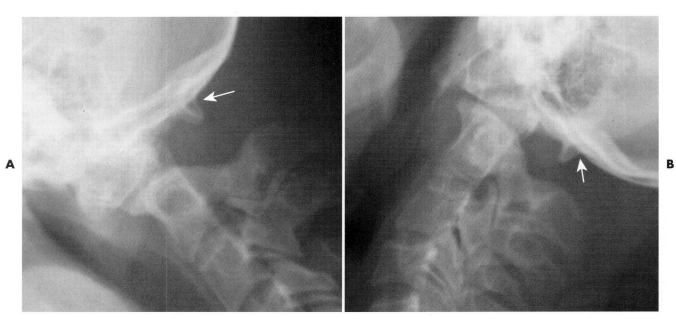

FIG. 7-9   The atlas is fused to the occiput evidenced by a lack of occipitoatlantal interval *(arrow)* on both **A,** the flexion and, **B,** extension radiographs.

TABLE 7-1 cont'd
Skeletal Variants, Anomalies, and Defects of the Skull

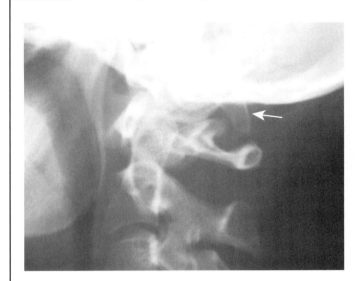

FIG. 7-10 A small, smooth bone projection extends from the base of the occiput toward the posterior tubercle of the atlas *(arrow)*, representing a paracondylar process.

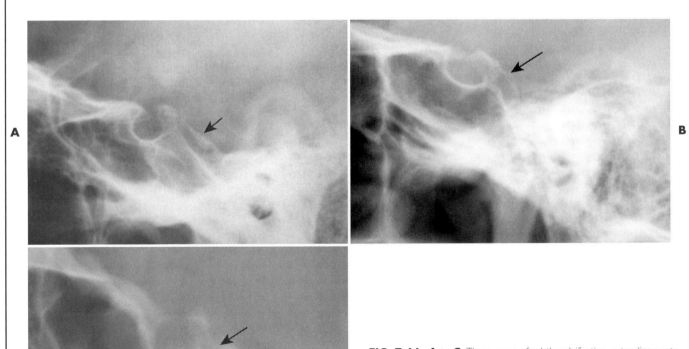

A

B

C

FIG. 7-11 **A** to **C,** Three cases of subtle calcification extending posterior from the free margin of the dorsum sellae, representing calcification in the petroclinoid ligaments *(arrows)*.

Continued

TABLE 7-1 cont'd
Skeletal Variants, Anomalies, and Defects of the Skull

Variant/Artifact	Comments
Petroclinoid ligament calcification (Fig. 7-11)	With calcification the petroclinoid ligaments appear as a horizontal, linear radiodense structure running from the dorsum sella to the petrous portion of the temporal bone, although commonly only the dorsum sella portion of the ligament actually calcifies.
Pineal gland calcification (Fig. 7-12)	Calcification of the pineal gland is present in approximately one third to one half of all adults and is a common finding on the lateral projection of the skull; it is even more common on CT scans of the region. Pineal calcification usually is without clinical significance; however, in children the finding is more concerning, at times suggesting the presence of neoplasm. The calcification may appear amorphous or homogenously radiodense, typically measuring 3 to 5 mm in size. Pinealoma is suggested by size greater than 1 cm. Displacement of the calcified pineal gland from its typical midline position, as noted on a frontal projection, is an indirect sign of a space-occupying lesion within the skull.[31]
Stylohyoid ligament ossification (Figs. 7-13 and 7-14)	Approximately 4% of the general population demonstrates elongated styloid processes and calcification of the stylohyoid ligaments, usually representing nothing more than an anatomic variant. However, rarely (estimated prevalence of 0.2 to 0.4%) the stylohyoid ligament thickens and ossifies, creating a more clinically relevant presentation (known as Eagle syndrome) as the enlarged structure compresses the external carotid artery, producing pain in the orbit and temporal region.[75] The ossification may result from persistence of a cartilaginous anlage. Associated symptoms include foreign body sensation in the throat, dysphagia, and intermittent facial pain.[6] Surgical consultation may be advised if related symptoms are identified.
Wormian (intrasutural or suture) bones (Fig. 7-15)	Wormian bones are small, irregular islands of bone located within sutures of the skull. The lambdoidal, posterior sagittal, and tympanosquamosal sutures are most often involved. They may regress into the adjacent bone over time. Although they commonly represent nothing more than a normal variant. There are diseases associated with wormian bones that are summarized in Chapter 16.

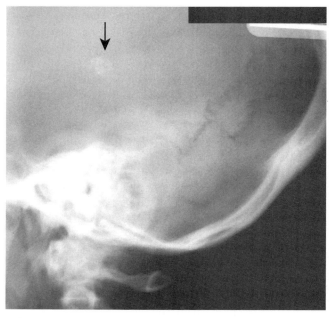

FIG. 7-12 A small focus of calcification is noted in the pineal gland (*arrow*).

TABLE 7-1 cont'd
Skeletal Variants, Anomalies, and Defects of the Skull

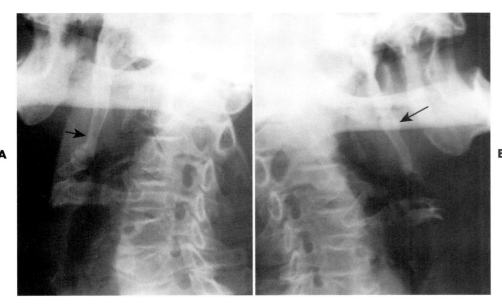

A

B

FIG. 7-13 **A** and **B,** Ossification of the stylohyoid ligament is noted as a linear radiodense shadow (*arrows*) on these oblique projections of the cervical spine.

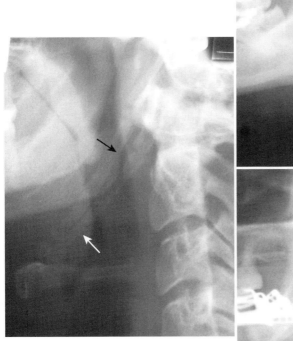

A

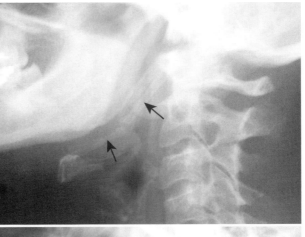

B

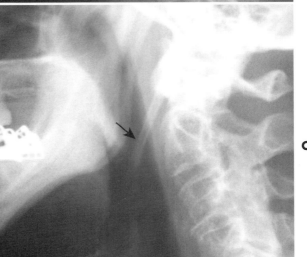

C

FIG. 7-14 **A** through **C,** Three cases of stylohyoid ligament ossification (*arrows*).

TABLE 7-1 cont'd
Skeletal Variants, Anomalies, and Defects of the Skull

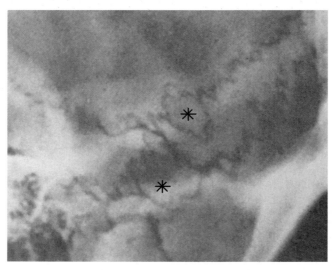

FIG. 7-15   Wormian (or intersutural) bones appearing as islands of bone formed within a skull fissure (*asterisks*).

TABLE 7-2
Skeletal Variants, Anomalies, Defects, and Artifacts of the Cervical, Thoracic, and Lumbar Spine

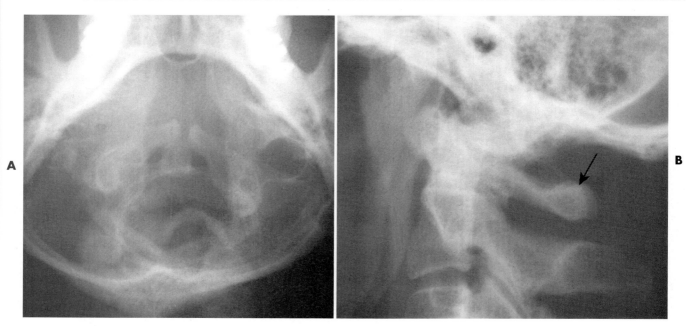

FIG. 7-16   **A,** The cervical base posterior projection demonstrates a midline cleft in the anterior and posterior arches of the atlas. **B,** The lack of a spinal laminal line confirms the cleft of the posterior arch of the atlas (*arrow*).

TABLE 7-2 cont'd
Skeletal Variants, Anomalies, Defects, and Artifacts of the Cervical, Thoracic, and Lumbar Spine

Variant/Artifact	Comments
Atlas	
Agenesis of the anterior arch of the atlas (Figs. 7-16 and 7-17)	Agenesis of the anterior arch of the atlas has been reported extremely rarely. Hypoplasia of the anterior arch is relatively more common but remains rare.
Agenesis of the posterior arch of the atlas (Figs. 7-18 and 7-19)	The posterior arch of the atlas begins to form from a secondary center of ossification during the second year of life, completely forming by the age of 3 or 4. Although typically viewed as a normal variant, there is a question of an associated defect of the transverse atlantal ligament, warranting flexion-extension radiographs in those affected. Enlargement of the C2 spinous process (megaspinous of C2) or enlargement of the anterior tubercle of atlas may be accompanying defects of agenesis of the posterior arch of the atlas. The latter is believed to be a stress response to the undeveloped portion of the atlas.
Atlantoaxial pseudojoint	Uncommonly the posterior tubercle of the atlas approximates the superior margin of the spinous process of C2. The resulting frictional sclerosis has been referred to as a *pseudojoint* or *Baastrup disease of the cervical spine.* Baastrup disease is more common to the lumbar spine associated with degenerative reduction of the disc height with resulting approximation of the spinous processes.
Down syndrome	Approximately 6% to 20% of those with Down syndrome demonstrate laxity of the transverse atlantal ligament and the ligaments from the lateral masses of the atlas to the occipital condyles,[109] jeopardizing the stability of the upper cervical spine and possibly resulting in irreversible spinal cord damage. Further discussion of this presentation is provided in Chapter 8.
Epitransverse process (Figs. 7-20 and 7-21)	An epitransverse (supratransverse) process arises from the superior aspect of the transverse process of the atlas and extends superiorly to or near the occiput.[49,64] It is of little clinical significance unless significance synostosis between the atlas and occiput exists that limits range of motion across the occipitoatlantal joint. It is opposite to a paracondylar process, which arises near or at the occipital condyle and extends inferiorly to the transverse process of the atlas.
Increased atlantodental interval (Figs. 7-22 and 7-23)	The atlantodental interval (ADI) defines the joint space created by the posterior surface of the anterior tubercle of the atlas and the anterior margin of the odontoid process. Normally the space measures less than 3 mm in adults, and less than 5 mm in children because of their greater joint laxity. Enlargement of the ADI indicates joint instability secondary to trauma, inflammatory joint disease, congenital defect, and so on. (See Chapter 17 for a more detailed differential list.) As a normal variant, the ADI may appear V-shaped, opened superiorly. In such cases the lower margin of the joint should be used as a reference to measure the joint space. Sagittal plane flexion-extension radiographs may be used to stress the joint on equivocal cases of instability.
Posterior ponticle of the atlas (Figs. 7-24 and 7-25)	A posterior ponticle (also known as *ponticulus posticus, foramen arcuale, Kimmerle anomaly,* or *Kimmerle variant*) represents a small bridge of bone arching over the arcuate rim of the atlas (forming an arcuate foramen). Although traditionally attributed to ossification of the anterior margin of the atlantooccipital membrane, some believe it to represent well-organized bone formed from a distinct ossification center.[86] It is seen in approximately 15% of the general population and often is bilateral. It is more common among women when it presents as a partial bridge of bone, and more common in men as a complete bridge of bone between the lateral mass and posterior arch.[104] Although controversial, it is generally felt to be a variant of normal. Associations with headaches, Barr-Liéou syndrome, photophobia, and migraine have been reported.[4,16] Also, given that the vertebral artery passes through the defect, there is some concern for ischemia of the posterior cerebral circulation. Posterior ponticles are visualized on lateral or oblique cervical projections. Rarely a lateral variation, known as *lateral ponticle,* is seen on the anteroposterior open-mouth projection as an osseous bridge from the superior-lateral margin of the lateral mass of atlas to the lateral portion of the transverse process of the atlas.

Continued

TABLE 7-2 cont'd
Skeletal Variants, Anomalies, Defects, and Artifacts of the Cervical, Thoracic, and Lumbar Spine

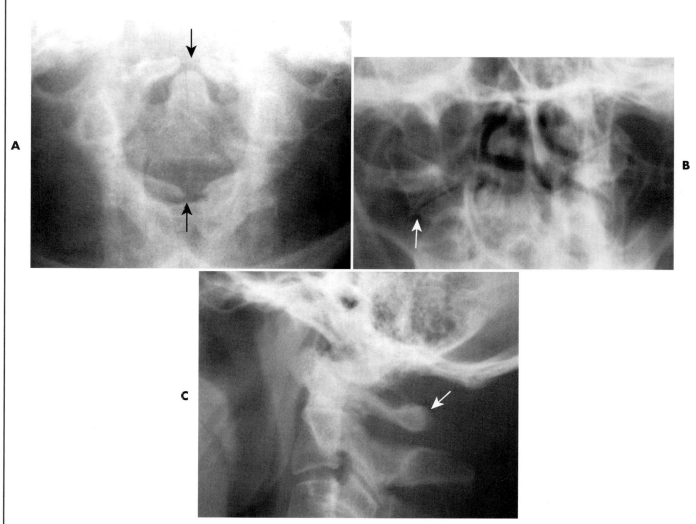

FIG. 7-17 Cleft of the anterior and posterior arch of the atlas. **A,** The cervical base posterior projection reveals a midline cleft in both the anterior and posterior arch of the atlas *(arrows)*. **B,** The anteroposterior open-mouth projection exhibits related lateral translation of the atlas' lateral masses secondary to the midline arch defects *(arrow)*. **C,** The lateral projection details absence of the spinolaminar line *(arrow)*. (Courtesy Kevin Cunningham, Eldridge, IA.)

TABLE 7-2 cont'd
Skeletal Variants, Anomalies, Defects, and Artifacts of the Cervical, Thoracic, and Lumbar Spine

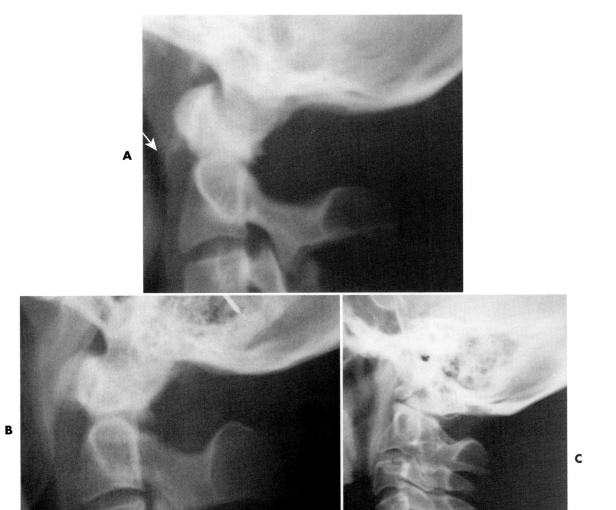

FIG. 7-18 Three patients in whom the posterior arch of the atlas failed to form. **A,** The first patient also demonstrates ossification of the stylohyoid ligament *(arrow).* All three patients also demonstrate the commonly associated finding of an enlarged spinous tubercle at C2 (most prominent in **B**). **C,** The odontoid process in this case is hypoplastic. (**A,** Courtesy William E. Litterer, Elizabeth, NJ; **B,** Courtesy Ron Firth, East Moline, IL.)

Continued

TABLE 7-2 cont'd

Skeletal Variants, Anomalies, Defects, and Artifacts of the Cervical, Thoracic, and Lumbar Spine

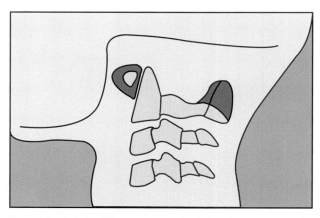

FIG. 7-19   Aplasia of the posterior arch of the atlas is often associated with a hyperplasia of the anterior tubercle of the atlas and the spinous process of C2 (megaspinous).

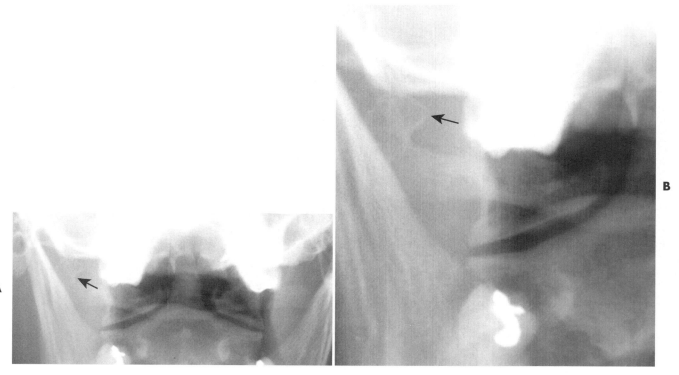

FIG. 7-20   A 27-year-old man with an epitransverse process extending superiorly from, **A,** the right transverse process of the atlas and, **B,** close-up view of the defect *(arrows)*. (Courtesy, J Todd Bish, New Bethlehem, PA.)

TABLE 7-2 cont'd

Skeletal Variants, Anomalies, Defects, and Artifacts of the Cervical, Thoracic, and Lumbar Spine

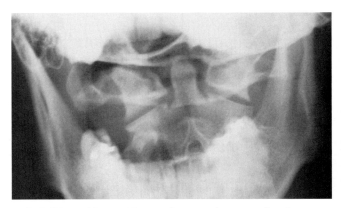

FIG. 7-21 A 25-year-old man demonstrating a small epitransverse process extending superiorly from the reading left transverse process. (Courtesy Jay Brammier, Durant, IA.)

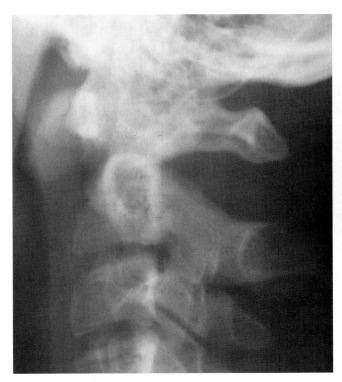

FIG. 7-22 A 16-year-old male patient demonstrating a superior wedged or V-shaped atlantodental interval (ADI). Typically the ADI should not exceed 3 mm in an adult or 5 mm in a child, measured on a 72-inch focal film distance lateral cervical projection. At times, as is the case here, the ADI demonstrates a wedge-shaped appearance that is open to the superior. The measure of the ADI should be taken at the base of the interval to avoid the influence of the variant wedged shape of the joint. An enlarged ADI suggests atlantoaxial instability secondary to trauma, Down syndrome, inflammatory arthritide, and so on.

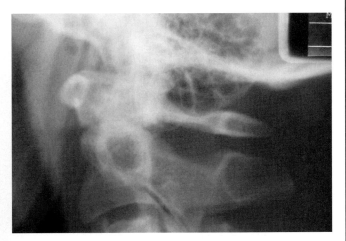

FIG. 7-23 The atlantodental interval measures 5 mm in this 25-year-old male patient. The enlarged measure is secondary to cervical trauma following an automobile accident. (Courtesy Frank C. Miramonti, Mt. Clemens, MI.)

Continued

TABLE 7-2 cont'd
Skeletal Variants, Anomalies, Defects, and Artifacts of the Cervical, Thoracic, and Lumbar Spine

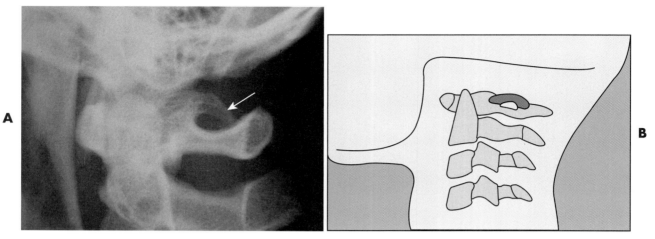

FIG. 7-24 **A** and **B,** Ponticulus posticus is an anomalous bar of bone across the superior margin of the posterior arch of the atlas, forming an arcuate foramen from the normal arcuate rim *(arrow).*

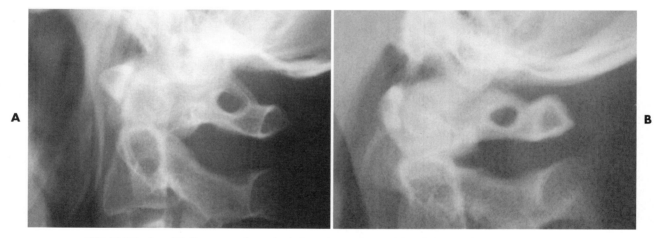

FIG. 7-25 **A** and **B,** Two cases of completely formed posterior ponticles of the atlas, forming arcuate foramen from arcuate rims.

TABLE 7-2 cont'd
Skeletal Variants, Anomalies, Defects, and Artifacts of the Cervical, Thoracic, and Lumbar Spine

Variant/Artifact	Comments
Spina bifida occulta (Fig. 7-26)	Spina bifida is a generalized term for congenital posterior midline defects of spine, alternatively known as spinal dysraphism, spondyloschisis, posterior rachischisis, or neural tube defects. Approximately 5% to 10% of the general population may have spina bifida occulta, the mildest form of midline defect. Spina bifida occulta usually is clinically insignificant; however, rarely (<0.1%) it may be associated with symptoms and other anatomic findings such as spinal lipomas, syringomyelia, and diastematomyelia. Rarely spina bifida occulta is associated with cervical spondylolisthesis, usually at C6. Spina bifida occulta is most common to the posterior arch of atlas or vertebral arch of S1, presenting as missing spinolaminar lines on lateral radiographic projections and as incomplete fusion of the posterior arch on the frontal projections. A complete discussion of this condition is found in Chapter 8.
Axis	
Odontoid process agenesis (Fig. 7-27)	Rarely a defect of ossification of the odontoid will result in an absent (agenesis) or small (hypoplasia) odontoid process of C2. Resulting instability of the atlantoaxial joint causes concern for spinal stenosis and spinal cord insult. Sudden death has been reported secondary to minor trauma. Atlantoaxial instability is more common among those with Down syndrome, Klippel-Feil syndrome, and skeletal dysplasias. The defect is well visualized on anteroposterior open-mouth projections. Computed tomography offers definitive evaluation.
Os odontoideum (Figs. 7-28 to 7-31)	Persistence of the odontoid synchondrosis leads to the formation of a separate odontoid bone (os odontoideum) instead of a normally united odontoid process. The underlying mechanism of the defect is disputed, with both developmental[57] and acquired[36] etiologies proposed. It is a clinically significant defect, potentiating cord pressure related to atlantoaxial instability. The defect is well visualized on the anteroposterior open-mouth projection, and noted to a lesser extent on the lateral cervical projection. See Chapter 8 for complete discussion of the os odontoideum.
Os terminale (Figs. 7-32 and 7-33)	The tip of the odontoid process forms from a secondary center of ossification that presents at 3 years of age and fuses to the odontoid process by 12 years. Rarely the tip of the odontoid fails to unite, creating an os terminale (also known as a Bergmann defect). It should not be mistaken for a fracture, which demonstrates irregular margins, or an os odontoideum, which occurs lower. On the anteroposterior open-mouth projection, the os terminale appears as a smooth-bordered round, oval, diamond-shaped ossicle separated from and cephalic to the odontoid process.
Pseudosubluxation of C2	Typically, significant vertebral misalignment raises concerns for trauma, advanced degeneration, and instability. However, in children and teenagers under the age of 15 it is common to see significant anterolisthesis of 2 mm or more at C2 on C3 (and less common at C3 on C4) without any signs of trauma or degeneration. The finding is believed to be the result of immature muscles and other connective tissues present in the young. Pseudosubluxation of C2 is seen only on lateral cervical projections that demonstrate a neutral or flexion position of the cervical spine. Pseudosubluxations tend to resolve with cervical extension. This helps differentiate a pseudosubluxation from a true injury of the upper cervical spine with resulting anterior displacement of C2 (e.g., hangman fracture). However, caution should be applied to avoid patient extension among those demonstrating significant indicators of fracture. Computed tomography is most helpful in such cases. Also, a Swischuk's line may be useful to differentiate pseudosubluxation from true injury. This line is drawn along the anterior margin of the posterior tubercle of C1 to the posterior aspect of the posterior arch (spinal laminar line) of C3. The posterior aspect of the posterior arch (spinal laminar line) of C2 should be within 1 to 2 mm of Swischuk's line. A true subluxation is indicated by posterior deviations of more than 2 mm and pseudosubluxation by deviation less than 2 mm.[105]
Spina bifida occulta (Fig. 7-34)	Spina bifida occulta is a small midline defect, sometimes occurring at C2. Spina bifida occulta is described in greater detail in the atlas or lumbar entries of this chapter, as well as in Chapter 8.

Continued

TABLE 7-2 cont'd
Skeletal Variants, Anomalies, Defects, and Artifacts of the Cervical, Thoracic, and Lumbar Spine

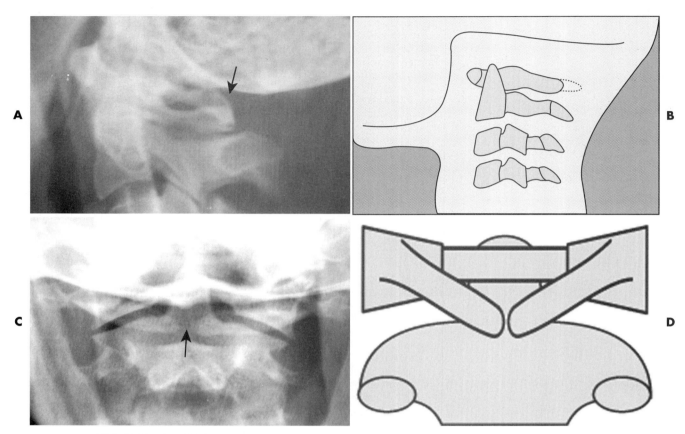

FIG. 7-26 **A** and **B,** Spina bifida occulta of atlas is indicated by the absence of the spinal laminal line in the lateral projection *(arrow)* and incompletely ossified posterior arch as seen in, **C** and **D,** the anteroposterior open-mouth projection. (Courtesy Troy Scheuermann, Farmington, IA.)

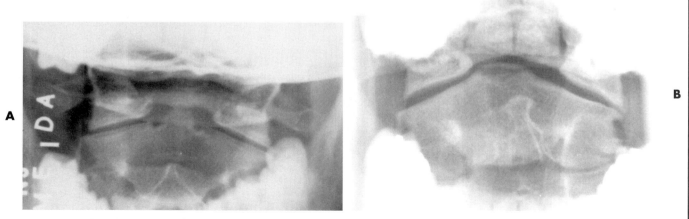

FIG. 7-27 **A** and **B,** Two cases of odontoid agenesis. At times, the incisors obstruct the view of the odontoid, making it difficult to definitively view the odontoid process. (**A,** Courtesy William E. Litterer, Elizabeth, NJ.)

TABLE 7-2 cont'd
Skeletal Variants, Anomalies, Defects, and Artifacts of the Cervical, Thoracic, and Lumbar Spine

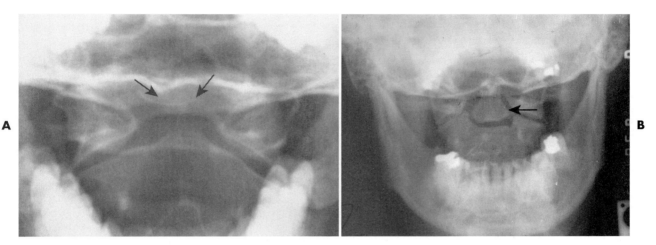

FIG. 7-28 **A** and **B,** The odontoid (arrows) is separated from the body of C2 in both cases. The margins surrounding the odontoid defect are smooth, indicating os odontoideum and mitigating against an acute fracture. (**B,** Courtesy Gary Longmuir, Phoenix, AZ.)

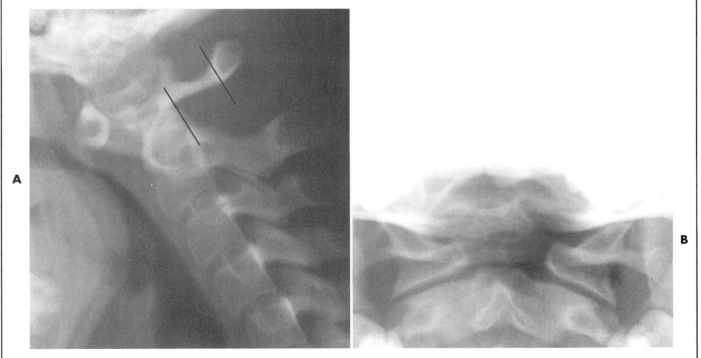

FIG. 7-29 Os odontoideum in a 20-year-old woman. **A** and **B,** The separated odontoid ossicle has smooth margin denoting its chronic presentation. (Courtesy Jeff Stackis, Dubuque, IA.)

Continued

TABLE 7-2 cont'd
Skeletal Variants, Anomalies, Defects, and Artifacts of the Cervical, Thoracic, and Lumbar Spine

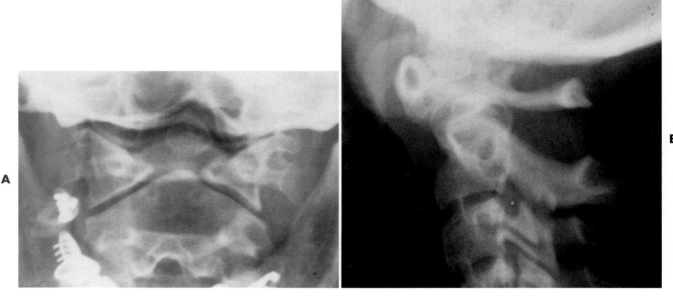

FIG. 7-30   Os odontoideum in a 32-year-old male patient. **A,** The anteroposterior open-mouth projection presents a smooth-margined defect of the odontoid process consistent with an os odontoideum. **B,** In the lateral projection, the posterior atlantodental interval is diminished, raising concern for spinal stenosis and instability. (Courtesy William E. Litterer, Elizabeth, NJ.)

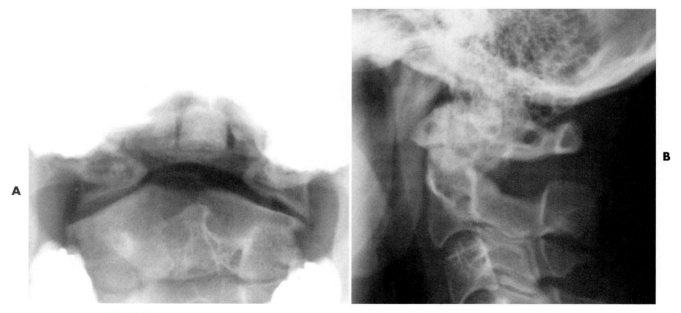

FIG. 7-31   **A** and **B,** Os odontoideum seen as a smooth defect of the odontoid process on the anteroposterior and lateral projection.

TABLE 7-2 cont'd
Skeletal Variants, Anomalies, Defects, and Artifacts of the Cervical, Thoracic, and Lumbar Spine

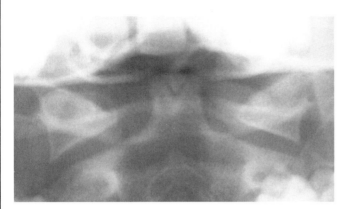

FIG. 7-32 There is a **V**-shaped defect of the tip of the odontoid process consistent with an os terminale. (Courtesy C. Robert Tatum, Davenport, IA.)

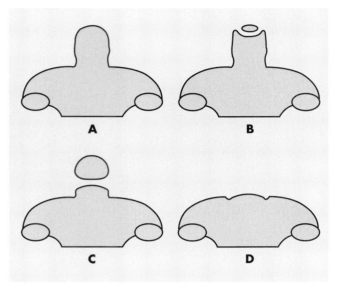

FIG. 7-33 **A,** Normal odontoid process of C2. **B,** Separation of the tip of the odontoid, representing an os terminale (or Bergmann defect). **C,** Separation of the larger portion of the odontoid process, representing an os odontoideum. **D,** Complete absence of the odontoid process secondary to congenital aplasia.

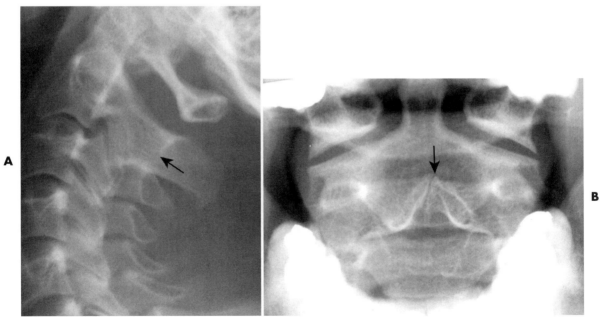

FIG. 7-34 **A,** The lack of spinal laminal line in the lateral projection *(arrow)* corresponds to spina bifida occulta. **B,** The midline spinous process defect is more obvious in the anteroposterior view *(arrow)*. (Courtesy Vince DeBono, Chicago, IL).

Continued

TABLE 7-2 cont'd
Skeletal Variants, Anomalies, Defects, and Artifacts of the Cervical, Thoracic, and Lumbar Spine

Variant/Artifact	Comments
C3-L5	
Agenesis of the pedicle (Figs. 7-35 to 7-40)	Aplasia of the pedicle is uncommon, and represents a unilateral developmental defect of the cartilage anlage dedicated to forming one half of the posterior arch of the vertebrae. Empiric evidence suggests that congenital absence is more common among males and at the L4 vertebrae.[103] In the cervical spine it is seen in decreasing prevalence at C6, C5, C4, and C7. Because aplasia interrupts the structural integrity of the posterior arch, spondylolisthesis may result from this defect. This is a classic finding at C6. The missing pedicle shadow is best seen radiographically, on the oblique projection, but is well demonstrated on the frontal radiograph. In adults, congenital agenesis often presents with an enlarged, radiodense contralateral pedicle, an appearance specific to the condition of aplasia. This is not typically the case among infants and children. If present, the enlarged radiodense contralateral pedicle may provide sufficient proof that the missing pedicle is associated with a congenital etiology as opposed to the more clinically relevant possibility of osteolytic bone disease. Metastasis or multiple myeloma ("winking owl" sign) should be of immediate concern in adult patients. Pathologic destruction of the pedicle by tumor, infection, or erosion seen with neurofibromatosis is not typically associated with hypertrophy or sclerosis of the opposite pedicle. If both pedicles are missing ("blind vertebra"), aggressive bone disease is clinically assumed until proved otherwise. Also, the vertebrae and lamina generally are not affected by developmental aplasia of the pedicle, where aggressive bone disease often has associated bone changes. Wilkinson syndrome describes a sclerotic pedicle with a contralateral pars defect.
Artifacts (Figs. 7-41 and 7-42)	Miscellaneous radiodense foreign objects, surgical implantations, and other features may be present in the field of view. Some of these may include: central venous port, tantalum mesh/hernia repair, portal stents, Pepto-Bismol in the stomach, gastric bypass staples, umbilical rings, gall bladder surgery, renal surgery, abdominal aorta surgery, Greenfield-Kinney filter, and so forth. Overlying anatomy may also mimic the appearance of disease.
Baastrup phenomenon (kissing spines) (Figs. 7-43 and 7-44)	Baastrup phenomenon, also known as *kissing spines,* refers to the approximation and resulting pseudoarthrosis of two or more spinous processes. It occurs secondary to intervertebral disc and posterior joint arthrosis but is also related to increased lumbar lordosis. The pseudoarthrosis is marked by a radiodense sclerotic zone subadjacent to the articulating portion of the spinous processes. In some patients it is postulated to be a source of regional pain. Although it is most common in the lumbar spine, a similar frictional sclerosis has been noted between the posterior tubercle of the atlas and the spinous process of C2.
Block vertebra (Figs. 7-45 to 7-55)	Block vertebra describes a union between adjacent segments. It can be the result of congenital nonsegmentation of vertebral somites during the third to eighth fetal week of life or acquired causes such as infections and surgery. A congenital block vertebra can occur anywhere in the cervical, thoracic, or lumbar region, but is most common to the C2-3 and C5-6 levels. Although several contiguous segments may be involved, usually only two vertebrae are affected. The intervening intervertebral disc may be missing or rudimentary in both a vertical and horizontal dimension, the latter producing a narrowed waist at the junction of the fused segments. Very often the posterior arches of the segments are also fused and the corresponding intervertebral foramina appear prominent.
Butterfly vertebra (Figs. 7-56 to 7-59)	This anomaly describes a persistent midline sagittal cleft of the vertebra body. When viewed from the frontal plane, the separated halves of the vertebra appear like the wings of a butterfly, or the full vertebra, like a sideways hourglass. It is common to note a slight triangular-shaped elevated area of bone that extends from the adjacent endplate of the normal segments above and below the butterfly defect that fits into the sagittal cleft of the anomalous segment. Disagreement exists over whether the configuration is an ossification defect of the right and left primary growth centers of the vertebral body, or results from a failure of notochordal regression. A butterfly vertebra is typically an isolated phenomenon and is of limited clinical significance.
Carotid calcification (Fig. 7-60)	Calcification of the carotid vessel is often seen as an age-related phenomenon. However, vessel calcification does play a role in the development of atherosclerosis. Therefore, when present, a review of the patient's history is advised to exclude clinical features of obstructive vessel disease. Severe calcification, especially in the area of the carotid siphon, correlates to vessel stenosis.

TABLE 7-2 cont'd
Skeletal Variants, Anomalies, Defects, and Artifacts of the Cervical, Thoracic, and Lumbar Spine

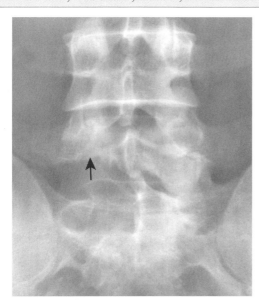

FIG. 7-35 The patient's right pedicle of L5 is missing *(arrow)*, confirmed as congenital etiology although the left pedicle shadow is not hypertrophic as is often the case with congenital absence of the contralateral side. (Courtesy William E. Litterer, Elizabeth, NJ.)

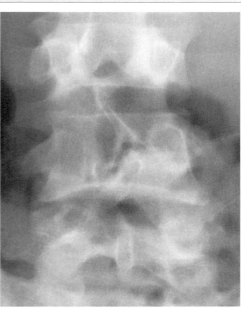

FIG. 7-36 There is congenital absence of the patient's right (reading left) L4 pedicle with a mild degree of contralateral hypertrophy of the left pedicle. (Courtesy Steven P. Brownstein, MD, Springfield, NJ.)

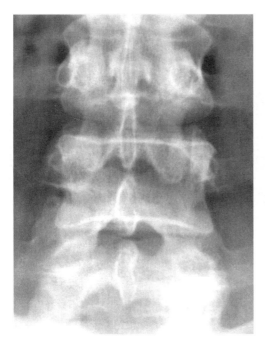

FIG. 7-37 The left pedicle shadow of L4 is not distinct, suggesting aggressive bone disease. (Courtesy Craig Petigout, Coralville, IA.)

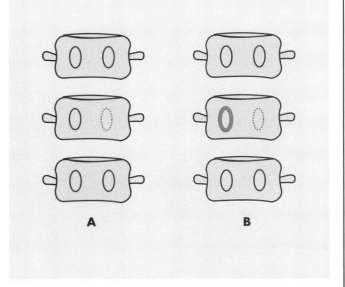

FIG. 7-38 A, Metastatic bone disease often involves the pedicle, causing destruction without hypertrophy of the opposite pedicle. **B,** When the etiology for a missing pedicle is congenital, the absence is most often associated with contralateral hypertrophy.

Continued

TABLE 7-2 cont'd
Skeletal Variants, Anomalies, Defects, and Artifacts of the Cervical, Thoracic, and Lumbar Spine

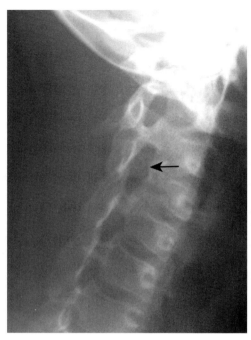

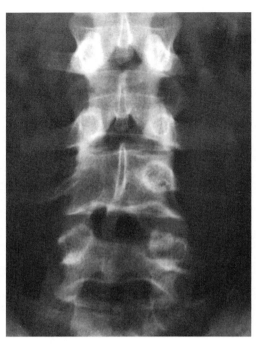

FIG. 7-39 Oblique cervical projection with missing pedicle shadow at C3 *(arrow)*. The intervertebral foramina appear enlarged because of the missing intervening pedicle.

FIG. 7-40 Missing L3 pedicle shadow resulting from congenital defect. (Courtesy Steven P. Brownstein, MD, Springfield, NJ.)

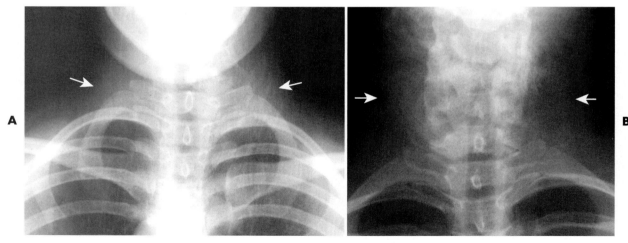

FIG. 7-41 **A** and **B,** The patient's hair may project as a peculiar radiodense shadow in the paravertebral soft tissues on the frontal projection *(arrows)*. (Courtesy Jamie and Lori Kirgis, Columbia City, IN.)

TABLE 7-2 cont'd
Skeletal Variants, Anomalies, Defects, and Artifacts of the Cervical, Thoracic, and Lumbar Spine

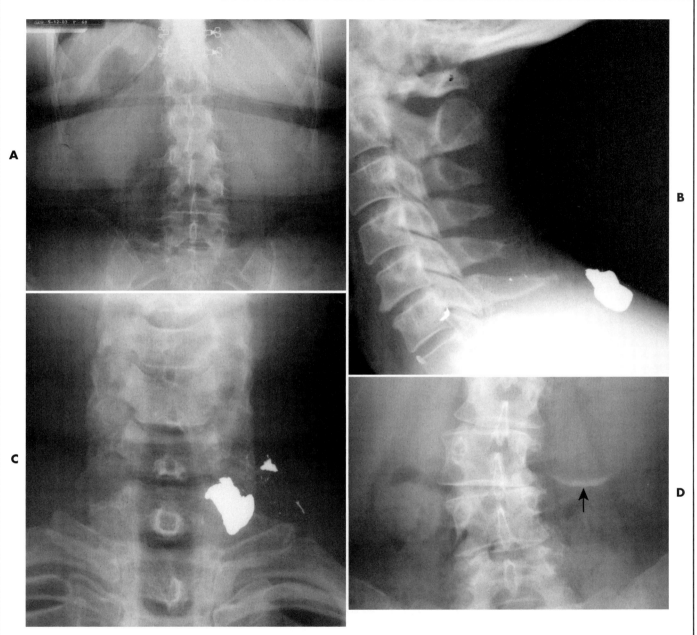

FIG. 7-42 At times, foreign bodies and artifacts can confuse the film interpretation. Some less confusing shadows include, **A,** skin folds; **B** and **C,** bullet; and, **D,** Pepto-Bismol in the body of the stomach (arrow). (**A,** Courtesy Brian Frank, Sunnyland, IL.)

Continued

TABLE 7-2 cont'd
Skeletal Variants, Anomalies, Defects, and Artifacts of the Cervical, Thoracic, and Lumbar Spine

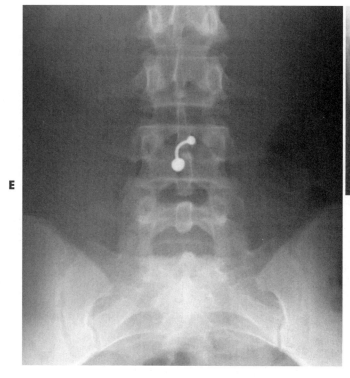

E

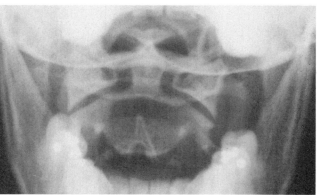

F

FIG. 7-42 cont'd   Other shadows include an, **E,** umbilical ring; and, **F,** anteroposterior open-mouth projection where the lip projects as a gray oval mass immediately inferior to the reading right transverse process of the atlas. (**E,** Courtesy Brian Frank, Sunnyland, IL.)

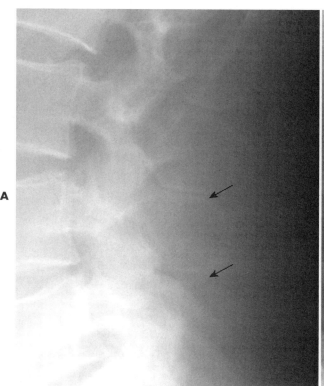

A

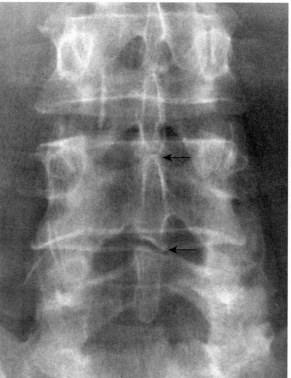

B

FIG. 7-43   **A** and **B,** These lower lumbar segments exhibit sclerosis and close approximation of the adjacent margins of the spinous processes as a feature of pseudoarthrosis (Baastrup disease) *(arrows)*.

TABLE 7-2 cont'd
Skeletal Variants, Anomalies, Defects, and Artifacts of the Cervical, Thoracic, and Lumbar Spine

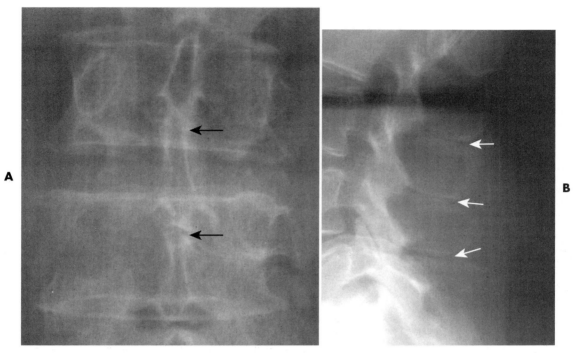

FIG. 7-44 **A** and **B,** Interspinous arthrosis (Baastrup disease) is noted by sclerotic margins of adjacent spinous processes of the lower lumbar spine *(arrows).*

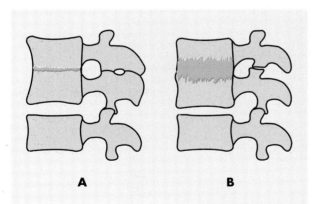

FIG. 7-45 **A,** Block segments are either congenital or acquired. **B,** Acquired segments are secondary to surgery or pathology. A congenital block segment often has a "wasp waist" transverse narrowing secondary to disc hypoplasia, commonly exhibits fusion of the posterior arch, and sometimes has a prominent appearance of the intervertebral foramen on the lateral projection. By contrast, surgical or pathologic block segments tend to appear more columnar, not as an hourglass, as do congenital block segments.

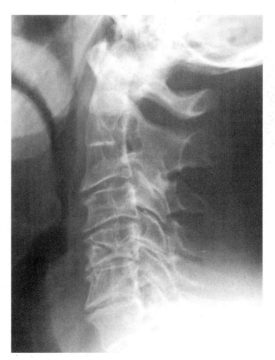

FIG. 7-46 Congenital block segment of C2-3 marked by a hypoplastic intervertebral disc, fusion of the posterior elements, prominent intervertebral foramina, and anterior concavity of the vertebral bodies. Moderate disc degeneration is noted from C3 to C7 by the degenerative osteophytes and thin intervertebral disc spaces. (Courtesy William E. Litterer, Elizabeth, NJ.)

PART ONE
Introduction to Imaging

Continued

TABLE 7-2 cont'd
Skeletal Variants, Anomalies, Defects, and Artifacts of the Cervical, Thoracic, and Lumbar Spine

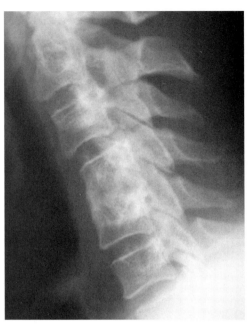

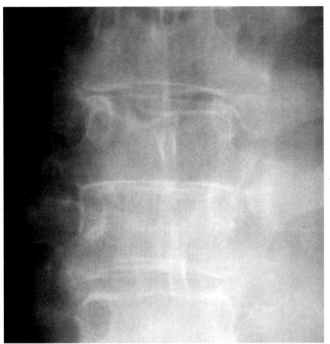

FIG. 7-47   Surgical block segment of C4-5. Surgical blocks appear columnar and are slightly taller than congenital block segments. Also, a patient history of surgery is helpful.

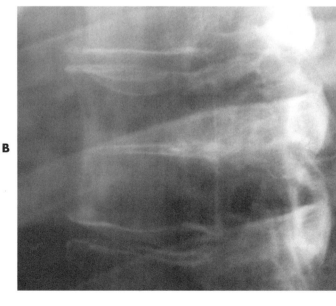

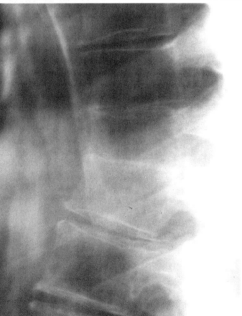

FIG. 7-48   **A** and **B,** A 48-year-old male patient exhibiting a congenital block segment of two middle thoracic vertebrae. **C,** Similar features are noted in a second patient.

TABLE 7-2 cont'd
Skeletal Variants, Anomalies, Defects, and Artifacts of the Cervical, Thoracic, and Lumbar Spine

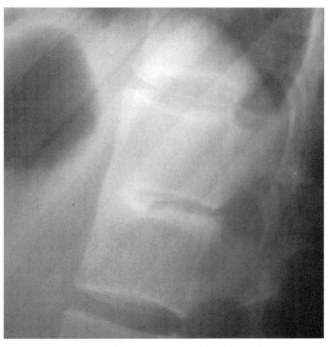

FIG. 7-49   Block segment created by hypoplasia of the T12 intervertebral disc.

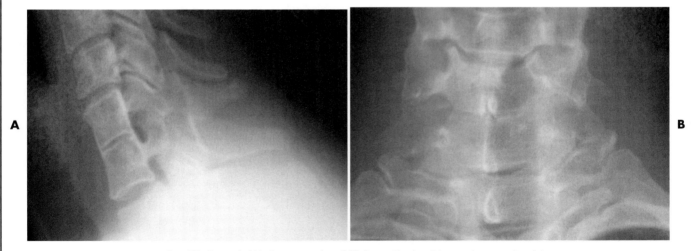

FIG. 7-50   **A** and **B,** Congenital block segmentation of C5-6 noted by the slight anterior concavity of the segments, hypoplastic disc space, prominent intervertebral foramina, and fused posterior arch.

Continued

TABLE 7-2 cont'd
Skeletal Variants, Anomalies, Defects, and Artifacts of the Cervical, Thoracic, and Lumbar Spine

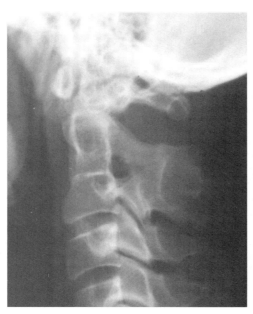

FIG. 7-51 Two congenital defects of segmentation, the first presenting at occiput-atlas and the second at C2-3. As exhibited in this case, it is not uncommon to see two levels of segmentation defect.

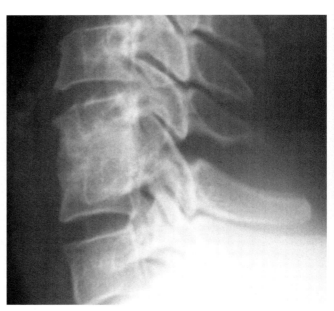

FIG. 7-52 Surgical block segment of C5-6. Notice the columnar appearance of the segment and preserved posterior joint space. (Courtesy Frank C. Miramonti, Mt Clemens, MI.)

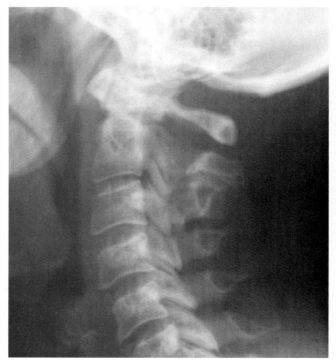

FIG. 7-53 Partial congenital block segment of C2-3 with an atypical presentation of fused posterior arch and near-normal formation of the intervertebral joint; there is only slight vertical hypoplasia of the intervertebral disc. (Courtesy Troy Scheuermann, Farmington, IA.)

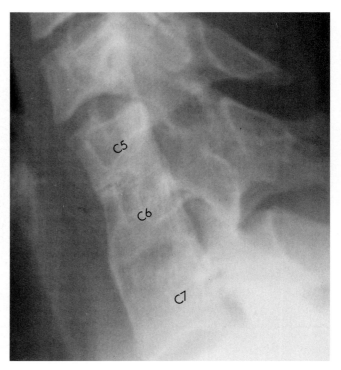

FIG. 7-54 Mixed presentation of a congenital block segment at C5-6 and surgical block segment at C6-7. Notice that the congenital block segment has an hourglass appearance from the anterior vertebral body concavity, in contrast to the more columnar appearance of the surgical block. (Courtesy, William E. Litterer, Elizabeth, NJ.)

TABLE 7-2 cont'd
Skeletal Variants, Anomalies, Defects, and Artifacts of the Cervical, Thoracic, and Lumbar Spine

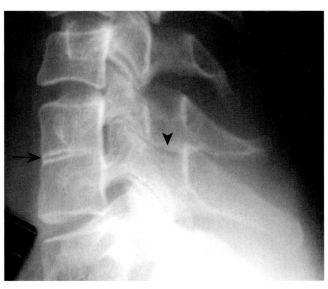

FIG. 7-55 Congenital block segment of C5-6 with minimal anterior concavity of the segment, hypoplasia of the intervertebral disc space *(arrow)*, and partial fusion of the posterior joints *(arrowhead)*.

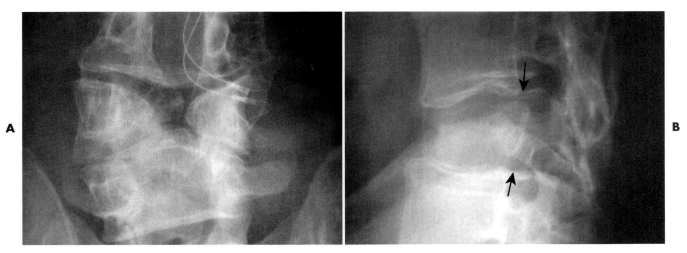

FIG. 7-56 **A,** Anteroposterior projection demonstrates a middle sagittal cleft and triangular halves of the vertebra representing a butterfly vertebra. **B,** The vertebra appears trapezoidal in the lateral projection. Notice that the butterfly segment is posteriorly displaced *(arrows)*.

Continued

TABLE 7-2 cont'd
Skeletal Variants, Anomalies, Defects, and Artifacts of the Cervical, Thoracic, and Lumbar Spine

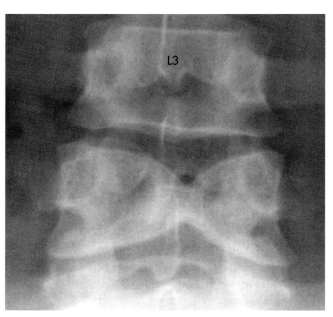

FIG. 7-57   Anteroposterior radiograph demonstrates a butterfly vertebra that appears with a central vertical cleft and mirror image triangular appearance of the right and left halves of the L4 segment. Notice the slight ridge deformity of the adjacent segments that forms into the sagittal cleft. (Courtesy William E. Litterer, Elizabeth, NJ.)

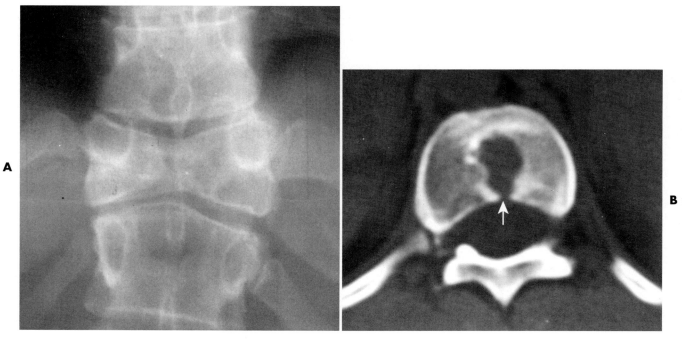

FIG. 7-58   Butterfly vertebrae at T11 noted on, **A,** the anteroposterior (AP) thoracolumbar projection and, **B,** corresponding computed tomography scan *(arrow)*. Notice the rhomboid shape of the adjacent segments on the AP radiographs as the adjacent vertebrae remodel to the butterfly segment. (Courtesy Gary Schultz, Los Angeles, CA.)

TABLE 7-2 cont'd
Skeletal Variants, Anomalies, Defects, and Artifacts of the Cervical, Thoracic, and Lumbar Spine

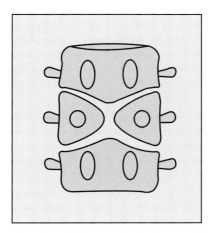

FIG. 7-59 A butterfly vertebra is constructed by a persistent sagittal cleft inhibiting fusion of the right and left halves of the involved vertebra. The right and left halves of the vertebra appear as the wings of a butterfly in the frontal projection. The adjacent endplates often deform slightly into the midline defect. The appearance of the clefted segment also mimics a sideways hourglass.

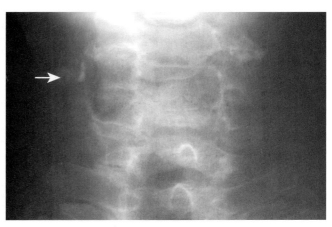

FIG. 7-60 Focal calcification of the carotid vessel is noted on the reading left (*arrow*). Calcification of the wall of the carotid arteries is common. By contrast, vertebral artery calcification is uncommon. When present, vertebral artery calcification appears as an upside-down V shape overlying the spine, whereas carotid vessel calcifications are noted in the paraspinal soft tissues.

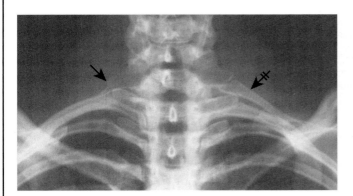

FIG. 7-61 The C7 segment has an enlarged transverse process on the reading left because it extends lateral to the margin of the T1 transverse process (*arrow*). The opposite side has a large cervical rib (*crossed arrow*).

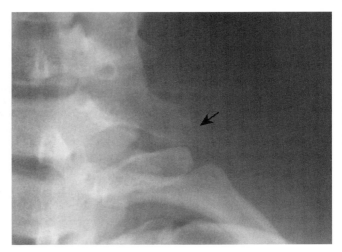

FIG. 7-62 The reading right C7 transverse process is enlarged, extending beyond the lateral margin of the T1 transverse process (*arrow*).

Continued

TABLE 7-2 cont'd

Skeletal Variants, Anomalies, Defects, and Artifacts of the Cervical, Thoracic, and Lumbar Spine

Variant/Artifact	Comments
Cervical ribs (Figs. 7-61 and 7-62)	Cervical ribs are supernumerary ribs arising from cervical vertebrae. About 1% of the population demonstrates radiographic evidence of ribs from the cervical vertebrae. Cervical ribs usually are isolated to the C7 segment, bilateral about two thirds of the time, and are less commonly seen at more cephalic levels of the cervical spine. They may fuse to the first thoracic rib (osseously or by a fibrous band) or end freely. For reference, the T1 segment is identified as the first segment with transverse processes directed cephalically, in contrast to the lower cervical vertebrae, which exhibit a caudal direction of their transverse processes. Cervical ribs should not be confused with C7 transverse process hyperplasia; the latter does not exhibit a costotransverse joint. Transverse hyperplasia is defined as a transverse process that expends laterally to the distal tip of the T1 transverse process with no evidence of a costotransverse joint. Clinically, cervical ribs are significant because they may promote thoracic outlet syndrome by compressing the brachial plexus or the subclavian vessels at the thoracic outlet. Specifically, cervical ribs may narrow the space between the posterior margin of the first thoracic rib and anterior scalene muscle, through which the nerves and subclavian artery pass to the upper extremity. Thoracic outlet syndrome is marked by upper extremity claudication or neurologic symptoms, especially pain and paresthesia along the ulnar borders of the hands and forearm. The thenar eminence demonstrates muscle weakness and wasting in some patients. Symptoms may be exacerbated by turning the head to the ipsilateral side or raising the involved arm overhead. Additionally, symptoms are more likely with postural changes of drooping shoulders and increased thoracic kyphosis. Cervical ribs may have cartilaginous extensions that are not seen on radiographs, making it difficult to appreciate the true size of the rib on plain film studies.
Clasp-knife deformity (Figs. 7-63 and 7-64)	Clasp-knife (or knife-clasp) deformity is the combination of a caudal elongation of the L5 spinous process and spina bifida occulta of S1. At times these individuals experience clinical symptoms (e.g., pain, bladder or bowel dysfunction) during lumbar extension, a presentation known as clasp-knife syndrome.
Cystic hygroma	Cystic hygromas are nonmalignant malformations of lymph vessels occurring in the neck and (less commonly) head region. They are typically present during childhood, may be single or multiple, and may regress over time. They appear as a large mass or soft-tissue density in the anterior region of the neck.
Diastematomyelia (Fig. 7-65)	This condition is marked by a fibrous, cartilaginous, or osseous bar, partially or completely extending across the vertebral canal. The bar may divide the cord, cauda equina, and meninges. It is most commonly found in the thoracolumbar region and is often accompanied by spina bifida occulta, hemivertebrae, and scoliosis. The impact of the bar on the neuroanatomy is best evaluated with magnetic resonance imaging.
Facet tropism (Figs. 7-66 and 7-67)	The lumbar zygopopyphyseal joint planes are normally J-shaped, with the longest part of the joint oriented symmetrically in the sagittal plane. Facet tropism (Greek for "turn") or facet asymmetry describes an asymmetric presentation of the joint planes, where one side is mostly in a sagittal plane and the contralateral side is mostly in a coronal plane. The clinical importance of this finding is debated in the related literature. Most studies trivialize facet joint asymmetry, although it may alter the application of chiropractic care given biomechanical concerns, as has been noted with upper cervical joint asymmetry.[92] The lumbar facet angle has been associated with disc degeneration and herniation.[24,35,77,109] However, other studies find no association with disc degeneration or disc herniation.[11,18,58,74,110]
Hahn's fissures (clefts)/vascular grooves (Fig. 7-68)	A single, thin, horizontal, radiolucent shadow traversing the middle of the vertebral body. It represents the channel for the segment's vascular plexus. It is often visualized on radiographic projections of the thoracic and lumbar regions, typically presenting at multiple levels. Hahn's fissures are common in young children, but the appearance may persist into adulthood. Vessels provide a similar appearance on the T2-weighted magnetic resonance scans, presenting as a small triangular focus of increased signal.

TABLE 7-2 cont'd
Skeletal Variants, Anomalies, Defects, and Artifacts of the Cervical, Thoracic, and Lumbar Spine

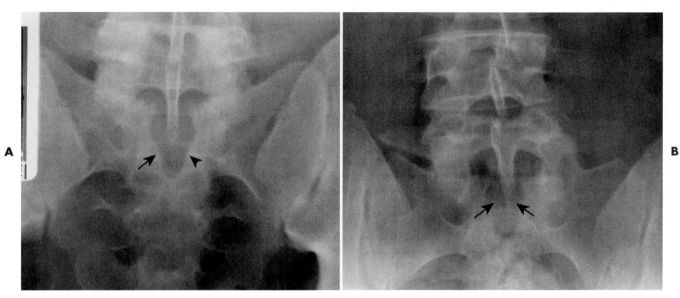

FIG. 7-63 **A** and **B,** The anteroposterior projection of the lumbosacral spine details a large spina bifida occulta defect of S1 and inferiorly enlarged spinous process of L5. Together these findings are known as a *clasp-knife* or *knife-clasp* deformity *(arrows)*. (**A,** Courtesy Gary Longmuir, Phoenix, AZ; **B,** Courtesy Brian Frank, Sunnyland, IL.)

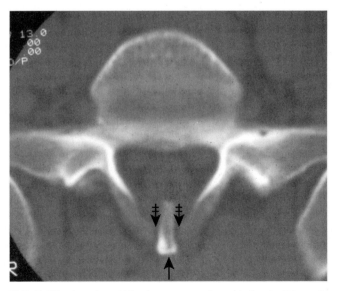

FIG. 7-64 An enlarged L5 spinous process *(arrow)* is found within a midline defect created by a cleft posterior arch of S1 *(crossed arrow)*. (Courtesy William E. Litterer, Elizabeth, NJ.)

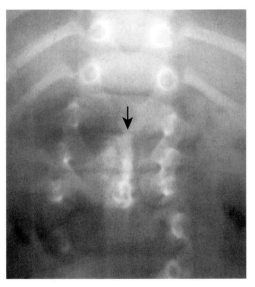

FIG. 7-65 This anteroposterior lumbar radiograph reveals a central osseous density representing an osseous bar crossing the spinal canal *(arrow)*, known as *diastematomyelia*. The degree of neurologic impact is best assessed with magnetic resonance imaging. (Courtesy Steven P. Brownstein, MD, Springfield, NJ.)

Continued

TABLE 7-2 cont'd

Skeletal Variants, Anomalies, Defects, and Artifacts of the Cervical, Thoracic, and Lumbar Spine

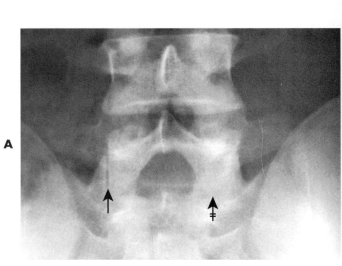

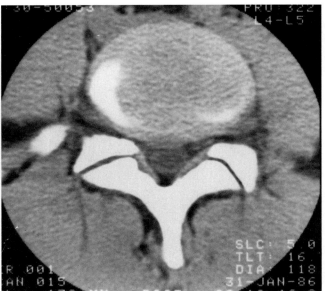

FIG. 7-66   **A,** There is facet tropism (turned facet) at the L5-S1 level. The joint plane is visible on the reading left *(arrow)*, indicating a sagittal alignment. The joint plane is not visible on the reading right *(crossed arrow)*, indicating a coronal plane of alignment. **B,** Axial computed tomography of another case exhibits the joint asymmetry to a better degree. Most facet joints appear J-shaped in the axial plane.

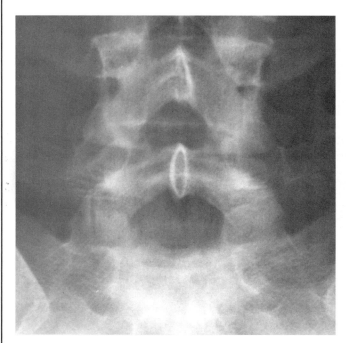

FIG. 7-67   Facet tropism at L5-S1, noted by a sagittal joint orientation on the reading left and a coronal orientation on the reading right.

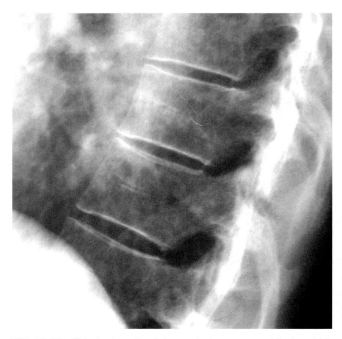

FIG. 7-68   Thin, horizontal radiolucent shadows are noted in the middle of the lower thoracic segments. These shadows are Hahn's fissures and represent vascular impressions of the vertebrae.

TABLE 7-2 cont'd
Skeletal Variants, Anomalies, Defects, and Artifacts of the Cervical, Thoracic, and Lumbar Spine

Variant/Artifact	Comments
Hemivertebra (Figs. 7-69 to 7-71)	The term *hemivertebra* describes a vertebra that is only half formed. These vertebrae usually appear in the thoracic region. Three varieties are noted based on the portion of the vertebral body that presents: lateral, dorsal, and ventral hemivertebrae. All hemivertebrae are trapezoidal or triangular in appearance in the frontal plane. They may be continuous with one or both of the adjacent segments (nonsegmented) or separated from the adjacent segments by an intervertebral disc (segmented). A singular lateral hemivertebra promotes a structural scoliosis with the lateral hemivertebra located at the apex of the curvature. Often lateral hemivertebrae are found in bilateral pairs, at differing spinal levels, forming a balanced **S** configuration of structural scoliosis that is usually only small in magnitude, because each compensates for the other. Dorsal hemivertebrae increase the thoracic kyphosis or decrease the lumbar lordosis. Ventral hemivertebrae create the opposite effect. The term *scrambled spine* has been applied to the presence of multiple levels of block vertebrae and hemivertebrae.
Hyoid fragmentation (Fig. 7-72)	The hyoid may appear fragmented as a variant of normal.
Iliolumbar ligament calcification (Fig. 7-73)	Calcification of the iliolumbar ligament appears as a radiodense band extending from the tip of the transverse process of the lowest lumbar vertebra laterally to the medial aspect of the iliac crest. It sometimes occurs with diffuse idiopathic skeletal hyperostosis (DISH), but more commonly is an isolated finding. Its relationship to clinical findings is ambiguous.
Intercalary ossicle (Figs. 7-74 and 7-75)	A small ossicle is sometimes found in the anterior margin of the intervertebral disc space representing calcification of the anterior longitudinal ligament. It is metaplastic in origin and represents a normal variant of no clinical significance, or is found in association with degenerative disc disease of the corresponding disc segment.
Intervertebral disc calcification (Figs. 7-76 to 7-78)	Intervertebral disc calcification occurs in the nucleus or, more commonly, the anulus fibrosus. It may appear linear, oval, or round. It is often seen in adults in association with degeneration, but idiopathic asymptomatic changes also can occur in children. A more lengthy discussion of intervertebral disc calcification is presented in Chapter 17.
Intervertebral disc hypoplasia	Underdevelopment (or hypoplasia) of the intervertebral disc is seen in several congenital defects such as blocked segmentation and sacralization or lumbarization. When the L5 disc space is slightly decreased, care should be taken not to misinterpret the changes as degenerative. That is, a narrowed L5 disc space, without features of degeneration (e.g., osteophytes, vacuum phenomena) should be interpreted as disc hypoplasia, assuming that infection and other causes can be excluded. Disc hypoplasia is a common cause of a narrow disc space at the L5 level in a younger patient who is not likely to exhibit degeneration.
Klippel-Feil syndrome (Figs. 7-79 and 7-80)	Klippel-Feil syndrome is a rare condition marked by one or multiple levels of blocked segmentation. Approximately half the patients with multiple blocked segments demonstrate a clinical triad of low hairline, limited range of motion, and a short webbed neck. (See Chapter 8 for a complete discussion of Klippel-Feil syndrome.)
Limbus bone (Figs. 7-81 to 7-85)	A limbus bone is a small (<1 cm), permanently separated portion of the vertebra's ring epiphysis that occurs secondary to a peripheral intravertebral herniation of disc material They are usually noted at the anterior-superior margin of a middle lumbar segment and are of little to no clinical significance. Limbus bones are caused by peripheral intravertebral disc herniations; by contrast, Schmorl's nodes are caused by central intravertebral disc herniations. Limbus bones are distinguished from a teardrop fracture by their usual presence of smooth, well-corticated margins, close proximity to the segment, and lumbar location (teardrop fractures are more common to the cervical spine). Intercalary bones are typically in the cervical spine and do not have a defect in the adjacent vertebra, differentiating them from limbus bones.
Lymph node calcification (Fig. 7-86)	Calcification of the lymph nodes is a common result of granulomatous diseases (e.g., tuberculosis or histoplasmosis). They usually appear mottled, but at times outer "eggshell" calcification is noted, a feature suggesting pneumoconiosis, treated lymphoma, and sarcoidosis as the etiology when presenting in the pulmonary tissue. Lymph node calcification often appears in the paraspinal soft tissues of the cervical spine.

TABLE 7-2 cont'd
Skeletal Variants, Anomalies, Defects, and Artifacts of the Cervical, Thoracic, and Lumbar Spine

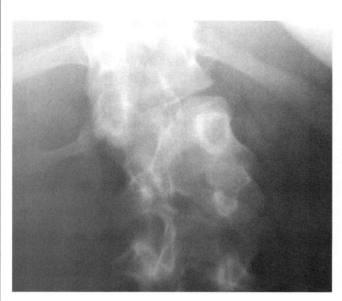

FIG. 7-69   Only the reading right side of the L1 vertebra is formed, creating a right lateral hemivertebra and right lateral thoracolumbar curvature.

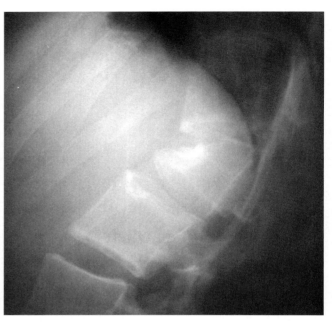

FIG. 7-70   Dorsal hemivertebra causing an acute kyphosis of the thoracolumbar spine.

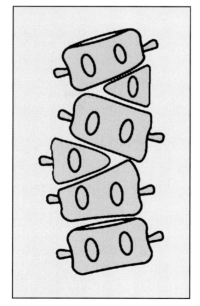

FIG. 7-71   Lateral hemivertebrae often occur in pairs, positioned on opposite sides of the spine; functionally, they tend to balance the congenital scoliosis that occurs secondary to their presence.

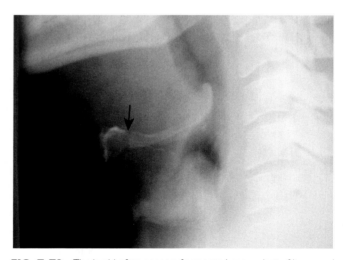

FIG. 7-72   The hyoid often appears fragmented as a variant of its normal configuration *(arrow)*.

TABLE 7-2 cont'd

Skeletal Variants, Anomalies, Defects, and Artifacts of the Cervical, Thoracic, and Lumbar Spine

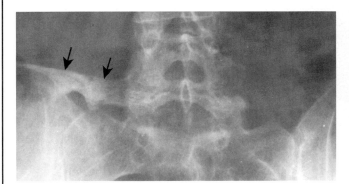

FIG. 7-73 There is prominent calcification of the iliolumbar ligament *(arrows)*. (Courtesy Steven P. Brownstein, MD, Springfield, NJ.)

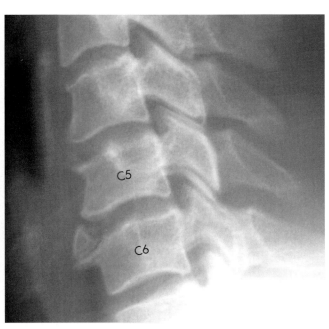

FIG. 7-74 A large intercalary ossicle is noted at the anterior margin of the C5 disc space.

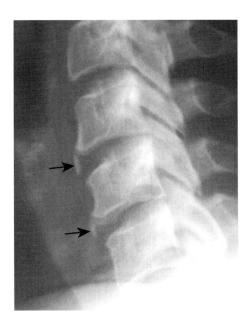

FIG. 7-75 Intercalary ossicles noted at two cervical levels *(arrows)*.

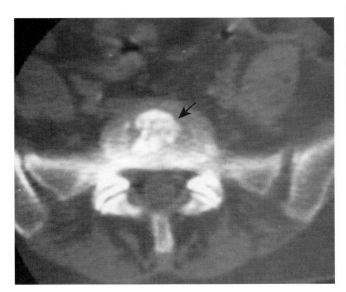

FIG. 7-76 Axial computed tomography image of demonstrating central calcification of the L5 disc *(arrow)*. (Courtesy Steven P. Brownstein, MD, Springfield, NJ.)

Continued

TABLE 7-2 cont'd
Skeletal Variants, Anomalies, Defects, and Artifacts of the Cervical, Thoracic, and Lumbar Spine

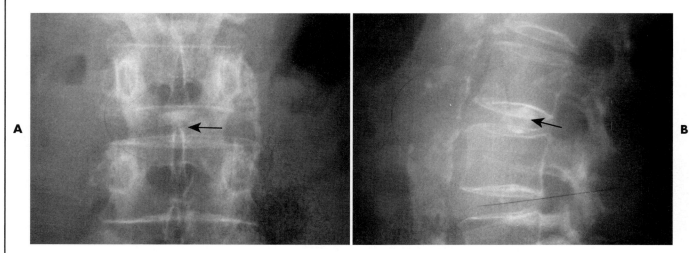

A

B

FIG. 7-77   **A** and **B,** A 63-year-old woman demonstrating calcification in the center of the L2 intervertebral disc *(arrows).*

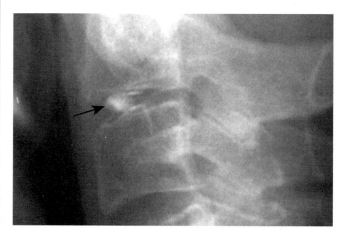

FIG. 7-78   Idiopathic focus of calcification in the anterior third of the C2 disc space *(arrow).* (Courtesy William E. Litterer, Elizabeth, NJ.)

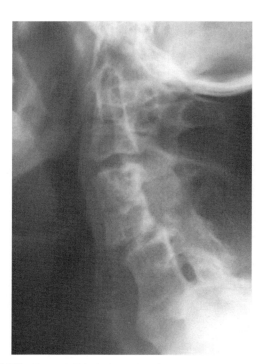

FIG. 7-79   Congenital blocked segmentation present at occiput-C1, C3-4, and C5-7. Generally, multiple block segments define Klippel-Feil syndrome. (Courtesy William E. Litterer, Elizabeth, NJ.)

TABLE 7-2 cont'd
Skeletal Variants, Anomalies, Defects, and Artifacts of the Cervical, Thoracic, and Lumbar Spine

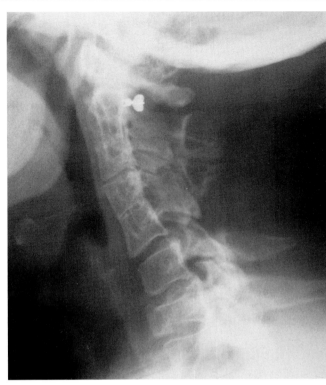

FIG. 7-80 A 29-year-old man exhibits multiple block vertebrae consistent with Klippel-Feil syndrome. Congenital block segments are noted at C2-3 and C4-5. Additionally, the C7 segment exhibits an altered appearance related to a past fracture. (Courtesy Darrell Petrey, Foley, AL.)

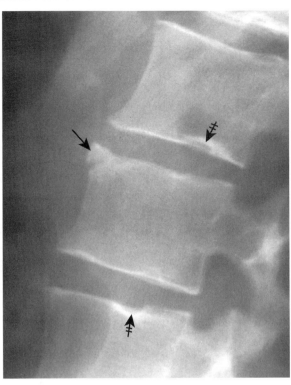

FIG. 7-81 There is a small fragment located at the anterosuperior aspect of L1 that represents a limbus bone *(arrow)*. Small inward endplate defects of the adjacent vertebrae represent Schmorl's nodes *(crossed arrows)*.

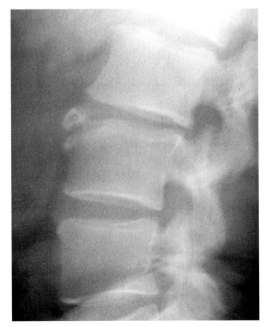

FIG. 7-82 A subepiphyseal herniation of nuclear material precluded the secondary growth center from uniting to the vertebral body, forming the limbus bone noted at the anterosuperior aspect of L2. (Courtesy Frank C. Miramonti, Walled Lake, MI.)

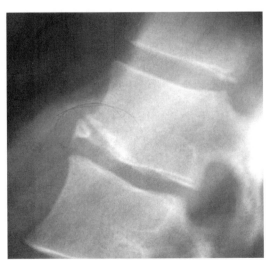

FIG. 7-83 Notice the smoothly corticated perimeter of the limbus bone, differentiating it from a fractured fragment. (Courtesy William E. Litterer, Elizabeth, NJ.)

TABLE 7-2 cont'd
Skeletal Variants, Anomalies, Defects, and Artifacts of the Cervical, Thoracic, and Lumbar Spine

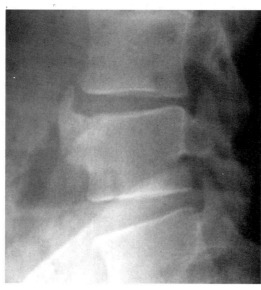

FIG. 7-84 Horn-shaped limbus bone formed at the anterosuperior corner of L4.

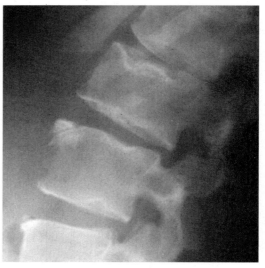

FIG. 7-85 Limbus bone formed at the anterosuperior margin of L2. Also, notice the prominent, paired Schmorl's nodes along the superior endplate of L1, and also at the superior and inferior endplates of L2.

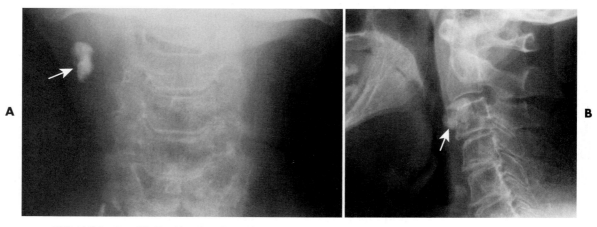

FIG. 7-86 A and **B,** Focal lymph node calcification is noted in this patient's paraspinal region *(arrows)*. Lymph node calcification most often represents residuum of past regional infection.

TABLE 7-2 cont'd

Skeletal Variants, Anomalies, Defects, and Artifacts of the Cervical, Thoracic, and Lumbar Spine

Variant/Artifact	Comments
Myelogram remnant	Some of the radiodense contrast may remain in the thecal sac following a myelographic procedure. The older oil-based residual contrast resorbs at approximately 5 ml/year until completely removed. The more contemporary water-based products resorb more quickly. Radiographically the contrast appears as multiple radiodense droplets in the lumbar dural sac.
Nuchal bone (Fig. 7-87)	A nuchal bone is a focal ossification of the nuchal ligament appearing as an oblong, vertically oriented, radiodense osseous structure that varies in size, but is often approximately 1 cm wide and 2 to 4 cm long. It is commonly seen among patients more than 40 years of age and is of limited clinical significance. A nuchal bone is sometimes confused with an ununited secondary growth center of the spinous process, which is typically smaller and has an associated defect of the spinous process, or a Clay shoveler's fracture, which usually is adjacent to a spinous fracture with ragged margins, is inferiorly displaced, and is accompanied by a history of trauma.
Nuclear impression (Figs. 7-88 to 7-90)	Nuclear impression, also known as *notochordal persistence*, is marked by subtle, gradual inward defects of the endplates that tend to involve most of the endplate. They appear as a concave deformity in a lateral radiographic projection. They may appear as two inward defects, creating a double hump appearance known as *cupid's bow* in a frontal radiographic projection. The two inward defects appear as radiolucent disc material on axial computed tomography scans, known as an *owl sign*. Nuclear impression is thought to be a normal variant of no importance, apparently related to a variation of notochordal development.
Oppenheimer ossicles (Figs. 7-91 and 7-92)	A persistent or ununited apophysis at the tip of the superior or inferior articular process is termed an Oppenheimer ossicle. They are most common to the lumbar region. Oppenheimer ossicles are differentiated from traumatic fragments by their smooth, well-corticated margins seen on either side of the intervening radiolucent defect, and by the fact that fractures of the articular processes are notably uncommon. Fractures are common in the region of the pars interarticularis but not confined to the articular processes.
Rima glottidis (Figs. 7-93 and 7-94)	The rima glottidis (true glottis, rima vocalis) is the fissure between the right and left true vocal folds of the larynx. In the frontal radiographic projection, it appears as a thin (1 to 2 mm), vertical, radiolucent shadow of 2 to 3 cm in length. It is inferiorly continuous with the tracheal air shadow and superiorly continuous with the piriform sinus. The appearance is often mistaken for spina bifida occulta, usually of the C4 segment. The narrow slit of the rima glottidis expands during respiration with abduction of the true vocal folds.
Salivary gland calcification (Fig. 7-95)	Calcification within the salivary glands may occur secondary to stone formation, infection, or, less commonly, tumor. Calculi occurring in a salivary gland are usually found in the submandibular gland, but also can occur in the parotid, sublingual, and minor salivary glands.
Schmorl's node (see also Figs. 7-81 and 7-85) (Figs. 7-96 and 7-97)	A Schmorl's node is an intravertebral body herniation of the nucleus pulposus common to the thoracic and lumbar regions of the spine. It is theorized that Schmorl's nodes occur through incomplete pores of the cartilaginous endplates formed by evacuated vascular loops that regress as part of the maturation process. Schmorl's nodes tend to appear during childhood. On imaging studies, they appear as abrupt, squared-off, U-shaped, focal defects of either (or both), the superior and inferior endplates. The margins of the defect are sclerotic. Large, usually peripheral Schmorl's nodes are sometimes associated with increased diameter of the vertebral body and narrowing of the intervertebral disc space. Schmorl's nodes are often multiple and sometimes associated with endplate irregularity and trapezoidal configuration of the vertebrae, together defined as Scheuermann's disease. Scheuermann's disease is discussed fully in Chapter 9. Schmorl's nodes are differentiated from nuclear impressions. Both represent inward defect of the vertebral endplate, but differ in that Schmorl's nodes are abrupt, focal defects and nuclear impressions are subtle, gradual defects. Schmorl's nodes are similar to limbus bones in that both represent defects arising from adjacent intervertebral disc herniations. However, a limbus bone defines a permanently separated fragment of the epiphysis secondary to a subepiphyseal disc herniation, and Schmorl's nodes develop from an intravertebral herniation of disc material.

Continued

TABLE 7-2 cont'd
Skeletal Variants, Anomalies, Defects, and Artifacts of the Cervical, Thoracic, and Lumbar Spine

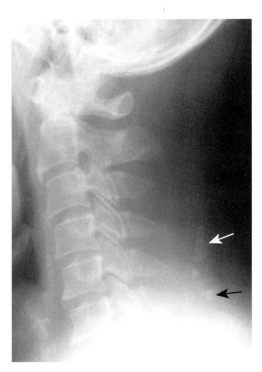

FIG. 7-87   A 46-year-old man demonstrating several radiodense shadows posterior to the lower cervical spinous processes *(arrows)*. The radiodense shadows represent calcification in the nuchal ligament (nuchal bones). (Courtesy Ryder M. Church, Peoria, IL.)

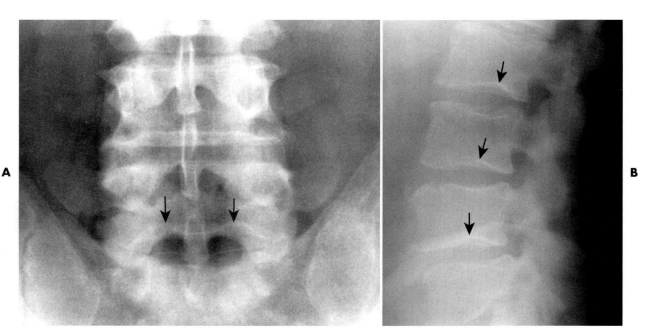

FIG. 7-88   **A,** Paired, smooth, inward deformities ("cupid's bow" sign) of the inferior endplate of L5 consistent with the developmental defect of nuclear impression (or notochordal persistence) *(arrows)*. **B,** The paired inward deformity of the anteroposterior projections appears as a single inward defect in the lateral projection *(arrows)*. (Courtesy Ian W. Shaw, Port Huron, MI.)

TABLE 7-2 cont'd
Skeletal Variants, Anomalies, Defects, and Artifacts of the Cervical, Thoracic, and Lumbar Spine

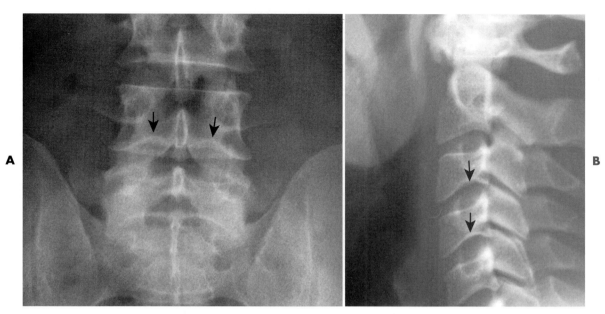

FIG. 7-89 A, Lumbar and, **B,** cervical spine presentation of nuclear impression *(arrows).* (Courtesy Jamie and Lori Kirgis, Columbia City, IN.)

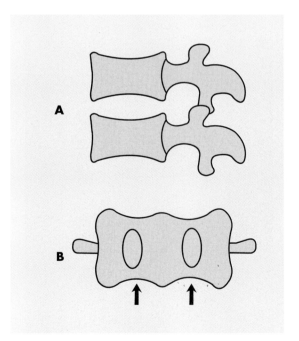

FIG. 7-90 A, Notochordal persistence (or nuclear impression) forms an inward deformity of the endplates, seen as a gradual sloping deformity on the lateral projection. **B,** The anteroposterior projection exhibits a bilobulate defect that has been likened to the appearance of "cupid's bow."

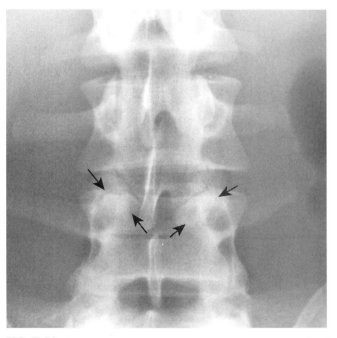

FIG. 7-91 The distal tip of the inferior articular process of L4 is not fused bilaterally. A persistent apophysis at this region is termed an *Oppenheimer ossicle (arrows).* (Courtesy C. Robert Tatum, Davenport, IA.)

Continued

TABLE 7-2 cont'd

Skeletal Variants, Anomalies, Defects, and Artifacts of the Cervical, Thoracic, and Lumbar Spine

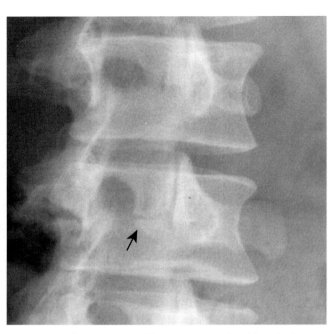

FIG. 7-92 Oppenheimer ossicle presenting on the oblique lumbar projection as a well-defined ossicle at the tip of the inferior articular process of a middle lumbar segment *(arrow)*. (Courtesy Ian D. McLean, Davenport, IA.)

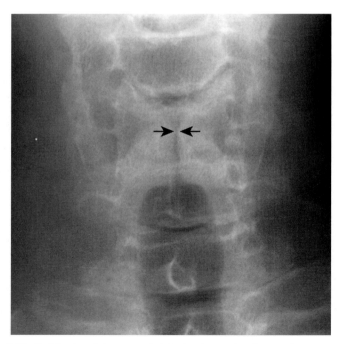

FIG. 7-93 A radiolucent vertical shadow is noted at the superior aspect of the tracheal air shadow that represents the space between the true vocal folds (rima glottidis) *(arrows)*. The space is *narrowed* when compared to the appearance in Figure 7-94. The rima glottidis appears wider during phonation or respiration than during rest. (Courtesy Kathy Skaggs, Farmington, IL.)

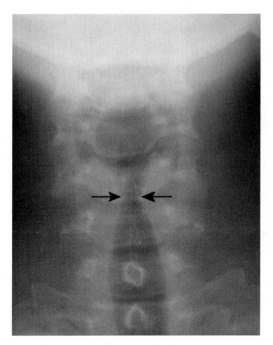

FIG. 7-94 The rima glottidis (true glottis) *(arrows)* is the radiolucent shadow between the right and left true vocal folds.

TABLE 7-2 cont'd
Skeletal Variants, Anomalies, Defects, and Artifacts of the Cervical, Thoracic, and Lumbar Spine

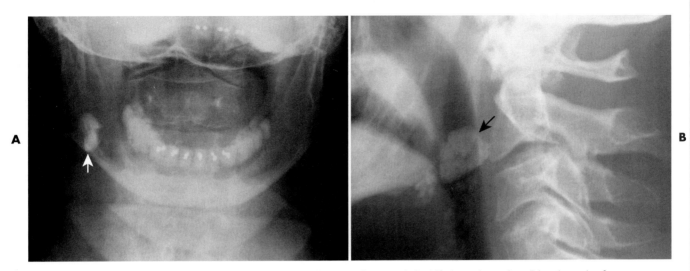

FIG. 7-95 **A** and **B,** A 41-year-old male patient demonstrating a mottled calcified mass located medial to the angle of the mandible *(arrows).* The mulberry appearance and location is consistent with submandibular calcification. (Courtesy Rodney Simmer, Rock Island, IL.)

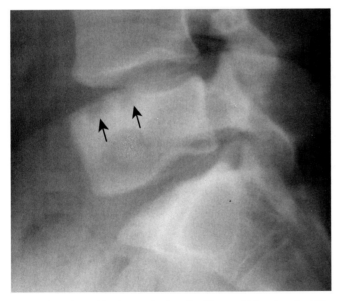

FIG. 7-96 Lateral lumbar projection of a 19-year-old female patient. The radiograph exhibits paired inward defects of the anterior third of the superior endplate of L5 *(arrows),* known as *Schmorl's nodes.* In this case the Schmorl's nodes have resulted in malformation of the vertebra manifesting as an increased anterior to posterior dimension of the segment. (Courtesy Lisa Jennings, Eldridge, IA.)

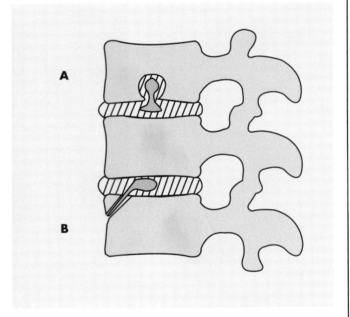

FIG. 7-97 **A,** Schmorl's nodes are intravertebral herniation of nuclear material occurring through remnant vascular pores of the cartilaginous endplate. **B,** In contrast, limbus bones are subepiphyseal herniations of nuclear material promoting a nonunion deformity of the secondary growth center of the epiphysis from the primary growth center of the vertebrae.

Continued

TABLE 7-2 cont'd

Skeletal Variants, Anomalies, Defects, and Artifacts of the Cervical, Thoracic, and Lumbar Spine

Variant/Artifact	Comments
Spina bifida occulta (Figs. 7-98 to 7-101)	Spina bifida occulta describes small, midline, osseous defects of the posterior arch. They are common to L5, S1, and the atlas, appearing as a radiolucent cleft on frontal radiographic projections and as a missing spinal laminal line on lateral projections.
Spinous apophysis (Figs. 7-102 and 7-103)	Persistence of the apical spinous apophysis is common at the C7 level. It may result from childhood trauma or represent a nontraumatic variant. It differs from a spinous process fracture in that the former is usually smooth and nondisplaced, and the latter has an irregular anterior margin and is usually inferiorly displaced secondary to muscle tension.
Supernumerary segments (Fig. 104)	A supernumerary segment is an extra segment. Variation in the number of cervical, thoracic, and lumbar segments is not uncommon. The lumbar region demonstrates the greatest variation.
Thyroid cartilage calcification (Figs. 7-105 to 7-107)	Physiologic calcification of the thyroid cartilage is common with increasing age. The finding appears as a mottled pattern of the calcification at the C5-6 level. It has the shape of a shield on anteroposterior film.
Transitional vertebra (Figs. 7-107 to 7-110)	A transitional vertebra (lumbarization and sacralization) is a segment that takes on the morphologic characteristics of an adjoining structure or region. Occipitalization, cervical ribs, lumbar ribs, or variations in the number of vertebrae are all types of transitional segments. The most common transitional segment occurs at the lumbosacral junction. For instance, at the lumbosacral junction, the S1 segment may appear with lumbar characteristics (lumbarization of S1) or the L5 segment may appear with sacral characteristics (sacralization of L5). Lumbarization and sacralization appear identical on imaging studies. The terms refer to whether the transitional segment represents the true L5 or S1 level. In other words, lumbarization is lumbar assimilation of S1 and sacralization is sacral assimilation of L5. Because of the variation in the number of segments in each region, it is not possible to definitively know whether a lumbosacral transitional segment is L5 (sacralization) or S1 (lumbarization) without counting down from the T1 segment. It is not always possible to obtain a true count of the vertebrae, leading most to prefer the inclusive term of transitional vertebra over the more specific terms of lumbarization or sacralization. The prevalence of a lumbosacral transitional vertebra is reported to be 0.6% to 25%.[89] Sacralization of L5 is approximately 30 times more common than lumbarization of S1.[67] Transitional segments have been reported to be more common among men,[67] but equal gender predisposition also has been reported.[62] Radiographically they are defined by the presence of a rudimentary, thin intervertebral disc below the transitional segment and broad transverse processes on one or both sides of the transitional segment (known as "batwing deformity" if bilateral). More specifically, there are four types of presentation of transitional vertebrae.[19] Each type has two subtypes. Type I appears with a dysplastic broad (or spatulated) transverse process that measures more than 19 mm in a vertical dimension. A type II transitional segment demonstrates a pseudojoint between the broad transverse process of the transitional segment and the superior margin of the sacrum. A type III transitional segment is marked by bone fusion between the transverse process of the transitional segment and the segment below. Types I, II, and III have subtypes A and B, denoting whether the morphologic changes defining the type are presenting unilaterally (subtype A) or bilaterally (subtype B). Type IV is a mixed presentation of type II on one side of the transitional segment and type III on the opposite side. There are suggested but not well-supported links between lumbosacral transitional vertebrae and clinical findings. Vergauwen and others found higher incidence of intervertebral disc degeneration, facet arthrosis, and spinal stenosis at the level above a transitional vertebrae than normally expected.[111] The type I and II transitional segments are associated with reduced intersegmental motion. No intersegmental motion is expected across type III and IV transitional vertebrae. Transitional segmentation often is mentioned as a possible cause of low back pain;[68] however, a strong empirical correlation is lacking.[62,67] When a lumbosacral transitional segment presents with scoliosis and *sciatica* it is termed *Bertolotti syndrome*.
Transverse process apophysis (Figs. 7-111 to 7-113)	Persistence of the apical apophysis of the transverse process is considered a normal variant, appearing most commonly at T1 or upper lumbar segments.

TABLE 7-2 cont'd
Skeletal Variants, Anomalies, Defects, and Artifacts of the Cervical, Thoracic, and Lumbar Spine

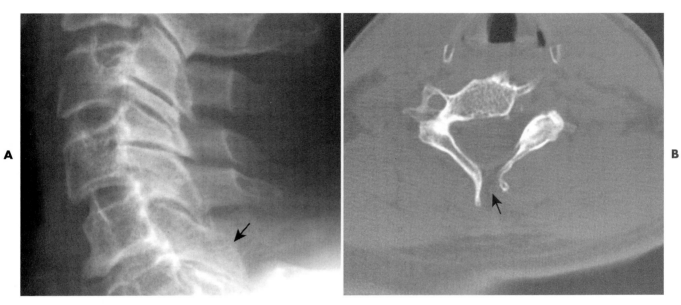

FIG. 7-98 Spina bifida occulta at C6. **A,** Lateral cervical projection of a 59-year-old man shows an absence of the spinal laminal line at C6 *(arrow)*. **B,** Computed tomography scan at the C6 level shows a clear defect in the posterior arch *(arrow)*.

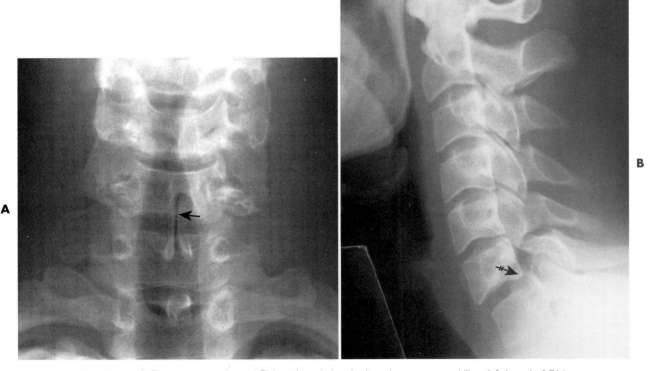

FIG. 7-99 **A,** The anteroposterior and, **B,** lateral cervical projections demonstrate a midline cleft *(arrow)* of C6 in this 21-year-old female patient. Spina bifida occurring at C6 is sometimes related to mild accompanying spondylolisthesis, as is noted in this case by the break in George's line *(crossed arrow)*. (Courtesy Beverly Harger, Portland, OR.)

TABLE 7-2 cont'd
Skeletal Variants, Anomalies, Defects, and Artifacts of the Cervical, Thoracic, and Lumbar Spine

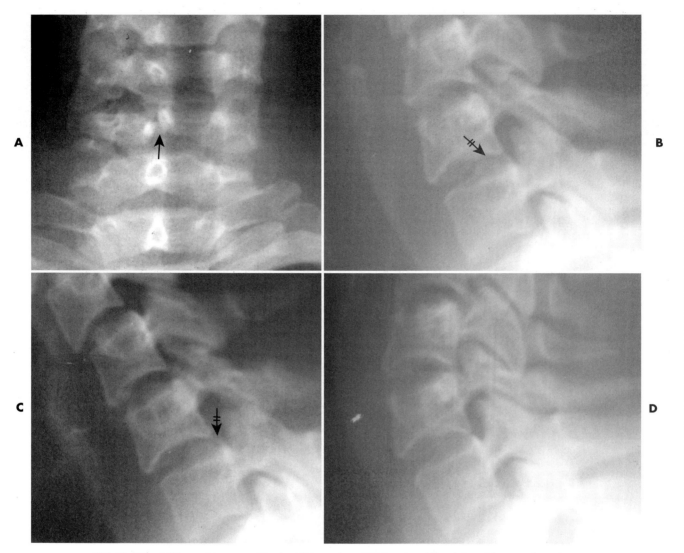

FIG. 7-100   A 27-year-old woman with spina bifida occulta at C6. Note the midline defect of the posterior arch seen in, **A,** the anteroposterior view *(arrow)*; **B,** the lateral flexion; **C,** neutral; and, **D,** extension projections exhibit only slight intersegmental translation during the sagittal movement *(crossed arrows)*. (Courtesy James Galyen, Scottsburg, IN.)

TABLE 7-2 cont'd
Skeletal Variants, Anomalies, Defects, and Artifacts of the Cervical, Thoracic, and Lumbar Spine

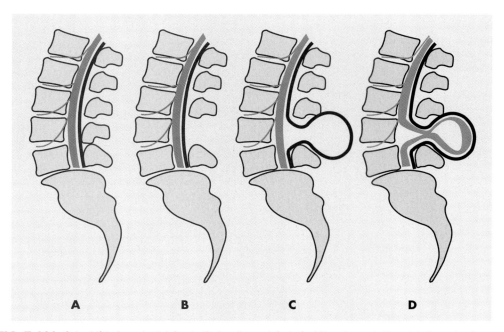

A   B   C   D

FIG. 7-101 Spina bifida (meaning "cleft spine") describes a defect of midline closure in the posterior arch of one or more vertebrae. There are two general expressions. *Spinal bifida occulta* describes, **B,** a "hidden" or subtle defect of the posterior arch of one or more vertebrae so that, **A,** the normal configuration is no longer maintained. The spinous process may be hypoplastic or missing, the latter depicted in this figure. *Spina bifida vera* (also known as *spina bifida manifesta*) is a "true" (or "manifesting") clinically significant defect of the posterior aspect of the vertebral column. There are two expressions of spina bifida vera. The first is a midline defect of the vertebral column with posterior extension of the meninges (**C,** spina bifida meningocele), noted here by the black line representing the meninges extending posteriorly through the midline defect. The second involves posterior extension of the cord or nerve roots and the meninges (**D,** spina bifida myelomeningocele) through the osseous midline defect, noted here by the black line (meninges) and blue lines (representing the nerve roots) extending posteriorly.

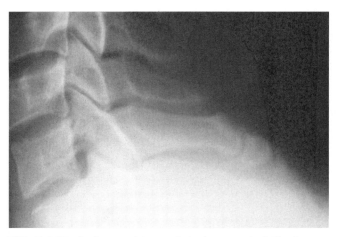

FIG. 7-102 Persistence of the terminal spinous apophysis. The fragment has a smooth, well-corticated perimeter that differentiates it from an acute traumatic etiology. However, most persistent apophyses are not inferiorly displaced, as exhibited here, suggesting that a traumatic etiology may be implicated in this case.

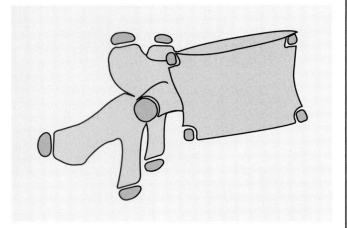

FIG. 7-103 This schematic demonstrates the secondary growth centers *(blue)* of the vertebra. Secondary growth centers are ossified by skeletal maturity. If a center remains unossified (or ununited) after this time, it will always persist. Persistent apophyses are differentiated from traumatic fractures in that the former is smooth, circumferentially corticated, usually not displaced, and typically without a corresponding history of trauma.

TABLE 7-2 cont'd
Skeletal Variants, Anomalies, Defects, and Artifacts of the Cervical, Thoracic, and Lumbar Spine

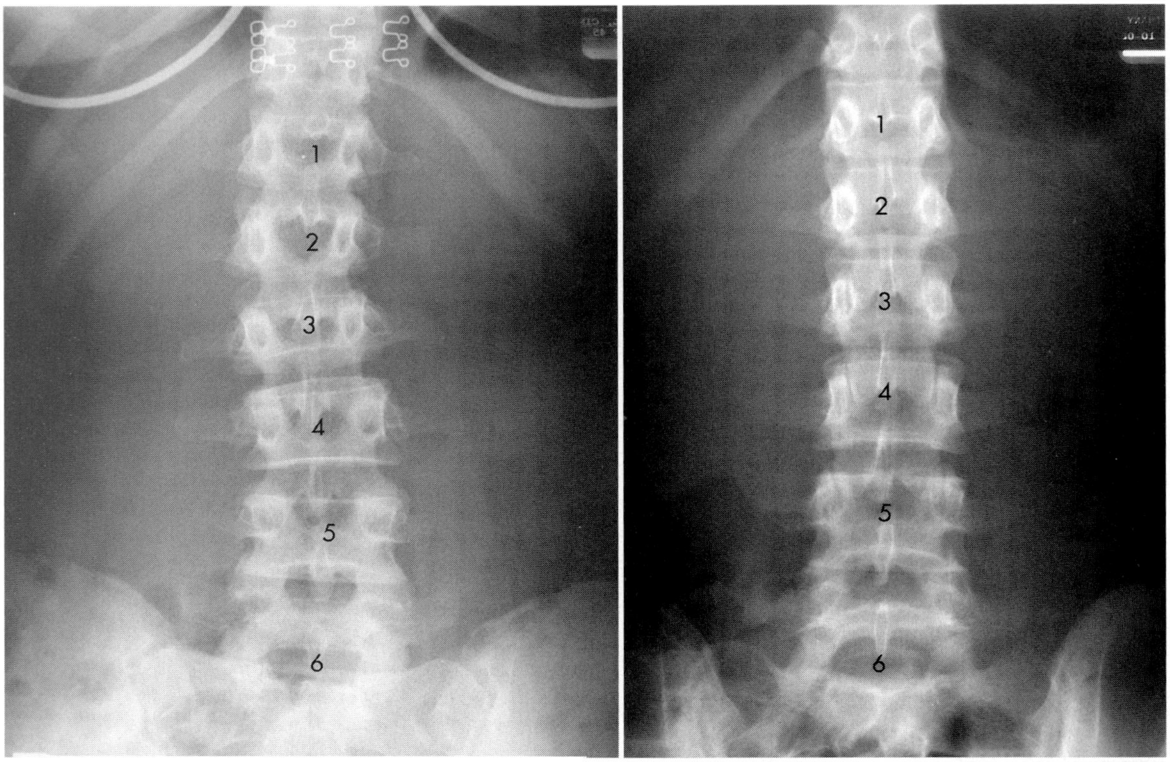

FIG. 7-104   **A** and **B,** Supernumerary or, **C,** missing segments may result in either six or four lumbar segments, respectively. (**A,** Courtesy Thomas Galli, Peoria, IL.)

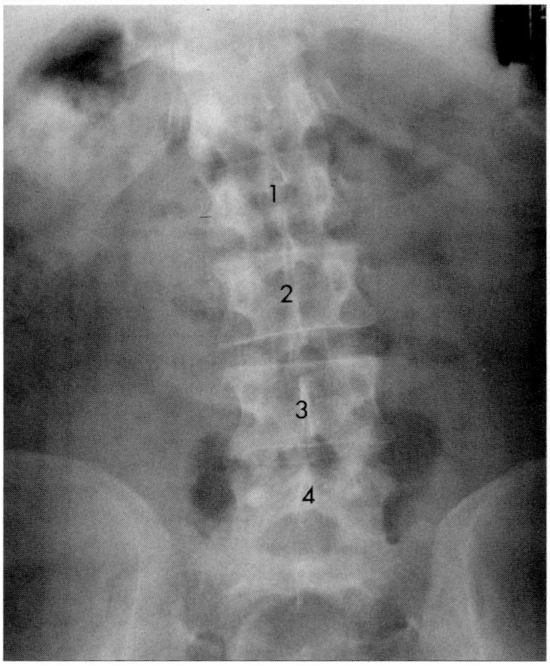

TABLE 7-2 cont'd
Skeletal Variants, Anomalies, Defects, and Artifacts of the Cervical, Thoracic, and Lumbar Spine

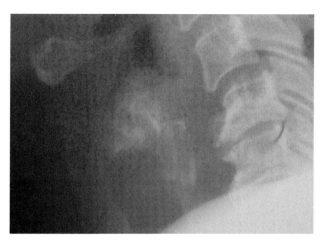

FIG. 7-105 Physiologic calcification of the thyroid cartilage of no clinical significance.

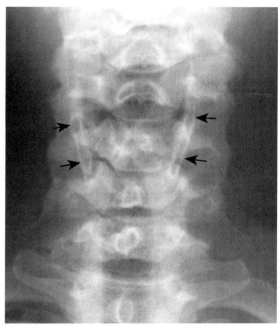

FIG. 7-106 Physiologic calcification of the thyroid cartilage of a 59-year-old woman. The calcification appears with a wide V-shaped radiodense appearance in the anteroposterior projection *(arrows)*.

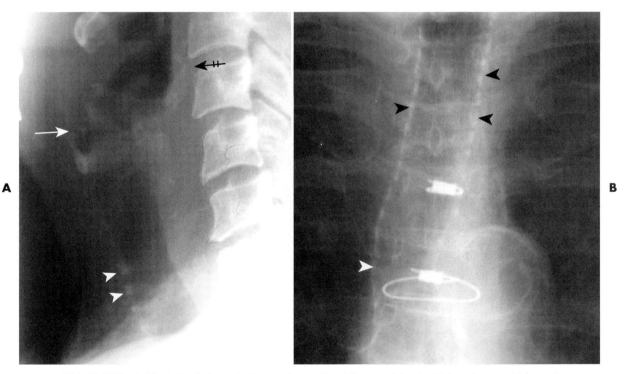

FIG. 7-107 **A,** Mottled radiodense shadow consistent with calcification of the thyroid *(arrow)*, arytenoid *(crossed arrow)*, and tracheal ring *(arrowheads)* cartilages. **B,** A second case exhibits prominent calcification of the tracheal ring cartilages. Metallic artifact is incidentally noted. (**A,** Courtesy Troy Scheuermann, Framington, IA; **B,** Courtesy Emanuel Vito, Scranton, PA.)

TABLE 7-2 cont'd
Skeletal Variants, Anomalies, Defects, and Artifacts of the Cervical, Thoracic, and Lumbar Spine

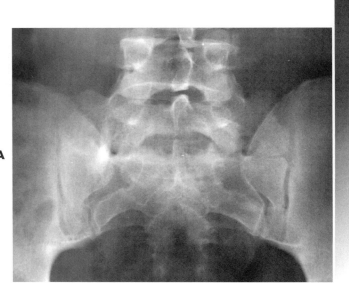

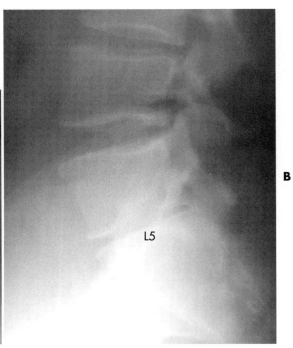

FIG. 7-108 **A,** Sacralization noted by the bilateral spatulated transverse processes of L5 that are nearly fused to the sacrum. **B,** The L5 disc space is rudimentary. (Courtesy William E. Litterer, Elizabeth, NJ.)

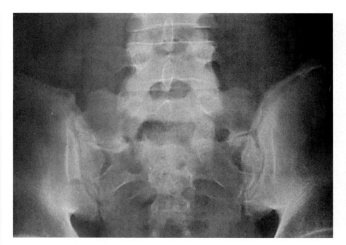

FIG. 7-109 Bilaterally enlarged transverse processes; both form articulations with the superior margin of the sacrum. The appearance is consistent with a transitional segment.

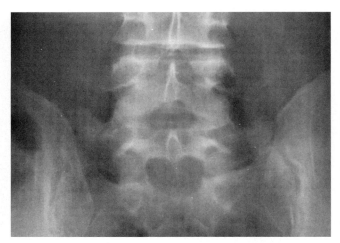

FIG. 7-110 Bilaterally enlarged transverse process; however, neither forms a pseudojoint with the superior aspect of the sacrum. Although the transverse processes appear approximated to the sacrum, there is no marginal bone sclerosis; therefore no articulation exists. (Courtesy Troy Scheuermann, Farmington, IA.)

TABLE 7-2 cont'd
Skeletal Variants, Anomalies, Defects, and Artifacts of the Cervical, Thoracic, and Lumbar Spine

Variant/Artifact	Comments
Transverse process pseudoarthrosis (Fig. 7-114)	The transverse process of adjacent cervical vertebrae may demonstrate enlarged anterior tubercles that articulate forming pseudoarthrosis. This finding is most common at C5-6.[3]
Trapezoidal segments (Figs. 7-115 and 7-116)	Not uncommonly, middle to lower thoracic and upper lumbar vertebrae present with a slight trapezoidal or wedged configuration, narrowed to the anterior, as a variant of normal, unrelated to accompanying disease. In such presentations, traumatic or pathologic compression fractures need to be excluded. A trapezoidal shape is clinically relevant if found at the level of spondylolisthesis. Trapezoidal segments, narrowed to the posterior, are more likely to continue to anteriorly displace.
VACTERL syndrome	VACTERL is an abbreviation for *V*ertebral anomalies (and vascular defects), *A*nal atresia, *C*ardiac anomalies, *T*racheoesophageal fistula, *E*sophageal atresia, *R*enal and *R*adial dysplasia, and *L*imb bud anomalies. The common link among the defects is that they all arise from a mesodermal defect occurring before the seventh week of fetal development.
Vertebral ring epiphysis (Fig. 7-117)	The vertebral bodies of infants and very young children appear oval on a lateral radiograph. As the child ages, the ossifying vertebral body demonstrates more of a rectangular appearance, but there remain "steplike" defects seen most prominently at the anterior corners of the lumbar vertebrae and slanted anterior corners of the thoracic vertebrae. This appearance is most notable between ages 6 and 9 years. Typically around the age of 12 years, the cartilaginous endplates begin to ossify, giving the appearance of small ossicles adjacent to the anterior margins of the vertebral bodies of the thoracic and lumbar segments. Fusion of the endplates begins around 15 years of age and is typically complete by 25 years of age.

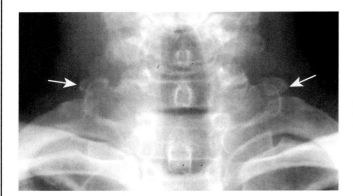

FIG. 7-111 A 13-year-old patient who exhibits the unossified apophyses at the distal aspect of the transverse processes *(arrows)*. This is a normal configuration in a patient of this age; however, sometimes this juvenile configuration persists into adulthood. (Courtesy Troy Scheuermann, Farmington, IA.)

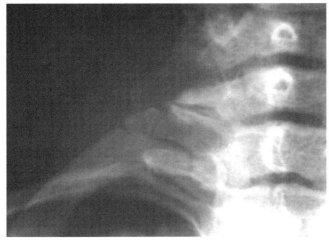

FIG. 7-112 Nonunion defect of the terminal end of the T1 transverse process.

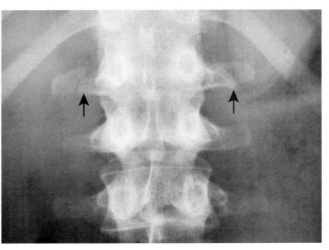

FIG. 7-113 Bilateral nonunion of the terminal end of the L1 transverse processes *(arrows)*.

TABLE 7-2 cont'd

Skeletal Variants, Anomalies, Defects, and Artifacts of the Cervical, Thoracic, and Lumbar Spine

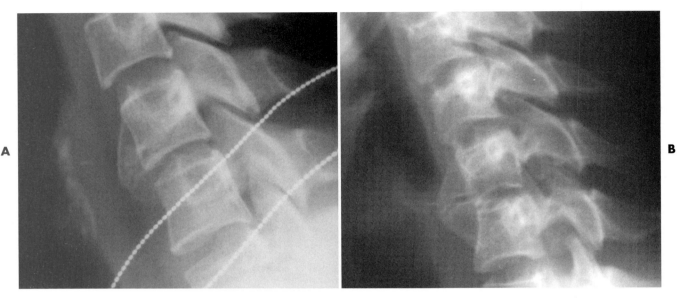

A

B

FIG. 7-114 **A** and **B,** Two cases of pseudoarthrosis formed between the transverse process of C5 and C6. (**B,** Courtesy William E. Litterer, Elizabeth, NJ.)

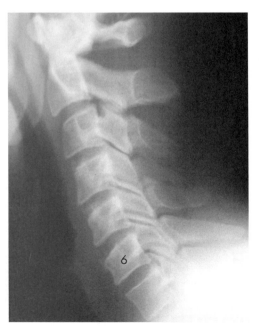

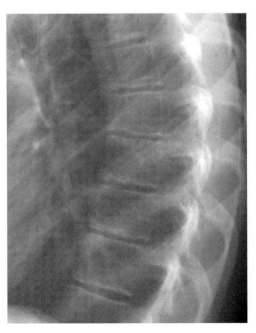

FIG. 7-115 The C6 segment appears trapezoidal. Although this is typically a sign of fracture, it also may represent a normal variant. (Courtesy Randy Hurt, Rock Island, IL.)

FIG. 7-116 The middle thoracic segments may be trapezoidal as a feature of developmental change and not fracture. (Courtesy Maureen Work, Ottawa, IL.)

TABLE 7-2 cont'd
Skeletal Variants, Anomalies, Defects, and Artifacts of the Cervical, Thoracic, and Lumbar Spine

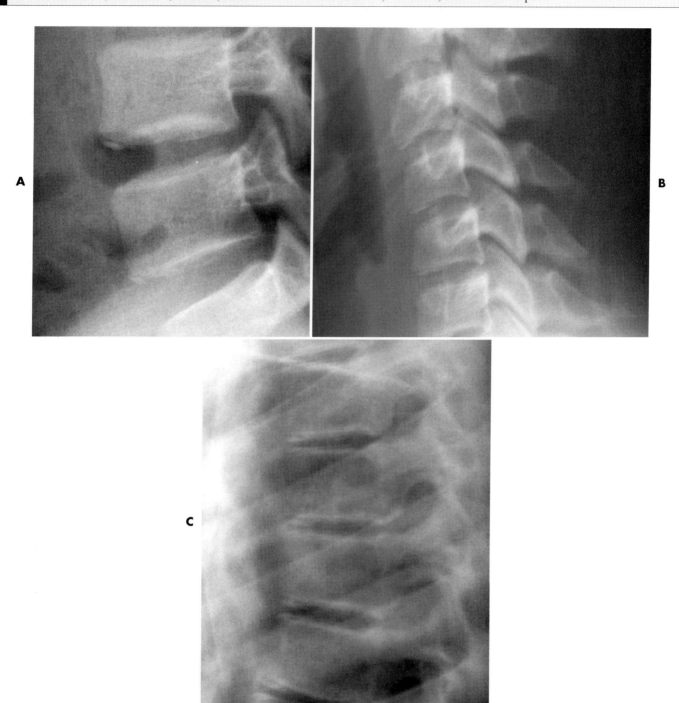

FIG. 7-117   The nonossified growth plate of the vertebrae should not be confused with traumatically induced fragments. The endplates typically close by age 17 in females and 20 in males. Examples of open growth plates are noted here in, **A,** a 15-year-old female, and, **B,** a 14-year-old female's cervical and, **C,** thoracic spine. Normally ossification begins during the third week of gestation. By the fourth month, most primary ossifications centers have appeared in the diaphyses of tubular bones. From birth to age 5 the secondary ossification centers appear in the epiphyses. Ossification continues from age 5 to 17 years. By 17 to 20 years the bones of the upper extremities, including scapulae, are completely ossified. By 18 to 23 years the bones of the lower extremities, including the pelvis, are completely ossified. Lastly, by 20 to 25 years the sternum, clavicles, and vertebrae demonstrate complete ossification. Ossification occurs earlier in females than in males.

TABLE 7-3

Normal Skeletal Variants and Defects of the Sacrum, Coccyx, and Pelvis

Variant	Comments
Acetabular protrusion (Fig. 7-118)	Inward migration of the medial wall of the acetabulum on one or both sides. Inward migration can be assessed with a Köhler line. See Chapter 19 for more detail on this condition.
Anterior deviation of the coccyx	Often the caudal end of the coccyx is significantly anteriorly deviated. This configuration is believed to be a normal variant in presentation but must be differentiated from trauma.
Artifacts (Fig. 7-119)	A wide variety of artifacts may be identified in the abdomen and pelvis. Commonly seen are tantalum mesh/hernia repair, abdominal aorta surgery, Greenfield-Kinney filter (Greenfield inferior vena cava filter, IVC), intrauterine device, Hulka clips for tubal ligation, and prostate seeding.
Gluteal striations (Fig. 7-120)	At times, the muscle striations of the gluleus major can be seen on the frontal radiographs of the pelvis.
Iliac horns (Fig. 7-121)	Bilateral, horn-shaped exostosis, of approximately 2 to 4 cm, may be noted from the posterior surface of the iliac fossae. These iliac horns are virtually pathognomonic of a rare inherited condition termed hereditary osteo-onychodysostosis (HOOD), or also known as Turner's-Fong syndrome or simply Fong syndrome. HOOD also demonstrates dysplastic brittle nails, small or absent patella, small or absent articular condyles of the knees and elbows, joint contracture (especially the elbow), clubfoot, "shamrock"-colored irises, renal dysplasia, and other bone and soft-tissue changes.
Iliac vascular channel (Fig. 7-122)	The normal iliac vessel may project as a Y-, J-, or V-shaped radiolucent tubular defect with sclerotic margins overlying the lower margin of the iliac fossa in the frontal projection. It should not be mistaken for a fracture. Iliac vascular channels are similar to the horizontal vascular (Hahn's) clefts of the vertebral body.
Injection granulomas (Fig. 7-123)	Intramuscular and subcutaneous injections may cause localized inflammatory response, necrosis, and resulting residual tissue calcification. The usual appearance is of homogenous, round densities, less than 2 cm in diameter, and common in the buttocks.
Ischiopubic synchondrosis (Fig. 7-124)	The normal ischiopubic synchondrosis may persist beyond adolescence, usually appearing as a bilateral bulbous defect at the predictable site of the normal synchondrosis.
Os acetabulum (Fig. 7-125)	In the radiology literature, a persistent marginal epiphysis of the acetabulum is referred to as an *os acetabulum*. In truth, they are more likely accessory ossicles located at the lateral margin of the acetabulum. An os acetabulum may be confused with the slightly more superior defect of an avulsion of the anterior inferior iliac spine (AIIS).
Osteitis condensans ilia (OCI) (Fig. 7-126)	Osteitis condensans ilia (hyperostosis condensans ilia) describes a triangular-shaped (apex superior, base inferior) hyperostosis of the lower, medial portion of the ilium immediately adjacent to the lower portion of the sacroiliac joint. It is uncommon in males, and most common in multiparous females. The defects are usually bilateral, and generally asymmetric. It is mostly a radiographic diagnosis, and is believed to represent a stress response of bone secondary to stresses across the sacroiliac joint[78] and pubic symphysis[14] secondary to pregnancy or other causes of joint instability. Osteitis condensans ilia can be differentiated from ankylosing spondylitis by the latter's tendency to be mostly found in males, involve the sacroiliac joint space, be present with marginal erosions, and cause sclerosis on both the sacral and iliac sides of the joint. An oblique film is invaluable to determine if both sides of the joint are involved, suggesting inflammatory arthritis. Osteitis condensans ilia has an ambiguous association with clinical complaints. Mild pain is noted in some patients but not all. Pain is likely associated with the degree of joint instability.[14] The condition of osteitis condensans ilia may resolve completely, yielding a normal appearance to the pelvis over time.
Paraglenoid sulci (Figs. 7-127 and 7-128)	Paraglenoid (preauricular) sulci usually are symmetric, semilunar notched defects about 1 cm deep and located in the lower margin of each ilium, immediately lateral to the caudal margins of the sacroiliac joints. Both men and women can demonstrate paraglenoid sulci, but in men they are uncommon and shallow. Women, especially those who have given birth, show deeper paraglenoid sulci. Because the sulcus develops at the site of attachment of the anterior sacroiliac ligament, some believe paraglenoid sulci represent a stress resorption of bone. Other sources suggest the sulci are created by the overlying superior gluteal artery; however, this is thought to be a less plausible cause.[94] Paraglenoid sulci are of no clinical significance.

TABLE 7-3 cont'd
Normal Skeletal Variants and Defects of the Sacrum, Coccyx, and Pelvis

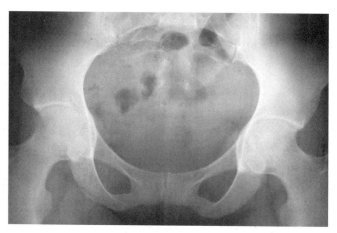

FIG. 7-118 Medial migration of the femoral head into the acetabular floor may occur secondary to bone-softening disease, inflammatory joint disease degeneration, or present as a normal variant. This anteroposterior radiograph of the pelvis exhibits bilateral protrusion of the medial walls of the acetabuli. When bilateral and idiopathic, acetabular protrusion is termed *Otto pelvis*.

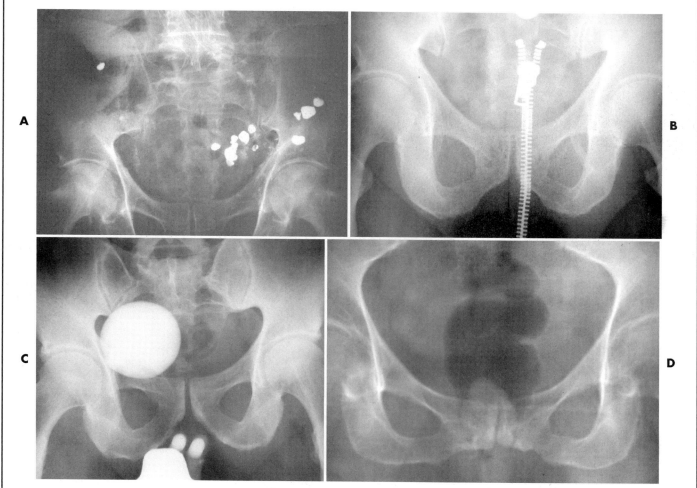

FIG. 7-119 Pelvic artifacts including, **A,** Residual barium; **B,** clothing; **C,** penile implant; and, **D,** bowel gas and fecal material. (**C,** Courtesy Julie-Marthe Grenier, Davenport, IA.)

TABLE 7-3 cont'd
Normal Skeletal Variants and Defects of the Sacrum, Coccyx, and Pelvis

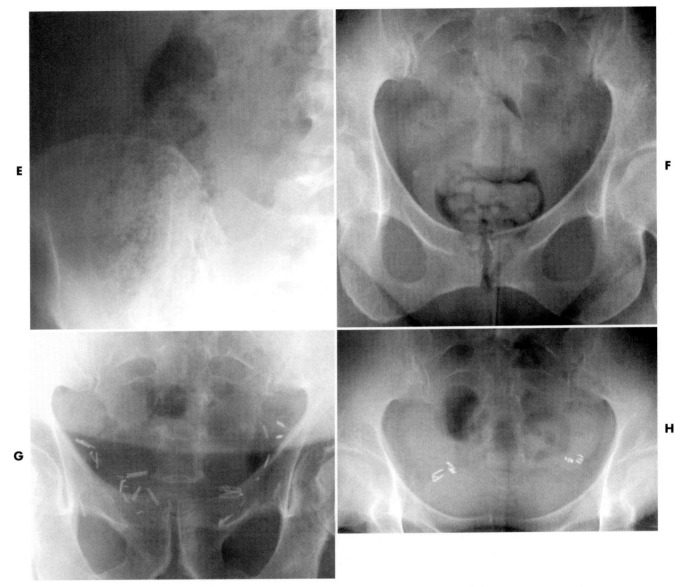

FIG. 7-119 cont'd   Pelvic artifacts including, **E** and **F,** bowel gas and fecal material; **G,** prostate surgery; and, **H,** Hulka clips of tubal ligation. (**E,** Courtesy John S. Urban, Beverly, OH; **F,** Courtesy Brad Stauffer, Gretna, NE.)

TABLE 7-3 cont'd
Normal Skeletal Variants and Defects of the Sacrum, Coccyx, and Pelvis

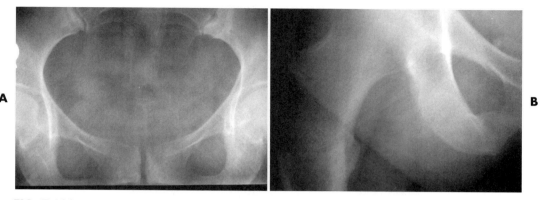

FIG. 7-120 **A** and **B,** Gluteal muscle striations can sometimes be seen as a normal finding of oblique shadows (oriented inferior and lateral) over the lower pelvis.

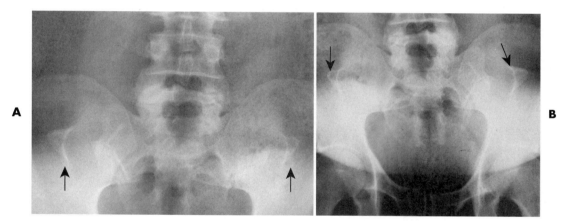

FIG. 7-121 **A** and **B,** Two cases of bilateral osseous extensions from the iliac fossae *(arrows)* known as *iliac horns.* (**B,** Courtesy Brad Stauffer, Gretna, NE.)

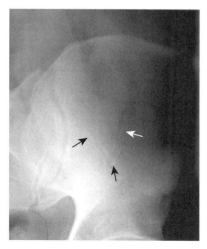

FIG. 7-122 A faint V-shaped radiolucent defect of the central ilium is noted *(arrows).* (Courtesy Aaron M. Hoffman, Bristol, RI.)

TABLE 7-3 cont'd
Normal Skeletal Variants and Defects of the Sacrum, Coccyx, and Pelvis

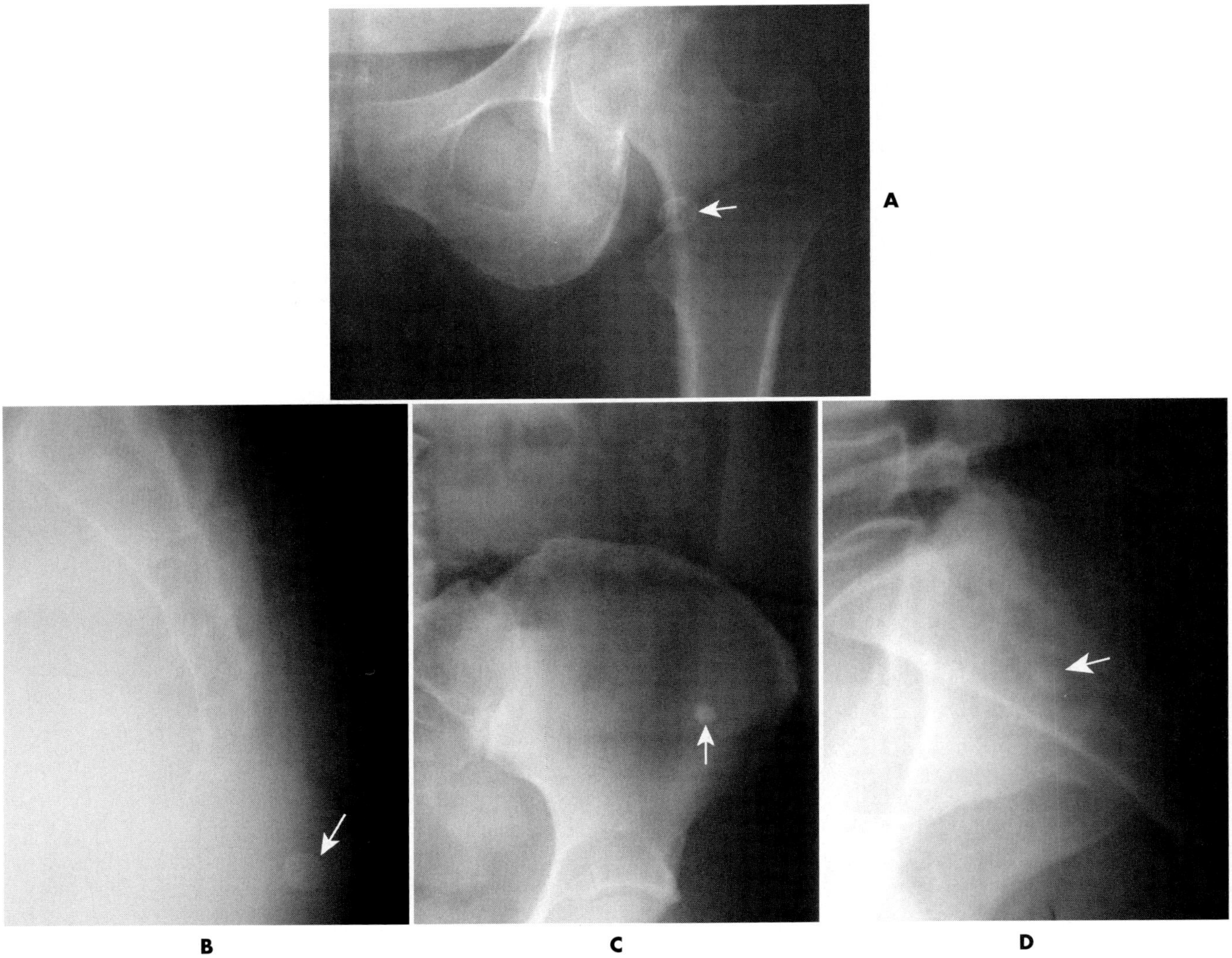

FIG. 7-123   A radiodense shadow noted overlying, **A,** the proximal femur and, **B,** posterior to the sacrum *(arrows)*. **C** and **D,** A second case exhibits a small radiodense shadow of the gluteal area also consistent with an injection granuloma *(arrows)*.

TABLE 7-3 cont'd

Normal Skeletal Variants and Defects of the Sacrum, Coccyx, and Pelvis

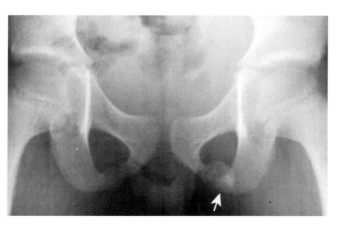

FIG. 7-124 Persistence of the ischiopubic synchondrosis *(arrow)*. (Courtesy Steven P. Brownstein, MD, Springfield, NJ.)

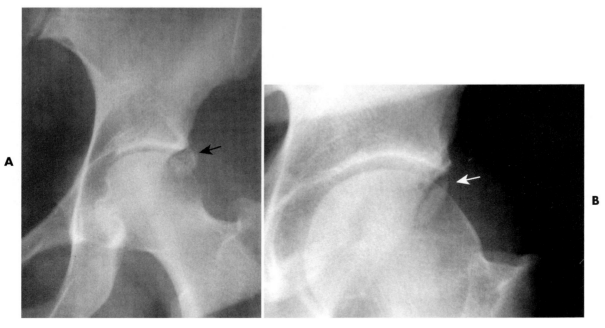

FIG. 7-125 **A** and **B,** Two cases of an accessory bone noted at the lateral aspect of the acetabulum, termed *os acetabuli (arrows)*. The appearance should not be confused with fracture. (Courtesy Gary Sclabassi, Walled Lake, MI.)

Continued

TABLE 7-3 cont'd
Normal Skeletal Variants and Defects of the Sacrum, Coccyx, and Pelvis

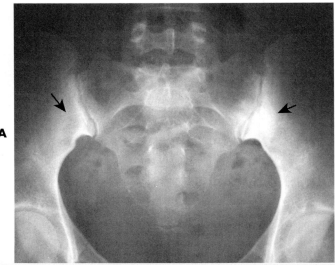

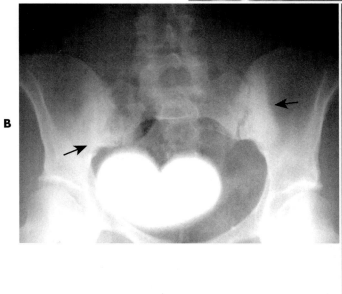

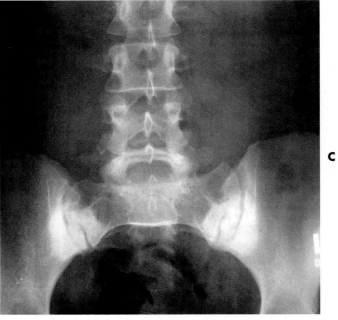

FIG. 7-126 **A** to **C,** Three cases of triangular-shaped (apex superior) regions of bone sclerosis involving the region of the iliac bone immediately adjacent to the sacroiliac joints, bilaterally *(arrows).* The appearance is known as *osteitis condensans ilia.*

TABLE 7-3 cont'd
Normal Skeletal Variants and Defects of the Sacrum, Coccyx, and Pelvis

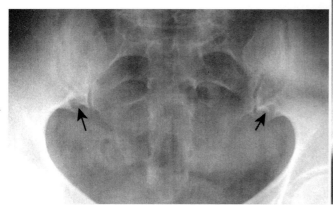

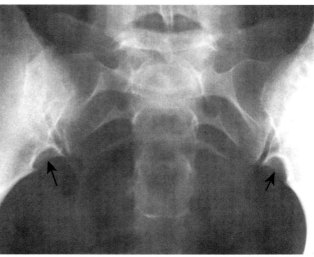

FIG. 7-127   **A** and **B,** Two cases of paraglenoid sulci appear as semilunar defects immediately lateral to the lower margin of the each sacroiliac joint *(arrows).* (**B,** Courtesy John Urban, Beverly, OH.)

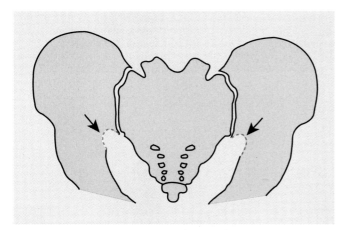

FIG. 7-128   Paraglenoid sulci appearing as bilateral, symmetric small defects of the lower medial margins of the ilia *(arrows).*

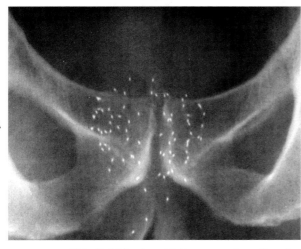

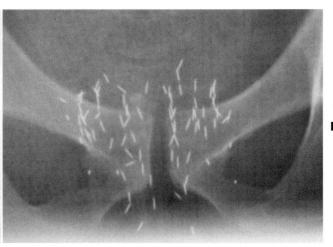

FIG. 7-129   **A** and **B,** Two cases of metallic radioactive implants placed about the prostate to deliver an internal dose of radiation. (**B,** Courtesy Julie-Marthe Grenier, Davenport, IA.)

Continued

TABLE 7-3 cont'd

Normal Skeletal Variants and Defects of the Sacrum, Coccyx, and Pelvis

Variant	Comments
Prostate brachytherapy (Fig. 7-129)	Permanent radioactive prostate seed implants are used alone or in combination with external radiation as a treatment for prostate cancer.
Prostate calcification (Fig. 7-130)	Prostate calcification is a common finding among older men. The calcification may be primary or secondary. Primary calcifications develop in the acini of the prostate's parenchyma. Although the etiology has not been identified, it may be related to desquamated epithelial cells. Secondary prostate calcification is associated with benign hyperplasia, infection, radiotherapy, or carcinoma.
Pseudosubluxation of S1 (Fig. 7-131)	The posterior aspect of the S1-2 interspace may appear widened in children. The appearance is a feature of the developing sacrum and should not be confused with trauma or other disease process.[17]
Pubic ears (Fig. 7-132)	A small (<1 cm) sessile exostosis may be noted from the inferior margin of the superior pubic ramus projecting into the obturator foramen on each side of the pelvis, forming a normal variant known as *pubic ears* or *pubic spurs*. Their small size and symmetric bilateral presentation distinguish them from osteochondromas.
Sacral agenesis (Figs. 7-133 and 7-134)	Sacral and lumbosacral agenesis describes an uncommon group of congenital disorders that present with a missing caudal portion of the sacrum. In severe cases, all of the sacrum and portions of the lumbar spine are missing, denoting the term *lumbosacral agenesis*. Four types have been described.[87] Type I is either partial or total unilateral sacral agenesis. Type II is partial sacral agenesis with bilateral symmetric defects, but intact sacroiliac joints with the first sacral segment. Type III is total sacral agenesis with the ilia articulating with the lowest vertebrae present. Lastly, type IV is variable sacral and lumbar agenesis with the caudal endplate of the lowest vertebrae articulating with the superior margin of the fused ilia or ilia pseudoarthrosis. The etiology of sacral agenesis is poorly defined. Maternal diabetes[10] and exposure to organic solvents have been implicated as causes.
Sacral fossae (Fig. 7-135)	Normal fossae of the sacral wings may mimic bone destruction.
Spina bifida occulta (Fig. 7-136)	Spina bifida occulta is a small midline defect of spine development. It is common at S1. The condition is discussed in more detail in Table 7-2.
Supernumerary coccygeal segments	Normally there are four coccygeal segments, but it is not uncommon to have five or six segments constituting the coccyx.
Vas deferens calcification (Fig. 7-137)	Calcification of the vas deferens may be seen in men, and is associated with long-standing diabetes. They appear as bilateral, tubelike structures that are present in the lower middle pelvis.

TABLE 7-3 cont'd
Normal Skeletal Variants and Defects of the Sacrum, Coccyx, and Pelvis

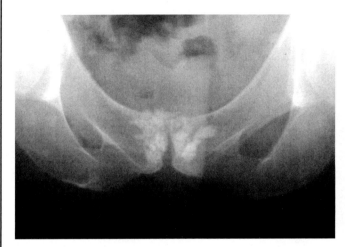

FIG. 7-130 Prostate calcification noted as a mottled pattern of radio-density overlying the pubic symphysis. (Courtesy Robert C. Tatum, Davenport, IA.)

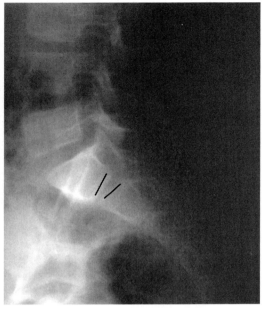

FIG. 7-131 Open posterior wedge of the S1 disc space *(lines)*, presenting as a normal variant in the developing spine. (Courtesy Frank C. Miramonti, Mt Clemens, MI.)

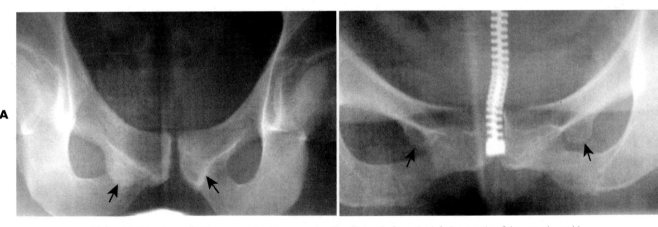

FIG. 7-132 **A** and **B**, Two cases of pubic ears extending bilaterally from the inferior margin of the superior pubic ramus as a common normal variant *(arrows)*.

Continued

TABLE 7-3 cont'd
Normal Skeletal Variants and Defects of the Sacrum, Coccyx, and Pelvis

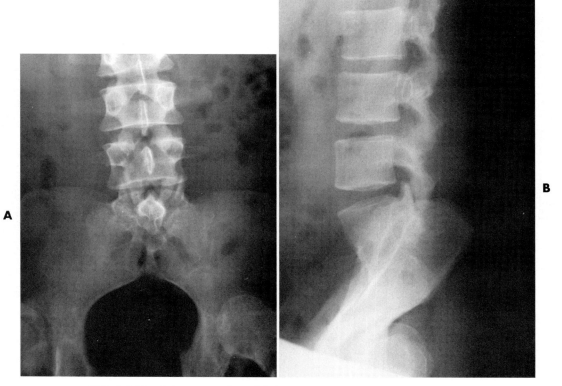

FIG. 7-133   A, Anteroposterior and, **B,** lateral projections demonstrate sacral aplasia.

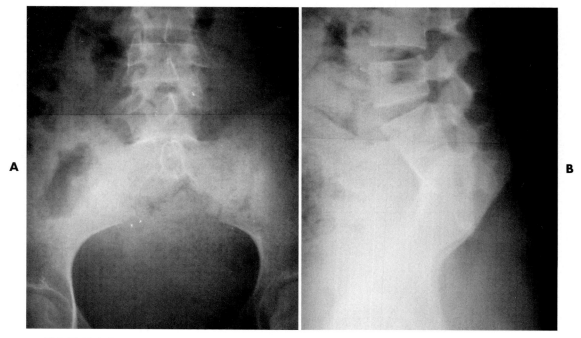

FIG. 7-134   The sacrum is hypoplastic on, **A,** the anteroposterior and, **B,** lateral projection. (Courtesy Geri Gangowski, Davenport, IA.)

TABLE 7-3 cont'd

Normal Skeletal Variants and Defects of the Sacrum, Coccyx, and Pelvis

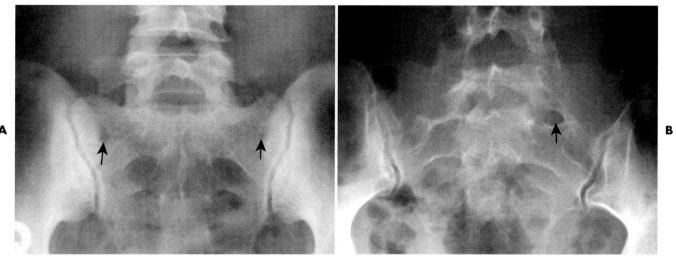

FIG. 7-135 **A** and **B,** Normal fossae of the sacrum may at times appear prominent, even mimicking a destructive process *(arrows).*

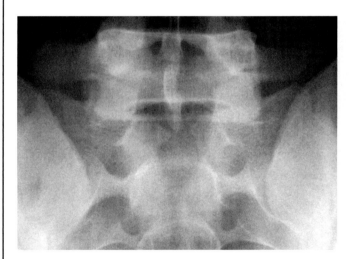

FIG. 7-136 Spina bifida occulta, presenting as a large V-shaped defect of the posterior arch of S1 and S2.

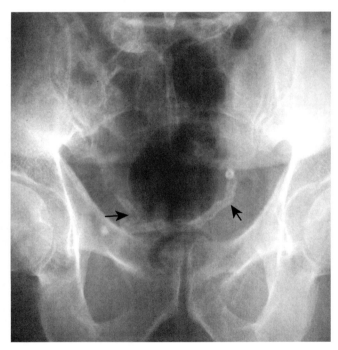

FIG. 7-137 Vas deferens calcification *(arrows)* is related to diabetes mellitus.

TABLE 7-4
Normal Skeletal Variants and Common Artifacts of the Thorax

Variant/Artifact	Comments
Artifacts (Fig. 7-138)	Commonly seen artifacts include: breast implants, prosthetic valves, pacemaker, and coronary artery bypass graft (CABG).
Clavicle companion shadow (Fig. 7-139)	The overlying skin of the clavicle may cause a radiodense shadow that parallels the shaft of the clavicle. The appearance should not be confused with a periosteal response.
Clavicle medial apophysis (Fig. 7-140)	Persistence of the medial clavicular apophysis presents as a thin osseous structure that may be confused with a fracture or apical calcification.
Costal cartilage calcification (Figs. 7-141 and 7-142)	Calcification of the costal cartilages is very common. It is slightly more common among men than women and has a definite positive correlation to age. It typically presents bilaterally and nearly symmetrically. The pattern of calcification generally begins at the first rib level and progresses to inferior levels. Men tend to demonstrate conduit-like calcification in the periphery of the costal cartilages. Women demonstrate central calcifications, likened to the appearance of a wagging tail or tongue. Calcification first rib's costal cartilage has been noted in 50%[43] to 88%[65] of subjects studied with computed tomography, with various ages sampled. The prevalence is less on plain films, but it remains as a very common finding. If the calcification of the first costal cartilage is prominent and isolated, it sometimes can be mistaken for a pulmonary mass in the lung apex (known as a *student tumor*). An apical lordotic projection (an anteroposterior projection of the lung apex taken with 15 to 20 degrees cephalic tube tilt) resolves any controversy, by projection of the first costal cartilage above the lung field.
Hypoplastic ribs	Smaller than normally expected ribs are sometimes noted, typically at T12.
Intrathoracic rib	Intrathoracic ribs are usually hypoplastic anomalous ribs that extend into the thoracic cavity, appearing as radiodense shadows appearing transverse or oblique to the normally formed ribs. They need to be distinguished from pulmonary lesions.
Pectus carinatum (Figs. 7-143 to 7-145)	Pectus carinatum (pigeon or keel chest) is a deformity where the anterior chest wall is sharply protruded anteriorly. At times a component of lateral deviation also can be seen. Pectus carinatum is significantly less common than pectus excavatum, the former with an overall prevalence estimated at 0.06% in the United States.[70] Although most patients exhibit some degree of thoracic rigidity and decreased inspiratory function, most individuals remain asymptomatic and typically present during adolescence for cosmetic or related psychologic concerns. Pectus carinatum may occur as an isolated anomaly, or in association with congenital heart disease (usually mitral valve prolapse), scoliosis, Morquio's syndrome, hyperlordosis, and increased kyphosis.[90] Bracing and surgical correction may be used to address significant presentations.[38,96]
Pectus excavatum	Pectus excavatum ("hollow," "funnel," or "sunken" chest) is an inward deformity of the anterior chest wall beginning at the manubrium and sloping posterior to its deepest point just before the xiphoid. The anterior portions of the lower ribs are also posteriorly curved. Pectus excavatum occurs in an estimated 0.3% births, and is three times more common among male patients.[40] It typically presents in the first year of life, but becomes most prominent during the rapid growth phase of adolescence.[40] It is associated with scoliosis, congenital heart disease, low bone density, rickets, and asthma. The psychologic impact related to the cosmetic deformity is a more common clinical concern than the possibility of cardiopulmonary compression.[33] Because clinical symptoms are uncommon in early childhood, surgical management has been controversial. However, long-term follow-up studies and less invasive surgical techniques confirm benefit of surgical correction in selected cases.[38,46] In the lateral projection, the anterior chest wall appears convex posteriorly. In the frontal projection, radiographic features include a straight left heart border, indistinct right heart border (false-positive silhouette sign), displaced cardiac shadow to the left, and a prominent pulmonary trunk. Assessment is best accomplished with computed tomography and quantified with the pectus index, calculated by dividing the thorax width (right to left dimension) by the depth (anterior to posterior dimension). The normal value for this index is 2.55 with a standard deviation of 0.35. Patients with an index of more than 3.25 may require surgical intervention.[47]

TABLE 7-4 cont'd
Normal Skeletal Variants and Common Artifacts of the Thorax

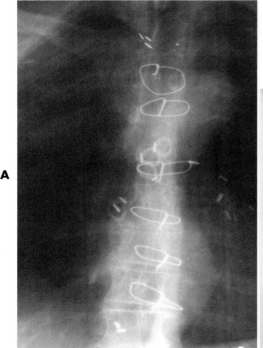

A

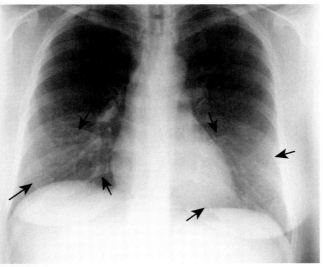

B

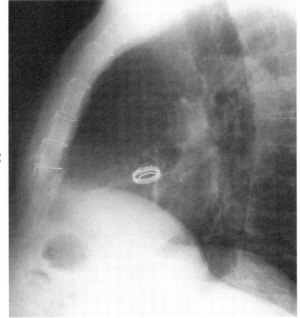

C

FIG. 7-138   Selected artifacts of the ribs and thorax, including, **A,** sternal wires; **B,** breast implants *(arrows)* and, **C,** mitral valve prosthesis. (**C,** Courtesy Julie-Marthe Grenier, Davenport, IA.)

Continued

TABLE 7-4 cont'd
Normal Skeletal Variants and Common Artifacts of the Thorax

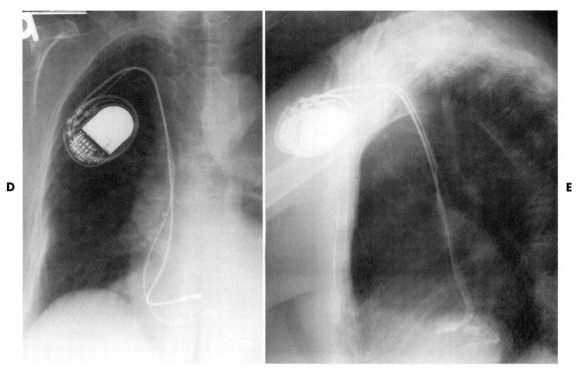

FIG. 7-138 cont'd   Selected artifacts of the ribs and thorax, including, **D** and **E,** pacemaker.

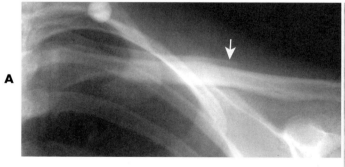

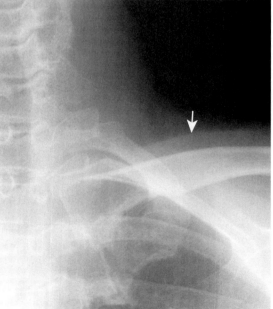

FIG. 7-139   **A** and **B,** The skin overlying the clavicle causes a parallel "companion" shadow to the bone *(arrows)*, seen here in two cases. (**A,** Courtesy Maureen Work, Ottawa, IL; **B,** Courtesy Randy Hurt, Rock Island, IL.)

TABLE 7-4 cont'd
Normal Skeletal Variants and Common Artifacts of the Thorax

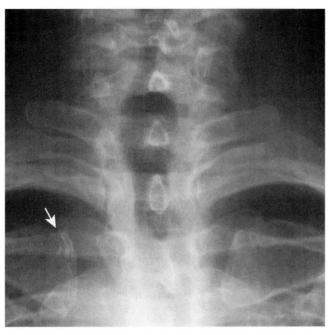

FIG. 7-140 Persistent medial clavicle apophysis on the patient's right side *(arrow)*.

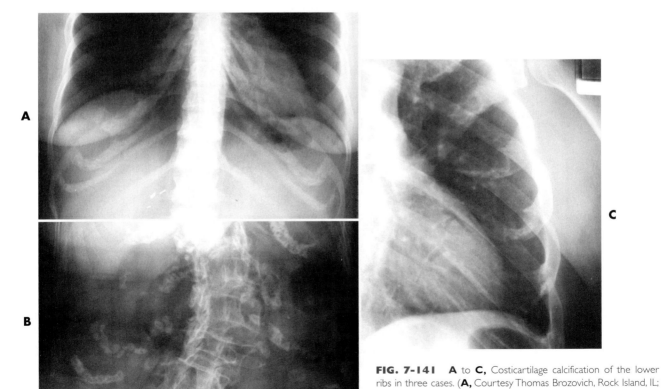

FIG. 7-141 **A** to **C,** Costicartilage calcification of the lower ribs in three cases. (**A,** Courtesy Thomas Brozovich, Rock Island, IL; **C,** Courtesy Troy Scheuermann, Farmington, IA.)

TABLE 7-4 cont'd
Normal Skeletal Variants and Common Artifacts of the Thorax

FIG. 7-142   A, Prominent calcification of the first costal cartilages that easily could be confused with pulmonary lesions (Student tumors *(arrows)*). An apical lordotic view would differentiate from a true pulmonary lesion in that the rib calcification would project above the pulmonary tissue. It is a more confusing appearance if the presentation is unilateral. **B,** A small (5 cm) intrathoracic rib is noted at an oblique superior angle from the proximal portion of the right fifth rib *(arrows)*.

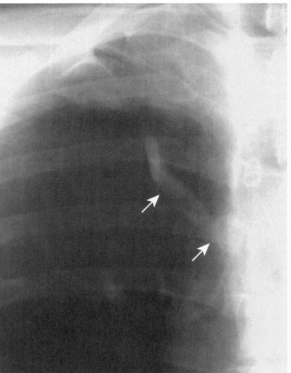

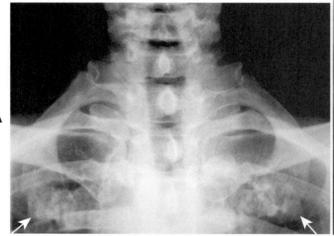

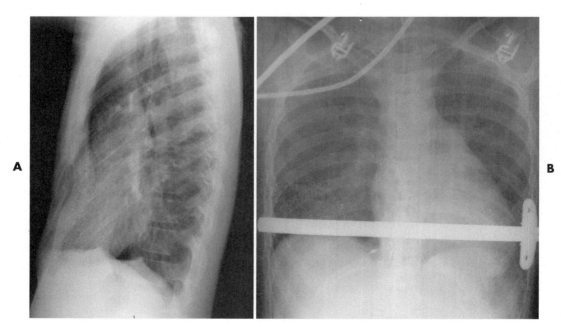

FIG. 7-143   Pectus excavatum. **A,** An 11-year-old boy exhibits inward deformity of the anterior chest wall. **B,** A curved bar is inserted across the posterior aspect of the anterior chest wall. After insertion, the bar is rotated 180 degrees, thereby applying anteriorly directed pressure to the deformed chest wall as a corrective measure. (Courtesy Thomas Brozovich, Rock Island, IL.)

TABLE 7-4 cont'd
Normal Skeletal Variants and Common Artifacts of the Thorax

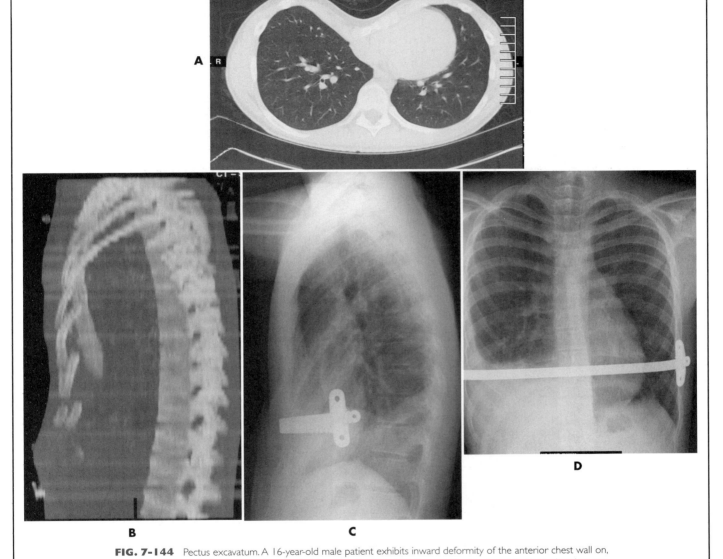

FIG. 7-144 Pectus excavatum. A 16-year-old male patient exhibits inward deformity of the anterior chest wall on, **A,** axial and, **B,** sagittal reformatted computed tomography. **C** and **D,** A corrective bar is put in place, aimed at correcting the deformity. This patient is the older brother of the patient appearing in Figure 7-143. Pectus excavatum is more common in males; however, contrary to the cases shown here, it does not exhibit a strong familial predisposition. (Courtesy Thomas Brozovich, Rock Island, IL.)

Continued

TABLE 7-4 cont'd
Normal Skeletal Variants and Common Artifacts of the Thorax

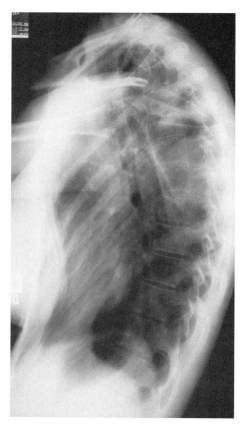

FIG. 7-145   Pectus excavatum. A 27-year-old woman exhibiting inward deformity of the anterior chest wall.

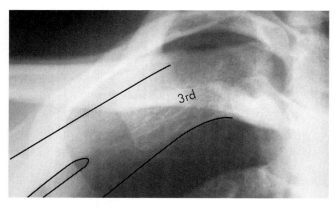

FIG. 7-146   The distal end of the third right rib is forked.

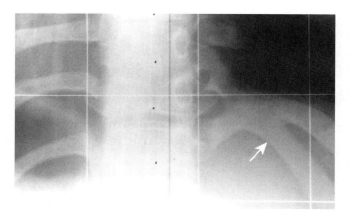

FIG. 7-148   Rib synostosis of two lower ribs *(arrow)*.

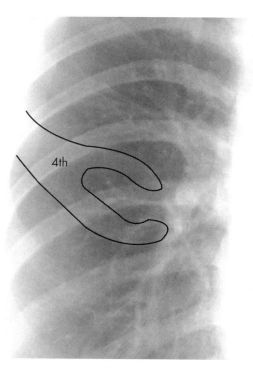

FIG. 7-147   The distal end of the fourth rib is forked, overlying the posterior portion of the sixth rib, in the center of the film.

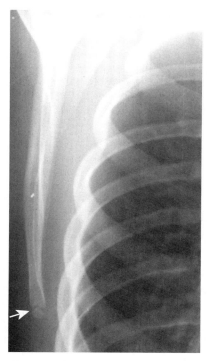

FIG. 7-149   Nonunion of the apophysis of the inferior angle of the scapula *(arrow)*. (Courtesy Steven P. Brownstein, MD, Springfield, NJ.)

TABLE 7-4 cont'd
Normal Skeletal Variants and Common Artifacts of the Thorax

Variant/Artifact	Comments
Rhomboid fossae	Rhomboid fossae define normal, bilateral, and symmetric irregularities along the lower margin of the medial ends of the clavicles. They mark the site of costoclavicular ligament insertion and should not be confused with fracture or tumor.
Rib bifurcation (Figs. 7-146 and 7-147)	A bifurcated (bicipital, bifid, or Luschka) rib is one that appears forked at its sternal end. They are nearly always of no clinical significance, but may be associated with Gorlin syndrome, a rare autosomal dominant cancer syndrome marked by the presence of basal cell carcinomas (or basal cell nevus syndrome where the nevi are basal cell carcinomas) and anomalies of multiple organ syndromes. At times the bifid end of the rib gives the false appearance of a pulmonary cyst.
Rib foramen	Variant formation of a radiolucent foramen within the body of a rib.
Rib synostosis (Fig. 7-148)	Adjacent ribs sometimes fuse, representing a variant of no direct significant clinical concern; however, there is a weak association with the presence of developmental foregut defects.
Scapula apophysis (Fig. 7-149)	The secondary ossification centers of the scapula typically fuse by the third decade; persistence may mimic a fracture.
Srb's anomaly	Srb's anomaly is partial longitudinal fusion of the first and second ribs to form a continuous osseous plate.
Straight back syndrome (Fig. 7-150)	Straight (or flat) back syndrome describes the coupled findings of reduced thoracic kyphosis (cobbler chest) and heart murmur. Traditionally, straight back syndrome was thought to be a "pseudo" heart disease; that is, that the heart murmur was secondary to the narrowed anteroposterior diameter of the thoracic and resulting compression of the heart. However, more current literature suggests that straight back syndrome is related directly to mitral valve prolapse.[4] Mitral valve prolapse also is associated with other structural deformities of the chest, including scoliosis and pectus excavatum.[60] Palpitations and chest pain are the most common symptoms. According to Davies,[27] straight back syndrome is defined on a lateral radiograph by measuring the interval between the anterior margin of T8 and a line constructed from the anterior margin of T4 to T12. An interval less than 1.2 cm is indicative of straight back syndrome.
Supernumerary ribs	Rib anomalies may occur in form and number. Too few or too many ribs can present as bilateral or unilateral phenomena. Supernumerary ribs are extra ribs, beyond the normal 12 pair, and typically present at C7 or L1.

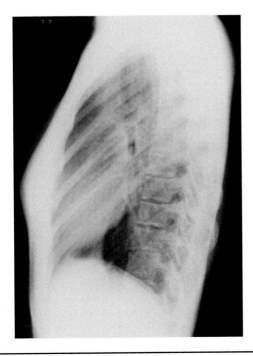

FIG. 7-150 Straight back syndrome noted by marked reduction of the anterior to posterior distance of the thorax. (Courtesy William E. Litterer, Elizabeth, NJ.)

TABLE 7-5
Normal Skeletal Variants of the Upper Extremities

Variant/Artifact	Comments
Accessory ossicle (Figs. 7-151 and 7-152)	An accessory ossicle (small bone) is either an anomalous congenital supernumerary ossicle, a normally present secondary ossification center that failed to unite, or occasionally an acquired ossification of posttraumatic degenerative etiology. They are commonly seen about the foot, hand, and wrist. Sesamoid bones are accessory ossicles formed in tendons and ligaments and are common in the first, second, and fifth digits. Although usually they are of no clinical significance, some accessory bones have been related to pain syndromes resulting from fracture, degenerative changes, avascular necrosis, and irritation or impingement of adjacent soft tissue.[71,85,88] At times accessory ossicles may be confused with traumatic fragments. Traumatic fragments typically are displaced from the host bone, are irregular, have a partially corticated periphery, and may demonstrate overlying soft-tissue edema. Accessory ossicles usually are smooth, have an entirely corticated periphery, are nondisplaced, and occur in typical locations. In addition, accessory ossicles are most often found to be bilateral and symmetric; fractures are not. Figure 7-151 maps some of the more common accessory bones of the hand.
Artifacts	Common artifacts include: interphalangeal joint prosthesis, shoulder prosthesis, and so on.
Brachydactyly	Brachydactyly refers to disproportionately short fingers and toes. It may present as an isolated autosomal dominant defect or in association with other findings (e.g., dwarfism, mental retardation). The short tubular bones develop as a consequence of premature epiphyseal closure. Radiographically, the involved epiphyses appear coned, with the apex directed into the corresponding metaphysis.
Calcification of the interosseous membrane	The margin of the interosseous membrane between the radius and ulna often ossifies, yielding an appearance that may mimic a periosteal reaction. Interosseous membrane calcification often occurs concurrently on adjacent bones.
Carpal boss	A carpal boss (carpe bossu), first described by Fiolle,[37] refers to a bony eminence at the base of the second or third metacarpal. Occasionally it extends to the dorsal aspect of the trapezoid and capitate. It is best visualized on the lateral wrist projection, appearing as a regular bony eminence at the carpometacarpal joint. The condition is usually symptom free; however, pain is associated with overuse syndromes of wrist flexion, and possibly subluxations of extensor tendons that overlie the carpal boss.[108] The discomfort and pain usually are treated by conservative means; surgery may be indicated in those cases that do not respond to conservative management. A review of 116 patients treated surgically for symptomatic carpal boss found complete symptomatic relief in 94% of patients within an average follow-up of 42 months.[41]
Carpal coalition (Fig. 7-153)	Carpal coalition refers to the uncommon occurrence when a portion of the carpal cartilaginous anlage fails to segment into separate carpal bones. Coalition is most typical between the lunate and triquetrum. Lunate-triquetral coalitions can be subdivided into four types according to the degree of union.[98] Previously considered completely asymptomatic, carpal coalition and associated degenerative arthritis of the incompletely involved joints has been proved as a cause of occult wrist pain.[69] At times coalition is found with round radiolucent shadows in the subarticular region of the fused bones. This appearance is attributed to abnormal differentiation of the joint space and remnants of misplaced synovial tissue residual to joint development.[45]
Clinodactyly	Clinodactyly refers to curvature of a finger in a mediolateral plane. Although it may involve any finger, radial deviation of the fifth digit toward the fourth digit is the most common presentation. It can occur as an isolated finding or in association with chromosomal abnormalities (e.g., Down syndrome), developmental disorders (e.g., macrodystrophia lipomatosa), electrical burns, and trauma.
Humerus pseudocyst (Fig. 7-154)	The on-end projection of the greater tuberosity during an anteroposterior shoulder projection with internal rotation can sometimes give the illusion of a cyst in the head of the humerus. Similar pseudocysts are seen with the tubercles of the proximal radius.
Kirner deformity	Kirner deformity is an uncommon palmoradial curvature of the distal phalanx of the fifth digit. It is usually bilateral. It is thought to result from an anomalous insertion of the deep flexor over the growth cartilage. No treatment is required in view of the absence of any clinical and functional symptoms.[28] Splinting may be beneficial for pain relief and, if used early, may retard progression of the deformity. (Disability usually is minimal, and treatment to correct the deformity may prevent recurrence.[95])

TABLE 7-5 cont'd
Normal Skeletal Variants of the Upper Extremities

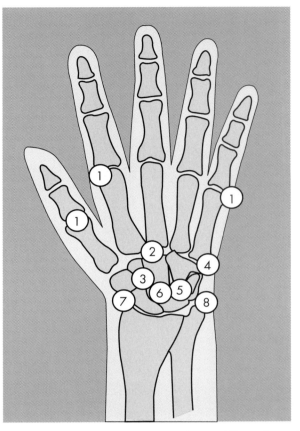

FIG. 7-151 Accessory ossicles of the hand: *1,* sesamoid bones; *2,* os styloideum; *3,* os centrale; *4,* os vesalianum manus; *5,* epipyramis; *6,* epilunatum; *7,* os radiale externum; *8,* os triangulare.

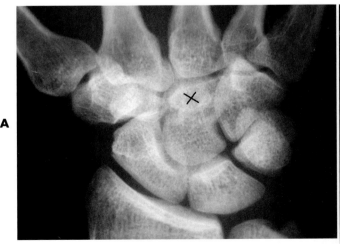

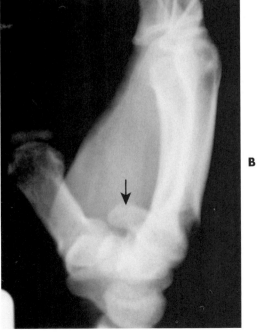

FIG. 7-152 Os centralis noted in the center of the wrist on, **A,** the posteroanterior and, **B,** lateral projections *(arrow).* (Courtesy Ron Firth, East Moline, IL.)

TABLE 7-5 cont'd
Normal Skeletal Variants of the Upper Extremities

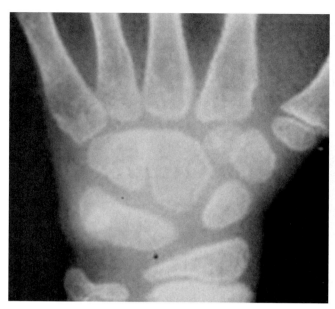

FIG. 7-153   Carpal coalition of the lunate and triquetrum is noted.

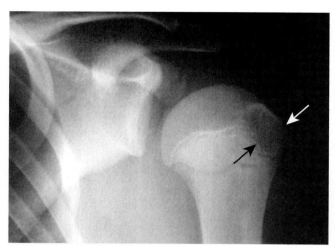

FIG. 7-154   On-end projections of a bone protuberance may simulate a cyst. In this case the greater tuberosity gives a pseudocyst appearance of the proximal humerus *(arrows)*. (Courtesy Robert Rowell, Davenport, IA.)

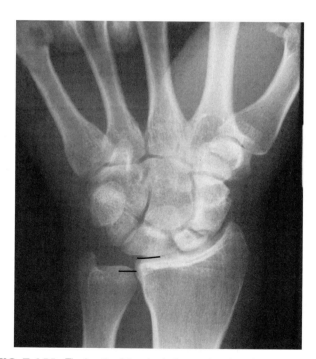

FIG. 7-155   The length of the ulna is shorter than that of the radius. This configuration is described as negative ulnar variance. At times there is associated avascular necrosis of the lunate. In this case unrelated avascular necrosis of the scaphoid is seen. (Courtesy Gary Longmuir, Phoenix, AZ.)

TABLE 7-5 cont'd
Normal Skeletal Variants of the Upper Extremities

Variant/Artifact	Comments
Madelung deformity	Madelung deformity is a congenital malformation of the wrist marked by dorsal and medial bowing of the radius and concurrent normal straight development of the ulna, resulting in a comparatively short radius. The carpal angle (formed by the intersection of two lines on the posteroanterior radiograph, one tangent to the proximal surfaces of the scaphoid and lunate and the other tangent to the proximal margins of the lunate and triquetrum) is decreased beyond the expected normal average value of 130 degrees.[48] Consistent with the decreased carpal angle, the proximal row of carpals appears V-shaped. The distal radial epiphysis demonstrates a triangular appearance with premature fusion of its medial half. Over time osteophytes tend to develop along the inferior ulnar aspect of the distal radius. The ulnar head is often enlarged with a tendency toward dorsal subluxation, leading to rupture of the extensor tendons of the fingers related to the deformity.[42] Most presentations of Madelung deformity are in association with dyschondrosteosis (Leri Weil disease), a mesomelic dwarfism, or less commonly with diaphyseal aclasis and Turner's syndrome. Cases of independent presentations have been reported.[7] Traumatic Madelung deformity may result from injury to the medial aspect of the radial epiphysis. Madelung deformity is more commonly bilateral than unilateral. The clinical impact ranges from little pain and cosmetic disturbance to moderate pain and functional impairment.[29] Treatment consisted of resection of the ulnar head, stabilization of the distal ulna, and repair of the extensor tendons by tendon transfers.[42] Radiographically it is recognized on the posteroanterior and lateral wrist projections by the volar and ulnar deviation of the distal end of the radius. Rarely some of the conditions named in the preceding may alternatively result in a "reverse" Madelung deformity marked by an anterior bowing and dorsal angulation of the distal end of the radius with dorsal displacement of the carpals.
Negative ulnar variance (Fig. 7-155)	Negative (−) ulnar variance describes the relative shortness of the ulna compared with the radius, as assessed at their distal ends. Negative ulnar variance has been associated with avascular necrosis of the lunate (Kienbock disease).[13] However, reports to the contrary exist,[22] leading to confusion in the literature. The mechanism for a proposed association is not causative but probably mechanical predisposition in which the relatively short ulna shifts the compressive and shear forces to the radiolunate joint, thereby promoting microfracture, focal avascularity, and subsequent necrosis of the lunate.[20] It is important to remember that most people with negative ulnar variance do not have Kienbock disease. Similarly, some reports suggest an association between negative ulnar variance and patient age; however, this finding is not consistent in the literature.[13,20,21,76]
Nutrient canal (Fig. 7-156)	Nutrient (or vascular) canals are a normal feature of all tubular bones. At times their presentation of an obliquely oriented radiolucent defect through the cortex of the shaft of a tubular bone may be confused with a fracture. Because nutrient canals are only small holes, they appear less radiolucent than fractures.
Polydactyly (Fig. 7-157)	Polydactyly is the presence of more than five fingers or toes. It is the most common congenital malformation of the hand[52] and has three presentations: preaxial (or duplication of the thumb), central (or duplication of the index, middle, or ring fingers), and postaxial (or duplication of the small finger). Postaxial polydactyly is further subdivided into type A, in which the extra digit is well developed, and type B, in which the extra digit is only rudimentary, without skeletal structure. Polydactyly can occur as an isolated condition or in conjunction with a large number of inherited and developmental disorders. Some of the more notable associations of preaxial polydactyly include acrocephalosyndactyly, acropectorovertebral dysplasia, Holt-Oram syndrome, and Fanconi syndrome. Postaxial polydactyly is associated with chondroectodermal dysplasia (Ellis-van Creveld syndrome), Laurence-Moon-Biedl syndrome, Jeunes syndrome, and Down syndrome.

Continued

TABLE 7-5 cont'd
Normal Skeletal Variants of the Upper Extremities

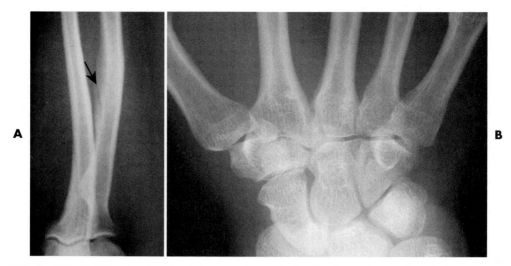

FIG. 7-156 **A,** Obliquely oriented radiolucent nutrient canal mimicking fracture in a long bone. **B,** Vascular channels often are mistaken for fractures. To differentiate between the two, vascular channels are less radiolucent than are fractures, the latter going through a greater portion of the cortex. The small notch noted at the lateral margin of the scaphoid represents the site where vessels enter and leave the waist of the scaphoid. This is commonly mistaken for fracture.

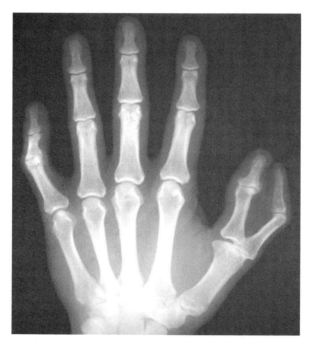

FIG. 7-157 The first digit is doubled, representing polydactyly. (Courtesy Ian D. McLean, Davenport, IA.)

TABLE 7-5 cont'd

Normal Skeletal Variants of the Upper Extremities

Variant/Artifact	Comments
Radioulnar synostosis	Congenital synostosis between the radius and ulna is an uncommon anomaly that develops after a failure of separation during the seventh fetal week. At least some cases are genetically transmitted, but spontaneous presentation often is noted. There are two broad presentations of radioulnar synostosis. The first occurs from the proximal border of the radius and ulna to about 3 to 6 cm distal, and the second presentation occurs as fusion between the ulna and radius just distal to the proximal radial epiphysis. Approximately 60% of cases are bilateral. The synostosis results in a fixed position of the forearm, which varies from neutral to full pronation. It can be severely disabling, especially if it is bilateral or severe hyperpronation (>60 degrees) exists.[99] Although there are marked limitations in pronation and supination, function of the hand is largely preserved.[5] Operative treatment consists of resection of the synostosis and interposition of fat, muscle, or an aponeurotic flap.[26,93] Radioulnar synostosis is often linked to sex chromosome abnormalities,[54] including XYY.[23] Associations are also reported with carpal coalition, Madelung deformity, clubfoot, Holt-Oram syndrome, acrocephalosyndactyly, Klinefelter syndrome (47, XXY), and Nievergelt (Pearlman) syndrome. Posttraumatic synostosis also has been described as an uncommon but serious complication of forearm fractures.[66,93]
Supracondylar process (Fig. 7-158)	A supracondylar process is a bony projection of varying length (usually 3 to 5 cm) that originates from the anteromedial surface of the distal humerus, approximately 5 cm from its distal end. At times, a fibrous band, known as Struthers ligament, extends from the process to the medial condyle of the humerus. A supracondylar process is seen in approximately 1% of the population, and is also seen in other mammals.[82] It is directed distally toward the elbow joint; a feature that is distinctive from a thin osteochondroma, which tends to project away from the joint. The supracondylar process is routinely of no clinical significance,[102] although a fractured supracondylar process does risk associated injury to the approximate neurovascular bundle.[56]
Syndactyly (Fig. 7-159)	Syndactyly is webbing between the fingers or toes. Syndactyly occurs as an isolated finding (type I) or with polydactyly (type II); the latter may be referred to as *synpolydactyly (SPD)*. Synpolydactyly generally is considered to be an autosomal dominant inherited trait with incomplete penetrance.[73]
Vacuum phenomenon	It is normal to see a vacuum phenomenon in a distracted synovial joint. However, vacuum phenomena are not normal features when seen in the disc space (see Chapter 9).

Continued

TABLE 7-5 cont'd
Normal Skeletal Variants of the Upper Extremities

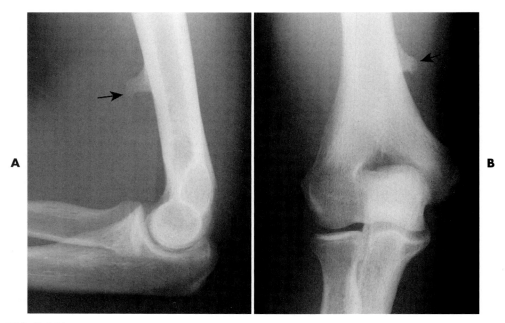

FIG. 7-158   A and **B,** A supracondylar process extends toward the elbow from the distal third of the humerus *(arrows).* (Courtesy Robert C. Tatum, Davenport, IA.)

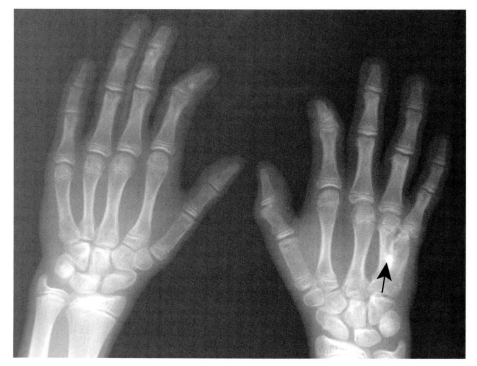

FIG. 7-159   Syndactyly presenting as fused fourth and fifth metacarpals *(arrow).* (Courtesy Steven P. Brownstein, MD, Springfield, NJ.)

TABLE 7-6

Normal Skeletal Variants of the Lower Extremities

Variant/Artifact	Comments
Accessory ossicles (Figs. 7-160 to 7-165)	An accessory ossicle (small bone) is either an anomalous congenital supernumerary ossicle, a normally present secondary ossification center that failed to unite, or occasionally an acquired ossification of posttraumatic degenerative etiology. Sesamoid bones are accessory ossicles formed in tendons and ligaments, common to the first, second, and fifth digits. Some accessory bones have been related to pain syndromes, but typically accessory bones are of no clinical significance. At times, they may be confused with traumatic fragments. Traumatic fragments are typically displaced from the host bone, are irregular, have a partially corticated periphery, and may demonstrate overlying soft-tissue edema. Accessory ossicles usually are smooth, have an entirely corticated periphery, are nondisplaced, and occur in typical locations. In addition, accessory ossicles are most often bilateral and symmetric; fractures are not. The os vesalianum and os peroneum are often mistaken for fractures of the styloid process at the base of the fifth metatarsal. To differentiate, the fracture is most often transverse to the long axis of the metacarpal and the line of separation between the accessory ossicle and the fifth metatarsal is oriented obliquely or longitudinally with the long axis of the metatarsal. Figure 7-160 maps some of the more common accessory bones of the foot. In the foot, some of the most common accessory bones include the os peroneum, accessory navicular, os trigonum, and os tibiale externum.[59]
Artifact (Fig. 7-166)	Common artifacts include: clothing artifact, skin folds, and so on.
Bipartite patella (Figs. 7-167 to 7-170)	Bipartite patella refers to a patella composed of two parts, the main body of the patella and a second fragment occurring inferior (type I), lateral (type II), or superolateral (type III), and connected by fibrous or cartilaginous tissue to the main body. Type III is most common. The fragments are in smooth and close approximation, maintaining the overall shape of the patella. Generally, the bipartite patella is described as a developmental variation seen in about 1% of the general population. Usually no symptoms are associated; however, the fragments can be traumatized, injuring the synchondrosis and promoting a painful syndrome, likely related to mobility of the synchondrosis.[79] Pain syndromes are more common among adolescents and adults who regularly participate in strenuous sports. Conservative management includes rest, stretching exercises of the quadriceps muscle, deep tissue massage, and patellar braces.[51,79] Occasionally the patella presents in three (tripartite) or more (multipartite) fragments.
Bone bars (Fig. 7-171)	Large, horizontally oriented trabeculations are often seen in the metaphysis of the long tubular bones, especially on radiographs taken of patients with osteoporosis or other causes of osteopenia.
Calcification of the interosseous membrane (Fig. 7-172)	Often the margins of the interosseous membrane between the tibia and fibula ossify, yielding an appearance that may mimic a periosteal reaction. Interosseous membrane calcification often occurs concurrently on adjacent bones. Similar changes are noted at the insertion of deltoid tendon into the lateral margin of the humerus.
Cavus foot	Cavus foot (or *pes cavus*) describes an exaggerated longitudinal arch of the foot involving either the entire foot (calcaneocavus) or isolated to the medial aspect (cavovarus) of the foot. The calcaneocavus variety is marked by dorsiflexion of the calcaneus and plantar flexion of the forefoot. Pes cavovarus appears with plantar flexion of the first metatarsal and pronation of the forefoot (metatarsals and phalanges). On the standing lateral foot project, the angle (Hibbs angle) of intersection created from a line drawn along the inferior margin of the calcaneus and a line through the long axis of the metatarsal should be greater than 155 degrees in normal presentations. Angles that measure less than 155 degrees suggest cavus foot. Cavus foot is associated with Charcot's-Marie-Tooth disease, syringomyelia, spinal cord tumor, diastematomyelia, and cerebral palsy.
Clubfoot deformity	Clubfoot deformity is also known as *talipes equinovarus*. It occurs in 1 in 800 live births, about half of the time is bilateral, and is twice as common among boys. Deformity is marked by plantar flexion of the hindfoot (calcaneus and talus), inversion of the hindfoot and midfoot (tarsal navicular, cuboid, and cuneiforms), and adduction of the midfoot and forefoot (metatarsals and phalanges). On the anteroposterior foot projection, clubfoot appears with nearly parallel lines of the long axis of the talus and calcaneus and marked medial deviation of the midfoot and forefoot. Similarly, the talus and calcaneus are abnormally parallel on the lateral projection. Clubfoot may lead to significant dysfunction if uncorrected.

Continued

TABLE 7-6 cont'd
Normal Skeletal Variants of the Lower Extremities

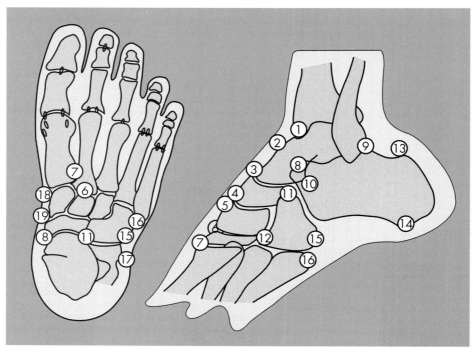

FIG. 7-160 Accessory ossicles of the foot: *1*, os talotibiale; *2*, os supratalare; *3*, os supranaviculare; *4*, os infran-aviculare; *5*, os intercuneiformes; *6*, os cuneometatarsal; *7*, os intermetatarsales; *8*, os tibiale externum; *9*, os trigonum; *10*, calcaneus secundarius; *11*, secondary cuboid; *12*, os unci; *13*, os accessorium supracalcaneum; *14*, os subcalcis; *15*, peroneal bone (os peroneum); *16*, os vesalianum; *17*, os trochleare calcanei; *18*, sesamum tibiale anterius; *19*, os cuneonavicular mediale.

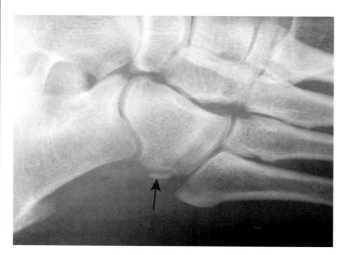

FIG. 7-161 Os perineum *(arrow)*.

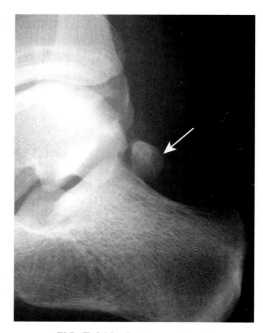

FIG. 7-162 Os trigonum *(arrow)*.

TABLE 7-6 cont'd
Normal Skeletal Variants of the Lower Extremities

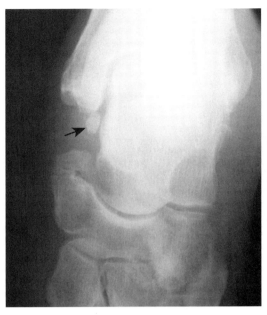

FIG. 7-163 Os tibialis externum *(arrow)*. (Courtesy Ron Simmer, Rock Island, IL.)

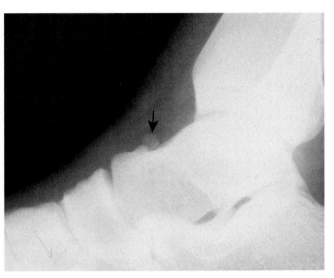

FIG. 7-164 Os supratalare *(arrow)*. (Courtesy Dale Fleming, Lacon, IL.)

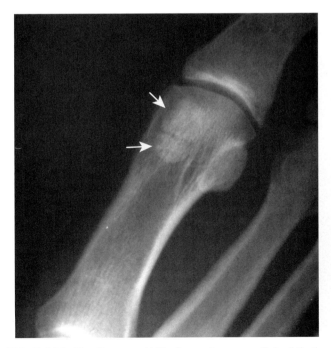

FIG. 7-165 Bipartite sesamoid. The fragments are smooth, in distinction to fracture fragments, which appear irregular *(arrows)*. (Courtesy Dustan Mattingly, Chillicothe, IL.)

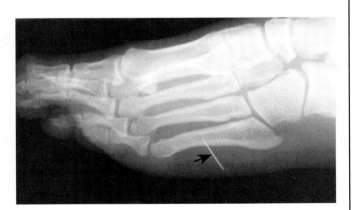

FIG. 7-166 Foreign body of a needle broken off in the foot *(arrow)*.

TABLE 7-6 cont'd
Normal Skeletal Variants of the Lower Extremities

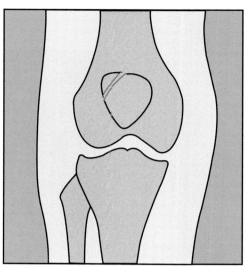

FIG. 7-167 A bipartite patella describes a patella formed from two pieces. At times, three (tripartite) or more (multipartite) fragments may be seen.

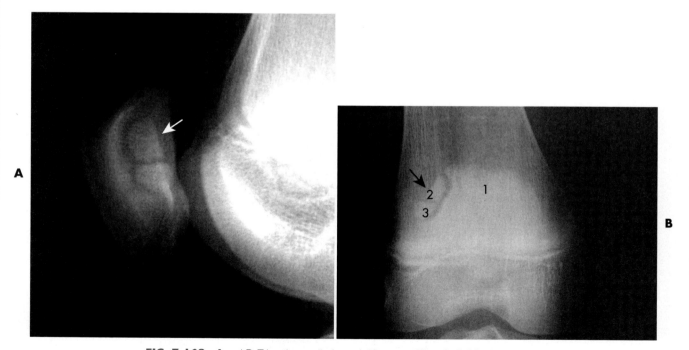

FIG. 7-168 **A** and **B,** Tripartite patella *(arrows).* (Courtesy Clifton Bethel, Rock Island, IL.)

TABLE 7-6 cont'd
Normal Skeletal Variants of the Lower Extremities

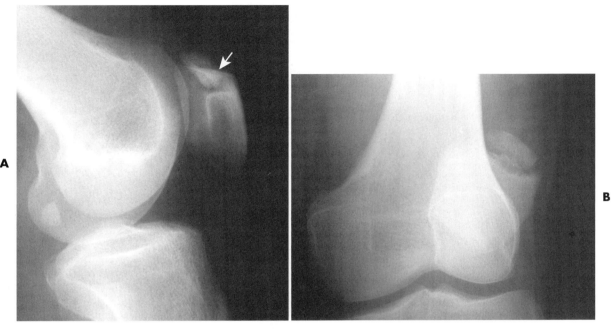

FIG. 7-169 **A** and **B,** The patella appears in two pieces *(arrow)*. (Courtesy Steven P. Brownstein, MD, Springfield, NJ.)

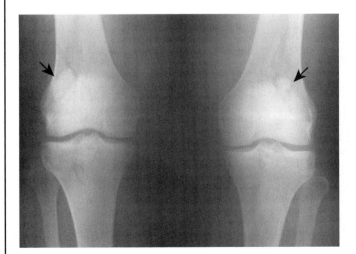

FIG. 7-170 Bilateral presentation of bipartite patella *(arrows)*.

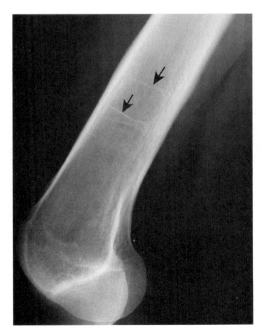

FIG. 7-171 Bone bars crossing the distal femur *(arrows)*.

TABLE 7-6 cont'd
Normal Skeletal Variants of the Lower Extremities

Variant/Artifact	Comments
Coxa valga	The angle of intersection formed by a line thorough the femoral shaft and a second line through the femoral neck is termed the *femoral angle*. Normally the femoral angle measures between 120 and 135 degrees. An angle less than 120 degrees is known as *coxa vara;* an angle larger than 135 degrees is *coxa valga*.
Coxa vara (Fig. 7-173)	The angle of intersection formed by a line through the femoral shaft and a second line through the femoral neck is termed the *femoral angle*. Normally the femoral degrees angle measures 120 to 135 degrees. An angle less than 120 degrees is known as *coxa vara;* an angle larger than 135 degrees is *coxa valga*. Coxa vara may occur as a congenital, acquired, or developmental defect. Congenital coxa vara is present at birth and results from a defect of the embryonic limb bud. It is associated with bowing and shortness of the femur. Acquired coxa vara occurs secondary to bone-softening disease (e.g., Paget's disease, rickets, fibrous dysplasia), bone dysplasias (e.g., Morquio's disease, metaphyseal, diaphyseal dysplasia), and trauma. Duncan[30] identified developmental coxa vara as a presentation that is not present at birth, but develops during the early childhood years. Progressive coxa vara deformity occurs secondary to defective enchondral ossification of the femoral neck.[52] A triangular section of the inferior-medial aspect of the femoral neck, vertically slanted epiphysis, shortened femoral neck, and relative overgrowth of the greater trochanter may be seen in advanced presentations. As an alternative to the femoral angle, Hilgenreiner epiphyseal angle may be helpful to recognize coxa vara. Hilgenreiner line is a horizontal line through the triradiate cartilages bilaterally (or a horizontal line parallel to the film can be drawn). An oblique line through the proximal femoral capital physes is drawn, and the angle of intersection with Hilgenreiner (or the film's parallel) line is measured. Normally this angle should measure 20 degrees, with normative values of 4 to 35 degrees. Patients with congenital coxa vara average 40 to 70 degrees and may be as high as 70 to 90 degrees.[113] Because of the progressive nature of the deformity, surgical correction is typically indicated for significant presentations of coxa vara.
Femoral herniation (Pitt's) pit (Figs. 7-174 and 7-175)	In 1982 Michael J. Pitt and associates described a round or oval radiolucent defect of approximately 1 to 2 cm in diameter appearing with a surrounding thin zone of sclerosis. It appears in the proximal, anterior, and superior quadrants of the adult femoral neck. In one review it was found to be more common among women and was rarely bilateral in approximately 5% of the cases reviewed.[50] The etiology remains to be explained. The herniation pit is theorized to represent a reaction area of degeneration with herniation of soft tissue into the defect.[83] It also has been described as the result of mechanical erosion by an irregularity of the overlying joint capsule.[50] Also, it has been theorized that the close approximation of the joint capsule and iliopsoas muscle are important in the pathogenesis of the herniation pit, especially in athletic persons.[25] Herniation pits typically are present without symptoms and as a normal variant. They may heal and disappear over time.[63] They are rarely hot on bone scan.[106] It is important not to mistake the herniation pit for more clinically relevant findings of osteoid osteoma, Brodie's abscess, intraosseous ganglion, or metastatic bone disease.
Flatfoot	Flatfoot (or pes planus) is a loss of the longitudinal arch of the foot. There are two presentations: flexible flatfoot, marked by mobile joints, and rigid flatfoot, in which the subtalar joint motion is limited and often related to tarsal coalition. Rigid flatfoot is more likely to be associated with pain and disability. An acquired variety of flatfoot presents in middle-aged women secondary to posterior tibial tendon pathology.
Hallux valgus/metatarsus primus varus (Fig. 7-176)	Hallux valgus is a lateral deviation of the first toe. It is associated with medial displacement of the first metatarsal (metatarsus primus varus) and bunion formation of the medial aspect of the first metatarsal head. It is caused by congenital malformation or can be acquired, for example, by ill-fitting shoes. Hallux valgus is noted by an angle of greater than 15 degrees created by lines through the longitudinal axis of the first metatarsal and the proximal phalanx of the first digit. Severe hallux valgus is suggested by an angle greater than 40 degrees. Metatarsus primus varus is suggested by an angle greater than 10 degrees between the long axes of the first metatarsal and the medial cuneiform.

TABLE 7-6 cont'd
Normal Skeletal Variants of the Lower Extremities

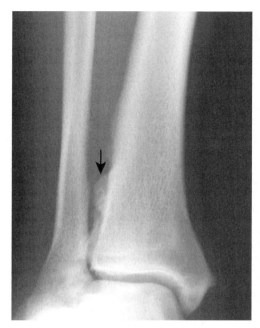

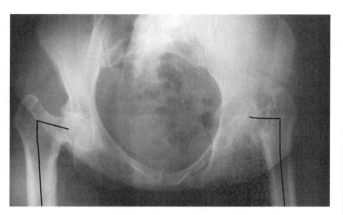

FIG. 7-173 Bilateral presentation of coxa vara. (Courtesy William E. Litterer, Elizabeth, NJ.)

FIG. 7-172 A 47-year-old woman exhibiting calcification of the distal tibia-fibula interosseous membrane *(arrow)*.

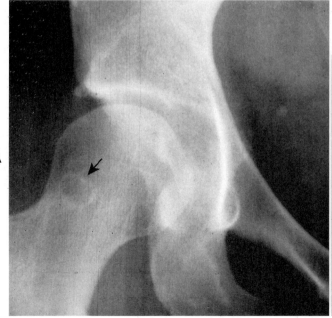

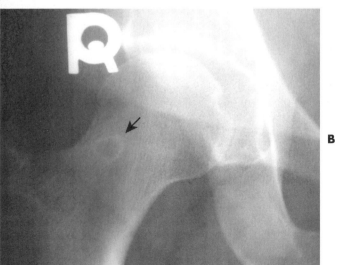

FIG. 7-174 **A** and **B,** A small, benign defect is noted in the central portion of the neck of the proximal femur in two cases. The defect is known as a *Pitt's pit (arrows)*. (**B,** Courtesy Brian Frank, Sunnyland, IL.)

Continued

TABLE 7-6 cont'd
Normal Skeletal Variants of the Lower Extremities

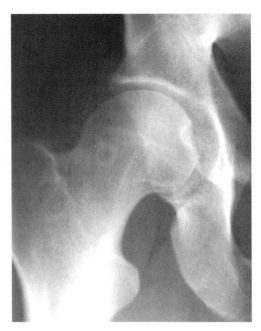

FIG. 7-175   Pitt's pit appearing as a small defect of the femoral neck.

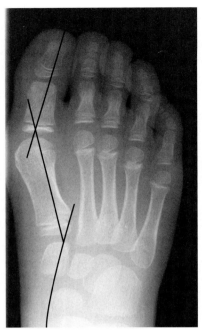

FIG. 7-176   This child demonstrates a slight degree of metatarsus primus varus, hallux valgus. (Courtesy Julie-Marthe Grenier, Davenport, IA.)

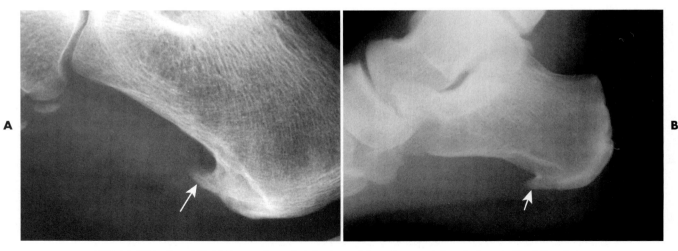

FIG. 7-177   **A** and **B,** Heel spurs formed at the base of the calcaneus at the attachment site of the plantar aponeurosis *(arrows)* in two cases.

TABLE 7-6 cont'd
Normal Skeletal Variants of the Lower Extremities

Variant/Artifact	Comments
Heel spur (Fig. 7-177)	The plantar fascia runs longitudinally along the sole of the foot, from the anterior-inferior margin of the calcaneus to the midfoot. Injury and inflammation at the point of origin of the plantar fascia results in calcium deposition, forming a heel spur. Heel spurs are noted on lateral radiographs of the ankle as osseous projections, about 1 to 2 cm in size, formed at the anterior-inferior margin of the calcaneus. Heel spurs may be clinically silent or associated with heel pain. They are promoted by biomechanical imbalance, running, ill-fitting shoes, obesity, or other cause of plantar fasciitis. Orthotics, deep massage, and biomechanical corrections may offer relief of pain syndromes.
Morton syndrome	Morton syndrome (also known as *Morton toe*) was first coined by Dudley Joy Morton.[72] It describes a hereditary presentation of a short first metatarsal, resulting in an increased proportion of body weight being borne by the second metatarsal. There is usually accompanying overpronation of the foot and prominent callosities under the second and third metatarsals. The second metatarsal may appear thickened or have a tendency toward stress fracture as a result of increased weight bearing. Clinical findings range from no symptoms to deep, dull, aching pain in the region of the stressed second metatarsal. Pain typically is worse while walking or standing and alleviated by rest. The condition usually is bilateral. Morton syndrome is alternatively described in the literature as intermetatarsal neuroma, usually between the third and fourth metatarsal heads.
Nutrient canal (Fig. 7-178)	Nutrient canals are a normal feature of all tubular bones. At times their presentation of an obliquely oriented radiolucent defect through the cortex of the shaft of a tubular bone may be confused with a fracture. Because nutrient canals are only small holes, they appear less radiolucent than a fracture.
Sever disease (Figs. 7-179 and 7-180)	Sever disease, or calcaneal apophysitis, refers to a painful heel in a growing child, usually 10 to 13 years of age. It may be bilateral. On a lateral radiograph, the calcaneal apophysis may appear radiodense, condensed, and fragmented. Pain is exacerbated by activity and alleviated with rest. Although in the past it was believed to be associated with an avascular necrosis etiology, it is now thought to be traumatically induced, secondary to microfracture of the growth plate and overuse syndrome in a typically very active child. The condition is self-limiting after decreased activity. At times, a radiodense, condensed, fragmented appearance of the calcaneus occurs without symptoms, representing a normal variant of no significance.
Tarsal coalition (Figs. 7-181 and 7-182)	Congenital tarsal coalition refers to a union of two or more tarsal bones as a result of failed segmentation of the primitive mesenchyme. The condition is generally inherited through autosomal dominant transmission. The union may be fibrous, cartilaginous, or bony. Fifty percent of all coalitions are bilateral. By far the most common sites of tarsal coalition are between the anterior process of the calcaneus and the lateral aspect of the tarsal navicular.[12] On the lateral foot projection of a patient with calcaneonavicular coalition, a tubular extension of the calcaneus can be seen anteriorly from the calcaneus. The appearance resembles the nose of an anteater ("anteater nose" sign). The tubular extension approaches or overlaps the midportion of the navicular. The finding invariably is present with calcaneonavicular coalition.[80] Talocalcaneal and, rarely, talonavicular coalitions also are seen.[8] Symptoms of tarsal coalition often follow ankle sprains or other minor injuries, sometimes leading to a rigid, painful foot made worse with continued activity. Oblique radiographs of the foot demonstrate the lack of joint space as the elongated anterior process of the calcaneus extends to the lateral aspect of the navicular, marking coalition. A small bony projection (known as a *talar beak*) occurring at the anterior-superior margin of the talus immediately proximal to the articular surface of the talar head represents a secondary radiographic sign of coalition. The talar beak should be differentiated from capsular osteophytes, the latter occurring more proximally, at the capsular insertion. Computed tomography and magnetic resonance imaging allow for better delineation of the coalition. Acquired coalitions may occur as a consequence of advanced degenerative joint disease, inflammatory arthritis, infection, and clubfoot deformities.

Continued

TABLE 7-6 cont'd
Normal Skeletal Variants of the Lower Extremities

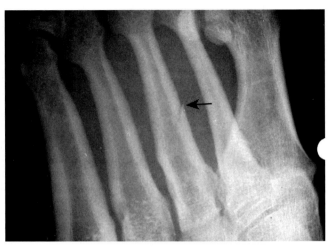

FIG. 7-178 Nutrient canal appearing as a faintly radiolucent defect *(arrow)* in the cortex of the third metatarsal shaft.

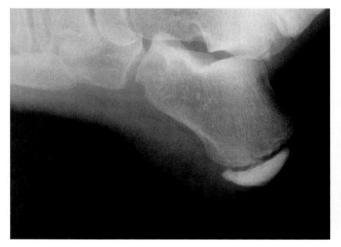

FIG. 7-179 The calcaneal apophysis is radiodense and irregular, consistent with a normal variant of the developing bone, known as *Sever phenomenon*. In the past this presentation was thought to result from avascular necrosis and be the cause of the patient's heel complaint (Sever disease).

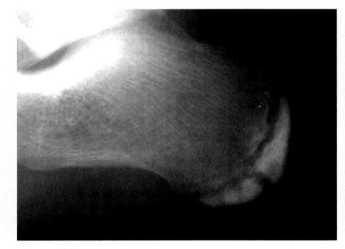

FIG. 7-180 Sever phenomenon presenting as a radiodense, fragmented calcaneal apophysis. (Courtesy Blair D. Hunt, Peoria, IL.)

TABLE 7-6 cont'd
Normal Skeletal Variants of the Lower Extremities

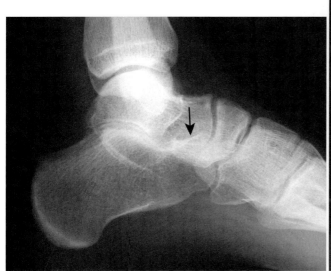

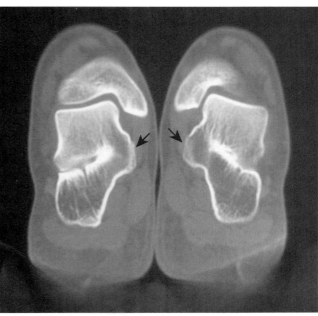

FIG. 7-181 Talocalcaneal coalition appearing on, **A,** plain film and, **B,** computed tomography with absence of the intervening joint space and continuous trabeculation *(arrows).* As noted in this case, coalition is often bilateral.

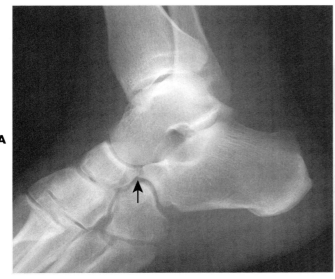

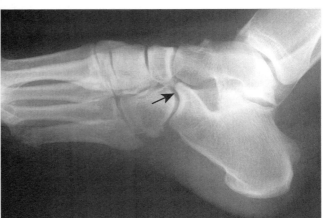

FIG. 7-182 Calcaneonavicular coalition. **A** and **B,** Both cases exhibit an osseous projection from the calcaneus to the navicular. The bony projection has been likened to an anteater's nose ("anteater nose" sign) *(arrows).* (**A,** Courtesy Julie-Marthe Grenier, Davenport, IA; **B,** Courtesy William E. Litterer, Elizabeth, NJ.)

Continued

TABLE 7-6 cont'd
Normal Skeletal Variants of the Lower Extremities

Variant/Artifact	Comments
Tibiotalar slant (Fig. 7-183)	A medial slant of the dome of the talus is associated with juvenile rheumatoid arthritis, hemophilia, and sickle-cell anemia.[1] A similar appearance can be induced by poor patient positioning.[9]
Vertical talus	A congenital vertically oriented talus typically is associated with a more widespread neuromuscular disorder. On the lateral projection of the foot, the arch of the foot is reversed, the talus is plantar flexed, and the cuboid is displaced dorsally.

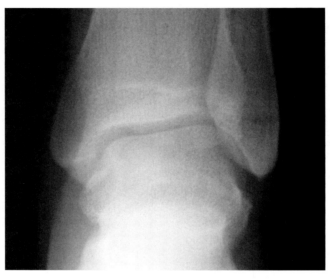

FIG. 7-183   Medial slant of the dome of the talus presenting as an isolated anomaly without hemophilia, juvenile rheumatoid, sickle-cell anemia, or other associated disease syndrome.

Surgical hardware is an often encountered residual feature of surgeries related to trauma, degenerative instability, or other pathologic changes of bone and joints. Closed operative fixation may involve the application of plates, pins, screws, and wires to selected regions of the anatomy. Some of the more common elements are listed in Table 7-7.

TABLE 7-7
Surgical Implants, Materials, and Devices

Variant/Artifact	Comments
Basket filters (Fig. 7-184)	Basket filters are advocated in patients at high risk for thromboembolic events. These baskets may be seen on radiographs as cone- or umbrella-shaped devices. There are many types of baskets, including the Mobin-Uddin umbrella filter, stainless steel Greenfield filter (SGF) (Kim-Ray-Greenfield filter), and titanium Greenfield filter (TGF), Filters are designed to trap thrombi while preserving flow in the inferior vena cava.
Cages (Figs. 7-185 and 7-186)	Cages are generally used as interbody fusion devices. They come in several varieties such as threaded cylinders (e.g., BAK cage) and vertical interbody rings or boxes (e.g., Harms mesh cage). Usually they are constructed from titanium and are visible on plain films of the region. Cages maintain the intervertebral disc space during spinal fusion. For example, the degenerative disc is removed and replaced with one (or paired) BAK cages. Bone grafts are packed around the segments, and the segments are fused in approximately 3 months. Bone grafting is a fundamental component of spinal fusion. Larger pieces of bone may be used as grafts to provide support by occupying the gaps between fused bones. Alternatively, bone that is ground into powder and packed around sites of fusion stimulates additional bone growth and speeds the healing process.[11] Bone grafts that are obtained from donor sites on the patient's own body are called *autografts*. Bone grafts taken from another person are called *allografts*.
Implants (Figs. 7-187 to 7-192)	Implants constructed of metal, plastics, or ceramics usually present prominently on radiographs of the region. Silicone elastomer (Silastic) implants are used with small joint arthroplasty. Polymethylmethacrylate (PMME) has been used for decades to cement orthopedic implants and generally fill space in bone.
	Complications of surgical implants should be examined on radiographs. The possibility of structure failure or movement of the orthopedic devices and associated hardware warrants close scrutiny. Infection and host bone response are other serious concerns that may present with radiographic evidence. Other than overt signs of failure of displacement, the interface among the implant, screw, rod, wire, and so on, and bone is a critical area of evaluation. Loosening and host bone response are suggested by a developing increased margin of radiolucency surrounding the hardware in question. Generally the radiolucent space between a femoral hip prosthesis and the surrounding bone should not exceed 1 to 2 mm, depending on whether the widening is focal or surrounding the majority of the prosthesis. A larger implant–bone space suggests loosening, infection, or host bone resorption. Infection is the most serious complication, necessitating immediate recognition and management. Infections also may demonstrate bone destruction, soft-tissue expansion, and clinical features of fever and unremitting pain.
	Magnetic resonance imaging and computed tomography imaging of orthopedic devices is associated with substantial limitations. Computed tomography images appear with spoke-formed streak hard beam artifacts within the vicinity of the metallic object because of the object's high-absorption, resulting in insufficient sampling numbers, saturation of projection data, and abrupt changes of the data. Plastics result in less beam hardening artifact and a clearer image. Magnetic resonance imaging suffers similar image degradation from orthopedic devices. The ferromagnetism of surgical hardware disrupts the homogeneity of the magnetic field and amplitude of the radiofrequencies, leading to significant image distortion. Titanium-based alloys are less problematic than cobalt-chromium or stainless steel devices.

Continued

TABLE 7-7 cont'd
Surgical Implants, Materials, and Devices

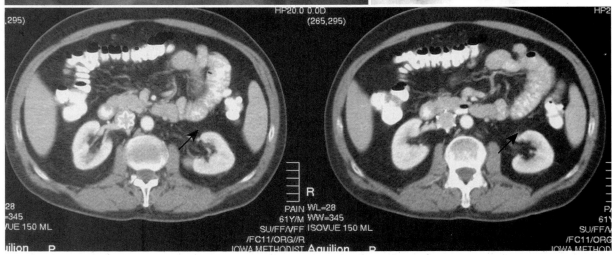

FIG. 7-184   A basket filter is noted on, **A,** the anteroposterior and, **B,** lateral lumbar radiograph of this 56-year-old man. Another basket filter is noted on, **C,** an abdominal computed tomography of a different patient (*arrows*). (**A,** Courtesy Julie-Marthe Grenier, Davenport, IA; **C,** Courtesy Troy Scheuermann, Farmington, IA.)

TABLE 7-7 cont'd
Surgical Implants, Materials, and Devices

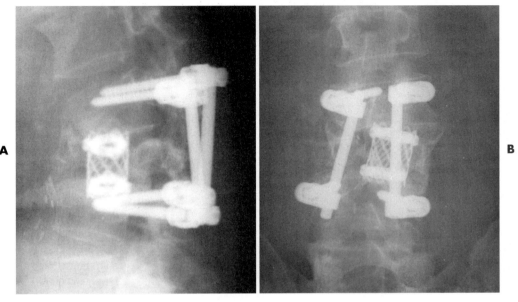

FIG. 7-185 **A** and **B,** spinal surgery was performed with a cage placed between the vertebrae, and stabilization rods were inserted along the posterior margins of the segment for this patient with a collapsed vertebra.

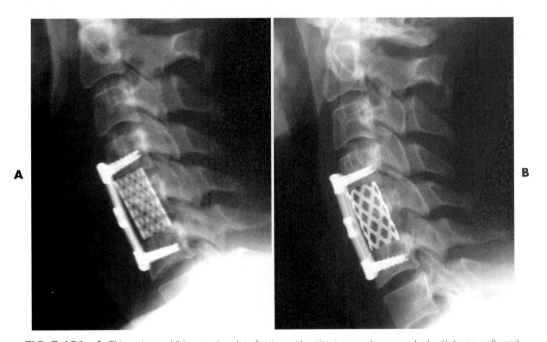

FIG. 7-186 **A,** This patient exhibits anterior plate fixation with a titanium mesh cage packed with bone grafts and placed between the C4 and C6 segments. The mesh cage is employed to maintain the space between segments. **B,** There is increased clarity of the mesh on the subsequent films taken 3 months later related to the resorption of the bone graft.

TABLE 7-7 cont'd
Surgical Implants, Materials, and Devices

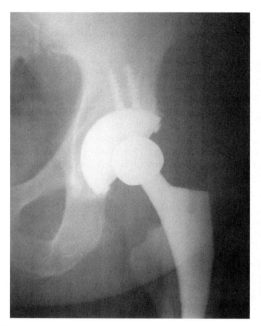

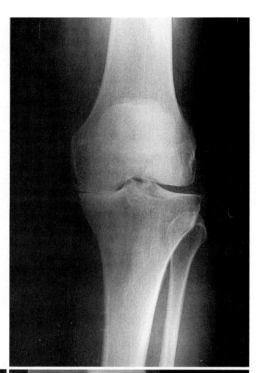

FIG. 7-187   Complete (femoral and acetabular) hip prosthesis.

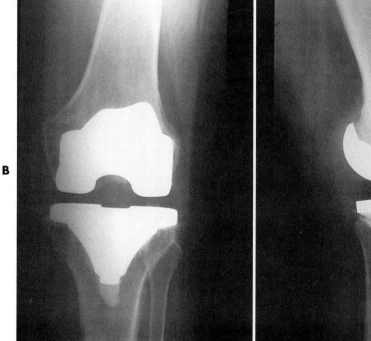

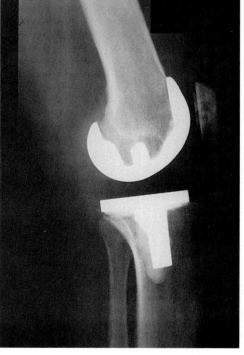

FIG. 7-188   **A,** Preoperative anteroposterior (AP) radiograph of a knee with varus arthritis and obliteration of the medial compartment with weight bearing. **B,** Postoperative AP and, **C,** lateral radiographs of an uncomplicated knee replacement. The femoral component's metal contour matches that of the bone, there is good bone coverage, the patella is at an appropriate height, and there is a mild anatomic posterior tibial slope. The limb alignment has been restored to slight valgus. (From Freiberg AA: The radiology of orthopaedic implants: an atlas of techniques and assessment, St Louis, 2001, Mosby.)

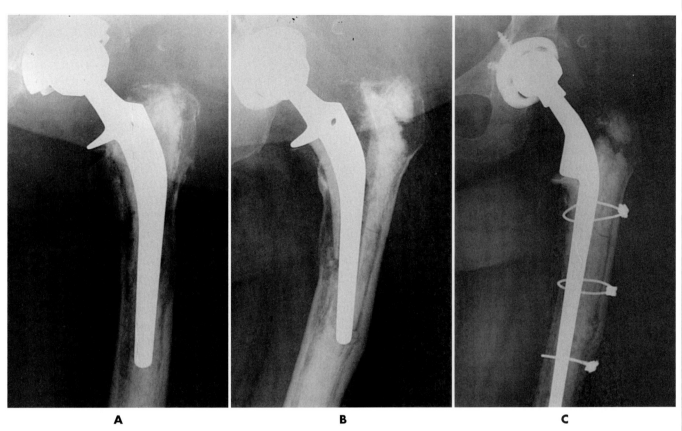

A   B   C

FIG. 7-189 **A,** Early postoperative radiograph of a hybrid total hip replacement. Poor cement technique has left voids near the inferior tip of the femoral prosthesis (known as *zone 4*) and along its lateral margin (*zone 2*). Around the proximal lateral aspect of the femoral implant (*zone 1*), there appears to be debonding of the cement from the implant. **B,** Second radiograph taken 1 year later demonstrates massive debonding of the implant and multiple cement fractures. There may be a pathologic fracture in the lower medial cortex about the prosthesis (*zone 5*) of the femur in the area of the osteolysis below the lesser trochanter. **C,** Because this patient was older and had low activity demands, she underwent revision to a cement stem. An extended trochanteric osteotomy was performed to fully expose the proximal femur, and a calcar replacement long stem was cemented. Cables were used to secure the osteotomy, which appears healed. Some areas of cement, such as that seen in the greater trochanter, could be left behind because there was no evidence of infection. (From Freiberg AA: The radiology of orthopaedic implants: an atlas of techniques and assessment, St Louis, 2001, Mosby.)

Continued

TABLE 7-7 cont'd
Surgical Implants, Materials, and Devices

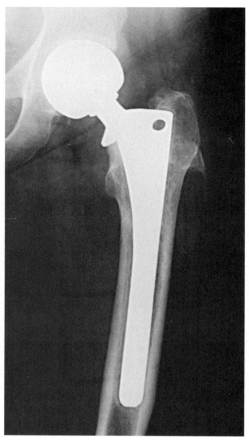

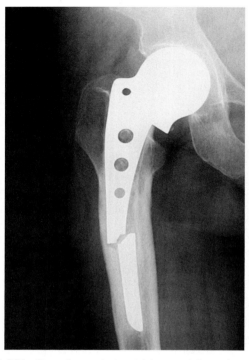

FIG. 7-191 Cementless, unipolar, stainless steel femoral component. Fatigue fracture of the stem has occurred secondary to cantilever bending in the presence of poor proximal and good distal fixation. (From Freiberg AA: The radiology of orthopaedic implants: an atlas of techniques and assessment, St Louis, 2001, Mosby.)

FIG. 7-190 Loose, cementless unipolar hemiarthroplasty performed for a displaced femoral neck fracture. The patient now presents with thigh pain. The femoral component shows several signs that suggest the presence of a loose implant, including a radiolucent line along the shaft of the stem of the prosthesis. The tip of the implant is up against the cortical bone laterally, and there is cortical hypertrophy at the tip. This is an example, in an older patient, of a press-fit implant that has settled into a slight varus position and has a very high likelihood of being loose. There are no definitive signs of loosening but several subtle signs that suggest this is the case, and that the features are related to the patient's thigh pain. (From Freiberg AA: The radiology of orthopaedic implants: an atlas of techniques and assessment, St Louis, 2001, Mosby.)

TABLE 7-7 cont'd
Surgical Implants, Materials, and Devices

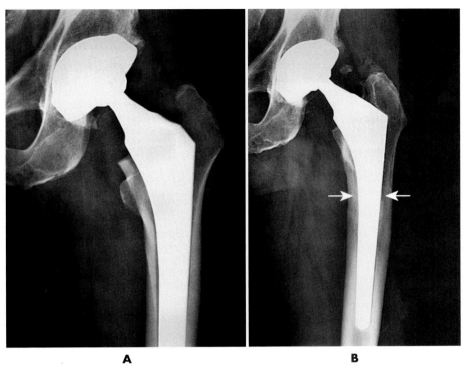

A   **B**

FIG. 7-192 A, Early postoperative radiograph taken after a hip arthroplasty that employed a hydroxyapatite-coated femoral component. **B,** Second radiograph taken 5 years after the total hip arthroplasty. The implant is stable. There are not radiolucent lines around the proximal stem where hydroxyapatite coating is present. Condensation of cancellous bone around the hydroxyapatite-coated portion of the stem is visible, particularly at the distal extent of the coating *(arrows).* The parallel radiolucent and radiodense lines around the distal, uncoated portion of the stem do not indicate loosening. There is mild bone atrophy of the femoral neck consistent with stress shielding. (From Freiberg AA: The radiology of orthopaedic implants: an atlas of techniques and assessment, St Louis, 2001, Mosby.)

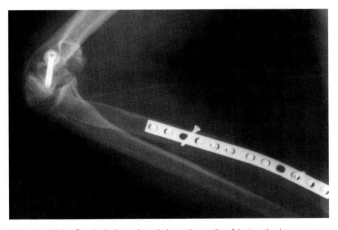

FIG. 7-193 Surgical plate placed along the radius. Notice the loose screw, third from the reading left. Also, there is a surgical screw placed in the distal humerus. (Courtesy Julie-Marthe Grenier, Davenport, IA.)

TABLE 7-7 cont'd
Surgical Implants, Materials, and Devices

Variant/Artifact	Comments
Plates (Figs. 7-193 to 7-196)	Plates are named by their appearance (e.g., T, T oblique, L, cloverleaf) and function (e.g., compression reconstruction). Static compression plates offer compression along the axial direction of the fracture by some included tension device on the plate. Alternatively, dynamic compression plates are identified by their oval screw holes with slanting beveled margins that draw the bone fragments together when the screws are tightened. Dynamic compression plates are used mostly for fractures that are stable during compression. A reconstruction plate is a thin, flexible plate convenient for extensive bone reconstruction often used during the repair of extensive pelvic fractures. Buttressing plates are substantial plates used to stabilize fractures that typically are not stable when compressed. Blade plates are L-shaped and often used to stabilized distal femoral fractures. Steffee plates are used with thoracolumbar stabilization surgeries. They are short plates placed vertically and in pairs along the posterior arch of the involved segments. They are attached to the vertebrae with screws placed through the pedicles and into the vertebral bodies, achieving fusion of the intervertebral disc and posterior joints with one apparatus.
Screws (Figs. 7-197 and 7-198)	Screws are commonly applied orthopedic hardware used for fixation.[14] Several types are noted, including cortical (long-threaded shaft), cancellous (threaded at the end), cannulated (hollow bore), Herbert, and inference. Herbert screws are cannulated screws with an opposite pitch of threads at either end, so that the screw draws the fragments closer together when tightened. Herbert screws are commonly used with scaphoid and other small bone fractures. Inference screws are employed to anchor cruciate ligament repairs and grafts.
Vascular clips, mesh, and sutures (Fig. 7-199)	Vascular clips, mesh, and sutures are employed with the wide variety of thoracic, abdominal, pelvic, and body wall surgeries. Often the location of the clips indicates what type of surgery was performed. For instance, a small cluster of clips appearing in the right upper abdominal quadrant on the anteroposterior lumbopelvic projection correlates to cholecystectomy. Tantalum mesh is a moldable, noncorrosive device used most often to repair inguinal hernias and other body wall lesions.
Washers (Fig. 7-200)	Generally washers are used to distribute stress to the head of the screw more evenly. Washers may be serrated to increase the grip on tendon and ligament they anchor.
Wires, pins, nails, and rods (Figs. 7-201 to 7-206)	Wires, pins, nails, and rods generally are differentiated from one another based on diameter; thinnest to thickest as listed. Kirschner wires (K-wires) may be used for percutaneous or open joint or bone fixation, often with small bones of the hands and feet. K-wires are also placed as guides for cannulated screws. Steinmann pins have similar application to K-wires, but are thicker and more substantial for added strength. Rush pins are placed in the medullary canal. They are slightly slanted (chisel-shaped) at the inserted end and hook-shaped for easy retraction at the external end. Ender nails are similar but without the hooked end. Knowles nails often are inserted into the femoral neck to stabilize the epiphysis with slipped capital femoral epiphysis. Intramedullary rods are placed into the medullary cavity of a long bone to establish and maintain the bone's alignment. In adjunct to the intramedullary rod, cerclage wire is wrapped around the displaced fragments to limit shear and rotational forces. The cerclage wire may be applied partially around the circumference of the fragments and then through a hole across the diameter of the bone (hemi-cerclage) or 360 degrees around the circumference (full cerclage). Tension band wiring is placed along the convex margin of fractures (e.g., posterior surface of the elbow with fractured olecranon). With this placement the muscle tension will leverage the bone fragment against the tightened wire and compress the bone fragments together, partially mitigating the tensile forces of the muscle tension and lessening the likelihood of reavulsion. Wire may be used for suturing bone and soft tissue together, as with sternal wiring following open thoracotomy. Harrington rods are spinal fixation devices most closely associated with scoliosis surgery. They are hooked to the lamina to either compress or distract the segments, lessening the degree of spinal curvature.

TABLE 7-7 cont'd
Surgical Implants, Materials, and Devices

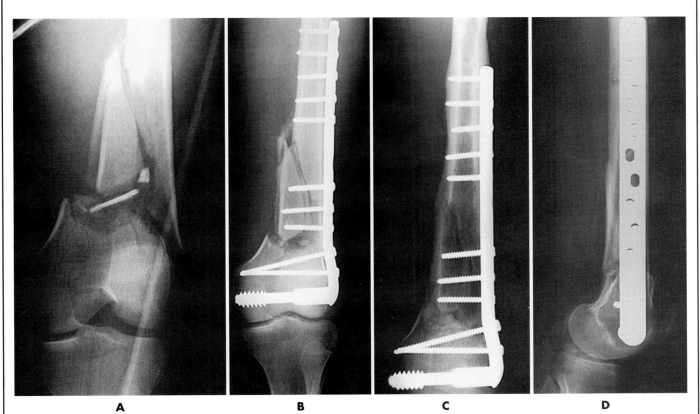

A **B** **C** **D**

FIG. 7-194 **A,** Comminuted supracondylar femur fracture. **B,** Fracture stabilized with a 95-degree dynamic condylar screw. The intercondylar split was first reduced with smaller lag screws. The large lag screw, which is placed parallel to the knee joint line, was then inserted. A barrel and sideplate attach to the lag screw and are secured to the femoral shaft. Screws have been inserted into the medial metaphyseal fracture fragment, but no attempt has been made to achieve an anatomic reduction of this fragment. This indirect reduction method minimizes further periosteal stripping so that blood supply to the fracture fragment is maintained. The two basic techniques for fracture reduction are direct and indirect reduction. Direct reduction requires extensive dissection in order to anatomically reduce each fracture fragment. This results in a biomechanically strong construct, but increases the possibility of infection. In indirect reduction, the articular surface is anatomically reduced and the correct limb alignment is achieved, but no attempt is made to reduce each of the individual fragments. Without periosteal stripping, these comminuted intervening fragments often heal rapidly. In these radiographs, taken 6 weeks postoperatively, early callus formation is seen. **C,** Fracture healed successfully. Some remodeling of the callus has occurred, as seen of these x-rays taken 10 months postoperatively. **D,** Lateral radiograph showing the correct axial alignment of the implant. (From Freiberg AA: The radiology of orthopaedic implants: an atlas of techniques and assessment, St Louis, 2001, Mosby.)

Continued

TABLE 7-7 cont'd
Surgical Implants, Materials, and Devices

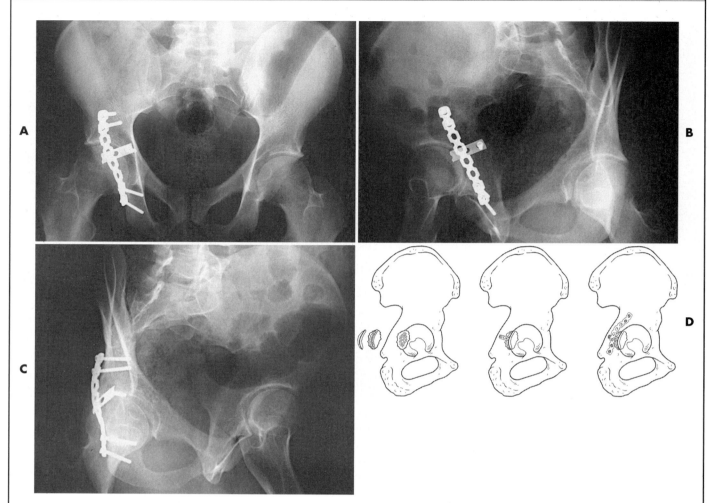

FIG. 7-195 Reconstruction plates are malleable and commonly used for the fixation of acetabular and distal humerus fractures. The plates may be shaped to fit irregular surfaces. They do not have the strength of standard compression plates; therefore they are rarely used for diaphyseal long-bone fractures, which require stronger implants. **A,** Anteroposterior pelvis radiograph showing the reconstruction plate. A portion of the third tubular plate has been fashioned to create a "spring plate." The teeth of the spring plate allow the fixation of small, marginal acetabular fragments. It is used in locations in which screws cannot be safely placed without violating the hip joint. **B,** Iliac oblique Judet view showing the posterior column of the pelvis most clearly. The reconstruction plate is located along the posterior column and is secured above and below the healed posterior wall acetabular fracture. (From Freiberg AA: The radiology of orthopaedic implants: an atlas of techniques and assessment, St Louis, 2001, Mosby.)

TABLE 7-7 cont'd
Surgical Implants, Materials, and Devices

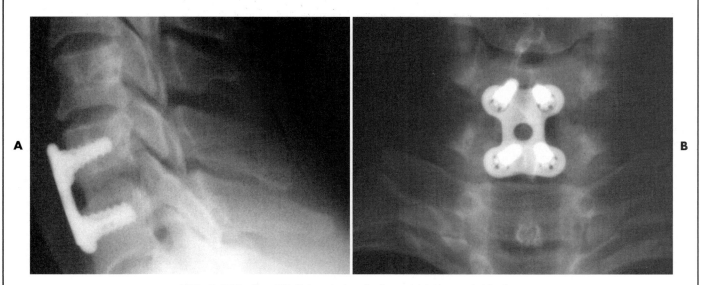

FIG. 7-196 **A** and **B,** Plate and screw fixation and anterior cervical fixation.

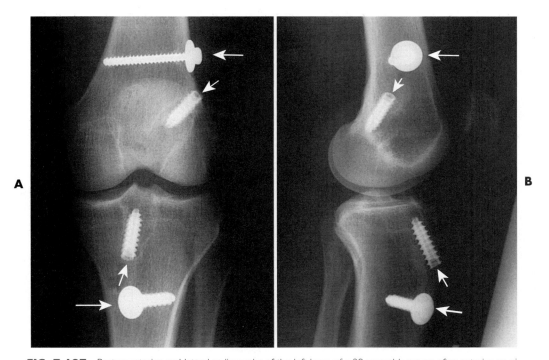

FIG. 7-197 Posteroanterior and lateral radiographs of the left knee of a 29-year-old woman after anterior cruciate ligament reconstruction with patellar tendon allograft. Interference screws (*small arrows*) fixate the graft through the femoral and tibial tunnels. The tibial interference screw has overpenetrated into the tunnel, partially engaging the tibial bone plug. Cancellous screws and washers (*large arrows*) are used as posts for sutures, which are threaded through the graft for additional stabilization of the proximal and distal ends. (From Freiberg AA: The radiology of orthopaedic implants: an atlas of techniques and assessment, St Louis, 2001, Mosby.)

TABLE 7-7 cont'd
Surgical Implants, Materials, and Devices

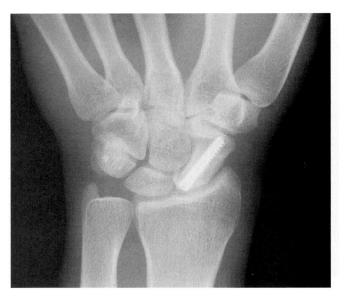

FIG. 7-198 A surgical screw is placed through the center of the scaphoid in an attempt to fixate the fractured bone. (Courtesy Julie-Marthe Grenier, Davenport, IA.)

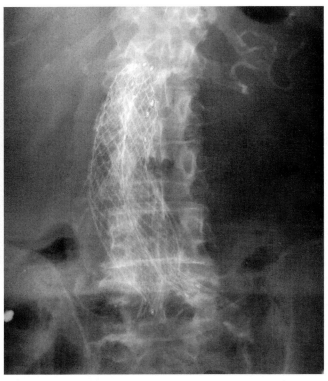

FIG. 7-199 Surgical mesh is used to reinforce the aorta and common iliac vessels.

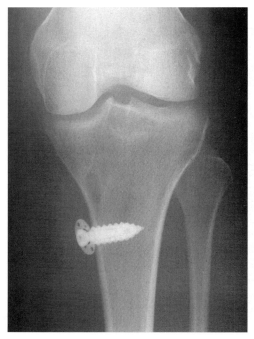

FIG. 7-200 A screw with washer is used to reattach the avulsed lateral collateral ligament in this patient. (Courtesy Julie-Marthe Grenier, Davenport, IA.)

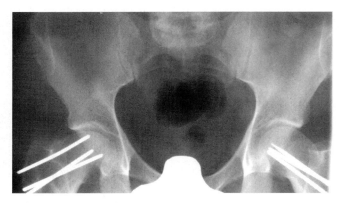

FIG. 7-201 Surgical pins are placed through the femoral neck bilaterally. (Courtesy Julie-Marthe Grenier, Davenport, IA.)

TABLE 7-7 cont'd
Surgical Implants, Materials, and Devices

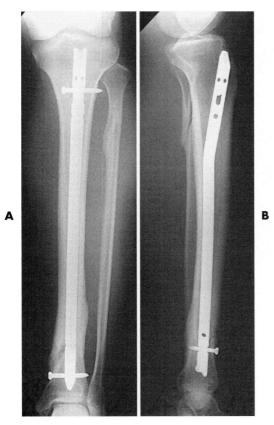

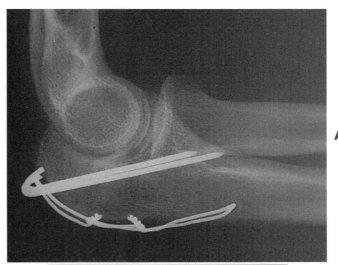

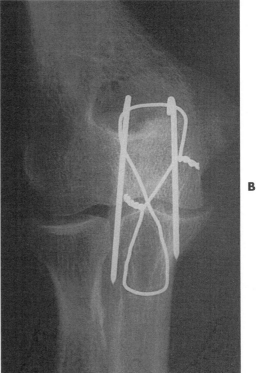

FIG. 7-202   A, Distal spiral tibial fracture treated with an intramedullary tibial nail. This particular intramedullary nail has several different proximal and distal interlocking options. Because of the very distal location of this fracture, distal interlocking has been performed with one medial-to-lateral screw and one anterior-to-posterior screw. The fracture has achieved a successful union. **B,** Lateral view showing the proximal and distal interlocking holes. A single proximal interlocking screw has been placed in the oval slot; this permits dynamic compression of the fracture site. That is, the interlocking screw can slide within the nail slot as the fracture compresses. (From Freiberg AA: The radiology of orthopaedic implants: an atlas of techniques and assessment, St Louis, 2001, Mosby.)

FIG. 7-203   A and **B,** A tension band wire technique has been used to repair this olecranon fracture. The malleable wire has been passed through a drill hole in the ulnar metaphysis and wrapped around the ends of the Kirschner wires. This construct converts the pull of the triceps into a compressive force across the fracture site. Tension band wiring is commonly used for fixation of olecranon and patella fractures, but it requires a stable fracture pattern. Plate fixation may be required in severely comminuted olecranon fractures. **B,** Anteroposterior view shows that the malleable wire has been placed in a figure-of-eight fashion around the Kirschner wire. This wire has been tightened by twisting it both medially and laterally. (From Freiberg AA: The radiology of orthopaedic implants: an atlas of techniques and assessment, St Louis, 2001, Mosby.)

TABLE 7-7 cont'd
Surgical Implants, Materials, and Devices

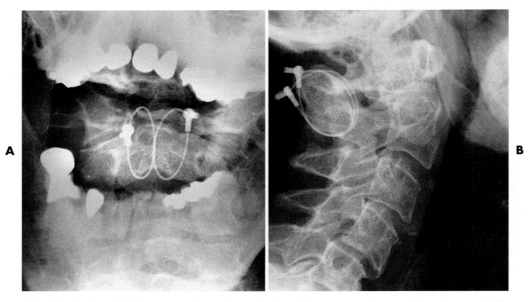

FIG. 7-204 **A** and **B,** Brooks posterior cervical wiring to stabilize an os odontoideum. (From Freiberg AA: The radiology of orthopaedic implants: an atlas of techniques and assessment, St Louis, 2001, Mosby.)

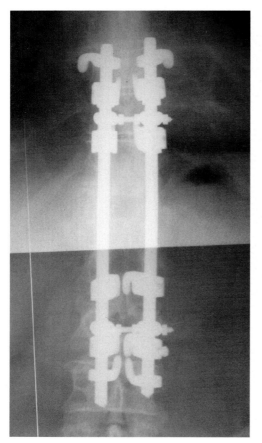

FIG. 7-205 Harrington rod instrumentation used for posterior fixation across the thoracolumbar spine. The hooks are facing centrally with respect to the rods, denoting that the rods are used for compression in this case, as opposed to distraction.

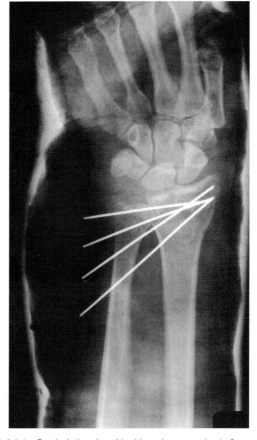

FIG. 7-206 Surgical pins placed in this patient to maintain fragment position during the healing process in this casted forearm.

References

1. Akamaguna AI et al: Tibial and fibular angles in homozygous sickle cell disease, *Eur J Radiol* 6:97, 1986.

2. Ansari A: The "straight back" syndrome: current perspective more often associated with valvular heart disease than pseudoheart disease: a prospective clinical, electrocardiographic, roentgenographic, and echocardiographic study of 50 patients, *Clin Cardiol* 8:290, 1985.

3. Applbaum G, Gerard P, Bryk D: Elongation of the anterior tubercle of a cervical vertebral transverse process: an unusual variant, *Skeletal Radiol* 10:265, 1983.

4. Arthur JT: Straight-back syndrome. A case report and review of the literature, *West African J Med* 14:61, 1995.

5. Bauer M, Jonsson K: Congenital radioulnar synostosis. Radiological characteristics and hand function: case reports, *Scand J Plast Reconstr Surg Hand Surg* 22:251, 1988.

6. Baugh RF, Stocks RM: Eagle's syndrome: a reappraisal, *Ear Nose Throat J* 72:341, 1993.

7. Beals RK, Lovrien EW: Dyschondrosteosis and Madelung's deformity. Report of three kindreds and review of the literature, *Clin Orthop Rel Res* 116:24, 1976.

8. Bhalaik V, Chhabra S, Walsh HP: Bilateral coexistent calcaneonavicular and talocalcaneal tarsal coalition: a case report, *J Foot Ankle Surg* 41:129, 2002.

9. Bigongiari LR: Pseudotibiotalar slant: a positioning artifact, *Radiology* 122:669, 1977.

10. Blumel J, Evans EB, Eggers GW: Partial and complete agenesis of malformation of the associated anomalies, *J Bone Joint Surg Am* 41:497, 1959.

11. Boden SD: Overview of the biology of lumbar spine fusion and principles for selecting a bone graft substitute, *Spine* 15:S26, 1996.

12. Bohne WH: Tarsal coalition, *Curr Opin Pediatr* 13:29, 2001.

13. Bonzar M et al: Kienbock diseassse and negative ulnar variance, *J Bone Joint Surg* 80A:1154, 1998.

14. Brockmeyer DL, York JE, Apfelbaum RL: Anatomical suitability of C1-2 transarticular screw placement in pediatric patients, *J Neurosurg* 92:7, 2000.

15. Brower AC: Arthritis in black and white, ed 2, Philadelphia, 1997, WB Saunders.

16. Buna M et al: Pontiles of the atlas: a review and clinical perspective, *J Man Phys Ther* 7:261, 1984.

17. Cacciarelli AA: Posterior widening of the S1-2 interspace in children: a normal variant of sacral development, *AJR Am J Roentgenol* 129:305, 1977.

18. Cassidy JD et al: Lumbar facet joint asymmetry. Intervertebral disc herniation, *Spine* 17:570, 1992.

19. Castellvi AE, Goldstein LA, Chan DPK: Lumbosacral transitional vertebrae and their relationship with lumbar extradural defects, *Spine* 9:493, 1984.

20. Chen WS: Kienbock disease and negative ulnar variance, *J Bone Joint Surg* 82A:143, 2000.

21. Chen WS, Shih CH: Ulnar variance and Kienböck's disease. An investigation in Taiwan, *Clin Orthop* 255:124, 1990.

22. Chung KC, Spilson MS, Kim MH: Is negative ulnar variance a risk factor for Kienbock disease? A meta-analysis, *Ann Plast Surg* 47:494, 2001.

23. Cleveland WW, Arias D, Smith GF: Radioulnar synostosis, behavioral disturbance, and XYY chromosomes, *J Pediatr* 74:103, 1969.

24. Cyron BM, Hutton WC: Articular tropism and stability of the lumbar spine, *Spine* 5:168, 1980.

25. Daenen B et al: Symptomatic herniation pits of the femoral neck: anatomic and clinical study, *AJR Am J Roentgenol* 168:149, 1997.

26. Dal Monte A et al: A critical review of the surgical treatment of congenital proximal radio-ulnar synostosis, *J Orthop Traumat* 13:181, 1987.

27. Davies MK et al: The straight back syndrome, *Q J Med* 49:443, 1980.

28. Dubrana F et al: Kirner's deformity. Four case reports and review of the literature, *Annales de Chirurgie de la Main et du Membre Superieur* 14:33, 1995.

29. Ducloyer P et al: Spontaneous ruptures of the extensor tendons of the fingers in Madelung's deformity, *J Hand Surg* 16B:329, 1991.

30. Duncan GA: Congenital and developmental coxa vara, *Surgery* 3:741, 1938.

31. Dyke CG: Indirect signs of brain tumor as noted in routine roentgen examinations. Displacement of the pineal shadow. (A survey of 3000 consecutive skull examinations), *AJR Am J Roentgenol* 23:598, 1930.

32. Dylkkanen PV: Coxa vara infantum, *Acta Orthop Scand* 48:7, 1960.

33. Einsiedel E, Clausner A: Funnel chest. Psychological and psychosomatic aspects in children, youngsters and young adults, *J Cardiovasc Surg* 40:733, 1999.

34. Eisenkraft BL, Som PM: The spectrum of benign and malignant etiologies of cervical node calcification, *AJR Am J Roentgenol* 172:1433, 1999.

35. Farfan HF, Huberdeau RM, Dubow HI: Lumbar intervertebral disc degeneration. The influence of geometrical features on the pattern of disc degeneration: a post mortem study, *J Bone Joint Surg* 54A:492, 1972.

36. Fielding WJ et al: Os odontoideum, *J Bone Joint Surg* 45A:1459, 1980.

37. Fiolle J: Le carpe Bossu, *Soc Nat de Chirugie* 57:1587, 1931.

38. Fonkalsrud EW et al: Repair of pectus deformities with sternal support, *J Thorac Cardiovasc Surg* 107:37, 1994.

39. Fonkalsrud EW, DeUgarte D, Choi E: Repair of pectus excavatum and carinatum deformities in 116 adults, *Ann Surg* 236:304, 2002.

40. Fonkalsrud EW et al: Repair of pectus excavatum deformities: 30 years of experience with 375 patients, *Ann Surg* 231:443, 2000.

41. Fusi S, Watson HK, Cuono CB: The carpal boss. A 20-year review of operative management, *J Hand Surg* 20B:405, 1995.

42. Gelberman RH, Bauman T: Madelung's deformity and dyschondrosteosis, *J Hand Surg* 5A:338, 1980.

43. Goodman LR, Teplik SK, Kay H: Computed tomography of the normal sternum, *AJR Am J Roentgenol* 141:219, 1983.

44. Griffiths HJ: Basic bone radiology, Norwalk, CT, 1987, Appleton & Lange.

45. Hadley MD: Carpal coalition and Sprengel's shoulder in Poland's syndrome, *J Hand Surg* 10B:253, 1985.

46. Haller JA et al: Evolving management of pectus excavatum based on a single institutional experience of 664 patients, *Ann Surg* 209:578, 1989.

47. Haller JA, Kramer SS, Lietman SA: Use of CT scans in selection of patients for pectus excavatum surgery: a preliminary report, *J Pediatr Surg* 22:904, 1987.

48. Harper HAS, Poznanski AK, Garn SM: The carpal angle in American population, *Invest Radiol* 9:217, 1974.

49. Hauser G, Stefano GF: Epigenetic variants of the human skull, Stuttgart, 1989, Schweizerbart.

50. Hedvabny Z, Zidkova H, Kofranek I: *Acta Chirurgiae Orthopaedicae et Traumatologiae Cechoslovaca*, 60:351, 1993.

51. Ishikawa H et al: Painful bipartite patella in young athletes. The diagnostic value of skyline views taken in squatting position and the results of surgical excision, *Clin Orthop Rel Res* 305:223, 1994.

52. Ivy RH: Congenital anomalies, *Plast Reconstr Surg* 20:400, 1957.

53. Izadi S: Intracranial calcifications, *Shiraz E-Med J* 3:4, 2002.

54. Jancu J: Radioulnar synostosis. A common occurrence in sex chromosomal abnormalities, *Am J Dis Child* 122:10, 1971.

55. Jong-Beom P et al: Facet tropism. A comparison between far lateral and posterolateral lumbar disc herniations, *Spine* 26:677, 2001.

56. Kahn G, Rath E, Atar D: Fracture of the supracondylar process of the humerus associated with Monteggia fracture, *Harefuah* 141:877, 2002.

57. Kirlew KA et al: Os odontoideum in identical twins: perspectives on etiology, *Skeletal Radiol* 22:525, 1993.

58. Ko HY, Park BK: Facet tropism in lumbar motion segments and its significance in disc herniation, *Arch Phys Med Rehabil* 78:1211, 1997

59. Kruse RW, Chen J: Accessory bones of the foot: clinical significance, *Military Med* 160:464, 1995.

60. Kumar UK, Sahasranam KV: Mitral valve prolapse syndrome and associated thoracic skeletal abnormalities, *J Assoc Phys India* 39:536, 1991.

61. Lakovlev VM, Nechaeva GI, Viktorova IA: Clinical function of the myocardium and cardiac hemodynamics in patients with pectus carinatum deformity, *Ter Arkh* 62:69, 1990.

62. Leboeuf C, Kimber D, White K: Prevalence of spondylolisthesis, transitional anomalies and low intercrestal line in chiropractic patient populations, *J Man Phys Ther* 12:200, 1989.

63. Leras JM et al: Spontaneous disappearance of herniation pit on the femoral neck, *J Radiol* 76:593, 1995.

64. Lombardi G: The occipital vertebra, *AJR Am J Roentgenol* 86:260, 1961.

65. Lucet L et al: Computed tomography of the normal sternoclavicular joint, *Skeletal Radiol* 25:237, 1996.

66. Maempel FZ: Post-traumatic radioulnar synostosis. A report of two cases, *Clin Orthop Rel Res* 186:182, 1984.

67. Magora A, Schwartz A: Relation between the low back pain syndrome and x-ray findings, *Scand J Rehabil Med* 10:135, 1978.

68. Mann DC, Keene JS, Drummond DS: Unusual causes of back pain in athletes, *J Spinal Disord* 4:337, 1991.

69. Marburger R, Burgess RC: Symptomatic lunate-triquetral coalition, *J South Orthop Assoc* 4:307, 1995.

70. Mielke CH, Winter RB: Pectus carinatum successfully treated with bracing. A case report, *Int Orthop* 17:350, 1993.

71. Miller TT: Painful accessory bones of the foot, *Semin MusculoSkeletal Radiol* 6:153, 2002.

72. Morton DJ: Metatarsus atavicus: the identification of a distinct type of foot disorder, *J Bone Joint Surg Bos* 9:531, 1927.

73. Muragaki Y: Altered growth and branching patterns in synpolydactyly caused by mutations in HOXD13, *Science* 272:548, 1996.

74. Murtagh FR, Paulsen RD, Rechtine GR: The role and incidence of facet tropism in lumbar spine degenerative disc disease, *J Spinal Disord* 4:86, 1991.

75. Murtagh RD, Caracciolo JT, Fernandez G: CT findings associated with Eagle syndrome, *Am J Neuroradiol* 22:1401, 2001.

76. Nakamura R et al: The influence of age and sex on ulnar variance, *J Hand Surg* 16B:84, 1991.

77. Noren R et al: The role of facet joint tropism and facet angle in disc degeneration, *Spine* 16:530, 1991.

78. Numaguchi Y: Osteitis condensans ilii, including its resolution, *Radiology* 98:1, 1971.

79. Ogden JA, McCarthy SM, Jokl P: The painful bipartite patella, *J Pediat Orthop* 2:263, 1982.

80. Oestreich AE et al: The "anteater nose": a direct sign of calcaneonavicular coalition on the lateral radiograph, *J Pediatr Orthop* 7:709, 1987.

81. Park JB et al: Facet tropism: a comparison between far lateral and posterolateral lumbar disc herniations, *Spine* 26:677, 2001.

82. Pecina M, Boric I, Anticervic D: Intraoperatively proven anomalous Struthers' ligaments diagnosed by MRI, *Skeletal Radiol* 31:532, 2002.

83. Pitt MJ et al: Herniation pit of the femoral neck, *AJR Am J Roentgenol* 38:1115, 1982.

84. Plafki C et al: Bilateral Madelung's deformity without signs of dyschondrosteosis within five generations in a European family: case report and review of the literature, *Arch Orthop Trauma Surg* 120:114, 2000.

85. Potter HG, Pavlov H, Abrahams TG: The hallux sesamoids revisited, *Skeletal Radiol* 21:437, 1992.

86. Pyo J, Lowman RM: The "ponticulus posticus" of the first cervical vertebra, *Radiology* 72:850, 1959.

87. Renshaw TS: Sacral agenesis, *J Bone Joint Surg Am* 60:378, 1978.

88. Requejo SM, Kulig K, Thordarson DB: Management of foot pain associated with accessory bones of the foot: two clinical case reports, *J Orthop Trauma Sports Phys Med* 30:580, 2000.

89. Resnick D: Diagnosis of bone and joint disorders, ed 4, Philadelphia, 2002, WB Saunders.

90. Robicsek F et al: Pectus carinatum, *J Thorac Cardiovasc Surg* 78:52, 1979.

91. Robin NH et al: Clinical and molecular studies of brachydactyly type D, *Am J Med Genet* 85:413, 1999.

92. Ross JK, Bereznick DE, McGill SM: Atlas-axis facet asymmetry implications in manual palpation, *Spine* 24:1203, 1999.

93. Sachar K, Akelman E, Ehrlich MG: Radioulnar synostosis, *Hand Clin*, 10:399, 1994.

94. Schmidt H et al: Borderlands of normal and early pathologic findings in skeletal radiography, New York, 1993, Thieme Medical Publishers.

95. Scott CE, Engber W: Kirner's deformity: a case report and review, *Iowa Orthop J* 16:167, 1996.

96. Shamberger RC, Welch KJ: Surgical correction of pectus carinatum, *J Pediatr Surg* 22:48, 1987.

97. Shopfner C, Jarboner EJT, Vallion RM: Craniolucania, *AJR Am J Roentgenol* 93:343, 1965.

98. Simmons BP, McKenzie WD: Symptomatic carpal coalition, *J Hand Surg Am Vol* 10(2):190, 1985.

99. Simmons BP, Southmayd WW, Riseborough EJ: Congenital radioulnar synostosis, *J Hand Surg* 8A:829, 1983.

100. Smoker WR: Congenital anomalies of the cervical spine, *Neuroimaging Clin N Am* 5:427, 1995.

101. Smoker WR: Craniovertebral junction: normal anatomy, craniometry and congenital anomalies, *Radiographic* 14:255, 1994.

102. Spinner RJ et al: Fractures of the supracondylar process of the humerus, *J Hand Surg* 19A:1038, 1994.

103. Stelling CB: Anomalous attachments of the transverse process to the vertebral body: an accessory finding in congenital absence of a lumbar pedicle, *Skeletal Radiol* 6:47, 1981.

104. Stubbs DM: The arcuate foramen: variability in distribution related to race and sex, *Spine* 17:1502, 1992.

105. Swischuk LE: Anterior displacement of C2 in children: physiologic or pathologic? A helpful differentiating line, *Radiology* 122:759, 1977.

106. Thomason CB et al: Focal bone tracer uptake associated with a herniation pit of the femoral neck, *Clin Nuclear Med* 8:304, 1983.

107. Tsuruta T et al: Radiological study of the accessory skeletal elements in the foot and ankle, *J Jpn Orthop Assoc* 55:357, 1981.

108. Urban J: Carpal bone protuberance, *Chirurgia Narzadow Ruchu i Ortopedia Polska* 61:339, 1996.

109. Van Schaik JP, Verbiest H, Van Schaik FD: The orientation of laminae and facet joints in the lower lumbar spine, *Spine* 10:59, 1985.

110. Vanharanta H et al: The relationship of facet tropism to degenerative disc disease, *Spine* 18:1000, 1993.

111. Vergauwen S et al: Distribution and incidence of degenerative spine changes in patients with a lumbosacral transitional vertebra, *Eur Spine J* 6:168, 1997.

112. Violas P et al: Acetabular protrusion in osteogenesis imperfecta, *J Pediatr Orthop* 22:622, 2002.

113. Weinstein JN, Kuo KN, Millar EA: Congenital coxa vara. A retrospective review, *J Pediatr Orthop* 4:70, 1984.

114. Wight S, Osbourne N, Breen A: The incidence of ponticulus posterior of the atlas in migraine and cervicogenic headache, *J Man Phys Ther* 22:15,1999.

115. Wilson MD: Special considerations for patients with Down's syndrome, *ODA J* 184:24, 1994.

116. Zimmer EZ, Bronshtein M: Fetal polydactyly diagnosis during early pregnancy: clinical applications, *Am J Obstet Gynecol* 183:755, 2000.

Bone, Joints, and Soft Tissues

chapter 8

Congenital Diseases

TIMOTHY J. MICK

Achondroplasia

BACKGROUND

Classic, heterozygous, autosomal-dominant achondroplasia is the most common dwarfing skeletal dysplasia and typically is evident at birth. The condition results from a defect at the 2.5 Mb locus of chromosome 4p16.3.[74] The name (*a-*, meaning "not," *chondroplasia*, meaning "formation of cartilage") implies that a complete lack of normal cartilage formation exists. This is not the case, although the hallmark of the condition is hypochondrogenesis, with a decreased rate of formation of essentially normal cartilage.

Achondroplasia usually is evident at birth and generally is compatible with a normal life expectancy; therefore patients with this condition may be seen at any age. Achondroplasia is recognized easily clinically and is differentiated from other dwarfing dysplasias readily.

IMAGING FINDINGS

General. Imaging findings in achondroplasia reflect gross anatomic changes. The ilia are broad and squared, with constricted sciatic notches. The pelvic inlet has a "champagne glass" configuration. The sacrum is horizontal and deeply seated in the pelvis. The ribs are broad and short, resulting in a diminished anteroposterior (AP) dimension of the thorax. The sternum is short and broad. The long and tubular bones are shortened and the developing metaphyses flared. Limb shortening is more profound proximally than distally (rhizomelic micromelia).[140]

Epiphyses. Epiphyseal changes may resemble a variety of epiphyseal dysplasias. Broad, short proximal phalanges, with short middle phalanges of the feet and (more classically) the hands may occur. This results in a clinically apparent, trident-shaped hand in infants. (The trident is a three-pronged spear wielded by the fish-god of classical mythology.)

Limb lengthening. As limb-lengthening procedures pioneered by the Russian physician Ilizarov have become more widely used, clinicians may encounter patients with atypical postoperative long bone changes.[29,53] A number of studies have shown impressive gains in limb length in patients treated with this procedure.[5,75,194]

Studies in growth hormone therapy for achondroplasia are not extensive, although subjects receiving growth hormone demonstrate sustained increases in rate of growth for 4 to 6 years.[30,109,179,293]

Spine. Plain films highlight most of the characteristic spinal abnormalities, including short pedicles and diminished central spinal canal dimensions (Fig. 8-1), with a cephalocaudal decrease in the coronal interpediculate distance. However, advanced, cross-sectional imaging (magnetic resonance imaging [MRI] or computed tomography [CT]) is necessary to directly identify the classic trefoil central spinal canal morphology and resultant compression of neural elements (Figs. 8-2 and 8-3). Posterior vertebral body scalloping results from vertebral dysplasia and dural ectasia. Platyspondyly is typical, although it may not be remarkable.

Degenerative disc disease and facet arthrosis are common in older adult patients because of biomechanical and gross anatomic factors. Degenerative disc and joint disease often is premature and may be unusually severe for age. Vertebral spondylophyte and hypertrophic degenerative facet joint changes may contribute significantly to central canal and nerve root canal stenosis, superimposed on a developmentally small canal dimension. The surgical approach to treatment may range from single-level laminectomy to complete craniospinal decompression from brainstem to cauda equina. This reportedly (and incredibly) does not produce spinal instability.[273]

CLINICAL COMMENTS

Achondroplastic dwarfs typically have macrocephaly and a broad, flat nasal bridge. Prominence of the frontal bone and frontal sinuses is described as "frontal bossing." Achondroplastic adults obviously are short, ranging in height from 112 to 145 cm. However, these are not the shortest of the dwarfs. Patients with spondyloepiphyseal dysplasia (SED) or spondyloepimetaphyseal dysplasia range from 94 to 132 cm and have much more apparent trunk than extremity shortening.[102]

Clinically and radiographically apparent angular thoracolumbar kyphosis with a classic "bullet-shaped" vertebra at the thoracolumbar junction is a hallmark of the condition and usually is present at birth. Lumbar hyperlordosis tends to develop in later childhood and into adulthood.[140]

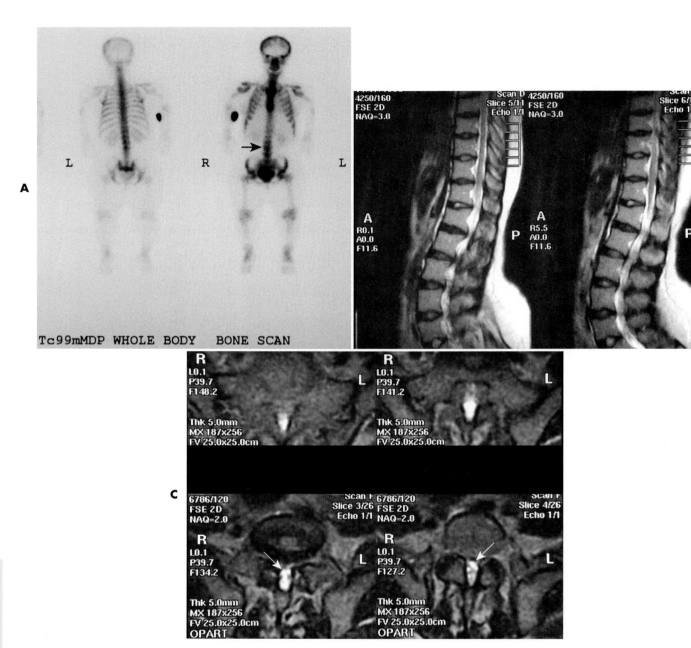

FIG. 8-1 A 42-year-old female achondroplastic patient with persistent low back pain. **A,** The bone scan exhibits mild radiotracer uptake secondary to the posterior joint disease *(arrow)*. The T2-weighted, **B,** sagittal and, **C,** axial images demonstrate a narrow spinal canal. Achondroplasia is the prototypical example of congenital spinal stenosis. Patients often experience clinical manifestations of spinal stenosis as the congenitally narrowed canal *(arrows)* is further affected by posterior joint degeneration and disc displacement, which inevitably occur during middle age.

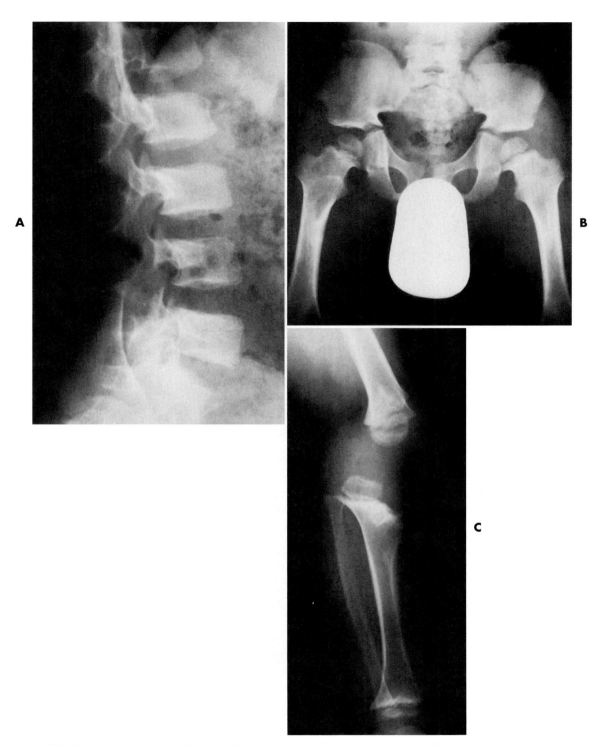

FIG. 8-2 Achondroplasia in a 5-month-old girl. **A,** Platyspondyly, posterior scalloping. **B,** Broad, square ilia, hemispheric capital femoral epiphyses, short femoral necks. **C,** Exaggerated tibial tubercle apophysis, fibulae overgrowth. (From Taybi H, Lachman RS: Radiology of syndromes, metabolic disorders, and skeletal dysplasias, ed 4, St Louis, 1996, Mosby.)

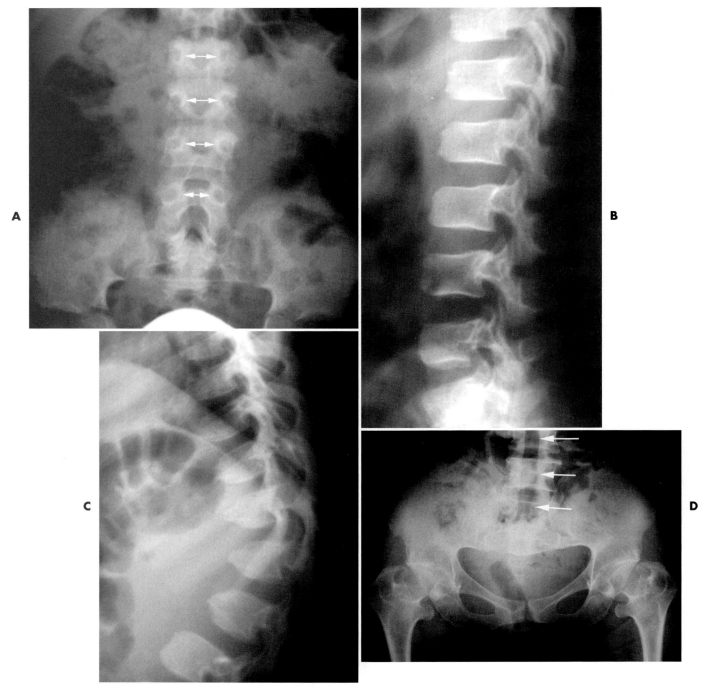

FIG 8-3   Achondroplasia. **A,** Anteroposterior spine shows narrow interpedicular distance in the lower lumbar spine *(arrows).* **B,** Lateral lumbar spine. Note the posterior vertebral body scalloping, mild anterior beaking, and short pedicles. **C,** Lateral spine, more severe dysplasia. Note the thoracolumbar kyphosis with prominent anterior beaking. **D,** Pelvis in an adult. Note the prior lumbar laminectomy *(arrows)* performed to relieve spinal stenosis. (From Manaster BJ, Disler DG, May DA: Musculoskeletal imaging, ed 2, St Louis, 2002, Mosby.)

As mentioned, achondroplasia is a prototypical cause of developmental spinal canal stenosis, often causing spinal cord, cauda equina, and nerve root compression. Stenosis of the foramen magnum also may lead to brainstem, cerebellar, or upper cervical cord compression, angulation, or displacement in addition to hydrocephalus, which commonly is diagnosed in infancy or early childhood. This may produce neurologic complications, including ataxia, incontinence, and depression of respiratory function, which occasionally is lethal.[191,225,278] Advanced diagnostic imaging has been valuable in identifying infants at risk for these complications and associated abnormalities, such as Arnold-Chiari malformation.[54] Abnormalities on polysomnography, as well as clinical findings of hyperreflexia and clonus, also have been considered to be indications for surgical decompression of the cervicomedullary junction. About 10% of infants fit this clinical picture. Achondroplastic infants should be screened for these findings.[192]

Achondroplastic patients often have a waddling gait because of hip joint involvement, frequently leading to advanced osteoarthritis early in life. Femoral epiphyseal changes may resemble those of Legg-Calvé-Perthes disease.

KEY CONCEPTS

- *Achondroplasia is the most common cause of dwarfism.*
- *A normal or near-normal trunk and marked rhizomelic micromelia are characteristic.*
- *A number of classic radiographic changes affect the axial and appendicular skeleton.*
- *Anomalies involving the skull and spine are particularly important because of the potential for neurologic complications.*
- *Achondroplasia is associated with developmental spinal canal stenosis, often causing spinal cord, cauda equina, and nerve root compression.*
- *In the peripheral skeleton, in addition to the obvious limb shortening, early, severe, and sometimes debilitating osteoarthritis may develop.*

Chondroectodermal Dysplasia

BACKGROUND

Chondroectodermal dysplasia (Ellis-van Creveld syndrome) is an autosomal recessive, short-limbed, dwarfing dysplasia characterized by polydactyly, congenital heart anomalies, and ectodermal dysplasia that are evident at birth. The condition, classified as a short-ribbed polydactyly syndrome (SRPS), is linked to consanguineous relationships. Previously this was particularly common among old-order Amish, but an awareness of this problem has prompted the Amish to encourage young adults to move away and seek a spouse from another Amish community.

IMAGING FINDINGS

Thoracic changes resemble those of Jeune asphyxiating thoracic dysplasia. Ribs are short and broad anteriorly, with an increased anteroposterior dimension of the thorax. Constriction of the thorax is caused by diminished coronal dimension. The ilia are hypoplastic. There is variation in shape, size, and number of tubular bones of the hands and feet. Hexadactyly (six digits on each hand and foot) is invariable with this condition and may be associated with syndactyly. There also may be supernumerary carpal bones, carpal coalition across carpal rows, and cone-shaped epiphyses. Congenital radial head dislocation and marked widening of the distal radial and proximal ulnar metaphyses occur, with metaphyseal flaring producing a so-called drumstick appearance.

More generalized alteration of bone formation in the epimetaphyseal region may be seen. Genu varum resulting from a hypoplastic medial tibial plateau may resemble Blount's disease. Tibiotalar slant and bony excrescences at the medial aspect of the proximal tibia also are commonly seen. The axial skeleton is largely spared, with generally normal skull and spine.[47,166] Coronal vertebral clefts may be seen.[283]

CLINICAL COMMENTS

Patients are short, with greater limb shortening distally (acromelic shortening). Skeletal anomalies of size, shape, and number, along with congenital synostoses, may be suspected clinically, but are best assessed radiographically. Nails and teeth are agenetic or markedly dysplastic. Cardiopulmonary complications often lead to death in early childhood, although some individuals survive into adulthood. Dandy-Walker malformation has been reported, but it is unclear whether this is directly related or a coincidental occurrence.[303]

KEY CONCEPTS

- *The classic clinical presentation of Ellis-van Creveld disease occurs in infancy or childhood as hexadactyly marked phalangeal and nail hypoplasia, congenital heart anomaly, typical thoracic anomalies, and genu varum.*
- *Radiologic changes include developmental metaphyseal alterations and congenital synostosis, especially carpal coalition.*

Cleidocranial Dysplasia

BACKGROUND

This rather rare, autosomal-dominant condition was first described in 1898, but only fairly recently was localized to the short arm of chromosome 6p,[66,81] refuting an earlier report that the chromosomal abnormality involved was the 8q locus.[32] One third of cases represent new mutations. Despite a name that implies a process limited to the clavicle and calvarium, cleidocranial dysplasia actually is a generalized autosomal dominant dysplasia combining developmental midline spinal defects, delayed skeletal maturity, dental anomalies, and the more widely recognized skull and clavicle abnormalities.

As with most skeletal dysplasias, identification of specific genetic markers has vastly enhanced the ability to distinguish between conditions that share many clinical and radiographic features. This led to identification of newly described dysplasias that otherwise would have been lumped together with another more familiar or common syndrome.[242,296] As a result, it may seem that the study of skeletal dysplasias has advanced from an esoteric and uncertain exercise undertaken by a small, erudite group of pediatric and bone radiologists to a more certain (perhaps still esoteric) exercise carried out by a small (perhaps still erudite) group of geneticists. A report of cleidocranial dysplasia occurring in three consecutive generations, but previously unrecognized in the first two, has prompted recommendation of assessment of family members in every case of what may appear to be a sporadic occurrence of the disorder.[37]

IMAGING FINDINGS

Skull. Cleidocranial dysplasia is characterized by multiple wormian (intrasutural) bones, especially within the lambdoid suture, frontal bossing of the calvarium, and variable hypoplasia and dysplasia of the clavicles (Fig. 8-4). Examination of the development of the cranium in neonates with this condition has revealed

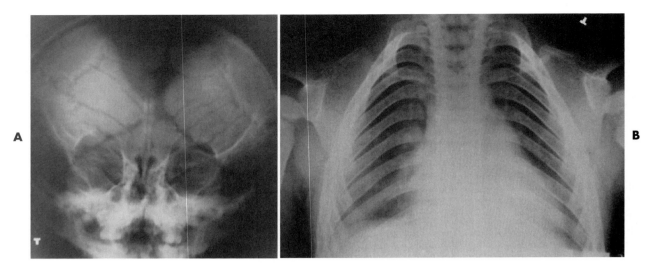

FIG. 8-4 Cleidocranial dysplasia in a 5-year-old boy with "soft shoulders," large head, prominent anterior fontanelle open down through forehead, and poor teeth. **A,** Widely open sutures and fontanelle, and wormian bones. **B,** Partial aplasia of clavicles, droopy shoulders, small scapulae, spina bifida, wide ribs. (From Taybi H, Lachman RS: Radiology of syndromes, metabolic disorders, and skeletal dysplasias, ed 4, St Louis, 1996, Mosby.)

a marked delay in skeletal maturity over the first 6 months of life. Also, normal mineralization of the calvarium typically is grossly reduced. Calvarial size may be relatively normal, considering marked postpartum deformity secondary to the poor mineralization. Widening of the skull has been reported in some cases. About 60% of patients have an inverted "pear-shaped" calvarium and a persistent anterior fontanelle, one of the midline defects typical of this disorder. The portion of the skull base formed through enchondral ossification is narrowed and shows delayed ossification. Also apparent is cephalad displacement of the clivus and sella turcica, with anteriorly facing foramen magnum, often accompanied by basilar invagination. The sphenooccipital synchondrosis is widened.[117,119]

Clavicles. Fewer than 10% of patients show complete agenesis of the clavicles.[32] Other clavicular anomalies involving hypoplasia and dysplasia are consistent and specific enough that the diagnosis may be at least suspected in utero.[95]

Face and sinuses. The paranasal sinuses are characteristically absent or hypoplastic, consistent with an abnormality predominating in bones formed, through intramembranous ossification. The sella turcica often is hypoplastic, and the dorsum sellae often is bulbous. Nasal bones almost always are hypoplastic or agenetic. Likewise the zygomatic arches are hypoplastic or absent.[119] All craniofacial regions are affected in cleidocranial dysplasia.[117] Even the hyoid bone may demonstrate decreased ossification.[210] The height and width of the mandible and maxilla are decreased, with anterior inclination of the mandible.[117] The coronoid process of the mandible is slender and obliquely oriented in a posterosuperior direction. Persistence of a midline suture at the mandibular symphysis is classic for cleidocranial dysplasia.[65] Facial abnormalities appear to progress with increasing age and may not be readily apparent in younger children.[119,120]

Other anomalies. Other anomalies include incompletely descended, hypoplastic scapulae with shallow glenoid fossae. The iliac wings are hypoplastic and ossification of the pubic bones and obturator rings is delayed and deficient. Pubic diastasis is a characteristic feature. Coxa vara or valga may occur, with the latter more common. Long bones may be overtubulated (excessively constricted at the diametaphyseal junctions). Fibular agenesis or congenital pseudoarthrosis of the femur may occur.

The predominant finding in the spine is spina bifida occulta, most commonly in the cervicothoracic region. Another potential anomaly is structural scoliosis resulting from vertebral segmentation anomalies, including hemivertebrae and asymmetric nonsegmentation (block vertebrae). The hands may demonstrate hypoplasia of carpal bones and distal phalanges, with relative hyperplasia of the epiphyses, especially of the distal phalanges.[211] The second and fifth metacarpals typically are long, and the second and fifth middle phalanges are short. Supernumerary ossification centers may be apparent.

CLINICAL COMMENTS

The clinical manifestations of cleidocranial dysplasia are highly variable. Affected individuals may be somewhat below average in height. The head is macrocephalic overall, but shortened in an anteroposterior dimension (brachycephalic), with frontal bossing and a small face. The shoulders may appear drooped and demonstrate an increased range of motion. Genu valgum and brachydactyly also may be seen. Respiratory dysfunction may result from a developmentally narrow thorax.[211]

Unlike other conditions involving midline defects and spinal dysraphism, cleidocranial dysplasia is not classically associated with neurologic deficit. When present, such a deficit should prompt assessment for other abnormalities of the central nervous system (CNS), such as neoplasm, syringomyelia, or other developmental anomaly.[58,190] Supernumerary and anomalous teeth are typical in cleidocranial dysplasia. A strategy has been devised to successfully predict the development of supernumerary teeth before the permanent teeth are fully developed. This allows extraction of the supernumerary teeth and, when indicated, of the primary teeth and overlying bone, improving eruption of the remaining permanent teeth.[118,213]

KEY CONCEPTS

- *Radiographic finding include wormian bones, clavicular deformity (aplasia [10%] and hypoplasia), mild spinal dysraphism (spina bifida occulta), delayed closure of the symphysis pubis, and supernumerary epiphyses.*
- *The patient's clinical appearance is marked by drooping shoulders, possible respiratory distress, large head, small face, and anomalous teeth.*

Congenital Insensitivity to Pain

BACKGROUND

Congenital insensitivity to pain is sometimes described as "indifference to pain." This is somewhat misleading, implying that pain is perceived but ignored. Instead an essential absence of or marked diminution of pain perception exists, whereas all other sensory findings are normal. The condition, first described in 1932, may spare sensation of light touch, and deep tendon reflexes also may be normal.

IMAGING FINDINGS

The radiographic findings of congenital insensitivity to pain are those seen in other neuropathic conditions and summarized as the classic 6 Ds of neuroarthropathy. As one of the classic causes of "degenerative joint disease with a vengeance," there is typically joint destruction, disorganization, diminished joint space, intraarticular debris (detritus), joint distention, and reactive subchondral sclerosis (increased density). Because of its presence from infancy, congenital insensitivity to pain typically leads to disruption of the physes, essentially representing stress fracture through the growth plate. This may be evident in children with spinal dysraphism as well. Extensive subperiosteal hemorrhage also may occur, along with periarticular disintegration and fragmentation, which may be mistaken for child abuse.[252] In the spine, radiographic changes are similar to those seen in neuroarthropathy (e.g., from syphilis or diabetic neuropathy), which may be thought of as "degenerative disc disease with a vengeance."[198]

Patients with congenital insensitivity to pain may have complicating infections of both the soft tissues and skeleton in addition to neuroarthropathy. This results from a chronic open wound resulting from an abrasion, burn, or other superficial injury.[188] Such infections may necessitate amputation. Other complications that may require extensive orthopedic or neurosurgical intervention include pathologic fracture, dislocation, autoamputation, and rapidly progressing scoliosis.[90,99]

CLINICAL COMMENTS

Generally, the abnormality is manifested in infancy or early childhood as a marked absence of reaction to pain stimuli, frequently with cutaneous manifestations of scars and burns, unnoticed by the child. Self-mutilation and aggressive behavior may occur, especially in conjunction with Lesch-Nyhan syndrome or familial dysautonomia (Riley-Day syndrome). Patients with these and related hereditary sensory neuropathies (HSN) or dysautonomic conditions also may suffer from mental deficits, anhidrosis (inability to sweat), and resultant alteration of thermoregulation.[57,185]

A distinct form of congenital insensitivity to pain with anhidrosis (CIPA) has been identified, also known as *hereditary sensory* and *autonomic neuropathy type IV*. Nearly 20% of patients with this disorder die within the first 3 years of life because of hyperpyrexia.[220] At least five variants of HSN exist; in some cases a precise distinction of one disorder from another may not be possible without prolonged follow-up and nerve biopsy. Reports detail patients who are initially diagnosed with congenital insensitivity to pain, and later determined to have a hereditary sensory and autonomic neuropathy.[141] Nerve biopsies reveal loss of nonmyelinated and small myelinated fibers.[220]

Recently, abnormalities of muscle also have been reported in patients with congenital insensitivity to pain. Muscle weakness and hyporeflexia or areflexia may be evident. Histologically and anatomically, the involved muscle demonstrates marked variation in fiber size. Some small fibers have central nuclei and a few small angulated fibers.[261]

KEY CONCEPTS

- *Congenital indifference to pain is suggested by an infant or young child presenting with a history of multiple traumas (e.g., burns, abrasions) that are unnoticed by the patient and, at least initially, also by the parents or guardians.*
- *Repeated traumas to joints and surrounding structures, resulting from a lack of protective proprioceptive feedback, lead to an appearance of advanced joint disease.*
- *Developing physes are particularly vulnerable to stress fractures, resulting in significant fragmentation and other architectural distortion.*
- *A loose periosteum in infants and children and subperiosteal hemorrhage may lead to remarkable periosteal reaction.*
- *Severe burns may be associated with joint contractures.*

Developmental Dysplasia of the Hip

BACKGROUND

Developmental dysplasia of the hip (DDH) is lateral displacement of the hip with varying degrees of acetabular dysplasia. In the past the condition was termed *congenital hip dysplasia* or *congenital hip dislocation*. The newer term reflects the fact that the condition may not be present at birth, but develops in infancy and early childhood. It appears six to nine times more frequently in females, slightly more often on the left, and occasionally bilaterally.

IMAGING FINDINGS

The proximal femur may be subluxated or dislocated. Displacement is difficult to detect on radiographs in neonates and young infants because of the incomplete mineralization of the hip and pelvis. Classic imaging findings are summarized in Putti's triad, consisting of lateral displacement of the femur, a small or radiographically invisible femoral capital epiphysis, and an increased acetabular angle (Figs. 8-5 through 8-8). The anteroposterior projection of the hip is used for radiographic assessment. The frog-leg

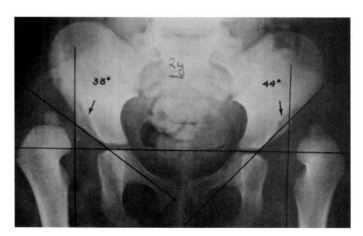

FIG. 8-5 Bilateral developmental dysplasia of the hip in a 2-year-old girl. Putti's triad is present on both sides; the right acetabular angle is enlarged to 38 degrees, the left to 44 degrees. The arrows point to bilateral false acetabulae. The acetabular angles should not exceed standards based on age (e.g., at birth they should measure less than 36 degrees in females and 30 degrees in males; see Chapter 4). (From Silverman FN, Kuhn JP: Caffey's pediatric x-ray diagnosis: an integrated imaging approach, ed 9, St Louis, 1993, Mosby.)

PART TWO Bone, Joints, and Soft Tissues

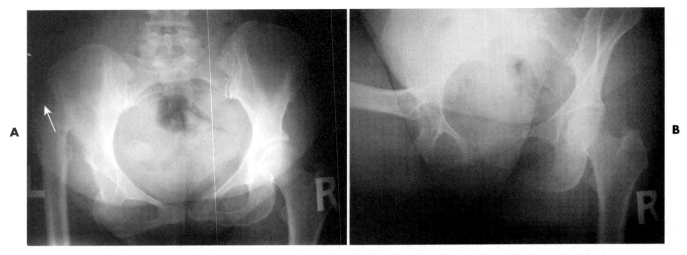

FIG. 8-6 **A** and **B,** Uncorrected developmental dysplasia of the hip *(arrow)* in a 41-year-old man. The femoral head has displaced laterally and superiorly, with residual deformity of the acetabulum. (Courtesy Matthew Rich, Clearfield, PA.)

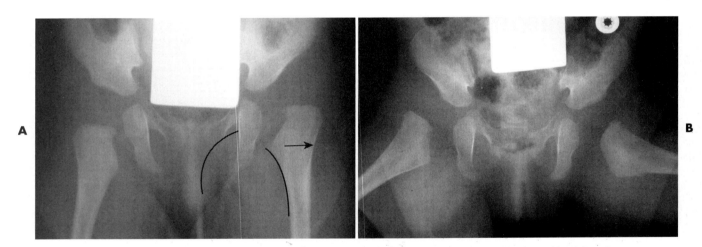

FIG. 8-7 **A** and **B,** Three-month-old infant with a subtle lateral dislocation of the reading right femoral head *(arrow).* Identifying the lesion is made easier by noticing the disruption of Shenton's line (drawn along the inferior surface of the superior pubic ramus and internal cortex of the femoral neck). (Courtesy Ian D. McLean, LeClaire, IA.)

view is not helpful, because the dislocation reduces during the abduction movement. In addition to Putti's triad, other radiographic features include acetabular sclerosis, shallow acetabulum, and delayed ossification of the femoral head.

Roentgenometrics are useful to assess the acetabular angle and determine whether lateral or superior displacement of the femur is present. The acetabular center-edge angle and acetabular index are useful in evaluating the acetabular angle. Shenton's line and the iliofemoral line are helpful to assess for femoral displacement. These roentgenometrics have been presented in greater detail in Chapter 4.

Diagnostic ultrasonography, arthrography, and CT are useful to delineate the anatomy of the hip and acetabulum in this disease. These modalities are particularly useful to locate the position of the acetabular labrum, which affects clinical outcome. The case is more difficult to resolve and often necessitates surgical correction if the labrum inverts during dislocation.

CLINICAL COMMENTS

Detection of displacement is accomplished largely through the application of appropriate imaging. Ortolani's and Barlow's orthopedic maneuvers are helpful, but there is a substantial false-negative rate. Asymmetry of rotation and apparent shortening of the affected leg may be evident when a patient is 3 months old. A waddling gait is typical.

Management is most effective when the condition is detected early, preferably in the neonatal period. Ultrasound is the technique of choice for assessing the immature hip in a neonate suspected of having developmental dysplasia. Mild cases may be successfully treated by maintaining the hips in a position of flexion and abduction. This may be accomplished by double or triple diapering the infant. In more advanced cases, a Pavlik harness (worn full-time for at least 6 weeks, then part-time for another 6 weeks) is used to maintain hip flexion and abduction.

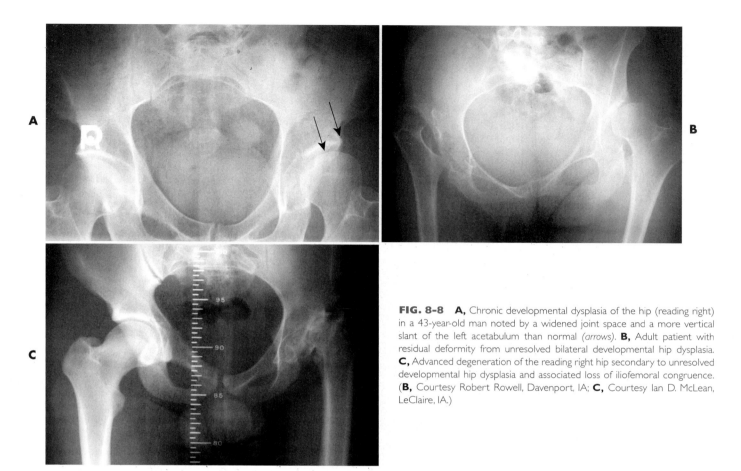

FIG. 8-8 A, Chronic developmental dysplasia of the hip (reading right) in a 43-year-old man noted by a widened joint space and a more vertical slant of the left acetabulum than normal *(arrows)*. **B,** Adult patient with residual deformity from unresolved bilateral developmental hip dysplasia. **C,** Advanced degeneration of the reading right hip secondary to unresolved developmental hip dysplasia and associated loss of iliofemoral congruence. (**B,** Courtesy Robert Rowell, Davenport, IA; **C,** Courtesy Ian D. McLean, LeClaire, IA.)

Surgery may be indicated to achieve reduction when conservative treatment fails. Successful reduction is largely dependent on the location of the acetabular labrum. Reduction is achieved with good outcome if the labrum is displaced lateral to the femoral head. However, successful reduction is more difficult if the labrum becomes inverted into the acetabulum during lateral displacement of the hip.

KEY CONCEPTS

- *Developmental hip dysplasia describes lateral displacement of the proximal femur with related dysplasia of the acetabulum.*
- *Basic imaging findings are summarized by Putti's triad: lateral displacement of the femur, small or absent femoral capital epiphysis, and increased acetabular angulation.*
- *Ultrasonography, arthrography, and computed tomography may be used to demonstrate the position of the acetabular labrum, the location of which affects clinical outcome.*
- *Management is most effective when the condition is detected early.*

Diastrophic Dysplasia

BACKGROUND

This autosomal recessive dwarfing dysplasia derives its name from the twisted appearance of the spine and extremities resulting from scoliosis, which may be progressive, as well as deformities, contractures, subluxations, and dislocations of the extremities. The condition is particularly common in Finland, although the reason is not clear. A study from the University of Helsinki demonstrated ankle and foot anomalies in 93% of cases, with the most common deformity involving combined metatarsus valgus and metatarsus adductus or equinovarus.[226]

IMAGING FINDINGS

General. Radiographic changes are consistent with the dwarfing and diffuse skeletal deformities seen clinically (Fig. 8-9). Severe peripheral deformities typically lead to early, advanced degenerative joint disease, which may necessitate arthroplasty.[193] Tubular bones are markedly shortened and metaphyses are widened, which does not help much in distinguishing this from other dwarfing conditions.

Hands. The first metacarpal is characteristically more severely affected and may be oval in shape. The carpal bones may demonstrate multiple accessory ossification centers, premature ossification, and deformity.

Epiphyses. The appearance of epiphyseal ossification centers is delayed, and other epiphyseal changes, which tend to be most marked at the proximal femora, resemble those of severe Legg-Calvé-Perthes disease. Developmental joint space narrowing may occur, and equinovarus deformity is common.[211]

Spine. Severe cervical kyphosis resulting from dysplastic vertebrae occurs in about one third of patients and may reach 180 degrees, with the spine literally folded in upon itself. Unlike extremity deformities, which typically increase as the child ages, some of these kyphoses completely resolve by adulthood.

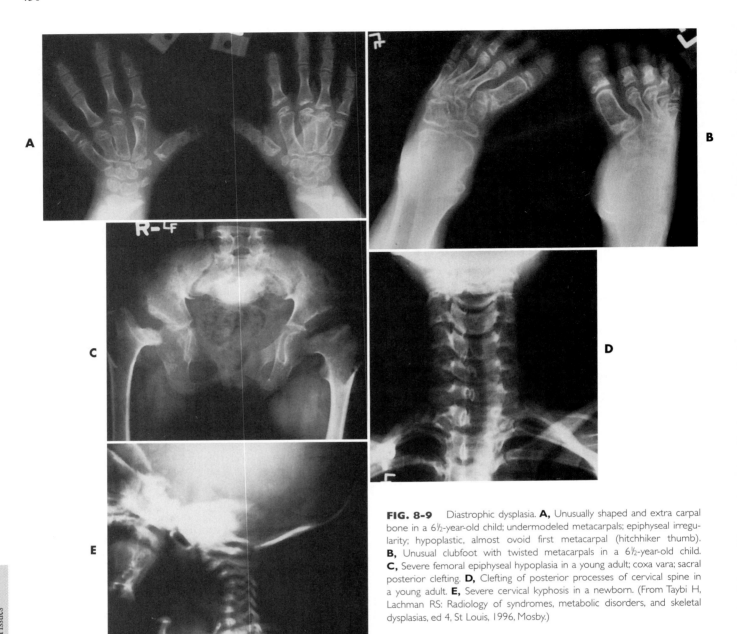

FIG. 8-9 Diastrophic dysplasia. **A,** Unusually shaped and extra carpal bone in a 6½-year-old child; undermodeled metacarpals; epiphyseal irregularity; hypoplastic, almost ovoid first metacarpal (hitchhiker thumb). **B,** Unusual clubfoot with twisted metacarpals in a 6½-year-old child. **C,** Severe femoral epiphyseal hypoplasia in a young adult; coxa vara; sacral posterior clefting. **D,** Clefting of posterior processes of cervical spine in a young adult. **E,** Severe cervical kyphosis in a newborn. (From Taybi H, Lachman RS: Radiology of syndromes, metabolic disorders, and skeletal dysplasias, ed 4, St Louis, 1996, Mosby.)

Others may lead to myelopathy or even death.[15] Scoliosis occurs in about one third of all patients, but it is more common in female patients (approximately 50%). Although they typically develop at a much younger age than idiopathic scolioses (usually apparent by 2 to 4 years of age), fewer than 15% of these curves progress beyond 50 degrees.[201] Diastrophic dysplasia represents a rare cause of atlantoaxial subluxation.[212] Congenital central spinal canal stenosis often occurs, with a narrowed interpediculate distance, although this is not as marked or consistent as in achondroplasia.

CLINICAL COMMENTS
Clubfoot deformity has been reported in the literature frequently, although a true clubfoot (talipes equinovarus) is actually not seen.

Hands and feet are short and broad, demonstrating a characteristic abduction or "hitchhiker" deformity of the thumbs and great toes. Peculiar cystic masses develop on the external ears, resulting in clinically apparent deformity. Cleft palate is seen in about 75% of cases, although only about half of these are open and clinically obvious.[214]

Expression is variable. Some patients attain a normal life span, and others die in infancy from respiratory complications. A milder form of diastrophic dysplasia has been referred to, probably inappropriately, as "diastrophic variant."[110,137] Conversely, particularly severe cases with cervical spine dislocations and congenital heart anomalies previously were considered by some to represent a unique, lethal form of the condition.[91]

Down Syndrome

BACKGROUND

Down syndrome was first described in 1959 in individuals with ocular abnormality, dystonia, mental and developmental retardation, brachycephaly, and macroglossia. Although most affected individuals demonstrate 47 chromosomes, this trisomy 21 configuration is absent in 5% to 10% of individuals with the typical phenotype. Such cases exhibit translocation and mosaicism.[289]

A well-known relationship exists between advancing maternal age and an increased incidence of trisomy 21. Women more than 35 years of age are typically offered prenatal testing. Maternal serum markers have been used recently, typically to detect unborn babies in the second trimester at risk for Down syndrome. The first of the serum markers to be used was maternal serum alpha-fetoprotein (MSAFP), but unconjugated estriol (uE3) and human chorionic gonadotropin (hCG) have been used as well. None of these is infallible, and there remains some controversy about which is the best method of detection in utero. Combining measurement of MSAFP and free-beta hCG with maternal age reportedly results in an 80% detection rate and a 5% false-positive rate. This still leaves mothers with a 1 in 20 chance of aborting a normal baby in response to a positive test and a 1 in 5 chance of having a baby with Down syndrome despite a negative test.[150]

IMAGING FINDINGS

Atlantoaxial instability. The single most important articulation to evaluate in a patient with Down syndrome is the atlantoaxial articulation, with anterior atlantoaxial dislocation or instability in approximately 20% of affected individuals.[170] The most critical ligamentous structure to assess is the transverse ligament. The most crucial plain film study is a lateral cervical film with head nod or flexion to evaluate for anterior atlantoaxial subluxation or the far less common occipitoatlantal instability. This is essential, especially with patients in whom activity, anticipated therapy (especially spinal manipulation), or past atlantoaxial surgical fusion may place the upper cervical complex or craniovertebral junction at increased risk.[221]

The relationship between Down syndrome and congenital laxity of the transverse portion of the cruciate ligament of C1 is well known, and is generally considered to be the primary etiology for most cases of atlantoaxial instability and subluxation. However, other factors such as odontoid hypoplasia and dysplasia along with upper respiratory infections and trauma are believed to contribute.[159,270] The atlantoaxial relationship in Down syndrome does not tend to change significantly over time, at least in asymptomatic individuals. Unless a clinical indication exists, serial lateral and flexion lateral cervical radiographs typically are not warranted.[205]

Atlas hypoplasia. A lesser-known, associated anomaly is a developmentally short posterior arch of C1, seen in more than one fourth of patients in one study.[160] This could present a sort of

"double jeopardy" in the presence of atlantoaxial instability. This anomaly is readily detected on lateral cervical radiographs and appears as an anterior displacement of the spinolaminar junction line of C1 relative to that of C2. When anterior atlantoaxial subluxation is present because of abnormality of the transverse ligament, it is difficult to estimate the potential contribution of a short posterior arch to spinal canal stenosis. As mentioned, Down syndrome patients also have an increased incidence of occipitoatlantal hypermobility and instability. Anteroposterior translation of the occiput between the neutral and fully flexed neck posture averages about 0.6 mm in normal individuals. A measurement of more than 1 mm in an adult implies instability. A study of 38 children with Down syndrome demonstrated an average of 2.3 mm, with a range from 0 to 6.4 mm. However, only one of these patients had symptoms that might be attributed to occipitoatlantal instability. The clinical implications are not entirely clear, but caution is indicated and cranioverterbral junction instability is possible, even in the presence of an apparently stable atlantoaxial articulation.[162]

Cervical spine. Other abnormalities of the cervical spine identified on plain film radiographs include an unusually high incidence of degenerative joint changes in the mid to upper cervical spine, congenital synostosis, and developmental platyspondyly. A relationship is reported between Down syndrome and small separate ossicles in the upper cervical region, which are thought to represent avulsions of the distal aspect of the dens rather than associated anomalies.[76] Partial or complete hypopneumatization of the sphenoid sinus also may be noted on the lateral cervical neutral view, although typically without clinical relevance.[170,265] Other abnormalities associated with Down syndrome include inconsequential but classic findings, such as a prominent conoid tubercle of the clavicle.[280]

Organ systems. A variety of other anomalies have been reported in individuals with Down syndrome, affecting virtually all organ systems. Plain film radiography may be used to identify infants with duodenal atresia, the most common gastrointestinal anomaly, or thoracic anomalies such as diaphragmatic hernia. Angiography may demonstrate anomaly of the radial, anterior interosseous, ulnar, subclavian, or vertebral artery.[149,209]

Other anomalies. Milder skeletal changes include rib anomalies, especially agenesis of the twelfth ribs, microcephaly with hypopneumatized sinuses, clinodactyly, and brachydactyly. Hypoplasia of the middle phalanx of the fifth digit is seen in about 60% of patients. Characteristics may include a short, arched hard palate, a small posterior fossa, and calcification of the basilar ganglia, best demonstrated on CT.[113,215] Accessory epiphyses and supernumerary ossification centers of the manubrium may be seen in as many as 90% of patients.[46,215] Knee pain and dysfunction should prompt an evaluation for patellofemoral dislocation, present in about 4% to 8% of individuals with Down syndrome, but rarely disabling.[60] Infants with Down syndrome demonstrate flared iliac wings and flat acetabular roofs. In ambulatory adult patients, this may contribute to hip instability and frequently, early, advanced osteoarthritis.[112]

SPECIALIZED IMAGING

Computed tomography and magnetic resonance imaging have demonstrated a variety of intracranial abnormalities, including abnormally large sylvian fissures, mega cisterna magna, and cerebellar hypoplasia. Hippocampal and neocortical structures are smaller, whereas the parahippocampal gyrus is larger than normal. CT may demonstrate intracranial calcification in as many as 85% of patients, most of which are not directly associated with clinical findings.

These calcifications affect the basal ganglia, choroid plexus, and pineal gland. However, some overlap is likely with normal physiologic calcification, because a high percentage of normal individuals demonstrate similar calcifications.[3] It does not appear that these calcifications are related to the increased incidence of seizure disorders in patients with Down syndrome.[254]

Older adult Down syndrome patients have greater cerebellar atrophy, related ventricular dilatation, and deep white matter lesions than the normal aging population. Vascular studies demonstrate decreasing cerebral perfusion, presumably related to altered blood–brain barrier permeability. Dynamic MRI shows a fluctuating cortical cerebrospinal (CSF) volume in aging Down syndrome patients similar to otherwise normal elderly individuals with shunted hydrocephalus. This finding, first reported in 1995, suggests a relationship between aging in Down syndrome and edematous states of the brain.[64]

CLINICAL COMMENTS

Leukemia. Leukemia is one of the most serious complications of Down syndrome. About 50% of cases represent acute megakaryoblastic leukemia (AMKL). This form typically occurs by age 4, and may be preceded by transient leukemia (TL), involving a megakaryoblastosis, which clears by 3 months of age. Between 20% to 30% of infants with TL develop AMKL.[306] Transient leukemoid reactions, myelofibrosis, and leukemia may all result from an increased sensitivity of cells to interferon in patients with Down syndrome. This results in aberrant antigen expression, which leads to autoimmune disease. In the bone marrow, this may manifest as premature egress of blast cells (as in TL inflammation) or incomplete repair (as in myelofibrosis and binding of autoantibodies to cell nuclei), resulting in malignant transformation and leukemia.[305]

Atlantoaxial instability. As mentioned, atlantoaxial subluxation and instability is a second potentially life-threatening complication commonly encountered. The only clinical finding that may have some predictive value for the presence of this condition in otherwise neurologically intact individuals is gait disturbance, but the sensitivity of this finding was only 50% in 180 children with Down syndrome, with a specificity of 81%.[234] This study failed to identify any reliable clinical indicators of atlantoaxial subluxation or instability and also concluded that x-rays, like clinical indicators, were not reliable for detecting this complication. Other studies have disputed this. Measurement of the anterior atlantodental interspace on neutral and flexion lateral cervical radiographs typically is still performed to identify at-risk individuals.[170,221,265] This includes patients being considered for spinal manipulation, participating in contact sports, and (preoperatively) being anesthetized, especially for otolaryngeal surgery.[97,171]

OTHER FINDINGS

In addition to the features in the original report of this syndrome, gastrointestinal anomalies, especially duodenal atresia, are typical.[246] Cardiac anomalies and pulmonary hypertension are frequent, with congenital heart disease found in some 40% to 50% of patients. Atrioventricular and ventriculoseptal defects and tetralogy of Fallot are among the most common, whereas certain other anomalies, including situs inversus and transposition of the great vessels, are distinctly uncommon.[158] In about a dozen reports, Down syndrome has been associated with moyamoya disease, an intracranial vascular anomaly.[14] About 40% of patients have developmental dysplasia of the hips.[142,215] Tracheal, anorectal, and esophageal anomalies also are seen.[271,282] A characteristic form of

subpleural cystic pulmonary disease has been reported, which typically is difficult to appreciate on plain films and may require high-resolution CT of the chest.[92]

Down syndrome is associated with celiac disease (gluten enteropathy). Because of other common abdominal complaints, considerable delay frequently occurs in diagnosing celiac disease in Down syndrome patients, versus otherwise normal patients. The length of time between initial symptoms and diagnosis averages 2.5 years in Down syndrome patients versus 8 months in non–Down syndrome patients.[104] This condition should be suspected in any child with Down syndrome who shows failure to thrive, especially when accompanied by chronic diarrhea.[104]

An increased incidence of a variety of autoimmune diseases occurs in Down syndrome, including thyroid disease. Although hypothyroidism is most common, reports exist of hyperthyroidism in the form of classic Graves disease.[264]

In addition to gastrointestinal and autoimmune diseases, males with Down syndrome appear to have an increased risk for testicular cancer.[72]

KEY CONCEPTS

- *Down syndrome, or trisomy 21, produces classic clinical features and is typically diagnosed or at least suspected before radiography.*
- *Plain film radiographs and other diagnostic imaging studies typically are obtained to assess for the multitude of associated anomalies seen in this condition.*
- *Approximately 20% of Down syndrome patients have instability or dislocation of the atlantoaxial joint.*
- *These anomalies affect most organ systems, including the gastrointestinal tract, cardiovascular system, and skeleton.*
- *Potentially life-threatening atlantoaxial subluxation and instability are special concerns even after other serious internal organ system anomalies have been ruled out in the prenatal and neonatal period.*

Epiphyseal Dysplasias

The epiphyseal dysplasias represent an overlapping group of diseases that express the common denominator involving growth deformities of the epiphyses. Three systemic and one localized form of epiphyseal dysplasia are presented in this chapter. The three system varieties include chondrodysplasia punctata, multiple epiphyseal dysplasia, and spondyloepiphysis dysplasia. Dysplasia epiphysealis hemimelica (Trevor disease) is the localized form.

Chondrodysplasia Punctata

BACKGROUND

Chondrodysplasia punctata is a rare familial disorder characterized by punctate or "stippled" calcification of developing epiphyses. As with other dysplasias, chondrodysplasia punctata is actually a heterogeneous group of disorders rather than a single disease entity, with at least four distinct forms reported.[143,253]

IMAGING FINDINGS

Radiographs illustrate marked shortening of tubular bones and expanded metaphyses, with marked rhizomelic shortening of long tubular bones (Fig. 8-10). Epiphyseal ossification is delayed and irregular, with characteristic "stippling" bilaterally and symmetrically. This gradually diminishes in infants who survive. Generalized decreased bone density also occurs over time. Similar stippled calcification occurs in the spine and pelvis, as well as in the ribs, laryngeal and tracheal cartilages, tarsal and carpal regions, and patellae.

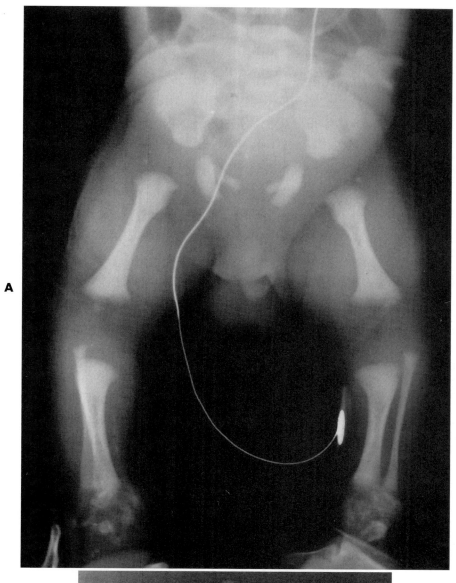

A

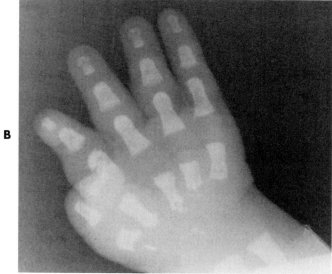

B

FIG. 8-10 Chondrodysplasia punctata, tibial-metacarpal type in the neonate. **A,** Diffuse areas of stippling in hips, ankles, and sacrum; short femurs, long fibulae with very short tibiae. **B,** Generalized brachydactyly with special shortening of the first, third, and fourth metacarpals and the proximal phalanx of the second digit combined with stippling in these areas and the carpus.

Continued

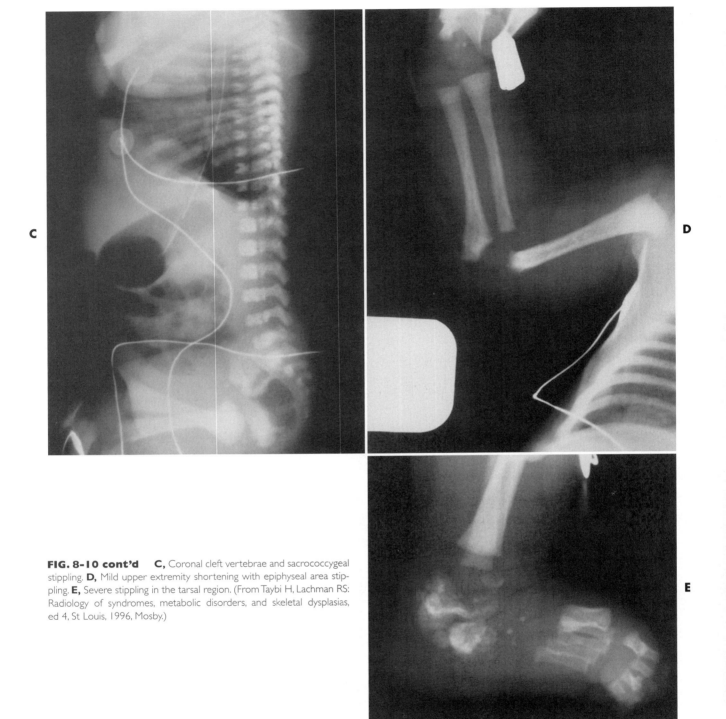

FIG. 8-10 cont'd   C, Coronal cleft vertebrae and sacrococcygeal stippling. **D,** Mild upper extremity shortening with epiphyseal area stippling. **E,** Severe stippling in the tarsal region. (From Taybi H, Lachman RS: Radiology of syndromes, metabolic disorders, and skeletal dysplasias, ed 4, St Louis, 1996, Mosby.)

Radiographic changes reflect histologic and gross anatomic changes resulting from altered development and alignment of chondrocytes.[85] Poznanski[202] has emphasized the fact that the presence of punctate or "stippled" epiphyses merely represents a radiographic sign, as opposed to a specific disease entity. In fact, the differential diagnosis for stippled epiphyses is extensive. The conditions most closely resembling chondrodysplasia punctata, radiographically, are Zellweger syndrome and warfarin or alcohol-related embryopathy. The presence of brain lesions distinguishes

Zellweger syndrome from chondrodysplasia punctata. A history of warfarin (Coumadin) treatment or alcoholism in the mother of an affected infant is a red flag for warfarin or alcohol-related embryopathy.[143,202] Evidence exists that warfarin-induced changes may result from the same deficiency of a novel sulfatase enzyme seen in chondrodysplasia punctata.[73]

Chondrodysplasia punctata, along with Kniest syndrome, metatropic dwarfism, and some forms of osteopetrosis, may demonstrate a coronal cleft in the vertebral bodies in utero, detectable with ultrasound. Generally this cleft is obliterated before birth. Dysplasia of vertebral bodies may result in kyphoscoliosis or other spinal deformity. Rare manifestations of chondrodysplasia have been reported, including asymmetric or unilateral involvement, which may overlap with the so-called CHILD syndrome, consisting of congenital hemidysplasia, ichthyosiform erythroderma, and limb defects.[96] Reported characteristics include a long bone, cone-shaped phalanges and metacarpal bones, brachydactyly, and bowing of the long bones.[143]

CLINICAL COMMENTS

The most readily identifiable form of chondrodysplasia punctata is an autosomal recessive type characterized by rhizomelic shortening of the extremities, microcephaly, a depressed nasal bridge, developmental delays, congenital cataracts, and joint contracture. Clinical features usually are apparent in infancy, and the condition typically is lethal. A milder, autosomal dominant form (Conradi-Hünermann syndrome) demonstrates similar but less severe changes, with patients more often experiencing a normal life span and no significant neurologic deficit.[44,238,241] An X-linked dominant form and a mild sporadic form (Sheffield type) also have been identified.[143,157] In addition to characteristic epiphyseal changes, seen radiographically, ichthyosiform (resembling fish scales) dermatitis exists.[143] There are few other classic clinical features.

> **KEY CONCEPTS**
> - *All forms of the disease are rare.*
> - *The classic radiographic feature of "stippled" epiphyses also may be seen in other conditions, such as warfarin or alcohol-induced embryopathy, and therefore are not pathognomonic for this condition.*
> - *Other radiographic findings, including dysplasia of long bones and vertebrae, are variable and nonspecific.*
> - *Clinical findings are not distinctive, with considerable overlap with other conditions.*

Multiple Epiphyseal Dysplasia

BACKGROUND

Multiple epiphyseal dysplasia (MED) is an autosomal dominant condition characterized by dwarfism, brachydactyly, altered appearance, and development of epiphyseal ossification centers, which commonly leads to early, severe osteoarthritis.[189]

The condition typically is apparent clinically by ages 5 to 14 and may necessitate bilateral total joint arthroplasties by early to middle adulthood (Fig. 8-11). Second only to the hips, other weight-bearing joints and the wrists are the most frequently and severely affected. Unlike spondyloepiphyseal dysplasia, the spine usually is normal or only minimally involved (Fig. 8-12).

IMAGING FINDINGS

Two distinct subtypes historically have been described based on the degree of abnormality of the developing hips. This classification may assist in prognosis and treatment planning. Both forms are inherited as an autosomal dominant disorder. Type I (Fairbank's form) is associated with more severe changes, including fragmented and flattened ossification centers and acetabular dysplasia. Markedly deformed femoral heads at skeletal maturity almost invariably lead to premature, severe osteoarthritis. Type II (Ribbing's form) shows no gross femoral head deformity at skeletal maturity and is less likely to demonstrate severe osteoarthritis.[272]

Similarly, a study of shoulders in 50 patients with MED demonstrated two distinct clinical and radiologic subtypes.[115]

The first group, with minor epiphyseal changes, developed painful osteoarthritis in middle age but retained shoulder movement until the osteoarthritis was determined to be severe radiographically. The other group demonstrated more severe deformity, described as a "hatchet head" epiphysis. These patients had markedly restricted glenohumeral motion early, but, like the other group, did not experience pain until they were in their forties or fifties.[115]

A limited focal epiphyseal dysplasia isolated to the femoral heads is termed *dysplasia epiphysealis capitis femoris* or *Meyer dysplasia*. This is bilateral in about 50% of cases and five times more common in male patients. Most cases are symptomatic, but a waddling gait sometimes occurs. Radiographs show a hypoplastic proximal femoral epiphysis, with the delayed appearance of single or multiple ossification centers. This improves with age; the separate ossification centers consolidate and develop a nearly normal appearance by 6 years. The only residual finding is a slightly diminished cephalocaudal dimension to the femoral head.[127]

CLINICAL COMMENTS

A patient with MED has normal intelligence. Joint pain and gait disturbance are among the most notable clinical manifestations. The joint involvement leads to osteoarthritis, usually by the second or third generation of life. Patients should avoid contact sports and high-impact activities (e.g., running). Weight control should be emphasized in conservative management. Osteotomies may be done to realign involved joints, and joint replacement surgery is common among adult patients. Urine and blood laboratory indices are within normal limits.

Avascular necrosis (AVN) of the hip may be superimposed on multiple epiphyseal dysplasias. AVN is suggested by an asymmetric presentation of hip involvement and the presence of metaphyseal subchondral cyst formation.

> **KEY CONCEPTS**
> - *Multiple epiphyseal dysplasia is a familial disorder that may show delayed and abnormal appearance and development of the epiphyseal ossification centers, although generally with a normal age of fusion.*
> - *Multiple epiphyseal dysplasia results in short, stubby digits and dwarfing, which is milder than in spondyloepiphyseal dysplasia because of lack of significant spinal involvement.*
> - *Because the end of the bone is altered, multiple epiphyseal dysplasia often results in early, often severe, and disabling osteoarthritis. Changes are most pronounced in the hips and knees.*

Spondyloepiphyseal Dysplasia

BACKGROUND

Spondyloepiphyseal dysplasia (SED) congenita is an autosomal dominant dwarfing chondrodysplasia that usually is evident at birth and demonstrates a short trunk, generalized platyspondyly, and epiphyseal dysplasia. This has been linked to the gene locus COL2AI for type II collagen production.[2,239] A Danish study of more than 450,000 people demonstrated a prevalence of SED tarda of 7 per million, as compared with 40 per million for MED tarda.[1]

The more familiar SED tarda was first described by Maroteaux, Lamy, and Bernhard in 1957 in 20 patients from three families, although reports as early as 1937 described what may have been SED tarda.[125] This is an X-linked recessive disorder characterized by epiphyseal and spinal apophyseal dysplasia, with spinal changes predominating. The condition is usually first suspected in boys 5 to 10 years of age who demonstrate impaired spinal growth.[139] Chest expansion may occur along with typical trunk shortening.

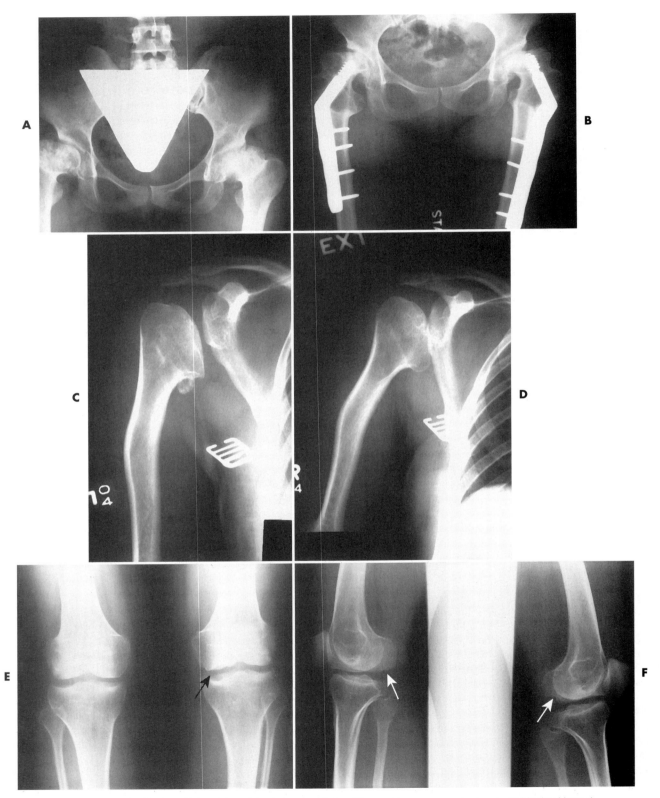

FIG. 8-11   Classic multiple epiphyseal dysplasia congenita in a 39-year-old woman experiencing severe hip, shoulder, and knee involvement. **A,** Initial hip films at age 25 years resembled severe bilateral Legg-Calvé-Perthes disease but with more significant acetabular involvement. Note the oversized triangular gonadal shield obscuring the lumbosacral region. **B,** Osteotomy and instrumentation was performed at age 31, in an attempt to alter weight-bearing stresses on the femoral heads. **C** and **D,** The glenoid fossae are markedly hypoplastic and shallow with chronic subluxation of the "hatched head" proximal humeri. **E** and **F,** The knees are only mildly affected, with changes resembling osteochondritis dissecans (arrows). Dwarfing has resulted from rhizomelic shortening, most prominent at the humeri.

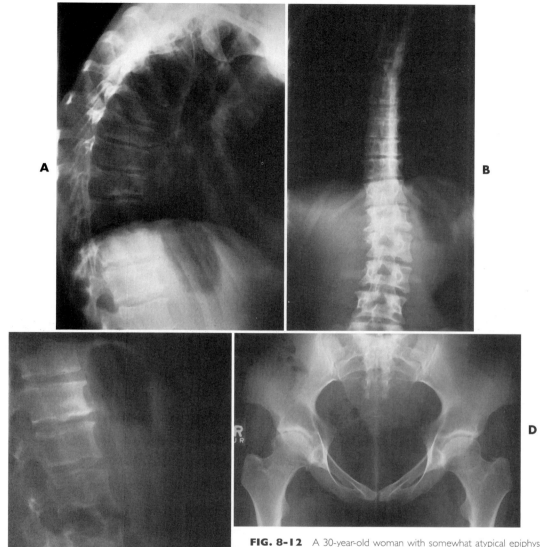

FIG. 8-12 A 30-year-old woman with somewhat atypical epiphyseal and spinal dysplasia, diagnosed previously as a form of multiple epiphyseal dysplasia (MED) (Fairbank disease). **A** and **B,** Unusually marked thoracic spine changes more reminiscent of spondyloepiphyseal dysplasia (SED), but with few classic changes in the, **C,** lumbar and cervical regions. **D,** Hips and shoulders only mildly affected, with the most apparent changes at the right hip, where moderate, painful osteoarthritis had developed. One might question the diagnosis of MED tarda and suggest the possibility that this represents one of the rare autosomal dominant variants of SED. However, even though by definition the spine is normal with MED, it is not uncommon to see Schmorl's nodes and irregular vertebral endplates with MED.

Rare variants of SED tarda have been reported, including a presumably autosomal recessive form occurring in female patients with mild to moderate mental retardation.[133] Another paper reported a case of localized SED apparently affecting only the proximal femora and thoracolumbar junction. This case was discovered, incidentally, in an 11-month-old infant and therefore was classified as SED congenita.[107] One case series from a family with several affected members involved autosomal dominant transmission and, in some instances, hearing deficit. The precise cause for the auditory complication was not indicated.[228] In another family, five patients in three generations demonstrated autosomal dominant SED tarda, associated with congenital hypotrichosis.[284]

In 1990 a report of a new form of SED tarda was published. This probably autosomal dominant condition, termed *spondyloepiphyseal dysplasia of Maroteaux,* demonstrated generalized platyspondyly as in Morquio's syndrome but without anterior vertebral body beaks. Also unlike Morquio's syndrome, no increase was noted in excretion of keratosulfate or corneal opacities. Patients were of normal intelligence and skeletal changes were not apparent at birth, which are features shared with Morquio's syndrome.[56] An interesting variant of SED has been reported in 19 white South Africans of German descent, with mild to moderate dysplasia, progressive infantile kyphoscoliosis, altered trabecular pattern, and generalized joint laxity.[134]

IMAGING FINDINGS

Spinal changes predominate in the lumbar region but may affect the entire spine. Characteristics include generalized endplate irregularity and platyspondyly, which may resemble changes of severe Scheuermann's disease. A characteristic "heaped up" appearance of the vertebral "endplates," especially superiorly, helps to distinguish SED tarda from other conditions, although a similar appearance may infrequently result from isolated Schmorl's node formation.

Degenerative disc space narrowing is asymmetric, affecting the posterior aspect of the disc to a greater extent and sometimes leading to false impression of a widened anterior disc space. In the pelvis, the innominate and femoral neck may be hypoplastic. The epiphyses of the larger joints (shoulders and hips) may be slightly flattened, and early, advanced osteoarthritis, especially of the hips, may occur.[134,135,200] The epiphyseal changes are much milder and the spinal changes considerably more pronounced than in MED.

CLINICAL COMMENTS

In addition to a short trunk, generalized platyspondyly, and epiphyseal dysplasia, patients with SED congenita demonstrate other clinical findings, including myopia, hypertelorism, frequent retinal detachment, short neck, mild thoracic kyphoscoliosis, and an expanded anteroposterior thoracic dimension. One case, involving a dysplastic and unstable cervical spine, required surgical management.[144]

Individuals affected with the tarda form of SED often complain of back and hip pain, especially in early adulthood. Early advanced degenerative disc disease begins in later adolescence and may be severe by 25 to 30 years of age.

A case series involving three boys with SED tarda and growth failure suggested an association with the nephrotic syndrome. Two of those patients showed focal and segmental glomerulosclerosis on renal biopsy.[62] Another report has appeared of three siblings with an autosomal recessive form of SED tarda, leading to severe, progressive arthropathy, mimicking juvenile rheumatoid arthritis.[216]

KEY CONCEPTS

- *With some rather isolated exceptions, spondyloepiphyseal dysplasia may be seen as an autosomal recessive (spondyloepiphyseal dysplasia congenita) form or as an autosomal dominant (spondyloepiphyseal dysplasia tarda) form, the latter being more common.*
- *Generalized platyspondyly with endplate irregularities and classic "heaped up" endplates is expected and is associated with significant short-trunk dwarfism.*
- *Epiphyseal regions are more mildly affected, especially when compared with multiple epiphyseal dysplasia.*

Dysplasia Epiphysealis Hemimelica

Also known as *Trevor disease,* dysplasia epiphysealis hemimelica is a rare congenital disorder marked by localized cartilage overgrowth causing asymmetric limb deformity. The condition usually is of the lower extremities, especially the medial aspect of the ankle (e.g., distal tibia, talus, tarsal navicular, and first cuneiform), but the proximal femur, wrist, and foot are other demonstrated locations. The cartilage overgrowth closely mimics osteochondroma. It affects male patients more often than female patients. The condition causes a lump, swelling, and painful joint. There also may be a limp, leg-length discrepancy, and muscle wasting. Surgical treatment often is applied to remove the lesion and reshape the deformed bone.

Homocystinuria

BACKGROUND

Homocystinuria is actually a group of three related genetic abnormalities that result in a deficiency of cystathionine synthetase, the enzyme that metabolizes methionine. The autosomal recessive condition was first described in the early 1960s as a variant of Marfan's syndrome and is most common in individuals of northern European descent.[35,83,84,168,245]

According to common belief, homocystinuria results in abnormal aldehyde cross-linkages and defective collagen synthesis, similar to the pathogenesis of Ehlers-Danlos syndrome, Marfan's syndrome, and osteogenesis imperfecta. Therefore it should be no surprise that these conditions share features, especially radiographically. However, homocystinuria actually has been classified with alkaptonuria (ochronosis), Menkes syndrome, and pseudoxanthoma elasticum because it secondarily affects the fibrous components of connective tissues.[123,167]

IMAGING FINDINGS

Osteopenia. The imaging findings in homocystinuria may be nonspecific and are not present at birth. Osteopenia is typical and is believed to result from deficiency of collagen cross-linking rather than a gross deficiency in collagen itself.[152] The presence of osteoporosis, often with multiple compression fractures, helps to distinguish homocystinuria from Marfan's syndrome.

Skeleton. Skeletal abnormalities occur in up to 60% of patients and closely resemble those of Marfan's syndrome. Extremities are long and thin, and patients are usually above average in height. Arachnodactyly typically is seen. Multiple growth resumption lines may be present. Scoliosis, pectus excavatum, and generalized joint laxity may appear to be identical to Marfan's syndrome. Joint contractures may occur in the knees, elbows, and digits, whereas such contractures are usually limited to the fifth digits in Marfan's syndrome. Ligamentous laxity may result in genu valgum, patella alta, and repeated subluxations. Infants and children may demonstrate metaphyseal flaring and irregularity of epiphyseal ossification centers.

Other reports include a variety of other less common or less classic imaging findings diffusely affecting the skeleton, in addition to vascular calcification and medullary sponge kidney.[28,31,45,168]

Skull and facial changes in homocystinuria include sinus expansion, a widened diploic space, prognathism, and dural calcification.[168,245] The spine may show early advanced degenerative disc disease, and posterior vertebral body scalloping. This appears to be a primary developmental abnormality rather than a pressure-related change, as from dural ectasia.[28,245]

The radiographic changes of homocystinuria may be distinguished from Marfan's syndrome primarily by osteoporosis, flared metaphyses, and joint contractures, which are absent in Marfan's syndrome.[28,245]

CLINICAL COMMENTS

Homocystinuria is generally asymptomatic in infants and very young children, although urinary levels of homocystine are increased. Skin lesions begin to develop, including a malar flush, striae over the extremities and buttocks, and scars described as having the appearance of "cigarette paper." The palate is high and arched, and dentition is poor. Hair usually is thin and sparse.[168]

Homocystinuria primarily affects the CNS, eyes, skeleton, and cardiovascular system. Increased homocystine levels are strongly correlated to atherosclerotic, coronary artery, and thromboembolic disease. Cardiopulmonary diseases are the most common causes of death.[49] Cystic medial necrosis occurs, as in Marfan's syndrome, but aortic dissection, a common cause of premature death in Marfan's syndrome, generally is not seen in homocystinuria. Accumulation of homocystine may adversely affect platelets, clotting factors, and vascular endothelial cells.

It is believed that individuals with deficiencies of vitamin B_6, B_{12}, or folic acid or who are heterozygous for cystathionine synthetase deficiency are at increased risk for occlusive vascular disease and that supplementation may lower the plasma homocystine levels in some affected individuals.[31,163,217] Diets low in methionine and supplementation with betaine or its precursor choline may be beneficial in management of homocystinuria.[248,287] Decision making, especially when considering elective surgery, must reflect the fact that surgeries increase the risk for vascular catastrophes.[28]

The most characteristic ocular lesion is dislocation of the lens, which also is seen in Marfan's syndrome. Lens dislocation may be detected in infancy in homocystinuria, but not in Marfan's syndrome.[28] Other optic anomalies also may occur, including congenital cataracts and glaucoma.

Unlike Marfan's syndrome, CNS involvement leading to mental deficit and seizures is seen in about 30% of patients, although the pathogenesis has not been delineated clearly. CNS complications may be modified by therapy.[245]

KEY CONCEPTS

- *Homocystine and methionine accumulate in the tissues as a result of an autosomal recessive deficiency of cystathionine synthetase.*
- *The accumulation of homocystine and methionine leads to mental deficit in 60% of patients and marfanoid features, including tall, thin stature, and arachnodactyly, as well as scoliosis, pectus excavatum or carinatum, and genu valgum.*
- *Vascular changes are similar to those of Marfan's syndrome, with medial degeneration of arteries.*
- *Lens subluxation, common to both conditions, typically occurs inferiorly in homocystinuria and superiorly in Marfan's syndrome.*
- *Osteoporosis is a distinctive feature of homocystinuria, as is the presence of flared metaphyses and diffuse joint contractures.*

Klippel-Feil Syndrome

BACKGROUND

As with so many other syndromes bearing the name of long-dead scholars who cannot defend or explain themselves, the Klippel-Feil syndrome gradually has evolved from a concise clinical triad to a confusing collection of loosely related vertebral anomalies. Purists may still apply the eponym only to the triad first described in 1912 by Klippel and Feil, without benefit of radiographs. They described patients with a short neck (often webbed at its base), low hairline, and restricted cervical range of motion, although these features were not carefully quantified. They also described anomalies of the skull base and thoracic cage, which have received little attention over the years.[131,132] Subsequently it was discovered that such patients typically demonstrate vertebral segmentation anomalies, primarily in the form of congenital nonsegmentation ("block vertebrae").

Today whether proper or improper, the term has been extended to include any patient with nonsegmentation of even a single vertebral motion unit, although it is most often implied to mean at least two vertebral motion units. In the context of this broadened definition, approximately 50% of individuals with the requisite segmentation anomalies demonstrate the complete clinical triad. A diagnosis that once was dictated by clinical findings is now made primarily on the basis of radiographic changes in the majority of cases.

IMAGING FINDINGS

Congenital nonsegmentation most commonly affects C2-3. About two thirds of cases involving C2-3 nonsegmentation also involve assimilation of C1 to occiput ("occipitalization" of C1). Nonsegmentation varies from minimal to extensive and may be continuous or intermittent, with intervening normal disc levels (Figs. 8-13 through 8-19). The anomaly may extend caudally to

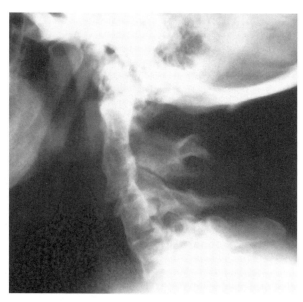

FIG. 8-13 Klippel-Feil syndrome. Note the congenital nonsegmentation and dysplasia of C2 through C4 and C5-6, with only two functional disc spaces in the cervical spine. Assimilation of the C1 posterior arch to occiput and marked hypoplasia of the dens also are noted. The neck appears to be short, which is more obvious clinically, along with a low hairline and diminished range of motion. Similar vertebral segmentation anomalies also may be seen as an isolated finding or in other syndromes, including neurofibromatosis.

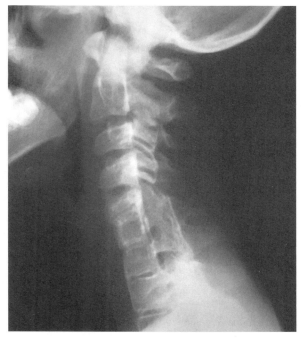

FIG. 8-14 Klippel-Feil syndrome in a young female patient marked by congenital nonunion defect extending from C5 to T1.

the mid to upper thoracic spine, and may involve similar non-segmentation in the lower thoracic and lumbar regions. Incomplete or abbreviated forms of congenital nonsegmentation may occur at some levels. Associated anomalies may exist, especially spina bifida occulta and hemivertebrae, which are seen in about 20% of cases and may be associated with structural scoliosis and kyphosis. Intraspinal anomalies such as syringomyelia and diastematomyelia may occur.[78]

Other skeletal anomalies commonly accompany the vertebral segmentation anomalies. Failure of descent (often improperly described as "elevation") of one or both scapulae is seen in about 25% of cases, described as Sprengel's deformity (see Fig. 8-16). This is more common in patients with extensive spine and, especially, upper cervical involvement and may be corrected surgically.[36,181] Between 30% and 40% of Sprengel's deformity cases are associated with an omovertebral "bone," an osseous, fibrous, or

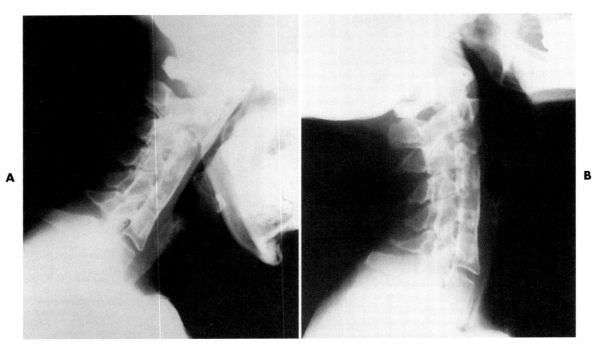

FIG. 8-15   **A** and **B,** Extensive congenital nonsegmentation of C3 through C6. The more normal C2-3 and C6-7 motion units at the cephalic and caudal ends of the nonsegmentation are prone to hypermobility or instability and subsequent premature degenerative disc disease and facet arthrosis. Notice that the range of cervical motion is reduced in this flexion and extension series.

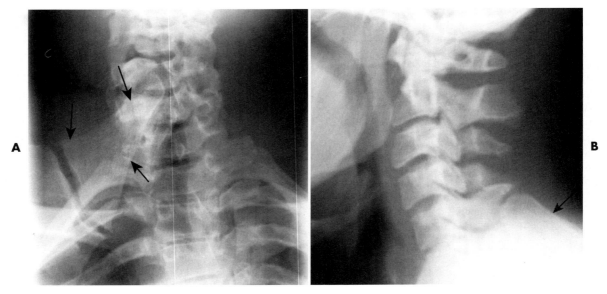

FIG. 8-16   Sprengel's deformity. **A,** Anteroposterior projection illustrates a large bar of bone extending from the medial border of the scapula to the spinous process of C5 *(arrows)*. The articulation with the spinous process is also noted on, **B,** the lateral projection *(arrows)*.

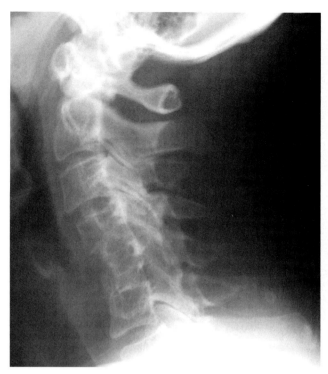

FIG. 8-17 Klippel-Feil syndrome presenting as a long block segment extending across two motion units (C4 to C6) in this 51-year-old man.

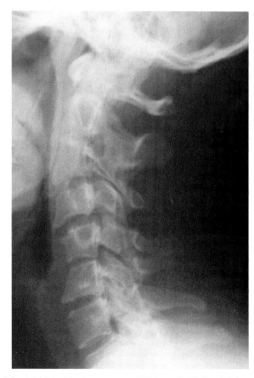

FIG. 8-18 Multiple block segments (C2-3 and C5-6), defining Klippel-Feil syndrome, appearing in a 52-year-old woman. Approximately half of patients who demonstrate multiple block segments express the associated clinical triad of a low hairline, webbed neck, and limited range of cervical motion. (Courtesy Nicole Poirier, Shelby Twp, MI.)

cartilaginous structure extending from the scapula (*omo-*, meaning "scapula") to the posterior vertebral elements, most often in the mid- to lower-cervical region. Solid fusion or an accessory articulation may exist at both the scapular and vertebral junctions.[181] Similar bones have been reported, extending from the upper ribs or clavicles to the vertebrae, although these are rare.[88] Cervical ribs, Srb's anomaly, and a variety of rib anomalies, including agenesis or synostosis, are common in Klippel-Feil syndrome.

Craniovertebral junction anomalies may be seen in Klippel-Feil syndrome. Basilar impression is common, with or without assimilation of C1 to occiput. Diagnosis of basilar impression is based upon observance of the tip of the dens projecting significantly above McGregor's line on a well-positioned lateral skull or lateral cervical neutral view. Arnold-Chiari type I malformation also may occur, in which the cerebellar tonsils project significantly below the foramen magnum, extending into the upper cervical canal. Dens anomalies also may be seen. Imaging of the thorax, abdomen, and pelvis may be ordered based upon clinical findings and may demonstrate cardiac anomalies (especially septal defects), enteric cysts, accessory lobes of the lung, and anomalies of the urinary tract.[101]

CLINICAL COMMENTS

Klippel-Feil syndrome affects males and females equally. The prevalence of congenital nonsegmentation of at least one spinal motion segment has been estimated to be as high as 0.5% in the general population.[236] The segmentation defects in Klippel-Feil syndrome tend to be more extensive and may be associated with neurologic deficit, most often seen with marked upper cervical and craniovertebral junction anomalies. However, many patients are relatively asymptomatic. Cosmetic concerns, including associated spinal curvatures, Sprengel's deformity, or pterygium colli (webbed neck) may first prompt the patient to seek attention.

Lateral flexion and rotation motion are most markedly restricted, with lesser decrease in sagittal plane rotation (flexion-extension). The head may appear to be resting on the shoulders. Patients may present with acute torticollis. Other signs and symptoms range from neck pain to paresis and paralysis. Hyperreflexia and pathologic reflexes may occur, such as upward-going toes on Babinski testing, signifying an upper motor neuron lesion. Neurologic deficit may be gradual in onset or may appear acutely, often secondary to trivial trauma. Cranial nerve dysfunction also may occur, including oculomotor disturbance. Some patients demonstrate cardiopulmonary, gastroenteric, or genitourinary tract anomalies.

> ### KEY CONCEPTS
> - *Klippel-Feil syndrome is most often defined as the presence of multiple block segments, usually in the cervical spine.*
> - *Approximately 50% of Klippel-Feil patients exhibit a classic clinical triad of a short neck, low hairline, and diminished cervical range of motion.*
> - *Additional anomalies of other organ systems occur, often affecting the genitourinary tract. These are often occult on plain films.*
> - *A wide variety of other clinically or radiographically apparent findings have been described in this heterogeneous syndrome.*

Marfan's Syndrome

BACKGROUND

Marfan's syndrome is an autosomal dominant disorder of connective tissues primarily affecting the ocular, cardiovascular, and musculoskeletal systems. As many as 30% of cases may result from sporadic mutations. The condition bears the name of Antonin Marfan's,

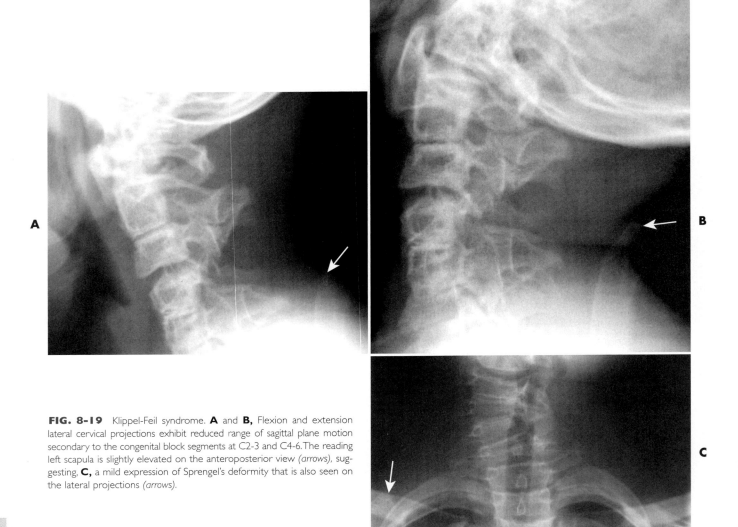

FIG. 8-19 Klippel-Feil syndrome. **A** and **B,** Flexion and extension lateral cervical projections exhibit reduced range of sagittal plane motion secondary to the congenital block segments at C2-3 and C4-6. The reading left scapula is slightly elevated on the anteroposterior view *(arrows),* suggesting, **C,** a mild expression of Sprengel's deformity that is also seen on the lateral projections *(arrows).*

who first described the phenotype in 1896. Marfan's syndrome is estimated to affect 4 to 6 people per 100,000.[154,304] At one time or another, several famous characters from history were thought to have had Marfan's syndrome, including Niccolo Paganini, Rachmaninov, and Mary, Queen of Scots.[33,156,298] Despite significant investigation and impressive advances in understanding this condition, Marfan's syndrome remains an enigma in many ways. Numerous questions have gone unanswered about the precise etiology of the ligamentous laxity, muscular hypotonia, and skeletal changes that characterize this disorder.[154]

IMAGING FINDINGS

In addition to clinically apparent scoliosis and other postural changes, protrusio acetabulum was reported in nearly half of a study group of 22 patients.[136] This was bilateral in 50% of cases. When the protrusio was unilateral, it occurred on the side of a scoliotic convexity 90% of the time. Presumably the inherent abnormality of formation of connective tissues in combination with altered stresses associated with scoliosis leads the protrusio acetabulum in this condition.[136]

Dural ectasia is another associated abnormality emphasizing the generalized effects of Marfan's syndrome on connective tissues. This may be suspected first on the basis of pedicle thinning and erosion with widening of the interpediculate distance and posterior vertebral body scalloping (Fig. 8-20). Although the condition may be asymptomatic and found incidentally, follow-up MRI is indicated to exclude other more serious space-occupying lesions of the central spinal canal associated with similar pedicle or vertebral body changes on plain films.[197,255] Multiple meningeal cysts also have been reported in Marfan's syndrome and may result in similar gradual pressure erosion of the neural arch or posterior vertebral body margin.[216,218] Also, tubular bones may appear long and thin (dolichostenomelic) (see Fig. 8-20).

CLINICAL COMMENTS

The clinical features overlap considerably in several related disorders characterized by dolichostenomelia (abnormally long limbs) and arachnodactyly (spiderlike digits). Patients may demonstrate marfanoid habitus, with tall stature and arachnodactyly, yet not truly have Marfan's syndrome. A biomolecular assay is valuable in differentiating

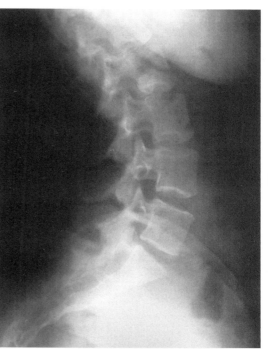

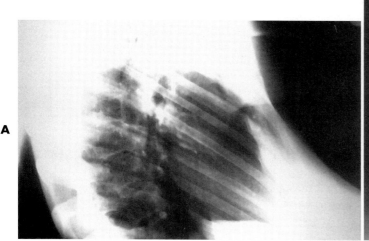

FIG. 8-20 Marfan's syndrome in a young adult black woman, not previously diagnosed. **A** and **B,** Note the "tall" lumbar vertebrae and gracile ribs along with pectus excavatum. The sacrum is also remarkably thin and elongated, a "tall" sacrum.

Marfan's syndrome from an otherwise normal patient with marfanoid features. In as many as 50% of cases, patients initially diagnosed as having Marfan's syndrome may be reclassified.[276] In some instances, patients may demonstrate an incomplete marfanoid phenotype, whereas other family members have unequivocal Marfan's syndrome.

Initially the most noticeable clinical features include tall stature, exceeding the 95th percentile for age, race, and gender in most cases. The condition is more common in black individuals. Long gracile limbs and digits are readily apparent, as well as hyperextendable joints (especially genu recurvatum), frequently with a history of subluxation, secondary to generalized ligamentous laxity. Scoliosis, an akyphotic thoracic spine, and pectus excavatum also are typical. Atrophy of subcutaneous fat and muscle exaggerates the skeletal changes. The arm span may equal or exceed the patient's height. The ratio of the upper body segment (from vertex of the skull to the symphysis pubis) versus the lower body segment (from symphysis pubis to the floor) often is greatly reduced, but this is variable and is significantly affected by scoliosis. This clinical feature is not diagnostic but suggestive of the diagnosis. The maximally apposed thumb overlaps the ulnar aspect of the hand ("thumb sign"), and when one hand grasps the opposite wrist, the first and fifth distal phalanges overlap ("wrist sign"). These latter signs also are not definitive and may be seen in some normal individuals.[154]

From 50% to 80% of patients have cephalic lens dislocation of the eyes. This is usually bilateral and typically present at birth. The zonules remain intact, and the eye accommodates normally. In contrast, homocystinuria, which resembles Marfan's syndrome in various ways, demonstrates caudal lens dislocation with zonular disintegration and lack of accommodation. Myopia and retinal detachment are frequent complications of Marfan's syndrome because of increased axial length of the globe. This condition, along with flattening of the corneas, contributes to impaired visual acuity.[43]

The cardiovascular complications of Marfan's syndrome are more serious and well known. These include mitral valve prolapse, mitral and aortic regurgitation, aortic root dilatation, and proximal aortic dissection, which is the most immediately life-threatening complication that commonly occurs in Marfan's syndrome. Sudden onset of severe chest pain should prompt consideration of either aortic dissection or spontaneous pneumothorax, another complication of Marfan's syndrome. Mitral valve prolapse and aortic root dilatation are the most common cardiovascular complications, with one or both present in at least 80% of patients. Although mitral prolapse frequently is associated with dyspnea, chest pain, palpitations, and lightheadedness, aortic root dilatation usually is asymptomatic, unless accompanied by aortic regurgitation or aortic dissection. Auscultation reveals most cases of regurgitation or nonejection systolic clicks.[106]

A rare complication of Marfan's syndrome reported in a father and his two sons is spontaneous bilateral pneumothorax. The precise etiology is uncertain.[297] Another rare complication is retroperitoneal fibrosis, apparently secondary to abnormality of the abdominal aorta. This may lead to hydronephrosis or other nephropathy.[38]

KEY CONCEPTS

- *Marfan's syndrome is an autosomal dominant connective tissue disorder, in which affected individuals are tall and thin, with gracile limbs and generalized joint laxity.*
- *Scoliosis and other postural alterations are common, seen in more than half of all patients, along with pectus excavatum or carinatum.*
- *Superior versus inferior lens dislocation and lack of osteoporosis help to distinguish Marfan's syndrome from homocystinuria.*
- *Dilatation and aneurysms of the ascending thoracic aorta are common, frequently with sudden onset and dissection, which is fatal in about 90% of cases. Aneurysms of other vessels are less frequent.*

PART TWO Bone, Joints, and Soft Tissues

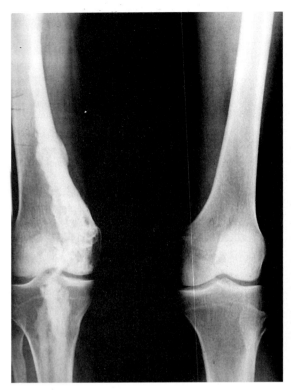

FIG. 8-21   Melorheostosis appearing as a unilateral thick endosteal sclerosis of the medial aspect of the distal femur and the proximal tibia. A second case exhibits similar changes along the anterior aspect of the distal tibia. (Courtesy Steven P. Brownstein, MD, Springfield, NJ.)

Melorheostosis

BACKGROUND

Melorheostosis was first described by Leri and Joanny in France in 1922 and also has been called Leri-Joanny syndrome. To date the precise etiology of this unusual syndrome is unknown, but theories include vascular insufficiency, inflammation or degeneration of connective tissues, and developmental abnormality of innervation.[211]

IMAGING FINDINGS

The classic radiographic appearance of melorheostosis is that of linear and curvilinear hyperostoses extending varying distances along the endosteal and periosteal surfaces, particularly of long and short tubular bones (Fig. 8-21). These may demonstrate a wavy or irregular margin, resembling candle wax flowing along the bone, from which the condition derives its name. The hyperostosis may predominate on the lateral aspects of the extremities and may extend across joints. Spinal, pelvic, and craniofacial involvement occurs less frequently.[288] In the extremities, the hyperostosis follows a single sclerotome in about two thirds of the cases, a feature first reported in 1979. Multiple sclerotomes appear to be affected in the remaining cases, leading to the theory that melorheostosis is a late result of a segmental sensory nerve lesion. However, the precise etiology is yet to be determined. An association with paraarticular ossification raises the question of involvement of the corresponding myotome in some cases.[55,175]

Melorheostosis is typically first discovered on plain films, but radiologists also should be familiar with its appearance on radionuclide imaging. A bone scan demonstrates asymmetric cortical uptake of radionuclide, which may extend across joints to affect contiguous bones.[48] The MR features of melorheostosis and its associated soft-tissue masses are characteristic. MRI is the optimal imaging study for assessing the extent of soft-tissue involvement.[301]

The occurrence of melorheostosis, in combination with radiographic changes of osteopoikilosis and osteopathia striata, has been termed mixed sclerosing bone dystrophy (MSBD). These patients may demonstrate diffuse sclerosis of the axial skeleton.[285] Although most cases of MSBD involve both upper and lower extremities, single limb involvement has been reported.[184] Isolated reports of regression of melorheostosis have appeared, and osteosarcoma arising in an affected femur also has been reported.[19,124]

CLINICAL COMMENTS

Melorheostosis varies in its clinical presentation and may be asymptomatic or may be associated with pain along its typically sclerotomal distribution. Joint contractures, growth disturbances, other gross postural or biomechanical alterations, and linear scleroderma may occur.[175,240] Other changes in the overlying soft tissues may include tight, shiny, erythematous skin, discoloration, induration, and fibrosis. Such changes, which may be present at birth, may precede obvious osseous abnormality. Paraspinal soft-tissue mass lesions and intrathecal lipoma were found in several patients with axial melorheostosis and linear cutaneous vascular malformation in one other patient with peripheral involvement; this emphasizes the fact that the disease affects mesenchymal tissue generally, rather than being confined to bone.[79,87,208] Single case reports exist of melorheostosis with hypophosphatemic rickets, minimal change nephrotic syndrome with mesenteric fibromatosis, and capillary hemangioma or renal artery stenosis.[114,145,219]

Although melorheostosis may not be discovered until adulthood, lesions are known to become apparent in children. Typical clinical findings include soft-tissue contractures, joint pain and stiffness, and anisomelia, which generally are resistant to surgical correction.[204] Pain is uncommon in children and when present is typically mild. In one study of melorheostosis in children, the average delay between onset of clinical findings and diagnosis was 6 years.[299] Case reports exist of carpal tunnel syndrome secondary to melorheostosis, including one apparently congenital case in an infant.[9,18,19] Pain may be severe and debilitating in adults. Nifedipine and a disodium salt of diphosphonic acid both have been used successfully for pain control.[126,235]

KEY CONCEPTS

- *Melorheostosis is characterized, radiographically, by thick, wavy periosteal new bone formation, usually after a spinal sclerotome, myotome or, less frequently, a dermatome and sometimes crossing a joint space.*
- *Although axial involvement may occur, the extremities are more typically affected.*
- *Variable changes of the overlying soft tissues and adjacent joints may be seen in this painful, sometimes deforming, idiopathic condition.*

Mucopolysaccharidoses

BACKGROUND

The mucopolysaccharidoses (MPSs) represent a heterogeneous group of conditions sharing the common feature of an abnormal sulfatase enzyme, leading to intralysosomal accumulation of partially degraded mucopolysaccharides. The first such condition was described in 1952 in individuals with physical features of gargoylism (coarse facies resembling the mythical gargoyle) and dwarfism. Histologic studies revealed collagen tissues and organs laden with water-soluble material also identified in the urine as mucopolysaccharide, in the form of glycosaminoglycans (GAGs).

Subsequently, at least eight different MPSs and a number of mucolipidoses (MLs), which result in similar clinical and radiographic changes, have been recognized.[26,59] Several of these also have been divided into subtypes that demonstrate considerable variation in clinical and radiographic changes. Other storage disorders that may show some resemblance to MPS include aspartylglycosaminuria, fucosidosis, gangliosidosis, and mannosidosis.[211]

Differentiation of the various MPSs is based upon examination of the pattern of inheritance and the urinary excretion of a particular acid mucopolysaccharide (GAGs). The originally reported screening urinalysis based upon the color reaction of GAGs with dimethylmethylene blue was modified to reduce protein interference and also may be used to determine GAGs in other body fluids.[50] The better known MPSs are Morquio's (Brailsford) syndrome (MPS IV) (Fig. 8-22), Hurler's syndrome (MPS IH), Hunter's syndrome (MPS II), and San Filippo syndrome (MPS III).

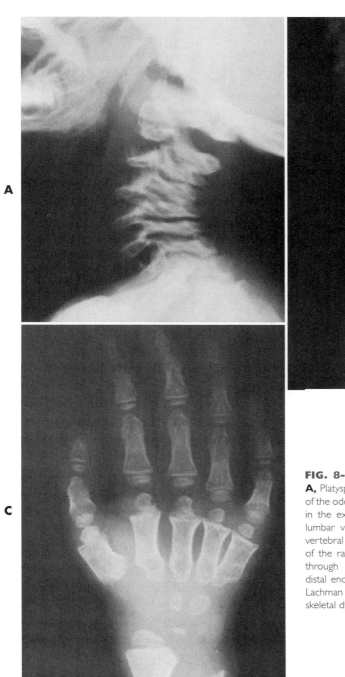
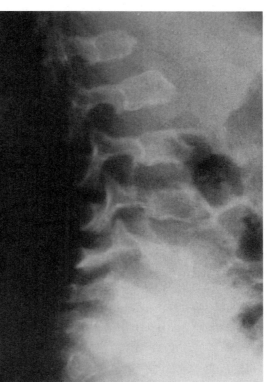

FIG. 8-22 Mucopolysaccharidosis IV in a 3-year-old girl. **A,** Platyspondyly of the cervical vertebrae, underdevelopment of the odontoid process of the axis, and atlantoaxial subluxation in the extension position. **B,** Universal platyspondyly of the lumbar vertebrae and a central beak protruding from the vertebral bodies. **C,** Marked irregularity of the distal metaphysis of the radius and ulna, pointed proximal end of the second through fifth metacarpals, short metacarpals, and pointed distal end of the middle and distal phalanges. (From Taybi H, Lachman RS: Radiology of syndromes, metabolic disorders, and skeletal dysplasias, ed 4, St Louis, 1996, Mosby.)

IMAGING FINDINGS

General. The skeletal changes common to the MPSs and MLs have been described as dysostosis multiplex. They include macrocephaly and dolichocephaly, related to premature closure of the sagittal suture and a characteristic J-shaped sella turcica and pituitary fossa. Widening of the diploic space and hypopneumatized sinuses typically are seen.

Intracranial. In patients with mental retardation, MRI has been used to demonstrate such abnormalities as deficient myelination, enlarged ventricles resulting from hydrocephalus, and widened fissures and sulci.[122,174,279] MRI also has been used to identify characteristic "cribriform" (multicystic or sievelike) changes in the periventricular and supraventricular parietal white matter, corpus callosum, and basal ganglia. These changes were most severe in Hunter's and Hurler's syndromes and were related inversely to the amount of atrophy, ventricular dilatation, and white matter abnormality. There appears to be a progression from cribriform changes to white matter changes and, finally, atrophy.[146] Bone marrow transplantation has shown promise in limiting CNS complications, when performed early, before demonstrable atrophy.[237]

Spine. The developing vertebrae are initially oval, with a beaklike appearance anteriorly, resulting from a combination of developmental deficiency, hypotonia, and anterior herniation of the nucleus pulposus. The beak is most frequently seen in Morquio's syndrome, in which it is centrally located (see Fig. 8-22). The beak is inferior in Hurler's syndrome, as well as other congenital syndromes, including Down syndrome and congenital hypothyroidism (cretinism). Beaked or hook-shaped vertebrae contribute to angular kyphosis or gibbus deformity, most typical in the thoracolumbar junction. In ambulatory patients, hyperkyphosis increases the altered stress on developing abnormal vertebrae and perpetuates the deformity. Developmental platyspondyly may result, which typically is not obvious until later childhood and resembles the changes of SED.

Advanced imaging may reveal dural ectasia, which may result in spinal cord or thecal sac compression.[251] Reported atlantoaxial subluxation and instability are caused by odontoid hypoplasia, os odontoideum, and other anomalies of the atlantoaxial articulation.[199,268]

Thorax. In the thorax, mucopolysaccharide deposition in the wall of the trachea may lead to luminal narrowing, which may be visible on plain films. In one series, 9 out of 56 patients demonstrated this finding, which is not necessarily symptomatic.[196] Ribs are widened generally, but with marked narrowing near their articulation with the spine, resulting in an oarlike appearance. The clavicles also are typically short and wide. Pectus carinatum may result from premature fusion of the sternal ossification centers.

Pelvis. The pelvis shows an increase in the acetabular angles and a widened appearance to the acetabular roofs. Characteristics include delayed ossification and dysplasia of the femoral heads.

Extremities. The long bones show delayed ossification of the epiphyses and cortical thinning with osteopenia. These changes are greater in the upper extremities. Initial undertubulation of the diaphyses and valgus joint deformity may later give way to overtubulation (overconstriction) and varus deformity, especially at the proximal humeri and femora. Other changes of the proximal femora resemble those of Legg-Calvé-Perthes disease. Premature osteoarthritis may be present.

The distal ulnae and radius are tapered, decreasing the carpal angle. The tubular bones of the hands and, to a lesser extent, the feet, may be affected. The metacarpal and metatarsal bones are tapered, proximally, with relative sparing of the first. The distal phalanges are hypoplastic, and the remaining phalanges are wide and short. In addition, dysplasia and hypoplasia of the carpal bones also may occur.

CLINICAL COMMENTS

These conditions share many features, such as macroglossia, adenoidal hyperplasia, and abnormal dentition. Patients may be short or average in height. Cardiomegaly and associated cardiac abnormality may occur, as well as hepatosplenomegaly. Cardiopulmonary complications, when severe, may lead to death in infancy or childhood. Pneumonia, upper airway obstruction, and aortic regurgitation are among the complications that frequently lead to death. Bone marrow transplantation has been shown to diminish or at least limit the progression of cardiac complications in about two thirds of patients.[80] In one study of 45 patients, chronic otitis media was reported in more than 70% of the cases. More than half of all the patients in that study underwent some type of operative management by an otolaryngologist; seven underwent tracheostomy to relieve upper airway obstruction.[27] Congenital umbilical and inguinal hernias are common. Joint stiffness and contractures occur in some individuals, whereas other individuals may demonstrate joint laxity. Joint deformities, including genu valgum, may be apparent clinically, as well as radiographically.

Carpal tunnel syndrome appears to be an unusually common complication of mucopolysaccharidosis or mucolipidosis and was reported in 17 of 18 patients in one case series.[292] In that study, the only patient without nerve conduction abnormality indicative of carpal tunnel syndrome was a 6-month-old infant.[292] Optic nerve head swelling and secondary optic atrophy have been reported as common complications of several of the MPSs.[41]

Mental deficit in these syndromes is highly variable both within and among the various disorders, ranging from absent to profound. Morquio's syndrome generally is associated with normal mentation. Behavior problems occur at high rates, especially among children with San Filippo and Hunter's syndromes. These include destructiveness, restlessness, and aggression, as well as sleep disturbance in about two thirds of patients.[10]

> ### KEY CONCEPTS
> - *Mucopolysaccharidoses have been classified along with the mucolipidoses and oligosaccharidoses as conditions of "dysostosis multiplex."*
> - *Mucopolysaccharidosis may demonstrate varying degrees of alteration of bone texture, including widening or undertubulation of the diaphyses, dysplasias of the distal radius and ulna (Madelung's deformity), tapered metacarpal bases, macrocephaly and thickening of the calvarium, a J-shaped sella turcica, and an anterior beak of a vertebral body at the thoracolumbar junction.*
> - *Macroglossia, adenoidal hyperplasia, abnormal dentition, short stature, cardiomegaly, and hepatosplenomegaly are clinical features seen with presentations of mucopolysaccharidosis.*

Os Odontoideum

BACKGROUND

Os odontoideum is a condition in which a variable portion of the ossification center for the odontoid process of C2 is separate from the body and often is associated with atlantoaxial subluxation and instability (Figs. 8-23 through 8-32). Before advanced diagnostic imaging, os odontoideum may have been misdiagnosed as agenesis or hypoplasia of the dens, because the separate ossicle may be

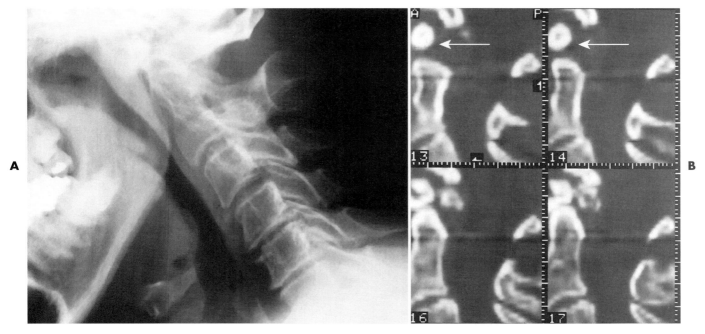

FIG. 8-23 Os odontoideum. **A,** The flexion lateral cervical projection does not show signs of instability, with a normal relationship maintained between the spinolaminar junction lines of C1 and C2. A congenital nonsegmentation exists at C2-3. **B,** Reformatted sagittal CT images demonstrate the separate dens to better advantage *(arrows).*

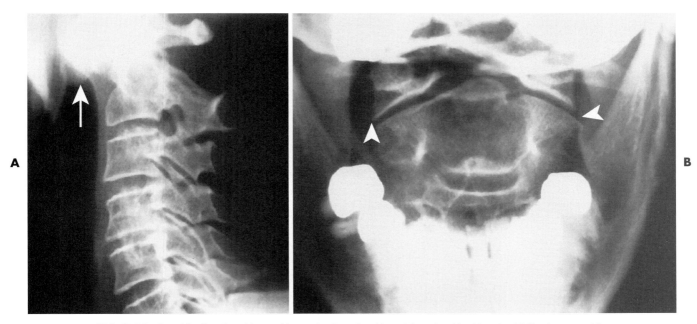

FIG. 8-24 **A** and **B,** Os odontoideum with anterior *(arrow)* and lateral *(arrowheads)* subluxation. Unlike the case exhibited in Figure 8-23, this patient reveals advanced anterior translation of the atlas, resulting in a marked decrease in the space available for the cord, measuring only 1 cm. A more typical measurement is 2 cm. Despite the narrowing, this 68-year-old man had only mild neck pain and stiffness, without clinical evidence of cord compression and myelopathy. Gradual onset of the upper cervical spinal stenosis and presumed compensatory changes of the cord help to explain his lack of symptoms. In addition, compressible tissue and cerebrospinal fluid occupy as much as one third of the central canal dimension; the other two thirds is occupied by cord and dens. The same degree of subluxation or dislocation occurring rapidly would likely be much more devastating.

PART TWO Bone, Joints, and Soft Tissues

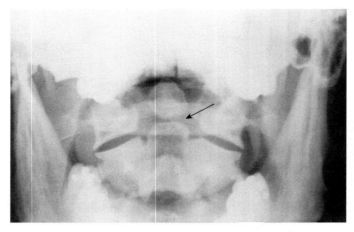

FIG. 8-25　Clearly separated odontoid ossicle (os odontoideum) from the superior margin of C2 *(arrow)* in this patient with a history of multiple traumas over the past 3 years.

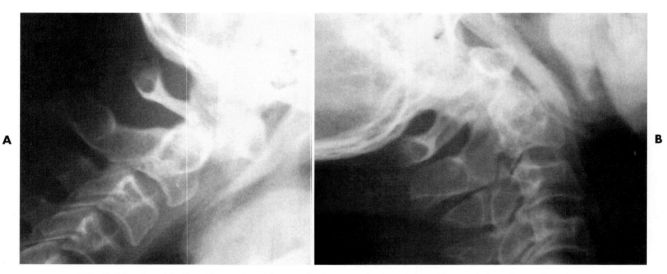

FIG. 8-26　**A** and **B,** Unstable os odontoideum on flexion-extension lateral views. Note typical angular configuration at the posterior margin of the anterior tubercle of C1, known as a *molding* defect (see Fig. 8-27).

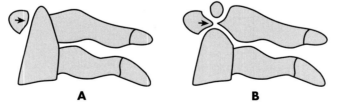

FIG. 8-27　Because os odontoideum is a long-standing defect, the posterior surface of the anterior tubercle of the atlas remodels into the gap between the os odontoideum and the odontoid process remnant of C2. **A,** Normally the posterior surface of the anterior tubercle is nearly flat *(arrow)*. **B,** The triangular molding defect *(arrow)* represents a classic associated developmental anomaly and helps to distinguish os odontoideum from acute dens fracture in patients with recent significant trauma.

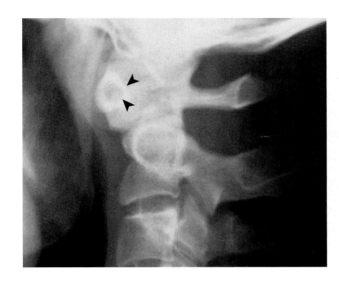

FIG. 8-28 Os odontoideum appearing on a lateral cervical radiograph exhibiting a rounded ("molding") defect (arrowheads) of the posterior surface of the anterior tubercle of the atlas.

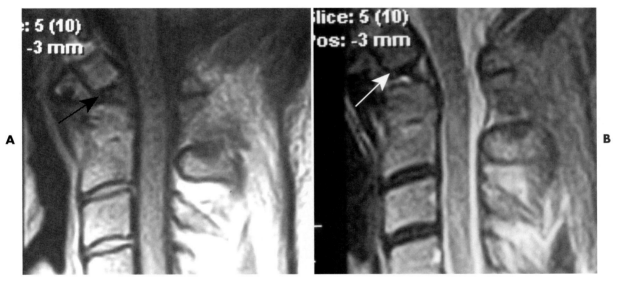

FIG. 8-29 Os odontoid appearing on, **A,** T1-weighted and, **B,** T2-weighted magnetic resonance imaging (MRI) sagittal scans. MRI has the ability to detail the impact of this structural defect on the adjacent spinal canal and contents (arrows).

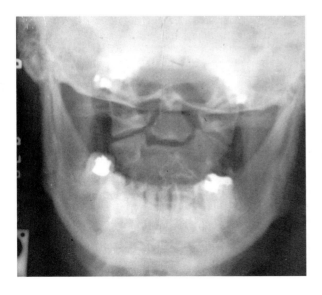

FIG. 8-30 Persistent defect of the odontoid after a type II fracture. A portion of os odontoideum defects are thought to represent nonunion consequence to odontoid fractures. (Courtesy Gary Longmuir, Phoenix, AZ.)

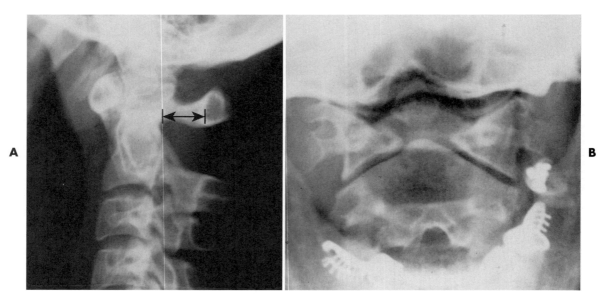

FIG. 8-31   Os odontoideum appearing with a wedged "molding defect" *(arrowheads)* of the posterior surface of, **A,** the anterior tubercle of the atlas and defect through, **B,** the lower odontoid process on the anteroposterior open mouth projection. Notice the narrowed spinal canal occurring secondary to anterior translation of the unstable segment. (Courtesy William E. Litterer, Elizabeth, NJ.)

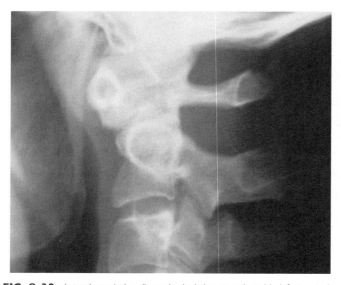

FIG. 8-32   Lateral cervical radiograph depicting an odontoid defect, anterior translation of the atlas, and rounded ("molding") defect of the posterior surface of the anterior tubercle of the atlas. (Courtesy Steven P. Brownstein, MD, Springfield, NJ.)

IMAGING FINDINGS

On plain films the os odontoideum often is overlooked or confused with a recent dens fracture. Plain films demonstrate a separate ossicle of varying conspicuity, frequently largely obscured on an anteroposterior open mouth view. On the lateral view, a helpful finding is hypertrophy and sclerosis of the anterior tubercle of the atlas. This finding, which also may be seen in other long-standing upper cervical abnormalities such as spina bifida occulta or rheumatoid arthritis, is caused by abnormal stresses concentrated on the anterior tubercle and may be helpful in distinguishing the os odontoideum from an acute dens fracture posttraumatically.[108]

Carefully positioned flexion lateral views usually reveal anterior atlantoaxial subluxation and instability (see Figs. 8-23, 8-24, and 8-26). The spinolaminar junction line of C1 is displaced anteriorly to that of C2 on flexion, yet the anterior atlantodental interspace (ADI) is normal, a very important sign of either os odontoideum or dens fracture. In instability resulting from disruption of the transverse ligament, both the ADI and the relationship of the spinolaminar junction lines at C1-2 are altered. The upper cervical relationship may be normal or altered in the neutral posture, and an extension lateral view illustrates typical posterior subluxation with the spinolaminar junction line of C1 now lying posterior to that of C2.

Another helpful plain film finding is a smooth, well-corticated margin at the inferior aspect of the separate odontoid and at the base of the dens. Of course, this does not definitively distinguish a long-standing ununited dens fracture from an os odontoideum, but it helps to exclude a recent dens fracture when this might otherwise be in question. A similar appearance is seen on the lateral view as an angular configuration to the posterior margin of the C1 anterior tubercle, because of remodeling related to the odontoid ossicle superiorly and the odontoid process remnant inferiorly (see Fig. 8-27). The angular appearance (apex directed to the posterior) to the posterior surface of the anterior tubercle is known as a "molding defect." The anterior tubercle also may be fused to the separate dens.

obscured by superimposed osseous structures or teeth on conventional plain films. It was long taught that the dens represents the embryologic derivative of the atlas body, but it is now known that it is merely a bony projection arising from the C2 body.

Abnormal motion, sometimes in the form of a specific acute trauma, appears to be essential to the development of the os odontoideum. This increased motion also may be in conjunction with a syndrome such as Down or Morquio's syndrome.[42,256] The first clear evidence that os odontoideum could be produced from a single traumatic event was found in a case report in 1991.[231] The lesion was considered to be congenital before that.

In addition to plain films, other potentially helpful diagnostic imaging techniques include plain film and CT, myelography, and MRI. CT may help in initial establishment of the diagnosis, especially when in doubt or occult on plain films. MRI is helpful in assessing possible cord compression and, with open scanning technology, may be performed with head nodding or cervical flexion. As with functional radiographs, this type of imaging requires careful monitoring to ensure the safety of the patient and prevent neurologic injury.[295]

CLINICAL COMMENTS

The clinical presentation of patients with os odontoideum varies considerably. The abnormality sometimes is discovered as an incidental finding on plain films of patients who are asymptomatic or whose symptoms are apparently unrelated. Symptoms may include headaches or upper cervical or suboccipital pain of varying severity. Os odontoideum also may be discovered in previously asymptomatic patients who experience trauma, in which case the findings may include significant neurologic deficit.

Given the previously mentioned role of abnormal motion or specific trauma in the development of os odontoideum, most authorities today favor an acquired etiology for the os odontoideum. However, compelling evidence still exists that at least some os odontoidea are congenital, including a report of identical twins with os odontoideum and a known association between os odontoideum and Down syndrome.[71,129] A case report from 1989 indicates that at least some cases may be familial and associated with syndromes involving spinal anomalies, such as Klippel-Feil syndrome.[173]

In some instances it is unclear whether the os odontoideum is congenital or acquired, especially when only relatively minor trauma has occurred.[103] Os odontoideum appears to be either congenital or acquired. The question of primary importance is not whether a given case of os odontoideum is congenital or traumatic, but rather how the condition should best be managed once discovered to ensure the best outcome for the patient. Of course, the question of traumatic or congenital etiology may still hold weight among academics and attorneys, and the debates continue.[40]

Surgical management for os odontoideum has included interlaminar wiring alone; posterior screw fixation, with or without bone graft; or combined bone graft and wire fixation. Procedures that do not involve sublaminar wiring are associated with a lower risk of neural injury.[257] Some have advocated the use of cineradiography to help determine the most appropriate means of surgical fixation.[111]

In addition to the obvious potential for upper cervical cord compression, a less widely recognized complication of the unstable os odontoideum is compromise of the vertebral artery, which may lead to brainstem, cerebellar, or cerebral infarction. This may be associated with neurologic deficit that ranges from permanent and profound to partially or completely reversible.[16,128,172,262]

KEY CONCEPTS

- Whether posttraumatic, developmental, or congenital, the os odontoideum represents a relatively uncommon but important abnormality of the upper cervical complex.
- Its presence may compromise the stability of the atlantoaxial articulation, which may be catastrophic, especially when a previously asymptomatic and seemingly normal individual experiences hyperflexion or other trauma to the upper cervical complex.
- The os odontoideum may be seen alone or in conjunction with other anomalies of the cervical spine and craniovertebral junction.

Osteogenesis Imperfecta

BACKGROUND

Osteogenesis imperfecta, also known as *Lobstein disease, Ekman syndrome,* and *osteopsathyrosis,* encompasses a heterogenous group of genetic disorders that are marked by abnormal collagen type I formation. Osteogenesis imperfecta may be inherited as a dominant or recessive defect, or it may arise from a mutation. At least four distinct types exist, ranging in clinical presentation from mild osteopenia with normal stature to severe dwarfing osteoporosis, with multiple fractures occurring in utero. The disease was dichotomized into congenita and tarda forms in the past; however, this is no longer thought to be valid.[266]

Type I is the most common form, marked by easily fractured bones, blue sclera, abnormal dentition, normal stature, joint hypermobility, and a tendency toward spinal curvature.

IMAGING FINDINGS

Radiographic studies may demonstrate osteopenia, one or more fractures, hypoplastic dentition, dwarfism, and kyphoscoliosis (Figs. 8-33 and 8-34). Bone cortices may be thin and most apparent in the long bones, which also may demonstrate bowing deformity. The skull may be large, exhibiting delayed ossification and wormian bones.

CLINICAL COMMENTS

Severe types of the disease are lethal at birth. Milder forms of the disease are characterized by weakened, easily fractured bones, but are compatible with a normal life span. Patients may exhibit blue sclera, translucent skin, and deafness.

No cure exists for osteogenesis imperfecta. Treatment is directed toward limiting deformity and injury. Conservatively this may entail limiting physical activity. More aggressive approaches involve placement of intramedullary rods to prevent long bone deformity and fracture.

KEY CONCEPTS

- Osteogenesis imperfecta is a heterogenous group of genetic disorders that are marked by abnormal collagen.
- The severity of the clinical presentation varies.
- Radiographic examination may reveal osteoporosis, fractures, abnormal dentition, dwarfism, kyphoscoliosis, thin cortices, delayed calvarial ossification, and wormian bones.
- Treatment is directed toward limiting deformity and injury.

Osteopetrosis

BACKGROUND

Rather than a single disease, osteopetrosis syndromes include at least four distinct entities, with varying clinical and radiographic features. These are grouped with a larger collection of diseases known as the *sclerosing bone dysplasias,* sharing a common feature of increased density of bone in varying patterns.

Severe and intermediate autosomal recessive forms of osteopetrosis exist. A third autosomal recessive form is associated with tubular acidosis and was recognized as a unique syndrome in 1972. It has been called "marble brain disease," owing to the typical intracranial calcifications, especially in the basal ganglia and cerebral hemispheres. This is similar to the term "marble bone disease," which has been used to describe the osseous changes.

Finally, a mild, autosomal dominant form exists, usually discovered incidentally in patients x-rayed for other reasons. This condition has been named *Albers-Schönberg's disease,* after the

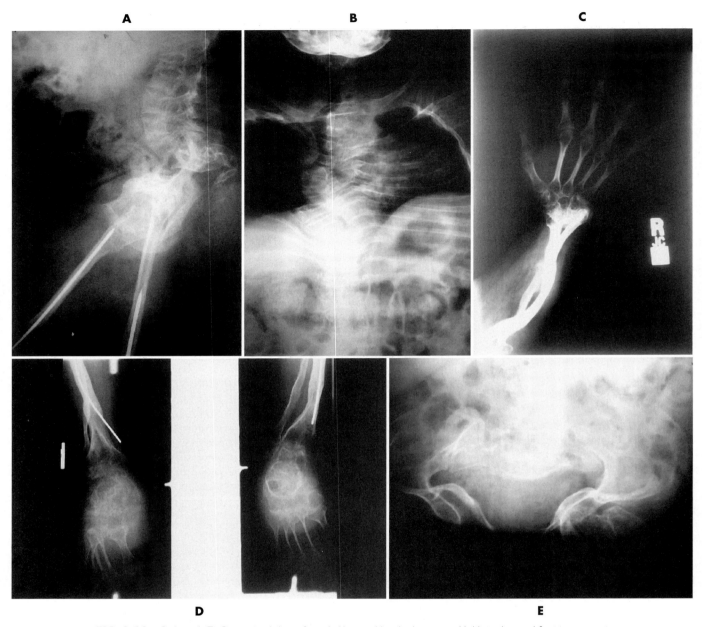

FIG. 8-33   A through **E,** Osteogenesis imperfecta. A 41-year-old male drummer with blue sclera and fractures present from birth. Diagnosis was first made at 7 months, and the patient had experienced more than 200 fractures before age 20. As is typical, the rate of new fracture decreased markedly after puberty. Note gracile, overtubulated long bones with multiple healed fractures and severe osteopenia. Marked protrusio acetabulum, multiple vertebral compression fractures, and sacral and rib fractures are present. Lifelong wheelchair confinement has contributed to deformity of the trunk, with scoliosis and short stature noted.

radiologist who first reported it. Previously osteopetrosis was separated grossly into benign and aggressive or "malignant" forms. This simplistic classification system is invalid because of the heterogeneity within the various forms.

IMAGING FINDINGS
Radiographic findings vary widely, both among and within the various forms of osteopetrosis, but the typical changes are a result of deficient osteoclastic activity. Although the number of osteoclasts generally is normal, most of the population is dysfunctional. As expected, this condition involves a lack of proper remodeling of

bones, especially the most metabolically active portions, the ends of long bones. Undertubulation with a widened appearance of the metaphyses and metadiaphyseal regions is described as an "Erlenmeyer flask" deformity, a finding also seen in hemolytic anemias, Gaucher's disease, and a variety of other conditions. A loss of distinction may occur between cortical and medullary bone and, in the most severe cases, may completely obliterate the medullary spaces.

A "bone-within-a-bone" appearance, or "endobone," is caused by persistence of infantile bone matrix within the medullary cavity and is often most striking in the spine (Figs. 8-35 through 8-37).

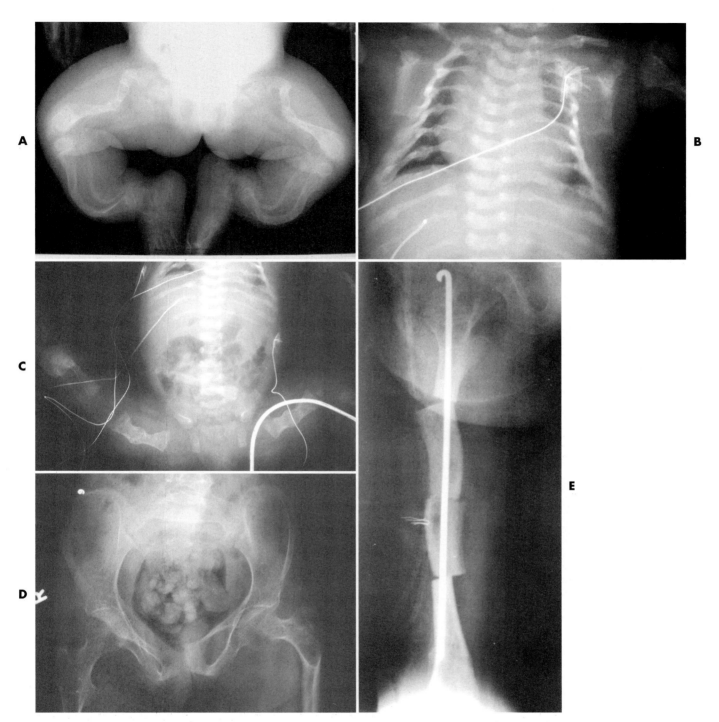

FIG. 8-34 Osteogenesis imperfecta. **A,** Osteogenesis imperfecta with severe bowing. **B,** Osteogenesis imperfecta in a newborn with multiple rib fractures. **C,** Lower body in same patient as **B.** There are numerous fractures but the bones are not bowed. **D,** Pelvis in an older child shows osteopenia, deformity caused by prior fractures, and gracile and deformed proximal femurs. **E,** Surgical intervention for a bowed femur. Multiple osteotomies were performed with intramedullary pin fixation. (From Manaster BJ, Disler DG, May DA: Musculoskeletal imaging, ed 2, St Louis, 2002.)

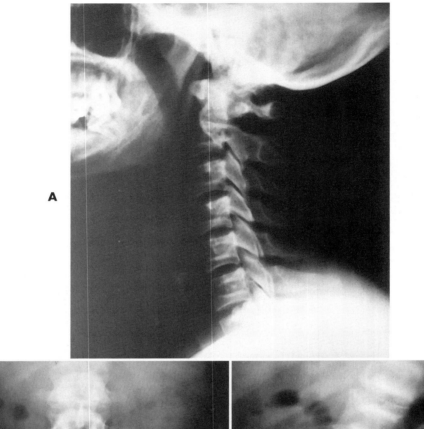

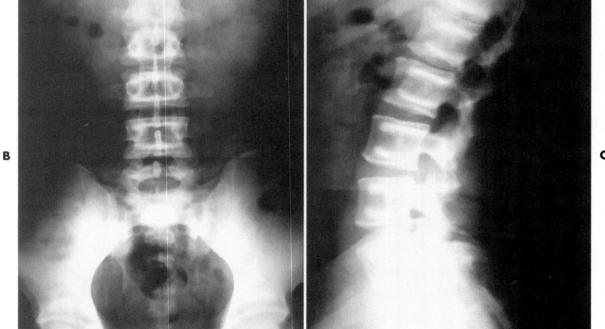

FIG. 8-35 A through **C,** Mild form of osteopetrosis with typical "bone-within-a-bone" appearance resulting from defective osteoclastic activity, which fails to fully remove the immature vertebral body anlage. Note also spondylolisthesis of L5 secondary to ununited stress fractures of the pars interarticularis. This is extremely common in osteopetrosis and attests to the fact that the bones are more prone to fracture than normal bones, despite the increased radiographic density. The vertebrae, sometimes described as *sandwich vertebrae,* might be confused with the "rugger jersey" appearance of renal osteodystrophy (secondary hyperparathyroidism). In the latter condition the bands of sclerosis are reactive, a response to resorption of bone at the discovertebral junction. They are therefore immediately adjacent to the endplates, as opposed to several millimeters away from the endplates as seen here in osteopetrosis.

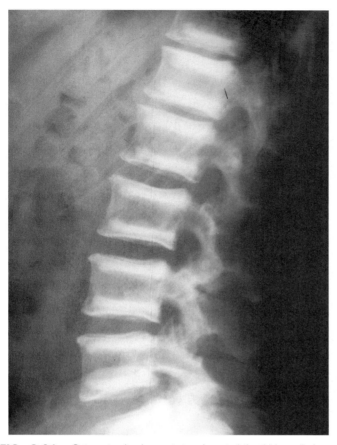

FIG. 8-36 Osteopetrosis demonstrate characteristic thick, radiodense, horizontal bands adjacent to the endplates of the lumbar vertebrae, known as *sandwich vertebrae.*

In the skull, changes predominate in the enchondral bone of the skull base. Paranasal sinuses are underdeveloped. Acute and insufficiency type of stress fractures may be seen. Other characteristics of osteopetrosis include an especially high incidence of lumbar spondylolysis and spondylolisthesis. Dental anomalies also may be seen, including supernumerary teeth, retention of infantile teeth, and impaction of permanent teeth.

Although all forms of osteopetrosis may show at least minimal regression of radiographic changes, this feature is most characteristic of the recessive form associated with renal tubular acidosis. The intracranial calcifications in this form of osteopetrosis are also unique and are most readily demonstrated on CT, predominating in the basal ganglia.[182,243,244] A relationship may exist between osteopetrosis and calcific tendinitis, although this remains uncertain.[206]

CLINICAL COMMENTS

The severe, autosomal recessive form of osteopetrosis often, although not invariably, is lethal in infancy and unlikely to be seen by most health care practitioners. Frequently osteopetrosis is marked by hydrocephalus and macrocephaly, failure to thrive, hepatosplenomegaly, and cranial nerve dysfunction resulting from stenosis of skull foramina. Death is typically caused by severe anemia, resulting from stenosis of the medullary, hematopoietic regions of bone. Thrombocytopenia, including leukocytopenia, predisposes to infections, which also may be fatal.

The intermediate, recessive form is associated with hepatomegaly, anemia, below-average height, and pathologic fractures.[12,130] The intermediate, recessive form with renal acidosis may be associated with mental deficit. Symptoms may include failure to thrive, muscle weakness, hypotonia, and other clinical findings of renal acidosis.[182,243,244]

Although many with the autosomal dominant form (Albers-Schönberg's) of the disease remain asymptomatic, some experience

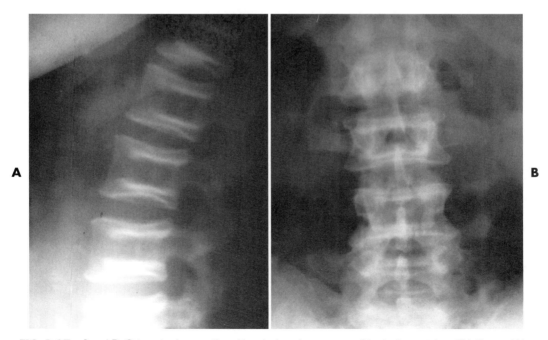

FIG. 8-37 **A** and **B,** Osteopetrosis presenting with a shadowed appearance of the lumbar vertebrae. This "bone-within-a-bone" appearance is typical of osteopetrosis.

anemia, cranial nerve dysfunction, and pathologic fractures, which may bring the condition to clinical light.[105,121,247]

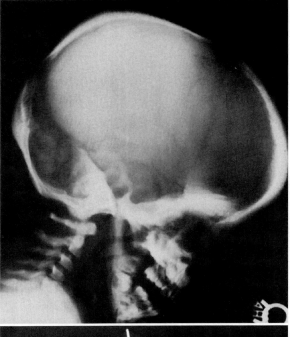

KEY CONCEPTS

- *Osteopetrosis is actually a combination of several related conditions, formerly divided simply into benign and malignant forms, all with an underlying decrease in osteoclastic activity, resulting in lack of normal bone resorption.*
- *Those with the more severe, autosomal recessive form die within the first decade from complications of severe anemia.*
- *An autosomal recessive form with renal tubular acidosis tends to improve radiographically, and bone density may appear to be relatively normal by later childhood. Intracranial calcifications are invariably seen, distinguishing this form from the others.*
- *The autosomal dominant, tarda form is the one most likely to be encountered by the typical clinician and may be found incidentally on radiographs performed for another reason.*
- *Those with the autosomal dominant, tarda form may experience mild anemia, cranial nerve compromise, pathologic acute and insufficiency fractures, and osteomyelitis resulting from dental extraction, although most who are affected remain asymptomatic throughout their life.*

Pyknodysostosis (Pycnodysostosis)

BACKGROUND

Pyknodysostosis is a rare, autosomal recessive syndrome consisting of diffuse osteosclerosis; below-average height; skull anomalies; broad, short hands; hypoplasia of the mandible; acroosteolysis; hypoplastic nails; and abnormal dentition. Although some have considered this to be a variant of osteopetrosis, it appears to be a distinct entity, first described by Maritoux and Lamy in 1962. Toulouse-Lautrec probably suffered from this condition.[45,63,300]

IMAGING FINDINGS

Craniofacial changes are most striking, with frontal and occipital bossing, a small face, and micrognathia (Fig. 8-38). The mandible is hypoplastic and the mandibular angle increased. Closure of skull sutures is delayed. The anterior fontanelle often persists into adulthood, and multiple wormian bones are common. As in osteopetrosis, the skull base is particularly sclerotic and dentition is abnormal. Unlike osteopetrosis, portions of the calvarium actually may be thinned and osteopenic and normal diploic markings generally are absent. Short tubular bones of the hands and feet are hypoplastic, and the distal phalangeal tufts often are marked by resorption or hypoplasia (see Fig. 8-38). In addition to sclerosis of the spine, segmentation anomalies, especially of the upper cervical spine, are common.

In contrast to osteopetrosis, in which skeletal changes remain static or may even improve over time, skeletal changes tend to progress in pyknodysostosis. As in osteopetrosis, characteristics of pyknodysostosis may include pathologic and insufficiency fractures, including cervical and lumbar pars interarticularis defects (spondylolysis).[45,63,300] Fracture complications arise most frequently in the second decade of life. Another associated complication is osteomyelitis of the mandible, which appears to be related to a combination of hypovascularity and abnormal dentition.[45,153]

CLINICAL COMMENTS

Although affected individuals often have a normal life span, hyperplasia of the uvula may lead to hypoventilation and subsequent cardiac or secondary hepatic failure.[4,300]

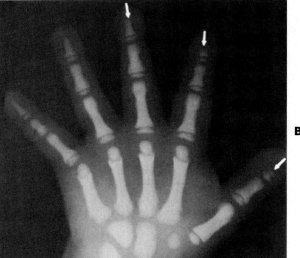

FIG. 8-38 Pyknodysostosis in a 5-year-old girl. **A,** Dense bones, widely open cranial sutures, prognathism (obtuse angle of mandible), lack of normal development of mastoids, and paranasal sinuses. **B,** Generalized osteosclerosis, partial absence of ossification of distal phalanx of thumb and middle and index fingers *(arrows)*. (From Taybi H, Lachman RS: Radiology of syndromes, metabolic disorders, and skeletal dysplasias, ed 4, St Louis, 1996, Mosby.)

KEY CONCEPTS

- *Autosomal recessive disorder that demonstrates generalized sclerosis of bone and short stature, without true dwarfism, along with dysplasia of the terminal tufts of the phalanges.*
- *Cranial, facial, spinal, and clavicular anomalies are common.*

Scheuermann's Disease

BACKGROUND

History. In 1921 Scheuermann's published the first report of the common spinal condition that bears his name, introducing the term *kyphosis dorsalis juvenilis*. This involved thoracic hyperkyphosis and characteristic morphologic changes of the discovertebral junctions somewhat resembling those of Legg-Calvé-Perthes disease of the proximal femur.[230] It seems that no other developmental spinal condition, with the possible exception of spondylolytic spondylolisthesis, has engendered as much confusion and controversy as Scheuermann's disease. In fact, the pathogenesis, epidemiology, and clinical relevance of these two conditions share some common features.

Both Scheuermann's disease and lumbar spondylolysis were first reported decades previously and have given rise to a perplexing array of etiologic hypotheses and revisions. Both are considered to be related, in some measure, to repetitive altered stresses on what may be inherently vulnerable developing structures in adolescents, the pars interarticularis for spondylolisthesis, and the osteocartilaginous endplate junction in Scheuermann's disease. Although both conditions seem to have some genetic component, lumbar spondylolysis should be considered to represent stress fracture of the pars interarticularis and is rarely, if ever, congenital.[93] Scheuermann's disease is best classified as a stress-related "apophysitis," rather than a congenital process, and is the result of combined genetics and environmental factors. Both conditions may be asymptomatic, and the severity of symptoms often is unrelated to the degree of abnormality demonstrated on diagnostic imaging and clinical examination. In both, more severe symptoms often are a result of associated or secondary abnormalities, such as intervertebral disc herniations, which are much more common in patients with these conditions than in the general population. Interestingly, an increased incidence of lumbar spondylolysis is seen in Scheuermann's disease, occurring in 32% to 50% of patients, as compared with about 7% in the general population.[89,183]

Terminology. Even the naming of Scheuermann's disease has led to confusion over the years. Scheuermann's disease has been called variably *vertebral epiphysitis, osteochondrosis juvenilis dorsi, adolescent kyphosis, osteochondrosis juvenilis Scheuermann's, juvenile kyphosis, spinal osteochondrosis,* and *osteochondritis.*[7,23,94,165,258] In fact, in some instances, the same author has published different articles using several different names for the same condition![7]

Diagnosis. The diagnosis of Scheuermann's disease typically is established on the basis of plain film radiographs, in conjunction with clinical findings of increasing kyphosis and variable back pain that develop in adolescence. Multilevel Schmorl's nodes, resulting from intravertebral disc protrusions through natural fissures (e.g., vascular channels) in the developing cartilaginous endplate, are an essential feature, along with more generalized endplate irregularity, anterior vertebral body wedging, diminished vertebral body height, and diminished disc height. Involvement usually is multilevel, typically in the lower thoracic or thoracolumbar region.

Although Scheuermann's did allow for the diagnosis in cases of isolated changes at one disc level, a stricter definition of Scheuermann's disease generally is used today, requiring three or more affected vertebral levels, each with at least 5 degrees of anterior vertebral body wedging, leading to hyperkyphosis.[211] This does not include minimal Schmorl's node formation even at more than one level if it is not accompanied by hyperkyphosis and alteration of vertebral body morphology. Because developmental and traumatic endplate changes occur on a continuum, some of these cases may be considered to be abbreviated forms of Scheuermann's disease.

As with idiopathic scoliosis, attention has been focused upon an alteration in biosynthesis of collagen and other ground substances as a fundamental abnormality leading to the typical gross anatomic and radiographic features of Scheuermann's disease.[7] Other authors have theorized that inadequate nutrition, structural weakness,

or a combination of these lead to Scheuermann's disease–like changes in the thoracolumbar region and premature degenerative disc disease in the lower lumbar spine. This constellation of findings has been described as "juvenile discogenic disease."[100] Studies demonstrating similar spinal changes in identical twins, sibling recurrence, and transmission over three generations lend credence to a fundamental genetic abnormality, with disease severity influenced by biomechanical stresses.[165,274] One researcher demonstrated disorganized enchondral ossification, resembling the changes of Blount's disease of the tibia and thought to be secondary to increased axial loading of the developing anterior vertebral body margin.[232]

Over the years, other theories about the cause or causes of Scheuermann's disease have included idiopathic osteochondrosis or avascular necrosis, hamstring tightness, a nonspecific myopathy, or even emotional stress.[67,70,164]

Prevalence. It is impossible to arrive at a precise estimate of the prevalence of Scheuermann's disease, because a specific figure demands a well-defined entity and many patients are mildly affected and never come to clinical light. A conservative estimate may be as low as 0.4%; however, this is based upon a study of adolescents between the ages of 11 and 13 years who were tracked for 3 years through their pubertal period.[180] As noted, one study calculated an incidence of 13%.[98] Another paper reported MRI changes of Scheuermann's disease in 38% of 90 asymptomatic subjects.[290] Still's another article, basing the diagnosis on a lateral plain film of the thoracic and lumbar spine, along with a questionnaire and assessment of passive stretch of the hamstrings, reported a prevalence of 60% of male and 23% of female students among 96 students 17 to 18 years old.[68] A later study by these same authors using a larger sample size of 500 subjects showed an incidence of 56.3% in male and 30.3% in female students 17 to 18 years old. Risk factors identified in this study included above-average height, more than 2 weeks spent in bed because of illness or injury, and hamstring tightness, which previously had been found in 85% of individuals with Scheuermann's disease.[67,69]

IMAGING FINDINGS

Plain film radiographs are the initial diagnostic imaging modality used in most cases, but Scheuermann's disease has been widely studied using CT, MRI, and even planar radionuclide imaging and single positron emission computed tomography (SPECT) (Figs. 8-39 through 8-42). These advanced imaging techniques may be indicated in atypical presentations of Scheuermann's disease that might mimic other more serious conditions (e.g., disc space infection) or when there is suspicion for associated intervertebral disc herniation or other complications.[6,155]

Advanced imaging also may be helpful in cases in which the patient has experienced substantial recent trauma, there is question of compression fracture versus changes related to Scheuermann's disease, and no prior studies are available for comparison.

Nonspecific studies such as radionuclide imaging, ordered for further evaluation of back pain unresponsive to conservative management, may be negative, but also may show abnormal findings that may resemble other processes such as disc space infection.[6,222] This fact, along with the similar sensitivity and greater specificity of MRI versus bone scan, makes MRI the diagnostic imaging procedure of choice in virtually all cases requiring further investigation beyond plain films, particularly when symptoms are localized.

CLINICAL COMMENTS

General. Scheuermann's described a condition of increased thoracic kyphosis in adolescents demonstrating unique, multilevel

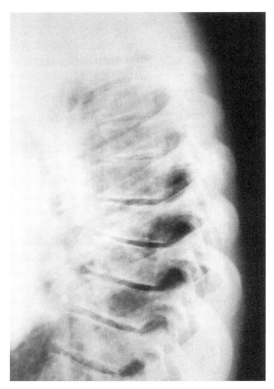

FIG. 8-39   Residuals of Scheuermann's disease in a 25-year-old man. Note the marked platyspondyly and increased kyphosis with less apparent endplate irregularities and Schmorl's node formation, as well as mild disc space narrowing.

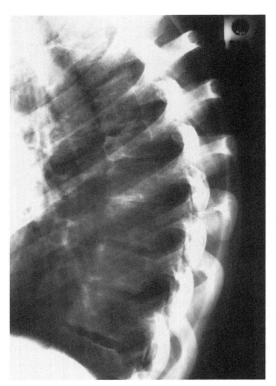

FIG. 8-40   Scheuermann's disease in a 14-year-old girl with moderate to severe progressive thoracic kyphosis. A markedly wedged midthoracic segment could be mistaken for a compression fracture, but no trauma occurred and symptoms were not more pronounced focally.

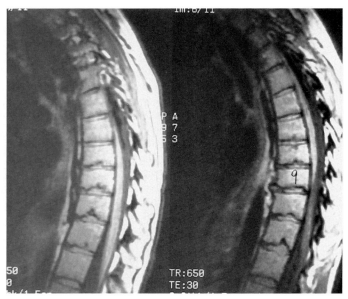

FIG. 8-41   With the exception of hyperkyphosis, the changes of Scheuermann's disease and its complications are generally much better seen on magnetic resonance imaging (MRI) than on plain films. Schmorl's node formation may appear to be minimal on plain films but substantial on MRI. Note the anterior disc protrusion at T9-10. There is a marked increase in the incidence of disc bulge and herniation in Scheuermann's disease patients versus a normal population.

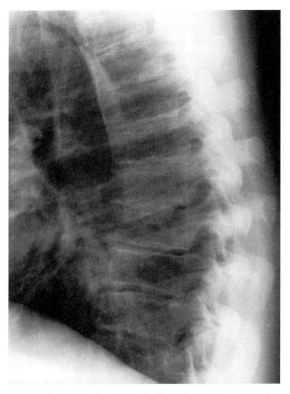

FIG. 8-42   Scheuermann's disease. The thoracic segments have a trapezoidal configuration with significant endplate irregularity.

thoracic endplate irregularities and Schmorl's nodes, along with anterior vertebral body wedging. Milder cases and abbreviated forms of Scheuermann's disease may be clinically occult and asymptomatic, with radiographic changes noted incidentally. Severe cases may lead to progressive deformity, pain, disability and, infrequently, acute neurologic deficit secondary to angular kyphosis with or without disc herniation.[224,294]

Patients with Scheuermann's disease may have associated, compensatory musculoskeletal abnormality, such as lumbar or cervical hyperlordosis, muscular imbalance, and hypertonicity, although a clear cause-and-effect relationship has not been established.[250]

As with idiopathic scoliosis, no clear predictive factors have been delineated to assist in determining which cases are likely to progress and which are likely to arrest with only mild or moderate hyperkyphosis. Reports conflict about the clinical significance of Scheuermann's disease–related endplate abnormality, especially chronic or residual changes in adults. A recent 25-year prospective cohort study of 640 schoolchildren failed to demonstrate a positive correlation between thoracolumbar changes of Scheuermann's disease and back pain, either in adolescence or adulthood. Thirteen percent of these children had radiographic evidence of Scheuermann's disease. Interestingly, these authors did find a strong correlation between adolescent back pain combined with a familial occurrence of back pain and pain in the same adolescents into adulthood, regardless of the presence or absence of radiographic abnormality.[98]

Activity. Historically Scheuermann's disease has been linked to activities that increase axial loading of the spine in adolescents, such as diving, gymnastics, weightlifting, or heavy lifting at work; however, this relationship has not been confirmed universally.[69,267] Although such activities have not been clearly demonstrated to cause the radiographic changes of Scheuermann's disease per se, the onset of symptoms in patients with this condition is often temporally linked to such activities.[89]

Scoliosis. Some authors have examined the relationship between Scheuermann's disease and idiopathic scoliosis and have concluded that they may share a common pathogenesis. One study found that 70% of patients with Scheuermann's disease had scoliosis, averaging 15 degrees. Just less than one third of these had an apex at the same level as the Scheuermann's kyphosis. The number of right convexities equaled that of left convexities. There was also an equal distribution among males and females, unlike scoliosis unrelated to Scheuermann's disease, which is far more common in females and results in a right convexity in approximately 90% of cases. The remaining lumbar curves, most commonly caudal to the kyphosis, averaged 16 degrees but were still felt to be compensatory. These curves were more often right-sided and far more common in females.[52] In this author's experience, many of the apparent mild "scolioses" seen in Scheuermann's disease patients, especially in the thoracic spine, actually are at least partially spurious. Such pseudoscolioses result on an AP radiograph positioned with some rotation of the patient, throwing the hyperkyphotic thoracic spine to one side of the midline. Observing for symmetry of the medial clavicles may help to eliminate misdiagnosis of some of these spurious "scolioses."

Osteoporosis. An apparent relationship has been noted between Scheuermann's disease and osteoporosis, developing in adolescence.[22,25] Osteoporosis limited to the axial skeleton, primarily the affected thoracic spine, could be explained by a combination of hyperemia and disuse. However, it has been subsequently shown that the osteoporosis is generalized, involving the appendicular skeleton as well and to roughly the same degree.[151] Another study found abnormal levels of serum alkaline phosphatase and urine hydroxyproline, as well as deficient dietary calcium intake in 12 adolescents with Scheuermann's disease and osteopenia.[22,25] In keeping with the controversial nature of Scheuermann's disease, yet another study found no evidence of a relationship between this condition and osteoporosis, even in the axial skeleton. However, the disparity may be explained by different inclusion criteria for defining Scheuermann's disease.[86]

Intervertebral disc disease. Thoracic disc herniation resulting in cord or nerve root compression is one of the more clinically significant lesions secondary to Scheuermann's disease, causing focal back and radicular intercostal pain, as well as occasional neurologic deficit such as gait disturbance or bowel and bladder dysfunction.[17] Individuals with Scheuermann's disease demonstrate MRI changes of thoracolumbar degenerative disc disease by their early twenties in approximately 55% of the cases, as compared with about 10% in asymptomatic controls.[186] Another study also found that plain film changes of Scheuermann's disease, with associated disc space narrowing, always were associated with MRI evidence of degenerative disc disease.[187] However, this study did not reveal a similar relationship between Scheuermann's disease and spondylolisthesis. A relationship has been noted between Scheuermann's disease and central spinal stenosis secondary to severe osteochondral changes, which may not be evident on plain films. Although these authors identified stenosis using myelography, today MRI or CT typically is indicated for this assessment.[263]

Treatment. Treatment of Scheuermann's disease depends largely upon the clinical findings. Although watchful monitoring is all that may be necessary in most cases, progressive deformity, intractable moderate to severe pain, or development of neurologic deficit warrant more aggressive treatment. This ranges from bracing and application of orthoses to surgery, although the efficacy of nonsurgical treatments has not been established and the complications of surgery generally should limit its application to debilitating pain, neurologic deficit, spinal cord compression, or severe deformity.[21,24,302]

KEY CONCEPTS

- *Scheuermann's disease and its abbreviated forms represent common developmental spinal abnormalities that may be asymptomatic or may lead to significant back pain and deformity.*
- *Physicians who encounter adolescents with back complaints certainly see many patients with this disorder and should be familiar with the clinical and diagnostic imaging findings, including multilevel endplate irregularity, Schmorl's nodes, disc space narrowing, and decreased anterior vertebral body height with hyperkyphosis.*
- *Patients with more severe pain should be considered for advanced imaging, specifically magnetic resonance imaging, to assess for the common complication of thoracic disc herniation, which is otherwise comparatively uncommon, in the general population.*
- *Patients with more severe kyphosis may require bracing or, in a few cases, surgery, to arrest or partially correct the deformity.*

Turner's Syndrome

BACKGROUND

The phenotype of females with infantile secondary sexual characteristics, webbed neck (pterygium colli), and cubitus valgus was first described by Henry Turner's more than 50 years ago. Shortly thereafter, gonadal dysgenesis was recognized as an integral part of the syndrome. It was not until about 20 years later, however, that Otto Ullrich identified the typical chromosomal abnormality, 45.XO, along with recognizing additional cases of mosaicism. Ullrich's name is sometimes assigned to the syndrome as well.[286]

IMAGING FINDINGS

The most widely recognized skeletal abnormality associated with Turner's syndrome is osteoporosis, which may be detectable before puberty. Turner's syndrome patients show below-average bone density relative to bone age, chronologic age, and body mass index (BMI) but normal density for height and age. Adolescents with Turner's syndrome show a predilection to fractures of the distal radius, although it is not clear that these are related to alteration of bone density.[223] Turner's patients receiving growth hormone replacement in adolescence do not demonstrate osteoporosis. Thus it appears that growth hormone therapy has the double benefit of preventing not only markedly shortened stature and delayed skeletal maturity, but also osteoporosis.[138,178]

Isolated reports of skeletal changes resembling spondyloepiphyseal dysplasia have appeared. These include platyspondyly and marked endplate irregularity, short femoral necks, coxa valga, coxa magna, and acetabular hypoplasia.[161,176] Anomalies of the sternum have been reported in Turner's syndrome. In addition to pectus excavatum, characteristics include shortening of the sternum, premature fusion of the manubriosternal joint or manubrium, and double manubrial ossification centers. These types of anomalies do not appear to be more common in patients with congenital heart disease, unlike isolated sternal anomalies in otherwise normal individuals.[169]

Radiographs of the hands may provide clues to the diagnosis. A classic, but by no means pathognomonic, radiographic finding in Turner's syndrome is shortening of one or more metacarpal bones, seen in approximately 50% of patients. The fourth metacarpal is the most commonly affected, although the third and fifth also may be involved. Other possible characteristics include carpal coalition, and, as in other syndromes producing coalition, the synostosis tends to be across rather than along carpal rows. Cubitus valgus generally is readily apparent clinically and seen in approximately 70% of patients. This may be confirmed and accurately quantified radiographically, allowing planning for orthopedic intervention when necessary. There is an increased incidence of Madelung's deformity of the forearm. The lower extremities may experience pes cavus and hyperplasia of the medial tibial plateau, with or without a small exostosis arising inferomedial to the tibial plateau.

CLINICAL COMMENTS

Turner's syndrome occurs in 1/2000 to 1/5000 live female births. The diagnosis is typically suspected early, on the basis of overt clinical findings, although some patients may show nothing more than markedly diminished height. Analysis of chromatin bodies in buccal smears was hoped to represent a helpful screening tool in this population, but this has not proved to be true.[51] Individuals with Turner's syndrome have a decreased life expectancy of approximately 10 to 12 years below average. This is primarily a result of increased mortality from cardiovascular complications of congenital heart disease and aortic dissections.[203]

Cardiovascular anomalies are present in approximately 20% of affected patients, 70% of which are aortic coarctation. Echocardiography may show an asymptomatic aortic root dilatation. Besides aortic coarctation, congenital cardiovascular anomalies include partial anomalous pulmonary venous return, bicuspid aortic valve, mitral valve prolapse, aortic sinus aneurysm, and hypoplastic left heart (HLH) syndrome.[177,260,275]

Hypertension also is seen frequently; it is present in childhood in about one quarter of patients and with at least episodic hypertension in nearly 50% of adults. Estrogen replacement therapy may initiate or exacerbate the hypertension.[277] Aortic dissection is typically related to cystic medial necrosis. This underlying abnormality, similar to that seen in Marfan's syndrome, may play an important role in the development of other cardiovascular complications.[260] Patients with Turner's syndrome and their families should be made aware of these potential complications and prophylaxis should be considered, to include methods of preventing bacterial endocarditis and monitoring and control of blood pressure. The onset of aortic dissection may be characterized by unexplained and often severe chest pain, dyspnea, or sudden hypotension.[147]

Renal anomalies are seen in approximately one third of patients and are typically screened for, using ultrasonography. The most common anomalies are horseshoe kidneys and duplication of the collecting system, accounting for somewhat less than half of all urinary tract anomalies (Fig. 8-43). Renal agenesis, crossed ectopia, or pelvic kidney may occur less often. These anomalies may lead to urinary tract obstruction and may play a role in the development of hypertension.[148] An association also may exist between renal anomalies and altered renal vitamin D metabolism. This may be an important factor in the development of osteoporosis, particularly because osteoblastic function has not been found to be impaired.[227] Turner's syndrome patients may have insulin-resistant diabetes mellitus. This appears to be related to abnormality at the muscular receptor site and may be partially overcome by increasing the insulin dose.[34,259]

Webbing of the neck (pterygium colli) is a frequent finding in Turner's syndrome, resembling some cases of Klippel-Feil syndrome. This may be corrected surgically, both for functional and

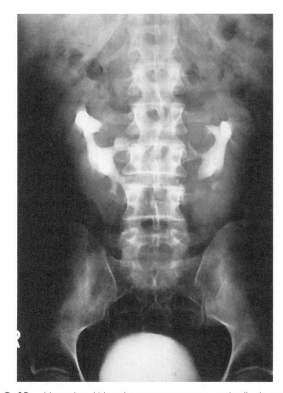

FIG. 8-43 Horseshoe kidney. Intravenous urogram optimally demonstrates typical renal morphology better than plain films. These and other renal anomalies may be seen in a variety of syndromes involving vertebral anomalies, including a distinctive "VATER syndrome," which consists of vertebral anomalies, anal atresia, tracheoesophageal fistula, and renal anomalies.

cosmetic reasons.[269] Turner's syndrome patients typically have a broad chest, with widely spaced nipples and mild pectus excavatum. A high incidence of chronic otitis media (approximately 80%) is noted, frequently with associated sensorineural hearing loss (approximately 35%), and routine otologic and audiologic assessment has been advocated.[233]

Turner's syndrome is related to other diseases. The incidence of autoimmune diseases is increased among Turner's syndrome patients, although a relationship between specific diseases such as juvenile rheumatoid arthritis and Turner's syndrome has not been firmly established.[8] A frequent association exists between Turner's syndrome and congenital lymphedema, which typically resolves in the first year of life. Persistence of lymphedema may signal congenital lymphangiectasia, which was not described until 1986.[195] Turner's syndrome is also reportedly associated with pedal angioma.[281] Some of the associated disorders seen in Turner's syndrome may be related to treatment rather than the disease itself. For example, an increased incidence of some types of uterine adenomyomas results from estrogen therapy.[39]

Because of the variety of abnormalities reported in Turner's syndrome, complications may be overlooked or receive little attention. This may be true of CNS dysfunction, which may result from intrinsic anomaly or may be secondary to a cerebrovascular anomaly. Cognitive abnormalities and seizure disorders may result. Turner's syndrome patients experience an increased incidence of malignant transformation of dysgenetic ovaries, prompting questions about the role of prophylactic oophorectomy.[249] Turner's syndrome is also accompanied by an increased incidence of melanocytic nevi. Particularly in patients with multiple nevi and those on growth hormone therapy (which has been shown to increase the rate of growth of nevi), periodic skin examinations and restriction of unprotected sun exposure are prudent to minimize the risk of malignant transformation to malignant melanoma.[11,20]

> **KEY CONCEPTS**
>
> - *Turner's syndrome is an inherited disorder of XO chromosomal pattern, associated with short stature, delayed skeletal maturity, osteoporosis, and varying multisystem anomalies.*
> - *Approximately 10% of patients have a mental deficit.*
> - *Classically associated anomalies of various organ systems include aortic coarctation, ovarian dysgenesis, and horseshoe kidney.*
> - *The skeleton may demonstrate, among other things, scoliosis, kyphosis, cubitus valgus, pes cavus, Madelung's deformity, and enlargement of the medial tibial plateau.*
> - *The most familiar anomaly of the skeleton is probably a short fourth metacarpal, although this is seen in only about half of all cases and also may be seen in a variety of other clinical settings, including as a normal variant.*

van Buchem's Disease

BACKGROUND

van Buchem's disease is a sclerosing bone dysplasia first described in 1955. The eponym was formerly used to describe what are now considered to be several separate and distinct entities.[116] Classic van Buchem's disease, an autosomal recessive condition, is characterized by the same endosteal hyperostosis as its autosomal dominant counterpart, Worth syndrome, and another autosomal recessive form known as sclerostenosis. In both conditions, the underlying histologic abnormality appears to be a defect in the endochondral modulatory step regulating transformation of osteoclasts to osteoblasts.[61]

The latter may be fatal in infancy or early childhood.[291] Sclerosteosis is more common among South African Afrikaners than in other regions of the world and is less common in Holland.[13] Although Worth syndrome becomes apparent clinically by early childhood, van Buchem's disease may not become apparent until puberty and demonstrates more severe skeletal changes, especially involving the mandible and skull. Frontal bossing and a broad nasal bridge are typical. Laboratory examination may be normal, or the serum alkaline phosphatase level may rise. Worth syndrome, on the other hand, invariably demonstrates normal alkaline phosphatase levels. Symptoms associated with the bony changes typically are mild, and the condition may be found incidentally.

Skull changes may result in headache and cranial nerve palsies, with the facial and auditory nerves most frequently affected. Cranial nerve compression resulting from sclerosis and thickening of bone around the foramina may occur in early infancy, even before sclerosis and thickening of the skull are apparent radiographically.[77] Basal foraminal encroachment is another feature absent in Worth syndrome, and this also may assist in distinguishing between these two very similar conditions.[82]

IMAGING FINDINGS

Characteristic imaging changes involve diffuse, symmetric sclerosis and cortical thickening, affecting both the axial and appendicular skeleton. The calvarium is thick and sclerotic, the mandible is enlarged, and a torus palatinum may exist. Unlike other syndromes affecting mandibular morphology, dental occlusion is unaltered.[229] Peculiar bony excrescences may be seen at the ends of long bones, a finding not seen with Worth syndrome. Sclerosis and expansion of bone is often most prominent at the clavicles and ribs. Although the differences are minimal, bony expansion and lack of abnormalities of bone remodeling also may help to distinguish between van Buchem's disease and Worth syndrome.[61,116]

> **KEY CONCEPTS**
>
> - *van Buchem's disease is a sclerosing bone dysplasia involving cranial and endosteal hyperostosis.*
> - *van Buchem's disease may be confused with other uncommon disorders, such as familial hyperphosphatasia, osteopetrosis, and diaphyseal dysplasia (Camurati-Engelmann disease).*
> - *Characteristic imaging changes involve diffuse, symmetric sclerosis and cortical thickening, affecting both the axial and appendicular skeleton.*

References

1. Andersen PE Jr et al: Bilateral femoral head dysplasia and osteochondritis. Multiple epiphyseal dysplasia tarda, spondyloepiphyseal dysplasia tarda, and bilateral Legg-Perthes disease, *Acta Radiol* 29:705, 1988.
2. Anderson IJ et al: Spondyloepiphyseal dysplasia congenita: genetic linkage to type II collagen (COL2AI), *Am J Hum Genet* 46:896, 1990.
3. Arai Y et al: Brain CT studies in 26 cases of aged patients with Down syndrome, *Brain Dev* 27:17, 1995.
4. Aronson DC et al: Cor pulmonale and acute liver necrosis, due to upper airway obstruction as part of pycknodysostosis, *Eur J Pediatr* 141:251, 1984.
5. Atar D et al: New method of limb deformities correction in children, *Bull NY Acad Med* 68:447, 1992.
6. Atkinson RN et al: Bone scintigraphy in discitis and related disorders in children, *Aust NZ J Surg* 48:374, 1978.
7. Aufdermauer M, Spycher M: Pathogenesis of osteochondrosis juvenilis Scheuermann's, *J Orthop Res* 4:452, 1986.

8. Balestrazzi P et al: Juvenile rheumatoid arthritis in Turner's syndrome, *Clin Exp Rheumatol* 4:61, 1986.

9. Barfred T, Ipsen T: Congenital carpal tunnel syndrome, *J Hand Surg* 10A:246, 1985.

10. Bax MC, Colville GA: Behaviour in mucopolysaccharide disorders, *Arch Dis Child* 73:77, 1995.

11. Becker B et al: Melanocytic nevi in Turner's syndrome, *Pediatr Dermatol* 11:120, 1994.

12. Beighton P et al: Osteopetrosis in South Africa. The benign, lethal and intermediate forms, *S Afr Med J* 55:659, 1979.

13. Beighton P et al: The syndromic status of sclerosteosis and van Buchem's disease, *Clin Genet* 25:175, 1984.

14. Berg JM, Armstrong D: On the association of moyamoya disease with Down syndrome, *J Ment Defic Res* 35:398, 1991.

15. Bethen D et al: Disorders of the spine in diastrophic dwarfism, *J Bone Joint Surg Am* 62:529, 1980.

16. Bhatnagar M et al: Pediatric atlantoaxial instability presenting as cerebral and cerebellar infarcts, *J Pediatr Orthop* 11:103, 1991.

17. Bhojraj SY, Dandawate AV: Progressive cord compression secondary to thoracic disc lesions in Scheuermann's kyphosis managed by posterolateral decompression, interbody fusion and pedicular fixation. A new approach to the management of a rare clinical entity, *Eur Spine J* 3:66, 1994.

18. Bostman OM, Bakalim GE: Carpal tunnel syndrome in a melorheostotic limb, *J Hand Surg* 10B:101, 1985.

19. Bostman OM et al: Osteosarcoma arising in a melorheostotic femur: a case report, *J Bone Joint Surg Am* 69:1232, 1987.

20. Bourguignon JP et al: Effects of human growth hormone therapy on melanocytic nevi, *Lancet* 341:1505, 1993.

21. Bradford DS: Juvenile kyphosis, Clin Orthop, 128:45, 1977.

22. Bradford DS et al: Scheuermann's kyphosis: a form of osteoporosis? *Clin Orthop* 118:10, 1976.

23. Bradford DS et al: Scheuermann's kyphosis and roundback deformity. Results of Milwaukee brace treatment, *J Bone Joint Surg Am* 56:740, 1974.

24. Bradford DS et al: Scheuermann's kyphosis. Results of surgical treatment by posterior spine arthrodesis in twenty-two patients, *J Bone Joint Surg Am* 57:439, 1975.

25. Bradford DS, Moe JH: Scheuermann's juvenile kyphosis. A histologic study, *Clin Orthop* 110:45, 1975.

26. Brante G: Gargoylism: a mucopolysaccharidosis, *Scand J Clin Lab Invest* 4:43, 1952.

27. Bredenkamp JK et al: Otolaryngologic manifestations of the mucopolysaccharidoses, *Ann Otol Rhinol Laryngol* 101:472, 1992.

28. Brenton DP, Dow CJ: Homocystinuria and Marfan's syndrome. A comparison, *J Bone Joint Surg Br* 54:277, 1972.

29. Bridgeman SA et al: Leg lengthening, *J R Coll Surg Edinb* 38:101, 1993.

30. Bridges NA, Brook CG: Progress report: growth hormone in skeletal dysplasia, *Hormone Res* 42:231, 1994.

31. Brill PW et al: Homocystinuria due to cystathionine synthetase deficiency: clinical roentgenologic correlation, *AJR Am J Roentgenol* 121:45, 1974.

32. Brueton LA et al: Apparent cleidocranial dysplasia associated with abnormalities of 8q22 in three individuals, *Am J Med Genet* 43:612, 1992.

33. Buchanan WW: The arthritis of Mary Queen of Scots: due to Marfan's syndrome? *Clin Rheumatol* 5:419, 1986.

34. Caprio S et al: Insulin resistance: an early metabolic defect of Turner's syndrome, *J Clin Endocrinol Metab* 72:832, 1991.

35. Carson NAJ et al: Homocystinuria: clinical and pathological review of ten cases, *J Pediatr* 66:565, 1965.

36. Carson WG: Congenital elevation of the scapula. Surgical correction by the Woodward procedure, *J Bone Joint Surg Am* 63:1199, 1981.

37. Chitayat D et al: Intrafamilial variability in cleidocranial dysplasia: a three generation family, *Am J Med Genet* 42:298, 1992.

38. Chong WK, al-Kutoubi MA: Retroperitoneal fibrosis in Marfan's syndrome, *Clin Radiol* 44:386, 1991.

39. Clement PB, Young RH: Atypical polypoid adenomyoma of the uterus associated with Turner's syndrome. A report of three cases, including a review of "estrogen-associated" endometrial neoplasms and neoplasms associated with Turner's syndrome, *Int J Gynecol Pathol* 6:104, 1987.

40. Clements WD et al: Os odontoideum: congenital or acquired? That's not the question, *Injury* 26:640, 1995.

41. Collins ML et al: Optic nerve head swelling and optic atrophy in the systemic mucopolysaccharidoses, *Ophthalmology* 97:1445, 1990.

42. Crockard HA, Stevens JM: Craniovertebral junction anomalies in inherited disorders: part of the syndrome or caused by the disorder, *Eur J Pediatr* 154:504, 1995.

43. Cross HE, Jensen AD: Ocular manifestations in the Marfan's syndrome: a heritable disorder of connective tissue, *Am J Ophthalmol* 75:405, 1973.

44. Curless RG: Dominant chondrodysplasia punctata with neurological symptoms, *Neurology* 33:1095, 1983.

45. Currarino G: Primary spondylolysis of the axis vertebra (C2) in three children, including one with pyknodysostosis, *Pediatr Radiol* 19:535, 1989.

46. Currarino G, Swanson GE: A developmental variant of ossification in manubrium sterni in mongolism, *Radiology* 82:916, 1964.

47. da Silva EO et al: Ellis-van Creveld syndrome: report of 15 cases in an inbred kindred, *J Med Genet* 17:349, 1980.

48. Davis DC et al: Melorheostosis on three-phase bone scintigraphy. Case report, *Clin Nucl Med* 17:561, 1992.

49. Davis JW et al: Amino acids and collagen-induced platelet aggregation. Lack of effect of three amino acids that are elevated in homocystinuria, *Am J Dis Child* 129:1020, 1975.

50. de Jong JG et al: Measuring urinary glycosaminoglycans in the presence of protein: an improved screening procedure for mucopolysaccharidoses based on dimethylmethylene blue, *Clin Chem* 38:803, 1992.

51. de Mel T et al: Screening for Turner's syndrome: how useful is the buccal smear test? *Ceylon Med J* 37:83, 1992.

52. Deacon P et al: Combined idiopathic kyphosis and scoliosis. An analysis of the lateral spinal curvatures associated with Scheuermann's disease, *J Bone Joint Surg Br* 67:189, 1985.

53. D'iachkova GV: X-ray diagnosis of the state of soft tissues in patients with achondroplasia in limb lengthening using Ilizarov technique, *Vestn Rentgenol Radiol* 2:46, 1995.

54. DiMario FJ et al: Brain morphometric analysis in achondroplasia, *Neurology* 45:519, 1995.

55. Dissing I, Zafirovski G: Para-articular ossifications associated with melorheostosis Leri, *Acta Orthop Scand* 50:717, 1979.

56. Doman AN et al: Spondyloepiphyseal dysplasia of Maroteaux, *J Bone Joint Surg Am* 72:1364, 1990.

57. Domingues JC et al: Congenital sensory neuropathy with anhidrosis, *Pediatr Dermatol* 11:231, 1994.

58. Dore DD et al: Cleidocranial dysostosis and syringomyelia. Review of the literature and case report, *Clin Orthop* 214:229, 1987.

59. Dorfman A, Lorincz AE: Occurrence of urinary acid mucopolysaccharides in the Hurler's syndrome, *Proc Natl Acad Sci USA* 43:443, 1957.

60. Dugdale TW, Renshaw TS: Instability of the patellofemoral joint in Down syndrome, *J Bone Joint Surg Am* 68:405, 1986.

61. Eastman JR, Bixler D: Generalized cortical hyperostosis (van Buchem's disease): nosological considerations, *Radiology* 125:297, 1977.

62. Ehrich JH et al: Association of spondylo-epiphyseal dysplasia with nephrotic syndrome, *Pediatr Nephrol* 4:117, 1990.

63. Elmore SM: Pycnodysostosis. A review, *J Bone Joint Surg Am* 49:153, 1967.

64. Emerson JF et al: Magnetic resonance imaging of the aging brain in Down syndrome, *Progr Clin Biol Res* 393:123, 1995.
65. Eppley BL et al: Developmental significance of delayed closure of the mandibular symphysis, *J Oral Maxillofac Surg* 50:677, 1992.
66. Feldman GJ et al: A gene for cleidocranial dysplasia maps to the short arm of chromosome 6, *Am J Hum Genet* 56:938, 1995.
67. Fisk JW, Baigent ML: Hamstring tightness and Scheuermann's disease: a pilot study, *Am J Phys Med Rehabil* 60:122, 1981.
68. Fisk JW et al: Incidence of Scheuermann's disease. Preliminary report, *Am J Phys Med Rehabil* 61:32, 1982.
69. Fisk JW et al: Scheuermann's disease. Clinical and radiological survey of 17 and 18 year olds, *Am J Phys Med Rehabil* 63:18, 1984.
70. Fitzsimons RB: Idiopathic scoliosis, Scheuermann's disease and myopathy: two case reports, *Clin Exp Neurol* 16:303, 1979.
71. Forlin E et al: Understanding the os odontoideum, *Orthop Rev* 21:1441, 1992.
72. Fountzilas G et al: Extragonadal choriocarcinoma in a patient with Down syndrome, *Am J Clin Oncol* 17:452, 1994.
73. Franco B et al: A cluster of sulfatase genes on Xp22.3: mutations in chondrodysplasia punctata (CDPX) and implications for warfarin embryopathy, *Cell* 81:15, 1995.
74. Francomano CA et al: Localization of the achondroplasia gene to the distal 2.5 Mb of human chromosome 4p, *Hum Mol Genet* 3:787, 1994.
75. Franke J et al: Ilizarov-Techniken zur Beinverlangerung. Probleme und Ergebnisse, *Orthopade* 21:197, 1992.
76. French HG et al: Upper cervical ossicles in Down syndrome, *J Pediatr Orthop* 7:69, 1987.
77. Fryns JP, Van den Bergh H: Facial paralysis at the age of 2 months as a first clinical sign of van Buchem's disease, *Eur J Pediatr* 147:99, 1988.
78. Gardner WJ, Collins JS: The Klippel-Feil syndrome. Syringomyelia, diastematomyelia and myelomeningocele: one disease? *Arch Surg* 83:638, 1961.
79. Garver P et al: Melorheostosis of the axial skeleton with associated fibrolipomatous lesions, *Skeletal Radiol* 9:41, 1982.
80. Gatzoulis MA et al: Cardiac involvement in mucopolysaccharidoses: effects of allogenic bone marrow transplantation, *Arch Dis Child* 73:259, 1995.
81. Gelb BD et al: Genetic mapping of the cleidocranial dysplasia (CCD) locus on chromosome band 6p21 to include a microdeletion, *Am J Med Genet* 58:200, 1995.
82. Gelman MI: Autosomal dominant osteosclerosis, *Radiology* 125:289, 1977.
83. Gerrittsen T, Waisman HA: Homocystinuria, an error in metabolism of methionine, *Pediatrics* 33:413, 1964.
84. Gibson JB et al: Pathological findings in homocystinuria, *J Clin Pathol* 17:427, 1964.
85. Gilbert EF et al: Chondrodysplasia punctata: rhizomelic form, *Eur J Pediatr* 123:89, 1976.
86. Gilsanz V et al: Vertebral bone density in Scheuermann's disease, *J Bone Joint Surg Am* 71:894, 1989.
87. Goldman AB et al: Case report 778. Melorheostosis presenting as two soft tissue masses with osseous changes limited to the axial skeleton, *Skeletal Radiol* 22:206, 1993.
88. Goodwin CB et al: Cervical vertebral-costal process (costovertebral bone): a previously unreported anomaly. A case report, *J Bone Joint Surg Am* 66:1477, 1984.
89. Greene TL et al: Back pain and vertebral changes simulating Scheuermann's disease, *J Pediatr Orthop* 5:1, 1985.
90. Guidera KJ et al: Orthopaedic manifestations in congenitally insensate patients, *J Pediatr Orthop* 10:514, 1990.
91. Gustavson KH et al: Lethal and non-lethal diastrophic dysplasia. A study of 14 Swedish cases, *Clin Genet* 28:321, 1985.
92. Gyves-Ray K et al: Cystic lung disease in Down syndrome, *Pediatr Radiol* 24:137, 1994.
93. Halal F et al: Dominant inheritance of Scheuermann's juvenile kyphosis, *Am J Dis Child* 132:1105, 1978.
94. Hall GS: A continuation to the study of melorheostosis: unusual bone changes associated with tuberous sclerosis, *Q J Med* 12:77, 1943.
95. Hamner LH et al: Prenatal diagnosis of cleidocranial dysplasia, *Obstet Gynecol* 83:856, 1994.
96. Happle R et al: The CHILD syndrome: congenital hemidysplasia with ichthyosiform erythroderma and limb defects, *Eur J Pediatr* 134:27, 1980.
97. Harley EH, Collins MD: Neurological sequelae secondary to atlantoaxial instability in Down syndrome. Implications in otolaryngologic surgery, *Arch Otolaryngol Head Neck Surg* 120:159, 1994.
98. Harreby M et al: Are radiologic changes in the thoracic and lumbar spine of adolescents' risk factors for low back pain in adults? A 25-year prospective cohort study of 640 school children, *Spine* 20:2298, 1995.
99. Heggeness MH: Charcot's arthropathy of the spine with resulting paraparesis developing during in a patient with congenital insensitivity to pain. A case report, *Spine* 19:95, 1994.
100. Heithoff KB et al: Juvenile discogenic disease, *Spine* 19:335, 1994.
101. Hensinger RN et al: Klippel-Feil syndrome. A constellation of associated anomalies, *J Bone Joint Surg Am* 56:1246, 1974.
102. Hertel NT, Muller J: Anthropometry in skeletal dysplasia, *J Pediatr Endocrinol* 7:155, 1994.
103. Heselson NG, Marus G: Chronic atlanto-axial dislocation with spontaneous bony fusion, *Clin Radiol* 39:555, 1988.
104. Hilhorst MI et al: Down syndrome and coeliac disease: five new cases with a review of the literature, *Eur J Pediatr* 152:884, 1993.
105. Hinkle CO, Beilard D: Osteopetrosis, *AJR Am J Roentgenol* 74:46, 1955.
106. Hirata K et al: The Marfan's syndrome: cardiovascular physical findings and diagnostic correlates, *Am Heart J* 123:743, 1992.
107. Hoeffel JC et al: Localized form of spondylo-epiphyseal dysplasia congenita, *Rontgen-Blatter* 41:20, 1988.
108. Holt RG et al: Hypertrophy of C1 anterior arch: useful sign to distinguish os odontoideum from acute dens fracture, *Radiology* 173:207, 1989.
109. Horton WA et al: Growth hormone therapy in achondroplasia, *Am J Med Genet* 42:667, 1992.
110. Horton WA et al: The phenotypic variability of diastrophic dysplasia, *J Pediatr* 93:609, 1978.
111. Hosono N et al: Cineradiographic motion analysis of atlantoaxial instability in os odontoideum, *Spine* 16:S480, 1991.
112. Hresko MT et al: Hip disease in adults with Down syndrome, *J Bone Joint Surg Br* 75:604, 1993.
113. Ieshima A et al: A morphometric CT study of Down syndrome showing small posterior fossa and calcification of basal ganglia, *Neuroradiology* 26:493, 1984.
114. Iglesias JH et al: Renal artery stenosis associated with melorheostosis, *Pediatr Nephrol* 8:441, 1994.
115. Ingram RR: The shoulder in multiple epiphyseal dysplasias, *J Bone Joint Surg Br* 73:277, 1991.
116. Jacobs P: van Buchem's disease, Postgrad Med, 53:479, 1977.
117. Jensen BL: Cleidocranial dysplasia: craniofacial morphology in adult patients, *J Craniofac Genet Dev Biol* 14:163, 1994.
118. Jensen BL, Kreiborg S: Dental treatment strategies in cleidocranial dysplasia, *Br Dent J* 172:243, 1992.
119. Jensen BL, Kreiborg S: Development of the skull in infants with cleidocranial dysplasia, *J Craniofac Genet Dev Biol* 13:89, 1993.
120. Jensen BL, Kreiborg S: Craniofacial growth in cleidocranial dysplasia: a roentgencephalometric study, *J Craniofac Genet Dev Biol* 15:35, 1995.
121. Johnson CC et al: Osteopetrosis. A clinical, genetic, metabolic and morphologic study of the dominantly inherited benign type, *Medicine* 47:149, 1968.

122. Johnson MA et al: Magnetic resonance imaging of the brain in Hurler's syndrome, *Am J Neuroradiol* 5:816, 1984.

123. Kang AH, Trelstad RL: A collagen defect in homocystinuria, *J Clin Invest* 52:2571, 1973.

124. Kanis JA, Thomson JG: Mixed sclerosing bone dystrophy with regression of melorheostosis, *Br J Radiol* 48:400, 1975.

125. Katona K et al: Spondyloepiphyseal dysplasia tarda, *Rontgen-Blatter* 38:397, 1985.

126. Kawabata H et al: Melorheostosis of the upper limb: a report of two cases, *J Hand Surg* 9:871, 1984.

127. Khermosh O, Wientroub S: Dysplasia epiphysealis capitis femoris. Meyer's dysplasia, *J Bone Joint Surg Br* 73:621, 1991.

128. Kikuchi K et al: Bilateral vertebral artery occlusion secondary to atlantoaxial dislocation with os odontoideum: implication for prophylactic cervical stabilization by fusion-case report, *Neurol Med Chir* 33:769, 1993.

129. Kirlew KA et al: Os odontoideum in identical twins: perspective on etiology, *Skeletal Radiol* 22:525, 1993.

130. Kivara N et al: Intermediate form of osteopetrosis, with recessive inheritance, *Skeletal Radiol* 9:47, 1982.

131. Klippel M, Feil A: Absence de colonne cervicale. Cage thoracique remontant jusqu'à la base du crane, *Presse Med* 20:411, 1912.

132. Klippel M, Feil A: Anomalie de la colonne vertebrale par absence des vertebres cervicales; cage thoracique remontant jusqu'à la base du crane, *Bull Mem Soc Anat Paris* 87:185, 1912.

133. Kohn G et al: Spondyloepiphyseal dysplasia tarda: a new autosomal recessive variant with mental retardation, *J Med Genet* 24:366, 1987.

134. Kozlowski K, Beighton P: Radiographic features of spondyloepiphyseal dysplasia with joint laxity and progressive kyphoscoliosis. Review of 19 cases, *Rofo Fortschr Rontgenstr Neuen Bildgeb Verfahr* 141:337, 1984.

135. Kozlowski K, Masel J: Spondyloepiphysial dysplasia tarda (report of 7 cases), *Australas Radiol* 27:285, 1983.

136. Kuhlman JE et al: Acetabular protrusion in the Marfan's syndrome, *Radiology* 164:415, 1987.

137. Lachman R et al: Diastrophic dysplasia: the death of a variant, *Radiology* 140:79, 1981.

138. Lanes R et al: Bone mineral density of prepubertal age girls with Turner's syndrome while on growth hormone therapy, *Horm Res* 44:168, 1995.

139. Langer LO: Spondyloepiphyseal dysplasia tarda. Hereditary chondrodysplasia with characteristic vertebral configuration in the adult, *Radiology* 82:833, 1964.

140. Langer LO et al: Achondroplasia, *AJR Am J Roentgenol* 100:12, 1967.

141. Larner AJ et al: Congenital insensitivity to pain: a 20 year follow up, *J Neurol Neurosurg Psychiatry* 57:973, 1994.

142. Laughlin GM et al: Sleep apnea as a possible cause of pulmonary hypertension in Down syndrome, *J Pediatr* 98:435, 1981.

143. Lawrence JJ et al: Unusual radiographic manifestations of chondrodysplasia punctata, *Skeletal Radiol* 18(1):15, 1989.

144. LeDoux MS et al: Stabilization of the cervical spine in spondyloepiphyseal dysplasia congenita, *Neurosurgery* 28:580, 1991.

145. Lee SH, Sanderson J: Hypophosphatemic rickets and melorheostosis, *Clin Radiol* 40:209, 1989.

146. Lee C et al: The mucopolysaccharidoses: characterization by cranial MR imaging, *Am J Neuroradiol* 14:1285,1993.

147. Lin AE et al: Aortic dilation, dissection and rupture in patients with Turner's syndrome, *J Pediatr* 109(5):820, 1986.

148. Lippe B et al: Renal malformations in patients with Turner's syndrome: imaging in 141 patients, *Pediatrics* 82:852, 1988.

149. Lo RN et al: Abnormal radial artery in Down syndrome, *Arch Dis Child* 61:885, 1986.

150. Loncar J et al: Advent of maternal serum markers for Down syndrome screening, *Obstet Gynecol* 50:316, 1995.

151. Lopez RA et al: Osteoporosis in Scheuermann's disease, *Spine* 13:1099, 1988.

152. Lubec B et al: Evidence for McKusick's hypothesis of deficient collagen cross-linking in patients with homocystinuria, *Biochim Biophys Acta* 1315:159, 1996.

153. Lyritis G et al: Orthopaedic problems in patients with pycnodysostosis, *Prog Clin Biol Res* 104:199, 1982.

154. Magid D et al: Musculoskeletal manifestations of the Marfan's syndrome: radiologic features, *AJR Am J Roentgenol* 155:99, 1990.

155. Mandell GA et al: Bone scintigraphy in patients with atypical lumbar Scheuermann's disease, *J Pediatr Orthop* 13:622, 1993.

156. Mantero R: The Marfan's hands of Niccolo Paganini, *Ann Chir Main Memb Super* 7:335, 1988.

157. Manzke H et al: Dominant sex-linked inherited chondrodysplasia punctata. A distinct type of chondrodysplasia punctata, *Clin Genet* 17:97, 1980.

158. Marino B: Congenital heart disease in patients with Down syndrome: anatomical and genetic aspects, *Biomed Pharmacother* 47:197, 1993.

159. Martel W, Tishler JM: Observations on the spine in mongoloidism, *AJR Am J Roentgenol* 97:630, 1966.

160. Martich V et al: Hypoplastic posterior arch of C1 in children with Down syndrome: a double jeopardy, *Radiology* 183:125, 1992.

161. Massa G, Vanderschueren-Lodeweyckx M: Spondyloepiphyseal dysplasia tarda in Turner's syndrome, *Acta Paediatr Scand* 78:971, 1989.

162. Matsuda Y et al: Atlanto-occipital hypermobility in subjects with Down syndrome, *Spine* 20:2283, 1995.

163. Mayer EL et al: Homocysteine and coronary atherosclerosis, *J Am Coll Cardiol* 27:517, 1996.

164. McCallum MJ: Scheuermann's disease the result of emotional stress? *Med J Austr* 140:184, 1984.

165. McKenzie L, Silence D: Familial Scheuermann's disease: a genetic and linkage study, *J Med Genet* 29:41, 1992.

166. McKusick VA et al: Dwarfism in the Amish. The Ellis-Van Creveld syndrome, *Bull Johns Hopkins Hosp* 115:306, 1964.

167. McKusick VA: The classification of hereditable disorders of connective tissue, *Birth Defects* 11:1, 1975.

168. McKusick VA: Hereditable disorders of connective tissues, ed 4, St Louis, 1972, Mosby.

169. Mehta AV et al: Radiologic abnormalities of the sternum in Turner's syndrome, *Chest* 104:1795, 1993.

170. Miller JD et al: Changes at the skull and cervical spine in Down syndrome, *Can Assoc Radiol J* 37:85, 1986.

171. Mitchell V et al: Down syndrome and anaesthesia, *Pediatr Anaesthes* 5:379, 1995.

172. Miyata I et al: Pediatric cerebellar infarction caused by atlanto-axial subluxation-case report, *Neurol Med Chir* 34:241, 1994.

173. Morgan MK et al: Familial os odontoideum. Case report, *J Neurosurg* 70:636, 1989.

174. Murata R et al: MR imaging of the brain in patients with mucopolysaccharidosis, *Am J Neuroradiol* 10:1165, 1989.

175. Murray RO, McCredie J: Melorheostosis and the sclerotomes: a radiological correlation, *Skeletal Radiol* 4:57, 1979.

176. Nakashima N et al: Two cases of Turner's syndrome with spondyloepiphyseal dysplasia like bone appearance, *Fukuoka Igaku Zasshi* 81:384, 1990.

177. Natowicz M, Kelley RI: Association of Turner's syndrome with hypoplastic left heart-syndrome, *Am J Dis Child* 141:218, 1987.

178. Neely EK et al: Turner's syndrome adolescents receiving growth hormone are not osteopenic, *J Clin Endocrinol Metab* 76:861, 1993.

179. Nishi Y et al: Growth hormone therapy in achondroplasia, *Acta Endocrinol* 128:394, 1993.

180. Nissinen M: Spinal posture during pubertal growth, *Acta Paediatr* 84:308,1995.

181. Ogden JA et al: Sprengel's deformity. Radiology of the pathologic deformation, *Skeletal Radiol* 4(2):204, 1979.

182. Ohlsson A et al: Marble brain disease: recessive osteopetrosis, renal tubular acidosis and cerebral calcification in three Saudi Arabian families, *Dev Med Child Neurol* 22:72, 1980.

183. Olgilvie JW, Sherman J: Spondylolysis in Scheuermann's disease, *Spine* 12:251, 1987.

184. Ostrowski DM, Gilula LA: Mixed sclerosing bone dystrophy presenting with upper extremity deformities. A case report and review of the literature, *Br J Hand Surg* 17:108, 1992.

185. Ozbarlas N et al: Congenital insensitivity to pain with anhidrosis, *Cutis* 51:373, 1993.

186. Paajanen H et al: Disc degeneration in Scheuermann's disease, *Skeletal Radiol* 18:523, 1989.

187. Paajanen H et al: Magnetic resonance study of disc degeneration in young low-back pain patients, *Spine* 14:982, 1989.

188. Parker RD, Froimson AI: Neurogenic arthropathy of the hand and wrist, *J Hand Surg* 11A:706, 1986.

189. Patrone NA, Kredich DW: Arthritis in children with multiple epiphyseal dysplasia, *J Rheumatol* 12:145, 1985.

190. Pattisapu J et al: Cleidocranial dysostosis and schwannoma, *Neurosurgery* 18:827, 1986.

191. Pauli RM et al: Apnea and sudden unexpected death in infants with achondroplasia, *J Pediatr* 104:342, 1984.

192. Pauli RM et al: Prospective assessment of risks for cervicomedullary junction compression in infants with achondroplasia, *Am J Hum Genet* 56:732, 1995.

193. Peltonen JI et al: Cementless hip arthroplasty in diastrophic dysplasia, *J Arthroplasty* 7(suppl):369, 1992.

194. Peretti G et al: Staged lengthening in the prevention of dwarfism in achondroplastic children: a preliminary report, *J Pediatr Orthop* 4:58, 1995.

195. Perry HD, Cossari AJ: Chronic lymphangiectasis in Turner's syndrome, *Br J Ophthalmol* 70:396, 1986.

196. Peters ME et al: Narrow trachea in mucopolysaccharidoses, *Pediatr Radiol* 15:225, 1985.

197. Peyritz RE et al: Dural ectasia is a common feature of the Marfan's syndrome, *Am J Hum Genet* 43:726, 1988.

198. Piazza MR et al: Neuropathic spinal arthropathy in congenital insensitivity to pain, *Clin Orthop* 236:175, 1988.

199. Pizzutillo PD et al: Atlantoaxial instability in mucopolysaccharidosis type VII, *J Pediatr Orthop* 9:76, 1989.

200. Poker N et al: Spondyloepiphyseal dysplasia tarda. Four cases in childhood and adolescence, and some considerations about platyspondyly, *Radiology* 85:474, 1965.

201. Poussa M et al: The spine in diastrophic dysplasia, *Spine* 16:881, 1991.

202. Poznanski AK: Punctate epiphyses: a radiological sign, not a disease, *Pediatr Radiol* 24:418, 1994.

203. Price WH et al: Mortality ratios, life expectancy, and causes of death in patients with Turner's syndrome, *J Epidemiol Commun Health* 40:97, 1986.

204. Pruitt DL, Manske PR: Soft tissue contractures from melorheostosis involving the upper extremity, *J Hand Surg* 17A:90, 1992.

205. Pueschel SM et al: A longitudinal study of atlanto-dens relationships in asymptomatic individuals with Down syndrome, *Pediatrics* 89:1194, 1992.

206. Quinn SF, Dyer R: Osteopetrosis with calcifying tendinitis, *South Med J* 77:400, 1984.

207. Qureshi F et al: Skeletal histopathology in fetuses with chondroectodermal dysplasia (Ellis-Van Creveld syndrome), *Am J Med Genet* 45:471, 1993.

208. Raby N, Vivian G: Case report 478: melorheostosis of the axial skeleton with associated intrathecal lipoma, *Skeletal Radiol*, 17:216, 1988.

209. Rathore MH, Sreenivasan VV: Vertebral and right subclavian artery abnormalities in the Down syndrome, *Am J Cardiol* 63:1528, 1989.

210. Reed MH, Houston CS: Abnormal ossification of the hyoid bone in cleidocranial dysplasia, *Can Assoc Radiol J* 44:277, 1993.

211. Resnick D: Diagnosis of bone and joint disorders, ed 4, Philadelphia, 2002, WB Saunders.

212. Richards BS: Atlanto-axial instability in diastrophic dysplasia. A case report, *J Bone Joint Surg Am* 73:614, 1991.

213. Richardson A, Deussen FF: Facial and dental anomalies in cleidocranial dysplasia: a study of 17 cases, *Int J Paediatr Dent* 4:225, 1994.

214. Rintala A et al: Cleft palate in diastrophic dysplasia. Morphology, results of treatment and complications, *Scand J Plast Reconstr Surg Hand Surg* 20:45, 1986.

215. Roberts GM et al: Radiology of the pelvis and hips in adults with Down syndrome, *Clin Radiol* 31:475, 1980.

216. Robinson D et al: Spondyloepiphyseal dysplasia associated with progressive arthropathy. An unusual disorder mimicking juvenile rheumatoid arthritis, *Arch Orthop Trauma Surg* 108:397, 1989.

217. Robinson K et al: Homocysteine and coronary artery disease, *Cleveland Clin J Med* 61:438, 1994.

218. Robinson L et al: Multiple meningeal cysts in Marfan's syndrome, *Am J Neuroradiol* 10:1275, 1989.

219. Roger D et al: Melorheostosis with associated minimal change nephrotic syndrome, mesenteric fibromatosis and capillary hemangiomas, *Dermatology* 188:166, 1994.

220. Rosemberg S et al: Congenital insensitivity to pain with anhidrosis hereditary sensory and autonomic neuropathy type IV, *Pediatr Neurol* 11:50, 1994.

221. Rosenbaum DM et al: Atlanto-occipital instability in Down syndrome, *AJR Am J Roentgenol* 146:1269, 1986.

222. Rosenshtein A, Negrin JA: Increased Tc-99MDP in multiple lumbar intervertebral disk spaces in Scheuermann's disease without concomitant radiographic calcification or discitis, *Clin Nucl Med* 19:863, 1994.

223. Ross JL et al: Normal bone density of the wrist and spine and increased wrist fractures in girls with Turner's syndrome, *J Clin Endocrinol Metab* 73:355, 1991.

224. Ryan MD, Taylor TK: Acute spinal cord compression in Scheuermann's disease, *J Bone Joint Surg* 64B:409, 1982.

225. Ryken TC, Menezes AH: Cervicomedullary compression in achondroplasia, *J Neurosurg* 81:43, 1994.

226. Ryoppy S et al: Foot deformities in diastrophic dysplasia. An analysis of 102 patients, *J Bone Joint Surg Br* 74:441, 1992.

227. Saggese G et al: Mineral metabolism in Turner's syndrome: Evidence for impaired renal vitamin D metabolism and normal osteoblast function, *J Clin Endocrinol Metab* 75:998, 1992.

228. Schantz K et al: Spondyloepiphyseal dysplasia tarda. Report of a family with autosomal dominant transmission, *Acta Orthop Scand* 59:716, 1988.

229. Schendel SA: van Buchem's disease: surgical treatment of the mandible, *Ann Plast Surg* 20:462, 1988.

230. Scheuermann HW: Kyphosis dorsalis juvenilis, *Z Orthop Chir* 41:305, 1921.

231. Schuler TC et al: Natural history of os odontoideum, *J Pediatr Orthop* 11:222, 1991.

232. Scoles PV et al: Vertebral alterations in Scheuermann's kyphosis, *Spine* 16:509, 1991.

233. Sculerati N et al: Otitis media and hearing loss in Turner's syndrome, *Arch Otolaryngol* 116:704, 1990.

234. Selby KA et al: Clinical predictors and radiological reliability in atlanto-axial subluxation in Down syndrome, *Arch Dis Child* 66:876, 1991.

235. Sembel EL et al: Successful symptomatic treatment of melorheostosis with nifedipine, *Clin Exp Rheumatol* 4:277, 1986.

236. Shands AR Jr, Bunden WD: Congenital deformities of the spine. An analysis of the roentgenograms of 700 children, *Bull Hosp Jt Dis* 17:110, 1956.

237. Shapiro EG et al: Neuropsychological outcomes of several storage diseases with and without bone marrow transplantation, *J Inherit Metab Dis* 18:413, 1995.

PART TWO Bone, Joints, and Soft Tissues

238. Sheffield LJ et al: Chondrodysplasia punctata: 23 cases of a mild and relatively common variety, *J Pediatr* 89:916, 1976.

239. Sher C et al: Mild spondyloepiphyseal dysplasia (Namaqualand type): genetic linkage to the type II collagen gene COL2AI, *Am J Hum Genet* 48:518, 1991.

240. Siegel A, Williams H: Linear scleroderma and melorheostosis, *Br J Radiol* 65:266, 1992.

241. Silengo MC et al: Clinical and genetic aspects of Conradi-Hunermann disease, *J Pediatr* 97:911, 1980.

242. Silverman FN, Reiley MA: Spondylo-mega-epiphyseal-metaphyseal dysplasia: a new bone dysplasia resembling cleidocranial dysplasia, *Radiology* 156:365, 1985.

243. Sly WS et al: Recessive osteopetrosis, a new clinical phenotype, *Am J Hum Genet* 24:34,1972.

244. Sly WS et al: Carbonic anhydrase II deficiency in twelve families with autosomal recessive syndrome of osteopetrosis and renal tubular acidosis and cerebral calcifications, *N Engl J Med* 313:139, 1985.

245. Smith GV, Teele RL: Delayed diagnosis of duodenal obstruction in Down syndrome, *AJR Am J Roentgenol* 134:937, 1980.

246. Smith SW: Roentgen findings in homocystinuria, *AJR Am J Roentgenol* 100:147, 1967.

247. Smith NH: Albers-Schönberg's disease (osteopetrosis). Report of a case and review of the literature, *Oral Surg Oral Med Oral Pathol Oral Radiol Endodl* 22:6, 699, 1966.

248. Smolin LA et al: The use of betaine for treatment of homocystinuria, *J Pediatr* 99:467, 1981.

249. Soh LT et al: Embryonal carcinoma arising in Turner's syndrome, *Ann Acad Med Singapore* 21:386, 1992.

250. Somhegyi A, Ratko I: Hamstring tightness and Scheuermann's disease, *Am J Phys Med Rehabil* 72:44, 1993.

251. Sostrin RD et al: Myelographic features in mucopolysaccharidosis: a new sign, *Radiology* 125:421, 1977.

252. Spencer JA, Grieve DK: Congenital indifference to pain mistaken for non-accidental injury, *Br J Radiol* 63:308, 1990.

253. Spranger JW et al: Heterogeneity of chondrodysplasia punctata, *Hum Genet* 11:190, 1971.

254. Stafstrom CE: Epilepsy in Down syndrome: clinical aspects and possible mechanisms, *Am J Ment Retard* 98(suppl):12, 1993.

255. Stern WE: Dural ectasia and the Marfan's syndrome, *J Neurosurg* 69:221, 1988.

256. Stevens JM et al: A new appraisal of abnormalities of the odontoid process associated with atlanto-axial subluxation and neurological disability, *Brain* 117:133, 1994.

257. Stillerman CB, Wilson JA: Atlanto-axial stabilization with posterior transarticular screw fixation: technical description and report of 22 cases, *Neurosurgery* 32:948, 1993.

258. Stoddard A, Osborn JF: Scheuermann's disease or spinal osteochondrosis: its frequency and relationship with spondylosis, *J Bone Joint Surg* 61B:56, 1979.

259. Stoppoloni G et al: Characteristics of insulin resistance in Turner's syndrome, *Diabetes Metab* 16:267, 1990.

260. Subramaniam PN: Turner's syndrome and cardiovascular anomalies: a case report and review of the literature, *Am J Med Sci* 297:260, 1989.

261. Tachi N et al: Muscle involvement in congenital insensitivity to pain with anhidrosis, *Pediatr Neurol* 12:264, 1995.

262. Takakuwa T et al: Os odontoideum with vertebral artery occlusion, *Spine* 19:460, 1994.

263. Talroth K, Schlenzka D: Spinal stenosis subsequent to juvenile lumbar osteochondrosis, *Skeletal Radiol* 19:203, 1990.

264. Tambyah PA, Cheah JS: Hyperthyroidism and Down syndrome, *Ann Acad Med Singapore* 22:603, 1993.

265. Tangerud A et al: Degenerative changes in the cervical spine in Down syndrome, *J Ment Defic Res* 34:179, 1990.

266. Taybi H, Lachman RS: Radiology of syndromes, metabolic disorders, and skeletal dysplasias, ed 4, St Louis, 1996, Mosby.

267. Tertti M et al: Disc degeneration in young gymnasts. A magnetic resonance imaging study, *Am J Sports Med* 18:206, 1990.

268. Thomas SL et al: Hypoplasia of the odontoid with atlanto-axial subluxation in Hurler's syndrome, *Pediatr Radiol* 15:353, 1985.

269. Thomson SJ et al: Web neck deformity; anatomical considerations and options in surgical management, *Br J Plast Surg* 43:94, 1990.

270. Tishler JM, Martel W: Dislocation of the atlas in mongoloidism. A preliminary report, *Radiology* 84:904, 1965.

271. Torfs CP et al: Anorectal and esophageal anomalies with Down syndrome, *Am J Med Genet* 44:847, 1992.

272. Treble NJ et al: Development of the hip in multiple epiphyseal dysplasias. Natural history and susceptibility to premature osteoarthritis, *J Bone Joint Surg* 72B:1061, 1990.

273. Uematsu S et al: Total craniospinal decompression in achondroplastic stenosis, *Neurosurgery* 35:250, 1994.

274. van Linhoudt D, Revel M: Similar radiologic lesions of localized Scheuermann's disease of the lumbar spine in twin sisters, *Spine* 19:987, 1994.

275. van Wassenaer AG et al: Partial anomalous pulmonary venous return in Turner's syndrome, *Eur J Pediatr* 148:101, 1988.

276. Viljoen D, Beighton P: Marfan's syndrome: a diagnostic dilemma, *Clin Genet* 37:417, 1990.

277. Virdis R et al: Blood pressure behaviour and control in Turner's syndrome, *Clin Exp Hypertens* 8:787, 1986.

278. Waters KA et al: Breathing abnormalities in sleep in achondroplasia, *Arch Dis Child* 69:191, 1993.

279. Watts RWE et al: Computed tomography studies on patients with mucopolysaccharidoses, *Neuroradiology* 21:9, 1981.

280. Weinberg B et al: The prominent conoid process of the clavicle: a new radiographic sign in Down syndrome, *AJR Am J Roentgenol* 160:591, 1993.

281. Weiss SW: Pedal hemangioma (venous malformation) occurring in Turner's syndrome: an additional manifestation of the syndrome, *Hum Pathol* 19:1015, 1988.

282. Wells TR et al: Association of Down syndrome and segmental tracheal stenosis with ring tracheal cartilages: a review of nine cases, *Pediatr Pathol* 12:673:1992.

283. Wells TR et al: Studies of vertebral coronal cleft in rhizomelic chondrodysplasia punctata, *Pediatr Pathol* 13:123, 1993.

284. Whyte MP et al: Hypotrichosis with spondyloepimetaphyseal dysplasia in three generations: a new autosomal dominant syndrome, *Am J Med Genet* 36:288, 1990.

285. Whyte MP et al: Mixed sclerosing bone dystrophy: report of a case and review of the literature, Skeletal Radiol, 6:95, 1981.

286. Wiedemann HR: Otto Ullrich and his syndromes, *Am J Med Genet* 41:128, 1991.

287. Wilcken DEL et al: Homocystinuria-the effects of betaine in treatment of patients not responsive to pyridoxine, *N Engl J Med* 309:448, 1983.

288. Williams JW et al: Craniofacial melorheostosis: case report and review of the literature, *Br J Radiol* 64:60, 1991.

289. Willich E et al: Skeletal manifestations in Down syndrome. Correlation between roentgenologic and cytogenetic findings, *Ann Radiol* 18:355, 1975.

290. Wood KB et al: Magnetic resonance imaging of the thoracic spine. Evaluation of asymptomatic individuals, *J Bone Joint Surg Am* 77:1631, 1995.

291. Worth HM, Wollin DG: Hyperostosis corticalis generalisata congenita, *J Can Assoc Radiol* 17:69, 1966.

292. Wraith JE, Alani SM: Carpal tunnel syndrome in the mucopolysaccharidoses and related disorders, *Arch Dis Child* 65:962, 1990.

293. Yablon JS et al: Thoracic cord compression in Scheuermann's disease, *Spine* 13:896, 1988.

294. Yamashita Y et al: Atlantoaxial subluxation. Radiography and magnetic resonance imaging correlated to myelopathy, *Acta Radiol* 30:135, 1989.

295. Yamate T et al: Growth hormone (GH) treatment in achondroplasia, *J Ped Endocrinol* 6:45, 1993.
296. Yang SS et al: Two lethal chondrodysplasias with giant chondrocytes, *Am J Med Genet* 15:615, 1983.
297. Yellin A et al: Familial multiple bilateral pneumothorax associated with Marfan's syndrome, *Chest* 100:577, 1991.
298. Young DA: Rachmaninov and Marfan's syndrome, *BMJ* 299:1624, 1986.
299. Younge D et al: Melorheostosis in children. Clinical features and natural history, *J Bone Joint Surg* 61B:415, 1979.
300. Yousefzadeh DK et al: Radiographic studies of upper airway obstruction with cor pulmonale in a patient with pycnodysostosis, *Pediatr Radiol* 8:45, 1979.
301. Yu JS et al: Melorheostosis with an ossified soft tissue mass: MR features, *Skeletal Radiol* 24:367, 1995.
302. Yucel M et al: Treatment of florid dorsal Scheuermann's disease with two new breathable plaster-of-paris casts and their biomechanical principles of action, *Z Orthop Ihre Grenzgeb* 119:292, 1981.
303. Zangwill KM et al: Dandy-Walker malformation in Ellis-van Creveld syndrome, *Am J Med Genet* 31:123, 1988.
304. Zettergvist P et al: The man behind the syndrome: Antonin Marfan's, *Lakartidningen* 86:2205, 1989.
305. Zihni L: Downs' syndrome, interferon sensitivity and the development of leukaemia, *Leuk Res* 18:1, 1994.
306. Zipursky A et al: Leukemia in Down syndrome: a review, *Pediatr Hematol Oncol* 9:139, 1992.

PART TWO Bone, Joints, and Soft Tissues

chapter 9

Arthritides

Inflammatory and Crystal-Induced Arthritides

TAWNIA L. ADAMS

Degenerative Arthritides

DENNIS M. MARCHIORI

INFLAMMATORY ARTHRITIDES **Rheumatoid Arthritis**	**CRYSTAL-INDUCED ARTHRITIDES** **Gouty Arthritis** **Calcium Pyrophosphate Dihydrate**	**DEGENERATIVE ARTHRITIDES** **Degenerative Joint Disease** **Intervertebral Disc Herniation**
JUVENILE IDIOPATHIC ARTHRITIS	**Crystals** **Hemochromatosis**	**Spinal Stenosis** **Diffuse Idiopathic Skeletal**
Seropositive and Connective Tissue **Arthropathies** **Seronegative Spondyloarthropathy**	**Hydroxyapatite Deposition** **Disease**	**Hyperostosis** **Neuropathic Arthropathy**

Arthritis is the most common self-reported chronic condition among whites, the second most common among Native Americans and Hispanics, the third most common among blacks, and the fourth most common condition among Asians. For all groups, arthritis is a more prevalent chronic condition than heart disease, hearing impairments, chronic bronchitis, asthma, and diabetes.[106] Arthritis and its related conditions have a significant impact on activities of daily living, such as housekeeping, sleeping, driving, and working. Early recognition and appropriate management of arthritis are important to limit its progression and related disabilities.

IMAGING

Plain film radiography is still the most widely used and useful imaging modality for diagnosing, differentiating, and evaluating the various arthropathies.[552] Despite some limitations (e.g., insensitivity to very early joint changes), it is difficult to imagine proceeding to more advanced imaging techniques without first evaluating the patient with plain film radiography. It adequately demonstrates bone erosions, osteophytes, alterations of joint space, and misalignment. Plain film radiographs yield a relatively low dose of radiation, are inexpensive, and are readily and rapidly obtained. These factors make it perfect for baseline and serial studies that can be used to provide important information about the progression of the disease and the effectiveness of any treatment regimen. The addition of intraarticular injections of air or contrast allows limited demonstrations of the internal components of joints.

Advanced imaging modalities are being used in conjunction with plain film radiography because they may provide early detection of subtle findings such as synovitis, periarticular osteoporosis, and early erosions, when plain films are negative or inconclusive. Advanced imaging also is useful in evaluating joints with complex anatomy such as the sacroiliac (SI) articulations, which may be difficult to evaluate by the use of plain film. Computed tomography (CT) provides excellent anatomic detail and images in an axial plane. Magnetic resonance imaging (MRI) is used to evaluate the cartilaginous and ligamentous joint structures and marrow of the adjacent bone. Scintigraphy provides a useful method of gathering functional information to aid in morphologic assessments provided by other imaging modalities. Ultrasonography has the capability to define joint effusions and identify edematous connective tissues.

CLASSIFICATION

In general, arthritis can be grouped into three major categories: inflammatory (rheumatoid), crystal-induced (gout), and degenerative (osteoarthritis). Inflammatory arthritides are subdivided into rheumatoid arthritis (and related diseases) and connective tissue disorders. They also can be subdivided into rheumatoid types (seropositive) and rheumatoid variants (seronegative) based on the likelihood of the serologic presence or absence of the rheumatoid factor, as established by the latex fixation test.

Arthritis may be monoarticular or polyarticular. All types of arthritis may be monoarticular early in their pathologic course. Joint abnormalities that are caused by trauma or infections usually remain monoarticular. Arthritides are differentiated on the basis of clinical data and imaging studies (Table 9-1 and Fig. 9-1). The most useful information about them comes from plain film radiographs coupled with clinical data that relate to skeletal distribution, patient age, patient gender, joint swelling, joint stiffness, joint range of motion, symptom response to physical activity, and laboratory tests (e.g., erythrocyte sedimentation rate [ESR], antinuclear antibodies [ANAs], human leukocyte antigen [HLA] typing).

TABLE 9-1
Summary of Selected Arthritides

Arthritis/mode	F:M ratio	Age of onset	Target joints	Distribution	Radiographic features	Clinical features	Lab	Extraticular manifestations
Rheumatoid/inflammatory	3:1	40–70	MTP, MCP, PIP, knees, hips, cervical spine	Bilateral, symmetric	Capsular swelling, symmetric joint space narrowing, juxtaarticular osteoporosis, marginal erosions; joint deformity	Morning stiffness, joint swelling	+RF (IgM), ↑ESR, 10%–50% ANA, ↑C-reactive (CR) protein	Rheumatoid subcutaneous nodules, pulmonary, cardiovascular
JIA/inflammatory	3.5:1	<16	Knees; ankles; elbows; wrists; cervical spine	Bilateral, symmetric if polyarticular	Capsular swelling, symmetric joint space narrowing, juxtaarticular osteoporosis, marginal erosions, ankylosis, growth abnormalities, periostitis	Varies with subtype: systemic-fever, adenopathy; arthralgia; rash; limp	±RF, HLA-B27 and ANA depending on subtype; ↑ESR and C-R protein; systemic = leukocytosis	Varies with subtype; hepatosplenomegaly subcutaneous nodules; iridocyclitis
SLE/inflammatory	9:1	30–50	MCP; PIP of the hands primarily	Bilateral, symmetric	Nonerosive, reversible, joint deformities; osteonecrosis as possible complication	Arthralgia; butterfly rash; constitutional signs and symptoms	ANA (98%); anti–DNA antibodies; LE cells (70%–85%); RF (20%–35%); ↑ESR and C-R protein	Rash; renal disease; interstitial lung disease
Scleroderma/inflammatory	8:1	35–65	Distal tufts; DIP; PIP of the hands primarily	Bilateral, symmetric or asymmetric	Acroosteolysis, erosions, subcutaneous calcifications	Raynaud phenomenon; skin fibrosis; arthralgia of hands; telangiectasia	ANA in 60%; +RF (30%); ↑ESR	Skin fibrosis; renal fibrosis; GI fibrosis; interstitial lung disease; pericarditis
Polymyositis/dermatomyositis/inflammatory	2:1	40–60	Large muscles of the proximal appendicular skeleton; DIP, PIP, and MCPs	Bilateral, symmetric muscle involvement	Muscle edema; subcutaneous, intermuscular, and periarticular calcifications; transient osteopenia, soft-tissue swelling	Muscle weakness and atrophy; rash; arthralgia of hands, wrists, and knees	↑CPK; muscle biopsy = inflammation and degeneration	Interstitial lung disease; pericarditis
AS/inflammatory	1:10	15–35	SI; spine: vertebral bodies and apophyseal articulations; hip; shoulder	Bilateral, symmetric	Erosions; periostitis; ankylosis; thin, marginal syndesmophytes	LBP and stiffness; limited chest expansion	+HLA-B27 (90%); –RF, ↑ESR, and C-R protein	Interstitial fibrosis; aortic insufficiency; iritis

Type	M:F	Age	Location	Distribution	Radiographic Findings	Clinical	Laboratory	Associated
Enteropathic/ inflammatory	Varies with underlying bowel disorder	Varies	SI; spine; knee	Symmetric in axial skeleton; asymmetric in extremities	Mimics AS in the axial skeleton; nonerosive in the extremities	LBP and stiffness; IBD	+HLA-B27; –RF; ↑ESR	Underlying bowel disorder
Psoriatic/ inflammatory	1:1	30–50	Predilection for upper extremity; DIP and PIP; SI; spine	Bilateral, symmetric, or asymmetric in SI joints; asymmetric in extremities	Sausage digit; marginal or central erosions with periostitis; early joint space widening with eventual narrowing; bulky, nonmarginal syndesmophytes; SI erosions and ankylosis	Psoriasis; nail changes (thickening, pitting, discoloration); LBP	+HLA-B27; –RF; ↑ESR	Psoriatic skin and nail changes
Reiter's/ inflammatory	1:5	15–35	Predilection for lower extremity; MTP; calcaneus; SI; spine	Asymmetric in foot; bilateral, symmetric, or asymmetric in SI joints	Mimics psoriatic in the spine and extremities; calcaneal enthesopathy	LBP; heel pain, urethritis; conjunctivitis	Leukocytosis; ↑ESR; HLA-B27 (75%); –RF	Pulmonary fibrosis; urethritis; conjunctivitis
Gout/crystal deposition	1:20	40–50	MTP of first digit; other MTPs, DIP, midfoot, ankle, DIPs of hand	Asymmetric; often monoarticular	Soft-tissue nodules (tophi) with calcification; paraarticular erosions; overhanging edge; preserved joint space; lack of osteopenia	Red, hot, swollen joint; usually monoarticular	Hyperuricemia; sodium urate crystals in synovial fluid	Tophus in bursa or helix of the ear
CPPD/crystal deposition	Varies with site of involvement	Varies; increases with age	Knee; wrist; hip; MCP	Often bilateral, asymmetric	Chondrocalcinosis; DJD-like changes; subchondral cysts	Varies from asymptomatic to acute goutlike pain.	Calcium pyrophosphate crystals in synovial fluid	None
HADD/ crystal deposition	1:1	40–70	Shoulder	Asymmetric; usually monoarticular	Cloudlike periarticular calcification	Varies from asymptomatic to acute joint pain	Hydroxyapatite crystals by electron microscopy	None

ANA, Antinuclear antibodies; *AS*, ankylosing spondylitis; *CPK*, creatinine phosphokinase; *CPPD*, calcium pyrophosphate dihydrate; *ESR*, erythrocyte sedimentation rate; *HADD*, hydroxyapatite deposition disease; *IBD*, inflammatory bowel disease; *JIA*, juvenile idiopathic arthritis; *LBP*, low back pain; *MCP*, metacarpophalangeal; *MTP*, metatarsophalangeal; *PIP*, proximal interphalangeal joint; *RF*, rheumatoid factor; *SI*, sacroiliac.

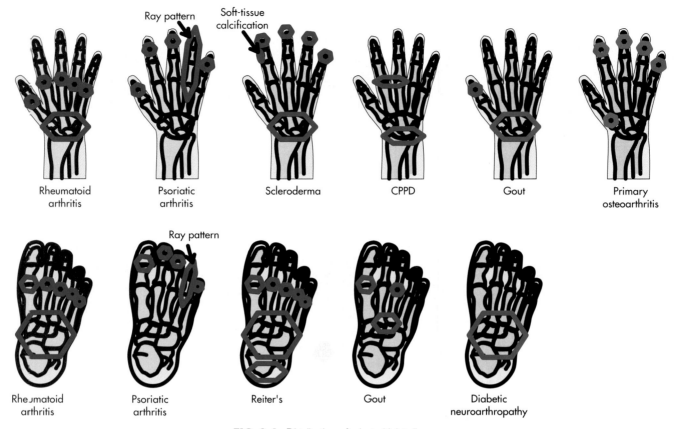

FIG. 9-1 Distribution of selected joint diseases.

Inflammatory Arthritides

Rheumatoid Arthritis

Adult Rheumatoid Arthritis

BACKGROUND

Rheumatoid arthritis (RA) is an autoimmune disorder, and the most common chronic inflammatory arthritide, affecting approximately 1% of the general population and 2% of the population over 60 years old.[243,607,610] However, studies indicate that the incidence may be on a decline in certain populations.[155,289,303,304,503] The disease primarily affects the synovial lined joints and is frequently associated with a variety of extraarticular manifestations. RA is characterized by an inflammatory, hyperplastic synovitis (pannus), resulting in cartilage and bone destruction and consequent loss of function. Although it is known that genetic and immunologic factors play a role in its pathogenesis, the underlying etiology remains uncertain.[316,537] Proposed etiologic theories revolve around a combination of genetic susceptibility, hormonal changes or imbalances (e.g., pregnancy), and environmental or biologic triggers or risk factors (e.g., smoking, obesity).[30,129,338,679] The T cell is involved in initiating and possibly propagating the chronic inflammatory disease process. Competing theories hold that the T cell initiates the disease process, but the chronic inflammation is self-perpetuated via macrophages and fibroblasts independent of the T cell.

Joint involvement typically is bilateral and symmetric, involving the peripheral and axial skeleton, with the small joints of the hands and feet, the wrists, knees, elbows, hips, and shoulders

particularly affected.[89] Changes in SI articulations are relatively infrequent. Although the peak occurrence of disease onset has previously been reported as 20 to 50 years of age, recent trends indicate an increased age of onset as 40 to 70 years old, with the peak occurrence at age 58.[155,303] Women are affected more often than men, and although some studies have shown a ratio as high as 7:1, it is generally accepted that women are affected two to three times more frequently than men.[63,129,406,610] If the disease onset occurs at a more advanced age (>60 years), this ratio approaches 1:1.[488,658]

IMAGING FINDINGS

Plain film radiography is an inexpensive tool and may be used by practitioners on a frequent basis in clinical practice to support clinical and laboratory findings consistent with a diagnosis of RA, aid in eliminating possible differential diagnoses, and follow the progression of RA and the effectiveness of its treatment.[568,590] Ultrasonography and MRI are superior in detecting synovitis, and many of the initial subtle joint changes are visible much earlier with MRI; however, it is not used routinely because of its high cost. Therefore this section focuses on plain film findings.[123,165,513]

RA is classically symmetric and may involve any synovial joint. The general radiographic findings reflect the underlying pathologic change of chronic synovial joint inflammation with associated hyperemia, edema, and pannus formation. The first feature, which is usually the sole finding for the first few months, is fusiform periarticular soft-tissue swelling arising from capsular

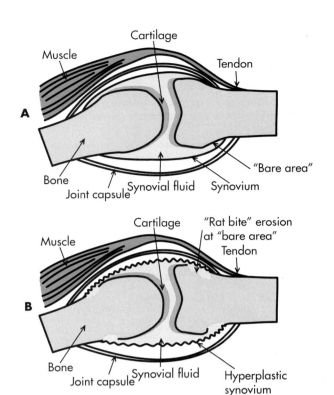

FIG. 9-2 **A** and **B,** Inflamed, hyperplastic synovitis of rheumatoid arthritis, known as *pannus,* classically demonstrates early osseous erosions at the margins of the synovial joint that are unprotected by articular cartilage ("bare area").

distention caused by excessive fluid accumulation seen clinically. Increased blood flow to the synovium leads to a second early radiographic finding of juxtaarticular osteoporosis, which later becomes more generalized because of patient inactivity.[298,380]

Joint spaces eventually narrow uniformly as the cartilage is destroyed by the enzymatic nature of pannus. Osseous erosions usually become apparent within the first 2 years of the disease,[84,212,512] first occurring at the unprotected bone margins or "bare areas" (Fig. 9-2) in which the pannus has direct osseous contact, and later involving the subchondral bone. The appearance of alternating pattern of erosions and normal cortical bone has been termed a "dot dash" appearance. Multiple, nonmarginated subchondral cysts or geodes typically develop and may communicate with the synovium.[400,652]

Later stages of the disease give rise to joint deformities resulting from tendon and ligament laxity, ruptures, and contractures. During periods of prolonged remission, radiographic signs of secondary osteoarthritis (OA) may develop, fibrous ankylosis may occur, and bony ankylosis may develop on rare occasions.

Hands and feet. The earliest clinical and radiographic changes are characteristically found in the hands and feet.[652] Although evaluation methods of RA focus on radiographs of the hands, the feet appear to show osseous erosions first and to a greater extent.[84,272,284,512,651] The initial involvement is of the head of the fifth metatarsal, with erosion and narrowing of the fifth metatarsophalangeal (MTP) joint.

The classic joint distribution of RA in the hands is bilateral and symmetric involvement of the metacarpophalangeal (MCP) and proximal interphalangeal joint (PIP) articulations. Some or all of the general radiographic features may be seen, with the earliest osseous erosions occurring at the MCP joints of the second and

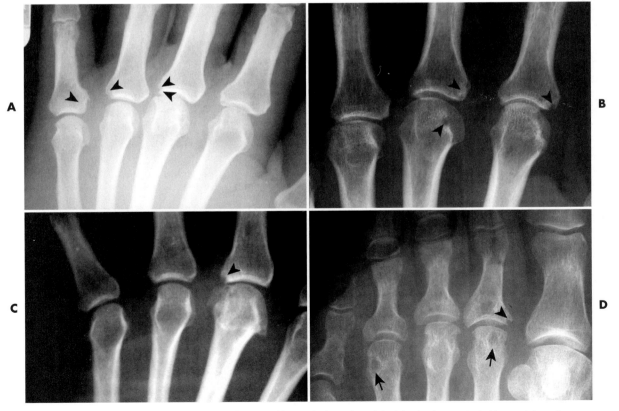

FIG. 9-3 Small marginal "rat bite" erosions *(arrowheads)* occur in the region of the joint that is unprotected by overlying articular cartilage, known as the *bare area.* **A** to **C,** Small marginal erosions of the metacarpophalangeal and, **D,** metatarsophalangeal joints are hallmark features of rheumatoid arthritis, noted here in three patients. Subchondral cysts also are noted in case **D** *(arrow).*

third digits of the dominant hand,[357] and at the radial aspect of the metacarpal heads (Fig. 9-3). Norgaard and Brewerton's views may aid in visualization of these early joint erosions, although it is difficult to duplicate the exact positioning on serial radiography.[652] In Norgaard's view, the hands are 45 degrees supine, with the fingers straight,[461] and in Brewerton's view *(ballcatcher's view)*, the MCP joints are flexed at 65 degrees.[79]

Characteristic joint deformities include the swan neck deformity, boutonnière deformity, ulnar deviation of the fingers *(doigts en coup de vent)*, and the hitchhiker's or Z-shaped deformity of thumb. The swan neck deformity results from hyperextension of the PIP and hyperflexion of the distal interphalangeal joint (DIP) (Figs. 9-4 to 9-7), whereas the boutonnière deformity represents the opposite configuration of hyperflexion of the PIP and hyperextension of the DIP. The hitchhiker's thumb is secondary to MCP flexion and interphalangeal (IP) extension (see Fig. 9-5). Ulnar deviation at the MCPs is called ulnar drift; when combined with radial deviation in the radiocarpal articulations it results in a "zigzag" deformity (see Fig. 9-5). Loosening or disruption of the distal attachment of the extensor tendon to the terminal phalanx leads to a "mallet" finger.

Changes in the feet tend to parallel those of the hands, with the MTP articulations commonly being affected first and other deformities, including lateral or fibular deviation at the MTPs of the first through fourth digits, flexion of the DIPs (hammer or claw toes), and extension of the MTPs eventually developing (Figs. 9-8 to 9-11).

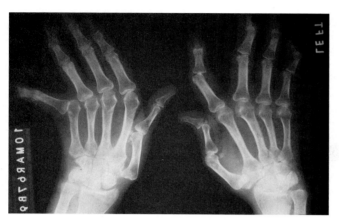

FIG. 9-4　Rheumatoid arthritis. The ulnar deviation of the fingers, especially prominent at the fifth digit of the right hand, and Z-deformity of the left thumb are the most obvious features of rheumatoid arthritis in this patient. (Courtesy Steven P. Brownstein, MD, Springfield, NJ.)

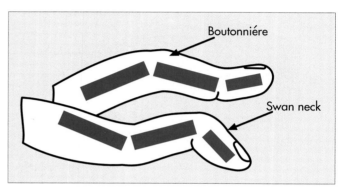

FIG. 9-6　Rheumatoid arthritis characteristically manifests with interphalangeal joint misalignments. The misalignments express either swan neck deformity (flexion of distal and extension of the proximal interphalangeal joints) or boutonnière deformity (extension of the distal and flexion of the proximal interphalangeal joints).

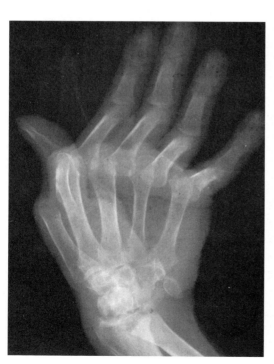

FIG. 9-5　Ulnar deviations of the fingers and advanced arthropathy of the metacarpocarpal joints and wrist are consistent with rheumatoid arthritis. (Courtesy Steven P. Brownstein, MD, Springfield, NJ.)

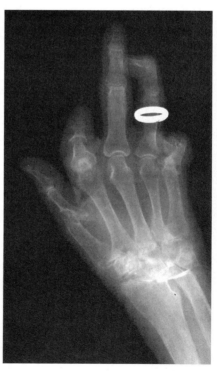

FIG. 9-7　Rheumatoid arthritis with ulnar deviation of the fingers, metacarpal joint involvement, and advanced destruction of the wrist. (Courtesy Gary Longmuir, Phoenix, AZ.)

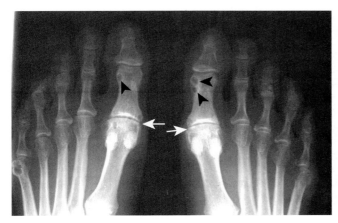

FIG. 9-8 Rheumatoid arthritis presenting with subchondral cysts *(arrowheads)* and reduction of the first metatarsophalangeal joint bilaterally *(arrows)*.

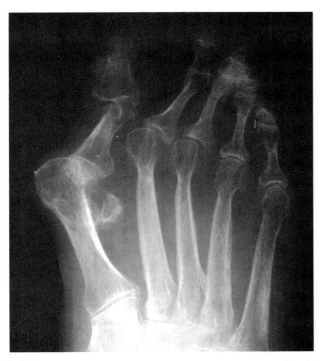

FIG. 9-9 Rheumatoid arthritis of the foot with advanced changes of the fibular misalignment of the toes, osteopenia (more pronounced in the periarticular regions), reduced joint spaces, and generalized atrophy of the bones.

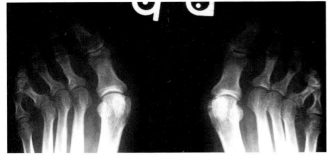

FIG. 9-10 Fifty-year-old male rheumatoid patient demonstrating marked symmetric and bilateral fibular deviation of the toes. (Fibular deviation with posterior subluxation of the metatarsophalangeal joints is termed *Lanois deformity*.)

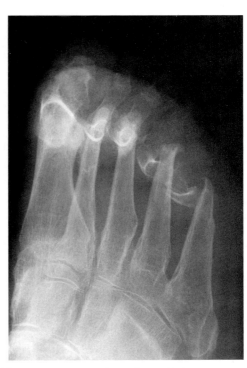

FIG. 9-11 Rheumatoid arthritis manifests with bone reapportion. In this 64-year-old woman, rheumatoid arthritis has caused a tapered appearance of the distal metatarsals.

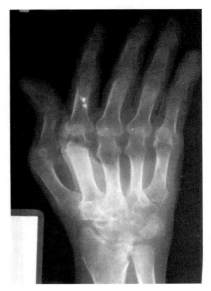

FIG. 9-12 Rheumatoid arthritis presenting with wrist and metacarpal destruction with slight ulnar deviation of the fingers. (Courtesy Steven P. Brownstein, MD, Springfield, NJ.)

Pathologic changes in the deep transverse tendons may lead to spreading of the metatarsals or forefoot. Pathologic changes in supporting ligaments also may lead to hallux valgus. Retrocalcaneal bursitis, plantar fasciitis, Achilles tendonitis, or Achilles tendon rupture may occur in the heel.

Wrist. Pancompartmental involvement typically is in the wrist, with the earliest erosions usually involving the radial and ulnar styloid processes; distal radioulnar and radiocarpal joints; and waist of the scaphoid, triquetrum, and pisiform (Figs. 9-12 to 9-16).[357] Ligamentous instability results in patterns that parallel posttraumatic lesions, such as scapholunate dissociation, distal radioulnar dissociation, and dorsiflexion or volar flexion instability.

Elbows. Joint effusion is recognized by a positive fat pad sign. Osseous erosions may be noted at each of the articulating surfaces.

Shoulders. The glenohumeral and acromioclavicular (AC) joints may be affected. Resorption of the distal clavicle, in addition to erosions at the coracoclavicular ligament insertion on the undersurface of the clavicle, is not uncommon. Erosion may be observed on the medial aspect of the humeral neck as it abuts the glenoid process from elevation of the humerus, which is caused by a rotator cuff tear secondary to a chronically inflamed supraspinatus tendon. The acromiohumeral distance narrows with progressive elevation of

the humeral head, and sclerosis and cyst formation are noted on the adjacent portions of the humeral head and acromion process.

Hips. Abnormalities of the hips generally are bilateral and symmetric. Axial migration of the femoral head and bilateral acetabular protrusion are common findings that accompany the other general features of concentric joint space narrowing, erosions, and subchondral cysts associated with RA (Figs. 9-17 and 9-18).[134] There is an absence of sclerosis and osteophyte formation unless secondary OA has developed.

Knees. Tricompartmental involvement that includes the general features of joint space narrowing and osseous erosions is typical (Figs. 9-19 and 9-20). A genu valgus deformity is more likely to develop than a varus joint deformity (Fig. 9-21). Soft-tissue swelling may be present in the form of suprapatellar effusion or a large popliteal (or Baker's) cyst. Subchondral sclerosis and osteophytes may be noted with the development of secondary osteoarthritis.

Cervical spine. RA involvement is rare in other regions of the axial skeleton but affects the cervical spine in more than half the patients within the first 10 years of disease onset,[531,652] with a preference for the apophyseal and atlantoaxial joints. The more chronic the disease, the greater is the likelihood of cervical involvement.[466] Radiographs of the cervical spine are a prudent consideration in all

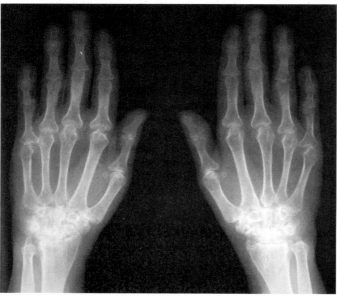

FIG. 9-13 Rheumatoid arthritis presenting with bilateral, symmetric destructive changes of the intercarpal joints of the wrist.

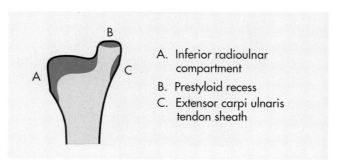

FIG. 9-14 Erosions of the ulnar styloid may manifest in each of the areas that have adjacent synovial tissue: radiocarpal joint, prestyloid recess, and extensor carpi ulnaris.

A. Inferior radioulnar compartment
B. Prestyloid recess
C. Extensor carpi ulnaris tendon sheath

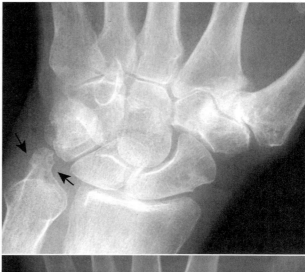

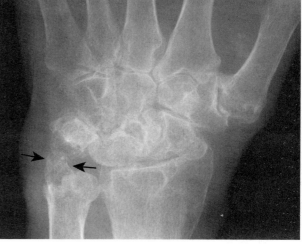

FIG. 9-15 **A** and **B,** Erosions of the styloid process in two patients *(arrows).*

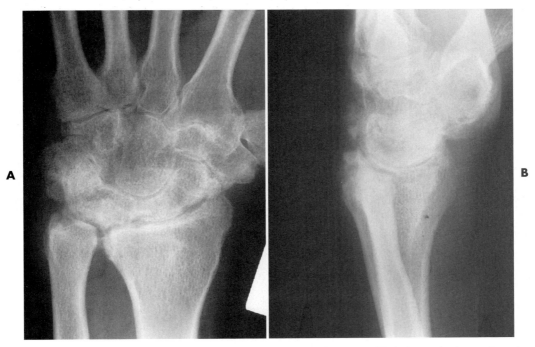

FIG. 9-16 **A** and **B,** Rheumatoid arthritis in the wrist. Inflammation is most notable in the proximal row of carpals, radiocarpal compartment, and distal ulna. Mild osseous proliferation is noted, suggesting clinical quiescence.

patients with RA regardless of symptoms, because many patients are asymptomatic despite cervical involvement.[117] These should include lateral views with the patient in flexion and extension.

Atlantoaxial subluxation or instability is the most common radiographic abnormality encountered in the cervical spine, with the prevalence varying from 19% to 70% depending on the patient selection and radiographic examination (Fig. 9-22).[311] Movement may occur in several directions (listed in order of decreasing frequency): anterior (most frequent, 9.5% to 36%), lateral, vertical, or posterior.[55,107] Movement is usually the result of odontoid erosions or transverse ligament laxity, although the alar and apical ligaments also may be involved.

The degree of anterior subluxation shown on conventional radiography correlates poorly with neurologic signs and the presence of cord compression, which is in part a result of the unknown thickness of the synovial pannus not visible on plain films.[55,542] The standard method for determining anterior atlantoaxial subluxation has been an anterior atlantodental interval* (ADI) of greater than 3 mm, but it has been shown that a posterior atlantodental interval† (PADI) of 14 mm or less may be a more reliable predictor for neural compression and necessitate an MRI for evaluation of true cord space (Fig. 9-23).[55]

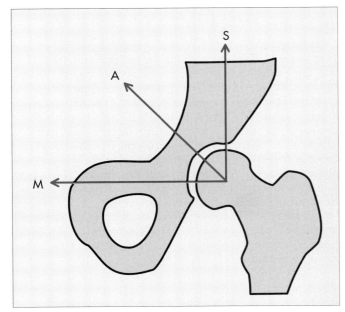

FIG. 9-17 The iliofemoral joint is divided into an, *M,* medial; *A,* axial; and, *S,* superior component. The inflammatory arthritides, inclusive of rheumatoid arthritis, tend to decreased all of these spaces symmetrically, whereas degenerative joint disease reduces the superior, weight-bearing aspect of the joint and increases the medial joint space.

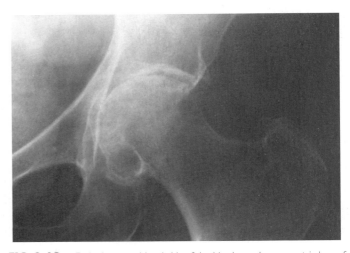

FIG. 9-18 Early rheumatoid arthritis of the hip shown by concentric loss of joint space, small erosions of the femoral head and acetabulum, and osteopenia. Note the lack of osteophytosis and eburnation.

PART TWO
Bone, Joints, and Soft Tissues

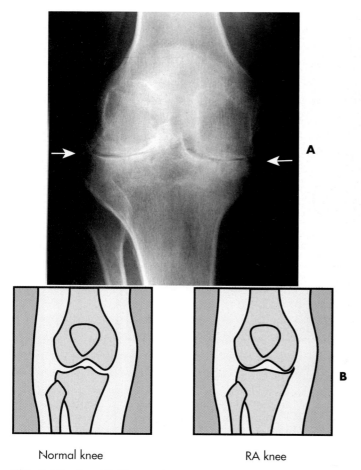

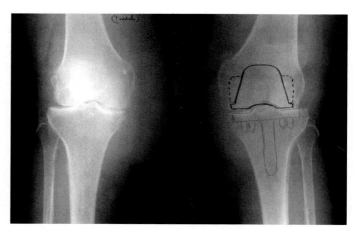

FIG. 9-21   Genu valgus deformity is noted in this 57-year-old woman. The film is annotated in preparation for surgical placement of a prosthesis.

FIG. 9-19   **A** and **B,** Rheumatoid arthritis noted by symmetric reduction of both the medial and lateral femorotibial joint spaces *(arrows).*

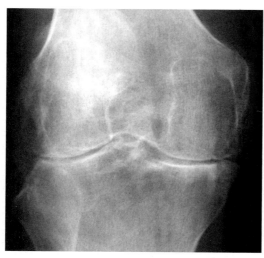

FIG. 9-20   Rheumatoid arthritis. In this case, rheumatoid manifests with osteoporosis and symmetric loss of the femorotibial joint spaces. The symmetric loss of joint space noted in these cases is contrary to what is expected with degenerative joint disease. Degeneration presents with asymmetric loss of joint space (more advanced in the medial femorotibial compartment) and osteophytes.

Vertical atlantoaxial subluxation also is known as cranial settling, atlantoaxial impaction, and pseudobasilar invagination. Superior migration of the odontoid occurs with erosion of the occiput-C1 and C1-2 articulations, resulting in approximation of the dens and brainstem, which can lead to direct compression or cause neurologic damage by excessive kyphosis.[92,542] McGregor's line may be used to assess superior migration, or the Sakaguchi-Kauppi method may be used, which was developed for screening purposes and evaluating the position of C1 in relation to C2.[312]

Subaxial subluxations may occur in 10% to 20% of patients and often are at multiple levels. C3-4 and C4-5 are the most common areas of involvement, producing a "stepladder" or "doorstep" deformity and associated kyphosis on the lateral radiograph.[478] Although these are less common than upper cervical spine subluxations, they are potentially more important neurologically because of the smaller spinal canal dimensions.[55,107] A canal measurement may be taken from the lateral radiograph in a similar way that the PADI is taken. If the subaxial canal diameter measures less than 14 mm, MRI is advised.[55]

Disc height narrowing, mild subchondral sclerosis, and erosions of the vertebral endplates, facet joints, and spinous processes are other less severe signs of rheumatoid involvement. These signs often are subtle and difficult to diagnose on plain film radiographs.

Lungs. Lung involvement is common, although not always clinically significant. Pleural involvement (e.g., pleurisy, pleural effusion) is the most common lung manifestation and usually is asymptomatic.[13] Other pulmonary manifestations include pulmonary fibrosis or honeycombing, constrictive bronchiolitis, bronchiectasis, pulmonary nodules, and subpleural micronodules (Fig. 9-24). High-resolution computed tomography (HRCT) is useful for this avenue of investigation. These findings have been observed on CT in patients with symptoms, and those asymptomatic patients with no abnormalities noted on chest plain film.[546] Caplan syndrome describes inflammation and scarring of pulmonary tissue in people with RA who have exposure to coal dust.

*The ADI is the distance between the posteroinferior aspect of the anterior arch of the atlas and the most anterior point of the odontoid process. Measurements of greater than 3 cm are considered abnormal. The measurement should be obtained from a lateral flexion radiograph.
†The PADI is measured from the posterior wall of the dens to the anterior aspect of the C1 lamina.

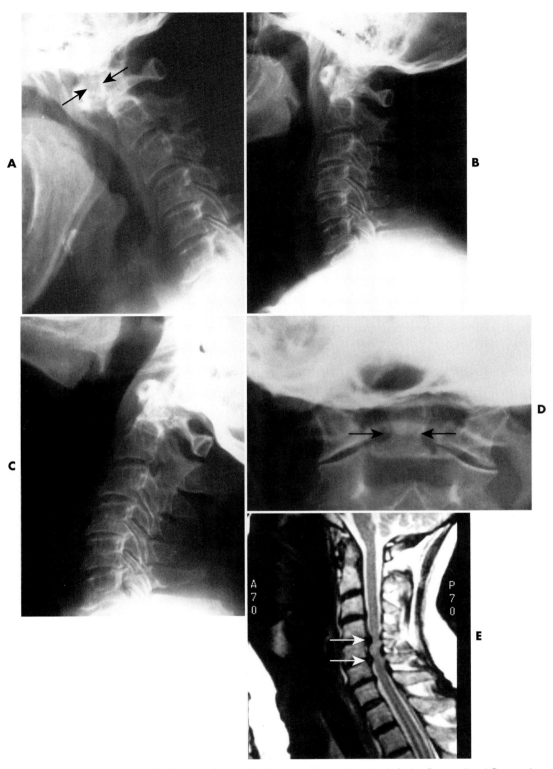

FIG. 9-22 Anterior atlantoaxial subluxation. **A,** Lateral radiographs of the cervical spine in flexion; **B,** neutral; and, **C,** extension positions revealing an atlantoaxial subluxation that is most notable on the flexion radiograph. Note the wide gap between the posterior surface of the anterior arch of the atlas and anterior aspect of the odontoid *(arrows)*. **D,** The anteroposterior open mouth radiograph of the same patient reveals rheumatoid erosions at the base of the odontoid process *(arrows)*. The lateral atlantoaxial joints appear unaffected. **E,** Sagittal T2-weighted magnetic resonance image (MRI) of same patient revealing marrow changes of the odontoid process, synovial inflammation, and multiple subaxial subluxations in the middle and lower regions of the cervical spine with disc protrusions *(arrows)* and resulting cord compression. Instability resulting from rheumatoid pannus is a concern for neck movement, including chiropractic adjustments, neck movement with spinal surgery, or placement of an endotracheal tube related to emergency medicine. If instability is suspected, flexion-extension studies, computed tomography, or MRI are warranted for further investigation.

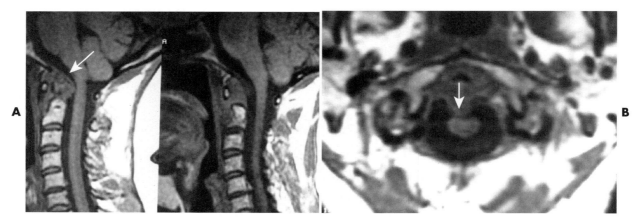

FIG. 9-23   **A,** Sagittal T1-weighted gradient echo and, **B,** axial gradient echo magnetic resonance images revealing prominent synovial inflammation (pannus) in the posterior median atlantoaxial joint *(arrow)* with apparent destruction of the dens and mild compression of the spinal cord *(arrow)*.

CLINICAL COMMENTS

The criteria for the diagnosis of RA, which were designed originally to aid in research consistency, have been revised and are now easier for the clinician to use.[22] The diagnosis can be made if the patient meets at least four of the following criteria established by the American College of Rheumatology. The first four must be present for at least 6 weeks.

1. Stiffness in the morning that lasts at least 1 hour
2. Swelling of at least three joints
3. Swelling of the wrist, MCP, or PIP joints
4. Symmetric swelling
5. Rheumatoid nodules
6. Positive rheumatoid factor test
7. Radiographic changes consistent with RA

The joint stiffness is sometimes termed *jelling phenomenon* and occurs in the morning or after periods of inactivity. Jelling also is described in fibromyalgia.

Although the main sites affected by RA are the joints, extraarticular manifestations are common. Rheumatoid nodules are the classic extraarticular lesions. These subcutaneous lesions are found in approximately 25% to 40% of patients and are typically located on the extensor surfaces at sites subject to trauma.[406,610] These nodules also can be present in visceral organs. Pulmonary and cardiovascular systems often are affected in patients with RA. Two syndromes associated with RA are Felty (a combination of RA, splenomegaly, and neutropenia) and Sjögren (marked by RA and dry eyes and mouth). A laboratory clue to Felty syndrome is decreased white blood cells, which occurs with splenomegaly.

Patients with RA tend to have reduced life expectancies and decreases in their ability to perform activities of daily living and work.[454,510] The disease course is variable, ranging from mild with periods of remission to severe and quickly progressive. The highest rate of joint damage and progression occurs early in the disease; therefore treatment should begin immediately after the diagnosis is made so that irreversible joint damage is prevented.[652] Known risk factors may increase the possibility of developing the severe stages of the disease and early mortality, so these patients may need a more aggressive treatment.[509,510,658,661]

Laboratory tests. Laboratory tests aid in establishing the diagnosis and assessing disease activity. The test for the presence of rheumatoid factor is positive in approximately 70% to 80% of patients with RA (95% if presenting with subcutaneous nodules) but also is positive in approximately 5% of individuals who do not

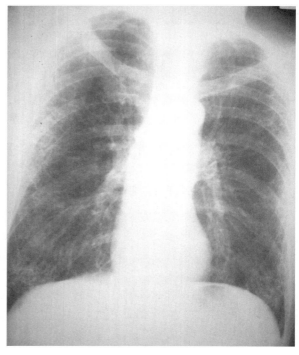

FIG. 9-24   Radiodense linear shadows most prominent in the lower lung fields as a feature of pulmonary fibrosis in a rheumatoid patient. (Courtesy Steven P. Brownstein, MD, Springfield, NJ.)

have RA, and in patients with other nonrheumatoid diseases.[368,384] Therefore a positive or negative rheumatoid factor test must be correlated closely with other clinical features. A complete blood count, ESR, C-reactive protein, and ANA assay also may be performed to initially evaluate and as follow-up for rheumatoid patients.[684]

Treatment and management. RA has become one of the most costly musculoskeletal disorders because of loss of work and limitations in daily activities caused by pain and functional disability,[6,10,194,693] and because of the associated treatment cost. More aggressive treatment is being used at the initial onset of RA to combat unfavorable long-term outcomes.[650,656]

Treatment is multifaceted and geared toward reducing pain and limiting or slowing the progression of deformities and associated disability. Conservative therapy should include patient education (inclusive of pain coping techniques) and emotional support;[318,367,645] rest; application of heat or cold; dietary changes or supplementation; and resistance training, exercise, and joint mobilization to improve joint range of motion, strengthen muscles, and minimize joint deformity.*

Pharmacologic treatment includes nonsteroidal antiinflammatory drugs (NSAIDs), corticosteroids, and more aggressive second-line of therapy or disease-modifying antirheumatic drugs (DMARDs), such as antimalarial drugs, intramuscular gold, and penicillamine. Infliximab and etanercept are biologic response modifiers that block specific immune factors leading to RA; these treatments

*References 2, 143, 151, 253, 532, 681.

have now been approved as second-line therapy. Third-line drugs or immunosuppressants inhibit the immune system and may have serious side effects.[65,610]

At the disease onset, radiographs of the hands, wrists, and feet should be obtained as a baseline and then repeated at 6-month intervals for a minimum of 2 years to aid in identifying those patients at risk for serious joint damage and deformity.[85,494] MRI of the spine should be performed on patients with radiographic abnormalities combined with neurologic deficits, and should be considered in patients with superior migration of the dens, a PADI of less than 14 mm, and a subaxial canal diameter of less than 14 mm regardless of symptoms. MRI with contrast (gadolinium) should be used to differentiate synovial fluid from pannus. Surgical intervention may be indicated to replace joints (Fig. 9-25), correct severe deformity,[229] or treat neurologic compromise.[207]

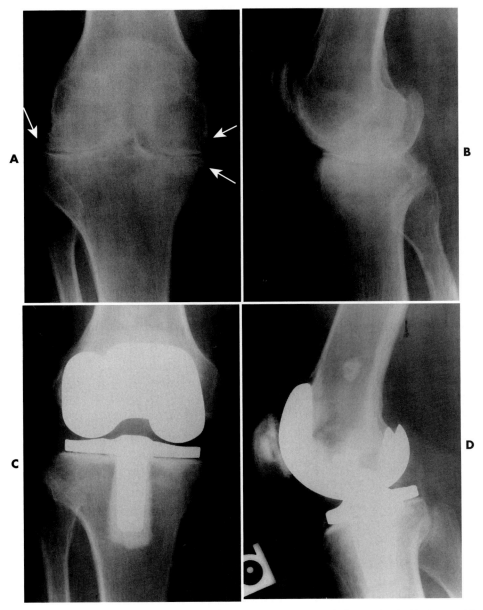

FIG. 9-25 **A,** Anteroposterior and, **B,** lateral radiographs showing changes typically associated with rheumatoid arthritis of the knee. The most striking finding is tricompartmental loss of joint space and joint effusion. Small marginal osteophytes indicate secondary osteoarthritis (arrows). **C** and **D,** Because of ongoing pain and disability related to the advanced rheumatoid arthritis, the patient underwent total resurfacing knee arthroplasty.

KEY CONCEPTS

- *Rheumatoid arthritis is the most common inflammatory arthritis.*
- *Females are more likely to develop the disease than men (two or three times more likely, less in older populations), with the peak incidence occurring between 40 and 70 years of age.*
- *The primary sites affected are the synovial tissues of the hands, feet, wrists, hips, knees, elbows, and shoulders. Affected metacarpophalangeal and proximal interphalangeal joints of the hand and atlantoaxial subluxation of the cervical spine are most characteristic. The sacroiliac articulations are rarely affected.*
- *This arthritide is marked by a bilateral symmetric distribution, periarticular soft-tissue swelling, initial juxtaarticular osteoporosis progressing to generalized uniform loss of joint space, marginal erosions (bare areas) progressing to subchondral erosions, subchondral cysts, and joint deformities.*
- *Hip involvement may lead to bilateral acetabular protrusion.*
- *Subluxations and joint deformities, including swan neck, boutonnière, and hitchhiker's thumb, are characteristic.*
- *Treatment is directed toward limiting pain and disability and may include surgery for joint replacement or to address neurologic complications.*

Juvenile Idiopathic Arthritis

BACKGROUND

In the United States *juvenile rheumatoid arthritis* (JRA) and *juvenile chronic arthritis* (JCA) are terms often used interchangeably to encompass the three major subsets of JRA, whereas in Europe the designation of JCA includes not only JRA (and its subsets), but also the addition of the *juvenile spondylarthropathies* (ankylosing spondylitis [AS], enteropathic arthritis, and psoriatic arthritis).[104,105,689] To unify these previous classifications and decrease confusion, which in turn would facilitate research and aid in identification of homogeneous groups of children, a new classification known as *juvenile idiopathic arthritis* (JIA) has been developed.[506,639] The definition of JIA basically is consistent with the definitions of JRA and JCA, although additional subsets have been added to the new classification system.

Classification according to the International League against Rheumatism: JIA

1. Systemic arthritis
2. Oligoarthritis
   a. Persistent
   b. Extended
3. Polyarthritis (rheumatoid factor negative)
4. Polyarthritis (rheumatoid factor positive)
5. Enthesitis-related arthritis
6. Psoriatic arthritis
7. Other or unclassified arthritis

Classification according to the American College of Rheumatology: JRA

1. Systemic
2. Pauciarticular or monoarticular
3. Polyarticular
   a. Seronegative
   b. Seropositive

Classification according to the European League against Rheumatism: JCA

1. Juvenile-onset adult type (seropositive)
2. Seronegative chronic arthritis (Still's disease)
   a. Classic systemic disease
   b. Polyarticular
   c. Pauciarticular or monoarticular

3. Juvenile spondyloarthropathy (AS, psoriatic arthritis, enteropathic arthritis)

The terms JIA, JRA, and JCA all indicate an inflammatory disease of unknown cause, occurring in childhood (<16 years of age), characterized primarily by arthritis (joint inflammation and stiffness) persisting for a minimum of 6 weeks (JCA symptoms must last at least 3 months). The term *juvenile idiopathic arthritis* (JIA) is used in this book.

JIA is the most common type of arthritis affecting children.[677] It is an autoimmune disorder with a prevalence that appears to range between 12 and 148 cases per 100,000,[503,601,646] and an incidence rate of 17 per 100,000, that appears to on the decline.[304,503] It targets predominantly the synovial joints, in which synovial proliferation leads to joint and soft-tissue destruction. It is suspected that genetics may predispose a patient to the disease, and an infectious or environmental factor may trigger its onset.

The first four subsets of the new classification system of JIA encompass the vast majority of cases and are essentially the same subsets listed by the American College of Rheumatology (ACR) as representative of JRA. They are the main focus of this section. They are divided according to the presence or absence of rheumatoid factor, systemic symptoms within the first 6 months of onset, and number of joints involved within the first 6 months of onset. Subsets 1, 2, and 3 comprise approximately 70% of all JIA patients. Subset 4 represents approximately 5% to 10% of all JIA cases.

1. Systemic arthritis (essentially classic systemic onset disease) is the most serious. It occurs in children under 5 years of age; affects males and females equally; and presents with spiking fevers, a characteristic salmon-colored rash on the trunk and thighs, hepatosplenomegaly, serositis, adenopathy, leukocytosis, and mild polyarthritis, usually of the wrist, knees, and ankles.
2. Oligoarthritis (essentially pauciarticular or monoarticular) is the most common variety, and is found in young children under 5 years of age and affects no more than four joints during the first 6 months, generally affecting large joints (e.g., knees, ankles, elbows, wrists). This form frequently is accompanied by asymptomatic chronic iridocyclitis, uveitis, cataracts, and (in a minority) blindness. There is a large association with antinuclear antibodies. Two additional subcategories are recognized: persistent oligoarthritis and extended oligoarthritis. Persistent oligoarthritis affects no more than four joints throughout the course of the disease. Extended oligoarthritis affects a cumulative total of five or more joints after the first 6 months of onset.
3. Polyarthritis (rheumatoid factor negative, essentially polyarticular seronegative) involves more than five joints during the first 6 months of the disease, is more prevalent among females between 12 and 16 years of age, and has an early onset between the ages of 1 and 3 years. Symmetric small joint involvement of the hands and feet is common, which is similar to the distribution of adult RA.
4. Polyarthritis (rheumatoid factor positive, essentially polyarticular seropositive) develops in teenage girls and is similar clinically and radiographically to adult RA.[15,572] Juvenile patients may present with subcutaneous nodules, although this symptom occurs less frequently in juveniles than adults. More than five joints are affected, most commonly the hands, wrists, feet, knees, hips, and cervical spine.
5. Enthesitis-related arthritis usually occurs in males over 8 years old and indicates the presence of arthritis and enthesitis, or arthritis or enthesitis with at least two of the following: SI tenderness or inflammatory spinal pain, presence of HLA-B27, or family history of confirmed HLA-B27 in at least one first- or second-degree relative.

6. Psoriatic arthritis indicates arthritis and psoriasis, or arthritis and at least two of the following: dactylitis, nail abnormalities (pitting or onycholysis), or family history of psoriasis in at least one first-degree relative.

7. Other or unclassified arthritis indicates childhood arthritis of unknown cause persisting for at least 6 weeks that does not fulfill criteria for subsets 1 to 6, or fulfills criteria for more than one of the other subsets.

IMAGING FINDINGS

Although other imaging modalities may be more sensitive for early detection of joint pathology, plain film radiography continues to be the primary method of imaging for the diagnosis and follow-up evaluation of JIA. The radiographic presentation in the majority of JIA cases is similar in appearance to adult RA with few exceptions (Table 9-2). Although features within each subset of JIA can differ, there are features that may be common to all. These include early manifestations such as fusiform periarticular soft-tissue swelling and juxtaarticular osteopenia (which may include growth recovery lines) that may become diffuse. Intermediate or later-stage manifestations may include joint space narrowing, osseous erosions, growth disturbances, bony ankylosis, joint contractures, subluxation,

or dislocation. Early plain film radiographs may be negative, and a technetium bone scan, CT, or MRI may be more helpful.

Distinct features of JIA include periostitis and growth abnormalities, which are the result of the disease process combined with skeletal immaturity. Periostitis commonly involves the diaphysis of the metacarpals, metatarsals, and proximal phalanges and may be an early and prominent finding that is likely explained by the exposure of loosely attached periosteum to an inflammatory and hyperemic process. Growth abnormalities result from hyperemia to the epiphysis and growth plates, causing an overgrown "ballooned" or "squared" epiphysis. Hyperemia also may lead to premature growth plate fusion, resulting in shortening of limbs or limb length discrepancies.

Overall joint involvement mimics that of adult RA in the majority of cases, although JIA has more of a predilection for large joints. Individual joint manifestations are noted in the following explanations.

Knees. The knee is the most commonly affected joint in JIA. Effusion; joint space narrowing; osteopenia and enlargement, or "ballooning" of the metaphysis and epiphysis of the distal femur and proximal tibia; widening or expansion of the intercondylar notch; and patellar squaring are the most distinctive findings associated with JIA in the knee (Fig. 9-26). Growth arrest lines may

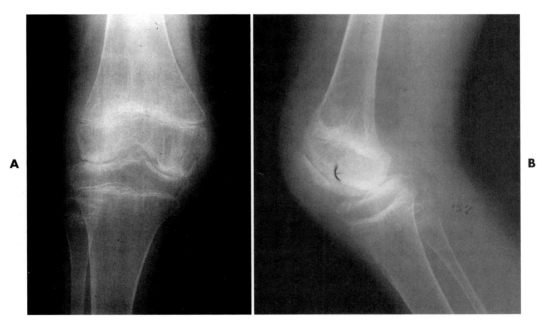

FIG. 9-26 **A,** Anteroposterior and, **B,** lateral knee radiograph in a patient with juvenile idiopathic arthritis. The femoral condyles are enlarged and the intercondylar notch is widened, both of which are common features of the disease in this joint. (Courtesy Steven P. Brownstein, MD, Springfield, NJ.)

TABLE 9-2
Radiographic Findings Associated with Juvenile and Adult Rheumatoid Arthritis

Radiographic finding	Juvenile rheumatoid	Adult rheumatoid
Joint space narrowing	Common in late stages of disease	Common in early stages of disease
Marginal bony erosion	Common in late stages of disease	Common in early stages of disease
Intraarticular fusion	Common	Uncommon
Growth abnormalities	Common	Absent
Periostitis	Common	Absent

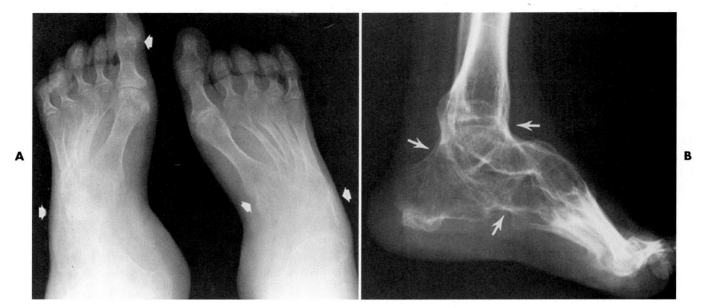

FIG. 9-27   Juvenile idiopathic arthritis. **A,** Symmetric findings include generalized osteopenia, diaphyseal overtubulation, widespread joint space narrowing, evolving ankylosis *(arrows)*, and diffuse muscle wasting. **B,** Another patient exhibits widespread ankylosis *(arrows)* in the hindfoot and midfoot with a cavus deformity secondary to the disease and stabilizing surgery. Osteopenia and muscle atrophy also are evident. Differential diagnosis should include consideration of other causes of disuse beginning in childhood, and certain congenital foot deformities. (From Sartoris DJ: Musculoskeletal imaging: the requisites, St Louis, 1996, Mosby.)

result from temporary reduction in growth velocity, and frequently are seen around the knee. A discrepancy in leg lengths may occur with knee inflammation. If the inflammation is controlled and occurs before the age of 9, the leg lengths equalize and no residual discrepancy remains. If involvement exists after the age of 9, early epiphyseal closure may occur and result in a permanently shorter leg on the involved side.[600]

Ankles and feet.   Swelling may be noted on the dorsum of the foot because of involvement of the subtalar and tibiotarsal joints (Fig. 9-27). Tibiotalar slant, valgus, and varus deformities may result.[545]

Hands and wrist.   Early findings include soft-tissue swelling and juxtaarticular osteoporosis of the carpals, MCPs, and PIPs; preservation of joint space; lack of erosions; and periosteal new bone formation, resulting in a widened midportion of the phalanges (Figs. 9-28 and 9-29). Accelerated skeletal maturation; osseous erosions in the carpus, distal radius, and ulna; joint space narrowing; carpal and carpometacarpal ankylosis; and boutonnière and swan neck deformities (see description in previous section of adult RA) may present in later stages. Growth defects may be seen in the ulna and the fourth and fifth metacarpal bones (positive metacarpal sign).

Hips.   JIA may be indicated by lack of growth of the iliac bone, femoral head flattening and enlargement, early growth plate closure, coxa valga deformity, and acetabular protrusion. Osteonecrosis also may develop as a complication of the disease but more often is related to treatment (corticosteroids).

Cervical spine.   Atlantoaxial subluxation and odontoid erosions occur, but not as frequently as in patients with adult-onset RA. Cervical spine flexion and extension radiographs should be a consideration. Apophyseal joint ankylosis may occur after facet erosions in the upper and middle cervical spine (Fig. 9-30), and

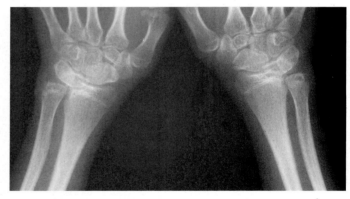

FIG. 9-28   Juvenile idiopathic arthritis demonstrating enlarged radial and ulnar epiphyses, carpals, osteoporosis, thin cortices, and soft-tissue swelling in this 14-year-old boy. (Courtesy Steven P. Brownstein, MD, Springfield, NJ.)

appears to be the most common abnormality of the cervical spine occurring more frequently at multiple levels than at a single level.[172,343,344,401] The ankylosis is thought to cause vertebral body and disc hypoplasia. The so-called juvenile cervical vertebra is more commonly found in patients with early-onset disease[172,344] than in those with late-onset disease.

Mandible.   Micrognathia may be observed clinically, but more often radiographically in children with JIA.

Radiographic changes in enthesitis-related arthritis.   The SI joint is involved, but usually not at the onset of the disease. There is widening of the joint space with erosions on the inferior aspects of both articulating surfaces. CT may best assess these changes given the presence of a normally wide SI joint space in children. In the feet, the MTP and IP joints of the first

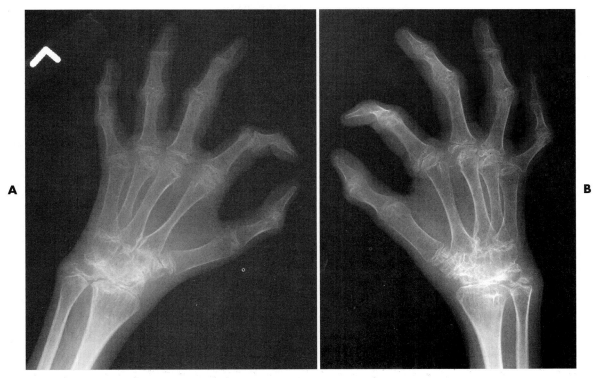

FIG. 9-29 **A** and **B,** Bilateral symmetric expression of osteoporosis, soft-tissue swelling, carpal and hand joint erosions, and enlarged epiphysis of the distal radius and ulna consistent with juvenile idiopathic arthritis. (Courtesy Steven P. Brownstein, MD, Springfield, NJ.)

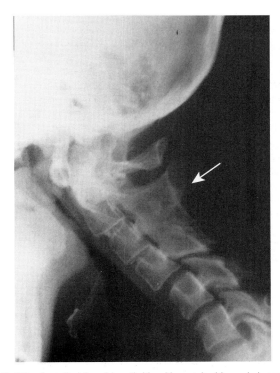

FIG. 9-30 Juvenile idiopathic arthritis with vertebral hypoplasia and fusion of the posterior joints (arrow) in the cervical spine. Although inflammation may affect the posterior facets in both adult and juvenile forms of rheumatoid arthritis, resultant apophyseal fusion is common in children and unlikely in adults. Vertebral body and disc hypoplasia also are prominent features in juvenile rheumatoid arthritis. (Courtesy Jack C. Avalos, Davenport, IA.)

digit frequently are affected. Plantar enthesitis also may be noted. Hip involvement may be noted with enlargement of the femoral epiphysis, iliofemoral joint space narrowing, and femoral neck osteophytosis (similar to that seen in adult AS).

CLINICAL COMMENTS

Presentation. Because there is no single test to diagnose JIA, it is considered a diagnosis of exclusion,[76] as other conditions such as infection; trauma; congenital, hematologic, and collagen vascular disorders; and malignancies are eliminated. The clinical presentation may be a child with persistent joint swelling, pain, and stiffness; a painless limp; or a presentation with systemic symptoms (e.g., fever, rash, lymphadenopathy). Symptoms should be present for 6 weeks before the diagnosis of JIA is made. Children with JIA may be undersized and have generalized or localized growth abnormalities.

Laboratory abnormalities. Laboratory abnormalities reflect the inflammatory process, and studies are used only to support the clinical suspicion of or monitor the progression of JIA. Depending on the subtype, anemia, leukocytosis, proteinuria, antinuclear antibodies, rheumatoid factor, HLA-B27, and an elevated ESR may be present.

Therapy and management. The approach to therapy is similar to that for adult-onset RA and varies depending on the course of the disease. It should focus on pain relief, preservation of joint function, maintenance of normal growth and muscle strength, and psychosocial development. Adequate nutrition is essential. Active exercise, maintaining joint range of motion, and physical therapy may aid in preserving or restoring joint space and leading to clinical improvements.[491] Aspirin and NSAIDs usually are given to help with inflammation, whereas the use of systemic corticosteroids initially is avoided because growth retardation is a major complication, but may be used in low doses, or for children with life-threatening complications, and topically for eye involvement. The more "hard-core" second- or third-line therapies are considered with unresponsive patients or those with life-threatening systemic disease. Ophthalmologic examinations should be given at least semiannually to detect asymptomatic iridocyclitis. Eye examinations are given more often in ANA-positive patients.

> ### KEY CONCEPTS
>
> - *Juvenile rheumatoid arthritis (JRA) and juvenile chronic arthritis (JCA) are often used synonymously in the United States, whereas the additional subset of juvenile spondylarthropathies is included with JRA to form JCA in Europe. For unification, a new classification, juvenile idiopathic arthritis (JIA), has been developed to encompass and expand on these two systems.*
> - *JIA is the most common childhood arthritis, affecting children under 16 years of age.*
> - *The subsets of JIA are based on the number of joints involved, systemic involvement, and the presence or absence of rheumatoid arthritis factor.*
> - *Although joint involvement mimics that of adult rheumatoid arthritis, JIA has a greater predilection for large joint involvement and intraarticular fusion. Periostitis and growth abnormalities are noted in juvenile-onset disease, and not adult-onset disease.*
> - *Hands, wrists, knees, hips, and the cervical spine are commonly affected.*
> - *Therapy is similar to that used for adult rheumatoid arthritis, although more caution is used with regard to use of corticosteroids and more "hardcore" lines of defense because of the potentially devastating side effects.*

Seropositive and Connective Tissue Arthropathies

Systemic Lupus Erythematosus

BACKGROUND

Systemic lupus erythematosus (SLE) is an inflammatory connective tissue disorder that involves multiple organ systems and is characterized by excessive immunoreactivity (an autoimmune disorder) in which the antibodies are directed against cell nuclei.[457,540] Although the factor that activates this immune response is unclear, a major element of the underlying pathogenesis is widespread vasculitis, which may be secondary to local deposition of immune complexes.[39] Virtually any tissue can be damaged, but the joints, skin, kidneys, and serosal membranes are most frequently affected.[70,346] There is a genetic predisposition or a familial link associated with SLE. In addition, factors known to trigger flare-ups include exposure to sunlight and certain medications.

SLE usually follows an irregular chronic course of exacerbations and remissions. The mean length of time between the initial onset of symptoms and diagnosis is 5 years. The prevalence of SLE is approximately 24 cases per 100,000,[288] with some evidence of an increasing incidence rate.[648] Recent population-based studies reveal that SLE may now occur at a later age of onset, 30 to 50 years,[268,295,418,648] than the previously reported range of 20 to 40 years. Women are affected up to nine times more often than men,[288] and the most significant ratio variance occurs during the childbearing years. The ratio appears to lessen if disease onset occurs in childhood or at more than 50 years of age. SLE typically occurs 5 to 10 years earlier in women than men, although this difference may be limited to white patients.[418] In the United States, blacks are at a higher risk than whites for the development of SLE; in addition, the age at diagnosis is approximately 7 years younger among blacks.[418]

IMAGING FINDINGS

Although up to 90% of patients complain of articular problems, prominent and severe radiographic changes are uncommon.[342] The most frequently affected joints are the hands, feet, wrists, and knees. Soft-tissue swelling and minimal periarticular osteoporosis are the earliest radiographic manifestations and usually present bilaterally and symmetrically. Joint deformities may ensue in later stages. Subcutaneous calcifications (calcinosis cutis) are not common in SLE, but when they occur they have a predilection for the lower extremities and can be diffuse or nodular.[675] These calcific densities are prone to ulceration and infection.

Hands. In the hands, SLE has a joint distribution similar to RA, affecting the MCPs and PIPs.[456,543] Joint spaces typically are not narrowed. Chronic joint inflammation and effusion may lead to ligamentous laxity and result in joint deformities. The most common deformities include ulnar deviation at the MCPs, flexion and extension deformities of the IP articulations resembling swan neck and boutonnière deformities, and malalignment of the first carpometacarpal joint. These deformities are typically nonerosive and reducible (Jaccoud's-type) and therefore are more visible on an oblique or lateral radiograph of the hand as compared with a posteroanterior radiograph, in which the pressure of the cassette may make the subluxations less pronounced. These nonerosive, flexible deformities are considered pathognomonic and are present in less than one half of patients with SLE who demonstrate articular abnormalities. Rarely these deformities eventually become permanent or fixed. Erosive changes may be seen with lupus, if subtle, and periarticular MRI may be needed for their detection.[474]

Axial skeleton. Although spinal changes are uncommon, atlantoaxial subluxation has been reported in patients with SLE. It is wise to obtain a lateral cervical flexion radiograph because this abnormality may be present and not apparent on a neutral lateral radiograph.[28]

Unilateral or bilateral sacroiliitis, with radiographic features that are similar to those associated with seronegative spondylarthropathies, has been reported as an uncommon manifestation of SLE.[337]

Chest. Plain film chest radiography may be normal, or may reveal pleural or pericardial effusion, acute infiltrate, interstitial reticulation, or cardiomegaly. High-resolution chest CT may find evidence of airway disease and interstitial lung disease in patients without respiratory symptoms and with normal chest radiographs.[31,191] Chronic interstitial changes appear to predominate in the lower lung fields.[471]

Osteonecrosis. Avascular necrosis is a common complication in patients with SLE. The radiographic features are identical to those associated with osteonecrosis caused by factors other than SLE (see Chapter 11). The femoral condyle, humeral head, and femoral head are the most common sites involved; the latter is most affected. Other common sites include the proximal tibia and distal tibia. Although high doses of corticosteroids can significantly increase the risk of osteonecrosis, some treatment regimens may reduce this risk.[260] The disease process itself also seems to increase risk for developing osteonecrosis, because patients not receiving steroids also develop this condition.[336]

CLINICAL COMMENTS

Presentation. The revised criteria for SLE must include four of the following:[629]

- Malar rash
- Discoid rash
- Photosensitivity
- Oral ulcers
- Arthritis
- Serositis
- Renal disorder
- Neurologic disorder
- Hematologic disorder
- Immunologic disorder
- Antinuclear antibody

The clinical presentation varies according to the distribution of lesions and extent of systemic involvement. Many patients initially present with constitutional signs and symptoms (malaise, fever, and weight loss), polyarthritis, or a skin rash. The classic malar "butterfly" erythema may be noted but is only one of several cutaneous lesions that may present intermittently during the course of the disease.[346] The renal system is almost always involved, but the extent differs widely from one patient to the next.[18] Manifestations in any organ system (e.g., respiratory, cardiac, gastrointestinal, central nervous) may appear eventually.[579] Associated life-threatening conditions may include intestinal perforation and vasculitis, seizures, stroke, pulmonary embolus, and nephritis. Pregnancy may be related to an increase in the disease morbidity.[504]

Laboratory tests. The screening test for SLE detects the presence of ANAs, which are present in virtually all patients with SLE. Although this test is sensitive for SLE, it is not specific and therefore may be positive in nonlupus conditions. However, the presence of antibodies to native (double-stranded [ds]) DNA and anti–Sm antibodies strongly suggests SLE. Lupus erythematosus cells* also may be observed. Rheumatoid factor is found in a minority of patients, which may indicate an overlap syndrome other than true SLE.

Treatment and management. The diagnosis of idiopathic lupus should be made only after ruling out the possibility of a drug-induced condition, which can be concluded if discontinuing use of a suspected drug alleviates all signs and symptoms.[260] Treatment depends on the location and severity of the disease. In mild cases it may involve counseling, use of sunscreen, exercise, and NSAIDs, whereas in more severe disease immediate corticosteroid or other immunosuppressive drug therapy may be necessary.[133,382] Unfortunately, the use of immunosuppressive drugs increases the risk of infection, which is currently a major cause of morbidity and mortality in these patients.[282] New drug therapies are being tested that may reduce disease activity.[263,642] Sex hormones are being investigated as potential therapeutic agents because of their immunomodulatory properties.[659]

> ## KEY CONCEPTS
>
> - *Systemic lupus erythematosus (SLE) is an inflammatory connective tissue disorder that affects many organs (skin; vascular endothelium; central nervous system; and renal, hematologic, musculoskeletal, cardiovascular, pulmonary, and gastrointestinal organs).*

---

*ANAs react with nuclei of damaged cells, which disrupt the cells' chromatin structures and transform them into lupus erythematosus bodies. These bodies undergo phagocytosis by neutrophils to form lupus erythematosus cells.

> - *The disease is more common in blacks, 90% of cases are in women, and the majority of cases develop between 30 and 50 years of age.*
> - *The metacarpophalangeal and proximal interphalangeal joints of the hands are affected, and nonerosive, flexible deformities are characteristic.*
> - *Although not common, atlantoaxial subluxation may occur; therefore lateral flexion-extension radiographs of the cervical spine should be a consideration.*
> - *The clinical presentation is marked by arthralgia, "butterfly" rash, ulcers in the nose and mouth, and constitutional signs and symptoms (e.g., fever and fatigue).*
> - *Infection and nephritis are major causes of mortality in all stages of SLE.*
> - *Laboratory tests include a test for the presence of antinuclear antibodies, anti–Sm antibodies, lupus erythematosus cells, and rheumatoid factor.*

Scleroderma

BACKGROUND

Scleroderma, which literally means "hard skin," describes progressive thickening of the skin from increased collagen deposits. The disease also is known as *progressive systemic sclerosis* (PSS), a term that more appropriately describes the entire disease process, because it is a connective tissue disorder characterized by small vessel disease, fibrosis, and excessive deposits of collagen that may affect not only the skin, but also the musculoskeletal system and internal organs (e.g., gastrointestinal tract, lungs, heart, kidneys). Scleroderma has been divided into two major classifications, localized and systemic, and subclassifications depend on the existence and extent of systemic involvement, as well as the rapidity of the disease progression. Localized scleroderma usually only involves the skin and may affect the musculoskeletal system to a limited degree. There are three subtypes: morphea (localized), generalized morphea, and linear scleroderma. Systemic sclerosis causes more widespread skin changes and may be associated with internal organ damage (lungs, heart, and kidneys). Systemic sclerosis has two subtypes: limited and diffuse. Systemic limited scleroderma also is known as CREST, an acronym for its most prominent features: *c*alcinosis, *R*aynaud's phenomenon, *e*sophageal dysfunction, *s*clerodactyly, and *t*elangiectasia. Systemic diffuse scleroderma is the most serious form of the disease because of its severe onset and rapid progression.

Although the etiology is unknown, genetics, hormonal events, the immune system, and an environmental agent or trigger are believed to play important roles in its pathogenesis.* A positive family history appears to be the greatest risk factor, although the familial risk is still relatively low (<1%).[23] The prevalence in the United States has been noted to be 4.4 to 27.6 cases per 100,000,[414,613] with an incidence rate reported to range between 1.4 to 1.9 cases per 100,000.[414,613] It is unclear as to whether this rate is stable or on the rise.[413,426] The female-to-male ratio has been reported as 3:1, although in the United States it is approximately 8:1,[414,612,613] with the highest rates occurring during the childbearing years. There is evidence to suggest that the age of onset is later than has been reported in earlier studies, with the age of occurrence typically 35 to 65[345,414] rather than 20 to 50.[611,612] In the United States African Americans are at a higher risk of developing scleroderma compared with whites, and young African American women appear to be stricken most often and most severely.[345,414,426,613]

---

*References 24, 45, 102, 250, 300, 423, 426.

PART TWO Bone, Joints, and Soft Tissues

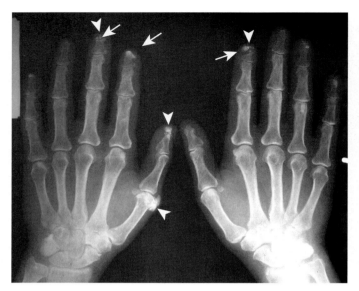

FIG. 9-31 Scleroderma presenting on a bilateral posteroanterior hand view demonstrating characteristic resorption of the distal margins of the distal phalanges (acroosteolysis) *(arrows)* and foci of radiodense soft-tissue calcifications *(arrowheads)*.

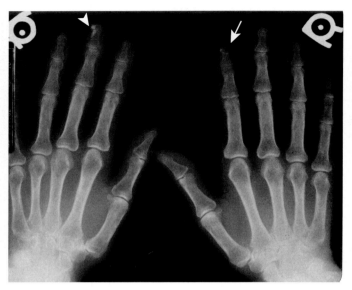

FIG. 9-32 Acroosteolysis *(arrow)* and soft-tissue calcifications *(arrowhead)* of scleroderma. (Courtesy Gary Longmuir, Phoenix, AZ.)

IMAGING FINDINGS

The majority of patients with scleroderma eventually develop joint involvement. The major abnormalities discovered on plain film examination are noted in the hands and include soft-tissue atrophy, osseous resorption, and subcutaneous calcification. Gastrointestinal contrast studies may reveal characteristic findings in the esophagus, small intestine, and large bowel that are primarily caused by fibrosis and atrophy. Plain film chest radiography may be negative or reveal signs of pulmonary hypertension or interstitial fibrosis.

Hands. Atrophy of the soft tissues of the fingertips (acral tapering) is a very common feature, the incidence of which increases if the patient has accompanying Raynaud's phenomenon.[35] Involved digits often have accompanying bony changes (acroosteosclerosis, acroosteolysis) and soft-tissue calcification. Bone resorption or erosion is noted frequently, primarily involving the tufts of the terminal phalanges (acroosteolysis) (Figs. 9-31 to 9-33).[581] Resorption may of lead to a "penciled" or pointed appearance of the phalanx; most of the entire distal phalanx may be destroyed with continued resorption. Erosions also involve the DIP and PIP articulations, but to a lesser degression distal tuft.[158] Erosion at the first carpometacarpal joint is a distinctive feature also,[582] and may lead to radial subluxation of the metacarpal base. Juxtaarticular or diffuse osteoporosis may be present. Joint space narrowing and marginal erosions are noted in up to 15% of patients.[51]

Subcutaneous calcifications. The presence of subcutaneous and periarticular calcinosis is prominent in the hands and also may develop around other joints and over bony eminences (Fig. 9-34).[158,178,670] These calcifications may have a varied appearance, ranging from punctate, to sheetlike, to large focal conglomerations. Ulcerations, especially over bony prominences, may be a complicating factor. Paraspinal calcifications may lead to localized pain, stiffness, dysphagia, or neurologic compromise.[505,580]

Gastrointestinal tract. The gastrointestinal tract is frequently involved in systemic scleroderma, with the esophagus being involved up to 85%. Smooth muscle dysfunction causes esophageal aperistalsis and reduced lower esophageal sphincter

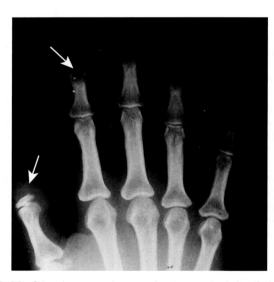

FIG. 9-33 Scleroderma causing prominent acroosteolysis of the hand *(arrows)*. (Courtesy Joseph W. Howe, Sylmar, CA.)

pressure, resulting in gastroesophageal reflux and an increased incidence of peptic stricture and Barrett's esophagus. The esophageal changes lead to dysmotility and may be reflected on plain film as air or air-fluid levels within the esophagus.[468] Esophageal involvement may be diagnosed by a barium swallow, which shows a "stiff glass tube" appearance. Barium studies initially may reveal rapid transit; esophageal reflux; dilatation of the esophagus and small bowel; and large-mouthed sacculations or pseudodiverticula in the colon, jejunum, and ileum. Over time barium studies reveal decreased motility and possibly obstruction.

Chest. The lung is the most commonly involved internal organ after the gastrointestinal tract. The two major pulmonary manifestations associated with scleroderma are pulmonary hypertension and interstitial lung fibrosis. Pulmonary arterial hypertension has a high mortality rate and may occur in approximately 15% of PSS patients. It may develop secondary to pulmonary

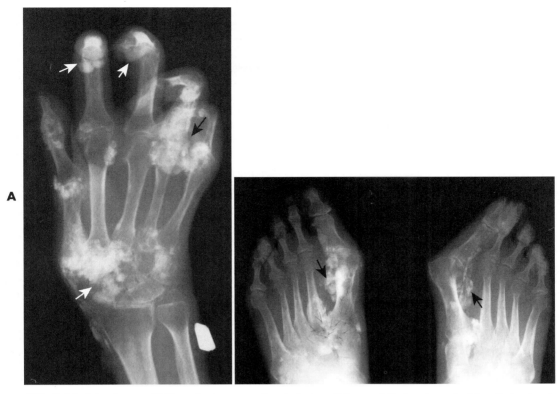

FIG. 9-34 Scleroderma exhibiting subcutaneous and periarticular soft-tissue calcification *(arrows)* of the, **A,** hand and, **B,** feet in this 62-year-old patient. Although fibular subluxations of the phalanges at the metatarsophalangeal articulations are evident, no signs of significant erosions are present.

fibrosis or as an isolated complication. Therefore screening procedures should include Doppler-echocardiography and pulmonary function tests.[145]

If the interstitial fibrosis is extensive enough to be visible on a plain chest radiograph, it will predominate in the lower lungs. The radiographic findings are characterized by fine reticular, partly nodular fibrosis. There may be thick linear radiopacities and thickened septae near the blood vessels. In later-stage or end-stage fibrosis, a more cystic or "honeycomb" pattern appears. HRCT significantly increases early detection of alveolitis and fibrosis, given that plain film chest radiography may appear unremarkable in the early stages.

Mandible. Thickening of the periodontal membrane may create an increase in the radiolucent area between the tooth and mandible that is best noted on dental radiographs. The involvement is most visible around the molars or posteriorly located teeth.

CLINICAL COMMENTS
The patient should fulfill the major criterion or two of the minor criteria as defined by the American College of Rheumatology.[619]
- Major criterion: proximal diffuse (truncal) sclerosis (skin tightness, thickening, nonpitting induration)
- Minor criteria:
  - Sclerodactyly
  - Digital pitting scars or loss of substance of the digital finger pads (pulp loss)
  - Bibasilar pulmonary fibrosis

Changes in the skin's appearance (e.g., thickness and fibrosis, tightening, shininess, atrophy), Raynaud's phenomenon,[299] and arthralgias of the fingers may be the first signs of systemic sclerosis, although visceral involvement may have occurred already.[147,280,628] A thorough, multisystem evaluation is necessary to detect serious problems that may exist in a seemingly asymptomatic patient.[359] As noted, the gastrointestinal tract is the most common internal site affected, with complications including dysphagia, gastroesophageal reflux, Barrett's esophagus, small bowel bacterial overgrowth, malnutrition, and intestinal pseudoobstruction.[26,206,602] Periodontal membrane thickening causes loose teeth, which further complicates maintaining good nutritional status. The heart, lungs, and kidneys also may become involved; pulmonary disease causes higher mortality than renal failure.[113,147,247,359] Scleroderma renal crisis, a condition that was considered almost certainly fatal, now is being treated successfully with angiotensin converting enzyme (ACE) inhibitors.[611]

Laboratory tests. No single test accurately and definitively determines a diagnosis of scleroderma. Laboratory tests may reveal an elevated ESR, the presence of rheumatoid factor in approximately 30% of patients, and the presence of serum ANAs in more than 90% of cases. A variety of disease-specific autoantibodies (e.g., anticentromere antibodies, anti–Schl-70) have been discovered, and are not only useful in the diagnosis of PSS, but also provide markers for certain clinical features.[24,264]

The nail fold capillary test is a useful noninvasive test that examines the skin beneath the fingernail to determine the presence or absence of normal capillary function. Absence of normal capillary function may aid in confirming a suspicion of scleroderma, given that an early sign of systemic scleroderma is the disappearance of the capillaries in the skin of the extremities.[392,573]

Treatment and management. Treatment includes patient education, avoidance of temperature extreme, cessation of smoking to reduce digital vascular complications,[245] dietary modification, physical therapy and exercise, drug therapy, and surgery. Treatment and management are directed toward the varied systemic manifestations of the disease.[427,448,459,602] No generalized therapy for progressive systemic sclerosis has been proved to be effective. Evidence suggests that drug therapy should target one or all of the involved disease processes: vascular disease, autoimmune disorder, and tissue fibrosis. The extent of specific organ involvement must be known to make an appropriate treatment decision.[621] The continuous accumulation of information about pathogenesis of fibrosis in scleroderma and the numerous therapies that are being studied provide hope for the development of a successful treatment or disease-modifying therapy for the complications of this condition.[335,343,459,570]

It should be noted that certain chemical compounds (vinyl chloride), solvents (aromatic hydrocarbons), minerals (silica), pesticides, and drugs can induce scleroderma-like disease.[249,251] This should be a consideration if exposure is a possibility in the patient's work environment or the patient's drug history is suspicious.

KEY CONCEPTS

- *Scleroderma is a connective tissue disorder that affects the skin, musculoskeletal system, and internal organs.*
- *It is divided into two major classifications, limited and systemic, based on the extent of involvement.*
- *In the United States, women are eight times more likely to develop the condition than men.*
- *The disorder typically develops between 30 and 50 years of age.*
- *The hands develop distal tuft resorption (acroosteolysis), acral tapering caused by soft-tissue atrophy, and subcutaneous calcinosis.*
- *Major pulmonary manifestations include hypertension and interstitial fibrosis.*
- *Gastrointestinal manifestations include esophageal dysmotility and large-mouthed (wide-mouthed) bowel sacculations.*
- *Laboratory tests may reveal an elevated erythrocyte sedimentation rate, the presence of rheumatoid factor in 30% of patients, and the presence of serum antinuclear antibodies in 90% of patients.*
- *Specific autoantibodies may aid in the diagnosis of lupus, and provide clues about the onset and prevalence of related clinical feature.*
- *Certain chemicals and drugs may produce scleroderma-like disease.*

Polymyositis and Dermatomyositis

BACKGROUND
Polymyositis and dermatomyositis are two of the three idiopathic inflammatory myopathies. The third, inclusion-body myositis, has most recently been discovered to be a separate entity from polymyositis. The incidence of polymyositis/dermatomyositis has been noted at 0.8 cases per 100,000, with a prevalence of 5.1 cases per 100,000,[288] although these estimates may not be not reliable because the criteria used likely failed to separate inclusion-body myositis from polymyositis.[130,407] The widely used classification system[61] was developed before these two entities were found to be distinct. The female-to-male ratio is approximately 2:1.[288] The age at the time of diagnosis typically ranges from 40 to 70 years, with 52 years of age being the mean onset.[393] Dermatomyositis may affect children and adults.[240] Polymyositis is rarely seen before the second decade of life.

The etiology is unknown. However, like most connective tissue disorders, it is believed that an autoimmune disorder[631] is responsible for the mechanism of damage, which revolves around a genetic predisposition (there is an association with HLA genes)[208,587] and an environmental trigger or initiating factor.[539] Failure of apoptosis, or programmed cell death, is believed to play a major role in the pathogenesis of inflammatory muscle disease.[507] Both polymyositis and dermatomyositis are nonsuppurative inflammatory disorders that lead to subsequent fibrosis and degeneration of striated muscle and result in muscle atrophy and weakness. Predominant muscle involvement is that of the large muscles of the proximal portions of the upper and lower extremities. In addition, dermatomyositis involves the skin.

IMAGING FINDINGS
The radiographic manifestations of polymyositis and dermatomyositis usually are discussed by dividing them into two major categories: soft-tissue and articular abnormalities.

Soft-tissue abnormalities. Initial soft-tissue changes are associated with swelling and edema in the subcutaneous tissue and muscle, particularly affecting the proximal appendicular skeleton in a bilaterally symmetric presentation.[616] Radiographically these changes appear as an increase in the soft-tissue density and poor delineation, blurring, or loss of the fascial plane lines. Extensive edema of the subcutaneous tissue may allow visualization of thickened septa. Chronic disease is associated with a loss of soft-tissue mass or bulk resulting from muscle atrophy and marked osteoporosis of the long bones and vertebral bodies.

Soft-tissue calcification is the most striking radiographic abnormality in polymyositis and dermatomyositis. It is uncommon in adults but occurs in approximately 25% to 50% of children (Fig. 9-35).[622] Soft-tissue calcifications can be subdivided by location into subcutaneous and intermuscular. Calcinosis cutis, or scleroderma-like subcutaneous calcifications, may appear as firm nodules or plaques commonly over bony prominences. These may be associated with skin ulcerations, infection, and pain,[132]

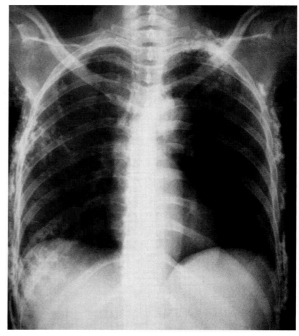

FIG. 9-35 Soft-tissue calcifications of dermatomyositis. (Courtesy Steven P. Brownstein, MD, Springfield, NJ.)

especially at sites of compression. Small, diffuse, linear or curvilinear subcutaneous calcifications also may be evident. Calcification at the fingertips may be associated with terminal tuft erosion.

Intermuscular calcifications generally are asymptomatic and predominate in the proximal large muscles of the upper and lower extremities. The classic radiographic appearance is large calcareous masses or "tumoral" deposits in the fascial planes. In severe forms they may cause loss of function or bone formation in place of calcification.

Joints. Joint involvement occurs but is infrequent. Typically the associated arthritis is transient and nondeforming. The most common abnormalities are periarticular osteoporosis and soft-tissue swelling. Destructive joint changes have been reported, although there is discussion as to whether this erosive presentation is representative of overlap syndromes. Radiographic changes that have been described include soft-tissue swelling, small periarticular calcifications and erosions involving the DIP, PIP, and MCP articulations of the hands, and radial subluxations or dislocation of the IP joint of the thumb ("floppy thumb" sign).[91] Joint contractures may occur and are most commonly associated with dermatomyositis.

Lungs. Pulmonary disease occurs in about 15% to 30% of patients with dermatomyositis and polymyositis. Diffuse interstitial lung disease may be noted in these patients and usually presents on chest radiographs as bilateral irregular linear opacities involving the lung bases.[19,157]

CLINICAL COMMENTS

Patients with polymyositis and dermatomyositis typically present with fatigue, myalgia, and varying degrees of proximal muscle weakness that is usually symmetric and develops over weeks or months. Gross movements such as lifting or climbing stairs are affected, whereas fine motor skills usually are not affected until late in the disease process. "Head drop" may occur if the extensor muscles of the neck are affected. Sensation and tendon reflexes remain normal, although the latter may be absent in severe cases of muscle atrophy. Pain is present in a minority of patients.[130] Dysphagia and pulmonary symptoms may be present depending on muscle involvement.

In patients with dermatomyositis, characteristic skin manifestations may precede or less commonly accompany the onset of muscle weakness. These include (a) a heliotrope rash that appears as a bluish-purple discoloration on the upper eyelids; (b) an erythematous rash that may occur on the face, "V" of the neck and chest ("V" sign), upper back and shoulders (shawl sign) or the knees, elbows, and malleoli; (c) a Gottron rash, which appears as papules over the bony prominences, especially the MCP and IP articulations;[98] and (d) dermatitis affecting the scalp.[310] Thickened and distorted cuticles and telangiectasis at the fingernail base also may occur.

Laboratory tests. Several tests are useful in evaluating muscle disorders, including serum muscle enzyme concentrations, urinary creatine and creatinine excretion, electromyogram, and muscle biopsy. The characteristic findings in patients with dermatomyositis and polymyositis are elevated serum enzyme and urinary creatinine levels, an abnormal electromyogram, and muscle biopsy findings consistent with inflammation (myositis). In addition, skin biopsy may be needed in certain cases of dermatomyositis.

Treatment and management. Treatment is directed toward increasing muscle strength and relieving other associated

manifestations of the disease (e.g., rash, arthralgia). A combination of pharmaceuticals and physical activity should be included in the treatment regimen. Studies have shown that patients may benefit from a therapeutic exercise program to improve function and increase strength.[9,170,254,374,680] Regarding drug therapy, Dalakas and Hohlfeld recommend a sequential, step-by-step, empiric, escalating approach (that may be modified) that successively employs corticosteroids, immunosuppressive therapy,[109] intravenous immunoglobulin therapy,[111,131] and an immunosuppressive drug.[130]

Other factors that must be considered in the management of polymyositis and dermatomyositis patients are the likelihood of dysphagia resulting from esophageal disease, cardiac abnormalities, pulmonary abnormalities,[260] and the increased risk of specific cancer types.[261,262,598] Patients should be assessed and monitored for these complications.

Ultrasound and MRI may be helpful in defining involved muscle groups and possible associated features such as tenosynovitis and tendon nodules, as well as assessing the degree of involvement and possible response to therapy.

> ### KEY CONCEPTS
>
> - *Polymyositis and dermatomyositis are forms of idiopathic inflammatory myopathies in which there is inflammation, fibrosis, and loss of muscle fiber leading to muscle atrophy that affects strength and function.*
> - *Involves the striated muscle; especially the large muscles of the proximal aspects of the upper and lower extremities.*
> - *Bilateral, symmetric muscle involvement.*
> - *Women are affected 2:1 more than men.*
> - *Dermatomyositis has characteristic skin manifestations that include a heliotrope rash and Gottron rash.*
> - *The most striking and characteristic radiographic features are soft-tissue calcifications, which present as subcutaneous or intermuscular.*
> - *Joint involvement usually is limited to soft-tissue swelling and periarticular osteoporosis, although erosive changes have been noted in the metacarpophalangeal, proximal interphalangeal, and distal interphalangeal joints of the hands.*
> - *Characteristic laboratory results are increased serum enzyme and urinary creatinine levels, an abnormal electromyogram, and muscle biopsy finding consistent with inflammation.*
> - *Exercise therapy, corticosteroids, immunosuppressants, and intravenous immunoglobulin therapy are part of the treatment protocol.*
> - *Polymyositis and dermatomyositis carry an increased association with certain cancer types.*
> - *Pulmonary and cardiac abnormalities may exist.*

Jaccoud's Arthropathy

BACKGROUND

Jaccoud's arthritis (arthropathy, disease, or syndrome) is a nonerosive, relatively asymptomatic deforming arthropathy of the hands and feet. It was initially described in 1867 (and for some time thereafter) as a rare complication of rheumatic fever (chronic postrheumatic fever arthritis).[287,595] Jaccoud's arthropathy has since been reported in patients without a previous history of rheumatic fever, and is now more commonly seen in association with connective tissue disorders, such as systemic lupus,[660] scleroderma[69] and dermatomyositis,[71] psoriatic arthritis,[641] sarcoidosis, Parkinson disease, and lung disease.* The condition often is called *deforming nonerosive arthropathy* or *Jaccoud's-type arthropathy* when it occurs in non–postrheumatic patients.

---

*References 29, 69, 70, 279, 296, 387, 403, 412, 487, 597, 620, 626, 641.

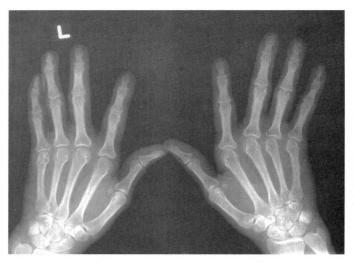

FIG. 9-36 Jaccoud's arthritis marked by ulnar deviation of the first to fourth digits at their metacarpophalangeal joints. (Courtesy Steven P. Brownstein, MD, Springfield, NJ.)

Although the etiology is unclear, biopsy studies reveal no evidence of synovial pathology and do not indicate the presence of a synovial inflammatory condition. Jaccoud's arthropathy is characterized by articular deformities believed to result from capsular inflammation and fibrosis, and in certain cases secondary degenerative changes are noted that presumably result from long-standing joint deformities.[215,646]

IMAGING FINDINGS

The hallmark of Jaccoud's arthropathy is nonerosive, reversible joint deformity, although eventually the deformities may become fixed (Fig. 9-36). The joint deformities cannot be actively corrected by the patient but can be corrected by an examiner if the patient relaxes the joint. Radiographic examination of the hands may reveal this passive reducibility; when the cassette puts pressure on the hand during the PA view, the hand is restored to nearly normal alignment, but the deformities become apparent during the oblique radiography procedure.

Hands and feet. The most common deformities in the hands are flexion and ulnar deviation of the MCP joints, which is most marked in the fourth and fifth digits, and in the foot, flexion and fibular deviation of the MTP articulations.[449] Hallux valgus also may be present in the foot. Swan neck and boutonnière deformities of the digits also are noted (see Rheumatoid Arthritis for descriptions of these deformities),[320] and are more common when associated with an autoimmune disorder such as RA or SLE. A Z-deformity is observed when the thumb is affected. The bone density may be normal or exhibit periarticular osteoporosis. Usually the joint space is preserved until late in the disease, when mechanical stress of the accompanying subluxation may cause secondary degeneration. Osseous erosions are rare, but when they occur they appear as "hook lesions" on the radial and palmar aspect of the metacarpal heads.[490]

CLINICAL COMMENTS

Jaccoud's arthropathy is no longer considered a rare condition and should be mentioned in the differential diagnosis of chronic arthritis.[449] The pattern of joint involvement mimics that of RA and SLE; therefore it may be misdiagnosed given that these diseases also lack erosions early in their course. Laboratory tests may help establish the correct diagnosis because patients with Jaccoud's arthropathy typically have negative tests for the rheumatoid factor and ANA. Patients with Jaccoud's arthropathy (despite its striking deformities) usually have no pain, little or no evidence of synovitis, and good functional capabilities. In fact, the arthropathy may not be the reason the patient is seeking care.

> **KEY CONCEPTS**
> - *Jaccoud's arthropathy is a chronic arthritis that follows rheumatic fever, although it is now seen more in association with connective tissue disorders such as systemic lupus erythematosus.*
> - *It is often an asymptomatic, nonerosive arthritis that is marked by reversible joint deformities.*
> - *It is characterized by ulnar deviation of the second to fifth fingers and subluxations of the metacarpophalangeal joints. Similar findings may involve the metatarsophalangeal joints of the feet.*

Seronegative Spondyloarthropathy

The seronegative spondyloarthropathies are a group of interrelated, sometimes overlapping but distinct inflammatory conditions of unknown cause that have a high prevalence of HLA-B27 antigen, and an affinity for the axial skeleton (spine and SI joints), entheses sites (bony attachments of tendons or ligaments), and to varying degrees the peripheral joints. In addition, they have several common extraarticular manifestations (e.g., iritis, skin lesions). This group of diseases is composed of AS, arthritis of inflammatory bowel disease (enteropathic arthritis), Reiter's syndrome, psoriatic arthritis, and undifferentiated spondyloarthropathy.

Ankylosing Spondylitis

BACKGROUND

Ankylosing spondylitis, also called *Bechterew disease* or *Marie-Strümpell disease,* is the most common of the seronegative spondyloarthropathies, affecting approximately 0.1% to 0.2% of white North Americans,[301] with a prevalence of 68 to 197 per 100,00 people in the United States.[655] It is a chronic, progressive, inflammatory condition involving predominantly the synovial and cartilaginous joints of the axial skeleton and often the large, proximal appendicular joints. Alterations at entheses, the sites where ligaments and tendons attach to bone, also are a prominent feature.

Although the etiology remains unknown, the high prevalence (>90%) of the genetic marker HLA-B27 in white patients with AS[57,78,227] as compared with the prevalence of the antigen in unaffected white patients (6% to 8%) suggests that the disease occurs in persons with a genetic predisposition,[77,301,450] and may be triggered by an environmental factor. The onset is usually between 15 and 35 years of age[186] and typically presents as an insidious onset of low back pain and stiffness. The time period between the first spondyloarthritic symptom and the diagnosis may be years, and is longer in those patients who are HLA-B27 negative.[186] The disease is more common and severe in men, with ratios of 1:1 to 10:1 reported.[142,163,170,294,655] There is the possibility of underreporting in women, in whom the clinical presentation is not as consistently "classic" as in men. The spinal involvement appears less severe in women. Sacroiliitis is more likely to be asymptomatic, and there is an increased frequency of peripheral arthritis.[174,226]

IMAGING FINDINGS

Plain film radiography is still the conventional mode of imaging for AS and all of the seronegative spondyloarthropathies, probably

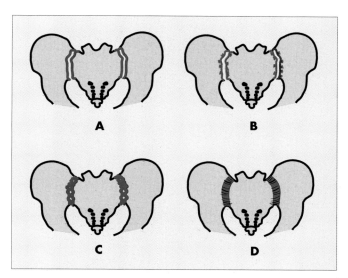

FIG. 9-37 A, Normally the sacroiliac joint margins are well defined. **B,** Inflammation may initially appear hazy with loss of cortical definition. Progression leads to joint space widening, **C,** erosions, and, **D,** fusion.

but predominate in the middle and lower two thirds of the articulation. The articulating surface of the ilium shows earlier and greater radiographic involvement than the sacral surface apparently resulting from less protection from the thinner iliac cartilage.[45] The early stages of the disease are characterized by subtle periarticular osteoporosis and loss of cortical bone definition. More obvious erosions develop, leading to irregular joint margins and joint space widening. Patchy and ill-defined reactive sclerosis accompanies the erosions and becomes more diffuse and uniform as the disease advances (Fig. 9-37). Bony bridges form across the joint, and lead to eventual fusion or ankylosis, which appears radiographically as obliteration of the SI articulation. After ankylosis occurs, the reactive sclerosis is resorbed, and generalized osteoporosis becomes a prominent feature. Approximately 50% of patients progress to complete SI fusion (Figs. 9-38 to 9-40).

Early changes in the SI joints are not well visualized, if at all, on plain film radiography. The diverging rays of a pelvic radiograph taken in the anterior to posterior direction directly opposes the plane line of the joint, and therefore cannot clearly define the subchondral bone or joint space because of superimposition. Two ways to optimize visualization are to (a) perform a posterior to anterior examination and decrease the tube distance to 90 cm, thereby attempting to parallel beam and joint divergence; and (b) perform two separate oblique radiographs (Figs. 9-38, *B*) for each joint with a caudocranial tube angulation. Plain film radiographs may still be negative given the subtlety of these findings in combination with the complexity of the SI joint surfaces, and other more sensitive modalities such as MRI or CT may be needed.[375,432]

Spine. Spondylitis occurs in about 50% of patients and as a rule develops after SI disease, with the thoracolumbar and lumbosacral junctions being the most common initial target sites.[152,220] The disease process typically ascends the spine contiguously without skip lesions and progresses bilaterally and symmetrically. The most characteristic spinal finding occurs at the discovertebral junction, but the inflammatory process also may affect the apophyseal joints, posterior ligamentous attachments, costovertebral joints, and atlantoaxial joint (Figs. 9-41 to 9-47).

Discovertebral junction. The classic spinal findings associated with AS are thin, vertical ossifications or syndesmophytes

because of its accessibility and cost. However, because of its lack of sensitivity to the early stages of the disease and consequent delay in disease diagnosis, other modalities such as MRI, CT, ultrasound, and bone scintigraphy may become more heavily used for diagnosis confirmation and monitoring disease progression, depending on the stage of the disease and area of involvement.[209,375,432]

Radiographic findings, regardless of the location, reflect the underlying inflammatory condition associated with AS, which is characterized by erosions, osseous proliferation, and bony ankylosis. Joint involvement in the axial and appendicular skeleton is typically bilateral and symmetric, although this may vary early in the disease process.

Sacroiliac joint. The SI joint is the classic site of initial involvement in AS and usually is symmetric. The ensuing changes may affect both the ligamentous and synovial portions of the joint,

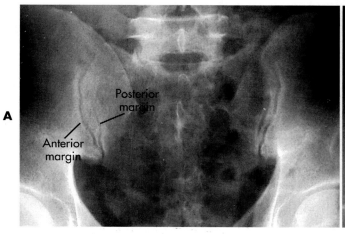
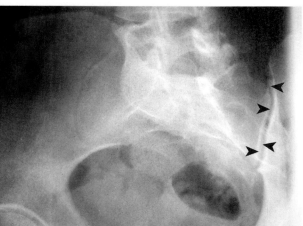

FIG. 9-38 Normal sacroiliac joint. **A,** Because of its obliquity, the normal sacroiliac joint appears as a double projection (anterior margin of the joint is lateral and posterior margin of the joint is medial) in the anteroposterior or, to a lesser extent, posteroanterior projection. **B,** An oblique projection of the joint allows the examiner to better visualize the joint without the confounding double projection. In all views, the cortical margins of the joints should be well defined and continuous *(arrowheads)*. Sacroiliitis presents with ill-defined and interrupted margins of the joint.

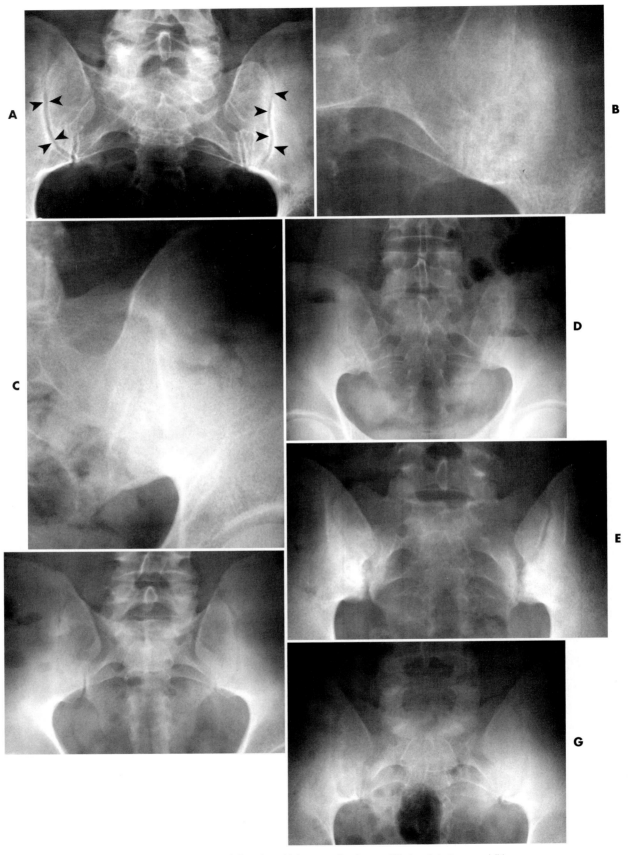

FIG. 9-39 A, Normal sacroiliac joints and, **B** to **I,** multiple cases of early sacroiliitis in ankylosing spondylitis.

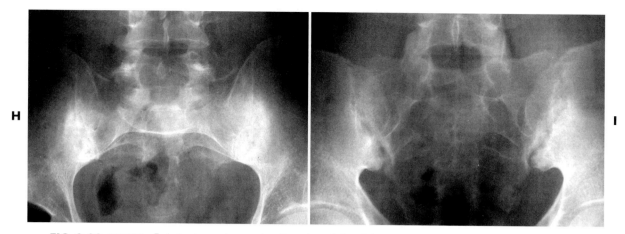

FIG. 9-39 cont'd Early involvement presents with an irregularity of the normally well-defined cortical margins of the joint. The erosions in the joint surface become noticeable as the disease progresses.

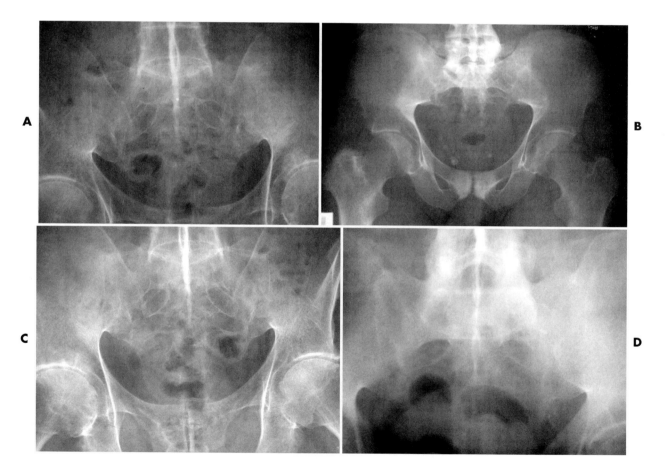

FIG. 9-40 **A** to **D,** Multiple cases of sacroiliac joint fusion in ankylosing spondylitis. Joint fusion results in an absence of the normal thin, radiodense, vertically curvilinear cortical margins and joint space (see Figs. 9-37, 9-38, and 9-39). (**B,** Courtesy Steven P. Brownstein, MD, Springfield, NJ.)

Continued

PART TWO Bone, Joints, and Soft Tissues

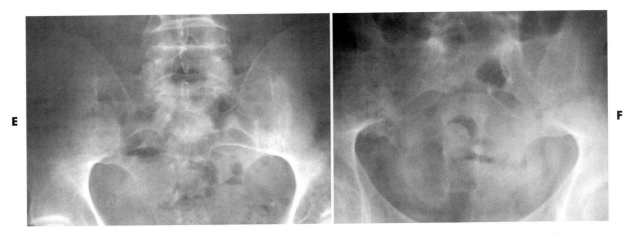

FIG. 9-40 cont'd   E to **F,** Multiple cases of sacroiliac joint fusion in ankylosing spondylitis. Joint fusion results in an absence of the normal thin, radiodense, vertically curvilinear cortical margins and joint space (see Figs. 9-37, 9-38, and 9-39).

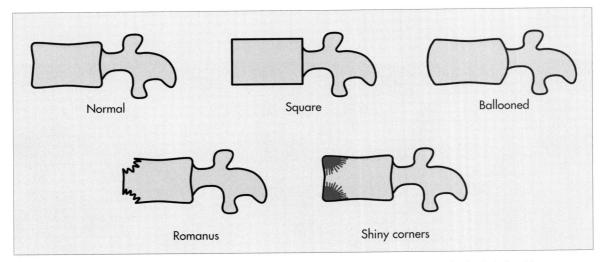

FIG. 9-41   Several key radiographic features of ankylosing spondylitis are noted in the lateral projection, including thin marginal syndesmophytes (see Fig. 9-42), a square or ballooned configuration of the vertebral body (as opposed to the normal slight concavity of the anterior and posterior margins of the vertebral body), sclerotic "shiny" corners of the vertebrae (representing reactive sclerosis to the enthesopathy), and small erosions at the corners of the vertebral body, known as *Romanus lesions.*

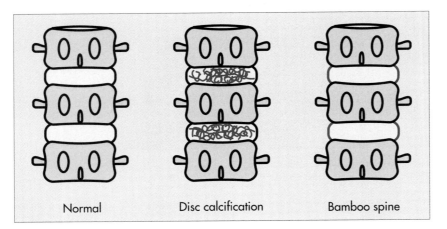

FIG. 9-42   As with other conditions of spinal hypomobility, dystrophic calcification of the intervertebral disc may occur with ankylosing spondylitis. A hallmark feature of ankylosing spondylitis is the formation of thin sydnesmophytes, connecting adjacent vertebrae. In the anteroposterior view the thin sydnesmophytes bow outward slightly, giving the spine the appearance of a bamboo stick.

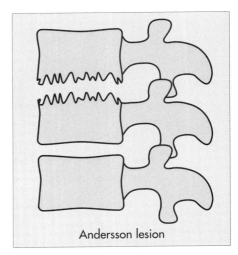

FIG. 9-43   Rarely ankylosing spondylitis manifests with advanced endplate destruction, known as an *Andersson lesion,* mimicking an infection.

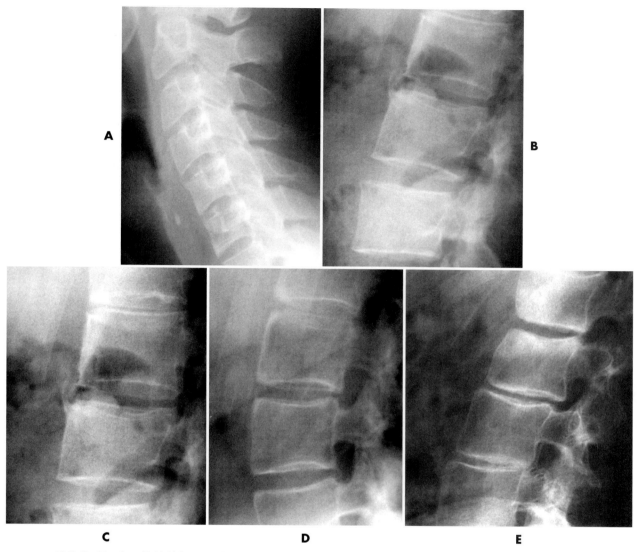

FIG. 9-44 **A** to **C,** Multiple cases of square and, **D** and **E,** ballooned vertebra in different patients with ankylosing spondylitis.

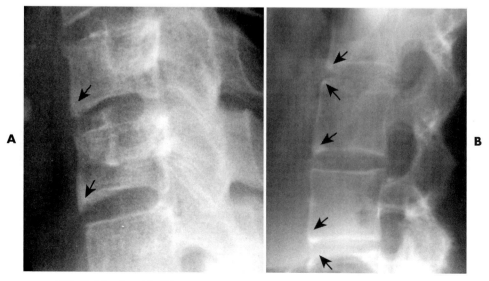

FIG. 9-45 **A** and **B,** Shiny corners in two patients with ankylosing spondylitis *(arrows).*

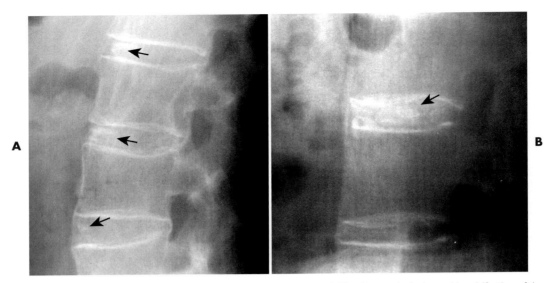

FIG. 9-46   **A** and **B,** The spinal fusion associated with ankylosing spondylitis often results in dystrophic calcification of the involved intervertebral discs *(arrows).*

that bridge adjacent vertebrae and cause ankylosis of multiple segments. Complete ankylosis occurs as the disease progresses, resulting in a distinctive, undulating spinal outline that radiographically resembles a piece of bamboo. The classic "bamboo spine" occurs in a minority of patients and takes an average of 10 years to develop (see Figs. 9-42 and 9-47).

A syndesmophyte begins as a focal osteitis or erosion with surrounding sclerosis at the anterior vertebral body margins. The small corner erosions, or Romanus lesions, combined with new bone formation in the anterior curve of the vertebrae, lead to a loss of the normal anterior body concavity and may cause vertebral "squaring," which is most apparent in the lumbar spine (see Figs. 9-41 and 9-45). This early finding often is overlooked, but new techniques are being designed to evaluate this subtle change in an attempt to aid early radiologic diagnosis and assess spinal progression.[533] The radiographic brightness of reactive sclerosis is intensified by the accompanying vertebral body osteoporosis and is appropriately called the *shiny corner sign.* Ossification then develops in the outer annular fibers and results in thin, marginal syndesmophytes that are predominantly found on the anterolateral aspects of the spine but can arise posteriorly and may cause symptomatic spinal stenosis.[239]

Other abnormalities occurring at the discovertebral junction include discal calcification (see Fig. 9-46), which is common to many conditions of spinal hypomobility; discal ballooning, which is found in the later stages of spinal ankylosis as osteoporosis causes the endplates to weaken and become biconcave (fish vertebrae) and the disc to appear "ballooned" or biconvex; and Andersson lesions, which are discovertebral erosions or a destructive process that result from inflammation and stress fractures in the ankylosed spine (posttraumatic pseudoarthrosis).[153]

Rarely the discovertebral junction undergoes advanced destruction and sclerosis, known as an Andersson lesion (see Fig. 9-43). The appearance is easily confused with an infection of the disc. The presence of radiographic features of AS of the posterior elements and other spinal levels is an important differential clue.

Apophyseal joints and posterior ligaments. Ankylosis of the apophyseal joints is secondary to an underlying erosive process followed by reactive sclerosis that leads to osseous fusion and capsular ossification. This process is considered a prerequisite for the postural changes of reduced lumbar and cervical lordosis, and the increased thoracic kyphosis associated with patients in the later stages of the disease (Fig. 9-48). One study that examined 50 radiographs of the cervical and lumbar spine demonstrated greater involvement of apophyseal joints than in bridging syndesmophytes, suggesting the possibility that the apophyseal joint is primarily involved in AS.[139] The lateral cervical radiograph well demonstrates the changes in the apophyseal articulations. Oblique radiographs may be needed in the thoracic and lumbar spine to better visualize these changes. Radiographically, bilateral apophyseal fusion resembles two thick, vertically oriented linear radiopacities, which are known as the railroad track sign on the anteroposterior (AP) radiograph. If this appearance is present in combination with ossification of the interspinous and supraspinous ligaments, the resulting three vertical stripes are called the *trolley track sign.* The single vertical stripe caused by ossification of only the supraspinous and interspinous ligaments is called the *dagger sign* (Figs. 9-49 to 9-53).

Costovertebral and costotransverse joints. Osseous fusion of the costovertebral and costotransverse joints is responsible for the limited chest expansion and chest or thoracic spine pain associated with AS.[356] It is difficult to visualize on plain film and may require specialized imaging such as radionuclide scintigraphy (hot scan initially, and cold once fused) or CT.[356,499] Involvement of the sternoclavicular joints also may be present.

Spinous processes. Spinous process involvement is most common at the cervicothoracic junction, and appears as "whittling" or "sharpening" of the spinous processes secondary to subligamentous erosions.

Cervical spine. Special attention should be given to the cervical spine, although involvement typically occurs later in the disease process than involvement in the thoracic and lumbar

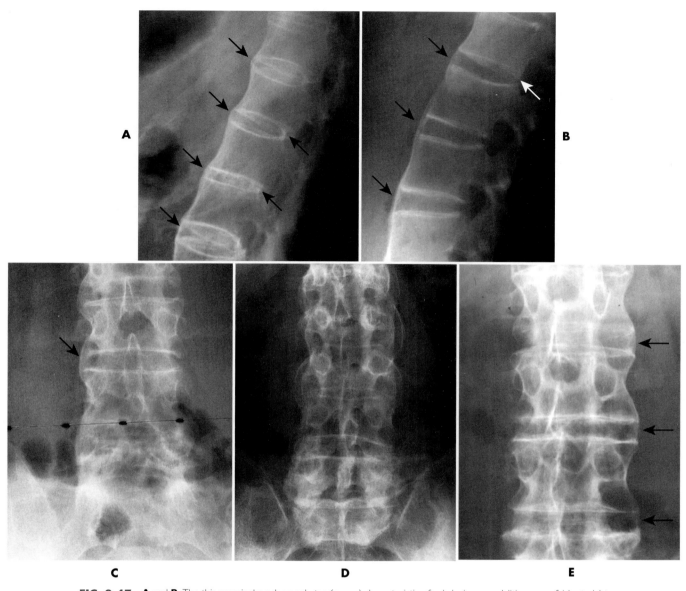

FIG. 9-47 **A** and **B,** The thin marginal syndesmophytes *(arrows)* characteristic of ankylosing spondylitis appear fairly straight in the lateral projection but are more curved in, **C,** the frontal projection. In the frontal projection, the curved syndesmophytes give the spine, especially the lumbar spine, an appearance that has been likened to a bamboo stick. **D,** A second and, **E,** third, slightly oblique, is presented.

regions (Fig. 9-54).[87,381] In addition to the universal changes noted throughout the spine, atlantoaxial instability may develop with a rate of occurrence that has been noted to range between 2% and 23%.[275,534] Atlantoaxial instability in AS is less frequent and severe, but mimics the atlantoaxial involvement seen in patients with RA. Inflammatory changes of the synovium and adjacent ligamentous and osseous structures may lead to atlantoaxial subluxation, cranial settling, odontoid erosions, or complete destruction of the dens. Anterior atlantoaxial subluxation appears to be the most common presentation.

Spinal fractures associated with AS usually are caused by extension injuries and may occur even after minor trauma.[262] Fractures may occur in any spinal region; however, they are most prevalent in the cervical spine. These may be difficult to detect with plain films and CT; MRI or bone scans may be necessary.[221]

With the ankylosed spine, fractures involve all three columns of the spine; therefore they are unstable with significant incidence of neurologic injury.[196,224] Resultant pseudoarthrosis in the cervical spine is extremely rare. It also is rare in the thoracolumbar spine, but not to the degree noted in the cervical spine.[140]

Appendicular skeleton. Peripheral arthritis occurs in approximately 40% of AS patients;[227] the hips, shoulders, knees, and small joints of the hands and feet are the most commonly affected sites.

Hips. AS has a particular affinity for the large proximal joints (rhizomelic spondylitis), primarily the hip, which it affects in approximately 25% of patients (Figs. 9-55 and 9-56).[87] The associated radiographic findings are consistent with any inflammatory disorder, and include concentric joint space narrowing, mild erosions, subchondral cysts, ankylosis, and rarely acetabular protrusion.

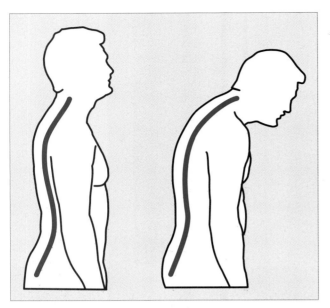

FIG. 9-48 Advanced ankylosing spondylitis results in an increased thoracic kyphosis, loss of lumbar lordosis, and an anterior weight-bearing posture of the cervical spine.

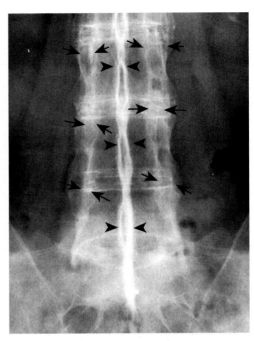

FIG. 9-50 Trolley track sign. In the frontal radiographic projection, ankylosing spondylitis may appear with three radiodense vertical bands. The appearance has been likened to the three rails of a trolley track, hence the term *trolley track sign* to describe the appearance. The outer vertical bands represent ossification of the posterior joints (known as a *railroad track sign* when present alone) *(arrows)*, and the midline radiodense band is secondary to ossification of the supraspinous and interspinous ligament (known as a *dagger sign* when found alone) *(arrowheads)*.

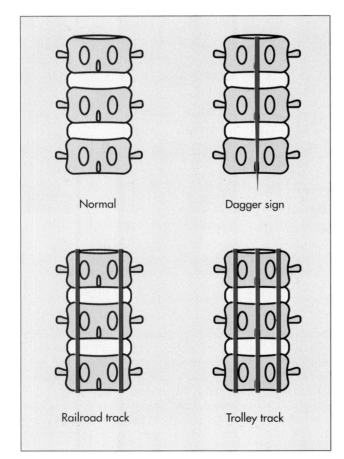

Normal

Dagger sign

Railroad track

Trolley track

FIG. 9-49 Ossification of the supraspinous and interspinous ligaments results in a midline, thin, vertical radiodense band running down the lumbar spine, known as a "dagger" sign. Fusion of the capsular ligament of the posterior joints causes similar bilateral radiodense vertical bands to be seen in the frontal radiographic projection. The appearance of only the capsular ligament bands is termed a "railroad track" sign. When the dagger sign and railroad track sign coexist, the configuration of the three vertical bands is termed a "trolley track" sign.

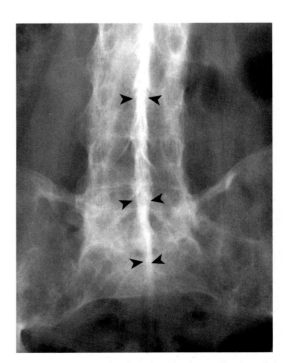

FIG. 9-51 Dagger sign. In the frontal projection, ossification of the interspinous and supraspinous ligaments appear as a midline radiodense vertical band in the lumbar spine known as the *dagger sign (arrowheads)*. (See also Fig. 9-49.)

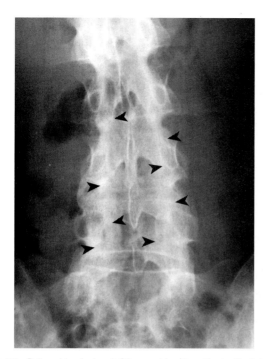

FIG. 9-52 Railroad track sign. A 26-year-old male patient with fusion of the posterior joints secondary to ankylosing spondylitis. The fused posterior joints appear as parasagittal radiodense vertical bands in the frontal projection, nicknamed a *railroad track sign (arrowheads)*.

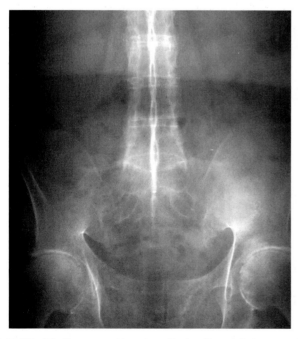

FIG. 9-53 Fifty-three-year-old male patient with ankylosing spondylitis. Characteristic features of the disease are noted by fusion of the sacroiliac joints, fusion of the posterior joints and ossification of the interspinous and supraspinous ligaments (trolley track sign), bilateral concentric loss of joint space of the hips, and osteopenia.

Bony proliferation may occur as femoral osteophytosis, which begins at the lateral margin of the femoral head and progresses to form a circumferential ring around the femoral neck (Fig. 9-56). Hip disease is more prevalent in patients with an early age of onset, and appears to be a prognostic marker for long-term severe disease and more severe cervical spine involvement.[86]

Shoulders. The glenohumeral joint is the second most common peripheral joint affected. Involvement is usually bilateral, and the osteoporosis, joint space narrowing, erosions, and proliferative changes typically mirror those in the hip. More severe erosions may occur on the lateral margin of the humeral head, and may progress to the appearance of a "hatchet" sign, in which the entire lateral aspect is destroyed. Chronic involvement also may lead to rotator cuff disruption, which is noted on the radiograph as elevation of the humeral head relative to the glenoid cavity.

Enthesopathy. Enthesopathy is an inflammation at the insertion of tendons and ligaments into bone, and appears to be the hallmark of inflammatory spondyloarthropathies such as AS.[40] These changes usually occur in a bilateral and symmetric manner.[220] Bony erosions and osseous proliferation at entheses are common and most notably affect the pelvis (upper portion of the SI joint, ischial tuberosities and spines, iliac crests, symphysis pubis, greater and lesser trochanters), the plantar or posterior aspect of the calcaneus, and the anterior aspect of the patella. This reactive new bone is termed *periostotic whiskering*, which describes its frayed radiographic appearance (Fig. 9-57). Similar changes may develop around the shoulders and involve the AC articulations, coracoid process, and greater tuberosity of the humerus.

Lungs. In addition to the characteristic skeletal changes associated with AS, pulmonary involvement also is a well-known feature. Pleuropulmonary disease has been reported to affect 1% to 2% of AS patients.[558] The classic manifestation is upper lobe interstitial fibrosis. The use of HRCT in addition to plain film chest radiography is revealing much more diverse involvement (nonapical interstitial lung disease, bronchiectasis, emphysema, mediastinal lymphadenopathy), as well as a higher percentage of affected patients.[190,329,583]

CLINICAL COMMENTS

Early diagnosis of patients with AS may be delayed because of the mild and vague clinical presentation, nonspecific laboratory findings, and subtle radiographic changes. The initial complaint usually includes an insidious onset of low back pain and morning stiffness, which is relieved with activity and aggravated by resting in the supine position. Fifteen percent of patients have shoulder or hip pain as the initial complaint.[544] Acute iritis is rarely the initial complaint, although eventually this becomes one of the most common extraarticular manifestations and occurs in 25% to 30% of patients.[544] Additional early physical findings may include limited range of motion, limited chest expansion, postural changes (to ease back pain), fever, fatigue, anorexia, weight loss, and anemia. Neurologic signs and symptoms may include radiating leg pain that does not extend below the knee, cauda equina syndrome, and myelopathic changes caused by stenosis or a fracture.[170,234,421] Extraskeletal manifestations include heart disease (especially aortic insufficiency), upper lobe pulmonary fibrosis, and inflammatory bowel disease.

Pain is intermittent in the early stages, but pain and stiffness become more constant as the disease progresses. It has been noted that symptoms actually diminish or disappear in late-stage disease, with ossification of the paraspinal ligaments and apophyseal joints.[353]

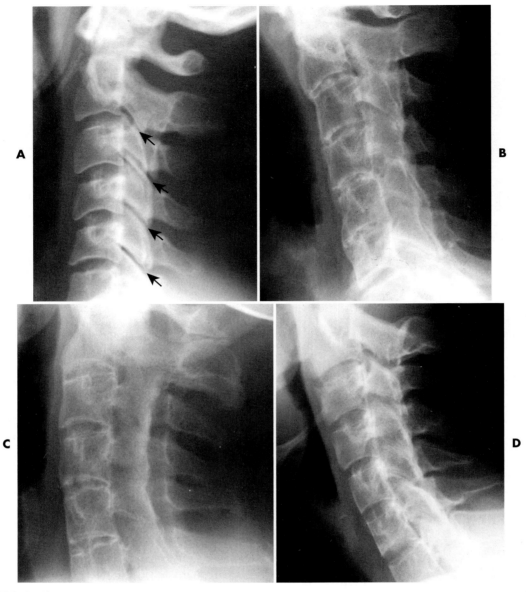

FIG. 9-54 A, Normal and, **B** to **D,** three cases of abnormal lateral cervical projections. The normal study exhibits loss of the normal cervical lordosis, but the vertebrae are of normal configuration and the posterior joints spaces are clearly seen *(arrows).* The abnormal cases reveal a loss of the posterior joint spaces secondary to joint fusion occurring with anklylosing spondylitis. (**B,** Courtesy Robert Tatum, Davenport, IA.)

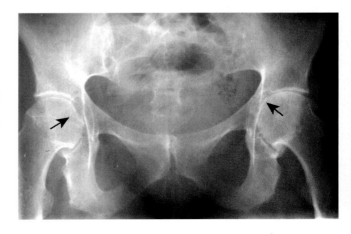

FIG. 9-55 Anteroposterior projection of the pelvis revealing bilateral fusion of the sacroiliac joints consistent with ankylosing spondylitis. The projection also demonstrates bilateral concentric joint space reduction of the hips (direction of *arrows*).

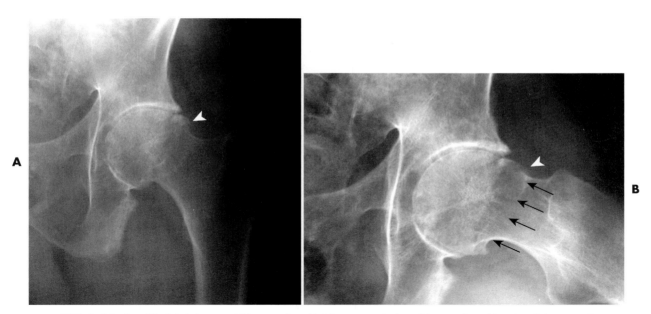

FIG. 9-56 **A** and **B,** Ankylosing spondylitis presenting with joint space reduction of the superior, axial, and medial aspects of the hip equally. In this case, a 58-year-old man with ankylosing spondylitis exhibits mostly even reduction of the illofemoral space, a feature of inflammatory joint disease. Also, a small osteophyte on the lateral aspect of the femoral head is present as an early finding associated with ankylosing spondylitis *(arrowheads)*. With disease progression a ring of osteophytes occurs around the femoral neck *(arrows)*.

Other studies do not concur and report continued daily pain and stiffness.[227] An increase or recurrence of pain after diminution may signal a superimposed complication such as a fracture.[489,551] Spinal or "carrot stick" fractures are common and usually are a result of seemingly minor trauma, such as slipping, to bone that has become severely osteoporotic because of disease-related ankylosis or surgical fusion.[435] Patients with AS are at an increased risk of spinal cord injury, which occurs most commonly in the cervical spine.[5]

Diagnosis of AS is confirmed by radiographic examination. Although plain film radiography is not the most sensitive for the early changes associated with AS, it is still the primary and most widely used imaging modality for the diagnosis and assessment. If a spinal plain film is being used for a baseline study, repeating the radiograph in 6 months may be beneficial to detect early changes. PA radiographs of the hands and feet should be included at baseline, and follow-up radiographs are based on clinical features. If assessing progressive structural damage, serial films of the pelvis and cervical, thoracic, and lumbar spine should not be taken more frequently than annually.[473] Several radiologic scoring systems have been developed for the evaluation of AS. The most commonly used system is the New York criterion, which scores the SI disease on a scale from 0 to 4: 0 is normal; 4 is severe.[41] A more recently proposed system is the Bath Ankylosing Spondylitis Radiology Index (BASRI), which not only grades the SI joints, but also the lumbar and cervical spine. SI grading with BASRI is based on the New York system.[377]

Because of its lack of sensitivity for early synovial and bony changes, use of plain film radiography alone may significantly delay the diagnosis. MRI, CT, and other imaging techniques are playing expanding roles to aid in earlier diagnosis and provide a better understanding of treatment response.[27,93,535,536] Investigators are discovering relationships between specific radiographic findings and how they relate to the patient's physical signs and symptoms and long-term prognosis.[86,358,632,665] One example is the

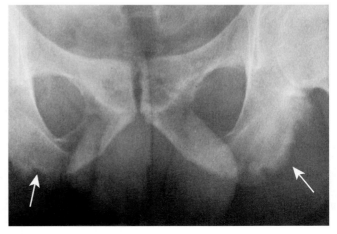

FIG. 9-57 Clearly visible periostotic "whiskering" of the ischial tuberosities on the radiograph of a man with ankylosing spondylitis *(arrows)*.

relationship of hip disease as an indicator of more progressive spinal changes and long-term severe disease.[86] These types of correlations will eventually aid assessment, treatment, and evaluation of disease progression while reducing the need for costly or invasive tests.

Laboratory tests. Laboratory studies may be helpful but are not specific for AS and must be considered only when significant clinical suspicion exists. HLA-B27, probably the most well-known laboratory finding associated with AS, may be found in patients with any of the seronegative spondyloarthropathies and in a small percent of unaffected patients (6% to 8%). The ESR also is nonspecific and may be increased in patients with any inflammatory or necrotic condition. Tests for rheumatoid factor and ANA are characteristically negative and are more useful for excluding seropositive disorders than diagnosing AS.

Treatment and management. Treatment should focus on pain relief; a long-range plan to prevent, decrease, or delay joint and postural deformities; and preventing or reducing other associated complications (fractures). Patients with AS should be screened for osteoporosis; however, patient selection, time interval, and an optimal screening method are yet to be determined.[42] Osteoporosis of the spine may not be detectable with most current bone density measuring techniques because the ossification of the spinal ligaments produces a falsely elevated reading.[452] Patient education should stress safety, avoidance of fractures and spinal cord injury, and information about factors known to increase functional disability, such as smoking and lack of social support.[671] A rehabilitation and exercise regimen has been shown to slow the progression of functional disability[671] and is necessary to maintain proper joint motion and function and promote proper posture by strengthening muscle groups that oppose the direction of the ensuing deformity. If joints are inflamed and painful, NSAIDs may be used to suppress pain, inflammation, and spasms in an effort to facilitate exercise. In the recent past, drug therapy has been fairly stagnant; however, the new tumor necrosis factor-alpha (TNF-α) antagonists appear not only to reduce signs and symptoms associated with AS, but also to reduce structural damage.[73,74,618]

KEY CONCEPTS

- *Ankylosing spondylitis is the most common seronegative spondyloarthropathy.*
- *It primarily involves the synovial and cartilaginous joints of the axial skeleton.*
- *Males are predisposed to developing the condition (1:1 to 10:1), with the usual onset from 15 to 35 years of age.*
- *The radiographic findings are characterized by erosions, osseous proliferation, and bony ankylosis.*
- *Involvement is bilateral and symmetric and targeted to the spine, hips, shoulders, and particularly the sacroiliac joints.*
- *Ankylosing spondylitis causes sacroiliac erosions, joint widening, sclerosis, and fusion.*
- *It is associated with vertebral changes such as body squaring, Romanus lesions, shiny corner sign, syndesmophytes, and apophyseal fusion.*
- *Clinical characteristics are vague and include pain, limited range of motion, limited chest expansion, fever, fatigue, and weight loss.*
- *The condition causes decreased cervical and lumbar lordosis and increased thoracic kyphosis.*
- *Diagnosis is confirmed by radiographic appearance, negative test for rheumatoid factor, positive test for HLA-B27 antigen marker, and an elevated erythrocyte sedimentation rate.*
- *Treatment includes pain relief, with a long-range plan to decrease or delay joint and postural deformities.*

Enteropathic Arthritis

BACKGROUND

Enteropathic arthritis, or arthropathy, is a disorder in which the articular alterations of the axial and appendicular skeleton are believed to be a direct pathogenic consequence of a group of bowel abnormalities, predominantly inflammatory bowel disorders. The condition is most frequently associated with ulcerative colitis and regional enteritis (Crohn's disease), but Whipple disease; enteritis

caused by *Salmonella, Shigella,* or *Yersinia* organisms; cirrhosis; hepatitis; pancreatic disease; and intestinal bypass surgery are all conditions that somehow can induce joint disease. The suspected mechanisms of the onset of arthritis include simultaneous joint and bowel infections or bowel infections that subsequently reach the joint (impaired barrier function), an immune response against a common bowel and joint antigen, and a genetic predisposition given the increased proportion of HLA-B27 in affected individuals as compared with unaffected individuals.[450]

The underlying bowel disorder has an influence on which joints are affected and the percentage of involvement. The axial and appendicular skeletons may be separately or simultaneously involved. In general, peripheral arthritis is seen in approximately 15% to 20% of patients with inflammatory bowel disease, and it is most common in the lower extremities. It typically develops after the onset of bowel disease, and peripheral arthritic flares correlate with the underlying disease activity.[228] Axial involvement is noted in 3% to 18% of patients with inflammatory bowel disease. It may precede or follow the onset of bowel disease, and shows no strong association with disease activity.[228]

In ulcerative colitis, peripheral arthritis occurs mostly in females and is noted in approximately 10% to 15% of patients, with the knees and elbow being the most common sites of involvement, respectively. Spondylitis occurs in 5% of ulcerative colitis patients, and they are predominantly male.

Peripheral arthritis is present in 15% to 20% and spondylitis in 5% of patients with Crohn's disease. The cervical spine is the most common region of spinal involvement. There does not appear to be a particular gender association.

IMAGING FINDINGS

Radiographic alterations reflect the underlying inflammatory disease process, showing peripheral joint involvement similar to RA and axial changes identical to AS.

Axial skeleton. Bilateral and symmetric SI erosions and sclerosis, joint space narrowing, and possible subsequent fusion occurs in combination with spinal changes or as isolated sacroiliitis in 4% to 18% of patients (Figs. 9-58 and 9-59).[228] The spondylitis that occurs in 3% to 6% of patients begins as a marginal vertebral

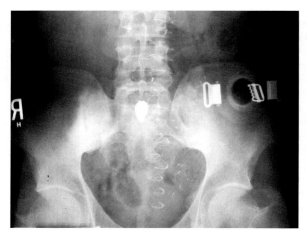

FIG. 9-58 Ulcerative colitis in a 49-year-old man presenting with evidence of bowel surgery (surgical clips and colostomy apparatus). The osseous changes of the sacroiliac joints result from associated enteropathic arthritis. Residual subdural contrast from a past myelogram is noted incidentally. (Courtesy Steven P. Brownstein, MD, Springfield, NJ.)

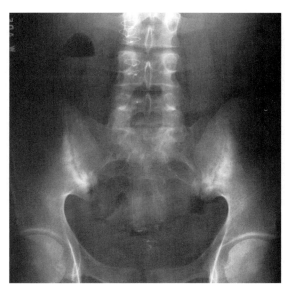

FIG. 9-59 Bilateral sacroiliitis occurring in a patient with ulcerative colitis. (Courtesy Steven P. Brownstein, MD, Springfield, NJ.)

body osteitis, progresses to the characteristic syndesmophytes that bridge adjacent vertebrae, and results in intersegmental fusion. (Please refer to the imaging section on AS for a more detailed description of the pathologic-radiographic changes that occur in the SI joints and the spine. As noted, these changes are identical.)

Appendicular skeleton. Initially the peripheral joint involvement associated with inflammatory bowel disease was thought to be RA caused by similar inflammatory episodes. However, enteropathic arthritis is usually nondestructive and asymmetric, consisting primarily of soft-tissue swelling and periarticular osteopenia. Osseous and cartilaginous destructive changes occur in rare cases. The arthropathy usually is self-limiting but tends to recur with a flare-up of the bowel disease. The most commonly affected joint is the knee, followed by the ankle, shoulder, wrist, elbow, and joints of the hands and feet, respectively.[47]

CLINICAL COMMENTS

Not only do the radiographic features mimic AS, but so may the clinical manifestations (in a young patient with low back pain). Obviously patients may complain of symptoms associated with inflammatory bowel disease, such as abdominal pain, malaise, weight loss, diarrhea, or constipation. However, arthropathy can precede the onset of bowel disease symptoms or the actual disease itself. An ileocolonic study may be useful if inflammatory bowel disease is a possibility in a patient with unusual peripheral arthropathy or radiographic features consistent with AS.[363] Skin lesions and eye infections also can parallel the bowel condition or may precede them and be of diagnostic value.[507]

Laboratory tests. Laboratory test findings typically reflect those of other seronegative spondyloarthropathies. The percentage of positive HLA-B27 enteropathic arthritis patients as a whole is approximately 60%; however, this varies with the underlying gut abnormality and arthritic distribution. For example, the antigen is present in approximately 75% of patients with ulcerative colitis or Crohn's disease who develop axial involvement but is not an associated genetic marker in patients with peripheral arthritis.[450] Tests for the rheumatoid factor typically are negative, and the ESR may be elevated.

Treatment and management. Treatment involves control of the intestinal inflammation, which may incorporate the use of NSAIDs, and conservative management of the arthralgia. Surgical removal of the diseased portion of the colon can result in improvement of the peripheral arthropathy but does not seem to affect the progression of axial involvement.[105]

Sacroiliitis is conventionally diagnosed with plain film radiography; however, the sensitivity to early joint change is low, and other imaging modalities may become more commonplace in the diagnosis and continued assessment of seronegative spondyloarthropathies. Imaging of sacroiliitis in the early or transient stage appears optimal with bone scan or MRI.[432] Detection of osseous erosions is best performed by HRCT, which also yields positive findings through "cold" or inactive periods when a bone scan may be negative.[432]

> ### KEY CONCEPTS
>
> - *Enteropathic arthritis is a seronegative spondyloarthropathy associated with disorders of the gut and most commonly related to inflammatory bowel disease.*
> - *The radiographic features of the axial skeleton mimic ankylosing spondylitis.*
> - *The radiographic features of the appendicular skeleton mimic rheumatoid arthritis but typically are not erosive.*
> - *Enteropathic arthritis has laboratory findings that are typical of other seronegative arthropathies.*

Psoriatic Arthritis

BACKGROUND

Psoriatic arthritis is an inflammatory arthritide that may affect 0.1% of the general population,[591] and approximately 5% to 7% of patients with the skin disorder psoriasis, although in certain studies it has been reported at a substantially higher incidence in those with psoriasis (30% to 40%).[81,230,571] In the majority of patients, the onset of arthritis usually follows the onset of the skin disease; however, it may precede it or they may occur relatively simultaneously.[128,511] Articular involvement is more common in those individuals with moderate or severe dermatologic involvement. Although the etiology is unclear, the pathogenesis of both skin and joint disease is believed to be triggered by environmental factors in those with a genetic susceptibility, and mediated by the immune system.[34,127,128,485,663]

The age of onset is usually between 30 and 50 years old; no significant gender bias is reported.[127,163] The main target areas are the distal joints of the hands and to a lesser degree the feet (2:1 hand-to-foot ratio).[529] Axial skeleton involvement occurs in up to half (and possibly more) of psoriatic arthritis patients.[37,163,325]

Several classification systems for subtyping psoriatic arthritis have been proposed.[256,396,422] One of the most widely accepted is the system described by Moll and Wright that divides the arthritis into five basic patterns of disease, including polyarthritis, asymmetric oligoarthritis, spondylitis psoriatic arthritis, DIP involvement, and arthritis mutilans (a term describing advanced joint destruction and end-stage changes of rheumatoid and other arthritides).[443] These classifications are not clear cut; patients often demonstrate overlapping involvement, or may present with one subtype and progress into another over time.

IMAGING FINDINGS

In the past psoriatic arthritis has been thought of as having a relatively mild disease course when considering the arthritides as a whole.

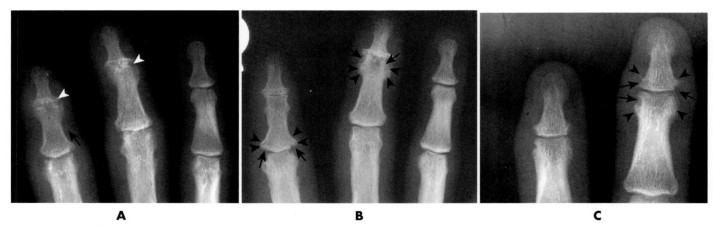

FIG. 9-60 The periarticular erosions of psoriatic arthritis *(arrows)* stimulate periostitis, appearing as fluffy bone growth adjacent the erosions *(arrowheads)*. **A** to **C,** The appearance of the bone growth on either side of the phalanx has been likened to the ears of a mouse *(mouse ear periostitis)*, seen here in three cases *(arrowheads)*. Periostitis is not limited to periarticular area, but also may be found on the shaft of the bone.

However, recent studies have shown that commonly severe joint damage may occur, and result in a deforming and debilitating disease.[216,529]

The radiographic changes in the appendicular and axial skeleton are similar to those associated with RA and AS, respectively, although there are some distinct differences. In general, characteristic radiographic features include erosions, well-maintained bone density (unless during an acute attack when osteopenia can be seen), periarticular and shaft periostitis, osteolysis (including acroosteolysis), initial joint space widening with eventual joint space narrowing, and ankylosis. Joint involvement tends be asymmetric, although up to 50% of those with polyarticular involvement may have a symmetric presentation.[216] Patients with peripheral and axial arthritis have a tendency toward more frequent and severe joint lesions.[627]

Hands and wrist. The bone density usually remains normal (lack of periarticular osteoporosis); however, it may appear osteopenic during an acute attack. The joint spaces may appear unchanged, or may appear to be widened. Swelling and inflammation or tenosynovitis of the entire length of a finger (dactylitis) gives the characteristic appearance of "sausage" digit. Patients with psoriatic arthritis typically have asymmetric small joint involvement, with erosions initially and predominantly involving the DIP joints. Erosions may start at the bone margins, involving the bare area, and be fairly well defined, mimicking the appearance of RA. The erosions then become irregular and ill defined because of the subsequent fluffy periosteal new bone formation or whiskering, which produces a "mouse ears" appearance (Figs. 9-60 to 9-62). In severe cases the erosions may progress centrally, forming a

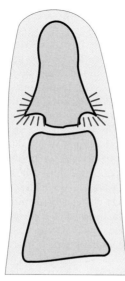

FIG. 9-61 Bone proliferations from marginal periostitis result in a "mouse ear" configuration of the end of the bone.

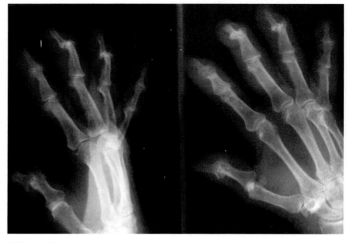

FIG. 9-62 Extensive erosions and disorganization of the distal interphalangeal joints in psoriatic arthropathy. Notice there is no appreciable osteopenia or involvement of the metacarpal phalangeal joints, features that are typical of rheumatoid arthritis, which facilitates differential diagnosis. (Courtesy Gary Longmuir, Phoenix, AZ.)

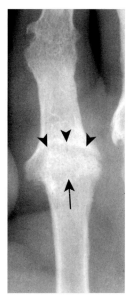

FIG. 9-63 The second metacarpal head inserts into the large central erosion of the base of the adjacent proximal phalanx, forming a "pencil-and-cup" deformity, in which the pencil is noted by the *arrow* and the cup outlined by the *arrowheads*. In this case, and almost always, it looks more like a "cup and saucer." This is the same patient as presented in Figure 9-74. (Courtesy Steven P. Brownstein, MD, Springfield, NJ.)

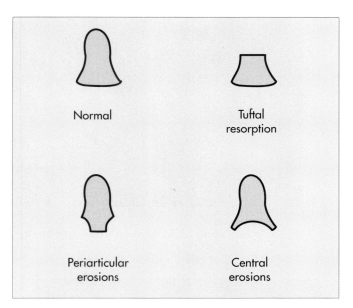

FIG. 9-64 The distal phalanges of the hands provide an important clue to the presence and differentiation of inflammatory arthritides. Normally the distal phalanges appear with a slight spade shape. Abnormality of this shape may occur with distal, central, or periarticular erosions.

"pencil-and-cup" or "cup-and-saucer" deformity (Figs. 9-63 to 9-65), so named because of the apparent expansion of bone at the distal articular surface and the sharpening of bone at the proximal articular surface. Acroosteolysis or tuftal resorption of the distal phalanx of the hands also may develop.[370] An advanced erosive course leads to the debilitating form of psoriatic arthritis known as *arthritis mutilans* (Fig. 9-66). The erosive and proliferative changes may be followed by intraarticular fusion (Fig. 9-67).[514]

In addition to DIP involvement, the MCPs, PIPs, and carpus may develop erosions (Fig. 9-68). If all joints of a single digit are affected, the pattern formed is called a *ray pattern*. Joint deformities and subluxations similar to those of RA may occur, such as ulnar deviation of the metacarpals and boutonnière and swan neck deformities, but are not as common. If severe erosive disease occurs at multiple joints, one phalanx may "slide" onto another or onto the metacarpal. The overlying excess skin develops overlapping folds

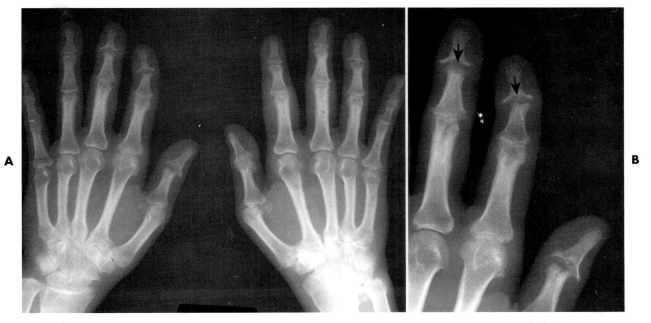

FIG. 9-65 A, Psoriatic arthropathy appearing with asymmetric wrist and distal interphalangeal involvement. **B,** A close-up view exhibits the central erosions to better advantage *(arrows).*

PART TWO Bone, Joints, and Soft Tissues

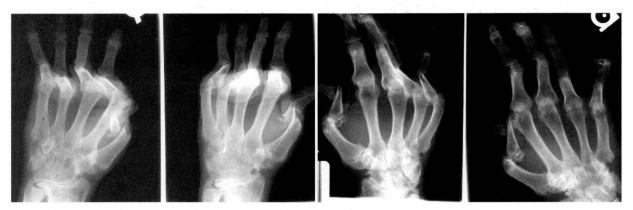

FIG. 9-66 Psoriatic arthritis of the hand resulting in severe erosions and misalignments, termed *arthritis mutilans*. Arthritis mutilans can be caused by other conditions, such as rheumatoid arthritis.

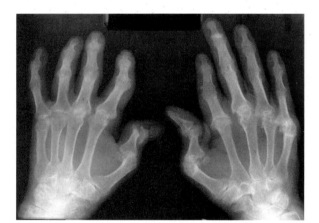

FIG. 9-67   End stage psoriatic arthropathy may present with joint fusion.

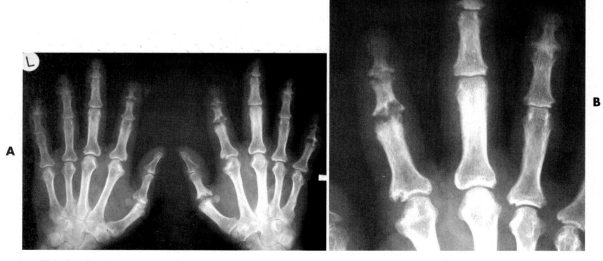

FIG. 9-68   A characteristic feature of psoriatic arthritis is its propensity to involve all of the joints in one digit, as opposed to a type of joint in all digits. This tendency toward a digit pattern is termed *ray pattern*, in which *ray* is a zoological term for finger. **A,** The tendency to distribute more pronounced changes in one finger leads to noticeable soft-tissue swelling more in one finger, known as a *sausage digit finger*. **B,** The ray pattern tendency of psoriatic arthropathy is in contrast to the metacarpophalangeal involvement of rheumatoid. The ray pattern may present in any digit, not just the second.

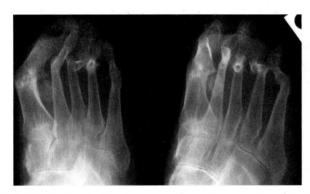

FIG. 9-69 Significantly affected metatarsophalangeal joints with fusion of multiple joints.

and is called an *opera glass hand*. Wrist abnormalities usually follow DIP involvement and may occur within any compartment.

Feet. Changes in the feet caused by psoriatic arthritis are similar to changes in the hand, although the feet are affected less often. The bone density usually remains normal, without evidence of significant osteoporosis. Dactylitis occurs, leading to the appearance of "sausage" digits. Joint erosions and osseous proliferation commonly take place at the IP joint of the great toe and the DIP articulations of all digits (Fig. 9-69). Tuftal resorption may occur. An "ivory" phalanx may result from exuberant periosteal and endosteal proliferation and sclerosis or the terminal phalanx, and has a predilection for the terminal phalanx of the first digit. This is an uncommon presentation, but one that is unique and specific for psoriatic arthritis; it is of diagnostic importance if tuft resorption and articular abnormalities are absent.[548]

Erosive and subsequent proliferative changes may take place at the calcaneal entheses (enthesitis), leading to findings similar to those associated with other seronegative spondyloarthropathies, particularly Reiter's disease.

Sacroiliac joints. It has been reported that 30% to 50% of psoriatic arthritis patients develop SI involvement (Fig. 9-70),[230,248] but a more recent study noted sacroiliitis at a substantially higher incidence of 78%.[37] The sacroiliitis occurring in patients with psoriatic arthritis mimics those changes noted in AS patients. Erosions, joint space widening, sclerosis, and possible fusion typically are bilateral and symmetric; however, other distributions

are seen and the bilateral symmetric distribution is less frequently seen with psoriatic arthropathy than with AS. Proliferative enthosopathic changes may be noted in the pelvis, predominantly affecting the ischium and iliac crests.

Spine. Spinal involvement usually but not always is associated with sacroiliitis. Erosions occur on the surface of the vertebrae, with subsequent ossification at the paramarginal site of erosion or in the adjacent soft tissue. In contrast to patients with AS, the spinal lesions or syndesmophytes associated with psoriatic arthritis are typically bulky, asymmetric, and nonmarginal ossifications that do not appear in consecutive vertebrae ("skip" lesions). These "skip" lesions develop most commonly at the lateral aspects of the vertebral bodies in the thoracolumbar junction (Fig. 9-71).[514] Radiographic changes in the cervical spine in patients with psoriatic arthritis have been reported to be 36% to 70% (Fig. 9-72).[292,569] Atlantoaxial subluxations and apophyseal involvement (joint space narrowing, sclerosis, possibly ankylosis) may occur, but these findings are not nearly as common as those noted in patients with AS.

Radiologic differentiation between the spondylitis caused by psoriatic arthritis and the spondylitis caused by Reiter's syndrome is impossible, although the latter may be less severe.[492]

CLINICAL COMMENTS

The majority of patients who present with joint pain as a result of psoriatic arthritis are aware of the psoriasis; however, some are not. They may have a single, hidden lesion and not realize they have any skin condition, or on presentation of their clinical history patients may fail to mention the skin disorder after it has cleared, assuming it is not related to their joint pain. Therefore if psoriatic arthritis is a diagnostic consideration, a prudent cutaneous search is needed, and the patient's dermatologic history should be directly questioned. Although the onset of arthritis usually follows the development of the skin lesions; up to 20% of patients develop arthritis before psoriasis, and the condition may present simultaneously in approximately 16%.[571]

Low back, hand, and foot pain may be the initial presenting complaints. Joint symptoms are similar to those of a patient with RA and may consist of pain and stiffness (especially in the morning), soft-tissue swelling, and limited range of motion. Physical examination of patients with psoriatic arthritis may reveal skin lesions, soft-tissue swelling of an entire digit ("sausage" digit),[100] and nail lesions (pitting, ridging, and onycholysis), the latter of

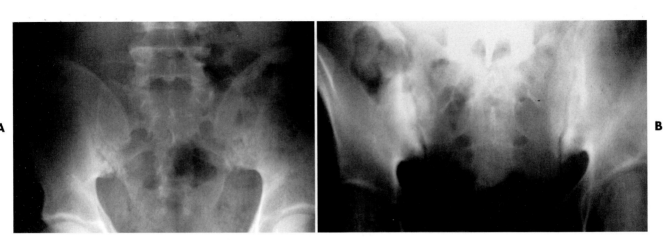

FIG. 9-70 **A** and **B,** Bilateral asymmetric sacroiliitis in different patients with psoriatic arthropathy.

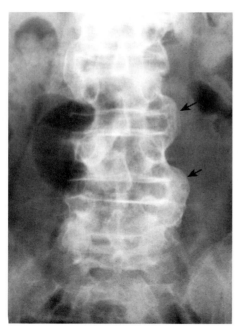

FIG. 9-71 Psoriatic arthropathy. Thick, bulky syndesmophyte formation (*arrows*) is noted along the lateral margins of the lumbar vertebra. Uncharacteristically these syndesmophytes appear continuous on the reading right side. Usually they skip segments. The appearance of this case would be impossible to separate from Reiter's syndrome without clinical data or other imaging, diffuse idiopathic skeletal hyperostosis, or an atypical presentation of degeneration. (Courtesy Trevor Ireland, Anchorage, AK.)

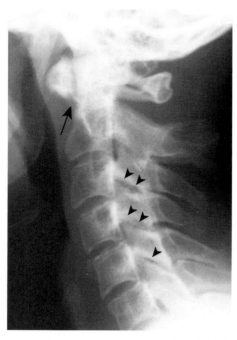

FIG. 9-72 The posterior joint margins are sclerotic and ill defined, consistent with involvement in this psoriatic arthropathy (*arrowheads*). In addition, although the region is underexposed, the atlantodental interval appears suspicious for enlargement (*arrow*), which is also suggested by the anterior offset of the spinal laminal lines of C1 on C2.

which seems to best correlate with the arthritis. Nail changes have been noted in 63% to 86% of patients with psoriatic arthritis, and in 37% of patients with psoriasis without arthritis.[163,354,571]

Laboratory tests. Laboratory tests usually reveal an increased sedimentation rate, are negative for rheumatoid factor, and possibly are positive for HLA-B27 (in 25% to 60% of patients).[77]

Treatment and management. Baseline PA radiographs of the hands, wrists, and feet, and radiographs of the spine and other symptomatic regions should be obtained. Serial radiographs then should be taken at 6-month intervals for the first 2 years after disease onset, depending on treatment regimen.[473]

Treatment is directed at controlling the joint inflammation and is dependent on the severity of joint involvement. Antiinflammatory agents such as NSAIDs may yield clinical improvement of joint pain, but they may exacerbate skin lesions,[520] and joint damage may continue to progress.[217,241] In these cases disease-modifying antirheumatic drugs (DMARDs), including methotrexate or cyclosporine, may be effective. Cyclosporine in low doses has been used because it aids in treating both skin and joint conditions.[563] High doses of vitamin D also may be beneficial.[270] Recently the Food and Drug Administration (FDA) approved etanercept for the treatment of psoriatic arthritis. This is the first FDA-approved treatment for psoriatic arthritis.[173,424,425] Etanercept is a biologic agent that has been used for the treatment of RA. It is designed to target specific mediators involved in the pathogenesis of psoriatic arthritis.

KEY CONCEPTS

- *Psoriatic arthritis is a seronegative spondyloarthropathy that develops in 5% to 7% of patients with psoriasis.*
- *The age of onset is between 30 and 50 years of age and does not develop more often in a particular gender.*
- *The changes in the axial skeleton mimic the changes in patients with ankylosing spondylitis, but often patients may have unilateral or asymmetric sacroiliac involvement.*
- *Syndesmophyte formation may be thick and asymmetric with "skip" lesions.*
- *The effects on the hands are similar to those caused by rheumatoid arthritis; however, the distal interphalangeal joints usually are affected first. Erosions may become central and more severe, and periostitis is a prominent feature.*
- *Physical examination may reveal nail pitting, skin lesions, and soft-tissue swelling of an entire digit.*

Reiter's Syndrome

BACKGROUND

Reiter's syndrome, a seronegative spondyloarthropathy, is an asymmetric polyarthritis that targets the large joints of the lower extremities, small joints of the feet, and axial skeleton. Incidence is estimated at 3 to 4 per 100,000, but values vary widely. Reiter's syndrome is commonly associated with eye disorders, skin rashes, and mouth sores. A minority of patients have the classic triad of symptoms (arthritis, urethritis, and conjunctivitis) that originally characterized the syndrome introduced by Hans Reiter's in 1916.[508]

Reiter's syndrome is considered a form of *reactive arthritis*, a term often used as a synonym. It is precipitated by a bacterial infection that initially involves mucosal surface. It is an aseptic or sterile, likely immune-mediated, inflammatory process that occurs distant to the primary focus of infection, which is generally in the genitourinary or gastrointestinal tract.[315] Its etiology appears to be linked to genetic factor(s), given the high incidence of HLA-B27 (80%), and to infection, given the frequent occurrence after an infectious episode.[315,528] Most cases follow genitourinary infections with *Chlamydia trachomatis,* although it may follow enteric infections with some strains of *Shigella, Yersinia,* and *Salmonella.* Males are affected five times more frequently than females, with the average age of onset from 15 to 35 years.[180]

IMAGING FINDINGS

Reiter's syndrome has a predilection for the lower extremities and is asymmetric in distribution. As with all of the seronegative spondyloarthropathies it is associated with sacroiliitis and spondylitis. The changes associated with Reiter's syndrome may be radiographically indistinguishable from those of psoriatic arthritis. However, the propensity for patients with Reiter's syndrome to have lower extremity involvement and patients with psoriatic arthritis to have upper extremity involvement is helpful. Differential diagnosis also may be accomplished through clinical distinction, not purely radiologic appearance:[197,316] for example, the presence of *balanitis circinata* and *keratoderma blennorrhagica* in patients with Reiter's syndrome or presence of nail pitting and psoriasis in patients with psoriatic arthritis.

Feet. The feet are the most commonly involved site of Reiter's syndrome, with the calcaneus, MTP, and IP articulations of the first digit being specifically affected. Calcaneal erosion followed by fluffy periosteal new bone occurs at the insertion of the plantar fascia and Achilles tendon (enthesitis) (Figs. 9-73 to 9-76).[596] These inflammatory heel spurs are typically bilateral, present in approximately 59% of patients, and are highly suggestive of Reiter's syndrome.[594] The erosive changes involving the MTPs are similar to those that occur in patients with RA. Lanois deformity is a term for resultant joint subluxations and deformities at the MTPs, often specifically defined as dorsal subluxation of the MTP joints and fibular deviation of the toes. In addition, these patients have periostitis, "sausage" digits, and relatively little osteopenia, findings that are similar to those of psoriatic arthritis (Figs. 9-77 and 9-78), although osteopenia may be present during acute attacks.

Tendons. Tenosynovitis is striking in patients with Reiter's syndrome, particularly in the tendons of the feet (Achilles). MRI is useful to demonstrate the distended tendon sheath.

Large joints of lower extremities. The knee and ankle are frequently affected in patients with Reiter's syndrome, whereas the hip is rarely affected. The radiographic findings are consistent with other inflammatory arthritides: soft-tissue swelling, joint effusion, loss of joint space, and erosions. In addition, mild bony productive changes usually are seen, and osteopenia typically does not develop. Severe joint destruction is uncommon.[399,594] Enthesitis may involve the tibial tubercle at the insertion of the patella tendon.

Sacroiliac joints. Sacroiliitis may be bilateral and symmetric, bilateral and asymmetric, or unilateral (Fig. 9-79). The joint changes mirror those of the other seronegative spondyloarthropathies. Subchondral erosions, adjacent sclerosis, and joint space widening are noted. Progression to complete joint fusion in patients with Reiter's syndrome is much less common than in patients with AS.[594] With chronic disease, more than 50% of Reiter's patients eventually develop sacroiliitis; in the early stages fewer than 10% demonstrate SI involvement.

Spine. The spine is involved less frequently in patients with Reiter's syndrome compared with patients with AS or psoriatic arthritis. The thoracolumbar junction is the most common spinal site affected.[508] Thick, nonmarginal syndesmophytes, identical to those associated with psoriatic arthritis, bridge the spine and commonly skip segments (Fig. 9-80).

If associated arthritic changes occur in the cervical spine (Figs. 71 and 72), they are less common and less severe than in patients with psoriatic arthritis.

CLINICAL COMMENTS

Reiter's syndrome presents most commonly as a polyarthritis in young men, and therefore should be a diagnostic consideration in any young man presenting with asymmetric oligoarticular polyarthritis. It typically develops within days or weeks after genitourinary infection or dysentery. The patient generally experiences lower extremity polyarthritis for at least 1 month in addition to one or more of the following: urethritis; conjunctivitis (less commonly uveitis); mucocutaneous lesions; nail changes; dysentery; heel pain; low back pain; or radiographic signs of sacroiliitis, periostitis, or heel spurs. Nonspecific cervicitis may occur in female patients.

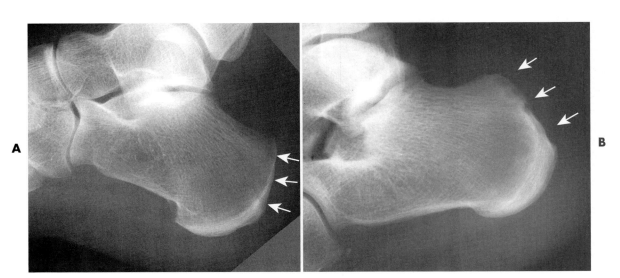

FIG. 9-73 Reiter's syndrome. **A,** The normal calcaneus exhibits a thin uninterrupted cortical margin *(arrows).* **B,** The cortex is interrupted by three small erosions *(arrows).* The posterior superior margin of the calcaneus is a targeted site of involvement for Reiter's syndrome. (Courtesy Arthur Holmes, Foley, AL.)

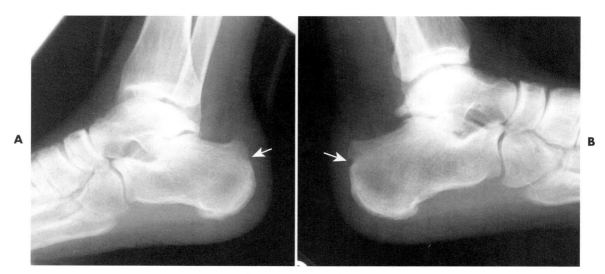

FIG. 9-74 Reiter's syndrome. **A** and **B,** Bilateral erosions at the insertion of the calcaneal tendon *(arrows)*. (Courtesy Steven P. Brownstein, MD, Springfield, NJ.)

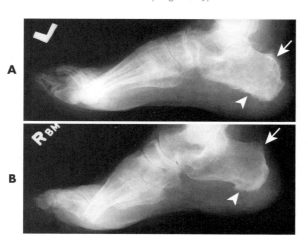

FIG. 9-75 Reiter's syndrome. **A,** Left and, **B,** right calcaneus exhibit extensive erosions at the attachment site of the calcaneal tendon *(arrows)* and plantar fascia *(arrowheads)* in this patient with Reiter's syndrome. (Courtesy Steven P. Brownstein, MD, Springfield, NJ.)

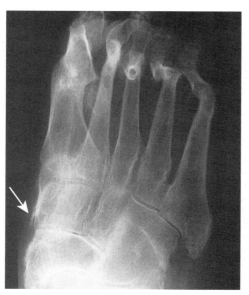

FIG. 9-76 Erosive changes and multiple subluxations affecting predominantly the metatarsophalangeal articulations. Mild periostitis can be seen along the medial aspect of the tarsals *(arrow)*. Bone density is usually relatively well preserved in Reiter's syndrome; however, in this patient, pain has caused disuse and resulting osteoporosis.

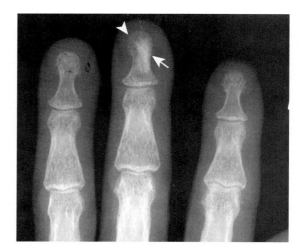

FIG. 9-77 Although the foot is more commonly involved, Reiter's syndrome can exactly mimic psoriatic disease. In this case there is distal tuft resorption *(arrowhead)* and sclerosis of the distal phalanx *(arrow)*. These features are more typical of psoriatic arthropathy. Because of the commonality in presentation, definitive differentiation of psoriatic arthropathy and Reiter's syndrome is done via clinical data, not radiographic presentation. (Courtesy Steven P. Brownstein, MD, Springfield, NJ.)

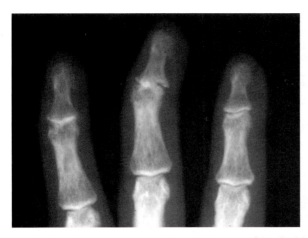

FIG. 9-78 Periarticular erosions and reduced joint space of the distal interphalangeal joints in a patient with Reiter's syndrome. Although it is not uncommon to see involvement of the distal interphalangeal joints in Reiter's syndrome, a presentation like the one seen here is more typical of primary degeneration or psoriatic arthropathy. (Courtesy Steven P. Brownstein, MD, Springfield, NJ.)

Patients also may present with a fever and significant weight loss. The initial disorder usually is self-limiting, but most patients have recurrent episodes of active arthritis.[528]

Reiter's syndrome may produce two characteristic cutaneous lesions. *Balanitis circinata* is present in about 25% of post–*Shigella*- and post–*Chlamydia*-infected patients and is characterized by small, painless ulcers on the glans penis and urethral meatus. *Keratoderma blennorrhagica,* which develops in 12% to 14% of patients, is characterized by hyperkeratotic skin lesions that usually are on the plantar surface of the feet, toes, penis, and trunk. Painless oral ulcers may be present as well.

Reiter's syndrome may occur in human immunodeficiency virus (HIV)–infected patients, and sometimes is the initial manifestation of the disease.[688] This should be considered if the etiology of reactive arthritis is unknown.

Laboratory tests. Laboratory findings are consistent with the other seronegative spondyloarthropathies. There is an increase in the erythrocyte sedimentation (SED) rate, rheumatoid factor is negative, and HLA-B27 is positive in approximately 75%.

Treatment and management. Tetracycline or erythromycin is the usual treatment for sexually transmitted chlamydial infections. Until recently, similar antibiotic therapy for the treatment of Reiter's syndrome was unsuccessful;[528] however, more

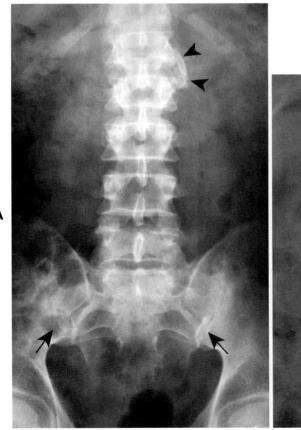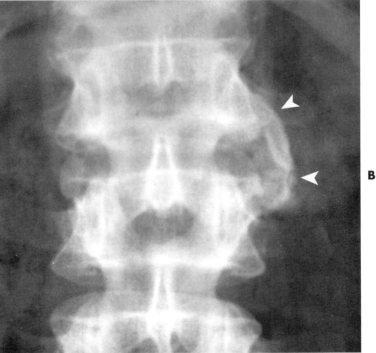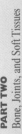

FIG. 9-79 **A,** Reiter's syndrome appearing with asymmetric bilateral sacroiliitis *(arrows)* and, **B,** a single thick syndesmophyte *(arrowheads).* (Courtesy Steven P. Brownstein, MD, Springfield, NJ.)

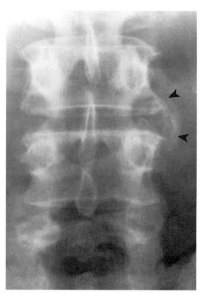

FIG. 9-80   Close-up view of a paravertebral ossification *(arrowheads)* characteristic of the spinal changes associated with Reiter's syndrome, or psoriatic arthritis. This patient is the same as the patient whose calcaneus is presented in Figure 9-73, and is a different patient than presented in Figure 9-79; note how typical these thick syndesmophytes can be. (Courtesy Arthur Holmes, Foley, AL.)

current studies have yielded favorable results.[32,33,352,485] It has been suggested that prophylactic antibiotics eventually may benefit individuals who are at risk for developing Reiter's syndrome.[33] At the onset, arthritic flare-ups usually respond to NSAIDs. Oral corticosteroids do not appear to be as effective. Intraarticular steroid injections may be necessary if the arthralgia is severe, especially in patients with large knee effusions.

KEY CONCEPTS

- *Reiter's syndrome is a seronegative spondyloarthropathy that predominantly affects the large joints of the lower extremities and small joints of the feet.*
- *Five times more men than women develop the syndrome. The average age of onset is between 15 and 35 years.*
- *The radiographic changes of the axial skeleton (sacroiliitis and spondylitis) may be identical to the changes seen in psoriatic arthritis.*
- *Inflammatory changes in the feet are similar to a combination of those associated with rheumatoid and psoriatic arthritis.*
- *Calcaneal enthesopathies (erosive and proliferative) are characteristic.*
- *Only a minority of patients develop the classic triad of arthritis, urethritis, and conjunctivitis that is associated with Reiter's syndrome.*
- *It is associated with nongonococcal genitourinary and enteric bacterial infections.*

■ Crystal-Induced Arthritides

Gouty Arthritis

BACKGROUND

Gout is the most common cause of inflammatory arthritis in men over 40 years old. It is a clinical disorder associated with elevated serum urate levels. Uric acid is the normal by-product of purine metabolism that is filtered and excreted by the kidneys. Hyperuricemia develops if overproduction of uric acid or underexcretion by the kidneys occurs. The excess urate crystallizes as monosodium salt, and is deposited into various connective tissues, including the articular and periarticular structures. When crystalline monosodium urate is deposited in the joint, an inflammatory response occurs, resulting in acute pain and swelling (gouty arthritis). These acute episodes are followed by asymptomatic periods. Chronic gout may result after approximately 10 years of recurrent intermittent acute attacks. A minority of patients (about 20%) with hyperuricemia develop gout. Its development is multifactorial; although hyperuricemia is requisite, it is not the sole determinant.

Gout is classified into two forms based on etiology: (a) an idiopathic or primary form that has no known underlying disorder, and is believed to result from an inborn error of purine metabolism, and (b) a much less common secondary form associated with an acquired disorder that is enzymatic, hereditary, hematologic, endocrine, renal, or associated with amyloidosis, multiple myeloma, or chemotherapy.[66] The first gouty attack of the idiopathic form occurs among individuals 40 to 50 years old; it is 20 times more common in men than women.[225] Women who develop gout generally are postmenopausal; only 17% are premenopausal.

Four phases of idiopathic gout are recognized:

1. *Asymptomatic gout.* The first phase is hyperuricemia, which may not lead to gout. Patients experiencing their first attack of acute gout have had sustained hyperuricemia for 20 to 30 years.

2. *Acute gouty arthritis.* The second phase involves acute inflammatory arthritis, which is classically monoarticular and usually involves the first MTP joint of the first toe, although oligoarticular or polyarticular involvement may occur. The ankle, tarsals, and knee also are commonly involved. Early attacks tend to subside without treatment in 7 to 10 days.

3. *Intercritical gout.* The third phase is the period between acute attacks. This stage may last for months or years, but tends to shorten with recurring episodes.

4. *Chronic tophaceous gout.* The fourth, or chronic, tophaceous gout phase is marked by the development of radiographically evident gross deposits of urate crystal or tophi in the subcutaneous tissues, synovium, subchondral bone, articular cartilage, joint capsule, and periarticular tissues such as the tendons (calcaneal), ligaments, and bursae (olecranon and prepatellar), and the classic extraarticular location, the helix of the ear. Often patients in the chronic phase of gout may not exhibit tophi for 10 to 12 years after the onset of joint pain.

IMAGING FINDINGS

Acute.   It is difficult for plain film to detect the early phases of gout, as the radiographic findings in the acute phase are nonspecific, presenting as soft-tissue swelling from capsular distention and adjacent soft-tissue edema, and not always easily recognized radiographically. In addition, these initial changes subside when the attacks remiss.

Chronic.   Chronic gout is well demonstrated on plain film with eccentric well-marginated osseous erosions that have overhanging edges of bone, central sclerotic erosions that may appear cystic, and soft-tissue deposits or tophi in and around the joint. These tophaceous deposits are the underlying mechanism for the radiographic appearance. The deposits appear as dense lobulated soft-tissue masses and may contain calcification. They are

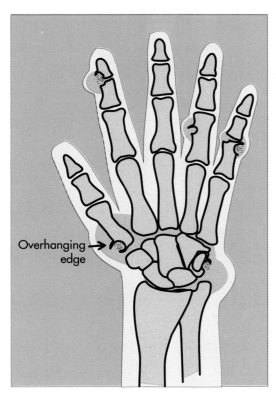

FIG. 9-81 Intraarticular or extraarticular deposits of gouty tophi cause mechanical erosion of the underlying bone. The mechanical nature of the erosion is marked by a sclerotic rim of cater, a feature not seen in inflammatory erosion of rheumatoid arthritis. At times the elevated margin of the erosion caused by the gouty tophus forms a shelf of bone that extends partially around the tophus. The shelf of bone is known as an *overhanging edge*.

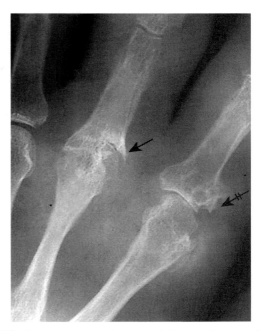

FIG. 9-82 Overhanging edge *(arrow)* partially extending around a gouty tophus of the fourth digit and two small but similar features present with the fifth digit *(crossed arrows)*.

asymmetric in distribution, and may cause bone erosions that are intraarticular, paraarticular, or located some distance from the joint. The tophi are directly deposited into the bone, or nestle into the bone via mechanical erosion. In the latter case, a thin "over-hanging edge" of bone with a sclerotic margin is left above and below the tophaceous deposit (Figs. 9-81 and 9-82). Even in

chronic gout, bone density usually remains normal. Osteoporosis is not characteristic of gout, unless severe pain causes disuse atrophy. Joint spaces usually are preserved until late in the disease, irrespective of adjacent large erosions. Bony ankylosis is not a feature; however, fibrous ankylosis may occur as a late manifestation of the disease.

Lower extremities. Gout tends to affect the peripheral joints of the lower the extremities, particularly the feet. The MTP articulation of the first toe is the most common initial site of gouty arthritis and when present in this location is called *podagra* (Fig. 9-83). Ninety percent of patients exhibit changes in this articulation during the course of the disease. Erosions of the first metatarsal head are most pronounced on the dorsal and medial

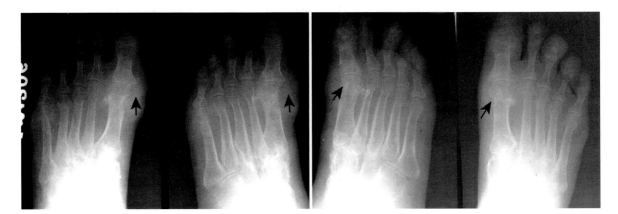

FIG. 9-83 Posteroanterior and oblique projections of both feet in a patient with gout. Gout is predisposed to the first metatarsophalangeal joint. Sometimes gout is called *podagra* at this site. As is typical, the erosions in this case are more pronounced on the medial and dorsal aspects of the joint *(arrows)*. However, the symmetry noted in this case is not a consistent feature of the disease. (Courtesy Steven P. Brownstein, MD, Springfield, NJ.)

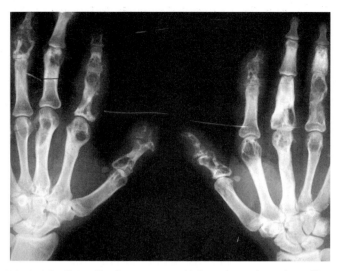

FIG. 9-84   *Gout.* The fingers appear with large destructive regions of bone on overlying soft-tissue masses.

aspects. There is associated soft-tissue swelling, and possibly a resultant valgus deformity. Soft-tissue swelling from tophaceous deposits and erosions may occur over the dorsum of the foot as a result of involvement of the tarsometatarsal, intertarsal, and talocalcaneal articulations. Tophi in the Achilles tendon and the adjacent structures are common.

Erosions may occur on the medial and lateral aspects of the knee, without visible joint space narrowing. Intraarticular tophaceous deposits in the knee may cause pain and swelling. MRI can be used to confirm their presence.[110] Erosive changes may involve

the patella, and tophi may lead to inflammation of the prepatellar bursa.

Upper extremities. Gout has a predilection toward the peripheral joints when the upper extremities are involved. Asymmetric joint changes may be noted in the wrists and hands, particularly involving the carpometacarpal joints, but the DIP, PIP, and to a lesser extent MCP articulations also may be affected (Figs. 9-84 and 9-85). Soft-tissue masses usually are located on the dorsum of the hand and wrist. Soft-tissue swelling, cystic defects, and joint destruction may be present in the wrist. Scapolunate dissociation also may occur.[530]

Large tophaceous deposits often are seen near the olecranon process of the elbow (Fig. 9-86). Adjacent bursal involvement may be bilateral, and presents as soft-tissue swelling over the extensor surface of the elbow.

Axial skeleton. Spinal involvement in gout is rare. SI involvement has been reported more commonly than spinal involvement, but is still considered infrequent.

CLINICAL COMMENTS

Acute gouty attacks present as joint pain, swelling, and erythema (Fig. 9-87). The presentation is usually monoarticular, although several joints may be involved. The presentation mimics cellulitis. The MTP of the great toe is the most commonly involved joint. Attacks are self-limiting, and usually subside within 3 to 10 days. The diagnosis often is presumed based on a classic presentation, but a definitive diagnosis for gouty arthritis depends on confirming the presence of monosodium urate crystals in the synovial fluid or tophi. Fluid samples are ordinarily drawn from the first MTP joint.

The kidneys are the most common extraarticular organ to be affected by gout. Urate nephropathy is an inflammation secondary to chronic hyperuricemia. Renal stones (uric acid nephrolithiasis) may occur in patients with long-standing gout.

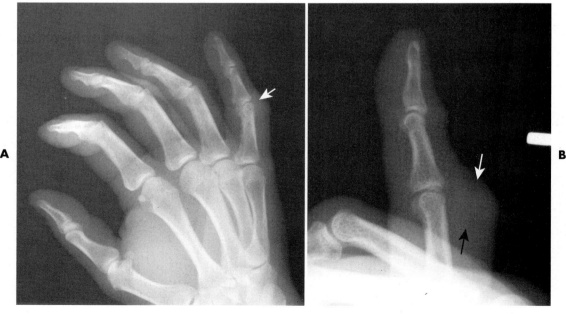

FIG. 9-85   Gout in one digit. **A,** The oblique hand reveals a small region of increased radiodensity of the proximal interphalangeal joint of the fifth digit. **B,** The large dorsal soft tissue mass is noted on the lateral view of the finger *(arrows).*

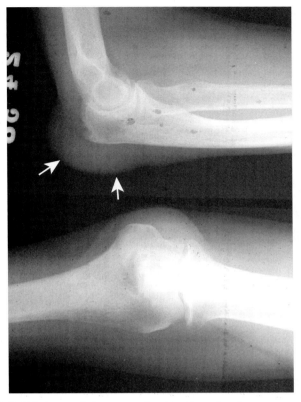

Laboratory tests. *Hyperuricemia* is defined as serum urate concentrations of more than 7 mg/dl in men and 6 mg/dl in women. Serum urate levels alone cannot be used to definitively diagnose gout because they may be high or low and therefore are often misleading. A normal level does not exclude the diagnosis of gout. However, serial uric acid measurements are useful in following the disease progression and treatment response.

Treatment and management. After diagnosis, the treatment objective is twofold. It is directed toward pain relief, consequent restoration of normal joint function, and the prevention of crystal accumulation within the joint that can lead to destruction and secondary degenerative disease. Any osseous changes noted radiographically usually are permanent, although minor improvement may be noted. Of course a search must be made for a possible underlying disorder (secondary gout) that may be treated directly. Acute pain and swelling usually responds well to the administration of NSAIDs, corticosteroids, and colchicine. Prophylactic use of NSAIDs and colchicine may be used in patients with severe, multiple, recurrent arthralgia. Patients should also be aware of factors that may contribute to or trigger the onset of an attack, such as alcohol or drug use, obesity, and high purine diets (e.g., all meats and seafood, meat extracts and gravies, yeast and yeast extracts, alcoholic beverages, beans). Low purine foods include pasta, flour, bread, milk, eggs, and fruits.

FIG. 9-86 Large soft-tissue mass of gout tophi near the olecranon process of the elbow *(arrows)*. (Courtesy Steven P. Brownstein, MD, Springfield, NJ.)

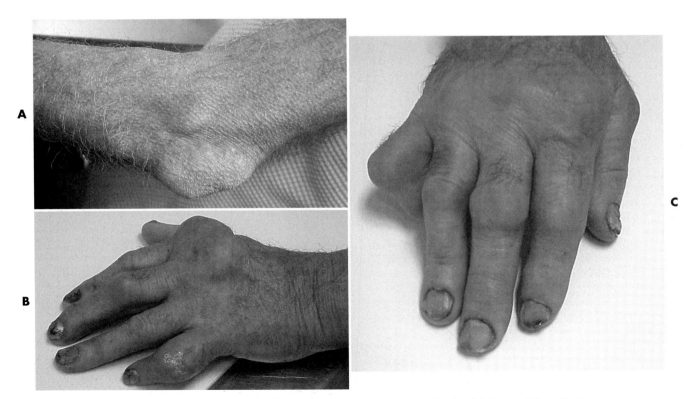

FIG. 9-87 Middle-aged male patient with large subcutaneous masses representing the clinical presentation of tophaceous gout in, **A,** the elbow and, **B** and **C,** both hands. (Courtesy Ian D. McLean, LeClaire, IA.)

PART TWO Bone, Joints, and Soft Tissues

- Gout is a clinical disorder resulting in monosodium urate crystal deposition into a variety of tissues, including the joints.
- Four gout phases are recognized: asymptomatic gout, acute arthritic gout, intercritical gout, and chronic tophaceous gout.
- The peripheral joints of the lower extremities are most commonly affected, and the first metatarsophalangeal joint is eventually affected in 90% of gout patients. This classic presentation is known as podagra.
- Early-stage radiographic features of gout are difficult to evaluate radiographically because they predominate as soft-tissue swelling resulting from capsular distention.
- Late-stage radiographic features of gout include randomly scattered eccentric nodular soft-tissue prominences or tophi that may contain calcium, and that have a predilection for the dorsum of the feet and hands and the extensor surfaces of the extremities; preservation of the joint space until very late stage; lack of osteoporosis; and intraarticular or periarticular bony erosions with a sclerotic well-defined "overhanging edge" whose formation is secondary to adjacent tophaceous deposits.

Calcium Pyrophosphate Dihydrate Crystals

BACKGROUND

The deposition of calcium pyrophosphate dihydrate (CPPD) crystals in and around joints results in an arthropathy with protean manifestations. The nomenclature relating to this process and disease is often confusing and incorrectly used. For the purposes of simplification, the text focuses on the following three major presentations of the calcium pyrophosphate deposition disease:

1. *Chondrocalcinosis.* The classic presentation of CPPD is radiographic evidence of calcified articular cartilage (chondrocalcinosis) involving characteristic sites, which include the knee, wrist, MCPs, and symphysis pubis. Less commonly, crystals also may be deposited and radiographically visible in the synovium, joint capsules, tendons, and ligaments.[499] The term *chondrocalcinosis* often is used incorrectly as a synonym for CPPD. Although calcium pyrophosphate is the most common crystal to cause chondrocalcinosis,[549] the terms *CPPD* and *chondrocalcinosis* are not truly interchangeable because crystals other than calcium pyrophosphates can be deposited in and around joints and lead to visible calcification; in addition, factors other than crystal deposition can lead to chondrocalcinosis or cartilage calcification (degeneration).

2. *Pyrophosphate arthropathy.* The intraarticular deposition of crystals may degrade the cartilage and lead to a second manifestation of CPPD that radiographically mimics severe joint degeneration, a condition called pyrophosphate arthropathy. The radiographic image is difficult to distinguish from primary OA or secondary OA after trauma; however, the location of joint involvement is helpful. Pyrophosphate arthropathy typically develops in an articulation or compartment that is unusual for primary OA, and there is lack of documented history of trauma that indicates secondary OA.

3. *Pseudogout.* The clinical presentation of CPPD varies; a patient can be completely asymptomatic or may present with an acute, painful, and inflamed joint that is similar to those associated with gout. The latter presentation has been appropriately called pseudogout.

The underlying cause of this CPPD is unknown, but its frequent association with other conditions such as gout, hyperparathyroidism, hemochromatosis, diabetes mellitus, and neurotrophic osteoarthropathy suggests that it may be secondary to metabolic or degenerative changes in the cartilage. It also has been proposed that the simultaneous occurrence of pseudogout and the aforementioned conditions is purely coincidental.

It is generally accepted that the prevalence of chondrocalcinosis increases with age, and that no particular gender develops the condition more often.[164,187,682] One study suggests that this increased prevalence with age and lack of gender bias may correlate with the affected tissues.[691] The study, which focused on structures of the knee, concluded that the prevalence of hyaline cartilage calcification increases with age and is not gender related, whereas meniscal calcification is not age related and is significantly more prevalent in men.

IMAGING FINDINGS

General radiographic features of CPPD can consist of a characteristic solitary finding such as chondrocalcinosis or a combination of features, which may include other intraarticular and periarticular calcifications, soft-tissue swelling, and progressive structural joint damage such as secondary degenerative joint disease (DJD) or mimic a neurotrophic arthropathy if severe.

Chondrocalcinosis. Cartilage calcification may involve hyaline or fibrocartilage (Figs. 9-88 to 9-93). Fibrocartilage calcification is most common in the menisci of the knees, triangular cartilage complex of the wrist, symphysis pubis, and acetabular labrum. The calcification presents radiographically as a thick, irregular radiopaque focus within the affected structure. Hyaline cartilage calcification also is common in the knee, wrist, hip, MCPs, elbows, and shoulders. On a radiograph it appears as a thin, linear radiopacity that runs adjacent and parallel to the articular surface of the bone.

Pyrophosphate arthropathy. Chronic pyrophosphate crystal deposition within hyaline cartilage may lead to intraarticular damage that radiographically simulate DJD. However, the joint *location* is unusual, or has an unusual intraarticular distribution when compared to DJD. These changes tend to be progressive and severe, with advanced joint space narrowing, prominent bony proliferation (sclerosis and osteophytosis), and often dramatic cyst formation. The articular and intraarticular (or compartmental) distribution classically differs from that of primary OA and should aid in the diagnosis. Non–weight-bearing joints such as the shoulder, elbow, wrist, and patellofemoral joint compartment are involved, as well as weight-bearing articulations such as the knee and hip. In a patient with no history of trauma, a DJD pattern in the mentioned non–weight-bearing joints suggests pyrophosphate arthropathy. Isolated involvement of the patellofemoral compartment (Fig. 9-94), advanced tricompartmental disease of the knee, and selective

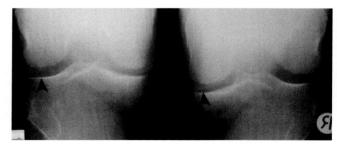

FIG. 9-88 Calcium pyrophosphate dihydrate presenting with chondrocalcinosis in the menisci bilaterally (*arrowheads*).

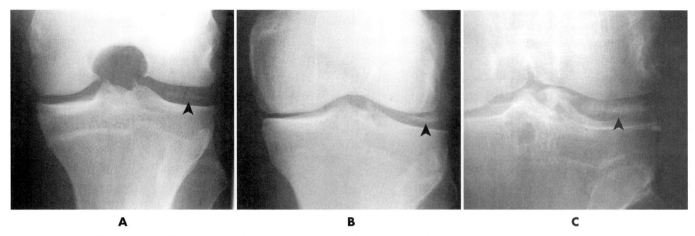

A   **B**   **C**

FIG. 9-89 **A** to **C,** Calcium pyrophosphate dihydrate meniscal chondrocalcinosis of the knee in multiple patients *(arrowhead).*

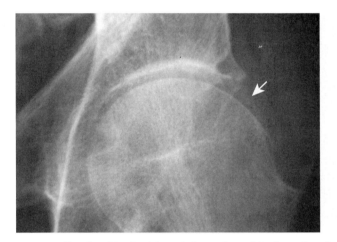

FIG. 9-90 Chondrocalcinosis of the articular cartilage of the femur *(arrow).*

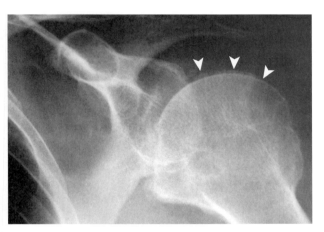

FIG. 9-91 Calcification of the articular cartilage of the humerus *(arrowheads)* in a patient with calcium pyrophosphate dihydrate chondrocalcinosis.

radiocarpal or trapezioscaphoid joint degeneration also are unusual for nontraumatic DJD and suggest that an underlying crystal deposition is responsible for the radiographic findings.

CLINICAL COMMENTS

The varied clinical presentations of CPPD can cause a diagnostic dilemma. CPPD may masquerade as primary DJD (chronic progressive joint pain, crepitus, and limited range of motion), manifest as an acute inflammatory disorder such as RA or gout (with intermittent attacks of painful, red, swollen joints), or appear as an asymptomatic condition in a patient with a concomitant disorder.

The diagnostic possibilities narrow if the clinical signs and symptoms are combined with radiographic evidence of chondrocalcinosis. This combination indicates that the patient probably has CPPD, and survey radiographs (such as an AP view of the knees, a PA view of the hands and wrists, and an AP view of the symphysis) perhaps should be taken. The clinician must keep in mind that chondrocalcinosis may not always develop, and as previously mentioned is not the only characteristic radiographic finding.

Laboratory tests. If clinical suspicion is high for CPPD, a diagnosis can be confirmed by synovial aspiration and

consequent microscopic identification of calcium pyrophosphate crystals. Other laboratory findings are not diagnostic but may reveal additional diseases such as diabetes, gout, hyperparathyroidism, or hemochromatosis.

Treatment and management. The treatment and prognosis for CPPD vary because they depend on the clinical presentation, radiographic findings, and presence of any underlying or associated disorders. The clinician must be aware that the patient may have an additional or underlying disease to make an appropriate investigation and provide the necessary treatment. The prognosis of CPPD without an associated underlying disease usually is excellent, although in some cases it may be poor (severe joint damage) and require the administration of intravenous colchicine or use of NSAIDs to control inflammatory episodes. Prophylactic use of oral colchicine may be used to prevent acute attacks.

A balance of exercise and rest is necessary to preserve the articular cartilage and control pain from active inflammation. Immobilization may help reduce overt inflammation, but it may have a more adverse affect on the articular cartilage than the inflammation itself; therefore joint mobility should be maintained to the patient's tolerance.[178]

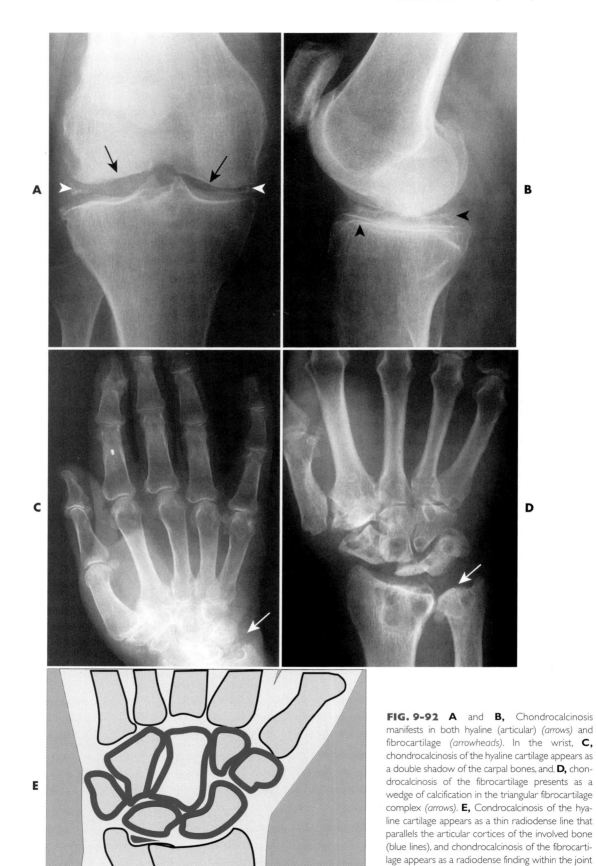

FIG. 9-92 A and **B,** Chondrocalcinosis manifests in both hyaline (articular) *(arrows)* and fibrocartilage *(arrowheads).* In the wrist, **C,** chondrocalcinosis of the hyaline cartilage appears as a double shadow of the carpal bones, and, **D,** chondrocalcinosis of the fibrocartilage presents as a wedge of calcification in the triangular fibrocartilage complex *(arrows).* **E,** Condrocalcinosis of the hyaline cartilage appears as a thin radiodense line that parallels the articular cortices of the involved bone (blue lines), and chondrocalcinosis of the fibrocartilage appears as a radiodense finding within the joint space (blue triangle).

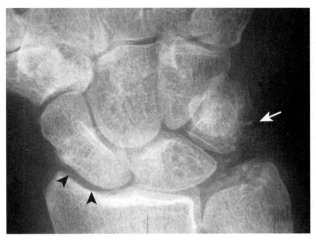

FIG. 9-93 Chondrocalcinosis of the triangular fibrocartilage complex *(arrow)* and faintly seen involvement of the hyaline cartilage *(arrowheads)*.

KEY CONCEPTS

- *Calcium pyrophosphate dihydrate (CPPD) is a disease in which calcium pyrophosphate dihydrate crystals are deposited in and around joints; the disease has three common presentations.*
- *The first presentation, which is marked by calcification of hyaline and fibrocartilage in and around joints (chondrocalcinosis), is considered classic.*
- *The second presentation involves progressive joint degeneration that radiographically mimics osteoarthritis or neurotrophic arthritis, and is called pyrophosphate arthropathy. Location is one key component in differentiating these disorders.*

- *The third presentation is characterized by acutely painful, swollen joints that simulate the clinical presentation of gout and is therefore called pseudogout.*
- *The sites commonly affected by CPPD are the knees, wrists, hips, and metacarpophalangeal joints.*
- *CPPD is often found with an underlying disorder (e.g., hemosiderosis, hyperparathyroidism, gout, amyloidosis).*
- *The prevalence of CPPD increases with advancing age, and in general does not demonstrate a male or female bias.*
- *Diagnosis is confirmed by joint aspiration.*
- *Wilson disease (associated with an accumulation of copper in tissues) is an extraordinarily rare condition that can result in chondrocalcinosis.*

Hemochromatosis

BACKGROUND

Primary hemochromatosis is an autosomal recessive disorder creating a mutated and abnormal protein that allows excessive cellular uptake of iron. It is the most common disease of iron overload. Patients with hemochromatosis have an increase in intestinal iron absorption. The excessive iron becomes stored in the body tissues, especially the liver, heart, and pancreas. Affected patients, most often nontreated children, may have abnormal bronze skin pigmentation and are at risk of developing diabetes mellitus because of pancreatic damage (bronze diabetes). These patients also are at increased risk for developing cirrhosis, which may lead to hepatocellular carcinoma.

Secondary hemochromatosis is seen in patients who receive multiple blood transfusions; however, this is of minimal clinical significance unless high volumes of blood are involved. Hemolytic anemias inclusive of thalassemia also may be implicated.

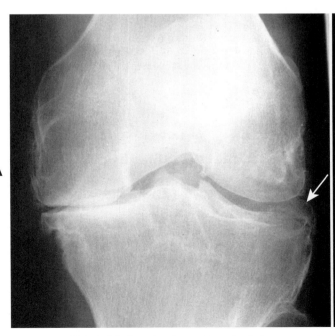
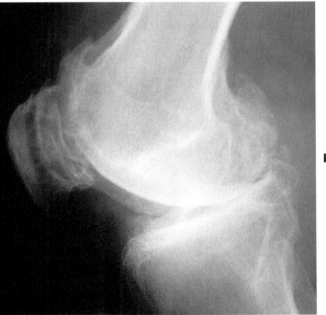

FIG. 9-94 Pyrophosphate arthropathy. **A,** Anteroposterior and, **B,** lateral knee radiographs revealing characteristic features of pyrophosphate arthropathy. Advanced femoropatellar compartment degenerative changes are present; the medial and lateral compartments of the knee are relatively spared. Meniscal calcification also is apparent *(arrow)*. Primary osteoarthritis has an affinity for the medial femorotibial compartment and tends to spare the lateral and retropatellar compartments.

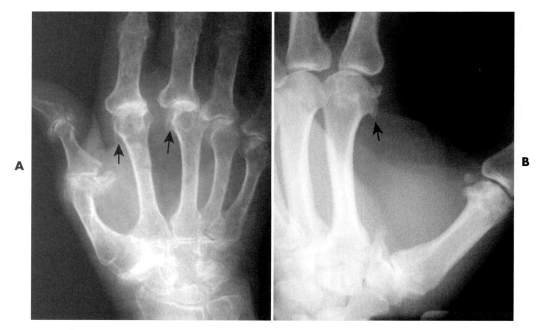

FIG. 9-95 A, Hemochromatosis with a characteristic hooklike osteophyte formed along the radial aspect of the metacarpal head and advanced joint degeneration *(arrows)* and, **B,** a second case of the hooklike osteophytes *(arrow)*. These peculiar osteophytes and the propensity for hemochromatosis to severely narrow joint spaces aid in differential diagnosis with other joint diseases.

IMAGING FINDINGS

The radiographic features of the arthropathy of hemochromatosis are similar to CPPD, with joint disease occurring in 25% to 50% of patients. However, hemochromatosis-related arthropathy has a predilection for the second and third MCPs (Fig. 9-95). Associated joint changes include joint space narrowing, sclerosis, and subchondral cysts. Beaklike osteophytes at the radial margins of the metacarpal heads are characteristic for hemochromatosis. As with CPPD, arthropathic features can be widespread with or without chondrocalcinosis. MRI is the best imaging examination to evaluate abnormal iron deposition in the liver. Liver parenchyma iron overload is characterized on MRI as a prominent decrease in signal intensity because of the paramagnetic effect of ferric ions that causes shortening of the T1 and T2 relaxation times. The pancreas also may exhibit a decrease in signal intensity on T2-weighted images. This is notable especially when comparing the signal intensity to the spleen, which typically remains normal. Complications of hemochromatosis also may be identified with this modality.

CLINICAL COMMENTS

Hereditary hemochromatosis is mainly associated with a defect of the HFE gene, which regulates iron absorption. Although primary hemochromatosis is present from birth, symptoms rarely appear before adulthood. Hereditary hemochromatosis is one of the most common genetic disorders in the United States, primarily affecting whites of Northern European descent (Celtic) and African Americans. Approximately 0.5% (1 in 200) of the U.S. white population is homozygous for hemochromatosis; one person in 8 to 12 is a carrier of the abnormal gene. Men are about five times more likely to be diagnosed with the effects of hereditary hemochromatosis than women. Men also tend to develop clinical symptoms at a younger age.

Diagnosis of hemochromatosis is performed with measurement of serum ferritin and transferring saturation. Definitive diagnosis of primary hemochromatosis can be made with genetic testing or liver biopsy with quantitative determination of liver iron concentration. Because of the prevalence of this disease, many suggest widespread screening; however, this is not practical at this time because the testing methods available are very costly.

Joint pain is the most common clinical complaint associated with the disease. Other common symptoms include fatigue, lethargy, abdominal cramping, impotence, and heart irregularities (Box 9-1).

Treatment and management. Phlebotomy is accomplished to rid the body of excess iron. Depending on disease severity,

---

BOX 9-1
Symptoms Related to Hemochromatosis

- Weakness
- Fatigue
- Abdominal pain
- General muscle aches
- Loss of sex drive
- Loss of body hair
- Impotence
- Cessation of monthly menstrual cycles
- Joint pain in the fingers
- Shortness of breath on exertion
- Increased skin pigmentation (a bronze color)

a unit of blood is obtained every 2 to 4 months and blood ferritin levels are monitored. Early management prevent organ system involvement, although joint disease still may occur with treatment.

Hydroxyapatite Deposition Disease

BACKGROUND

Calcium hydroxyapatite crystal deposition disease, often called *hydroxyapatite deposition disease* or HADD, is a disorder in which abnormal deposits of basic calcium phosphate crystals (predominantly hydroxyapatite) are present in and around the tissues of the joint. These deposits are frequently asymptomatic; however, they may give rise to a number of clinical syndromes caused by crystal-induced inflammation and degeneration. When a tendinous structure is involved, the term *calcific tendinitis* is often used as a descriptor or synonym for the condition. Although the etiology is unknown, it has been suggested that trauma, tissue necrosis, or degeneration and decreased vascularity play a role in its pathogenesis.[101,237,498,649] However, these alone do not explain the familial associations found,[351,391] nor the increased prevalence of the histocompatibility antigens HLA-A2 and HLA-BW35,[21] both of which lend themselves to the idea of a genetic predisposition or susceptibility to the disorder. Investigations of the mechanisms governing cartilage calcification and underlying pathogenesis of crystal deposition disorders are ongoing.[495]

There does not appear to be a significant gender association. The age at the time of involvement is usually 40 to 70, although it has been noted in children.[567] The condition is characteristically monoarticular, although polyarticular presentations do occur.[668]

IMAGING FINDINGS

Calcium hydroxyapatite crystals usually are deposited in periarticular structures, classically affecting the tendons, but also involving the joint capsule, or bursae, and to a lesser degree may be present in the intraarticular structures.[150] This periarticular predilection is an important differentiating feature in contrast to CPPD crystal deposition that has a primary tendency toward deposition in hyaline and fibrocartilage (intraarticular structures). The shoulder is the number one site of periarticular crystal deposition, although the wrist, hand, foot, elbow, hip, cervical spine, and lumbar spine also are commonly affected.

The radiographic features of HADD depend on the site and the structure involved (e.g., tendon, ligament, bursae), but classically appear as a cloudlike amorphous radiodensity in a periarticular location (Fig. 9-96). Over time the deposit may appear more distinct, well defined, or linear. On serial radiographs it may appear unchanged, or it may change shape, size, or even location. The calcific densities also may completely disappear[214] or reappear.[185]

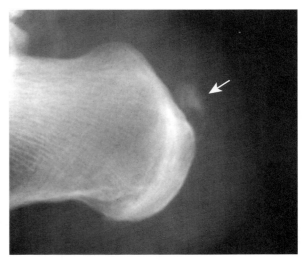

FIG. 9-96 Calcium hydroxyapatite crystals are deposited in the Achilles (calcaneal) tendon *(arrow)*.

The adjacent bony structures of the joint usually are unaffected; however, osteopenia, sclerosis, or cysts may occur.[179] Osteoporosis may be a feature because of disuse if the disorder is long-standing and associated with painful range of motion.

Shoulders. The supraspinatus tendon is the classic site of involvement for HADD, but deposits are also commonly seen in the adjacent capsule, bursa, ligaments, and other tendons.[267] The location of the deposit on plain film depends on the involved structure and the radiographic view (Fig. 9-97). Calcific deposits in the supraspinatus tendon are visible directly above the greater tuberosity of the humerus on external rotation, and overlie the humeral head on internal rotation.

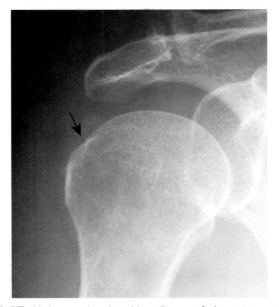

FIG. 9-97 Hydroxyapatite deposition disease of the rotator cuff. The supraspinatus tendon usually is involved, typically in its area of relative avascularity (known as the critical zone) near its insertion on the greater tubercle *(arrow)*. There also is advanced degeneration of the acromioclavicular joint, a common related finding to supraspinatus tendinopathy. (A similar case is noted in Fig. 9-141.)

Elbows. Calcific deposits may be seen in the various structures of the elbow (collateral ligaments, triceps tendon, and olecranon bursa). Calcification may have a classic cloudlike or linear appearance in these locations.

Hands and wrist. Calcification may be seen within the flexor and extensor tendons of the wrist and adjacent to the MCP articulations.

Hips. In the hip, calcific deposits frequently are noted adjacent to the greater trochanter of the femur involving the gluteal insertions and the surrounding bursae (Fig. 9-98).[306] In this location, they typically demonstrate the classic cloudlike appearance.

Knees. Calcific deposits have been described involving various structures of the knee. Equal propensity for involvement is noted with most structures. However, the quadriceps tendon is noted to be rarely affected.[148] The first case of popliteus tendon involvement was reported recently (Fig. 9-99).[636]

Cervical spine. Hydroxyapatite crystal deposition in the tendinous insertion of the longus colli muscle presents as a prevertebral calcific deposit usually at the level of C2, and may have accompanying soft-tissue swelling (Fig. 9-100). It can be asymptomatic or be the cause of acute neck pain. The latter presentation is called *acute calcific retropharyngeal tendonitis* or *longus colli tendonitis*.[25,557] Eventual resorption of the calcium deposit is common.

A rare presentation of hydroxyapatite in the cervical spine is called the *crowned dens syndrome*.[383] This is defined as calcification in the periodontic space with associated acute cervical spine pain. This peculiar and rare presentation is believed to only affect adult women.

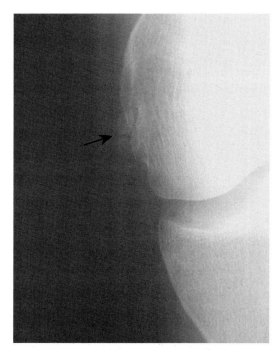

FIG. 9-99 Calcification in the region of the medial collateral ligament of the knee *(arrow)*. Pellegrini-Stiedi is an eponym for ossification of the medial collateral ligament after trauma, hematoma formation, and resulting dystrophic calcification.

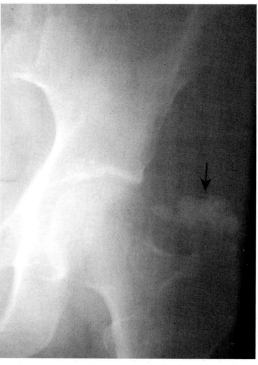

FIG. 9-98 Calcific deposit adjacent to the greater trochanter *(arrow)*.

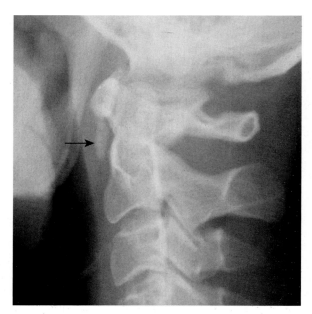

FIG. 9-100 Hydroxyapatite deposition disease of the longus colli muscle noted as amorphous calcification anterior to the C1 and C2 vertebrae *(arrow)*.

CLINICAL COMMENTS

Acute symptoms may include pain, tenderness, and localized swelling or edema. The clinical onset may mimic the presentation of a monoarticular arthritis or septic arthritis.[379] However, it is not uncommon to discover these calcific deposits in asymptomatic regions when ordering a radiograph for another, unrelated complaint (e.g., taking a chest film, noting calcium deposits in the shoulder). Chronic symptoms usually consist of mild pain and possibly limited range of motion.

Laboratory tests. Laboratory studies typically are unremarkable.

Treatment and management. Treatment may vary depending on the affected location. NSAIDs may be used, or corticosteroids may be prescribed if severe symptoms are present. Transcutaneous electric nerve stimulation (TENS) therapy, extracorporeal shock wave therapy (ESWT),[482] and a combination of phonophoresis, cross-friction massage, and range-of-motion exercises have all been reported to yield improvement.[214] A more

invasive treatment, arthroscopic débridement,[306,636] also has produced symptomatic improvement in the treatment of calcific tendinitis.

KEY CONCEPTS

- *Hydroxyapatite deposition disease is characterized by basic calcium phosphate crystals in the periarticular soft tissues, especially the tendons (calcific tendinitis).*
- *The age of presentation is typically between 40 and 70, and there is no significant gender bias.*
- *The shoulder is the major site of involvement, with the supraspinatus tendon being classic.*
- *The general radiographic appearance is a periarticular amorphous, cloudlike radiopacity. The adjacent bony structures typically are not affected.*
- *Laboratory tests usually are unrevealing.*
- *Clinical presentation ranges from asymptomatic to an appearance consistent with an acute monoarticular arthritis.*

Degenerative Arthritides

Degenerative Joint Disease

BACKGROUND

DJD (osteoarthritis, osteoarthrosis [OA]) is the most common of the arthropathies. It exhibits a slowly progressive nature, primarily affecting joint cartilage,[385] and represents the first[694] or second most common cause of disability in the adult (after cardiovascular disease).[433] Although the term *degenerative joint disease* presumes a synovial joint, similar changes occur in cartilaginous joints (e.g., AC, intervertebral disc) and therefore are included in the following discussion.

Etiology. Degeneration has a multifactorial etiology, representing a heterogenous collection of processes that affect the joints and periarticular tissues. Traditionally degeneration is divided into primary (or idiopathic) and secondary forms, based on the identification of an underlying condition or traumatic event. Primary degeneration represents a de novo process without causative factors; secondary follows a predisposing condition. However, the literature does not exhibit a uniform application of these categories. Many if not most cases of degeneration do not exhibit an obvious underlying etiology, prompting some authors to refer to these presentations as *primary degeneration*. However, other authors assume these cases are caused by unrecognized causative factors such as minute congenital malformation, microtrauma, and senescence, and therefore should be termed *secondary degeneration*. In other words, some authorities question the validity of the primary classification altogether, asserting that some type of underlying process or mechanical deviation nearly always precedes degeneration; one cannot identify it.[554] The primary OA designation will become increasingly obsolete as underlying causes of degeneration are researched and identified.

When the cause of secondary degeneration is identified, it usually entails trauma (acute or repetitive), avascular necrosis, diabetes mellitus, Paget's disease, slipped capital femoral epiphysis, chondrocalcinosis, neuropathy, acromegaly, ochronosis, hereditary disorders of collagen, and a variety of other conditions, especially those that lead to mechanical incongruity of the joint.

There are several etiologic theories of degeneration,[49] including repetitive trauma,[386] altered function of the synovium,[160,218] or subchondral bone. The most widely held theory implicates changes in the microenvironment of joint cartilage.[96,236] Chondrocytes facilitate the production of extracellular proteolytic enzymes that degrade the upper layers of the articular cartilage. Reparative processes respond, but are dominated by the degradation side of the equation. Because they are interdependent, cartilage degradation eventually leads to similar degenerative changes of the synovium and subchondral bone.

Risk factors. Many risk factors for developing degeneration have been identified. They are often grouped as systemic or local influences. Age is a systemic influence, and represents the strongest and most consistent correlate to degeneration.[137] Heredity, hormones, gender, and diet are other systemic influences.[566] Mechanical influences, including trauma, are the most important local influences, resulting in site-specific degeneration.[137] Risk factors are not equal in all people and for all joints; individual variations are common.

Bone density. Studies have shown a decrease in the incidence of degeneration among osteoporotic individuals. It has been postulated that osteoporotic bone may function as a better shock absorber, protecting the joint from trauma. However, this concept is not universally accepted. Other investigators have found an inverse relationship between bone density and the incidence of degeneration.[451] The influence of bone density on the incidence of degeneration remains unclear.

Age. Increasing age is a strong determinant to the occurrence and progression of degeneration.[433,657] Lawrence and associates found that all patients more than 65 years of age exhibited DJD in either the hands, feet, knees, hips, or spine.[355] Other studies indicate that 63% to 85% of Americans more than 65 years of age demonstrate radiographic findings of degeneration, 35% to 50% of whom have associated pain.[112,566,694] Although age is a major risk factor, degeneration is not necessarily a consequence of aging.[385,451,525,644] This is evidenced by the fact that degenerative cartilage differs structurally and biochemically from the normal cartilage found in elderly patients.[624] Therefore degeneration is age related, but not age dependent.[235]

Gender. Differences in the prevalence of degeneration are noted in men and women. Women are at greater risk than men for developing DJD in the knees,[604] hands, and feet. A hereditary influence of DJD appears to occur in the hands of women, whereas the influence of inheritance is less obvious in men.

Obesity. Obesity is a positive risk factor for DJD of the knees, hips, and probably hands.[189] Obesity appears to be a greater risk factor for females.[607] Weight loss reduces the risk of symptomatic DJD in the knees.[112,188]

Physical activity. Exercise and occupation influence the distribution of the disease; athletes and workers frequently develop characteristic patterns.[8,122,210,274] For example, degeneration is common in the feet of ballet dancers,[82] ankles of soccer players,[666] knees of football players, shoulders of baseball pitchers, hands of boxers, and elbows of pneumatic drill operators.[527]

A growing concern has developed about the potential of routine exercise as a risk factor for degeneration. Research suggests that normal joints tolerate prolonged vigorous low-impact exercise without accelerated development of degeneration.[265,347,348] However, the risk of developing degeneration appears to increase in high-impact activities, biomechanical alterations, sports played at the professional or elite levels, activities with torsional loading, and among individuals who continue exercise programs while injured.[265,348,349]

Exercise should not be discouraged in osteoarthritic patients. Evidence suggests that stretching, muscle strengthening, and aerobic conditioning can improve functional deficits in these patients.[696]

Trauma. Trauma is probably the single most important local factor predisposing a joint to degeneration.[373] The process of wear and tear explains many of the manifestations of DJD, but it does not account for all of the biochemical changes noted in degenerative cartilage.

Heredity. There is a significant body of evidence linking genetic factors to OA. This evidence is found in epidemiologic studies of family history and family clustering, twin studies, adoption studies, and detailed study of genetic disorders that express advanced OA (e.g., chondrodysplasias).[606]

IMAGING FINDINGS

The radiographic features of DJD are characterized by nonuniform reduction of the joint spaces, osteophytes, subchondral sclerosis, subchondral cysts, intraarticular loose bodies, joint misalignment, and deformity (Figs. 9-101 to 9-105 and Table 9-3). Narrowing of the joint spaces is the most often selected criterion variable for assessing DJD in research trials.[538] A traditional radiographic grading system of the severity of joint degeneration is presented in Table 9-4. Some of the radiographic features are more prominent in specific regions of the skeleton.

Although weight-bearing joints are most often involved, there is no consistent relationship to weight-bearing joints, because the ankles are rarely involved.[525] Nontraumatic OA occurring in the shoulder, elbows, wrists, or midfoot should raise suspicion of an underlying disease such as calcium pyrophosphate arthropathy or hemochromatosis.[433] Some of the more common locations of joint degeneration are listed in more detail in the following explanations.

Spine. Degeneration of the spine may affect the posterior joints (facets), intervertebral disc (IVD), uncovertebral joints,

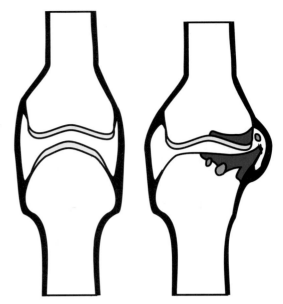

FIG. 9-101 Normal and degenerating joints. Degenerative joint disease is marked by nonuniform reduction of joint space, osteophytes, subchondral sclerosis, subchondral cysts, intraarticular loose bodies, joint misalignment, and deformity.

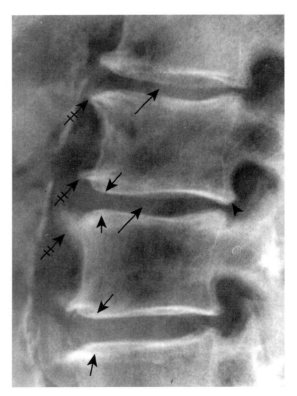

FIG. 9-102 Degenerative disc disease of the lumbar spine with reduced disc spaces (*large arrows*), osteophytes (*crossed arrows*), retrolisthesis (*arrowhead*), and endplate sclerosis (*small arrows*).

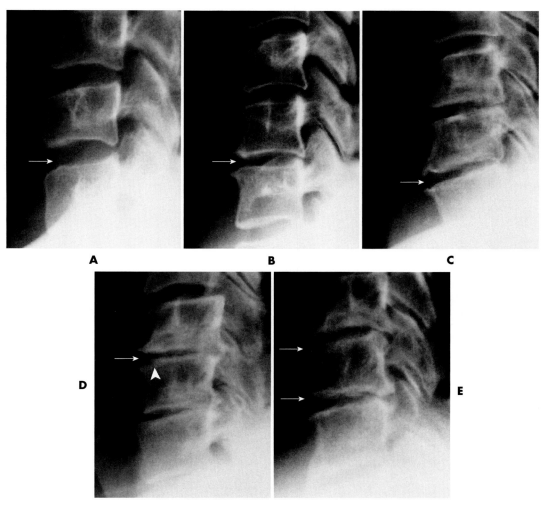

FIG. 9-103 Lateral cervical projections of different patients showing increasing stages of spinal degeneration. **A,** Disc spaces are well maintained without evidence of facet or disc degeneration *(arrow).* **B,** Small osteophytic processes extend from the anterior vertebral body margins, and disc space has been slightly reduced *(arrow).* **C,** Slightly larger osteophytes *(arrow)* than those in **B** and disc space reduction and endplate irregularity *(arrow).* **D,** Moderate disc space narrowing and osteophyte formation *(arrow)* of advanced degeneration. In addition, a degenerative radiolucent vacuum phenomenon is noted in the anterior disc region *(arrowhead).* **E,** The involvement of the disc space is less advanced than in **D,** but the osteophytes are more advanced, as shown by the fact that they are beginning to cross over the anterior disc space *(arrows).*

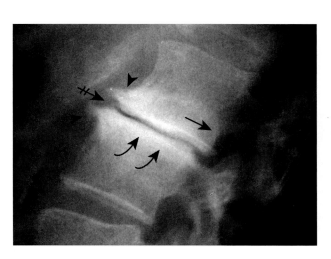

FIG. 9-104 Degenerative disc disease resulting in retrolisthesis *(arrow)*, reduction of the disc space *(crossed arrow)*, radiolucent vacuum phenomenon, endplate sclerosis *(curved arrows)*, and osteophytes *(arrowheads)*.

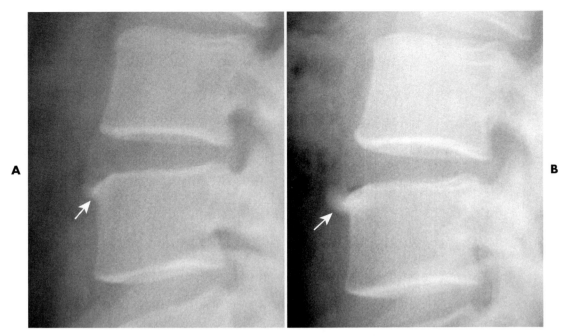

FIG. 9-105   A, A horizontal ("traction") osteophyte is formed at the anterior superior margin of L3 *(arrow).* **B,** Four years later, the osteophyte has progressed to a curved ("claw") appearance *(arrow).* The terms *traction* and *claw* should be avoided. Their use implies a meaningful difference between the two when no meaning difference exists.

costovertebral joints, and costotransverse joints (Figs. 9-106 to 9-121). Indirect findings of IVD degeneration are well demonstrated on radiographs. In the purest sense, because the disc is not a synovial joint, the use of *DJD* or *osteoarthritis* is inappropriate to describe IVD degeneration. Instead the terms *spondylosis* or *degenerative disc disease* (DDD) are used. Because the disc and facets are closely related anatomically and physiologically, degeneration affecting one will eventually affect the other.[58] Although the temporal direction of the relationship is difficult to detail, there is limited evidence that suggests, in general, that degeneration may first appear in the IVD and progress to the facets.[95] The working hypothesis suggests that increased loss of disc height leads to increased loading and subsequent degeneration of the facet joints.

Although individual segments degenerate at different rates depending on individual factors, in broad terms the process of spinal degeneration occurs in three stages. The first stage marks joint dysfunction and occurs in young adults. It involves anular tears and early synovitis of the posterior joints. The second stage is instability, occurring in those of middle to older age. The instability stage entails internal disc disruption and posterior joint degeneration and ligamentous laxity. The third and last stage, stabilization, occurs in patients more than 60 years of age and is characterized by osteophyte proliferation and joint stiffening.[333]

Intervertebral disc. Spondylosis (or DDD) presents with a narrowed disc space, osteophytes, misalignment, and eburnation; all similar findings to DJD. However, in addition DDD also presents with vacuum phenomena and Schmorl's nodes, which are both unique to degeneration of the IVD (see Table 9-3). Intercalary bones, representing calcifications within the anterior longitudinal ligament, may occur in association with degeneration. Only rarely,

TABLE 9-3	
Radiographic Grading of Osteoarthritis	
Grade	**Radiographic features**
0 (normal)	No features
1 (doubtful)	Minute osteophytes, doubtful significance
2 (minimal)	Definite osteophytes, unimpaired joint space
3 (moderate)	Definite osteophytes, moderate loss of joint space
4 (severe)	Definite osteophytes, advanced loss of joint space, with sclerosis of subchondral bone

From Kellgren JH, Lawrence JS: Radiological assessment of osteoarthrosis, *Ann Rheum Dis,* 16:494, 1957.

Text continued on p. 537.

TABLE 9-4

Pathophysiology of Radiographic Features Associated with Degeneration

Radiographic features	Description
Reduced joint space	Widely used criteria for radiographically assessing degeneration. This feature develops secondary to degenerative thinning of the articular cartilage or intervertebral disc.
Osteophytes	Osteophytes represent degenerative osteochondral nodules formed at the enthesis or attachment of ligaments or tendons into bone near a joint. It appears that both mechanical and humoral influences stimulate the formation of osteophytes from tissue at the chondrosynovial junction or progenitor cells residing in the perichondrium.[3,361,411] Osteophyte formation appears to be triggered by joint trauma and is an important part of the stabilization process. Osteophytes develop via enchondral bone formation along the internal (central) and external (marginal) aspects of the joint or through intramembraneous bone growth along the margin of the cortex (periosteal osteophytes or "buttressing"). Capsular osteophytes result from capsular tension.[521] Osteophytes are common in the spine, resulting from traction forces on the Sharpey's fiber insertions of the outer anulus into the compact bone of the outer vertebral rim.[553] Some authors divide spinal osteophytes into curved "claw" and horizontal "traction" types based on appearance. However, other than their difference in appearance, there is no clinically important difference between the "claw" and "traction" designation, and the practice should be avoided to limit confusion. It has been postulated that osteophytes tend to develop in a marginal location in an attempt to stabilize and reduce the range of joint motion[537] or as a feature to increase the surface area of the articular surface, thereby reducing joint load. Others postulate that the common marginal location of osteophytes is merely the default growth pattern occurring in the direction of least resistance.[7,212,246,398] Similar marginal bony outgrowths occur secondary to traction forces applied to the insertion of ligaments and tendons into bone (enthesis). Osteophytes should be distinguished from the thinner syndesmophytes that develop in patients with inflammatory arthropathies (e.g., ankylosing spondylitis, rheumatoid arthritis) or thick syndesmophytes that develop in patients with Reiter's syndrome and psoriatic arthropathy.
Vacuum phenomena*	Knuttson's sign—radiolucent defects indicating the presence of nitrogen gas accumulations in annular and nuclear degenerative fissures. The nitrogen gas is thought to arise from the extracellular spaces; because the gas accumulates in areas of lower pressure, it is often seen in fissures of the anterior disc on extension radiographs. The presence of a vacuum phenomenon virtually excludes the possibility of an infection causing a narrow intervertebral disc (except in the rare cases in which a patient has a gas-forming infection). Vacuum phenomena are normal in synovial joints under slight distraction[204] (e.g., vacuum often is seen in the anteroposterior projection of the glenohumeral joint because of the weight of the arm slightly distracting the joint).
Cartilaginous (Schmorl's) nodes*	Abrupt, focal, radiolucent intravertebral disc displacements. Schmorl's nodes usually are normal variants that develop in weakened areas of the vertebral endplate where a blood vessel or the chordal dorsalis has regressed from the cartilaginous endplate; they usually develop in young patients. The more clinically significant Schmorl's nodes, which typically develop in a patient's thirties or forties, are related to intervertebral osteochondrosis, or are the result of an endplate fracture (and are called traumatic Schmorl's nodes).
Subchondral sclerosis	Also known as eburnation; represents infraction, compression, and necrosis of stressed subchondral bone trabeculae.[99,252] At times subchondral vertebral sclerosis may appear exaggerated (hemispheric spondylosclerosis), mimicking an infection. Absence of bone destruction, paravertebral mass, and historic indicators assist the exclusion of an infection.
Subchondral cysts	Also known as geodes—regions in which synovial fluid has been forced through degenerative cartilaginous fissures in the subchondral bone.
Joint misalignment	Misalignment of articular surfaces occurring secondary to reduced joint space and laxity of surrounding ligaments; in the spine, advanced facet arthrosis may lead to anterior displacement of the vertebral body (degenerative spondylolisthesis). Degenerative spondylolisthesis is common in the "three Fs"—females over 40 at the fourth lumbar level, and the degree of displacement partially depends on the severity of concurrent intervertebral disc and facet degeneration; another example of joint misalignment occurs as muscle tension laterally displacing the first metacarpal secondary to joint laxity associated with advanced first carpometacarpal joint degeneration.
Joint deformity	Redistribution of forces across the joint surfaces and secondary bone remodeling that can be caused by advanced degeneration.
Intraarticular fragments	Also referred to as loose bodies or joint mice—intraarticular postdegenerative fragments of bone, cartilage, meniscus, and synovium.
Degenerative enthesopathies	Degenerative enthesopathies occurring at a joint are termed osteophytes. However, degenerative enthesopathies are not limited to the proximity of joints, or degenerative joint disease. For instance, enthesopathy is a prominent feature of several seronegative inflammatory joint diseases. Degenerative enthesopathies are common to the inferior margin of the calcaneus, at the insertion of the plantar aponeurosis; commonly termed a heel spur.

*Characteristics of degenerative disc disease (DDD) only.

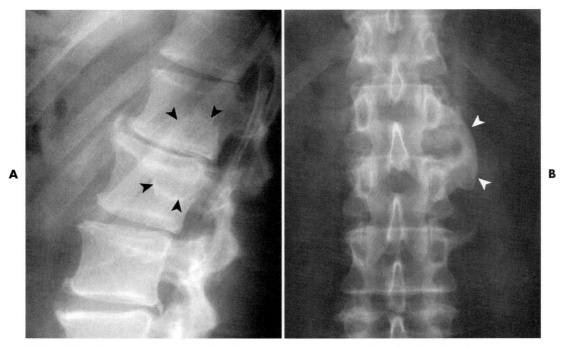

FIG. 9-106   A, Large osteophytes are formed along the reading right side of L1-2 *(arrowheads).* **B,** It appears as a radio-dense shadow over the vertebrae and disc space in the lateral projection. Large osteophytes, as noted here, are not typical. In the absence of other data, the appearance is difficult to separate from diffuse idiopathic skeletal hyperostosis, psoriatic arthropathy, or Reiter's syndrome.

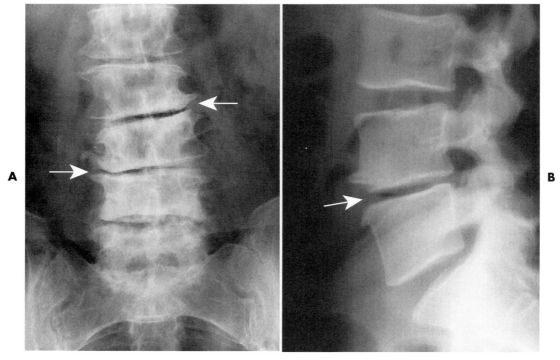

FIG. 9-107   A, Anteroposterior and, **B,** lateral lumbar radiographs on different patients with, **A,** advanced and, **B,** moderately advanced intervertebral disc degeneration and vacuum phenomena *(arrows).*

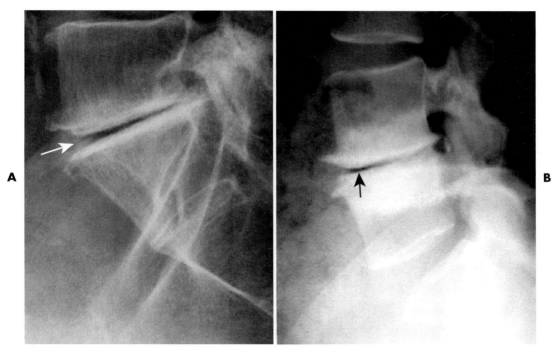

FIG. 9-108 Degenerative vacuum phenomenon at, **A,** L4 and, **B,** L5 *(arrows)*.

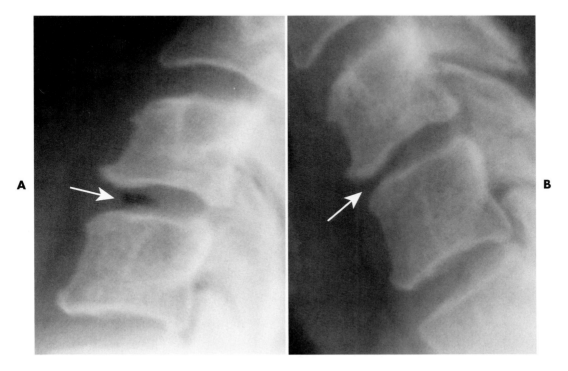

FIG. 9-109 A, Lateral cervical radiograph with the patient in extension revealing intradiscal vacuum phenomena *(arrows)* that, **B,** disappear during flexion. The extension movement decreases the intradiscal pressure, which makes vacuum phenomena more easily seen.

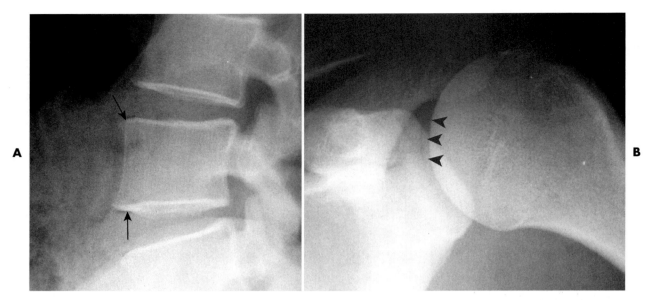

FIG. 9-110   A, Small vacuum clefts representing defects at the anulus insertion into the endplate *(arrows).* **B,** An intraarticular vacuum phenomenon is normal when found in an extremity joint under slight distraction, as often occurs in the shoulder joint as patients hold a weight to distract the acromioclavicular joint, testing the joint's integrity *(arrowheads).* They are not normal when found in the intervertebral disc.

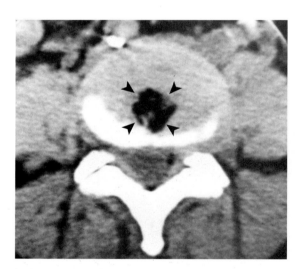

FIG. 9-111 Intradiscal vacuum phenomenon *(arrowheads)* seen as a central radiolucent defect on a computed tomography scan. (Courtesy Steven P. Brownstein, MD, Springfield, NJ.)

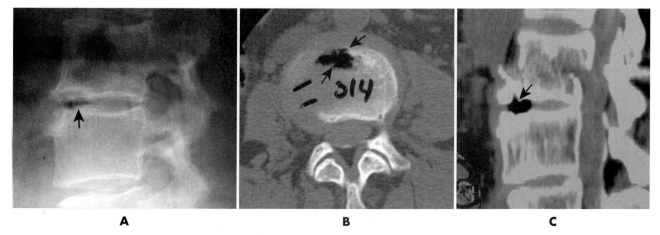

A   **B**   **C**

FIG. 9-112 The anterior intradiscal vacuum phenomenon of L3 is seen, **A,** on plain film; **B,** axial; and, **C,** sagittal reformatted computed tomography scans *(arrows).*

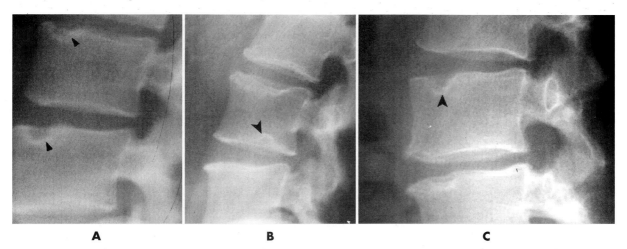

A   **B**   **C**

FIG. 9-113 A to **C,** Schmorl's node herniations seen in a lateral lumbar projection as abrupt focal intravertebral endplate intrusions on three patients *(arrowheads)*. (**A,** Courtesy Steven P. Brownstein, MD, Springfield, NJ.)

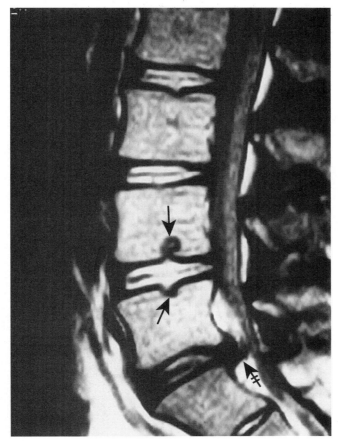

FIG. 9-114 T2-weighted sagittal lumbar magnetic resonance imaging scan demonstrating a Schmorl's node herniation at the superior endplate of L5 and inferior endplate of L4 *(arrows)*, and an L5 disc herniation *(crossed arrow)*.

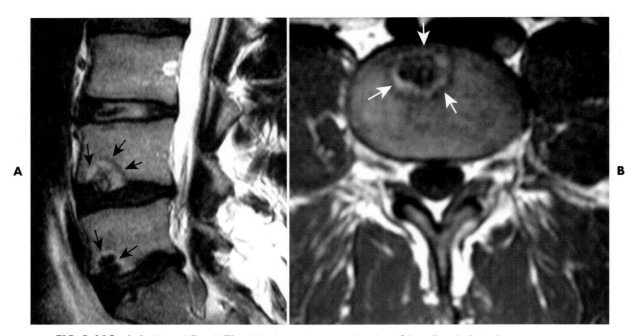

FIG. 9-115 **A,** Sagittal and, **B,** axial T2-weighted scans demonstrating a large Schmorl's node *(arrows)*.

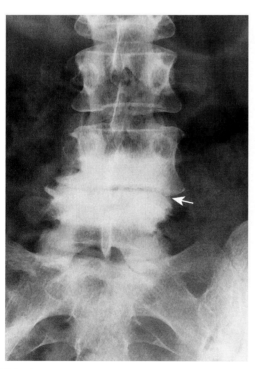

FIG. 9-116 Anteroposterior lumbar projection showing advanced intervertebral disc degeneration of L4 marked by reduced L4 disc space by surrounding osteophytes from the vertebral margins and dense radiopacity of the subchondral bone in response to the degeneration *(arrow)*. Laterolisthesis of L4 on L5 developed because of the advanced degeneration and subsequent joint laxity. (Courtesy Joseph W. Howe, Sylmar, CA.)

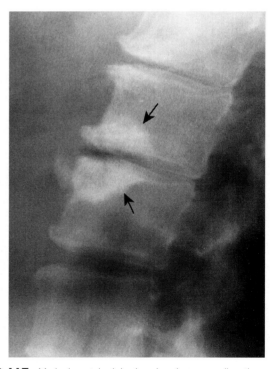

FIG. 9-117 Marked vertebral body sclerosis surrounding the narrowed degenerative disc *(arrows)* with vacuum phenomena. Vertebral sclerosis may be visually confused with an infection. However, the presence of vacuum phenomena virtually excludes non–gas-producing infection as a cause for the vertebral sclerosis. In theory, an infection replaces the air-filled vacuum with pus and edema, eliminating the air density on the radiograph. (Courtesy Ronnie Firth, East Moline, IL.)

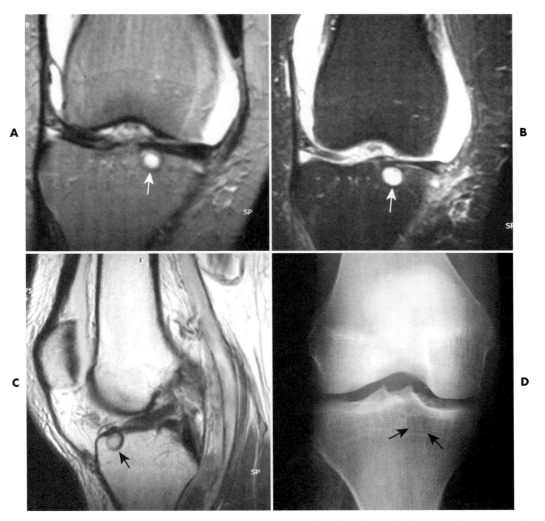

FIG. 9-118 A degenerative cyst *(arrows)* is noted incidentally in this patient who suffered a recent knee trauma that produced a large amount of joint effusion on, **A,** the T2-weighted coronal; **B,** short tau inversion recovery; and, **C,** T1-weighted sagittal scans. **D,** The effusion is not seen on plain film, and the cyst is barely visible. An intraosseous ganglion also explains the features; the two are impossible to distinguish without observing a communication to the joint or other degenerative features to aid in differentiation. (Courtesy Ian McLean, LeClaire, IA.)

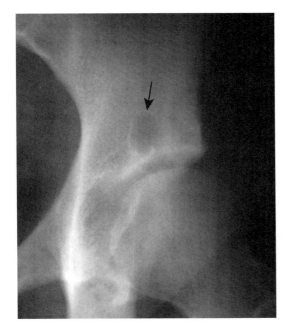

FIG. 9-119 Small subchondral cyst in the supraacetabular region *(arrow).* Typically the degenerative subchondral cyst is not an early manifestation of degeneration; however, this may be the case in the hip, in which it is often the first feature of degeneration. As is the case in this example, subchondral cysts often have a thin rim of sclerosis. Similar to the case presented in Fig. 9-118, in the absence of osteophytes or reduced joint space, this finding also could represent an interosseous ganglion.

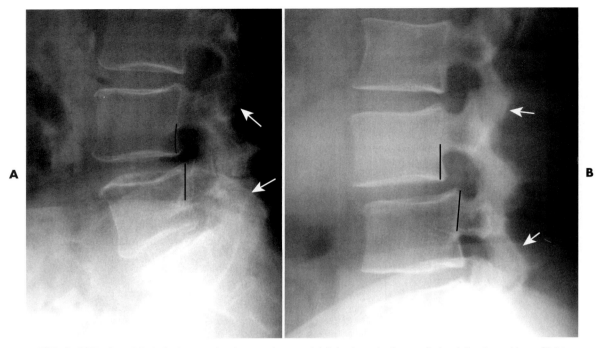

FIG. 9-120   **A** and **B,** In both examples degenerative spondylolisthesis results from articular deformity and loss of joint space associated with posterior joint and disc degeneration *(arrows).*

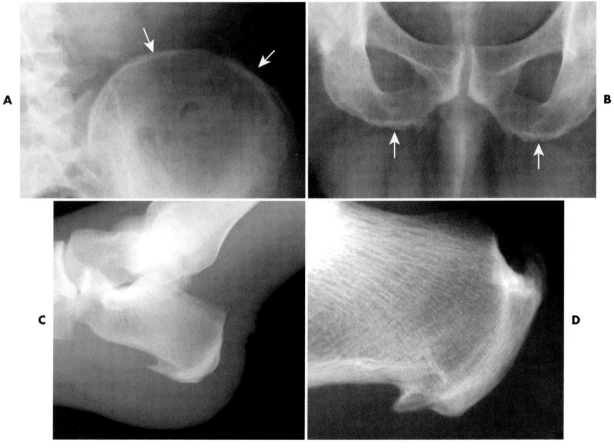

FIG. 9-121   Degenerative enthesopathy appears as irregularity of, **A,** the iliac crest; **B,** ischial tuberosities; or, **C,** a bone spur at the insertion of the plantar aponeurosis, or additionally at, **D,** the insertion of the calcaneal tendon *(arrows).*

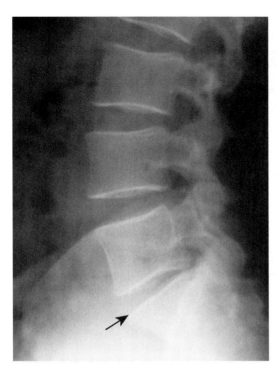

FIG. 9-122 Decreased L5 disc space. Because no other signs of degeneration are present (e.g., osteophytes, vacuum phenomena), the narrowing of the L5 disc (arrow) probably is not degenerative, especially in young patients. Disc hypoplasia is a common cause of a narrow disc space.

and usually in very advanced cases, are all of the radiographic findings present concurrently. Marginal osteophytes and IVD narrowing are the most common and reliable degenerative radiographic findings. Osteophytes are less pronounced on the left side throughout the middle to lower levels of the thoracic spine because of the pulsations of the adjacent descending aorta.[588] Narrowing of the posterior lumbosacral disc height below 5.5 mm on plain film is associated with degenerative changes.[115] However, because the fifth lumbar disc space is often developmentally narrow (Fig. 9-122), do not interpret a narrow disc space without osteophytes (or other concurrent signs of degeneration) as degenerative at the L5 level.

At times, it is more descriptive to divide spondylosis into two often parallel loci of degeneration. Degeneration of the outer portion of the anulus fibrosus, marked by marginal osteophytes, has been termed *spondylosis deformans*.[388,553] Degeneration of the innermost portion of the anulus fibrosus, together with dehydration of the nucleus pulposus and breakdown of the cartilaginous endplate, is called *intervertebral chondrosis*. The term *intervertebral osteochondrosis* is applied if the adjacent vertebrae appear to be involved, suggested by vertebral endplate sclerosis (or eburnation). Degeneration of the inner disc is demonstrated radiographically by reduction of the IVD height[388,553] and intradiscal vacuum phenomena.

MRI is particularly helpful to image the IVD. The normally well-hydrated nucleus pulposus has high signal intensity on the sagittal T2-weighted spin-echo MRI sequence. Loss of nuclear signal intensity indicates dehydration and alterations in the macromolecule content and distribution in the nucleus pulposus.[440,577] These changes are the result of senescence and degeneration (Figs. 9-123 and 9-124).*

*References 52, 211, 261, 291, 360, 436, 438, 440, 442, 477, 483, 497, 574, 577, 586, 687.

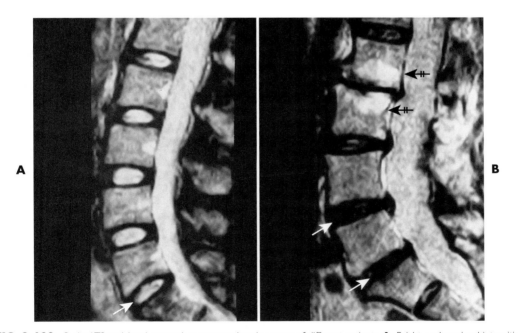

FIG. 9-123 Sagittal T2-weighted magnetic resonance imaging scans of different patients. **A,** Bright nuclear signal intensities at the L1 to L4 levels and a slight decrease in intensity at the L5 level (arrow). High signal intensity indicates that the water content is high and the inner disc is healthy. **B,** Low signal intensity indicating loss of water and degeneration of the inner disc (arrows). High signal intensity is noted in the region of the vertebral body marrow subjacent to the endplates surrounding the L2 disc (crossed arrows). Bright signal intensity corresponds to vascularized tissue formed in response to degeneration (Modic type I). The region of the vertebra was less intense on the T1-weighted scans (not shown).

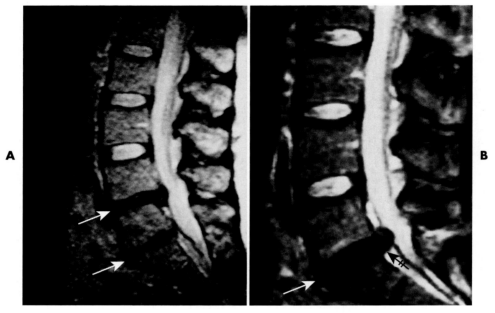

FIG. 9-124   Sagittal lumbar magnetic resonance imaging scans of two different patients exhibiting decreased nuclear signal intensity, which indicates disc degeneration. **A,** Degeneration involving the L4 and L5 levels *(arrows)*. **B,** Degeneration only of the L5 level *(arrow)*. A large disc herniation is noted at the L5 disc level *(crossed arrow)*.

In addition to delineating the IVD anatomy directly, MRI exhibits characteristic vertebral body changes that occur in response to IVD degeneration. These changes have been categorized into three types based on the vertebral appearance on a spin-echo MRI sequence (Figs. 9-125 to 9-127 and Table 9-5).[17,146,404,438] Any relationship between these marrow changes and patient symptoms remains unclear.

Uncovertebral joints.   The bilateral posterolateral uncinate processes of the third through seventh cervical vertebrae articulate with the corresponding grooves of the vertebra above to form cartilaginous uncovertebral (Luschka, neurocentral) joints. Uncovertebral degeneration presents as pointed or bulbous osteophytes extending from the uncinate processes that may encroach on the intervertebral foramina, possibly causing radiculopathy (Figs. 9-128 and 9-129).[365,683] It is possible that hypertrophic uncinate processes compromise the vertebral artery blood flow.[121,592]

Degeneration is most common in the middle and lower cervical levels. Uncinate degeneration is readily demonstrated on the frontal or oblique radiographic projections. In the lateral radiographic projection, uncinate process hypertrophy may give the appearance of a radiolucent fracture line (pseudofracture) extending horizontally across the lower cervical body at the level above the degeneration (Figs. 9-130 and 9-131).[561] CT may be useful to further delineate clinically relevant levels.

Zygapophyseal joints.   The zygapophyseal (apophyseal, facet, posterior) joints are synovial articulations formed between the paired superior and inferior articular processes of adjacent vertebrae from C2-S1. Radiographically, degeneration is most often observed in the middle cervical, upper and middle thoracic, and lower lumbar regions.[331,390] It is recognized by joint irregularity, increased sclerosis, vertebral anterolisthesis (degenerative spondylolisthesis), and osteophytosis (Figs. 9-132 to 9-135). The AP and oblique views are best to demonstrate these changes of the zygapophyseal joints. The axial images provided by CT and MRI

are particularly helpful to assess degenerative changes and existing soft-tissue complications (Fig. 9-136).

Factors influencing zygapophyseal degeneration are similar to those affecting other joints. In particular, altered stresses across the articulations increase the incidence of zygapophyseal degeneration. This occurs with kyphosis, scoliosis, and probably facet tropism.[54,633]

Costovertebral joints.   The costovertebral joints are the articulations between the rib heads and transverse processes. The costotransverse joints (Fig. 9-137) are the articulations between the rib tubercles and transverse processes. Both joints are synovial and exhibit osteophytosis, sclerosis, and irregularity when they become degenerative. Degeneration most often affects costovertebral joints at the lower thoracic levels.

Sacroiliac joints.   Degeneration of the SI joints appears as increased sclerosis and irregularity of the joint margins. Degeneration has a propensity to the middle third of the SI joint, distinguishing it from the propensity of inflammatory arthritides (e.g., AS) to target the lower third of the joint (Figs. 9-138 and 9-139). In advanced cases, portions of the joint space may not be seen clearly because of bridging osteophytes. Intraobserver and interobserver error is a limiting factor for reliably interpreting degeneration of such an irregularly shaped joint on radiographs.[559]

Shoulders.   The AC joint is more commonly involved than the glenohumeral joint (Figs. 9-140 and 9-141). Large osteophytes may project from the inferior margin of the AC joint producing rotator cuff tendinopathy, usually of the supraspinatus tendon. Inflammation and compromise of the tendon lead to superior migration of the humeral head because of the unopposed action of the deltoid, with consequential narrowing of the acromiohumeral space (shoulder impingement syndrome). Advanced degeneration of the glenohumeral joint often results from complete rupture of the supraspinatus tendon, disruption of the joint capsule, and loss of synovial fluid. MRI is particularly valuable to evaluate the integrity of the supraspinatus tendon. Radiographic evidence of dystrophic

Text Continued on p. 549.

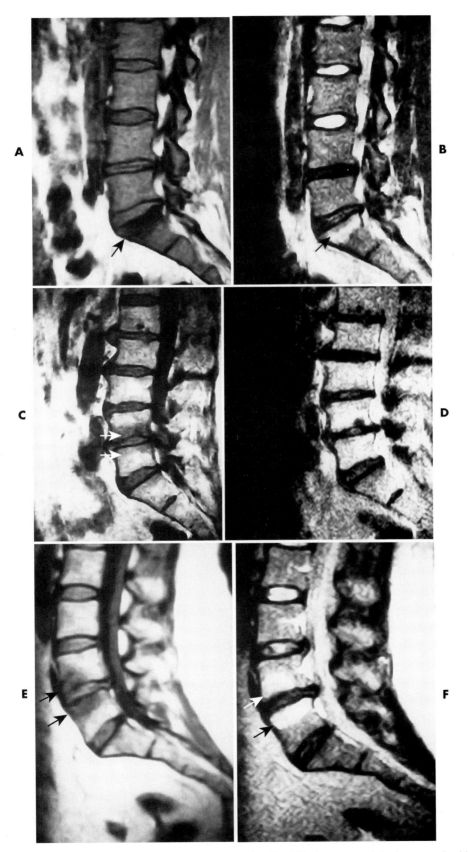

FIG. 9-125 Modic type I vertebral changes. Three patients who all exhibit decreased vertebral marrow signal intensity *(arrows)* on, **A, C,** and **E,** the T1-weighted studies that increased on, **B, D,** and **F,** the corresponding T2-weighted images, indicating the presence of highly vascularized fibrous tissue.

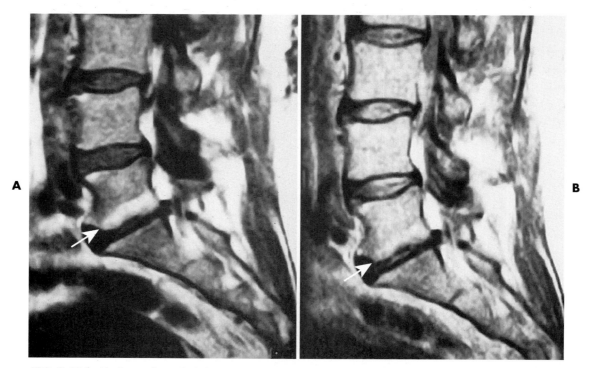

FIG. 9-126   Modic type II vertebral changes. Vertebral bands of increased signal intensity *(arrows)* on, **A,** the T1-weighted image remain increased on, **B,** the T2-weighted image, indicating the presence of yellow bone marrow.

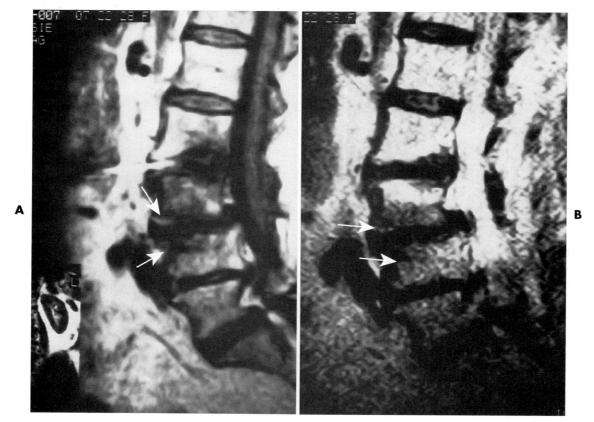

FIG. 9-127   Modic type III vertebral changes. Vertebral bands of decreased signal intensity *(arrows)* on, **A,** the T1-weighted image remain decreased on, **B,** the T2-weighted image, indicating bone sclerosis.

TABLE 9-5

Classification of the Magnetic Resonance Imaging (MRI) Appearance of Vertebral Body Marrow Patterns Resulting from Degenerative Disc Disease

Classification (Modic)	Appearance on MRI	Histology and significance
Type I	Decreased signal intensity (appearing dark) on T1-weighted images and increased signal intensity (appearing bright) on T2-weighted images	Highly vascularized fibrous tissue in the vertebral body corresponding to acute stages of disc degeneration
Type II	Increased signal intensity (appearing bright) on T1-weighted images and equal to slightly increased signal intensity (medium) on T2-weighted images	Continuation of type I vertebral changes in which vascularized fibrous tissue is replaced by yellow bone marrow
Type III	Decreased signal intensity (appearing dark) on both T1- and T2-weighted images	Extensive body sclerosis that is associated with long-standing degeneration and correlates with radiographic evidence of vertebral sclerosis

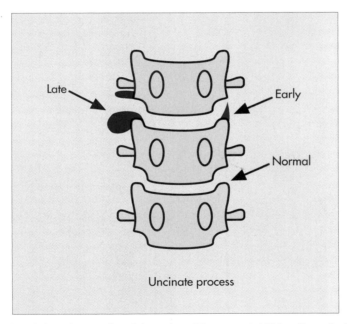

FIG. 9-128 In the frontal plane, degeneration of the uncinate joints presents initially with small spikes from the uncinate processes, progressing to a bulbous enlargement that directs posterolaterally, potentially encroaching on the adjacent intervertebral foramen.

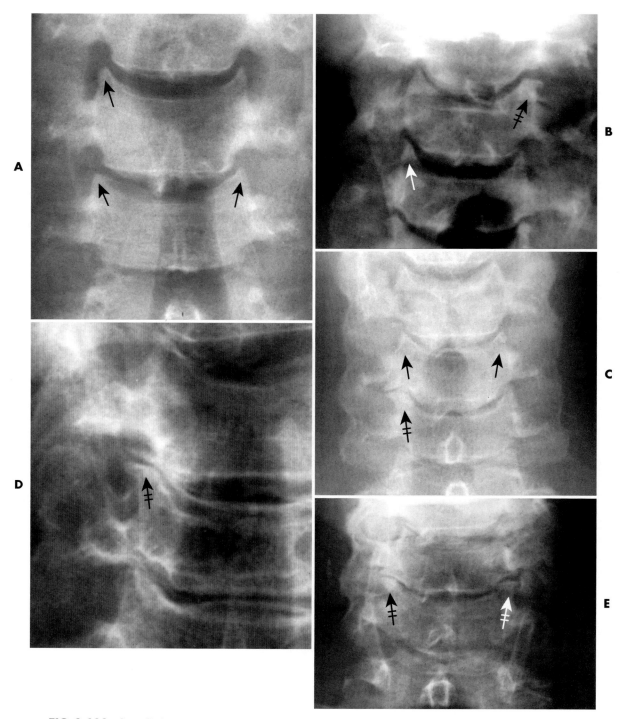

FIG. 9-129   A to **E,** Anteroposterior projections of the middle cervical region of different patients showing normal *(arrows)* and degenerative *(crossed arrows)* changes of the uncinate processes.

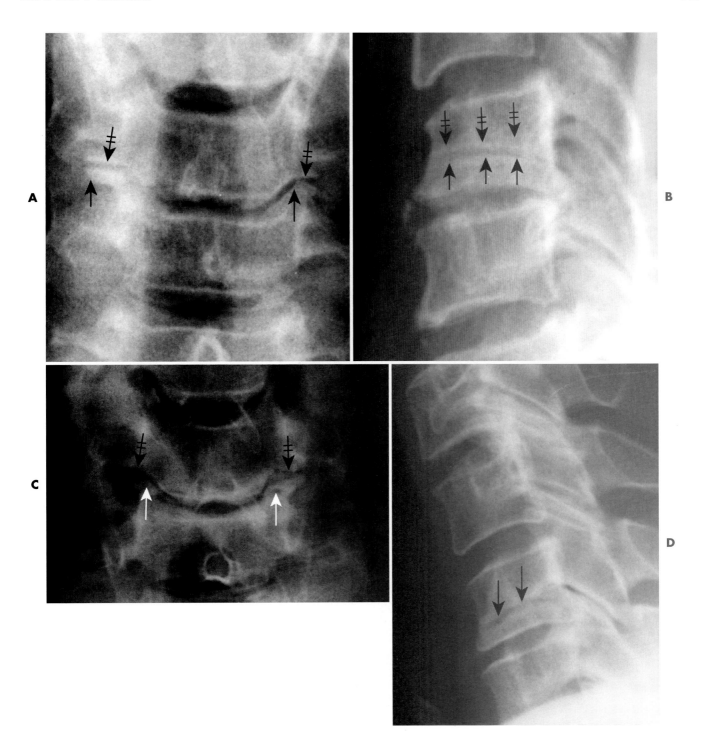

FIG. 9-130 **A** through **D,** Pseudofracture line of uncinate hypertrophy in two cases. **A** and **C,** The uncinate hypertrophy *(arrows)* and marginal osteophytes of the grooves that receive the uncinates on the vertebrae above *(crossed arrows)* present as two thin horizontal radiodense lines in, **B** and **D,** the lateral projection. In, **B** and **D,** the lateral projection, a thin horizontal radiolucent line is perceived between the two radiodense lines, mimicking a fracture (pseudofracture line) *(arrows).*

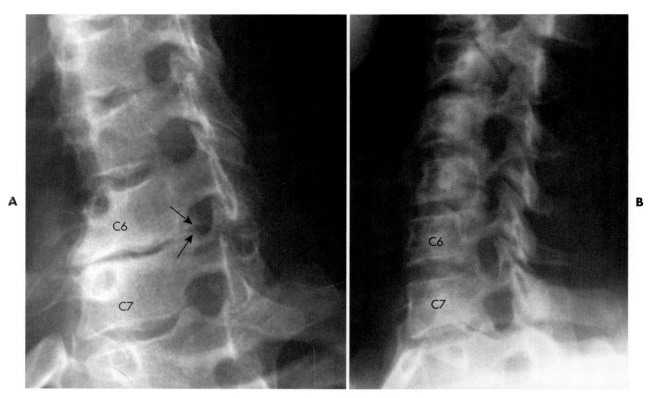

FIG. 9-131   A and **B,** Significant narrowing of the C6-7 intervertebral foramina secondary to marginal osteophytes of unci-nate hypertrophy *(arrows).* Because the narrowing osteophytes may have cartilage caps of varying degrees and the soft-tissue canal and foramen features are not seen, the true degree of intervertebral foramina stenosis is best assessed with magnetic resonance imaging or computed tomography, with clinical correlation indicated to determine the importance of any abnormalities found.

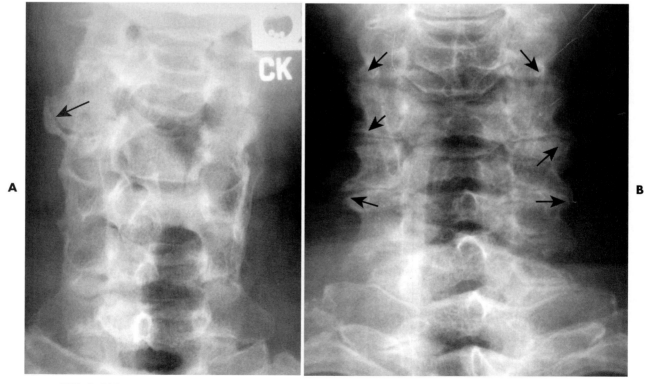

FIG. 9-132   A and **B,** Posterior joint degeneration of the cervical spine is noted in the anteroposterior projection as osteo-phytes projecting laterally from the articular pillars of the cervical spine, best seen with a hotlight *(arrows).*

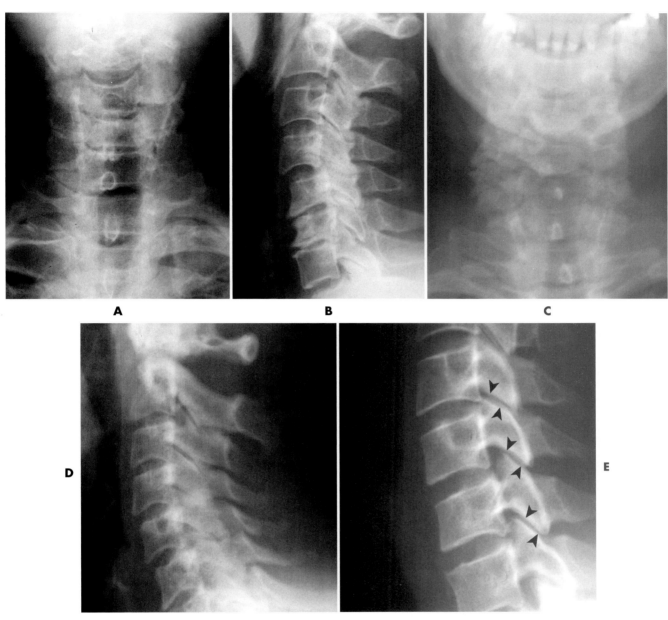

FIG. 9-133 On radiographs, posterior joint degeneration is noted by degenerative osteophytes projecting from the articular pillars in, **A** and **C,** the anteroposterior projection, and as increased radiodensity and irregularity of the articular pillars, **B** and **D,** blurring the, **E,** normally clear *(arrowheads)* posterior joint spaces in the lateral projection.

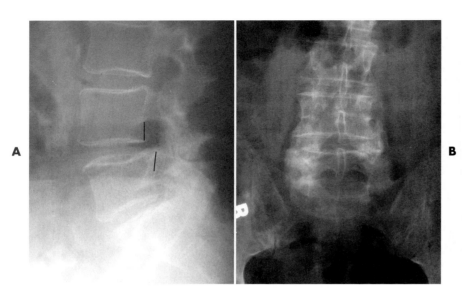

FIG. 9-134 A and **B,** Posterior joint disease in the lumbar spine noted by increased radiodensity and irregularity of the joints in both the anteroposterior and lateral projections. Posterior joint degeneration often is accompanied by anterior displacement of the lower lumbar segments (degenerative spondylolisthesis) or degenerative retrolisthesis of the upper lumbar segments.

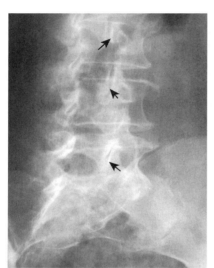

FIG. 9-135   Posterior joint degeneration noted by osteophytes and increased bone density of the articular processes. Degeneration of the lumbar posterior joints is demonstrated to a better degree on the oblique radiographs than the anteroposterior or lateral radiograph *(arrows).*

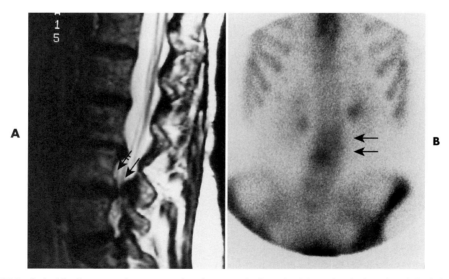

FIG. 9-136   Sagittal lumbar magnetic resonance imaging scans. **A,** Posterior joint arthrosis *(arrow)* and disc bulge *(crossed arrow)* narrow the sagittal dimension of the spinal canal. **B,** The posterior joint arthrosis causes increased radionuclide uptake on the bone scan *(arrows).*

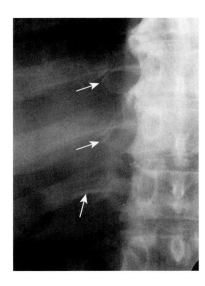

FIG. 9-137 Degeneration of the costotransverse joints *(arrows)*.

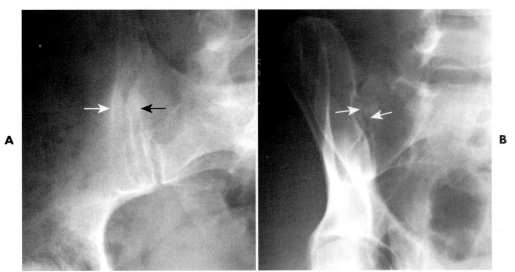

FIG. 9-138 Degeneration of the sacroiliac joint is usually unilateral and targets the middle of the joint. Also, as noted in this case on, **A,** the anteroposterior and, **B,** oblique radiographs, degeneration typically involves a focal region of the joint *(arrows)*.

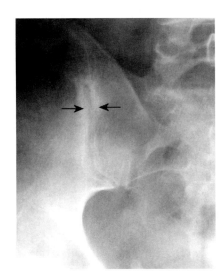

FIG. 9-139 Degeneration of the central region of the sacroiliac joint, presenting with marginal sclerosis *(arrows)*.

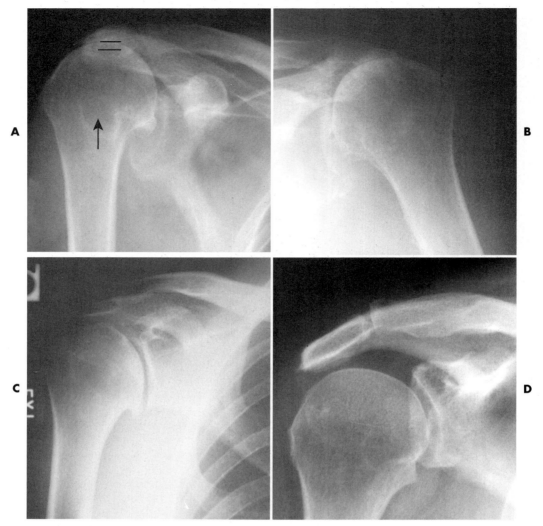

FIG. 9-140 A to **D,** Four cases of degeneration of the glenohumeral joint of the shoulder. The humerus elevates with degeneration *(arrow),* narrowing the distance between the humerus and acromion *(lines).*

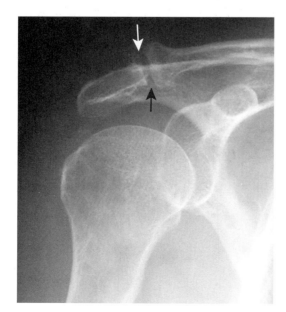

FIG. 9-141 Degeneration of the acromioclavicular joint presenting with osteophytes at the superior and inferior margins of the joint and reduction of the joint space *(arrows).*

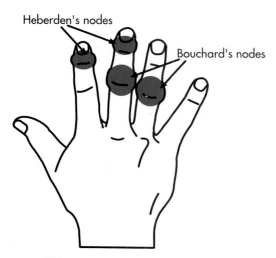

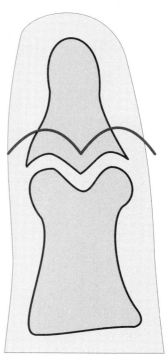

FIG. 9-142 Clinical evaluation of the painful nontraumatic hand begins with close inspection for signs of inflammation (edema, redness), changes in alignment, and changes in the contour of the soft tissues. Patients with chronic rheumatoid arthritis present with muscle atrophy, especially noticeable in the thenar eminence and bony protuberance near the metacarpophalangeal joints. Bony enlargements are also noted in osteoarthritis, occurring near the proximal (Bouchard's nodes) or distal (Heberden's nodes) interphalangeal joints. Although these names apply to the hand, similar nodes are noted in the feet.

FIG. 9-143 Central erosions of the phalanges give the appearance of a gull's wings. Most commonly, the gull is seen at the proximal articular surface of the distal phalanx, which develops a flattened M appearance as the center of the M (or body of the gull) fits into the central erosion of the distal articular surface of the middle phalanx.

calcification or HADD may be seen in the supraspinatus tendon, usually seen just proximal to its insertion on the greater tuberosity.

Hands. As with all joints, degeneration of the hands can be of primary or secondary etiology. Primary degeneration of the IP joints may be called *Kellgren arthritis*. Typically it expresses in more than three joints, is more common in females, is more likely to express accompanying clinical features, is more advanced in appearance, and tends to present in slightly younger patients than the typical secondary etiology of degeneration. IP joint degeneration reveals characteristic nodes on physical examination. The nodes about the DIP joints are termed *Heberden's nodes,* and those about the PIP joints are termed *Bouchard's nodes* (Fig. 9-142). These nodes are not exclusive to a primary etiology of degeneration. Also they compare with *Haygarth's nodes* of the MCP joints that occur in rheumatoid arthritis patients.

Erosive arthritis is a distinct variant of primary DJD, also more common among postmenopausal women, presenting most commonly bilaterally in the IP joints (more distal than proximal) and occasionally the first carpometacarpal joint. Erosive DJD is differentiated from typical DJD by the former's bilateral symmetric pattern of distribution and its greater tendency to be painful.[38] As the name implies, the diagnosis depends on the presence of central (subchondral) joint erosions. The central erosions resemble "gull wings" on the PA radiograph (Figs. 9-143 to 9-145).[38,560] It is not clear whether erosive DJD is a separate disease, or simply a

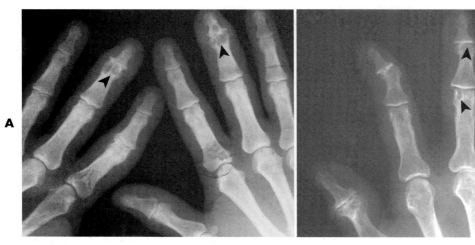

FIG. 9-144 A and **B,** Two cases of primary degeneration noted by subchondral cysts *(arrowheads),* osteophytes, and central erosions of the distal interphalangeal joints.

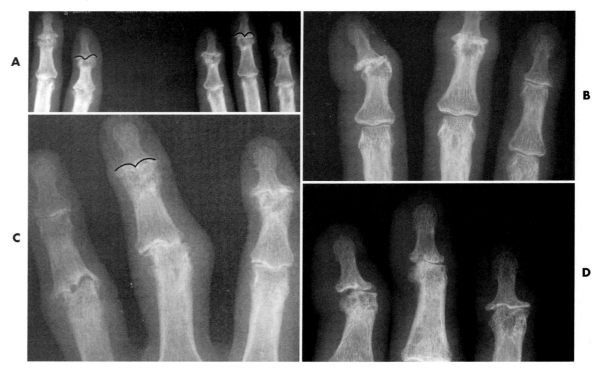

FIG. 9-145   **A** to **D,** Gull wing deformities consistent with primary degeneration of the distal interphalangeal joints in four cases.

variant expression of DJD.[114] As a general rule, erosive DJD is distinguished from RA in that the former involves the IP joints initially and the latter involves the MCP joints before progressing distally. Erosive DJD is distinguished from psoriatic arthritis (with its propensity for DIP involvement) by the former's central erosions of the proximal articular surface, compared with the marginal proliferations of the distal articular surface seen in psoriatic arthritis ("mouse ears"). Psoriatic arthritis has central erosions, but of the distal articular surface ("cup and saucer" deformity).

Secondary degeneration also occurs in the small joints of the hands, especially common to the first carpometacarpal articulation (Fig. 9-146).

Hips.   Asymmetric reduction in the joint space with subsequent superior, axial, or medial migration of the femoral head is the earliest sign of degeneration involving the hip (Figs. 9-147 to 9-149). Superior migration is by far the most common pattern and accompanies an increased distance between the medial margin of the femoral head and the lateral margin of the acetabulum

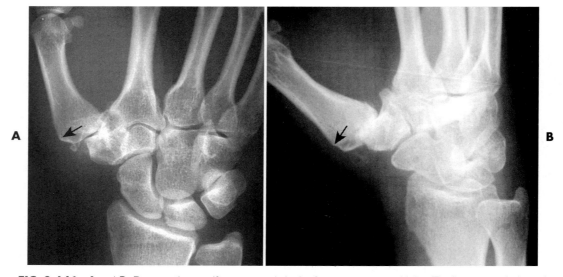

FIG. 9-146   **A** and **B,** Degeneration manifests commonly in the first carpometacarpal joints. The ligamentous laxity and jo nt instability associated with the degenerative process promote lateral movement of the base of the first metacarpal on trapezium (arrows).

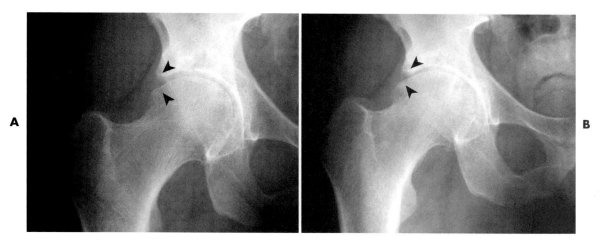

FIG. 9-147 A and **B,** Hip degeneration progressing over a 3-year period. Notice the developing osteophytes *(arrowheads)* and relative reduction in the superior joint space *(arrowheads).*

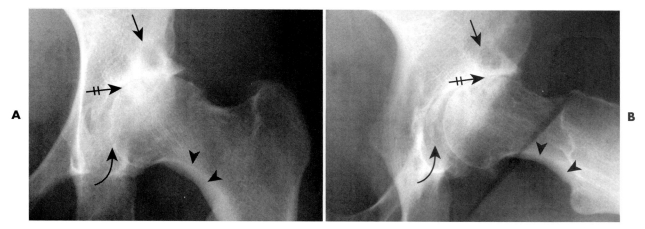

FIG. 9-148 A, Anteroposterior and, **B,** frog-leg projection of hip degeneration exhibiting an enlarged medial joint space *(curved arrows),* decreased superior joint space *(crossed arrows),* subchondral cysts *(arrows),* and buttressing (or thickening) of the medial femoral cortex *(arrowhead).*

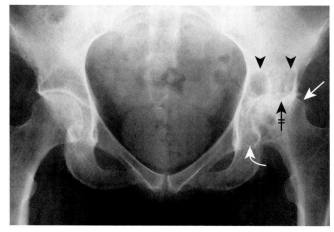

FIG. 9-149 Unlike rheumatoid arthritis, degeneration does not demonstrate bilateral symmetry. In this case, the patient has dramatically different presentation in the right hip than the left. The patient's left hip exhibits the typical features of advanced degeneration, including marginal osteophytes *(arrow),* reduced superior joint space *(crossed arrow),* increased medial joint space *(curved arrow)* occuring secondary to superior and lateral migration of the femoral head, and subchondral cysts *(arrowheads).*

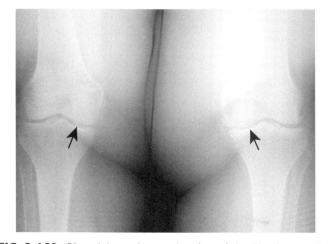

FIG. 9-150 Bilateral knee degeneration *(arrows)* in this obese patient. Obesity is a positive predictive factor of knee degeneration.

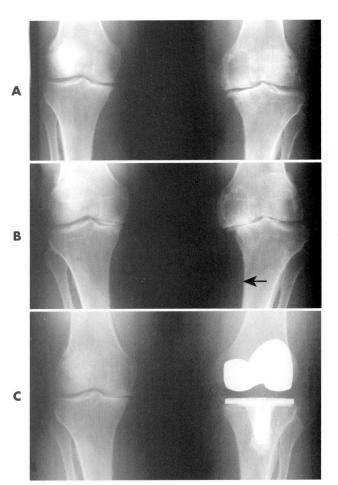

FIG. 9-151 Radiographic evaluation of the knee joint space is a commonly used index of degeneration. This case of a man in his early sixties demonstrates reduced joint space in his left (reading right) and less advanced changes in his right knee. As is typical with degeneration, there is asymmetric involvement bilaterally, and asymmetric involvement within each joint as well. **A,** The medial femorotibial joint spaces are more reduced than are the lateral femorotibial spaces. This film is taken in a recumbent posture. **B,** This film is taken on the same day in an upright, weight-bearing posture and is more informative because it now demonstrates marked varus deformity *(arrow)* and near-absence of medial femorotibial joint space and thereby provides a more accurate assessment of joint space reduction. **C,** After years of related pain and disability, often associated with advanced knee degeneration, the patient underwent joint replacement surgery on his left knee and is now considering similar surgery on his right knee. Since his first surgery, the patient has responded well, regaining function and suffering only mild discomfort instead of the severe pain of the past. However, the degree of knee degeneration is not directly predictive of the amount of pain and disability the patient is suffering. In other words, surgery is based on function, disability, and pain, not the amount of degeneration. (Courtesy Don Gran, Bluegrass, IA.)

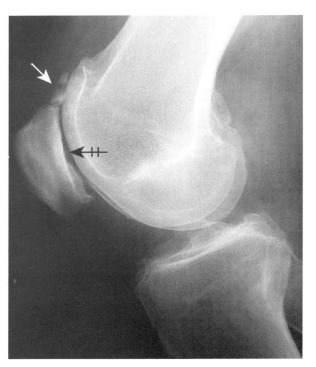

FIG. 9-152 Degenerative fragments within the suprapatellar space of the knee *(arrow)* accompanying reduced patellofemoral joint space *(crossed arrows).*

(Waldenström's sign). Axial migration indicates concentric loss of joint space more typical of an inflammatory arthropathy (e.g., RA). Medial migration occurs in fewer than 20% of cases and may be accompanied by a mild degree of acetabular protrusion.[328] Periosteal osteophytes (or buttressing) are noted on the medial and, less commonly, lateral side of the femoral neck.[521]

Knees. The knee is one of the most common joints to degenerate. Of the three compartments in the knee, the medial femorotibial joint compartment is most often involved (Figs. 9-150 to 9-156). Internal or central osteophytes may be seen extending from the tibial eminence (see Fig. 9-154).[1,519] Osteophytes arising from the proximal pole of the patella may cause an erosion defect of the anterior distal femur. Occasionally in the tangential projection, tiny bony proliferative projections extend from the external proximal surface of the patella near the insertion of the patellar tendon (patellar "tooth" sign).

Isolated DJD of the patellofemoral compartment is unusual. In this case, underlying conditions (e.g., CPPD disease, hemochromatosis, chondromalacia patella, previous trauma) should be considered. When compared with other joints, DJD of the knee less commonly exhibits subchondral sclerosis and cysts (see Fig. 9-155),[475] and more commonly exhibits intraarticular loose bodies.

Feet. The first MTP joint is a common site of DJD. Often it is accompanied with clinical findings of pain and stiffness secondary to the hypertrophic changes, a presentation termed *hallux rigidus.* First metatarsal varus, hallux valgus joint misalignment, often is present (Fig. 9-157).

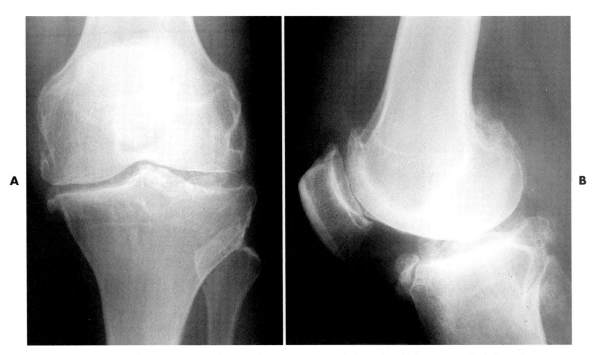

FIG. 9-153 **A** and **B,** Advanced knee degeneration noted by osteophytes, reduced joint space, and misalignment.

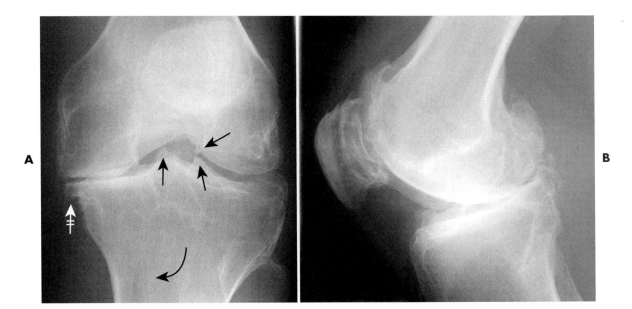

FIG. 9-154 **A,** Internal *(arrows)* and external *(crossed arrows)* osteophytes, reduced joint spaces, and varus deformity of the knee *(curved arrow)* consistent with degeneration. **B,** The lateral film demonstrates advanced degeneration of the patellofemoral joint.

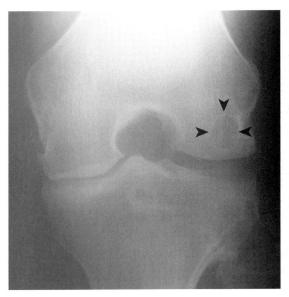

FIG. 9-155 Knee degeneration with subchondral cysts *(arrowheads)*. Subchondral cysts are not common findings of knee degeneration relative to other joints.

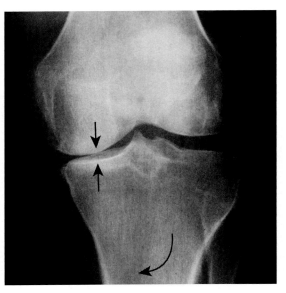

FIG. 9-156 Greater reduction of the medial femorotibial joint space *(arrows)* relative to the lateral space promotes a varus misalignment of the knee *(curved arrow)*.

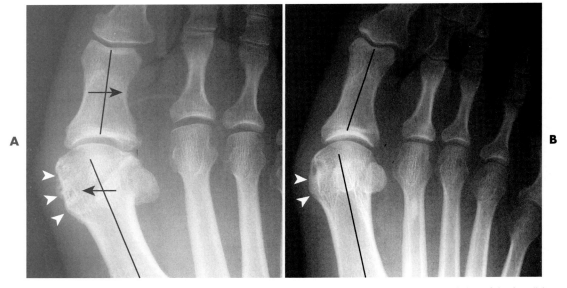

FIG. 9-157 **A** and **B,** Metatarsus primus varus, hallux valgus deformity *(lines)* caused by lateral deviation of the first digit and medial deviation of the first metatarsal *(arrows)* with bunion formation *(arrowheads)* along the lateral margin of the first metatarsal head in two cases. Both patients exhibit reduced joint space, osteophytes, and marginal sclerosis consistent with degeneration.

Advanced imaging. Plain film radiography is the most widely used modality to assess the presence and progression of an arthropathy. However, soft-tissue limitations of this procedure must be recognized. MRI is a valuable adjunctive modality because it offers superior imaging of the cartilage and detects the presence of synovitis in addition to the reaction of the bone to the arthropathy.[62] MRI has the advantages of providing true multiplanar imaging and superior soft-tissue contrast, and it is noninvasive as well.[48,192]

Radionuclide bone scintigraphy, CT, arthrography, and arthroscopy represent some of the other methods for joint assessment. Each has advantages and disadvantages depending on its application and the clinical situation.

CLINICAL COMMENTS

DJD is associated with joint pain, which usually is related to activity. Because cartilage has no nerve endings, symptoms arise from

TABLE 9-6	
Treatment Options for Degenerative Joint Disease	
Treatment	**Uses**
Chiropractic adjustments; improvement of muscle strength, range of motion, and balance and flexibility	Used to restore joint function
Pharmacology	Used to decrease inflammation (aspirin, NSAIDs) and pain (acetaminophen)
Surgery	Used for joint replacement, joint fusion, osteotomy, arthroscopic débridement, and joint space wash
Social support	Used to encourage social interaction, improve coping skills, manage stress, and coordinate support services
Reduction of body weight, modification of activities, use of walkers or canes, use of orthotics to shift weight	Used to protect joint
Physiotherapy (ice, heat [paraffin baths, diathermy], hydrotherapy)	Used to alter circulation and as palliative relief

NSAIDs, Nonsteroidal antiinflammatory drugs.

other components of the joint.[11] Multiple mechanisms have been proposed to explain the production of pain, including distention of joint capsule, joint inflammation, muscle spasm, contracture of joint capsule, periosteal elevation, or direct pressure on subchondral bone resulting from loss of articular cartilage.

The pain limits activity, leading to loss of muscle strength (deconditioning), reduced range of motion (contracture), limited function (disability), crepitus, occasional joint effusion, and localized inflammation. The pain worsens with activity in the early stages of the disease, and with rest in the late stages.[451] Not all degenerative joints are painful or disabling.[389,501,503] Disability is more likely to result if concurrent psychologic disorders of depression or anxiety are present, or in cases of insufficient social support.[617,623]

Treatment is aimed at limiting pain, maintaining function, continuing independence, and avoiding complications. Treatment plans are individualized to the patient and are directed in multiple areas (Table 9-6). Treatment is often directed at the maintenance of joint motion. Cartilage does not have a blood supply and depends on joint motion to provide nutrition and eliminate toxins.[49]

Pain control is crucial to the continuance of activity and motion. However, there is little evidence to support the long-term use of NSAIDs, which may interfere with normal repair mechanisms.[112,415] In addition, chronic ingestion of NSAIDs is linked to systemic complications (including gastric ulceration),[75] one third of which are asymptomatic. NSAIDs should be given only when inflammation is present.[200] Joint replacement surgery may be necessary if the pain and disability are severe. In fact, more than 70% of total hip and knee replacements are for osteoarthritis.[189]

Practitioners should keep in mind that it is very difficult to predict the presence or severity of a patient's clinical complaint from the degree of spondylosis and facet degeneration present on radiographs.* However, the chronicity of the patient's complaint is associated with the degree of spondylosis.[390] Limited evidence has suggested that spondylosis is associated with changes in lifestyle activities, at least in women.[390] Further study is needed.

Spondylotic radiculopathy usually responds to conservative management.[420] Spondylotic myelopathy, the most serious complication of spondylosis, is more complex and difficult to resolve with a conservative approach. Surgical intervention is warranted in patients with progressive neurologic deficits.[420]

Laboratory findings usually are within normal limits, but are helpful to exclude other disease.[451]

KEY CONCEPTS

- *Degenerative joint disease ([DJD], osteoarthritis, osteoarthrosis [OA]) is the most common of the arthropathies.*
- *Multifactorial etiology, influenced by local and systemic factors: trauma, aging, obesity, genetics, activity, gender, bone density, and nutrition.*
- *The spine, hips, knees, first metatarsal, and phalanges are most commonly involved.*
- *Classic radiographic findings include narrowing of the joint spaces, osteophytosis, subchondral bone sclerosis, subchondral cysts, intraarticular loose bodies, joint misalignment, and deformity.*
- *Intervertebral disc degeneration (spondylosis or degenerative disc disease [DDD]) also has findings of vacuum phenomena and Schmorl's nodes.*
- *Erosive DJD affects middle-aged women and is characterized by central joint erosions ("gull wing" sign).*
- *Magnetic resonance imaging (MRI) is a valuable adjunctive modality to plain film radiography because it offers superior imaging of the cartilage and detects the presence of synovitis and reaction of the bone to the arthropathy.*
- *The axial images provided by computed tomography (CT) and MRI are helpful to assess intricate joints of the spine, ankle, wrist, and so on.*
- *Pain is a common clinical complaint, although the severity of pain does not correlate well to the radiographic appearance.*
- *The pain limits activity leading to loss of muscle strength (deconditioning), reduced range of motion (contracture), limited function (disability), crepitus, occasional joint effusion, and localized inflammation.*
- *Treatment is aimed at limiting pain, maintaining function, continuing independence, and avoiding complications; pain control is crucial to the continuance of activity and motion.*
- *Laboratory findings usually are within normal limits, but are helpful to exclude other diseases.*

*References 163, 198, 199, 222, 223, 255, 390.

Intervertebral Disc Herniation

BACKGROUND

Intervertebral disc anatomy. IVD herniation represents only one manifestation of an ongoing process of IVD degeneration.[259] Because herniated discs are degenerative, this discussion continues and expands on the previous discussion of IVD degeneration listed in the degenerative joint disease section of this chapter. It is worth elaborating on the structure and cellular metabolism of the intervertebral components in the present topic to provide a more complete picture of the pathophysiology of IVD herniations.

Intervertebral discs unite adjacent vertebrae from C2 through S1. Each disc is named for the vertebra immediately above it. The IVD is composed of a central nucleus pulposus, surrounding anulus fibrosus, and cartilaginous endplates above and below the majority of the IVD (Fig. 9-158). The cross-sectional anatomy of the spinal canal is illustrated with CT and MRI (Figs. 9-159 and 9-160).

Nucleus pulposus. The semifluid nucleus pulposus is composed of a loose network of cells of notochordal origin interspersed within a collagen and proteoglycan matrix. Nuclear proteoglycans have a strong affinity for water, giving the nucleus a positive swelling pressure or turgor.[634] The nucleus is abneural and avascular.

Anulus fibrosus. The anulus fibrosus consists of about 20 concentric lamellae that surround the nucleus. Each lamella is composed of obliquely oriented bundles of collagen fibers. The exact orientation of the fibers differs with spinal location. Lumbar and thoracic annular fibers are oriented approximately 30 degrees from the horizontal plane. Cervical annular fibers are more perpendicular in orientation. Another difference noted in the cervical spine is that the anulus does not completely surround the nucleus pulposus. The anulus is thick in the anterior, somewhat thinner in the posterior, and thin or lacking on the lateral borders of the cervical spine. Structural support is likely compensated for this deficit by the uncinate processes.[429] The direction of obliquity of the bundles alternates with each successive lamella. The inner third of the lamellae are anchored into the cartilaginous endplates, forming a retaining envelope around the nucleus. The outer two thirds of the lamellae are functionally and histologically more similar to ligaments and are firmly attached to the vertebrae.[273] The outer lamellae are innervated posteriorly by the sinuvertebral nerve, posterolateral by ventral rami, and anteriorly by gray rami communicantes.[57] Blood vessels are found in the outermost lamellae.[634]

Cartilage endplates. The cartilage endplates are homologous to unossified epiphyses and cover each end of the vertebrae.[634] They are encircled by the ossified ring apophysis of the vertebrae. Endplates are about 1 mm thick, and facilitate fluid exchange between the vertebrae and IVD.[177] Although there is a blood supply during early phases of development, it subsequently regresses, leaving the cartilaginous endplates completely avascular by adulthood.[634] No neural elements are present.

Intervertebral disc health*. Intervertebral discs have low cellular density (~5 million cells/ml),[394] yet these cells are critical in maintaining disc health. A characteristic finding in degenerated discs is a loss of cellularity.[372] In a very simplistic sense, cells determine both structure and function of the disc. The cells produce extracellular matrix. The extracellular matrix contains many hydrophilic "water-loving" molecules; therefore the extracellular matrix creates osmotic pressure. Osmotic pressure pulls water into the disc. Water comprises the majority of soft-tissue structure, including intervertebral discs. This maintenance of structure allows optimal function. Realizing this relationship puts an appropriate focus on factors influencing IVD cell viability.

IVD cell viability is dependent on cellular demand and nutrient supply. Either an increase in demand or a decrease in supply can decrease the cells' viability.[269] When the cells are placed in either situation, they react by altering their metabolism or committing cellular suicide, apoptosis. The following sections examine both nutrient supply and cellular demand alterations and their influence on disc health and injury.

Nutrient supply. Cells of the IVD function much as other cells of the body. Their main activity is reproducing adenosine triphosphate (ATP) for use as the cell's universal energy currency. The sodium or potassium pump uses much of cellular ATP within cells. Glucose plays a primary role in creating ATP for IVD cells. Nuclear cells of the disc survive fewer than 3 days without glucose.[269] The cells also have mitochondria requiring oxygen during aerobic metabolism of macronutrients. Low oxygen[283] and acidic pH[267] decrease IVD cell protein and proteoglycan synthesis. IVD cells may survive under low oxygen conditions, but produce little extracellular matrix.[269] If low oxygen concentration is maintained, the cells will survive fewer than 2 weeks.[269] The low pH can be a result of elevated glycolytic rates producing lactic acid. This occurrence is further discussed in the section on increased cellular demand.

---

*This section on intervertebral disc health is authored by Dan Weinert, DC, MS, DACRB, Davenport, IA.

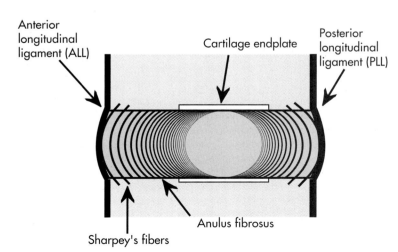

Anterior longitudinal ligament (ALL)

Cartilage endplate

Posterior longitudinal ligament (PLL)

Sharpey's fibers

Anulus fibrosus

FIG. 9-158 The intervertebral disc comprises a central nucleus pulposus, surrounding anulus fibrosus, and cartilaginous endplates above and below.

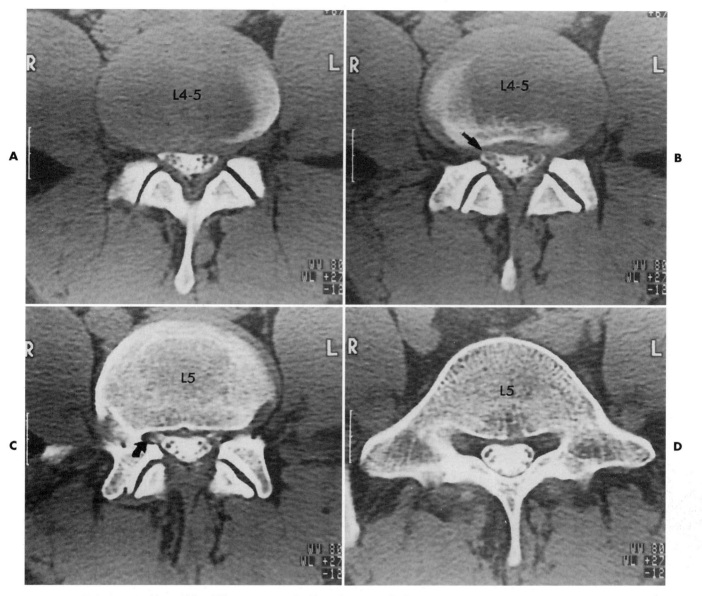

FIG. 9-159 Normal L5 and S1 nerve roots and exiting spinal nerves. **A,** Computed tomography myelogram axial slice just below the inferior endplate of L4. Descending roots are found in the dural sac anterolaterally; however, the L5 roots have not separated from the sac yet. **B,** Axial slice at the superior endplate of L5. The L5 descending roots are just budding. The arrow points to the right L5 root. **C,** Four millimeters below **B.** The descending lumbar roots are completely separated from the dural sac and are within the sleeves. The arrow points to the right L5 root. **D,** A slice that is distal to the end of the L5 dural sleeve. The descending L5 roots are visible in the lateral recess of L5. The descending sacral roots are close to the anterolateral corners of the dural sac.   *Continued*

The mature disc is mostly avascular, yet it still must receive nutrition. Therefore the cells of the disc rely on the surrounding structures of the spine for nutrient supply. The outer perimeter of the anulus is supplied with nutrients via the surrounding soft tissue. The inner nucleus must receive its nutrition from the vertebra above and below. Capillaries that penetrate the subchondral plate of the vertebral body bring the nutrients in approximation with the cartilaginous endplate. Nutrients must diffuse across this endplate for inner nuclear cells to receive nutrition. The central portion of the disc becomes the most vulnerable area to decreased nutrient supply. This is because of distance. The centralized cells are the furthest from the nutrient supply, therefore limiting their supply.

When endplate permeability decreases, blood and nutrient supply are compromised, creating unfavorable living conditions for IVD cells.

A relationship between an individual's aerobic capacity and IVD cell viability seems to exist. Stepping back from directly looking at the cell, atherosclerosis is known to be associated with low back pain.[341] More specifically, aortic atherosclerosis is associated with increased risk of developing disc degeneration.[313] The spine's ability to function is affected by aerobic conditioning. A person's aerobic capacity has been shown to be an independent predictor of lift capacity.[408] Lift capacity is the maximum acceptable weight that the subject is able to lift on a safe and dependable basis eight to twelve times per day.

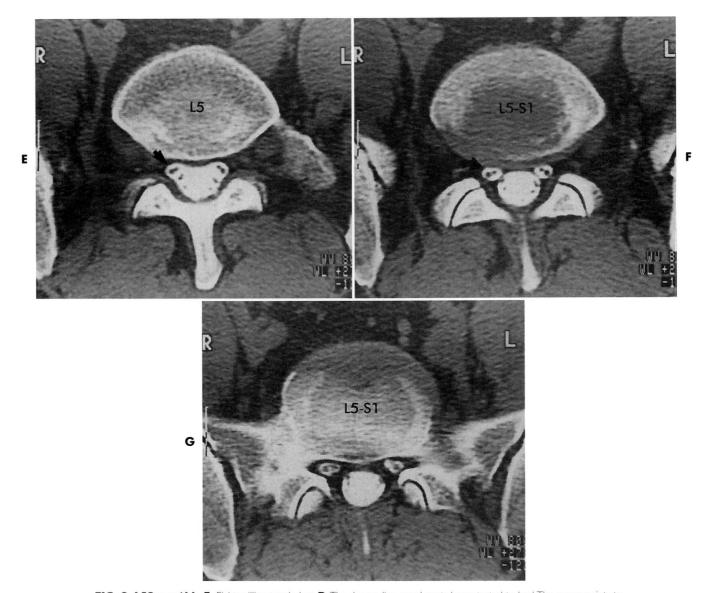

FIG. 9-159 cont'd **E,** Eight millimeters below **D.** The descending sacral roots have started to bud. The arrow points to the right S1 root. **F,** Four millimeters below **E.** The sacral roots are in the anterior epidural space posterior to the L5-S1 disc. **G,** Eight millimeters below **F.** The descending sacral roots can be seen in the lateral recess of S1. (From Firooznia H et al: MRI and CT of the musculoskeletal system, St Louis, 1992, Mosby.)

Nicotine treatment is an excellent example showing how compromised nutrient supply creates detrimental IVD effects. When nicotine is taken in, it creates stenosis of vascular buds, perivascular calcification, hypertrophy of vascular walls, and a decreased number of vascular buds.[286] Nicotine treatment causes necrosis and hyalinization of the nucleus and a disruption of the annular fiber pattern, including clefts and separations.[286]

The aerobic characteristics of the surrounding spinal tissue also are worth noting. Paraspinal muscles are predominantly involved in maintaining posture. In unsupported sitting or standing, much of the musculature is in a continuous level of activity.[465] Paraspinal muscle contains predominantly slow-twitch oxidative fibers. Vascularity is high. For example, a single multifidus fiber or cell contacts, on average, approximately five capillaries.[555] Any spinal or aerobic deconditioning may have a dual destructive role: (a) the compromised supply of nutrient—the surrounding structures'

vasculature supplies the disc's nutrition; (b) deconditioning's role in altering biomechanics and loading of the spine.

Increased cellular demand. Although the disc commonly experiences compressive force, there are conditions in which loading may exceed optimal levels or duration. For example, individuals with low back pain produce greater spinal loads during normal activities.[395] Compression results from gravity, yet a significant contribution results from muscular activity.[493] Stress profilometry has shown that the highest compressive stresses occur in the anulus, not the nucleus.[154] Typically the highest forces are posterior to the nucleus, in the middle of the anulus. Younger, more fully hydrated discs are less sensitive to posture changes and are less likely to have focused stress areas.[154]

Even though the spine deals with compression well, the degree of cell death is dependent on magnitude and duration of compressive loading.[372] Compression increases hydrostatic pressure.

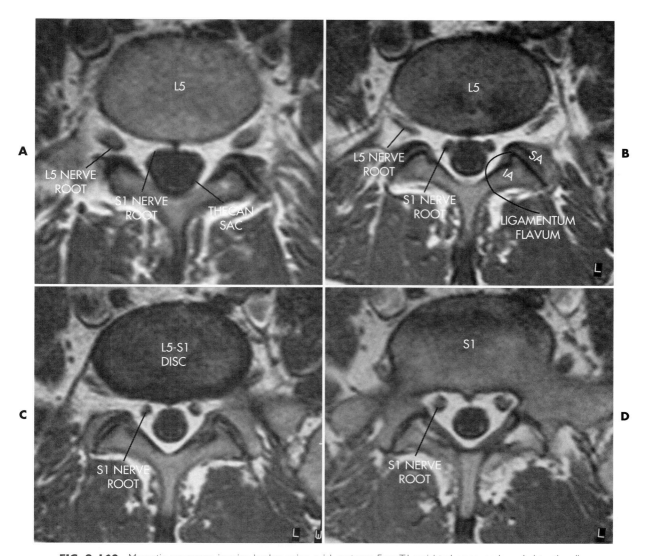

FIG. 9-160 Magnetic resonance imaging lumbar spine axial anatomy. Four T1-weighted scans, each angled to the disc plane, demonstrate the contents of the vertebral canal. **A,** This image is a slice through the lower margin of the L5 vertebrae. **B,** This image is a slice through the inferior endplate of L5. **C,** This image is a slice through the L5-S1 disc. **D,** This image is a slice through the superior portion of the sacrum. Notice that the nerve roots begin to bud off of the thecal sac and move laterally at descending levels, **A** to **D,** to exit the intervertebral foramen of the segment below. Collectively, the configuration of the thecal sac and nerve roots transforms from the appearance of a "bear's head," **A,** in which the nerve roots move laterally and the configuration appears more like a "mouse's head," **B** and **C,** Note that the configuration of the thecal sac and nerve roots is normal. Disc lesions, congenital defects, and other space-occupying lesions may distort these normal configurations. The superior (SA) and inferior (IA) articular processes are in close approximation to the canal; their degenerative hypertrophy may have consequences of spinal canal stenosis.

This places a larger demand on IVD cells, especially in maintaining sodium/potassium gradients. Larger ATP consumption creates demands on glycolysis, resulting in increased lactic acid and a lower pH. These conditions result in decreased production of extracellular matrix and possibly apoptosis of the IVD cells. Cells of the disc cannot survive at a pH of less than 6.0 for extended durations.[269]

Endplate chondrocytes undergo apoptosis when significantly loaded, whereas apoptosis is absent without loading.[23] When compressed, IVD cell genetic expression changes.[378] Anabolic pathways are downregulated, whereas catabolic pathways are upregulated. The net result is disc degradation. Long-term loading results in microscopic changes including decreased proteoglycan in the nucleus and inner anulus.[278] Immobilization also has been shown to alter the phenotype of IVD cells. Just 72 hours of immobilization result in significant upregulation of catabolic enzymes (aggrecanase, collagenase, and stromelysin) within the anulus.[378] Immobilization also decreases production of type I and II collagen.[378]

Scoliosis is an example of alternative loading from one side of the disc to the other. The convex side of the curvature exhibits elevated synthetic activity.[16] When tension or stress is applied to the disc, nucleus pulposus cells increase synthesis rates of protein and promote the proliferation of cells.[410]

If external conditions limit nutrient supply, or excessive loading or immobilization exists, the cells of the disc suffer and produce little matrix or die. IVD cell viability is dependent on cellular demand and nutrient supply. Either an increase in demand or a decrease in supply can decrease the cells' viability.[269]

Injury and intervertebral disc motion. Intervertebral discs allow for 6 degrees of freedom, meaning they allow both rotation and translation about and along the *x, y,* and *z* axes. This motion can be affected by injury. Radial tears, concentric tears, and rim lesions all result in decreased torsional stiffness.[640] Both radial and concentric tears result in increased flexion and extension stiffness, whereas rim lesions correlate with increased flexion stiffness.[640]

Disc degeneration also is associated with motion changes. The changes in motion tend to mirror the effect of creep. Creep is a normal temporary phenomenon that discs and other soft tissues experience daily. *Creep* is defined as deformation created by loading of longer duration and is primarily the movement of water when the definition is applied to soft tissue. Creep results in temporary decreased fluid content and a respective loss in disc height. Creep of a healthy disc and disc degeneration both result in increased disc range of motion.[205] IVD degeneration most significantly affects axial rotation in the lumbar spine.[205] The lumbar spine traditionally allows very little axial rotation, but IVD degeneration can increase this motion by 100% to 300%. Decreased facet cartilage thickness also contributes to the increased motion.

In a five-level model of degeneration, lumbar segmental motion increases until level four and decreases thereafter. This is true for flexion, extension, and axial rotation. Lateral bending motion tends to peak at stage three degeneration.[205]

Motion and intervertebral disc injury. Motion and loading can affect IVD health because injury affects motion. The disc most prone to degeneration tends to be the disc with the highest loading. Remember that cell viability is highly dependent on loading. The L5-S1 disc is traditionally the most prone to degeneration. It is relatively mobile and adjacent to the fixed segments of the sacrum. Proteoglycan and water loss associated with disc aging is accelerated in discs adjacent to fused segments.[635] Because of its location at the base of the spine, it also carries the greatest gravitational load. When cell metabolism is investigated, the L5-S1 disc shows greater turnover of proteoglycans compared with adjacent discs.[635]

An interesting finding is the correlation between the thickness of the iliolumbar ligament and the amount and location of degeneration in the lumbar spine. If the iliolumbar ligaments are shorter and thicker, the L5-S1 disc tends to have less degeneration than the L4-5 disc.[4] This supports the theory that more motion creates more degeneration and that increasing stability tends to decrease degeneration.

Increased range of motion of the lumbar spine is not a singular predictor of the incidence of low back pain. Increased range of motion if combined with low strength becomes a good predictor of the incidence of concurrent and future low back pain,[603] as is demonstrated by the sequence of events occurring with initial injury. After initial injury, segmental motion within the motor unit's neutral zone increases[476] and an inflammatory process begins. Inflammation acts to destabilize the area by decreasing certain muscular activity. An unstable spine creates abnormal loading. The perpetuation of disc degeneration is likely if a combination of more motion and low strength exists.

Pathophysiology of the disc

Normal function. The healthy disc is remarkably resilient to injury. The anulus fibrosus and nucleus pulposus work together to resist spinal loads. Forces applied to the nucleus become attenuated when dispersed peripherally to the surrounding anulus. Also, the centrally placed and well-hydrated nucleus pulposus retains the shape and function of the anulus fibrosus. Maintaining the function of the IVD is largely dependent on the ability of cells to maintain their matrix, as described. Mechanical, chemical, or nutritional factors may affect the viability of these cells, and degenerative changes ensue.[266] Cellular death and matrix alterations create more stressors, and a vicious cycle of degeneration develops. Like degeneration in other joints, many of these changes are age related; however, degeneration becomes rapidly progressive, resulting in spinal pain and disability in some individuals. As a result of degeneration, altered function, and impaired metabolism, the IVD becomes susceptible to injury from axial, shear, and rotational forces.

Injury to anulus fibrosus. Injury to the anulus progressively decreases its effectiveness to resist spinal loading. Circumferential, radial, and transverse fissures develop, signifying anular breakdown (Fig. 9-161).[182,183] The cleft of a circumferential tear is oriented in the same direction as the lamellae, extending in an arc around the center of the IVD. Radial tears represent disruption of adjacent anular lamellae, with the cleft of the tear oriented perpendicular to the fibers of the lamellae. Transverse tears occur at the rim of the disc, at the interface of the outer anulus with the vertebral ring apophysis.[259]

The posterior and posterolateral anulus is particularly susceptible to tearing for two reasons. First, it is thin. Second, the posteriorly concave design of the lumbar disc places posterolateral fibers at a mechanical disadvantage.[184] The latter is particularly true if a combined flexion and rotation posture is assumed.[496]

As portions of the anulus begin to tear and fragment, greater loading is placed on the remaining healthy anulus, leading to further breakdown. The resulting large radial fissures that develop provide a pathway for displacement of the nucleus pulposus into the spinal canal.

Injury to nucleus pulposus. The evolution of a herniated disc is more complicated than simply developing a radial fissure that provides a pathway for displacement to occur.[515] If a pathway resembling a radial fissure is experimentally cut into the anulus and the spinal segment is then loaded, a posterior disc herniation will not occur.[80,496,667] Some authors attribute this phenomenon to the lack of concurrent breakdown of the nucleus pulposus.[56,60,647] They contend that a healthy nucleus pulposus exhibits natural cohesive properties that prevent herniation. They further propose that these cohesive properties become denatured as a consequence of vertebral endplate fractures. Endplate fractures expose the avascular and immunologically unfamiliar nucleus to the ample blood supply found in the vertebral body. The ensuing autoimmune reaction denatures the cohesive properties, permitting herniation of the nucleus through existing anular defects.

Alternatively, if nuclear degradation occurs without a concurrent anular defect, the inner IVD becomes disrupted, but herniation will not occur.[126] Internal disc disruption is marked by narrowing of the disc height and slight anular bulge, but not herniation. The interested reader is referred to the referenced citations[56,60] for a more complete discussion of this model.

Inflammation and intervertebral disc injury. Herniation of the IVD changes the physiology and chemistry of the area. The inflammatory result of injury can have far-reaching

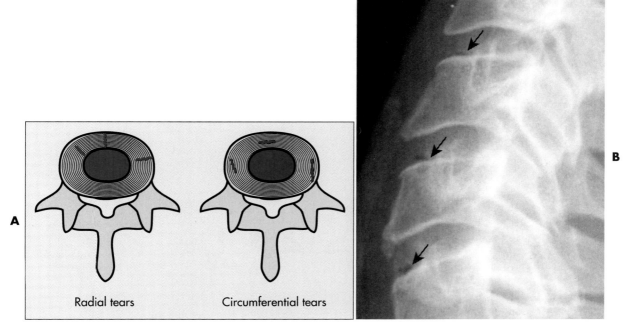

FIG. 9-161 Tears of the anulus fibrosus develop in three patterns: radial, circumferential, and transverse. **A,** Radial tears are oriented perpendicular to the direction of the anular lamellae. Circumferential tears are aligned longitudinal to the anular lamellae. **B,** Transverse tears are disruptions of the anulus at their interface with the vertebral endplate *(arrows)*.

consequences. An inflammatory stimulus to the multifidi has been shown to evoke a somatosympathetic reflex that can affect sympathetic outflow to the spleen and kidney.[307] Low back pain is associated with a less refined lumbosacral position sense.[90] Disc herniations have been shown to impair the feed-forward activation of paraspinal musculature.[362] Activation of paraspinal muscles is an important event during limb movement.[136] Both decreased position sense and lack of stabilizing feed-forward contraction have the potential to further injure the spine.

Within the inflammatory process associated with disc injury, TNF-α is a molecule of particular interest. TNF-α is a proinflammatory cytokine found within herniated intervertebral discs[470] and is important in producing hyperalgesia associated with intervertebral disc herniation. When TNF-α is applied to a nerve root, nociceptive specific neurons increase spontaneous discharge rates, neurons show enhanced responses to other noxious stimuli, and the ganglion shows inflammatory changes.[470] When antibodies targeting TNF-α are introduced into the injured disc area, there is a partial prevention of nociception.[469] TNF-α antibodies also have been shown to dramatically abate sciatica.[309]

Although the ability to reduce pain via TNF-α antibodies is impressive, TNF-α may be critical in the process of disc resorption. During resorption, the size of the disc is progressively decreased after the initial injury. When an IVD herniates, neovascularization begins and macrophage and lymphocyte infiltration is evident. The amount of resorption is correlated to the amount of vascularization.[242] It should be recalled that a healthy disc is avascular. The inflammatory process causes enzymes responsible for degrading disc material to become active. Matrix metalloproteinases, not normally expressed in uninjured intervertebral discs, are an example of degradative enzymes that are active during resorption. They are

highly expressed in surgical samples of herniated discs.[242] A relationship appears to exist between TNF-α and matrix metalloproteinase. After the initial injury, nuclear material becomes exposed to macrophages. Macrophages produce TNF-α. TNF-α induces the production of matrix metalloproteinases, which act as chemoattractants and degradative enzymes. It could be argued that this is a beneficial process despite the production of nociception. Much more information is necessary to get a clearer picture, defining the process of inflammation related to disc injury.

Intervertebral disc herniation. An IVD herniation describes the extension of nucleus pulposus substance through the anulus fibrosus and beyond the adjacent vertebral margins.[213] Fragments from the anulus fibrosus and cartilaginous endplate may accompany the displaced nucleus pulposus.

Disc herniations are more common among males, smokers, obese persons, and those exposed to vehicular vibration.[201-203,321] The contribution of genetics is less certain.[201-203] Herniations are rare before 20 and after 65 years of age. The most common age group is 25 to 45 years old.[321] Although many risk factors have been identified, it is difficult to assess which are causative and which are merely symptom aggravating.[556]

Classifying disc displacements. IVD herniations occur on a continuum, from very small focal protrusions to large sequestered fragments (Figs. 9-162 to 9-166). This continuum usually is categorized into subtypes based on the extent of nuclear displacement: protrusion (contained herniation), extrusion (noncontained herniation), or sequestration (free fragment) (Table 9-7). An IVD bulge is not a herniation. Bulge describes a broad-based extension of the anulus fibrosus without nuclear displacement. No system of classification is universally applied. Often the definitions of terms are not consistent between the individual interpreting the imaging

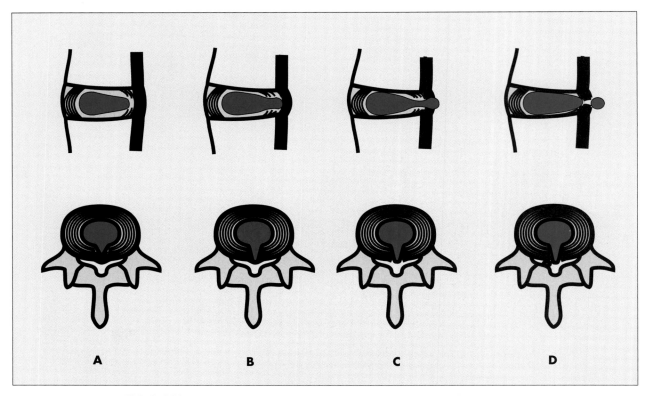

FIG. 9-162   Disc displacements: **A,** Bulge; **B,** protrusion; **C,** extrusion; and, **D,** sequestration.

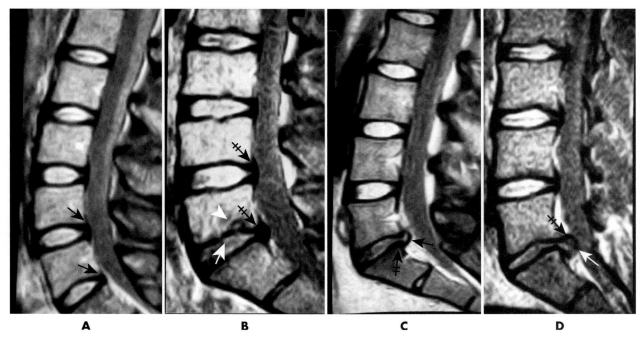

FIG. 9-163   Sagittal T2-weighted magnetic resonance imaging scans demonstrating classifications of intervertebral disc displacement in different patients. **A,** Normal scan. The nucleus has high signal intensity. The anulus is intact and has a normal configuration *(arrow)*. **B,** Disc bulges at the L4 and L5 levels *(crossed arrows)*. In addition, decreased nuclear signal intensity *(arrow)* and a Schmorl's node at L5 *(arrowhead)* are noted. **C,** L5 disc protrusion is indicated by the thinned but intact anulus *(arrow)* and posteriorly displaced nuclear material *(crossed arrow)*. Although the nucleus is posteriorly displaced, it is still contained by the thinned anulus; therefore it is alternatively called a *contained disc herniation*. **D,** L5 disc extrusion is indicated by the disrupted posterior anulus *(arrow)* and posteriorly displaced nucleus *(crossed arrow)*, which is no longer contained by the anulus (a noncontained herniation).

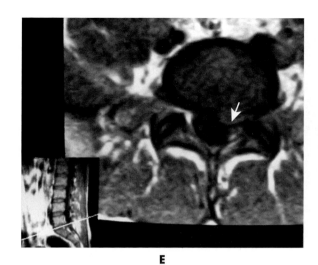

FIG. 9-163 cont'd   E, T1-weighted axial magnetic resonance imaging scan of the same patient in **D.** The herniation effaces the thecal sac as it projects left of the midline *(arrow)*.

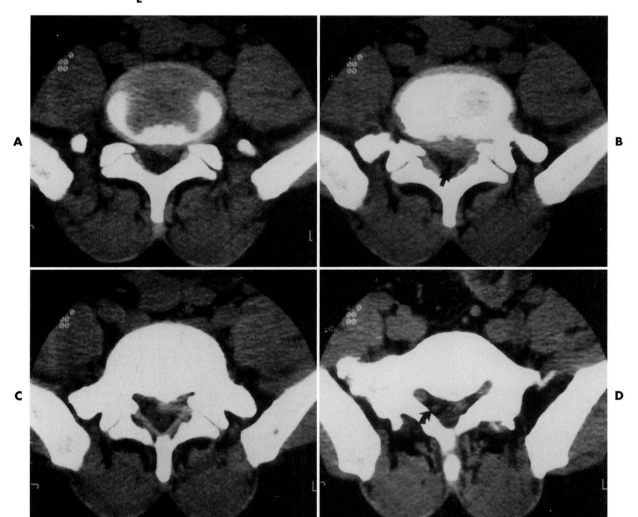

FIG. 9-164 An L4-5 herniated disc with extension inferiorly and migration of a free fragment affecting the left S1 descending nerve root. **A** and **B,** Axial computed tomography slices show large herniations with a major component on the left *(arrow in **B**)*. **C,** An axial slice through the upper part of the L5 pedicle shows extension inferiorly on the left side. Note the obliteration of epidural fat anteriorly and anterolaterally on the left. **D,** Axial slice 8 mm below **C,** through the lower portion of the L5 pedicles. The arrow points to the normal right descending S1 nerve root. A small migrated free fragment is present on the left, engulfing the left S1 descending root. There was no abnormality 4 mm above this level indicating detachment of the fragment (visible in **D**) from the extended herniated disc (visible in **C**). (From Firooznia H et al: MRI and CT of the musculoskeletal system, St Louis, 1992, Mosby).

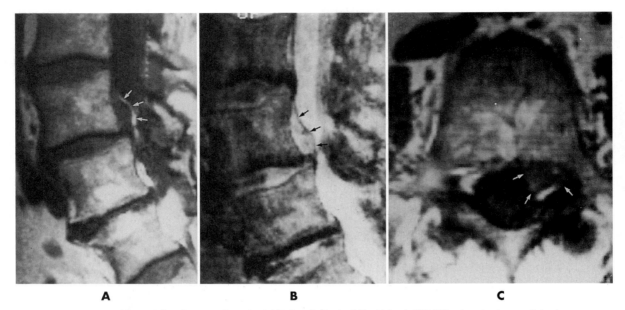

FIG. 9-165 Migrated free fragment from the L4-5 disc. **A,** Sagittal T1-weighted (500/17) spin-echo image of the lower lumbar spine showing narrowing of the L4-L5 and L5-S1 disc spaces with type II vertebral body changes at the latter level. A soft-tissue density fragment is seen posterior to the inferior aspect of L4 *(arrows).* The high signal intensity surrounding probably is epidural fat. Surgery revealed that the fragment was posterior to the vertebral body but anterior to the posterior longitudinal ligament. **B** and **C,** Sagittal T2-weighted (2000/90) spin-echo and axial T1-weighted (500/17) spin-echo images. The migrated fragment is indicated by the small arrows. (From Modic M et al: Magnetic resonance imaging of the spine, ed 2, St Louis, 1994, Mosby.)

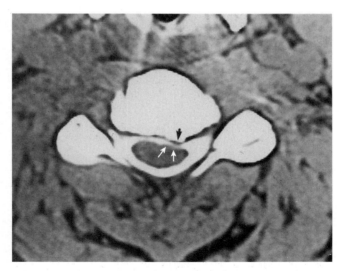

FIG. 9-166 Hard disc. Computed tomography myelography demonstrating a small left-sided osteophytic ridge *(black arrow).* Note the mild flattening on the left side of the anterior cord *(white arrows).* (From Firooznia H et al: MRI and CT of the musculoskeletal system, St Louis, 1992, Mosby.)

TABLE 9-7

Classification and Terms of Lumbar Intervertebral Disc Displacement

Terms	Description
Bulge/bulging disc	Concentric outward overhang of the anulus fibrosus beyond the margins of the vertebral endplate involving 50% (180 degrees) of the disc. The extent of overhang generally is less than 3 mm from the margins of the vertebrae (exclusive of osteophytes). Bulge is a form of disc displacement, but is not a form of disc herniation. Bulges are common among individuals more than 40 years old.
Protrusion/prolapse/ contained herniation	Focal (<25% or 90 degrees of the disc circumference) displacement of nuclear, annular, or endplate material beyond the peripheral margin of the IVD (defined by the osseous boundaries of the adjacent vertebral endplates exclusive of osteophytes). However, the protruded material remains "contained" by some portion of intact outer anulus; that is, the displaced nuclear material does not penetrate all layer of the anulus.
Extrusion/true herniation/noncontained herniation	Focal (<25% or 90 degrees of the disc circumference) displacement of nuclear, annular, or endplate material beyond the peripheral margin of the IVD (defined by the osseous boundaries of the adjacent vertebral endplates exclusive of osteophytes). In distinction to protrusion, extrusion focally disrupts all the layers of the anulus, thereby permitting displaced nuclear material to enter the spinal canal. If a central disc herniation does not extend past the PLL, the term *subligamentous herniation* is appropriate, whereas if the herniation passes through the PLL, the term *transligamentous herniation* is used. Contained and noncontained refer to the anulus fibrosus, not the PLL. (Although some sources disagree, contending that distinction between the anulus and PLL is not possible on available imaging systems and that the term extrusion implies extension beyond the PLL.)
Sequestration	Migration of a "free fragment" of herniated material that has no connecting bridge to the IVD. Fragments (in decreasing order of frequency) migrate laterally, superiorly, or inferiorly; stay in the midline; or disperse in multiple directions.
Hard disc	Colloquialism used to describe the presence of osteophytosis from the posterior margin of the vertebral endplate or uncinate process, which mimics the clinical presentation of a herniation or "soft disc."
High-intensity zone	Refers to a focus of high signal intensity on a T2-weighted MRI image occurring in the normally low signal intensity substance of the anulus. High-intensity zones may denote a focal tear of the anulus, but its association to symptoms is not well defined.

From Fardon DF et al: Nomenclature of lumbar disc disorders. In Garfin SR, Vaccaro AR, editors: Orthopaedic knowledge update: spine, Rosemont, IL, 1997, American Academy of Orthopaedic Surgeons; Kieffer SA et al: Bulging lumbar intervertebral disc: myelographic differentiation from herniated disc with nerve root compression, *AJR Am J Roentgenol,* 138:709, 1982; Herzog RJ: The radiologic assessment for a lumbar disc herniation, *Spine* 21:19, 1996.
IVD, Intervertebral disc; *PLL,* posterior longitudinal ligament.

studies and the practitioner who reads the radiology report. Confusion can be avoided by emphasizing an accurate anatomic description of the imaging findings and not overrelying only on the use of categories. Also, the terms listed in Table 9-7 are best applied to the lumbar spine. Because only a rudimentary nucleus is present in the cervical discs, large frank nuclear displacements do not develop. Instead, cervical disc displacements typically are discussed as bulges for small, broad-based lesions and herniations for more extensive focal lesions.

Distribution of herniations. Disc herniations are most common in the lumbar spine and are uncommon in the thoracic spine. Ninety percent of lumbar herniations occur at the L4 and L5 disc levels, 5% to 7% at the L3 level, and only rarely at the L1 or L2 levels.[271,502] Most herniations are directed in a posterolateral direction; only 5% are posterocentral.

Thoracic disc herniations of sufficient size to encroach on the thecal sac are rare. When they do occur, they are typically posterocentral and much more likely to cause myelopathy than radiculopathy.

Ninety percent of cervical disc herniations occur at the C5 and C6 levels, with the remainder mostly in the lower cervical spine. Similar to the lumbar spine, the direction is usually posterolateral. Because the epidural space is less capacious than that of the lower lumbar spine, a small herniation in the cervical spine is more apt to cause symptoms. Because there is a less substantial nucleus pulposus, large herniations such as those of the lumbar spine are not seen in the cervical spine. Most cervical disc herniations result in radiculopathy, although myelopathy is much more common than in the upper lumbar spine.

IMAGING FINDINGS

The appearance of IVD herniation is dependent on the imaging modality employed, the level of involvement, presence of concurrent degeneration, and chronicity of the lesion.

Plain films. Because the IVD is not demonstrated directly, disc herniations are not seen on plain film radiographs.[502] Disc bulging accompanies degeneration and can be inferred from extensive marginal osteophytosis and narrowing of the disc height. Rarely a calcified sequestration is noted as a radiopaque ossicle in the spinal canal.

Myelography. Myelography depends on the introduction of a water-based (e.g., Metrizamide, Omnipaque, Isovue) or oil-based (Pantopaque) contrast agent into the subarachnoid space.[36] If a herniation is present and of sufficient size, the column of contrast demonstrates a slight indentation and possibly amputation of the nerve root sleeve.[323,324] Herniations at the L5 level may be missed or underrepresented because of the large epidural space (Fig. 9-167).

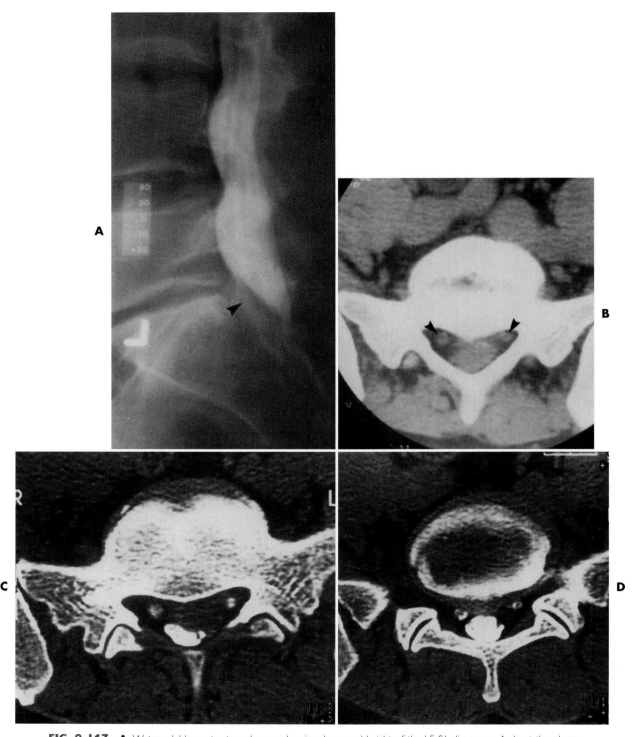

FIG. 9-167 **A,** Water-soluble contrast myelogram showing decreased height of the L5-S1 disc space. A short thecal sac can be seen, and an insensitive ventral epidural space also is present *(arrowhead)*. **B,** Computed tomography (CT) slice without intrathecal contrast obtained at the vertebral endplate level of S1 shows the descending roots in the lateral S1 recesses *(arrowheads)*. The thecal sac is present centrally and appears unremarkable. A small fleck of calcification is visible to the left of midline anteriorly within the thecal sac. **C,** Postmyelographic CT scan at the same level reveals a large epidural defect indicative of an extruded herniated disc situated anterolaterally to the left of midline and displacing the left S1 root laterally. It compresses the thecal sac focally (especially to the left of midline). **D,** Another postmyelographic CT slice, this time through the disc space of L5-S1, demonstrates a mild focal epidural defect centrally without distortion of the thecal sac or right S1 root sleeve. The left S1 root sleeve is displaced laterally. (From Firooznia H et al: MRI and CT of the musculoskeletal system, St Louis, 1992, Mosby.)

Although myelography was the procedure of choice for many years, it is currently inferior to either CT or MRI for locating and defining disc pathology. CT myelography (CTM) provides anatomic detail beyond that of either study alone. It is most often performed in the cervical and thoracic regions.

Myelography has the advantage of providing a large field of study and allows provocation of patients with spinal stenosis. It is used in place of CT and MRI with patients who are too large to fit in the scanners or if the patient has a large metallic construct, which may cause excessive image artifact.[259]

Discography. Discography entails injecting radiopaque contrast into the nucleus pulposus and imaging the morphology of the dye with plain films or CT (Fig. 9-168). The injected dye disperses throughout the substance of the nucleus and into those anular fissures that communicate with the nucleus. If a disc herniation is present, the injected dye enters the spinal canal and an anular fissure is clearly delineated by the trail of contrast extending to the spinal canal. For the most part, discography has been superseded by CT and MRI. Its only common use is before chemonucleolysis or percutaneous nucleotomy.

In addition to its application in imaging, discography offers the only provocative method to determine if a disc is painful.[116,118,119,169,176] Contrast injected into the nucleus pulposus distends the anulus and, if the patient's pattern of pain is reproduced or amplified, it provides evidence of a discogenic pathogenesis. Discography may be helpful in determining the symptomatic level of disc herniation if multiple herniation levels are demonstrated on CT or MRI.

Computed tomography. CT is advantageous for evaluating patients with suspected herniations for several reasons. It is available in most hospitals, offers an axial plane of imaging, is quick, and yields excellent visualization of the bony anatomy and good visualization of possible disc herniations (Figs. 9-169 to 9-171).

The disadvantages are that radiation is used, true multiplanar imaging is not possible, it only provides limited region of examination, and it does not demonstrate components of the IVD or contents of the thecal sac. These structures can be seen only if contrast is introduced.

Advantages of CT over MRI include the short examination times, higher resolution of cortical bone, and usual capacity to obtain thinner sections than MRI. The latter is particularly advantageous when imaging the cervical spine.

Magnetic resonance imaging. Twenty years ago MRI images were of poor quality, but substantial improvements have occurred in recent years. At present, most agree that MRI has become the primary imaging modality for investigating the spine and spinal canal.* In some spinal imaging circumstances (in which visualization of osseous detail is paramount), MRI remains inferior to CT. Some examiners prefer CTM to MRI for imaging the intricate details of the cervical spine and canal. However, as advances continue, the application and superiority of MRI will most likely broaden and become more certain.

The advantages of MRI are that it is noninvasive, provides true three-dimensional imaging, has a field of examination from the conus to the sacrum, and provides visualization of the bone marrow and intrathecal contents. Disadvantages are the long examination times, unavailability in some areas, expense, and low cortical bone resolution.

Both CT and MRI show excellent morphologic changes of an IVD herniation. However, only MRI provides information on the physiochemical changes within the disc. On T2-weighted MRI images, it is possible to differentiate the high signal intensity (bright) of the nucleus pulposus and inner anulus from the low signal intensity (dark) of the outer anulus.[698] Commonly a dark

---

*References 36, 232, 384, 439, 441, 605.

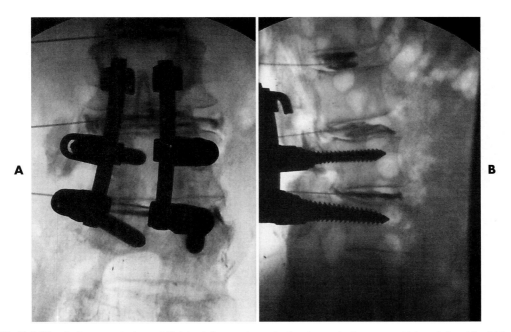

FIG. 9-168 **A,** Anteroposterior and, **B,** lateral discography projection demonstrating a normal internal disc at the L1 level and disc herniation at the L2 and L3 levels. Pedicle screws and stabilization bars also are noted.

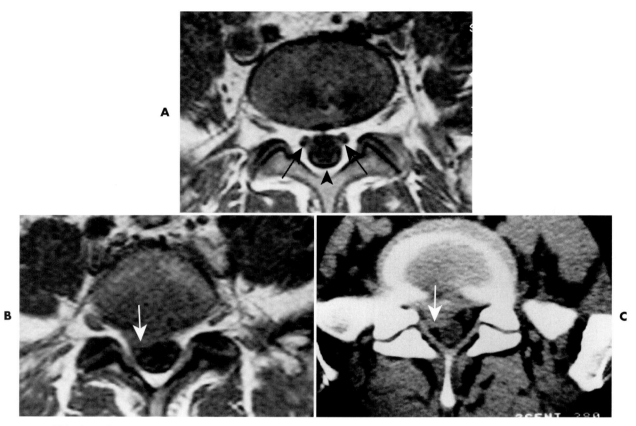

FIG. 9-169   Disc herniation in axial plane. **A,** T1-weighted axial magnetic resonance imaging (MRI) slice exhibiting the normal configuration of the thecal sac *(arrowhead)* and branching nerve roots *(arrows)*. Notice the hyperintense epidural fat interposed between the thecal sac and the vertebra. **B,** T1-weighted axial MRI slice in a different patient reveals a large disc herniation to the right of midline projecting into the thecal sac *(arrow)* with loss of the interposed epidural fat. **C,** Computed tomography scan of soft-tissue window of a third patient with a large right-sided L5 disc herniation *(arrow)*. The right nerve root is not visualized. (**C,** Courtesy Steven P. Brownstein, MD, Springfield, NJ.)

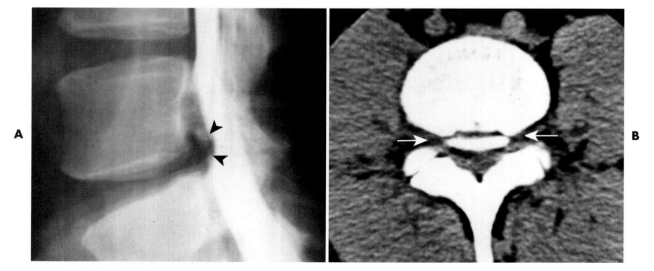

FIG. 9-170   **A,** The myelogram demonstrated a defect in the contrast column at the level of the L4 disc *(arrowheads)*. **B,** The corresponding axial computed tomography slice demonstrates a calcified disc fragment *(arrows)* in this nontrauma patient. (Courtesy Steven P. Brownstein, MD, Springfield, NJ.)

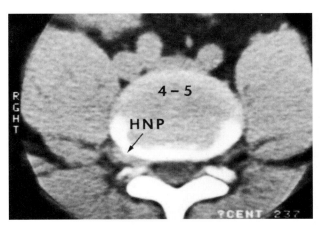

FIG. 9-171 Far right side herniated nucleus pulposus *(arrow)*. (Courtesy Steven P. Brownstein, MD, Springfield, NJ.)

Anular tears. Transverse and radial anular tears have been visualized on MRI images (Fig. 9-173).[698] They are seen as small foci of increased signal intensity on the T2-weighted image. They are best seen when hydrated nuclear material fills the cleft of the tear. If adequate neovascularity is present, anular tears may enhance brightly on the T1-weighted image after administration of an intravenous contrast agent (e.g., gadolinium diethylenetriamine pentaacetic acid [Gd-DTPA]). The observation of anular tears is highly dependent on their orientation.

Intervertebral disc herniations. The sagittal proton density image is probably most helpful to assess the integrity of the anulus fibrosus and posterior longitudinal ligament.[326] Axial images give the best information about the direction of the herniation (e.g., midline, parasagittal, posterolateral) and any resulting effacement of the thecal (neural or dural) sac or encroachment of the nerve roots (Figs. 9-174 to 9-180). *Thecal effacement* is an abnormal morphology of the thecal sac, usually best seen on the T2-weighted axial image. *Cord effacement* describes the additional finding of deformity of the spinal cord. Last, *cord compression* designates a posterior deviation of the spinal cord that obliterates the interval of T2-weighted high signal intensity cerebrospinal fluid located between the spinal cord and posterior confines of the spinal canal.

Disc extrusions and sequestered fragments may exhibit a high-intensity signal on the T2-weighted images.[405] It is not clear if these lesions represent acute herniations that have not desiccated completely or whether the high signal intensity has something to do with neovascularity or inflammation of the disc pathology.

MRI is helpful to differentiate recurrent disc herniations from surgical scars or tumors in the same location. Postoperative scars typically demonstrate lower signal intensity on T1-weighted images and higher signal intensity on the T2-weighted images than the surrounding epidural fat. The appearance is difficult to separate

horizontal band representing an intranuclear cleft can be seen in the middle of the nucleus in healthy individuals more than 30 years of age (Fig. 9-172). It represents ingrowth of fibrous tissue and is thought to be a natural consequence of aging. The nuclear signal intensity on the T2-weighted image is dependent on the hydration and macromolecular composition of the nucleus.[674] The normal disc exhibits high signal intensity on the T2-weighted middle sagittal scan. The signal intensity or brightness of the nucleus inversely correlates to aging and degeneration.*

---

*References 52, 211, 261, 291, 360, 436, 438, 440, 442, 477, 497, 574, 577, 586, 687.

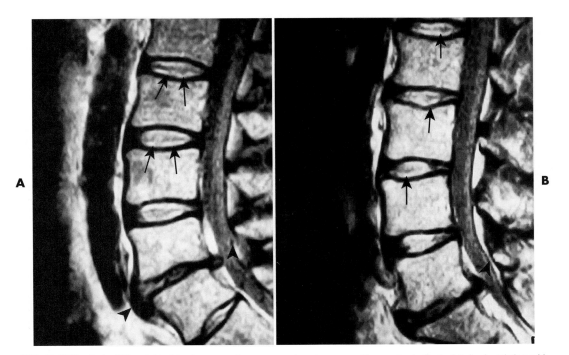

FIG. 9-172 Sagittal T2-weighted lumbar magnetic resonance imaging scans of two patients. **A,** An L4 disc herniation with anterior and posterior displacement *(arrowheads)*. **B,** A posterior L5 herniation is noted. Both patients demonstrate high nuclear signal ntensity, with dark horizontal bands indicating intranuclear clefts created by fibrous tissue invaginations *(arrows)*.

Text continued on p. 574.

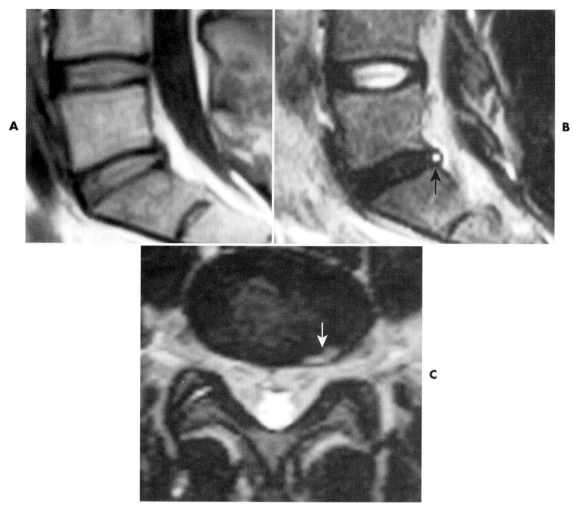

FIG. 9-173   **A** to **C,** High-intensity zone. At times, a focus of high signal intensity presents in the anulus fibrosus on the lumbar T2-weighted and gadopentetate dimeglumine–enhanced axial or sagittal scans *(arrows).* A high-intensity zone is thought to represent an area of inflammation secondary to anular tearing. The clinical importance of a high-intensity zone is not entirely clear in the related literature. Most authors feel the finding indicates internal disc disruption, but there is not the same level of agreement that high-intensity zones represent a reliable indicator of an accompanying discogenic pain pattern.

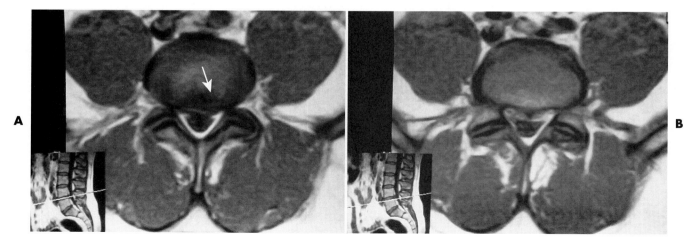

FIG. 9-174   **A,** T1-weighted (TR 750, TE 25) axial magnetic resonance imaging (MRI) scans denoting left parasagittal disc protrusion at the L4 level *(arrow).* **B,** The lesion is nearly gone on MRI scan of one slice below.

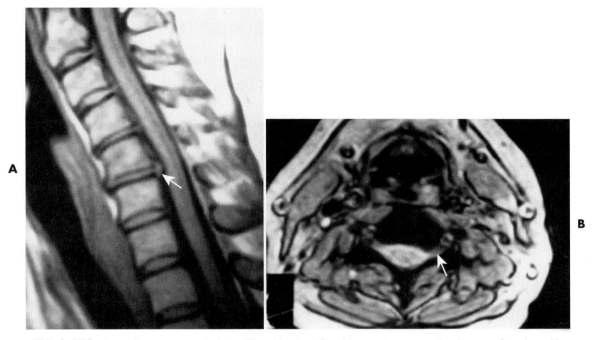

FIG. 9-175 Cervical disc herniation. **A,** Sagittal T1-weighted and, **B,** axial magnetic resonance imaging scan of a patient with focal disc herniation at the C5 *(arrows)*. The axial images demonstrate an uncinate osteophyte encroaching on the left intervertebral foramen.

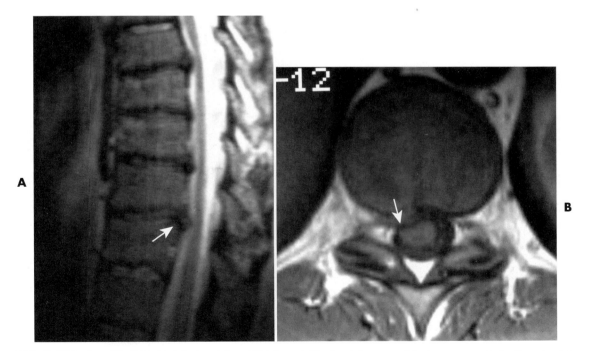

FIG. 9-176 **A** and **B,** Right-sided disc herniation at T11 *(arrows)*. Disc herniations are relatively uncommon in the thoracic spine.

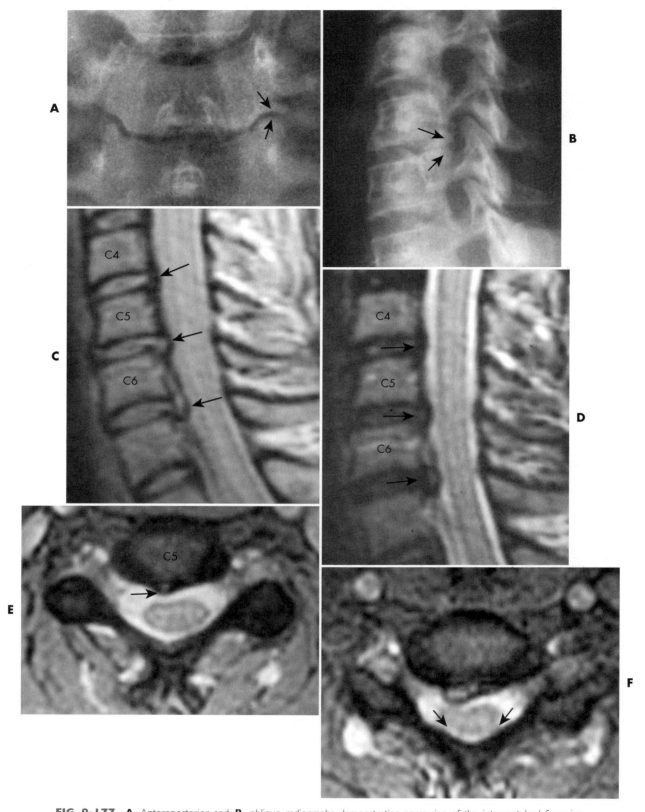

FIG. 9-177 A, Anteroposterior and, **B,** oblique radiographs demonstrating narrowing of the intervertebral foramina. A corresponding magnetic resonance imaging study exhibits disc bulge at C4 and disc herniations at C5 and C6 *(arrows)* noted on, **C,** the T1-weighted and, **D,** T2-weighted sagittal images. The axial scans demonstrated effacement of the thecal sac and cord at C5 noted by, **E,** the narrowed subdural space *(arrows)*. The thecal sac is effaced at C6, the cord is effaced, and the cord is slightly compressed as, **F,** the posterior subdural space is obliterated *(arrows)*. No edema is seen in the cord on, **D,** the sagittal T2-weighted image.

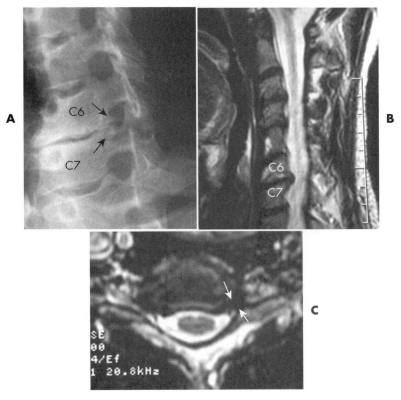

FIG. 9-178 The extent of intervertebral foramina narrowing is estimated with, **A,** plain film, but, **B** and **C,** magnetic resonance imaging relates much greater detail about the degree from the uncinate hypertrophy *(arrows).*

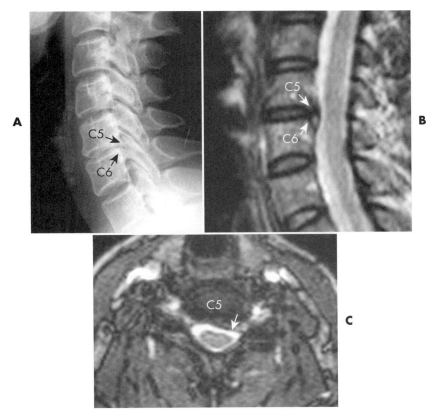

FIG. 9-179 A disc lesion cannot be visualized on plain film. However, as in this case, **A,** the presence of posterior marginal osteophytes *(arrows)* often correlates to, **B** and **C,** disc lesions seen on accompanying magnetic resonance imaging scans *(arrows).*

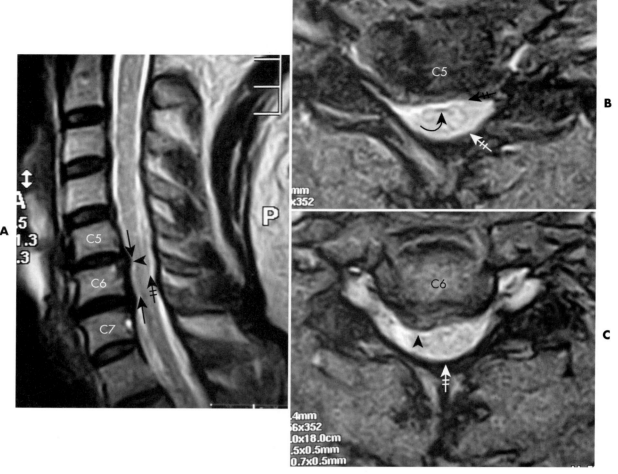

FIG. 9-180   A, Sagittal T2-weighted magnetic resonance imaging scan exhibiting disc lesion at C5 *(arrowhead)* and C6 noted by the posterior displacement of disc material and narrowing of the normally bright cerebrospinal fluid tract running parallel to the spinal cord *(arrows).* **B,** The T2-weighted axial image at C5 reveals normal shape of the spinal cord *(curved arrow),* but narrowed subdural space *(crossed arrows).* **C,** The T2-weighted axial image at C6 reveals an effaced (shape change) of the spinal cord *(arrowhead)* and absence of the anterior and posterior normally bright subdural space *(crossed arrow).*

from recurrent disc herniation. However, distinction is easier after the administration of intravenous contrast (Gd-DTPA). Postoperative scars and tumors exhibit diffuse enhancement on postcontrast T1-weighted images; by contrast, recurrent herniations enhance only peripherally (Fig. 9-181).

CLINICAL COMMENTS

Clinical complaint. The most common clinical complaint of a patient with a disc herniation is severe low back pain with or without leg pain. However, only about 5% of all acute low back pain cases are caused by disc herniation.[46] The pain typically occurs immediately or within a few hours of an injury. The pain is typically exaggerated by flexion, sneezing, bowel movement, and sitting.

Pain types. Pain may be local, referred, or radicular. Local pain is limited to the area of the lesion (Fig. 9-182). The painful structure must be innervated for local pain to occur. Referred (sclerotomal) pain is limited to anatomy of similar embryologic origin. Referred pain usually is described as deep, dull, and poorly

localized, and it does not extend beyond the knees or elbows.[669] Radicular (dermatomal) pain is located along dermatomal nerve root distributions. It may be accompanied by predicable sensory or motor deficits (Table 9-8). It is usually described as superficial, sharp, and well defined.

Radicular pain is thought to be related to nerve root inflammation.[625] Loss of muscle strength and muscle atrophy is typically attributed to nerve root pressure. Local and referred spinal pain patterns may arise from irritation of the spinal dura, paravertebral muscles, ligaments, and joints (e.g., IVD, facet, SI).[59,125] It is difficult to pinpoint the offending tissue.

The displaced disc typically affects the nerve root exiting at the same level in the cervical spine and one segment below in the lumbar spine (see Table 9-8). For instance, an L4 disc herniation affects the L5 nerve root, not the L4 nerve root, unless it is a far lateral herniation or laterally migrated sequestration.

Myelopathy. IVD displacement in the cervical, thoracic, and upper lumbar spine may produce long tract deficits secondary to cord pressure (myelopathy). Symptoms include bilateral complaints

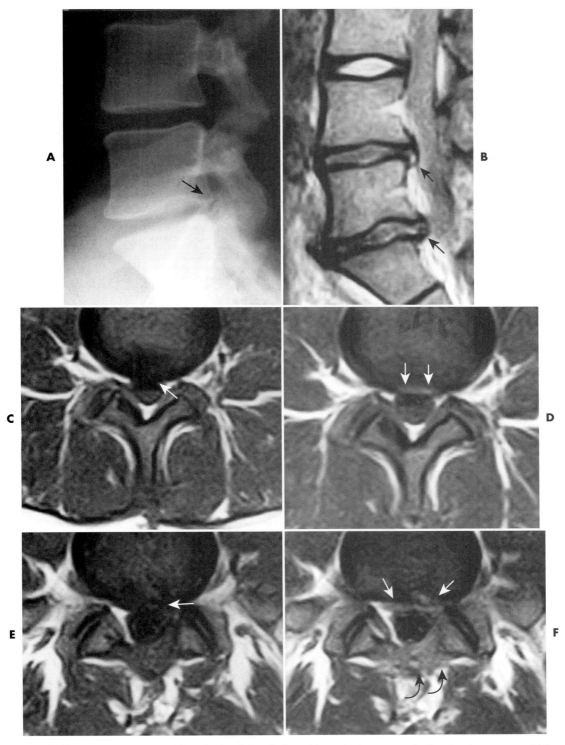

FIG. 9-181 Scar formation mimicking disc herniation. **A,** Lateral lower lumbar spot projection showing a narrowed L5 disc space and small osteophyte extending from the posterior aspect of L5 *(arrow).* **B,** T1-weighted (TR 700, TE 25) sagittal lumbar magnetic resonance imaging scan demonstrating two levels of disc herniations *(arrows).* **C,** The preconstrast T1-weighted axial image demonstrates a midline L4 disc herniation that appears to contact but not flatten the thecal sac *(arrow).* **D,** The mass becomes enhanced along its periphery after administration of gadopentetate dimeglumine contrast *(arrows),* indicating L4 disc herniation. **E,** Larger mass extending from the disc spaces is noted at the L5 level to the left of the midline effacing the thecal sac *(arrow).* **F,** Suspected disc herniation becomes diffusely enhanced after gadopentetate dimeglumine contrast administration *(arrows).* This pattern of enhancement is associated with the highly vascular nature of scar formation, not disc herniation, which tends to become only peripherally enhanced. In addition, enhancement of a surgical scar from a previous laminectomy is noted in the region of the posterior arch of L5 *(curved arrows).* (Courtesy Ian D. McLean, Davenport, IA.)

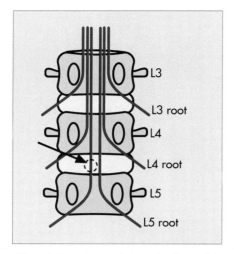

FIG. 9-182 The spinal cord extends from the base of the brain to the L1-L2 disc level. Therefore intact middle and lower lumbar disc lesions do not have the potential to compress the cord. Instead they may compromise nerve roots, whereas the cervical and thoracic disc may involve the cord or nerve roots, depending on the direction and degree of disc displacement. In the cervical spine, the nerve root is named for the segment below (e.g., C6 nerve root exits the C5-6 intervertebral foramen adjacent the C5 disc). However, in the thoracic and lumbar spine, the nerve is named for the segment above (e.g., the L4 nerve root extis the L4-5 intervertebral foramen). Cervical nerve roots exit horizontally, and therefore cervical dissc herniations tend to involve nerve roots exiting at the adjacent intervertebral foramen level, which is the nerve root at the same level, but is named for the segment below (e.g., a C5 disc lesion impacts the immediately adjacent C6 nerve root). By contrast, lumbar nerve roots travel obliquely from medial superior to lateral inferior from the thecal sac to their exiting intervertebral foramen, causing middle to lower lumbar lesions to involve the nerve root exiting the subadjacent intervertebral foramen (e.g., the L4 disc tends to involve the L5 nerve root [see arrow in above figure], not the L4 nerve root). In the lumbar spine, only far lateral disc displacements or sequestered disc fragments involve the same level nerve root.

40 years of age.[53] Jensen and co-workers studied 98 asymptomatic individuals with an average age of 48 years and found a lumbar disc bulge in 58%, protrusion in 27%, and extrusion in 1%.[293] Anular tears were noted in 14%.[293] The prevalence of disc herniations on MRI, CT, and myelographic studies is estimated to be 20% to 35% in asymptomatic subjects.[259]

The size of the spinal canal and presence of concurrent facet joint arthrosis or ligamentum flavum hypertrophy are important features determining who will experience symptoms; however, currently it is not clear why some herniations are painful and others are not.[464] Prospective data are needed to determine the long-term consequences of disc herniations.

Physical examination. Abdominal and erector spinal muscle spasm is common on physical examination. Apprehension and tenderness to palpation usually are present, and are reported more on one side. Functional scoliosis is common.[669] A positive straight-leg raising orthopedic test is positive in 95% of patients with disc herniations.[149] A positive straight-leg raising test lifting the asymptomatic leg (contralateral straight-leg raising test) is positive less often, but more accurate for disc herniation when the test is positive.[149]

Clinical course. IVD herniations usually are associated with a favorable prognosis.[565] Cauda equina syndrome represents one of the most serious complications and is marked by altered bowel and bladder function, impotence, progressive muscle atrophy, and saddle paresthesia. It is uncommon, occurring in 1% to 16% of patients.[213] When present, it is widely regarded as a surgical emergency to alleviate nerve pressure and restore function.

The use of serial imaging studies to assess the impact of applied treatments on the size of a disc lesion is confounded by the natural history of disc herniations. Over time, herniations undergo cicatrization and retraction, as part of their normal healing process.[281,564,637] Moreover it is theorized that exposure of disc herniations to the epidural blood supply facilitates phagocytosis of the extruded material. Apparently the larger the lesion, the greater is the resorption.[409] Extrusions demonstrate greater reduction in size over time than prolapses (contained herniations).[285] The degree of sequestration resorption is positively associated with its distance of migration.[327]

Management. Generally it is not necessary to order imaging studies to evaluate the IVD or spinal canal during the initial 4 to 6 weeks after onset of symptoms that suggest disc herniation.[259]

of numbness, muscle weakness, and spasticity. The pain and numbness does not follow dermatomal patterns, differentiating it from radiculopathy.

Asymptomatic herniations. Not all patients who exhibit disc herniation are symptomatic.[53,66,120,638] Boden and associates found cervical disc herniations in five (10%) of 40 asymptomatic patients under 40 years of age, and in one (5%) of 23 patients more than

---

TABLE 9-8
Clinical Findings Associated with Disc Herniations

Disc level	Nerve root	Reflex affected	Muscle affected	Location of sensation
C4-5	C5	Biceps	Deltoid, biceps	Lateral arm
C5-6	C6	Brachioradialis	Wrist extensors, biceps	Lateral forearm
C6-7	C7	Triceps	Wrist flexors, triceps	Middle finger
C7-T1	C8	None reliable	Finger flexors	Medial forearm
L1-2	L2	None reliable	Iliopsoas	Anterior thigh, groin
L2-3	L3	Patellar	Quadriceps	Anterior and lateral thigh
L3-4	L4	Patellar	Anterior tibialis	Medial leg and foot
L4-5	L5	None reliable	Extensor hallucis	Lateral leg and foot
L5-S1	S1	Achilles	Peroneus longus	Lateral foot and fifth toe

From Andersson GBJ, Deyo RA: History and physical examination in patients with herniated lumbar discs, *Spine* 21:10, 1996; Weinstein JN, Rydevik BL, Sonntag VKH: Essentials of the spine, New York, 1995, Raven Press.

TABLE 9-9

Management of Intervertebral Disc Herniations

Type of management	Comments
Chiropractic	Judicious application of side posture and flexion distraction adjustments for lumbar discs and other approaches for cervical herniations; chiropractic care is beneficial for many patients with confirmed disc herniations.
Other conservative measures	NSAIDs and other analgesics, muscle relaxants, epidural steroid injections, oral steroids, traction, ice biofeedback, limited bed rest, braces, acupuncture.
Chemonucleolysis	Injection of the enzyme chymopapain into the nucleus pulposus; indiscriminate destruction of the disc often results in poor outcome; generally, surgery is preferable for patients who do not respond to conservative care.
Surgery	Some options include: (a) removing the offending disc through a needle without the aid of an incision (percutaneous discectomy); (b) using a small incision to make a hemilaminotomy and removing the offending disc material (microdiscectomy); (c) removing a larger portion of the lamina (laminectomy) and possibly removing a portion of the disc (discectomy—most common approach); and (d) performing central or lateral decompression, or spinal fusion. In general, surgical techniques are directed toward alleviating nerve root or cord pressure or stabilizing the vertebral segments.

Exceptions include suspected cauda equina syndrome, progressive neurologic deficit, intractable pain, or constitutional signs and symptoms suggesting tumor, fracture, infection, or other aggressive pathology.[673] If the patient is unresponsive to conservative therapy, imaging studies usually are warranted to determine if the management plan should be altered.[259] Management approaches are listed in Table 9-9.

Conservative management. The management paradigm should begin with conservative measures, typically for at least 2 or 3 months.[371,518] If agreed to by the patient, slow recoveries can be managed even longer.[371] However, the use of muscle relaxants, analgesic, and bed rest for more than 2 weeks may further complicate the patient's status.[213] Activities that exacerbate back pain (e.g., heavy lifting, repetitious axial rotation, flexion) should be avoided.[149,669] Often psychological counseling is helpful.[669] Chiropractic care has been shown to be beneficial by many investigators and a few experimental studies.* Serious complications to the judicious application of chiropractic care are rare.[103,124,584]

Surgery. Immediate surgery may be indicated if intractable pain, significant or progressive neurologic deficit, and loss of bowel and bladder function (cauda equina syndrome) develop.[371] Surgery is most often done on the basis of symptoms, not neurologic deficits. This accounts for the wide variation in surgical rates among different geographic areas.[202] Surgery may provide immediate and dramatic relief of symptoms, but symptoms often return[518] and may be worse than the original complaint. Only about 5% to 10% of patients with radicular pain require surgery.[213]

The mere presence of a disc herniation is not an absolute indication of surgery. Appropriate patient selection is the key to surgical success.[445] The failure of a few selective conservative measures is not an appropriate criterion for surgical intervention.[565] Surgery is most successful on patients who have exhausted all other options.[625,669]

---

*References 64, 103, 124, 235, 286, 332, 340, 526, 593.

KEY CONCEPTS

- An intervertebral disc herniation describes the extension of nuclear, anular, or endplate substance through the anulus fibrosus.
- It is more common among males, smokers, the obese, those exposed to vehicular vibration, and those 25 to 45 years old.
- Herniations represent a continuum of displacement that may be categorized into protrusions (contained herniations), extrusions (noncontained herniations), and sequestrations (free fragments).
- Bulges are not herniations, but rather represent broad-based extension of the anulus fibrosus without nuclear displacement.
- Herniations are most common in the lumbar spine, followed by the cervical and then thoracic regions; 90% of lumbar herniations occur at the L4 and L5 levels, and 90% of cervical herniation occur at the C5 and C6 levels.
- Plain films do not demonstrate disc herniations.
- Myelography is antiquated except for specific circumstances.
- Discography precedes chemonucleolysis and provides a provocative test for suspected discogenic pain syndromes.
- Computed tomography (CT): axial images, rapid examination, excellent osseous detail, and the capability of very thin sections; may be combined with myelography to offer visualization of the thecal sac.
- Magnetic resonance imaging (MRI): widely regarded as the best imaging modality for the spine and canal contents, noninvasive, provides true three-dimensional imaging, field of examination from the conus to the sacrum, and provides excellent visualization of the intervertebral disc, bone marrow, and intrathecal contents.
- Many disc herniations produce no symptoms; when symptoms are present, they are usually described as severe low back pain with or without leg pain, exaggerated by flexion, sneezing, bowel movement, and sitting.
- The prevalence of disc herniations on MRI, CT, and myelographic studies is estimated to be 20% to 35% in asymptomatic subjects.
- The size of the spinal canal and presence of concurrent facet joint arthrosis or ligamentum flavum hypertrophy are important features determining who will experience symptoms.

- *Ipsilateral straight-leg raising test is positive in 95% of patients with disc herniation, contralateral straight-leg raising test is less often positive but more accurate.*
- *Cauda equina syndrome represents one of the most serious complications and is marked by altered bowel and bladder function, impotence, progressive muscle atrophy, and saddle paresthesia.*
- *The use of serial imaging studies to assess the impact of applied treatments on the size of a disc lesion is confounded by the natural history of disc herniations to resorb over time.*
- *The management paradigm should begin with conservative measures, typically for at least 2 or 3 months.*
- *The use of muscle relaxants, analgesics, and bed rest for more than 2 weeks may further complicate the patient's status.*
- *Chiropractic care has been shown to be beneficial; complications are rare.*
- *Immediate surgery may be indicated if intractable pain, significant or progressive neurologic deficit, and loss of bowel and bladder function develop.*
- *Appropriate patient selection is the key to surgical success; surgery is most successful on patients who have exhausted all other options.*

Spinal Stenosis

BACKGROUND

Spinal stenosis refers to narrowing of the spinal canal or intervertebral foramen (IVF, neuroforamen) secondary to adjacent soft-tissue or bone enlargement.[156,166,479] Stenosis may involve one or more levels.[446]

Demographics. Spinal stenosis appears to involve men more than women[479,589] except for cases related to degenerative spondylolisthesis, which are more common in women. Stenosis is more common among middle-aged people (40 to 50 years).[108,589] There is no clear relationship to occupation or body size. Valid incidence and prevalence data are difficult to obtain because of the lack of specific diagnostic criteria for spinal stenosis.[402,692] Stenosis occurs most commonly in the cervical and lumbar regions of the spine. Central lumbar stenosis is most common at the L4 level.

Classification system. Stenosis is classically divided into congenital (e.g., achondroplasia, Morquio's syndrome, Down syndrome) and acquired (e.g., intervertebral disc herniation, zygapophyseal arthrosis, postsurgical) types based on etiology (Fig. 9-183 and Table 9-10). Another classification system divides

TABLE 9-10
Conditions Related to Spinal Stenosis

Condition	Description
Congenital stenosis	
Achondroplasia (see Chapter 8 for more detail)	Narrowing of interpeduncular distance and all components of the spinal canal secondary to aberrant enchondral bone formation; the condition is most severe in the lumbar spine.[447,522]
Idiopathic stenosis	Usually characterized by uniform narrowing of the lumbar spinal canal and neuroforamina of congenital origin (usually) but not associated with a congenital syndrome;[67] symptoms typically begin in middle-aged patients.
Morquio's mucopolysaccharidosis	Metabolic disease associated with spinal stenosis secondary to altered vertebral shape, posterior segmental displacements, and thoracolumbar kyphosis.[43]
Acquired stenosis	
Calcification or ossification of ligamentum flavum or posterior longitudinal ligament	Condition that may lead to spinal canal stenosis; ossification of the posterior longitudinal ligament is more common among Japanese men[455] and is a characteristic complication of diffuse idiopathic skeletal hyperostosis;[547] calcification or ossification of the ligamentum flavum is less common and is usually secondary to calcium pyrophosphate dihydrate or degeneration.[305,314]
Spondylolisthesis	Degenerative (nonspondylolytic) spondylolisthesis results from zygapophyseal joint degeneration and up to 33% forward displacement of the vertebra; degenerative spondylolistheses most commonly occur among middle-aged women at the L4 level;[458] by contrast, because of the pars defect, spondylolytic spondylolisthesis is rarely associated with spinal stenosis. Because of the pars defect, the zygapophyseal joints maintain normal alignment and the vertebrae slip forward, effectively enlarging the spinal canal, although advanced forward displacement may encroach on the thecal sac from the segment above.[686]
Spondylosis (see Fig. 9-58)	Degeneration of the intervertebral disc, zygapophyseal joints, and uncovertebral joints of the cervical spine; it is marked by proliferative osteophytic changes, decreased joint space, segmental misalignment, disc bulging, and associated hypertrophy and forward buckling of the ligamentum flavum,[516-518] which narrows the spinal canal; neuroforamina are most affected by degeneration of the uncovertebral and zygapophyseal joints.
Postsurgical	Spinal stenosis following laminectomy, fusion, or chemonucleolysis occurs in 30 to 40% of cases;[83,277,524] chemonucleolysis narrows the intervertebral disc space and projects the superior articular facet into the neuroforamina.[141]
Metabolic/endocrine/other	Acromegaly: associated with spinal stenosis secondary to advanced osteophytosis;[167] calcium pyrophosphate dihydrate: affecting the spinal ligaments, particularly the ligamentum flavum;[314] bone overgrowth associated with Paget's disease narrowing the spinal canal[678] and neuroforamina; deformity caused by trauma may lead to spinal stenosis.

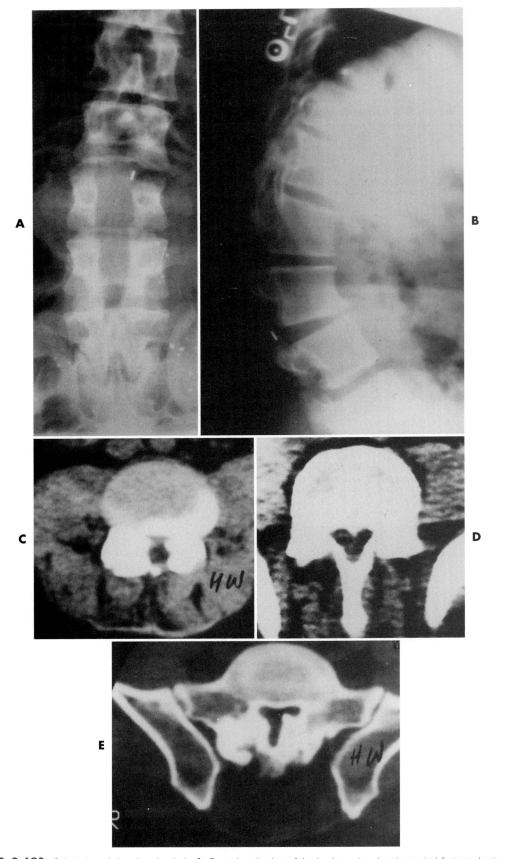

FIG. 9-183 Spinal stenosis in achondroplasia. **A,** Frontal projection of the lumbar spine showing typical features; laminectomy has been performed. **B,** Lateral projection of the thoracolumbar region showing the exaggerated concavity of the posterior vertebral surfaces. **C,** Axial computed tomography at L3-4. Note the marked stenosis of the canal after the laminectomy. Superimposed degenerative disease of the facet joints also is present, which has contributed to the stenosis. **D** and **E,** Note the triangular configuration of, **D,** the spinal canal and degenerative disease of, **E,** the facet joints at S1. The protruding hypertrophied facets have caused further distortion and stenosis of the canal. (From Firooznia H et al: MRI and CT of the musculoskeletal system, St Louis, 1992, Mosby.)

spinal stenosis into three types based on the anatomic locale involved: central (narrowing of the spinal canal), neuroforaminal (narrowing of the intervertebral foramen), and lateral recess (narrowing of the lateral zone, the distance between the thecal sac and the intervertebral foramen) stenosis.[156] Combined narrowing of the lateral recess and neuroforamen is termed *peripheral stenosis.*

IMAGING FINDINGS

Plain film. Plain film radiographs are of limited value in the diagnosis of spinal stenosis.[516,517] Because of gender, race, and age differences, radiographic measures of spinal canal or neuroforamina lack specificity.[161,162,234,257,296] Variations of the shape of the canal appear to be more important than size variations.[578]

Projectional distortion may alter the appearance of the canal or neuroforamina, leading to spurious conclusions. This is a particularly common pitfall when observing the neuroforamina on the lateral lumbar radiograph. The lower lumbar neuroforamina are directed anterolaterally and appear narrower than their actual anteroposterior dimension (Fig. 9-184).

Plain film radiographs are very helpful to exclude conditions often associated with spinal stenosis (e.g., achondroplasia, Paget's disease, spondylosis, spondylolisthesis).

Advanced imaging. CT and MRI are the most helpful procedures to assess spinal stenosis and have essentially eliminated the use of myelography. Both CT and MRI yield axial images to assess the size and shape of the spinal canal and neuroforamen (Figs. 9-185 to 9-189). CT seems to have an advantage over MRI for diagnosing spondylosis. Contrast-enhanced CT is preferred by some for evaluating stenosis in the cervical spine.[290] MRI is advantageous for assessment of the thecal sac and contents. T2-weighted images are best to assess for spinal canal (central)

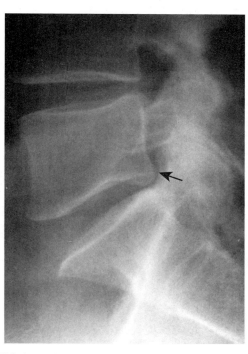

FIG. 9-184 Lateral lumbosacral spot projection demonstrating a narrow L5-S1 intervertebral foramen (IVF) *(arrow).* The IVF is directed anterolaterally in the lower lumbar spine; therefore a lateral projection underestimates the anteroposterior dimension of the foramen. Care should be taken not to interpret this projectional phenomenon incorrectly as neuroforaminal stenosis.

stenosis, because the cerebrospinal fluid of the thecal sac is well contrasted with the epidural fat. The epidural fat, which is best for evaluating peripheral stenosis, is best seen on a T1-weighted image.

CLINICAL COMMENTS

Clinical symptoms. Spinal stenosis results in compression of the nerves, arteries, capillaries, and veins.[330,334] It is theorized that pain results from arterial obstruction, venous hypertension, and pressure on the primary rami and recurrent meningeal nerves (sinuvertebral nerves).[159,339,444]

The presenting pain patterns are related to the region of stenosis. Neuroforaminal stenosis is associated with well-defined pain patterns that correspond to the level of stenosis. Conversely, spinal stenosis typically produces vague, poorly defined pain patterns. Both patterns usually are preceded by a long history of intermittent spinal complaints.[234] Stenosis is typically multifactorial, resulting from a combination of congenital hypoplasia, disc degeneration, facet hypertrophy, ligamentum flavum hypertrophy, ossification of the surrounding ligaments, and other changes and involvement of the related anatomy. It is difficult to tease out the major factor or involvement.

Spinal region. The findings in the cervical spine differ from the lumbar spine. In the cervical spine, long tract and radicular signs and symptoms are present in many cases.[99,156,291,407] Headaches and neck pain usually are experienced.[479] Often, cervical spine flexion may bring about sudden electric-like shocks extending down the spine and extremities (Lhermitte's sign). Cervical spine stenosis may mimic the clinical presentation of multiple sclerosis, syringomyelia, and amyotrophic lateral sclerosis (ALS).[662] Concurrent cervical and lumbar spinal stenosis produces a perplexing clinical presentation marked by gait disturbance, mixed and multiple level myelopathy, and radiculopathy that is particularly suspicious of ALS or other motor neuron disease.[168]

Neurogenic claudication. Neurogenic claudication (pseudoclaudication) is a common clinical presentation of patients with lumbar spinal canal stenosis.[234] It is marked by poorly defined leg pain accompanied by limb numbness and muscle weakness. The pain is exacerbated by walking or standing, and alleviated by trunk flexion.[156,234,330,479,608] Patients are often seen in a posture of trunk, hip, and knee flexion (simian stance).[599] Although vascular claudication appears with similar symptoms, clinical differentiation is possible on the basis of symptom-aggravating movements. Vascular claudication worsens with exercise, and improves with standing and lying. Neurogenic claudication is exacerbated by standing and spinal extension, and not dramatically changed by exercise.

Differentiating disc herniation. Differentiating spinal stenosis from discogenic pain is difficult because the two conditions often coexist.[156,686] Disc herniation is a common cause of stenosis. If differentiation is possible, symptom-aggravating movements may be useful. Sitting, bending, lifting, and Valsalva maneuvers aggravate discogenic back pain and have no affect on pain resulting from spinal stenosis.[156,234,330] Conversely, walking may aggravate spinal stenosis complaints and alleviate discogenic pain.[156,234,330] Symptoms of spinal stenosis are more chronic in nature than symptoms associated with intervertebral disc herniation.[479]

Treatment and management. Treatment for spinal stenosis usually is based on symptoms. Most patients with intermittent or mild symptoms can be managed by nonsurgical means.[481,700] If the patient does not respond, surgical decompression with or without fusion is considered.[108]

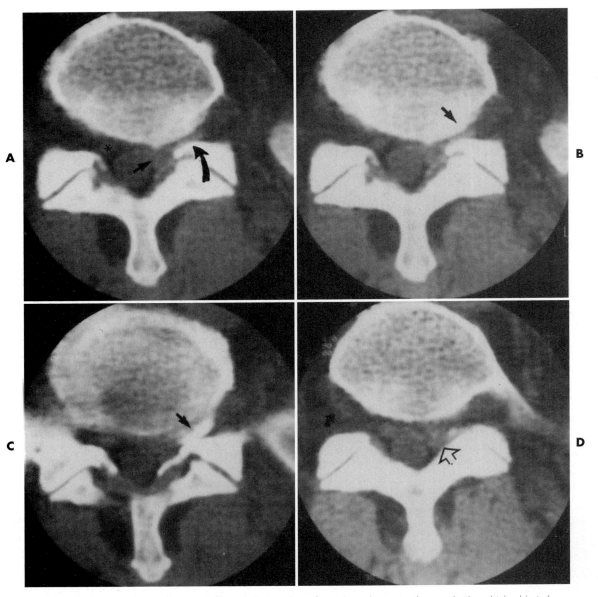

FIG. 9-185 Neuroforaminal stenosis. Two window settings of a computed tomography examination obtained just above the inferior endplate of L5. There are hypertrophic changes of the posterolateral border of L5 on the left, which have caused stenosis of the lower portion of the L5-S1 foramen. **A,** The *curved arrow* denotes the stenotic foramen. The normal descending right S1 nerve root *(asterisk)* already has separated from the dural sac. A soft-tissue density *(straight arrow)* in the epidural space occupies the anterolateral portion of the spinal canal on the left; it is a migrated fragment of herniated disc. The left descending S1 nerve root is obscured by the herniated disc. **B,** Hypertrophic changes on the posterolateral border of L5 *(arrow).* **C,** Axial slice obtained 4 mm below **A** and **B,** showing the hypertrophic changes and a calcified ridge *(arrow).* A soft-tissue density, which is herniated disc material obscuring the left anterior epidural fat and extending laterally, also obscures the left descending S1 nerve root and lateral recess. **D,** Axial slice just below the L5 pedicle showing that the neuroforamen is normal at this level. The dorsal root ganglion also is normal *(curved arrow).* The fragment of herniated disc obscures the descending left S1 nerve root *(open arrow).* This patient has marked stenosis in the lower portion of the neuroforamen but no evidence of compression of the L5 dorsal root ganglion in the upper part of the foramen. The exiting L5 spinal nerve is more anterior and lateral to the site of the stenosis and is not involved. (From Firooznia H et al: MRI and CT of the musculoskeletal system, St Louis, 1992, Mosby.)

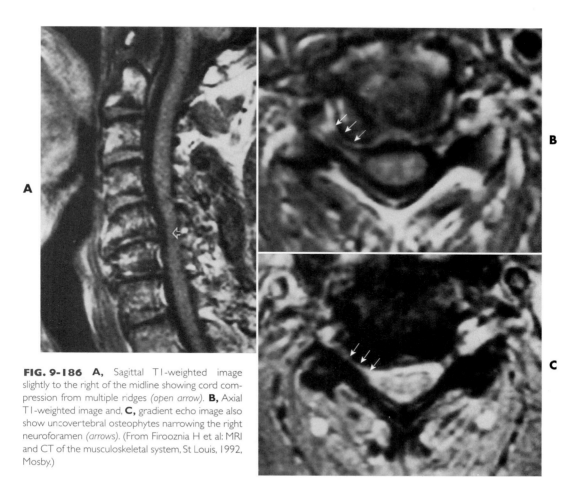

FIG. 9-186 A, Sagittal T1-weighted image slightly to the right of the midline showing cord compression from multiple ridges *(open arrow).* **B,** Axial T1-weighted image and, **C,** gradient echo image also show uncovertebral osteophytes narrowing the right neuroforamen *(arrows).* (From Firooznia H et al: MRI and CT of the musculoskeletal system, St Louis, 1992, Mosby.)

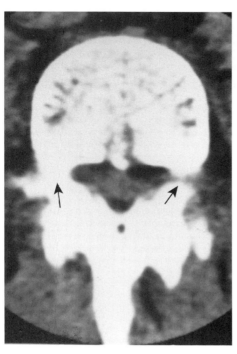

FIG. 9-187 Lumbar computed tomography scan revealing a narrowed intervertebral canal secondary to short, thick pedicles *(arrows).* (Courtesy Steven P. Brownstein, Springfield NJ.)

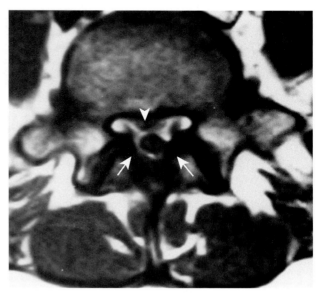

FIG. 9-188 Axial T1-weighted lumbar magnetic resonance imaging scan at the lower margin of the L5 disc. The development of spinal stenosis is multifactorial, influenced by posterior joint arthrosis and ligamentum flavum hypertrophy *(arrows),* disc lesions *(arrowhead),* and predisposing congenital size of the canal. Patients with a capacious canal can tolerate disc and posterior joint degeneration without developing stenosis, whereas the presence of only small lesions can bring about clinical findings in those predisposed by a small canal.

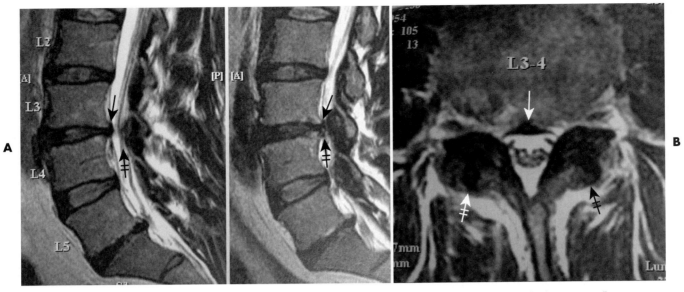

FIG. 9-189 A and **B,** This patient has a congenitally small spinal canal, which predisposes to spinal stenosis when even small disc lesions *(arrows)* and moderate facet joint degeneration develop *(crossed arrows).*

KEY CONCEPTS

- *Spinal stenosis refers to narrowing of the spinal canal or intervertebral (IVF, neuroforamen) foramen secondary to adjacent soft-tissue or bone enlargement.*
- *Overall stenosis is more common in men and middle-aged (40 to 50 years old) people.*
- *Stenosis is more common in the cervical and lumbar regions of the spine than the thoracic region.*
- *It is divided by etiology into congenital (e.g., achondroplasia, Morquio's, and Down syndromes) and acquired (e.g., intervertebral disc herniation, zygapophyseal arthrosis, and postsurgical) types.*
- *It is categorized by location into central (narrowing of the spinal canal), neuroforaminal (narrowing of the intervertebral foramen), and lateral recess (narrowing of the lateral zone, the distance between the thecal sac and the intervertebral foramen) types.*
- *Plain film radiographs are helpful in evaluating related conditions (e.g., spondylolisthesis, Paget's disease, and achondroplasia).*
- *Computed tomography and magnetic resonance imaging provide axial images and the ability to evaluate deformity of the thecal sac.*
- *Neuroforaminal stenosis is associated with a well-defined pain pattern.*
- *Spinal stenosis produces vague, poorly defined pain patterns.*
- *Stenosis usually has a chronic history; disc herniations do not.*
- *Cervical spine stenosis commonly is associated with myelopathy and diffuse symptoms.*
- *Neurogenic claudication (pseudoclaudication) is a common clinical presentation of patients with lumbar spinal canal stenosis, marked by poorly defined leg pain accompanied by limb numbness and muscle weakness that tends to resolve on trunk flexion.*
- *Treatment for spinal stenosis usually is based on symptoms; most patients with intermittent or mild symptoms can be managed by nonsurgical means; failure of conservative management is followed by decompressive surgery and possible fusion.*

Diffuse Idiopathic Skeletal Hyperostosis

BACKGROUND

Diffuse idiopathic skeletal hyperostosis (DISH) (ankylosing hyperostosis of the spine, Forestier disease) is a common rheumatologic abnormality characterized by exuberant proliferation of bone at osseous sites of ligamentous and tendinous attachments throughout the body. Both spinal and extraspinal sites are affected, but the most notable occurrence involves the anterior longitudinal ligament of the spine.

A high prevalence of the disease is noted among diabetics (13% to 49%)[195] and the general population (8.5% to 20%).[581,664] An association between DISH and diabetes traditionally has been reported by authors in the field, but focused controlled research is limited and contrary to popular opinion. For example, a case control study by Daragon and associates[138] could not establish a link between DISH and diabetes, suggesting that the precept of an association reported in the past may be an artifact of confounding factors (e.g., obesity). However, because research in the field is limited and diabetes prevalent, continued screening for diabetes among DISH patients is arguably prudent and probably warranted. Further controlled investigation is necessary to inform such practices.

The incidence of DISH increases with age,[195] is most common in middle-aged and elderly people, and is more frequent in men. The etiology of this bone-forming disorder remains unknown despite several avenues of investigation: growth hormone (GH), insulin, and vitamin A or retinoid derivatives[138,630] and associated metabolic syndromes.[664]

Initial studies evaluating levels of GH in patients with DISH were unrewarding, but more recent investigations support the hypothesis that GH may act as a bone growth–promoting factor in DISH similar to its role in promoting tissue growth in patients with acromegaly.[12,144]

Insulin also has been suggested to play a role in the new bone formation associated with DISH, because it may act as a growth factor. Elevated insulin levels[144] and marked hyperinsulinemia after

glucose challenge[369] have been reported. Although a high incidence of diabetes has been reported in the past (as cited), a more recent study revealed no difference compared with the control group.[135]

IMAGING FINDINGS

Spine. The diagnosis of spinal involvement is based on the following three strict radiographic criteria,[550] which aid in distinguishing DISH from spondylosis deformans (degeneration) and AS (Figs. 9-190 and 9-191).

1. Flowing ossification of the anterolateral aspect of at least four contiguous vertebral bodies.
2. Relative preservation of disc height over the involved segments, and absence of radiographic changes associated with DDD (vacuum sign or discogenic sclerosis).
3. Absence of sacroiliitis and facet ankylosis.

The anterior ossification can be subtle or dramatic depending on its thickness and contour. The hyperostotic outline may be smooth or bumpy, continuous or interrupted, and range from 1 or 2 mm to more than 20 mm in thickness. There may be lucent defects through the ossification anterior to the disc space, representing discal extrusions, not fractures, through the new bone formation (Fig. 9-190, *A, B,* and *D*).

The most common site of involvement is the middle to lower thoracic spine, in which the new anterolateral bone formation is more often on the right, apparently resulting from the pulsating descending thoracic aorta on the left. Upper lumbar hyperostosis is noted almost as frequently as in the lower thoracic segments, with the ossification occurring bilaterally and predominantly on the anterior aspect. Lower cervical spine abnormalities also are common, and include posterior alterations (e.g., posterior spinal osteophytes, ossification within the nuchal ligament and the posterior longitudinal ligament) in addition to the more common anterior deposition of bone.

Ossification of the posterior longitudinal ligament (OPLL), once known as the "Japanese disease" because of its predilection for the Asian race, is a condition that may occur alone or in conjunction with DISH. OPLL is twice as common among men, and usually forms during the fifth to seventh decade. It is a common contributor to canal stenosis, with up to 25% of patients presenting with cervical myelopathy demonstrating OPLL rather than spondylotic and stenotic myelopathy or disc disease alone.[168] Resnick and co-workers[547] reported that 50% of the DISH patients they radiographed revealed evidence of calcification or ossification in the PLL. Other reports indicated that DISH was present in approximately 40% of patients with OPLL. However, in practical experience, most patients with DISH do not demonstrate visible features of OPLL on their radiographs.

If visible on plain film radiography, OPLL is best seen on the lateral view, and appears as a thin (1- to 5-mm) linear calcification running parallel and posterior to the vertebral bodies (Figs. 9-192 to 9-194). There may be a lucent cleft sandwiched between the dense ligament and vertebral bodies. The cervical spine is most commonly involved (C3 to C5), with thoracic and lumbar involvement rarely present (see Fig. 9-195). OPLL may be missed on plain film because of overlying anatomy.[453] CT is the recommended procedure of choice if OPLL is suspected, or to determine the extent of ossification and possible cord compression.[416,462,699]

Sacroiliac joints. The synovial portion, or lower two thirds of the SI joint, is not commonly affected; however, the upper one third may become blurred or indistinct; in addition, the superior and inferior portions of the joints are often bridged by paraarticular ligamentous calcification (Fig. 9-196).

Extraspinal enthesopathy. The typical sites of involvement include the pelvis, calcaneus, and patella. The enthesopathic changes that ensue are purely productive; there are no erosive components. Radiographically, this is reflected by initial roughening or fraying of the bone and later by more extensive proliferation (Fig. 9-197).

CLINICAL COMMENTS

The clinical findings of mild pain and stiffness that accompany the majority of patients with DISH are much less remarkable than extensive radiographic changes suggest. Patients may demonstrate dyspnea and hoarseness,[308] dysphagia,[417] aspiration pneumonia,[672] myelopathies,[350,685] peripheral nerve entrapment,[417] or tendonitis. Although these complications are uncommon, they may result from direct compression in which surgical intervention may be necessary, or may manifest because of associated tissue inflammation.[417] Given the lack of clinical relevance associated with spinal and extraspinal hyperostosis,[44,575] other causes should be investigated before the presence of DISH is assumed to be responsible for the patient's complaint.

Although most patients with limited presentations of OPLL remain asymptomatic, extensive presentations can result in significant neurologic complications. Symptoms are more likely if OPLL occupies more than 40% of the normal diameter of the spinal canal. Posterior decompression may be warranted for presentations of OPLL that span more than three segments.

Spinal fractures in DISH patients are rarely reported, but can occur in patients with spinal ankylosis who sustain even trivial trauma.[94,97,258,480,523] These patients should be carefully evaluated to prevent a delay in diagnosis and minimize possible complications, which include pseudoarthrosis, neurologic injury, and death.[94,258,480,523]

KEY CONCEPTS

- *Diffuse idiopathic skeletal hyperostosis represents a variant of degenerative disease marked by exuberant proliferation of bone at osseous sites of ligament and tendon attachments.*
- *It is more common among men, and usually presents during the fourth decade; the incidence increases with age.*
- *It is radiographically marked by ossification of the anterior longitudinal ligament (ALL) with relative maintenance of the disc height and absence of posterior joint fusion or sacroiliitis.*
- *It is associated with ossification of the posterior longitudinal ligament and possibly diabetes mellitus.*
- *It may lead to dysphagia and dysphasia.*

Neuropathic Arthropathy

BACKGROUND

Neurogenic, neuropathic, or neurotrophic arthritis is a destructive arthropathy resulting from impaired pain perception or proprioception (position sense).[585] The joint's normal protective reflexes and muscle tone are lost, allowing a cycle of repeated unrecognized episodes of trauma and resultant joint damage to occur. Distribution usually is monarticular and dependent on the underlying etiology of the arthropathy.

The epidemiology also is etiology dependent. Today diabetes and syringomyelia are the two most common causes, respectively. Tabes dorsalis resulting from syphilis is no longer a leading cause. Traditionally, neurogenic arthropathy resulting from tabes dorsalis

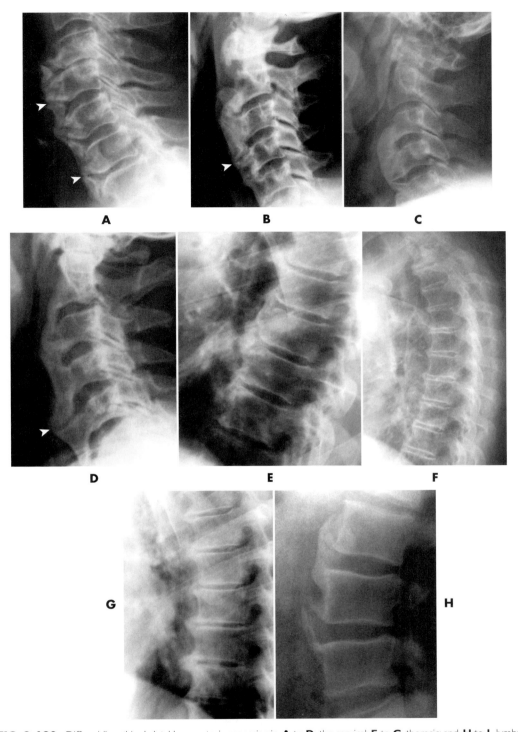

FIG. 9-190 Diffuse idiopathic skeletal hyperostosis appearing in, **A** to **D,** the cervical; **E** to **G,** thoracic; and, **H** to **J,** lumbar regions of different patients. Definitively, *diffuse idiopathic skeletal hyperostosis* is defined as flowing hyperostosis at three or more contiguous levels, with well-maintained disc spaces, and noninvolvement of the posterior joints or sacroiliac joints. However, slight involvement of the sacroiliac joints is seen occasionally at the superior aspect of the joint. It is common to see concurrent features of posterior joint or disc degeneration in older patients causing a mixed presentation of diffuse idiopathic skeletal hyperostosis and degeneration. The intermittent radiolucent interruptions of the flowing hyperostosis are typical, representing fibrous extensions of the anulus fibrosus *(arrowheads).*

Continued

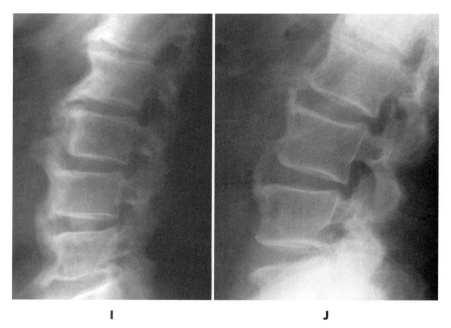

I   J

FIG. 9-190 cont'd

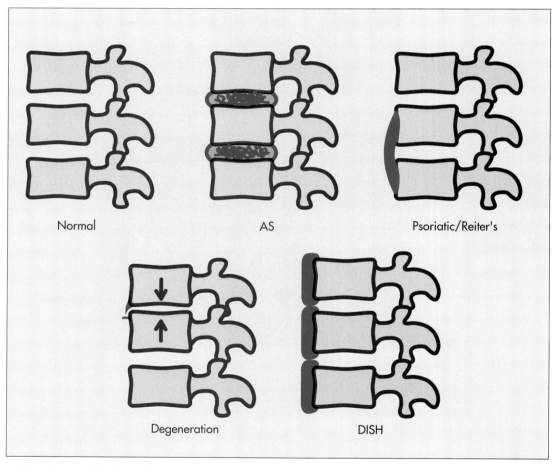

FIG. 9-191   The shape of the bony outgrowths of the spine provides a clue to the underlying condition. For instance, ankylosing spondylitis produces characteristic thin syndesmophytes; degeneration usually is indicated by nonmarginal curving or horizontal bone projections; and diffuse idiopathic skeletal hyperostosis produces thick flowing bone growth along the anterior margins of the involved segments.

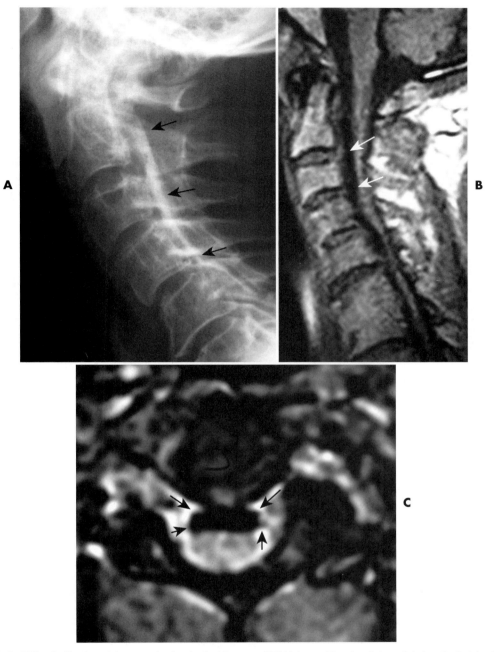

FIG. 9-192 Ossification of the posterior longitudinal ligament (OPLL) is considered a distinct clinical entity that is often found in association with diffuse idiopathic skeletal hyperostosis. Patients with OPLL may exhibit a range of clinical complaints, including syndromes of pain, numbness, and muscle weakness in the extremities. Paralysis has been described in severe presentations. In this case, OPLL is clearly noted on the lateral cervical radiograph as, **A,** a radiodense strip and on the magnetic resonance imaging images as, **B** and **C,** a signal void *(arrows)*. Magnetic resonance imaging provides an assessment of related canal stenosis.

was termed a Charcot's joint. However, now the term *Charcot's joint* has a broader definition and is used interchangeably with *neuropathic joints,* regardless of the underlying disease process.

IMAGING FINDINGS
Radiographic changes may be divided into two major categories. The hypertrophic or bone-forming variety is likely to occur in weight-bearing joints such as the spine and lower extremities, whereas the atrophic or resorptive form develops more often in the

non–weight-bearing joints of the upper extremities. These two forms may occur separately or in combination (Figs. 9-198 and 9-199).[88]

Hypertrophic. The radiographic features manifest as a severely aggressive OA. The classic description of these proliferative joint changes is often called the *six Ds* (dense subchondral bone, joint distention, debris or loose bodies, joint disorganization, dislocation, and destruction of articular cortex), or an abbreviated version, *Distention in 3D* (dislocation, destruction, and degeneration).[585] Patients suffering from diabetes, syphilis, and spinal cord trauma

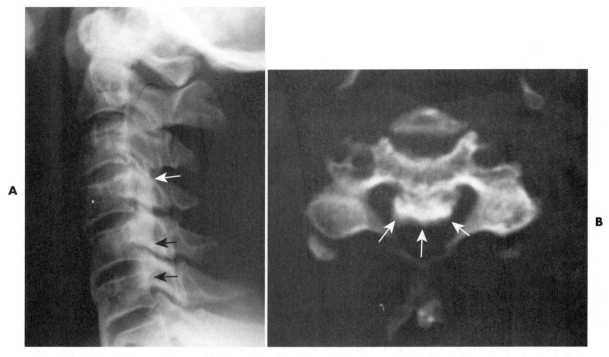

FIG. 9-193 A 68-year-old man with bilateral hand numbness demonstrates ossification of the posterior longitudinal ligament (OPLL) on, **A,** the lateral plain film *(arrows)* and, **B,** computed tomography (CT) scan. On an axial CT or magnetic resonance imaging image, the segment of OPLL may produce a "hill"-shaped (seen here, *arrows*) or "mushroom"-shaped ossified mass. (Courtesy Steven P. Brownstein, MD, Springfield, NJ.)

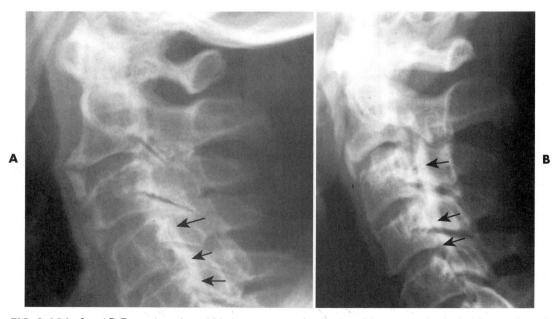

FIG. 9-194 A and **B,** Two patients that exhibit short segments of ossification of the posterior longitudinal ligament *(arrows).*

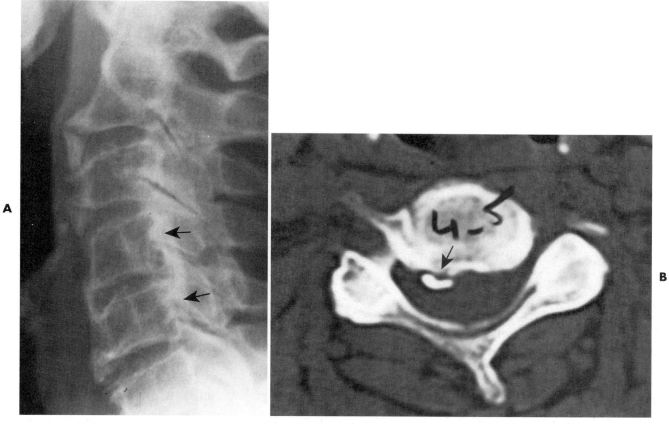

FIG. 9-195 Diffuse idiopathic skeletal hyperostosis patient with ossification of the posterior longitudinal ligament noted on, **A,** plain film anc, **B,** computed tomography *(arrows)*.

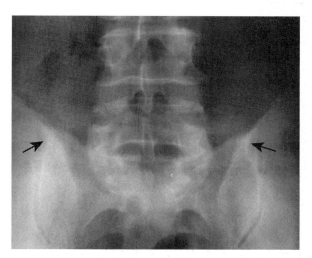

FIG. 9-196 Hyperostosis of the upper portion of the sacroiliac joints *(arrows)* in a patient with diffuse idiopathic skeletal hyperostosis.

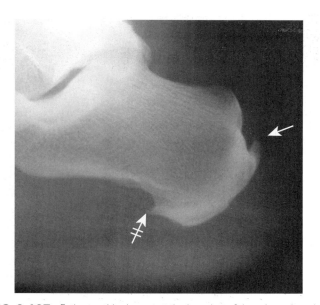

FIG. 9-197 Enthesopathic changes at the insertion of the calcaneal tendon *(arrow)* and plantar aponeurosis *(crossed arrow)*. Diffuse idiopathic skeletal hyperostosis is associated with enthesopathic changes of the calcaneus as seen in this case. Differential diagnosis includes degeneration, diffuse idiopathic skeletal hyperostosis, acromegaly, hypoparathyroidism, fluorosis, and vitamin D–resistant osteomalacia.

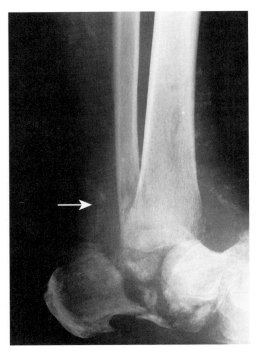

FIG. 9-198   A 52-year-old woman with diabetes developed a neurotrophic ankle joint. Destruction of the joint and bony debris is evident; vascular calcification *(arrow)* also is apparent. Diabetes is the most common cause of a neurotrophic arthropathy.

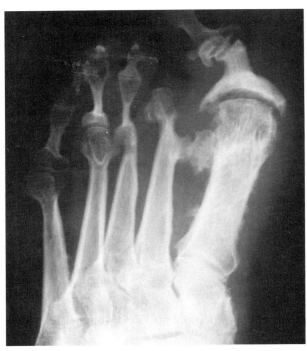

FIG. 9-199   Mixed atrophic and hypertrophic neurotrophic arthropathy of the foot in a patient with diabetes. (Courtesy Steven P. Brownstein, MD, Springfield, NJ.)

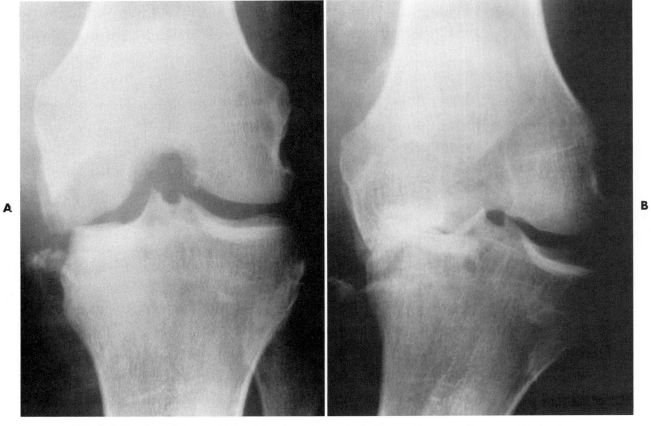

FIG. 9-200   **A** and **B,** Sequential films (taken 4 months apart) of a 65-year-old woman with neurosyphilis showing features consistent with a Charcot's joint: destruction of the articulating bone ends, joint disorganization and subluxation, bony debris, and joint distention.

are prone to develop this form of neurotrophic arthropathy in the feet, knees, and spine, respectively (Figs. 9-200 and 9-201).

Atrophic. The noted radiographic changes may be depicted as an osteolytic process that (a) completely resorbs the articulating bone end, leaving a sharp transverse demarcation at the metadiaphysis which has been likened to surgical amputation, or (b) tapers the bone end to a sharp "pencil point." The former is most frequently described in syringomyelia, with osteolysis affecting the proximal humerus (Fig. 9-202). The latter reflects findings that more commonly involve the metatarsals and phalanges of a diabetic patient (Figs. 9-203 and 9-204).

CLINICAL COMMENTS

Obviously the diagnosis of Charcot's joint should be suspected in a patient with an appropriate neurologic disorder who develops a painless swollen joint accompanied by radiographic signs of bony destruction. However, consideration also must be given to the fact that one third of affected patients may have no demonstrable neurologic deficit,[585] one third may experience pain, and the osseous radiographic findings initially may be unremarkable or resemble early OA.

Joint infection and a crystal deposition disease, such as CPPD, may mimic the clinical and radiographic features of a neuropathic joint, presenting a possible diagnostic dilemma. Joint sepsis also may be a complication of a Charcot's joint.

Treatment is directed toward the underlying disease, because this may slow or reverse the destructive arthropathy; in addition, antiinflammatories, splints, braces, and other devices to prevent further weight-bearing trauma may aid in limiting joint damage.

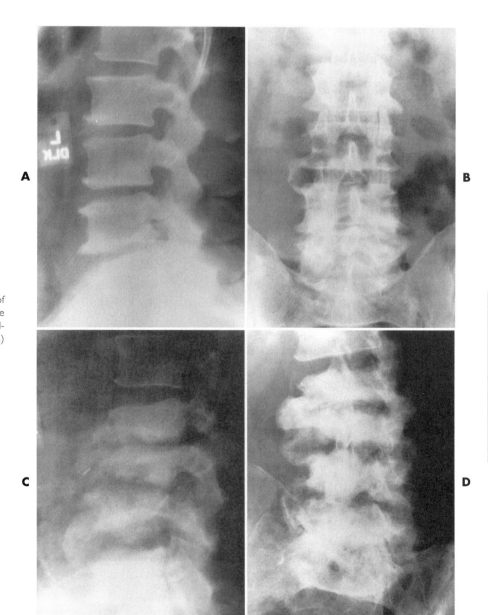

FIG. 9-201 Hypertrophic neurotrophic disease of the spine, **A** and **B,** before and, **C** and **D,** after the changes have occurred. The neuropathies are secondary to syphilis. (Courtesy Joseph W. Howe, Sylmar, CA.)

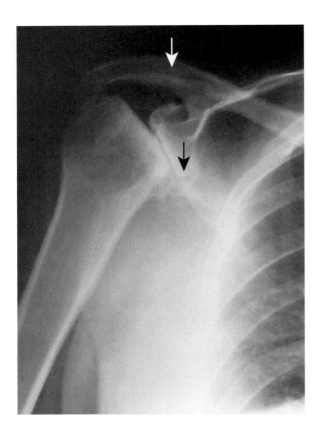

FIG. 9-202   A 47-year-old woman with syringomyelia developed an extremely swollen and mildly uncomfortable shoulder joint. Anteroposterior shoulder radiograph reveals joint destruction, debris *(arrows)*, and subluxation of the humeral head.

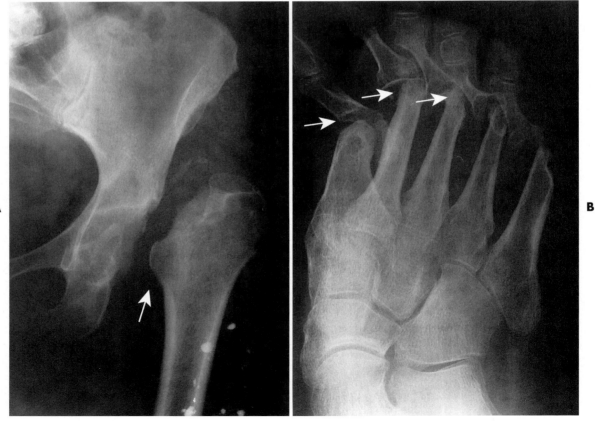

A

B

FIG. 9-203   Atrophic neurotrophic arthropathy *(arrows)* of, **A,** the hip and, **B,** foot secondary to syphilis. (Courtesy Joseph W. Howe, Sylmar, CA.)

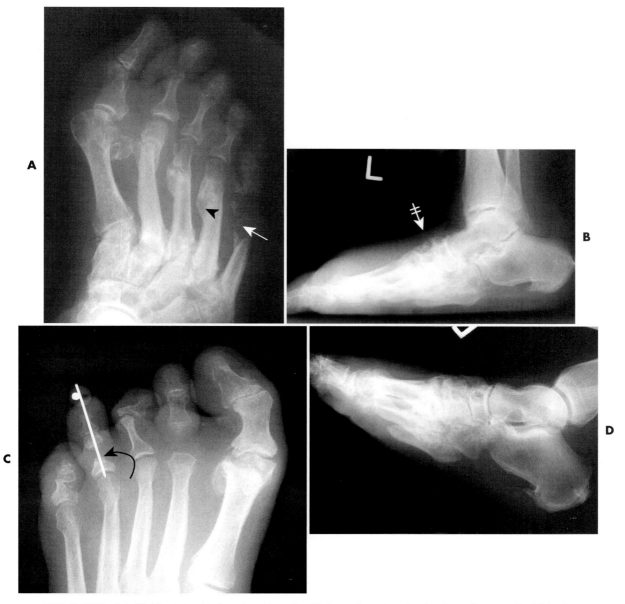

FIG. 9-204 A to **D,** Mixed atrophic *(arrow)* and hypertrophic *(crossed arrow)* neutropic arthropathy presenting bilaterally in a diabetic patient. Note the bone callus from past fractures *(arrowhead)* and Kirschner wire placed to provide stability to the partially resorption digit *(curved arrows).* (Courtesy Rodney Simmer, Rock Island, IL.)

KEY CONCEPTS

- *Destructive arthropathy results from impaired pain perception or proprioception.*
- *Diabetes (foot and ankle) and syringomyelia (upper extremity) are the most common causes.*
- *Radiographic changes may be divided into hypertrophic and atrophic varieties, although some degree of crossover is recognized.*
- *Hypertrophic (dense subchondral bone, joint distention, debris or loose bodies, joint disorganization, dislocation, and destruction of articular cortex) are common to weight-bearing joints.*
- *Atrophic (pseudoamputation, tapered bone ends) occurs more often in non–weight-bearing joints of the upper extremity.*

References

1. Abrahim-Zadeh R, Yu JS, Resnick D: Central (interior) osteophytes of the distal femur. Imaging and pathologic findings, *Invest Radiol* 29:1001, 1994.
2. Adam O: Nutrition as adjuvant therapy in chronic polyarthritis, *Z Rheumatol* 52:275, 1993.
3. Aigner T et al: Differential expression of collagen types I, II, III, and X in human osteophytes, *Lab Invest* 73:236, 1995.
4. Aihara T et al: Does the morphology of the iliolumbar ligament affect lumbosacral disc degeneration? *Spine* 27:1499, 2002.
5. Alaranta H, Luoto S, Konttinen YT: Traumatic spinal cord injury as a complication to ankylosing spondylitis. An extended report, *Clin Exp Rheumatol* 20(1):66, 2002.

6. Albers JMC, et al: Socio-economic consequences of rheumatoid arthritis in the first years of the disease, *Rheumatology* 38:423, 1999.
7. Alexander CJ: Osteoarthritis: a review of old myths and current concepts, *Skeletal Radiol* 19:327, 1990.
8. Alexander CJ: Relationship between utilization profile of individual joints and their susceptibility to primary osteoarthritis, *Skeletal Radiol* 18:199, 1989.
9. Alexanderson H, Stenstrom CH, Lundberg I: Safety of a home exercise regimen programme in patient with polymyositis and dermatomyositis: a pilot study, *Rheumatology* 38:608, 1999.
10. Allaire SH, Prashker MJ, Meenan RF: The costs of rheumatoid arthritis, *Pharmacoeconomics* 6:513, 1994.
11. Altman RD et al: Future therapeutic trends in osteoarthritis, Scand J Rheumatol 77(suppl):37, 1988.
12. Altomonte L et al: Growth hormone secretion in diffuse idiopathic skeletal hyperostosis, *Ann Ital Med Int* 7(1):30, 1992.
13. Anaya JM, Diethelm L, Ortiz LA: Pulmonary involvement in rheumatoid arthritis, *Semin Arthritis Rheum* 24:242, 1995 (review).
14. Andersson GBJ, Deyo RA: History and physical examination in patients with herniated lumbar discs, *Spine* 21(suppl 24):10, 1996.
15. Ansell BM: Joint manifestations in children with juvenile chronic polyarthritis, *Arthritis Rheum* 20:204, 1977.
16. Antoniou J et al: Elevated synthetic activity in the convex side of scoliotic intervertebral discs and endplates compared with normal tissues, *Spine* 26:E198, 2001.
17. Aoki J et al: Endplate of the discovertebral joint: degenerative change in the elderly adult, *Radiology* 164:411, 1987.
18. Appel GB, Valeri A: The course and treatment of lupus nephritis, *Annu Rev Med* 45:525, 1994.
19. Arakawa H et al: Nonspecific interstitial pneumonia associated with polymyositis and dermatomyositis: serial high-resolution CT findings and functional correlation, *Chest* 123(4):1096, 2003.
20. Ariga K et al: mechanical stress-induced apoptosis of endplate chondrocytes in organ-cultured mouse intervertebral discs, *Spine* 28:1528, 2003.
21. Armor B et al: Hydroxyapatite rheumatism and HLA markers, *J Rheumatol* 4(suppl 3):101, 1977.
22. Arnett FC et al: The American Rheumatism Association 1987 revised criteria for the classification of rheumatoid arthritis, *Arthritis Rheum* 31:315, 1988.
23. Arnett FC et al: Familial occurrence frequencies and relative risks for systemic sclerosis (scleroderma) in three United States cohorts, *Arthritis Rheum* 44(6):1359, 2004.
24. Arnett FC: HLA and autoimmunity in scleroderma (systemic sclerosis), *Int Rev Immunol* 12:107, 1995.
25. Artenian DJ et al: Acute neck pain due to tendinitis of the longus colli: CT and MRI findings. *Neuroradiology* 31(2):166, 1989.
26. Attar A: Digestive manifestations in systemic sclerosis, *Ann Med Interne (Paris)* 153(4):260, 2002.
27. Azouz EM, Duffy CM: Juvenile spondylarthropathies: clinical manifestations and medical imaging, *Skeletal Radiol* 24:399, 1995.
28. Babini SM et al: Atlantoaxial subluxation in systemic lupus erythematosus: further evidence of tendinous alterations, *J Rheumatol* 17:173, 1990.
29. Babini SM et al: Tendinous laxity and Jaccoud's syndrome in patients with systemic lupus erythematosus. Possible role of secondary hyperparathyroidism, *J Rheumatol* 16:494, 1989.
30. Baker GHB, Brewerton DA: Rheumatoid arthritis: a psychiatric assessment, *Br Med J* 282:2014, 1981.
31. Bankier AA et al: Discrete lung involvement in systemic lupus erythematosus: CT assessment, *Radiology* 196(3):835, 1995.
32. Bardin T, Enel C, Lathrop GM: Treatment of tetracycline and erythromycin of urarthritides allows significant prevention of post-venereal arthritic flares in Reiter's syndrome patients, *Arthritis Rheum* 33(suppl):26, 1990.
33. Bardin T, Lathrop GM: Postvenereal Reiter's syndrome in Greenland, *Rheum Dis Clin North Am* 18:81, 1992.
34. Barker JN: The immunopathology of psoriasis, *Baillieres Clin Rheumatol* 8:429, 1994.
35. Basset L et al: Skeletal findings in progressive systemic sclerosis (scleroderma), *AJR Am J Roentgenol* 136:1121, 1981.
36. Bates D, Ruggeri P: Imaging modalities for evaluation of the spine, *Radiol Clin North Am* 29:675, 1991.
37. Battistone MJ et al: The prevalence of sacroiliitis in psoriatic arthritis: new perspectives from a large, multicenter cohort. A Department of Veterans Affairs Cooperative study, *Skeletal Radiol* 28(4):196, 1999.
38. Belhorn LR, Hess EV: Erosive osteoarthritis, *Semin Arthritis Rheum* 22:298, 1993.
39. Belmont HM, Abramson SB, Lie JT: Pathology and pathogenesis of vascular injury in systemic lupus erythematosus, *Arthritis Rheum* 39:9, 1996.
40. Benjamin M, McGonagle D: The anatomical basis for disease localisation in seronegative spondylarthropathy at entheses and related sites, *J Anat* 199:503, 2001.
41. Bennett PH, Wood PHN, editors: Proceedings of the Third International Symposium, New York, June 1966, Excerpta Medica Foundation, Amsterdam, 1968:456.
42. Bessant R, Keat A: How should clinicians manage osteoporosis in ankylosing spondylitis? *J Rheumatol* 29(7):1511, 2002.
43. Bethem D et al: Spinal disorders of dwarfism, *J Bone Joint Surg Am* 63:1412, 1981.
44. Beyeler C et al: Diffuse idiopathic hyperostosis (DISH) of the elbow: a cause of elbow pain? A controlled study, *Br J Rheumatol* 31:319, 1992.
45. Bezrodnyhk AA, Karelin AP: Systemic lupus erythematosus and systemic scleroderma in patients from the aboriginal people and the newcomers of Yakutia under the extreme conditions of the far north, *Alaska Med* 36:102, 1994.
46. Bigos SJ et al: The new thinking on low back pain, *Patient Care* 29:140, 1995.
47. Bjorkengren AG, Resnick D, Sartoris DJ: Enteropathic arthropathies, *Radiol Clin North Am* 25:189, 1987.
48. Blackburn WD, Chivers S, Bernreuter W: Cartilage imaging in osteoarthritis, *Semin Arthritis Rheum* 25:273, 1996.
49. Bland JH: The reversibility of osteoarthritis: a review, *Am J Med* 74:16, 1983.
50. Blane CE et al: Patterns of calcification in childhood dermatomyositis, *AJR Am J Roentgenol* 142(2):397, 1984.
51. Block KL, Bassett LW, Furst DE: The arthropathy of advanced progressive systemic sclerosis: a radiographic survey, *Arthritis Rheum* 24:874, 1981.
52. Bobest M et al: Hydrogen nuclear magnetic resonance study of intervertebral discs: a preliminary report, *Spine* 11:709, 1986.
53. Boden SD et al: Abnormal magnetic resonance scans of the cervical spine in asymptomatic subjects, *J Bone Joint Surg Am* 72:1178, 1990.
54. Boden SD et al: Orientation of the lumbar facet joints: association with degenerative disc disease, *J Bone Joint Surg Am* 78:403, 1996.
55. Boden SD: Rheumatoid arthritis of the cervical spine. Surgical decision making based on predictors of paralysis and recovery, *Spine* 19:2275, 1994.
56. Bogduk N, Twomey LT: Clinical anatomy of the lumbar spine, ed 2, Melbourne, 1991, Churchill Livingstone.
57. Bogduk N, Tynan W, Wilson AS: The nerve supply to the human lumbar intervertebral discs, *J Anat* 132:39, 1981.
58. Bogduk N: Pathology of lumbar disc pain, *J Manual Med* 5:72, 1990.
59. Bogduk N: The anatomical basis for spinal pain syndromes, *J Man Physiol Ther* 18:603, 1995.
60. Bogduk N: The lumbar disc and low back pain, *Neurosurg Clin N Am* 2:791, 1991.
61. Bohan A, Peter JB: Polymyositis and dermatomyositis, *N Engl J Med* 1975;292:344.
62. Bohndorf K, Schalm J: Diagnostic radiography in rheumatoid arthritis: benefits and limitations, *Baillieres Clin Rheumatol* 10:399, 1996.

63. Boki DA et al: Examination of HLA-DR4 as a severity marker for rheumatoid arthritis in Greek patients, *Ann Rheum Dis* 52:517, 1993.

64. Boos N et al: The diagnostic accuracy of magnetic resonance imaging, work perception and psychosocial factors in identifying symptomatic disc herniations, *Spine* 20:2613, 1995.

65. Borenstein DG, Silver G, Jenkins E: Approach to initial medical treatment of rheumatoid arthritis, *Arch Fam Med* 2:545, 1993.

66. Boss GR, Seegmiller JE: Hyperuricemia and gout. Classification, complications and management, *N Engl J Med* 300:1459, 1979.

67. Bowen V, Cassidy JD: Macroscopic and microscopic anatomy of the sacroiliac joint from embryonic life until the eighth decade, *Spine* 6:620, 1981.

68. Bowen V, Shannon R, Kirkaldy-Willis WH: Lumbar spinal stenosis: a review, *Childs Brain* 4:257, 1978.

69. Bradley JD, Pinals RS: Jaccoud's arthropathy in scleroderma, *Clin Exp Rheumatol* 2:337, 1984.

70. Bradley JD, Pinals RS: Jaccoud's arthropathy in scleroderma, *Clin Exp Rheumatol* 2:337, 1984.

71. Bradley JD: Jaccoud's arthropathy in adult dermatomyositis, *Clin Exp Rheumatol* 3:273, 1986.

72. Bradley JD: Jaccoud's arthropathy in adult dermatomyositis, *Clin Exp Rheumatol* 4:273, 1986.

73. Brandt J, Haibel H, Sieper J, et al: Infliximab treatment of severe ankylosing spondylitis: one-year follow-up, *Arhtritis Rheum* 44:2936, 2001.

74. Brandt J, Sieper J, Braun J: Treatment of ankylosing spondylitis and undifferentiated spondyloarthritis with TNF alpha-antagonists, *Z Rheumatol* 62(3):218, 2003.

75. Brandt KD: Nonsurgical management of osteoarthritis, with an emphasis on nonpharmacologic measures, *Arch Fam Med* 4:1057, 1995.

76. Brewer EJ: Pitfalls in the diagnosis of juvenile rheumatoid arthritis, *Pediatr Clin North Am* 33:1015, 1986.

77. Brewerton DA et al: HL-A 27 and the arthropathies associated with ulcerative colitis and psoriasis, *Lancet* 1:956, 1974.

78. Brewerton DA et al: Ankylosing spondylitis and HL-A27, *Lancet* 1:904, 1973.

79. Brewerton DA: A tangential radiographic projection for demonstrating involvement of metacarpal heads in rheumatoid arthritis, *Br J Radiol* 40:233, 1967.

80. Brinckmann P: Injury of the anulus fibrosus and disc protrusions: an in vitro investigation on human lumbar discs, *Spine* 11:149, 1986.

81. Brockbank JE et al: Psoriatic arthritis (PsA) is common among patients with psoriasis and family medicine clinical attendees, *Arthritis Rheum* 44:S94, 2001.

82. Brodelius A: Osteoarthrosis of the talar joints in footballers and ballet dancers, *Acta Orthop Scand* 30:309, 1960.

83. Brodsky AE: Post-laminectomy and post-fusion stenosis of the spine, *Clin Orthop* 15:130, 1976.

84. Brook A, Corbett M: Radiographic changes in early rheumatoid disease, *Ann Rheum Dis* 36:71, 1977.

85. Brook A, Corbett M: Radiographic changes in early RA, *Ann Rheum Dis* 36:71, 1977.

86. Brophy S, Calin A: Ankylosing spondylitis: interaction between genes, joints, age at onset, and disease expression, *J Rheumatol* 28(1):2283, 2001.

87. Brophy S et al: The natural history of ankylosing spondylitis as defined by radiological progression, *J Rheumatol* 29(6):1236, 2002.

88. Brower A, Allman R: Pathogenesis of the neurotrophic joint: neurotraumatic vs neurovascular, *Radiology* 139:349, 1981.

89. Brown JH, Deluca SA: The radiology of rheumatoid arthritis, *Am Fam Physician* 52:1372, 1995.

90. Brumagne S et al: The role of paraspinal muscle spindles in lumbsacral position sense in individuals with and without low back pain, *Spine* 25:989, 2000.

91. Bunch TW, O'Duffy JD, McLeod RA: Deforming arthritis of the hands in polymyositis, *Arthritis Rheum* 19:243, 1976.

92. Bundschuh C et al: Rheumatoid arthritis of the cervical spine: surface-coil MR imaging, *AJR Am J Roentgenol* 151:181, 1988.

93. Burgos-Vargas R, Pineda C: New clinical and radiographic features of the seronegative spondylarthropathies, *Curr Opin Rheumatol* 3:562, 1991.

94. Burkus JK, Denis F: Hyperextension injuries of the thoracic spine in diffuse idiopathic hyperostosis. Report of four cases, *J Bone Joint Surg Am* 76:237, 1994.

95. Butler D et al: Discs degenerate before facets, *Spine* 15:111, 1990.

96. Byers PD, Contepomi CA, Farkas TA: Post-mortem study of the hip joint. Part III, Correlations between observations, *Ann Rheum Dis* 35:122, 1976.

97. Callahan EP, Aguillera H: Complications following minor trauma in a patient with diffuse idiopathic skeletal hyperostosis, *Ann Emerg Med* 22:1067, 1993.

98. Callen JP: Dermatomyositis, *Lancet* 355:53, 2000.

99. Cameron HU, Fornasier VL: Trabecular stress fractures, *Clin Orthop* 11:266, 1975.

100. Cantini F et al: Distal extremity swelling with pitting edema in psoriatic arthritis: a case-control study, *Clin Exp Rheumatol* 19(3):291, 2001.

101. Carroll RE, Sinton W, Garcia A: Acute calcium deposits in the hand, *JAMA* 157(5):422, 1955.

102. Casciola-Rosen L, Wigley F, Rosen A: Scleroderma autoantigens are uniquely fragmented by metal-catalyzed oxidation reactions: implications for pathogenesis, *J Exp Med* 185:71, 1997.

103. Cassidy JD, Thiel HW, Kirkaldy-Willis WH: Side posture manipulation for lumbar intervertebral disk herniation, *J Man Physiol Ther* 16:96, 1993.

104. Cassidy JE, Levinson JE, Brewer JE: The development of classification criteria for children with juvenile rheumatoid arthritis, *Bull Rheum Dis* 38:1, 1989.

105. Cassidy JT et al: A study of classification criteria for a diagnosis of juvenile arthritis, *Arthritis Rheum* 29:274, 1986.

106. Centers for Disease Control: Prevalence leisure-time physical activity among persons with arthrithis and other rheumatic conditions, *MMWR* 9:18, 1997.

107. Chang DJ, Paget SA: Neurologic complications of rheumatoid arthritis, *Rheum Dis Clin North Am* 19(4):955, 1993.

108. Chase JA: Spinal stenosis. When arthritis is more than arthritis, *Nurs Clin North Am* 26:53, 1991.

109. Chaudhry V et al: Mycophenolate mofetil: a safe and promising immunosuppressant in neuromuscular diseases. *Neurology* 56:94, 2001.

110. Chen CKH et al: Intra-articular gouty tophi of the knee: CT and MRI imaging in 12 patients, *Skeletal Radiol* 28(2):75, 1999.

111. Cherin P et al: Efficacy of intravenous immunoglobulin therapy in chronic refractory polymyositis and dermatomyositis: an open study with 20 adult patients, *Am J Med* 91:162, 1991.

112. Cicuttini FM, Spector TD: Osteoarthritis in the aged. Epidemiological issues and optimal management, *Drugs Aging* 6:409, 1995.

113. Clements P: Clinical aspects of localized and systemic sclerosis, *Curr Opin Rheumatol* 4:843, 1992.

114. Cobby M et al: Erosive osteoarthritis: is it a separate disease entity? *Clin Radiol* 42:258, 1990.

115. Cohn EL et al: Plain film evaluation of degenerative disk disease at the lumbosacral junction, *Skeletal Radiol* 26:161, 1997.

116. Colhoun E et al: Provocation discography as a guide to planning operations on the spine, *J Bone Joint Surg Br* 70:267, 1988.

117. Collins DN, Barnes CL, FitzRandolph RL: Cervical spine instability in rheumatoid patients having total hip or knee arthroplasty, *Clin Orthop* 272:127, 1991.

118. Collins HR: An evaluation of cervical and lumbar discography, *Clin Orthop* 107:133, 1975.

119. Collins JS, Gardner WJ: Lumbar discography—an analysis of 1,000 cases, *J Neurosurg* 19:452, 1962.

120. Connell MD, Wiesel SW: Natural history and pathogenesis of cervical disk disease, *Orthop Clin North Am* 23:369, 1992.

121. Constantin P, Lucretia C: Relations between the cervical spine and the vertebral arteries, *Acta Radiol* 11:91, 1971.

122. Cooper C: Occupational activity and the risk of osteoarthritis, *J Rheumatol* 43:10, 1995.

123. Corvetta A et al: MR imaging of rheumatoid hand lesions: comparison with conventional radiology in 31 patients, *Clin Exp Rheumatol* 10:217, 1992.

124. Cox JM, Feller J, Cox-Cid J: Distraction chiropractic adjusting: clinical application and outcome of 1,000 cases, *Top Clin Chiro* 3:45, 1996.

125. Cramer GD, Darby SA: Clinical pathoanatomy related to low back pain, *Top Clin Chiro* 3:1, 1996.

126. Crock HV: Internal disc disruption: a challenge to disc prolapse 50 years on, *Spine* 11:650, 1986.

127. Cuellar ML, Espinoza LR: Psoriatic arthritis. Current developments, *J Fla Med Assoc* 82:338, 1995.

128. Cuellar ML, Silveira LH, Espinoza LR: Recent developments in psoriatic arthritis, *Curr Opin Rheumatol* 6:378, 1994.

129. Da Silva JA, Spector TD: The role of pregnancy in the course and aetiology of rheumatoid arthritis, *Clin Rheumatol* 11:189, 1992.

130. Dalakas MC, Hohlfeld R: Polymyositis and dermatomyositis, *Lancet* 362(9388):971, 2003.

131. Dalakas MC et al: A controlled trial of high-dose intravenous immunoglobulin infusions as treatment for dermatomyositis, *N Engl J Med* 329:1993, 1993.

132. Dalakas MC: Calcifications in dermatomyositis, *N Engl J Med* 333:978, 1995.

133. Daltroy LH et al: Effectiveness of minimally supervised home aerobic training in patients with systemic rheumatic disease, *Br J Rheumatol* 34:1064, 1995.

134. Damron TA, Heiner JP: Rapidly progressive protrusio acetabuli in patients with rheumatoid arthritis, *Clin Orthop* 289:186, 1993.

135. Daragon A et al: Vertebral hyperostosis and diabetes mellitus: a case-control study, *Ann Rheum Dis* 54:375, 1995.

136. Davey N et al: Activation of back muscles during voluntary abduction of the contralateral arm in humans, *Spine* 27:1355, 2002.

137. Davis MA: Epidemiology of osteoarthritis, *Clin Geriatr Med* 4:241, 1988.

138. De Bandt M et al: Ossifcation of the posterior longitudinal ligament, diffuse idiopathic skeletal hyperostosis, abnormal retinol and retinol binding protein: a familial observation, *J Rheumatol* 22:1395, 1995.

139. de Vlam K, Mielants H, Veys EM: Involvement of the zygapophyseal joint in ankylosing spondylitis: relation of the bridging syndesmophyte, *J Rheumatol* 26(8):1738, 1999.

140. Deburge A et al: Cervical pseudarthrosis in ankylosing spondylitis, *Spine* 21:2801, 1996.

141. Deburge A, Rocolle J, Benoist M: Surgical findings and results of surgery after failure of chemonucleolysis, *Spine* 10:812, 1985.

142. Deesomchok U, Tumrasvin T: Clinical comparison of patients with ankylosing spondylitis, Reiter's syndrome, and psoriatic arthritis, *J Med Assoc Thai* 76:61, 1993.

143. Denisov LN et al: Therapeutic nutrition and sparing diet therapy in the combined treatment of rheumatoid arthritis, *Klin Med (Mosk)* 71:46, 1993.

144. Denko CW, Boja B, Moskowitz RW: Growth promoting peptides in osteoarthritis and diffuse idiopathic skeletal hyperostosis-insulin, insulin-like growth factor-I, growth hormone, *J Rheumatol* 21:1725, 1994.

145. Denton CP, Black CM: Pulmonary hypertension in systemic sclerosis, *Rheum Dis Clin North Am* 29(2):335, 2003.

146. ceRoos A et al: MR imaging of marrow changes adjacent to endplates in degenerative lumbar disc disease, *AJR Am J Roentgenol* 149:531, 1987.

147. Desai Y et al: Renal involvement in scleroderma, *J Assoc Phys India* 38:768, 1990.

148. Deshmukh NV, Deshmukh RG, Greenough C: Acute calcific quadriceps tendonitis: a case report, *Knee* 7(1):45, 2000.

149. Deyo RA, Loeser JD, Bigos SJ: Herniated lumbar intervertebral disc, *Ann Intern Med* 112:598, 1990.

150. Dieppe PA et al: Apatite deposition disease. A new arthropathy, *Lancet* 307(7954):266, 1976.

151. Diethelm U: Nutrition and chronic polyarthritis, *Schweiz Rundsc Med Prax* 82:359, 1993.

152. Dihlmann W: Current radiodiagnostic concept of ankylosing spondylitis, *Skeletal Radiol* 4:179, 1979.

153. Dihlmann W: Current radiodiagnostic concept of ankylosing spondylitis, *Skeletal Radiol* 4:179, 1979.

154. Dolan P, Adams M: Recent advances in lumbar spinal mechanics and their significance for modelling, *Clin Biomechan* 16:S8, 201.

155. Doran MF et al: Trends in incidence and mortality in rheumatoid arthritis in Rochester, Minnesota, over a forty-year period, *Arthritis Rheum* 46:625, 2002.

156. Dorwart RH, Vogler JB, Helms CA: Spinal stenosis, *Radiol Clin North Am*, 21:301, 1983.

157. Douglas WW et al: Polymyositis-dermatomyositis-associated interstitial lung disease, *Am J Respir Crit Care Med* 164(7):1182, 2001.

158. Doyle T et al: The radiographic changes of scleroderma in the hands, *Australas Radiol* 34:53, 1990.

159. Edgar MA, Ghadially JA: Innervation of the lumbar spine, *Clin Orthop* 115:35, 1976.

160. Ehrlich MG: Degradative enzyme systems in osteoarthritic cartilage, *J Orthop Res* 3:170, 1985.

161. Eisenstein S: Measurement of the lumbar spinal canal in 2 racial groups, *Clin Orthop* 115:42, 1976.

162. Eisenstein S: The morphometry and pathological anatomy of the lumbar spine in South African negroes and caucasoids with specific reference to spinal stenosis, *J Bone Joint Surg Br* 59:173, 1977.

163. El-Khoury GY, Kathol MH, Brandser EA: Seronegative spondylarthropathies, *Radiol Clin North Am* 34:343, 1996.

164. Ellman MH, Brown NL, Levin B: Prevalence of knee chondrocalcinosis in hospital and clinic patients aged 50 and older, *J Am Geriatr Soc* 29:189, 1981.

165. Eng BJ et al: Use of MRI with 3-dimensional reconstruction to measure changes in the synovium and joints in rheumatoid arthritis, *Arthritis Rheum* 35(suppl):196, 1992.

166. Epstein BS, Epstein JA, Jones MD: Lumbar spinal stenosis, *Radiol Clin North Am* 15:227, 1977.

167. Epstein H, Whelan M, Benjamin V: Acromegaly and spinal stenosis, *J Neurosurg* 56:145, 1982.

168. Epstein NE et al: Ossification of the posterior longitudinal ligament: diagnosis and surgical management, *Neurosurgery* 2:223, 1992.

169. Errico TJ: The role of diskography in the 1980s, *Radiology* 162:285, 1987.

170. Escalante A, Miller L, Beardmore TD: Resistive exercise in the rehabilitation of polymyositis/dermatomyositis, *J Rheumatol* 20:1340, 1993.

171. Escalante A: Ankylosing spondylitis. A common cause of low back pain, *Postgrad Med* 94:153, 1993.

172. Espada G et al: Radiologic review: the cervical spine in juvenile rheumatoid arthritis, *Semin Arthritis Rheum* 17:185, 1988.

173. Etanercept (package insert). Seattle, WA, 2002, Immunex Corporation and Wyeth-Ayerst Pharmaceuticals.

174. Eustace S, Coughlan RJ, McCarthy C: Ankylosing spondylitis. A comparison of clinical and radiographic features in men and women, *Irish Med J* 86:120, 1993.

175. Eustace SJ et al: Whole-body MR imaging. Practical issues, clinical applications, and future directions, *Magn Reson Imaging Clin N Am* 7(2):209, 1999.

176. Executive Committee of the North American Spine Society: Position statement on discography, *Spine* 13:1343, 1988.

177. Eyring EJ: The biochemistry and physiology of the intervertebral disc, *Clin Orthop* 67:16, 1969.

178. Fam AG, Pritzker KP: Acute calcific periarthritis in scleroderma, *J Rheumatol* 19:1580, 1992.

179. Fam AG: Calcium pyrophosphate crystal deposition disease and other crystal deposition diseases, *Curr Opin Rheumatol* (4):364, 1995.

180. Fan PT, Yu DTY: Reiter's syndrome. In Schumacher HR Jr, Klippel JH, Koopman WJ, editors: Primer on rheumatic disease, ed 10, Atlanta, 1993, Arthritis Foundation.

181. Fardon DF et al: Nomenclature of lumbar disc disorders. In Garfin SR, Vaccaro AR, editors: Orthopaedic Knowledge Update: Spine, Rosemont, IL, 1997, American Academy of Orthopaedic Surgeons.

182. Farfan HF et al: The effects of torsion on the lumbar intervertebral joints: the role of torsion in the production of disc degeneration, *J Bone Joint Surg Am* 52:468, 1970.

183. Farfan HF, Gracovetsky S: The nature of instability, *Spine* 9:174, 1984.

184. Farfan HF: A reorientation in the surgical approach to degenerative lumbar intervertebral joint disease, *Orthop Clin North Am* 8:9, 1977.

185. Faure G, Daculsi G: Calcified tendonitis: a review, *Ann Rheum Dis* 42:49, 1983.

186. Feldtkeller E et al: Age at disease onset and diagnosis delay in HLA-B27 negative vs. positive patients with ankylosing spondylitis, *Rheumatol Int* 23(2):61, 2003.

187. Felson DT et al: The prevalence of chondrocalcinosis in the elderly and its association with knee osteoarthritis: the Framingham study, *J Rheumatol* 16:1241, 1989.

188. Felson DT et al: Weight loss reduces the risk for symptomatic knee osteoarthritis in women: the Framingham study, *Ann Intern Med* 116:535, 1992.

189. Felson DT: Weight and osteoarthritis, *Am J Clin Nutr* 63:4305, 1996.

190. Fenlon HM et al: Plain radiographs and thoracic high-resolution CT in patients with ankylosing spondylitis, *AJR Am J Roentgenol* 168(4):1067, 1997.

191. Fenlon HM et al: High-resolution chest CT in systemic lupus erythematosus, *AJR Am J Roentgenol* 166(2):301, 1996.

192. Fernandez-Madrid F et al: MR features of osteoarthritis of the knee, *Magn Reson Imaging* 12:703, 1994.

193. Fessel JW: Systematic lupus erythematosus in the community, *Arch Intern Med* 134:1027, 1974.

194. Fex E, Larsson BM, Nived K, Eberhardt K: Effect of rheumatoid arthritis on work status and social and leisure time activities in patients followed 8 years from onset, *J Rheumatol* 25:44, 1998.

195. Forgacs SS: Diabetes mellitus and rheumatic disease, *Clin Rheum Dis* 12:279, 1986.

196. Fox MW, Onofrio BM, Kilgore JE: Neurological complications of ankylosing spondylitis, *J Neurosurg* 78:871, 1993.

197. Fox R et al: The chronicity of symptoms and disability in Reiter's syndrome, *Ann Intern Med* 91:190, 1979.

198. Friedenberg AH, Miller WF: Degenerative disc disease of the cervical spine, *J Bone Joint Surg Am* 45:1171, 1963.

199. Friedenberg ZB et al: Degenerative disc disease of the cervical spine: clinical and roentgenographic study, *JAMA* 174:375, 1960.

200. Fries JF et al: Nonsteroidal anti-inflammatory drug-associated gastropathy: incidence and risk factor models, *Am J Med* 91:213, 1991.

201. Frymoyer JW: Can low back pain disability be prevented? *Baillieres Clin Rheumatol* 6:595, 1992.

202. Frymoyer JW: Lumbar disk disease: epidemiology, *Instr Course Lect* 41:217, 1992.

203. Frymoyer JW: Predicting disability from low back pain, *Clin Orthop* 279:101, 1992.

204. Fuiks DM, Grayson CE: Vacuum pneumarthrography and the spontaneous occurance of gas in the joint spaces, *J Bone Joint Surg Am* 32:933, 1950.

205. Fuiwara A et al: The effect of disc degeneration and facet joint osteoarthritis on the segmental flexibiity of the lumbar spine, *Spine* 25:3036, 2000.

206. Fulp SR, Castell DO: Scleroderma esophagus, *Dysphagia* 5:204, 1990.

207. Garfin SR, Ahlgren BD: Current management of cervical spine instability, *Curr Opin Rheumatol* 7:114, 1995.

208. Garlepp MJ: Genetics of the idiopathic inflammatory myopathies, *Curr Opin Rheumatol* 8:514, 1996.

209. Geijer M et al: The role of CT in the diagnosis of sacro-iliitis, *Acta Radiol* 39(3):265, 1998.

210. Genti G: Occupation and osteoarthritis, *Baillieres Clin Rheumatol* 3:193, 1989.

211. Gibson MJ et al: Magnetic resonance imaging and discography in the diagnosis of disc degeneration, *J Bone Joint Surg* 68B:369, 1986.

212. Gilbertson EMM: Development of peri-articular osteophytes in experimentally induced osteoarthritis in the dog, *Ann Rheum Dis* 34:12, 1975.

213. Gilmer HS, Papadopoulos SM, Tuite GF: Lumbar disc disease: pathophysiology, management and prevention, *Am Fam Phys* 47(5):1141, 1993.

214. Gimblett PA, Saville J, Ebrall P: A conservative management protocol for calcific tendonitis of the shoulder, *J Man Physiol Ther* 22(9):622, 1999.

215. Girgis FL, Popple AW, Bruckner FE: Jaccoud's arthropathy. A case report and necropsy study, *Ann Rheum Dis* 37(6):561, 1978.

216. Gladman DD et al: Psoriatic arthritis (PsA)—an analysis of 220 patients, *Q J Med* 62:127, 1987.

217. Gladman DD, Stafford-Brady F, Chang CH, et al: Longitudinal study of clinical and radiological progression in psoriatic arthritis, *J Rheumatol* 17:809, 1990.

218. Glynn LE: Primary lesion in osteoarthrosis, *Lancet* 1(8011):574, 1977.

219. Goffe B, Cather JC: Etanercept: an overview, *J Am Acad Dermatol* 49(2):105, 2003.

220. Gold RH, Bassett LW, Seeger LL: The other arthritides. Roentgenologic features of osteoarthritis, erosive osteoarthritis, ankylosing spondylitis, psoriatic arthritis, Reiter's disease, multicentric reticulohistiocytosis, and progressive systemic sclerosis, *Radiol Clin North Am* 26:1195, 1988.

221. Goldberg AL et al: Ankylosing spondylitis complicated by trauma: MR findings correlated with plain radiographs and CT, *Skeletal Radiol* 22:333, 1993.

222. Gore DR et al: Neck pain: a long-term follow-up of 205 patients, *Spine* 12:1, 1987.

223. Gore DR, Sepic SB, Gardner GF: Roentgenographic findings of the cervical spine, in asymptomatic people, *Spine* 11:521, 1986.

224. Graham B, Van Peteghem: Fractures of the spine, in ankylosing spondylitis: diagnosis, treatment and complications, *Spine* 14:803, 1989.

225. Grahame R, Scott JT: Clinical survey of 354 patients with gout, *Ann Rheum Dis* 29:461, 1970.

226. Gran JT, Husby G, Hordvik M, et al: Radiological changes in men and women with ankylosing spondylitis, *Ann Rheum Dis* 43:57, 1984.

227. Gran JT, Skomsvoll JF: The outcome of ankylosing spondylitis: a study of 100 patients, *Br J Rheumatol* 36:766, 1997.

228. Gravallese EM, Kantrowitz FG: Arthritic manifestations of inflammatory bowel disease, *Am J Gastroenterol* 83(7):703, 1988.

229. Graziano G, Hensinger R, Patel C: The use of traction methods to correct severe cervical deformity in rheumatoid arthritis patients, *Spine* 26:1076, 2001.

230. Green L et al: Arthritis in psoriasis, *Ann Rheum Dis* 40(4):366, 1981.

231. Grishman E, Venkatasehan VS: Vascular lesions in lupus nephritis, *Mod Pathol* 1:235, 1988.

232. Hackney DB: Degenerative disk disease, *Top Magn Reson Imaging* 4(2):12, 1992.

233. Hadler NM et al: A benefit of spinal manipulation and adjunctive therapy for acute low back pain: a stratified controlled trial, *Spine* 12(7):703, 1987.

234. Hall S et al: Lumbar spinal stenosis: clinical features, diagnostic procedures, and results of surgical treatment in 68 patients, *Ann Intern Med* 103:271, 1985.

235. Hamerman D: Current leads in research on the osteoarthritic joint, *J Am Geriatr Soc* 31:299, 1983.

236. Hamerman D: The biology of osteoarthritis, *N Engl J Med* 320:1322, 1989.

237. Hamilton AR: Calcinosis, *J Bone Joint Surg Br* 33:572, 1951.

238. Hamilton MG, MacRae ME: Atlantoaxial dislocation as the presenting symptom of ankylosing spondylitis, *Spine* 18:2344, 1993.

239. Hammoudeh M, Rahim Siam A, Khanjar I: Spinal stenosis due to posterior syndesmophytes in a patient with seronegative spondyloarthropathy, *Clin Rheumatol* 14:464, 1995.

240. Hanlon R, King S: Overview of the radiology, of connective tissue disorders in children, *Eur J Radiol* 33(2):74, 2000.

241. Hanly JG, Russell ML, Gladmann DD: Psoriatic spondyloarthropathy. A long-term prospective study. *Ann Rheum Dis* 47:386, 1998.

242. Haro H et al: Matrix metalloproteinase-7-dependent release of tumor necrosis factor-a in a model of herniated disc resorption, *J Clin Invest* 105:143, 2000.

243. Harris EDJ: Rheumatoid arthritis: pathophysiology and implications for therapy, *N Engl J Med* 322:1277, 1990.

244. Harris P: Cervical spine stenosis, *Paraplegia* 15:125, 1977.

245. Harrison BJ et al: Cigarette smoking as a significant risk factor for digital vascular disease in patients with systemic sclerosis, *Arthritis Rheum* 46(12):3312, 2002.

246. Harrison MHM, Schajowicz F, Trueta J: Osteoarthritis of the hip: study of the nature and evolution of the disease, *J Bone Joint Surg Br* 35:598, 1953.

247. Harrison NK et al: Insulin-like growth factor-I is partially responsible for fibroblast proliferation induced by bronchoalveolar lavage fluid from patients with systemic sclerosis, *Clin Sci (Colch)* 86:141, 1994.

248. Harvie JN, Lester RS, Little AH: Sacroiliitis in severe psoriasis, *AJR Am J Roentgenol* 1976;127:579.

249. Haustein UF, Anderegg U: Silica induced scleroderma: clinical and experimental aspects, *J Rheumatol* 25:1917, 1998.

250. Haustein UF, Herrmann K: Environmental scleroderma, *Clin Dermatol* 12:467, 1994.

251. Haustein UF, Ziegler V: Environmentally induced systemic sclerosis-like disorders, *Int J Dermatol* 24:147, 1985.

252. Havdrup T, Huth A, Telhag H: The subchondral bone in osteoarthritis and rheumatoid arthritis of the knee: a histologic and microradiographical study, *Acta Orthop Scand* 47:345, 1976.

253. Hayes KW: Heat and cold in the management of rheumatoid arthritis, *Arthritis Care Res* 6:156, 1993.

254. Heikkila S, Viitanen JV, Kautiainen H, et al: Rehabilitation in myositis, *Physiotherapy* 87:301, 2001.

255. Heller CA et al: Value of x-ray examinations of the cervical spine, *BMJ* 287:1276, 1983.

256. Helliwell P et al: A re-evaluation of the osteoarticular manifestations of psoriasis, *Br J Rheumatol* 30:339, 1991.

257. Helms CA: CT of the lumbar spine-stenosis and arthrosis, *Comput Radiol* 6:359, 1982.

258. Hendrix RW et al: Fracture of the spine in patients with ankylosis due to diffuse skeletal hyperostosis: clinical and imaging findings, *AJR Am J Roentgenol* 162:899, 1994.

259. Herzog RJ: The radiologic assessment for a lumbar disc herniation, *Spine* 21:19, 1996.

260. Hess EV, Mongey AB: Drug-related lupus, *Bull Rheum Dis* 40:1, 1991.

261. Hickey DS et al: Analysis of magnetic resonance images from normal and degenerated lumbar intervertebral discs, *Spine* 11:702, 1986.

262. Hill CL et al: Frequency of specific cancer types in dermatomyositis and polymyositis: a population-based study, *Lancet* 357(9250):96, 2001.

263. Hirohata S, Ohnishi K, Sagawa A: Treatment of systemic lupus erythematosus with lobenzarit: an open clinical trial, *Clin Exp Rheumatol* 12:261, 1994.

264. Ho KT, Reveille JD: The clinical relevance of autoantibodies in scleroderma, *Arthritis Res Ther* 5(2):80, 2003.

265. Hoffman DF: Arthritis and exercise, *Primary Care,* 20:895, 1993.

266. Holm S: Pathophysiology of disc degeneration, *Acta Orthop Scand* 64(suppl 251):13, 1993.

267. Holt PD, Keats TE: Calcific tendonitis: a review of the usual and unusual, *Skeletal Radiol* 1993;22:1.

268. Hopkinson ND, Doherty M, Powell RJ: The prevalence and incidence of systemic lupus erythematosus in Nottingham, UK, 1989–1990, *Br J Rheumatol* 32:110, 1993.

269. Horner HA, Urban JPG: Effect of nutrient supply on the viability of cells from the nucleus pulposus on the intervertebral disc, *Spine* 26:2543, 2001.

270. Huckins D, Felson DT, Holick M: Treatment of psoriatic arthritis with oral 1,25-dihydroxyvitamin D3: a pilot study, *Arthritis Rheum* 33:1723, 1990.

271. Hudgins WR: The predictive value of myelography in the diagnosis of ruptured lumbar discs, *J Neurosurg* 32:152, 1970.

272. Hulsmans HMJ et al: The course of radiologic damage during the first six years of rheumatoid arthritis, *Arthritis Rheum* 43:1927, 2000.

273. Humzah MD, Soames RW: Human intervertebral disc: structure and function, *Anat Rec* 220:337, 1988.

274. Hunter D, McLaughlin AIG, Perry KMA: Clinical effects of the use of pneumatic tools, *Br J Intern Med* 2:10, 1945.

275. Hunter T: The spinal complications of ankylosing spondylitis, *Semin Arthritis Rheum* 19:172, 1989.

276. Husch Pereira ER, Brown RR, Resnick D: Prevalence and patterns of tendon calcification in patients with chondrocalcinosis of the knee. Radiologic study of 156 patients, *Clin Imag* 22(5):371, 1998.

277. Hutter CG: Spinal stenosis and posterior lumbar interbody fusion, *Clin Orthop* 193:103, 1985.

278. Hutton WC: Does long-term compressive loading on the intervertebral disc cause degeneration? *Spine* 25:2993, 2000.

279. Ignaczak T et al: Jaccoud's arthritis, *Ann Intern Med* 135:577, 1975.

280. Ihn H et al: Ultrasound measurement of skin thickness in systemic sclerosis, *Br J Rheumatol* 34:535, 1995.

281. Ikeda T et al: Pathomechanism of spontaneous regression of the herniated lumbar disc: histologic and immunohistochemical study, *J Spinal Disord* 9:136, 1996.

282. Iliopoulos AG, Tsokos GC: Immunopathogenesis and spectrum of infections in systemic lupus erythematosus, *Semin Arthritis Rheum* 25:318, 1996.

283. Ishihara H, Urban JP: Effects of low oxygen concentrations and metabolic inhibitors on proteoglycan and protein synthesis rates in the intervertebral disc, *J Orthop Res* 17:829, 1999.

284. Isomaki HA, Kaarela K, Martio J: Are hand radiographs the most suitable for the diagnosis of rheumatoid arthritis? *Arthritis Rheum* 31:1452, 1988.

285. Ito T, Yamada M, Ikuta F: Histologic evidence of absorption of sequestration-type herniated disc, *Spine* 21:230, 1996.

286. Iwahashi M et al: Mechanism of intervertebral disc degeneration caused by nicotine in rabbits to explicate intervertebral disc disorders caused by smoking, *Spine* 27:1396, 2002.

287. Jaccoud S: Vingt-troisieme leçon, sur une forme de rhumatisme chronique. Leçons de Clinique Medicale faites á l'Hôpital de la Charité, ed 1, Paris, 1867, Adrien Delahaye.

288. Jacobson DL et al: Epidemiology and estimated population burden of selected autoimmune diseases in the United States, *Clin Immunol Immunopathol* 84:223, 1997.

289. Jacobsson LT et al: Decreasing incidence and prevalence of rheumatoid arthritis in Pima Indians over a twenty-five-year period, *Arthritis Rheum* 37:1158, 1994.

290. Jahnke RW, Hart BL: Cervical stenosis, spondylosis, and herniation disc disease, *Radiol Clin North Am* 29:777, 1991.

291. Jenkins JPR et al: MR imaging of the intervertebral disc: a quantitative study, *J Bone Joint Surg Br* 58:705, 1985.

292. Jenkinson T et al: The cervical spine in psoriatic arthritis: a clinical and radiological study, *Br J Rheumatol* 33(3):255, 1994.

293. Jensen MC et al: Magnetic resonance imaging of the lumbar spine in people without back pain, *N Engl J Med* 331:69, 1994.

294. Jimenez-Balderas FJ, Mintz G: Ankylosing spondylitis: clinical course in women and men, *J Rheumatol* 20:2069, 1993.

295. Johnson AE et al: The prevalence and incidence of systemic lupus erythematosus in Birmingham, England. Relationship to ethnicity and country of birth, *Arthritis Rheum* 38:551, 1995.

296. Johnson JJ, Leonard-Segal A, Nashel DJ: Jaccoud's-type arthropathy: an association with malignancy, *J Rheumatol* 16:1278, 1989.

297. Jones RAC, Thomson JLG: The narrow lumbar canal: a clinical and radiological review, *J Bone Joint Surg Br* 50:595, 1968.

298. Jones SM, Bhalla AK: Osteoporosis in rheumatoid arthritis, *Clin Exp Rheumatol* 11:557, 1993.

299. Kahaleh B, Matucci-Cerinic M: Raynaud's phenomenon and scleroderma. Dysregulated neuroendothelial control of vascular tone, *Arthritis Rheum* 38:1, 1995.

300. Kahaleh B: Immunologic aspects of scleroderma, *Curr Opin Rheumatol* 5:760, 1993.

301. Kahn MS: Pathogenesis of ankylosing spondylitis, *J Rheumatol* 20:1273, 1993.

302. Kaipiainen-Seppanen O et al: Incidence of rheumatoid arthritis in Finland during 1980–1990, *Ann Rheum Dis* 55:608, 1996.

303. Kaipiainen-Seppanen O et al: Shift in the incidence of rheumatoid arthritis toward elderly patients in Finland during 1975–1990, *Clin Exp Rheumatol* 14:537, 1996.

304. Kaipiainen-Seppanen O, Savolainen A: Changes in the incidence of juvenile rheumatoid arthritis in Finland, *Rheumatology Oxford* 40:928, 2001.

305. Kamakura K et al: Cervical radiculomyelopathy due to calcified ligamenta flava, *Ann Neurol* 5:193, 1979.

306. Kandemir U et al: Endoscopic treatment of calcific tendinitis of gluteus medius and minimus, *Arthroscopy J Arthroscop Rel Surg* 19(1):4, 2003.

307. Kang YM et al: Somatosympathetic reflexes from the low back in the anesthetized cat, *J Neurophysiol* 90:2559, 2003.

308. Karlins NL, Yagan R: Dyspnea and hoarseness. A complication of diffuse idiopathic skeletal hyperostosis, *Spine* 16:235, 1991.

309. Karppinen J et al: Tumor necrosis factor a monoclonal antibody, infliximab, used to manage severe sciatica, *Spine* 28:750, 2002.

310. Kasteler JS, Callen JP: Scalp involvement in dermatomyositis: often overlooked or misdiagnosed, *JAMA* 272:1939, 1994.

311. Kauppi M et al: Pathogenetic mechanism and prevalence of the stable atlantoaxial subluxation in rheumatoid arthritis, *J Rheumatol* 23:831, 1996.

312. Kauppi M et al: A new method of screening for vertical atlantoaxial dislocation, *J Rheumatol* 17:167, 1990.

313. Kauppila LI et al: Disc degeneration/back pain and calcification of the abdominal aorta, *Spine* 22:1642, 1997.

314. Kawano N, Yoshida S, Ohwada T: Cervical radiculomyelopathy caused by deposition of calcium pyrophosphate dihydrate crystals in the ligamenta flava, *J Neurosurg* 52:279, 1980.

315. Keat A, Thomas BJ, Taylor-Robinson D: Chlamydial infection in the aetiology of arthritis, *Br Med Bull* 39:168, 1983.

316. Keat A: Reiter's syndrome and reactive arthritis in perspective, *N Engl J Med* 309:1606, 1983.

317. Keat A, Rowe I: Reiter's syndrome and associated arthritides, *Rheum Dis Clin North Am* 17(1):25, 1991.

318. Keefe FJ et al: Recent advances and future directions in the biopsychosocial assessment and treatment of arthritis, *J Consult Clin Psychol* 70:640, 2002.

319. Kellgren JH, Lawrence JS: Radiological assessment of osteoarthrosis, *Ann Rheum Dis* 16:494, 1957.

320. Kelly WL: Textbook of rheumatology, Philadelphia, 1997, WB Saunders.

321. Kelsey JL, Golden AL, Mundt DJ: Low back pain/prolapsed lumbar intervertebral disc, *Rheum Dis Clin North Am* 16:699, 1990.

322. Khan MA, van der Linden SM: Ankylosing spondylitis and other spondylarthropathies, *Rheum Dis Clin North Am* 16:551, 1990.

323. Kieffer SA et al: Bulging lumbar intervertebral disc: myelographic differentiation from herniated disc with nerve root compression, *AJR Am J Roentgenol* 138:709, 1982.

324. Kieffer SA, Cacayorin ED, Sherry RG: The radiological diagnosis of herniated lumbar intervertebral disc: a current controversy, *JAMA* 251:1192, 1984.

325. Killebrewk, Gold RH, Sholkoff SD: Psoriatic spondylitis, *Radiology* 108:9, 1973.

326. Kim KY et al: MRI classification of lumbar herniated intervertebral disc, *Orthopedics* 15:493, 1992.

327. Kimori H et al: The natural history of herniated nucleus pulposus with radiculopathy, *Spine* 21:225, 1996.

328. Kindyns P et al: Osteophytes of the knee. Anatomic, radiologic, and pathologic investigation, *Radiology* 174:841, 1990.

329. Kiris A et al: Lung findings on high resolution CT in early ankylosing spondylitis, *Eur J Radiol* 47(1):71, 2003.

330. Kirkaldy-Willis WH et al: Lumbar spinal stenosis, *Clin Orthop* 99:30, 1974.

331. Kirkaldy-Willis WH et al: Pathology and pathogenesis of lumbar spondylosis and stenosis, *Spine* 3:319, 1978.

332. Kirkaldy-Willis WH, Cassidy JD: Spinal manipulation in the treatment of low-back pain, *Can Fam Phys* 31:535, 1975.

333. Kirkaldy-Willis WH, Hill RJ: A more precise diagnosis for low-back pain, *Spine* 4:102, 1979.

334. Kirkaldy-Willis WH: The relationship of structural pathology to the nerve root, *Spine* 9:49, 1984.

335. Kissin EY, Korn JH: Fibrosis in scleroderma, *Rheum Dis Clin North Am* 29(2):351, 2003.

336. Klipper AR et al: Ischemic necrosis of bone in systemic lupus erythematosus, *Medicine* 55:251, 1976.

337. Kohli M, Bennett RM: Sacroiliitis in systemic lupus erythematosus, *J Rheumatol* 21:170, 1994.

338. Krishnan E: Smoking, gender and rheumatoid arthritis: epidemiological clues to etiology, *Bone Joint Spine* 70(6):496, 2003.

339. Kubota M, Baba I, Sumida T: Myelopathy due to ossification of the ligamentum flavum of the cervical spine. A report of two cases, *Spine* 6:553, 1981.

340. Kuo P, Loh Z: Treatment of lumbar intervertebral disc protrusion by manipulation, *Clin Orthop* 215:47, 1987.

341. Kurunlahti M et al: Association of atherosclerosis with low back pain and the degree of disc degeneration, *Spine* 24:20, 1999.

342. Labowitz R, Schumacher HR Jr: Articular manifestations of systemic lupus erythematosus, *Ann Intern Med* 74:911, 1971.

343. Laiho K et al: Cervical spine in patients with juvenile chronic arthritis and amyloidosis, *Clin Exp Rheumatol* 19:345, 2001.

344. Laiho K et al: The cervical spine in juvenile chronic arthritis, *Spine J* 2:89, 2002.

345. Laing TJ et al: Racial differences in scleroderma among women in Michigan, *Arthritis Rheum* 40:734, 1997.

346. Laman SD, Provost TT: Cutaneous manifestations of lupus erythematosus, *Rheum Dis Clin North Am* 20:195, 1994.

347. Lane NE et al: Long-distance running, bone density, and osteoarthritis, *JAMA* 255:1147, 1986.

348. Lane NE: Exercise: a cause of osteoarthritis, *J Rheumatol* 43:3, 1995.

349. Lane NE: Physical activity at leisure and risk of osteoarthritis, *Ann Rheum Dis* 55:682, 1996.

350. Laroche M et al: Lumbar and cervical stenosis. Frequency of the association, role of the ankylosing hyperostosis, *Clin Rheumatol* 11:533, 1992.

351. Lassere MN, Jones JG: Recurrent calcific periarthirits, erosive osteoarthritis and hypophosphatasia: a family study, *J Rheumatol* 17:1244, 1990.

352. Lauhio A et al: Double-blind, placebo-controlled study of three-month treatment with lymecycline in reactive arthritis, with special reference to chlamydia arthritis, *Arthritis Rheum* 34:6, 1991.

353. Laurent-Haupt L, Westmark KD: Long-standing ankylosing spondylitis with back pain, *Rheum Dis Clin North Am* 17:813, 1991.

354. Lavaroni G et al: The nails in psoriatic arthritis. *Acta Derm Venereol Suppl (Stockh)* 1994;186:113.

355. Lawrence JS, Bremner JM, Bier F: Osteoarthrosis: prevalence in the population and relationship between symptoms and x-ray changes, *Ann Rheum Dis* 25:1, 1966.

356. Le T et al: Costovertebral joint erosion in ankylosing spondylitis, *Am J Phys Med Rehabil* 80(1):62, 2001.

357. Leak R, Rayan G, Arthur RE: Longitudinal radiographic analysis of rheumatoid arthritis in the hand and wrist, *J Hand Surg* 28:427, 2003.

358. Lee HS et al: Radiologic changes of cervical Spine, in ankylosing spondylitis, *Clin Rheumatol* 20(4):262, 2001.

359. Lee P: Clinical aspects of systemic and localized sclerosis, *Curr Opin Rheumatol* 5:785, 1993.

360. Lee SH, Coleman PE, Hahn FL: Magnetic resonance imaging of degenerative disc disease of the spine, *Radiol Clin North Am* 26:949, 1988.

361. Lefkoe TP et al: Gene expression of collagen types IIA and IX correlates with ultrastructural events in early osteoarthrosis: new applications of the rabbit meniscectomy model, *J Rheumatol* 24:1155, 1997.

362. Leinonen V et al: Disc herniation-related back pain impairs feedforward control of paraspinal muscles, *Spine* 26:E367, 2001.

363. Leirisalo-Repo M: Enteropathic arthritis, Whipple's disease, juvenile spondyloarthropathy, and uveitis, *Curr Opin Rheumatol* 5:385, 1994.

364. Lerud C, Frost A, Bring J: Spinal fractures in patients with ankylosing spondylitis, *Eur Spine J* 5:51, 1996.

365. Lestini WF, Wiesel SW: The pathogenesis of cervical spondylosis, *Clin Orthop* 239:69, 1989.

366. Lias F: Roentgen findings in the asymptomatic cervical spine, *NY State J Med* 58:3300, 1958.

367. Linton SJ: The relationship between activity and chronic back pain, *Pain* 21:289, 1985.

368. Lisse JR: Does rheumatoid factor always mean arthritis? *Postgrad Med* 94:133, 1993.

369. Littlejohn GO, Smythe HA: Marked hyperinsulinemia after glucose challenge in patients with diffuse idiopathic skeletal hyperostosis, *J Rheumatol* 8:965, 1981.

370. Loebl DH et al: Psoriatic arthritis, *JAMA* 42:2447, 1979.

371. Long DM: Decision making in lumbar disc disease, *Clin Neurosurg* 39:36, 1992.

372. Lotz JC, Chin JR: Intervertebral disc cell death is dependent on the magnitude and duration of spinal loading, *Spine* 25:1477, 2000.

373. Lukoschek M et al: Synovial membrane and cartilage changes in experimental osteoarthritis, *J Orthop Res* 6:475, 1988.

374. Lundberg IE et al: Exercise is beneficial for patients with myositis. Both pharmaceuticals and physical activity should be included in the therapy of chronic rheumatic muscle inflammation, *Lakartidningen* 100(36):2754, 2003.

375. Luong AA, Salonen DC: Imaging of the seronegative spondyloarthropathies, *Curr Rheumatol Rep* 2(4):288, 2000.

376. Mackay K et al: The Bath Ankylosing Spondylitis Radiology, Index (BASRI): a new validated approach to disease assessment, *Arthritis Rheum* 41:2263, 1998.

377. MacKay K et al: The development and validation of a radiographic grading system for the hip in ankylosing spondylitis: the bath ankylosing spondylitis radiology hip index, *J Rheumatol* 27(12):2866, 2000.

378. MacLean JJ et al: Effects of immobilization and dynamic compression on intervertebral disc cell gene expression in vivo, *Spine* 28:973, 2003.

379. Macurak RB et al: Acute calcific quadriceps tendonitis, *South Med J* 73(3):322, 1980.

380. Magaro M et al: Generalized osteoporosis in non-steroid treated rheumatoid arthritis, *Rheumatol Int* 11:73, 1991.

381. Maghraoui AE et al: Cervical spine involvement in ankylosing spondylitis, *Clin Rheumatol* 22(2):94, 2003.

382. Maisiak R et al: The effect of person-centered counseling on the psychological status of persons with systemic lupus erythematosus or rheumatoid arthritis: a randomized, controlled trial, *Arthritis Care Res* 9:60, 1996.

383. Malca SA et al: Crowned dens syndrome: a manifestation of hydroxy-apatite rheumatism, *Acta Neurochir Wien* 135(3-4):126, 1995.

384. Manelfe C: Imaging of degenerative processes of the spine, *Curr Opin Radiol* 4:63, 1992.

385. Mankin HJ, Brandt KD, Shulman LE: Workshop on etiopathogenesis of osteoarthritis, *J Rheumtol* 13:1130, 1986.

386. Mankin HJ, Treadwell BV: Osteoarthritis: a 1987 update, *Bull Rheum Dis* 36:1, 1986.

387. Manthorpe R et al: Jaccoud's syndrome. A nosographic entity associated with systemic lupus erythematosus, *J Rheumatol* 7:169, 1980.

388. Marchiori DM et al: A comparison of radiographic signs of degeneration to corresponding MRI signal intensities in the lumbar spine, *J Man Physiol Ther* 17:238, 1994.

389. Marchiori DM, Henderson CNR: A cross-sectional study correlating cervical radiographic degenerative findings to pain and disability, *Spine* 21:2747, 1996.

390. Marchiori DM: A survey of radiographic impressions on a selected chiropractic patient population, *J Man Physiol Ther* 19:109, 1996.

391. Marcos JC et al: Idiopathic familial chondrocalcinosis due to apatite crystal deposition, *Am J Med* 71(4):557, 1981.

392. Maricq H: Comparison of quantitative and semiquantitative estimates of nailfold capillary abnormalities in scleroderma spectrum disorders, *Microvasc Res* 32:271, 1986.

393. Marie I et al: Influence of age on characteristics of polymyositis and dermatomyositis in adults, *Medicine Balt* 78:139, 1999.

394. Maroudas A et al: Factors involved in the nutrition of the human lumbar intervertebral disc: cellularity and diffusion of glucose in vitro, *J Anat* 120:113: 1975.

395. Marras WS et al: Spine loading characteristics of patients with low back pain compared with asymptomatic individuals, *Spine* 26:2566, 2001.

396. Marsal S et al: Clinical, radiographic and HLA associations as markers for different patterns of psoriatic arthritis, *Rheumatology* 38:332, 1999.

397. Marschalko M et al: Dermatomyositis: clinical study of 23 patients, *Orv Hetil* 141(5):225, 2000.

398. Marshall JL: Periarticular osteophytes, *Clin Orthop* 62:37, 1969.

399. Martel W et al: Radiologic features of Reiter's disease, *Radiology* 132:1, 1979.

400. Martel W, Hayes JT, Diff IF: The pattern of bone erosion in the hand and wrist in rheumatoid arthritis, *Radiology* 84:206, 1965.

401. Martel W, Holt JF, Cassidy JT: Roentgenologic manifestations of juvenile rheumatoid arthritis, *AJR Am J Roentgenol* 88:400, 1962.

402. Martinelli TA, Wiesel SW: Epidemiology of spinal stenosis, *Instr Course Lect* 41:179, 1992.

403. Martini A et al: Systemic lupus erythematosus with Jaccoud's arthropathy mimicking juvenile rheumatoid arthritis, *Arthritis Rheum* 30:1062, 1987.

404. Masaryk TJ et al: Effects of chemonucleolysis demonstrated by MR imaging, *J Comput Assist Tomogr* 10:917, 1986.

405. Masaryk TJ et al: High-resolution MR imaging of sequestered lumbar intervertebral disks, *AJNR* 150:1155, 1988.

406. Massardo L et al: Clinical expression of rheumatoid arthritis in Chilean patients, *Semin Arthritis Rheum* 25:203, 1995.

407. Mastaglia FL, Phillips BA: Idiopathic inflammatory myopathies: epidemiology, classification, and diagnostic criteria, *Rheum Dis Clin North Am* 28(4):723, 2002.

408. Matheson LN et al: The contribution of aerobic fitness and back strength to lift capacity, *Spine* 27:1208, 2002.

409. Matsubara Y et al: Serial changes on MRI in lumbar disc herniations treated conservatively, *Neuroradiology* 37:378, 1995.

410. Matsumoto T et al: Cyclic mechanical stretch stress increases the growth rate and collagen synthesis of nucleus pulposus cells in vitro, *Spine* 24:315, 1999.

411. Matyas JR, Sandell LJ, Adams ME: Gene expression of type II collagens in chondro-osteophytes in experimental osteoarthritis, *Osteoarthritis Cart* 5:99, 1997.

412. Mavrikakis M et al: Optic neuritis and Jaccoud's syndrome in a patient with systemic lupus erythematosus, *Scand J Rheum* 12:367, 1983.

413. Mayes MD et al: Epidemiology of scleroderma in Detroit tricounty area 1989-1991: prevalence, incidence, and survival rates. Proceedings of the American College of Rheumatology meeting, Orlando, Florida, 1996.

414. Mayes MD et al: Prevalence, incidence, survival, and disease characteristics of systemic sclerosis in a large US population, *Arthritis Rheum* 48(8):2246, 2003.

415. Mazzuca SA et al: Therapeutic strategies distinguish community based primary care physicians from rheumatologists in the management of osteoarthritis, *Br J Rheumatol* 20:80, 1993.

416. McAffee PC, Regan JJ, Bohlman HH: Cervical cord compression from ossification of the posterior longitudinal ligament in non-orientals, *J Bone Joint Surg Br* 89:569, 1987.

417. McCafferty RR et al: Ossification of the anterior longitudinal ligament and Forestier's disease: an analysis of seven cases, *J Neurosurg* 83:13, 1995.

418. McCarty DJ et al: Incidence of systemic lupus erythematosus. Race and gender differences, *Arthritis Rheum* 38:1260, 1995.

419. McCarty DJ, McCarthy GM: Valvular heart disease and systemic lupus erythematosus, *N Engl J Med* 336(18):1324, 1997.

420. McCormack BM, Weinstein PR: Cervical spondylosis. An update, *West J Med* 165:43, 1996.

421. McFadden JW: The stress lumbar discogram, *Spine* 13:931, 1988.

422. McGonagle D, Conaghan PG, Emery P: Psoriatic arthritis. A unified concept twenty years on, *Arthritis Rheum* 42:1080, 1999.

423. McHugh NJ et al: Anti-topoisomerase I in silica-associated systemic sclerosis. A model for autoimmunity, *Arthritis Rheum* 37:1198, 1994.

424. Mease P et al: Improvement in disease activity in patients with psoriatic arthritis receiving etanercept (ENBREL): results of a phase 3 multicenter clinical trial, *Arthritis Rheum* 44:226, 2001.

425. Mease PJ et al: Etanercept in the treatment of psoriatic arthritis and psoriasis: a randomized trial, *Lancet* 356:385, 2000.

426. Medsger TA Jr: Epidemiology of systemic sclerosis, *Clin Dermatol* 12:207, 1994.

427. Medsger TA Jr: Treatment of systemic sclerosis, *Ann Rheum Dis* 50:877, 1991.

428. Medsger TA, Masi AT: The epidemiology of systemic sclerosis (scleroderma), *Ann Intern Med* 74:714, 1971.

429. Mercer SR, Bogduk N: Joints of the cervical vertebral column, *J Orthop Sports Phys Ther* 31:174, 2001.

430. Mercer SR, Bogduk N: Joints of the cervical vertebral column, *J Orthop Sports Phys Ther* 31:174, 2001.

431. Mercola J: Protocol for using antibiotics in the treatment of rheumatic disease. Presentation at the first annual meeting of the American Academy of Environmental Medicine, Boston, MA, October, 1996.

432. Mester AR et al: Enteropathic arthritis in the sacroiliac joint. Imaging and differential diagnosis, *Eur J Radiol* 35(3):199, 2000.

433. Michet CJ: Osteoarthritis, *Arthritis* 20:815, 1993.

434. Migliaresi S et al: Avascular osteonecrosis in patients with SLE: relation to corticosteroid therapy and anticardiolipin antibodies, *Lupus* 3:37, 1994.

435. Miller FH, Roger LF: Fractures of the dens complicating ankylosing spondylitis with atlantooccipital fusion, *J Rheumatol* 18:771, 1991.

436. Miller JAA, Schmatz C, Schultz AB: Lumbar disc degeneration: correlation with age, sex, and spine level in 600 autopsy specimens, *Spine* 13:173, 1988.

437. Modic MT et al: Degenerative disk disease: assessment of changes in vertebral body marrow with MR imaging, *Radiology* 166:193, 1988.

438. Modic MT et al: Imaging of degenerative disc disease, *Radiology* 168:177, 1988.

439. Modic MT et al: Lumbar herniated disk disease and canal stenosis: prospective evaluation by surface coil MR, CT, and myelography, *AJNR* 7:709, 1986.

440. Modic MT et al: Magnetic resonance imaging of intervertebral disc disease, *Radiology* 152:103, 1984.

441. Modic MT et al: Nuclear magnetic resonance imaging of the spine, *Radiology* 148:757, 1983.

442. Modic MT, Herfkens RJ: Intervertebral disk: normal age-related changes in MR signal intensity, *Radiology* 177:332, 1990.

443. Moll JMH, Wright V: Psoriatic arthritis, *Semin Arthritis Rheum* 3:55, 1973.

444. Mooney V, Robertson J: The facet syndrome, *Clin Orthop* 115:149, 1976.

445. Mooney V: When is surgery appropriate for patients with low back pain? *J Musculoskeletal Med* 7:61, 1990.

446. Moreland LW, Lopez-Mendez A, Alarcon GS: Spinal stenosis: a comprehensive review of the literature, *Semin Arthritis Rheum* 19:127, 1989.

447. Morgan DF, Young RF: Spinal neurological complications of achondroplasia. Results of surgical treatment, *J Neurosurg* 52:463, 1980.

448. Morita A et al: Successful treatment of systemic sclerosis with topical PUVA, *J Rheumatol* 22:2361, 1995.

449. Moro C et al: Jaccoud's arthropathy in patients with chronic rheumatic valvular heart disease, *Eur J Cardiol* 6:459, 1978.

450. Morris R et al: HLA-B27 a useful discriminator in the arthropathies of inflammatory bowel disease, *N Engl J Med* 290:1117, 1974.

451. Moskowitz RW: Primary osteoarthritis: epidemiology, clinical aspects, and general management, *Am J Med* 83:5, 1987.

452. Mullaji AB, Upadhyay SS, Ho EK: Bone mineral density in ankylosing spondylitis. DEXA comparison of control subjects with mild and advanced cases, *J Bone Joint Surg Br* 76:660, 1994.

453. Murakami J et al: Computed tomography of posterior longitudinal ligament ossification: its appearance and diagnostic value with special reference to thoracic lesions, *J Comput Tomogr* 6:41, 1982.

454. Myllykangas-Luosujarvi RA, Aho K, Isomaki A: Mortality in rheumatoid arthritis, *Semin Arthritis Rheum* 25:193, 1995.

455. Nakanishi T et al: Symptomatic ossification of the posterior longitudinal ligament of the cervical spine, *Neurology* 24:1139, 1974.

456. Nalebuff EA: Surgery of systemic lupus erythematosus arthritis of the hand, *Hand Clin* 12:591, 1996.

457. Naparstek Y, Plotz PH: The role of autoantibodies in autoimmune disease, *Annu Rev Immunol* 11:79, 1993.

458. Newman PH: Stenosis of the lumbar spine in spondylolisthesis, *Clin Orthop* 115:116, 1976.

459. Ng SC, Clements PJ, Paulus HE: Management of systemic sclerosis: a review, *Singapore Med J* 31:269, 1990.

460. Niepel GA, Sitaj S: Enthesopathy, *Clin Rheum Dis* 5:857, 1979.

461. Norgaard F: Earliest roentgenological changes in polyarthritis of the rheumatoid type: rheumatoid arthritis, *Radiology* 85:325, 1965.

462. Nose T et al: Ossification of the posterior longitudinal ligament: a clinio-radiological study of 74 cases, *J Neurol Neurosurg Psych* 50:321, 1987.

463. Nwuga VCB: Relative therapeutic efficacy of vertebral manipulation and conventional treatment in back pain management, *Am J Phys Med* 61:273, 1982.

464. O'Donnell JL, O'Donnell AL: Prostaglandin E2 content in herniated lumbar disc disease, *Spine* 21:1653, 1996.

465. O'Sullivan PB et al: The effect of different standing and sitting postures on trunk muscle activity in pain-free population, *Spine* 27:1238, 2002.

466. Oda T et al: Natural course of cervical spine lesions in rheumatoid arthritis, *Spine* 20:1128, 1995.

467. Ohshima J, Urban JPG: Effect of lactate concentrations and pH on matrix synthesis rates in the intervertebral disc, *Spine* 17:1079, 1992.

468. Olive A et al: Air in the oesophagus: a sign of oesophageal involvement in systemic sclerosis, *Clin Rheumatol* 14:319, 1995.

469. Onda A et al: Effects of neutralizing antibodies to tumor necrosis factor a on nucleus pulposus-induced abnormal nociresponses in rat dorsal horn neurons, *Spine* 28:967, 2003.

470. Onda A et al: Exogenous tumor necrosis factor a induces abnormal discharges in rat dorsal horn neurons, *Spine* 37:1618, 2002.

471. Ooi GC et al: Systemic lupus erythematosus patients with respiratory symptoms: the value of HRCT, *Clin Radiol* 52(10):775, 1997.

472. Oriente CB et al: Psoriasis and psoriatic arthritis: dermatological and rheumatological co-operative clinical report, *Acta Derm Venereol (Stockh)* 146:69, 1989.

473. Ory PA: Radiography in the assessment of musculoskeletal conditions, *Best Pract Res Clin Rheumatol* 17(3):495, 2003.

474. Ostendorf B et al: Jaccoud's arthropathy in systemic lupus erythematosus: differentiation of deforming and erosive patterns by magnetic resonance imaging, *Arthritis Rheum* 38(9):1260, 1995.

475. Ostlere SJ, Seeger LL, Eckhardt JJ: Subchondral cysts of the tibia secondary to osteoarthritis of the knee, *Skeletal Radiol* 19:287, 1990.

476. Oxland TR, Panjabi MM: The onset and progression of spinal instability: a demonstration of neutral zone sensitivity, *J Biomechan*, 25:1165, 1992.

477. Paajanen H et al: Magnetic resonance study of disc degeneration in young low back pain patients, *Spine* 14:982, 1989.

478. Paimela L et al.: Progression of cervical spine changes in patients with early rheumatoid arthritis, *J Rheumatol* 24:1280, 1997.

479. Paine KWE: Clinical features of lumbar spinal stenosis, *Clin Orthop* 29:315, 1976.

480. Paley D et al: Fractures of the spine in diffuse idiopathic skeletal hyperostosis, *Clin Orthop* 267:22, 1991.

481. Palumbo MA, Lucas P, Akelman E: Lumbar spinal stenosis: a review, *Rhode Island Med* 78:321, 1995.

482. Pan P et al: Extracorporeal shock wave therapy for chronic calcific tendonitis of the shoulders: a functional and sonographic study, *Arch Phys Med Rehabil* 84(7):988, 2003.

483. Panangiotacopulos ND et al: Water content in human intervertebral discs, *Spine* 12:912, 1987.

484. Panayi GS, Clark B: Minocycline in the treatment of patients with Reiter's syndrome, *Clin Exp Rheumatol* 7:100, 1989.

485. Panayi GS: Immunology of psoriasis and psoriatic arthritis, *Baillieres Clin Rheumatol* 8:419, 1994.

486. Panayi GS: The pathogenesis of rheumatoid arthritis and the development of therapeutic strategies for the clinical investigation of biologics, *Agents Actions* 47:1, 1995.

487. Panichewa S, Chitrabamrung S, Vatanasuk M: Hand deformities in a patient with chronic lung disease: Jaccoud's arthropathy, *Clin Rheumatol* 2:65, 1983.

488. Papadopoulos IA et al: Early rheumatoid arthritis patients: relationship of age, *Rheumatol Int* 23(2):70, 2003.

489. Park WM et al: The detection of spinal pseudoarthrosis in ankylosing spondylitis, *Br J Radiol* 54:467, 1981.

490. Pastershank SP, Resnick D: "Hook" erosions in Jaccoud's arthropathy, *J Can Assoc Radiol* 31:174, 1980.

491. Patriquin HB, Camerlain M, Trias A: Late sequelae of juvenile rheumatoid arthritis of the hip: a follow-up study into adulthood, *Pediatr Radiol* 14:151, 1984.

492. Patton JT: Differential diagnosis of inflammatory spondylitis, *Skeletal Radiol* 1:77, 1976.

493. Patwardhan A et al: Load-carrying capacity of the human cervical spine in compression is increased under a follower load, *Spine* 25:1548, 2000.

494. Paulus HE et al: Monitoring radiographic changes in early rheumatoid arthritis, *J Rheumatol* 23:801, 1996.

495. Pay S, Terkeltaub R: Calcium pryophosphate dihydrate and hydroxyapatite crystal deposition in the joint: new developments relevant to the clinician, *Curr Rheumatol Rep* 5(3):235, 2003.

496. Pearcy MJ: Inferred strains in the intervertebral discs during physiological movements, *J Manual Med* 5:68, 1990.

497. Pech P, Haughton VM: Lumbar intervertebral disk: correlative MR and anatomic study, *Radiology* 156:699, 1985.

498. Pedersen HE, Key JA: Pathology of calcareous tendonitis and subdeltoid bursitis, *Arch Surg* 62:50, 1951.

499. Peh WC, Ho WY, Luk KD: Applications of bone scintigraphy in ankylosing spondylitis, *Clin Imaging* 21(1):54, 1997.

500. Peterson C et al: A cross-sectional study correlating degeneration of the cervical spine, with disability and pain in United Kingdom patients, *Spine* 28:129, 2003.

501. Peterson CK, Bolton JE, Wood AR: A cross-sectional study correlating lumbar spine degeneration with disability and pain, *Spine* 25:218, 2000.

502. Peterson HO, Kieffer SA: Radiology, of intervertebral disk disease, *Semin Roentgenol* 7:260, 1972.

503. Peterson LS et al: Juvenile rheumatoid arthritis in Rochester, Minnesota 1960–1993. Is the epidemiology changing? *Arthritis Rheum* 39:1385, 1996.

504. Petri M: Systemic lupus erythematosus and pregnancy, *Rheum Dis Clin North Am* 20:87, 1994.

505. Petrocelli AR et al: Scleroderma: dystrophic calcification with spinal cord compression, *J Rheumatol* 15:1733, 1988.

506. Petty RE et al: Revision of the proposed classification criteria for juvenile idiopathic arthritis: Durban 97, *J Rheumatol* 25:1991, 1998.

507. Pignone A et al: The pathogenesis of inflammatory muscle diseases: on the cutting edge among the environment, the genetic background, the immune response and the dysregulation of apoptosis, *Autoimmunity Rev* 1(4):226, 2002.

508. Pinals RS: Polyarthritis and fever, *N Engl J Med* 330:769, 1994.

509. Pincus T, Callahan LF: What is the natural history of rheumatoid arthritis? *Rheum Dis Clin North Am* 19:123, 1993.

510. Pincus T: Long-term outcomes in rheumatoid arthritis, *Br J Rheumatol* 34:59, 1995.

511. Pitzalis C et al: Cutaneous lymphocyte antigen-positive T lymphocytes preferentially migrate to the skin but not to the joint in psoriatic arthritis, *Arthritis Rheum* 39:137, 1996.

512. Plant MJ et al: Patterns of radiological progression in early rheumatoid arthritis: results of an 8-year prospective study, *J Rheumatol* 25:417, 1998.

513. Poleksic L et al: Magnetic resonance imaging of bone destruction in rheumatoid arthritis: comparison with radiography, *Skeletal Radiol* 22:577, 1993.

514. Porter GG: Psoriatic arthritis. Plain radiology and other imaging techniques, *Baillieres Clin Rheumatol* 8:465, 1994.

515. Porter RW: Pathology of symptomatic lumbar disc protrusion, *J R Coll Surg Edinb* 40:200, 1995.

516. Postacchini F et al: Ligamenta flava in lumbar disc herniation and spinal stenosis, *Spine* 19:917, 1994.

517. Postacchini F: Lumbar spinal stenosis and pseudostenosis, definition, and classification of pathology, *Ital J Orthop Traumatol* 9:339, 1983.

518. Postacchini F: Results of surgery compared with conservative management for lumbar disc herniations, *Spine* 21:1383, 1996.

519. Pottenger LA, Phillips FM, Draganich LF: The effect of marginal osteophytes on reduction of varus-valgus instability in osteoarthritic knee, *Arthritis Rheum* 30:853, 1990.

520. Powles AV et al: Exacerbation of psoriasis by indomethacin, *Br J Dermatol* 117:799, 1987.

521. Preidler KW, Resnick D: Imaging of osteoarthritis, *Radiol Clin North Am* 34:259, 1996.

522. Pyeritz RE, Sack GLH, Udvarhely GB: Genetics clinics of the Johns Hopkins Hospital. Surgical intervention in achondroplasia. Cervical and lumbar laminectomy for spinal stenosis in achondroplasia, *Johns Hopkins Med J* 146:203, 1980.

523. Quagliano PV, Hayes CW, Palmer WE: Vertebral pseudoarthrosis associated with diffuse idiopathic skeletal hyperostosis, *Skeletal Radiol* 23:353, 1994.

524. Quencer RM et al: Postoperative bone stenosis of the lumbar spinal canal: evaluation of 164 symptomatic patients with axial radiography, *AJR Am J Roentgenol* 131:1059, 1978.

525. Quinet RJ: Osteoarthritis: increasing mobility and reducing disability, *Geriatrics* 41:36, 1986.

526. Quon JA et al: Lumbar intervertebral disc herniation: treatment by rotational manipulation, *J Man Physiol Ther* 12:220, 1989.

527. Radin EL, Paul IL, Rose RM: Role of mechanical factors in pathogenesis of primary osteoarthritis, *Lancet* 1:519, 1972.

528. Rahman MU, Hudson AP, Schumacher HR: Chlamydia and Reiter's syndrome (reactive arthritis), *Rheum Dis Clin North Am* 18:67, 1992.

529. Rahman P et al: Comparison of radiological severity in psoriatic arthritis and rheumatoid arthritis, *J Rheumatol* 28:1041, 2001.

530. Raimbeau G et al: Arthropathie goutteuse du poignet a propos de cinq cas, *Chirurgie de la Main* 20(5):325, 2001.

531. Rajangam K, Thomas IM: Frequency of cervical spine involvement in rheumatoid arthritis, *J Indian Med Assoc* 93:138, 1995.

532. Rall LC et al: The effect of progressive resistance training in rheumatoid arthritis, *Arthritis Rheum* 39:415, 1996.

533. Ralston SH et al: A new method for the radiological assessment of vertebral squaring in ankylosing spondylitis, *Ann Rheum Dis* 51:330, 1992.

534. Ramos-Remus C et al: Frequency of atlantoaxial subluxation and neurologic involvement in patients with ankylosing spondylitis, *J Rheumatol* 22:2120, 1995.

535. Ramos-Remus C, Russell AS: Clinical features and management of ankylosing spondylitis, *Curr Opin Rheumatol* 5:408, 1993.

536. Ramos-Remus C, Russell AS: New clinical and radiographic features of ankylosing spondylitis, *Curr Opin Rheumatol* 4:463, 1992.

537. Rankin JA: Pathophysiology of the rheumatoid joint, *Orthop Nurs* 14:39, 1995.

538. Ravaud P: Quantitative radiography in osteoarthritis: plain radiographs, *Baillieres Clin Rheumatol* 10:409, 1996.

539. Reed AM, Ytterberg SR: Genetic and environmental risk factors for idiopathic inflammatory myopathies, *Rheum Dis Clin North Am* 28:891, 2002.

540. Reichlin M: Systemic lupus erythematosus. Antibodies to ribonuclear proteins, *Rheum Dis Clin North Am* 20:29, 1994.

541. Reijnierse M et al: The cervical spine in rheumatoid arthritis: relationship between neurologic signs and morphology on MR imaging and radiographs, *Skeletal Radiol* 25:113, 1996.

542. Reijnierse M, Dijkmans BA, Hansen B, Pope TL, Kroon HM, Holscher HC, et al: Neurologic dysfunction in patients with rheumatoid arthritis of the cervical spine. Predictive value of clinical, radiographic and MR imaging parameters, *Eur Radiol* 11(3):467, 2001.

543. Reilly PA et al: Arthropathy of hands and feet in systemic lupus erythematosus, *J Rheumatol* 17:777, 1990.

544. Reiter MF, Boden SD: Inflammatory disorders of the cervical spine, *Spine* 23:2755, 1998.

545. Remedios D et al: Juvenile chronic arthritis: diagnosis and management of tibio-talar and sub-talar disease, *Br J Rheumatol* 36:1214, 1997.

546. Remy-Jardin M et al: Lung changes in rheumatoid arthritis: CT findings, *Radiology* 193:375, 1994.

547. Resnick D et al: Association of diffuse idiopathic skeletal hyperostosis (DISH) and calcification and ossification of the posterior longitudinal ligament, *AJR Am J Roentgenol* 131:1049, 1978.

548. Resnick D, Broderick TW: Bony proliferation of terminal toe phalanges in psoriasis: the "ivory" phalanx, *J Can Assoc Radiol* 28:187, 1977.

549. Resnick D et al: Clinical, radiographic and pathologic abnormalities in calcium pyrophosphate dihydrate crystal deposition disease (CPPD): pseudogout, *Radiology* 122:1, 1977.

550. Resnick D, Niwayama G: Radiographic and pathologic features of spinal involvement in diffuse idiopathic skeletal hyperostosis (DISH), *Radiology* 119:559, 1976.

551. Resnick D, Williamson S, Alazraki N: Focal spinal abnormalities on bone scans in ankylosing spondylitis, *Clin Nucl Med* 6:213, 1981.

552. Resnick D: Common disorders of synovium-lined joints: pathogenesis, imaging abnormalities, and complications, *AJR Am J Roentgenol* 151:1079, 1988.

553. Resnick D: Degenerative diseases of the vertebral column, *Radiology* 156:3, 1985.

554. Resnick D: Diagnosis of bone and joint disorders, ed 4, Philadelphia, 2000, WB Saunders.

555. Richardson C et al: Therapeutic exercise for spinal segmental stabilization in low back pain. New York, 1999, Churchill Livingstone.

556. Riihimaki H: Low-back pain: its origin and risk indicators, *Scand J Work Environ Health* 17:81, 1991.

557. Ring D et al: Acute calcific retropharyngeal tendinitis. Clinical presentation and pathological characterization, *Bone Joint Surg Am* 76:1636, 1994.

558. Rosenow EC III et al: Pleuropulmonary manifestations of ankylosing spondylitis, *Mayo Clin Proc* 52:641, 1977.

559. Rothschild BM et al: Inflammatory sacroiliac joint pathology: evaluation of radiologic assessment techniques, *Clin Exp Rheumatol* 12:267, 1994.

560. Rovetta G, Bianchi G, Monteforte P: Joint failure in erosive osteoarthritis of the hands, *Int J Tissue React* 17:33, 1995.

561. Rowe LJ: The split vertebral body: a pseudofracture, *J Austral Chiro Assoc* 29:5, 1990.

562. Russell A et al: Current and emerging therapies for rheumatoid arthritis, with a focus on infliximab: clinical impact on joint damage and cost of care in Canada, *Clin Ther* 23(11):1824, 2001.

563. Ruzicka T: Psoriatic arthritis. New types, new treatments, *Arch Dermatol* 132:215, 1996.

564. Saal JA, Saal JS, Herzog RJ: The natural history of lumbar intervertebral disc extrusions treated non-operatively, *Spine* 15:683, 1990.

565. Saal JA: Natural history and nonoperative treatment of lumbar disc herniations, *Spine* 21(suppl 24):2, 1996.

566. Sack KE: Osteoarthritis. A continuing challenge, *West J Med* 163:579, 1995.

567. Sakamoto K, Kozuki K: Calcific tendinitis at the biceps brachii insertion of a child: a case report, *J Shoulder Elbow Surg* 11(1): 88, 2002.

568. Salaffi M et al: L'analisi quantitativa della progressione radiologica dell'artrite reumatoide: controversie e prospettive, *Radiol Med* 93:174, 1997.

569. Salvarani C et al: The cervical spine in patients with psoriatic arthritis: a clinical, radiological and immunogenetic study, *Ann Rheum Dis* 51(1):73, 1992.

570. Sattar MA, Guindi RT, Sugathan TN: Penicillamine in systemic sclerosis: a reappraisal, *Clin Rheumatol* 9:517, 1990.

571. Scarpa R et al: Psoriatic arthritis in psoriatic patients, *Br J Rheumatol* 23(4):246, 1984.

572. Schaller JG: Chronic arthritis in children. Juvenile rheumatoid arthritis, *Clin Orthop* 182:79, 1984.

573. Scheja A, Akesson A, Niewierowicz I: Computer based quantitative analysis of capillary abnormalities in systemic sclerosis and its relation to plasma concentration of von Willebrand factor, *Ann Rheum Dis* 55:52, 1996.

574. Schiebler ML et al: Normal and degenerated intervertebral disk: in vivo and in vitro MR imaging with histopathologic correlation, *AJR Am J Roentgenol* 157:93, 1991.

575. Schlapbach P et al: Diffuse idiopathic skeletal hyperostosis of the spine: a cause of back pain? *Br J Rheumatol* 28:299, 1989.

576. Schlosstein L et al: High association of an HL-A antigen, W27, with ankylosing spondylitis, *N Engl J Med* 288:704, 1973.

577. Schneiderman G et al: Magnetic resonance imaging in the diagnosis of disc degeneration: correlation with discography, *Spine* 12:276, 1987.

578. Schonstrom NS, Bolender NF, Spengler DM: The pathomorphology of spinal stenosis as seen on CT scans of the lumbar spine, *Spine* 10:806, 1985.

579. Schwab EP et al: Pulmonary alveolar hemorrhage in systemic lupus erythematosus, *Semin Arthritis Rheum* 23:8, 1993.

580. Schweitzer ME et al: Cervical paraspinal calcification in collagen vascular diseases, *AJR Am J Roentgenol* 157:523, 1991.

581. Scutellari PN, Orzincolo C, Castaldi G: Association between diffuse idiopathic skeletal hyperostosis and multiple myeloma, *Skeletal Radiol* 24:489, 1995.

582. Scutellari PN et al: Radiology, of the hand in progressive systemic sclerosis, *Radiol Med Torino* 72(7–8):528, 1986.

583. Senocak O et al: Lung parenchyma changes in ankylosing spondylitis: demonstration with high resolution CT and correlation with disease duration, *Eur J Radiol* 45(2):117, 2003.

584. Senstad O, Leboeuf-Yde C, Borchgrevink C: Frequency and characteristics of side effects of spinal manipulative therapy, *Spine* 22:435, 1997.

585. Sequeira W: The neuropathic joint, *Clin Exp Rheumatol* 12:325, 1994.

586. Sether LA, Yu S, Haughton VM: Intervertebral disk: normal age-related changes in MR signal intensity, *Radiology* 177:385, 1990.

587. Shamin EA, Rider LG, Miller FW: Update on the genetics of the idiopathic inflammatory myopathies, *Curr Opin Rheumatol* 12:482, 2000.

588. Shapiro R, Balt H: Unilateral thoracic spondylosis, *AJR Am J Roentgenol* 83:660, 1960.

589. Sharma S et al: Spinal stenosis: diagnosis and management: a clinical and radiological study, *Int Surg* 67:565, 1982.

590. Sharp JT: Radiologic assessment as an outcome measure in rheumatoid arthritis, *Arthritis Rheum* 32:221, 1989.

591. Shbeeb M et al: The epidemiology of psoriatic arthritis in Olmsted County, Minnesota, USA, 1982–1991, *J Rheumatol* 27:1247, 2000.

592. Sheehan S, Bauer R, Meyer J: Vertebral artery compression in cervical spondylosis, *Neurology* 10:968, 1960.

593. Shekelle P et al: Spinal manipulation for low back pain, *BMJ* 117:590, 1992.

594. Sholkoff SD, Glickman MG, Steinbach HL: Roentgenology of Reiter's syndrome, *Radiology* 97:497, 1970.

595. Short CL, Bauer W, Reynolds WE: Rheumatoid arthritis, Cambridge, MA, 1957, Harvard University Press.

596. Shumacher TM et al: HLA-B27 associated arthropathies, *Radiology* 126:289, 1978.

597. Siam AR, Hammoudeh M: Jaccoud's arthropathy of the shoulders in systemic lupus erythematosus, *J Rheumatol* 19:980, 1992.

598. Sigurgeirsson B et al: Risk of cancer in patients with dermatomyositis or polymyositis: a population based study, *N Engl J Med* 326:363, 1992.

599. Simkin PA: Simian stance: a sign of spinal stenosis, *Lancet* 2:652, 1982.

600. Simon S, Whitten J, Shapiro F: Leg-length discrepancies in monarticular and pauciarticular juvenile rheumatoid arthritis, *J Bone J Surg* 63A:209, 1981.

601. Singsen BH: Rheumatic diseases of childhood, *Rheum Dis Clin North Am* 16:581, 1990.

602. Sjogren RW: Gastrointestinal motility disorders in scleroderma, *Arthritis Rheum* 37:1265, 1994.

603. Sjolie AN, Ljunggren AE: The significance of high lumbar mobility and low lumbar strength for current and future low back pain in adolescents, *Spine* 26:2629, 2001.

604. Slemenda CW: The epidemiology of osteoarthritis of the knee, *Curr Opin Rheumatol* 4:546, 1992.

605. Smoker WRK et al: The role of MR imaging in evaluating metastatic spinal disease, *AJNR* 8:901, 1987.

606. Spector TD: Rheumatoid arthritis, *Rheum Dis Clin North Am* 16:513, 1990.

607. Spector TD: The fat on the joint. Osteoarthritis and obesity, *J Rheumatol* 17:284, 1990.

608. Spengler DM: Degenerative stenosis of the lumbar spine, *J Bone Joint Surg Am* 69:305, 1987.

609. Spilberg I: Current concepts of the mechanism of acute inflammation in gouty arthritis, *Arthritis Rheum* 18:129, 1975.

610. Starz TW, Miller EB: Diagnosis and treatment of rheumatoid arthritis, *Primary Care* 20:827, 1993.

611. Steen VD et al: Twenty-year incidence survey of systemic sclerosis, *Arthritis Rheum* 31(suppl) 57, 1988.

612. Steen VD, Medsger TA Jr: Epidemiology and natural history of systemic sclerosis, *Rheum Dis Clin North Am* 16:1, 1990.

613. Steen VD et al: Incidence of systemic sclerosis in Allegheny County, Pennsylvania. A twenty-year study of hospital-diagnosed cases, 1963–1982, *Arthritis Rheum* 40:441, 1997.

614. Steen VD: Scleroderma renal crisis, *Rheum Dis Clin North Am* 29:315, 2003.

615. Steen VD: Systemic sclerosis, *Rheum Dis Clin North Am* 16:641, 1990.

616. Steiner RM et al: The radiological finding in dermatomyositis of childhood, *Radiology* 111:385, 1974.

617. Stewart AL et al: Functional status and well-being of patients with chronic conditions, Results from the Medical Outcomes Study, *JAMA* 262:907, 1989.

618. Stone M et al: Clinical and imaging correlates of response to treatment with infliximab in patients with ankylosing apondylitis, *J Rheumatol* 28:1605, 2001.

619. Subcommittee for Scleroderma Criteria of the American Rheumatism Association Diagnostic and Therapeutic Criteria Committee: Preliminary criteria for the classification of systemic sclerosis (scleroderma), *Arthritis Rheum* 23:581, 1980.

620. Sukenik S et al: Jaccoud's-type arthropathy: an association with sarcoidosis, *J Rheumatol* 18:915, 1991.

621. Sule SD, Wigley FM: Treatment of scleroderma: an update, *Expert Opin Investig Drugs* 12:471, 2003.

622. Sullivan DB et al: Dermatomyositis in a paediatric patient, *Arthritis Rheum* 20:327, 1977.

623. Summers MN et al: Radiographic assessment and psychologic variables as predictors of pain and functional impairment in osteoarthritis of the knee or hip, *Arthritis Rheum* 31:204, 1988.

624. Swedberg JA, Steinbauer JR: Osteoarthritis, *Am Fam Phys* 45:557, 1992.

625. Swezey RL: Pathophysiology and treatment of intervertebral disk disease, *Rheum Dis Clin North Am* 19:741, 1993.

626. Szczepanski L, Targonska B, Piotrowski M: Deforming arthropathy and Jaccoud's syndrome in patients with systemic lupus erythematosus, *Scand J Rheumatol* 21:308, 1992.

627. Taccari E, Spadaro A, Riccieri V: Correlations between peripheral and axial radiological changes in patients with psoriatic polyarthritis, *Revue du Rhumatisme (English edition)* 63:17, 1996.

628. Takehara K, Soma Y, Ishibashi Y: Early detection of scleroderma spectrum disorders in patients with Raynaud's phenomenon, *Dermatologica* 183:164, 1991.

629. Tan EM et al: The 1982 revised criteria for the classification of systemic lupus erythematosus, *Arthritis Rheum* 25:1271, 1982.

630. Tangrea JA et al: Skeletal hyperostosis in patients receiving chronic, very low-dose isotretinoin, *Arch Dermatol* 128:921, 1992.

631. Targoff IN: Laboratory testing in the diagnosis and management of idiopathic inflammatory myopathies, *Rheum Dis Clin North Am* 28:859, 2002.

632. Taylor HG et al: The relationship of clinical and laboratory measurements to radiological change in ankylosing spondylitis, *Br J Rheumatol* 30:330, 1991.

633. Taylor JR, Twomey LT: Age changes in lumbar zygopophyseal joints. Observations on structure and function, *Spine* 11:739, 1986.

634. Taylor JR: The development and adult structure of lumbar intervertebral discs, *J Manual Med* 5:43, 1990.

635. Taylor TKF et al: Spinal biomechanics and aging are major determinants of the proteoglycan metabolism of intervertebral disc cells, *Spine* 25:3014, 2000.

636. Tennent TD, Goradia VK: Arthroscopic management of calcific tendonitis of the popliteus tendon, *J Arthroscop Rel Surg* 19:35, 2003.

637. Teplick JG, Haskin ME: Spontaneous regression of herniated nucleus pulposus, *AJR Am J Roentgenol* 145:371, 1985.

638. Teresi LM et al: Asymptomatic degenerative disc disease and spondylosis of the cervical spine: MR imaging, *Radiology* 164:83, 1987.

639. Thomas E et al: Subtyping of juvenile idiopathic arthritis using latent class analysis. British Pediatric Rheumatology group, *Arthritis Rheum* 43:1496, 2000.

640. Thompson RE et al: Disc lesions and the mechanics of the intervertebral joint complex, *Spine* 25:3026, 2000.

641. Tishler M, Yaron, M: Jaccoud's arthropathy and psoriatic arthritis, *Clin Exp Rheumatol* 11:663, 1993.

642. Tokuda M et al: Effect of low-dose cyclosporin A on systemic lupus erythematosus disease activity, *Arthritis Rheum* 37:551, 1994.

643. Torres MA, Furst DE: Treatment of generalized systemic sclerosis, *Rheum Dis Clin North Am* 16:2217, 1990.

644. Tsang IK: Update on osteoarthritis, *Can Fam Phys* 36:539, 1990.

645. Turk DC, Okofuji A: Psychological factors in chronic pain: evolution and revolution, *J Consult Clin Psychol* 70:678, 2002.

646. Twigg HL, Smith BF: Jaccoud's arthritis, *Radiology* 80:417, 1963.

647. Twomey L, Taylor TR: Structural and mechanical disc changes with age, *J Manual Med* 5:58, 1990.

648. Uramoto KM et al: Trends in the incidence and mortality of systemic lupus erythematosus, 1950–1990, *Arthritis Rheum* 42:46, 1999.

649. Uthoff HK, Sarkar K: Classification and definition of tendinopathies, *Clin Sports Med* 10(4):707, 1991.

650. van de Putte LBA, van Gestel AM, van Riel PLCM: Early treatment of rheumatoid arthritis: rationale, evidence, and implications, *Ann Rheum Dis* 57:511, 1998.

651. van der Heijde DM et al: Biannual radiographic assessments of hands and feet in a three-year prospective followup of patients with early rheumatoid arthritis, *Arthritis Rheum* 35:26, 1992.

652. van der Heijde DM: Radiographic imaging: the gold standard for assessment of disease progression in rheumatoid arthritis, *Rheumatology* 39S:9, 2000.

653. van der Heijde DM et al: Radiographic progression on radiographs of hands and feet during the first 3 years of rheumatoid arthritis measured according to Sharp's method (van der Heijde modification), *J Rheumatol* 22(9):1792, 1995.

654. van der Heijde DM: Joint erosions and patients with early rheumatoid arthritis, *Br J Rheumatol* 34:74, 1995.

655. van der Linden SF et al: The risk of developing ankylosing spondylitis in HLA-B27 positive individuals, *Arthritis Rheum* 27:241, 1984.

656. van Jaarsveld CHM et al: Aggressive treatment in early rheumatoid arthritis: a randomized controlled trial, *Ann Rheum Dis* 59:468, 2000.

657. Van Saase JL et al: Epidemiology of osteoarthritis: Zoetermeer survey. Comparison of radiological osteoarthritis in a Dutch population with that of 10 other populations, *Ann Rheum Dis* 48:271, 1989.

658. Van Schaardenburg D, Breedveld FC: Elderly-onset rheumatoid arthritis, *Semin Arthritis Rheum* 23:367, 1994.

659. Van Vollenhoven RF, McGuire JL: Estrogen, progesterone, and testosterone: can they be used to treat autoimmune diseases? *Cleve Clin J Med* 61:276, 1994.

660. van Vugt RM et al: Deforming arthropathy or lupus and rhupus hands in systemic lupus erythematosus, *Ann Rheum Dis* 57:540, 1998.

661. van Zeben D, Breedveld FC: Prognostic factors in rheumatoid arthritis, *J Rheumatol* 23:31, 1996.

662. Veidlinger OF et al: Cervical myelopathy and its relationship to cervical stenosis, *Spine* 6:551, 1981.

663. Veys EM, Mielants H: Current concepts in psoriatic arthritis, *Dermatology* 189:35, 1994.

664. Vezyroglow G et al: A metabolic syndrome in diffuse idiopathic skeletal hyperostosis. A controlled study, *J Rheumatol* 23:672, 1996.

665. Viitanen JV et al: Correlation between mobility restrictions and radiologic changes in ankylosing spondylitis, *Spine* 20:492, 1995.

666. Vincelette P, Laurin CA, Levesque HP: The footballer's ankle and foot, *Can Med Assoc* 107:872, 1972.

667. Virgin WJ: Experimental investigations into the physical properties of the intervertebral disc, *J Bone Joint Surg Br* 33:607, 1951.

668. Vizkelety T, Aszodi I: Bilateral calcareous bursitis of the elbow, *J Bone Joint Surg Br* 50:644, 1968.

669. Vlok GJ, Hendrix MR: The lumbar disc: evaluating the causes of pain, *Orthopedics* 14:419, 1991.

670. Walden CA et al: Case report 620. Progressive systemic sclerosis (PSS) with paraspinous and intraspinous calcifications, *Skeletal Radiol* 19:377, 1990.

671. Ward MM: Predictors of the progression of functional disability in patients with ankylosing spondylitis, *J Rheumatol* 29(7):1420, 2002.

672. Warnick C, Sherman MS, Lesser RW: Aspiration pneumonia due to diffuse cervical hyperostosis, *Chest* 98:763, 1990.

673. Weber H: The natural history of disc herniation and the influence of intervention, *Spine* 19:2234, 1994.

674. Weidenbaum M et al: Correlating magnetic resonance imaging with the biochemical content of the normal human intervertebral disc, *J Orthop* 10:552, 1992.

675. Weinberger A, Kaplan JG, Myers AR: Extensive soft tissue calcification (calcinosis universalis) in systemic lupus erythematosus, *Ann Rheum Dis* 38:384, 1979.

676. Weinstein JN, Rydevik BL, Sonntag VKH: Essentials of the spine, New York, 1995, Raven Press.

677. Weissman BN: Juvenile rheumatoid arthritis. In Feldman F, editor: Radiology, pathology, and immunology of bones and joints: a review of current concepts, New York, 1978, Appleton-Century-Croft.

PART TWO Bone, Joints, and Soft Tissues

678. Weisz GM: Lumbar spinal canal stenosis in Paget's disease, *Spine* 8:192, 1983.

679. Weyand CM, Goronzy JJ: Inherited and noninherited risk factors in rheumatoid arthritis, *Curr Opin Rheumatol* 7:206, 1995.

680. Wiesinger FG et al: Improvement of physical fitness and muscle strength in polymyositis/dermatomyositis patients by a training program, *Br J Rheumatol* 37:196, 1998.

681. Wilhelmi G: Potential influence of nutrition with supplements on healthy and arthritic joints, *J Rheumatol* 52:191, 1993.

682. Wilkin E et al: Osteoarthritis and articular chondrocalcinosis in the elderly, *Ann Rheum Dis* 42:280, 1983.

683. Wilkinson HA, LeMay ML, Ferris EJ: Roentgenographic correlations in cervical spondylosis, *AJR Am J Roentgenol* 105:370, 1969.

684. Williams RC: Rheumatoid arthritis: using laboratory tests in diagnosis and follow-up, *J Musculoskel Med* 13:14, 1996.

685. Wilson FM, Jaspan T: Thoracic spinal cord compression caused by diffuse idiopathic skeletal hyperostosis (DISH), *Clin Radiol* 42:133, 1990.

686. Wiltse LL, Kirkaldy-Willis WH, Melvor GWD: The treatment of spinal stenosis, *Clin Orthop* 115:83, 1976.

687. Wiltse LL: The effect of the common anomalies of the lumbar spine upon disc degeneration and low back pain, *Orthop Clin North Am* 2:569, 1971.

688. Winchester R et al: The co-occurrence of Reiter's syndrome and acquired immunodeficiency, *Ann Intern Med* 106:19, 1987.

689. Wood PH: Nomenclature and classification of arthritis in children. In Munthe E, editor: The care of rheumatoid children, Basel, Switzerland, 1978, EULAR Publishers.

690. Wortman RL: Gout and other disorders of purine metabolism. In Fauci AS, Braunwald E, Isselbachjer KJ, et al, editors: Harrison's principles of internal medicine, ed 14, New York, 1998, McGraw-Hill.

691. Yang BY et al: Calcium pyrophosphate dihydrate crystal deposition disease: frequency of tendon calcification about the knee, *J Rheumatol* 23:883, 1996.

692. Yates DAH: Spinal stenosis, *J R Soc Med* 74:334, 1981.

693. Yelin E, Callahan LF: The economic cost and social and psychological impact of musculoskeletal conditions, *Arthritis Rheum* 38:1351, 1995.

694. Yelin E: Impact of musculoskeletal conditions on the elderly, *Geriatr Med Today* 8:103, 1989.

695. Yonezawa T, Tsuji H, Matsui H, Hirano N: Subaxial lesions in rheumatoid arthritis. Radiographic factors suggestive of lower cervical myelopathy, *Spine* 20:208, 1995.

696. Ytterberg SR, Mahowald ML, Krug HE: Exercise for arthritis, *Baillieres Clin Rheumatol* 8:161, 1994.

697. Yu S et al: Progressive and regressive changes in the nucleus pulposus, *Radiology* 169:93, 1988.

698. Yu S et al: Tears of the anulus fibrosus: correlation between MR and pathologic findings in cadavers, *AJNR* 9:367, 1988.

699. Yusof ZB, Pratap RC: Cervical cord compression due to ossified posterior longitudinal ligament associated with diffuse idiopathic skeletal hyperostosis, *Aust N Z J Med* 29:697, 1990.

700. Zdeblick TA: The treatment of degenerative lumbar disorders, *Spine* 20:126S, 1995.

Trauma

DENNIS M. MARCHIORI

CHAPTER FORMAT

This chapter reviews trauma to the skeleton. The emphasis is presented under the heading of bone and joint trauma. Multiple tables list fractures and soft-tissue injuries stratified by body region. Other topics related to trauma, such as battered child syndrome, spondylolisthesis, and osteochondritis dissecans, also are presented in this chapter under separate headings.

IMAGING

Imaging of skeletal trauma is largely dominated by plain film radiology. Plain film offers excellent evaluation of small or simple anatomy, and provides a first step in imaging more complex anatomy, to be followed by more sophisticated modalities.

Computed tomography (CT) is beneficial for exhibiting complex anatomy, especially the head, calcaneus, acetabulum, and spine. CT provides imaging directly in an axial plane and is commonly reformatted to view the anatomy in other planes. CT is particularly adept at demonstrating cortical bone. Linear tomography is useful for detailing fractures and is often applied to the upper cervical spine and wrist.

Magnetic resonance imaging (MRI) is performed if a significant soft-tissue component is seen indirectly or suspected clinically, if visualization of bone marrow is needed, or neurologic findings are present. Like CT, MRI also provides axial imaging, but goes further to offer true multidimensional imaging in other planes (e.g., frontal, sagittal). MRI is noninvasive and has the advantage of being able to evaluate a wide range of both intraarticular and extraarticular anatomy.

Bone and Joint Trauma

BACKGROUND

Bone injuries. Traumatic lesions of the skeleton are common to all ages and patient populations. Traumatic bone insult may be fairly innocuous, manifesting with little more than a bone bruise or may be severe enough to break the bone producing a fracture. A fracture is defined as an interruption of the structural integrity and anatomic continuity of bone, manifesting as minor cracks, crumpling, splintering, or complete disruption of the cortex. If the overlying skin remains intact, the fracture is closed (or simple); if the skin is disrupted, the fracture is open (or compound).

Fractures are oriented transverse, longitudinal, or oblique to the long axis of the bone, largely dictated by the force applied to the bone. Spiral fractures result from rotational stresses and have an oblique fracture plane that encircles the long axis of the bone. Complete fractures extend through the bone and produce at least two fragments. Those with more than two fragments are termed *comminuted fractures*. Because of the pliability of long bones in children, a fracture may not appear to extend through the entire bone. If a portion of the bone remains intact, the fracture is incomplete. Incomplete fractures of long bones present with either distraction (greenstick) or impaction (buckle or torus) of the completely fractured cortical side of the bone (Table 10-1). Incomplete fractures are named according to their radiographic appearance. That is, they may extend completely thorough the bone anatomically, but routinely appear to only "incompletely" extend through the bone on the corresponding radiograph.

Reporting on fractures and dislocations should encompass such information as which bone is involved, where in the bone the fracture is found, fragment apposition (shift), alignment (tilt), rotation (twist), distraction (separation), and any resulting alteration in limb length. Descriptive terms for long bone and vertebral injuries are presented in Figures 10-1 to 10-3.

Types of fractures. Fractures develop from a single application of stress outside of the normal range of physiologic limits (traumatic, acute, or strain fracture), repetitive application of stress within the normal range of physiologic limits (fatigue or stress fracture), or the single (pathologic) or repeated (insufficiency) application of stress within the normal range of physiologic limits but applied to bone that has been weakened by underlying pathology (e.g., Paget's disease, metastatic bone disease). Tables 10-2 through 10-10 are constructed to provide examples and more detail of

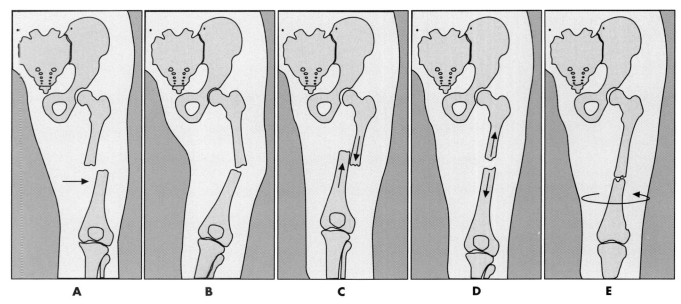

FIG. 10-1 Common descriptive terms of injury and fracture to the long bones include, **A,** translation, apposition or shear; **B,** varus (shown above) or valgus angulation; **C,** telescoping or bayonet deformity; **D,** distraction; and, **E,** rotation.

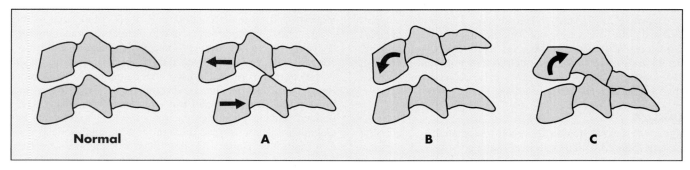

FIG. 10-2 Common descriptive terms of sagittal spinal injury include, **A,** translation; **B,** flexion; and, **C,** extension.

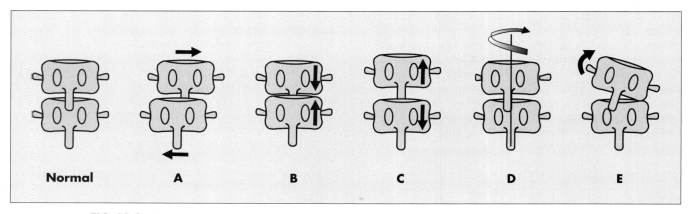

FIG. 10-3 Common descriptive terms of coronal spinal injury include, **A,** translation; **B,** compression; **C,** distraction; **D,** axial rotation; and, **E,** lateral flexion.

stress fractures (Table 10-2), Salter-Harris fractures (Table 10-3), and selected topics of bone and joint injury sorted by anatomic region: skull and face (Table 10-4), cervical spine (Tables 10-5 and 10-6), thoracic spine and thorax (Table 10-7), lumbar spine (Table 10-8), upper extremity (Table 10-9), and pelvis and lower extremity (Table 10-10).

Stress fractures. As noted, stress fractures are the consequence of repetitive applications of compressive, rotational, or tensile force to bone (see Table 10-2). Each application of stress is sub-threshold to cause a frank fracture, but results in microfracture injuries to bone. The microfractures stimulate reactive bone hypertrophy, evident radiographically as increased sclerosis and noted on bone scans and single photon emission computed tomography (SPECT) imaging as regions of radiotracer uptake (hot spots). A macrofracture results when the rate of osteoclastic resorption from microfractures outpaces the osteoblastic healing. Stress fractures are responsible for approximately 1% to 16% of all athletic injuries,[13,153] and have been associated with a variety of work and sport activities;[12] most of them involve running. Without question, the pars interarticulares of L5 are the most common sites of stress fractures. Excluding this region, approximately 95% of stress fractures involve the lower extremities.[209] Patients with stress fractures often report a change in the amount of activity tolerated, and report pain of a diffuse nature. Radiographs often are negative for abnormality during the early stages of stress fracture formation. In later stages they present as a linear band of sclerosis.

Epiphyseal injuries (Salter-Harris classification). The epiphysis is a susceptible site of injury in the growing skeleton. Approximately 6% to 15% of long bone fractures occurring in children under 16 years of age involve the epiphysis.[183,205,225] Because the epiphysis is responsible for longitudinal bone growth, injury disrupting vascular supply to the epiphysis or metaphysis affects bone growth. The distal tibia, fibula, ulna, and radius are the most common sites affected. Several variations of epiphyseal injury have been identified. The Salter-Harris classification is the most widely used system used to describe these injuries (see Table 10-3).[210] The classification of epiphyseal injury is important because it relates to the treatment of the patient and correlates to expected long-term clinical outcomes.

Joint injuries. Joint injury may result in subluxation, dislocation, diastasis, or fracture. Subluxation ("sub" under, "luxation" dislocation) is a displacement of a bone in relation to the apposing bone, resulting in *partial* loss of articulation of the opposing bone ends. Subluxation involves less joint misalignment than is seen with a dislocation. This generic use of the term *subluxation* differs from the chiropractic context of the term. A chiropractic subluxation describes a clinical entity that involves both an anatomic and physiologic component (Box 10-1). A dislocation is a displacement of a bone in relation to the apposing bone, producing a complete loss of articulation between the opposing bone ends. Simple or comminuted intraarticular fractures may involve only the articular cartilage (chondral) or extend into the subjacent bone (osteochondral fractures). Intraarticular fragments may dislodge or remain in situ. Diastasis describes separation of the adjacent joint surfaces of a fibrous or cartilaginous joint.

Fracture healing. Successful fracture healing is dependent on fragment apposition, fracture fixation, and ample blood supply. For purposes of exposition, bone healing often is divided arbitrarily into five stages (Fig. 10-4):

1. *Hematoma.* After trauma, vessels are damaged with subsequent bleeding from the damaged bone ends and surrounding soft tissues. A blood clot develops. Osteocytes, imprisoned in their lacunae near the fracture site, lose their blood supply and undergo necrosis (Fig. 10-4, *A*).

2. *Inflammation.* An acute inflammatory reaction develops within several hours of the injury with proliferation of cells from beneath the periosteum and endosteum of the traumatized area. Proliferating granulation tissue surrounds and bridges the fracture fragments. The hematoma is slowly resorbed and new capillary buds invaginate into the injured areas (Fig. 10-4, *B*).

3. *Callus.* The proliferating fibroblasts of the granular tissue show metaplasia to collagenoblasts, chondroblasts, and osteoblasts approximately 3 weeks after the initial trauma. This cellular reaction raises the periosteum away from the bone cortex and an osteoblastic collar is formed around the bone fragments, representing primitive woven bone laid down in a haphazard fashion. Although still mobile, the callus causes the fracture to become more stable. It is visible on a radiograph and may be felt as a firm mass on palpation (Fig. 10-4, *C*).

4. *Consolidation.* Osteoclasts are introduced by the penetrating capillary buds and assist the osteoblasts to alter the bone callus from woven to lamellar bone. The healing bone can withstand normal loads and there should be no detectable movement, a state called "clinically united" (Fig. 10-4, *D*).

5. *Remodeling.* Over a period of months to years, the bony bridge is remodeled to the pretrauma size and shape, or as near to it as possible. Excessive callus is removed and the medullary canal is recanalized. Children have greater powers of remodeling and may correct deformities and even discrepancies of length after a fracture (Fig. 10-4, *E*).

The time it takes for union varies depending on the age, health status, and bone injured. Generally a weak bone callus is formed by weeks 3 to 6, becoming thicker over months. This callus may be faintly seen on radiographs. Healing continues as the bone

---

BOX 10-1

Classification Scheme of Chiropractic Subluxation (ACA, 1984)

Static intersegmental subluxation
- Flexion malposition
- Extension malposition
- Lateral flexion malposition
- Rotation malposition
- Anterolisthesis
- Retrolisthesis
- Altered interosseous spacing (increased or decreased)
- Osseous foraminal encroachment

Kinetic intersegmental subluxation
- Hypomobility (flexion subluxation)
- Hypermobility (unstable subluxation)
- Aberrant motion (paradoxic motion)

Sectional subluxation
- Scoliosis or alteration of curves secondary to muscle imbalance
- Scoliosis or alteration of curves secondary to structural asymmetry
- Decompensation of adaptational curves
- Abnormalities of motion

Paravertebral subluxation
- Costovertebral or costotransverse disrelationships
- Sacroiliac subluxation

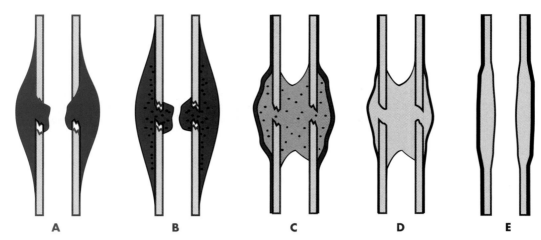

FIG. 10-4 Stages of fracture healing: **A,** hematoma; **B,** inflammation; **C,** callus; **D,** consolidation; **E,** remodeling (see text for description).

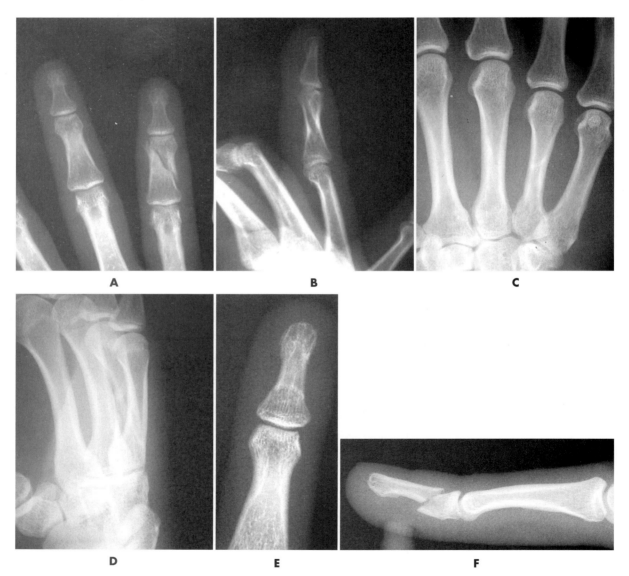

FIG. 10-5 Often fractures, especially oblique fractures, do not materialize equally well on all views of a radiographic series. For this reason it is very important to take all necessary views of a series, usually at least two opposing views of the area of interest. In case 1 (**A** and **B**) the fracture is clearly seen on, **A,** one view and nearly occult on, **B,** the opposing view. If only the lateral projection is taken, the fracture may be missed. In case two (**C** and **D**), another example of this tendency is exhibited with a fracture of the shaft of the fourth metacarpal. The fracture is not evident on, **C,** the posteroanterior (PA) projection but is seen on, **D,** the lateral view, although viewing is difficult because of adjacent bone imposition. Last, in a third case (**E** and **F**) the fracture of the distal phalanx is not seen clearly on, **E,** the PA view. Only a thin transverse radiodense band is noted. (**A** through **E,** courtesy Ian D. McLean, LeClaire, IA.)

regains much of its initial strength by 3 to 6 months. Cancellous bone heals about twice as quickly as does cortical bone. Children demonstrate healing more quickly and elderly people more slowly than adults. Cigarette smoking, malnutrition, diabetes, osteoporosis, steroid medications, and a variety of other systemic factors negatively affect the rate of fracture healing.

Fracture complications. Fracture complications are divided into early or late consequences. For the most part, early complications affect soft tissues and late complications affect bone. Early complications are noted within a few days after the injury, whereas late complications take months to appear. Some of the more common complications are listed in Table 10-11. Predictive factors of poor healing include severe tissue injury, interposition of soft-tissue elements, delayed vascularity, poor alignment, motion, and inadequate immobilization.

IMAGING FINDINGS

When considered alone, the patient's clinical presentation is not reliable in determining the presence or absence of skeletal injury. Radiographic examination is necessary to determine the presence or absence of clinically suspected fractures. Radiographic examination should involve at least two opposing projections of the region of interest (Fig. 10-5). Often the clinical circumstances warrant a second radiographic examination to exclude suspected occult fractures. Reexamination should occur after a 10-day period that gives the osteoclasts time to remove necrotic bone from around the fracture site, producing a more visible radiolucent fracture line than may have been present on the initial radiographs.

To exclude related joint injuries, minimal radiographic studies should include the joint closest to the patient's region of pain in the field of view. Tomography (linear and computed) and MRI are especially helpful to define areas of complex anatomy (e.g., spine, wrist, ankle). Radionuclide bone scintigraphy is helpful to locate fractures and is especially useful in evaluating the presence of stress fractures.

The radiographic features vary depending on the interval between the injury and radiographic examination. Initial radiographic findings may lag 2 to 6 weeks behind the onset of symptoms. Radionuclide bone scintigraphy more accurately denotes the presence of fracture during this interval.

For the most part, fractures appear radiographically as radiolucent lines traversing bone. There is often concurrent finding of soft-tissue swelling. Stress fractures or overlapping or impacted fractured fragments appear as radiodense bands indicating the bony proliferation occurring in response to the repetitive stress.

CLINICAL COMMENTS

Immediate clinical concern is directed toward first aid of the patient. Measures should be taken to limit pain and prevent further damage by limiting movement of the fragments by supporting or splinting the area. Fractures to long bones may be associated with considerable blood loss requiring compression.

In general, there are four levels of treatment: reduction, immobilization or fixation, bony union, and functional restoration. Closed reduction refers to nonsurgical manipulation or traction of the fracture fragments. Open reduction involves internal manipulation of the fragments. K-wires, plates, intramedullary rods, and bone screws may be inserted for internal fixation at the fracture site. Most fractures are treated initially with closed reduction. To be successful a soft-tissue bridge (e.g., periosteum) has to be in place for good outcome. Although stabilization is the key to initial management, the patient should undergo a vigorous rehabilitation program to achieve rapid and full recovery from the injury once bony union occurs.

KEY CONCEPTS

- Plain film is the first modality for most skeletal trauma, CT offers better osseous detail and provides rapid intracranial imaging, and MRI visualizes bone marrow and soft-tissue injuries best.
- A fracture is a break in the structural continuity of bone manifesting as minor cracks, crumpling, splintering, or complete disruption of the cortex. Fractures are often described on the basis of skin puncture (closed or open), etiology (acute, stress, pathologic, or insufficiency) or direction of the fracture plane (oblique, spiral, or transverse).
- Description of a fracture should include which bone, location in the bone, fragment apposition, alignment, rotation, distraction, and any resulting alteration in limb length.
- Epiphyseal injuries are described with the Salter-Harris (types I to V) and Rang-Ogden (VI to IX) classifications.
- Joint injury may result in subluxation (partial misalignment), dislocation (complete misalignment), diastasis (separation), or fracture (chondral, osteochondral, or osseous).
- Healing phases include hematoma, inflammation, callus, consolidation, and remodeling.
- There are four levels of treatment: reduction, immobilization or fixation, bony union, and functional restoration.

Text continued on p. 733.

TABLE 10-1
Descriptive Terminology of Fractures

Types of fracture	Comments
Avulsion (Figs. 10-6 and 10-7)	An avulsion fracture occurs as the attachment of a ligament or tendon is pulled from the bone, taking a small bone fragment with it. The fragments are often highly serrated.
Closed (simple)	A closed fracture does not penetrate the skin.
Comminuted (Fig. 10-8)	A comminuted fracture has more than two fragments. A butterfly fragment describes a triangular-shaped bone fragment split from one of the main fragments.
Complicated	A complicated fracture may be "complicated" by damage to nerves, vessels, and viscera.
Corner (chip) (Fig. 10-9)	A corner fracture describes a fracture of the articular margin of a bone, releasing a small fragment.

Continued

TABLE 10-1 cont'd
Descriptive Terminology of Fractures

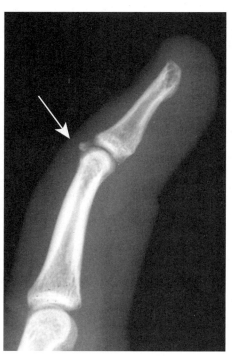

FIG. 10-6 Small avulsion of the dorsal, proximal margin of the distal phalanx. Although these fractures appear trivial, they may involve a significant defect of the extensor tendons, manifesting as a functional defect *(arrow)*.

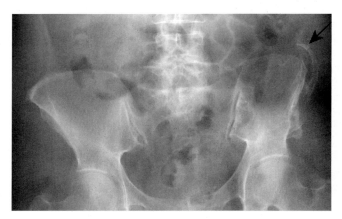

FIG. 10-7 Old avulsion fracture of the iliac crest with fingerlike appearance of avulsed fragment *(arrow)*. (Courtesy Steven P. Brownstein, MD, Springfield, NJ.)

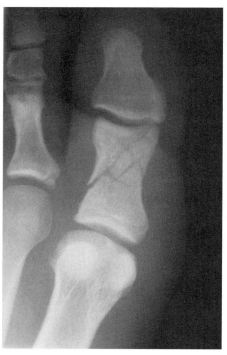

FIG. 10-8 The fractured proximal phalanx of the first pedal digit appears in multiple pieces. A fracture is termed *comminuted* if it results in more than two fragments (the original bone is fragment one and the fractured fragment is number two). (Courtesy Gary Longmuir, Phoenix, AZ.)

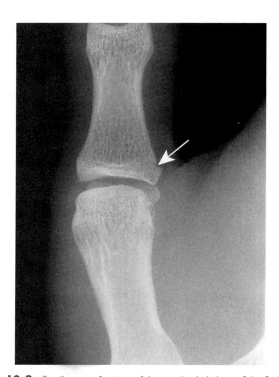

FIG. 10-9 Small corner fracture of the proximal phalanx of the first digit *(arrow)*.

TABLE 10-1 cont'd Descriptive Terminology of Fractures	
Types of fracture	**Comments**
Diastatic (Fig. 10-10)	A diastatic fracture is a separation injury of synarthrodial joints (e.g., pubic symphysis, proximal, and distal tibiofibular joints).
Greenstick (Fig. 10-11)	A greenstick fracture is an incomplete fracture of long bones that is seen in children. The concave side of the bending bone is intact and the opposite convex cortex is distracted with an obvious ragged fracture line.
Impaction (crush) (Fig. 10-12)	An impaction fracture occurs when one fragment is driven or telescoped into the cancellous bone of the adjacent fragment. There are two types: (a) *Depression fractures,* in which one bone is driven into the adjacent bone (e.g., occurs when the femoral condyle is driven into the softer tibial plateau), and (b) *compression fractures,* in which the articular surfaces of a bone approximate one another (e.g., compression fracture of the vertebral body). Like stress fractures, impaction fractures present as radiodense, not radiolucent, defects.
Incomplete	In this fracture, the fracture line radiographically appears not to traverse or penetrate the entire bone (periosteum may be intact); most often occurs in children in whom the soft, pliable bones bow in response to the applied force. Greenstick and torus are two examples of incomplete fractures (see entries in this table and also in Table 10-9).
Insufficiency (Fig. 10-13)	This is a stress fracture of diseased bone; that is, repeated application of normal loads resulting in an abnormal response of bone.
Intraarticular (Fig. 10-14)	An intraarticular fracture extends through the articular surface of a joint. Fractures that penetrate the joint may be complicated by the chondrolytic consequences of intraarticular blood.
Oblique	This is a fracture line that is oriented oblique to the long axis of the bone but does not exhibit a spiral path.
Occult	This is clinical, but not radiographic, evidence of fracture. Radiographic evidence usually develops within 1 to 2 weeks of injury.
Open (compound)	An open fracture penetrates the skin.
Pathologic (Figs. 10-15 and 10-16)	A pathologic fracture occurs in bone that has been weakened by disease. The disease may be localized (e.g., infection, tumor, disuse) or more generalized (e.g., osteogenesis imperfecta, osteoporosis, rickets, osteomalacia). Pathologic fractures often are oriented transverse to the long axis of the bone. An insufficiency fracture is a pathologic fracture that results from repeated application of normal subthreshold forces.
Pseudoarthrosis	Pseudoarthrosis describes the articulation that develops between bone fragments after nonunion.
Spiral (Fig. 10-17)	A spiral fracture is a fracture line that is obliquely oriented and coils around the long axis of the bone.
Stellate	Stellate describes a fracture seen in flat bones or the patella where the fracture lines extend radially from a central point.
Stress	There are two types of stress fractures: fatigue and insufficiency. *Fatigue fractures* result from repeated applications of abnormal stresses on bones of normal elastic resistance. *Insufficiency fractures* result from repeated application of normal stresses on bones of abnormal elastic resistance. Common stress fractures are listed in Table 10-2.
Torus (buckle)	A torus fracture is an incomplete fracture of long bones seen in children. It presents as a cortical bulge on the concave side of a bending long bone and is common in the distal radius.
Transverse	A transverse fracture line is oriented perpendicular to the long axis of the bone. Fracture of transverse orientation suggests underlying osseous pathology (e.g., Paget's disease, metastatic bone disease).
Unstable/Stable	A biomechanically unstable fracture tends to displace once it has been reduced nonsurgically and immobilized; a stable fracture does not. A neurologically unstable fracture has a propensity for neurologic insult.

PART TWO Bone, Joints, and Soft Tissues

Continued

TABLE 10-1 cont'd
Descriptive Terminology of Fractures

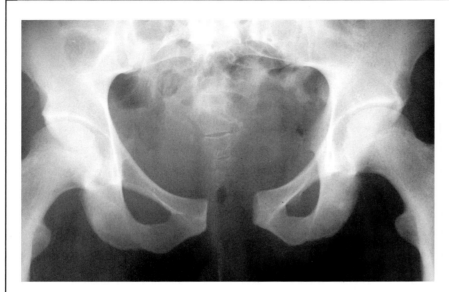

FIG. 10-10 A traumatic joint separation is termed a *diastatic* injury or fracture. This case exhibits pubic diastasis resulting from trauma. (Courtesy Steven P. Brownstein, MD, Springfield, NJ.)

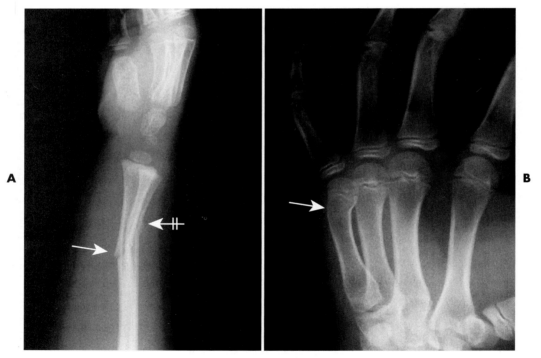

FIG. 10-11   A, Child with a greenstick fracture of the distal radius *(crossed arrow)* and torus fracture of the distal ulna *(arrow).* Both bones are posteriorly angulated without evidence that each fracture extends through the entire bone. **B,** Incomplete fracture of the fifth metacarpal denoting cortical disruption without clear fracture through the entire bone *(arrow).* (Courtesy Steven P. Brownstein, MD, Springfield, NJ.)

TABLE 10-1 cont'd

Descriptive Terminology of Fractures

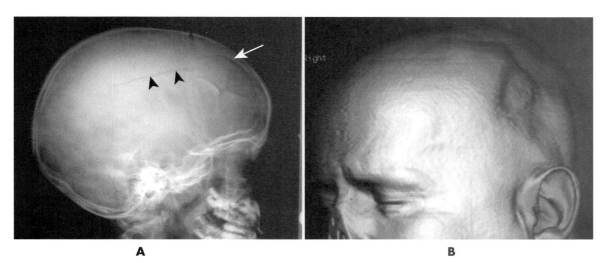

FIG. 10-12 A, Depression *(arrow)* and linear *(arrowheads)* fracture of the skull. **B,** In another example, the three-dimensional computed tomography reconstruction reveals an inward deformity of the skull. (**B,** Courtesy Sean Mathers, Pittsburgh, PA.)

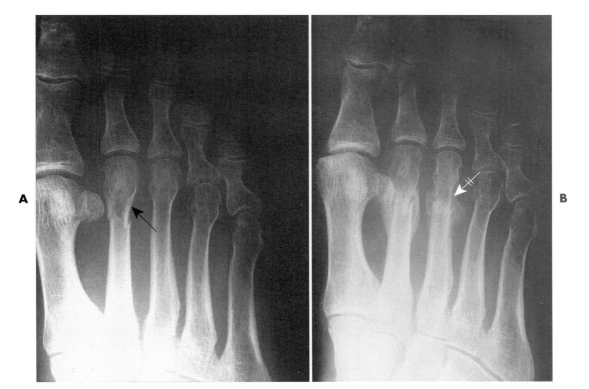

FIG. 10-13 A, This patient demonstrates advanced osteoporosis that has weakened the bone and promoted fracture of the shaft of the second metacarpal after trauma *(arrow).* **B,** Continued ambulation caused an insufficiency fracture of the third digit *(crossed arrow).* Repeated application of force on weakened bone (in this case the weakened bone is a result of osteoporosis) is termed an *insufficiency fracture.*

Continued

TABLE 10-1 cont'd
Descriptive Terminology of Fractures

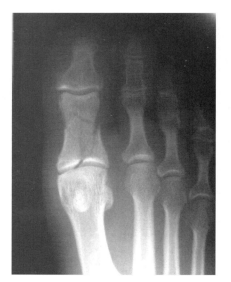

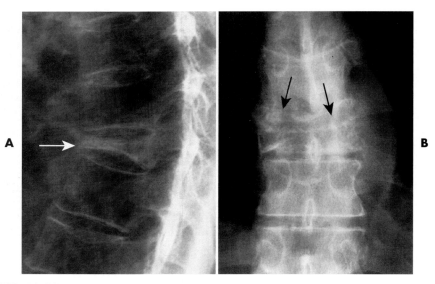

FIG. 10-14 Intraarticular comminuted fracture of the proximal phalanx of the big toe. Fractures are more clinically significant when they extend into the joint. Intraarticular fractures are associated with precocious degeneration, because the blood that is now free to enter the joint has a destructive effect on the cartilage of the joint.

FIG. 10-15 **A,** Lateral and, **B,** anteroposterior thoracic radiograph demonstrating pathologic compression fracture. **A,** Both the anterior and posterior body height is decreased. Further, **B,** the interpeduncular distance is widened *(arrows),* a sign of neurologic instability.

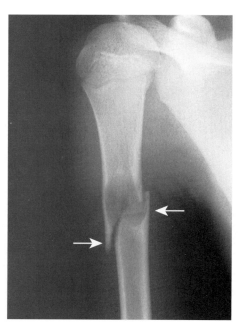

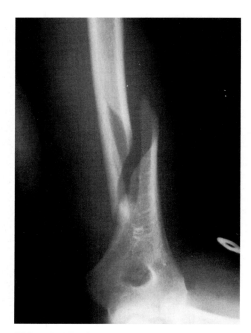

FIG. 10-16 Pathologic fracture through a simple bone cyst in the proximal diaphysis of the humerus *(arrows).* (Courtesy Steven P. Brownstein, MD, Springfield, NJ.)

FIG. 10-17 Spiral fracture of the distal humerus.

TABLE 10-2

Common Stress Fractures and Associated Causes[198]

Skeletal location	Related activities
Calcaneus (Fig. 10-18)	Jumping, parachuting, prolonged standing, recent immobilization
Cervical and thoracic vertebrae (spinous processes)	Shoveling action, classically clay shoveling
Femur (shaft and neck) (Fig. 10-19)	Ballet, long-distance running, marching, gymnastics
Fibula (shaft)	Long-distance running, jumping, parachuting
Hamate (hook)	Golfing, racquet sports, baseball batting
Humerus (distal shaft)	Throwing a ball
Lumbar vertebrae (pars interarticularis)	Ballet, weightlifting, football, scrubbing floors, lumbar hyperextension
Metatarsal shaft (Fig. 10-20)	Marching, prolonged standing, ballet
Navicular	Marching, long-distance running
Patella	Hurdling
Pelvis (obturator ring) (Fig. 10-21)	Stooping, bowling, gymnastics, ballet
Ribs (Fig. 10-22)	Carrying heavy pack, golfing, coughing
Scapulae (coracoid process)	Trapshooting
Sesamoid bones	Prolonged standing
Tibia (shaft) (Fig. 10-23)	Long-distance running
Ulna (coronoid process)	Pitching a ball, using a pitchfork, propelling a wheelchair

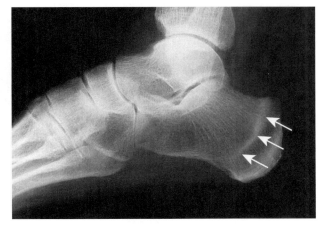

FIG. 10-18 Radiodense line traversing the posterior portion of the calcaneus representing a stress fracture (arrows).

Continued

TABLE 10-2 cont'd
Common Stress Fractures and Associated Causes

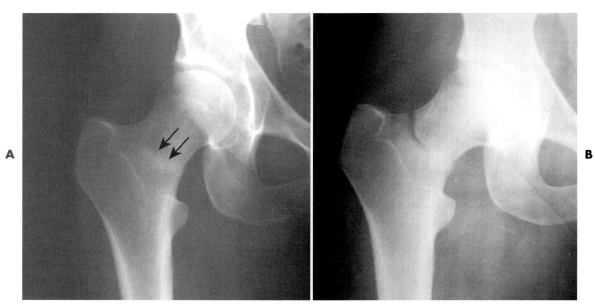

FIG. 10-19　A, Film demonstrates a radiodense line correlating to a stress fracture oriented parallel to the intertrochanteric line/crest *(arrows)*. **B,** A second film taken 1 month later shows a frank fracture of in the region. (Courtesy Steven P. Brownstein, MD, Springfield, NJ.)

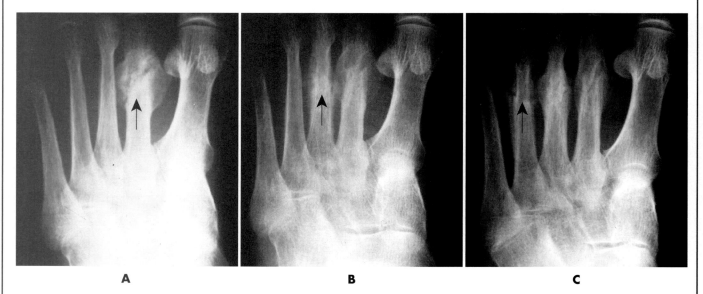

FIG. 10-20　Serial studies of stress fractures in one patient. **A,** The first film demonstrates one stress fracture of the second metatarsal's shaft. **B,** Nineteen days later, a second stress fracture is noted in the shaft of the third metatarsal *(arrow)*. **C,** Forty days after the second film, a third radiograph demonstrates another stress fracture in the fourth metatarsal *(arrow)*. (Courtesy Steven P. Brownstein, MD, Springfield, NJ.)

TABLE 10-2 cont'd
Common Stress Fractures and Associated Causes

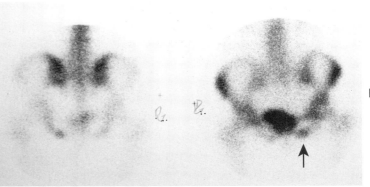

FIG. 10-21 Stress fracture of the reading right ischiopubic rami in a ballet dancer *(arrow)*. **A,** The plain film exhibits the defect and, **B,** the bone scan reveals a slight increase in the radiotracer *(arrow)*. (Courtesy Steven P. Brownstein, MD, Springfield, NJ.)

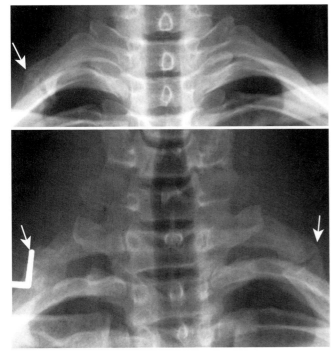

FIG. 10-22 A, Stress fracture of the *(reading left)* first rib *(arrow)*. **B,** Another patient exhibits bilateral first rib stress fractures *(arrows)* in an elite power lifter secondary to repetitive trauma related to the squatting lift (front squats).

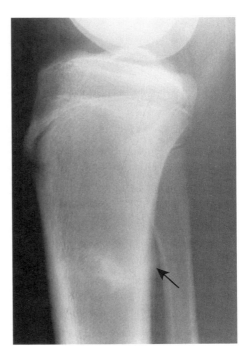

FIG. 10-23 Radiodense line indicating stress fracture extending into the posterior aspect of the proximal tibia *(arrow)*. (Courtesy Joseph W, Howe, Sylmar, CA.)

Continued

TABLE 10-3

Classifications of Epiphyseal Injuries (Salter-Harris I–V and Rang-Ogden VI–IX)*

Classification	Description and comments
Type I (Figs. 10-24 and 10-25)	Tansverse fracture through the physis. The physis is widened. Usually the widening is imperceptible on radiographs. No residual growth deformity is expected.
Type II (Fig. 10-26)	Transverse fracture through most of the physis and a small portion of the metaphysis. The separated portion of the metaphysis (known as a *Thurston-Holland fragment*) remains in contact with the epiphyseal fragment. It does not result in residual functional deficient of limb length. Type II is the most common Salter-Harris type.
Type III (Fig. 10-27)	Transverse fracture through a portion of the physis and a portion of the epiphysis. Because this fracture extends into the joint space, it can introduce blood with chondrolytic joint derangement from the hemarthrosis. Type III fractures pass through the hypertrophic layer of the physis, leading to damage of the reproductive layers of cartilage and resulting in possible growth retardation. Although serious consequences are possible, usually the type III fracture heals with little real deficit. Surgery may be required.
Type IV	Oblique or spiral fracture through the metaphysis, physis, and epiphysis. Along with the type III, the type IV fracture extends into the joint with possible joint destruction as a consequence of hemarthrosis. It may cause bone deformity of the bone growth by injuring the growing layers of the physis.
Type V	Compression injury of the physis with no associated fracture to the epiphysis or metaphysis. It may result in serious injury with common residual shortening of the involved limb because of injury to the growing layers of cartilage. Type V fractures are practically impossible to see with plain film radiography initially. Retrospectively they are suggested by the findings of limb shortening or premature closure of the physis. MRI, bone scan, or CT is warranted for initial detection.
Type VI	Rare injury to the perichondral elements (portion of physis shears off) promoting reactive bone formation.
Type VII	Injury to the epiphysis and articular cartilage without involving the adjacent physis or metaphysis (e.g., osteochondritis dissecans).
Type VIII	Rare injury exclusive to the metaphysis, with potential implications to endochondral bone formation.
Type IX	Rare injury to the periosteum, with potential implications to intramembranous bone growth.

*SALTR is a commonly applied mnemonic to remember the order of the first five classifications. The mnemonic only works if one visualizes a bone where the epiphysis is below the metaphysis (e.g., distal femur or radius in anatomic position). The SALTR letters stand for *simple*, *above*, *lower*, *together*, and *reduction* (of physis).

TABLE 10-3 cont'd

Classifications of Epiphyseal Injuries (Salter-Harris I–V and Rang-Ogden VI–IX)*

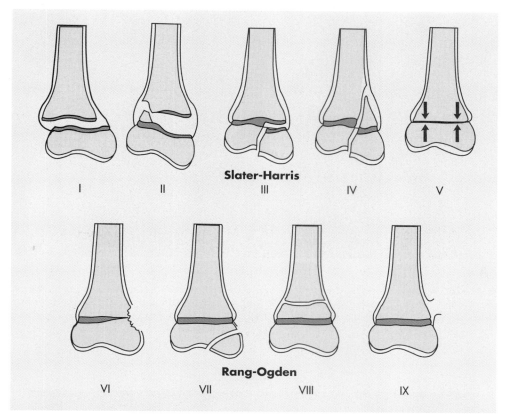

FIG. 10-24 Physeal injuries described by, *I* to *IV,* the Salter-Harris and, *VI* to *IX,* Rang-Ogden classifications, defined by, *I,* fracture through the physis; *II,* fracture through the physis and metaphysis; *III,* fracture through the physis and epiphysis; *IV,* fracture through the metaphysis, physis, and epiphysis; *V,* compression injury of the physis; *VI,* injury to the perichondrium; *VII,* osteochondritis dissecans; *VIII,* injury to the metaphysis; and, *IX,* injury to the periosteum.

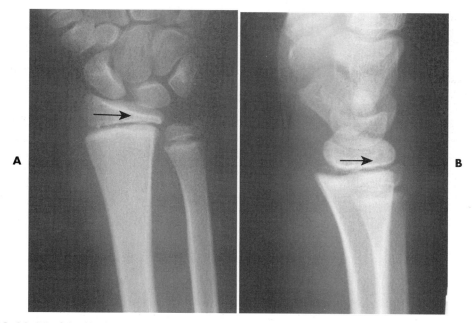

FIG. 10-25 Salter-Harris type I. **A,** The posteroanterior and, **B,** lateral projections of the wrist demonstrate medial and posterior translation of the epiphysis (direction noted by the *arrows*) consistent with a type I fracture. (Courtesy Kevin Cunningham, Eldridge, IA.)

Continued

TABLE 10-3 cont'd
Classifications of Epiphyseal Injuries (Salter-Harris I–V and Rang-Ogden VI–IX)*

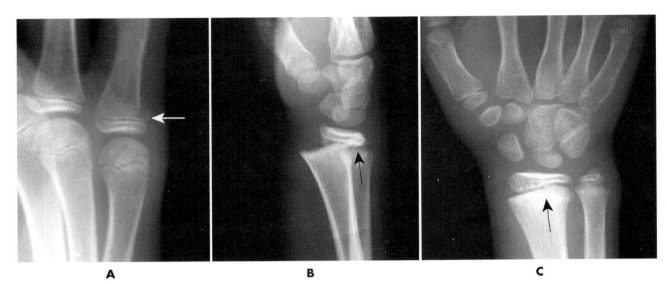

FIG. 10-26 A, Salter-Harris type II fracture at the base of the proximal phalanx of the fifth digit *(arrow).* **B** and **C,** A second case is noted of the distal radius, with a metaphyseal fragment *(arrows)* consistent with a Salter-Harris type II fracture. (Courtesy Steven P. Brownstein, MD, Springfield, NJ.)

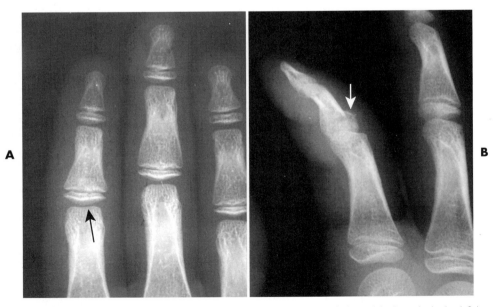

FIG. 10-27 Salter-Harris type III fracture. **A,** There is a subtle defect of the epiphysis and physis defining a Salter-Harris type III fracture *(arrow).* **B,** The fracture is better seen on the oblique projection *(arrow),* although it is difficult to categorize from this angle.

TABLE 10-4

Fractures of the Skull and Face

Fracture	Comments
Skull	
Basilar skull fracture	Results from a blow to front of skull; difficult to detect with plain film radiography. As is the case with all skull and face fractures, CT is usually needed to demonstrate the injury. The air-fluid level or opacification of sphenoid sinus is the most reliable sign of basilar skull fractures.[201]
Depressed fracture (see Fig. 10-12)	Results from an impact injury to the cranial vault causing depression of fragments, and represents 15% of all skull fractures; usually it is located in the frontoparietal area. Thirty-three percent are associated with dural tears that are suggested when fragments are depressed beyond 5 mm of the skull surface or beyond the level of the inner table.[241] The plasticity of a child's skull allows depression without obvious fracture, known as a *ping-pong fracture.*
Diastatic fracture (see Fig. 10-10)	A diastatic fracture results from trauma that causes widening of the cranial sutures, and accounts for 5% of skull fractures,[100] most commonly lambdoid and sagittal sutures. They often are associated with, or are extensions of, linear fractures.
Leptomeningeal cyst	Represents fracture complication resulting from arachnoid mater extending through a tear in the dural mater, into a skull fracture. The pulsatility of the cerebrospinal fluid may inhibit fracture healing and, at times, erode the perimeter of the fracture, giving the appearance of a "growing fracture."
Linear fracture	A linear fracture represents a lucent line of several centimeters, and represents 80% of all skull fractures; usually occurs in the parietal or temporal bone and may cross sutures and vascular grooves. It does not exhibit a branching pattern as is seen with normal vascular channels.[204]
Pneumocephalus	Pneumocephalus is a fracture complication resulting from air in the subarachnoid space. Trauma to the walls of the air-filled paranasal sinus or mastoid air cells permits dissection of air into the subarachnoid space. Other causes include infection, neoplasm, or surgery.
Face	
LeFort fractures (Fig. 10-28)	LeFort fractures occur along three planes of weakness in the facial skeleton. All types are unstable, bilateral, involve the pterygoid processes, and separate a fragment of bone from the face. LeFort type fracture I is a transverse fracture through the maxilla separating the upper dentition from the rest of the head (floating palate).[63] LeFort type fracture II is an oblique fracture through the maxilla separating a pyramid-shaped segment of the midface.[62] LeFort type fracture III is a nearly vertical fracture through the nasal bones and septum, maxilla, and orbits completely separating the face from the skull.[62]
Mandible fracture	A mandible fracture is the third most common facial fracture (after nasal and maxilla), usually occurring in the body (40%), angle (30%), and condyloid process (20%) of the mandible,[158] presenting bilaterally[17,247] and often is multiple. Mandible fractures are seen well with CT or a panoramic projection with linear tomography. Physical assault and automobile accidents account for 80% of mandibular fractures.[17,158]
Nasal bone fracture (Figs. 10-29 and 10-30)	Fracture of the nasal bones are the most frequent facial fracture.[122,218] They nearly always exhibit a transverse orientation. Fragments usually are depressed and displaced. Nasofrontal sutures or longitudinal grooves often are mistaken for fractures.
Orbital fracture (Fig. 10-31)	Orbital fracture occurs as an isolated fracture to the rim or walls (blowout) of the orbit, or as components of more complex tripod or LeFort fractures. Orbital floor fractures may be complicated by entrapment of the inferior rectus and inferior oblique muscles. Medial wall fractures may be complicated by entrapment of the medial rectus. Closed cavity traumas correlate to eye injuries. Open cavity injuries have a risk of infection via communication with the sinuses.
Tripod (trimalar) fracture (Fig. 10-32)	Conflicting reports exist as to whether the tripod fracture is the most common fracture of the face[204] or second most common fracture of the face (following nasal bones).[122,218] The term *tripod* is used to describe the three limbs of the zygoma that are fractured, separating the zygoma from its frontal, temporal, and maxillary attachments by a direct blow to the malar prominence.[138] They are isolated and usually comminuted. Fractures of the zygomatic arch are caused commonly by a direct blow to the side of the face.

Continued

TABLE 10-4 cont'd
Fractures of the Skull and Face

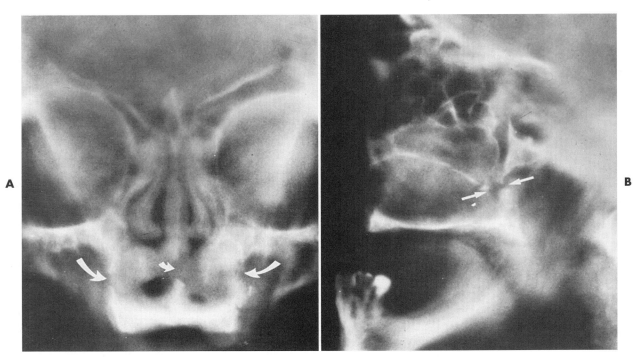

FIG. 10-28   A, Coronal multidirectional tomogram shows a LeFort I fracture *(arrows).* **B,** Lateral multidirectional tomogram shows a LeFort I fracture. The extension of the fracture through the pterygoid plates is seen *(arrows).* From Som PM, Bergeron RT: Head and neck imaging, ed 2, St Louis, 1991, Mosby.)

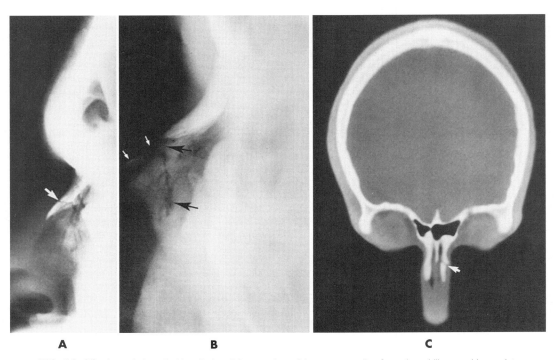

FIG. 10-29   Lateral view. **A,** Nondisplaced fracture *(arrow)* is seen extending from the midline nasal bones laterally. **B,** Lateral view shows comminuted nasal bone fracture *(small arrows)* with extension of the fracture into the lateral nasal bones and frontal processes of the maxilla *(large arrows).* **C,** Coronal computed tomography scan shows isolated minimally depressed left nasal fracture *(arrow).* (From Som PM, Bergeron RT: Head and neck imaging, ed 2, St Louis, 1991, Mosby.)

TABLE 10-4 cont'd
Fractures of the Skull and Face

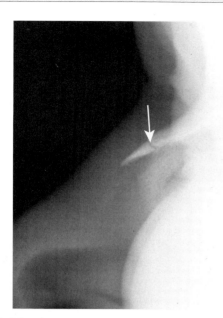

FIG. 10-30 Nondisplaced fracture of the nasal bone (arrow). (Courtesy Patty Litwiler-Britt, East Moline, IL.)

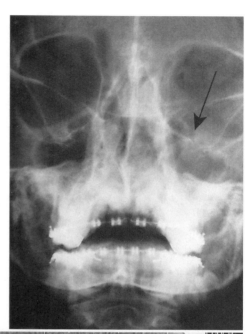

A

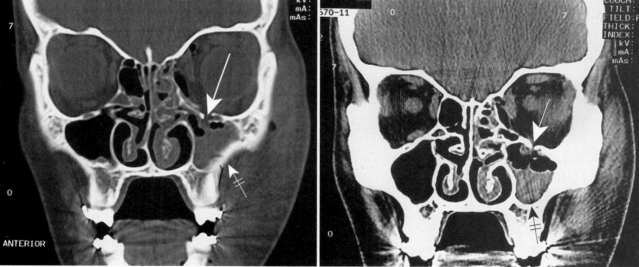

B   **C**

FIG. 10-31 Fracture of the orbital floor (arrow) seen on, **A**, plain film; **B**, bone; and, **C**, soft-tissue computed tomography windows. The left maxillary sinus is opacified secondary to accumulations of blood and edema (crossed arrows). (Courtesy Jack C. Avalos, Davenport, IA.)

Continued

PART TWO
Bone, Joints, and Soft Tissues

TABLE 10-4 cont'd
Fractures of the Skull and Face

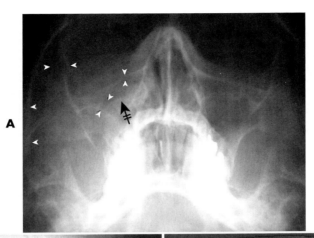

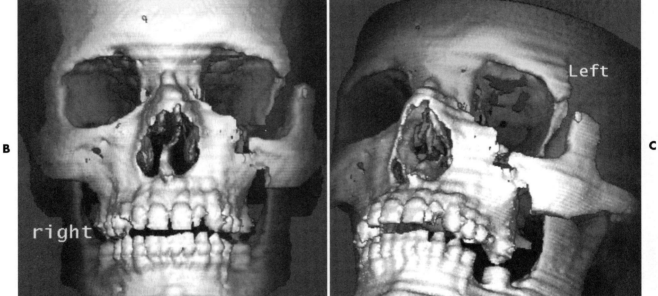

FIG. 10-32 Tripod fractures. **A,** Fracture of the orbit with filling of the maxillary sinus *(crossed arrow)* on plain film. All three limbs (frontal, temporal, and maxillary) of the zygoma are involved *(arrowheads)*, designating this as a tripod fracture. **B** and **C,** Another patient exhibits a tripod fracture of his left side, detailed very well with these three-dimensional reconstructions of the computed tomography scan. (**A,** Courtesy Gary Longmuir, Phoenix, AZ; **B** and **C,** Courtesy Sean Mathers, Pittsburgh, PA.)

TABLE 10-5

Fractures and Dislocations of the Cervical Spine

Injury	Comments
Fractures	
Occipital condyle fracture	A combination of axial compression and lateral bending may result in avulsion or compression fractures of the occipital condyles. These injuries are associated with cranial nerve deficits. This area of complex anatomy is difficult to visualize on plain film, requiring CT to determine if fracture is present.
Atlas posterior arch fracture (Fig. 10-33)	Fracture of the posterior arch of the atlas is defined by vertical fractures secondary to a cervical hyperextension injury and resulting compression of the weaker posterior arch of the atlas between the larger anatomic structures of the spinous process of C2 and occiput. Generally the mechanism of cervical trauma provides a clue to the type of resultant injury (Box 10-2). The fracture line is seen on the lateral cervical view, and the anteroposterior (AP) open-mouth projection appears normal. Because the transverse atlantal ligament and anterior arch of the atlas are intact, posterior arch fractures are stable and generally without risk of neurologic deficit. They are the most common fractures of the atlas.[223]
Jefferson's fracture (Figs. 10-34 through 10-38)	A Jefferson's fracture is a bursting fracture of the atlas involving both the posterior and anterior arches secondary to an axial force.[120] It is indicated by lateral offset of lateral masses on the C2 articulations as seen in the frontal projection. Offset of more than 7 mm may indicate rupture of the transverse atlantal ligament and resulting instability (Box 10-3),[204] a common accompanying injury and strong positive predictor of associated neurologic involvement. There is usually a marked distention of the precervical soft tissue as noted on the lateral cervical projection. At times its diagnosis may be missed because of lack of marked neurologic signs, or the AP open-mouth radiograph, which is typically pathognomonic for the diagnosis, is often inadequate or not obtained.[129]
Odontoid process fracture (Figs. 10-39 through 10-43)	Odontoid fractures represent about 50% of all C2 fractures[204] and are divided into three types based on location. Type I is an avulsion of the tip of the odontoid process. Type II is a transverse fracture at the base of the odontoid process and is the most common type. Type III is a fracture of the C2 body, below the base of the odontoid process. Type I is mechanically stable. Type II often is associated with nonunion because of poor regional blood supply. Types II and III may result in cord compression from posterior migration of the odontoid fragment directly, or from the resulting guillotine effect on the cord from the anterior translation of the posterior arch of the atlas.
Hangman's fracture (traumatic spondylolisthesis) (Figs. 10-44 through 10-46)	Hangman's fracture describes a bilateral fracture of the posterior arch of axis, usually the pedicles or pars interarticularis (fracture to the latter is also termed *traumatic spondylolisthesis*).[212] Hangman's fracture occurs from cervical hyperextension, usually from a car accident, although the historic example is hanging a person at the gallows (hence the name). Hangman's fractures represent about 25%[204] of all C2 fractures, and are difficult to detect radiographically at times. They typically result in anterior displacement of C2 on C3 that can be classified into three types: type 1 is minimal to 3 mm of anterior displacement with no evidence of focal kyphosis; type 2 is more than 3 mm of anterior displacement and focal kyphosis; type 2a is severe angulation but less than 3 mm anterior displacement; and type 3 is severe angulation and unilateral or bilateral dislocation of the C2-3 facets.[145] Generally displacement of more than 3 mm indicates instability; cord compression is a concern, but does not commonly realize because the spinal canal is maintained or enlarged.[167] Angiography to detect intimal injury of the vertebral arteries, and possibly anticoagulation therapy, may be necessary when the fracture involves the transverse foramina.[167]
Teardrop fracture (Figs. 10-47 and 10-48)	Teardrop fractures most often occur at C2, produced from hyperflexion or hyperextension forces that avulse and displace a small, usually triangular segment, of the inferior, less commonly superior, vertebral body.[18] Although both the flexion and extension mechanisms are serious injuries, the flexion injury disrupts the posterior ligament system, promotes instability, and is more often associated with neurologic deficient, resulting in acute anterior cord syndrome in nearly 90% of cases.[103] The extension teardrop fracture involves the anterior longitudinal ligament and anterior annulus fibrosis, yet the posterior ligament system remains intact; therefore it is a stable injury with flexion and unstable with extension.

Continued

TABLE 10-5 cont'd
Fractures and Dislocations of the Cervical Spine

BOX 10-2
Types of Forces Applied to the Cervical Spine
and Resultant Injury

Rotational hyperflexion mechanism
- Facet dislocation (unilateral or bilateral)
- Wedged compression fracture

Hyperextension mechanism
- Posterior arch fracture
- Hangman's fracture

Hyperflexion or hyperextension mechanism
- Teardrop fracture
- Spinous process fracture
- Odontoid process fracture

Lateral flexion mechanism
- Transverse process fracture
- Uncinate process fracture

Axial compression mechanism
- Burst fracture of atlas (Jefferson's fracture)
- Burst or vertical fractures of C2-C7

BOX 10-3
Listing of Selected Cervical Injuries from Most
Unstable to Most Stable[246]

1. Transverse atlantal ligament rupture
2. Odontoid fracture (type II)
3. Flexion teardrop
4. Bilateral facet dislocation
5. Burst fracture (intact posterior ligaments)
6. Hangman's fracture
7. Extension teardrop
8. Jefferson's fracture
9. Unilateral facet dislocation
10. Compression fracture of the vertebral body (stability depends on severity of compression and any posterior migration of fragments)
11. Pillar fracture
12. Posterior arch of atlas fracture
13. Clay shoveler's fracture

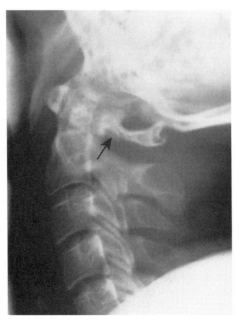

FIG. 10-33   Linear fracture of the posterior arch of the atlas. (Courtesy Tim Mick, St Paul, MN.)

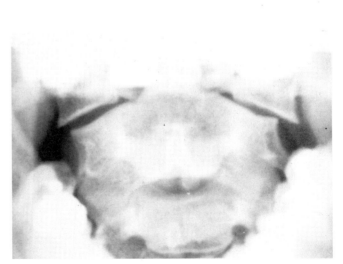

FIG. 10-34   Jefferson's fracture. This anteroposterior open-mouth projection demonstrates a Jefferson's fracture noted by lateral overhanging of the lateral mass beyond the lateral margins of the C2 superior articular processes. (Courtesy Gary Longmuir, Phoenix, AZ.)

TABLE 10-5 cont'd
Fractures and Dislocations of the Cervical Spine

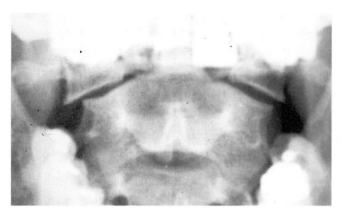

FIG. 10-35   Jefferson's fracture. Note the overhanging margins of the lateral masses of the atlas. (Courtesy Steven P. Brownstein, MD, Springfield, NJ.)

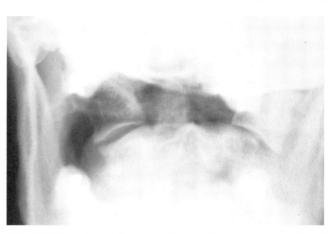

FIG. 10-36   Jefferson's fracture. A 67-year-old woman who experienced an axial force secondary to a fall, and now demonstrates several millimeters of offset along the right atlantoaxial margin, consistent with a Jefferson's fracture.

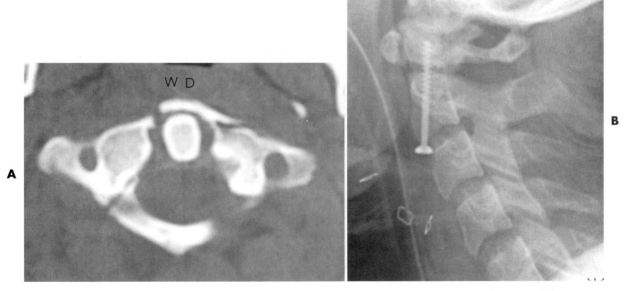

FIG. 10-37   A, Jefferson's fracture noted by defects of the anterior and posterior arches of the expanded circumference of the atlas. This 20-year-old man also sustained an odontoid fracture from the same injury. **B,** The odontoid fracture was repaired with surgical fixation. (Courtesy Sean Mathers, Pittsburgh, PA.)

PART TWO   Bone, Joints, and Soft Tissues

Continued

TABLE 10-5 cont'd

Fractures and Dislocations of the Cervical Spine

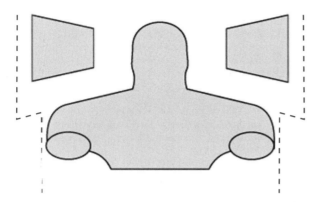

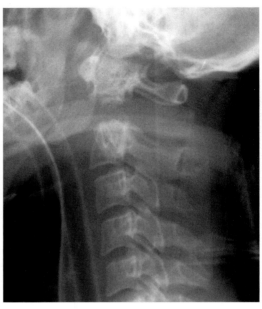

FIG. 10-38 Jefferson's fracture is indicated by lateral displacement of the lateral masses on the anteroposterior open-mouth projection (*dotted lines*). Normally, in the adult patient, the lateral lower margins of the lateral masses do not extend past the lateral upper margins of the superior articular processes of C2.

FIG. 10-39 Lateral cervical radiograph exhibiting a fracture at the base of the odontoid process (type II) and resulting anterior displacement of the atlas.

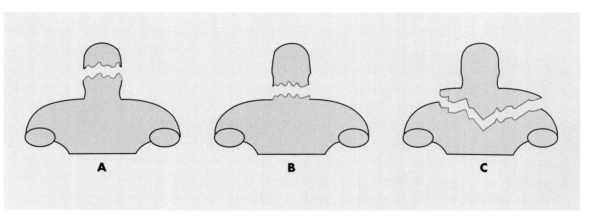

FIG. 10-40 Odontoid fracture are classified as, **A,** type I (upper odontoid); **B,** type II (base of the odontoid); and, **C,** type III (extends into the body of the C2 segment).

TABLE 10-5 cont'd

TABLE 10-5 cont'd
Fractures and Dislocations of the Cervical Spine

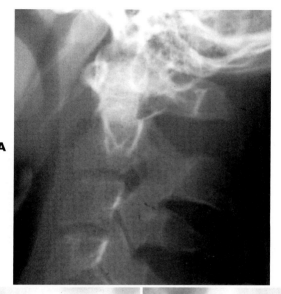

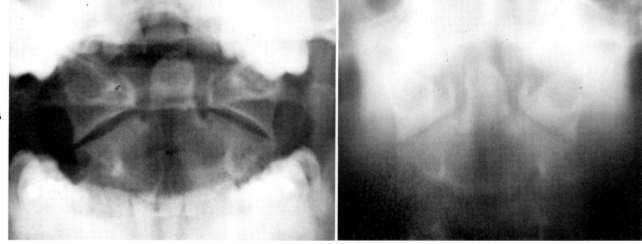

FIG. 10-41 A, Type II fracture of the base of the odontoid process with anterior displacement of the atlas. **B,** The anteroposterior projection does not reveal a clear defect on the plain film study; however, **C,** the linear tomography scan details a clear defect at the base of the odontoid. (Courtesy Steven P. Brownstein, MD, Springfield, NJ.)

Continued

TABLE 10-5 cont'd
Fractures and Dislocations of the Cervical Spine

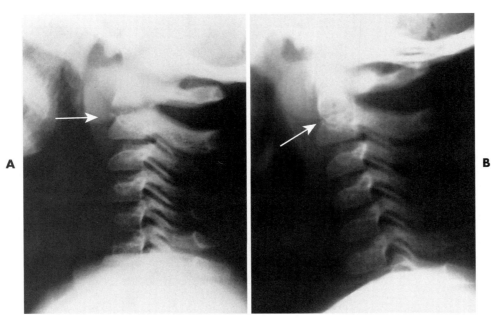

FIG. 10-42 **A,** Initial film demonstrating a type II odontoid fracture *(arrow)*. **B,** The fracture line is less prominent one month later *(arrow)*. (Courtesy Jack C. Avalos, Davenport, IA.)

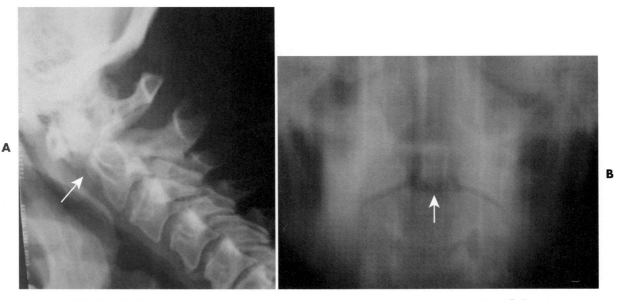

FIG. 10-43 Type II odontoid fracture demonstrated on, **A,** the flexion lateral cervical radiograph and, **B,** frontal linear tomography scan *(arrows)*.

TABLE 10-5 cont'd
Fractures and Dislocations of the Cervical Spine

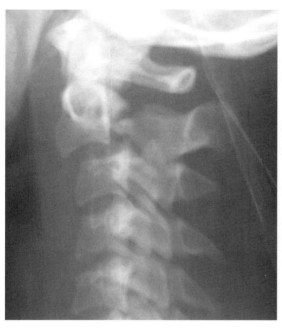

FIG. 10-44 Hangman's fracture noted through the articular pillar of C2, accompanied by anterior translation of the C2 body.

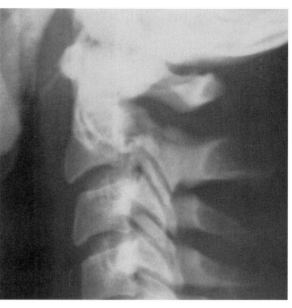

FIG. 10-45 Hangman's fracture appearing as a disrupted articular pillar of C2, anterior translation of C2, and retropulsion of the fracture posterior arch noted by the offset of the spinolaminar line.

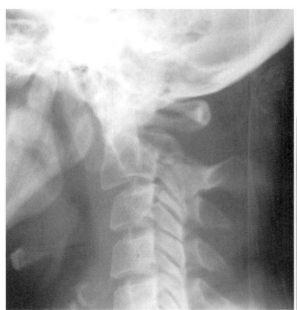

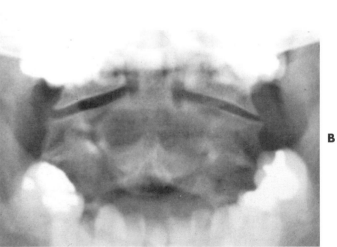

FIG. 10-46 **A,** Hangman's fracture through the articular pillar of C2 and, **B,** subtle radiolucent defect in the frontal projection. (Courtesy Steven P. Brownstein, MD, Springfield, NJ.)

Continued

PART TWO Bone, Joints, and Soft Tissues

TABLE 10-5 cont'd
Fractures and Dislocations of the Cervical Spine

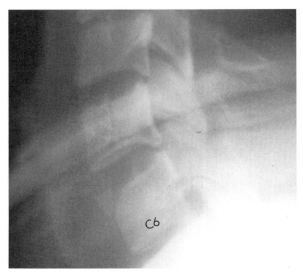

FIG. 10-47   Teardrop fracture of the anterior superior margin of C6. (Courtesy Robert Tatum, Davenport, IA.)

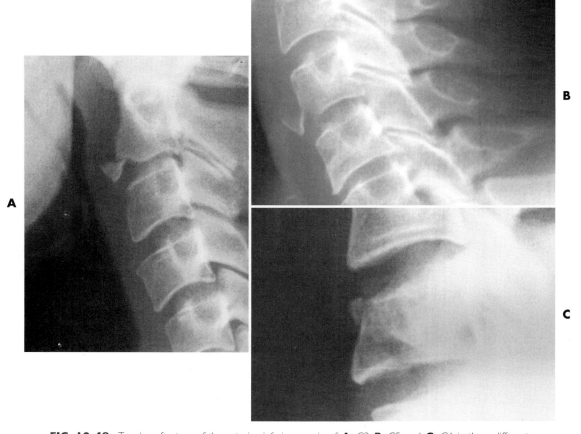

FIG. 10-48   Teardrop fracture of the anterior inferior margin of, **A,** C2; **B,** C5; and, **C,** C6 in three different cases. (**A,** Courtesy Robert Tatum, Davenport, IA. **B,** Courtesy Steven P. Brownstein, MD, Springfield, NJ.)

TABLE 10-5 cont'd
Fractures and Dislocations of the Cervical Spine

Injury	Comments
Articular pillar fracture (Fig. 10-49)	Fracture of the articular pillar usually follows a hyperextension and rotation injury. Most commonly it occurs at the C6 and C7 levels. In the lateral cervical projection, the articular pillar may appear as a double shadow ("double outline" sign), also a feature of unilateral facet dislocation.
Burst fracture (Figs. 10-50 and 10-51)	A burst fracture is a compression fracture in which axial loads drive portions of the intervertebral disc into the adjacent vertebra, producing a comminuted, circumferentially expanded fracture that may demonstrate posterior displacement of fracture fragments into the vertebral canal, often producing neurologic deficits.[6] These fractures usually have a sagittal component,[130] and often demonstrate an increased interpeduncular distance in the frontal projection.[6] Nearly 50% occur at the L1 level.[6]
Clay shoveler's fracture (coal shoveler's) (Figs. 10-52 through 10-56)	Clay shoveler's fracture is an oblique avulsion of the spinous process, occurring at the level of C6-T1. It is best seen in the lateral projection, and appears as a "double-spinous" sign in the AP projection. Irregularity and distraction of the fragment differentiate fracture from nonunion of secondary growth center of the spinous process that often occurs at lower cervical levels, or dystrophic calcification of the nuchal ligament (nuchal bones).

Dislocations

Injury	Comments
Atlantoaxial dislocation (Fig. 10-57)	An atlantoaxial dislocation results from acquired or congenital damage of the transverse atlantal ligament that produces anterior translation of the atlas, producing a guillotine effect on the cord. When trauma is the cause, the force is typically from hyperflexion. Atlantoaxial dislocation is indicated radiographically by an atlantodental interval larger than 3 mm in adults or 5 mm in children.
Atlantooccipital dislocation	Dislocation of the atlantooccipital joint is rare, usually occurring secondary to cervical hyperextension injury. An anterior direction of dislocation is most common, and usually results in immediate death from respiratory failure associated with brainstem injury.
Facet dislocation (Figs. 10-58 through 10-64)	Unilateral facet dislocation usually is a stable lesion resulting from a flexion rotation injury. It occurs most often at a C4 to C7 level. The dislocated inferior facet appears "locked" or "perched" anterior to the superior articular process of the segment below. The articular pillars of the dislocated segment simulate a "bow tie" appearance in the oblique projection and "fanning" spinous processes in the lateral projection; decreased range of motion, accompanying fractures (e.g., pillar fracture),[18] and radicular symptoms may be present.[268] Bilateral facet dislocation is a usually unstable lesion resulting from a hyperflexion injury. It occurs most often at the C4 to C7 level. In the lateral projection, bilateral facet dislocation exhibits "fanning" of the spinous processes, narrowed disc space and anterolisthesis usually are evident, and cord damage is common.[103] Bilateral and unilateral dislocation have a similar incidence rate.[88] However, unilateral facet dislocation is more likely to present to private chiropractic, orthopedic, or other nonemergent practice settings.

Continued

TABLE 10-5 cont'd
Fractures and Dislocations of the Cervical Spine

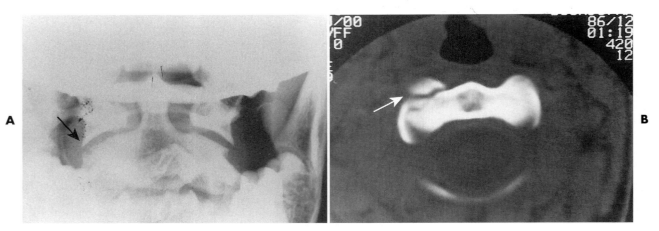

FIG. 10-49 **A,** Plain film and, **B,** computed tomography of a fracture through the articular pillar of C2. (Courtesy Tim Mick, St Paul, MN.)

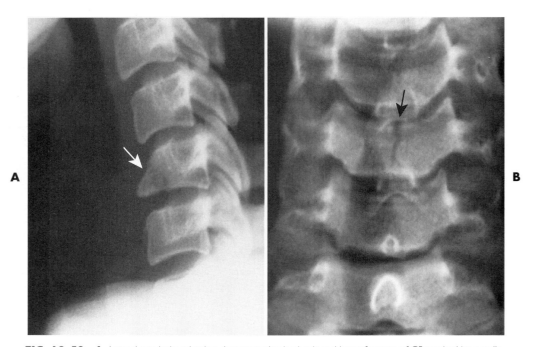

FIG. 10-50 **A,** Lateral cervical projection demonstrating kyphosis and burst fracture of C5 marked by a radiolucent fracture extending through the anterior lower margin of the vertebrae *(arrow)*. **B,** In the frontal projection, the lucent fracture line is noted to extend vertically through the C5 vertebra *(arrow)*.

TABLE 10-5 cont'd
Fractures and Dislocations of the Cervical Spine

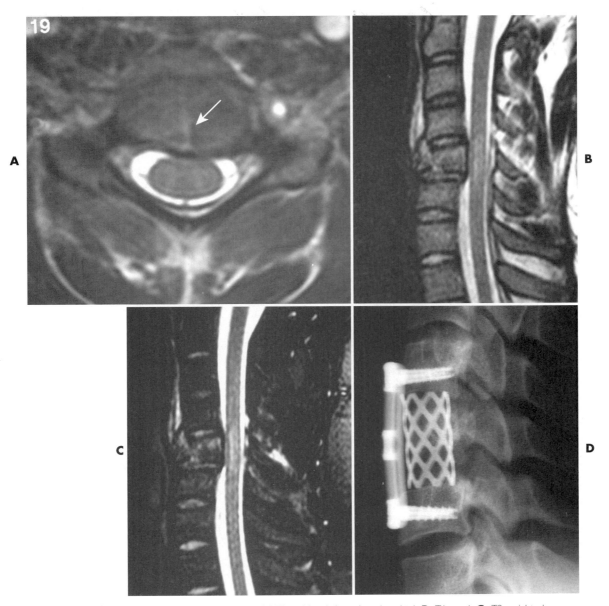

FIG. 10-51 **A,** Burst fracture seen on axial T2-weighted *(arrow)* and sagittal, **B,** T1- and, **C,** T2-weighted magnetic resonance imaging scans. Note the slight sagittal plane defect and expansion. **D,** The resulting segmental instability necessitated anterior cervical fusion, with plate and cage.

Continued

TABLE 10-5 cont'd
Fractures and Dislocations of the Cervical Spine

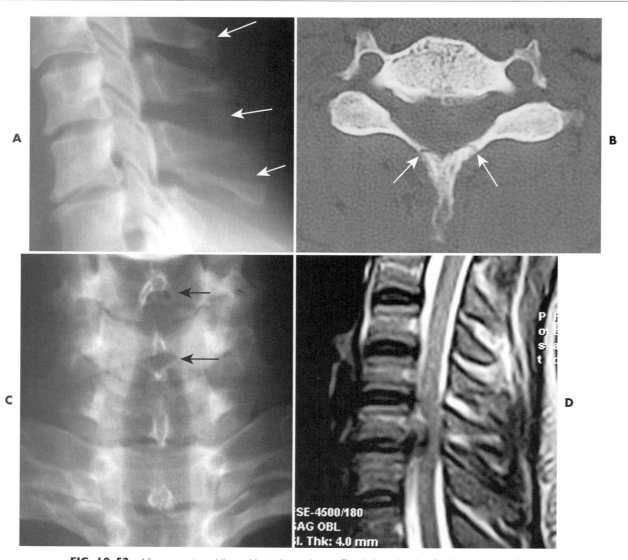

FIG. 10-52 After an automobile accident, the patient suffered three levels of spinous process fracture. **A,** The lateral plain film reveals defects at C5, C6, and C7 *(arrows)*. **B,** At the C6 level, the defect is noted extending into the lamina bilaterally *(arrows)*. **C,** A spinous process fracture often presents with a "double-spinous" sign because of the offset of the spinous process fragment and the remaining base of the spinous process. **A** through **C,** The plain films and noncontrasted computed tomography images do not reveal the degree of spinal stenosis. **D,** Magnetic resonance imaging scans demonstrate the degree of soft-tissue injury and spinal stenosis. (Courtesy Robert Rowell, Davenport, IA.)

TABLE 10-5 cont'd
Fractures and Dislocations of the Cervical Spine

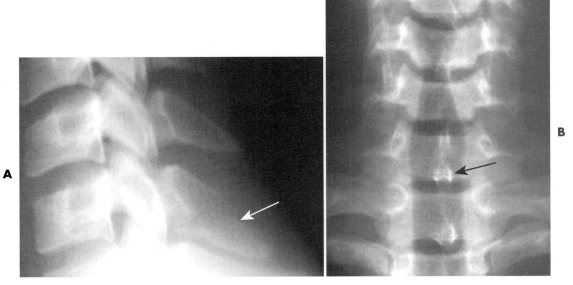

FIG. 10-53 Acute Clay shoveler's fracture of the C6 vertebra, appearing with inferior displacement of the distal fragment on, **A,** the lateral and, **B,** anteroposterior projection *(arrows)*.

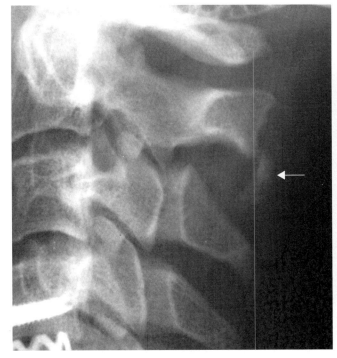

FIG. 10-54 Acute fracture of the C2 spinous process *(arrow)*.

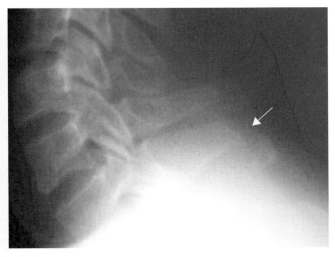

FIG. 10-55 Clay shoveler's fracture of the C7 spinous process *(arrow)*. The corticated margins of the fractured fragment indicate that the fracture is not acute. This chronic fracture is differentiated from an unossified apophysis by the fact that it is inferiorly displaced.

PART TWO
Bone, Joints, and Soft Tissues

Continued

TABLE 10-5 cont'd
Fractures and Dislocations of the Cervical Spine

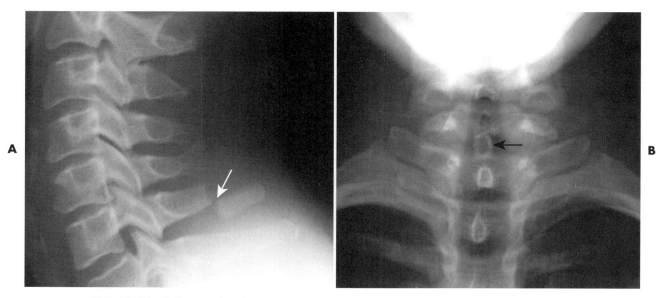

FIG. 10-56   **A,** Fracture of the C6 spinous process with, **B,** an obvious double projection of the spinous process on the anteroposterior projection. (**A,** Courtesy Steven P. Brownstein, MD, Springfield, NJ.)

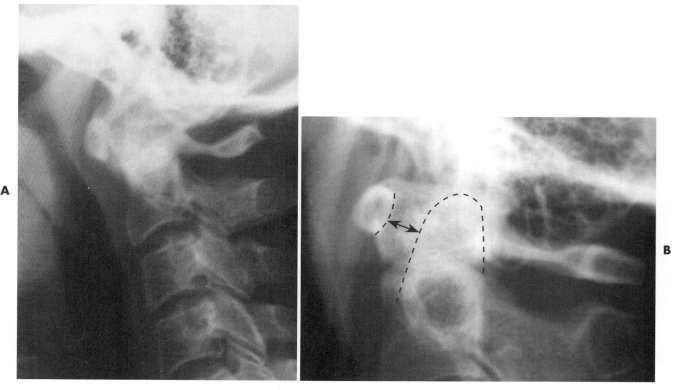

FIG. 10-57   **A** and **B,** Enlarged atlantodental interval indicating atlantoaxial instability in two cases *(arrows).*

TABLE 10-5 cont'd

Fractures and Dislocations of the Cervical Spine

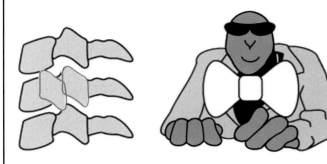

FIG. 10-58 Unilateral facet dislocation presents with axial rotation of the dislocated segment that produces a double shadow of the articular pillars in the lateral projection. The double shadow appearance has been likened to the configuration of a bow tie.

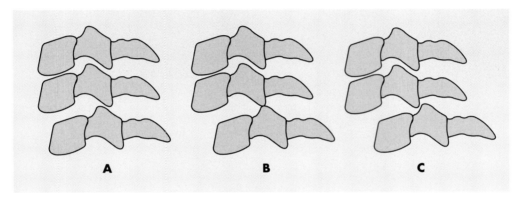

A   **B**   **C**

FIG. 10-59 The degree of facet dislocation is expressed as, **A,** partial dislocation; **B,** perched facets; and, **C,** complete dislocation.

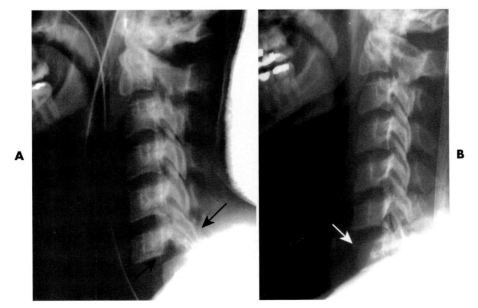

FIG. 10-60 **A,** This film taken on a backboard and exhibiting some motion reveals a frank bilateral dislocation of the facets of C6-7 *(arrows).* **B,** The second film is taken after reduction of the dislocation. The second film also demonstrates a small teardrop fracture of C7 *(arrow).* (Courtesy Steven P. Brownstein, MD, Springfield, NJ.)

Continued

TABLE 10-5 cont'd

Fractures and Dislocations of the Cervical Spine

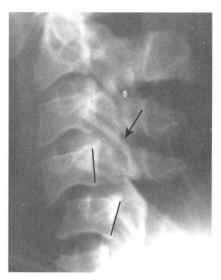

FIG. 10-61 Unilateral facet dislocation at C4-5. The rotated C4 segment causes an offset of the articular pillars in the lateral projection. The offset appearance has been likened to a bow tie ("bow tie sign") *(arrow)*.

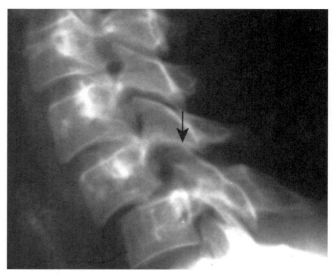

FIG. 10-62 Partial bilateral dislocation of the C5-6 facets. A portion of the facets remain in articulation *(arrow)*. (Courtesy Steven P. Brownstein, MD, Springfield, NJ.)

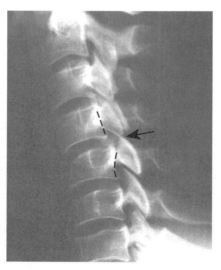

FIG. 10-63 Unilateral facet dislocation noted by an interruption of the facet alignment at the C4-5 level *(arrow)*. (Courtesy Julie-Marthe Grenier, Port Orange, FL.)

TABLE 10-5 cont'd
Fractures and Dislocations of the Cervical Spine

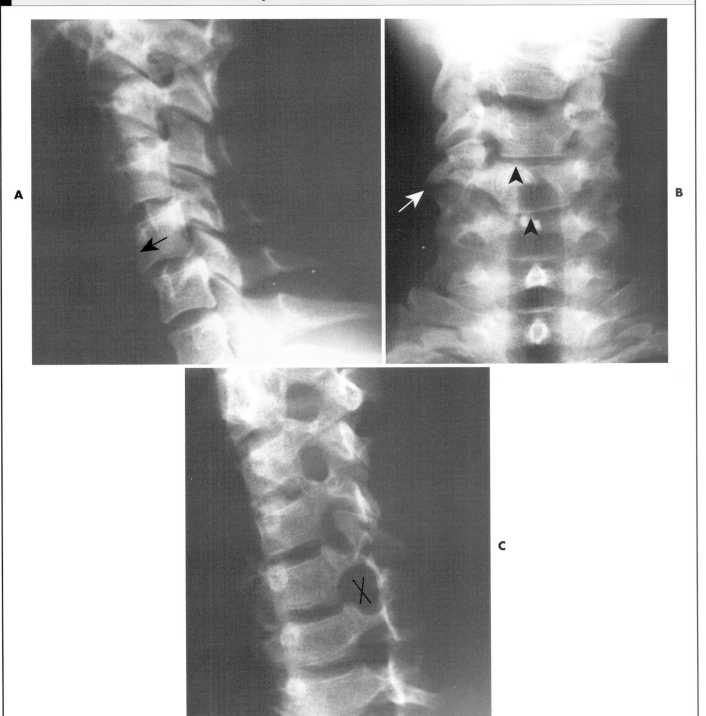

FIG. 10-64 Unilateral facet dislocation of C5 on C6. **A,** The lateral film appears normal, except for a slight anterior translation of C5 *(arrow)*. **B,** The anteroposterior lower cervical projection exhibits lateral deviation of the spinous process *(arrowheads)* and irregular appearance of the right articular pillar *(arrow)*. **C,** The oblique projection illustrates an enlarged intervertebral foramen *(X)*. (Courtesy Julie-Marthe Grenier, Port Orange, FL.)

PART TWO Bone, Joints, and Soft Tissues

Continued

TABLE 10-6

Cervical Acceleration-Deceleration Syndrome or "Whiplash Syndrome"

Injury	Comments
Cervical "whiplash" syndrome or cervical acceleration-deceleration syndrome (CADS) (Figs. 10-65 through 10-68)	*Whiplash* is a medicolegal term first used by Crowe in 1928 to describe the effects of rapid acceleration-deceleration mechanism of energy transfer to the neck.[48] It may result in bony or soft-tissue injuries. According to the Quebec Task Force,[227] there are four grades of whiplash injury:

0: No complaint about the neck
I: Neck complaint of pain and stiffness, no signs
II: Neck complaint, musculoskeletal signs
III: Neck complaint, neurologic signs
IV: Neck complaint plus fracture or dislocation

Imaging assessment of the cervical trauma patient begins with plain film radiography. Generally clues to cervical spine injury include obvious fracture or dislocation, axial rotation of a vertebra, increased atlantodental interval beyond 3 mm (>5 mm in children), loss or reversal of the normal cervical lordosis, acute angular kyphosis, interspinous process gapping, widened retropharyngeal space (>6 mm at C2), widened retrotracheal space (>22 mm at C6), displacement of the prevertebral fat stripe, lateral tracheal deviation, and soft-tissue emphysema. The S-shape curvature—defined as hypolordosis in the upper region and kyphosis in the lower region of the sagittal cervical curvature—of the cervical spine has been qualitatively associated with whiplash injuries; however, it has not been subjected to detailed quantitative analyses.[96] Griffiths found high sensitivity (81%) and specificity (76%) to whiplash injuries when the radiographs exhibited greater than 10 degrees of intersegmental motion or over 12 mm of spinous process fanning.[98] These measures are difficult to directly apply to the young patient where ligamentous laxity is the norm and abnormally large measures may be physiologic, not pathologic.

White and Panjabi[260] describe cervical injury with subsequent neurologic damage as a clinical unstable situation. Clinical instability is defined on the neutral 72-inch focal film distance lateral radiograph as more than 3.5 mm of displacement of one segment relative to the position of the subadjacent vertebra or greater than 11 degrees intersegmental rotation relative to the rotation of the adjacent vertebrae.[260] With use of flexion-extension radiographs, relative translations greater than 3.5 mm or more than 20 degrees of sagittal plane rotation is abnormal. Clinical instability generally is regarded as a contraindication to same-level chiropractic adjustment and relative contraindication to distal, but related areas. Dai[51] found that cervical segmental instability may be associated with early degeneration of the involved intervertebral disc.

Radiographs remain as the modality of choice for the initial evaluation of whiplash-type injuries;[72] however, plain film radiographs may not reveal significant trauma. For example, up to 20% of fractures are missed on initial plain film studies; therefore it is important to proceed to a CT scan if there are significant historic indicators of trauma and suspicious clinical presentation.[131,150,269] CT is particularly useful for reviewing complex anatomy and clinically suggested fracture, and in circumstances where quality radiographs are difficult to obtain (e.g., large body habitus or structural deformity as with scoliosis), MRI and bone scans may be useful to exhibit radiographically occult fractures.

Disc pathology is a contributing factor in the development of chronic symptoms after whiplash injury. However, because of the high proportion of false-positive results, it is best to reserve MRI examination for patients with persistent upper extremity pain and neurologic deficits.[21,189] Therefore MRI is most useful for chronic pain syndromes (>6 months) and to evaluate the soft-tissue elements of the spine, including the cord, disc, and ligaments.

According to the National Emergency X-Radiography Utilization Study (NEXUS) study criteria, the patient's cervical spine injury is considered low risk for fracture if it exhibits the following criteria: no posterior midline cervical spine tenderness, no evidence of intoxication, normal level of alertness, no focal neurologic deficit, and no painful distracting injuries.[107] If radiographs are indicated, evaluation begins with the standard three-view series (AP lower cervical, AP open-mouth, and lateral). The lateral view is most helpful.

TABLE 10-6 cont'd

Cervical Acceleration-Deceleration Syndrome or "Whiplash Syndrome"

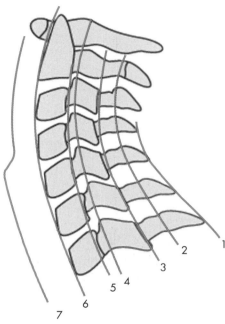

FIG. 10-65 When viewing the lateral cervical spine radiograph for abnormality, check the vertical alignment of seven anatomic lines. From posterior to anterior the lines include: line 1 (along posterior tips of spinous processes), line 2 (along spinal laminal lines), line 3 (along posterior margins of posterior joints), line 4 (along anterior margins of posterior joints), line 5 (along posterior margins of bodies C2 to C7, known as *George's line*), line 6 (along anterior margins of bodies C2 to C7), and line 7 (along posterior margin of pharynx and tracheal air shadows). Most significant injury disrupts one or more of these lines, making them an important and efficient check of the structural integrity of the anatomy.

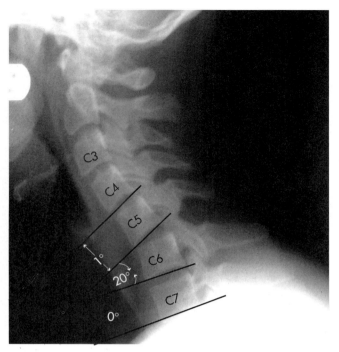

FIG. 10-66 Clinical instability (relative rotation). After drawing endplate lines on C4, C5, C6, and C7, the C4 segment is 1 degree in extension with respect to C5, the C5 segment is 20 degrees in flexion with respect to C6, and the C6 segment is parallel to the C7 segment (0 degrees). Using these values, the C5 segment exhibits 21 degrees of intersegmental rotation of C5 relative to the C4 segment and 20 degrees of intersegmental rotation of C5 relative to the C6 segment. Both values of relative rotation are beyond the accepted upper limit of 11 degrees, denoting clinical instability. Relative rotations are employed to correct for the expected contribution of the normal cervical lordosis.

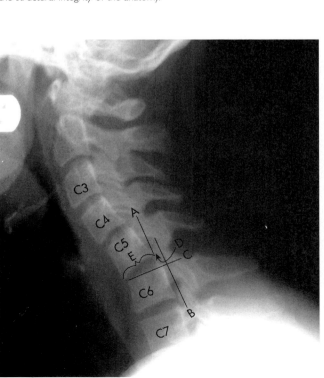

FIG. 10-67 Clinical instability (displacement). *A,* The posterior inferior margin of the C5 segment is 2.5 mm anterior to, *B,* the posterior superior margin of C6. Displacement is measured by the interval between lines intersecting points *A* and *B* that are constructed perpendicular to, *C,* the endplate line. If, *D,* the value of displacement exceeds 3.5 mm (it does not in this case), clinical instability is present. Another method of assessment compares, *D,* the degree of displacement to, *E,* the anteroposterior length of the vertebral body above. Clinical instability is present if more than 20% displacement is noted. The same radiograph is used for Figures 10-66 and 10-67. As in this case, at times clinical instability can be noted in rotation, but not translation, or vice versa.

PART TWO Bone, Joints, and Soft Tissues

Continued

TABLE 10-6 cont'd
Cervical Acceleration-Deceleration Syndrome or "Whiplash Syndrome" Spine

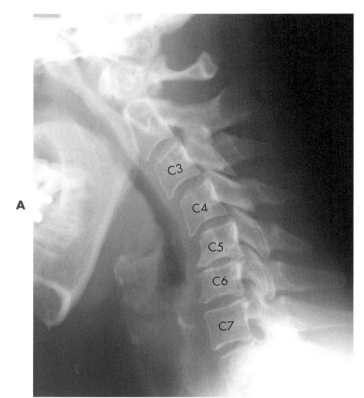

A

FIG. 10-68   A, Flexion; **B,** neutral; and, **C,** extension lateral cervical radiographs. The neutral lateral cervical projection shows 9 degrees of flexion of C4, 4 degrees of extension of C3, and 2 degrees of extension of C5, yielding 11 degrees of relative rotation with the segment below and 13 degrees of relative rotation with the segment above. These values are marginally beyond the upper limit of 11 degrees and suggest clinical instability. Using the same procedure (not shown), the flexion-extension radiographs note 8 degrees of extension and 13 degrees of flexion relative to C5, combining for 21 degrees of relative intersegmental motion. This value is beyond the upper limit of 20 degrees. Therefore this case exhibits a visible alteration in the intersegmental motion pattern of C5 that constitutes marginal evidence of clinical instability given the values of relative rotation.

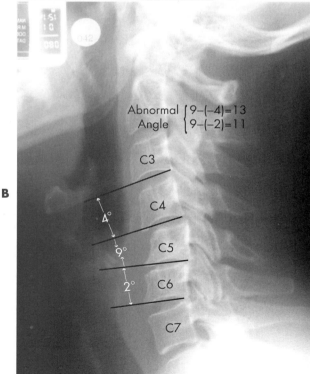

B

Abnormal ⎰ 9−(−4)=13
Angle   ⎱ 9−(−2)=11

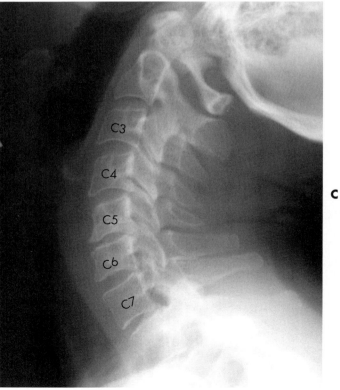

C

TABLE 10-6 cont'd
Cervical Acceleration-Deceleration Syndrome or "Whiplash Syndrome"

Injury	Comments
Cervical "whiplash" syndrome—cont'd	Additional views such as oblique, swimmer's, flexion-extension, and odontoid may be included. Oblique projections often are added if there is a neurologic component to the clinical presentation. Flexion-extension views are indicated if assessment of intersegmental biomechanics is warranted. When performing flexion-extension views, care should be taken on the part of the examiner not to force the injured patient in either flexion or extension, and possibly injuring the patient further. The traditional seven views (neutral lateral, AP lower cervical, AP open-mouth, right and left oblique, flexion, and extension) are no longer routinely advocated. If plain film imaging is warranted, a three-view series (lateral, AP open-mouth, and AP lower cervical) with possible helical CT is likely to be more informative. If warranted, flexion and extension views are best applied 7 to 10 days after injury, at which time confounding muscle spasm has largely subsided. However, MRI is more accurate in evaluating ligamentous injury and very useful for examining any associated neurologic involvement.
	The expected clinical outcomes to whiplash injury are difficult to accurately predict. Typically patients recover completely.[22] However, as many as 20% to 60% of patients exhibit clinical features 6 months after the injury.[9,235] Age, gender, baseline pain intensity, and radicular signs and symptoms are important prognostic factors for the outcome of whiplash trauma.[43] In addition, there is a significant correlation between a narrowed sagittal dimension of the spinal canal (secondary to fragment retropulsion and edema) and increased severity of concurrent neurologic symptoms.[71] A small cervical canal predisposes to an adverse clinical outcome after whiplash injury.[124]
	Spinal cord injury without radiographic abnormality (acronym SCIWORA) can be a fatal or disabling condition developing from childhood injuries, and most often affects those under the age of 8 or 9 years. A contributing mechanism of injury appears to be the poorly developed cervical musculature that offers little protection to the injured cervical spine. The injuries can be focused on the cervical or thoracic spine, including whiplash-type mechanisms from automobile accidents, sports, and falls. SCIWORA most often represents a diagnosis of exclusion, necessitating a high index of clinical suspicion. The neurologic signs may be delayed or evolve slowly. SCIWORA is a pre-MRI diagnosis of exclusion. By definition, plain film radiographs are negative. MRI is the standard assessment, commonly exhibiting central disc herniation, spinal stenosis, and spinal cord edema.[228]

TABLE 10-7
Fractures of the Thoracic Spine and Thorax

Fracture	Comments
Compression fracture Flail chest	Flail chest describes the occurrence of multiple fractures of the same ribs, isolating a plate of one or more ribs that are now free to move inward and outward in response to respiration. Posterior flail segments are easier to manage because they are stabilized by the strong scapular musculature, and the patient can rest for longer periods of time more comfortably on his or her back than any other position. (see discussion in Table 10-8).
Golfer's fracture	This describes a lateral rib fracture that occurs when a golf club strikes the ground instead of striking the ball.
Rib fracture (Figs. 10-69 through 10-76)	Rib fracture is a common sequela of blunt trauma to the thorax. Motor vehicle accidents are particularly common among adults, whereas physical abuse and falls are common causes among children. Most commonly the sixth, seventh, and eighth levels are involved, more frequent in the posterior and middle two thirds of the rib. Stress fracture can result from sports (e.g., golf) or chronic coughing. Rib fracture may compromise proper ventilation, or penetrate pleura or lungs, resulting in hemothorax (usually from lacerated intercostal vessels) or pneumothorax. About 60% of rib fractures involve multiple levels; 40% involve only one level. There is a direct correlation between the number of ribs fractured and the associated clinical impact of the injury. When one or two ribs are fractured, mortality is estimated at 5%, but increases to nearly 30% when more than six ribs are fractured.[273] There is a 13% to 69% lung-related morbidity rate with multiple rib fractures. Because of their elasticity, a child's ribs are less likely to fracture. Conversely, senior patients are more likely to experience fractures. Senior women are the most common group to demonstrate nontraumatically induced rib fractures (e.g., coughing). Fractures of the first three ribs are associated with brachial plexus and major vessels; arteriography may be considered. Lower rib fractures are associated with solid organ injury; CT may be considered. Fractures of the upper ribs indicate that the patient has experienced severe trauma.[190,202] Treatment consists of chest wall stabilization, reduction of the respiratory dead space, and management of any associated pulmonary contusion, pneumothorax, effusion, or other features. It is important to search for visceral complications, which are of more clinical concern than the fractured ribs themselves. Also, costicartilage and costochondral injuries often mimic rib fractures clinically but are invisible on radiographs.
Sternal fracture (Fig. 10-77)	Direct frontal force (e.g., steering wheel during automobile accident) most often results in transverse fracture of the sternal body. Hyperflexion injury of the spine most often results in a posterior dislocation of the manubrium at the manubriosternal joint. Forty percent of sternal fractures occur with associated spinal fractures.[121] A sternal fracture has a 25% to 45% mortality rate secondary to associated cardiac and great vessel injury. Although sometimes seen on radiographs, CT is needed to detail sternal injuries.

TABLE 10-7 cont'd
Fractures of the Thoracic Spine and Thorax

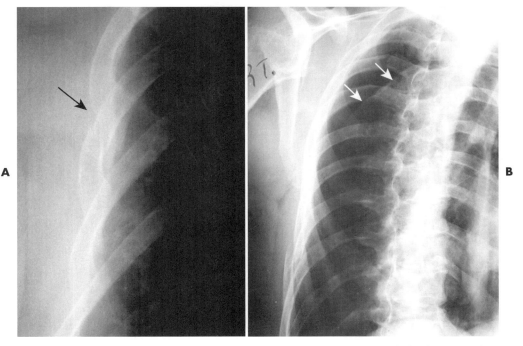

FIG. 10-69   Rib fracture at the lateral margin of a middle rib in a 61-year-old woman. **A,** Rib fractures are best discovered by focusing on the cortices of the ribs *(arrow)*. Usually, as is the case here, there is a cortical offset that indicates fracture. **B,** Another case shows offset of the rib cortices and a faint linear shadow of pleura consistent with pneumothorax accompanying the rib fracture. (**B,** Courtesy Steven P. Brownstein, MD, Springfield, NJ.)

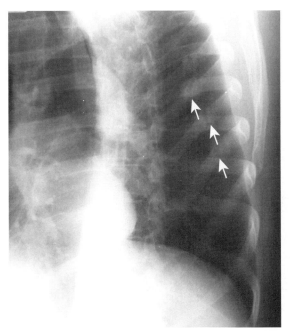

FIG. 10-70   Several levels of rib fracture noted on this oblique projection *(arrows)*. (Courtesy Gary Longmuir, Phoenix, AZ.)

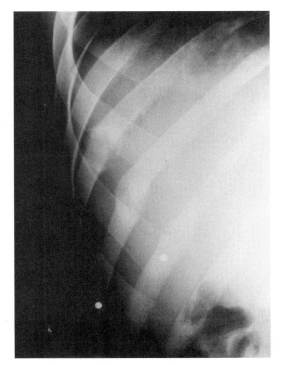

FIG. 10-71   Multiple rib fractures with some early callus formation noted, consistent with a subacute stage of fracture. Sometime it is helpful to place a small metallic marker at the point of patient tenderness or complaint to facilitate close scrutiny of the area, as was done in this case.

Continued

TABLE 10-7 cont'd
Fractures of the Thoracic Spine and Thorax

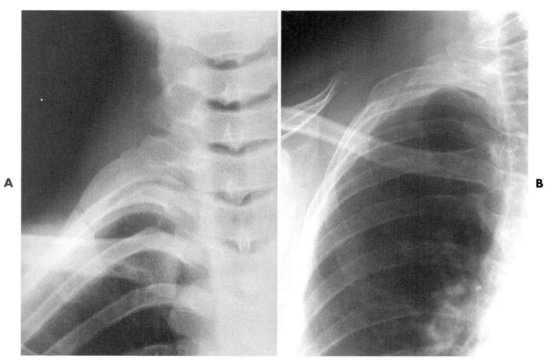

FIG. 10-72   A, There is a fracture of the first rib on the reading right obtained in an automobile accident. The clavicle and upper ribs may be injured from pressure of the shoulder seat belt. **B,** Fracture of the second right rib in another patient.

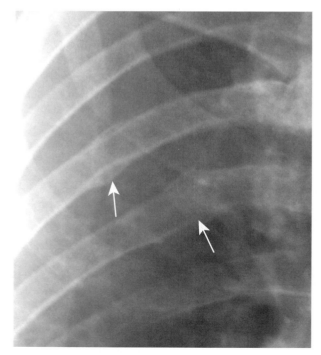

FIG. 10-73   Note the residual deformity of several healed rib fractures (arrows).

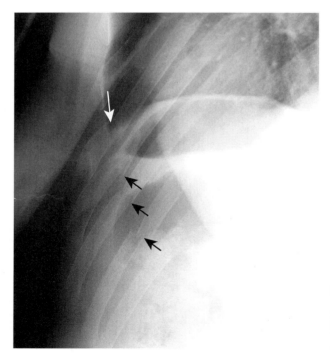

FIG. 10-74   Multiple rib fractures presenting below the diaphragm obtained when this passenger struck the dashboard during a car accident (arrows). (Courtesy Robert Percuoco, Long Grove, IA.)

TABLE 10-7 cont'd
Fractures of the Thoracic Spine and Thorax

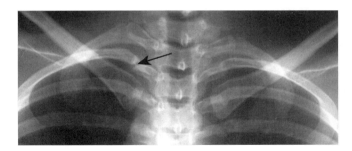

FIG. 10-75 Isolated fracture of the proximal portion of the patient's right second rib *(arrow)*.

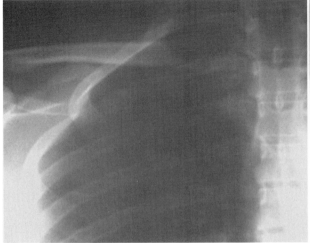

A

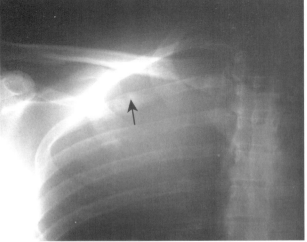

B

FIG. 10-76 Because the ribs are usually overexposed on radiographs taken with a spine technique, abnormalities of the ribs are difficult to see on plain film radiographs of the spine. Evaluate the overexposed areas of the spine film using a hotlight. **A,** Notice that the film illuminated by the view box does not reveal a rib fracture. **B,** However, when the hotlight is applied, a subacute rib fracture is seen *(arrow)*.

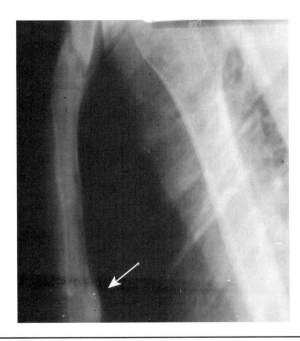

FIG. 10-77 Fracture of the lower sternum, noted on this anteroinferior portion of the lateral thoracic projection *(arrow)*. (Courtesy Steven P. Brownstein, MD, Springfield, NJ.)

Continued

TABLE 10-8

Fractures and Dislocations of the Lumbar Spine

Injury	Comments
Chance (seatbelt, lap belt, fulcrum) fracture (Figs. 10-78 and 10-79)	Chance fracture describes a transverse fracture through the spinous process and neural arch that extends into and possibly through the vertebral body. It is named for the British radiologist with the same name.[34] Classically it develops from an automobile accident in which flexion forces are applied to the spine while the patient is held down by a lap seatbelt, which acts as a fulcrum to cause the fracture. In the frontal projection a radiolucent region ("empty vertebra") is created by the separation of the vertebrae. About 50% of cases have associated intraabdominal injuries at the time of presentation. It most often presents at L1 and L2; however, T11 and T12 sometimes are seen. Children have a low center of gravity, causing the middle lumbar levels to be involved more often.
Pars interarticularis fracture (Fig. 10-80)	Acute fracture of the pars interarticularis is uncommon, develops from hyperextension injury, and is best seen in the oblique projection. Stress fractures of the region are common, typically occur at L5, are usually bilateral, and promote spondylolisthesis at the same level.
Transverse process fracture (Figs. 10-81 and 10-82)	Transverse process fracture is common and often occurs at multiple levels. It is typically present in the upper lumbar levels and in either a vertical or oblique direction. Irregularity of the fracture line and distraction of the fragment differentiate it from nonunion of the transverse process. There is usually an associated history of direct blunt trauma, violent lateral flexion injuries, or avulsion of the psoas muscle. Generally there is little clinical concern for fractures of the transverse process itself. They are considered stable and minor, but there is clinical interest for associated soft-tissue defects to the abdominal or pelvic viscera, particularly renal injury. Approximately 20% of patients with transverse process fractures demonstrate concurrent injury to the abdominal viscera.[236] Because of overlying bowel gas and so on, CT may be necessary to fully evaluate the presence of fracture and any associated visceral injury.
Vertebral body compression fracture (Figs. 10-83 through 10-92)	Compression fracture most frequently occurs at T12, L1, or L2. Generally compression fracture is noted by a loss of more than 2 mm of anterior vertebral body height compared with the posterior; however, a history of trauma is essential, and differentiates a traumatically induced wedged vertebral configuration from a normal trapezoidal variant in configuration that is common to the T11-L1 levels. The wedged appearance results from forward rotation forces of the traumatic event. In general terms, flexion produces wedge fractures, compression causes burst fractures, shear causes Chance fractures, and rotation causes fracture-dislocations. Compression fracture also may exhibit depression of the vertebral endplates secondary to forces of axial loading. Four classifications (A to D) of compression fracture have been described: involvement of both endplates (A), involvement of superior endplate (B), involvement of inferior endplate (C), and buckling of the anterior cortex of the vertebral body with both endplates intact (D).[57] The stability of the lumbar spine after trauma is predicted by the anatomic region of injury, described by three columns (see Fig. 10-91).
	In a patient over 40 years of age, there is increased suspicion of a pathologic etiology of the compression fracture related to metastatic bone disease, multiple myeloma, and so on. These aggressive etiologies need to be excluded from fractures caused by osteoporosis or acute injury alone. Differentiation of a pathologic fracture from acute injury alone is aided by a history of malignancy, past radiographs, other sites of involvement (e.g., pedicles), cortical bone destruction, associated soft-tissue mass, collapse of posterior margin of the vertebral body, advanced collapse of the segment (vertebra plana), specialized imaging, and occasionally laboratory work (e.g., multiple myeloma).

TABLE 10-8 cont'd

Fractures and Dislocations of the Lumbar Spine

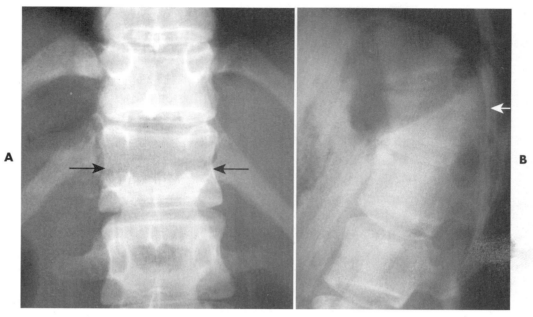

FIG. 10-78 **A** and **B,** Chance fracture of T12 noted on the anteroposterior projection as a separated superior and inferior portion of the vertebra, leaving a radiolucent "ghost vertebra" appearance between the halves of the segment (arrows). (Courtesy Steven P. Brownstein, MD, Springfield, NJ.)

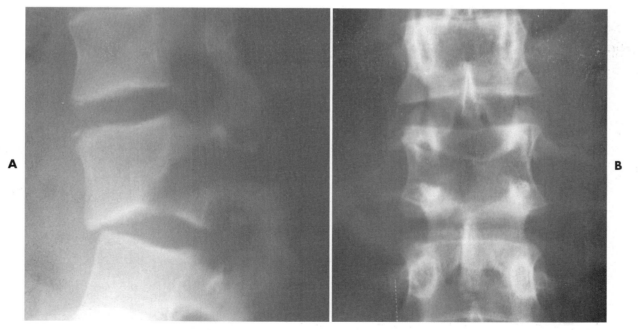

FIG. 10-79 **A** and **B,** Chance fracture of L3 marked horizontal slit of the vertebra. Dr. Chance first described this fracture that is notoriously related to a car lap belt, which functions as a fulcrum to split the vertebra.

Continued

TABLE 10-8 cont'd
Fractures and Dislocations of the Lumbar Spine

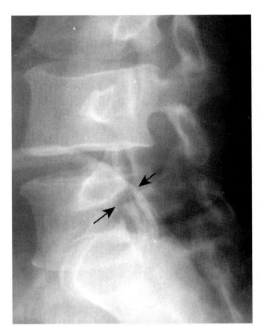

FIG. 10-80 Oblique projection of the lumbar spine demonstrating a fracture of the pars interarticularis. The pars interarticularis appears as the neck of a Scottie dog, and when fracture is present, the dog appears to be wearing a collar *(arrows)*.

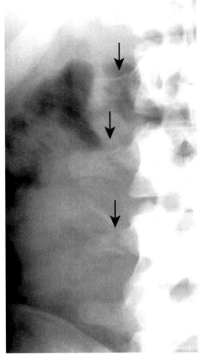

FIG. 10-81 Transverse process fractures *(arrows)*. Notice the rough margins of each fragment, which differentiate it from a persistent apophysis defect. (Courtesy Steven P. Brownstein, MD, Springfield, NJ.)

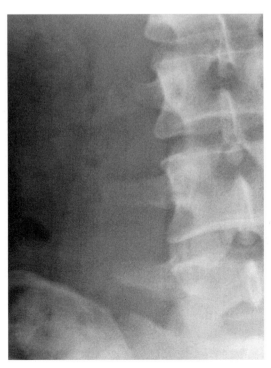

FIG. 10-82 Fracture, without displacement, of the patient's right third and fourth lumbar transverse processes.

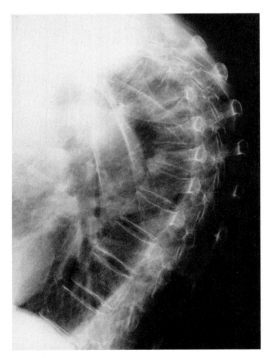

FIG. 10-83 Osteoporotic patient with advanced trapezoidal configuration of several middle thoracic segments. The presentation of multiple levels involved, middle thoracic location, and extensive loss of body height all suggest that an underlying pathology is present.

TABLE 10-8 cont'd

Fractures and Dislocations of the Lumbar Spine

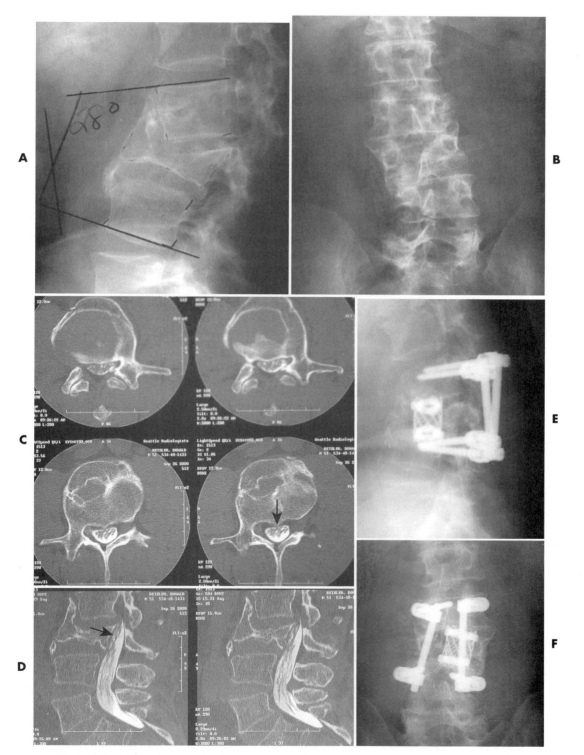

FIG. 10-84 Advanced compression fracture of L3. **A,** The lateral lumbar projection demonstrates marked reduction of the vertebral body causing an acute kyphosis. **B,** The fracture results in an increased interpeduncular distance. **C** and **D,** Computed tomography scans better define the trauma, clearly exhibiting the radial expansion (consistent with a burst fracture) and fragment retropulsion into the spinal canal narrowing the thecal sac as noted by deformity of the subarachnoid column of contrast *(arrows)*. **E** and **F,** Surgical rods, pedicle screws, and a cage spacer are placed to stabilize the segment.

Continued

TABLE 10-8 cont'd
Fractures and Dislocations of the Lumbar Spine

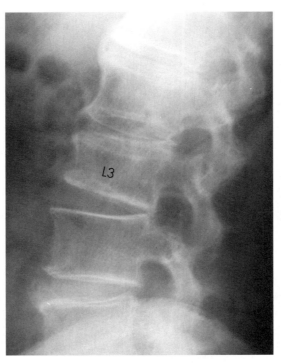

FIG. 10-85   Trapezoidal configuration of the L3 segment consistent with a compression fracture.

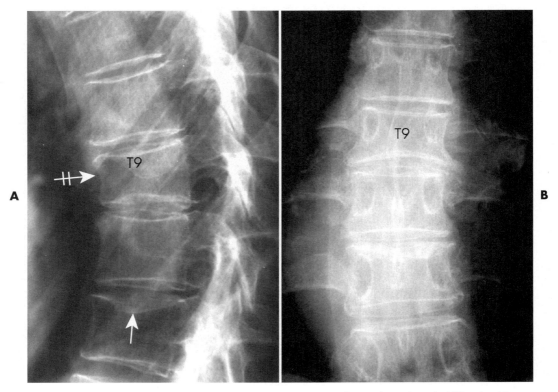

FIG. 10-86   **A** and **B,** Multiple fractures, manifesting as a compression fracture *(crossed arrow)* of T9 and endplate impaction *(arrow)* of T11 in a patient with advanced osteoporosis. (Courtesy Kevin Cunningham, Eldridge, IA.)

TABLE 10-8 cont'd
Fractures and Dislocations of the Lumbar Spine

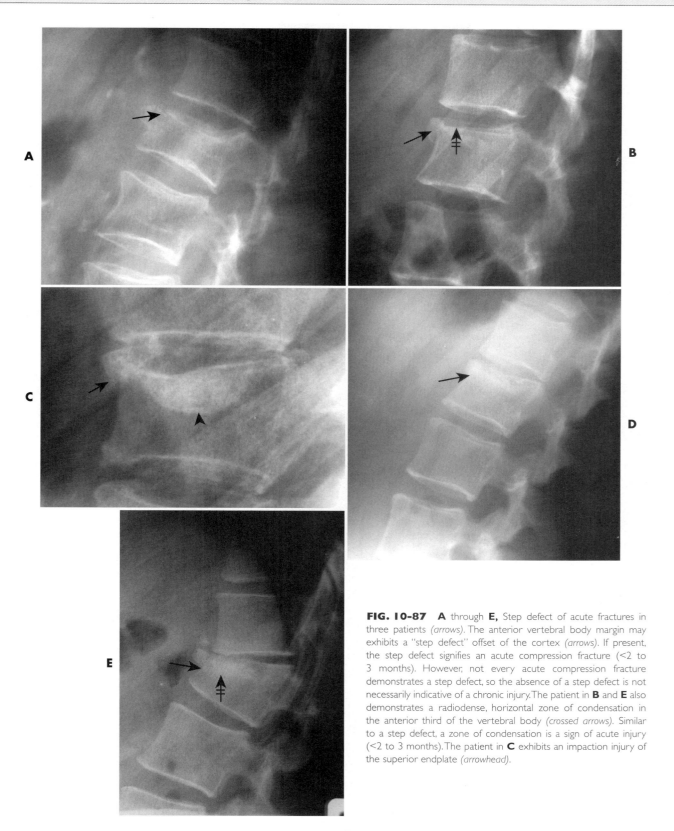

FIG. 10-87 **A** through **E,** Step defect of acute fractures in three patients *(arrows).* The anterior vertebral body margin may exhibits a "step defect" offset of the cortex *(arrows).* If present, the step defect signifies an acute compression fracture (<2 to 3 months). However, not every acute compression fracture demonstrates a step defect, so the absence of a step defect is not necessarily indicative of a chronic injury. The patient in **B** and **E** also demonstrates a radiodense, horizontal zone of condensation in the anterior third of the vertebral body *(crossed arrows).* Similar to a step defect, a zone of condensation is a sign of acute injury (<2 to 3 months). The patient in **C** exhibits an impaction injury of the superior endplate *(arrowhead).*

TABLE 10-8 cont'd
Fractures and Dislocations of the Lumbar Spine

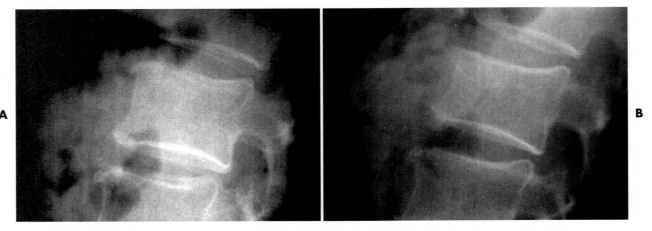

FIG. 10-88 Lateral lumbar projections, **A,** before and, **B,** after trauma. The first film shows normal vertical dimension of the L1 segment. L1 is fractured on the second film, taken immediately after injury, demonstrated by impaction of the anterior margin of the endplate.

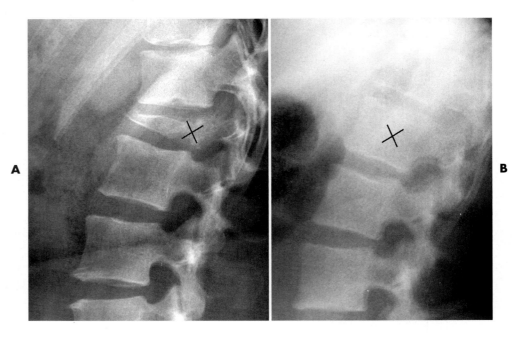

FIG. 10-89 A, The lateral lumbar radiograph exhibits marked compression of the L1 segment secondary to underlying bone metastasis. The patient is a 35-year-old woman diagnosed with breast cancer. **B,** There is no disease represented on films of 3.5 years earlier.

FIG. 10-90 Pathologic compression fractures occur when an aggressive pathology such as metastasis or multiple myeloma compromises the structural integrity of the normal vertebral body. A pathologic compression fracture is suggested by the presence of biconcave endplates, significant wedged configuration, narrowed posterior body margin, and substantial reduction of the body height. Each of these configurations also may occur with nonaggressive underlying pathology, such as osteoporosis.

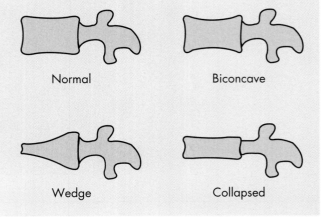

Normal   Biconcave

Wedge   Collapsed

TABLE 10-8 cont'd
Fractures and Dislocations of the Lumbar Spine

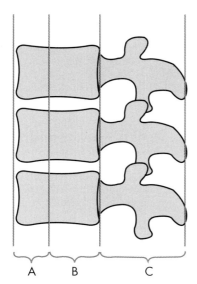

A   B   C

FIG. 10-91 The three-column concept of spine stability. The anatomic integrity of the injured spine can be categorized by identifying which region of the vertebral is traumatized. Denis[57,58] described the stability of the spine using a three-column model, as defined in a sagittal plane. *A,* The first column consists of the anterior longitudinal ligament and anterior portion of the vertebral bodies. *B,* The middle column consists of the posterior portion of the vertebral body and posterior longitudinal ligament. The posterior column is composed of the vertebral arch and all ligaments posterior to the posterior longitudinal ligament. *C,* Injuries to the anterior or posterior columns generally are regarded as stable. Injury of the middle, any two, or all three columns is considered unstable. The middle column is important. If it is not involved, the fracture is a simple wedge compression. If the middle column is involved via a compressive force, a burst fracture is present. If the middle column is involved via a tension force, a flexion-distraction injury is present. Last, a flexion-rotation injury occurs when the middle column is damaged by a shear force. Further, instability can be described as mechanical (first degree), neurologic (second degree), or mechanical and neurologic (third degree).

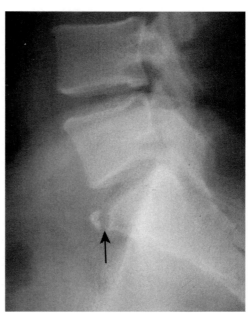

FIG. 10-92 A small teardrop fracture of the anterosuperior margin of S1 *(arrow).*

Continued

TABLE 10-8 cont'd

Fractures and Dislocations of the Lumbar Spine

Injury	Comments
Vertebral body compression fracture—cont'd	Plain film radiographs usually constitute the first step in imaging; the lateral view is most informative. Up to 20% of patients exhibit multiple levels of fracture. CT is used to define the osseous anatomy. MRI is used to assess for underlying pathology, ligamentous injury, and neurologic involvement. On the lateral radiograph, the presence of a horizontal radiopaque *zone of condensation* and cortical offset "*step defect*" along the anterior body margin indicate that the fracture is recent (<2-3 months);[270] vertebral compression fractures with less than 20 degrees of local kyphosis generally are stable and typically do not manifest with neurologic compromise. Surgical treatment may be considered for patients with documented progression or neurologic compromise; vertebroplasty, first described in 1987, involves the forced injection of low-viscosity polymethylmethacrylate cement into the center of the collapsed vertebral body. Once solidified, the cement significantly improves the structural strength of the vertebral body. Kyphoplasty involves the additional step of using an inflatable balloon inserted into the fractured segment to restore the normal configuration of the segment before injecting the cement.

TABLE 10-9

Fractures, Dislocations, and Soft-Tissue Injuries of the Upper Extremities

Injury	Comments
Shoulder	
Fractures	
Clavicle (Figs. 10-93 through 10-96)	The clavicle is the most common bone fractured during birth (3% of live births) and childhood;[270] 80% of fractures occur in the middle, 15% in the lateral, and 5% in the medial third of the bone. Nonunion often results in hypertrophic callus formation that may impinge on the neurovascular bundle exiting the root of the neck (thoracic outlet syndrome). Management is based on immobilization with a figure-eight brace or sling. A stress defect may occur to the distal clavicle as it presents with focal osteolysis after acute injury or repetitive stress, as in weightlifting.
Proximal humerus (Figs. 10-97 through 10-99)	Fracture of the proximal humerus occurs at the surgical neck (distal to tuberosities). Proximal humerus fractures are commonly the result of a fall on outstretched hand (acronym FOOSH injury) in an osteoporotic patient. A proximal humerus fracture can be described using the four-part Neer classification system, based on the number of fragments that are displaced. A 1-part Neer describes a proximal humerus fracture (comminuted or not) without any displaced fragments and is treated with a sling. A 2-part Neer has displacement of one fragment (creating two parts) and is treated with closed reduction. A 3-part Neer has two displaced fragments in which at least one tuberosity is in contact with the humeral head and is treated with closed reduction. Last, a 4-part Neer exhibits three displaced segments, necessitating open reduction and fixation. Several fractures of the proximal humerus are associated with an anterior dislocation of the proximal humerus, including avulsion of the greater tuberosity ("flap" fracture) and impaction of the posterolateral surface on the inferior glenoid tubercle (Hill-Sachs or "hatchet" defect).
Scapula (Figs. 10-100 through 10-103)	A fracture of the scapula is uncommon (about 1% of all fractures), usually as a result of direct impact. Most scapular fractures involve the body and neck of the scapula. They are rarely isolated; therefore they may be overlooked because attention is focused on more severe accompanying injuries.[104] Fractures can be described using four classifications.[99,116] I: Glenoid fossa (IA-anterior and IB-posterior). II: Fracture through the glenoid fossa that extends to the lateral border of the scapula. III: Fracture through the glenoid fossa that extends to the superior border of the scapula. IV: Fracture through the glenoid fossa that extends to the medial border of the scapula. V: Combination of II-IV, and VI-comminuted fracture. Avulsion of the inferior glenoid rim ("Bankart") is related to anterior dislocation of the humerus. The transscapular ("Y-view") is usually best to view a scapular fracture. Even if a fracture does not manifest, regional trauma and dislocations may create complex soft-tissue injuries of the related anatomy, warranting MRI follow-up.
Dislocations	
Acromioclavicular joint dislocation (Figs. 10-104 through 10-106)	Acromioclavicular dislocation is most often caused by a fall onto the lateral margin of the shoulder or as a result of severe arm traction, usually occurring without an associated fracture. Six grades of acromioclavicular injury are recognized. Grade I is a ligamentous sprain with no radiographic evidence of injury. Grade II is rupture of the joint capsule and acromioclavicular ligaments with radiographic evidence of joint space widening and mild elevation of the distal clavicle (<25% displacement). With Grade III the stronger coracoclavicular ligaments are also torn, resulting in increased coracoclavicular distance (>1.3 cm or 40% asymmetry from side to side) and superior displacement (25 to 100% displacement). Grade IV is total dislocation with posterior displacement of the distal clavicle into the trapezius muscle. Grade V is total dislocation with marked superior displacement (>100% displacement) of the distal clavicle. Grade VI is total dislocation with inferior (subacromial or subcoracoid) position of the distal clavicle. Commonly in casual clinical application of the grades, only three grades are used where Grades I and II are similar to the above description, and Grade III may encompass severe strains with extensive elevation of the clavicle. Separation of the joint is enhanced when the patients holds a 10- to 20-lb weight in the hand during the radiographic examination (AP with 15 degrees cephalic tube tilt) to draw the arm downward. Depending on the grade, the injury usually is treated conservatively; however, if a patient is physically active (e.g., manual worker or athlete) or does not wish to have the usual step-off bump as a residual cosmetic deformity that is characteristic of the injury, a screw may be surgically placed through the clavicle into the acromion.

Continued

TABLE 10-9 cont'd
Fractures, Dislocations, and Soft-Tissue Injuries of the Upper Extremities

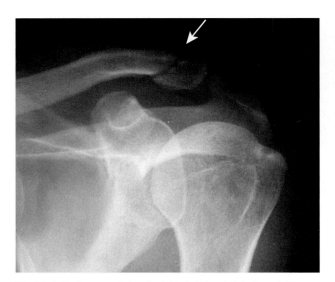

FIG. 10-93   Fracture of the distal third of the clavicle *(arrow)*. (Courtesy Steven P. Brownstein, MD, Springfield, NJ.)

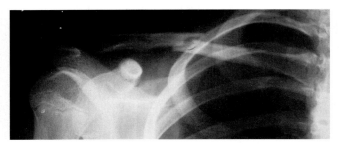

FIG. 10-94   Fracture of the middle third of the clavicle. Approximately 80% of fractures occur in its middle third. (Courtesy Steven P. Brownstein, MD, Springfield, NJ.)

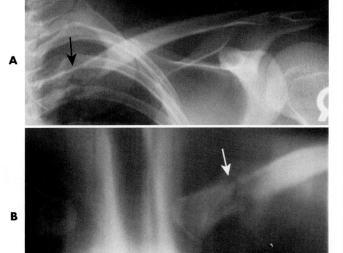

FIG. 10-96   Fracture of the medial third of the clavicle on, **A,** plain film and, **B,** linear tomography *(arrows)*. (Courtesy Steven P. Brownstein, MD, Springfield, NJ.)

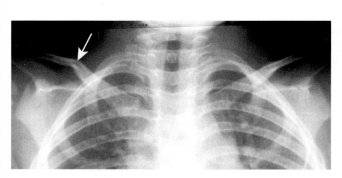

FIG. 10-95   Incomplete fracture of the middle third of the reading left clavicle, noted by abrupt angulation when compared with the contralateral side *(arrow)*. (Courtesy Steven P. Brownstein, MD, Springfield, NJ.)

Fractures, Dislocations, and Soft-Tissue Injuries of the Upper Extremities

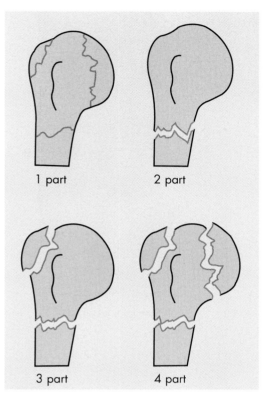

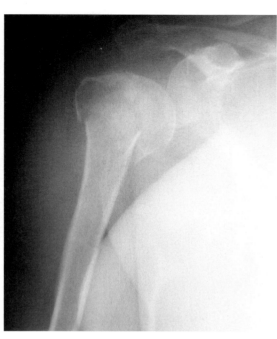

FIG. 10-98 Three-part Neer fracture of the proximal humerus in a 65-year-old woman. (Courtesy Steven P. Brownstein, MD, Springfield, NJ.)

FIG. 10-97 Fractures of the proximal humerus can be classified by the number of parts the humeral head presents with: 1 part (no fragments); 2 part (two fragments); 3 part (three fragments); and 4 part (four fragments). This system is known as the *Neer classification*. The threshold of separation is defined as 1 cm or 45 degrees of fragment rotation.

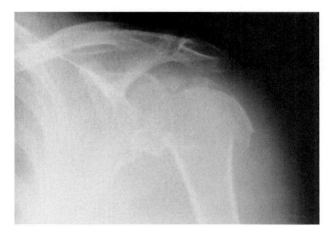

FIG. 10-99 The proximal humerus is fractured into three fragments (3-part Neer) classification.

Continued

TABLE 10-9 cont'd
Fractures, Dislocations, and Soft-Tissue Injuries of the Upper Extremities

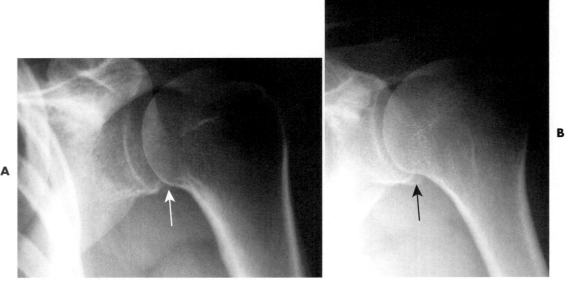

FIG. 10-100   A and **B,** Bankart fracture occurring as a small defect of the infraglenoid tubercle in two patients *(arrows).*

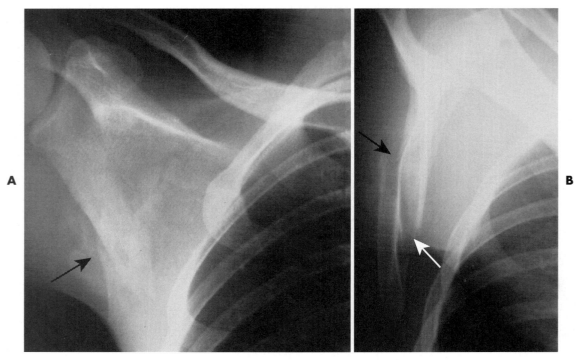

FIG. 10-101   A and **B,** Comminuted fracture of the scapula seen on the anteroposterior and Y projection of the scapula *(arrows).* (Courtesy Steven P. Brownstein, MD, Springfield, NJ.)

TABLE 10-9 cont'd

Fractures, Dislocations, and Soft-Tissue Injuries of the Upper Extremities

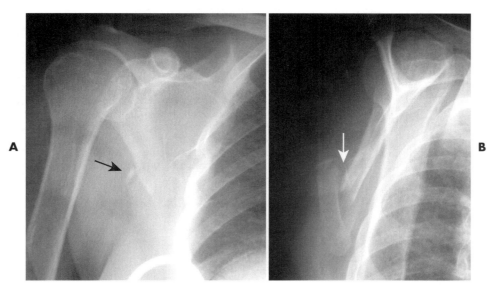

FIG. 10-102 A and **B,** Fracture and posterior displacement of the lower portion of the scapula *(arrows)*. (Courtesy Steven P. Brownstein, MD, Springfield, NJ.)

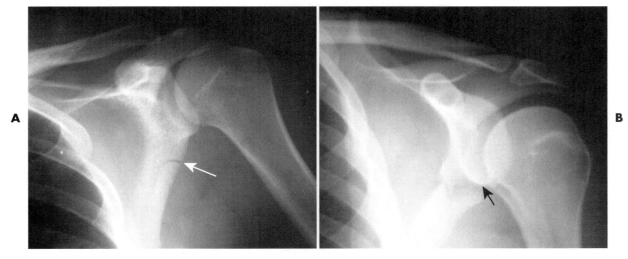

FIG. 10-103 A and **B,** Scapular fracture in two different patients. In both cases the fracture appears as a horizontal defect of the lateral margin of the bone *(arrows)*. (Courtesy Steven P. Brownstein, MD, Springfield, NJ.)

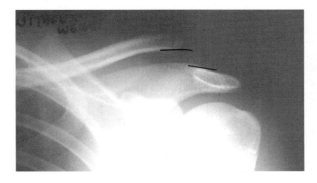

FIG. 10-104 Marked superior displacement of the distal clavicle consistent with a grade V dislocation of the acromioclavicular joint. Some authorities apply only a three-category system to describe acromioclavicular dislocations. If a three-category system is applied, this case is a Grade III. (Courtesy Steven P. Brownstein, MD, Springfield, NJ.)

Continued

TABLE 10-9 cont'd
Fractures, Dislocations, and Soft-Tissue Injuries of the Upper Extremities

Injury	Comments
Glenohumeral dislocation (Figs. 10-107 through 10-109)	Ninety-five percent of glenohumeral dislocations are directed anteriorly, of which 60% are associated with impaction fractures of the posterolateral surface of the humeral head (Hill-Sachs lesion), 15% with avulsion of the greater tuberosity (flap fracture), and less commonly a fracture of the infraglenoid tubercle (Bankart). The radiographic appearance of an anterior humeral dislocation is marked by an intrathoracic (between ribs), subclavicular, subcoracoid (most common), or subglenoid position of the humeral head. Posterior glenohumeral dislocations are less common (about 5%) and anecdotally associated with epileptic or electric shock convulsions. Posterior humeral dislocations are marked by joint widening between the humeral head and anterior glenoid rim (>6 mm, "rim" sign); an impaction of the medial humeral head may be seen ("trough line").[37] Rarely the humeral head becomes inferiorly displaced under the glenoid process (*luxatio erecta*), which most often is related to extreme hyperabduction injury.
Sternoclavicular joint dislocation	The medial end of the clavicle typically dislocates anteriorly, usually from a blow to the posterior shoulder. A direct anterior blow will dislocate the medial end of the clavicle posteriorly, which is potentially lethal if it encroaches on the great vessels. In those under 25 years old, many of these lesions represent separation of the growth plate (Salter-Harris type I) and not true dislocations.[204]

Soft-tissue injuries (ligaments and cartilage)

Injury	Comments
Biceps tendon injury (Fig. 10-110)	The tendon of the long head of the biceps usually appears as a round, low signal intensity structure within the intertubercular groove on the axial MRI images of the shoulder. When not seen within its expected location, rupture or dislocation should be considered; fluid also may be observed within the biceps tendon sheath, representing edema associated with trauma.
Glenoid labral tear (Fig. 10-111)	The glenoid labrum often tears when it becomes injured. These tears are most commonly of two types: Bankart lesions and SLAP lesions. Bankart tears involve the anteroinferior portion of the labrum, usually secondary to an anterior shoulder dislocation when the joint capsule avulses from its glenoid insertion. Bankart lesions predispose to recurrent anterior shoulder dislocations. SLAP (acronym for superior labral anterior-posterior) lesions occur in the superior margin of the labrum at the point where the long head of the biceps tendon attaches. SLAP lesions occur most commonly from falls on an outstretched hand. SLAP lesions have four expressions. Type I is fraying of the superior margin of the labrum. Type II is detachment of the labral-bicipital complex. Type III is a tear of the inner rim of the superior portion of the glenoid labrum (bucket handle tear). Type IV is a tear of the inner rim of the superior portion of the glenoid labrum (bucket handle tear) with extension of the tear into the labral-bicipital complex. At times a labral tear can develop gradually. Risk factors for this occurrence include repetitive movements, such as occur with throwing and strong muscle contractions of the biceps muscles, such as occur with weightlifting.
Rotator cuff tear (Figs. 10-112 and 10-113)	Any of the rotator cuff muscle group (subscapularis, supraspinatus, infraspinatus, or teres minor) can be involved with partial (more common) or full-thickness tears. Tears may be acute, but are more often chronic, appearing in patients over the age of 40 years. The radiographic appearance of rotator cuff tears manifests as an inferior concavity and sclerosis (Sourcil or eyebrow sign) to the inferior margin of the acromion along with elevation of the humerus, the latter observed as narrowing of the acromiohumeral space. MRI is accurate in diagnosing full-thickness tears of the rotator cuff to nearly 90%. The principal finding of a rotator cuff tear is a hyperintense signal on the T2-weighted image extending through the rotator cuff with discontinuity of the tendon and communicating with the subacromial or subdeltoid space. Retraction of the musculotendinous junction of the supraspinatus muscle also can be seen along with significant fluid accumulation in the subacromial bursa. Secondary signs of injury include loss of the subdeltoid fat, atrophy of the supraspinatus muscle, and cystic changes of the humeral head principally at the site of the supraspinatus tendon insertion. Partial thickness tears can involve either the articular or bursal surface of the tendon or the substance of the tendon and are seen as high signal intensity lesions on T2-weighted images. Articular surface lesions are the most common and are associated with impingement syndrome.

TABLE 10-9 cont'd

Fractures, Dislocations, and Soft-Tissue Injuries of the Upper Extremities

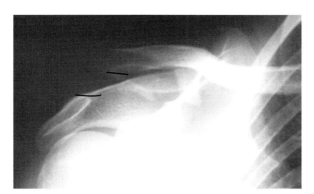

FIG. 10-105 Grade V dislocation of the acromioclavicular joints. Some authorities apply only a three-category system to describe acromioclavicular dislocations. If a three-category system is applied, this case is a Grade III.

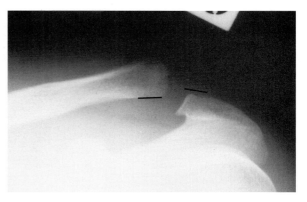

FIG. 10-106 The distal margin of the clavicle is elevated above the lower margin of the acromion, but not above the acromion, indicating a Grade II separation of the acromioclavicular joint.

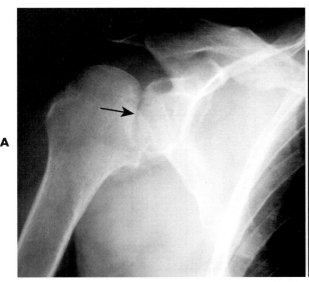

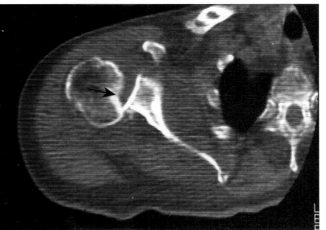

FIG. 10-107 **A,** Plain film and, **B,** computed tomography scan of a posterior dislocation of the humerus with impaction fracture of the medial humeral head on the posterior aspect of the glenoid rim *(arrows)*. (Courtesy Steven P. Brownstein, MD, Springfield, NJ.)

Continued

PART TWO Bone, Joints, and Soft Tissues

TABLE 10-9 cont'd

Fractures, Dislocations, and Soft-Tissue Injuries of the Upper Extremities

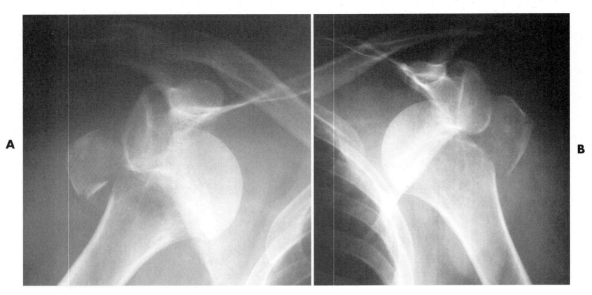

FIG. 10-108   A and **B,** Two cases of anterior shoulder dislocation and accompanying flap fracture of the posterior lateral humeral. The accompanying flap fracture is less common than an impaction or Hill-Sachs fracture of the same region of the humerus. (**A,** Courtesy Steven P. Brownstein, MD, Springfield, NJ.)

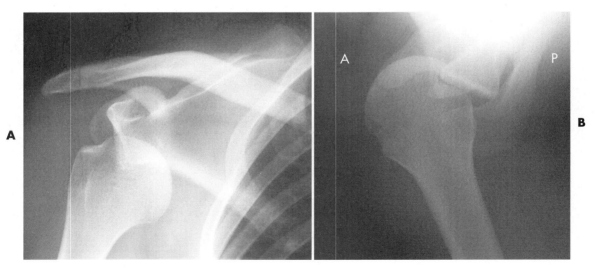

FIG. 10-109   A, After trauma, this 28-year-old man sustained an anterior subcoracoid dislocation of the humerus. There is no evidence of an associated fracture. **B,** The axial projection exhibits an anterior displacement of the humerus with respect to the glenoid cavity.

TABLE 10-9 cont'd
Fractures, Dislocations, and Soft-Tissue Injuries of the Upper Extremities

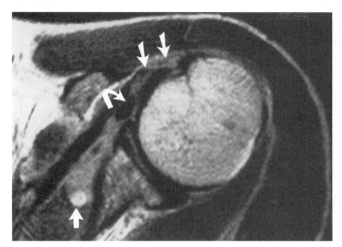

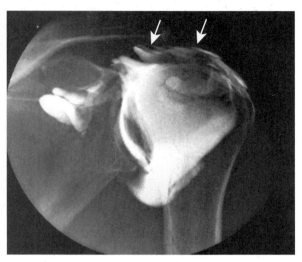

FIG. 10-110 Dislocated biceps tendon, left shoulder. Axial proton density (1800/30) image. The long head of the biceps tendon *(curved arrow)* is displaced out of the bicipital groove and into the glenohumeral joint through the torn transverse ligament and subscapularis tendon *(slanted arrows)*. A high-signal loose body is visible in the distended subscapularis bursa *(straight arrow)*. (From Firooznia H et al: MRI and CT of the musculoskeletal system, St Louis, 1992, Mosby.)

FIG. 10-112 Arthrogram demonstrating migration of injected contrast from the glenohumeral joint to the subacromial space *(arrows)*, which implies a tear in the supraspinatus tendon. (Courtesy Tim Mick, St Paul, MN.)

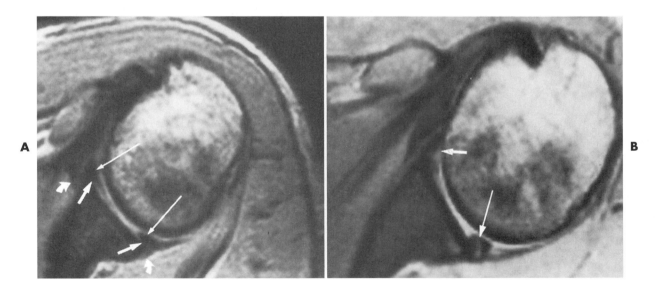

FIG. 10-111 Normal glenoid labrum morphology and magnetic resonance patterns of glenoid labral tears. **A,** Axial gradient echo sequence (400/191/65 degrees). The anterior and posterior glenoid labrum is visualized as a signal void structure *(long arrows)*. The medium-signal hyaline glenoid articular cartilage extends beneath the labrum to the glenoid margin *(short arrows)*. Note the smooth contour of the capsule and the clearly visualized anterior and posterior glenoid insertions *(curved arrows)*. **B,** Axial gradient echo sequence (400/19/65 degrees). Tearing of the anterior labrum is evidenced by contour abnormality *(short arrow)*. A linear tear of the posterior labrum is manifested by a band of medium signal through the labral substance *(long arrow)*. (From Firooznia H et al: MRI and CT of the musculoskeletal system, St Louis, 1992, Mosby.)

Continued

TABLE 10-9 cont'd
Fractures, Dislocations, and Soft-Tissue Injuries of the Upper Extremities

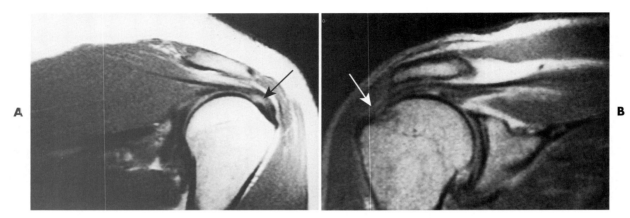

FIG. 10-113 A and **B,** Supraspinatus tendinopathy exhibited by increased signal intensity in the normally hypointense substance of the tendon *(arrows)*.

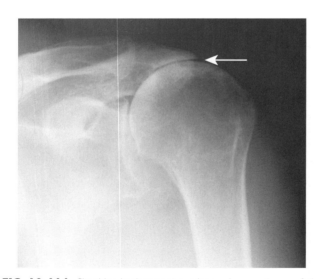

FIG. 10-114 Shoulder impingement syndrome. Incompetence of the rotator cuff allows superior elevation of the humerus because of the unopposed muscle tension of the deltoid. The acromiohumeral space is narrowed *(arrow)* and evidence of arthrosis, marked by bone sclerosis, is also present.

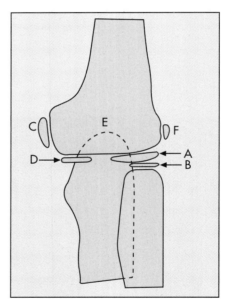

FIG. 10-115 The traumatized pediatric elbow can be difficult to interpret. At times the presence of multiple ossification centers can be confused with trauma fragments. Attention to the sequential order of the appearance of the ossification centers of the elbow can eliminate confusion and overinterpretation of the radiograph. In males, the ossification centers appear in the following order: *A* (1 year), capitellum; *B* (5 years), radial head; *C* (7 years), internal or medial epicondyle; *D* (10 years), trochlea; *E* (10 years), olecranon; and, *F,* external or lateral epicondyle. The sequence spells out the mnemonic CRITOE, and the chronology is slightly earlier for females than the values in the preceding list. CRITOE may resolve questionable presentations of fracture. For instance, if there is a small bone fragment next to the olecranon, one should also see growth centers at the capitellum for it to represent (C) a growth center, (R) radial head, (I) internal or medial epicondyle, and (T) trochlea. If the olecranon fragment is noted without the C-R-I-T, it probably represents a fracture, not a growth center. In other words, if a fragment is noted before the ossification center is scheduled to appear, then it probably represents a fracture.

TABLE 10-9 cont'd
Fractures, Dislocations, and Soft-Tissue Injuries of the Upper Extremities

Injury	Comments
Shoulder impingement syndrome (Fig. 10-114)	Shoulder impingement syndrome can be secondary to narrowing of the subacromial space, which includes changes in the shape and slope of the acromion process, subacromial osteophytes, and degenerative joint disease of the acromioclavicular articulation. These changes create chronic effacement of the rotator cuff tendon and often are precursors to rotator cuff tears. In older patients the combination of repetitive overhead activity along with a congenitally narrowed subacromial space is a common cause of osteophytes on the undersurface of the acromion. In younger patients, involvement in sports that require high arm velocity and overhead throwing can be an additional cause of instability. The Neer system is one of several that exist to classify the degree of impingement. Neer stage I describes edema or hemorrhage in the supraspinatus tendon, usually in young adult patients. Stage II is more advanced tendonitis and fibrosis, presenting in middle-aged patients. Stage III describes the long-term presence of degeneration leading to rupture in middle-aged and older patients.
Elbow *Fractures* Distal humerus fracture (Figs. 10-115 through 10-118)	Supracondylar fracture is the most common fracture about the elbow in children.[45,75] Comminuted intracondylar fracture of a T or Y configuration is common in adults.[133,166] There are three types of supracondylar fractures. Type I is nondisplaced. Type II is an angulated fracture with minimal displacement (portion of cortex retains continuity). Type III is total displacement (complete loss of cortical continuity). A small osteochondral flake fractured off the convex surface of the capitellum is termed *Kocher's fracture*. Malunion deformity (most often cubitus varus), nerve and vessel injury, and Volkmann's contracture are complications to distal humeral fractures. In children the appearance of normal secondary ossification centers may be mistakenly interpreted as fractures; the acronym CRITOE describes the order of appearance of the secondary ossification centers about the elbow: capitellum, radial head, internal epicondyle, trochlea, olecranon, and external epicondyle. If the trochlea is seen, there also must be an internal epicondyle; otherwise what is thought to be the trochlea is probably a fracture fragment.
Little Leaguer's elbow (Figs. 10-119 and 10-120)	Little Leaguer's elbow is an avulsion of the medial epicondyle resulting from traction forces of the flexor-pronator tendons.[27,36] Injury is related to chronic muscles strain placed on immature bone and cartilage. As the name implies, it is common among young baseball players from the throwing action of the baseball. Clinical presentations include pain and a hesitation or "catching" of the joint during its range of motion.
Olecranon (Fig. 10-121)	An olecranon fracture is the second most common elbow fracture, following the proximal radius.[204] Fractures usually are oriented transversely[111] and are easily noted in the lateral projection, usually occurring as isolated injuries. A fall on a semiflexed supinated forearm is the most common mechanism of injury, in which the triceps muscles leverage the olecranon over the fulcrum of the distal humerus. Other mechanisms of injury include hyperextension and a direct blow to the region.
Coronoid fracture (Fig. 10-122)	Fracture of the coronoid process is uncommon generally, and rare as an isolated injury. Fractures of the coronoid process usually are associated with either a posterior elbow dislocation or a radial head fracture.
Radial head fracture (Figs. 10-123 through 10-125)	A radial head fracture is the most common elbow fracture in the adult,[204] and typically is difficult to detect on radiographs. One hint to the diagnosis of an intracapsular injury (inclusive of the radial head) is the observation of the thin fat pads ("fat pad" sign) located between the synovial and fibrous layers of the joint capsule of the elbow. In the lateral flexed elbow position, an elbow injury with resulting joint effusion may cause elevation of the normally slightly visible anterior fat pad and visibility of the normally invisible posterior fat pad (an elevated fat pad is termed a *sail sign*).[20,135] A fracture oriented with the long axis of the bone is termed a *chisel fracture*. Radial head fractures are classified according to the degree of displacement. Type I fractures are generally small and nondisplaced. Type II fractures are larger and displaced. Type III fractures are comminuted. Displaced fragments may require surgery.

Continued

TABLE 10-9 cont'd

Fractures, Dislocations, and Soft-Tissue Injuries of the Upper Extremities

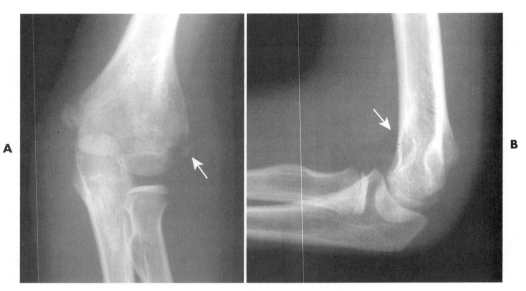

FIG. 10-116   A, Avulsion fracture of the lateral epicondyle of the distal humerus *(arrow)*. On occasion, normal growth centers can be misinterpreted as fractures. As in this case, the fracture fragment is typically irregular and distracted from its parent bone. **B,** The lateral view of the elbow exhibits an elevated anterior fat pad *(arrow)*. (Courtesy Steven P. Brownstein, MD, Sprinfield, NJ.)

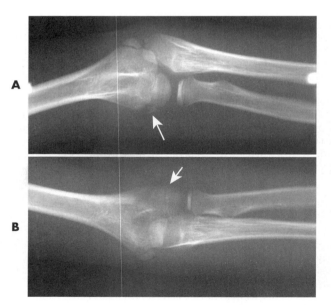

FIG. 10-117   A, An oblique projection of a child's elbow with an avulsion fracture of the lateral epicondyle *(arrow)*. **B,** Notice that the child's contralateral elbow is normal *(arrow)*. Although some advocate taking a radiograph of contralateral anatomy for comparison, it should not be a routine practice in the light of concerns for added cost and radiation exposure. A comparison with an atlas of normal skeletal development would provide the same information without these associated drawbacks. (Courtesy Steven P. Brownstein, MD, Springfield, NJ.)

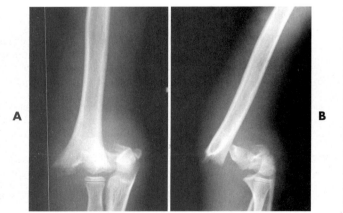

FIG. 10-118 There are three categories of supracondylar fractures: type I (nondisplaced), type II (mild displacement with continuity of the posterior cortex), and type III (total displacement). **A** and **B,** The fracture exhibited here is a type III. (Courtesy Steven P. Brownstein, MD, Springfield, NJ.)

TABLE 10-9 cont'd
Fractures, Dislocations, and Soft-Tissue Injuries of the Upper Extremities

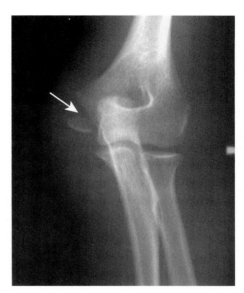

FIG. 10-119 Avulsion of the medial epicondyle of the distal humerus (*arrow*). (Courtesy Steven P. Brownstein, MD, Springfield, NJ.)

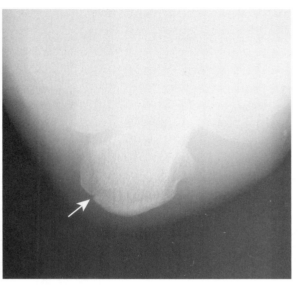

FIG. 10-121 Tangential view of the elbow revealing a fracture of the olecranon (*arrow*).

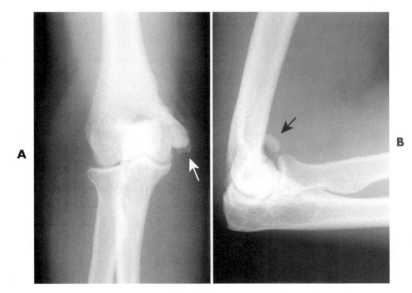

FIG. 10-120 **A,** An old avulsion of the medial epicondyle (*arrows*) that appears enlarged secondary to poor fragment union. **B,** The appearance on the lateral projection is differentiated from the more proximal supracondylar process and the "away from joint" projection of an osteochondroma. (Courtesy Martin Stine, Windsor, CO.)

Continued

TABLE 10-9 cont'd

Fractures, Dislocations, and Soft-Tissue Injuries of the Upper Extremities

Injury	Comments
Dislocations	
Elbow dislocation (Fig. 10-126)	Elbow dislocation is the third most common dislocation in adults, following those of the shoulder and interphalanges, and is the most common dislocation in children. Overall it is more common in children than adults.[5] The direction of dislocations of both the radius and ulna usually (90%) is posterior.[193] There is a high rate of concurrent fractures. On a normal lateral projection of the elbow, a line through the center of the shaft of the radius should intersect the center of the capitellum; failure to do so may indicate dislocation.[234] The anterior humeral line describes a line drawn along the anterior border of the humerus in the lateral projection. Under normal circumstances the line should intersect the middle third of the capitellum.[204] Anterior displacement of the line may indicate supracondylar fracture.
Pulled elbow (nursemaid's elbow)	A sudden jerk or pull on a toddler's pronated elbow may cause dislocation of the proximal radius with entrapment of the annular ligament within the joint space.[211] Radiographs typically are negative.
Forearm	
Fractures	
Essex-Lopresti injury (Fig. 10-127)	Essex-Lopresti fracture is a comminuted fracture of the radial head with dislocation of the distal radioulnar joint.[50,70,74] This complex injury usually results from a fracture-dislocation of the elbow or radial head impaction on the capitellum from longitudinal application of force associated with a fall on an outstretched hand.
Galeazzi (Piedmont, reversed Monteggia) injury (Fig. 10-128)	Galeazzi fracture is a fracture of the distal radius with dislocation of the distal radioulnar joint.[114,165] It is associated with a fall in which an axial load is placed on the hyperpronated forearm.[196,254] Sometimes the fracture is complicated by compartment syndrome. Anterior interosseous nerve (branch of the median nerve) palsy may arise, presenting with a loss in pinch strength of the thumb (flexor pollicis longus) and index finger (flexor digitorum profundus). A Galeazzi fracture usually is treated with open reduction.
Monteggia injury (Fig. 10-129)	Monteggia fracture involves the proximal ulna with dislocation of the radial head.[7] Although dislocation may occur in any direction, anterior dislocation of the radius was first described and is most common.[28] Monteggia fracture occurs in both children and adults. In adult patients, this fracture is historically notorious for its poor clinical outcome; however, modern techniques of plate-screw fixation have improved anatomic reduction and functional outcomes substantially.[200] In children, the ulna fracture typically is incomplete and therefore more stable.
Nightstick (parry) fracture	A nightstick fracture occurs to the distal third[65] or (less often) middle third of the ulnar shaft. Often it is secondary to raising the forearm overhead in an attempt to protect the victim's head or face from a nightstick or club strike.
Both bone (BB) fracture (Fig. 10-130)	Concurrent fractures of the radius and ulna (or tibia and fibula) most often are found in the middle third of the bones and often result in marked limb angulation and rotation.
Wrist	
Fractures	
Chauffeur's (backfire, Hutchinson) fracture (Figs. 10-131 and 10-132)	A chauffeur's fracture is an undisplaced fracture of the radial styloid. It is named for the occupational hazard of experiencing a backfire while attempting to start an automobile with a hand crank.[33]
Colles' fracture (Figs. 10-133 through 10-136)	A Colles' fracture results most often from a fall on an outstretched hand (acronym Foosh) with the forearm pronated in dorsiflexion.[257] It consists of a fracture of the distal radius with posterior angulation of the distal fragment producing a "dinner fork" or "silver fork" deformity. There is an increased incidence with advanced age; it is more common among women; and 60% are accompanied by fracture of the ulnar styloid process.[3]

TABLE 10-9 cont'd

Fractures, Dislocations, and Soft-Tissue Injuries of the Upper Extremities

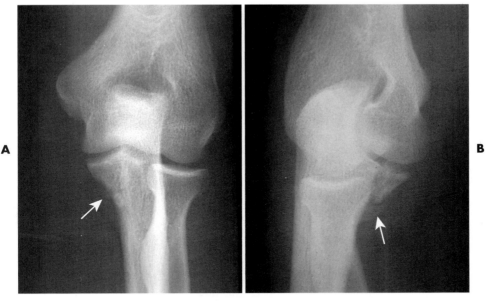

FIG. 10-122 A, Anteroposterior and, **B,** oblique views of the elbow. A mildly displaced coronoid process fracture is seen in the oblique projection *(arrows)*.

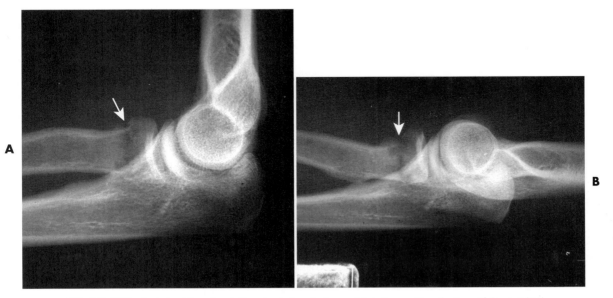

FIG. 10-123 A, Lateral flexed and, **B,** extended projections of the elbow with a fracture of the proximal radius seen on both views *(arrows)*.

Continued

TABLE 10-9 cont'd
Fractures, Dislocations, and Soft-Tissue Injuries of the Upper Extremities

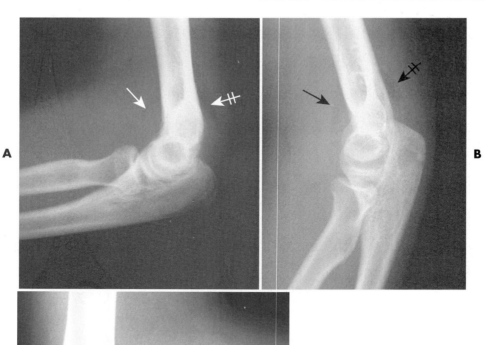

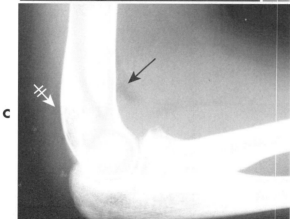

FIG. 10-124 **A** through **C,** Fat pads of the distal humerus in three cases. The anterior *(arrows)* and posterior *(crossed arrows)* fat pads of the distal humerus are elevated, although no evidence of osseous defect is seen. (**B** and **C,** Courtesy Steven P. Brownstein, MD, Springfield, NJ.)

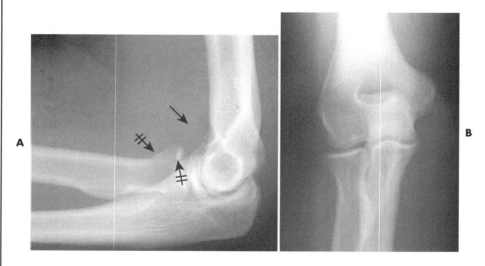

FIG. 10-125 Radial head fracture in a 64-year-old man *(crossed arrows)*. The fracture is seen in, **A,** the lateral projection but not in, **B,** the anteroposterior projection. As in this case, closely examine both views for defects. An anterior fat pad is visible *(arrow)*.

TABLE 10-9 cont'd

Fractures, Dislocations, and Soft-Tissue Injuries of the Upper Extremities

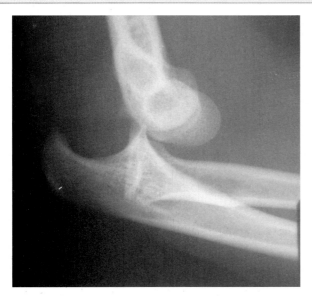

FIG. 10-126 Posterior dislocation of the elbow. Dislocations are named for the direction the distal fragment displaces in reference to the proximal fragment. (Courtesy Steven P. Brownstein, MD, Springfield, NJ.)

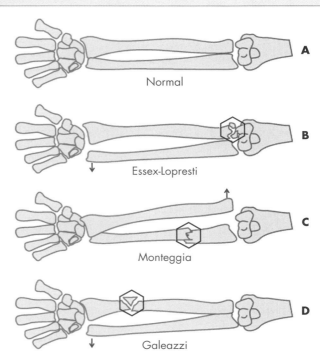

FIG. 10-127 The forearm functions as an oblong osseous-ligamentous ring. Injury to one area or the ring usually is accompanied by additional injuries to the ring. Essex-Lopresti, Monteggia, and Galeazzi fractures are three examples of complex injuries to the forearm.

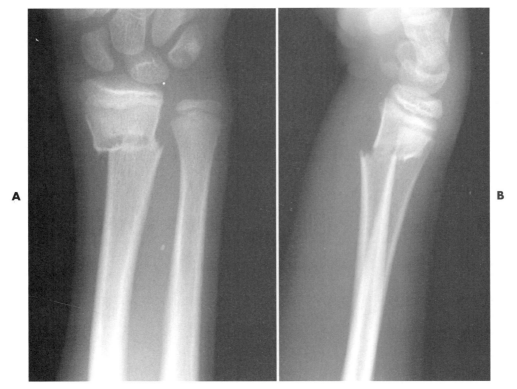

FIG. 10-128 A and **B,** A transverse fracture is noted through the distal radius with accompanying mild dislocation of the distal ulna-radial articulation. The configuration is generally consistent with Galeazzi fracture, but not specifically. Most sources define the radial fracture of Galeazzi occurring at the junction of the distal and middle thirds of the radius. The radial fracture noted in this figure is more distal than classically described.

Continued

TABLE 10-9 cont'd

Fractures, Dislocations, and Soft-Tissue Injuries of the Upper Extremities

Injury	Comments
Greenstick fracture (Fig. 10-137)	A greenstick fracture is an incomplete fracture occurring in a long bone of a child. The fracture occurs on the convex side of a bowing bone, demonstrating marked angulation at the site of fracture. It is common, but not limited, to the radius.
Hamate fracture	A hamate fracture is common to golf,[245] baseball,[32] and racquet sports,[229] and usually involves the hamulus, which appears sclerotic, ill defined, or absent if injured.[180]
Rim (Barton's) fracture	A Barton's fracture is an intraarticular fracture of the posterior rim of the distal radius. The carpals usually deviate posteriorly with the fractured fragment, often blurring the posterior distal forearm fat pad. A reversed Barton's fracture involves the anterior rim of the distal radius.
Scaphoid (navicular) fracture (Figs. 10-138 through 10-141)	A scaphoid fracture is the most common carpal fracture. It usually occurs in persons between 15 and 40 years of age, is rare in children, and is a common occult fracture.[97] Seventy percent of fractures occur at the waist of the bone, 20% in the proximal pole, and 10% are in the distal pole.[97] Scaphoid fractures often are subtle and overlooked on radiographs. Care must be exercised with radiographic positioning. It is helpful to distract the wrist to the ulnar side via the ulnar flexion view, which elongates the scaphoid for a better view of the bone on the posteroanterior wrist projection. Because the principal blood supply for the scaphoid enters at its waist, more proximal fractures risk avascular necrosis (up to 15%),[270] or nonunion (up to 30%)[204] of the proximal pole. Scaphoid fractures often are difficult to detect. The presence of carpal injury is suggested by distortion of the fat pad associated with the pronator quadratus along the ventral carpus. Ninety percent of scaphoid fractures have overlying obliteration of fat stripe.[242] MRI is helpful in the detection of radiographically occult scaphoid fractures and also helps delineate the complication of osteonecrosis. MRI is the most sensitive modality for the detection of osteonecrosis and is more sensitive than radionuclide studies in the early detection of this pathology.[253] MRI findings of osteonecrosis are variable, depending on the stages of ischemia. Typical findings include low signal intensity within the bone marrow on T1-weighted images with regions of increased signal intensity on the T2-weighted images, with the T2 feature thought to represent hemorrhage or edema.
Smith (reversed Colles') fracture (Figs. 10-142 and 10-143)	A direct blow to the back of the wrist results in a fracture of the distal radius with anterior (volar) angulation of the distal fragment. There are three categories of fracture. Type I is a horizontal fracture line through the distal radius. Type II is an oblique fracture line not extending to the articular surface. Type III is an oblique fracture line with intraarticular extension (representing a reversed Barton's fracture).
Torus fracture (Figs. 10-144 through 10-146)	A torus fracture is an incomplete fracture of the distal radius that appears as a bulged, buckled, or folded cortex along the concave side of a bowing long bone. It is probably the most common fracture of children 6 to 10 years old, and often results from a fall on an outstretched hand. Similar to greenstick fractures, it is common, but not limited to the radius.
Triquetrum (Figs. 10-147 and 10-148)	A triquetrum (Fisher) fracture is the second most common carpal bone fracture.[68] Usually it presents as a dorsal avulsion of the radiotriquetral and ulnotriquetral ligaments via hyperflexion motion of the wrist. It is visualized best in the lateral view.

TABLE 10-9 cont'd
Fractures, Dislocations, and Soft-Tissue Injuries of the Upper Extremities

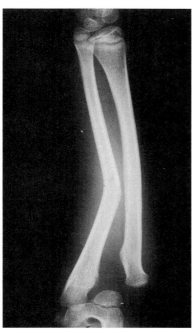

FIG. 10-129 Fracture through the proximal diaphysis of the ulna with dislocation of the radial head (Monteggia fracture-dislocation). (Courtesy of Jack C. Avalos, Davenport, IA.)

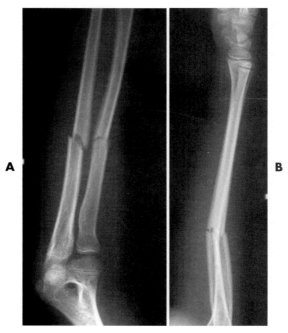

FIG. 10-130 **A** and **B,** A both bone fracture describes a fracture involving both the tibia and fibula (or radius and ulna as in this case). (Courtesy Steven P. Brownstein, MD, Springfield, NJ.)

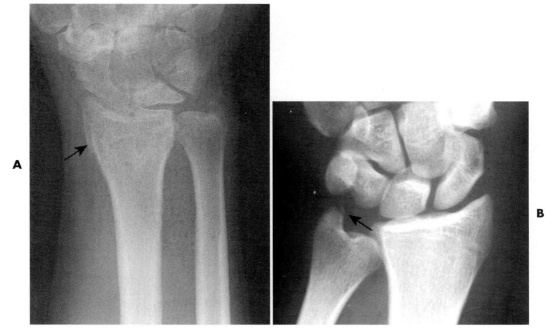

FIG. 10-131 **A,** Fracture of the radial styloid *(arrow)* and, **B,** another case that shows a fracture of the ulnar styloid *(arrow)*. Ulnar styloid fractures must be differentiated from an accessory ossicle, which is common to this location. Usually differentiation is possible by correlating to the patient's history and observing any edema or irregularity of the fragment that suggests fracture. (Courtesy Steven P. Brownstein, MD, Springfield, NJ.)

Continued

TABLE 10-9 cont'd

Fractures, Dislocations, and Soft-Tissue Injuries of the Upper Extremities

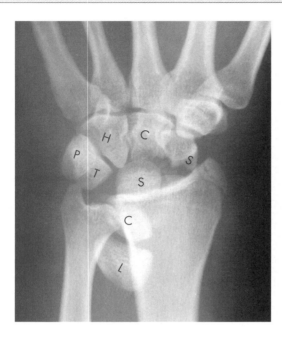

FIG. 10-132   Fracture of the radial styloid process and capitate with complete dislocation of the lunate and proximal fragment of the capitate. The patient fell from a ladder. *C,* Capitate; *H,* hamate; *L,* lunate; *P,* pisiform; *S,* scaphoid; and *T,* triquetrum. (Courtesy Steven P. Brownstein, MD, Springfield, NJ.)

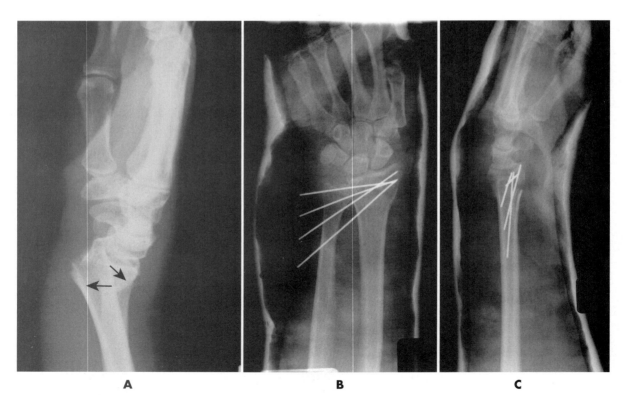

A   **B**   **C**

FIG. 10-133   A through **C,** Colles' fracture marked by a fracture through the distal radius with posterior displacement of the distal fragment with respect to the proximal fragment *(arrows).* The fracture was pinned and cast, as is the usual management for this fracture.

TABLE 10-9 cont'd

Fractures, Dislocations, and Soft-Tissue Injuries of the Upper Extremities

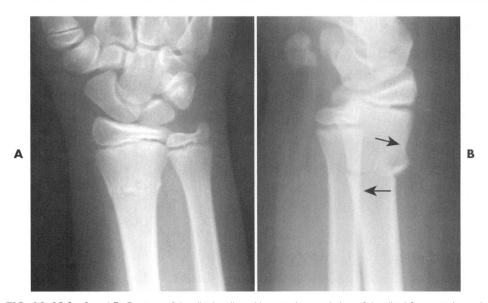

FIG. 10-134 **A** and **B,** Fracture of the distal radius with posterior angulation of the distal fragment *(arrows).* The configuration is generally consistent with a Colles' fracture, although definitively, a Colles' fracture is in the distal few centimeters of the radius. (Courtesy Steven P. Brownstein, MD, Springfield, NJ.)

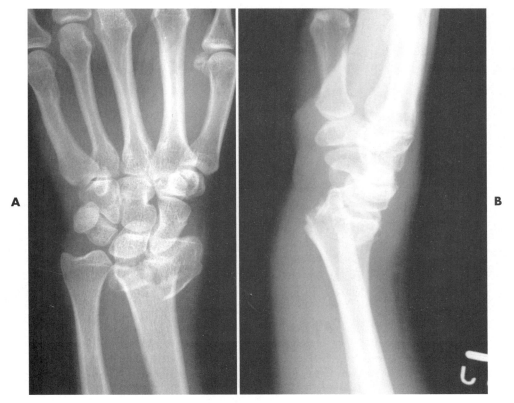

FIG. 10-135 **A** and **B,** Colles' fracture of the distal radius.

Continued

TABLE 10-9 cont'd

Fractures, Dislocations, and Soft-Tissue Injuries of the Upper Extremities

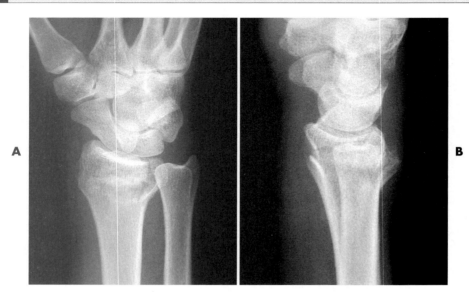

A

B

FIG. 10-136   **A** and **B,** Colles' fracture of the distal radius marked by dorsal angulation of the distal radial fracture.

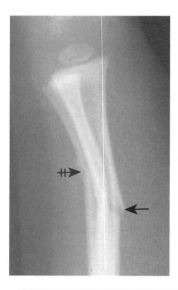

FIG. 10-137   Injury to the distal radius in a child that has resulted in a greenstick fracture on the distracted convex side of the bending bone *(arrow)* and a torus fracture on the compressed concave side of the bending bone *(crossed arrow).*

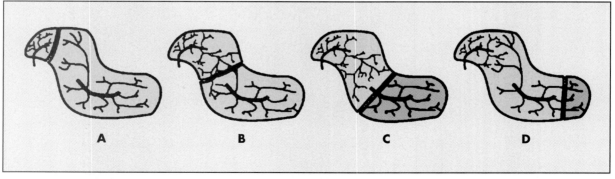

A   **B**   **C**   **D**

FIG. 10-138   The scaphoid is nourished by two vessels, one entering its distal pole and one entering its waist. **A** and **B,** Fracture through the distal pole does not interrupt blood flow to any part of the scaphoid, making avascular necrosis unlikely. However, **C,** a fracture through the waist or, **D,** proximal portion of the scaphoid interrupts the main blood supply to the portion of the scaphoid proximal to the fracture. Because of the altered perfusion, the proximal fragment has a tendency to undergo avascular necrosis when the fracture is proximal to the waist. (Modified from Rogers LF: Radiology of skeletal trauma, ed 2, vol 2, New York, 1992, Churchill Livingstone.)

TABLE 10-9 cont'd

Fractures, Dislocations, and Soft-Tissue Injuries of the Upper Extremities

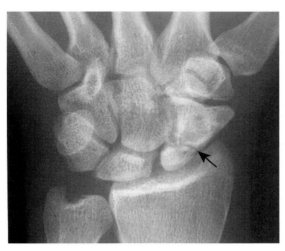

FIG. 10-139 Fracture through the waist of the scaphoid *(arrow)*. The condensed, slightly radiodense appearance of the proximal pole of the scaphoid is consistent with avascular necrosis.

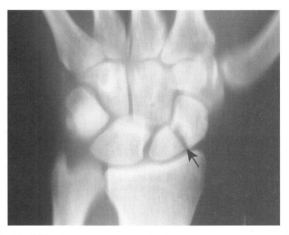

FIG. 10-141 Linear tomograph of a fracture through the waist of the scaphoid. Occult or ambiguous presentations on plain film radiographs can be more closely scrutinized with linear or computed tomography (CT). As the cost of examination continues to comparatively reduce, CT is becoming more routine for such applications.

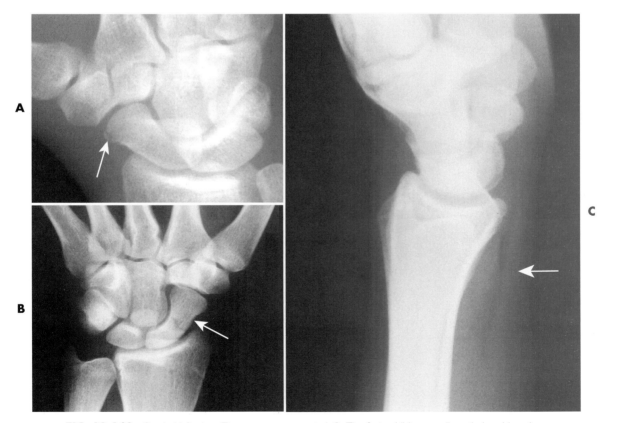

FIG. 10-140 Scaphoid fracture. Two cases are presented. **A,** The first exhibits a small cortical avulsion along the lateral margin of the scaphoid *(arrow)*. **B,** The second case is a fracture through the waist of the scaphoid *(arrow)*. **C,** On the lateral view that corresponds to **B,** there is no sign of edema in the proximal wrist. The degree of edema in this region can be assessed by observing if the fat pad overlying the pronator quadratus is distended *(arrow)*. The fat pad appears normal in **C.** If there were localized edema, as is often the case with a Colles' fracture or other injury of the distal radius, ulna, or carpals, there likely would be some degree of anterior distention or bulging of the radiolucent fat pad (a feature known as the *pronator sign*).

Continued

TABLE 10-9 cont'd

Fractures, Dislocations, and Soft-Tissue Injuries of the Upper Extremities

Injury	Comments
Dislocations	
Carpal dislocation (Figs. 10-149 through 10-155)	Detecting carpal dislocation is made easier by examining three carpal arcs for discontinuity in the posteroanterior (PA) projection:[92] Arc I is along the proximal articular surfaces of the proximal row of carpals. Arc II is along the distal articular surfaces of the proximal row of carpals. Arc III is along the proximal articular surfaces of the distal row of carpals (mostly hamate and capitate). One or several bones may be involved with dislocations. The lunate is the most common single bone dislocation, appearing triangular in shape ("pie", "C", or "spilled tea cup" sign) in the PA wrist projection. Rotational subluxations of the scaphoid present with a classic ringlike radiodensity of cortex ("signet ring" or "cortical ring" sign) and wide scapholunate joint space (>2 to 3 mm) in the PA projection ("Terry Thomas" sign, so-called because of the gap between this famous actor's front teeth). Normally in the lateral projection, the curved proximal surface of the capitate aligns with the curved surfaces of the lunate and distal radius, similar to three stacked saucers or three sideways "Cs." The appearance in the lateral projection of multiple carpal dislocations is described in three patterns: (a) perilunate dislocations involve dorsal dislocation of the capitate on the lunate, (b) midcarpal dislocations involve dorsal dislocation of the capitate on the lunate and partial anterior dislocation of the lunate on the radius, and (c) lunate dislocation is complete dislocation of the lunate with the radius and the capitate while the capitate remains in axial alignment with the radius. The three patterns are interrelated. Over time some patients progress in severity from perilunate to midcarpal to lunate patterns of dislocation.
Carpal instability (Fig. 10-156)	Several patterns of carpal instability have been described subsequent to ligamentous injury, usually of the proximal row of carpals.[77,93,146] The most common is scapholunate disassociation noted by a gap of more than 2 to 3 mm on the PA wrist radiograph ("Terry Thomas" or "David Letterman" sign, named for the gap in these celebrities' teeth). Increased dorsal flexion of the lunate on the lateral radiograph suggests a dorsal instability termed dorsal intercalated segment instability (DISI). Increased palmar flexion of the lunate on the lateral radiograph suggests a ventral instability termed ventral intercalated segment instability (VISI).[87] DISI and the less common VISI[93] may or may not accompany scapholunate disassociation. Instability patterns are best detailed by stress fluoroscopy. Carpal angles measured from the lateral radio-graph also are helpful. The scapholunate angle is formed from an axial line drawn through the center of the lunate and scaphoid. A second angle is formed by axial lines through the capitate and lunate (capitolunate angle). Scapholunate dissociation is suggested if the scapholunate angle measures greater than 60 degrees. VISI is indicated by a scapholunate angle less than 30 degrees and a capitolunate angle greater than 20 degrees. DISI is indicated by a scapholunate angle greater than 60 degrees and a capitolunate angle greater than 20 degrees.
Scapholunate advanced collapse	Chronic scapholunate advanced collapse (SLAC) is a common and specific pattern of degeneration marked by an increased scapholunate gap and narrowed radioscaphoid space. The progressive proximal migration of the capitate is related to disruption of the scapholunate ligaments. Ligament damage occurs from scaphoid nonunion advanced collapse (SNAC), calcium pyrophosphate dihydrate, trauma, Preiser disease, Kienböck disease, degeneration, and other conditions. Uncorrected SLAC deformity can lead to joint pain and limited range of wrist motion. PA radiographs of the wrist reveal reduced intercarpal joint spaces, bone sclerosis, subchondral cysts, osteophytes, scapholunate dislocation, and proximal displacement of the capitate.

TABLE 10-9 cont'd
Fractures, Dislocations, and Soft-Tissue Injuries of the Upper Extremities

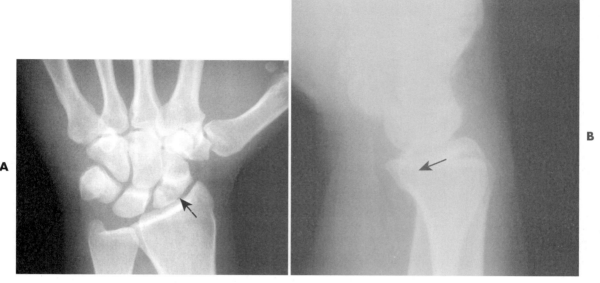

FIG. 10-142 A, Posteroanterior view reveals a scaphoid fracture *(arrow)*, whereas the distal radius appears normal. **B,** However, on the lateral projection, the distal radius has an anterior angulation consistent with a Smith fracture *(arrow)*.

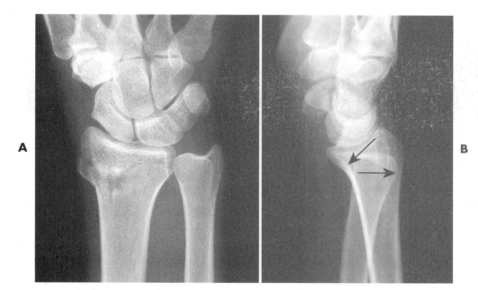

FIG. 10-143 A and **B,** Fracture of the distal radius with anterior angulation of the distal fragment, consistent with a Smith fracture *(arrows)*.

Continued

TABLE 10-9 cont'd
Fractures, Dislocations, and Soft-Tissue Injuries of the Upper Extremities

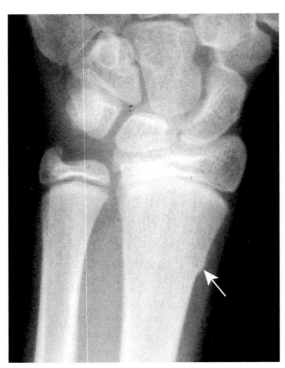

FIG. 10-144   Torus fracture of the distal radius noted by the slight cortical bulge *(arrow)*.

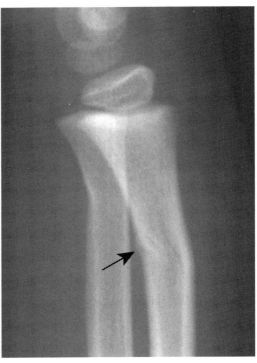

FIG. 10-145   Torus fracture along the lateral margin of the distal radius *(arrow)*. (Courtesy Steven P. Brownstein, MD, Springfield, NJ.)

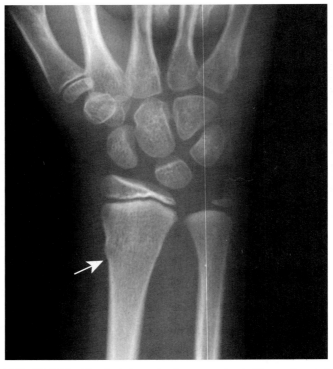

FIG. 10-146   The distal ulna and radius are angulated with a small cortical buckle (torus fracture) noted at the concave side of the deviation *(arrow)*.

TABLE 10-9 cont'd
Fractures, Dislocations, and Soft-Tissue Injuries of the Upper Extremities

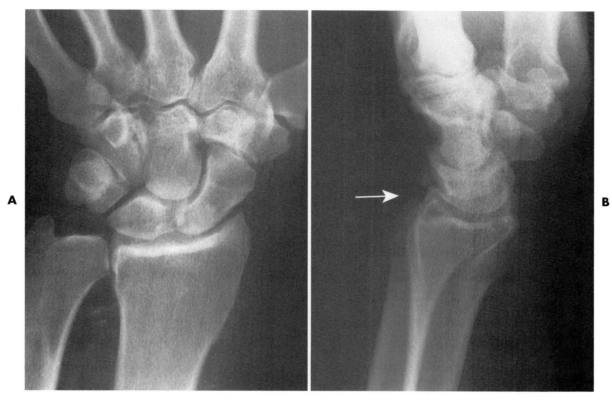

A

B

FIG. 10-147 Fragment at the posterior aspect of the wrist representing fracture of the triquetrum *(arrow)*. The lunate is dorsally flexed, consistent with dorsal intercalated segment instability. The posteroanterior view is essentially normal. (Courtesy Tim Mick, St Paul, MN.)

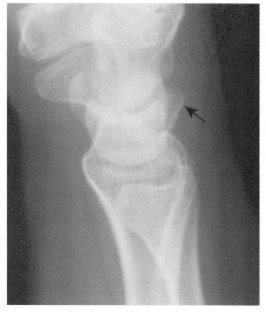

FIG. 10-148 Fragment of the posterior margin of the triquetrum *(arrow)*. (Courtesy Steven P. Brownstein, MD, Springfield, NJ.)

PART TWO Bone, Joints, and Soft Tissues

Continued

TABLE 10-9 cont'd
Fractures, Dislocations, and Soft-Tissue Injuries of the Upper Extremities

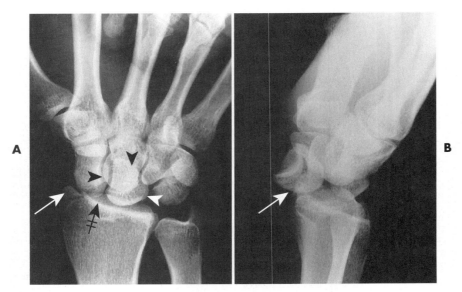

FIG. 10-149 Radial styloid fracture with lunate dislocation. **A,** Posteroanterior projection of the wrist denoting fracture of the radial styloid process *(arrow)* with a triangular "pie sign" appearance to the lunate *(arrowheads)*. The scapholunate joint space is increased, suggesting intercarpal ligament damage *(crossed arrow)*. **B,** The lateral projection reveals anterior displacement of the lunate *(arrow)* from its normal alignment with the distal radius and capitate. (Courtesy Jack C. Avalos, Davenport, IA.)

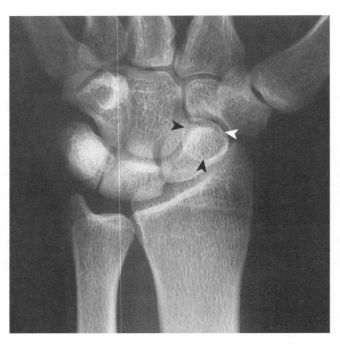

FIG. 10-150 Posteroanterior wrist projection with apparent foreshortening of the longitudinal axis of the scaphoid and noticeable circular density present ("signet ring" sign) *(arrowheads)*; both findings are suggestive of rotatory subluxation of the scaphoid. However, in this patient there is no subluxation. The appearance is an artifact caused by radial deviation of the wrist. The wrist should be slightly ulnar deviated to correctly assess for rotatory subluxation. Also, the scapholunate joint is not diastatic, a common finding in scaphoid subluxation. (Courtesy of Arthur W. Holmes, Foley, AL.)

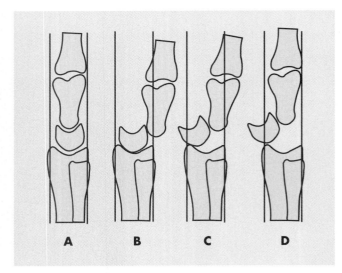

FIG. 10-151 **A,** Normally the longitudinal axes of the radius, lunate, and capitate align. **B,** Perilunate dislocation is marked by posterior dislocation of the capitate-lunate joint and normal alignment of the lunate-radius joint. **C,** Midcarpal dislocation is noted by posterior dislocation of the capitate-lunate joint and anterior dislocation of the lunate-radial joint. **D,** Lunate dislocation is noted by anterior dislocation of the lunate with normal alignment of the capitate and radius.

TABLE 10-9 cont'd
Fractures, Dislocations, and Soft-Tissue Injuries of the Upper Extremities

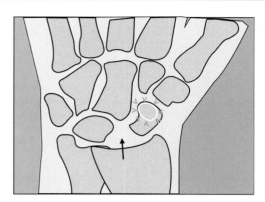

FIG. 10-152 On the posteroanterior radiograph, a scaphoid dislocation is accompanied by scapholunate dissociation ("Terry Thomas" or "David Letterman sign") *(arrow)*. The dislocated scaphoid rotates, causing it to appear shortened and appear as a cortical "signet" ring *(arrowheads)*.

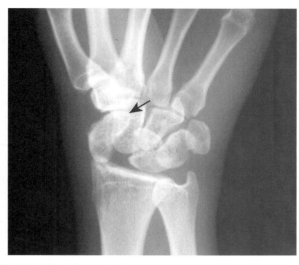

FIG. 10-153 The scaphoid appears shortened and with a cortical ring overlying its distal pole *(arrow)*. (Courtesy Steven P. Brownstein, MD, Springfield, NJ.)

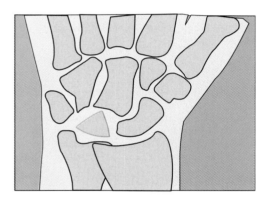

FIG. 10-154 On the posteroanterior radiograph, a lunate dislocation presents with rotation of the segment, causing it to appear as a big wedge of pie.

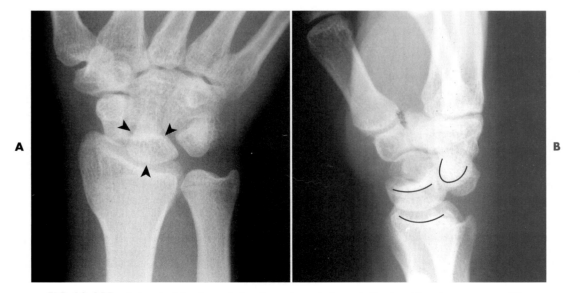

FIG. 10-155 **A,** Lunate dislocation noted on the posteroanterior projection by a triangular appearance of the lunate *(arrowheads)*. **B,** On the lateral projection, there is a loss of normal alignment of the three "Cs" of the distal radius, lunate, and capitate. (Courtesy Steven P. Brownstein, MD, Springfield, NJ.)

Continued

TABLE 10-9 cont'd

Fractures, Dislocations, and Soft-Tissue Injuries of the Upper Extremities

Injury	Comments
Soft-tissue injuries (ligaments and cartilage)	
Carpal tunnel syndrome (Fig. 10-157)	Carpal tunnel syndrome occurs from repetitive flexing and extension of the wrist, resulting in a thickening of the protective sheaths that surround each of the tendons. The inflamed tendon sheaths cause a narrowed carpal tunnel and median nerve deficiency. MRI clearly delineates the structure within the carpal tunnel that is the location of the most common of the nerve compression syndromes. MRI features of compression of the median nerve include flattening, swelling, increased signal intensity of this structure, and volan (palmer) bowing of the transverse ligament. Tingling, burning, numbness, and loss of grip strength may be present, rarely leading to permanent deficiency. Carpal tunnel syndrome is complicated by pregnancy, obesity, and diabetes.
Intercarpal ligament injury	The scapholunate and lunotriquetral ligaments are the most important intrinsic ligaments of the wrist. Injury to these structures may lead to instability syndromes such as dorsal or volar intercalated segmented instability (DISI and VISI).
Triangular fibrocartilage injury (Fig. 10-158)	The triangular fibrocartilage absorbs axial loading and lends stability to the ulnar aspect of the wrist joint. Most tears of the triangular fibrocartilage result from a degenerative etiology that makes the ligament vulnerable to biomechanical forces. High-resolution MRI shows tears of the triangular fibrocartilage, with the T2-weighted images providing the most information to differentiate degenerative from traumatic etiologies of the tear. Tears of the triangular fibrocartilage are associated with a positive ulnar length variance. Ulnar variance increases with pronation and grip. Patients exhibit ulnar-sided wrist pain that is exacerbated by activity and often accompanied by joint crepitus and a history of trauma.
Hand	
Fractures	
Metacarpal fracture (Figs. 10-159 through 10-162)	A metacarpal fracture is typically transverse in orientation. It is referred to as a *boxer fracture* if it occurs in the second or third metacarpal and a *barroom fracture* if the fourth or fifth metacarpals are involved. A Bennett fracture is an intraarticular fracture at the base of the first metacarpal with posterolateral dislocation of the first metacarpocarpal joint. A small medial fragment of the metacarpal remains in contact with the trapezium.[14] Rolando fracture is a comminuted Bennett fracture, exhibiting a Y, T, or V configuration.[188]
Phalangeal fracture (Figs. 10-163 through 10-167)	The phalanx is probably the most common site of skeletal injury.[203] The distal phalanx is more commonly fractured than the middle or proximal phalanx. A dorsal chip fracture at the site of the inserting extension tendon of the distal phalanx results in a flexion deformity of the finger, known as a "mallet" or "baseball" finger.[156] A swan neck deformity also may develop, appearing as simultaneous flexion of the distal interphalangeal joint and extension of the proximal interphalangeal joint.[258] Fracture of the palmar surface (or volar plate) of the middle phalanges may result in loss of digit flexion and proximal interphalangeal joint hyperextension. Acute fractures should be splinted and evaluated by an orthopedic specialist. Boutonnière (buttonhole) deformity results from rupture of the middle slip of the extensor tendons and appears as flexion of the proximal interphalangeal joint with extension of the distal interphalangeal joint.
Dislocations	
Metacarpal and phalangeal dislocation (Figs. 10-168 and 10-169)	Phalangeal dislocation may occur in any location. Posterior dislocation following hyperextension injury is most common. Interphalangeal dislocations are rarely multiple.[255] Metacarpal dislocations most often occur in a posterior direction.
Gamekeeper's thumb (Fig. 10-170)	Gamekeeper's thumb describes disruption of the ulnar collateral ligament of the first metacarpophalangeal joint with resulting joint instability, and often is associated with a fracture at the base of the proximal phalanx. Anecdotally this injury has been attributed to breaking the neck of game animals (rabbits and birds) between the thumb and forefinger.[30] In the modern era, it is more likely related to an incorrect grasp of a ski pole. Valgus stress views are indicated in the presence of clinical indicators and negative plain films. A Stenner's lesion occurs when a torn ulnar collateral ligament of the first metacarpophalangeal joint displaces superficial to the adductor tendon, and is an indication for surgical repair.

TABLE 10-9 cont'd
Fractures, Dislocations, and Soft-Tissue Injuries of the Upper Extremities

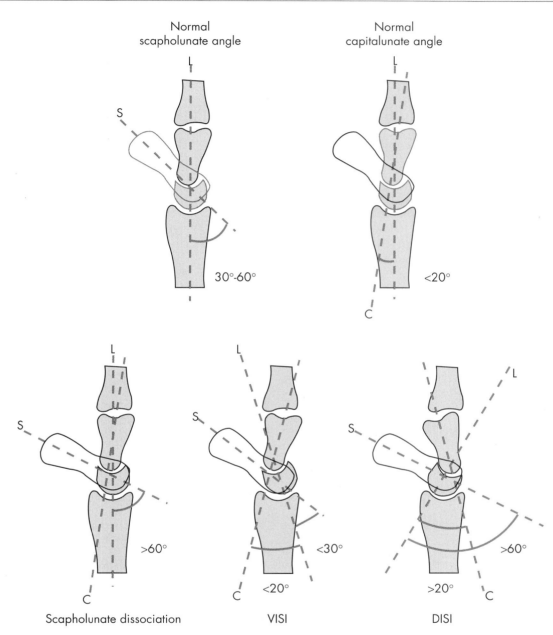

Normal scapholunate angle 30°-60°

Normal capitalunate angle <20°

Scapholunate dissociation >60°

VISI <30° <20°

DISI >60° >20°

FIG. 10-156 Normally, the scapholunate angle is between 30 and 60 degrees and the capitolunate angle less than 20 degrees. Scapholunate dissociation is marked by in increased scapholunate angle (>60 degrees). Volar intercalated segmental instability (VISI) is defined as a reduced scapholunate angle (<30 degrees) and increased capitolunate angle (>20 degrees). Dorsal intercalated segmental instability (OISI) is defined by increased scapholunate angle (>60 degrees) and increased capitolunate angle (>20 degrees).

Continued

TABLE 10-9 cont'd

Fractures, Dislocations, and Soft-Tissue Injuries of the Upper Extremities

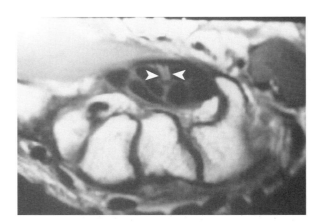

FIG. 10-157 Axial T1-weighted magnetic resonance imaging scan of the wrist demonstrating alteration of the normally oval median nerve (*arrowheads*) suggesting compression within the carpal tunnel.

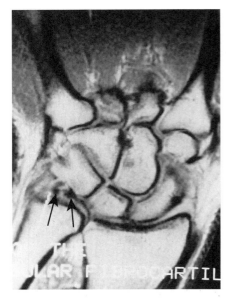

FIG. 10-158 Coronal T1-weighted magnetic resonance imaging scan of the wrist demonstrating hyperintense linear defects, signifying tears (*arrows*) through the normal hypointense triangular fibrocartilage.

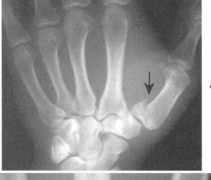

A

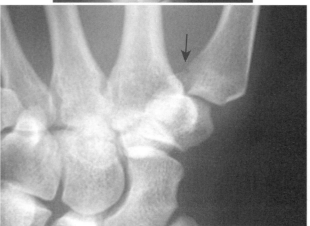

B

FIG. 10-159 **A** and **B**, Bennett fracture through the base of the first metacarpal with posterolateral dislocation of the first digit in two cases (*arrows*). (**A,** Courtesy Steven P. Brownstein, MD, Springfield, NJ.)

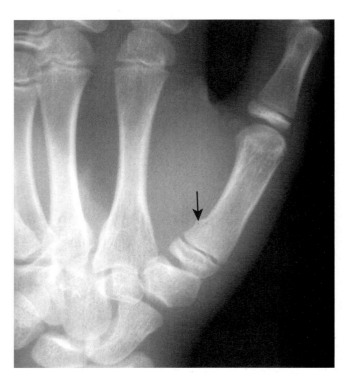

FIG. 10-160 Small defect at the medial base of the first metacarpal (*arrow*). (Courtesy Steven P. Brownstein, MD, Springfield, NJ.)

TABLE 10-9 cont'd
Fractures, Dislocations, and Soft-Tissue Injuries of the Upper Extremities

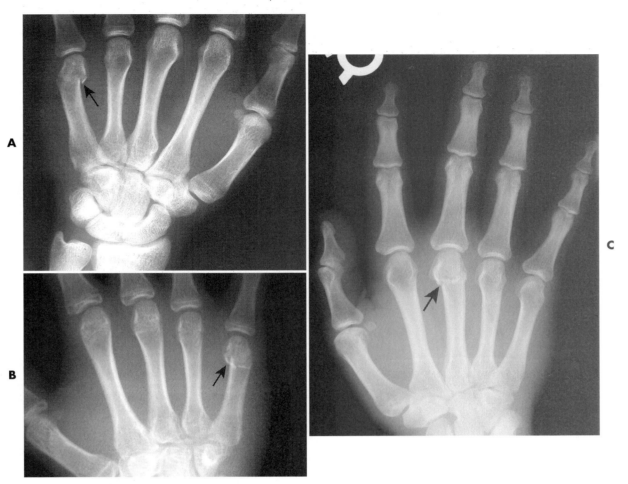

FIG. 10-161 **A** through **C,** Fracture of the metacarpal neck in three cases *(arrows).* (Courtesy Steven P. Brownstein, MD, Springfield, NJ.)

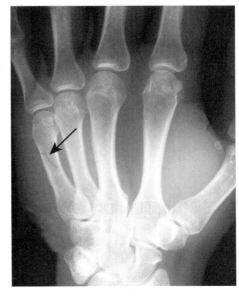

FIG. 10-162 Oblique fracture of the shaft of the fifth metacarpal *(arrow).*

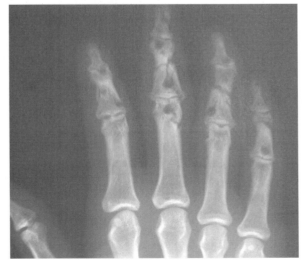

FIG. 10-163 Crush injury resulting in many comminuted fractures of the phalanges. (Courtesy Steven P. Brownstein, MD, Springfield, NJ.)

Continued

TABLE 10-9 cont'd

Fractures, Dislocations, and Soft-Tissue Injuries of the Upper Extremities

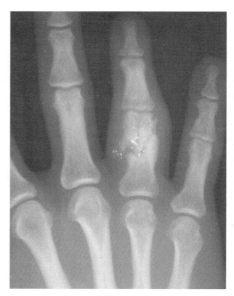

FIG. 10-164 Comminuted fracture, impacted metallic fragments, and soft-tissue distention of the proximal phalanx of the fourth digit.

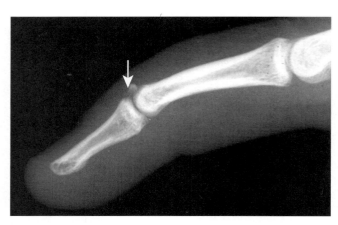

FIG. 10-165 Small avulsion at the dorsal, proximal corner of the distal phalanx from an avulsion injury of the extension tendon, with slight residual flexion of the finger *(arrow)*. This injury occurs from a sudden resisted flexion of the finger, as may occur when a baseball strikes the end of a finger; hence the injury is known as a "baseball" (or "mallet") finger. (Courtesy Steven P. Brownstein, MD, Springfield, NJ.)

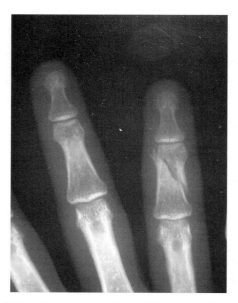

FIG. 10-166 Oblique fracture of the middle phalanx of the fourth digit.

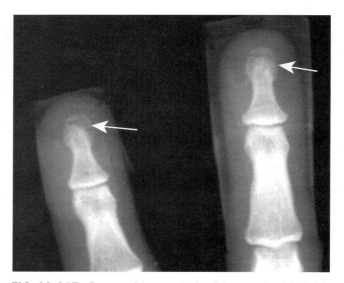

FIG. 10-167 Fracture of the ungual tufts of the second and third digits *(arrows)*.

TABLE 10-9 cont'd
Fractures, Dislocations, and Soft-Tissue Injuries of the Upper Extremities

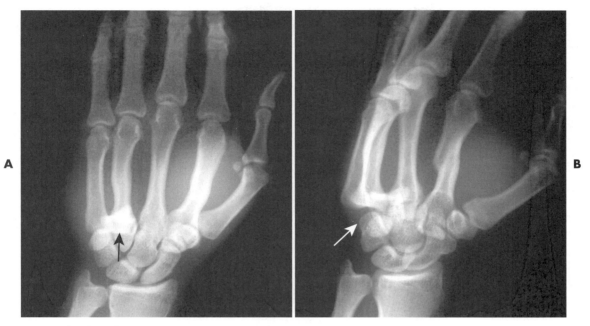

FIG. 10-168   A, Posteroanterior and, **B,** oblique projections of the hand that reveal a posterior dislocation of the fourth carpometacarpal articulation (arrows). An old fracture of the second metacarpal is also noted. (Courtesy Steven P. Brownstein, MD, Springfield, NJ.)

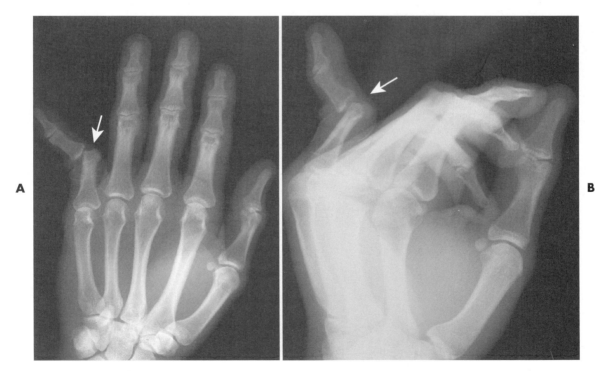

FIG. 10-169   A, Posteroanterior and, **B,** oblique projections of the hand showing posterior dislocation of the middle phalanx of the fifth digit (arrows). (Courtesy Steven P. Brownstein, MD, Springfield, NJ.)

Continued

TABLE 10-9 cont'd
Fractures, Dislocations, and Soft-Tissue Injuries of the Upper Extremities

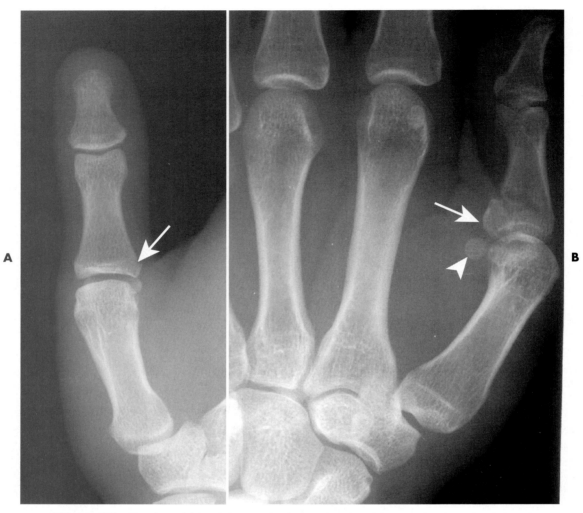

FIG. 10-170　Gamekeeper's injury defines a strain of the medial collateral ligament of the metacarpophalangeal joint. **A** and **B,** These cases show a small avulsion at the site of the ligament insertion *(arrows).* There is a small sesamoid bone just below the fracture in case B *(arrowhead).*

TABLE 10-10

Fractures, Dislocations, and Soft-Tissue Injuries of the Pelvis and Lower Extremities

Injury	Comments
Pelvis	
Fractures	
Acetabular fracture (Figs. 10-171 and 10-172)	There are five types of acetabular fractures: anterior (iliopubic) column, posterior (ilioischial) column, acetabular rim (anterior, posterior, and superior), transverse, and central or explosion.[144,243] Central fracture-dislocation describes displacement of the femoral head into the pelvis. Most fractures of the acetabulum fit into more than one category.[108] Acetabular fractures typically require great forces, such as those associated with auto accidents. Specifically, a "dashboard" fracture refers to fracture of the posterior rim of the acetabulum that occurs secondary to forces applied to the knee when the femur is flexed and adducted during auto accidents.
Double vertical contralateral (bucket handle) fracture-dislocation (Fig. 10-173)	A bucket handle fracture of the pelvic ring is composed of individual fractures of the superior and inferior pubic rami and fracture near or separation of the contralateral sacroiliac joint.[67]
Double vertical ipsilateral (Malgaigne) fracture-dislocation (Fig. 10-174)	A Malgaigne fracture of the pelvic ring is composed of individual fractures of the superior and inferior pubic rami and a fracture near or separation of the ipsilateral sacroiliac joint. It represents the most common fracture of the pelvis.[204]
Double vertical pubic (straddle) fracture (Figs. 10-175 and 10-176)	A straddle fracture describes fractures of all four pubic rami. Patients often have concurrent injury to the pelvic viscera.[41]
Iliac wing (Duverney's) fracture	A Duverney's fracture is a transverse, oblique, or vertical fracture of the iliac wing. Because it does not involve the pelvic ring, it is not associated with pelvic instability. The most common cause is a direct lateral blow to the ilium.
Pelvic avulsion fracture (Figs. 10-177 through 10-180)	An avulsion fracture of the pelvis is most common at the sites of open apophyses, occurring secondary to muscular traction. Common sites include avulsion of anterior superior iliac spine (ASIS) at the insertion of the sartorius muscle, avulsion of the anterior inferior iliac spine (AIIS) at the insertion of the rectus femoris, avulsion of the pubic symphysis at the insertion of femoral adductors, and avulsion of the ischial tuberosity at the insertion of the leg flexors (hamstrings). Avulsion injuries are most often related to athletes, such as hurdlers, cheerleaders, long jumpers, and sprinters. Continued muscle tension causes distraction of the avulsed fragment, which may enlarge to a notable bulbous deformity.
Ramus fracture	A single fracture to the pelvic rim generally is stable, and most often represents a fracture of the superior or inferior pubic ramus. Ramus fractures are common, representing 20%[159] to 50%[115] of pelvic fractures. They usually are seen in osteoporotic individuals following minor falls. Bilateral double ramus fractures are straddle fractures, as discussed in the preceding.
Sacral fracture (Figs. 10-181 through 10-184)	Sacral fractures occur in a transverse plane secondary to direct trauma (e.g., fall on the buttocks), and usually present in the lower margin of the sacrum. A transverse fracture of the upper sacrum is more closely related to a high fall (a "suicidal jumper" fracture). A vertical sacral fracture is often found in combination with other fractures of the pelvic ring[168,261] and often is associated with damage to the pelvic viscera. Vertical fractures occur in three zones, as defined by the Denis classification. Zone I is lateral to the sacral foramina. A fracture that involves the sacral foramen and not the sacral canal occurs in zone II. Zone III is medial to the sacral foramen, involving the sacral canal. A zone I fracture is more common; zone III has a greater association with neurologic deficits. A stress fracture of the sacrum usually is vertical. A sacral fracture is difficult to detect on plain film radiographs because the overlying gas and fecal matter often obstruct a clear view of the anatomy. Tracing the cortices of the sacral foramina helps to recognize abnormality. CT examination may be indicated to better define the osseous anatomy and evaluate for associated injury to the viscera.

Continued

TABLE 10-10 cont'd
Fractures, Dislocations, and Soft-Tissue Injuries of the Pelvis and Lower Extremities

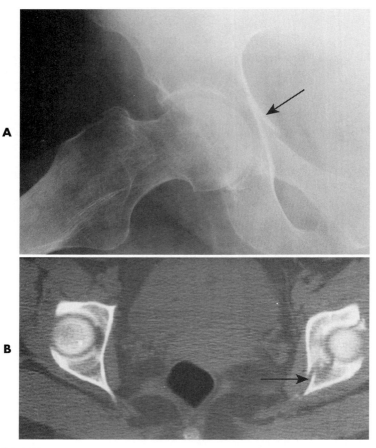

FIG. 10-171   Acetabular fracture noted on, **A,** plain film and, **B,** computed tomography *(arrows)*. (Courtesy Steven P. Brownstein, MD, Springfield, NJ.)

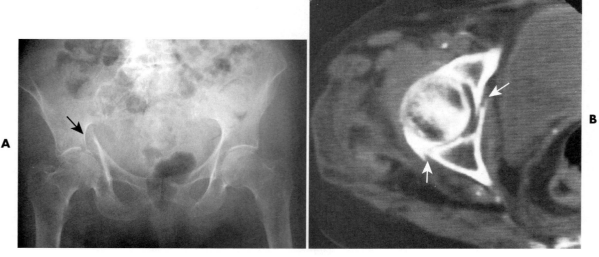

FIG. 10-172   Acetabular fracture noted on, **A,** plain film and, **B,** computed tomography *(arrows)*.

TABLE 10-10 cont'd

Fractures, Dislocations, and Soft-Tissue Injuries of the Pelvis and Lower Extremities

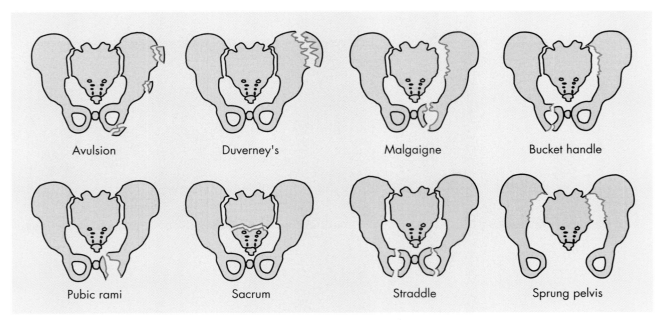

FIG. 10-173 Fractures and dislocations of the pelvis. From superior to inferior, avulsion fractures involve the sartorius at the anterior superior iliac spine, rectus femoris at the anterior inferior iliac spine, and femoral hamstring muscles at the ischial tuberosity. Duverney's fracture involves the iliac wing. Malgaigne's fractures are double vertical ipsilateral fractures of the pelvis. Bucket handle fractures are double vertical contralateral fractures of the pelvis. Straddle fractures are bilateral fractures of the pubic rami. A sprung (or open book) pelvis describes pubic diastasis and sacroiliac joint dislocation.

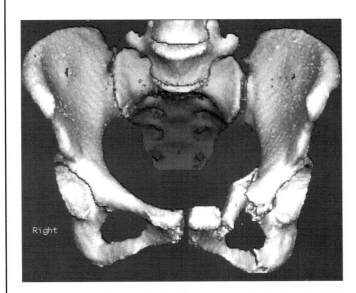

FIG. 10-174 Malgaigne fracture. Three-dimensional reformed computed tomography scan revealing fractures of the superior and inferior pubic rami and an accompanying ipsilateral separation of the sacroiliac joint. (Courtesy Sean Mathers, Pittsburgh, PA.)

Continued

TABLE 10-10 cont'd
Fractures, Dislocations, and Soft-Tissue Injuries of the Pelvis and Lower Extremities

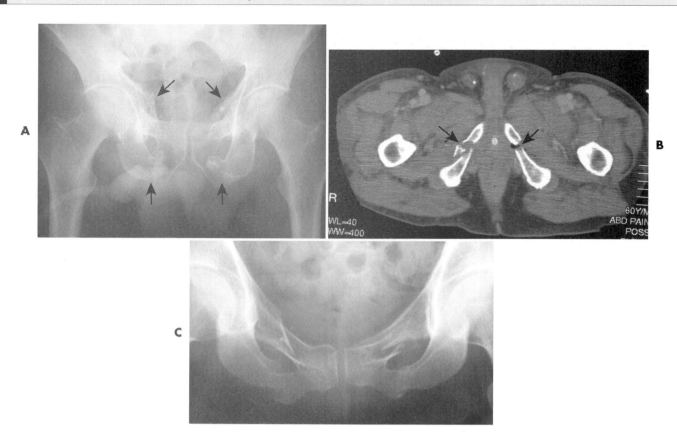

A

B

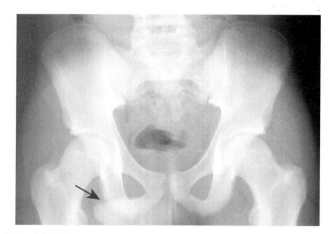

C

FIG. 10-175   **A,** A 62-year-old man with a straddle fracture noted on plain film. **B,** Lower ischiopubic rami fractures are evident on this computed tomography scan *(arrows)*. **C,** A second case of straddle fracture is noted. (**A** and **B,** Courtesy Troy Scheuermann, Farmington, IA.)

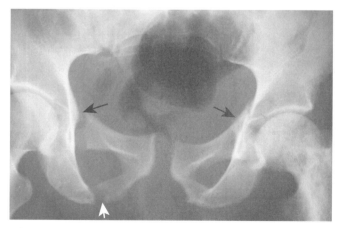

FIG. 10-176   A variation of straddle fracture noted by a double fracture of the pubic rami and contralateral fracture of the acetabulum *(arrows)*. (Courtesy Steven P. Brownstein, MD, Springfield, NJ.)

FIG. 10-177   Adolescent patient with a small avulsion fracture noted in the region of the sartorius insertion *(arrow)*. (Courtesy Steven P. Brownstein, MD, Springfield, NJ.)

TABLE 10-10 cont'd
Fractures, Dislocations, and Soft-Tissue Injuries of the Pelvis and Lower Extremities

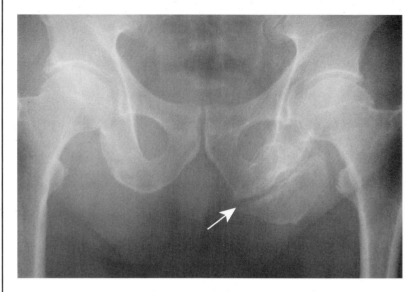

FIG. 10-178 Healed avulsion of the ischial tuberosity. The large bulbous appearance is sometimes mistaken for a sessile osteochondroma. The history of injury, such as hamstring muscles pull, and location help in differentiation *(arrow)*. (Courtesy Martin Stine, Windsor, CO.)

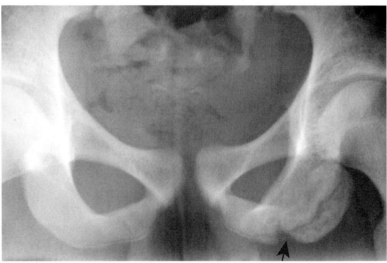

FIG. 10-179 Avulsion and resulting deformity of the left ischial tuberosity *(arrow)*. (Courtesy Markus Kirk, Findlay, OH.)

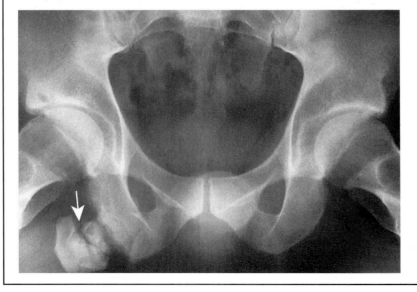

FIG. 10-180 Old avulsion fracture of the right ischial apophysis with residual bulbous deformity *(arrow)*. (Courtesy Jack C. Avalos, Davenport, IA.)

Continued

TABLE 10-10 cont'd
Fractures, Dislocations, and Soft-Tissue Injuries of the Pelvis and Lower Extremities

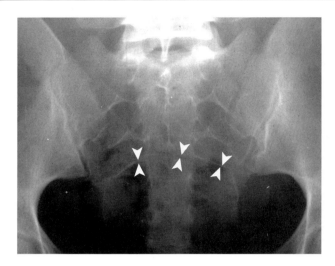

FIG. 10-181   Transverse (horizontal) fracture of the sacrum *(arrowheads).* (Courtesy Steven P. Brownstein, MD, Springfield, NJ.)

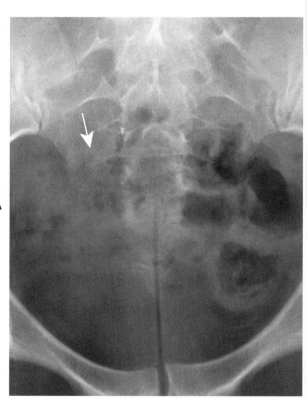

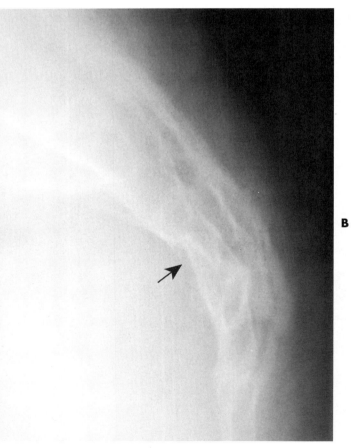

FIG. 10-182   **A** and **B,** Sacral fracture *(arrows).* Often sacral fractures are obstructed by overlying fecal material. Computed tomography and magnetic resonance imaging may assist in the patient evaluation. (Courtesy Clifton Bethel, Rock Island, IL.)

TABLE 10-10 cont'd
Fractures, Dislocations, and Soft-Tissue Injuries of the Pelvis and Lower Extremities

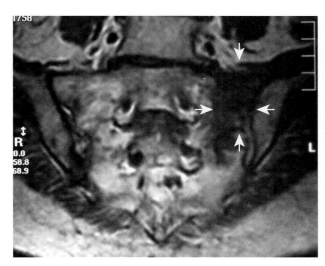

FIG. 10-183 Sacral fracture depicted on magnetic resonance imaging. The fracture is noted by the hypointense regions of edema replacing the normally hyperintense signal from the normal bone marrow on this T1-weighted image (arrows). (Courtesy Robin Canterbury, Davenport, IA.)

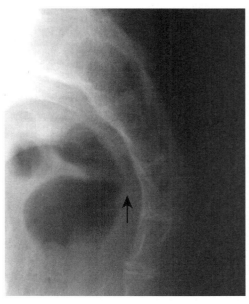

FIG. 10-184 An expanded presacral space provides a clue of the presence of fracture. The presacral space is normally less than 1 cm (arrow). The case shown here is normal.

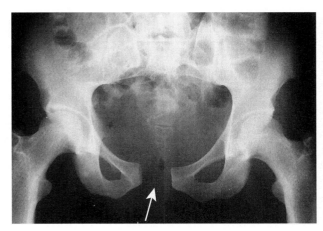

FIG. 10-185 Sprung pelvis noted by the widened pubic symphysis (arrow) and probable dislocation of one or both sacroiliac joints. The width of the pubic symphysis joint space should not exceed 6 mm in female and 7 mm in male patients. (Courtesy Steven P. Brownstein, MD, Springfield, NJ.)

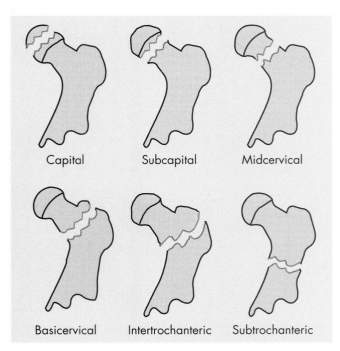

FIG. 10-186 Hip fractures are classified as intracapsular or extracapsular. Intracapsular fractures include capital, subcapital, midcervical, and basocervical. Extracapsular fractures include intertrochanteric, trochanteric, and subtrochanteric.

Capital Subcapital Midcervical

Basicervical Intertrochanteric Subtrochanteric

Continued

PART TWO Bone, Joints, and Soft Tissues

TABLE 10-10 cont'd
Fractures, Dislocations, and Soft-Tissue Injuries of the Pelvis and Lower Extremities

Injury	Comments
Coccygeal fracture	A coccygeal fracture is usually transverse in orientation and often anteriorly angulated with the presence of soft-tissue swelling (noted by a presacral space in excess of 1 cm as measured on the lateral 40-inch focal-spot-to-film distance film). Anterior angulation often occurs as a normal variant; this finding alone does not indicate trauma.
Sprung (open book) pelvis (Fig. 10-185)	A sprung pelvis describes diastasis of the pubic symphysis with dislocation of one or both of the sacroiliac joints. It occurs secondary to an anterior compression injury and often is associated with damage to the pelvic viscera.
Hip	
Fractures	
Hip fracture (Figs. 10-186 through 10-194)	Each year more than one third of adults over the age of 65 years fall.[105,110] Injury is common. In fact, falls are the leading cause of injury-related deaths among older adults.[172] Although a wide variety of injuries are associated with these falls, hip fractures cause the greatest number of deaths, disability, and reduced quality of life.[102,267] An estimated 17% of white women in the United States sustain a hip fracture after the age of 50 years.[95] Depending on age and other factors, mortality related to complications of immobility, embolism, nosocomial infection, and pneumonia is estimated at 12% to 40% within 1 year. Female gender, decreased bone density, and advancing age are all predictors of hip fractures. As a group, women sustain 75% to 80% of all hip fractures.[49,232] The rate of hip fracture increases exponentially with age.[213] People over the age of 85 are 10 to 15 times more likely to sustain hip fractures than people between 60 and 65 years of age.[219] It has been estimated that for each standard deviation (SD) decrease in bone mass density at the femoral neck there is a 2.6-fold increase in risk of hip fracture.[4]

Fractures are classified as intracapsular (occurring proximal to the trochanters) or extracapsular. Intracapsular fractures include fractures through the femoral head (capital), just below the femoral head (subcapital, most common type),[86] through the femoral neck (midcervical, rare), and at the base of the femoral neck (basocervical, uncommon). Pathologic fractures commonly occur at the femoral neck, usually in a basicervical location. The circumflex arteries may tear with capsular damage associated with intracapsular fractures, resulting in complication of avascular necrosis and nonunion.[8,10,118] Extracapsular fractures include fractures of the greater and lesser trochanters, and intertrochanteric and subtrochanteric regions. Because the arterial supply remains intact, extracapsular fractures are less often complicated by avascular necrosis and nonunion than are intracapsular fractures. Intertrochanteric femoral fractures are associated with age-related osteoporosis. Sometimes they are classified by the number of fragments. The state of the posteromedial cortex is particularly important because it relates to fracture stability.

Early detection of hip fractures is related to patient outcome; therefore it is increasingly important economically and legally in the changing health care environment.[160] Assessment often begins with AP and frog-leg plain film images. On the AP radiographs, there may be a coxa varus deformity because the patient often ambulates or places some body weight on the fractured proximal femur. Fractures, particularly those in a subcapital and midcervical location, exhibit a zone of condensation (radiopaque band) along the medial margin of the femoral neck and zone of rarefaction (radiolucent band) along the lateral margin of the femoral neck. Another hint to the presence of fracture, particularly in a subcapital location, is the offset of the femoral head on the neck. It looks lopsided or inferiorly sheared. |

TABLE 10-10 cont'd

Fractures, Dislocations, and Soft-Tissue Injuries of the Pelvis and Lower Extremities

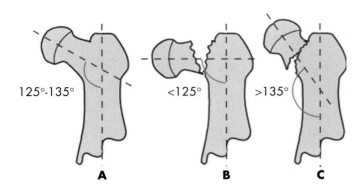

125°-135°   <125°   >135°

A   **B**   **C**

FIG. 10-187 Normally the femoral angle is between 125 to 135 degrees. Fractures of the proximal femur may cause the angle to deform, providing a film interpretation hint to the presence of fracture. An increased angle is associated with a valgus deformity and a decreased angle with a varus deformity.

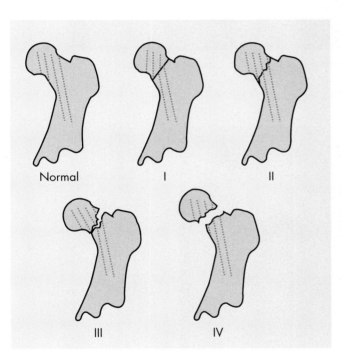

Normal   I   II

III   IV

FIG. 10-188 Garden classification of proximal femur fracture displacement. Garden type I is an incomplete fracture with valgus impaction. Garden type II is a complete fracture without displacement. Garden type III is a complete fracture with partial displacement (usually varus). Garden type IV is a complete fracture with total displacement and rotation of the femoral head. Garden types I and II are nondisplaced, and Garden types III and IV are displaced.

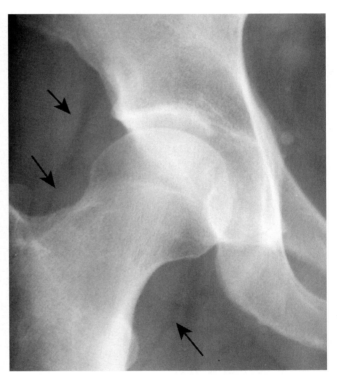

FIG. 10-189 Possible hip effusion is suggested by deviation of the lateral (gluteos medios) and medial fat (iliopsoas) planes of the hip. In this figure, the normal appearance of the fat planes is shown *(arrows)*. Effacement or displacement of these fat pads correlates to hip effusion. False-positive presentations may occur with hip abduction or external rotation. A prominent hip effusion also may widen the medial space of the hip joint.

Continued

TABLE 10-10 cont'd
Fractures, Dislocations, and Soft-Tissue Injuries of the Pelvis and Lower Extremities

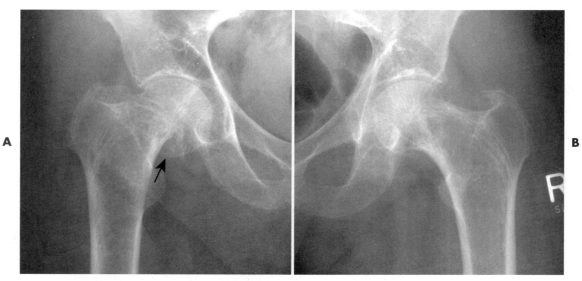

FIG. 10-190 A, Subcapital fracture in an osteoporotic patient. **B,** The contralateral side is not fractured. (Courtesy Steven P. Brownstein, MD, Springfield, NJ.)

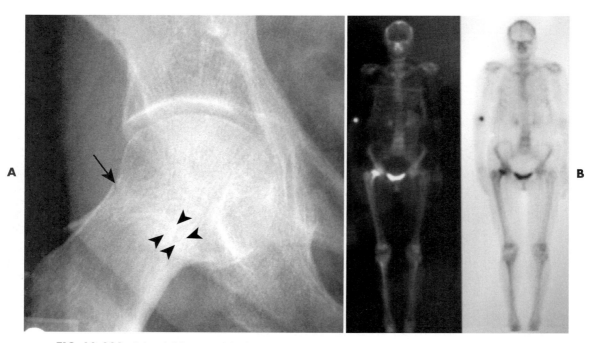

FIG. 10-191 Subcapital fracture of the femoral neck. **A,** Notice the compressed trabeculation and resulting radiodense band on the inferior margin of the femur *(arrowheads)* and cortical disruption on the distracted superior margin of the fractured femur *(arrow).* **B,** A bone scan reveals uptake of the radiotracer consistent with fracture and injection site on the arm. (Courtesy Cheryl E. Crawford, Clarion, PA.)

TABLE 10-10 cont'd
Fractures, Dislocations, and Soft-Tissue Injuries of the Pelvis and Lower Extremities

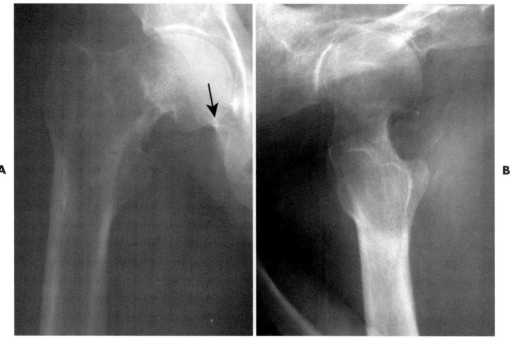

FIG. 10-192 **A** and **B,** Subcapital fracture with inferior translation in the direction of the arrow. Often fractures of the proximal femur, especially subcapital fractures, do not demonstrate an obvious radiolucent defect. In this case the fracture is noted by an offset of the femoral head on the femoral neck.

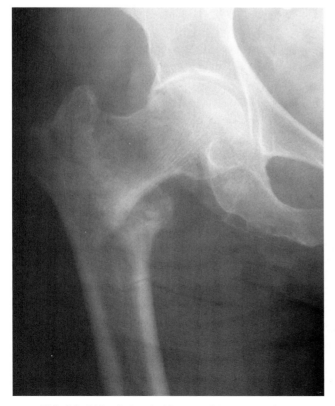

FIG. 10-193 Basicervical fracture of the proximal femur.

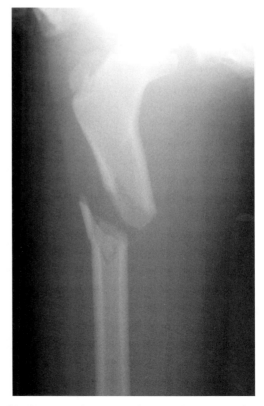

FIG. 10-194 Comminuted fracture of the proximal femur.

Continued

TABLE 10-10 cont'd
Fractures, Dislocations, and Soft-Tissue Injuries of the Pelvis and Lower Extremities

Injury	Comments
Hip fracture—cont'd	The degree of displacement is classified by Garden (I to IV). The degree of displacement is a key indicator of the expected patient prognosis.[15] Garden type I is an incomplete fracture with valgus impaction. Garden type II is a complete fracture without displacement. Garden type III is a complete fracture with partial displacement. Garden type IV is a complete fracture with total displacement and rotation of the femoral head. Garden types I and II are nondisplaced, and Garden types III and IV are displaced.
	The difficulty of diagnosing hip fractures increases with increasing patient age, mostly as a factor of osteoporosis. Nondisplaced femoral neck fractures are particularly difficult to diagnose.[221] Because hip fractures often are occult or equivocal on plain film, a bone scan, linear tomography, CT, or MRI examination should be considered when clinical features exist and plain films are negative for abnormality. Bone scans may not exhibit fractures until 72 hours after the traumatic event. After 72 hours a negative bone scan virtually excludes hip fracture. An MRI examination reveals decreased signal intensity of the bone marrow soon after injury, and is probably the best choice to exclude a hip fracture based on its high sensitivity, bilateral field of view, and noninvasive methods. The sensitivity of the plain film examination sometimes can be augmented by using 30-degree internal (or less often external) rotation of the leg in question to increase the radiographic sensitivity.
	The common clinical features of hip fracture include limited range of motion, acute or chronic pain with weight bearing in the hip or groin, external rotation and shortening of the leg, and being unable to put full weight on the foot after acute trauma with impact to the hip joint or pelvic region.[272]
	Treatment is dependent on the location, type, and severity of the fracture, as well as patient demographic and clinical factors. Long periods of bed rest, or any prolonged immobility, increase the patient's risk of thromboembolism, pneumonia, and cardiac deconditioning. Therefore nonoperative treatment typically is not indicated or successful for complete fractures, and is reserved for patients who cannot tolerate the risks associated with surgery and anesthesia. Surgical pinning (Knowles pins) and hip replacement surgery are typical treatment strategies. For those at risk for hip fracture, calcium, vitamin D, calcitonin, bisphosphonates, exercise, and hormone (e.g., estrogen and parathyroid) replacement therapy may prove beneficial.
Dislocations Hip dislocation (Figs. 10-195 through 10-197)	Most hip dislocations are posterior (80% to 85%), most often resulting from a force to the knee while the hip is in flexion, as occurs during a motor vehicle accident when the knee strikes the dashboard.[73,215] Fracture of the posterior column (or posterior rim of the acetabulum), sciatic nerve injury, degeneration,[73] or avascular necrosis[139] often accompanies a posterior dislocation. Anterior dislocations are caused by hyperextension and abduction injuries, displacing the femoral head into the obturator, pubic, or iliac region. On the AP radiograph, anterior dislocation often leaves the femur adducted, and posterior dislocation exhibits abduction of the femur. Internal dislocation defines a central acetabular fracture with displacement of the femoral head into the pelvis.
Knee *Fractures* Distal femur	Supracondylar fractures result from axial loading with varus or valgus stress forces. Fractures are oblique or transverse, often comminuted, and may extend into joint fractures[90,177,178] involving the condyles that often appear T or Y shaped with varying degrees of comminution.
Fibula fracture (Fig. 10-198)	Isolated fracture of the proximal fibula is uncommon. It is usually accompanied by ligamentous injury or other fractures about the knee and ankle. Fracture is more common in the middle and distal third of the bone. Compartment syndrome may develop secondary to accumulations of hemorrhage and edema within the anterior, posterior, or lateral compartment.

TABLE 10-10 cont'd

Fractures, Dislocations, and Soft-Tissue Injuries of the Pelvis and Lower Extremities

Injury	Comments
Flake fracture	Flake fracture describes a small fracture, typically of the posterior surface of the patella, associated with patellar dislocation.
Floating knee	A floating fracture is the combination of a supracondylar fracture of the femur and a fracture of the proximal tibia, allowing the knee to freely float without osseous attachment.
Patella fracture (Figs. 10-199 and 10-200)	Patella fracture occurs secondary to a direct trauma, or secondary to an indirect force such as that generated by contraction of the quadriceps.[148] A patella fracture may present in a vertical, transverse (50% to 90%), or stellate (comminuted) configuration. It is distinguished from the bipartite or multipartite normal variants by a history of trauma, nonbilateral presentation, better fit of the pieces than a variant, and lack of well-corticated margins characteristic of the variant.
Proximal tibia (Figs. 10-201 and 10-202)	Fracture of the proximal tibia occurs in the medial (10%) or lateral (80%) portion of the tibial plateau, related to the varus or valgus strain, respectively, with vertical and rotational forces also present. About 10% of fractures involve both the medial and lateral tibia. Twenty-five percent of fractures result from pedestrians being struck by an automobile (hence the nickname "bumper" or "fender" fractures to describe them). Ligamentous injuries often accompany plateau fractures.[222] Occasionally fractures about the knee, shoulder, and elbow extend into the subarticular space, allowing fatty marrow elements to enter the joint space. When this occurs, often a fat–blood interface (FBI) sign is noted in the lateral projection, indicating lipohemarthrosis. It appears as a linear change in radiodensity separating the radiolucent intraarticular fat from the more radiodense intraarticular blood. Lipohemarthrosis is most common in the knee, shoulder, and elbow.
Segond's fracture (Fig. 10-203)	A Segond's fracture is an avulsion of the lateral capsular ligament secondary to internal tibial rotation while the knee is flexed. It should be distinguished from the more anterior and inferior fragment created by avulsion of the iliotibial band from Gerdy's tubercle. A Segond's fracture is characterized by the presence of a fracture donor site on the tibial condyle in the frontal projection, and occurs more posteriorly on the tibia than avulsion of the iliotibial band.[204] Segond's fractures are found with concurrent tears of the anterior cruciate ligament more than 90% of the time and meniscal tears more than 75% of the time.
Trampoline fracture	Trampoline fracture is a greenstick fracture of the proximal tibial metaphysis occurring in a child.
Dislocations Knee dislocation	Knee dislocation occurs only rarely, resulting from severe trauma. There is an associated high morbidity secondary to torn ligaments, vessels, and so on.[128,154,182,197] Dislocations are classified by the position of the tibia with respect to the femur: anterior (most common, 50%), posterior, medial, lateral, and rotary varieties are possible.
Patellar dislocation	Dislocation of the patella from its normal trochlear location most often occurs in a lateral direction,[109] often associated with osteochondral flake fracture of the articular surfaces of the patella.[206] Lateral dislocation is associated with rapidly changing directions while running.[99] MRI diagnosis of patellar dislocation consists of a typical triad of patellar bone bruise, femoral bone bruise, and associated tearing of the medial retinacular attachments. A large degree of effusion is seen with acute dislocation. Generally dislocation is associated with hypoplastic lateral femoral condyle, genu valgum, abnormal lateral insertion of the patellar tendon, and patella alta.
Soft-tissue injuries (ligaments and cartilage) (Anterior) Cruciate ligament tear (Figs. 10-204 and 10-205)	Normally the anterior cruciate ligament (ACL) is of intermediate to low signal intensity on MRI, best seen on the sagittal images. The most common site for tear is within the midsubstance of the ligament. On occasion, avulsion occurs at the femoral attachment, but usually the tibial attachment is involved. Coexistent injuries to the meniscus and medial collateral ligament should be considered. The diagnostic accuracy of MRI reaches 95% in the evaluation of ACL tears.[78] ACL injury can be categorized as mild ligament strain, moderate ligament strain, and ligament rupture.

Continued

TABLE 10-10 cont'd
Fractures, Dislocations, and Soft-Tissue Injuries of the Pelvis and Lower Extremities

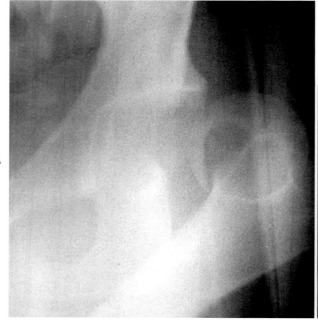

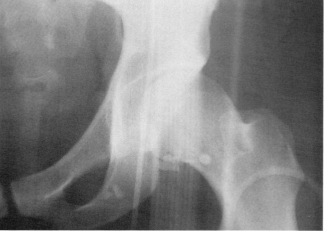

FIG. 10-195   A and **B,** Posterior dislocation of the femur. **A,** Initial radiograph taken at the time of injury shows a widened medial iliofemoral joint space and varus deformity. Anterior dislocations tend to exhibit valgus angulation, so the angulation is a hint to the direction of dislocation. **B,** Second image taken immediately after reduction represents normal alignment.

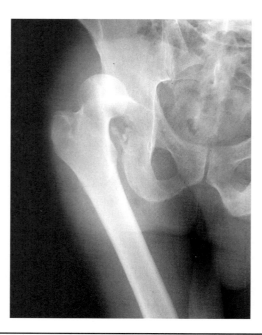

FIG. 10-196   Posterior hip dislocation, evidenced by the superior location of the femora head in relation to the acetabulum and varus deformity of the hip with the shaft of the femur deviated medially. (Courtesy Steven P. Brownstein, MD, Springfield, NJ.)

TABLE 10-10 cont'd
Fractures, Dislocations, and Soft-Tissue Injuries of the Pelvis and Lower Extremities

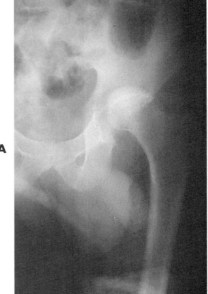

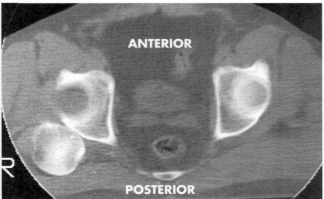

FIG. 10-197 Anterior hip dislocation. **A,** The hip is inferior in relationship to the acetabulum, and the shaft of the femur deviates medially (coxa varus). **B,** The computed tomography scan confirms a posterior direction of dislocation. (Courtesy Steven P. Brownstein, MD, Springfield, NJ.)

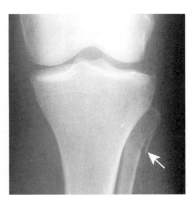

FIG. 10-198 Fracture through the neck of the fibula *(arrow).* (Courtesy Steven P. Brownstein, MD, Springfield, NJ.)

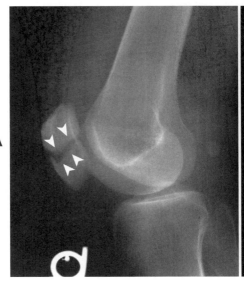

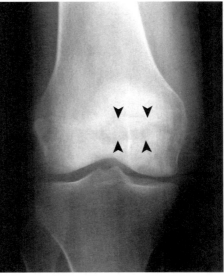

FIG. 10-199 **A** and **B,** Transverse fracture of the patella *(arrowheads).* (Courtesy Gary Longmuir, Phoenix, AZ.)

Continued

TABLE 10-10 cont'd
Fractures, Dislocations, and Soft-Tissue Injuries of the Pelvis and Lower Extremities

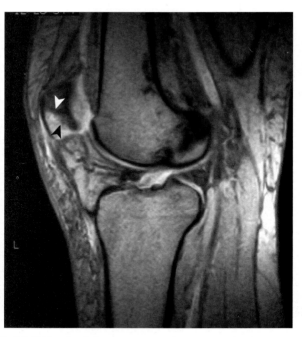

FIG. 10-200 Patella fracture seen on a T1-weighted magnetic resonance imaging scan of the midsagittal plane. The superior pole of the patella exhibits hypointense signal intensity consistent with marrow replacement with bone edema secondary to fracture (*arrowheads*).

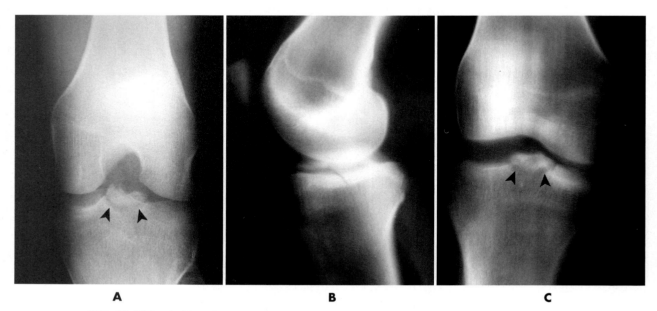

A   B   C

FIG. 10-201 Avulsion of the tibial eminence seen on, **A,** frontal; **B,** lateral plain film projections; and, **C,** linear tomography (*arrowheads*). (Courtesy Ronnie Firth, East Moline, IL.)

TABLE 10-10 cont'd

Fractures, Dislocations, and Soft-Tissue Injuries of the Pelvis and Lower Extremities

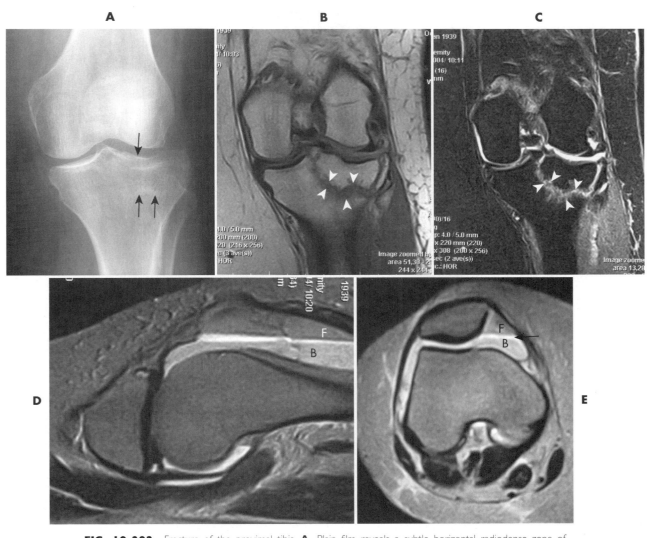

FIG. 10-202 Fracture of the proximal tibia. **A,** Plain film reveals a subtle horizontal radiodense zone of impacted trabeculae *(arrowheads)* and increased concavity of the lateral condyle *(arrows).* **B,** T1-weighted and, **C,** short tau inversion recovery sequence of the magnetic resonance imaging examination details the extent of the fracture *(arrowheads).* Because the fracture is intraarticular, a lipohemarthrosis develops. **D,** T2-weighted sagittal scan performed with the patient in a supine position displays the laying of *F,* the intraarticular fat and, *B,* blood occurring in a gravity-dependent orientation. The fat–blood interface, *FBI* sign, is a general indication that a fracture has extended into the joint, complicating the patient's outcome. There is a linear bright signal separating the hypointense fat, *F,* above and isointense blood, *B,* below. **E,** The axial T2-weighted scan demonstrates the layering effect of fat, *F,* and blood, *B,* to a better degree. The arrow denotes the hyperintense interface. On plain film and computed tomography, a lipohemarthrosis appears as a single interface (two layers). However, on magnetic resonance imaging lipohemarthrosis appears with at least three layers in which the superior layer is fat, the most inferior layer is blood, and the middle layer (usually hyperintense, as in this case) is a chemical shift artifact. Chemical shift artifacts occur when the protons in water experience a different magnetic field than the protons in fat, causing the magnetic resonance imaging system to "mislocate" the position of the protons. The mislocated protons cause the extra linear interface shadow between the fat and blood. At times the lowest layer (blood) appears as two layers instead of one, in which the cellular component of the blood settles to the most gravity-dependent portion of the space. (Courtesy Ian D. McLean, LeClaire, IA).

Continued

TABLE 10-10 cont'd
Fractures, Dislocations, and Soft-Tissue Injuries of the Pelvis and Lower Extremities

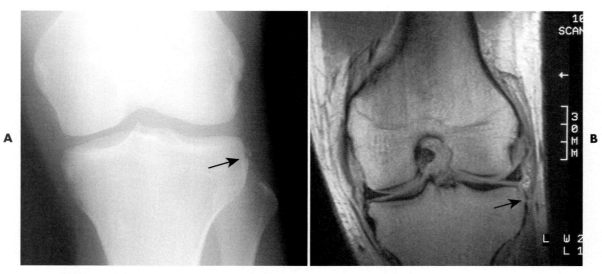

FIG. 10-203   Segond's fracture appearing as a small cortical avulsion on, **A,** plain film and, **B,** magnetic resonance imaging *(arrows).*

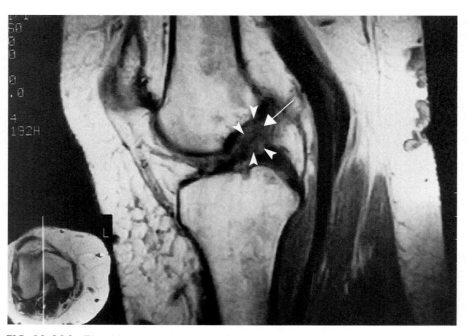

FIG. 10-204   T1-weighted magnetic resonance image with disruption of the anterior cruciate ligament *(arrow).* The anterior cruciate normally ligament appears as a smooth hypointense (black) oblique band. This case shows disruption of the band and surrounding mixed signal of hemorrhage and edema *(arrowheads).* (Steven Brownstein, Springfield, NJ.)

TABLE 10-10 cont'd
Fractures, Dislocations, and Soft-Tissue Injuries of the Pelvis and Lower Extremities

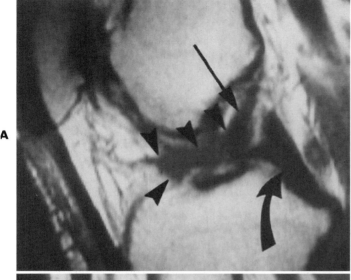

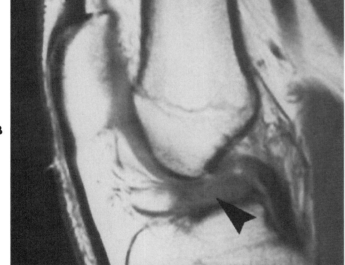

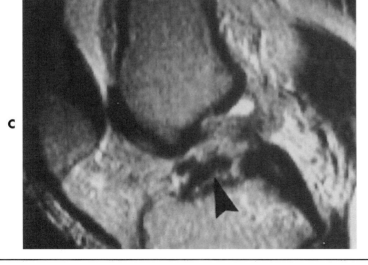

FIG. 10-205 Tear of the anterior cruciate ligament (ACL) in three patients. **A,** T1-weighted anatomic sagittal view. The curved arrow points to the posterior cruciate ligament. The arrow points to the proximal portion of the ACL, which is displaced posteriorly. The arrowheads point to hemorrhage-edema surrounding the torn lower half of the ACL. **B,** T1-weighted anatomic sagittal view. The arrowhead indicates hemorrhage-edema in the expected position of the ACL. **C,** T2-weighted oblique sagittal view. The arrowhead points to the torn distal half of the ACL, which is displaced inferiorly. (From Firooznia H et al: MRI and CT of the musculoskeletal system, St Louis, 1992, Mosby.)

Continued

TABLE 10-10 cont'd
Fractures, Dislocations, and Soft-Tissue Injuries of the Pelvis and Lower Extremities

Injury	Comments
(Anterior) Cruciate ligament tear—cont'd	*Mild* ACL strain may reveal a central hyperintense appearance within the substance of the tendon on the T2-weighted images. *Moderate* sprain correlates to the presence of hemorrhage and edema within the ligament with possible findings of posterior cruciate ligament (PCL) buckling, and altered angulation of the ACL. *Rupture* of the ACL exhibits a wavy contour, edema, bone bruise of the lateral plateau of the tibia, anterior displacement of the femur, medial collateral ligament injury, and medial meniscal injury.
(Posterior) Cruciate ligament tear (Fig. 10-206)	The PCL is moderately thicker and approximately twice as strong as the ACL. Consequently, PCL tears are less common than ACL tears. The PCL is of lower signal intensity than the ACL and normally assumes a slightly arcuate course. Tears of the PCL are most common in the midsubstance of the ligament, with avulsion occurring at the tibial insertion. Isolated PCL tears are uncommon, and associated injuries to the ACL or the menisci should be sought. Bone contusions often are noted about the knee, are associated with complete tears of the ACL, and are located on the posterolateral tibial plateau and the lateral femoral condyle because of impaction of the lateral femoral condyle into the posterior tibia.
Chondromalacia patella	Chondromalacia patella presents clinically with patellofemoral joint pain accentuated on flexion of the knee. The condition commonly affects young adults and adolescents. An axial MRI study may demonstrate cartilage thinning or erosion of the cartilaginous surface and hyperintensity corresponding to focal regions of edema and later marked hypointensity on T1- and T2-weighted (sclerosis) of the subchondral bone.
Collateral ligament injury	Medial collateral ligament (MCL) injury is secondary to a valgus stress applied to the flexed knee. Injury of the MCL is best evidenced on coronal T2-weighted images, demonstrating edema and hemorrhage about the usually low signal intensity fibers of the ligament. A complete tear exhibits a loss of continuity of the ligament fibers. Lateral collateral ligament (LCL) injury often occurs with the leg in internal rotation and resulting varus stress.
Meniscal tear (Figs. 10-207 through 10-210)	There are two menisci associated with the knee, medial and lateral. Each is a semilunar wedge of fibrocartilage, convex on the femoral side and flat on the tibial side, that functions to lubricate, stabilize, and distribute forces applied to the knee. The medial meniscus is larger, more mobile, and several times more likely to tear than is the lateral meniscus. Concurrent tears of the medial and lateral menisci are uncommon. Tears of the lateral meniscus often are concurrent to injury to the ACL. Meniscal tears are characterized by pain, joint swelling, joint locking, and limited motion, with a correlative history of trauma. It is typical for the patient to exhibit marked tenderness when the examiner palpates on the joint line.
	Several clinical examinations are predictive of meniscal injury, including McMurray's test (examiner straightens internally rotated and flexed injured leg of supine patient, where pain or click indicates a medial meniscus injury), Apley's test, Steinmann test, and ballottement test. Some meniscus tears respond to conservative management, although surgical repair or excision is usual, depending on the patient's age, proximity of the tear to the well-vascularized periphery (termed the "red zone"), and so on.
	A meniscus tear can result from multiple etiologies: degenerative joint disease, direct trauma, joint tracking disorders, intraarticular fractures, and other joint disease. Degeneration is more closely associated with causing flap or horizontal tears in the meniscus. By contrast, trauma, especially rotational forces, is more likely to cause longitudinal tears. Tears may occur in the posterior horn, body, or anterior horn of the meniscus.
	One of the greatest impacts of articular musculoskeletal MRI has been in the evaluation of the knee, and in many circumstances MRI has replaced knee arthrography and is probably the examination of choice for patients when the symptoms are severe enough to warrant arthroscopy.[208] MRI is very accurate in the evaluation of meniscal tears, with the diagnostic certainty reaching approximately 95% with the likelihood of MRI to fail to detect a clinically significant meniscal tear being quite low.[47]

TABLE 10-10 cont'd
Fractures, Dislocations, and Soft-Tissue Injuries of the Pelvis and Lower Extremities

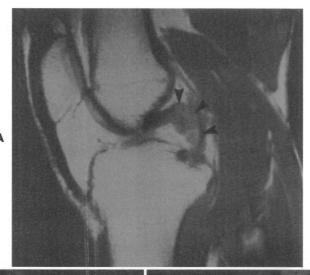

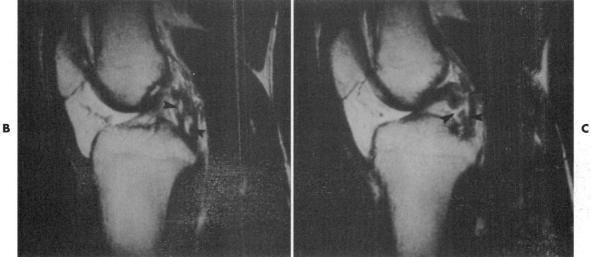

FIG. 10-206 Posterior cruciate ligament (PCL) tear. **A,** A sagittal anatomic T1-weighted image. Note the markedly irregular, thickened, and buckled PCL *(arrowheads)*, with its nonhomogeneously increased internal signal intensity (SI). The ACL was also torn in this patient. **B** and **C,** Sagittal anatomic T2-weighted images. The multiple zones of increased SI in the substance of the PCL indicate tears of the ligament *(arrowheads)*. (From Firooznia H et al: MRI and CT of the musculoskeletal system, St Louis, 1992, Mosby.)

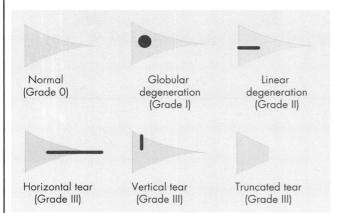

Normal
(Grade 0)

Globular
degeneration
(Grade I)

Linear
degeneration
(Grade II)

Horizontal tear
(Grade III)

Vertical tear
(Grade III)

Truncated tear
(Grade III)

FIG. 10-207 Magnetic resonance imaging categorization of meniscal tears as seen in a sagittal or coronal scan.

PART TWO
Bone, Joints, and Soft Tissues

Continued

TABLE 10-10 cont'd
Fractures, Dislocations, and Soft-Tissue Injuries of the Pelvis and Lower Extremities

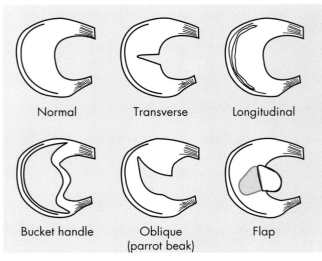

Normal   Transverse   Longitudinal

Bucket handle   Oblique (parrot beak)   Flap

FIG. 10-208   Meniscal tears as seen in an axial plane.

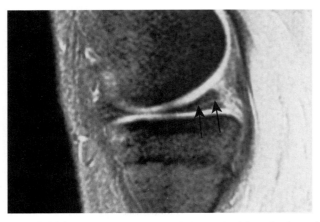

FIG. 10-209   Grade II meniscal signal. Linear signal intensity (arrows), which may communicate with the capsular margin but not with an articular surface, is seen on this radial gradient echo image (SE 700/14/25 degrees). (From Stark DD, Gradley WG: Magnetic resonance imaging, ed 2, St Louis, 1992, Mosby.)

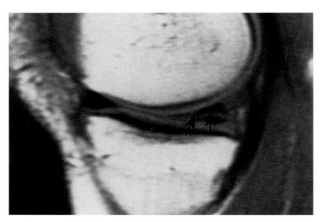

FIG. 10-210   Grade III meniscal signal. Horizontal cleavage tear of the posterior horn of this medial meniscus is visualized as a region of Grade III signal (arrows) (SE 2000/20). (From Stark DD, Gradley WG: Magnetic resonance imaging, ed 2, St Louis, 1992, Mosby.)

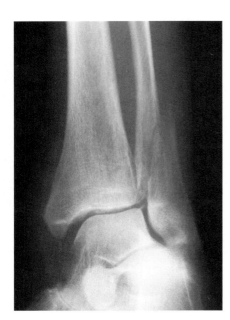

FIG. 10-211   Dupuytren's fracture presenting as an oblique fracture of the lower fibula and lateral displacement of the talus in reference to the distal tibia.

TABLE 10-10 cont'd

Fractures, Dislocations, and Soft-Tissue Injuries of the Pelvis and Lower Extremities

Injury	Comments
Meniscal tear—cont'd	The intact meniscus has low signal intensity, appearing uniformly dark on all sequences. A meniscus tear or degeneration appears with bright areas within the meniscus. The diagnosis of meniscal tear requires evidence of an abnormal linear signal intensity extending to an articular surface of the meniscus. Three grades of abnormal signal intensity are described:
	Grade 0 (normal): Uniformly dark.
	Grade I (degeneration): Globular foci of abnormal high-signal intensity correlating with mucinous degeneration. The signal does not extend to the meniscal articular surface.
	Grade II (degeneration): A linear, horizontal region of increased signal intensity that does not extend to the articular surface. Grade I and II menisci are arthroscopically normal, and are common in older patients as part of the degenerative aging process.
	Grade III (tear): An abnormal high-signal intensity (often linear) that extends to an articular surface.
	MRI-arthroscopic correlation produces categories of meniscus tear appearing in meniscal cross section (horizontal and vertical) and circumferentially or from the surface (longitudinal, transverse, oblique or parrot beak, bucket handle, and flap). A bucket handle tear is a displaced longitudinal tear. With MRI, horizontal tears are the most common. MRI is noninvasive, has a high negative predictive value (estimates are above 95%), and has the ability to demonstrate concurrent injuries, such as bone bruising and ligament damage.
Osteochondritis dissecans	Osteochondritis dissecans affects young patients; primarily the non–weight-bearing lateral surface of the medial femoral condyle and medial portion of the dome of the talus, appearing as a low signal intensity and subchondral foci on both the T1- and T2-weighted images. Conventional radiographic findings usually are absent early in the disease. Later, a small osteochondral defect may be seen that is either in location (in situ) or displaced. See the entry later in this chapter for more information.
Ankle	
Fractures	
Cotton's fracture	A Cotton's fracture is a trimalleolar fracture involving the medial and lateral malleolus and posterior lip of the distal tibia (sometimes referred to as the *third malleolus*).[155]
Dupuytren's fracture (Fig. 10-211)	Dupuytren's[69] described fibular fractures associated with outward movement of the foot (abduction). A low Dupuytren's fracture is a spiral fracture of the distal portion of the fibula. A high Dupuytren's fracture is a transverse or oblique fracture of the fibula occurring at the junction of the middle and distal third of the bone, with accompanying tearing of the syndesmosis.
Maisonneuve fracture	A Maisonneuve fracture is a fracture of the proximal fibula[151] with rupture of the distal tibiofibular ligaments and interosseous membrane extending proximal to the fibular fracture; secondary to external rotation of foot. Because of its proximal location, it is often missed on radiographs of the ankle.[186]
Malleolar fractures (Figs. 10-212 through 10-217)	Ankle injury usually results from indirect forces applied to the foot in internal rotation, external rotation, inversion, or eversion. A key feature to the seriousness of the injury is the stability of the ankle mortise. If there is abnormal movement of the talus with respect to the distal tibia, the injury is more serious. Two main classification systems are used to describe ankle fractures: the simpler Danis-Weber system and the more complex Lauge-Hansen system. Some clinicians employ a straightforward approach by describing ankle fractures on the basis of the number of malleoli fractured: unimalleolar (medial or lateral), bimalleolar (medial and lateral), and trimalleolar (medial, lateral, and posterior rim of the distal articular surface of the tibia).

Continued

TABLE 10-10 cont'd
Fractures, Dislocations, and Soft-Tissue Injuries of the Pelvis and Lower Extremities

Injury	Comments
Malleolar fractures—cont'd	The Danis-Weber system (A to C) is based on the location of the fibular fracture in reference to the height of the ankle joint (below, at, or above).
	Type A: Fracture below the ankle joint.
	Type B: Fracture at the level of the ankle joint (the tibiofibular ligaments are intact)
	Type C: Fracture above the ankle joint that tears the tibiofibular ligaments
	The Lauge-Hansen ("Continental") system is based on cadaveric studies and employs two word descriptions: the first word describes the position of the foot relative to the leg, and the second word describes the motion of the foot (talus) relative to the leg (distal tibia), the most common of which is the supination-external rotation injury.
	Supination-adduction: (a) Transverse fracture of the lateral malleolus below the tibial plafond, and (b) vertical shearing fracture of the medial malleolus.
	Supination-external (eversion) rotation: (a) Anteroinferior tibiofibular injury, (b) oblique or spiral lateral malleolar fracture at the level of the plafond, (c) medial malleolar fracture or deltoid avulsion, and (d) posterior malleolar and posteroinferior tibiofibular injury.
	Pronation-abduction: (a) Rupture of the deltoid ligament or transverse fracture of the medial malleolus, (b) rupture of the anterior and posteroinferior tibiotalofibular ligaments or bony avulsions, and (c) oblique fracture of the lateral malleolus at the level of the syndesmosis.
	Pronation-external (eversion) rotation: (a) Transverse fracture of the medial malleolus or rupture of the deltoid ligament, (b) injury of the anteroinferior tibiofibular ligaments, (c) spiral or oblique fracture of the fibular above the level of syndesmosis, and (d) rupture of the posteroinferior tibiofibular ligament or fracture of the posterior malleolus.
	Pronation-dorsiflexion: (a) Fracture of the medial malleolus, (b) fracture of the anterior rim of the distal articular surface of the tibia, (c) fracture of the supramalleolar aspect of the fibula, and (d) rupture of the posteroinferior tibiofibular ligament or fracture of the posterior rim of the distal articular surface of the tibia (known as the third malleolus).
	These classification systems guide management. For instance, closed reduction is based on reversing the forces of injury described by the Lauge-Hansen system. The necessity of open reduction of the fracture increases the higher the syndesmotic injury, or Danis-Weber classification. Last, the basic classification system of unimalleolar, bimalleolar, or trimalleolar has prognostic value, correlating to a better clinical outcome with unimalleolar fractures.
	Approximately 15% of ankle injuries produce malleolar fractures. Clinical signs and symptoms include a history of trauma to the ankle or foot, swelling, ecchymoses, tenderness, and pain on weight bearing. Clinical features have been incorporated into decision rules regarding radiographic examination. For example, the Ottawa ankle rule suggests that the patient's inability to bear weight on an acutely injured ankle and to walk for four consecutive steps with the presence of pain on digital palpation of the region closely correlates with the presence of fracture.
Pilon (pestle) fracture	Compression injury that drives the talus into the tibial plafond similar to a pestle into a mortar.[152] It most often accompanies other ankle or skeletal trauma.
Pott's fracture	In 1768 Pott's[191] described a fracture of the fibula occurring approximately 2 to 3 inches proximal to the distal tip of the fibula with associated tear of the deltoid ligament and lateral displacement of the talus.

TABLE 10-10 cont'd

Fractures, Dislocations, and Soft-Tissue Injuries of the Pelvis and Lower Extremities

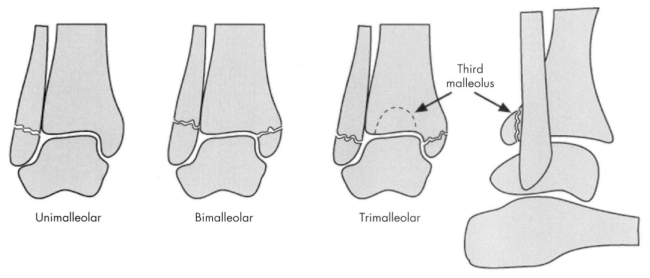

Unimalleolar   Bimalleolar   Trimalleolar   Third malleolus

FIG. 10-212 A basic categorization of malleolar fracture is to simply designate the fracture as unimalleolar, bimalleolar, or trimalleolar, whereas the third malleolus is the posterior, inferior tubercle of the distal tibia.

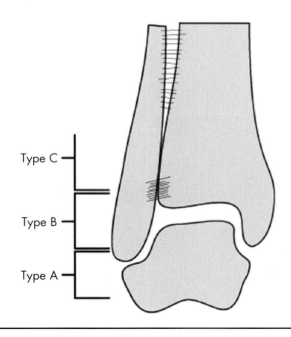

Type C

Type B

Type A

FIG. 10-213 The Danis-Weber system of categorizing malleolar fractures concentrates on the location of the fibular fracture. Using this system, a type A fracture is below the tibiotalar joint, type B is at the joint, and type C is above the joint.

Continued

TABLE 10-10 cont'd

Fractures, Dislocations, and Soft-Tissue Injuries of the Pelvis and Lower Extremities

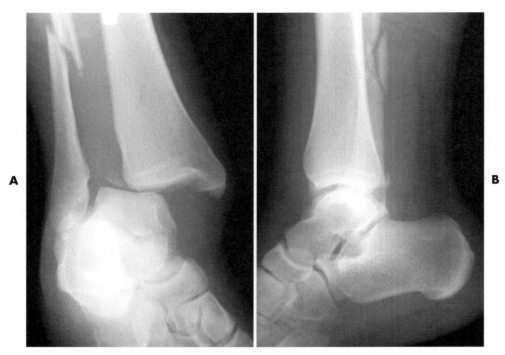

FIG. 10-214 A and **B,** Bimalleolar fracture with lateral dislocation of the tibiotalar (ankle) joint. This fracture categorized as a type C fracture using the Danis-Weber system and a pronation-external rotation fracture using the Lauge-Hansen system. (Courtesy Steven P. Brownstein, MD, Springfield, NJ.)

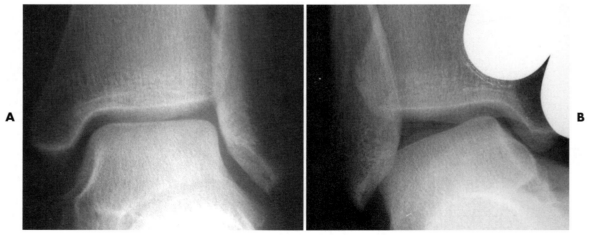

FIG. 10-215 A and **B,** Ankle injury without obvious fracture, but when stressed, the ankle inverts excessively, consistent with a diagnosis of instability. Normally, the ankle should not tilt more than 5 degrees. When instability is present, the ankle tilts 15 to 20 degrees.

TABLE 10-10 cont'd

Fractures, Dislocations, and Soft-Tissue Injuries of the Pelvis and Lower Extremities

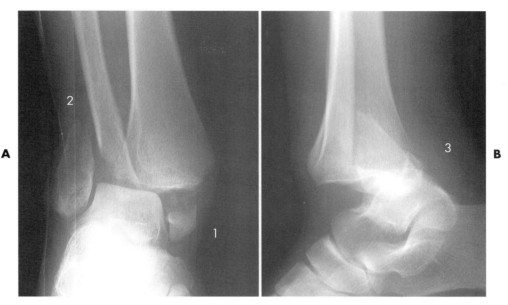

FIG. 10-216 Trimalleolar fracture with dislocation. **A** and **B,** Transverse fracture of the medial malleolus *(1),* oblique fracture of the lateral malleolus, *(2)* posterior fracture of the distal tibia, and *(3)* posterior dislocation of the talus. The configuration of fracture is consistent with an eversion injury that produces the oblique fracture on the compression (push) side of the injury and an avulsion or transverse fracture line on the distraction (pull) side of the injury.

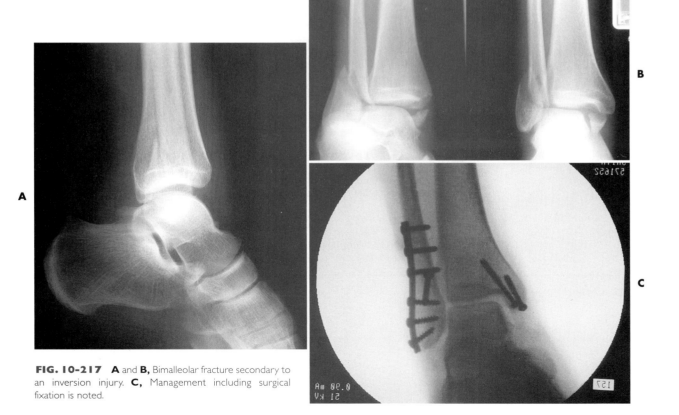

FIG. 10-217 **A** and **B,** Bimalleolar fracture secondary to an inversion injury. **C,** Management including surgical fixation is noted.

PART TWO Bone, Joints, and Soft Tissues

Continued

TABLE 10-10 cont'd

Fractures, Dislocations, and Soft-Tissue Injuries of the Pelvis and Lower Extremities

Injury	Comments
Tillaux fracture (Fig. 10-218)	Tillaux[244] described a fracture of the anterolateral corner of the lower tibia secondary to a rotational injury and avulsion of the anterior tibiofibular ligament. Tillaux fractures occur in adolescence,[66] representing a Salter-Harris type III injury. It is important to assess for displacement of the articular surface fragment.
Triplane fracture (Fig. 10-219)	As the name implies, a distal tibial triplane fracture occurs in three planes: transverse fracture within the epiphyseal plate, sagittal fracture of the epiphysis, and a coronal (or oblique) fracture in the posterior distal tibial metaphysis.[60] It occurs most commonly during adolescence.
Dislocations	
Ankle dislocation	Ankle dislocations usually are posterior; anterior dislocations are less frequent. Medial and lateral dislocations may accompany malleolar fractures.
Soft-tissue injuries (ligaments and cartilage)	
Achilles tendon (Fig. 10-220)	The Achilles tendon represents the largest tendon in the body and is formed from the gastrocnemius and soleus muscles. Partial tears and complete rupture are clearly demonstrated on MRI, whereas clinical examination can miss rupture of the Achilles tendon in up to 25% of cases. Radiography is not effective in identifying abnormalities in the Achilles tendon. Injuries to the tendon often are secondary to athletic activity and are frequently observed in middle-aged men. With rupture, MRI can demonstrate both a proximal and distal portion of the torn tendon. Associated hemorrhage within the tendon sheath also can be appreciated. Because tendon tears can be managed conservatively, the MRI examination is critical in documenting the degree of apposition in the disrupted tendon and allows early identification of patients who are candidates for surgical intervention.
Foot	
Fractures	
Calcaneal fracture (Figs. 10-221 through 10-223)	The calcaneus is the most common tarsal fracture, and usually is related to compressive injuries. The arc along the superior margin of the calcaneus (Boehler angle, normally 28 to 40 degrees) may be the most obvious sign of fracture. Beak fractures involve the superior margin of the calcaneal tuberosity, often secondary to avulsion of the Achilles tendon.[149] Approximately 5% to 10% of patients demonstrate a bilateral presentation of calcaneal fracture, and a similar proportion exhibit a concurrent vertebral compression fracture.
Metatarsal fracture (Figs. 10-224 and 10-225)	A metatarsal fracture often is the result of a heavy object falling on the foot. Stress fractures are common at the second or third metatarsal (*March fractures*). A *Dancer's* or *Jones'* fracture describes a fracture of the base of the fifth metatarsal that appears transverse in orientation to the long axis of the metatarsals. This is contrary to the normal longitudinal radiolucency often noted at the base of the metatarsal representing a nonunion defect of the secondary growth center in children.
Phalangeal fracture (Figs. 10-226 through 10-228)	A phalangeal fracture occurs secondary to a kicking or "stubbing" injury (*bedroom fracture*), or when the foot is struck by a heavy falling object. An oblique, transverse, or comminuted configuration may occur. *Hallux rigidus* refers to a stiff, painful first digit after trauma.

TABLE 10-10 cont'd
Fractures, Dislocations, and Soft-Tissue Injuries of the Pelvis and Lower Extremities

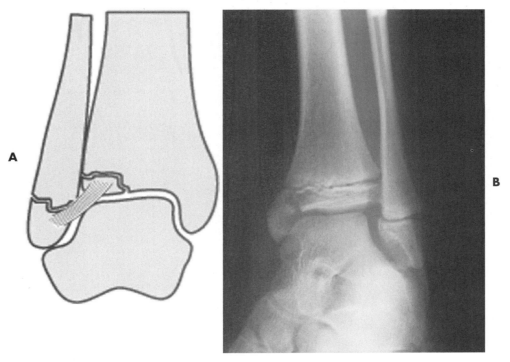

FIG. 10-218 **A** and **B,** Tillaux fracture is a Salter-Harris III fracture of the distal tibia.

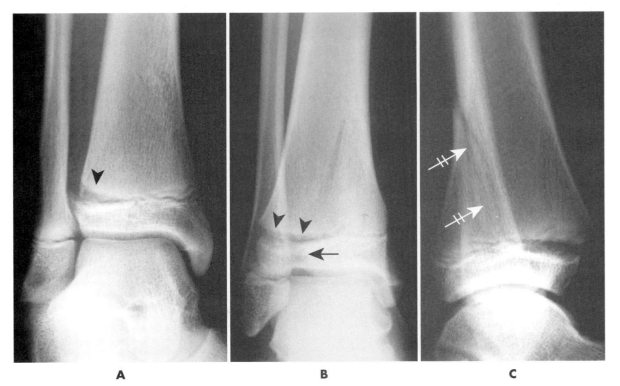

A **B** **C**

FIG. 10-219 **A** through **C,** Triplane fracture comprising transverse fracture within the epiphyseal plate *(arrowheads),* sagittal fracture of the epiphysis *(arrow),* and an oblique fracture in the posterior distal tibial metaphysis *(crossed arrows).*

Continued

TABLE 10-10 cont'd
Fractures, Dislocations, and Soft-Tissue Injuries of the Pelvis and Lower Extremities

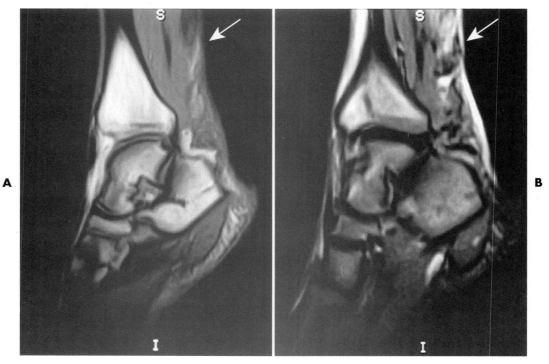

FIG. 10-220   A, T1- and, **B,** T2-weighted magnetic resonance imaging scan of a calcaneal (Achilles) tendon rupture. The arrows point to tissue remnants and the area in which the hypointense (dark) tendon should be found. (Courtesy Joseph W. Howe, Sylmar, CA.)

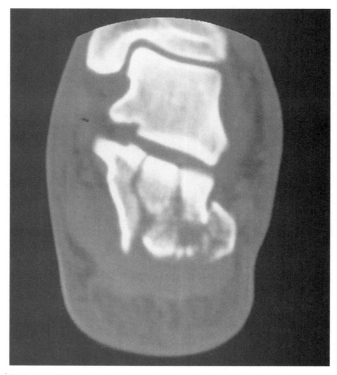

FIG. 10-221   Comminuted fracture of the calcaneus noted on computed tomography.

TABLE 10-10 cont'd

Fractures, Dislocations, and Soft-Tissue Injuries of the Pelvis and Lower Extremities

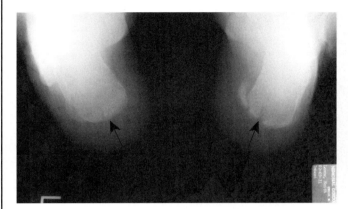

FIG. 10-222 Bilateral tangent view of the right and left calcaneus exhibiting fracture *(arrows)*. (Courtesy Steven P. Brownstein, MD, Springfield, NJ.)

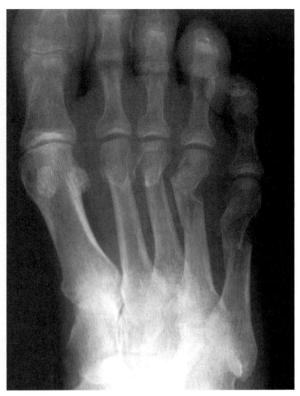

FIG. 10-224 Comminuted fractures of the second to fifth metatarsal shafts. (Courtesy Charles Wachob, Dubois, PA.)

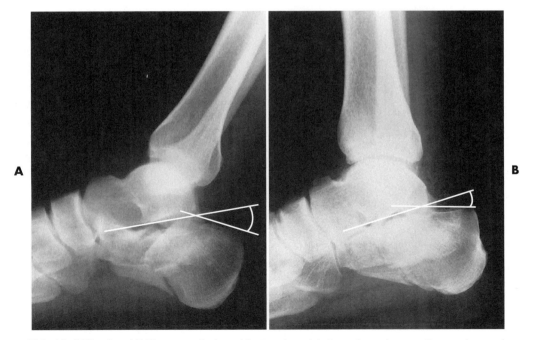

FIG. 10-223 **A** and **B,** Two cases of calcaneal fracture. In each instance the angle across the superior margin of the calcaneus (Boehler angle) is reduced to less than 28 degrees, from its normal value between 28 to 40 degrees. (Courtesy Steven P. Brownstein, MD, Springfield, NJ.)

Continued

TABLE 10-10 cont'd
Fractures, Dislocations, and Soft-Tissue Injuries of the Pelvis and Lower Extremities

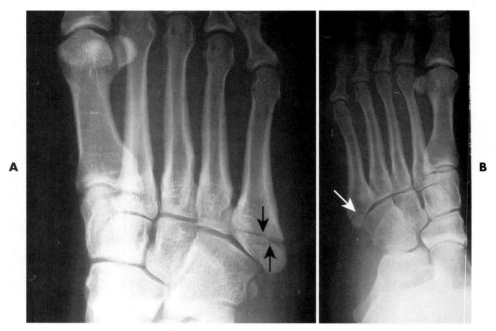

FIG. 10-225 **A** and **B,** Dancer's fracture at the base of the fifth metatarsal *(arrows).* A Dancer's fracture is oriented perpendicular to the long axis of the metatarsal. This is in contrast to the orientation of the growth center, which is parallel to the long axis of the metatarsal. (Courtesy Melody Dittmer, Blue Grass, IA.)

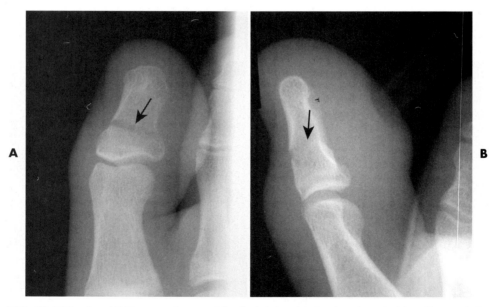

FIG. 10-226 **A** and **B,** Transverse fracture of the distal phalanx in a female patient who injured her toe during a track event *(arrows).*

TABLE 10-10 cont'd

Fractures, Dislocations, and Soft-Tissue Injuries of the Pelvis and Lower Extremities

Injury	Comments
Talus fracture	The talus fracture is the second most common tarsal fracture. The mechanism usually is avulsion. An *aviator's fracture* or *aviator's astragalus* refers to a fracture through the neck of the talus that may occur as the pilot's foot impacts on the steering pedals during an aircraft crash. A subcortical radiolucent line within the dome of the talus (Hawkins' sign) after injury indicates good vascularity and that avascular necrosis is unlikely to complicate the injury.
Dislocation	
Midtarsal (Chopart's) dislocation	This describes a rare separation of the hindfoot from the midfoot at the talonavicular and calcaneocuboid joints. The distal foot typically is displaced medially.
Phalangeal, metatarsal dislocation (Fig. 10-229)	Most of these dislocations are posterior and may be found in combination with fractures of the phalanges and metatarsals.
Subtalar dislocation	Subtalar dislocation describes simultaneous dislocations of the talonavicular and talocalcaneal joints produced by compression injuries applied while the foot is inverted,[29] usually displacing the calcaneus, navicular, and forefoot medially respective to the talus.
Tarsometatarsal (Lisfranc's) dislocation (Fig. 10-230)	A tarsometatarsal dislocation is a lateral displacement of the metatarsal's base at its articulation with the tarsals. The separation may be associated with fractures, particularly the base of the second metatarsal.[87,263] Convergent (or homolateral) dislocations consist of lateral dislocation of the first to fifth or second to fifth metatarsals. Divergent dislocations are lateral dislocations of the second to fifth metatarsals and medial dislocation of the first metatarsal.

Continued

TABLE 10-10 cont'd
Fractures, Dislocations, and Soft-Tissue Injuries of the Pelvis and Lower Extremities

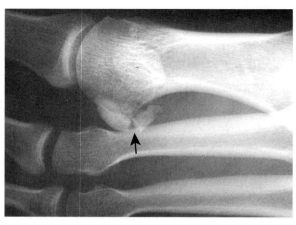

FIG. 10-227   Fracture of the lateral sesamoid bone associated with the first digit (*arrow*).

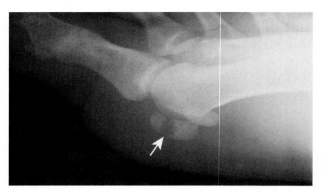

FIG. 10-228   Fracture of the sesamoid bone in a 22-year-old man (*arrow*).

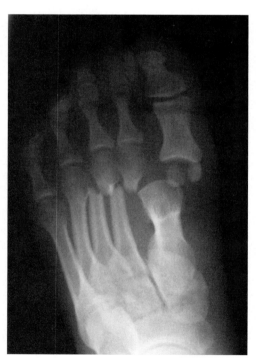

FIG. 10-229   Fracture of the shafts of the second and third metatarsals with dislocation of the first metatarsophalangeal joint. (Courtesy Steven P. Brownstein, MD, Springfield, NJ.)

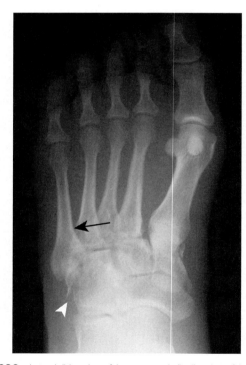

FIG. 10-230   Lateral dislocation of the metatarsals (in direction of the *arrow*) at their metatarsotarsal joints (Lisfranc's dislocation). A small fracture is noted of cuboid (*arrowhead*). (Courtesy Steven P. Brownstein, MD, Springfield, NJ.)

TABLE 10-11
Early and Late Fracture Complications

Complications	Description
Early	
Compartment (Volkmann) syndrome	Hemorrhage or edema may increase the osteofascial intracompartmental pressure after trauma, thereby reducing arterial flow that may produce avascular muscle ischemia. A vicious cycle results as the ischemia causes more edema, which in turn causes more ischemia. Ischemic contracture results from damaged, contracted muscle after prolonged ischemia.
Hemarthrosis	Bleeding into the joint space results in chondrolysis and early arthritis.
Infection	Occurs in 12%[230] to 16%[56] of open fractures; femur and tibia are most common sites; the dominant organism is *Staphylococcus aureus.*
Loss of function	Avulsions of tendons and ligaments may lead to loss of limb or digit mobility; notoriously, loss of function follows apparently innocuous chip fractures of the phalanges that represent avulsions of the extensor or flexion tendon groups.
Nerve injury	Nerves more often are severed with open fractures.
Spinal cord injury	With any fracture of the spine, however trivial it may appear to be, a meticulous neurologic examination is essential, to establish whether the spinal cord or nerve roots have been damaged, and to obtain a baseline for later comparison if neurologic signs should develop.
Vascular injury	Vessels may be compressed, cut, or contused by associated trauma. Vascular injury most often occurs in the extremities about the knee and elbow.
Visceral injury	Often abdominal and pelvic viscera are injured during trauma to the trunk, namely, puncture of the lung with development of pneumothorax after rib fractures, and rupture of the bladder or urethra with pelvic fractures. It is important to inquire about urinary function. Diagnostic urethrography may be necessary if a urethral or bladder injury is suspected.
Late	
Algodystrophy (Sudeck's atrophy)	Algodystrophy (Sudeck's atrophy) is a form of reflex sympathetic dystrophy syndrome (RSDS) and follows slight trauma, and typically is seen in the hand or foot after trivial injury.
Avascular necrosis	After trauma some areas of the skeleton are notorious for developing ischemic necrosis, such as the femoral head and scaphoid.
Delayed union	Delayed healing results from an inadequate blood supply or fixation of fragments. If there is no radiographic evidence of bone callus within 3 months, internal fixation and bone grafting may be necessary.
Growth disturbance	Trauma to the epiphyseal growth plates in children may manifest in abnormal growth and deformity.
Joint stiffness	Joint stiffness is characterized by reduced joint motion, most often developing in the knee, elbow, and small joints of the hand and resulting from adhesions after hemarthrosis or prolonged immobilization.
Malunion (Fig. 10-231)	Malunion is characterized by unsatisfactory healing, usually referring to poor alignment, unacceptable deformity, or fibrous union.
Myositis ossificans (Fig. 10-232)	Heterotropic bone formation develops in soft tissues, although most often it is related to injury. It is also seen in nontraumatic conditions such as paraplegia or coma.
Nonunion (Fig. 10-233)	Nonunion is characterized by incomplete healing, resulting from an inadequate blood supply, fixation, or apposition; and the presence of interposed cartilage, muscle, or periosteum between bone fragments. The fracture site is filled in with fibrous tissue that may form a rudimentary joint (pseudoarthrosis) if motion continues at the fracture site. Nonunion that appears with large callous formation is termed *hypertrophic nonunion,* whereas nonunion with little callous is termed *atrophic nonunion.*
Osteoarthritis	Hemorrhage or trauma may alter the smooth articular joint surfaces.

PART TWO Bone, Joints, and Soft Tissues

Continued

TABLE 10-11 cont'd
Early and Late Fracture Complications

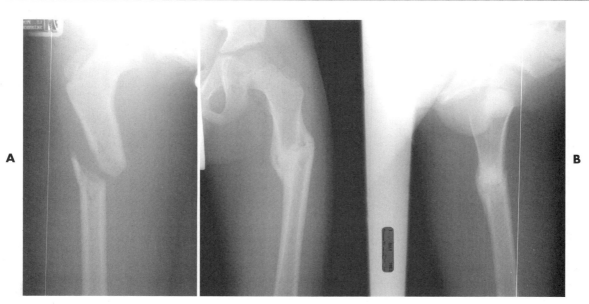

FIG. 10-231   **A,** Fracture through the proximal shaft of the femur. The displacement of the fragments was not properly reduced; **B,** therefore the fracture healed with deformity as seen in this image taken 4.5 months after image **A.**

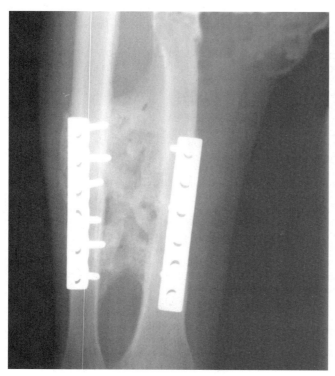

FIG. 10-232   Hypertropic bone formation noted within the interosseous space.

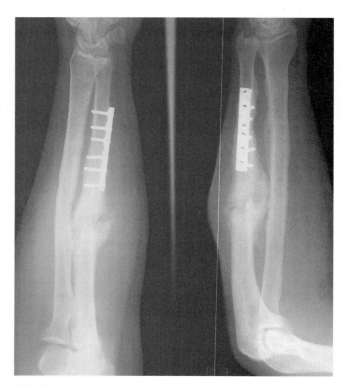

FIG. 10-233   Hypertropic nonunion is seen of the fracture in the middle region of the shaft of the ulna.

Battered Child Syndrome

BACKGROUND

Battered child syndrome describes nonaccidental trauma to children, representing a major cause of morbidity and mortality during childhood.[85] The abuse usually is inflicted by boyfriends, stepparents, baby sitters, and others responsible for the child's care. Abuse is more common among stepchildren, handicapped, and first-born children. Most victims are under 2 years of age,[194] with a reported average age of 16 months.[147]

IMAGING FINDINGS

Although uncommon,[147] the presence of multiple fractures in various stages of healing is a classic radiographic presentation of battered child syndrome. Fractures of the skull, spinous processes, scapula, posterior ribs, and sternum are suspicious for abuse. Metaphyseal corner fractures secondary to twisting action of the distal limb, and avulsion of the metaphyseal arcuate rim that overlies the lucent physis appearing as a "bucket handle" fracture are particularly indicative of abuse (Fig. 10-234).[133] Pulmonary infiltrate without fever is suspicious of lung contusion.

Exuberant periosteal reaction often is present. Radionuclide bone scans or skeletal surveys are useful to detect other sites of injury,[119,132,237] Osteogenesis imperfecta, scurvy, syphilis, and other diseases that may mimic the radiographic findings of battered child syndrome usually are differentiated by clinical data and specific radiographic findings.[59]

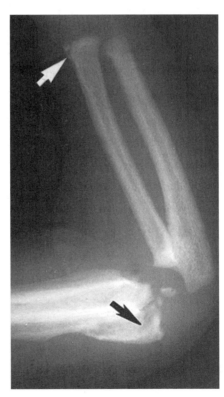

FIG. 10-234 Metaphyseal corner fractures *(arrows)* of differing ages in battered child syndrome. Similar findings may occur in Menkes' kinky hair syndrome and scurvy. (From Sartoris DJ: Musculoskeletal imaging: the requisites, St Louis, 1993, Mosby.)

CLINICAL COMMENTS

Often the reported patient history of trauma is inadequate to explain the presenting injuries. Concurrent burns, bruises, retinal damage, subdural hemorrhages, pulmonary infiltrates without fever representing lung confusion, and other soft-tissue injuries may accompany the osseous injuries.

> ### KEY CONCEPTS
> - *Multiple fractures in various stages of healing.*
> - *Corner and bucket-handle metaphyseal fractures.*
> - *Usually under the age of 2 years.*

Myositis Ossificans

BACKGROUND

Myositis ossificans (heterotopic bone formation) presents in two forms: circumscripta and progressiva. The circumscribed form is a benign, solitary, self-limiting disorder representing metaplasia of soft tissue to bone.[137] Usually it is related to trauma (myositis ossificans traumatica), but also may be idiopathic in nature (myositis ossificans idiopathica). The trauma is most often to the muscle; fascia, tendon, and joint capsules are involved less commonly. Only rarely is fatty tissue implicated. The exact pathogenesis is unknown, and, contrary to the name, no primary muscle inflammation is present.[137]

The progressive form, also known as *Münchmeyer disease* or *fibrodysplasia ossificans progressiva,* is a rare hereditary connective tissue disorder of unknown etiology. The disease is believed to be an autosomal dominant trait with complete penetrance and variable expressivity.[26]

IMAGING FINDINGS

In its early stages, myositis ossificans may appear similar to osteosarcoma or other bone malignancies. Therefore one should recognize the radiographic features of circumscribed myositis ossificans to aid its differentiation. On plain film radiographs, myositis ossificans circumscripta may be present as faint tissue calcifications within 2 to 6 weeks after the onset of symptoms.[1] Within 6 to 8 weeks the center of the lesion becomes more radiolucent as the periphery develops a surrounding radiodense ring (Fig. 10-235). This is called a *zonal phenomenon* and is more easily noted on CT. A reversal of this zonal pattern is noted in some malignancies, such as osteosarcoma. A malignancy may present with a more radiodense center and with a surrounding radiolucent periphery about the lesion. In addition, malignancies are not clearly separated from their parent bone, as is myositis ossificans.

Myositis ossificans circumscripta may occur anywhere but is most common in the brachialis (fencer's bone), adductor longus (rider's bone), soleus (dancer's bone), and adductor magnus tendon.[248]

The progressive form appears as extensive ossification of the connective tissues of the limbs and spine with microdactyly, usually of the big toe (90%) and thumbs (50%) (Figs. 10-236 and 10-237). Fusion of the vertebrae and ossification of the voluntary muscle may be complete by age 20. The hands, sphincters, diaphragm, and viscera are spared.[46] The progressive form of the disease results in severe complications, disabilities, and early death.

CLINICAL COMMENTS

A history of trauma is present in up to 60% of circumscribed presentations. Supportive care (e.g., ice, reduced mobility) is the accepted conservative management.[31,52] However, surgical removal of ectopic bone occasionally is necessary.[161] The progressive form

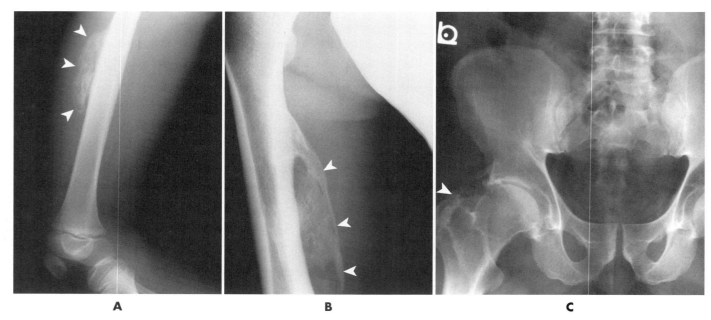

FIG. 10-235 Myositis ossificans appearing as a calcific soft-tissue mass in, **A,** the anterior; **B,** medial; and, **C,** lateral regions of the femur in different patients *(arrowheads).* The perimeter of the mass in **B** appears more radiodense than the center identifying the zonal phenomena characteristic of myositis ossificans. (**A,** Courtesy Steven P. Brownstein, MD, Springfield, NJ.)

usually presents in the first year of life as neck stiffness with concurrent edematous subcutaneous nodules. The symptoms progress to the shoulders, upper limbs, and, later, lower extremities. Commonly paraplegics demonstrate circumscribed areas of myositis ossificans in the paralyzed regions, usually the hips or thighs.

KEY CONCEPTS

- *Myositis ossificans traumatica is related to the history of trauma, presenting with zonal phenomena, separation from bone, and predictive development of radiographic pattern that helps to differentiate from malignancy.*
- *Zonal phenomena are marked by the appearance of a radiolucent center and radiodense periphery of the involved region.*
- *Reverse zonal phenomena are apparent in some malignancies.*
- *Myositis ossificans idiopathica appears similar to the traumatica variety.*
- *Myositis ossificans progressiva is rare, beginning in the first year of life with neck stiffness and advancing to near-total body ossification by age 20.*

Osteochondritis Dissecans

BACKGROUND

Osteochondritis dissecans describes fragmentation of a portion of the articular surface of a joint, involving articular cartilage and possibly subjacent bone. It follows acute osteochondral fracture, or may be a consequence of repeated stresses, representing a fatigue fracture.[2] However, because many of the separated fragments appear necrotic, some authorities question a purely traumatic etiology, believing instead that avascular necrosis is a primary reason for the development of osteochondritis dissecans.[174] The fragment of bone and cartilage may remain in place (in situ) or dislodge to become a free fragment within the joint space (loose body). Occasionally those remaining in situ renew their blood supply and heal.

Osteochondritis dissecans may present in adult form (occurring after the growth plates have closed) or juvenile form (occurring before the growth plates have closed). Together these forms occur in approximately 15 to 60 cases per 100,000 persons.[113,181] It presents most often during the ages of 5 to 50 with peak incidence in young adults immediately after the closure of the growth plates. It is the most common cause of a loose body in adolescent patients. Traditionally the disease has been reported to be more common in males; however, recent reports note increasing frequency among young female athletes.[264]

IMAGING FINDINGS

Osteochondritis dissecans is predisposed to target areas of the skeleton. The most common site is the distal femur, involving the medial condyle (usually lateral portion) 85% of the time and the lateral condyle 15% of the time. The knee accounts for nearly 75% of the overall cases.[38] Approximately 20% of presentations are bilateral. Less common sites include the patella, tibial plateau, and convex surfaces of the metatarsals, talus, capitellum, and femoral head. The appearance typically is marked by a small saucer defect of the articular cortex (Figs. 10-238 through 10-244). If radiographs are negative and clinical symptoms are strongly suggestive, an MRI is warranted as follow-up. Staging is presented in Table 10-12. Of those listed, MRI is the most accurate method for staging the disease.[61]

Injury to the articular surface has a variety of presentations (Fig. 10-245). If the underlying bone is not involved, radiographs typically are normal. MRI and arthroscopy provide a more sensitive assessment (see Table 10-12).

Spontaneous osteonecrosis of the knee (SONK) is a related appearance of the knee, usually involving the medial femoral condyle. It occurs as an idiopathic presentation, usually in patients over the age of 50 years, and is more common among women. Patients present clinically with knee pain, often of rapid onset, and

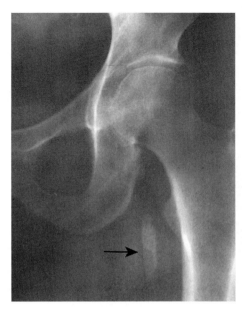

FIG. 10-236 A focus of ossification is noted in the adductors of the thigh *(arrow).*

generally the clinical syndrome mimics those of joint degeneration or meniscal injury. Radiographs often are normal, but may demonstrate a flattening segment of the articular surface with either subchondral radiolucency or sclerosis. The defect appears with surrounding edema on the T2-weighted MRI scan and with increased radioisotope uptake on the bone scan.

CLINICAL COMMENTS

Symptoms are variable, ranging from completely asymptomatic to pain on movement with limitations of motions, joint locking, joint aching related to activity, and resulting stiffness. Because clinical features may be subtle, at times presenting with nothing more than slight restriction in the range of motion, clinicians should have a low threshold for obtaining radiographs when the condition is

suspected. Usually it is not possible to trace the presenting defect to a single traumatic event.

MRI is valuable in assessing the stability of the fragment,[270] which has implications for the viability of healing. Although many MRI stage I and II lesions respond well to conservative therapy, the more advanced stages (III and IV) usually necessitate surgical intervention, usually done via arthroscopy.[176] Because it lacks blood, lymph, or neural elements, mature articular cartilage exhibits limited to no ability to heal once injured.

In addition to the immediate management of the condition, further clinical interest should be directed to concerns for future joint degeneration. For example, moderate to severe knee degeneration has been reported in up to 32% of patients over the age of 34 who experienced an episode of osteochondritis dissecans as an adolescent.[250]

> **KEY CONCEPTS**
> - *Traumatic or avascular etiology.*
> - *Predisposed to target areas of the skeleton.*
> - *Most common at the lateral margin of the medial femoral condyle.*
> - *Usually occurs before 50 years of age with peak incidence during adolescence.*

Slipped Capital Femoral Epiphysis

BACKGROUND

Slipped capital femoral epiphysis (SCFE) is a posteromedioinferior[112] displacement of the proximal femoral epiphysis occurring during childhood. The defect represents a type I Salter-Harris epiphyseal injury. Although the etiology is not clearly defined, trauma, hormonal influences,[261] adolescent growth spurt,[101] body weight,[25,192] vertical orientation of the growth plate,[192] retroversion of the proximal femur,[89,192] renal osteodystrophy,[64] and physical activity all have been implicated.

The condition is more prevalent among blacks,[106,127] males, those who are overweight,[15] and those of short stature.[125,126] The peak age is during early adolescence. Males present between the ages of 10 and 17, with peak incidence at 12; females present between the ages of 8 and 15, with peak incidence at age 11 or 12.[198]

IMAGING FINDINGS

Slipped capital femoral epiphysis is more common on the left and is noted bilaterally in 20% to 35% of individuals.[226] The lateral (frog-leg) projection is more sensitive than the frontal projection for demonstrating early changes (Figs. 10-246 and 10-247). To aid

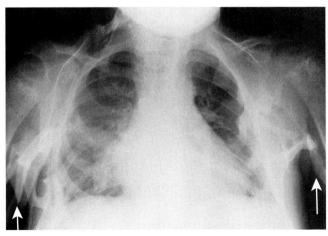

FIG. 10-237 Soft tissue ossifications most prominent in the axillary regions *(arrows)* of a patient with myositis ossificans progressiva. (Courtesy Jack C. Avalos, Davenport, IA.)

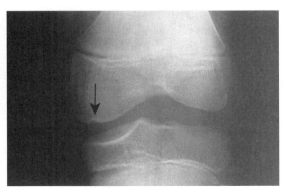

FIG. 10-238 Osteochondritis dissecans of the central medial femoral condyle *(arrow).* (Courtesy Joseph W. Howe, Sylmar, CA.)

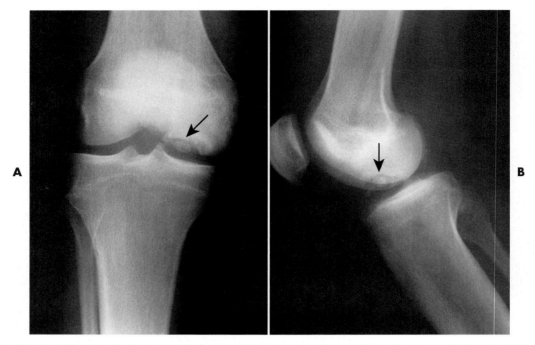

FIG. 10-239   **A** and **B,** Osteochondritis dissecans of the knee *(arrow).* (Courtesy Steven P. Brownstein, MD, Springfield, NJ.)

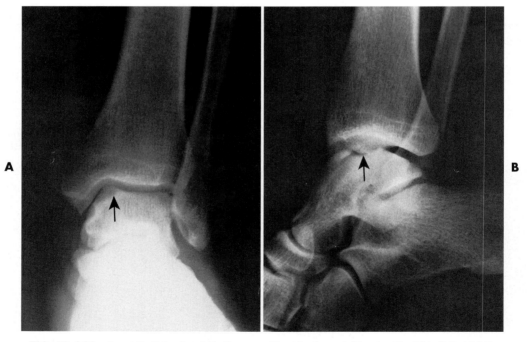

FIG. 10-240   **A** and **B,** Osteochondritis dissecans of the talus *(arrows).* (Courtesy Tim Mick, St Paul, MN.)

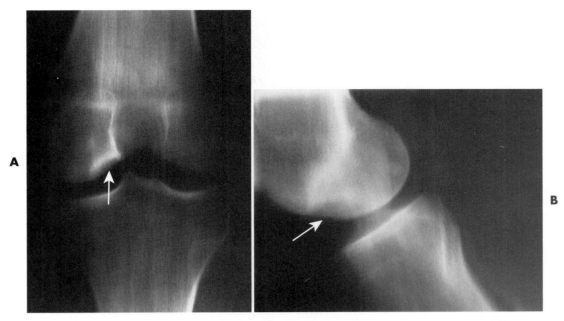

FIG. 10-241 **A** and **B,** Linear tomograms demonstrating osteochondritis dissecans of the knee *(arrows)*. (Courtesy Tim Mick, St Paul, MN.)

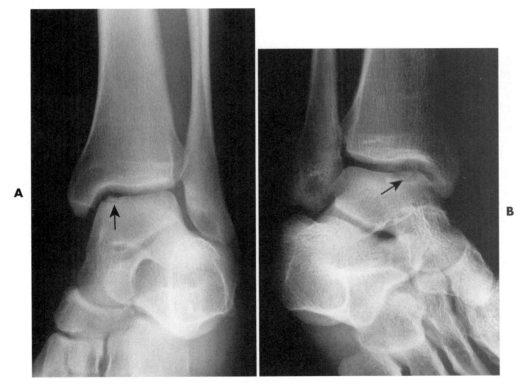

FIG. 10-242 **A** and **B,** Two cases of osteochondritis dissecans of the talus *(arrows)*. (**A,** Courtesy Steven P. Brownstein, MD, Springfield, NJ.)

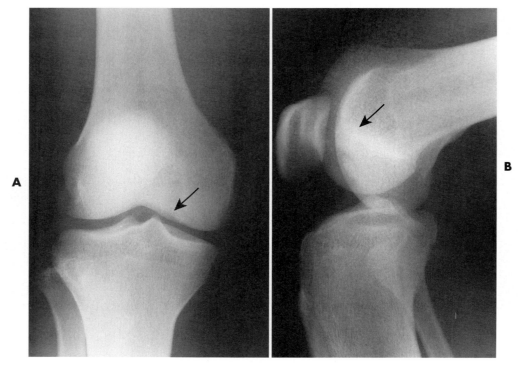

FIG. 10-243 **A,** Anteroposterior and, **B,** lateral projections of the knee with revealing osteochondritis dissecans on the lateral aspect of the medial femoral condyle *(arrows)*. (Courtesy Joseph W. Howe, Sylmar, CA.)

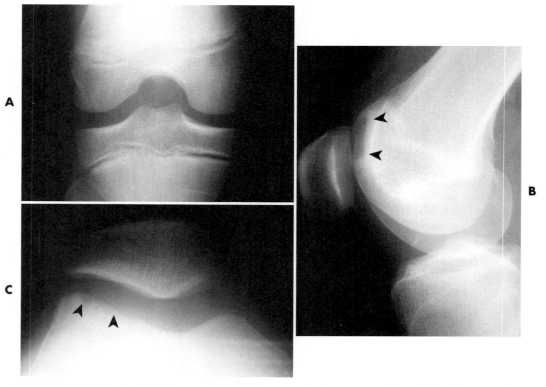

FIG. 10-244 Osteochondritis dissecans. **A,** Defect is not seen in the anteroposterior projection. However, a large defect of the articular cortex is noted on, **B,** the lateral and, **C,** tangent projections *(arrowheads)*. It is often the case that the articular defect is not seen in all projections.

TABLE 10-12
Staging Osteochondritis Dissecans

Stage	Features
Radiographs[16]	
I	Normal radiograph
II	Partial detached osteochondral fragment
III	Complete, nondisplaced osteochondral fragment
IV	Detached, loose osteochondral fragment
CT[76]	
I	Cystic defect in the subchondral bone
II	Cystic defect extending to the articular surface
III	Nondisplaced osteochondral defect
IV	Displaced osteochondral defect
MRI[181]	
I	Bone marrow edema (stable defect)
II	Cystic defect of the articular cartilage and subchondral bone with a rim of low signal intensity behind the fragment at its interface with bone (stable defect)
III	Defect of the articular cartilage with a rim of high signal intensity behind the fragment at its interface with bone, representing surrounding fluid (unstable defect)
IV	Loose body representing an displaced osteochondral fragment (unstable defect)
Arthroscopy[35]	
A	Smooth, but soft surface of the articular cartilage
B	Irregular surface of the articular cartilage
C	Fissure of the articular cartilage
D	Flap defect of the articular cartilage
E	Loose, nondisplaced osteochondral fragment
F	Displaced osteochondral fragment

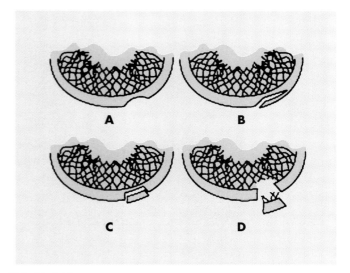

FIG. 10-245 Injuries to the articular surface of a joint appear as, **A,** indented; **B,** hinged; or, **C** and **D,** detached. **D,** Detached fractures of the articular cartilage and underlying bone are known as osteochondral fractures. Detached chondral and osteochondral fractures may remain in situ or dislodge to become free bodies within the joint. (Modified from Rogers LF: Radiology of skeletal trauma, ed 2, New York, 1992, Churchill Livingstone.)

CLINICAL COMMENTS

Ninety percent of patients present with clinical symptoms and only half of this group relate a history of trauma. The usual presentation is that of hip pain and limp. Referred pain to the knee is less common. Limitations of hip motion, particularly in abduction and internal rotation, are usual. SCFE is classified as acute symptoms are present for 3 weeks or less, and chronic if longer than 3 weeks. The goal of treatment is stabilization and reduction of further slippage. In situ pinning is the most common treatment.[170,238] A poor outcome may lead to one or more identifiable complications: severe varus deformity, shortened and broadened femoral neck, osteonecrosis,[164] chondrolysis,[117] and precocious degenerative joint disease.[42]

> **KEY CONCEPTS**
> - *Posteromedioinferior displacement of the proximal femoral epiphysis occurring during early adolescence, representing a Salter-Harris type I fracture.*
> - *Frog-leg (lateral) projection is more sensitive to early slippage.*
> - *Hip pain with a limp is the usual clinical presentation.*
> - *Higher incidence among males, blacks, and those who are overweight.*

Spondylolisthesis and Spondylolysis

BACKGROUND

Definition. Spondylolisthesis is an anterior displacement of a vertebra (and those above it) in relation to a vertebra immediately below (Fig. 10-248). Descriptions of partial dislocation of vertebrae are found as early as the year 1741, but Kilian usually is given credit for adopting the term "spondylolisthesis" in 1853 to describe these changes.[240,259]

The term *spondylolisthesis* should not be confused with spondylosis, which denotes degeneration of the spine (Table 10-13). Another term, *spondylolysis*, defines disruption of the pars interarticularis (the anatomy between the superior and inferior articular processes in the thoracic and lumbar region; known as the articular

recognition some advocate the use of a line drawn along the lateral cortical margin of the femoral neck (Klein's line). Normally this line should intersect the lateral portion of the femoral capital epiphysis. Failure to do so indicates medial slippage of the epiphysis. When compared with the normal side, the slipped epiphysis may appear irregular with decreased vertical height. Buttressing (e.g., thickening) of the lateral femoral neck (Herndon's hump), rounded deformity of the proximal femur (pistol-grip femur), and beaking of the medial epiphysis are other radiographic clues of SCFE.

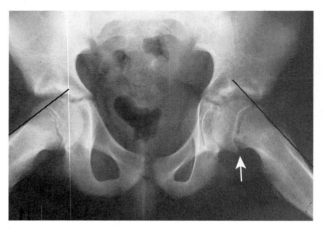

FIG. 10-246 Frog-leg projection demonstrating slipped capital epiphysis on the left *(arrow)*. Klein's line, drawn along the lateral margin of the femoral neck, is a useful aid in the determination of slipped capital femoral epiphysis. (Courtesy Jack C. Avalos, Davenport, IA.)

pillar in the cervical region of the spine). Defects of the pars inter-articulares may occur unilaterally or bilaterally and with (spondylolytic spondylolisthesis) or without (prespondylolisthesis) anterior displacement of the same vertebral body.

Spondylolysis. The incidence of spondylolysis is estimated at 5% to 7%, and occurs most commonly between the ages of 8 and 20 years.[40,157] The risk of spondylolysis decreases through middle age and demonstrates a slight second peak between 60 and 80 years of age.[120] Higher incidence occurs among males,[175] whites,[202] native Alaskans,[233] Japanese,[136] and those involved in gymnastics, football, weightlifting, pole-vaulting, diving, and other activities.[207] Some authors feel that precocious weight-bearing posture caused by infant carriers and walkers may be a precipitant factor for developing spondylolysis.[268] Nearly 70% of spondylolysis occurs at L5.[198]

Classification. Wiltse, Newman, and MacNab developed a widely used classification system that is based on the etiology and anatomy involved:[263]

Type I: Dysplastic, congenital abnormalities of the neural arch resulting in deformity and anterior vertebral displacement (Fig. 10-249). For example, a congenital etiology may include

spina bifida occulta and an abnormally increased angle of the inferior articular process. Hereditary traits are thought to be important predictive factors for congenital spondylolisthesis.[240] Dysplastic spondylolisthesis is uncommon.

Type II: Isthmic, defect of the pars interarticularis (Figs. 10-250 and 10-251)

  a. Fatigue fracture through pars interarticularis. This is the most common type of spondylolisthesis in young patients. Spondylolysis is not seen among infants, prompting the hypothesis that pars defects are acquired through repetitive weight-bearing stress. Defects are thought to occur from repeated direct loading during hyperextension movements or increased shear stresses applied during flexion movements.[120,171]

  b. Elongated pars interarticularis. An elongated pars interarticularis is probably another expression of repeated applications of stress to the region, in addition to the type IIa stress fracture, which is thought to occur from this mechanism.

  c. Acute fracture of the pars interarticularis (rare).

Type III: Degenerative, intersegmental laxity secondary to advanced degeneration of the intervertebral disc and posterior joints (Figs. 10-252 and 10-253). The resulting anterior displacement is secondary to the loss of joint space and morphologic changes in the angle of the facet joints. This is the most common type of spondylolisthesis in patients over the age of 40 years and may result in spinal stenosis.[239]

Type IV: Traumatic, acute fractures involving the neural arch other than at the pars interarticularis (e.g., pedicle).

Type V: Pathologic, osseous deformity secondary to local or systemic pathology (e.g., Paget's disease, metastatic bone disease, osteopetrosis) (Fig. 10-254).

A sixth category, known as *iatrogenic spondylolisthesis* or *spondylolisthesis acquisita,* may be used to describe those lesions developing secondary to spinal surgery (e.g., laminectomies, spinal fusions).[268]

With the various etiologies, spondylolisthesis may present across a broad age range. However, when spondylolisthesis presents before the age of 30 years, it is usually a type IIa (stress fracture of the pars interarticularis) defect at L5, with a mean age of presentation of 16 years.[53] In patients over the age of 50 years, spondylolisthesis usually is a type III (degenerative) etiology, typically occurring at L4, and is more common among women.[23]

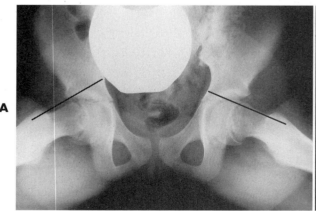
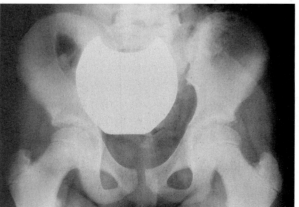

FIG. 10-247   A, Frog-leg projection demonstrating a bilateral presentation of slipped capital femoral epiphysis *(arrows)*.
B, The anteroposterior projection appears normal. (**A,** Courtesy Steven P. Brownstein, MD, Springfield, NJ.)

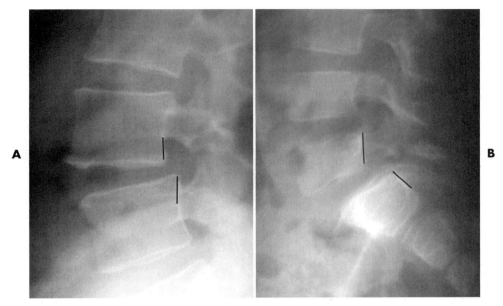

FIG. 10-248 Spondylolisthesis defines anterior displacement of a vertebra with respect to the vertebra below, usually determined by an offset of the posterior body lines (George's line). **A** and **B**, In each of theses cases, there is an anterior displacement of the superior segment. (Courtesy Christine Velos, Ottawa, IL.)

IMAGING FINDINGS

The presence of anterior displacement is best evaluated in a lateral projection. The most noteworthy finding is disruption of the posterior body (George's) line at the level of anterior displacement. An alternative, less sensitive method involves constructing a line along the sacral base and a second line perpendicular to the sacral base line (Ulmann's line). A spondylolisthesis is present if the second line intersects the vertebral body of L5.

The degree of anterior displacement is most often measured by Meyerding's grading system (Fig. 10-255).[162] This system divides the sacral base (or whatever segment is subadjacent to the spondylolisthesis) into four equal divisions. The degree of spondylolisthesis is described by which of the imaginary sacral base divisions the posterior body line intersects. For example, if the body of L5 slips forward between 0% and 25% of the total length of the sacral base so that a line drawn along the posterior margin of the L5 body interrupts the most posterior division of the sacral base, it is designated as a Grade I spondylolisthesis. A Grade II spondylolisthesis represents anterior displacement of 26% to 50% of the total sacral base length so that the posterior body line of L5 intersects the second from most posterior quadrant of the sacral base. If the L5 vertebra extends beyond the front of the sacrum and into the pelvic cavity it is designated as a Grade V spondylolisthesis, also termed a *spondyloptosis.* A more informative but less often used method to

TABLE 10-13	
Terms Related to Spondylolisthesis	
Term	**Description**
Spondylolisthesis	Anterior displacement of a vertebra (and those above it) on the vertebra below.
Spondylolysis	Unilateral or bilateral defects of the pars interarticularis.
Spondylolytic spondylolisthesis	Unilateral or bilateral pars defects and anterior displacement of the same segment.
Nonspondylolytic spondylolisthesis	Anterior displacement without accompanying defects of the same level pars interarticularis.
Lytic spondylolisthesis	Another term for spondylolytic spondylolisthesis.
Isthmic spondylolisthesis	Another term for spondylolytic spondylolisthesis.
Pseudospondylolisthesis	Another term for a degenerative spondylolisthesis.
Prespondylolisthesis	Unilateral or bilateral pars defects without same-level anterior displacement. The prefix "pre" implies that displacement is expected, but this is misleading because displacement is not inevitable.

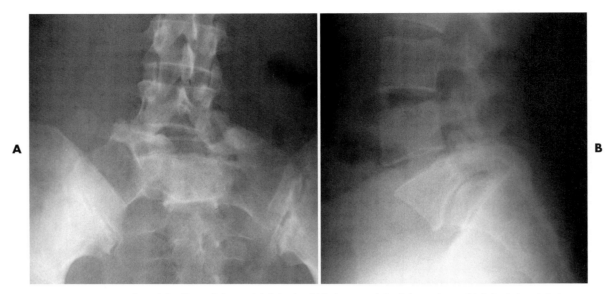

FIG. 10-249　A and B, Congenital spondylolisthesis of L5. A congenital etiology of spondylolisthesis is relatively uncommon and is caused by underdevelopment of the posterior vertebral arch. In this case the vertebral is trapezoidal, the anterosuperior corner of the sacrum is rounded, and there is degeneration of the subadjacent disc, all predictive features that further progression of the displacement is likely to occur. (Courtesy Thomas Galli, Peoria, IL.)

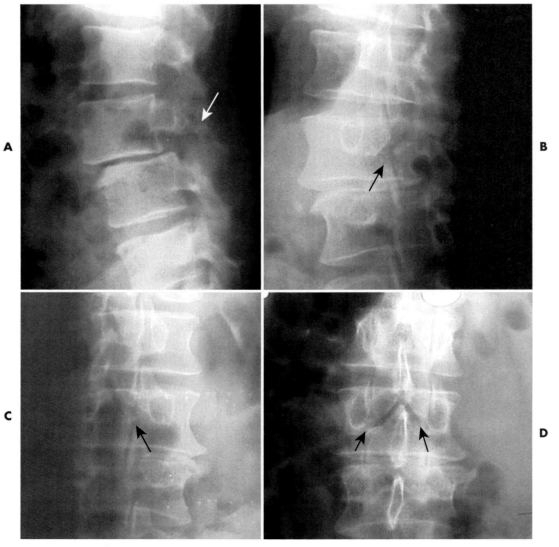

FIG. 10-250　A through D, Isthmic spondylolisthesis with bilateral defects of the pars interarticularis of L3 *(arrows).*

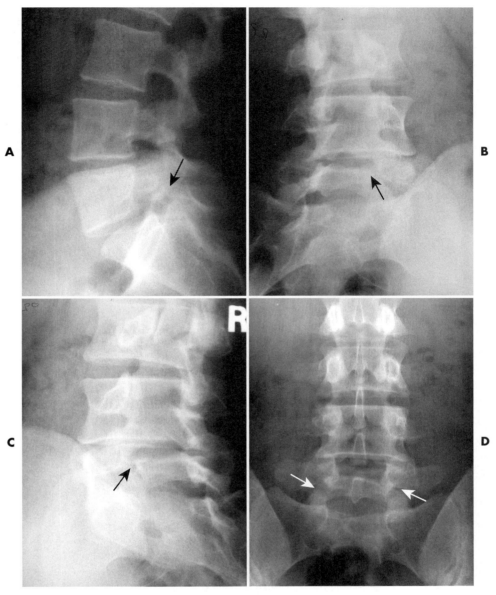

FIG. 10-251   A, Spondylolisthesis with bilateral defects of the pars interarticularis noted on, **B** and **C,** the oblique and, to a lesser degree, **D,** the anteroposterior projection at L5 *(arrows).*

describe the degree of displacement is to record the displacement as a percentage. This is done by dividing the amount of displacement by the total length of the inferior endplate of the slipped vertebra.

In addition to the amount of slippage, it may be important to document the amount of sagittal angular rotation, with the notion that increased rotation complicates the case. This is accomplished by recording the angle of intersection between a line drawn along the anterior margin of the slipped segment (e.g., L5) and a second line along the posterior body margin of the segment below (e.g., S1) the slipped segment.

In the frontal projection, advanced spondylolisthesis of L5 may demonstrate a characteristic configuration in which the vertebral body resembles an inverted Napoleon hat or inverted bow (Bowline of Brailsford) (Figs. 10-256 and 10-257). The spinous process at the level of spondylolisthesis often is deviated.[195]

Often the transverse processes of an L5 spondylolisthesis overlaps the upper sacrum (Fig. 10-258).

In the oblique lumbar projection the neural arch resembles a "Scottie dog" in which the dog's neck represents the pars interarticularis (Fig. 10-259). Disruption of the pars interarticularis appears as a "collared" dog. An additional clue to the presence of spondylolisthesis in the oblique projection is a disruption of the normal progression of each facet joint placed slightly anterior to the segment immediately above ("stepladder sign").

Radionuclide bone scanning is helpful in determining if a spondylolysis is active in patients with chronic low back pain.[249] If the region of the pars interarticularis demonstrates increased uptake of the radiopharmaceutical, an active stress fracture or healing fracture is suspected. SPECT relates better detail than conventional radionuclide bone scanning. Specialized imaging

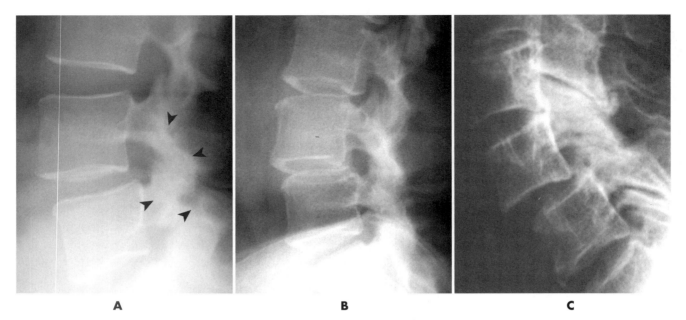

FIG. 10-252 Degenerative spondylolisthesis. **A** through **C,** The degenerative etiology of these cases is reflected by the disc and facet degeneration. Disc degeneration is noted by the reduced disc space and osteophytes. Posterior joint arthrosis is recognized by the increased radiopacity and irregularity of the facet region *(arrowheads)*.

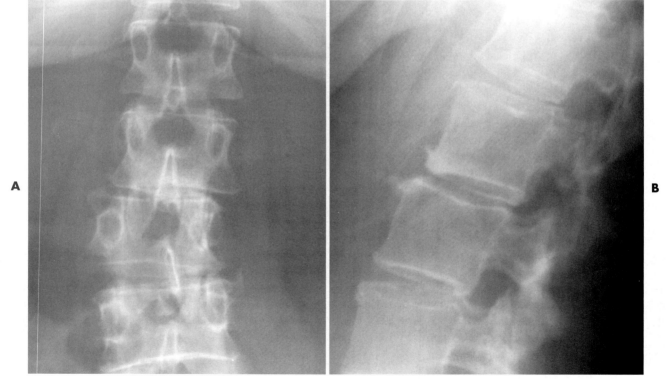

FIG. 10-253 Disc and posterior joint degeneration tend to promote spondylolisthesis of the middle cervical and lower lumbar segments. However, not all degenerative joint laxity leads to an anterior displacement. **A,** Lateral displacement is common when scoliosis is present, and, **B,** posterior displacement of the upper lumbar segments is seen with spinal degeneration.

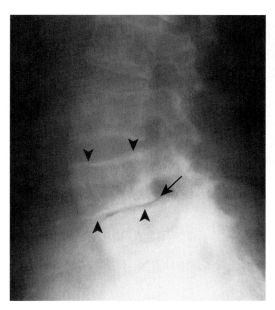

FIG. 10-254 Pathologic (type V) spondylolisthesis of L4 on L5 in a patient with Paget's disease *(arrow)*; observe the picture frame vertebra *(arrowheads)* and degenerative disc disease with vacuum phenomena of the L4 disc. (Courtesy Robert C. Tatum, Davenport, IA.)

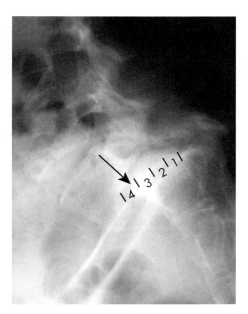

FIG. 10-255 Meyerding's grading system divides the superior endplate of the segment below into quadrants. The grade of spondylolisthesis is determined by the quadrant intersected by a posterior body line *(arrow)* drawn along the slipped segment. In this case, a Grade IV spondylolisthesis is noted.

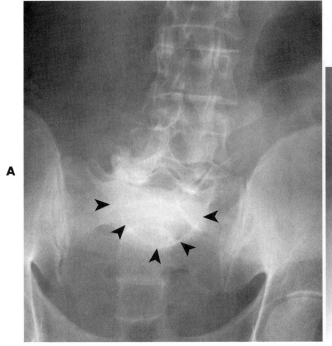

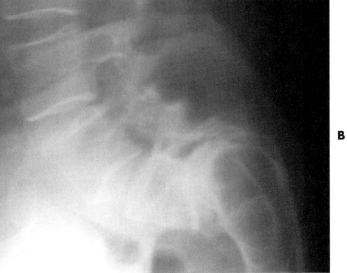

FIG. 10-256 **A** and **B,** "Napoleon hat" sign noted with Grade III spondylolisthesis *(arrowheads)*. With advanced grades of spondylolisthesis and forward sacral rotation, the anteroposterior lumbopelvic radiograph may project the slipped segment in a superoinferior orientation instead of a normal anteroposterior orientation. The resulting configuration has been likened to the appearance of an upside-down hat, specifically the hat that Napoleon wore. The anterior margin of the vertebra forms the top of the inverted hat. The posterior margin of the slipped segment appears as the bottom of the hat. The lateral margins of the hat are formed from the transverse processes of the slipped segment. The Napoleon hat sign becomes more obvious with increasing grades of spondylolisthesis and forward sacral rotation. It is not typically seen with Grade I or II spondylolisthesis.

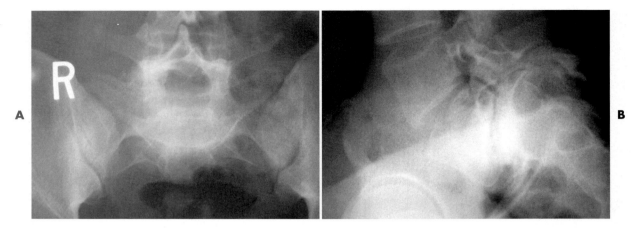

FIG. 10-257   **A** and **B,** Bowline of Brailsford is the curved anterior radiodense shadow that represents the anterior margin of the spondylolisthesis segment. Bowline of Brailsford is the top of the inverted Napoleon hat.

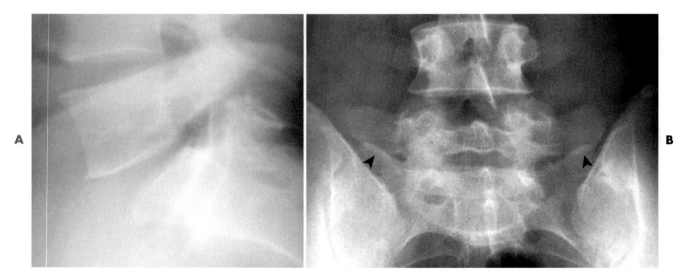

FIG. 10-258   **A** and **B,** An overlap of the L5 transverse processes with the superior margins of the sacrum in the anteroposterior or posteroanterior projection provides a clue to the presence of spondylolisthesis. In this case there is a minimal spondylolisthesis in the lateral projection and corresponding slight overlap of the transverse processes and the sacrum in the anteroposterior projection *(arrowheads).*

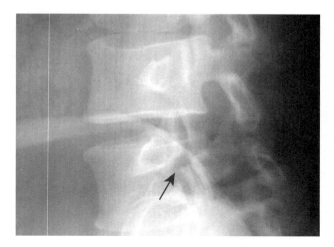

FIG. 10-259   The posterior arch of the lumbar vertebrae resembles a Scottie dog in the oblique projection (see Chapter 6 for more detail). The pars interarticularis is the neck of the dog. A pars defect appears with a radiolucent "collar" across the dog's neck, as is seen in this case *(arrow).*

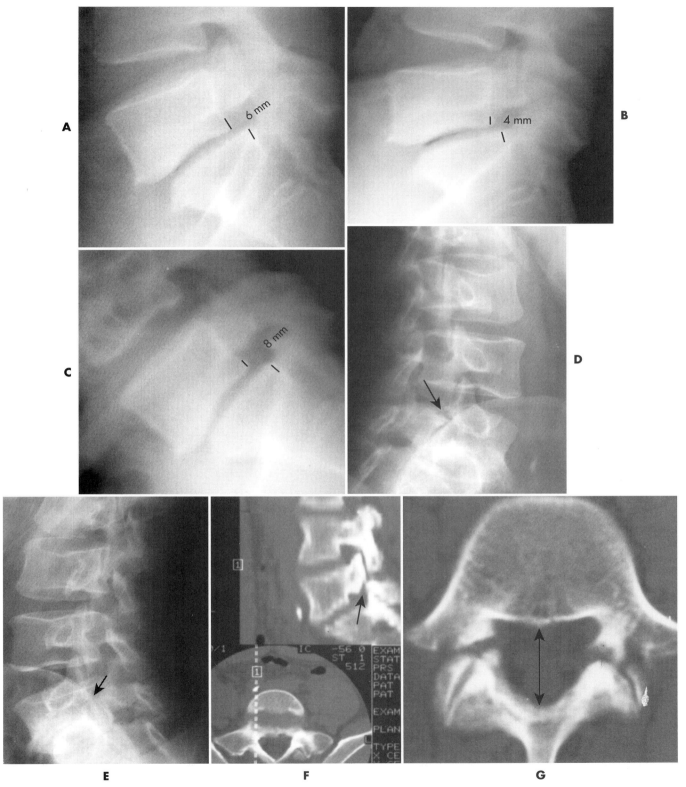

FIG. 10-260 Spondylolisthesis. **A,** Lateral lumbar projection reveals 6 mm of spondylolisthesis. The amount of displacement, **B,** reduces in extension and, **C,** exaggerates in flexion. The net translation of 4 mm (8-4 mm) is within the limits of normal intersegmental motion; often reported at 4.5 mm. **D** and **E,** Oblique projections exhibit bilateral pars defects at L5 *(arrows)*, probably representing stress fractures that occurred in early adolescence (type IIa). **F,** Computed tomography with sagittal reformatted images demonstrates the pars defect to a better degree *(arrow)*. **G,** Spondylolisthesis is associated with an enlarged sagittal dimension of the spinal canal at the level of the slipped segment *(arrow)*. A degenerative etiology, in which the pars interarticularis is intact, is associated with forward movement of the posterior arch and hence a narrowed canal at the level below the slipped segment. (Courtesy Frank Bemis, St Louis, MO.)

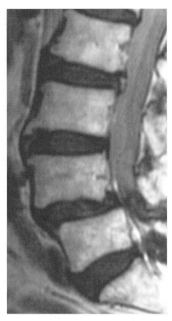

FIG. 10-261   Magnetic resonance imaging details the spinal canal and the impact of spinal deformity such as spondylolisthesis on the neurology contained within.

of displacement.[268] However, radiographic detection is usual, and often leads to a spurious association between back pain and spondylolisthesis. In reality, the association between low back pain and spondylolisthesis is ambiguous and poorly documented.

Spondylolisthesis may or may not be painful. It is poorly understood why some patients remain asymptomatic throughout their life and others do not.[252] Moreover, a general relationship between the degree of anterior displacement (spondylolisthesis) and back pain is lacking.[249] About 50% of those with spondylolisthesis develop symptoms, usually back pain or sciatica.[118] The clinical outcome and functional disability of adult spondylolisthesis and in low back pain of nonspecific origin are similar.[169] Although spondylolisthesis exhibits an ambiguous association to back pain, spondylolysis has been more directly implicated as a possible source of back pain, at least around the time when the defect develops.[217]

Most spondylolistheses occurs in the lumbar spine, usually at L5 secondary to pars fractures (spondylolysis), and may heal if the patient is immobilized by bracing.[11,163,187] Unfortunately, spontaneous healing is rarely the outcome because the spondylolysis may go unnoticed for some time. Also, if healing occurs after bracing, the pars fractures often recur when activity is resumed. Spondylolisthesis can occur at any vertebrae, including the cervical spine, where degenerative and congenital etiologies are most common (Fig. 10-261).

The degree of spondylolisthesis may progress over time. The majority of progression is thought to occur during early adolescence. Predisposing factors for progression include rounded sacrum promontory,[240] trapezoidal configuration of the displaced vertebra,[240] narrowed disc space,[214] increased sacral angle, and advanced degree of displacement. However, others feel that these are the result of slippage and not the cause of it,[198] and that no radiographic findings exist that can accurately predict future displacement.[83]

For adults, the rate of progression has been reported at 2% per year in one cohort study that followed patients over 7 years.[79] Another cohort study failed to show any progression over a

demonstrates a same-level enlarged spinal canal in the axial plane in patients with spondylolytic spondylolisthesis (Fig. 10-260).[251]

CLINICAL COMMENTS

Spondylolytic spondylolisthesis usually is discovered during the period from childhood to early adulthood. Physical examination may reveal joint crepitus and palpatory "step defect" at the level

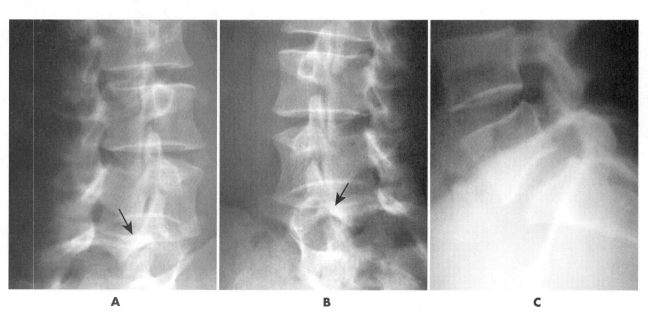

FIG. 10-262   Impending stress fractures. **A** and **B,** The oblique lumbar projections exhibit a radiodense focus in the middle region of each pars interarticularis *(arrows).* The appearance correlates to impending stress fractures. **C,** The lateral projection details a Grade I spondylolisthesis.

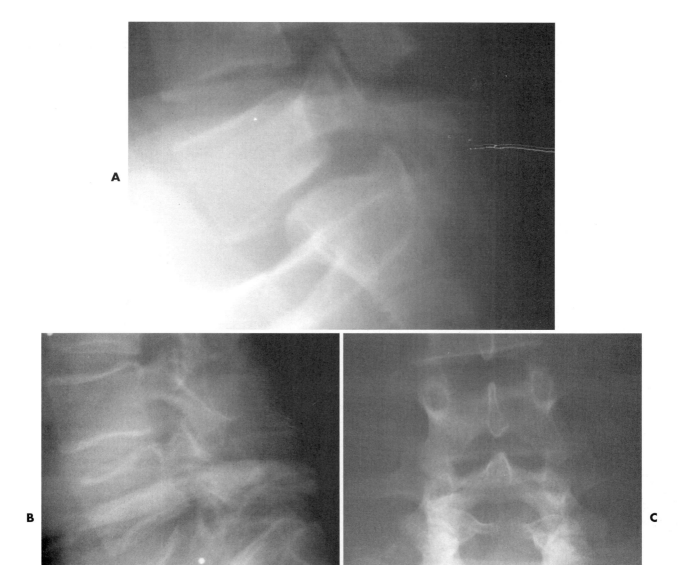

FIG. 10-263 **A,** Late Grade II spondylolisthesis is noted at L5. **B,** Forty years later, the spondylolisthesis has progressed to nearly a spondyloptosis. The patient also suffered a gunshot (notice the pellets) during this time. **C,** The anteroposterior projection correlating to **B** exhibits a Napoleon hat sign *(arrowheads)*. The progression of a spondylolisthesis is difficult to predict (see text).

45-year period when the patients demonstrated unilateral pars defects.[19] When progression does occur, usually it is related to disc and facet joint degeneration, and not necessarily an increase in symptoms.[19] Advanced grades of spondylolisthesis necessitate spondylolysis (Figs. 10-262 and 10-263). It is rare for spondylolisthesis with degenerative etiology to progress beyond a Grade I category.

In general, patients who demonstrate a spondylolisthesis beyond the age of 10 years may continue athletics without fear of further displacement.[82,220,268] In patients under the age of 10 years it is best advised to curtail activity until serial flexion and extension lateral lumbar radiographs rule out instability.[268] However, all patients who demonstrate persistent symptoms, an active pars interarticularis defect as noted by a positive SPECT bone scan, and instability as defined by excessive translation ($\geq$4.5) on flexion-extension or compression-traction[123] lateral radiographs may warrant further clinical evaluation.[268]

KEY CONCEPTS

- *Spondylolisthesis is an anterior displacement of a vertebra in relation to the segment immediately below.*
- *Spondylolysis denotes unilateral or bilateral disruption of the pars interarticularis.*
- *Spondylolisthesis are classified by etiology (type I, congenital; type II, pars interarticularis defect; type III, degenerative; type IV, traumatic; type V, pathologic; type VI, surgical) and degree of anterior displacement (Grade I, 0% to 25%; Grade II, 26% to 50%; Grade III, 51% to 75%; Grade IV, 76% to 100%).*
- *Spondylolisthesis usually results from a stress fracture of the pars interarticularis when presenting in younger individuals and degeneration of the facet and intervertebral disc when presenting in older individuals.*
- *Disruption of the posterior body (George's) line on the lateral projection is the best method of assessment.*
- *There does not appear to be a correlation between the presence or degree of anterior displacement and back pain.*

References

1. Ackerman LV: Extra-osseous localized non-neoplastic bone and cartilage formation (so-called myositis ossificans), *J Bone Joint Surg (Am)* 40:279, 1958.
2. Aichroth PM: Osteochondritis dissecans of the knee. A clinical survey, *J Bone Joint Surg* 53B:440, 1971.
3. Alffram P, Bauer GCH: Epidemiology of fractures of the forearm, *J Bone Joint Surg (Am)* 44:105, 1962.
4. Aloia JF, Flaster ER: Estimating the risk of fracture in osteopenic patients, *Endocrinologist* 5:397, 1995.
5. Asher MA: Dislocations of the upper extremity in children, *Orthop Clin North Am* 7:583, 1976.
6. Atlas SW et al: The radiographic characterization of burst fractures of the spine, *AJR Am J Roentgenol* 147:575, 1986.
7. Bado JL: The Monteggia lesion, *Clin Orthop* 50:71, 1967.
8. Barnes R et al: Subcapital fractures of the femur, *J Bone Joint Surg (Br)* 58:2, 1976.
9. Barnsley L, Lord S, Bogduk N: Whiplash injury: clinical review, *Pain* 58:283, 1994.
10. Bayliss AP, Davidson JK: Traumatic osteonecrosis of the femoral head following intracapsular fracture: incidence and earliest radiological features, *Clin Radiol* 28:407, 1977.
11. Bellah RD et al: Low back pain in adolescent athletes: detection of stress injury to the pars interarticularis with SPECT, *Radiology* 180:509, 1991.
12. Bennell KL, Brukner PD: Epidemiology and site specificity of stress fractures, *Clin Sports Med* 16(2):179, 1997.
13. Bennell KL et al: The incidence and distribution of stress fractures in competitive track and field athletes: a twelve-month prospective study, *Am J Sports Med* 24(2):211, 1996.
14. Bennett EH: On fracture of the metacarpal bone of the thumb, *Clin Orthop* 220:3, 1987.
15. Bentley G: Treatment of nondisplaced fractures of the femoral neck, *Clin Orthop* 152:93, 1989.
16. Berndt AL, Harty M: Transchondral fracture (osteochondritis dissecans) of the talus, *J Bone Joint Surg (Am)* 41(A):988, 1959.
17. Bernstein L, McClurg FL: Mandibular fractures: a review of 156 consecutive cases, *Laryngoscope* 87:957, 1976.
18. Berquist TH: Imaging of orthopedic trauma and surgery, Philadelphia, 1986, WB Saunders.
19. Beutler WJ et al: The natural history of spondylolysis and spondylolisthesis: 45-year follow-up evaluation, *Spine* 28(10):1027; discussion 1035, 2003.
20. Bledsoe RC, Izenstark JL: Displacement of fat pads in disease and injury of the elbow. A new radiographic sign, *Radiology* 73:717, 1959.
21. Boden SD et al: Abnormal magnetic-resonance scans of the cervical spine in asymptomatic subjects. A prospective investigation, *J Bone Joint Surg* 72A:1178, 1990.
22. Bogduk N: Summary of the WAD Congress. International Congress on Whiplash Associated Disorders, Berne, Switzerland, 2001.
23. Bolesta MJ, Bohlman HH: Degenerative spondylolisthesis (review), *Instr Course Lect* 38:157, 1989.
24. Brenkel IJ et al: Hormone status in patients with slipped capital femoral epiphysis, *J Bone Joint Surg (Br)* 71:33, 1989.
25. Brenkel IJ et al: Thyroid hormone levels in patients with slipped capital femoral epiphysis, *J Pediatr Orthop* 8(1):22, 1988.
26. Bridges AJ et al: Fibrodysplasia (myositis) ossificans progressiva (review), *Semin Arthritis Rheum* 24(3):155, 1994.
27. Brogdon BG, Crow NE: Little leaguer's elbow, *AJR Am J Roentgenol* 83:671, 1960.
28. Bruce HE, Harvey JP Jr, Wilson JC Jr: Monteggia fractures, *J Bone Joint Surg (Am)* 56:1563, 1974.
29. Buckingham WW: Subtalar dislocation of the foot, *J Trauma* 13:753, 1973.
30. Campbell CS: Gamekeeper's thumb, *J Bone Joint Surg (Br)* 37:148, 1955.
31. Carlson WO, Klassen RA: Myositis ossificans of the upper extremity: a long-term follow-up, *J Pediatr Orthop* 4(6):693, 1984.
32. Carter PR, Eaton RG, Littler JW: Un-united fracture of the hook of the hamate, *J Bone Joint Surg (Am)* 59:583, 1977.
33. Cautilli RA et al: Classifications of fractures of the distal radius, *Clin Orthop* 103:163, 1974.
34. Chance GQ: Note on a flexion fracture of the spine, *Br J Radiol* 21:452, 1948.
35. Cheng MS, Ferkel RD, Applegate GR: Osteochondral lesion of the talus: A radiologic and surgical comparison. Paper presented at the annual meeting of the Academy of Orthopaedic Surgeons, New Orleans, February 1995.
36. Chessare JW et al: Injuries of the medial epicondylar ossification center of the humerus, *AJR Am J Roentgenol* 129:49, 1977.
37. Cisternino SJ et al: The trough line: a radiographic sign of posterior shoulder dislocation, *AJR Am J Roentgenol* 130:951, 1978.
38. Clanton TO, DeLee JC. Osteochondritis dissecans: history, pathophysiology and current treatment concepts, *Clin Orthop* 167:50, 1982.
39. Cohn I: Observations of the normally developing elbow, *Arch Surg* 2:455, 1921.
40. Comstock CP, Carraggee EJ, O'Sullivan GS: Spondylolisthesis in the young athlete, *Phys Sports Med* 22:39, 1994.

41. Conolly WB, Hedberg EA: Observations of fractures of the pelvis, *J Trauma* 9:104, 1969.

42. Cooperman DR et al: Post-mortem description of slipped capital femoral epiphysis, *J Bone Joint Surg (Br)* 74:595, 1992.

43. Côté P et al: A systematic review of the prognosis of acute whiplash and a new conceptual framework to synthesize the literature, *Spine* 26:E445, 2001.

44. Cotton FJ: A new type of ankle fracture, *JAMA* 64:318, 1915.

45. Crawley DB, Reckling FW: Supracondylar fracture of the humerus in children, *Am Fam Phys* 5:113, 1972.

46. Cremin B, Connor JM, Beighton P: The radiological spectrum of fibrodysplasia ossificans progressiva, *Clin Radiol* 33(5):499, 1982.

47. Crotty JM, Monu JU, Pope TL: Magnetic resonance imaging of the musculoskeletal system, *Clin Orthop Rel Res* 330:288, 1996.

48. Crowe H: Injuries to the cervical spine, Presented at the annual meeting of the Western Orthopaedic Association, San Francisco, 1928.

49. Cummings SR, Melton III LJ: Epidemiology and outcomes of osteoporotic fractures, *Lancet* 359(9319):1761, 2002.

50. Curtis RJ Jr, Corley FG Jr: Fractures and dislocations of the forearm, *Clin Sports Med* 5:663, 1986.

51. Dai L: Disc degeneration and cervical instability. Correlation of magnetic resonance imaging with radiography, *Spine* 23(16):1734, 1998.

52. Danchik JJ, Yochum TR, Aspegren DD: Myositis ossificans traumatica, *J Man Physiol Ther* 16(9):605, 1993.

53. Danielson BI, Frennered AK, lrstam LK: Radiologic progression of isthmic lumbar spondylolisthesis in young patients, *Spine* 16(4):422, 1991.

54. Danis R: Les fractures malleolaires. In Danis R, editor: Theorie et practique de l'osteosynthese, Paris, 1949, Masson et Cie.

55. DeBehnke DJ, Havel CJ: Utility of prevertebral soft tissue measurements in identifying patients with cervical spine fractures, *Ann Emerg Med* 24:1119, 1994.

56. Dellinger EP et al: Risk of infection after open fracture of the arm or leg, *Arch Surg* 123:1320, 1988.

57. Denis F: Spinal instability as defined by the three column spine concept in acute trauma, *Clin Orthop* 189:65, 1984.

58. Denis F: The three column spine and its significance in the classification of acute thoracolumbar spinal injuries, *Spine* 8(8):817, 1983.

59. Dent JA, Paterson CR: Fractures in early childhood: osteogenesis imperfecta or child abuse? *J Pediatr Orthop* 11:184, 1991.

60. Dias LS, Giegerich CR: Fractures of the distal tibial epiphysis in adolescence, *J Bone Joint Surg (Am)* 65:438, 1983.

61. Dipaola JD, Nelson DW, Colville MR: Characterizing osteochondral lesions by magnetic resonance imaging, *Arthroscopy* 7:101, 1991.

62. Dolan D, Jacoby C, Smoker W: The radiology of facial fractures, *Radiography* 4:577, 1984.

63. Dolan KD, Jacoby CG: Facial fractures, *Semin Roentgenol* 13:37, 1978.

64. Drake DG, Griffiths HJ: Radiologic case study. Slipped epiphysis associated with renal osteodystrophy, *Orthopedics* 12(11):1489, 1989.

65. Du Toit FP, Grabe RP: Isolated fractures of the shaft of the ulna, *S Afr Med J* 56:21, 1979.

66. Duchesneau S, Fallat LM: The Tillaux fracture, *J Foot Ankle Surg* 35:127, 1996.

67. Dunn AW, Morris HD: Fractures and dislocations of the pelvis, *J Bone Joint Surg (Am)* 50:1639, 1968.

68. Dunn AW: Fractures and dislocations of the carpus, *Surg Clin North Am* 52:1513, 1972.

69. Dupuytren G: Of fractures of the lower extremity of the fibula, and luxations of the foot, *Med Classics* 4:151, 1939.

70. Edwards GS Jr, Jupiter JB: Radial head fractures with acute distal radioulnar dislocation, Essex-Lopresti revisited, *Clin Orthop* 234:61, 1988.

71. Eismont FJ et al: Cervical sagittal spinal canal size in spine injury, *Spine* 9(7):663, 1984.

72. El-Khoury GY, Kathol MH, Daniel WW: Imaging of acute injuries of the cervical spine: value of plain radiography, CT, and MR imaging, *AJR Am J Roentgenol* 164:43, 1995.

73. Epstein HC: Traumatic dislocations of the hip, *Clin Orthop* 92:116, 1973.

74. Essex-Lopresti P: Fractures of the radial head with distal radioulnar dislocation, *J Bone Joint Surg (Br)* 33:244, 1951.

75. Fahey JJ: Fractures of the elbow in children, *Instr Course Lect* 17:13, 1960.

76. Ferkel RD, Sgaglione NA: Arthroscopic treatment of osteochondral lesions of the talus: long-term results, *Orthop Trans* 17:1011, 1993.

77. Fischer SP et al: Accuracy of diagnoses from magnetic resonance imaging of the knee, *J Bone Joint Surg* 73A:2, 1991.

78. Fisk GR: The wrist, *J Bone Joint Surg (Br)* 66:396, 1984.

79. Floman Y: Progression of lumbosacral isthmic spondylolisthesis in adults, *Spine* 25:342, 2000.

80. Follow-up study, *J Pediatr Orthop* 11(2):209, 1991.

81. Foster SC, Foster RR: Lisfranc's tarsometatarsal fracture-dislocation, *Radiology* 120:79, 1976.

82. Fredrickson BE et al: The natural history of spondylolysis and spondylolisthesis, *J Bone Joint Surg (Am)* 66:669, 1984.

83. Frennered AK, Danielson BI, Nachemson AL: Natural history of symptomatic isthmic low-grade spondylolisthesis in children and adolescents: a seven-year follow-up study. *J Pediatr Orthop* 11:209, 1991.

84. Jefferson G: Fracture of the atlas vertebra: report of four cases, and a review of those previously recorded, *Br J Surg (London)* 7:407, 1920.

85. Garcia C, Zaninovic A: Battered child syndrome, X-ray findings, *Revista Chilena de Pediatria* 62(4):273, 1991.

86. Garden RS: Reduction and fixation of subcapital fractures of the femur, *Orthop Clin North Am* 5:683, 1974.

87. Garth WP, Hofammann DY, Rooks MD: Volar intercalated segment instability secondary to medial carpal ligamental laxity, *Clin Orthop* 201:94, 1985.

88. Gehweiler JA, Osborne RL, Becker RF: The radiology of vertebral trauma, Philadelphia, 1980, WB Saunders.

89. Gelberman RH et al: The association of femoral retroversion with slipped capital femoral epiphysis, *J Bone Joint Surg (Am)* 68:1000, 1968.

90. Giles JB et al: Supracondylar-intercondylar fractures of the femur treated with a supracondylar plate and lag screw, *J Bone Joint Surg (Am)* 64:864, 1982.

91. Gilula LA, Weeks PM: Post-traumatic ligamentous instabilities of the wrist, *Radiology* 129(3):641, 1978.

92. Gilula LA, Weeks PM: Wrist arthrography. The value of fluoroscopic spot viewing, *Radiology* 146(2):555, 1983.

93. Gilula LA: Carpal injuries: analytic approach and case exercises, *AJR Am J Roentgenol* 133:503, 1979.

94. Goss TP: Scapular fractures and dislocations: diagnosis and treatment, *J Am Acad Orthop Surg* 3(1):22, 1995.

95. Gourlay M, Richy F, Reginster J-Y: Strategies for the prevention of hip fracture, *Am J Med* 115:309, 2003.

96. Grauer JN: Whiplash produces an S-shaped curvature of the neck with hyperextension at lower levels, *Spine* 22:2489, 1997.

97. Green DP, Terry GC: Complex dislocation of the metacarpophalangeal joint, *J Bone Joint Surg (Am)* 55:1480, 1972.

98. Griffiths HJ et al: Hyperextension strain of "whiplash" injuries to the cervical spine, *Skeletal Radiol* 1995:24, 263.

99. Gross RM: Acute dislocation of the patella: the Mudville mystery, *J Bone Joint Surg (Am)* 68:780, 1986.

100. Grossart KWM, Samuel E: Traumatic diastasis of cranial sutures, *Clin Radiol* 12:164, 1961.

101. Hägglund G et al: Growth of children with physiolysis of the hip, *Acta Orthop Scand* 58:117, 1987.

102. Hall SE et al: Hip fracture outcomes: quality of life and functional status in older adults living in the community. *Aust NZ J Med* 30(3):327, 2000.

103. Harris JH, Edeiken-Monroe B: The radiology of acute cervical spine trauma, ed 2, Baltimore, 1987, Williams & Wilkins.

104. Harris RD, Harris JH: The prevalence and significance of missed scapular fractures in blunt chest trauma, *AJR Am J Roentgenol* 151:747, 1988.

105. Hausdorff JM, Rios DA, Edelber HK: Gait variability and fall risk in community-living older adults: a 1-year prospective study, *Arch Phys Med Rehabil* 82(8):1050, 2001.

106. Henrikson B: The incidence of slipped capital femoral epiphysis, *Acta Orthop Scand* 40:365, 1969.

107. Hoffman JR: Validity of a set of clinical criteria to rule out injury to the cervical spine in patients with blunt trauma, *N Engl J Med* 343:94, 2003.

108. Hofmann AA, Dahl CP, Wyatt RWB: Experience with acetabular fractures, *J Trauma* 24:750, 1984.

109. Hohl M, Luck JV: Fractures of the tibial condyle. A clinical and experimental study, *J Bone Joint Surg (Am)* 38:1001, 1956.

110. Hornbrook MC et al: Preventing falls among community-dwelling older persons: results from a randomized trial, *Gerontologist* 34(1):16, 1994.

111. Horne JG, Tanzer TL: Olecranon fractures: a review of 100 cases, *J Trauma* 21:469, 1981.

112. Howorth B: History of slipping of the capital femoral epiphysis, *Clin Orthop* 48:11, 1966.

113. Hughston JC, Hergenroeder PT, Courtenay BG: Osteochondritis dissecans of the femoral condyles, *J Bone Joint Surg (Am)* 66:1340, 1984.

114. Hughston JC: Fracture of the distal radial shaft, *J Bone Joint Surg (Am)* 39:249, 1957.

115. Huittinen VM, Slatis P: Fractures of the pelvis. Trauma mechanism, types of injury and principles of treatment, *Acta Chir Scand* 138:563, 1972.

116. Ideberg R: Unusual glenoid fractures: a report on 92 cases, *Acta Orthop Scand* 58:191, 1987.

117. Ingram AJ et al: Chondrolysis complicating slipped capital femoral epiphysis, *Clin Orthop* 165:99, 1982.

118. Iversen BJ, Aalberg, JR, Naver LS: Complications of fractures of the femoral neck, *Ann Chir Gynaecol* 75:341, 1986.

119. Jaudes PK: Comparison of radiography and radionuclide bone scanning in the detection of child abuse, *Pediatrics* 73:166, 1984.

120. Johnson RJ: Low back pain in sports, *Phys Sports Med* 21:53, 1993.

121. Jones HK, McBride GG, Mumhy RC: Sternal fractures associated with spinal injury, *J Trauma* 29:360, 1989.

122. Juhl JH, Crummy AB: Paul and Juhl's essentials of radiologic imaging, ed 6, Philadephia, 1993, JB Lippincott.

123. Kalebo P et al: Stress views in the comparative assessment of spondylolytic spondylolisthesis, *Skeletal Radiol* 17(8):570, 1989.

124. Kang JD, Figgie MP, Bohlman HH: Sagittal measurements of the cervical spine in subaxial fractures and dislocations. An analysis of two hundred and eighty-eight patients with and without neurological deficits, *J Bone Joint Surg (Am)* 76(11):1617, 1994.

125. Kelsey JL, Acheson RM, Keggi KJ: The body build of patients with slipped capital epiphysis, *Am J Dis Child* 124:276, 1972.

126. Kelsey JL, Keggi KJ, Southwick WO: The incidence and distribution of slipped capital femoral epiphysis in Connecticut and Southwestern United States, *J Bone Joint Surg (Am)* 52:1203, 1970.

127. Kelsey JL: Epidemiology of slipped capital femoral epiphysis: a review of the literature, *Pediatrics* 51:1042, 1973.

128. Kennedy JC: Complete dislocation of the knee joint, *J Bone Joint Surg (Am)* 45:889, 1963.

129. Kesterson L et al: Evaluation and treatment of atlas burst fractures (Jefferson fractures), *J Neurosurg* 75:231, 1991.

130. Kilcoyne RF et al: Thoracolumbar spine injuries associated with vertical plunges: reappraisal with computed tomography, *Radiology* 146:137, 1982.

131. Kirshenbaum KJ et al: Unsuspected upper cervical spine fractures associated with significant head trauma: role of CT, *J Emerg Med* 8:183, 1990.

132. Kleinman PK, Marks SC, Blackbourne B: The metaphyseal lesion in abused infants: a radiologic histopathologic study, *AJR Am J Roentgenol* 146:895, 1986.

133. Kleinman PK: Diagnostic imaging in infant abuse, *AJR Am J Roentgenol* 155:703, 1990.

134. Knight RA: Fractures of the humeral condyles in adults, *South Med J* 48:1165, 1955.

135. Kohn AM: Soft tissue alterations in elbow trauma, *AJR Am J Roentgenol* 82:867, 1959.

136. Kono S, Hayashi M, Kashahara T: A study on the etiology of spondylolysis with reference to athletic activities (Japanese), *J Jpn Orthop Assoc* 49:125, 1975.

137. Kransdorf MJ, Meis JM, Jelinek JS: Myositis ossificans: MR appearance with radiologic-pathologic correlation, *AJR Am J Roentgenol* 157:1243, 1991.

138. Kristensen S, Tveteras K: Zygomatic fractures: classification and complications, *Clin Otolaryngol* 11:123, 1986.

139. Larsen CB: Fracture dislocations of the hip, *Clin Orthop* 92:147, 1973.

140. Lauge-Hansen N: Fractures of the ankle: combined experimental-surgical and experimental-roentgenologic investigations, *Arch Surg* 60(5):957, 1950.

141. Lauge-Hansen N: Fractures of the ankle: III. Genetic roentgenologic diagnosis of fractures of the ankle, *AJR Am J Roentgenol* 71:456, 1954.

142. Lauge-Hansen N: Fractures of the ankle: IV. Clinical use of the generic roentgen diagnosis and genetic reduction, *AMA Arch Surg* 64:488, 1952.

143. Lauge-Hansen N: Fractures of the ankle: V. Pronation-dorsiflexion fracture, *AMA Arch Surg* 67:813, 1963.

144. Letournel E: Acetabulum fractures: classification and management, *Clin Orthop* 151:81, 1980.

145. Levine AM, Edwards C: The management of traumatic spondylolisthesis of the axis, *J Bone Joint Surg (Am)* 67:217, 1985.

146. Linscheid RL et al: Traumatic instability of the wrist, diagnosis, classification and pathomechanics, *J Bone Joint Surg* 54-A:1612, 1972.

147. Loder RT, Bookout C: Fracture patterns in battered children, *J Orthop Trauma* 5(4):428, 1991.

148. Lotke PA, Ecker ML: Transverse fractures of the patella, *Clin Orthop* 158:180, 1981.

149. Lowy M: Avulsion fractures of the calcaneus, *J Bone Joint Surg (Br)* 51:494, 1969.

150. Mace SE. Emergency evaluation of cervical spine injuries: CT versus plain radiographs, *Ann Emerg Med* 14:973, 1985.

151. Maisonneuve JG: Recherches sur la fracture du perone, *Arch Gen Med* 7:165, 1840.

152. Mast JW, Spiegel PG, Pappas JN: Fractures of the tibial pilon, *Clin Orthop* 230:68, 1988.

153. Matheson GO et al: Stress fractures in athletes: a study of 320 cases, *Am J Sports Med* 15(1):46, 1987.

154. McCutchan JDS, Gillham NR: Injury to the popliteal artery associated with dislocation of the knee: palpable distal pulses do not negate the requirement for arteriography, *Br J Accident Surg* 20:307, 1989.

155. McDaniel WJ, Wilson FC: Trimalleolar fractures of the ankle. An end result study, *Clin Orthop*, 122:37, 1977.

156. McMinn DJW: Mallet finger and fractures, *Injury* 12:477, 1981.

157. McTimoney CA, Micheli LJ: Current evaluation and management of spondylolysis and spondylolisthesis (review), *Curr Sports Med Rep* 2(1):41, 2003.

158. Melmed EP, Koonin AJ: Fractures of the mandible: a review of 909 cases, *Plast Reconstr Surg* 56:323, 1975.

159. Melton LJ et al: Epidemiologic features of pelvic fractures, *Clin Orthop* 155:43, 1981.

160. Melton LJ: Hip fractures: a worldwide problem today and tomorrow, *Bone* 14:1, 1993.

161. Merchan EC et al: Circumscribed myositis ossificans. Report of nine cases without history of Injury, *Acta Orthop Belg* 59(3):273, 1993.

162. Meyerding HW: Low backache and sciatic pain associated with spondylolisthesis and protruded intervertebral disc, *J Bone Joint Surg (Am)* 23:461, 1941.

163. Micheli LJ, Hall JE, Miller ME: Use of modified Boston brace for back injuries in athletes, *Am J Sports Med* 8:5, 1980.

164. Mickelson MR et al: Aseptic necrosis following slipped femoral epiphysis, *Skeletal Radiol* 4:129, 1979.

165. Mikic ZDJ: Galeazzi fracture-dislocations, *J Bone Joint Surg (Am)* 57:1071, 1975.

166. Miller WE: Comminuted fractures of the distal end of the humerus in the adult, *J Bone Joint Surg (Am)* 46:644, 1964.

167. Mirvis SE et al: Hangman's fracture: radiologic assessment in 27 cases, *Radiology* 163:713, 1987.

168. Moed BR, Morawa LG: Displaced midline longitudinal fracture of the sacrum, *J Trauma* 24:435, 1984.

169. Möller H, Sundin A, Hedlund R: Symptoms, signs, and functional disability in adult spondylolisthesis, *Spine* 25:683, 2000.

170. Moreau MJ: Remodeling in slipped capital femoral epiphysis, *Can J Surg* 30(6):440, 1987.

171. Motley G et al: The pars interarticularis, stress reaction, spondylolysis, and spondylolisthesis progression, *J Ath Train* 33:351, 1998.

172. Murphy SL: Deaths: final data for 1998. National Vital Statistics Reports, Hyattsville, MD, 2000, National Center for Health Statistics.

173. Muschik M et al: Competitive sports and the progression of spondylolisthesis, *J Pediatr Orthop* 16(3):364, 1996.

174. Nambu T et al: Deformation of the distal femur: a contribution towards the pathogenesis of osteochondrosis dissecans in the knee joint, *J Biomechan* 24(6):421, 1991.

175. Nathan H: Spondylolysis, *J Bone Joint Surg (Am)* 41:303, 1959.

176. Navid DO, Myerson MS: Approach alternatives for treatment of osteochondral lesions of the talus (review), *Foot Ankle Clin* 7(3):635, 2002.

177. Neer CS, Shelton ML: Supracondylar fractures of the adult femur. A study of one hundred and ten cases, *J Bone Joint Surg (Am)* 49:591, 1967.

178. Newman JH: Supracondylar fractures of the femur, *Injury* 21:280, 1990.

179. Newman PH, Stone KH: The etiology of spondylolisthesis, *J Bone Joint Surg (Br)* 45:39, 1963.

180. Norman A, Nelson, Green S: Fracture of the hook of the hamate: radiographic signs, *Radiology* 154:49, 1985.

181. Obedian RS, Grelsamer RP: Osteochondritis dissecans of the distal femur and patella, *Clin Sports Med* 16:157, 1997.

182. Ogden JA: Dislocation of the proximal fibula, *Radiology* 105:547, 1972.

183. Ogden JA: Injury to the growth mechanisms of the immature skeleton, *Skeletal Radiol* 6:237, 1981.

184. Ogilvie-Harris DJ, Hons CB, Fornaiser VL: Pseudomalignant myositis ossificans: heterotropic new-bone formation without a history of trauma, *J Bone Joint Surg (Am)* 62:1274, 1980.

185. Panjabi M et al: Cervical spine curvature during simulated whiplash, *Clin Biomechan* 19:1, 2004.

186. Pankovich AM: Maisonneuve fracture of the fibula, *J Bone Joint Surg (Am)* 58:337, 1977.

187. Papanicolaou N et al: Bone scintigraphy and radiography in young athletes with low back pain, *AJR Am J Roentgenol* 145:1039, 1985.

188. Pellegrini VD Jr: Fractures at the base of thumb, *Hand Clin* 4:87, 1988.

189. Pettersson K et al: Disc pathology after whiplash injury. A prospective magnetic resonance imaging and clinical investigation, *Spine* 22:283, 1997.

190. Pierce GE, Maxwell JA, Boggan MD: Special hazards of first rib fractures, *Trauma* 15:264, 1975.

191. Pott P: Some few general remarks on fractures and dislocations, London, 1768, Hawes, Clarke, Collins.

192. Pritchett JW, Perdue KD: Mechanical factors in slipped capital femoral epiphysis, *J Pediatr Orthop* 8(4):385, 1988.

193. Protzman RR: Dislocation of the elbow joint, *J Bone Joint Surg (Am)* 60:539, 1978.

194. Radkowski MA, Merten DF, Leonidas JC: The abused child: criteria for the radiologic diagnosis, *Radiographics* 3:262, 1983.

195. Ravichandran G: A radiological sign in spondylolisthesis, *AJR Am J Roentgenol* 134:113, 1980.

196. Reckling FW, Peltier LF: Riccardo Galeazz and Galeazzi's fracture, *Surgery* 58:453, 1965.

197. Reckling JW, Peltier LF: Acute knee dislocations and their complications, *J Trauma* 9:181, 1969.

198. Resnick D: Diagnosis of bone and joint disorders, ed 3, vol 5, Philadelphia, 1995, WB Saunders.

199. Richardson JD, McElvein RB, Trinkle JK: First rib fracture: a hallmark of severe trauma, *Ann Surg* 181:251, 1975.

200. Ring D, Jupiter JB, Waters PM: Monteggia fractures in children and adults, *J Am Acad Orthop Surg* 6:215, 1998.

201. Robinson AE, Meares BM, Goree JA: Traumatic sphenoid sinus effusion: an analysis of 50 cases, *AJR Am J Roentgenol* 101:795, 1967.

202. Roche MB, Rowe GG: The incidence of separate neural arch and coincidental bone variations, *Anat Rec* 109:233, 1951.

203. Rockwood C, Green D: Fractures, Philadelphia, 1975, JB Lippincott.

204. Rogers LF: Radiology of skeletal trauma, ed 2, New York, 1992, Churchill Livingstone.

205. Rogers LF: The radiography of epiphyseal injuries, *Radiology* 96:289, 1970.

206. Rorabeck CH, Bobechko WP: Acute dislocation of the patella with osteochondral fracture. A review of 18 cases, *J Bone Joint Surg (Br)* 58:237, 1976.

207. Rossi F: Spondylolysis, spondylolisthesis and sports, *Sports Med* 18:317, 1978.

208. Ruwe PA et al: Can MR imaging effectively replace diagnostic arthroscopy? *Radiology* 183:335, 1992.

209. Sallis RE, Jones K: Stress fractures in athletes: how to spot this underdiagnosed injury, *Postgrad Med* 89(6):185, 1991.

210. Salter RB, Zaltz C: Anatomic investigations of the mechanism of injury and pathologic anatomy of "pulled elbow" in young children, *Clin Orthop* 77:134, 1971.

211. Salter RB, Harris WR: Injuries involving the epiphyseal plate, *J Bone Joint Surg (Am)* 45:587, 1963.

212. Samaha C et al: Hangman's fracture: the relationship between asymmetry and instability, *J Bone Joint Surg (Br)* 82:1046, 2000.

213. Samelson EJ et al: Effect of birth cohort on risk of hip fracture: age-specific incidence rates in the Framingham study, *Am J Pub Health* 92(5):858, 2002.

214. Saraste H: Long-term clinical and radiological follow-up of spondylolysis and spondylolisthesis, *J Pediatr Orthop* 7(6):631, 1987.

215. Sarmiento A, Laird CA: Posterior fracture-dislocation of the femoral head, *Clin Orthop* 92:143, 1973.

216. Schafer RC: Basic chiropractic procedural manual, ed 4, Arlington, VA, 1984, American Chiropractic Association.

217. Schneiderman GA et al: The pars defect as a pain source. A histologic study, *Spine* 20(16):1761, 1995.

218. Schultz RC, Oldham RJ: An overview of facial injuries, *Surg Clin North Am* 57:987, 1977.

219. Scott JC: Osteoporosis and hip fractures, *Rheum Dis Clin North Am* 16(3):717, 1990.

220. Semon RL, Spengler D: Significance of lumbar spondylolisthesis in college football players, *Spine* 6:1972, 1981.

221. Shearman CM: Pitfalls in the radiologic evaluation of extremity trauma: part II. The lower extremity, *Am Fam Phys* 57:1314, 1998.

222. Shelton ML, Neer CS, Grantham SA: Occult knee ligament ruptures associated with fractures, *J Trauma* 11:853, 1971.

223. Sherk HH, Nicholson JT: Fractures of the atlas, *J Bone Joint Surg (Am)* 52:1017, 1970.

224. Siegel S, White LM, Brahma S: Magnetic resonance imaging of the musculoskeletal system, Part 5. The wrist, *Clin Orthop Rel Res* 332:281, 1996.

225. Siffert RS: The effect of trauma to the epiphysis and growth plate, *Skeletal Radiol* 2:21, 1977.

226. Sorensen KH: Slipped upper femoral epiphysis, clinical study on aetiology, *Acta Orthop Scand* 39:499, 1968.

227. Spitzer WO et al: Scientific monograph of the Quebec Task Force on Whiplash-Associated Disorders: redefining "whiplash" and its management, *Spine* 20(suppl 8);1S, 1995.

228. Spivack B: SCIWORA in childhood. Spinal cord injury without radiographic abnormality, *J Trauma* 53(6):1198, 2002.

229. Stark HH et al: Fracture of the hook of the hamate in athletes, *J Bone Joint Surg (Am)* 59:575, 1977.

230. Stevens DB: Postoperative orthopaedic infections, *J Bone Joint Surg (Am)* 46:96, 1964.

231. Stevens JA, Olson S: Reducing falls and resulting hip fractures among older women. In CDC Recommendations about Selected Conditions Affecting Women's Health, *MMWR* 49(RR-2):3, 2000.

232. Stevens JA, Olson S: Reducing falls and resulting hip fractures among older women. In CDC Recommendations about Selected Conditions Affecting Women's Health, *MMWR* 49(RR-2):3, 2000.

233. Stewart TD: The age incidence of neural-arch defects in Alaskan natives, considered from the standpoint of etiology, *J Bone Joint Surg (Am)* 35:937, 1953.

234. Store G: Traumatic dislocation of the radial head as an isolated lesion in children. Report of one case with special regard to roentgen diagnosis, *Acta Chir Scand* 116:144, 1958.

235. Stovner LJ: The nosologic status of the whiplash syndrome: a critical review based on a methodological approach, *Spine* 21:2735, 1996.

236. Sturm JT, Perry JF Jr: Injuries associated with fractures of the transverse processes of the thoracic and lumbar vertebrae, *J Trauma* 24:597, 1984.

237. Sty JR, Starshak RJ: The role of bone scintigraphy in the evaluation of the suspected abused child, *Radiology* 146:369, 1983.

238. Swiontkowski MF: Slipped capital femoral epiphysis, complications relative to internal fixation, *Orthopaedics* 6:705, 1983.

239. Szpalski M, Gunzburg R: Lumbar spinal stenosis in the elderly: an overview, *Eur Spine J* 12:S170, 2003.

240. Taillard WF: Etiology of spondylolisthesis, *Clin Orthop* 117:30, 1976.

241. Taveras JM, Wood EH: Diagnostic neuroradiology, ed 2, Baltimore, 1976, Williams & Wilkins.

242. Terry DW, Ramin JE: The navicular fat stripe. A useful roentgen fracture for evaluating wrist trauma, *AJR Am J Roentgenol* 124:25, 1975.

243. Thaggard A, Harle TS, Carlson V: Fractures and dislocations of bony pelvis and hip, *Semin Roentgenol* 13:117, 1978.

244. Tillaux P: Traite de chirurgie clinique, vol 2 Paris, 1848, Asselin et Houseau.

245. Torisu T: Fracture of the hook of the hamate by a golf swing, *Clin Orthop* 83:91, 1972.

246. Trafton PG: Spinal cord injuries, *Surg Clin North Am* 62:61, 1982.

247. Trapnell DH: The "magnification sign" of the triple mandibular fracture, *Br J Radiol* 50:97, 1977.

248. Tsuno MM, Shu GJ: Myositis ossificans (review), *J Man Physiol Ther* 13(6):340, 1990.

249. Turner RH, Bianco AJ: Spondylolysis and spondylolisthesis in children and teenagers, *J Bone Joint Surg (Am)* 53:1298, 1971.

250. Twyman RS, Desai K, Aichroth PM: Osteochondritis dissecans of the knee. A long-term study, *J Bone Joint Surg* 73B:461, 1991.

251. Ulmer JL et al: Distinction between degenerative and isthmic spondylolisthesis on sagittal MR images: importance of increased anteroposterior diameter of the spinal canal ("wide canal sign"), *AJR Am J Roentgenol* 163(2):411, 1994.

252. Virta L, Rönnemaa T: The association of mild-moderate isthmic lumbar spondylolisthesis and low back pain in middle-aged patients is weak and it occurs only in women, *Spine* 18:1496, 1993.

253. Vlarkisz JA et al: Segmental patterns of avascular necrosis of the femoral heads: early detection with MR imaging, *Radiology* 162:717, 1987.

254. Walsh HPJ, McLaren CAN, Owen R: Galeazzi fractures in children, *J Bone Joint Surg (Br)* 69:730, 1987.

255. Watson FM: Simultaneous interphalangeal dislocation in one finger, *J Trauma* 23:65, 1982.

256. Weber BG: Die Verletzungen des oberen Sprunggelenkes, ed 2, Bern, Switzerland, 1972, Verlag Hans Huber.

257. Weber ER: A rational approach for the recognition and treatment of Colles' fracture, *Hand Clin* 3:13, 1987.

258. Wehbe MA, Schneider LH: Mallet fractures, *J Bone Joint Surg (Am)* 66:658, 1984.

259. Wertzbarger K, Peterson HA: Acquired spondylolysis and spondylolisthesis in the young child, *Spine* 5:437, 1980.

260. White AA, Panjabi MM: Clinical biomechanics of the spine, ed 2, Philadelphia, 1990, JB Lippincott.

261. Wiesel SW, Zeide MS, Terry RL: Longitudinal fractures of the sacrum: case report, *J Trauma* 19:70, 1979.

262. Wilcox PG, Weiner DS, Leighley B: Maturation factors in slipped capital femoral epiphysis, *J Pediatr Orthop* 8(2):196, 1988.

263. Wiley JJ: The mechanism of tarso-metatarsal joint injuries, *J Bone Joint Surg (Br)* 53:474, 1971.

264. Williamson LR, Albright JP: Bilateral osteochondritis dissecans of the elbow in a female pitcher, *J Fam Pract* 43:489, 1996.

265. Wiltse LL, Newman PH, Macnab I: Classification of spondylolysis and spondylolisthesis, *Clin Orthop* 117:23, 1976.

266. Wiltse LL, Widell EH, Jackson DW: Fatigue fracture: the basic lesion in isthmic spondylolisthesis, *J Bone Joint Surg* 57A:17, 1975.

267. Wolinsky FD, Fitzgerald JF, Stump TE: The effect of hip fracture on mortality, hospitalization, and functional status: a prospective study, *Am J Public Health* 87(3):398, 1997.

268. Woodring JH, Goldstein SJ: Fractures of the articular processes of the cervical spine, *AJR Am J Roentgenol* 139:341, 1982.

269. Woodring JH, Lee C: Limitations of cervical radiography in the evaluation of acute cervical trauma, *J Trauma* 34:32, 1993.

270. Yochum TR, Rowe LJ: Essentials of skeletal radiology, ed 2, Baltimore, 1996, Williams & Wilkins.

271. Yulish BS et al: MR imaging of osteochondral lesions of the talus, *J Comput Assist Tomogr* 11:296, 1987.

272. Zacher J, Gursche A: Hip' pain, *Best Pract Res Clin Rheumatol* 17(1):71, 2003.

273. Ziegler DW, Agarwal NN: The morbidity and mortality of rib fractures, *J Trauma* 37:975, 1994.

chapter 11

Hematologic Bone Diseases

GARY D. SCHULTZ

Avascular Necrosis
Hemochromatosis
Hemophilia
Hereditary Spherocytosis
Leukemia
Sickle Cell Anemia
Thalassemia

Vascular conditions that affect bone may manifest through alterations in the blood supply or changes in the skeletal architecture because of abnormal activation of the hematopoietic potential within bone marrow. Unfortunately, the slow metabolic rate of bone significantly delays visualization of quantitative, qualitative, and morphologic changes in the skeleton. The limited number of skeletal responses to hematologic alterations often impairs the physician's ability to render a specific diagnosis based on plain films alone. In general, vascular conditions of the skeleton often have a chronic history of development and nonspecific radiographic findings. Consequently, all radiographic clues must be correlated with historic and laboratory findings. Typically the clinical findings suggest the correct diagnosis long before plain film radiographs are useful.

Avascular Necrosis

BACKGROUND

Avascular necrosis is the most common hematologic condition affecting the skeleton. Pathologically, this condition is simply bone death resulting from an inadequate blood supply. Avascular necrosis is more likely to develop when the blood supply to bone is tenuous or little collateral circulation is present. Many conditions and disorders can be responsible for the interruption of blood supply to a segment of bone.[10]

The many conditions known to be responsible for avascular necrosis include trauma, alcoholism, infections, dysbaric trauma, marrow infiltration disorders, hypercoagulability states, autoimmune diseases, and idiopathic etiology.[3] These causes may be divided into three categories: (a) conditions resulting in external blood vessel compression near or within the bone, (b) disorders resulting in blood vessel occlusion because of thickening of the vessel wall, and (c) disorders resulting in blood vessel blockage from a thromboembolic process (Box 11-1).[11]

For conditions that result in external blood vessel compression, the mechanism is either marrow edema causing compression of the vessel in an enclosed region or excessive packing of the marrow through the deposition of abnormal tissue or material (e.g., fat in steroid administration or hyperlipidemia).[15,19,39] Box 11-2 lists in

descending order of frequency the common causes of ischemic necrosis in children and adults.

Bone ischemia can have several presentations. Infarction affecting a focal segment of the articular surface is termed *osteochondritis dissecans* in the growing skeleton. This defect may occur in adults and children, and it more frequently affects weight-bearing bones. The lateral aspect of the medial femoral condyle is the most common location of the infarction, followed by the talar dome. Trauma is believed to be the precipitating mechanism, although patients commonly report no history of trauma.

BOX 11-1
Causes of Skeletal Ischemic Necrosis

External vessel compression
Trauma or surgery
Steroid administration
Idiopathic
Regional infection
Neuropathic joint
Gaucher disease
Hyperlipidemia

Vessel wall disorders
Systemic lupus erythematosus
Polyarteritis nodosa
Giant cell arteritis
Radiation therapy

Thromboembolic disorders
Alcoholism
Arteriosclerosis
Steroid administration
Thromboembolic syndrome
Diabetes
Trauma
Sickle cell disease

BOX 11-2
Most Frequent Causes of Ischemic Necrosis

Children
Idiopathic origin
Trauma
Infection

Adults
Drugs and other substances (steroids, alcohol, immuno-suppressants)
Trauma
Inflammatory arthritis
Metabolic conditions (diabetes, Cushing's syndrome, pregnancy)

BOX 11-3
Legg-Calvé-Perthes Disease

Background
Idiopathic osteonecrosis of the proximal femoral capital epiphysis in children
Trauma, endocrine abnormality, and infection implicated as possible causes
More common among boys, whites, and those between 3 and 5 years of age

Imaging
Bilateral in approximately 15% of patients
Magnetic resonance imaging (MRI) and bone scans more sensitive to early disease than plain film radiographs
Bone scans cold during avascular phase and hot during revascularization phase
MRI scans revealing replacement of normal marrow by necrosis
Plain film findings of capsular distention, a small fragmented epiphysis, osteosclerosis (snowcap sign), subchondral collapse (crescent sign), radiolucent defect of the lateral margin of the involved epiphysis (Cage's sign), curved radiodense cortical line at the base of the femoral neck representing the margin of the deformed femoral head (sagging rope sign), and growth deformity leading to a wide, short femoral neck with an enlarged (coxa magna), flattened (coxa plana) femoral head (mushroom) deformity

Clinical
Slowly evolving painless limp with limited abduction and internal rotation
Clinical outcome worse if weight-bearing area of bone involved
Osteoarthritis secondary to incongruent articular surfaces representing a significant complication
Treatment options of avoidance of full weight-bearing, bracing, and possible surgical realignment

The term *medullary bone infarction* is used to describe ischemic necrosis localized to the medullary portion of a long bone. This infarction generally is not of primary therapeutic interest because it causes no significant symptoms or alterations in osseous shape or integrity. However, the medullary bone infarction is associated with metabolic conditions such as alcoholism, diabetes, and chronic renal disease.

An infarction that affects the entire epiphysis of a skeletally immature long bone is termed *epiphyseal ischemic necrosis*. The proximal femur is by far the most common location for this event.[29] When the proximal femur is affected, the condition is called *Legg-Calvé-Perthes disease* (Box 11-3) in the child and *Chandler disease* in the adult. Early diagnosis of Legg-Calvé-Perthes disease is important in prevention of postischemic deformity and functional impairment.[24] Most cases of Legg-Calvé-Perthes disease have an idiopathic origin, although slipped femoral capital epiphysis, trauma, developmental dysplasia of the hip, and other pathologies also are associated with this process.

Although ischemia of any segment of a bone is possible, certain locations are more likely to be affected because of their vascular supply (Table 11-1). An avascular etiology has been disproved for some epiphyseal conditions previously attributed to an avascular origin (Table 11-2).

The histologic changes in bone necrosis are essentially the same, regardless of location. Pathologically, absence of a blood supply results in bone death within 48 hours; a predictable sequence of events then ensues: inflammatory reaction to the dead bone, neovascular infiltration into the dead segment of bone, resorption of dead bone and deposition of new bone, and remodeling of the resultant bone.[25] This process may take 1 to 8 years to complete.

IMAGING FINDINGS

Osteochondritis dissecans. Osteochondritis dissecans (local subchondral infarction) generally first manifests radiographically, the plain film showing a subarticular defect accompanied by a free-floating fragment of bone that formerly filled the defect. The defect is characteristically smooth and regular, corresponding to the borders of the fragment (Fig. 11-1). The fragment may be displaced from the parent bone defect, or remain in site (in situ, meaning in itself). Marginal sclerosis is always present at the defect and blends into the subchondral bone peripherally (Fig. 11-2). These findings assist in differentiation of focal subchondral infarction from an acute, traumatic insult. Intraarticular swelling is often noted, but its severity varies considerably (Figs. 11-3 and 11-4).

TABLE 11-1
Common Locations for Ischemic Necrosis

Location	Disorder
Metatarsal head	Freiberg disease
Tarsal navicular	Köhler bone disease
Talus	Diaz's disease
Patella (secondary ossification center)	Sinding-Larsen-Johansson disease
Medial femoral condyle	Spontaneous osteonecrosis of the knee (SONK)
Femoral head (child)	Legg-Calvé-Perthes disease
Phalanges of hand	Thiemann's disease
Metacarpal head	Mauclaire disease
Carpal lunate	Kienböck disease
Carpal scaphoid	Preiser disease
Capitellum of the humerus	Panner disease
Humeral head	Hass disease
Vertebral body	Kümmel disease

TABLE 11-2

Epiphyseal Conditions Unrelated to Avascular Necrosis

Condition	Etiology	Description
Blount's disease (tibia vara)	Trauma	Local growth alteration of the medial portion of the proximal tibial epiphysis; infantile and adolescent presentation; depressed medial metaphysis of the tibia with an osseous overgrowth noted; shortening of involved leg; usually a tibia vara deformity
Osgood-Schlatter disease	Trauma	Altered appearance of the tibial tuberosity occurring mostly between the ages of 11 and 15 years; more common among boys and girls who participate in sports such as soccer and weight lifting; fragmentation and soft-tissue swelling of the tibial tuberosity evident on radiographs; pain and tenderness over the region; tibial tuberosity possibly fragmented as a normal variant and distinguishable from Osgood-Schlatter disease by lack of pain and soft-tissue swelling
Scheuermann's disease*	Trauma	Posttraumatic defect of vertebral endplate maturation first seen during adolescence with three or more levels of wedged vertebrae, narrowed anterior disc space, multiple Schmorl's nodes, and vertebral endplate irregularity; middle and lower thoracic spine are the usual locations; back pain is common; more severe kyphosis possibly necessitates bracing or, in a few cases, surgery to arrest or partially correct the resulting deformity
Sever's phenomenon	Variation in ossification	Irregularity and fragmentation of the secondary ossification center of the calcaneus; generally considered a normal variant and unrelated to any heel pain in the adolescent
Sinding-Larsen-Johansson disease	Trauma	Fragmented appearance of the lower pole of the patella, most commonly occurring between 10 and 14 years of age; soft-tissue swelling and tenderness common and exacerbated by activity

*See Chapter 8.

Medullary bone infarction. The plain film radiograph generally demonstrates no evidence of a medullary bone infarction in the acute phase. After resolution and revascularization, the infarction is seen radiographically as discontinuous, longitudinally oriented, and wavy or serpiginous calcific opacities that lie centrally in the medullary cavity (Figs. 11-5 and 11-6). The infarction does not result in periosteal reaction, alteration in the cortical thickness, or expansion of the bone. Differentiating a medullary bone infarction from a benign enchondroma of bone can be impossible on plain film images. However, definitive differentiation generally is unnecessary because both conditions are benign.

Epiphyseal necrosis

Avascular phase. From both therapeutic and prognostic standpoints, epiphyseal necrosis is a significantly more important condition than medullary bone infarction. During the avascular phase of epiphyseal necrosis, plain film radiographic skeletal changes are absent (Fig. 11-7).[21] Intraarticular effusion may be visible, but the degree of effusion varies, making it an unreliable sign.

Changes in marrow signal can be identified with magnetic resonance imaging (MRI), which is considered the most sensitive imaging modality for the detection of early bone infarction.[5] MRI demonstrates loss in the epiphyseal marrow signal, particularly on T1-weighted images, even in the earliest phases of the disease (Fig. 11-8).[17,38]

Early epiphyseal infarction also can be detected by radionuclide scintigraphy, which demonstrates focal photopenia affecting the avascular segment. Generally a zone of increased radionuclide uptake is present in the region surrounding the avascular segment, presumably resulting from hyperemia (Fig. 11-9).[8]

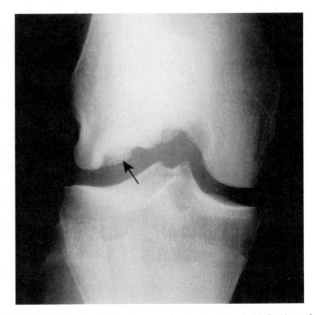

FIG. 11-1 Osteochondritis dissecans. Focal osteochondral infarction of the lateral femoral condyle demonstrating smooth margins and a clear articular defect *(arrow).*

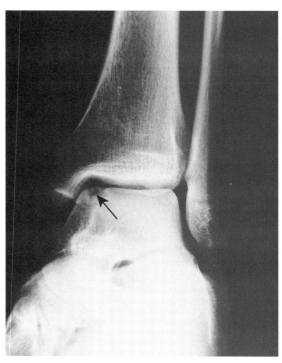

FIG. 11-2   Osteochondritis dissecans of the ankle. Note the in situ osseous fragment at the superomedial aspect of the talar dome (arrow). (From Deltoff MN, Kogon PL: The portable skeletal x-ray library, St Louis, 1998, Mosby.)

Inflammatory phase. As the avascular phase gives way to the inflammatory response in epiphyseal necrosis, plain films may demonstrate periarticular osteopenia affecting all but the involved segment of bone. This may create the plain film appearance of sclerosis of the avascular segment, but it is not an infallible radiographic finding (Fig. 11-10). The inflammatory phase may persist for weeks.

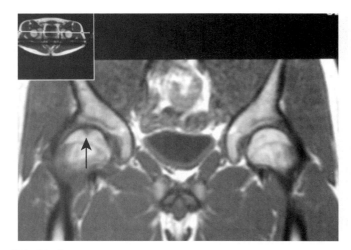

FIG. 11-4   A small defect is noted at the top of the reading left femoral head, consistent with osteochondritis dissecans (arrow).

During this time the dead bone begins to soften and may collapse under the stresses of use. With this collapse the involved articular surface becomes deformed (Figs. 11-11 and 11-12). Subchondral fractures allowing joint fluid to intrude into the subchondral ischemic bone may produce the "crescent" sign on plain films. This sign appears as a lucent defect in the subchondral bone that parallels the subchondral cortical surface (Fig. 11-13). The crescent sign is considered the most reliable early plain film sign of epiphyseal infarction.[21] Larger regions of bone collapse may develop, appearing as semilunar radiolucent defects extending from the articular cortex. The defects have been likened to configuration of a bite mark, known as *bite sign.* A variation of this is designated by the Gage's sign, a radiolucent defect of bone (often shaped as a V) appearing at the lateral margin of the involved epiphysis in patients with Legg-Calvé-Perthes disease.

Revascularization phase. As revascularization continues, the dead bone is resorbed while new bone matrix is being deposited

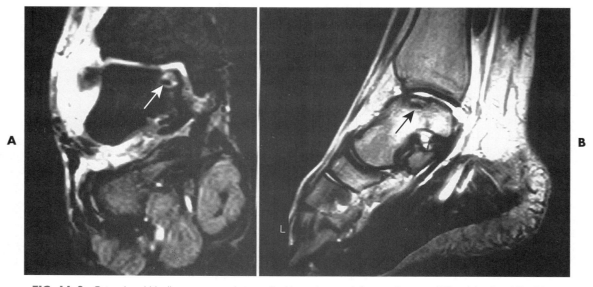

FIG. 11-3   Osteochondritis dissecans appearing as a focal hyperintense defect on, **A,** coronal T2-weighted and, **B,** oblique T1-weighted sequences (arrows). Osteochondritis dissecans is a traumatic defect of the articular surface, common to the dome of the talus, particularly on the medial side. It is suggested clinically by persistent symptoms after an ankle strain. (Courtesy Robert Rowell, Davenport, IA.)

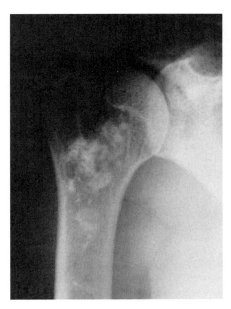

FIG. 11-5 Irregular patchy sclerosis of a medullary bone infarction.

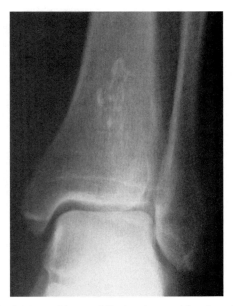

FIG. 11-6 Subtle serpiginous calcifications in a medullary bone infarction.

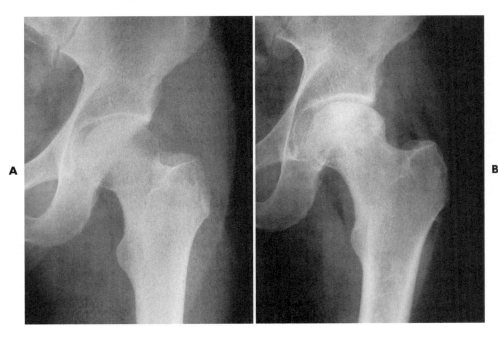

FIG. 11-7 **A,** Normal plain films in a patient with a painful hip. **B,** Plain films 3 months later demonstrating increased radiodensity and a mottled appearance of the femoral head. These are typical signs of avascular necrosis of the femoral head.

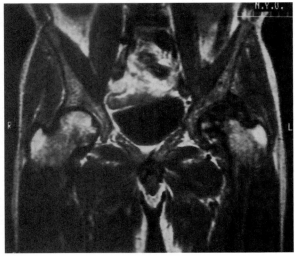

FIG. 11-8 Avascular necrosis of the patient's left *(reading right)* hip with severe secondary osteoarthritis on a coronal T1-weighted magnetic resonance imaging scan. (From Firooznia H et al: MRI and CT of the musculoskeletal system, St Louis, 1992, Mosby.)

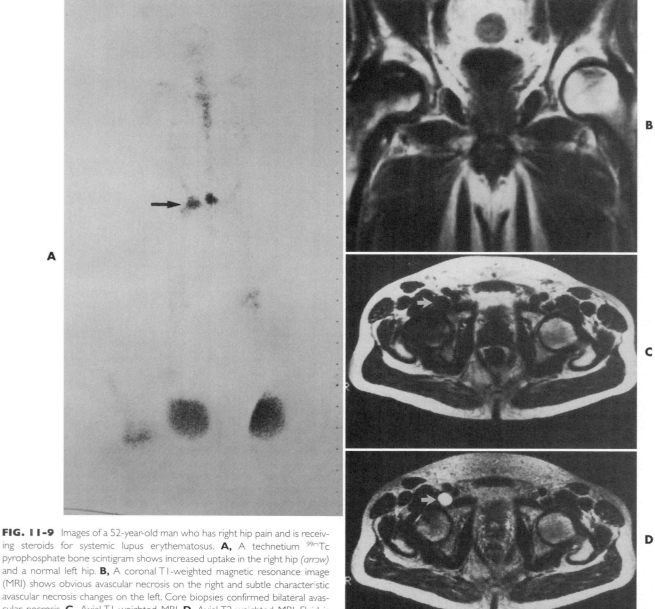

FIG. 11-9 Images of a 52-year-old man who has right hip pain and is receiving steroids for systemic lupus erythematosus. **A,** A technetium ^{99m}Tc pyrophosphate bone scintigram shows increased uptake in the right hip *(arrow)* and a normal left hip. **B,** A coronal T1-weighted magnetic resonance image (MRI) shows obvious avascular necrosis on the right and subtle characteristic avascular necrosis changes on the left. Core biopsies confirmed bilateral avascular necrosis. **C,** Axial T1-weighted MRI. **D,** Axial T2-weighted MRI. Fluid is shown *(arrows)* in the right iliopsoas bursa. Iliopsoas bursitis may accompany avascular necrosis and cause a variety of symptoms. (From Firooznia H et al: MRI and CT of the musculoskeletal system, St Louis, 1992, Mosby.)

FIG. 11-10 Anteroposterior projection of the pelvis demonstrating a small radiodense epiphysis on the reading right. These changes indicate ischemic necrosis of the epiphysis (Legg-Calvé-Perthes disease) in this child.

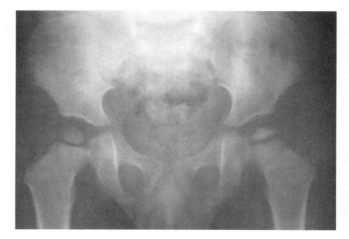

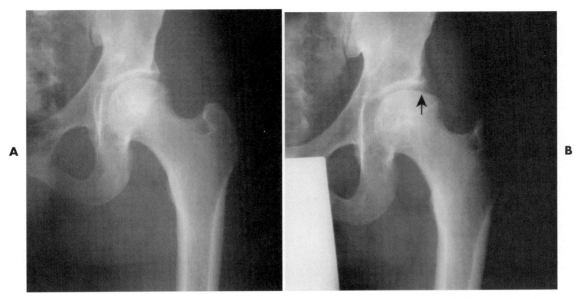

FIG. II-II Avascular necrosis. **A,** The first radiograph of this 32-year-old woman appears normal. **B,** However, I year later, clear signs of necrosis are evident by the increased radiodensity of the femoral head and the flattened appearance of the femoral head's articular cortex *(arrow).*

to replace it. On radiographs this process is seen as apparent fragmentation of the epiphysis. In addition, sclerosis begins to appear at the margin of the necrotic segment, producing a mottled appearance (Figs. 11-14 to 11-17). Articular collapse is common (Fig. 11-18). The fragmentation gradually recedes as the new epiphyseal bone ossifies.

Any deformity that has occurred during the process of necrosis or early revascularization forms the substrate for the new epiphyseal

bone. The result is deformity of the repaired epiphysis in the general shape left by the necrotic segment of bone. In most cases the deformity manifests as a flattened and widened epiphysis. Widening of the metaphysis of the involved bone may accompany the epiphyseal deformity. In the adult skeleton, subchondral infarctions can result in significant deformity of the articular morphology. Figures 11-19 to 11-24 exhibit selected defects of avascular necrosis and trauma in various body regions.

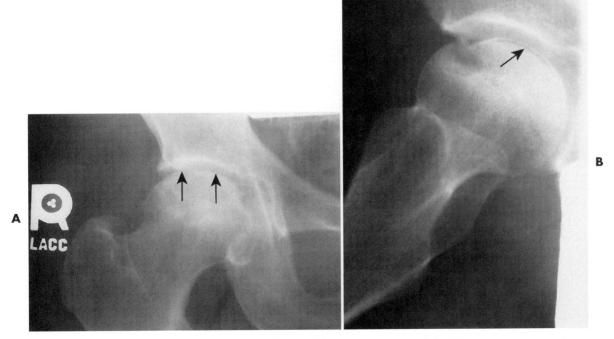

FIG. II-I2 **A** and **B,** Ischemic necrosis indicated by a radiolucent crescent sign is faintly visible on the anteroposterior view of the hip but is obvious on the frog-leg lateral view *(arrows).* Mottled bone sclerosis of the femoral head is also noted.

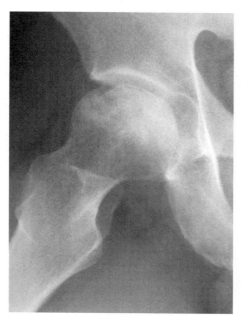

FIG. 11-13   *Articular collapse in a patient with adult-onset ischemic necrosis of the femoral head.*

CLINICAL COMMENTS

The earliest clinical signs of avascular necrosis of the epiphysis are related to the synovitis and inflammatory response or a mechanical deformity. Children complain of hip or knee pain. In either location the pain is generally dull, achy, and boring and is exacerbated with activity. Orthopedic testing of the involved joint often suggests an intraarticular problem. The pain is generally intense enough to cause ambulation with a limp, and it worsens with activity. A child with bilateral Legg-Calvé-Perthes disease has a "waddling" gait because of the abduction and external rotation of the hips. (Patients with osteonecrosis may be staged using the systems listed in

Table 11-3. These systems typically are applied to avascular necrosis of the femoral head.)

Patients with osteochondritis dissecans generally first report swelling and pain in the involved joints. The symptoms may develop gradually, or they may become apparent after a specific episode or traumatic event. The severity of the symptoms can vary considerably. Objective signs may be difficult to demonstrate if the joint is difficult to palpate or muscular dysfunction accompanies the joint disease. Crepitus, clicking, or locking of the joint occur if cartilage integrity is violated or the ischemic segment is displaced.

Medullary bone infarctions are asymptomatic conditions that may not be detected on radiographs for months to years. Although these infarctions generally are considered self-limited problems, they can indicate the presence of more serious underlying conditions. The clinician should search for an underlying metabolic or vascular cause when medullary bone infarctions are bilateral and symmetric.

KEY CONCEPTS

- *Avascular necrosis is bone death secondary to an inadequate blood supply.*
- *Pathophysiologic changes are marked by stages of ischemia, revascularization, repair, deformity, and osteoarthritis.*
- *Osteochondritis dissecans is a focal region of bone necrosis, usually secondary to trauma; commonly occurring at the lateral aspect of the medial femoral condyle.*
- *Medullary bone infarcts appear radiographically as serpiginous calcifications after avascularity within the medullary canal.*
- *Epiphyseal necroses occurring in the skeletally immature (Legg-Calvé-Perthes disease) are potentially serious clinical conditions that may lead to subchondral fracture, bone deformity, and premature joint degeneration.*
- *No reliable radiographic signs exist during the avascular stage of epiphyseal necrosis, but signs during later stages may include increased sclerosis, fragmentation, altered bone contour, and osteoarthritis.*
- *Magnetic resonance imaging demonstrates a loss of marrow signal in the region of bone ischemia early in the disease.*

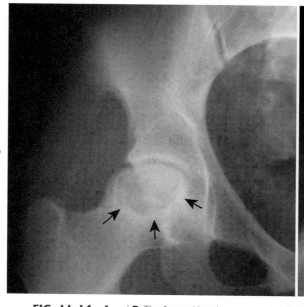

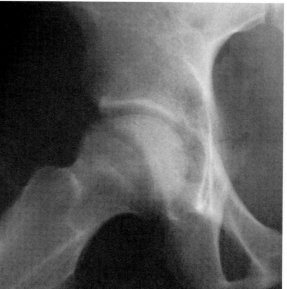

FIG. 11-14   **A** and **B,** The femoral head appears mottled, with a semicircular defect extending into the femoral head from the superior cortical margin ("bite sign") *(arrows).*

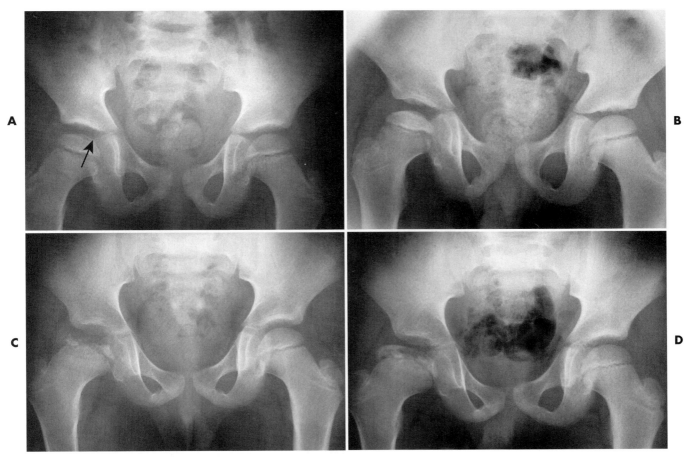

FIG. 11-15 Legg-Calvé-Perthes disease. **A,** Early changes of Legg-Calvé-Perthes disease. Note the lucent crescent sign *(arrow)* at the superior aspect of the femoral epiphyseal surface. **B** through **D,** Six-month progression of Legg-Calvé-Perthes disease. Note the progression of articular collapse. The fragmentation of the epiphysis is evidence of revascularization.

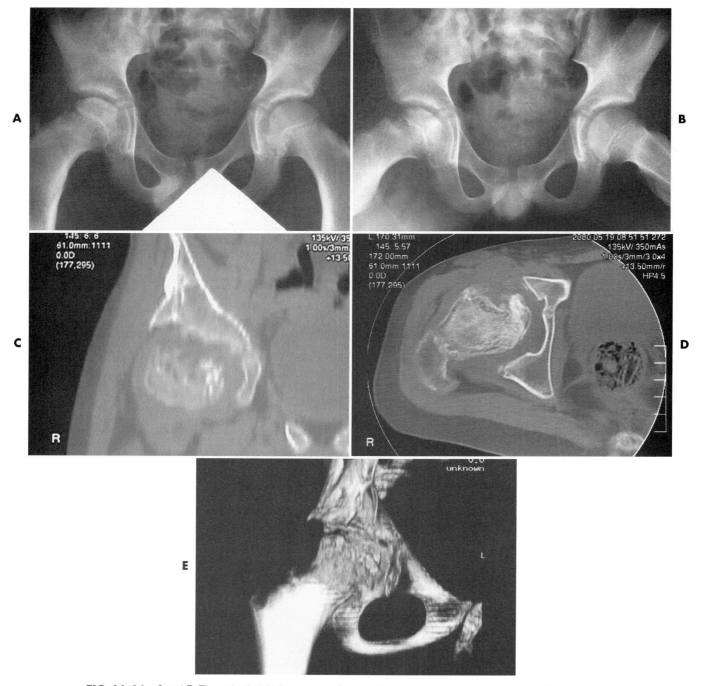

FIG. 11-16   A and **B,** The patient's right femoral head *(reading left)* appears small, fragmented, and with increased radio-density on the anteroposterior and frog-leg projections, consistent with Legg-Calvé-Perthes disease. **C** through **E,** Coronal, axial, and reformatted computed tomography scans exhibit further detail of the involved femoral head and adjacent acetabulum. (Courtesy James Owens, Davenport, IA.)

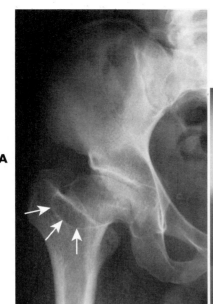

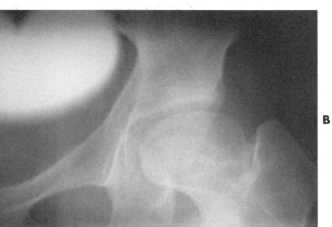

FIG. II-17 **A** and **B,** Two cases of healed Legg-Calvé-Perthes disease exhibiting a broad, flattened femoral head as residuum to past osteonecrosis. Case **A** exhibits a curved radiodense band that represents the rim of the deformed femoral head, known as a *sagging rope sign.* (**A,** Courtesy Gary Longmuir, Phoenix, AZ).

FIG. II-18 Ischemic necrosis of the third, and possibly second, metacarpal head (Feiberg disease). The involvement of the third metacarpal is obvious, evidenced by flattening and irregularity of the metatarsal head *(arrow).* The mild flattening of the articular surface of the second metacarpal head is suspicious for a second digit of involvement *(arrow).*

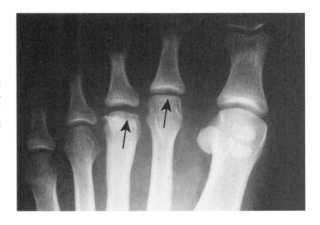

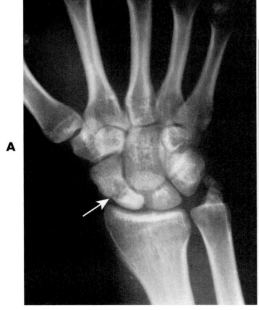

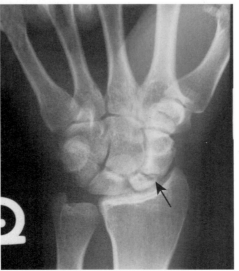

FIG. II-19 **A** and **B,** Two cases of ischemic necrosis of the proximal pole of the scaphoid secondary to fracture through the waist of the scaphoid *(arrows).*

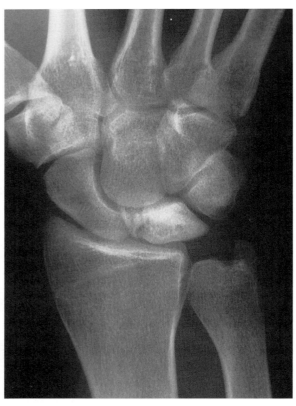

FIG. 11-20   Ischemic necrosis of the lunate (Kienböck disease) marked by increased radiodensity and fissures.

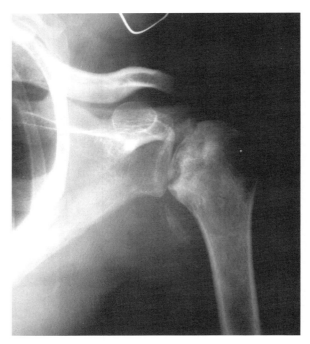

FIG. 11-21   The articular portion of the humeral head appears fragmented and radiodense in this patient who has systemic lupus erythematosus, a risk factor for developing osteonecrosis. Osteonecrosis of the humeral head is known as *Hass disease*. (Courtesy Steven P. Brownstein, MD, Springfield, NJ.)

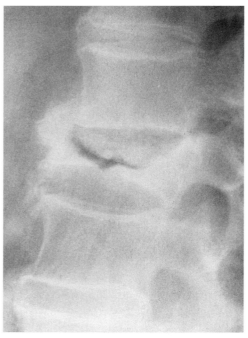

FIG. 11-22   Kümmell disease is a rare phenomenon of delayed vertebral collapse from osteonecrosis secondary to vascular injury. The collapse occurs 6 weeks or more after the traumatic incident.

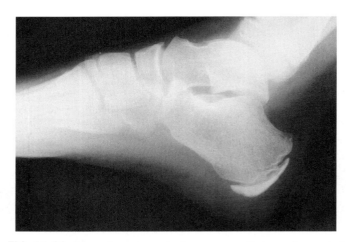

FIG. 11-23   The calcaneal apophysis appears radiodense, fragmented, and small; all features of avascular necrosis. This presentation was originally thought to be a presentation of osteonecrosis (Sever disease), but is now known to be a normal variant that resolves over time (Sever's phenomenon).

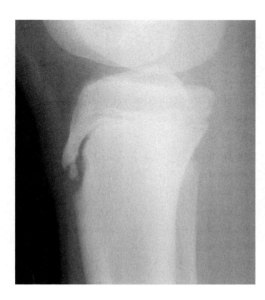

FIG. 11-24 Osgood-Schlatter disease presenting as a fragmented tibial apophysis radiographically, with pain and tenderness clinically. Osgood-Schlatter disease is a common cause of knee pain in the adolescent patient (ages 10 to 14 years, most commonly), related to localized weakness in the growing skeleton. Although the early literature attributed this finding to avascular necrosis, it is now known to be a microavulsion traction apophysitis of the tibial tuberosity. However, at times, the tibial tuberosity appears fragmented as a normal finding, necessitating the confirmation of radiographic fragmentation by the presence of pain and swelling clinically. The condition usually heals within a few months of cessation of the aggravating activities. (Courtesy, Steven P. Brownstein, MD, Springfield, NJ.)

TABLE 11-3
Staging Osteonecrosis of the Femoral Head

Categories	Findings
Based on radiographs	
*Ficat stages**	
Stage 0	No clinical manifestations, normal radiographs
Stage I	Clinical manifestations, normal to regions of slight osteopenia on the radiographs
Stage II	Clinical manifestations, regions of osteopenia and osteosclerosis on the radiograph
Stage III	Clinical manifestations, early subchondral bone collapse (crescent sign)
Stage IV	Clinical manifestations, late bone collapse and flattened deformity
Ponseti classes	
Class I	Involves less than 50% of femoral head
Class II	Involves at least 50% of the femoral head
Herring groups†	
Group A	The femoral head is divided into three parts as it appears on the anteroposterior projection: lateral, central, and medial. In group A, the femoral head is involved, but not in the lateral region.
Group B	Group B describes less than 50% of reduction in its original height
Group C	Group C describes 50% or greater reduction in the original height
Catterall classes	
Class I	Involves anterior portion of the femoral head as seen on the frog-leg view (good prognosis)
Class II	Involves anterior and some of the lateral portion of the femoral head (good prognosis)
Class III	Involves anterior and lateral portion of the femoral head (poor prognosis)
Class IV	Involves all portions of the femoral head (poor prognosis)
Based on MRI‡	
Class A	Normal marrow, high signal intensity on T1-weighted scans and intermediate signal intensity on T2-weighted scans
Class B	Subacute hemorrhage, high signal intensity on both T1- and T2-weighted scans
Class C	Fluid accumulation, low signal intensity on T1-weighted scans and high signal intensity on T2-weighted scans
Class D	Fibrosis and sclerosis, low signal intensity on both T1- and T2-weighted scans

*Mont M, Hungerford D: Non-traumatic avascular necrosis of the femoral head, *J Bone Joint Surg Am* 77: 459, 1995.
†Herring JA: Current concepts review. The treatment of Legg-Calvé-Perthes Disease. A critical review of the literature, *J Bone Joint Surg* 76A:448, 1994.
‡ARCO (Association Research Circulation Osseous): Committee on Terminology and Classification, *ARCO News* 4:41, 1992.

Hemochromatosis

BACKGROUND

Hemochromatosis is an autosomal recessive, inherited (the result of hepatic xanthene oxidase deficiency), or acquired disorder of excessive iron deposition within tissues. The disease is most frequently encountered in northern European lineages, and is rare in Asian and African ethnicities.[18] Patients with this condition generally have liver disease that is of greater long-term significance than the articular disease.[20]

IMAGING FINDINGS

Articular manifestations of hemochromatosis are present in 20% to 50% of cases. The metacarpophalangeal joints of the second and third digits are the most common location, with the wrists, elbows, and shoulders less frequently affected. The radiographic manifestations of this disorder are the result of degenerative disease secondary to calcium pyrophosphate dihydrate (CPPD) deposition disease. Hemochromatosis is suspected when unusual distributions of degenerative disease are encountered. Chondrocalcinosis is commonly present and is the result of CPPD within the afflicted joints. The exact association between CPPD and hemochromatosis remains unclear. Morphologically, degenerative disease associated with hemochromatosis demonstrates as flattening of the metacarpal heads along with prominent cyst formation and small beaklike osteophytes, most prominently in the metacarpophalangeal joints (Figs. 11-25 and 11-26).[2]

CLINICAL COMMENTS

Genetic testing has become the confirmatory test of choice for inherited forms of the disease.[23] The articular manifestations of hemochromatosis clinically are typical of secondary degeneration. Symptoms are intermittent, and joint function generally is impaired. Considerable joint destruction may be encountered.[1]

> ### KEY CONCEPTS
> - *Hemochromatosis represents excessive iron deposits within tissues.*
> - *Articular manifestations are common and include both osteoarthritis and chondrocalcinosis.*

Hemophilia

BACKGROUND

The term *hemophilia* is applied to a class of recessive X-linked disorders that are the result of insufficient clotting factors. Only males manifest clinically evident disease, whereas females classically are carriers of the disease.

Several types of hemophilia have been identified. Hemophilia A (classic hemophilia) is a deficiency of clotting factor VIII and is the most common type. The second most common type is hemophilia B (Christmas disease), which is a deficiency of clotting factor IX. The clinical manifestations of hemophilia generally become apparent in the first year of life and have the most severe impact during childhood. Radiographic manifestations may appear in infancy but generally are not present until the childhood years.[35]

IMAGING FINDINGS

The earliest plain film finding of hemophilia is intraarticular soft-tissue swelling, with the large joints usually affected initially and most significantly. In decreasing order of frequency, the knees, elbows, and ankles are the most commonly affected joints. Joint changes consisting of articular irregularity, epiphyseal overgrowth,

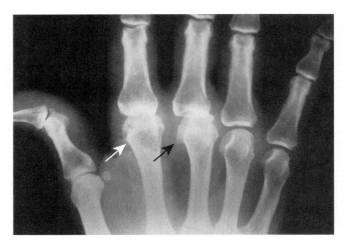

FIG. 11-25   Narrowing and subchondral sclerosis of the second and third metacarpophalangeal joints accompanied by subtle chondrocalcinosis (of the third metacarpophalangeal joint) and subchondral cyst formation (of the second metacarpal head). Small beaklike osteophytes are noted from the second and third metacarpal heads *(arrows)*.

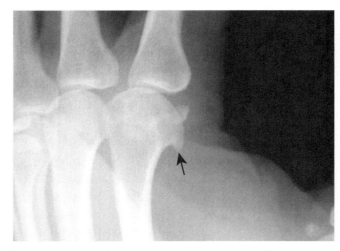

FIG. 11-26   Hemochromatosis appearing with small, beaklike osteophytes of the metacarpal heads *(arrow)*.

and early physeal closure make the femoral condyles and inferior patella appear "squared."[35] Generalized osteopenia is present (Figs. 11-27 and 11-28). The synovium increases in thickness and density because of hemosiderin deposition, which accompanies resolution of intraarticular hemorrhagic episodes.

Soft-tissue changes outside the joints generally relate to hemorrhage and its resolution. Myositis ossificans is relatively unusual at the location of previous hematomas, but it can be present. Intramuscular hemorrhage most commonly occurs in the iliopsoas muscles.

In rare cases the skeleton demonstrates rapidly expanding lytic lesions of bone called *pseudotumors of hemophilia*. The etiology of these lesions is obscure, but their development is probably related to unabated hemorrhage in an intraosseous location.[16] Pseudotumors tend to be painless masses in the pelvis and femur. However, when the lesions are intramuscular or affecting the peripheral skeleton, they may produce painful deformity of the extremity.[34]

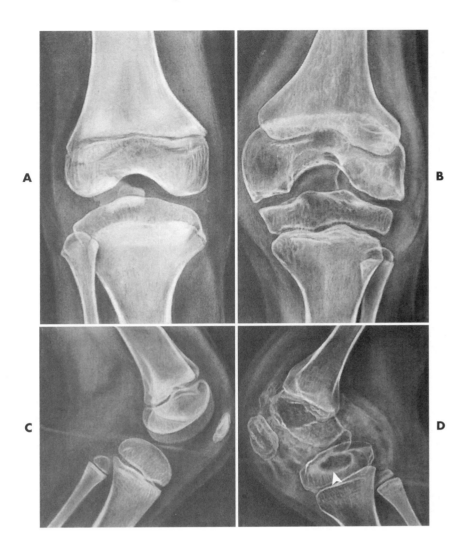

FIG. 11-27 Hemophilia panarthritis in a 7-year-old boy. **A** and **C,** Normal right knee. **B** and **D,** Hemarthrotic left knee—frontal and lateral projections. In the left knee the soft tissues are swollen and denser. In addition, marked generalized rarefaction of the epiphyses and shafts and atrophy of the shafts is present. However, the epiphyseal centers and patella are enlarged on the left side; the intercondylar notch is deepened and the juxtaarticular surfaces of the bones are ragged. **D,** Large intraosseous hematoma visible in the tibial epiphysis (*arrowhead*). (From Caffey J: Pediatric x-ray diagnosis: an integrated imaging approach, St Louis, 1993, Mosby.)

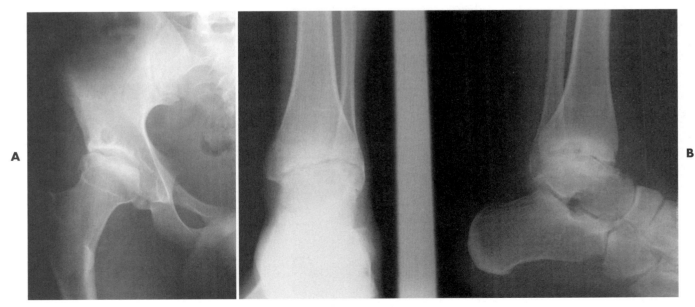

FIG. 11-28 Hemophilia presenting with, **A,** avascular necrosis of the hip and, **B,** cartilaginous and osseous destruction of the ankle joint. (Courtesy Gary Longmuir, Phoenix, AZ.)

CLINICAL COMMENTS

Patients with hemophilia are seen early in life with excessive and spontaneous bleeding. Bone pain and arthralgia with swelling are common complaints. As the disease becomes chronic, degenerative disease may greatly affect articulations. Osteophytic growth is not prominent, but joint thinning and subchondral cyst formation are obvious. Chronic inflammatory reactions lead to fibrosis and scarring of the synovium. As a consequence, the joints become stiff.

> ### KEY CONCEPTS
> - *Hemophilia results from insufficient clotting factors. Females are carriers for disease; clinically significant disease develops only in males.*
> - *Knees, elbows, and ankles are the most commonly affected joints in hemophilia.*
> - *Joint changes include articular irregularity, epiphyseal overgrowth, epiphyseal squaring, generalized osteopenia, radiodense effusions, and degenerative changes.*

Hereditary Spherocytosis

BACKGROUND

Hereditary spherocytosis is a curious condition in which the red blood cells are spherical rather than biconcave. Because of their shape, the cells are fragile and have a reduced capacity to carry oxygen. Consequently, the life span of red blood cells is considerably shortened, resulting in anemia of varying severity.

IMAGING FINDINGS

Radiologic findings are uncommon in hereditary spherocytosis. However, if the disorder is severe, mild changes of marrow hyperplasia, including osteopenia and expansion of the marrow cavity in the proximal extremities and the axial skeleton, may be seen. The most severe cases may demonstrate extramedullary hematopoiesis resulting from severe, protracted anemia.[12,36]

CLINICAL COMMENTS

The spleen may be enlarged, and laboratory values may reflect elevated hemolysis. Additionally, patients may demonstrate cholelithiasis as a part of their hemolytic anemia.[37]

> ### KEY CONCEPTS
> - *Hereditary spherocytosis is a condition marked by morphologic alterations of red blood cells that reduce their ability to carry oxygen.*
> - *Radiographic findings are uncommon, but changes may develop secondary to marrow hyperplasia in severe cases.*

Leukemia

BACKGROUND

Leukemia, the most common childhood cancer, has both acute and chronic forms. Although adults also may develop this cancer, the vast majority of leukemia patients are younger than 5 years of age. Lymphoblastic leukemia is the histologic variety in approximately 80% of cases.

IMAGING FINDINGS

Plain film findings are abnormal in nearly 50% of children with leukemia. The most common radiologic manifestation of this cancer is generalized osteopenia. The earliest radiographic findings are transmetaphyseal lucent bands near the physes of long bones such as the femur and tibia (Fig. 11-29). Rather than leukemic infiltrates, these bands appear to represent a metabolic reaction to

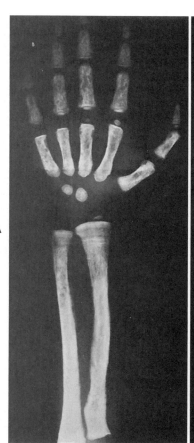

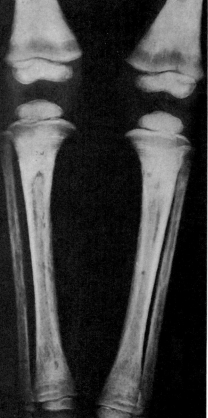

FIG. 11-29 Leukopenic lymphatic leukemia in a 2-year-old boy. **A,** Hand and forearm. **B,** Lower limbs; irregular destruction of all the bones is evident. Deep transverse zones of diminished density occupy the ends of the shafts. In addition to these destructive features, numerous large and small irregular patches of sclerosis are present, indicating a massive osteoblastic reaction. (From Caffey J: Pediatric x-ray diagnosis: an integrated imaging approach, St Louis, 1993, Mosby.)

the process. Alternatively, they may develop because pressure on the physis from the neoplastic infiltrates alters bony maturation at the zone of provisional calcification.

Discrete bony lesions may be present in the metaphysis or diaphysis in which they create a "moth-eaten" or permeative pattern of destruction. Periostitis also may develop with the discrete bone lesions. In some cases, focal, spotty sclerosis is noted after chemotherapy or radiation treatment. Diffuse sclerosis of the bones has been encountered, but it is thought to be secondary myelofibrosis resulting from therapeutic interventions.[7]

Infiltration of the meninges of the brain creates a separation of the skull sutures in a small percentage of patients with leukemia. Based on the radiographic findings alone, differentiation of infiltration of the meninges from neuroblastoma metastasis to the skeleton can be challenging because both conditions cause periostitis and separations of the sutures.

Focal accumulations of leukemic cells have been identified in a small number of patients with acute myelogenous leukemia. Because of their green color, these cells have been termed *chloromas*. Most commonly, chloromas accumulate outside the skeleton.[27,40] Skeletal accumulations most often occur in the face, sternum, and ribs.[30]

CLINICAL COMMENTS

Patients with leukemia generally have a number of systemic complaints, including fever, malaise, and weakness. The musculoskeletal findings in leukemia include diffuse bone and joint pain, similar to the findings in juvenile rheumatoid arthritis. Joint and soft-tissue swelling should alert the physician to the presence of a more serious condition. The laboratory finding of blast cells in the peripheral blood smear is strongly suggestive of leukemia, and bone marrow biopsy is diagnostic.

> **KEY CONCEPTS**
> - *Leukemia is the most common childhood cancer.*
> - *Radiographic findings include generalized osteopenia, transmetaphyseal lucent bands, and, occasionally, osteolytic bone lesions with a moth-eaten or permeative pattern of destruction.*
> - *Clinical findings include fever, malaise, weakness, and joint pain.*

Sickle Cell Anemia

BACKGROUND

Sickle cell anemia is the most common disorder in a class of hemoglobinopathies known as hemolytic anemias.[32] This autosomal dominant condition is caused by the substitution of valine for glutamic acid at position 6 on the β-globin molecule. The clinically relevant result of this substitution is that red blood cells flatten and become sickle shaped during episodes of low oxygen tension. The sickling is reversible in mild cases but not in more severe cases.

The worldwide prevalence of sickle cell disease is considerable, with as many as 50% of East Africans having some variant of the disease. In North America the prevalence of sickle cell anemia is estimated to be nearly 9% of African Americans, the most commonly affected ethnicity. The homozygous form of sickle cell disease is present in approximately 1 in 600 African Americans in the United States.[14]

Pathologically, sickle cells aggregate into clumps of deformed red cells that obstruct blood vessels. Not only do these cells tend to deform, but also they are fragile, and their life span is dramatically shortened. This in turn necessitates accelerated hematopoiesis.

IMAGING FINDINGS

The frequency and severity of the skeletal manifestations in sickle cell anemia depend on the degree of genetic penetrance of the disease. More pronounced radiographic changes are demonstrated at an earlier phase in patients who are homozygous for sickle cell disease than in those who are heterozygous.

The radiographic findings of sickle cell disease relate to marrow hyperplasia and infarction.[39] Marrow hyperplasia appears as an accentuation of the marrow, particularly in the long bones. Long bones demonstrate varying degrees of undertubulation (widening of the diaphysis), and the marrow takes on a somewhat lacelike or reticulated appearance (Fig. 11-30).

In sickle cell anemia, bone density is universally reduced because of cortical thinning and reduced concentration of trabeculae in the medullary bone. In the skull, marrow hyperplasia results in a widening of the diploë with accentuation of the trabeculae. This imparts a "hair-on-end" appearance to the calvarium. In the spine, marrow hyperplasia causes coarsening of the trabeculae and overall osteopenia. The osteopenia may be severe enough to increase the likelihood of spinal compression deformities.[26,33]

Because of the protective presence of hemoglobin F in the blood, infarctions rarely occur before the age of 6 months in infants with sickle cell anemia. Infarctions begin to occur as hemoglobin F recedes from the blood and is replaced by hemoglobin S. Hemoglobin S may constitute 70% to 99% of circulating hemoglobin if sickle cell anemia is severe. Infarctions occur early in life in these instances. In milder sickle cell anemia, infarctions may be less numerous and they may occur much later in life.

Sickle cell infarctions affect the tubular bones of the hands and feet, most commonly in young patients.[6] Within these bones, infarctions generally affect the diaphysis or metaphysis. In larger bones such as the humerus and femur, epiphyseal infarction is more common and produces the typical changes of epiphyseal ischemic necrosis (Fig. 11-31). Epiphyseal infarctions also can

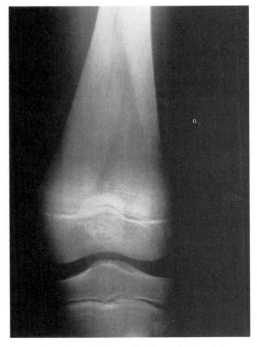

FIG. 11-30 Marrow hyperplasia manifesting as flaring of the metaphysis in a child with sickle cell disease.

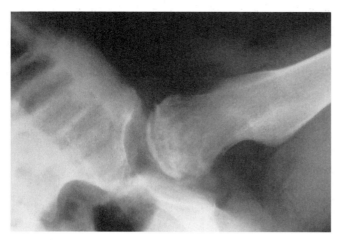

FIG. 11-31 Epiphyseal ischemic necrosis in a patient suffering from sickle cell disease.

occur in other long bones and the spine. Interestingly, the skull is an unusual site for sickle cell infarctions.

The earliest plain film evidence of skeletal infarction in the young is an aggressive-appearing lytic destructive process at the site of infarction. At this early stage, differentiation of an infarction from an infection or a neoplasm is difficult based on the radiographic appearance. Radionuclide scintigraphy is useful because infarctions demonstrate focal photopenia, whereas other destructive processes generally increase radiopharmaceutical uptake. Once periostitis develops days to weeks later, the differential diagnosis of infection is more difficult, even with scintigraphy.[22] Likewise, distinguishing acute infarction from acute infection with MRI remains difficult.[31] Skeletal deformity and pathologic fracture may occur as the infarction progresses.

Old, quiescent infarctions are characterized by mottled sclerosis and irregularity of the medullary bone architecture. Large infarctions may develop marginal sclerosis parallel to the outer surface of the bone, which creates a "bone-within-a-bone" appearance. Quiescent diaphyseal infarctions may extend through a considerable length of bone and generally demonstrate parallel tracks of sclerosis adjacent to but distinct from the diaphyseal cortex. When infarctions are epiphyseal or pathologic fracture has occurred, the deformity that is present when the bone begins to revascularize persists as a permanent alteration in the bone structure. A classic but not pervasive example of this phenomenon occurs in the spine, where endplate infarctions result in central collapse of the vertebral bodies, which, when healed, are accentuated by focal sclerosis at the infarction. These central depressions can alter the overall appearance of the vertebral segments, with the term *H vertebrae* used to describe the biconcavity of the phenomenon (Fig. 11-32). However, this finding is present in only about 50% of sickle cell cases.[33]

CLINICAL COMMENTS

The clinical manifestations of sickle cell disease usually are related to the hemolytic aspect of the disorder.[9] Skeletally bilateral pain and swelling in the hands and feet are characteristic of the "hand-foot syndrome," which is the result of infarctions in the small tubular bones of the distal extremities. This syndrome generally occurs between the first and second years of life in patients with severe sickle cell disease. In the gastrointestinal tract, infarctions of the mesenteric arteries create symptoms of bowel perforation or obstruction. These bowel infarctions predispose patients to infections at distant sites in the body by allowing gastrointestinal flora, particularly *Salmonella paratyphi,* entrance to the circulatory system. Salmonella osteomyelitis, which tends to affect the diaphysis of the long bones, is considered a classic complication of sickle cell disease. Jaundice and hyperbilirubinemia are constant findings that result from high red cell turnover. Hepatosplenomegaly may be present but usually is minor. Eventually, the infarctions cause involution of the spleen that will progress to autosplenectomy. Renal papillary necrosis and high-output cardiac failure also may result from sickle cell disease.

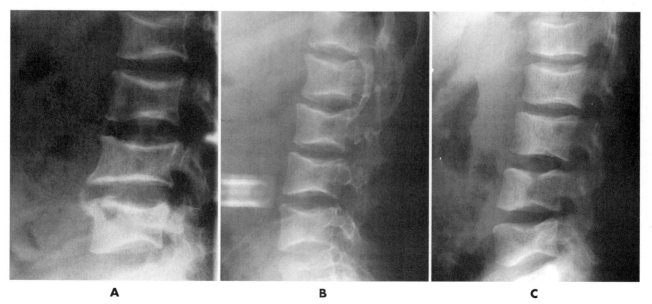

A   B   C

FIG. 11-32   **A** through **C,** Central endplate invaginations (*H vertebrae sign*) with sclerotic margins in three different patients with sickle cell anemia. (**B,** Courtesy Steven P. Brownstein, MD, Springfield, NJ; **C,** Courtesy Ronnie Firth, East Moline, IL.)

Thalassemia

BACKGROUND

Thalassemia represents a spectrum of hematologic disorders that are characterized by varying degrees of hypochromic microcytic anemia. The principal abnormality in thalassemia is an excess of hemoglobin F. The disorder is inherited through autosomal dominant transmission. Severe (homozygous) thalassemia is also known as *Cooley's anemia* or *Mediterranean anemia*. Patients with severe manifestations of thalassemia generally die during childhood.

IMAGING FINDINGS

The primary radiographic manifestations of thalassemia are the result of marrow hyperplasia. Signs of the disease often are present on plain films obtained in the first year of life. In the peripheral skeleton, severe osteopenia is the most common and consistent finding. Expansion of the marrow cavity is recognized through undertubulation of the long bones, as well as cortical thinning. With severe thalassemia, remodeling of long bones may include

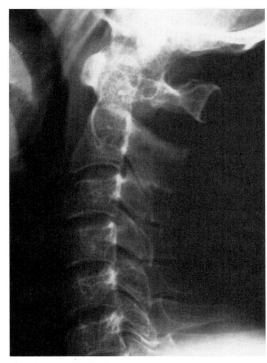

FIG. 11-33 Severe osteopenia in a young adult with thalassemia. The trabecular pattern is coarse, and there is mild expansion (ballooning) of the C2 vertebral body from marrow hyperplasia.

"Erlenmeyer flask" deformities of the metaphyseal regions. The trabecular pattern, particularly in the small tubular bones of the hands and feet, has a lacelike appearance typical of severe osteopenia.[4]

In the axial skeleton, signs of profound osteopenia include trabecular paucity, cortical thinning, and overall loss of bone density (Fig. 11-33). Insufficiency fractures may occur. In severe thalassemia, ballooning of the vertebral bodies may be a manifestation of marrow hyperplasia. Extramedullary hematopoiesis, seen by computed tomography, arises from the vertebral bodies or ribs.[13]

The changes in the skull are characteristic. Because of severe marrow proliferation, the sinuses fail to pneumatize but are filled with a proliferation of marrow. This creates overgrowth of the maxillary region and protrusion of the maxillary incisors, producing the "rodent facies" of thalassemia. Hypertelorism resulting from marrow proliferation in the frontal bones also is noted. Diploic marrow proliferation causes the calvaria to demonstrate varying degrees of the "hair-on-end" appearance,[28] which terminate abruptly at the external occipital protuberance and do not extend into the petrous portion of the occipital bone because the bone segment has no active marrow potential. Infarctions are distinctly unusual. Radiographically this helps to distinguish thalassemia from Gaucher's disease and sickle cell anemia.

CLINICAL COMMENTS

Patients with severe thalassemia do not have a normal life span. Growth is retarded, and epiphyses may close early as a result of marrow proliferation across the physis and pressure on the physeal margin by the marrow. Skeletal deformities generally are the result of insufficiency fractures; these fractures may be spontaneous or may be a consequence of minor trauma. Hepatosplenomegaly is present, and jaundice is a constant finding. Increased levels of the by-products of red blood cell catabolism are present in the stool, blood, and urine.

References

1. Adams P, Speechley M: The effect of arthritis on the quality of life in hereditary hemochromatosis, *J Rheumatol* 23:707, 1996.
2. Adamson TC et al: Hand and wrist arthropathies of hemochromatosis and calcium pyrophosphate deposition disease: distinct radiographic features, *Radiology* 147:377, 1983.
3. Assouline-Dayan Y et al: Pathogenesis and natural history of osteonecrosis, *Semin Arthritis Rheum* 32:94, 2002.
4. Baker D: Roentgen manifestations of Cooley's anemia, *Ann NY Acad Sci* 119:641, 1964.
5. Barr M, Anderson M: The knee: bone marrow abnormalities, *Radiol Clin North Am* 40:1109, 2002.
6. Bennet O, Namnyak S: Bone and joint manifestations of sickle cell anemia, *J Bone Joint Surg Br* 72:494, 1990.
7. Benz G, Brandeis W, Wilich E: Radiological aspects of leukemia in childhood: an analysis of 89 children, *Rediatr Radiol* 4:201, 1976.

8. Bonnarenz F, Hernandez A, D'Ambrosia R: Bone scintigraphic changes in osteonecrosis of the femoral head, *Orthop Clin North Am* 16:697, 1985.

9. Childs J: Sickle cell disease: the clinical manifestations, *J Am Osteopath Assoc* 95:593, 1995.

10. Crues R: Osteonecrosis of bone: current concepts as to etiology and pathogenesis, *Clin Orthop* 208:30, 1986.

11. Cushner M, Friedman R: Osteonecrosis of the humeral head, *J Am Acad Orthop Surg* 5:339; 1997.

12. De Backer A et al: The body packer syndrome, *JBR-BTR* 85: 312, 2002.

13. El Bahri-Ben Mrad F et al: A new case report of spinal cord compression secondary to beta thalassemia, *Rev Neurol* 159:574, 2003.

14. Gaston M: Sickle cell disease: an overview, *Semin Roentgenol* 22:150, 1987.

15. Gebhard K, Maibach H: Relationship between systemic corticosteroids and osteonecrosis, *Am J Clin Dermatol* 2:377, 2001.

16. Gilbert M: Characterizing the hemophilic pseudotumor, *Ann NY Acad Sci* 240:311, 1975.

17. Gillespy T, Genant H, Helms C: Magnetic resonance imaging of osteonecrosis, *Radiol Clin North Am* 24:193, 1986.

18. Hash R: Hereditary hemochromatosis, *J Am Board Fam Pract* 14:266, 2001.

19. Hungerford D, Lennox D: The importance of increased intraosseous pressure in the development of osteonecrosis of the femoral head: implications for treatment, *Orthop Clin North Am* 16:635, 1985.

20. Jager H et al: Radiological features of the visceral and skeletal involvement of hemochromatosis, *Eur Radiol* 7:1199, 1997.

21. Kenzora J, Glimcher M: Pathogenesis of idiopathic osteonecrosis: the ubicuitous crescent sign, *Orthop Clin North Am* 16:681, 1985.

22. Kim H et al: Differentiation of bone and bone marrow infarcts from osteomyelitis in sickle cell disorders, *Clin Nucl Med* 14:249, 1989.

23. Kohli M et al: Use of the HFE mutation analysis for hereditary hemochromatosis: the need for physician education in the translation of basic science to clinical practice, *South Med J* 93:469, 2000.

24. Madan S, Fernandes J, Taylor J: Radiological remodeling of the acetabulum in Perthes disease, *Acta Orthop Belg* 69:412, 2003.

25. Milner P, Kraus S, Sebes J: Osteonecrosis of the humeral head in sickle-cell disease, *Clin Orthop* 289:136, 1993.

26. Nelson D et al: Trabecular and integral bone density in adults with sickle cell disease, *J Clin Denistom* 6:125, 2003.

27. Ooi G et al: Radiologic manifestations of granulocytic sarcoma in adult leukemia, *AJR: Am J Roentgenol* 176:1427, 2001.

28. Orzincolo C et al: Circumscribed lytic lesions of the thalassemia skull, *Skeletal Radiol* 17:344, 1988.

29. Pavelka K: Osteonecrosis, *Baillieres Best Pract Res Clin Rheumatol* 14:399, 2000.

30. Pomeranz S et al: Granulocytic sarcoma (chloroma): CT manifestations, *Radiology* 155:167, 1985.

31. Rao V et al: Painful sickle cell crisis: bone marrow patterns observed with MR imaging, *Radiology* 161:211, 1986.

32. Reed M: Pediatric skeletal radiology, Baltimore, 1992, Williams & Wilkins.

33. Reynolds J: Sickle cell disease: the skull and spine, *Semin Roentgenol* 22:168, 1987.

34. Rodriguez-Merchan E: Haemophilic cysts (pseudotumours), *Haemophilia* 8:393, 2002.

35. Stein H, Duthie R: The pathogenesis of chronic hemophilic arthropathy, *J Bone Joint Surg Br* 63:601, 1981.

36. Sutton C et al: Pelvic extramedullary haematopoiesis associated with hereditary spherocytosis, *Eur J Haematol* 70:326, 2003.

37. Tamary H et al: High incidence of early cholelithiasis detected by ultrasonography in children and young adults with hereditary spherocytosis, *J Pediatr Hematol Oncol* 25:952, 2003.

38. Toby E, Kiman L, Bechtold R: Magnetic resonance imaging of pediatric hip disease, *J Pediatr Orthop* 5:665, 1985.

39. Vande Berg B et al: Fat conversion of femoral marrow in glucocorticoid treated patients: a cross sectional and longitudinal study with magnetic resonance imaging, *Arthritis Rheum* 42:1405, 2001.

40. Velasco F et al: Meningioma-like intracranial granulocytic sarcoma (chloromas), radiologic and surgical findings, *Rev Invest Clin* 45:473, 1993.

chapter 12

Infections

D. ROBERT KUHN

NONSUPPURATIVE INFECTIONS
Blastomycosis
Coccidioidomycosis
Maduromycosis (Mycetoma or
 Eumycetoma)
Syphilis
Tuberculosis

SUPPURATIVE INFECTIONS
Brodie's Abscess
Septic Arthritis
Suppurative Osteomyelitis

Nonsuppurative Infections

Blastomycosis

BACKGROUND

Blastomycosis, also called *Gilchrist disease* or *North American blastomycosis,* is produced by the fungus *Blastomyces dermatitidis.*[1,13] *B. dermatitidis* is inhaled by the patient into the lungs and causes pneumonitis.[13,40] Although blastomycosis affects immunocompromised individuals, it can affect healthy individuals as well. Hematogenous spread may lead to involvement of the skin and osseous structures. The disease also can cause the patient to develop asymptomatic bone lesions.

Blastomycosis is endemic to the central and Great Lakes regions and the Ohio and Mississippi River valleys[46] of the United States and to regions of Canada.[1] African Americans and Native Americans are more commonly affected than whites.[46] Men are affected more often than women, with the ratio of men to women ranging from 4:1 to 15:1.[46] Infections often develop in people who have contact with soil, work outside, or frequently engage in outdoor activities[13,32,46]; some cases of human–human infection transmission have been noted. Blastomycosis develops less frequently than other dimorphic fungi infections in immunocompromised individuals.[13]

IMAGING FINDINGS

Skeletal infections develop in up to 60% of blastomycosis cases, representing 25% of the extrapulmonary infections.[1,13] Bone is the third most commonly infected site after the pulmonary system and skin[32]; in some cases the disease may spread to the prostate.[13] The vertebral bodies, ribs, and skull are the most commonly affected bones. Features of blastomycosis bone invasion include eccentric, well-circumscribed lesions that cause no significant periosteal reactions and have little cortical penetration.[32] Punched-out lesions occasionally are reported, but sequestration rarely occurs.[32] Whereas the vertebrae may be significantly damaged, the intervertebral discs may be spared. The infection may spread along the anterior longitudinal ligament and skip a vertebral level—a feature that also is associated with tuberculosis.[46]

Blastomycosis joint involvement usually is monoarticular; however, polyarticular presentations may be seen. Systemic or pulmonary disease may develop concurrently.[13] The knee is most commonly infected, followed by the ankle, elbow, wrist, and hand.[1,13] In some cases, blastomycosis presents as a soft-tissue mass that is solid, has punctate calcifications, and is similar to a synovial cell sarcoma.[1] A soft-tissue neoplasm cannot be differentiated from this fungal lesion by plain film radiography.[3,46] In addition, neither ultrasound, magnetic resonance imaging (MRI), nor bone scanning can properly diagnose blastomycosis. Accurate diagnosis is based on a combination of radiographic localization, biopsy, and culture.[32]

CLINICAL COMMENTS

Signs and symptoms of blastomycosis include subclinical infections and signs and symptoms that are similar to those of acute histoplasmosis. Typical features include joint and muscle pain, a productive cough, and chest pain that resolves spontaneously.[13] Other signs and symptoms include fever, weight loss, night sweats, and pleuritic pain.[40] Patients with blastomycosis who have essentially normal laboratory profiles (e.g., normal complete blood count [CBC], erythrocyte sedimentation rate [ESR], and differential count) may have draining ulcers.[46] In certain cases the hematocrit values may indicate the presence of chronic infection. No skin test exists for blastomycosis—biopsy and culture are the keys to the diagnosis. Silver methenamine is used to detect the fungus. The culture may take 1 to 2 weeks to grow. Historically, mortality rates in treated patients in whom the disease had disseminated were as high as 23%.[46] Patients with untreated disease have an 80% mortality rate.[1]

Treatment protocols for blastomycosis include débridement and administration of oral imidazole, ketoconazole, itraconazole, or amphotericin B. A 6-month course of treatment is typical. Patients who are prescribed amphotericin B must be closely monitored[1]; side effects include anorexia, nausea and vomiting, fever with chills, anemia, and nephrotoxicity. In spite of the numerous side effects, the benefits of using amphotericin B outweigh the risks.

KEY CONCEPTS

- *Blastomycosis is produced by the fungus Blastomyces dermatitidis.*
- *The fungus is inhaled by the patient and produces pneumonitis.*
- *Hematogenous transport is the likely means by which the infection is disseminated to the skin and osseous structures.*
- *It is endemic to the central and Great Lakes regions of the United States, the Ohio and Mississippi River valleys, and Canada.*
- *Radiographic features include a geographic region of lytic destruction and in some cases punched-out lesions.*
- *The vertebrae may be severely damaged even when the discs are not.*
- *The infection may skip a vertebral level and involve an adjacent segment.*
- *Radiographic localization followed by biopsy and culture are the most accurate methods of diagnosis.*
- *Clinical features include joint and muscle pain, a productive cough, and chest pain that resolves spontaneously.*

Coccidioidomycosis

BACKGROUND

Coccidioidomycosis, which is also called *valley fever* and *desert rheumatism,*[4,51] is a systemic infection caused by the soil fungus *Coccidioides immitis.* It is endemic to the southwestern United States, San Joaquin Valley, Mexico, and regions of Central and South America.* The fungus spores typically are inhaled into the lungs, which are the primary site of infection.[39,59] Many patients have mild or no symptoms, so the infection is found incidentally.[26]

Individuals who are older than 65 years of age or have acquired immunodeficiency syndrome (AIDS) are the primary populations at risk of becoming infected.[39] Other individuals at risk are those being treated with steroids or chemotherapy. Some evidence suggests that individuals may be genetically predisposed to contracting the infection.[24] Although dissemination is rare, an increased risk for spread of the disease exists among Filipinos, blacks, Mexicans, pregnant women, children younger than 5 years of age, adults older than 50 years of age, and immunosuppressed individuals.[13,59] The skin and subcutaneous tissues are the most common sites of dissemination from pulmonary disease. The next most common site is the mediastinum, followed by the skeletal system.[59] The incidence of coccidioidomycosis has dramatically increased since 1991.[24] Currently 50,000 patients a year are diagnosed with the infection.[13]

IMAGING FINDINGS

Skeletal lesions are seen in 10% to 50% of the cases in which the disease has spread. Coccidioidomycosis may affect multiple sites, producing osteolytic lesions in cancellous and cortical bone and soft-tissue swelling. A periosteal reaction is possible but uncommon.[13,24,59] Previously, bony prominences were considered common sites for coccidioidomycosis infection. More recent studies have failed to document this association and have found that involvement of the axial skeletal is more common.[13,26] In the appendicular skeleton the ankles and knees are more frequently affected; remission occurs in 2 to 4 weeks, and no residual damage remains.[13]

Plain film radiography may not detect infection during the initial stages. Findings of decreased joint space and areas of localized osteopenia may be early signs.[13,26] Ankylosis can be an end result of joint infection.[13] A bone scan is sensitive and typically can

detect the infection in the early stages.[26,59] MRI may demonstrate a large, poorly marginated mass with an intermediate signal and lower central signal. MRI also typically demonstrates a decreased signal on T1-weighted images and an increased signal on T2-weighted images, together a sign of abscess or necrosis.[33] MRI and computed tomography (CT) are useful for detection and surgical planning.[35] A positive bone scan should be followed by CT or MRI. A decreased disc space and gibbous formation may be seen, but are much less common than they are in patients with tuberculosis.[59] CT demonstrates low-attenuation lesions that may appear bubbly and expansile.[59]

Septic arthritis secondary to coccidioidomycosis may develop and is usually seen as: (a) synovitis with joint effusion, (b) periarticular bone destruction similar to that in patients with tuberculosis or neuropathic joints, and (c) well-defined periarticular erosions resembling pigmented villonodular synovitis. Periosteal reactions typically are associated with a permeative destructive pattern.[59] Soft-tissue swelling and osteoporosis also may be seen in conjunction with permeative destructive lesions. A periosteal reaction is not commonly associated with punched-out lesions. Some lesions demonstrate a thin, sclerotic margin surrounding the area of bone involvement that indicates reactive sclerosis.[47]

CLINICAL COMMENTS

Coccidioidomycosis infection of bone and joints is uncommon; therefore it is frequently overlooked as an initial diagnostic option, resulting in frequent delays in diagnosis.[26] The clinical presentation may closely mimic that of tuberculosis.[5] Two thirds of the patients recover uneventfully and may be asymptomatic throughout the course of their infection. One third develops symptoms that usually include a self-limiting pneumonitis caused by the inhaled air-borne spores. Of those, 40% of patients present with the symptoms within 2 to 3 weeks of exposure. The signs and symptoms reported by 80% of the infected patients are fatigue, coughing, night sweats, and fever, a presentation that can significantly resemble the flu.[51] Pneumonia that does not respond to antibiotics may be part of an infected patient's history.[24] Other signs and symptoms are a general achiness, sore throat, peripheral eosinophilia, erythema nodosum, and erythema multiform.[13] If arthralgia develops it is usually polyarticular and migratory; tenderness and pain are common when the affected joint is moved through its range of motion, but effusion is not typical.[13] In approximately 1% of the cases the disease spreads to the skin, bones, joints, lymph nodes, and in rare cases the central nervous system.[13,24,26,38] Spread of the disease has been reported to occur months to years after the primary infection.[13]

A brief visit to an area in which coccidioidomycosis is endemic is all that is needed to contract the infection. In one study, 24 out of 25 patients with symptomatic coccidioidomycosis lived in endemic regions or were immunocompromised.[26] Exposure and subsequent infection can begin insidiously.

An effective skin test can be used to detect previous coccidioidomycosis infection.[24] A definitive diagnosis of an emerging case of coccidioidomycosis requires biopsy and culture.[26] A tissue biopsy of an infected individual contains necrotic debris composed of polymorphonuclear leukocytes and often Langerhans cells. A culture takes 2 to 5 days to yield results. A microscopic examination is quicker but less sensitive.[26] Methenamine silver is used during the laboratory examination to blacken the capsules of spherical fungi such as *Coccidioides.*[5,24] Laboratory findings may include elevations in the white blood cell (WBC) count and ESR, but these results are not consistent.[26]

---

*References 4, 6, 24, 28, 53, 59.

Surgical débridement is mandatory once the diagnosis of coccidioidomycosis in osseous or joint structures is made.[26] Itraconazole is slow but effective, and fluconazole was found to be effective in nonmeningeal coccidioidomycosis. Amphotericin B should be reserved for severe infections with skeletal involvement.[13] Open drainage, synovectomy, arthrodesis, and sometimes amputation are reserved for later stages of severe cases. If a timely diagnosis is made and proper treatment is instituted, patients with coccidioidomycosis have excellent outcomes, although fatalities do occur in rare instances of treated individuals.[26]

> **KEY CONCEPTS**
> - *Coccidioidomycosis, also called valley fever or desert rheumatism, is caused by the fungus Coccidioides immitis.*
> - *Individuals at risk are individuals older than 65 years of age or who have AIDS.*
> - *Many patients demonstrate no symptoms and signs; the infection is found incidentally.*
> - *When the disease spreads, it most commonly affects the skin, subcutaneous tissues, mediastinum, and skeleton.*
> - *Plain film radiography often does not detect the early stages of infection but does reliably demonstrate the later changes of decreased joint space and osteopenia.*
> - *Performing a tissue biopsy and staining biologic samples with silver methenamine are diagnostic methods.*
> - *Early diagnosis and treatment are associated with excellent outcomes.*

Maduromycosis (Mycetoma or Eumycetoma)

BACKGROUND

Maduromycosis was first discovered in Madura, India, some time between 1842 and 1846.[47] It predominantly affects the feet,[30,43] which are infected by a penetrating trauma.[53] Eumycetoma is a disease that is usually found in the tropics; only a few cases have been reported in temperate climates.[30,44] The organism that causes the disease has been isolated in soil and on thorns, the most likely sources of infection. Mycetoma is produced by a number of organisms that are distributed in two distinct groups:[12] eumycetes, or true fungi, and actinomycetes, or false fungi, which is a filamentous bacteria. The organism that is usually responsible for maduromycosis in the United States and Canada is *Petriellidum boydii;* in Africa and India, it is *Madurella mycetomi;* in Mexico, it is *Nocardia brasiliensis,* and in Japan, it is *Nocardia asteroides.*[12] Maduromycosis is rare in the United States; it is slightly more common in Mexico, Guatemala, and other parts of South America.[43] Because pharmacologic treatments are frequently unsuccessful, surgical resection or amputation is often necessary.[4]

IMAGING FINDINGS

Radiographic characteristics of maduromycosis include mottled osseous destructive patterns with a periosteal reaction[12,43] and marked soft-tissue swelling, often resulting in permanent deformities.[43] When the periosteum is breached, a laminated, or spiculated, periosteal reaction typically is seen. The cortex often is eroded. Eumycotic lesions tend to be fewer in number and produce larger bone cavities that are greater than 1 cm, and a periosteal reaction occurs in about 50% of cases.[30] Actinomycetes produce more numerous, smaller lesions, and a periosteal reaction is seen in approximately 75% of cases.[30] In all cases, a soft-tissue mass is seen.

The sequestrum associated with other types of osteomyelitis is not a feature of maduromycosis.[12] Loss of cortical margins followed by erosion and adjacent sclerosis is more typical. If the infection develops near a joint, the cartilage is typically spared; however, ankylosis may develop as an end result of this process.[12] Osteopenia is rare, possibly because patients can walk on even a severely infected foot, evidence that this type of infection typically is painless.[30]

CLINICAL COMMENTS

General signs and symptoms of maduromycosis include the presence of multiple, crusted nodules surrounded by hyperpigmented tissue. The common clinical triad consists of a sinus track, granules (colonies), and nodular enlargements of infected body parts.[43] Hematologic laboratory values usually are normal. Patients with maduromycosis often have long histories associated with the development of the disease; one documented case lasted for 18 years.[43]

The disease is almost painless, and few constitutional symptoms are seen unless a secondary infection has developed.[44] The bacteria initially invade soft tissue around superficial and deep fascia. The first sign typically is a small bump; the foot then becomes swollen (but not painful).[12] The affected limb becomes deformed as a result of microbial colonies forming grains and intercommunicating sinuses that may drain onto the skin's surface.[30] The grains extrude and form colonies that vary in color according to the infecting species.[30] The lesion is usually confined to the soft tissues for years before bone infection occurs.[30] When the disease breaks into the bone in the much later stages, it is usually painless. Hematogenous spread is rare.[12]

An antimicrobial treatment may be sufficient while the infection is limited to the soft tissues.[30] Once the bones are involved, a cure may be impossible and amputation may be necessary, although it is considered to be a last resort.[12,30] Differentiation between eumycetoma and an actinomycetoma is important because the most effective treatments for each type are different.[44] Some actinomycetomas respond to high doses and long-term usage of antibiotics.[12] In particular, *Nocardia* organisms seem to be sensitive to some of the sulfonamides. Use of solely surgical débridement and resection rarely cures the infection. Some recent progress has been made using itraconazole for 6 months.[43]

> **KEY CONCEPTS**
> - *Maduromycosis is the most common fungal infection worldwide.*
> - *The organism that causes the infection has been isolated in soil and on thorns, the typical sources of infection.*
> - *The feet usually are involved.*
> - *Painless soft-tissue swelling is one of the early findings.*
> - *A painless swollen foot often reveals sinus tract formation and extrusion of grain colonies, with various colors depicting the primary infecting species.*
> - *Treatment consists of antimicrobial agents and amputation.*

Syphilis

BACKGROUND

Syphilis is a chronic systemic infection caused by the spirochete *Treponema pallidum.*[45] Infections are capable of involving any organ or tissue and are classified as either congenital or acquired.[41] Congenital syphilis is contracted by transplacental exposure of the fetus to the infection after about the fourth month of pregnancy. It is categorized into early and late presentations. Early congenital syphilis is diagnosed in children who are younger than 2 years of age, whereas late congenital syphilis is diagnosed in children who are 2 years and older.[41] Acquired syphilis is contracted by close physical (usually sexual) contact with an infected individual's skin lesions or mucous membranes. The disease initially develops as a chancre with local lymphadenopathy. The infection progresses over a period of several months and becomes systemic, or secondary, syphilis. After a latent period of 5 to 15 years, the disease progresses to the tertiary stage, which is characterized by gumma formation. Gummas are rubbery, soft, destructive lesions of various sizes that contain necrotic caseous material and affect bone, skin, viscera, the central nervous system, and other organs and tissues.

Although the incidence of syphilis decreased for many years after World War II, it increased through the 1970s and 1980s and peaked in 1988.[9,20] It has been on the decline since 1997. The increase in the number of congenital syphilis cases has been attributed to an associated rise in the number of women with syphilis who subsequently became pregnant but did not receive adequate prenatal care.[9] Drug addiction also has been associated with the increase, because individuals who abuse drugs have impaired immune systems and are less likely to take protective measures against sexually transmitted diseases while engaging in sexual activity.[20] A clear association has been described between the use of crack cocaine and an increased incidence of syphilis.[20] It was reported in 1988 that congenital syphilis had reached its highest levels since widespread use of penicillin began.[45] The increase is particularly high among homosexual men. Many cases of congenital and especially acquired syphilis are never reported. It is likely that morbidity and mortality figures for both varieties are underestimated.[45]

Yaws is caused by another species of *Treponema, Treponema pertenue,* which is very similar to *T. pallidum.* Yaws primarily develops in children, is an acquired disease through direct contact, but is rarely transmitted sexually. The radiographic findings are similar to those of syphilis, but symptoms tend to be more severe.

IMAGING FINDINGS
Congenital syphilis
Early. Some radiographic evidence of the disease usually can be obtained from most symptomatic newborns with syphilis.[9] Early manifestations of congenital syphilis include osteochondritis or metaphysitis, periostitis, and diaphyseal osteitis. Polyostotic, symmetric bone involvement is characteristic of congenital syphilis.[18,41,48,56] The long bones, pelvis, vertebrae, and small tubular bones are involved.[18]

The first stage of osteochondritis, or metaphysitis, leads to fragmentation of the metaphysis, with transverse lucencies arising subjacent to the epiphyseal plate (Fig. 12-1). Invading granulation tissue is responsible for the metaphysitis[48] and is particularly common around the large joints, knees, shoulders, and elbows. Horizontal radiolucent metaphyseal bands are seen in the early stages of the disease. The ossification of the epiphyseal cartilage may be impeded, and a zone of rarefaction may be present at the epiphyseal line, indicating the presence of syphilitic granulation tissue.[55] This tissue can weaken the bone and cause a pathologic fracture. Metaphyseal abnormalities are seen in more than 90% of infants with symptomatic congenital syphilis.[9] The most common radiographic finding in patients with congenital syphilis is lucent metaphyseal bands.[20]

Metaphysitis results in erosive bone destruction, producing a characteristic sawtooth pattern of bone destruction. Although the

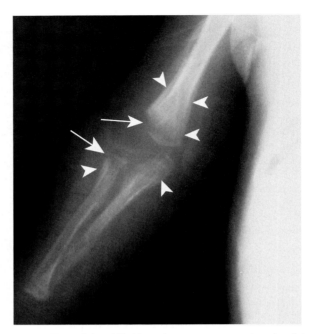

FIG. 12-1 Congenital syphilis. Note the transverse metaphyseal radiolucent band *(arrows)* and solid periostitis along the metadiaphyseal shaft of the humerus, ulna, and radius *(arrowheads).* (Courtesy Gary M. Guebert, Maryland Heights, MO.)

sawtooth appearance of the metaphyseal margin is characteristic, it is generally uncommon.[41] Radiographic examination of the destructive pattern of metaphysitis (which follows longitudinal bone growth) may reveal streaking radiolucent bands extending centrally from the physis, an appearance that resembles a celery stalk. Destructive metaphysitis is particularly common along the medial margin of the proximal tibia, a finding known as Wimberger's sign (Fig. 12-2).[41] Although this sign is a characteristic of syphilis, it is not pathognomonic.

The second stage of early congenital syphilis is marked by bilateral, symmetric, diffuse periostitis that affects the long tubular bones but usually spares the short tubular bones of the hands and feet.[6,41,56] Although it is less common, a third stage may develop that exhibits radiolucent long bone defects consistent with osteitis. Osteitis is commonly associated with a diffuse region of the diaphysis that has a moth-eaten appearance.[41] These changes can occur in any bone, but the femur and humerus are most commonly affected.[56] Reparative periostitis during this phase may produce prolific changes along the anterior margin of the tibia, creating a saber shin deformity.

Late. Late manifestations of congenital syphilis include destruction of and periostitis in the tibia, skull, jaw, nose, maxilla, and other superficial osseous structures. These changes are noted in patients in their late teens or early twenties. Periostitis is most pronounced along the anterior surface of the tibia bilaterally, creating a saber shin deformity. The destructive changes result from osteomyelitis, which may be associated with gumma formations. *Clutton's joints* refer to the joints that undergo the particular pattern of destruction. The abnormally peg-shaped teeth secondary to syphilis are known as *Hutchinson's teeth.*

Acquired syphilis. Radiographic findings are mostly confined to the tertiary stages of acquired syphilis. Less than 10% of

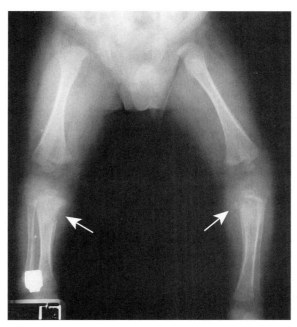

FIG. 12-2 Congenital syphilis. Bilateral periosteal reaction with medial, proximal erosion of the tibia known as Wimberger's sign *(arrows)*. (Courtesy Gary M. Guebert, Maryland Heights, MO.)

patients with acquired syphilis ever develop an osseous lesion. The changes that do occur mimic those associated with late congenital syphilis. The most pronounced radiographic findings consist of proliferative and destructive changes affecting superficial osseous structures, particularly the tibia, clavicle, jaw, maxilla, and skull. It is extremely uncommon to encounter disseminated skeletal lesions in either infants or adults, and it is particularly rare to encounter them in patients who live in developed countries.[55] The proliferative changes manifest as prolific periostitis that is especially prominent along the anterior surface of the tibia, producing bilateral anterior bowing or a saber shin deformity. Destructive changes are secondary to gumma formations that most commonly appear in the skull, nose, and diaphysis of long bones.

CLINICAL COMMENTS

Congenital syphilis should be suspected in a newborn whose mother has positive serologic evidence of syphilis and is receiving inadequate or no treatment.[20] Anemia, hepatosplenomegaly, skin lesions, and rhinitis are the predominant signs and symptoms of affected newborns. Some infants also have gastroenteritis, bronchopneumonia, septicemia, meningitis, pseudoparalysis, and joint swelling. A small number of children may have polydactylism, pathologic fractures, and signs and symptoms mimicking brachial plexus lesions.[41] Thermal instability, mucocutaneous lesions, snuffles, hepatosplenomegaly, adenopathy, anemia, hydrops fetalis, pathological jaundice, and pseudoparalysis are consistent with syphilis.[9]

Babies with congenital syphilis are four times more likely to have low birth weights than babies without syphilis. Approximately 62% of patients with congenital syphilis are symptomatic at birth.[48] Microhemagglutination tests usually are used to make a diagnosis,[20] but patients who have none of the typical gummatous lesions or spirochetes are diagnosed by exclusion.[55] The periostitis

and osteochondritis seen are often self-limiting and usually heal within a few months even with no treatment.[56]

> **KEY CONCEPTS**
> - *The organism associated with syphilis is* Treponema pallidum.
> - *The highest rate of increase is in drug-addicted individuals.*
> - *There are two forms of syphilis, congenital and acquired.*
> - *Congenital syphilis is divided into early and late categories.*
> - *Radiographic signs of congenital syphilis include metaphysis fragmentation and transverse lucencies subjacent to the epiphyseal plate; the most common radiographic finding is bilateral symmetric periostitis.*
> - *The osteitis stage may produce the classic saber shin deformity.*
> - *Congenital syphilis should be suspected in any newborn whose mother has positive serologic evidence of syphilis.*
> - *Chronic signs and symptoms of congenital syphilis include anemia, hepatosplenomegaly, skin lesions, and rhinitis.*
> - *Infants born with syphilis are four times more likely to have low birth weights.*
> - *Microhemagglutination tests are fundamental to the diagnosis.*
> - *The neurotrophic disease associated with syphilis is secondary to the damage done to the nervous system.*

Tuberculosis

BACKGROUND

Mycobacterium tuberculosis, Mycobacterium bovis, and *Mycobacterium africanum* are all capable of producing tuberculosis in humans.[20] The infection is spread almost exclusively by human–human air-borne transmission, and the lungs are its primary target.[19]

Tuberculosis has been a documented human disease for centuries. Hippocrates described features consistent with tuberculosis as early as 450 BC, and typical characteristics were seen in a mummy whose remains dated 3000 BC. After a long period of decline, the incidence of tuberculosis has been increasing since 1985, with its current rate being 14% in the United States.[48,58] The largest increase has been among Hispanics and African Americans.[45]

Several factors are related to the increased incidence, including the human immunodeficiency virus (HIV) epidemic and introduction of tuberculosis cases of a foreign origin.[45] The cities with the highest incidences of AIDS have had a concomitant increase in the incidence of tuberculosis. The incidence of tuberculosis infection in AIDS patients is 500 times the incidence in the general population.[58] In the late 1980s and early 1990s, 60% of tuberculosis cases were of a foreign origin. Some evidence suggests that the number of foreign tuberculosis cases is beginning to decline.[58]

Skeletal tuberculosis develops in 1% to 3% of all patients with tuberculosis and comprises about 10% of all extrapulmonary forms reported.[46] Skeletal tuberculosis is slightly more common in females than males. All races are affected equally, but a higher incidence has been found among adults living in developed countries.[46] In less developed countries, all ages are equally affected.[2]

IMAGING FINDINGS

Despite its nonspecific findings, plain film radiography is the best initial imaging modality for detecting tuberculosis.[58] Tuberculosis can involve any of the bones or joints but is often confined to one location. In long bones, it begins in the epiphysis and results in a secondary infection of the trabeculae. As the infected mass

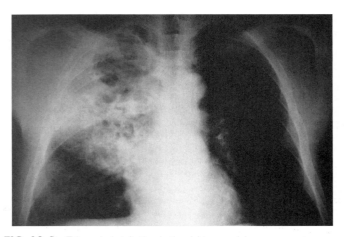

FIG. 12-3 Tuberculosis infection in the right upper lobe.

enlarges, the trabecular fibers are resorbed and tuberculosis granulation tissue is formed.[58] Over time caseation and liquefaction may develop and produce an abscess cavity containing pus and bone fragments.

Skeletal tuberculosis is secondary to hematogenous dissemination from a lesion that is usually pulmonary in origin. The lung lesion often is located in the upper or apical regions (Fig. 12-3). The spine is affected in 50% of cases (Fig. 12-4), the hip in 15%, and the knee in 15%.[21] Various bones are affected in the remaining 20% of the cases (Figs. 12-5 and 12-6).[58] Joint involvement is similar to the pattern associated with septic arthritis of causes other

than tuberculosis. However, the following triad (Phemister's triad) of findings historically have suggested tubercular arthritis:[42]
1. Juxtaarticular osteoporosis
2. Peripherally located osseous erosions
3. Gradually narrowing joint space

In cases involving the spine the anterior portion of the vertebral body is the most commonly affected region.[31] The most common spinal joint affected is the intervertebral disc.[6] Tuberculosis osteomyelitis in the thoracic or thoracolumbar region can produce an angular kyphosis called a *gibbous formation* (Fig. 12-7).[6] The average value of the gibbous angle is 113 degrees, as compared with normal kyphotic angles of 20 to 40 degrees (depending on the patient's age).[52] A characteristic paraspinal cold abscess develops as a result of slow development and little inflammation.[6] Healed paraspinal abscesses may calcify, making them readily visible on plain film (Fig. 12-8). If the cervical spine is involved, the soft-tissue mass that forms may become large enough to produce dysphagia.

In the majority of cases the lesion spreads and produces an inflammatory reaction that is followed by granulation tissue (pannus) formation (Fig. 12-9). Subligamentous spread of tuberculosis produces scalloping of the vertebral bodies. An effusion can develop, and rice bodies or fibrin precipitates may be seen. The pannus then erodes and destroys cartilage, eventually affecting the underlying bone and leading to progressive, local demineralization. The cartilage is destroyed peripherally, so relatively normal joint spaces can remain for a period of time.[58]

CLINICAL COMMENTS
The most remarkable clinical feature of tuberculosis sometimes can be its lack of symptoms. When the presenting signs and symptoms

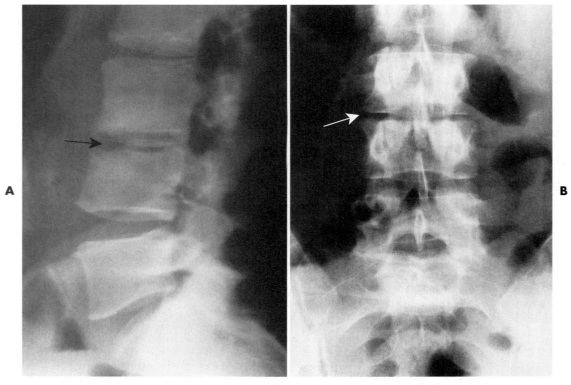

FIG. 12-4 Tuberculosis spondylitis (Pott's disease) with intervertebral disc involvement. Shown are the typical features of disc space narrowing (*arrows*) and endplate destruction on, **A,** the lateral and, **B,** frontal radiographs.

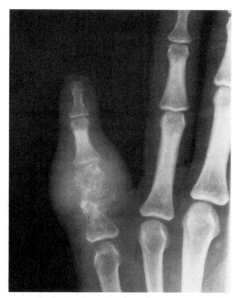

FIG. 12-5 Tuberculosis dactylitis (spina ventosa) demonstrating an expanded proximal phalanx of the fifth digit with marked surrounding soft-tissue enlargement.

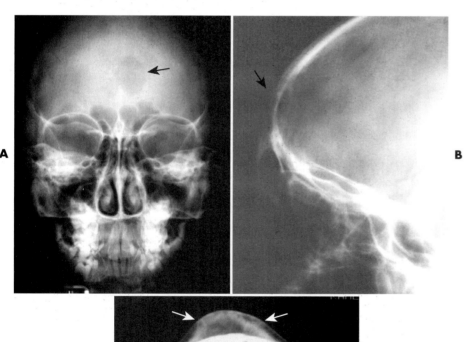

FIG. 12-6 **A** and **B,** Tuberculosis of the frontal bone (Pott's puffy tumor) seen in radiographs and, **C,** computed tomography *(arrows).* (Courtesy Ronnie Firth, East Moline, IL.)

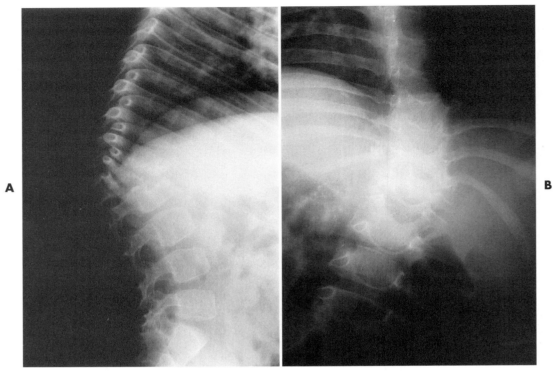

FIG. 12-7   **A,** Gibbous formation. Marked vertebral destruction, **A** and **B,** followed by formation of this angular deformity is a hallmark. Compressive myelopathy may result in Pott's paraplegia. (Courtesy Gary M. Guebert, Maryland Heights, MO.)

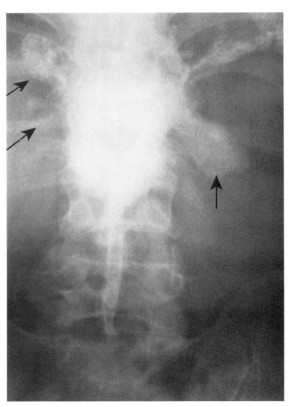

FIG. 12-8   Cold abscess. Healed paraspinal abscess in the thoracolumbar region *(arrows).*

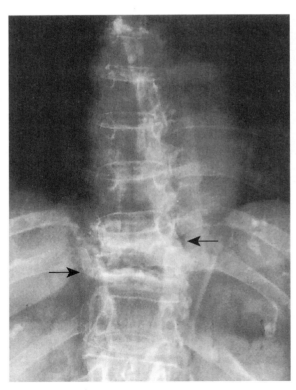

FIG. 12-9   An anteroposterior view of the thoracolumbar junction in a patient with a known paraspinal tuberculosis abscess. Note the loss of height of the T10 and T11 vertebral bodies, as well as the marked bony sclerosis *(arrows).* These findings suggest a relatively chronic destructive process.

of tuberculosis are insidious, diagnosis often is delayed. Associated drug addiction or chronic alcoholism also may delay diagnosis.[45] When symptoms are present, they are nonspecific and include anorexia, weight loss, night sweats, and fever.[2,58] Pulmonary complaints become more prominent as the disease progresses.[2] A small percentage of patients have extrapulmonary symptoms such as back pain. Tenderness may develop in the affected bones and joints,[2] and stiffness and a change in range of motion may be noted.

The tuberculosis skin test is positive in 90% to 100% of non-anergic patients.[2,58] Chest radiographs show some evidence of previous or active pulmonary tuberculosis in approximately 50% of cases. Definitive diagnosis depends on bone biopsies and synovial fluid cultures. Bone biopsies are 90% sensitive to tuberculosis, whereas synovial fluid cultures are 95% sensitive.[58]

Without proper treatment, tuberculosis can produce a cold abscess in surrounding tissues.[58] Fibrous or osseous ankylosis of the joint may occur as healing takes place.[15] Once an accurate diagnosis has been made, treatment must begin as soon as possible to be effective. Treatment durations typically are between 9 and 12 months; in some cases surgery may be used to débride or repair the deformity.[58] Acquired drug resistance can be caused by unsuccessful therapy, a situation that usually arises because therapy is inadequate or a patient is not compliant.[28] Forms of tuberculosis

that are resistant to multiple drugs are significant concerns because they increase the risk of mortality.[45]

KEY CONCEPTS

- *Skeletal tuberculosis is a relatively uncommon indolent infection that develops secondary to hematogenous spread of pulmonary infections.*
- *Disseminated osteomyelitis involving the skeleton affects the spine in 50% of cases, hip in 15%, and knee in 15%. Various other bones are affected in the remaining 20% of cases.*
- *Tubercular osteomyelitis may be surrounded by prominent abscess formation. Young children and debilitated elderly patients usually account for the bulk of tuberculosis cases.*
- *The most remarkable clinical feature of tuberculosis can be its lack of symptoms.*
- *Symptoms are not specific and include anorexia, weight loss, night sweats, and afternoon fevers.*
- *As the disease progresses, pulmonary complaints increase.*
- *Definitive diagnosis of tuberculosis involving osseous structures depends on synovial samples or bone biopsy and culture.*
- *Once tuberculosis is diagnosed, treatment must begin immediately. Treatments last between 9 and 12 months.*
- *Surgery may be used to débride the wound or repair an acquired deformity.*

■ Suppurative Infections

Brodie's Abscess

BACKGROUND

A Brodie's abscess, or "cystic osteomyelitis," is a distinct presentation of subacute or chronic osteomyelitis. It is believed to result from a lack or inadequate treatment of osteomyelitis.[10,47] The infection is named after Sir Benjamin Brodie's, who in 1832 described localized lesions of tibial metaphyses of children and young adults.[47] *Staphylococcus* organisms are the most common cause of infection.[7] Most affected patients are younger than 25 years of age, and males are slightly more likely than females to become infected.[37]

IMAGING FINDINGS

Imaging studies reveal a Brodie's abscess to be an area of radiolucency surrounded by varying degrees of bone reaction or surrounding sclerosis (Fig. 12-10). The surrounding sclerosis is usually well defined on the inside and less well defined outside. The lesion usually is slightly eccentric, metadiaphyseal, varies in size, and is located in intramedullary bone, but it also affects the cortex (Fig. 12-11).[47] The femur and tibia are the bones most commonly involved.[49]

MRI of a Brodie's abscess reveals well-demarcated lesions with low signal intensity on T1-weighted sequences that brighten on T2-weighted sequences. The sclerotic edge of a Brodie's abscess has a low signal on both T1- and T2-weighted images. Bone marrow edema surrounding the lesion exhibits a poorly defined high signal band on T2-weighted images. The bright/dark/bright appearance on T2-weighted images is known as the *double line sign*, a sign also found in patients with avascular hip necrosis.[15,47] CT reveals a

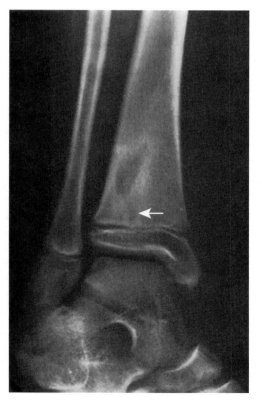

FIG. 12-10 Brodie's abscess. An example of a walled-off or aborted form of suppurative osteomyelitis *(arrow)*. (From Blickman JG: Pediatric radiology: the requisites, St Louis, 1994, Mosby.)

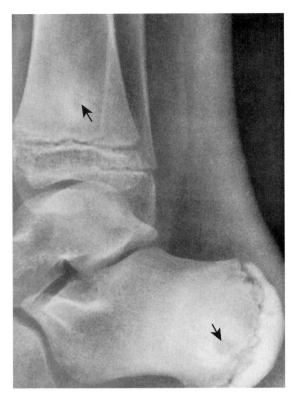

FIG. 12-11   Brodie's abscess in the distal tibia *(upper arrow)* and calcaneus *(lower arrow)*. (From Silverman FN, Kuhn JP: Caffey's pediatric x-ray diagnosis: an integrated imaging approach, ed 9, St Louis, 1993, Mosby.)

region of trabecular destruction of low attenuation surrounded by bone sclerosis.

CLINICAL COMMENTS

Patients with a Brodie's abscess may have no fever or leukocytosis and often have no signs or symptoms whatsoever.[33] One of the symptoms patients may have is an affected limb that is warm to the touch and tender when palpated.[33] Pain is the most common complaint associated with a Brodie's abscess. The pain is often persistent, but it may increase and decrease in severity and often worsens at night. Aspirin may dramatically relieve the pain, making it more difficult to differentiate an osteoid osteoma from a Brodie's abscess based solely on clinical symptoms. Although it is not a characteristic that can be used to definitively distinguish the two, the radiolucent nidus and surrounding sclerosis of a Brodie's abscess are more pronounced than those of an osteoid osteoma. Angiography can be used to confidently distinguish a Brodie's abscess from an osteoid osteoma. Osteoid osteomas demonstrate an opaque vascular blush that is not associated with a Brodie's abscess.

Progressive, nocturnal pains that may waken patients are classic features of a Brodie's abscess.[34] Biopsy and examination of fluid from an abscess may help in its diagnosis, but if the sample is purulent or mucoid, it may be impossible to detect the infective organism.[33] Classic treatment for a Brodie's lesion involves aseptic drainage, curettage, and administration of systemic antibiotics. Three consecutive negative cultures are a sign of resolution.[33]

KEY CONCEPTS

- A Brodie's abscess is caused by subacute or chronic osteomyelitis that has resulted from lack of or inadequate treatment for preexisting osteomyelitis.
- Plain film radiographic evidence of a Brodie's abscess consists of a geographic region of osteopenia surrounded by a rim of sclerosis, with lesions that are typically slightly eccentric, metadiaphyseal, and varied in size.
- The femur and tibia are most commonly involved.
- The most common chief complaint is persistent pain with periods of exacerbation and remission.
- Patients often describe the pain as being worse at night; it may be dramatically alleviated by aspirin (as can the pain caused by osteoid osteomas).
- In some cases the patient may have no fever, evidence of leukocytosis, or any other symptoms.
- The classic treatment for a Brodie's abscess is aseptic drainage, curettage, and administration of systemic antibiotics.

Septic Arthritis

BACKGROUND

Septic arthritis is an articular manifestation of an infection. A joint may become infected as a result of hematogenous dissemination or contiguous spread (e.g., from epiphyseal osteomyelitis) or directly through surgery or trauma. Hematogenous dissemination is the most common means by which the infection spreads. Septic arthritis causes joint damage and disability, with the knee, hip, shoulder, and wrist being common sites. Usually only one joint is involved.

Septic arthritis tends to affect young children and elderly individuals. Although *Staphylococcus aureus* is the most common causative agent, certain populations are predisposed to becoming infected by a particular microbe. For instance, individuals who abuse drugs intravenously are predisposed to *Pseudomonas aeruginosa* infections of the axial skeleton joints.[8] Salmonellae commonly cause septic arthritis in patients with sickle cell disease. However, *S. aureus* is still the most common causative agent in each of these populations overall. Although uncommon, infections in prosthetic joints are devastating, leading to loosening, failure, and advanced derangement of the joints.

IMAGING FINDINGS

Early radiographic findings of patients with joint infection include distention of the joint capsule, soft-tissue swelling, and osteopenia. Intermediate and late changes are marked by the less distinct cortical bone, permeative or moth-eaten bone destruction, loss of joint space, joint derangement, and bony ankylosis. Hip involvement may distend the lateral (gluteus medius), superomedial (obturator internus), or inferomedial (iliopsoas) muscle–fat interfaces. Waldenström's sign may be seen. Waldenström's sign is defined as lateral displacement of the femoral head from the medial wall of the acetabulum (also known as the *teardrop distance*) by more than 11 mm (or >2 mm from the contralateral side) secondary to hip effusion. This finding does not specifically indicate the presence of infection and may be seen in association with other causes of hip effusion (e.g., trauma).[25]

CLINICAL COMMENTS

Joint infections typically cause pain and tenderness, loss of function, and possibly a fever. A high degree of clinical suspicion and proper radiographic evaluation usually lead to the appropriate diagnosis. Administration of antibiotics is the first component of therapy, with surgical débridement, joint replacement, or amputation indicated for advanced or unresponsive disease. Antibiotic selection is based on the patient's age and history and results of a culture. The duration and modification of the antibiotic therapy is based on the patient's response. The duration of the symptoms, age of the patient, and degree of immunocompetence are all important factors that are used to predict the patient's outcome.

> **KEY CONCEPTS**
> * *Septic arthritis is a joint infection that is transmitted directly through surgery or trauma, through contiguous spread, or most commonly through hematogenous dissemination.*
> * *The knee, hip, shoulder, and wrist are the most typically affected sites.*
> * *Young children and elderly individuals are most commonly affected.*
> * *Staphylococcus aureus is the most common infecting organism.*
> * *Radiographic findings include joint space alterations, bone destruction, and, in later stages, ankylosis.*
> * *Conservative management entails antibiotic therapy. In rare cases, amputation may be necessary.*

Suppurative Osteomyelitis

BACKGROUND

Osteomyelitis is an infection of bone and bone marrow. Although it is usually caused by bacteria, it also can be caused by fungi and other microbes.[15] Osteomyelitis is categorized as either suppurative (pyogenic, or pus producing) or nonsuppurative (nonpyogenic, or non–pus producing). Suppurative osteomyelitis is further classified as acute, subacute, or chronic based on its clinical progression.

Region of involvement. Normal bone is generally extremely resistant to infection, which usually develops when a large population of microbes is introduced by trauma or surgery.[29] Although any bone can develop an infection (Fig. 12-12),[50] the bones of the knee (Figs. 12-13 and 12-14), hip, and shoulder

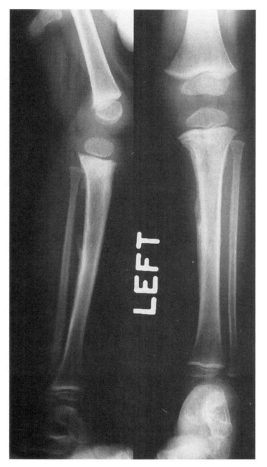

FIG. 12-13 Lateral and anteroposterior views of the lower leg demonstrating cortical and medullary destruction associated with periosteal reaction.

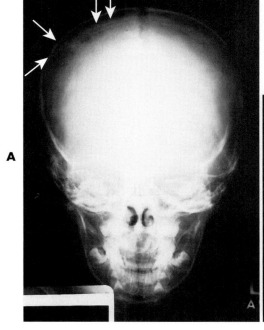

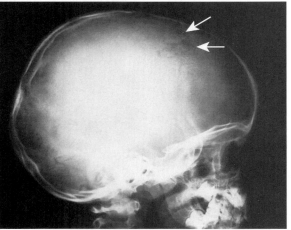

FIG. 12-12 **A,** Posteroanterior and, **B,** lateral views of the skull showing focal osteopenia caused by osteomyelitis *(arrows).*

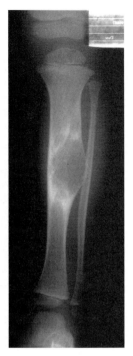

FIG. 12-14   Osteomyelitis presenting as a cystic defect of the shaft of the tibia. (Courtesy Gary Longmuir, Phoenix, AZ.)

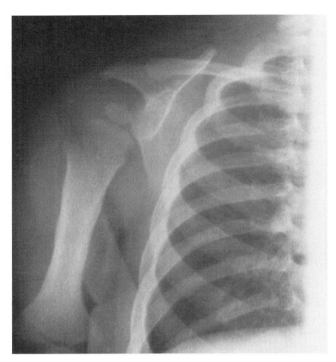

FIG. 12-15   Anteroposterior view of a shoulder with osteomyelitis involving the metaphysis of the proximal humerus.

(Fig. 12-15) are more commonly affected.[50] Osteomyelitis tends to affect long bones, particularly those in the lower extremities.[45] In children, hematogenous osteomyelitis usually is located in the metaphyseal region of long bones (Fig. 12-16), with the most commonly affected bones being the femur and tibia.[6] The epiphysis is more commonly involved in neonates and adults than in

children. From the first year of life until skeletal maturity, the physis acts as a barrier to circulatory vessels and therefore limits epiphyseal infections (Fig. 12-17). Infections of the epiphysis increase the likelihood of developing a septic joint.[15]

Suppurative osteomyelitis involves flat bones in about 30% of cases. Infective spondylitis, a combined infection of the vertebrae

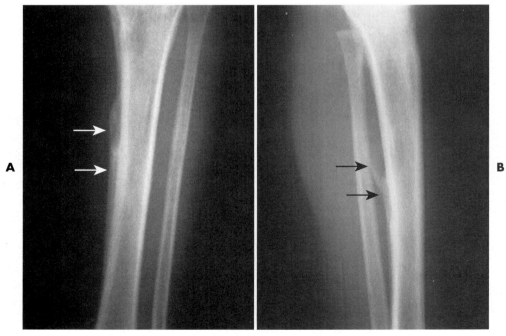

FIG. 12-16   **A,** Frontal and, **B,** lateral leg projections demonstrating hematogenous osteomyelitis with early osseous destruction and prominent periosteal lifting caused by periostitis *(arrows)*.

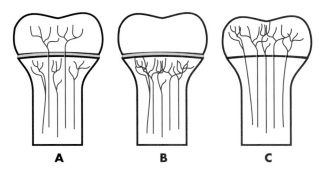

FIG. 12-17 Age-related vascular supply patterns. **A,** Before the age of 1 year, a few vessels extend from the metaphysis to the epiphysis. **B,** During childhood and adolescence, the growth plate isolates the epiphysis from metaphyseal blood vessels. **C,** Skeletal maturity leads to closure of the growth plate, allowing revascularization of the epiphysis by metaphyseal vessels. Because of the blood vessel patterns, hematogenous extensions of infections develop less often in the epiphysis while the physis is open. (From Resnick D: Diagnosis of bone and joint disorders, ed 4, Philadelphia, 2002, WB Saunders.)

and intervertebral disc space, is a rare condition that affects older individuals (Fig. 12-18).[16] The average age of a patient with suppurative osteomyelitis of the spine is 61.5 years.[7] Vertebral osteomyelitis may lead to conditions such as cauda equina syndrome that involve neurologic compression secondary to a fracture or large infective mass that compresses the neuroanatomic structures.[16,36] Like the symphysis pubis and sacroiliac joints, the apophysis, articular cartilage, and fibrocartilage are all potential targets. Although only one site is typically infected, multiple sites can become infected, especially in neonates.[6,19]

In adults the location of the infection depends on the mechanism by which the infection is established and the presence of an underlying disorder. For instance, diabetes mellitus is more commonly associated with osteomyelitis in lower extremities, whereas patients with spinal cord injuries may develop decubitus ulcers and subsequent pelvic osteomyelitis. Batson's plexus, the valveless venous network in the spine, provides an entryway for spinal infections secondary to urinary tract infections, intravenous drug abuse, abscesses, and bacterial endocarditis.[15]

Causative agents. The organisms that cause osteomyelitis vary according to age and health status. *S. aureus* is the most common cause of osteomyelitis among all individuals.[6,14,16,35] Some strains of *S. aureus* have an excellent ability to lodge in bone marrow, which may explain why this bacteria is frequently identified as the infectious agent in patients with osteomyelitis.[35] Other causes include *M. tuberculosis,* various fungi, and pneumococcal disease secondary to chronic respiratory infection.[15] Neonates usually develop *S. aureus* and streptococci infections,[6] whereas *S. aureus* is usually the source of infection in elderly persons. Fungal osteomyelitis may develop as a complication of a fungal infection caused by catheterization, drug abuse, or prolonged neutropenia.

The presence of underlying conditions or diseases and external factors also influence the type of organism that causes osteomyelitis. Examples include the following:

- *P. aeruginosa* has been isolated from patients who develop osteomyelitis from dwelling catheters.
- *Bartonella henselae* has been associated with infection in patients with HIV.
- Aspergilli, mycobacteria, or *Candida albicans* can infect immunocompromised patients.[21]
- *P. aeruginosa, Klebsiella pneumoniae,* and *C. albicans* commonly infect individuals who are abusing drugs.
- Gram-negative microorganisms usually are the cause of nosocomial osteomyelitis.
- Urogenital surgery is associated with *Escherichia coli* infections.
- Patients with diabetes mellitus or a history of long-term antibiotic therapy may develop *C. albicans* infections; premature infants also may develop *C. albicans* osteomyelitis.

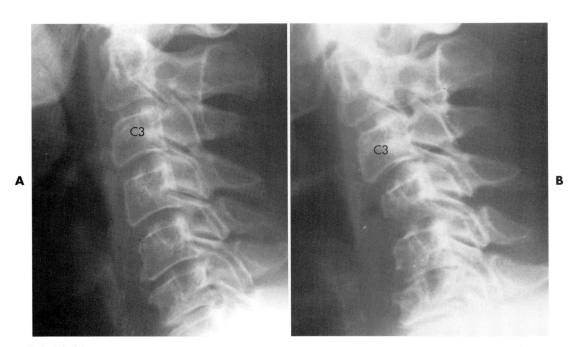

FIG. 12-18 Infection of the disc and vertebrae. **A,** First and, **B,** second lateral projections are taken 1 month apart. During this period of time, notable loss of C4 and C5 disc space, expansion of the precervical soft tissue, and endplate destruction of the surrounding segments is evident.

PART TWO Bone, Joints, and Soft Tissues

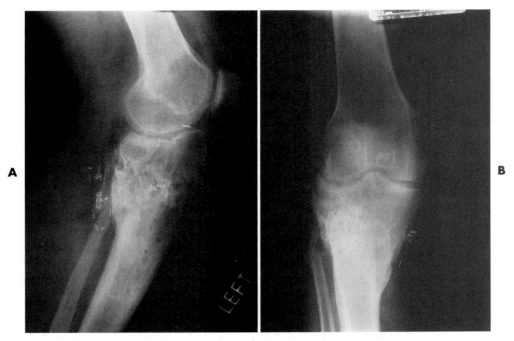

FIG. 12-19 **A,** Lateral and, **B,** anteroposterior views of a knee that has developed osteomyelitis as a complication of surgery.

Dissemination. Osteomyelitis is spread by three major routes: (a) hematogenous, (b) direct (e.g., implantation by trauma or surgery) (Fig. 12-19), and (c) contiguous.[15,54] Infections of joints or long bones usually are a result of hematogenous spread, with the common primary sources including urinary tract infections, pneumonia, and skin abscesses.[50] Hematogenous osteomyelitis introduces viable organisms into the medullary portion of the bone. If the infected medullary cavity lies within a joint capsule, septic arthritis is more likely to develop, a phenomenon that occurs in the hips and shoulders. In adults, it is less common for hematogenous osteomyelitis to develop in the tubular bones; it commonly spreads to the spine and pelvis, as compared with the pattern of dissemination in children, which is usually in the metaphysis of long bones.

The two most common types of trauma that produce osteomyelitis are open fractures and surgical bone reconstruction (Fig. 12-20) In addition, infections associated with prosthetic implantation are common, and staphylococcal organisms cause 75% of these infections.[29]

Risk factors. Individuals who have had urinary tract infections are predisposed to developing osteomyelitis. Approximately 40% of infective spondylitis cases are secondary to urinary tract infections. The lumbar spine is commonly involved and considered to be the result of spread through Batson's venous plexus. Neurologic abnormalities and paraplegia are also risk factors for osteomyelitis, as are sickle cell anemia and diabetes mellitus. Patients with a compromised immune system caused by conditions such as lymphoma or a connective tissue disease or who have overused broad-spectrum antibiotics may develop osteomyelitis from atypical organisms.[6,50] Patients who are elderly, are alcoholics, have active rheumatoid arthritis, or have recently received a prosthetic joint all have higher rates of osteomyelitis.[50] Drug addiction is also highly associated with spondylitis, and individuals who use the drugs intravenously seem to develop *P. aeruginosa* infections more often than individuals of other subpopulations. Pseudomonas

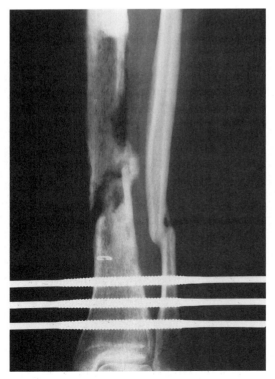

FIG. 12-20 Posttraumatic osteomyelitis. In this case, it is unclear whether the bone infection was caused by the surgery or the compound fracture. (Courtesy Gary M. Guebert, Maryland Heights, MO.)

tends to affect the "S" joints, which include the spine, sacroiliac, symphysis pubis, and sternoclavicular joints.[45,50]

Garré chronic sclerosing osteomyelitis. In 1893 a Swiss surgeon named Garré described the sclerosing type of osteomyelitis found in young adults that is now known as *Garré osteomyelitis*.[23] This form of osteomyelitis is characterized by an insidious onset of pain and marked sclerotic lesions on radiographic images. The absence of central radiolucent nidus helps distinguish it from osteoid osteoma or a Brodie's abscess. The shafts of the femur and tibia are commonly affected.

IMAGING FINDINGS

Plain film radiography. Plain film radiography (Fig. 12-21) may not detect the early stages of bone infection, the features of which often do not appear for several weeks or even months after implantation;[6] repeat examinations usually are necessary.[29] One of the earliest signs of osteomyelitis is deep soft-tissue swelling. Distortion or obliteration of fat planes and subcutaneous edema may be evident 3 to 10 days after infection.[6,15] Focal osteopenia within the medullary cavity typically occurs first, followed by cortical destruction in a focal or multifocal presentation.

During the middle stage of osteomyelitis, a cortical breach develops and leads to periostitis approximately 3 to 6 weeks after infection (Fig. 12-22). As suppurative osteomyelitis develops, pus moves into the vascular channels, raising the intramedullary pressure and impairing blood flow.[6,29] Ischemic necrosis hastens the damage and results in pockets of dead bone called *sequestra* (Fig. 12-23).[29]

In the late stages of osteomyelitis the remaining sequestra may be surrounded by a florid periosteal reaction called an *involucrum*

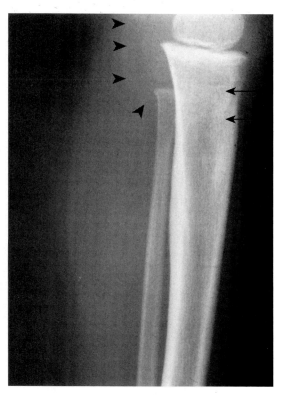

FIG. 12-21 Plain film radiography often does not detect early stages of osteomyelitis. Retrospectively, capsular swelling *(arrowheads)* and localized osteopenia *(arrow)* were noted in the case of known osteomyelitis.

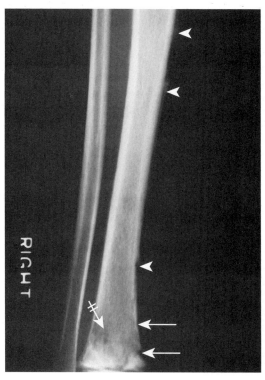

FIG. 12-22 Anteroposterior view of osteomyelitis of the tibia. Note the periosteal reaction *(arrowheads)* and cortical *(arrows)* and medullary *(crossed arrow)* osseous destruction.

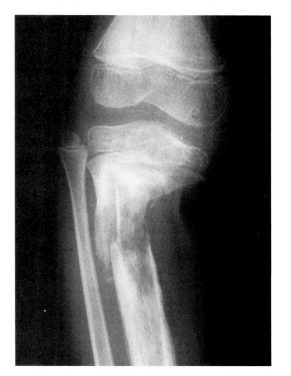

FIG. 12-23 Anteroposterior view of the knee showing residual dead bone, or sequestra *(arrow)*, and the florid periosteal response, or involucrum *(arrowheads)*. A sample was taken, and the culture that was performed revealed the presence of *P. aeruginosa*. (Courtesy Gary M. Guebert, Maryland Heights, MO.)

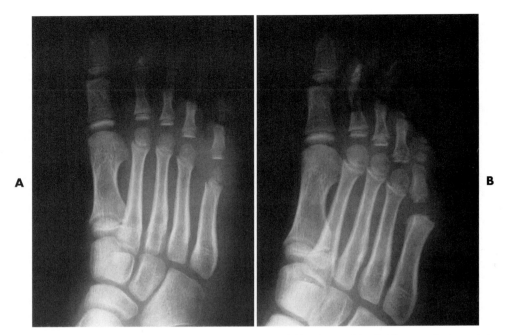

FIG. 12-24   A, Anteroposterior projection of a foot with no visible abnormalities. **B,** Two months later, destructive bone changes and periostitis secondary to infection of the fifth metatarsophalangeal joint can be seen.

(see Fig. 12-23). An opening in the involucrum is called a *cloaca*. The sequestra and involucrum appear no earlier than 3 weeks after infection.[6] Communication with the skin surface occurs through sinus tracts, and pus and bony debris may migrate to the surface. A rare complication of osteomyelitis is a Marjolin ulcer, which develops as the tissue associated with the cloaca and sinus tract degenerate into a squamous cell carcinoma. The latent period may be as long as 20 to 30 years.[6]

Chronic osteomyelitis can be used to describe osteomyelitis in a patient who has had the disease for many years or chronic osteomyelitis that is revealed for the first time. The disease typically presents as bony sclerosis. Viable organisms capable of producing infection can survive in necrotic abscesses or fragments of necrotic bone for months or years.[47] Continuous bouts with mild infections are typical.

Infections have the ability to cross joint spaces, whereas other aggressive bone diseases such as bone tumors typically do not exhibit this ability. Spinal infections usually involve the intervertebral disc. The vertebral body is more commonly affected and may develop endplate erosion.[11] In cases of spondylitis, the facet joints are rarely involved. Although the discs of some young children heal after the infection, residual deformities are typical in the elderly.

The radiographic differentiation of pyogenic infection from a tuberculosis infection or a tumor may not be possible.[6] Unlike tuberculosis, pyogenic spinal infections demonstrate less paravertebral soft-tissue involvement.[7] The paravertebral involvement is seen as a cuff around the involved vertebrae and discs.[7] Plain film radiography has a high incidence of false negative examinations (Fig. 12-24). Bone scanning and CT have improved sensitivity rates, but delays in diagnosis remain a problem.

Specialized imaging. Specialized imaging provides a more sensitive evaluation of a clinically suspected infection than is possible with plain film radiography. Whereas plain films of the early stages of infection may be essentially normal, bone scanning and MRI detect abnormalities.[45] Detection with plain film radiographs

may lag 10 to 14 days behind the onset of clinical symptoms,[15] whereas bone scans typically detect abnormalities within 24 hours of clinical onset. The classic positive sign of osteomyelitis from a three-phase bone scan is increased blood flow during the angiogram phase, focal hyperemia in the blood pool phase, and increased bony uptake in the bone activity phase. Bone scintigraphy is useful during the early stages of infection, but clinical correlation is essential (Fig. 12-25).[6,12] Some authors have suggested that a bone scan is not cost-effective in cases of suspected osteomyelitis. Seldom are surgeons satisfied with the ability of bone scans to define an image; therefore MRI or CT is needed to define the lesions' dimensions and features.[22]

CT is useful in assessing the extent of damage and detecting soft-tissue extensions (Fig. 12-26).[6] CT and MRI provide excellent resolution and can provide information about medullary and cortical destruction, articular damage, and periosteal and soft-tissue involvement.[29] MRI may detect osteomyelitis before a bone scan because of its superior ability to monitor bone marrow changes.[29]

The typical MRI findings associated with osteomyelitis during standard T1- and T2-weighted images are low signal intensity on T1-weighted images and an abnormally bright signal on T2-weighted images (Fig. 12-27).[29,33] With regard to osteomyelitis, MRI sensitivity is 88% and specificity is 93%, whereas bone scan sensitivity is 61% and specificity is 33%.[22] MRI also may detect articular involvement and the presence of sinus tracts (cloaca) during the early stages.[15] Evidence of epidural infection extension may be best seen using gadolinium-enhanced imaging.[7] MRI shows intervertebral disc involvement as a decreased signal on T1-weighted images and an increased signal on T2-weighted images, characteristics similar to other findings related to osteomyelitis.[15,24] However, a decreased signal from an intervertebral disc on a T2-weighted image does not rule out osteomyelitis.[14]

Other MRI findings include joint effusion, thickened synovium, and ill-defined margins of the lesion. The synovium is typically enhanced with gadolinium infusion. Articular cartilage destruction

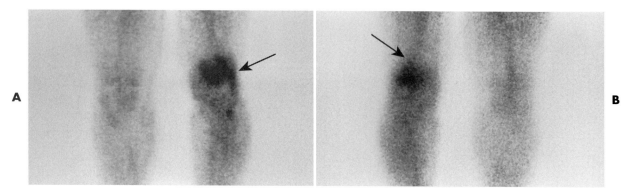

FIG. 12-25 A, Anterior and, **B,** posterior bone scans demonstrating evidence of increased bony uptake in a patient with osteomyelitis *(arrows).*

also may be seen on MRI images. Acutely evolving neuropathic arthropathy has a presentation that is similar to osteomyelitis. Chronic neuropathic arthropathy is easily distinguished from osteomyelitis by a decreased signal intensity that is not affected by pulse sequencing.[33]

Performing a proper workup of patients with suspected osteomyelitis requires cooperation between the clinician and radiologist.[6] In equivocal cases or cases in which abscess formation is suspected, radionuclide imaging using white blood cells tagged with gallium 67 is useful to investigate the presence of osteomyelitis.[6,15] In patients with diabetes, scans using leukocytes labeled with ^{111}In have shown great sensitivity and specificity.[15,54] Some large studies have suggested that an ^{111}In scan is superior to a three-phase ^{99m}Tc scan.[54] However, MRI usually is less costly than the combined cost of a bone scan and an ^{111}In or a ^{67}Ga scan.[15]

CLINICAL COMMENTS

Signs and symptoms of osteomyelitis often are vague and may be present for a long time. Subacute presentations are becoming more common, possibly because of the increased use of antibiotics.

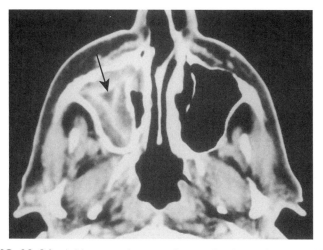

FIG. 12-26 Axial computed tomography scan showing an obstructed right maxillary sinus *(arrow).* In the center of the sinus is a triangular area of dense mucus composed of trapped sinus *(arrow)* secretions. The inflamed sinus mucosa surrounds this region and is seen on the scan as a thin, uniform enhancement. Between the mucosa and bony sinus wall is a zone of submucosal edema. (From Som PM, Curtin HD: Head and neck imaging, ed 4, St Louis, 2003, Mosby.)

In particular, patients with pyogenic spinal infections often experience a long delay in receiving their diagnosis.[11] The symptoms are not specific, and the disease is often not considered when the infection is in its early stages. A delay in diagnosis may cause excessive and extensive tissue destruction and abscess formation.[11,50]

The most common complaint from patients with vertebral osteomyelitis is back pain that has been increasing in severity for several days. Laboratory data such as WBCs and ESR elevations may indicate the presence of an inflammation, but these findings are variable and nonspecific.[11,49] Most studies report an average delay in diagnosis of 2 to 6 months after the onset of symptoms.[11] The nonspecific nature of laboratory and radiographic findings and the ubiquitous nature of back pain make diagnosis a challenge.

The classic clinical features of hematogenous suppurative osteomyelitis are chills, fever, malaise, local pain, and swelling. Loss of function or decreased range of motion in the affected region often develops.[29] Skin lesions are clear evidence of septicemia and vasculitis.[50] Possible osteomyelitis should be viewed as a medical emergency and be addressed immediately.

The major objective of a workup for a bone or joint infection is identification of the infectious organism,[50] which is essential for proper treatment.[29] Surgical sampling or a needle biopsy provides indispensable information. Information provided by swabs from ulcers or fistulae may be misleading. Assessment of stained histopathologic bone biopsy samples is the most reliable way to accurately identify the infectious agent.[29]

Attempting to diagnose osteomyelitis in a patient with a diabetic foot is difficult both from a clinical and an imaging point of view (Fig. 12-28). A concomitant neuropathic osteoarthropathy may be present and could produce a delay in diagnosis. Neuropathic joint destruction may simulate infection, and to further complicate the presentation, osteomyelitis can coexist with the neuropathy. The infection often starts as an ulcer in the dermal layer that later burrows into the underlying bone.[29,33,50] Osteomyelitis caused by vascular insufficiency or diabetes is found exclusively in the feet.[29] A physical examination may reveal that patients with neuropathy have little or no pain, whereas patients whose pain sense is intact and have rapid osseous destruction may experience excruciating pain. MRI may provide early information, and a bone biopsy is confirmatory of disease.[29] Fifteen percent of diabetic patients develop osteomyelitis as a result of a combination of vascular insufficiency and peripheral neuropathy.[33] Early diagnosis of osteomyelitis in patients with diabetes may help prevent the need for amputation. More limb-saving procedures are currently being used in an effort to improve patients' quality of life.[15]

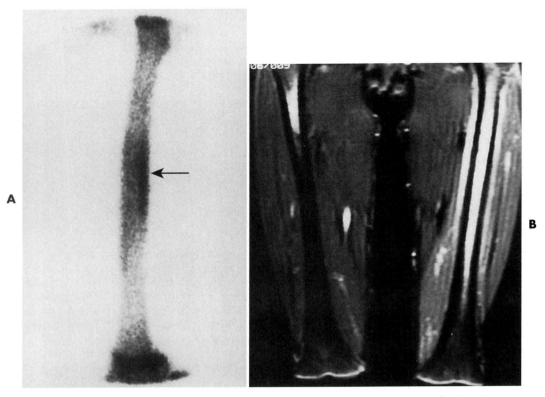

FIG. 12-27   Acute osteomyelitis. **A,** Increased radionuclide uptake as a result of infection *(arrow).* **B,** Magnetic resonance imaging shows the marrow and soft-tissue involvement and more accurately detects the multiple sites of infection. (From Blickman JG: Pediatric radiology: the requisites, St Louis, 1994, Mosby.)

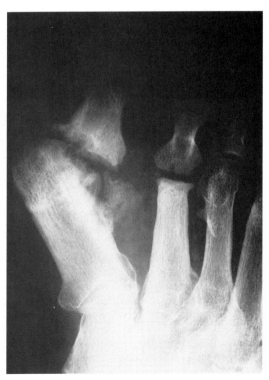

FIG. 12-28   Advanced arthropathy associated with diabetic osteomyelitis of the foot.

KEY CONCEPTS

- *Osteomyelitis is an infection of bone and bone marrow that usually is caused by bacteria but also can be caused by fungi and other microbes.*
- *Staphylococcus aureus is the most common cause.*
- *Populations at risk for osteomyelitis include infants and young children, elderly persons, and those who have diabetes or are immunocompromised.*
- *Radiographic findings include disruption of the surrounding fat planes and intramedullary bone and eventually endosteal scalloping, cortical destruction, and periosteal reactions.*
- *Sequestra are pockets of dead bone; an involucrum is the result of a florid periosteal response and surrounds the infective mass.*
- *The cloaca is a channel through the involucrum that may connect to a sinus and allow migration of pus and bloody bone debris onto the skin surface.*
- *The bone and joint structures of some young children heal after infection, whereas older patients usually have residual deformities.*
- *There is often a delay of 3 to 6 weeks between implantation and expression of signs and symptoms.*
- *A rare complication of osteomyelitis that can develop in later stages is a Marjolin ulcer-cloaca and sinus tract tissue that has developed into a squamous cell carcinoma; the latent period for carcinoma development may be as long as 20 to 30 years.*
- *Classic clinical features of suppurative osteomyelitis are chills, fever, malaise, local pain and swelling, and loss of function or decreased range of motion in the affected region.*

References

1. Albert MC, Zachary SV, Alter S: Blastomycosis of the forearm synovium in a child, *Clin Orthop* 317:223, 1995.
2. Antunes JL: Infections of the spine, Acta Neurochir, 116:179, 1992.
3. Banner AS: Tuberculosis. Clinical aspects and diagnosis, *Arch Intern Med* 139:1387, 1979.
4. Batra P, Batra RS: Thoracic coccidioidomycosis, *Semin Roentgenol* 31:28, 1996.
5. Bharucha NE et al: All that caseates is not tuberculosis, *Lancet* 348:1313, 1996.
6. Bonakdar-Pour A, Gaines VD: The radiology of osteomyelitis, *Orthop Clin North Am* 14:21, 1983.
7. Brailsford JF: Brodie's abscess and its differential diagnosis, *Br Med J* 120:119, 1938.
8. Brankos MA et al: Septic arthritis in heroin addicts, *Semin Arthritis Rheum* 21:81, 1991.
9. Brion LP et al: Long-bone radiographic abnormalities as a sign of active congenital syphilis in asymptomatic newborns, *Pediatrics* 88:1037, 1991.
10. Brodie BC: An account of some cases of chronic abscess of the tibia, *Trans Med Chiro Soc* 17:239, 1832.
11. Carragee EJ: The clinical use of magnetic resonance imaging in pyogenic vertebral osteomyelitis, *Spine* 22:780, 1997.
12. Ching BY, Maraczi G, Urbina D: Madura foot. A case presentation, *J Am Podiatr Med Assoc* 81:443, 1991.
13. Cuellar ML et al: Other fungal arthritides, *Rheum Dis Clin North Am* 19:439, 1993.
14. Dagirmanjian A et al: MR imaging of vertebral osteomyelitis revisited, *AJR Am J Roentgenol* 167:1539, 1996.
15. Deely DM, Scheitzer ME: MR imaging of bone marrow disorders, *Radiol Clin North Am* 35:193, 1997.
16. Faraj A, Krishna M, Mehdian SMH: Cauda equina syndrome secondary to lumbar spondylodiscitis caused by *Streptococcus milleri*, *Eur Spine J* 5:134, 1996.
17. Foster MR, Friedenberg ZB, Passero F: Lumbar Petriellidum boydii osteomyelitis with a systemic presentation, *J Spinal Disord* 7:356, 1994.
18. Giacola GP, Wood BP: Radiological case of the month. Congenital syphilis, *Am J Dis Child* 145:1045, 1991.
19. Gold R: Diagnosis of osteomyelitis, *Pediatr Rev* 12:292, 1991.
20. Greenberg SB, Bernal DV: Are long bone radiographs necessary in neonates suspected of having congenital syphilis? *Radiology* 182:637, 1992.
21. Gropper GR, Acker JD, Robertson JH: Computed tomography in Pott's disease, *Neurosurgery* 10:506, 1982.
22. Haygood TM: Magnetic resonance imaging of the musculoskeletal system: part 7, the ankle, *Clin Orthop* 336:318, 1997.
23. Jacobsson S, Heyden G: Chronic sclerosing osteomyelitis of the mandible, Histologic and histochemical findings, *Oral Surg Oral Med Oral Pathol* 43:357, 1977.
24. Johnston JO, Genant HK, Rosenam W: Ankle pain and swelling in a 30-year-old man, *Clin Orthop* 314:281, 1995.
25. Keats TE: Atlas of roentgenographic measurement, ed 6, St Louis, 1990, Mosby.
26. Kushwaha VP et al: Musculoskeletal coccidioidomycosis. A review of 25 cases, *Clin Orthop* 332:190, 1996.
27. Leff A, Geppert EF: Public health and preventive aspects of pulmonary tuberculosis. Infectiousness, epidemiology, risk factors, classification, and preventive therapy, *Arch Intern Med* 139:1405, 1979.
28. Lester TW: Drug-resistant and atypical mycobacterial disease. Bacteriology and treatment, *Arch Intern Med* 139:1399, 1979.
29. Lew DP, Waldvogel FA: Osteomyelitis, *N Engl J Med* 336:999, 1997.
30. Lewall DB, Ofole S, Bendl B: Mycetoma, *Skeletal Radiol* 14:257, 1985.
31. Lin-Greenberg A, Cholankeni J: Vertebral arch destruction in tuberculosis: CT feature, *J Comput Assist Tomogr* 14:300, 1990.
32. MacDonald PB, Black GB, MacKenzie R: Orthopaedic manifestations of blastomycosis, *J Bone Joint Surg Am* 72:860, 1990.
33. Marcus CD et al: MR imaging of osteomyelitis and neuropathic osteoarthropathy in the feet of diabetics, *Radiographics* 16:1337, 1996.
34. Mascola L et al: Congenital syphilis revisited, *Am J Dis Child* 139:575, 1985.
35. Matsushita K et al: Experimental hematogenous osteomyelitis by *Staphylococcus aureus, Clin Orthop* 334:291, 1997.
36. McHenry MC et al: Vertebral osteomyelitis presenting as spinal compression fracture, *Arch Intern Med* 148:417, 1988.
37. Miller WB, Murphy WA, Gilula LA: Brodie's abscess. Reappraisal, *Radiology* 132:15, 1979.
38. Mirels LF, Stevens DA: Update on treatment of coccidioidomycosis, *West J Med* 166:58, 1997.
39. Mosley D et al: From the Centers for Disease Control and Prevention. Coccidioidomycosis, Arizona, 1990–1995, *JAMA* 277: 104, 1997.
40. Proctor ME, Davis JP: Blastomycosis, Wisconsin, 1986–1995, *MMWR*, 45:601, 1996.
41. Rasool MN, Goender S: The skeletal manifestations of congenital syphilis. A review of 197 cases, *J Bone Joint Surg Br* 71:752, 1989.
42. Resnick D: Diagnosis of bone and joint disorders, ed 3, Philadelphia, 1995, WB Saunders.
43. Resnik BI, Burdick AE: Improvement of eumycetoma with itraconazole, *J Am Acad Dermatol* 33:917, 1995.
44. Restrepo A: Treatment of tropical mycoses, *J Am Acad Dermatol* 31(suppl):91, 1994.
45. Richter RW: Infections other than AIDS, *Neurol Clin* 11:591, 1993.
46. Riegler HF, Goldstein LA, Bett RF: Blastomycosis osteomyelitis, *Clin Orthop* 100:225, 1974.
47. Rogoff RS Tinkle JD, Bortis DG: Unusual presentation of calcaneal osteomyelitis. Twenty-five years after inoculation, *J Am Podiatr Med Assoc* 87:125, 1997.
48. Rosenfeld SR, Weinert CR, Kahn B: Congenital syphilis. A case report, *J Bone Joint Surg Am* 65:115, 1983.
49. Ruppert D, Barron BJ, Madewell JE: Osteomyelitis, acute and chronic, *Radiol Clin North Am* 25:1171, 1987.
50. Schmid FR: Infectious arthritis and osteomyelitis, *Prim Care* 11:295, 1984.
51. Schneider E et al: A coccidioidomycosis outbreak following the Northridge, Calif, earthquake, *JAMA* 277:904, 1997.
52. Smith IE et al: Kyphosis secondary to tuberculosis osteomyelitis as a cause of ventilatory failure. Clinical features, mechanisms, and management, *Chest* 110:1105, 1996.
53. Stevens DA: Coccidioidomycosis, *N Engl J Med* 332:1077, 1995.
54. Sutter CW, Shelton DK: Three-phase bone scan in osteomyelitis and other musculoskeletal disorders, *Am Fam Phys* 54:1639, 1996.
55. Ushigome S et al: Case report 308. Diagnosis: disseminated syphilitic osteomyelitis (presumptively proved), *Skeletal Radiol* 13:239, 1985.
56. Waldrogel FA, Vasey H: Osteomyelitis: the past decade, *N Engl J Med* 303:360, 1980.
57. Winer-Muram HT, Vargus S, Slabod K: Cavitary lung lesions in an immunosuppressed child, *Chest* 106:937, 1994.
58. Wright T, Sundaram M, McDonald D: Radiologic case study. Tuberculosis osteomyelitis and arthritis, *Orthopedics* 19:699, 1996.
59. Zeppa MA: Skeletal coccidioidomycosis: imaging findings in 19 patients, *Skeletal Radiol* 25:337, 1996.
60. Zimmerman MR: Pulmonary and osseous tuberculosis in an Egyptian mummy, *Bull NY Acad Med* 55:604, 1979.

chapter 13

Bone Tumors and Related Diseases

DENNIS M. MARCHIORI

Bone tumors are one of the most serious diagnostic possibilities in patients with musculoskeletal complaints. Bone tumors are categorized as either *primary* or *secondary*. Primary bone tumors arise from bone and related soft tissues directly in their site of involvement and may be either benign or malignant. Secondary bone tumors arise "secondary" to a primary lesion and also may be benign (e.g., secondary aneurysmal bone cyst arising in an area of past trauma) or malignant (e.g., bone metastasis from a lung carcinoma).

Benign tumors usually are designated as such by the suffix -*oma* (e.g., enchondroma) and generally are not regarded as cancers. Malignant primary tumors of bone and other connective tissues are designated by the use of the term, or suffix, *sarcoma* after the tissue type involved (e.g., osteosarcoma).

Metastatic bone disease describes a malignant tumor that secondarily seeds to bone, usually from a primary malignancy of the epithelial tissue (designated as *carcinomas*) of the lung, breast, prostate, kidney, liver, and so on. For instance, if the patient has a bronchogenic carcinoma that metastasizes to the thoracic spine,

the lung lesion is the primary lesion and the thoracic spine lesion is bone metastasis of the lung lesion.

In general terms both benign tumors of bone and bone metastasis are many times more common than primary malignancies of bone. Primary malignancy of bone is uncommon. Malignancy in general is thought to affect about 1 in 3 people over their lifetime. Approximately 1.2 million Americans are diagnosed with a malignancy each year. By comparison, fewer than 1 in 100,000 people are diagnosed with a true primary malignancy of bone. In fact, the incidence of primary malignant bone lesions (excluding multiple myeloma) is estimated at 8 per million persons.[61] The most common sarcomas include osteosarcoma (35.1%), chondrosarcoma (25.8%), Ewing's sarcoma (16.0%), chordoma (8.4%), and fibrosarcoma (5.7%). Because it arises from the plasma cell of bone marrow, many sources do not consider multiple myeloma as a primary malignancy of bone, instead naming osteosarcoma as the most common primary malignancy of bone. However, multiple myeloma is by far the most common primary malignancy of bone if considered in the group of primary bone malignancies. With an

PART TWO
Bone, Joints, and Soft Tissues

incidence of about 4.1 per 100,000[135] it is considerably more common than osteosarcoma.

The evaluation of a bone tumor necessitates careful assessment of the patient's history and application of clinical studies to develop a concise list of differential possibilities. Diagnostic imaging plays a major role in developing and narrowing this list. With advances in technology, biologic tissue assessments have added a valuable tool to the arsenal of the investigator. Therefore the diagnosis of tumors is accomplished along three dimensions of assessment: clinical (e.g., gender, age, symptoms), imaging (e.g., location, appearance), and pathologic (e.g., microscopic cell type and molecular assessment).

Imaging Modalities

Imaging studies should define the lesion, determine its location, grade its aggressiveness, decide if the lesion is limited to one bone (monostotic) or if multiple bones are involved (polyostotic), assess soft-tissue involvement, and identify the lesion's matrix. Plain film radiography remains the chief imaging modality for the initial assessment of bone tumors. Sometimes the radiographic presentation reveals a lesion that is nonaggressive with classic characteristics, necessitating no further examination and leading to an immediate diagnosis. However, further assessment often is necessary when lesions are poorly defined or accompanied by significant clinical signs and symptoms.

Computed tomography (CT) provides direct thin axial slices of anatomy, allowing for a more detailed assessment of complex anatomy (e.g., spine) than can be accomplished with plain film. CT demonstrates calcification well and therefore is capable of demonstrating calcification within the lesion's matrix and the cortical response of the lesion's host bone. Plain film radiographs and CT scans of the chest help to assess the possibility of pulmonary metastasis, the presence of which may alter the treatment plan.

Although radionuclide bone scans lack specificity, they are sensitive to the presence of early disease and are widely used to assess the possibility of multiple lesions, a finding that substantially limits the diagnostic list of possibilities. There is one notable exception to the sensitivity of bone scans. Bone scans often are falsely negative in the presence of multiple myeloma and purely lytic lesions. In this and other cases it may be best to apply radiographic surveys or multiregional magnetic resonance imaging (MRI) studies.

MRI has the ability to demonstrate abnormality of the bone marrow and delineate extraosseous involvement. Replacement of normal marrow by pathologic processes (e.g., metastasis, multiple myeloma, osteomyelitis) is readily demonstrated and provides an early sign of disease. However, MRI remains inferior to both plain film and CT for detailing calcification, ossification, cortical destruction, and periosteal reaction. MRI is especially valuable to assess the neurologic impact of the lesion. Plain film radiographs efficiently provide information about the rate of growth and aggressiveness of a lesion but do not establish a histologic diagnosis with the same accuracy as a biopsy. On MRI studies, most bone tumors are dark on T1-weighted images and bright on T2-weighted images. Fibrous tissue, cortical bone, desmoids, and scar tissue are dark on both T1- and T2-weighted images. Hemangiomas, lipomas, and liposarcomas are bright on both T1- and T2-weighted images because of the blood components of these lesions.

The information offered by imaging is coupled with clinical data, laboratory studies, and possibly biopsy to identify the specific lesion present.

Laboratory Tests

Laboratory tests generally are less helpful than imaging studies to diagnose bone tumors. Benign bone tumors demonstrate normal laboratory values, and malignant tumors often demonstrate normal laboratory values. However, a few characteristic laboratory findings may be noted with malignancy. For example, increased serum calcium levels and increased hydroxyproline in the urine are associated with massive bone osteolysis, as seen in generalized lytic metastasis or multiple myeloma. Some osteosarcoma, osteoblastic metastasis, and other bone-proliferating malignancies often are accompanied by increased serum alkaline phosphatase levels. Multiple myeloma is associated with monoclonal immunoglobulins "M-spike" on serum electrophoresis, Bence Jones proteins in the urine, hyperglobulinemia (reversed albumin-globulin [A/G] serum ratio), elevated creatine, and decreased hematocrit levels.

Bone Biopsy

Bone biopsy is the removal of suspect tissue from the body for examination by a pathologist. In most circumstances a biopsy provides the most accurate diagnosis possible, typically more accurate than can be obtained by imaging. However, biopsy is not especially helpful to determine the lesion's rate of growth and aggressiveness. The latter qualities are best assessed by conventional and specialized imaging modalities; therefore a biopsy and imaging studies are complementary, leading to an end diagnosis.

The accuracy of the biopsy results depends on which region of the lesion is collected, the skill of the person performing the biopsy, and the clinical circumstances in which the biopsy takes place. It is generally most accurate if the biopsy is taken from the most aggressive and viable portion of the lesions. This often necessitates an open biopsy approach. However, an open biopsy is associated with higher complication rates than is a closed (percutaneous) biopsy approach.[171] Open biopsy procedures may contaminate malignant cells in normal tissue, interfering with otherwise successful limb-sparing procedures. Closed biopsy procedures generally are safer, but may not produce enough tissue for accurate diagnosis. Biopsy of highly vascular lesions is cautioned generally, given the risk of massive hemorrhage.

Tumor Staging

Tumor staging is integral to patient management. Once a tumor is found, the extent of disease is defined along three parameters. The first parameter defines the size of the tumor (T) and whether it has invaded surrounding tissues. The second parameter examines the extent of lymph node involvement (N). Lastly, one must know

BOX 13-1
Tumor Staging

Tumor staging is the process of characterizing the extent of the patient's disease along three parameters: tumor (T), lymph nodes (N), and metastasis (M).
T: Indicates the size and regional involvement of the tumor
  TX: Primary tumor cannot be assessed
  T0: No evidence of a primary tumor
  Tis: Carcinoma in situ (the tumor cells are restricted to the epithelial layer of the involved tissue)
  T1: Localized tumor; diameter is 2 cm or less
  T2: Localized tumor; diameter is 5 cm or less and mild involvement of same organ tissue
  T3: Advanced tumor; diameter is greater than 5 cm and there is extensive involvement of same organ tissue
  T4: Massive tumor; diameter is greater than 5 cm and there is involvement of nerves, blood vessels, bone, or other organs
N: Indicates the extent of lymph node involvement
  NX: Regional lymph nodes cannot be assessed
  N0: No evidence of metastasis to regional lymph nodes
  N1: Small tumor in one lymph node
  N2: Medium tumor in one or more lymph nodes
  N3: Large tumor in one or more lymph nodes
M: Indicates the presence or absence of distant metastasis
  MX: Distal metastasis cannot be assessed
  M0: No evidence of distal metastasis
  M1: Evidence of distal metastasis present
A tumor stage (I to IV) can be calculated once the T, N, and M parameters are determined. In general, the higher the tumor stage, the lower the patient's chance of survival.
Stage I: T1 N0 M0
Stage II: T2 N1 M0
Stage III: T3 N0 M0, T1–3 N1 M0
Stage IV: T4 N0–1 M0, T0–4 N2–3 M0, T0–4 N0–4 M1

whether the tumor has metastasized to other regions of the body (M). These three parameters define the "TNM" system of staging lesions. Although some variation in the stages exists depending on the source and type of tumor being staged, a general presentation of the TNM method is presented in Box 13-1.

Signs and Symptoms

Clinically important lesions usually are detected secondary to the patient's complaint of pain or attention to a palpable mass. Aggressive bone lesions generate signs and symptoms directly, secondary to bone and tissue destruction. Classically the bone pain experienced is more dramatic at night and unrelated to physical activity. The patient may exhibit fever, impaired mobility, and cachexia with aggressive lesions. In contrast, most benign lesions are clinically asymptomatic, but commonly are recognized after pathologic fracture. This concept has been termed *traumatic determinism;* that is, the presence of the benign lesion is only determined as a result of trauma and subsequent fracture. Less frequently asymptomatic bone lesions are detected serendipitously on radiographs obtained for unrelated reasons.

Tumor Discriminators

Many tumors and tumorlike conditions produce similar imaging findings. The following list of radiologic and clinical parameters assists in narrowing the usually broad number of pathologic possibilities for a given radiographic appearance. In addition, the following parameters assist in evaluating the aggressiveness and clinical importance of a lesion.

PATIENT AGE

The age of the patient is an important clue to assist the examiner in differentiating between lesions that may look the same but are unique to certain age groups. Conversely, the patient's age may suggest a diagnostic possibility that would not otherwise be considered from the radiographic appearance because of an atypical presentation. Age is more helpful when the age range associated with the tumor is narrow. Given only the patient's age, an examiner can determine which tumor is present with a high degree of accuracy.[69] (Tables 13-1 and 13-2 present the ages at which common benign and malignant tumors develop, respectively.) Generally with malignant tumors, Ewing's sarcoma and osteosarcoma are present in children, and metastatic bone disease and multiple myeloma are found in patients over 40 years of age. Benign tumors are most common in patients 10 to 30 years of age, slightly younger for simple bone cysts and slightly older for lipomas and hemangiomas.

LOCATION

Individual tumors often predispose to certain bones (Table 13-3). Even more suggestive is the longitudinal (diaphysis, metadiaphysis, metaphysis, and epiphysis) (Fig. 13-1) and transverse (central or eccentric medullary, cortical, periosteal, and parosteal) (Fig. 13-2) location within bone (Table 13-4 and Fig. 13-3).

SOFT-TISSUE INVOLVEMENT

A soft-tissue mass, created when the tumor mass breaks through the host bone's cortex, suggests an aggressive tumor. Soft-tissue masses related to tumors distort but do not disrupt intramuscular soft-tissue planes; soft-tissue masses secondary to infections may. Tumors tend to respect soft-tissue boundaries; infections may not.

HOST BONE REACTION

A number of pathologic processes are capable of accentuating or reviving normal mechanisms of bone growth resulting in periosteal or endosteal reactions. The appearance of the periosteal and endosteal reactions relates to the aggressiveness, intensity, and duration of the inciting process.

TABLE 13-1
Typical Ages for the Development of Selected Benign Tumors

Age (in years)	Tumor
5 to 10	Simple bone cyst
10 to 20	Chondroblastoma, nonossifying fibroma, osteoid osteoma
10 to 30	Aneurysmal bone cyst, chondromyxoid fibroma, osteoblastoma, osteochondroma
15 to 35	Enchondroma, osteoma
20 to 40	Giant cell tumor
30 to 50	Lipoma
40 to 50	Hemangioma

TABLE 13-2

Typical Ages for the Development of Selected Malignant Tumors

Age (in years)	Tumor
Less than 1	Metastatic neuroblastoma
1 to 30	Ewing's sarcoma, osteosarcoma
20 to 40	Giant cell tumor, parosteal osteosarcoma
30 to 50	Fibrosarcoma, malignant fibrous histiocytoma, primary lymphoma of bone
More than 40	Chordoma, chondrosarcoma, metastatic bone disease, multiple myeloma

Periosteal and endosteal reactions must mineralize to be visible on radiographs; several patterns are identified (Fig. 13-4). Mineralization takes between 1 and 3 weeks. If the inciting process is indolent (e.g., vascular stasis), a thick, wavy periosteal reaction develops. Layered or lamellar periosteal reactions indicate a mildly aggressive underlying pathology (e.g., acute osteomyelitis). Aggressive pathology (e.g., osteosarcoma, Ewing's tumor) may disrupt the periosteum, producing a radiating (sunburst) or parallel (hair-on-end) spiculated pattern (Fig. 13-5). The disrupted periosteum may form an acute angle with the cortex of the bone (Codman's triangle) (see Fig. 13-4). Endosteal reactions are more limited, appearing thickened or scalloped in response to pathology within the medullary canal. Radiologic tumor grades based on the reaction of the host bone are presented in Table 13-5.

The tumor grade ultimately is derived from microscopic appearance of the tumor, as performed by a pathologist in association with the imaging findings and clinical data. Tumor staging (see Box 13-1) and grading relate inversely to the patient's chance of survival.

PATTERN OF BONE DESTRUCTION

A number of explanations exist as to why tumors produce bone destruction. Tumors may stimulate osteoclastic activity by direct pressure, local hyperemia, or invasion. Bone destruction may be permeative, moth-eaten, or geographic (Fig. 13-6). Geographic lesions generally are less aggressive than the more subtle moth-eaten–pattern lesions, which generally are less aggressive than the nearly imperceptible permeative pattern.

An observer's ability to recognize bone destruction depends primarily on the size and location of the lesion. Destructive lesions in cortical bone are more easily recognized than those in cancellous bone because greater contrast exists between osteolytic lesions and compact bone than osteolytic lesions and cancellous bone. Although technical factors should be considered, in general, lesions in cancellous bone that are less than 1 cm in diameter are difficult to recognize. Moreover, 30% to 50% of cancellous bone may be destroyed before an osteolytic lesion is recognized on the most optimally exposed and processed radiographs.[36,41,71,101] Osteolytic lesions in the diaphysis are more easily recognized because of the higher proportion of compact bone.

SIZE OF THE LESION

Each tumor has a unique growth rate influenced in part by the nature of the lesion and the response of the host bone. Markedly expansile lesions result when endosteal bone reabsorption of the inner cortex occurs in concert with periosteal appositional,

intramembranous new bone growth of the outer cortex (Fig. 13-7). Although generally it is true that larger lesions are more aggressive than smaller ones, one should be careful not to judge a tumor's clinical importance by size alone.

RATE OF GROWTH

The rate of growth is a very important characteristic for assessing the aggressiveness of a lesion. Benign lesions grow slowly and have thick margins. Malignant lesions grow quickly and have less defined margins. Although highly important, the assessment of a lesion's growth rate is difficult because of the usual lack of available serial studies.

MARGINATION AND ZONE OF TRANSITION

The appearance of the zone of transition between a lesion and the host bone is probably the single best indicator of a lesion's aggressiveness. An abrupt transition from normal to abnormal is a feature of benignancy. A wide transition is a feature of malignancy. The zone of transition is a direct reflection of the lesion's aggressiveness and the response of the host bone to the lesion infiltration (Fig. 13-8). Margination describes the presence and thickness of the rim around the lesion. Malignant tumors typically are nonmarginated, a feature of their wide zone of transition (Figs. 13-8 and 13-9). Conversely, a lesion is most likely benign if surrounded by a sclerotic rim of varying thicknesses producing a narrow zone of transition. The presence of a thick margin is always accompanied by a short zone of transition and represents an attempt of the host bone to surround and limit a lesion's growth. However, a short zone of transition is not always accompanied by a thick margin (e.g., giant cell tumor). The zone of transition should not be used as the sole criteria for determining the aggressiveness of the lesion. Even a well-marginated lesion can prove to be malignant in selected clinical circumstances. For example, a painful lesion presenting with a narrow zone of transition in a 60-year-old patient who has a previous history of a primary tumor should be considered bone metastasis until proved otherwise.

TUMOR MATRIX

The matrix is the internal tissue, or substance, of a tumor. The radiographic appearance of the tumor's matrix assists its categorization as primarily bone-, fibrous-, or cartilage-forming. Most bone tumors have a radiolucent matrix correlating to soft tissue. Only when the matrix is sufficiently mineralized with hydroxyapatite crystals will it become radiographically visible. Bone-producing tumors are radiodense. Highly aggressive bone-producing tumors appear less dense, with poorly formed osteoid material, than do nonaggressive bone-producing tumors. Tumors with a purely fibrous matrix appear radiolucent or slightly hazy (because of interspersed small bone fragments). Cartilage tumors usually are accompanied by irregular ringlike, flocculent, stippled, or flecklike radiodensities within the matrix (Figs. 13-10 and 13-11).

MULTIPLICITY

The presence of multiple lesions suggests different diagnostic possibilities than the presence of a single lesion. Generally radionuclide bone scanning determines if multiple lesions exist. Because radionuclide imaging is sensitive but not specific, plain film radiographs usually are taken at regions of increased radionuclide uptake. Radiographs usually are directed at evaluating a lesion rather than finding it. MRI and CT are applied less commonly to resolve uncertain findings of the radionuclide bone scan and plain films. The presence of multiple lesions limits the differential diagnosis. Common aggressive polyostotic diseases include metastatic

Text continued on p. 804.

TABLE 13-3
Summary of Common Benign and Malignant Lesions

Tumor	Frequency	Age (median) at diagnosis	Typical location	Radiologic features	Comments
Benign					
Aneurysmal bone cyst	Uncommon	10–30	Metaphysis of long bones; sometimes posterior arch of vertebrae	Widely expansile defect of the cortex with cortical buttressing at the region of expansion from the host bone and very thin cortices at outer edge of the lesion. The lesions are osteolytic and exhibit "a soap bubble" appearance	The lesion represents cavities filled with extravasated blood. Lesions may occur secondary to trauma, or concurrent to other tumors (e.g., giant cell tumor). Pain and swelling at the site of involvement
Bone island	Very common	Any age	Any location but skull	Homogenously radiodense focus with spiculated "brush" border	The lesion represents a hamartoma of bone. They are painless, usually small, and of no clinical significance except for their differentiation from blastic metastasis. Multiple bone islands are termed *osteopoikilosis*. Osteomas are similar lesions found in the skull
Chondroblastoma	Rare	10–20	Proximal femur, about the knee, and proximal humerus	Small (<5 cm) osteolytic subarticular lesion with a well-defined margin of sclerosis	A rare lesion composed of chondroblasts and immature cartilage. They appear in the secondary centers of enchondral ossification of skeletally immature patients
Chondromyxoid fibroma	Rare	10–30	Proximal tibia and fibula	Radiolucent, oval, eccentric lesion	Tumor involving the cartilage-forming connective tissue of marrow space
Enchondroma	Common	15–35	Small tubular bones of the hands and feet; however, possible in any enchondrally formed bone	Small round or oval cystic defects, typically with stippled matrix calcification and endosteal scalloping	Discrete islands of cartilage surrounded by layered bone. Enchondromas occur within a bone; periosteal chondromas occur next to the cortex and under the periosteum. Long bone lesions are more likely to be painful. Multiple enchondromas is termed *Ollier's disease*, and if soft-tissue hemangiomas are also presenting, it is termed *Maffucci's syndrome*. Solitary enchondromas have a malignant potential of <1%; this rate rises to 30% for Ollier's disease and greater for Maffucci's syndrome

Continued

TABLE 13-3 cont'd
Summary of Common Benign and Malignant Lesions

Tumor	Frequency	Age (median) at diagnosis	Typical location	Radiologic features	Comments
Fibrous cortical defect	Very common	4–8		Well-marginated, eccentric cortex-based osteolytic defect smaller than 3 cm	Nonaggressive fibrous lesion of bone, usually healing spontaneously
Fibrous dysplasia	Common	<20	Femur, tibia, craniofacial bones, ribs, and pelvis	Wide variety in appearance depending on the bone involved. Long bones demonstrate a mildly expansile medullary lesion that may be mildly sclerotic ("smoky" or "ground glass" appearance.). "Shepherd's crook" deformity is a lateral bowing and coxa vara deformity occurring in the proximal femur. Individual lesions often exhibit a thick "rind" of marginal sclerosis	Nonneoplastic disturbance of bone maintenance resulting in fibrous tissue replacing normal bone. Albright's syndrome is the triad of polyostotic fibrous dysplasia, precocious puberty, and cutaneous hyperpigmentations (café-au-lait spots)
Giant cell tumor	Common (18% of benign bone tumors)	20–40	Distal radius, distal femur, proximal tibia	Subarticular, osteolytic, mildly expansile, eccentric, no marginal sclerosis, and sometimes with internal septation	Tumor of the supportive tissues of bone marrow; composed of large mononuclear stromal cells and interspersed osteoclastic-like multinucleated giant cells. About 5% to 10% may be malignant, marked by pain, swelling, and aggressive radiographic appearance
Hemangioma	Common	40–50	Craniofacial bones and vertebral bodies	Osteolytic defect with characteristic coarsened, honeycomb trabeculae; or vertical striations ("corduroy cloth")	Represent vascular lesion of bone; typically asymptomatic; rarely expanding vertebral lesion may relate to spinal stenosis
Nonossifying fibroma	Very common	10–20	Metaphysis of tibia and femur	Well-marginated, eccentric cortex-based osteolytic defect >3 cm. Malignant lesions show cortical breakthrough and soft-tissue mass	Nonaggressive fibrous lesion of bone, usually healing spontaneously
Osteoblastoma	Uncommon	10–30	Posterior elements of the vertebrae; less commonly in proximal femur and tibia	Geographic, osteolytic, eccentric, mildly expansile lesion	Same as osteoid osteoma; highly vascular connective tissue nidus with interlaced osteoid tissue. Lesions may be painful
Osteochondroma	Common	10–30	Metaphyses of long bones, mostly lower extremities. Hereditary multiple exostoses of the proximal	Sessile or pedunculated ("coat hanger" exostosis or "cauliflower cap") cartilage capped bony outgrowth	Abnormal outgrowth of lateral portion of the growth plate; affects epiphyseal growth. Multiple osteochondromas are referred to as

Lesion	Frequency	Age (yr)	Location	Radiographic appearance	Comments
			femora and pelvis is common	that is continuous with underlying bone	hereditary multiple exostoses (HME), and are associated with a higher rate of malignancy (up to 25%) compared with solitary lesions (1% to 2%)
Osteoid osteoma	11% of benign bone tumors	10–20	Cortex of proximal femur or tibia; less commonly the posterior elements of the vertebrae	Small radiolucent nidus surrounded by radiodense reactive sclerosis	Highly vascular connective tissue nidus with interlaced osteoid tissue. Classically pain at night that is alleviated by aspirin. Spine lesions present on the concave side of a painful scoliosis. Low recurrence following excision
Simple bone cyst	Common	5–10	Proximal humerus and proximal femur	Oblong, central, expansile, radiolucent subepiphyseal (less frequently diaphyseal) osteolytic lesion. At times the partial internal septations may fracture and inferiorly migrate ("fallen fragment" sign)	Fluid-filled lesion of uncertain etiology; clinically silent unless fractured
Malignant					
Bone metastasis	Very common	>40	Spine, ribs, skull, and pelvis; rarely distal to the knees and elbows	Individual lesions appear osteolytic, less commonly osteoblastic, and characteristically with no or small soft-tissue mass or periosteal reaction	The most common mechanism is hematogenous seeding from primary tumors; the breast gives rise to 70% of female lesions, and prostate 60% of male lesions. Advanced osteolytic destruction may exhibit increased serum calcium. Osteoblastic lesions may reveal increased levels of alkaline phosphatase
Multiple myeloma	Common	>40 (60)	Vertebrae, rib, innominate, femur	Osteopenia, "punch-out" lesions, "raindrop" skull	Malignant plasma cell proliferation; with abnormal laboratory findings of Bence Jones proteins, anemia, thrombocytopenia, Rouleaux formation, Mott cell
Osteosarcoma	35.1*	Bimodal: first mode 1–30 (19); second mode in elderly	Metaphyses of long bones (distal femur, proximal tibia, and proximal humerus)	Osteolytic (25%), osteoblastic (50%), or mixed (25%) lesion with poorly defined margins, aggressive periosteal reaction ("onion skin" or Codman's triangle), and soft-tissue mass	Aggressive lesion of mesenchymal bone-producing cells. Lesions are painful, rapidly expanding, with malignant potential usually requiring amputation

Continued

TABLE 13-3 cont'd
Summary of Common Benign and Malignant Lesions

Tumor	Frequency	Age (median) at diagnosis	Typical location	Radiologic features	Comments
Chondrosarcoma	25.8*	>40 (53)	Femur, innominate, humerus	Destructive lesions appearing as a central lesion in bone with stippled calcifications, and cortical scalloping, or as a peripheral lesion extending from the bone's surface appearing as an exploded osteochondroma	Malignancy of mesenchymal cartilage-producing cells exhibiting varying degrees of malignancy. Lesions are painful and expanding with malignant potential. They may be primary malignant lesions of bone, or secondary to benign cartilage lesions (e.g., enchondroma, osteochondroma)
Ewing's sarcoma	16.0*	1–30 (15)	Femur, innominate, vertebrae, humerus	Permeative osteolytic eccentric pattern of bone destruction, often presenting as a scalloped deformity of the diaphyseal cortex ("saucerization"); in flat bones it appears as a mildly expansile, soap-bubble, osteolytic defect	Small round cell malignancy of bone. The patient exhibits a tender, warm, swollen limb
Chordoma	8.4*	30–70 (59)	Skull, sacrum, and C2 vertebral body	Appear as midline lesions, characterized by the presence of bone destruction and a large soft-tissue mass; calcification is noted in up to 40% of lesions on plain films	Develops from remnant portions of the notochord; patients complain of pain and enlarging soft-tissue mass, and regional visceral and neurologic involvement, such as headaches and diplopia for sphenooccipital lesions, and bowel and bladder dysfunction for sacrococcygeal lesions. Radiation is applied to those lesions that cannot be resected
Fibrosarcoma and malignant fibrous histiocytoma	5.7*	30–50 (59)	Distal femur and proximal tibia	Lesions appear as osteolytic destruction in the metaphysis, often extending to the diaphysis marked by cortical destruction and soft-tissue mass	Malignancy of deep fibrous tissue; patient complains of pain and tenderness in the region of involvement (usually around the knee)

*This percentage reflects the portion of primary malignant tumors of bone, excluding multiple myeloma.
From Dorfman HD, Czerniak B: Bone tumors, St Louis, 1998, Mosby; Dorfman HD, Czerniak B: Bone cancer, *Cancer* 75:2003, 1995.

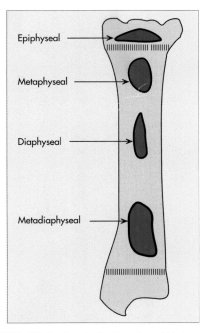

FIG. 13-1 Longitudinal location within bone.

Epiphyseal

Metaphyseal

Diaphyseal

Metadiaphyseal

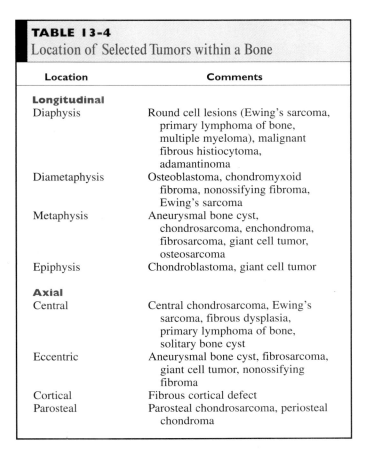

TABLE 13-4
Location of Selected Tumors within a Bone

Location	Comments
Longitudinal	
Diaphysis	Round cell lesions (Ewing's sarcoma, primary lymphoma of bone, multiple myeloma), malignant fibrous histiocytoma, adamantinoma
Diametaphysis	Osteoblastoma, chondromyxoid fibroma, nonossifying fibroma, Ewing's sarcoma
Metaphysis	Aneurysmal bone cyst, chondrosarcoma, enchondroma, fibrosarcoma, giant cell tumor, osteosarcoma
Epiphysis	Chondroblastoma, giant cell tumor
Axial	
Central	Central chondrosarcoma, Ewing's sarcoma, fibrous dysplasia, primary lymphoma of bone, solitary bone cyst
Eccentric	Aneurysmal bone cyst, fibrosarcoma, giant cell tumor, nonossifying fibroma
Cortical	Fibrous cortical defect
Parosteal	Parosteal chondrosarcoma, periosteal chondroma

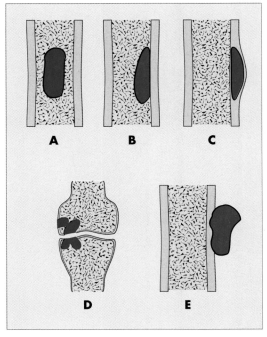

FIG. 13-2 Axial location within bone. **A,** Central. **B,** Eccentric. **C,** Cortical. **D,** Intraarticular. **E,** Parosteal. (From Juhl JH, Crummy AB: Paul and Juhl's essentials of radiologic imaging, ed 6, Philadelphia, 1993, JB Lippincott.)

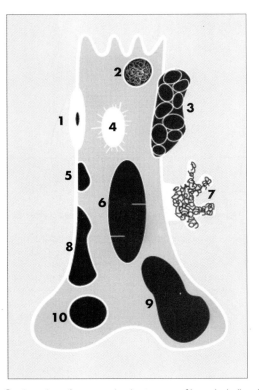

FIG. 13-3 Location of common benign tumors of bone including: *1,* osteoid osteoma; *2,* enchondroma; *3,* aneurysmal bone cyst; *4,* bone island; *5,* fibrous cortical defect; *6,* simple bone cyst; *7,* pedunculated osteochondroma; *8,* nonossifying fibroma; *9,* giant cell tumor; and *10,* chondroblastoma.

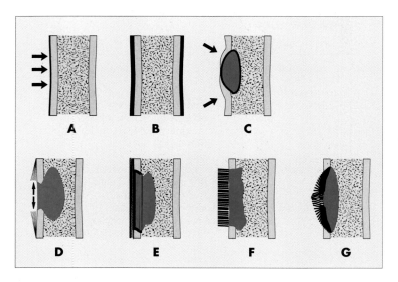

FIG. 13-4   Periosteal reaction of bone. **A,** Thin lamellar. **B,** Thick lamellar. **C,** Cortical buttressing *(arrows)*. **D,** Codman's triangles *(arrows)*. **E,** Aggressive lamellar. **F,** Hair-on-end spiculated. **G,** Sunburst. Patterns **A** through **C** are associated with benign lesions of bone. Patterns **D** through **G** are associated with aggressive lesions of bone (e.g., Ewing's sarcoma and osteosarcoma). (From Juhl JH, Crummy AB: Paul and Juhl's essentials of radiologic imaging, ed 6, Philadelphia, 1993, JB Lippincott.)

bone disease and multiple myeloma. Less common possibilities include multicentric osteosarcoma and multifocal infections. Common nonaggressive polyostotic lesions include fibrous dysplasia, Paget's disease, histocytosis, hereditary multiple exostoses (HME), multiple enchondromas (Ollier's disease), and osteomyelitis.

Treatment Options

Treatment options include surgery, chemotherapy, radiation, or pain management; all may be applied alone or in combination.

Surgical options extend from curettage for benign lesions to wide resection and possible amputation for highly malignant lesions. Each treatment approach is associated with complications, tumor recurrence, and varying success rates dependent on the patient's clinical status and the type and stage of the lesions (Table 13-6). Often the treatment plan is aimed at offering the patient only palliative relief.

TABLE 13-5
Radiographic Characteristics of Tumor Grades

Aggressiveness	Characteristics
Low grade—nonaggressive	Geographic destruction surrounded by sclerotic rim of bone
Medium grade—moderately aggressive	Geographic destruction, short transition zone, possible sclerotic rim, possible bone expansion, possible thick periosteal reaction
High grade—highly aggressive	Permeative or moth-eaten destruction, wide transition zone, no surrounding sclerosis, possible bone expansion, aggressive periosteal reaction

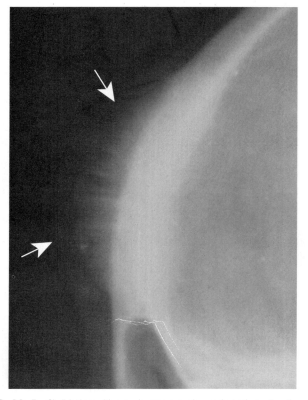

FIG. 13-5   Skull lesion with a sunburst aggressive periosteal reaction *(arrows)*. (Courtesy Steven P. Brownstein, MD, Springfield, NJ.)

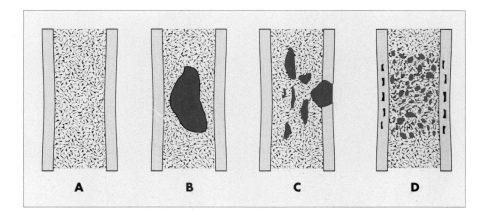

FIG. 13-6 Patterns of bone destruction. **A,** Normal bone. **B,** Geographic. **C,** Moth-eaten. **D,** Permeative. (From Juhl JH, Crummy AB: Paul and Juhl's essentials of radiologic imaging, ed 6, Philadelphia, 1993, JB Lippincott.)

FIG. 13-7 Cortical bone reaction. **A,** Expansile. **B,** Endosteal scalloping. **C,** Thin, nearly imperceptible. **D,** Destructive. **E,** Saucerization. (From Juhl JH, Crummy AB: Paul and Juhl's essentials of radiologic imaging, ed 6, Philadelphia, 1993, JB Lippincott.)

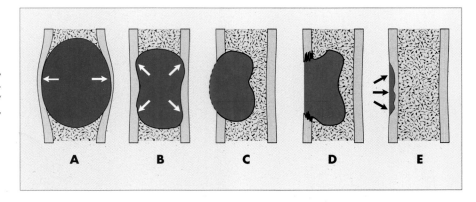

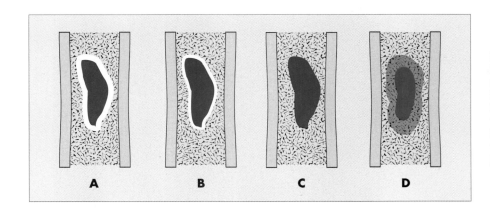

FIG. 13-8 Margination of bone lesions. **A,** Thick. **B,** Thin. **C,** Absent. **A** through **C** demonstrate a short zone of transition between normal bone and the lesion. **D,** Ill-defined. Demonstrates a long zone of transition between normal bone and the lesion. A long zone of transition is most often associated with an aggressive lesion. (From Juhl JH, Crummy AB: Paul and Juhl's essentials of radiologic imaging, ed 6, Philadelphia, 1993, JB Lippincott.)

FIG. 13-9   A, Well-defined benign defect of fibrous dysplasia characteristically exhibiting a thick surrounding margin and short zone of transition between the defect and the normal bone. **B,** Osteosarcoma with a wide zone between the center of the lesion and the normal bone. (Courtesy Steven P. Brownstein, MD, Springfield, NJ.)

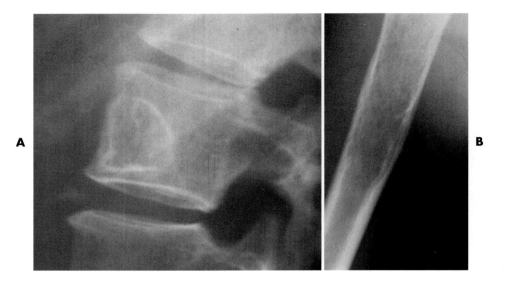

A

B

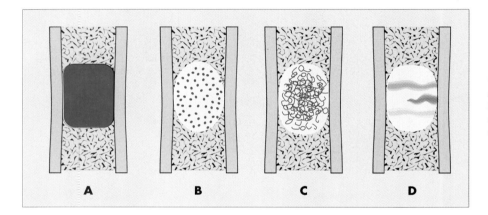

A   **B**   **C**   **D**

FIG. 13-10   Matrix appearance of the bone lesion. **A,** Solid pattern of radiodensity indicates a bone matrix. **B,** Stippled appearance or, **C,** rings and arcs suggest a cartilage matrix. **D,** Hazy, smoky, or ground glass appearance correlates to a fibrous matrix of the lesion.

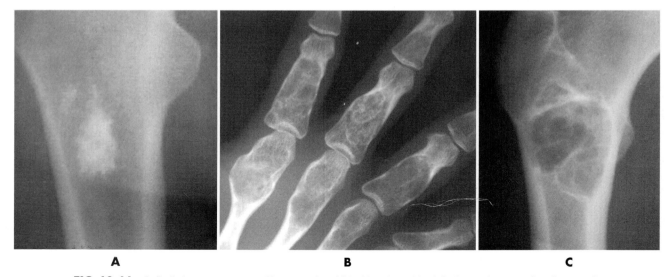

A   **B**   **C**

FIG. 13-11   A, Radiodense appearance of bone matrix exhibited by a bone island. **B,** Arcs and curves of cartilage matrix exhibited by an enchondroma. **C,** Hazy or smoky appearance of fibrous matrix exhibited by a fibrous dysplasia. (**B,** Courtesy Gary Longmuir, Phoenix, AZ.)

TABLE 13-6
Treatment Options

Treatment	Description
Chemotherapy	Chemotherapy involves the intravenous or oral application of anticancer drugs Many agents are not selective to cancer cells, and may produce significant side effects (e.g., low blood count, vomiting, loss of appetite, loss of hair, mouth sores)
Complementary and alternative therapies	Complementary or alternative management strategies may be applied to reduce malignant lesions or offer palliative relief
Hormone therapy	The growth of some forms of cancer is enhanced by circulating hormones. For instance, estrogen promotes the growth of some breast cancers and testosterone promotes the growth of most prostate cancers. In an attempt to limit the growth of cancers, surgical removal of the ovaries or testes may be considered. More often drugs can be administered to limit the production of tumor-enhancing hormones or limit their effect on the tumor cells (e.g., tamoxifen)
Immunotherapy	Immunotherapy describes efforts to facilitate the patient's immune system to recognize and destroy cancer cells by focusing on cytokines, monoclonal antibodies, and various tumor vaccines
Radiation therapy	Radiation therapy employs high-energy rays or particles to limit cancer growth, with the aim of either destroying the tumor, or at least shrinking its size, thereby giving the patient some palliative relief Radiation is most commonly applied via an external beam. Internal methods of delivering the radiation, for instance, the implantation of small seeds of radioactive material near the cancer, are less often used
Radiopharmaceuticals	Radiopharmaceuticals are radioactive substances most often applied to manage the bone pain of patients who have skeletal metastasis; agents include venous injections of strontium 89 (Metastron), samarium 153, and rhenium 186
Surgical	*Biopsy* is performed, with either closed or open methods, to gather tissue specimens for laboratory evaluation. *Curettage* is the use of hand instruments to gently remove medullary bone. *En bloc* means the lesion is removed altogether as a whole. *Wide resection* implies that a surround margin of normal tissue is removed with the lesion. *Limb-sparing surgery* describes efforts to preserve limb function by the use of a metal endoprosthesis to reconstruct bone and joint function after wide resection. *Amputation* is the surgical removal of all or part of a limb or body part and is reserved for the most aggressive lesions

 # Bone Origin

Benign

Bone Island (Enostosis), Osteoma, and Osteopoikilosis

BACKGROUND

A bone island (enostosis) is a commonly encountered entity, representing a region of compact bone located in cancellous bone (Fig. 13-12).[128] Their etiology is not well documented, but most sources list them as developmental hamartomatous or dysplastic lesions. They may appear as a single defect or multiple defects with a variety of shapes. Bone islands are estimated to appear in 1% to 14% of the adult population without a demonstrated gender, age, or racial disposition.

Osteopoikilosis (spotted bone disease) is a relatively uncommon condition of skeletal dysplasia that is marked by a symmetric presentation of multiple bone islands. Each lesion is microscopically identical to a bone island.

Osteomas differ from enostoses in that the former protrude from the surface of the affected bone and are found in the skull. Also, bone islands are encountered in all age groups, whereas osteomas typically are discovered in the adult patient. Multiple osteomas may be one component of Gardner syndrome, comprising colonic polyposis, osteomatosis, dental lesions, and soft-tissue tumors.[3,217]

IMAGING FINDINGS

Enostoses are small (usually 0.1 to 2.0 cm), radiodense lesions that occur in all bones, although they are more common in the pelvis, proximal femora, and ribs. They have a characteristic thorny or spiculed border that blends into normal trabeculae, producing a typical whiskered or "brush border" periphery of the lesion (Fig. 13-13), a feature best seen on CT. Usually they are slightly oblong with their long axis running parallel to that of the host bone. Bone islands larger than 2 cm in diameter are less common, and are called giant bone islands. Larger lesions may exhibit active bone remodeling, evidenced by increased uptake of radiotracer with bone scintigraphy.[53] Although most bone islands are stable in size, some do exhibit slow growth over time.[19] Bone islands appear as hypointense signals on MRI.

Osteopoikilosis exhibits a symmetric presentation common to the metaphyses of long bones, or commonly diffusely scattered in the carpals or tarsals. They may appear periarticular less commonly, especially about the hips (Fig. 13-14).

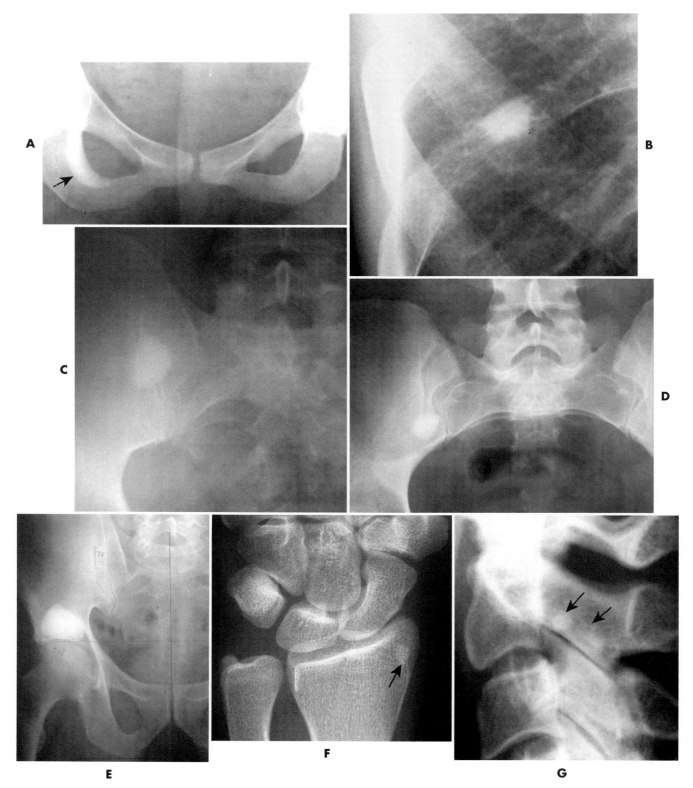

FIG. 13-12 Well-defined focal radiopaque lesions representing bone islands of the **A,** pelvis *(arrow);* **B,** rib; **C, D,** and **E,** ilium; **F,** radial styloid *(arrow);* and **G,** spine *(arrows).* (**E,** Courtesy Steven P. Brownstein, MD, Springfield, NJ.)

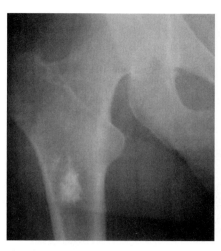

FIG. 13-13 Bone island of the femur exhibiting a spiculated periphery that is known as a *brush border.*

Osteomas appear as dense radiopacities found almost exclusively in the skull and facial bones, especially near the frontal sinuses (Figs. 13-15 and 13-16).

CLINICAL COMMENTS

A bone island usually is identified readily because it occurs without symptoms and has a characteristic appearance on imaging. However, if bone islands are multiple, large, growing, or present in patients with clinical red flags of aggressive bone disease (e.g., pain at night, personal history of past malignancy), differentiation from an entity such as osteoblastic metastasis may be warranted. Past radiographs may help in this differential. If past radiographs are unavailable, a bone scan represents the traditional method of differentiating bone islands from more aggressive entities.[96,183,215] However, it is possible that bone islands (especially large lesions) may appear active on bone scans, necessitating other methods of differentiation. MRI usually is definitive. Similar to a bone island, osteopoikilosis is not associated with clinical symptoms. Osteomas may become clinically significant if they enlarge and interfere with sinus drainage.

Osteoid Osteoma and Osteoblastoma

BACKGROUND

An osteoid osteoma and osteoblastoma are histologically similar benign bone lesions that differ in size and (usually) radiographic appearance. Each consists of a highly vascularized nidus of connective tissue with interlacing trabeculae of osteoid and calcified bone surrounded by osteoblasts. Reactive bone response is variable and most often more pronounced on the cortical side of the lesions (less pronounced in osteoblastoma). Trabeculae merge into a mass of calcified bone toward the center of the lesion. Osteoid osteomas and osteoblastomas usually occur in patients between the ages of 10 and 25 years, with a 2:1 male predominance.

IMAGING FINDINGS

Osteoid osteoma appears as a small (<1.5 cm in diameter) osteolytic lesion with surrounding reactive sclerosis (Fig. 13-17). The central radiolucent nidus (Figs. 13-18 to 13-20) may be only a few millimeters in diameter and often contains a small focus of calcification. The surrounding reactive sclerosis may become so prominent that it completely obscures the radiolucent nidus, a feature that is particularly common when the lesions present in the vertebrae. The surrounding sclerosis represents a secondary finding and therefore may reverse after removal of the nidus. Osteoid osteomas are most commonly located in the cortex of long bones, usually the proximal femur (see Fig. 13-18) or tibia. Other locations include the posterior elements of the spine (e.g., concave side of painful scoliosis), humerus, hand, and talus. Osteoid osteomas usually are based in the cortex, but medullary, subperiosteal, and intracapsular locations do occur.[122]

Osteoblastoma appears as a larger (≥1.5 cm in diameter), geographic, expansile, generally nonaggressive, eccentric medullary lesion. It may exhibit a sclerotic component. Osteoblastomas are

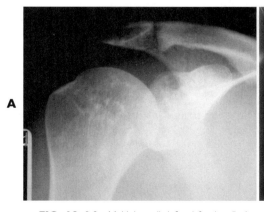
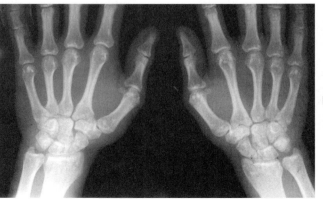

FIG. 13-14 Multiple well-defined focal radiodense shadows distributed symmetrically near the joints representing multiple bone islands, known as osteopoikilosis of, **A,** the shoulder and, **B,** hands. (**A,** Courtesy Texas Chiropractic College, Pasadena, TX; **B,** Courtesy Steven P. Brownstein, MD, Springfield, NJ.)

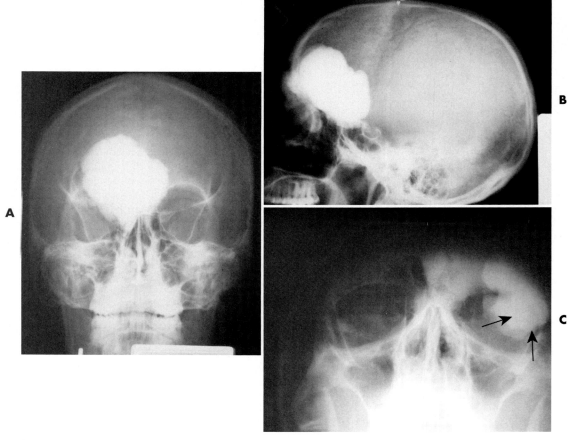

FIG. 13-15   Large radiodense lesion of the skull consistent with an osteoma projected on, **A,** the anteroposterior; **B,** lateral; and, **C,** water's *(arrows)* view. (Courtesy Steven P. Brownstein, MD, Springfield, NJ.)

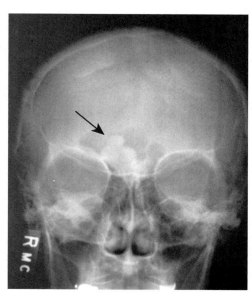

FIG. 13-16   Irregular radiodense lesion of the right frontal sinus representing an osteoma *(arrow)*.

most commonly located in the posterior elements of the spine[157] (Fig. 13-21) and less frequently in the proximal femur, tibia, talus, ribs, and hands.[161]

Because osteoid osteomas and osteoblastomas are richly vascularized, an intense uptake is noted on radionuclide bone scans. CT is valuable to further delineate the lesions and demonstrate a radiolucent nidus. This is particularly true when imaging areas of complex anatomy, such as the spine.

On MRI the central nidus shows low to intermediate signal intensity on both T1- and T2-weighted MRI scans, and enhancement after contrast administration.[246]

CLINICAL COMMENTS

Patients with osteoid osteomas and osteoblastomas often describe pain in the affected region. The pain begins as intermittent and vague, progressing to a dull and boring quality, which typically is not related to activity. Approximately 80% of patients with osteoid osteomas report a worsening of pain at night, which is characteristically alleviated by aspirin or other nonsteroidal antiinflammatory agents.[106,209]

Osteoid osteomas of the spine typically are located on the concave side of a painful scoliosis, and should be excluded in all children and young adults who present with unexplained back pain or painful scoliosis.[124] Osteoblastomas also are associated with scoliosis but do not exhibit a predilection for the concave side.[134]

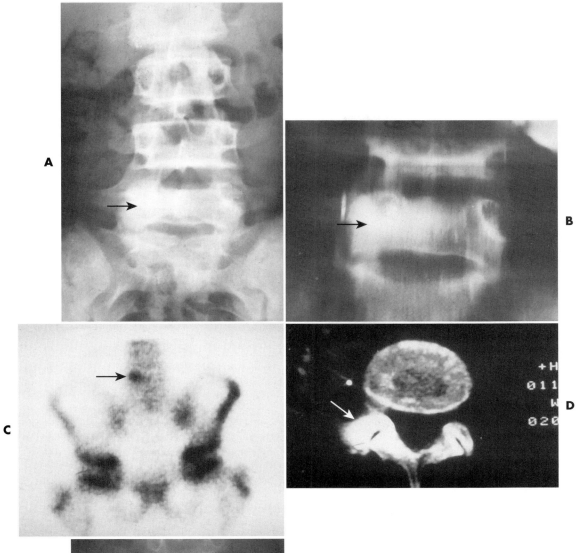

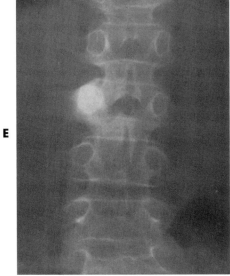

FIG. 13-17 A, The pedicle is a predilectory site for the development of an osteoid osteoma of the spine *(arrow).* **B,** Tomogram manifesting the homogenous sclerosis associated with an osteoid osteoma, suggesting a "bright" pedicle *(arrow).* **C,** Increased radioisotopic uptake is noted in the presence of a pedicular osteoid osteoma *(arrow).* **D,** Computed axial tomographic scan exhibiting the presence of an osteoid osteoma in the vertebral arch *(arrow).* **E,** Note the dense, homogeneous sclerosis, representing the "bright" pedicle associated with an osteoid osteoma of the neural arch. (From Deltoff MN: The portable skeletal x-ray, St Louis, 1997, Mosby.)

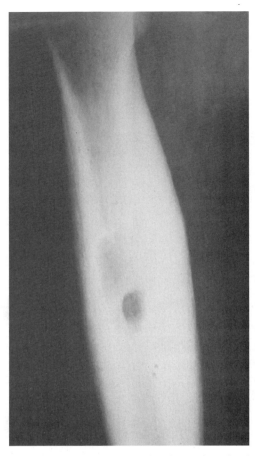

FIG. 13-18 The femur represents another frequent site for the development of an ostecid osteoma. (From Deltoff MN: The portable skeletal x-ray, St Louis, 1997, Mosby.)

Markedly expansile osteoblastomas may cause canal stenosis. An osteoid osteoma in a cortical location of the medial femoral neck may mimic clinically an impeding stress fracture or infection. En bloc surgical excision of the nidus and some surrounding sclerosis is the preferred treatment for both lesions. Often the excision of the radiolucent nidus of an osteoid osteoma is followed by dramatic relief of the patient's complaint.[170] Alternatively, long-term antiinflammatory treatment of 3 to nearly 4 years' duration has been shown to regress the size of the lesion and provide permanent relief of symptoms.[129] Cryotherapy has been applied successfully as adjuvant treatment.

KEY CONCEPTS

- *Osteoid osteomas and osteoblastomas are histologically similar.*
- *Osteoid osteomas appear sclerotic, small (<1.5 cm), and cortically based in the femur or tibia, associated with pain that is dramatically alleviated with aspirin.*
- *Osteoid osteomas are most common to the lower extremities, particularly the neck of the femur.*
- *Osteoblastomas are larger (≥1.5 cm), expansile, medullary lesions of the spine, femur, and tibia.*
- *Both are noted in patients between 10 and 25 years of age.*

Ossifying Fibroma

BACKGROUND

Ossifying fibromas are lesions that closely resemble fibrous dysplasia, both radiographically and pathologically. They present as two pathologically distinct lesions, one that occurs in the mandible derived from periodontal ligament (also termed *cementifying fibroma*) and a second that occurs in the tibia and fibula representing osteofibrous dysplasia. Osteofibrous dysplasia is marked by fibrous tissue and bone trabeculae circumscribed by osteoblasts, and occurring exclusively in the tibia and fibula.[31,125]

Long bone ossifying fibromas typically occur within the first two decades of life and undergo a self-healing process until puberty and then stabilize. The mandibular lesions occur in the

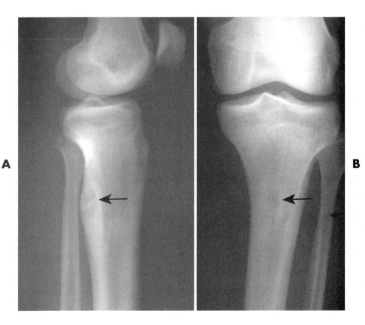

FIG. 13-19 **A** and **B,** Osteoid osteoma presenting in the tibia (arrows). (Courtesy Steven P. Brownstein, MD, Springfield, NJ.)

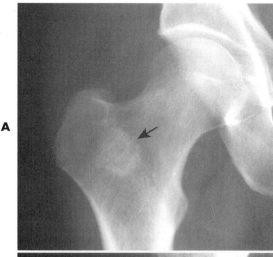

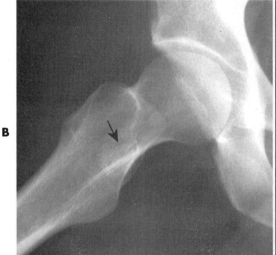

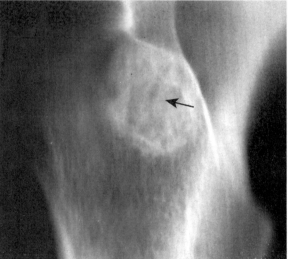

FIG. 13-20 Osteoid osteoma of the intertrochanteric region of the proximal femur. The lesion appears as a radiodense region of reactive bone sclerosis surrounding a more radiolucent central nidus on, **A,** the anteroposterior; **B,** frog-leg; and **C,** linear tomogram (*arrows*). (Courtesy Gary Longmuir, Phoenix, AZ.)

third and fourth decades and are much more common in females.[77] There is no gender predilection for the long bone presentation. The long bone lesions occur de novo or in association with an adamantinoma.

IMAGING FINDINGS

Whether they are in the mandible or long bones, ossifying fibromas initially present as radiolucent lesions, stabilize, and then become sclerotic over time (Fig. 13-22). In the long bones, lesions present in the tibia, fibula, or both. In fact, synchronous lesions of the tibia and fibula that appear on one side of the body are common presentations. Individual lesions appear radiolucent, circumscribed, expansile, and eccentric. Lesions in the tibia have a propensity to locate in the anterior or anterolateral cortex, creating an anterior bowing deformity of the bone's shaft. The mandibular lesions likewise may deform the lower margin of the mandible and may contain a target, central opacification.

CLINICAL COMMENTS

Clinical concern for these rare lesions centers on differentiating them from typical fibrous dysplasia. Most lesions are treated conservatively.

KEY CONCEPTS

- *In long bones, ossifying fibromas are rare lesions of osteofibrous dysplasia occurring in the tibia or fibula during the first two decades of life.*
- *Ossifying fibromas initially appear radiolucent, becoming radiodense over time.*
- *Mandibular lesions typically are tissues in the molar or premolar area.*
- *Both lesions usually begin as painless masses and may exhibit bone deformity.*

Malignant

Osteosarcoma

BACKGROUND

Osteosarcomas are highly aggressive malignant bone tumors. They are the second most common primary malignant bone tumors after multiple myelomas. However, because of their hematopoietic origin, some sources do not categorize multiple myeloma lesions as true bone tumors. In which case, osteosarcomas become the most common primary malignant bone tumors.

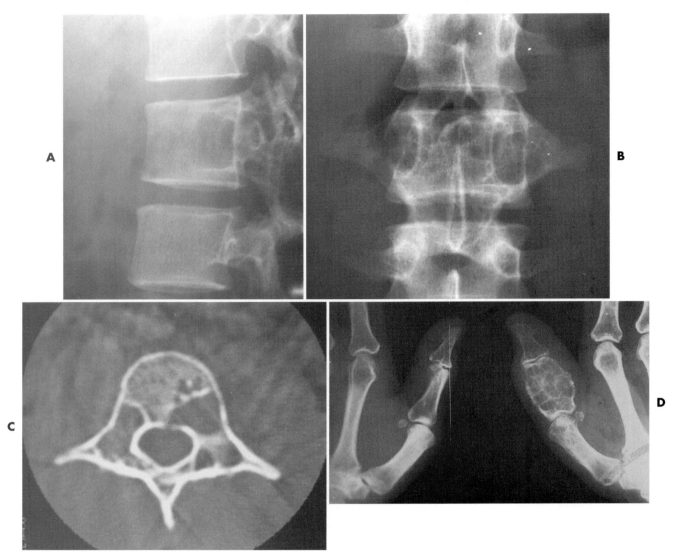

FIG. 13-21 Expansile lesion of the neural arch and posterior body present on, **A,** the lateral; **B,** anteroposterior; and **C,** axial computed tomography image. The lesion is most consistent with an osteoblastoma. **D,** Another patient demonstrates similar bone expansion of the right thumb's proximal phalanx, consistent with osteoblastoma. (Courtesy Steven P. Brownstein, MD, Springfield, NJ.)

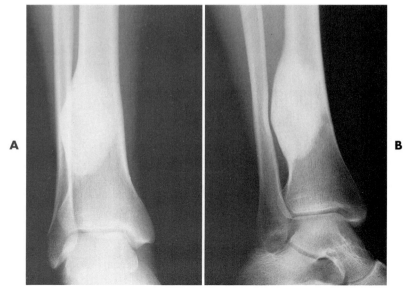

FIG. 13-22 **A** and **B,** Ossifying fibroma of the distal tibia. (Courtesy Ian D. McLean, LeClaire, IA.)

Although all osteosarcomas produce osteoid matrix, the proportion of chondroid and fibroid histologic constituents is variable. Only about 50% of osteosarcomas contain predominantly osteoid matrix, appearing osteoblastic on the radiographs. Osteosarcoma can be classified into intraosseous, surface, extraosseous, secondary, and multicentric types.[20]

Intraosseous osteosarcoma. Conventional and telangiectatic osteosarcomas are subtypes of the intraosseous classification. Conventional osteosarcomas account for 75% to 85% of all osteosarcomas. Conventional osteosarcomas arise within cancellous bone and then grow aggressively, extending into the medullary canal and penetrating the cortex to invade the soft tissues. Telangiectatic osteosarcoma is an aggressive, rare variant of osteosarcoma. It is characterized by large, blood-filled cavities and thin septations.[112]

Surface osteosarcoma. Periosteal and parosteal (juxtacortical) osteosarcomas are subtypes of surface osteosarcoma classification that arise from the cortex, subperiosteal tissue, or periosteum. They are marked by outward growth toward the soft tissues of the involved limb. Parosteal osteosarcoma is more common and exhibits large amounts of osteoid production. Periosteal osteosarcoma is rare and difficult to distinguish from periosteal chondrosarcoma because of the large amounts of chondroid and scant osteoid tissue that may be present in the lesion.

Other osteosarcomas. Extraosseous osteosarcomas are soft-tissue tumors with the same histologic composition as conventional osteosarcomas. Secondary osteosarcoma most commonly occurs in elderly patients with Paget's disease, infarcts, fibrous dysplasia, or regions of previous radiation therapy.[204,247] Multicentric osteosarcoma defines symmetrically distributed, multiple synchronous osteosarcomas of similar size and development.[190]

Patient age. Conventional and telangiectatic osteosarcomas have a slight male predominance and occur most commonly in people 10 to 25 years old; the median is 19 years. The occurrence of a second peak of incidence has been noted among those over the age of 60 years.[113] Periosteal osteosarcomas are seen most often in people 10 to 20 years old, and occur more commonly in female patients. Parosteal osteosarcomas occur in a slightly older age group than conventional or periosteal osteosarcomas. The average age of patients with extraosseous osteosarcomas is 45 years. Multicentric osteosarcoma occurs during the first decade.

IMAGING FINDINGS

Conventional osteosarcomas most commonly arise in the metaphysis of long bones, usually the distal femur (40%) (Fig. 13-23), proximal tibia (20%), humerus (9%), pelvis (5%), facial bones (5%), fibula (4%), and patella (<1%). Older patients exhibit a higher incidence of osteosarcoma in flat bones. The radiographic appearance of conventional osteosarcomas begins with a medullary osteolytic (25%), osteoblastic (25%), or mixed (50%) lesion in the metaphysis, often extending into the epiphysis or diaphysis. Ninety percent have a large, cloudlike density representing tumor bone and an aggressive (laminated, sunburst, "hair-on-end," or Codman's triangles) periosteal reaction (Fig. 13-24). The aggressive periosteal reaction occurs from tumor invasion lifting the periosteum of the bone, and subsequent reactive bone formation. A large soft-tissue mass is typical.

Telangiectatic osteosarcoma usually appears as an osteolytic, expansile lesion in the diaphysis of the femur, tibia, or humerus.

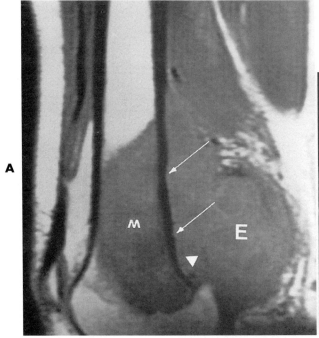

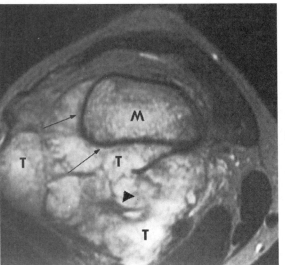

FIG. 13-23   Distal femoral osteosarcoma. **A,** Sagittal T1-weighted magnetic resonance imaging demonstrates low signal intensity marrow involvement (M) with prominent posterior extension (E). **B,** Transaxial T2-weighted image reveals predominantly high signal intensity within both the marrow (M) and soft-tissue (T) components of the lesion. Areas of intact cortex (arrows) are evident on both images, along with tumor bone formation (arrowheads), suggesting the correct diagnosis. (From Sartoris DJ: Musculoskeletal imaging: the requisites, St Louis, 1993, Mosby.)

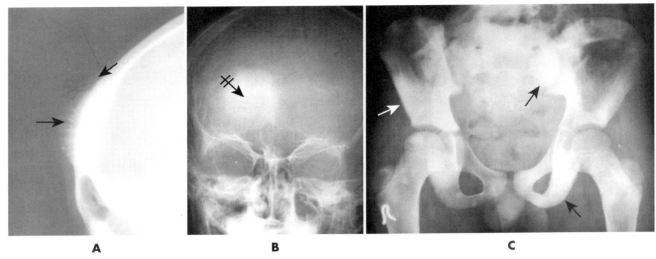

FIG. 13-24 **A** and **B,** Osteosarcoma of the frontal bone with increased radiodensity (arrows) and aggressive periostitis (crossed arrow). **C,** Additional regions of increased radiodensity are noted in the pelvis (arrows), representing metastasis. (Courtesy Steven P. Brownstein, MD, Springfield, NJ.)

It is characterized by periosteal reaction with a large soft-tissue mass and lack of visible bone production. The periosteal reaction often is layered, appearing as an "onion skin." Parosteal osteosarcoma usually appears as a lobular, radiodense mass arising from a sessile base to surround the metaphysis of the host bone (Figs. 13-25 to 13-29). A thin radiolucent line is present but rarely seen, separating the tumor from the host bone. Nearly 70% of parosteal osteosarcomas are metaphyseal, arising from the posterior surface of the distal femur; other sites include the proximal tibia and humerus. Periosteal reaction is rare. Periosteal osteosarcomas present as soft-tissue masses extending from the diaphysis of long bones, usually the femur or tibia, which may have small perpendicular bone spicules or amorphous calcification within the tumor mass. The endosteal margin is not involved.

Secondary osteosarcomas appear as destructive lesions usually indistinguishable from conventional osteosarcomas, occurring in the region of primary disease. Extraosseous osteosarcomas appear as large soft-tissue masses, most often in the buttocks and thigh.[79] More than half of the lesions demonstrate radiographic evidence of calcification. These lesions are best demonstrated by MRI.[234] Multicentric osteosarcoma is accompanied by multiple, symmetrically distributed radiodensities in the metaphyses.

For the most part, primary osseous lesions are well defined on conventional radiographs. CT and MRI are used to assess the extent

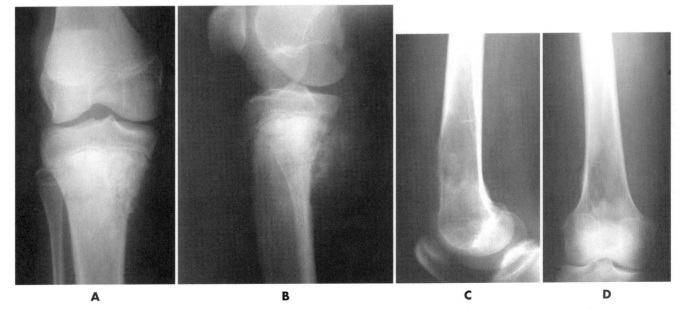

FIG. 13-25 Osteosarcoma is most common around the knee. Two cases: **A** and **B,** the first presents osteosarcoma of the proximal tibia presenting the typical aggressive appearance and radiodense matrix. **C** and **D,** The second presents osteosarcoma of the distal femur appearing with a radiolucent destructive matrix. (**C** and **D,** Courtesy Steven P. Brownstein, MD, Springfield, NJ.)

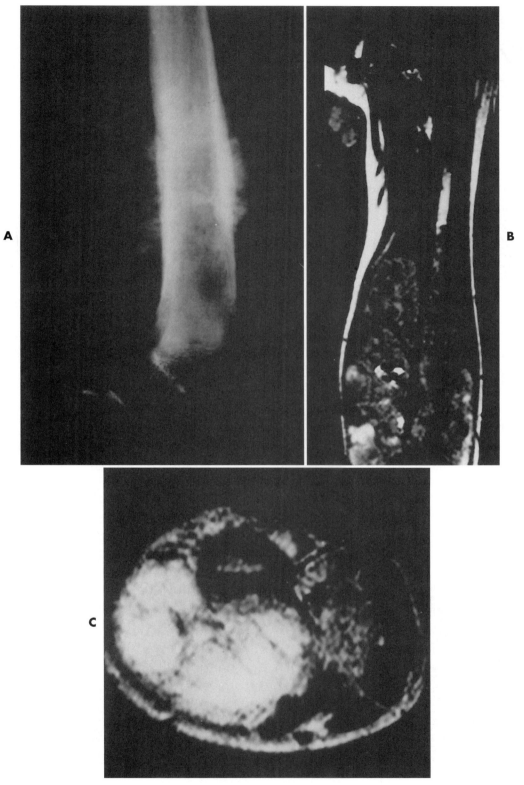

FIG. 13-26 Characteristic appearance of osteosarcoma in the distal femur of a 15-year-old boy. **A,** Involved portion of bone has a mixed sclerotic and lytic appearance with periostosis and a soft-tissue mass. Note the sunburst appearance caused by radially oriented linear ossification. **B,** Coronal T1-weighted image demonstrates the relatively low signal tumor extending to the middiaphysis. The signal intensity of the tumor contrasts well with the normal bright signal of the yellow marrow. The rather low signal from the proximal diaphysis is caused by partial volume averaging of the cortical and medullary signal. The low signal in the proximal metaphysis is secondary to the presence of the normal red marrow. Note the loss of the signal void of the distal femoral cortex resulting from destruction (and replacement) by a tumor. The signal intensity of the tumor is only marginally different than the normal skeletal muscle. The bright signal areas represent areas of hemorrhage. **C,** T2-weighted image better defines the high signal intensity of the tumor from the surrounding low signal muscle vessels. (From Firooznia H et al: MRI and CT of the musculoskeletal system, St Louis, 1992, Mosby.)

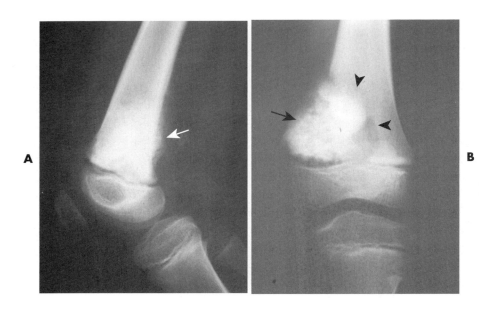

FIG. 13-27 **A,** Osteosarcoma in the distal femur with aggressive spiculated periostitis *(arrow)* present in an 8-year-old boy. **B,** A band of osteolytic destruction *(arrowheads)* surrounding the radiodense matrix of the lesion *(arrow)* in the frontal projection.

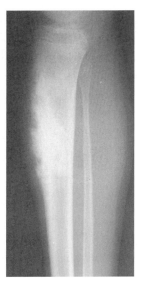

FIG. 13-28 Aggressive periostitis outlining a radiodense matrix of a lesion within the proximal tibia in a 12-year-old patient. The lesion is consistent with osteosarcoma. (Courtesy Steven P. Brownstein, MD, Springfield, NJ.)

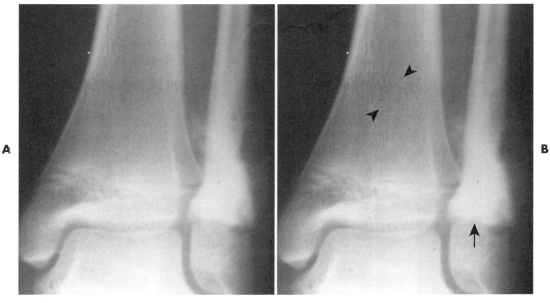

A

B

FIG. 13-29 Osteosarcoma. **A,** Anteroposterior and, **B,** oblique ankle projections reveal an aggressive osteosclerotic lesion of the distal fibula. Aggressive periosteal and soft-tissue extension is noted on the medial side of the fibula *(arrow)*. **B,** Incidentally noted is a nonossifying fibroma in the distal tibia, best seen on the oblique projection *(arrowheads)*.

of the lesion and evaluate its relationship to adjacent anatomy to aid surgical planning.

CLINICAL COMMENTS

Patients with osteosarcoma present with pain, swelling, and sometimes limited joint motion of the involved limb. Symptoms usually are present a few months before presentation. Serum alkaline phosphatase levels may be elevated. An initial complaint of pathologic fracture is more common with telangiectatic osteosarcoma. Multicentric, telangiectatic, and conventional osteosarcomas have poorer prognoses than surface osteosarcomas.

Conventional treatment includes the application of one or some combination of the following: excision, amputation, chemotherapy, and radiation.[52,164,194,227,244] Patient survival rates range from promising (with parosteal osteosarcoma) to poor (with multicentric

osteosarcoma) and depend on the type of osteosarcoma, applied treatment, and general patient health status.

KEY CONCEPTS

- *Osteosarcoma is the second most common primary malignant tumor of bone after multiple myeloma.*
- *Osteosarcoma has a bimodal age distribution. Most lesions occur in patients between the ages of 10 and 25, with a later age group for the parosteal subtype.*
- *Osteosarcomas are aggressive, including bone, periosteal, and soft-tissue manifestations; 50% have radiodense matrices.*
- *These tumors most commonly arise from the metaphysis of long bones around the knee.*
- *Symptoms include pain, swelling, and limited motion of the limb that is involved.*

Bone Marrow Origin

Malignant

Plasmacytoma and Multiple Myeloma

BACKGROUND

Multiple myeloma (MM) is a malignant monoclonal proliferation of plasma cells occurring predominantly in the red marrow of various bones. Plasma cells are mature B lymphocytes that produced immunoglobulins (antibodies). Therefore the proliferation of plasma cells results in increased amounts of circulating immunoglobulins (Ig) that have the potential to affect multiple organ systems.

Numerous diffuse foci or larger nodular accumulations of malignant plasma cells are surrounded by areas of increased osteoclastic activity. MM represents the most common primary tumor of bone, although some consider MM a hematologic disease, making osteosarcoma the most common primary tumor of bone. In any case, MM is the most common malignancy to present as a primary skeletal site. A solitary lesion of plasma cell myeloma is termed *plasmacytoma* (Fig. 13-30).

It is believed that the abnormal plasma cells produce osteoclastic-activating factors[203] and osteoblastic inhibitory factors, which leads to increased bone resorption and decreased bone formation.[11,67] Initially MM invades the axial skeleton, progressing to the appendicular skeleton over time. It represents the most common primary malignant tumor of bone. Most patients with MM are 50 to 70 years old; rarely are those under the age of 30 years affected.[115] The median age is 60 years. A slight male predominance is often reported, and the lesions are twice as common among blacks as whites.

IMAGING FINDINGS

Approximately 80% of MM patients demonstrate radiographic features. Most commonly, MM occurs as multicentric (polyostotic) lesions of punched-out or moth-eaten patterns of bone destruction. Less commonly, MM presents as diffuse osteopenia without focal bone destruction; probably this is the most difficult presentation to recognize because it mimics osteoporosis.[34]

Up to 30% of MM patients initially exhibit only a solitary lesion of bone known as a plasmacytoma (Figs. 13-31 to 13-33). Plasmacytomas appear as large (typically >4 cm in diameter), expansile, and cystic lesions. About 70% of patients with solitary plasmacytomas progress to multifocal disseminated MM.[243]

Rarely, MM presents as one or more sclerotic lesions, typically part of a larger syndrome known as POEMS (polyneuropathy, organomegaly, endocrinopathy, myeloma, and skin changes).

MM lesions exhibit a short zone of transition and no surrounding sclerosis, have no visible matrix (except for lesions in POEMS), and usually are less than 4 cm in diameter. MM originates in bones that are high in red marrow content. The skull, vertebral bodies, ribs, and proximal humerus and femur are most commonly involved (Figs. 13-34 to 13-36). Extraosseous manifestations are rare; they are found in fewer than 5% of patients.[95,177] Ribs and other small bones may be slightly expanded when involved.

Neoplastic plasma cells produce an osteoclastic activating factor that stimulates massive osteolysis with only minimal bone reaction; therefore MM frequently is associated with a negative bone scan. Plain film radiography appears more sensitive than radionuclide bone scanning; however, both miss a significant portion of cases. MRI is highly sensitive and is used in cases of negative radiographs and radionuclide imaging.[229]

CLINICAL COMMENTS

Clinical findings are secondary to excessive plasma cell production. Pain is the most common patient complaint, reported in up to 70% of cases. Pathologic fractures are common and may be the presenting sign, especially collapsed vertebrae. MM is associated with multifocal bone pain (especially in the weight-bearing bones), amyloidosis, renal failure, hemorrhages, recurrent infections, and general weakness.[136] Amyloidosis and related organ impairment is seen in association with about 10% to 15% of MM patients.[130] Involvement of the kidneys and heart is most serious. In rare instances, patients with MM may remain asymptomatic.[59,60]

Laboratory examination may reveal hypercalcemia, hyperuricemia, elevated creatine levels, anemia, and thrombocytopenia. The plasma cells can accumulate in renal cells, causing dysfunction and renal failure. The amount of Bence Jones proteins in the urine is an indicator of the degree of renal involvement. Elevated serum renal chemistries such as BUN (blood urea nitrogen) and creatinine point to renal impairment from the deposition of immunoglobulins in the kidney.

The corresponding serum abnormality consists of hyperglobulinemia with a reversal of the albumin-globulin (A/G) ratio.

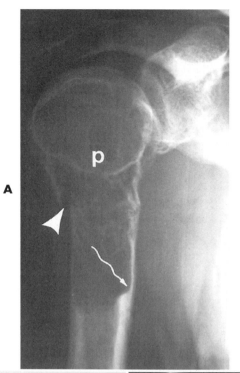

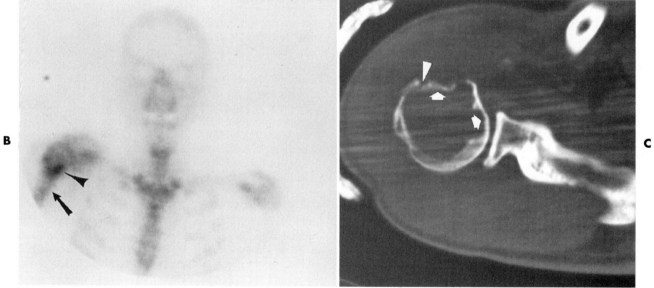

FIG. 13-30   Plasmacytoma of the proximal humerus. **A,** Radiography reveals a septate lytic lesion *(p)* with endosteal scalloping *(wavy arrow)* and pathologic fracture *(arrowhead)*. **B,** Increased activity is present within the lesion *(arrow)* and particularly at the site of fracture *(arrowhead)* as seen on a radionuclide bone scan. **C,** Computed tomography optimally demonstrates the degree of cortical thinning *(arrows)*, as well as the fracture *(arrowhead)*. (From Sartoris DJ: Musculoskeletal imaging: the requisites, St Louis, 1993, Mosby.)

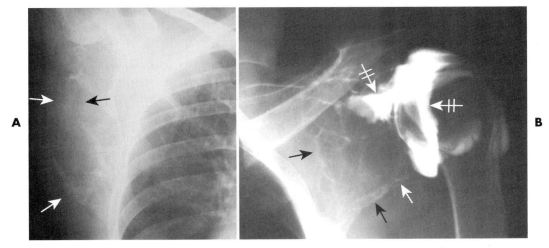

FIG. 13-31   A and **B,** Two cases of plasmacytoma presenting in the scapula *(arrows).* Both lesions exhibit the characteristic expansile, multiseptated lesions characteristic of the disease. **B,** This case is a arthrogram, exhibited by the injected contrast *(crossed arrows).* (Courtesy Steven P. Brownstein, MD, Springfield, NJ.)

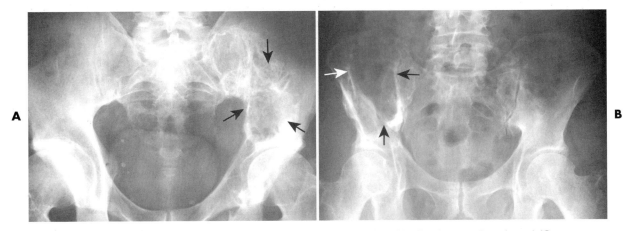

FIG. 13-32   A and **B,** Plasmacytoma presenting as an expansile cystic defect of the ilium in two patients *(arrows).* (Courtesy Steven P. Brownstein, MD, Springfield, NJ.)

Most patients produce an overabundance of the immunoglobulin G (IgG) type. Serum abnormalities are recognized by electrophoresis and are considered central to the diagnosis of the disease. The increased levels of monoclonal immunoglobulins (M component) can be detected by protein electrophoresis as an abnormal "M spike" or "M component spike." The level of M component reflects the tumor's burden and can be used as a surrogate index to monitor the course of the disease and its therapeutic outcome. For example, 0.5 g/dl of M component in the serum estimates 10 g of neoplastic tissue in the body. High levels of M component are seen with MM and Waldenström macroglobulinemia. Usually MM patients who exhibit only an isolated plasmacytoma do not exhibit the M component abnormality in their serum.

The peripheral blood smear reveals rouleaux formations, defined by red blood cells appearing stacked on top of one another like a roll of coins. This appearance is from the immunoglobulins, which act as "glue" and stick the red blood cells together.

Mott cells are found on bone marrow aspiration. Mott cells represent immature plasma cells with numerous intercellular vacuoles filled with immunoglobulins.

MM is diagnosed by a high index of clinical suspicion, with radiographic and laboratory correlation. A biopsy for histologic examination is necessary once a lesion is identified. Although variable, the usual course of the disease is that of gradual progression with a median survival of 3 years.[137] Treatment includes radiation and chemotherapy.

> ### KEY CONCEPTS
>
> - *Multiple myeloma (MM) is the most common primary malignant tumor of bone.*
> - *Most patients are between 50 and 70 years of age.*
> - *Bone scans are notoriously insensitive because of suppressed osteoblastic activity.*
> - *MM exhibits a predilection for the axial skeleton.*
> - *Most commonly, MM presents as multicentric (polyostotic) lesions of punched-out or moth-eaten patterns of bone destruction.*
> - *Solitary lesions are termed plasmacytomas, appear less aggressive, and are expansile.*

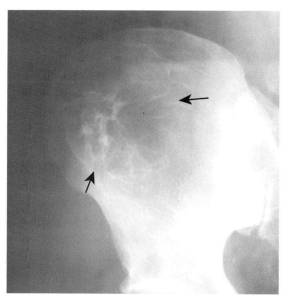

FIG. 13-33   Plasmacytoma of the ilium appearing as a cystic, radiolucent lesion with mild expansion *(arrows)*.

Ewing's Sarcoma

BACKGROUND

In 1921 James Ewing's described a small, malignant round cell neoplasm of uncertain origin that bears his name.[78] Traditionally Ewing's sarcoma was thought to originate from noncommitted mesenchymal cells; however, more recent studies suggest an

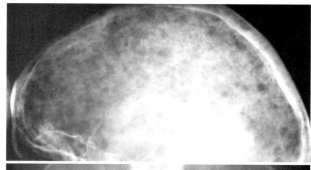

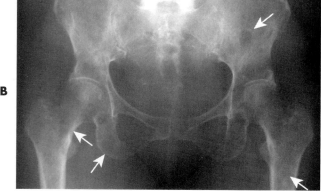

FIG. 13-34   Multiple myeloma of, **A,** the skull and, **B,** pelvis. Both locations demonstrate the punched-out lesions characteristic of the disease *(arrows)*. In the skull, the punched-out lesions give a raindrop skull appearance.

association between Ewing's sarcoma and a neuroectodermal origin.[55,150,248] Ewing's sarcoma is the fourth most common primary malignant tumor of bone after multiple myeloma, osteosarcoma, and chondrosarcoma.

Ewing's sarcoma of bone and soft tissue is one of four distinct histologic subtypes of a group of lesions known as the Ewing's family of tumors. The three other subtypes include peripheral neuroepithelioma (arising from the peripheral nervous system), esthesioneuroblastoma (developing from olfactive placode in the nasal vault), and Askin's tumor (thoracopulmonary pediatric tumor).

Although Ewing's sarcoma has been reported in patients from 5 months to 79 years old, 90% of cases involve patients younger than 30 years of age.[72,182] It exhibits a strong predilection for whites[143,167] and a slight predilection for males.

IMAGING FINDINGS

Ewing's sarcoma may occur in any bone of the body, although the majority of cases occur in the pelvis and long bones of the lower extremities (Figs. 13-37 to 13-40). A diaphyseal location is classic, but a metadiaphysis is more common.[51,72]

The radiographic appearance is marked by ill-defined, permeative, osteolytic bone destruction, cortical erosion (known as *saucerization*), laminated or "hair-on-end" periosteal reaction, and a large soft-tissue mass.[199] Ewing's sarcoma is less commonly a mixed osteolytic and sclerotic lesion (see Fig. 13-39). Only rarely does Ewing's sarcoma appear as a predominantly sclerotic lesion. A Ewing's tumor may appear similar to other round cell tumors, including lymphoma and metastatic neuroblastoma radiologically, but is differentiated from them easily with molecular probes and immunohistochemical techniques.

CLINICAL COMMENTS

Ewing's sarcoma is very aggressive; usually patients experience a history of diffuse pain and swelling involving the affected region. Other symptoms frequently include an elevated sedimentation rate, erythema, leukocytosis, and fever, mimicking osteomyelitis, a main differential diagnosis. It has a high likelihood of metastasis, especially common to the pulmonary tissue. The prognosis has been very poor traditionally, but recent combinations of irradiation, surgical resection, and multidrug chemotherapy have elevated the 5-year survival to nearly 70%.[3] Survival rates are influenced by the age of onset, location, gender, and size of the lesion.

KEY CONCEPTS

- Ewing's sarcoma is the fourth most common primary malignant tumor.
- Patients are usually younger than 30 years of age.
- The clinical presentation may mimic an infection.
- Ewing's sarcoma typically presents as a metadiaphyseal permeative osteolytic lesion with cortical saucerization and aggressive periosteal changes and less commonly appears as an osteosclerotic lesion.

Lymphoma of Bone

BACKGROUND

A lymphoma is a malignant tumor composed of lymphocytes, and (less commonly) histiocytes, that arise from lymph nodes, the spleen, or other sites of lymphoid tissue anywhere in the body. Lymphomas are classified by cell type, degree of differentiation, and nodular or diffuse pattern of distribution. Hodgkin's disease (HD) is a distinctive form of lymphoma, separated from the larger, more common spectrum of non–Hodgkin lymphoma (NHL), by the presence of Reed-Sternberg cells. Reed-Sternberg cells are

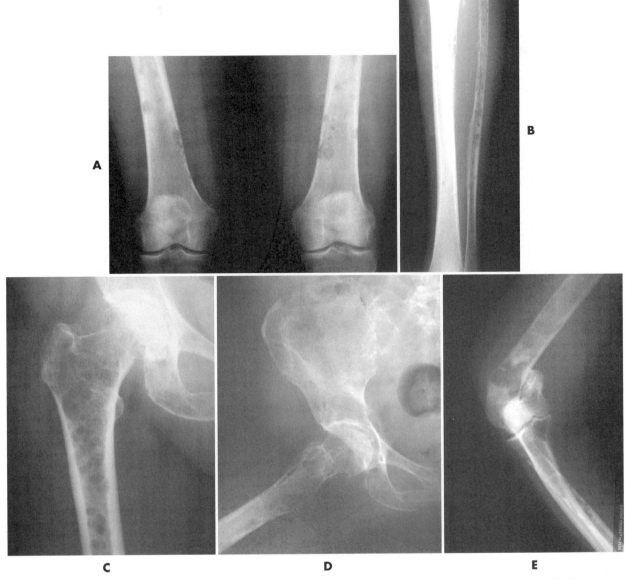

FIG. 13-35 Multiple myeloma presenting with characteristic findings of osteopenia and "punched-out" lesions of, **A,** the femora; **B,** tibia and fibula; **C,** proximal femur; **D,** ilium; and **E,** elbow. (**C,** Courtesy Steven P. Brownstein, MD, Springfield, NJ.)

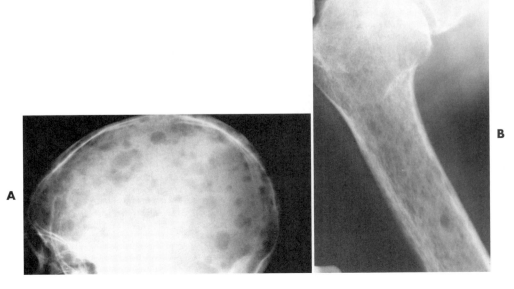

FIG. 13-36 "Punched-out" lesions in, **A,** the skull (raindrop skull) and, **B,** proximal femur in different patients with multiple myeloma. (Courtesy Joseph W. Howe, Sylmar, CA.)

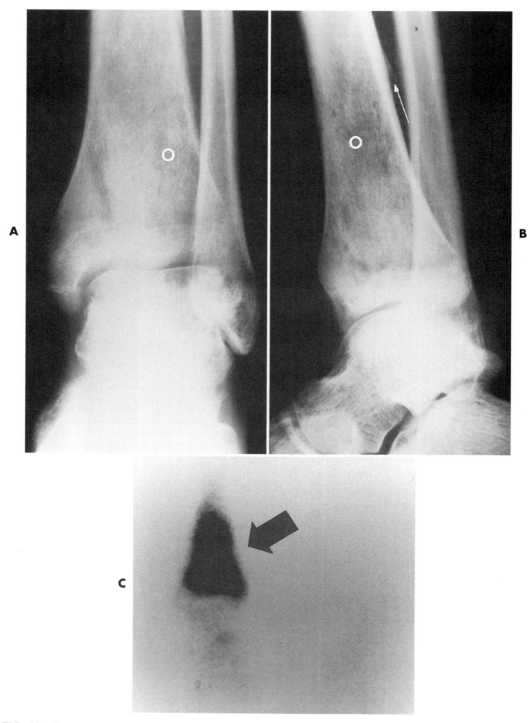

FIG. 13-37   Ewing's sarcoma. **A** and **B,** Frontal and lateral radiographs reveal permeative osteolysis *(o)* in the distal tibia with an associated Codman's triangle *(arrow)*. **C,** The process exhibits increased activity *(arrow)* on a radionuclide bone scar. (From Sartoris DJ: Musculoskeletal imaging: the requisites, St Louis, 1993, Mosby.)

giant connective tissue cells, usually multinucleated, and characteristic of HD.

Lymphoma involves bone as either a primary focus or secondary to systemic lymphoma. Lymphoma is classified as a primary bone lesion if the single osseous lesion, with occasional minimal regional metastasis, is the only lymphoma lesion found in the body.

Therefore primary lymphoma of bone is nonsystemic by definition. Primary lymphoma of bone is incorporated within the NHL classification and often is called *reticulum* cell sarcoma of bone. Primary NHL lymphoma of bone is microscopically identical to the nodal form of the disease; it differs only in its bone location. Burkitt's lymphoma is a type of primary bone lymphoma.

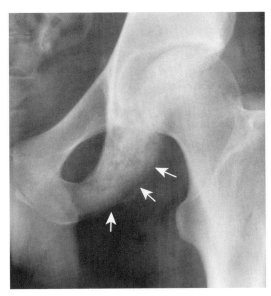

FIG. 13-38 Ewing's sarcoma appearing as a mixed radiodense and osteolytic lesion of the ischial tuberosity with aggressive periostitis *(arrows)*. (Courtesy Jack C. Avalos, Davenport, IA.)

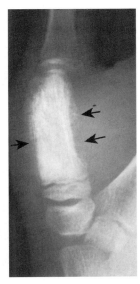

FIG. 13-39 Mixed radiodense and osteolytic lesion of the first metacarpal. Aggressive periostitis is noted *(arrows)* and is consistent with Ewing's tumor. (Courtesy Ian D. McLean, LeClaire, IA.)

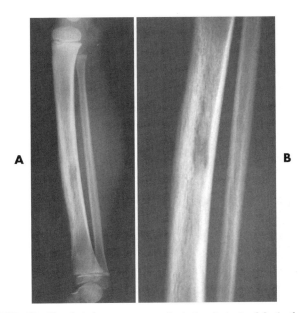

FIG. 13-40 Ewing's sarcoma appearing in the diaphysis of, **A,** the femur and, **B,** close-up. (Courtesy Ian D. McLean, LeClaire, IA.)

Secondary bone involvement can occur from either systemic NHL or HD. HD involves bone only as a secondary lesion.

Bone involvement with lymphoma occurs at any age and affects men more often than women.[191] The average age is 34 years; 50% of patients are between 10 and 30 years of age.[25,45,83,213]

IMAGING FINDINGS
Eighty-eight percent of patients with primary lymphoma of bone present with a single osseous lesion that fulfills the definition

of primary NHL of bone (Figs. 13-41 through 13-43).[45] The remaining cases are polyostotic at presentation. Four percent of all patients with systemic NHL present with a concurrent skeletal lesion. Twenty percent of patients with HD demonstrate concurrent osseous lesions.[14,236]

Osseous lesions caused by primary NHL of bone are radiographically indistinguishable from metastatic osseous lesions caused by systemic NHL and HD.[153] All types of lymphoma usually exhibit a permeative or moth-eaten pattern of osteolytic bone destruction (Figs. 13-42 and 13-43). In the long bones, the diaphysis is preferentially involved. Soft-tissue masses are common, and periosteal reactions are infrequent.[202] CT and MRI are useful to define the extent of the lesion, especially its soft-tissue component. Osteoblastic lesions are more common secondary to HD, often presenting as an "ivory vertebra" (Fig. 13-41).

Primary lymphoma of bone predominates in the lower extremities. Secondary (metastatic) bone involvement from systemic NHL and HD most commonly involves the spine, pelvis, and ribs. Burkitt's lymphoma is most common in the mandible and maxilla (Fig. 13-44).[29]

CLINICAL COMMENTS
Patients with osseous lymphoma typically complain of pain in the region of involvement but otherwise appear healthy. Radiation therapy, with or without adjuvant chemotherapy, may control the local bone lesions for years.

KEY CONCEPTS
- *Primary lymphoma of bone and secondary lymphoma of bone (systemic non–Hodgkin lymphoma and Hodgkin lymphoma) appear as permeative radiolucent lesions of the lower extremities, pelvis, and spine.*
- *Although generally osteolytic, bone lesions secondary to Hodgkin lymphoma are the most common to appear osteosclerotic ("ivory vertebra").*
- *Lymphoma of bone occurs in patients over a wide age range.*

Leukemia

BACKGROUND

Leukemia, the most common childhood cancer, has both acute and chronic forms. Although adults also may develop this cancer, the vast majority of leukemia patients are younger than 5 years of age. Lymphoblastic leukemia is the histologic variety in approximately 80% of cases in children.

IMAGING FINDINGS

Plain film findings are abnormal in nearly 50% of children with leukemia. The most common radiologic manifestation of this cancer is generalized osteopenia. The earliest radiographic findings are transmetaphyseal lucent bands near the physes of long bones such as the femur and tibia (Fig. 13-45). Rather than leukemic infiltrates, these bands appear to represent a metabolic reaction to the process. Alternatively, they may develop because

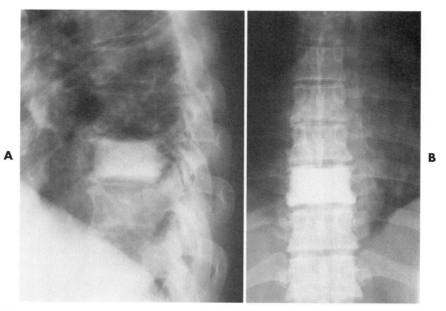

FIG. 13-41   Lymphoma presenting as a radiodense "ivory vertebra" lesion of the lower thoracic spine in, **A,** the lateral and, **B,** anteroposterior projection. (Courtesy Steven P. Brownstein, MD, Springfield, NJ.)

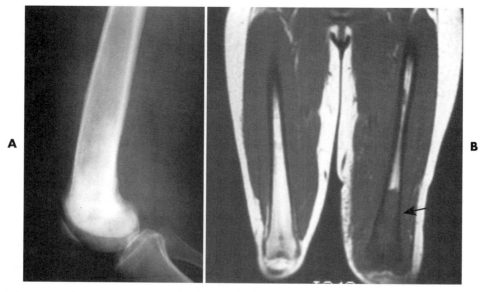

FIG. 13-42   Lymphoma presenting as a sclerotic lesion in, **A,** the lower femur and demonstrating decreased marrow signal intensity on, **B,** the T1-weighted magnetic resonance imaging consistent with marrow replacement in the distal region of the left femur secondary to lymphoma *(arrow)*. (Courtesy Ian D. McLean, LeClaire, IA.)

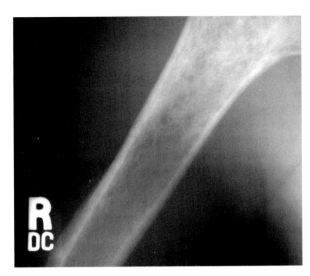

FIG. 13-43 Lymphoma of bone appearing as a rarefied region of bone destruction in the proximal humerus. (Courtesy Joseph W. Howe, Sylmar, CA.)

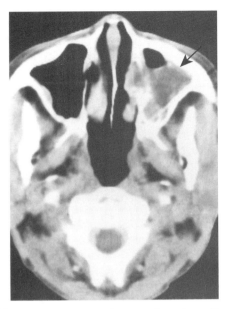

FIG. 13-44 Computed tomography scan of a patient with Burkitt's lymphoma. The scan demonstrates partial filling of the left maxillary sinus with thickening and irregularity of the medial sinus wall (arrow). (Courtesy Steven P. Brownstein, MD, Springfield, NJ.)

pressure on the physis from the neoplastic infiltrates alters bony maturation at the zone of provisional calcification.

Discrete bony lesions may be present in the metaphysis or diaphysis, where they create a moth-eaten or permeative pattern of destruction. Periostitis also may develop with discrete bone lesions. In some cases, focal, spotty sclerosis is noted after chemotherapy or radiation treatment. Diffuse sclerosis of the bones has been encountered, but it is thought to be secondary myelofibrosis resulting from therapeutic interventions.[3]

Infiltration of the meninges of the brain creates a separation of the skull sutures in a small percentage of patients with leukemia.

Based on the radiographic findings alone, differentiation of infiltration of the meninges from neuroblastoma metastasis to the skeleton can be challenging because both conditions cause periostitis and separations of the sutures.

Focal accumulations of leukemic cells have been identified in a small number of patients with acute myelogenous leukemia.

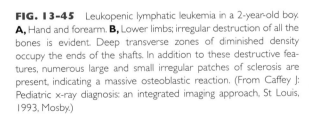

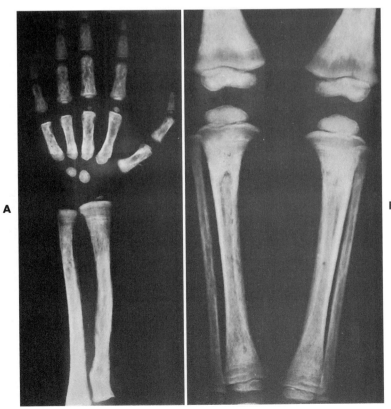

FIG. 13-45 Leukopenic lymphatic leukemia in a 2-year-old boy. **A,** Hand and forearm. **B,** Lower limbs; irregular destruction of all the bones is evident. Deep transverse zones of diminished density occupy the ends of the shafts. In addition to these destructive features, numerous large and small irregular patches of sclerosis are present, indicating a massive osteoblastic reaction. (From Caffey J: Pediatric x-ray diagnosis: an integrated imaging approach, St Louis, 1993, Mosby.)

Because of their green color, these cells have been termed *chloromas,* and are more common in adults. Most commonly chloromas accumulate outside the skeleton. Skeletal accumulations most often develop in the face, sternum, and ribs.[16]

CLINICAL COMMENTS

Patients with leukemia generally have a number of systemic complaints, including fever, malaise, and weakness. The musculoskeletal findings in leukemia include diffuse bone and joint pain, similar to the findings in juvenile rheumatoid arthritis. Joint and soft tissue swelling should alert the physician to the presence of a more serious condition. In leukemic patients the complete blood count (CBC) may be increased, normal, or decreased. However, the laboratory finding of blast cells in the peripheral blood smear is strongly suggestive of leukemia, and bone marrow biopsy is diagnostic.

Cartilage Origin

Benign

Chondroma, Ollier's Disease, and Maffucci's Syndrome

BACKGROUND

A chondroma is a cartilage tumor involving enchondrally formed bones. If the chondroma is located within the medullary canal, it is called an enchondroma (Fig. 13-46). Less commonly it is found adjacent to the cortex beneath the periosteal membrane, known as a periosteal chondroma, juxtacortical chondroma, or perichondroma. Chondromas represent discrete islands of hyaline cartilage surrounded by lamellar enchondral bone. Enchondroma is the most common tumor occurring in the phalanges and is the second most common benign cartilage neoplasm of bone after osteochondroma.[91]

Enchondromas most often present in patients 20 to 30 years old, with an equal gender distribution.

The presence of multiple enchondromas (enchondromatosis, or Ollier's disease) increases the risk of malignant transformation by 30%.[16,44,211] The combination of multiple enchondromas and subcutaneous hemangiomas is termed *Maffucci's syndrome* and is associated with a 30% or greater increased risk for malignant transformation than occurs with solitary enchondromas.[4,121,232] Malignant transformation is usually to a chondrosarcoma.

Juxtacortical chondromas are found in patients predominantly before the age of 30 years,[23] appearing more commonly in males than females, at a ratio of 2:1.

IMAGING FINDINGS

Chondromas, whether medullary or juxtacortical, solitary or multiple, usually are found in the small bones of the hands, particularly the proximal phalanges (Figs. 13-47 and 13-48), and less commonly the feet (Fig. 13-49). The humerus, femur, and tibia also are involved.

An enchondroma appears as a well-defined medullary lesion, most often with some degree of calcification, endosteal scalloping (see Fig. 13-48), and bone expansion. Enchondromas are usually small, less than 3 cm in diameter (Fig. 13-50). On MRI the calcific foci appear as minute signal voids (Fig. 13-51). Enchondromas often are not as clearly outlined in long bones as when they appear in small tubular bones.

Malignant transformation to a chondrosarcoma is a rare event, occurring in less than 1% of patients. Malignant transformation occurs more often in proximal lesions (e.g., humerus versus phalanx), and is suggested by the disappearance of a previously noted pattern of matrix calcification.

Juxtacortical chondromas appear as soft-tissue masses with erosion or saucerization of the adjacent cortex (Figs. 13-52 and 13-53). Calcification is noted in 50% of juxtacortical chondromas.[240]

Ollier's disease appears with multiple (usually many) cystic defects of the hands, and less commonly the feet (Figs. 13-54 to 13-57). Soft-tissue hemangiomas are signified radiographically as soft-tissue masses with multiple phleboliths (Fig. 13-58).

CLINICAL COMMENTS

Chondromas typically are asymptomatic. The presence of associated pain increases the clinical suspicion for the presence of pathologic fracture, malignant transformation, or a low-grade de novo chondrosarcoma. In addition, any chondroma that exhibits continued growth in a skeletally mature patient should be closely scrutinized to exclude malignancy because lesions typically stop

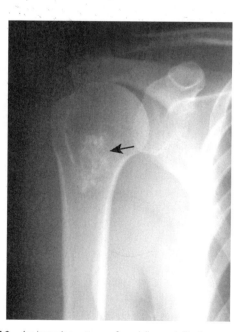

FIG. 13-46　An irregular pattern of medullary calcification appearing in the proximal humerus *(arrow)* of an asymptomatic middle-aged adult. The presentation is consistent with an enchondroma. Other consideration should be given to intramedullary bone infarct or central chondrosarcoma. The latter usually is accompanied by pain.

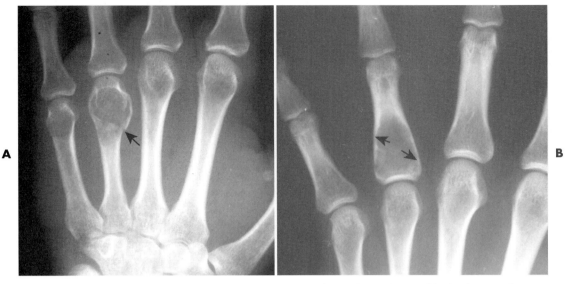

FIG. 13-47 Enchondroma. **A,** Fractured enchondroma of the hand *(arrow)*. Enchondromas of the hand commonly appear as slightly expansile, geographic lesions, usually with a well-defined pattern of matrix calcification. **B,** Faint, mildly expansile cystic defect noted in the proximal aspect of the proximal phalanx of the fourth digit *(arrows)*. These lesions do not exhibit prominent matrix calcification that is common for enchondromas in this location.

growing in adult patients. Surgical curettage usually is indicated for substantial lesions.

KEY CONCEPTS

- *Chondromas are the most common tumor of the phalanges.*
- *Chondromas have a medullary (enchondroma) or juxtacortical (perichondroma) location.*
- *They usually occur in patients younger than age 30 years.*
- *Matrix calcification occurs in 50% of patients with chondromas.*
- *Malignant transformation to a chondrosarcoma is a rare occurrence (1% of patients) unless multiple lesions are present (30% of patients).*

Chondroblastoma

BACKGROUND

A chondroblastoma (Codman's tumor) is a rare, benign primary bone tumor usually occurring in secondary centers of enchondral ossification. Lesions appear most frequently in long, tubular bones and less frequently in short tubular and flat bones.[27,70,235] Up to 15% of lesions are found in combination with an aneurysmal bone cyst.[46] Ninety percent of lesions occur in patients who are between the ages of 5 and 25 years. Men are affected more than women, at a 1.5 or 2:1 ratio.[70]

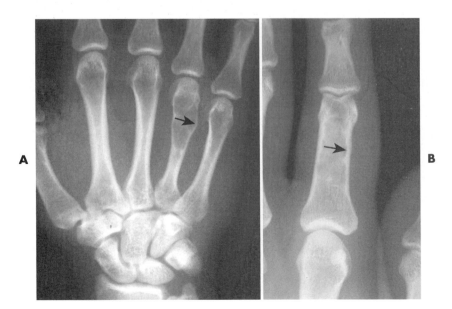

FIG. 13-48 **A,** Oblong enchondroma with scalloping of the inner cortex of the lesion *(arrow)*, a characteristic feature, in a 12-year-old boy. **B,** Faint lesion in a second patient demonstrates similar endosteal scalloping. (**B,** Courtesy Robert C. Tatum, Davenport, IA.)

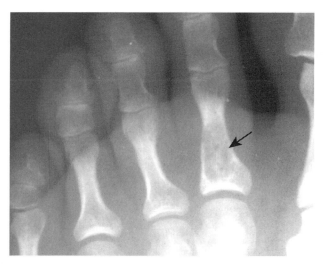

FIG. 13-49 Small cystic defect of the proximal phalanx of the foot's second digit *(arrow)*. This lesion exhibits a faint punctate pattern of matrix calcification consistent with the cartilage origin of the lesion. (Courtesy Jay Brammier, Durant, IA.)

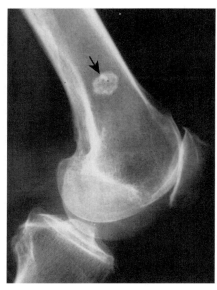

FIG. 13-50 Calcific enchondroma of the distal femur *(arrow)*. (Courtesy Jack Avalos, Davenport, IA.)

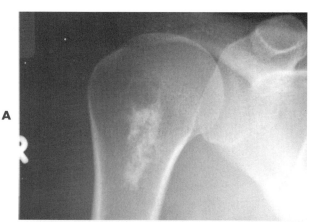

FIG. 13-51 Enchondroma appearing on, **A,** plain film. **B,** T1- and, **C,** T2-weighted magnetic resonance imaging of the proximal humerus. The lesion is well circumscribed radiographically. The T2-weighted coronal image demonstrates small lobulated foci of increased signal intensity separated by a collagen mesh of decreased signal intensity. (Courtesy John Rizzo, Edensburg, PA.)

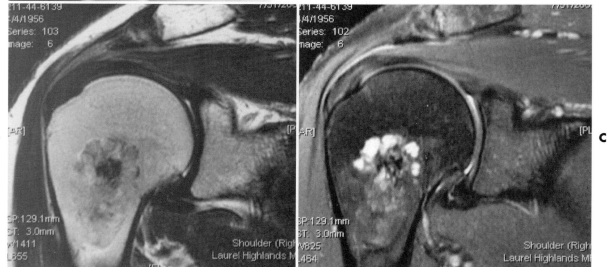

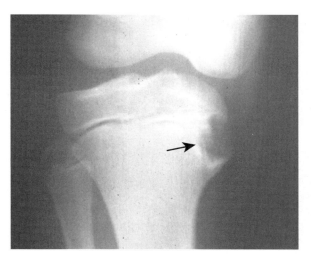

FIG. 13-52 Periosteal chondroma *(arrow)* of the medial portion of the proximal tibia. (Courtesy Steven P. Brownstein, MD, Springfield, NJ.)

IMAGING FINDINGS

The imaging findings of those lesions within long bones are highly characteristic, consisting of a sharply demarcated, centric or eccentric, osteolytic region of less than 5 cm, well defined by a thin rim of sclerosis, and located within an epiphysis or apophysis (Figs. 13-59 to 13-62). The proximal femur, distal femur, proximal tibia, and proximal humerus are the most common sites of involvement. Less commonly chondroblastoma occurs in the patella or acral skeleton (most often the calcaneus or talus). The matrix typically is radiolucent, but commonly minute or larger foci of calcification are present, producing a radiodense matrix of varying degrees.

Microscopically the pattern of calcification appears as a fine linear honeycomb pattern that has been likened to the appearance of "chicken wire," a feature that identifies the lesion after biopsy or excision. The appearance of chondroblastoma in a nontubular bone is less characteristic.

Chondroblastoma is many times less common than giant cell tumor; therefore the latter should be considered first when encountering an epiphyseal lesion, especially around the knee.

CLINICAL COMMENTS

Local pain, tenderness, and swelling of the involved region often are reported, and present early in the course of the tumor's development. Complete curettage with bone grafting is the preferred treatment, with uncommon reoccurrence. [231]

KEY CONCEPTS

- This rare, benign bone tumor is located within an epiphysis or apophysis.
- It is most commonly found around the knee.
- Chondroblastoma usually presents between 5 and 25 years of age and is more common among men.

Chondromyxoid Fibroma

BACKGROUND

A chondromyxoid fibroma is the least frequent benign cartilage neoplasm, representing less than 2% of benign bone tumors. [147,185] It forms from the cartilage-forming connective tissue of marrow space. Histologically the basic composition is cartilage, but varying degrees of myxoid and fibrous tissues also are present. Chondromyxoid fibroma most often occurs in patients before the age of 30 years and has a slight male predilection.

IMAGING FINDINGS

Long, tubular bones of the lower extremity, namely the proximal tibia and fibula and proximal and distal femur, are involved most often (Fig. 13-63). Chondromyxoid fibromas characteristically appear as 2- to 10-cm oval, eccentric, metaphyseal, noncalcified, osteolytic lesions. Because of the scalloped inner margins of the host bone, the lesions may appear chambered by thick trabeculation. [81] The lesion is difficult to distinguish from an aggressive malignancy when it is not well defined. Chondromyxoid fibromas are devoid of matrix calcification. The presence of calcification is more likely

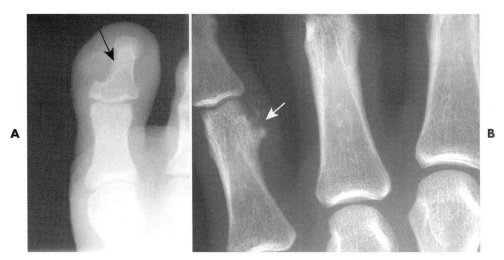

FIG. 13-53 **A,** Patient exhibiting periosteal chondroma of the distal phalanx of the first pedal digit *(arrow)*. **B,** Second patient exhibiting involvement in the proximal phalanx of the hand *(arrow)*. (**A,** Courtesy Ian D. McLean, LeClaire, IA.)

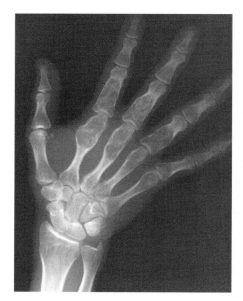

FIG. 13-54 Ollier's disease, defined as multiple enchondromas. Each lesion presents as a slightly expansile cystic defect with well-defined central matrix calcification. (Courtesy Gary Longmuir, Phoenix, AZ.)

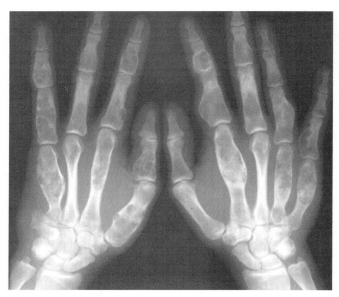

FIG. 13-55 Ollier's disease. A 28-year-old male patient with a bilateral presentation of multiple enchondromas throughout the small bones of the hands. A patient with Ollier's disease is at greater risk of experiencing malignant transformation to a chondrosarcoma than is someone with a solitary enchondroma presentation.

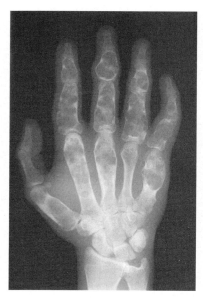

FIG. 13-56 Ollier's disease defined by the multiple enchondromas, that in this case appear symmetrically placed within the small bones of the hands. (Courtesy Beverly Harger, Portland, OR.)

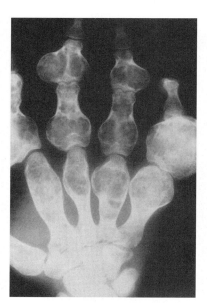

FIG. 13-57 Ollier's disease exhibiting individual lesion with marked expansile appearance and characteristic stippled matrix calcification. At quick glance, the appearance is reminiscent of gout, except the former has interosseous lesions, the latter soft-tissue tophi. (Courtesy Joseph W. Howe, Sylmar, CA.)

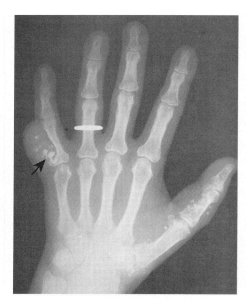

FIG. 13-58 Maffucci's syndrome describes the concurrent presentation of multiple enchondromas (Ollier's disease) and soft-tissue hemangiomas within (arrow). (Courtesy Steven P. Brownstein, MD, Springfield, NJ.)

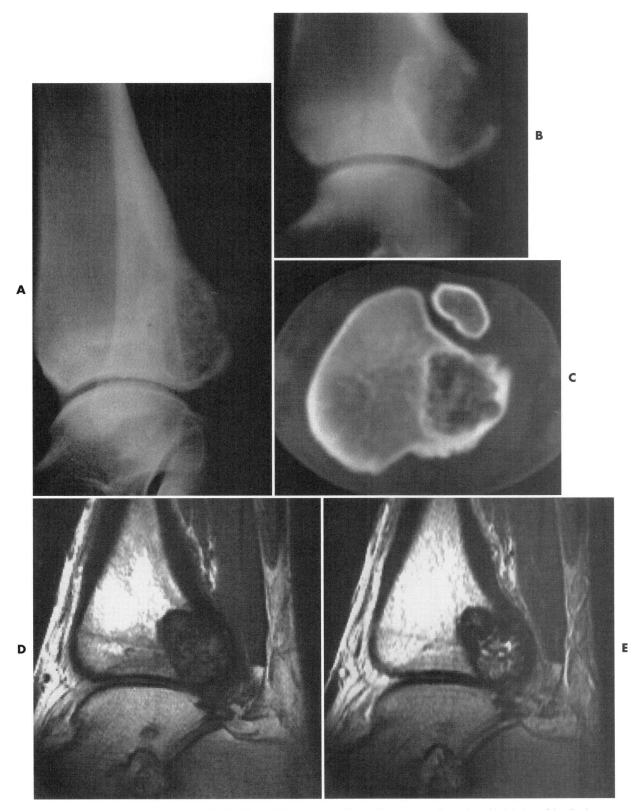

FIG. 13-59 Chondroblastoma. **A,** Plain film and, **B,** tomogram of the ankle reveal a well-marginated lytic lesion of the distal tibial epiphysis with prominent lesional calcification. **C,** Computed tomography scan defines the cortical expansion. **D,** T1-weighted magnetic resonance images demonstrate diffuse low signal intensity. **E,** T2-weighting reveals mixed areas of high and low signal intensity. The high signal intensity probably represents uncalcified cartilage, and the low signal corresponds to areas of calcified matrix. (From Stark DD, Gradley WG: Magnetic resonance imaging, ed, 2 St Louis, 1992, Mosby.)

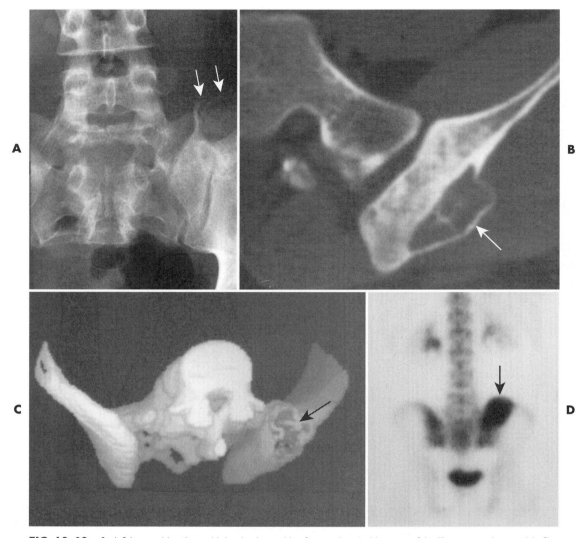

FIG. 13-60 **A,** A 24-year-old patient with local pain resulting from a chondroblastoma of the ilium presenting on plain film as a well-circumscribed radiolucent defect in the iliac crest *(arrows).* The lesion appears expansile on, **B,** conventional and, **C,** reformatted computed tomography *(arrows).* **D,** The ilium appears as a hot spot on the posterior view of the radionuclide bone scan *(arrow).* This is not a common location of chondroblastoma.

in chondroblastoma, conventional chondrosarcoma, or another cartilaginous lesion.

CLINICAL COMMENTS

Pain, tenderness, swelling, and restricted motion of the involved region are common clinical complaints. Lesions rarely undergo malignant transformation, and less than 5% demonstrate pathologic fracture.[91] En bloc excision is the treatment of choice.

KEY CONCEPTS

- *Chondromyxoid fibroma is a rare tumor of mixed histology.*
- *Chondromyxoid fibroma is usually located in the proximal tibia and usually occurs in patients before the age of 30 years.*
- *Chondromyxoid fibroma is a 2- to 10-cm, eccentric, oval, osteolytic lesion.*

Osteochondroma and Hereditary Multiple Exostoses

BACKGROUND

An osteochondroma (exostosis) is a benign outgrowth of bone covered by a cartilaginous cap of varying thickness. Osteochondromas are the most common benign skeletal neoplasms[103] and may arise in any bone that is preformed in cartilage. However, osteochondromas are not truly tumors, but rather develop from a small dysplastic fragment of the epiphyseal growth plate. Consistent with the dysplastic etiology, osteochondromas can be experimentally induced in animals by transplanting growth plate tissue beneath their periosteum.[165]

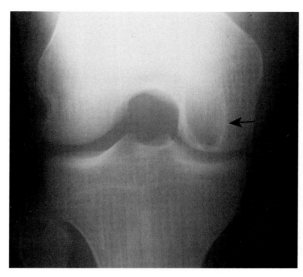

FIG. 13-61 Chondroblastoma located in the subarticular region of the distal femur (*arrow*).

Because they are composed of displaced growth plate tissue, osteochondromas typically stop growing when the patient reaches skeletal maturity. Growth beyond skeletal maturity suggests malignant degeneration. Malignant degeneration has been reported to occur in 1% to 2% of solitary lesions and from 1% to 3% or up to 25% of multiple lesions.[68,192,241] As measured on MRI or CT, a cartilage cap of greater than 2 cm strongly suggests malignant transformation.[109]

Multiple autosomal dominant inherited lesions are called hereditary multiple exostoses (HMEs) or diaphyseal aclasis. The term diaphyseal aclasis refers to the altered growth patterns of the involved bones.

Single or multiple osteochondromas usually are discovered in patients before they reach the age of 20 years.[23] A slight male predominance is noted. Multiple lesions are most often discovered earlier than solitary lesions.

IMAGING FINDINGS

Osteochondromas are found in the metaphyses of long bones, affecting the lower extremities more commonly than the upper extremities (Figs. 13-64 to 13-67).[111,138] Most lesions occur around the knee and virtually never involve the craniofacial bones.

Osteochondromas arise from the cortex and grow outward, pointing away from the nearest joint. They most often appear pedunculated, with a pedicle or stalk measuring several centimeters along its long axis and blending smoothly with the host bone's cortex. Less often the lesion appears broad and flat, which is known as a sessile osteochondroma. The base of a sessile osteochondroma is broader than the sessile variety, measuring up to 10 cm. It has been reported that the pedunculated configuration is more closely related to the possibility of malignant transformation.[175]

MRI and CT are useful to define the extent of the lesion, especially if malignant transformation is suspected or the lesion originates from regions that are difficult to image with plain film (e.g., vertebral arch, ribs). Radionuclide bone imaging may not accurately differentiate benign osteochondroma from malignant transformation to chondrosarcoma.[111,138]

HME appears with multiple osteochondromas and growth deformities (Fig. 13-68). Wrist and ankle deformities are associated with relative shortening and bowing of the ulna and fibula.[192] Specifically, shortening of the ulna and outward bowing of the radius are called a *bayonet deformity*, or *pseudo–Madelung's deformity* (Figs. 13-69 to 13-71). Multiple lesions usually are polyostotic and only rarely occur as multiple lesions within a single bone. The individual lesions of HME tend to be larger and are more likely to be of the sessile variety than when a solitary lesion presentation occurs.

Osteochondromas appear with mixed signal intensity on both T1- and T2-weighted MRI. MRI is useful to delineate the overlying cartilage cap of the tumor during phenomena of malignant transformation. Neurologic involvement, such as cord compression, also is well presented by MRI.[173]

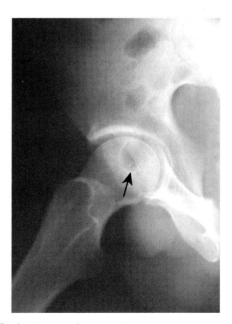

FIG. 13-62 Small cystic defect located in the subarticular region of the proximal femur (*arrow*) representing a chondroblastoma. (Courtesy Gary Longmuir, Phoenix, AZ.)

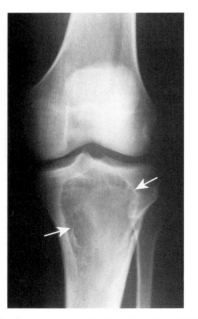

FIG. 13-63 Chondromyxoid fibroma of the proximal tibia (*arrows*).

Text continued on p. 842.

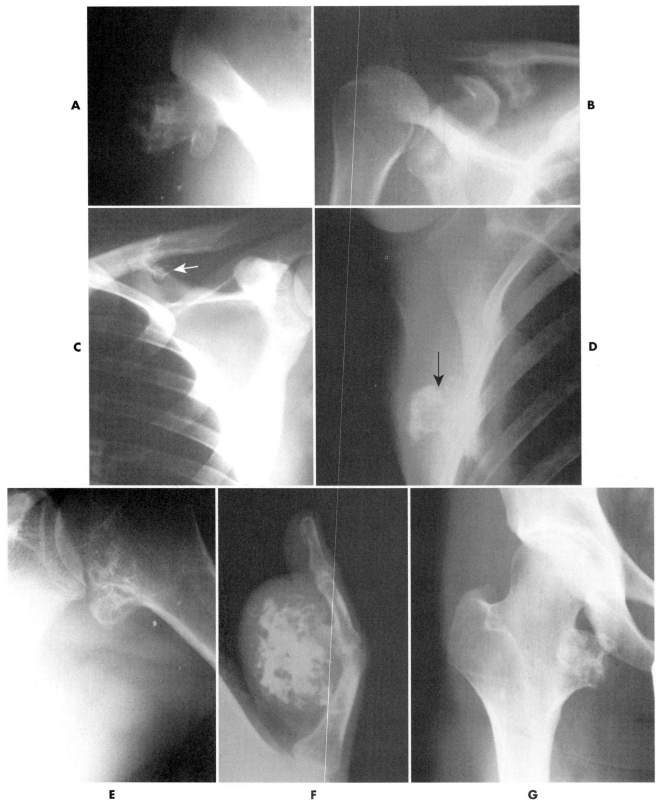

FIG. 13-64   Solitary pedunculated osteochondromas projecting from, **A,** the ilium; **B,** inferior margin of the clavicle; **C** and **D,** scapula *(arrows)*; **E,** proximal humerus; **F,** distal phalanx; **G** and **H,** proximal femur; and **I** and **J,** distal femur. (**B,** Courtesy Gary Longmuir, Phoenix, AZ; **C,** Courtesy Steven P. Brownstein, MD, Springfield, NJ; **H** and **I,** Courtesy William E. Litterer, Elizabeth, NJ.)

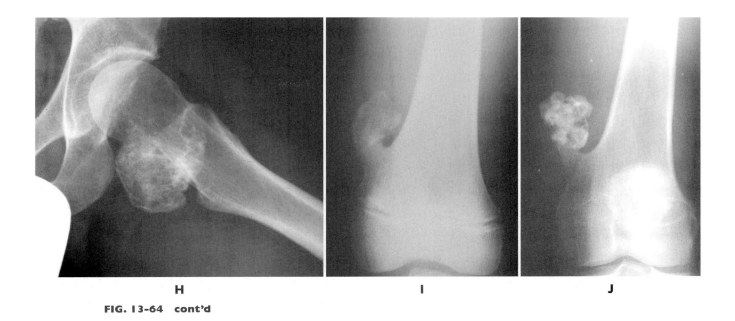

H   **I**   **J**

FIG. 13-64   cont'd

FIG. 13-65   Solitary sessile osteochondromas projecting from, **A,** the ischial ramus *(arrow);* **B,** proximal tibia *(arrow);* and **C,** fibula.

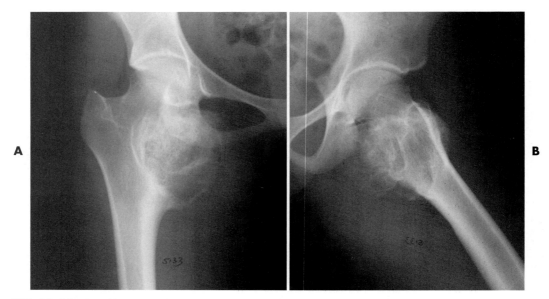

FIG. 13-66   A and **B,** Lesion of the proximal femur appearing as a slight exostosis with cartilage matrix consistent with osteochondroma. Often the matrix of cartilaginous lesions appears partially mineralized as rings and arcs, corresponding to calcifications around the lobules of cartilage that constitute the lesion.

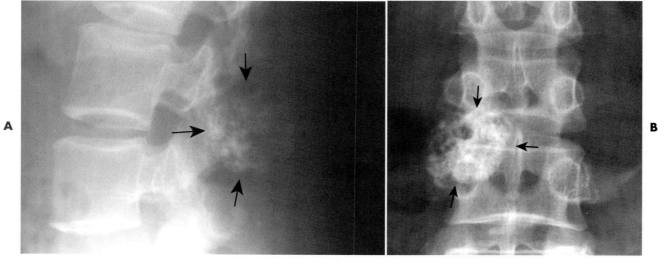

FIG. 13-67   A and **B,** Pedunculated osteochondroma of the lumbar spine *(arrows).*

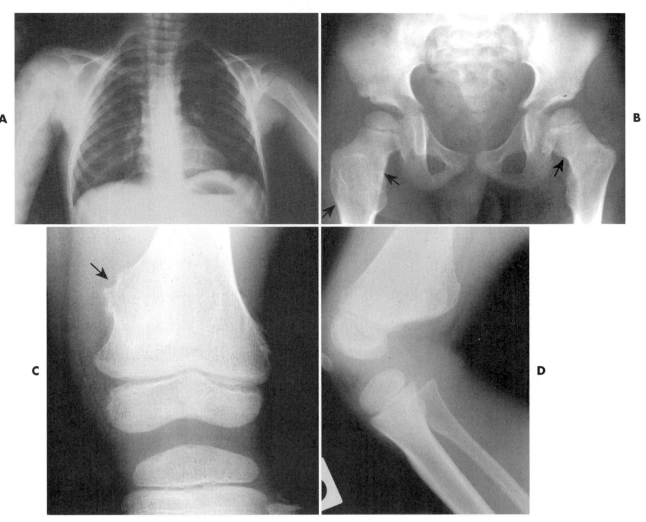

FIG. 13-68 A 4-year-old patient with hereditary multiple exostoses, exhibited in, **A,** the proximal humeri; **B,** proximal femora (appearing as wide femoral necks, *arrows*); and, **C** *(arrow)* and **D,** knee.

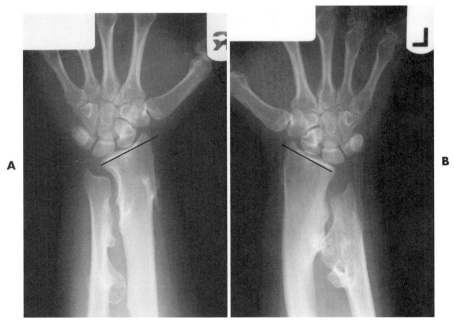

FIG. 13-69 **A,** Right and, **B,** left forearm of a patient with hereditary multiple exostoses (HME). In addition to the multiple osteochondromas, notice the shortened ulna and medial slant of the distal articular surface of the radius (bayonet deformity). (Courtesy Gary Longmuir, Phoenix, AZ.)

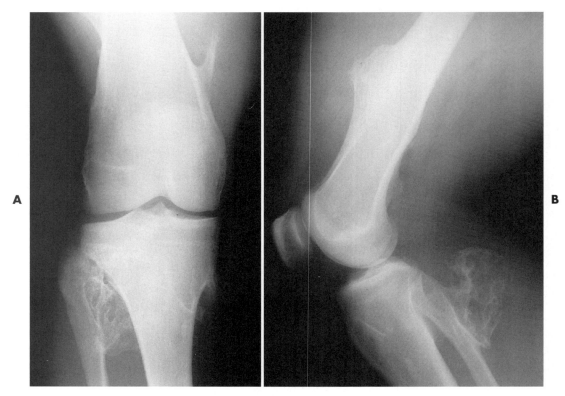

FIG. 13-70 **A** and **B,** Knee radiographs of a 29-year-old man with multiple osteochondromas, known as *hereditary multiple exostoses (HME)*.

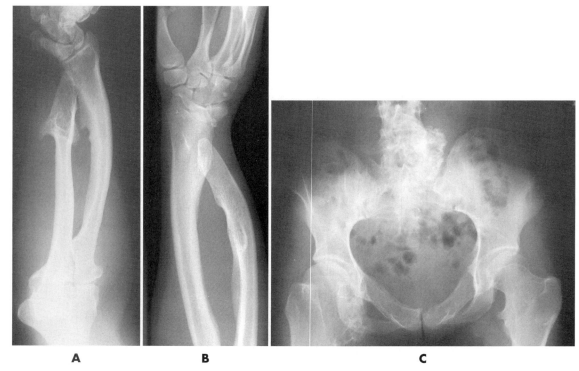

FIG. 13-71 Multiple sessile and pedunculated osteochondromas of, **A,** the right and, **B,** left forearm; **C,** pelvis; **D,** proximal femur; **E,** proximal humerus; **F** and **G,** right knee; and, **H** and **I,** left knee of a patient with hereditary multiple exostoses (HME) *(arrows)*. (Courtesy Ian D. McLean, LeClaire, IA.)

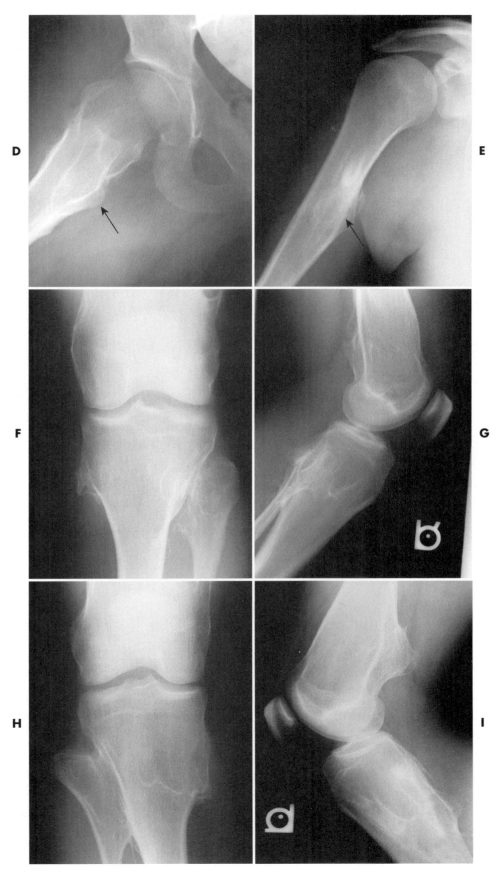

FIG. 13-71 cont'd

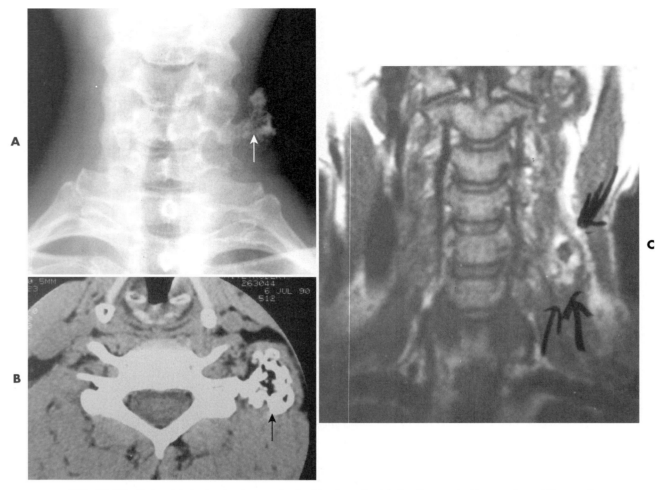

FIG. 13-72 Pedunculated osteochondroma extending laterally on, **A,** plain film; **B,** computed tomography; and **C,** magnetic resonance image *(arrows)*. Osteochondromas are clinically important because they may cause pressure on surrounding anatomy (e.g., vessels and nerves) and have the potential for malignant degeneration to chondrosarcoma. (Courtesy Ian D. McLean, LeClaire, IA.)

CLINICAL COMMENTS

Patients typically present with a palpable mass, sometimes of many years' history, and with or without pain. Pressure on the adjacent neurovascular bundle may produce neuropathy or vascular disturbance (Figs. 13-72 and 13-73). [22,73] Overlying ectopic bursa may become inflamed, causing the initial clinical attention. An enlarging painful osteochondroma suggests malignant degeneration. Treatment consists of surgical excision when necessary.

KEY CONCEPTS

- *Osteochondromas are the most common primary skeletal neoplasms.*
- *They are found in metaphyses of long bones, particularly around the knee.*
- *Osteochondromas usually are discovered in patients younger than 20 years of age.*
- *Hereditary multiple exostoses (HME) describes the presentation of multiple osteochondromas.*
- *HME is associated with a higher (up to 25%) rate of malignant transformation than seen with a solitary osteochondroma (1% to 2%).*

Malignant
Chondrosarcoma

BACKGROUND

Chondrosarcomas are a heterogeneous group of bone neoplasms of which the basic neoplastic tissue is cartilaginous. [58] They represent the third most common primary malignant tumor of bone, after multiple myeloma and osteosarcoma. The higher the histologic grade, the more likely metastasis is to occur.

Chondrosarcomas are classified by primary or secondary lesions. Primary chondrosarcomas arise de novo. Secondary chondrosarcomas develop from solitary or multiple enchondromas (Ollier's disease), solitary or multiple osteochondromas (hereditary multiple exostoses), synovial osteochondrometaplasia, chondromyxoid fibromas, and chondroblastomas. Because of this association, growing or painful preexisting benign cartilaginous tumors warrant particular clinical attention. The secondary chondrosarcoma is the most malignant of the chondrosarcomas, associated with an extremely high risk of distant metastasis.

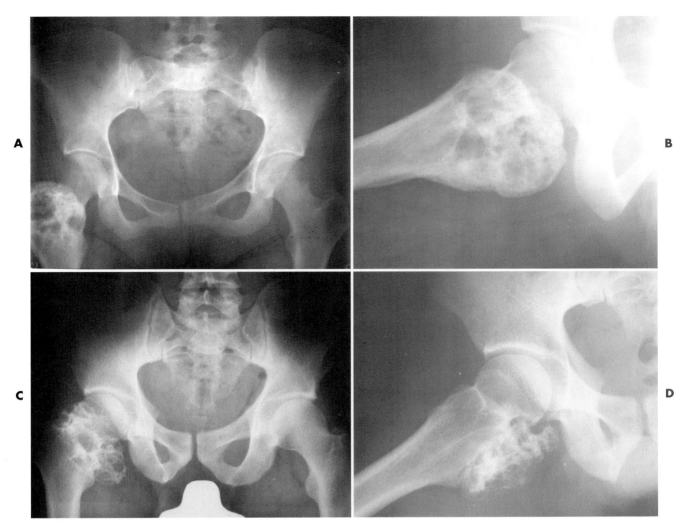

FIG. 13-73 **A** through **D,** Osteochondroma extending from the proximal femur in two different patients. In each case the frontal radiographs, **A** and **C,** exhibit the lesions to lesser advantage than, **B** and **D,** the frog-leg projections. Osteochondromas typically are asymptomatic, but may become clinically important if they place pressure on surrounding nerves and arteries.

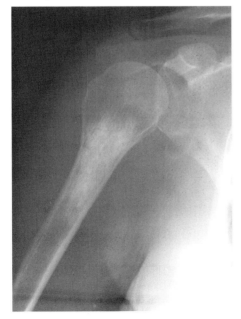

FIG. 13-74 Suspected chondrosarcoma presenting as an irregular, radiodense lesion is noted in the central region of the proximal humerus. The patient is an 89-year-old woman with dull, aching pain that is unrelated to activity. (Courtesy Robin Canterbury, Davenport, IA.)

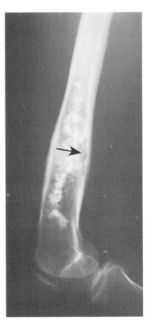

FIG. 13-75 Central chondrosarcoma of the distal femur. The lesion demonstrates stippled calcification and endosteal cortical bone destruction *(arrow).* (Courtesy Steven P. Brownstein, MD, Springfield, NJ.)

Primary chondrosarcomas occur within the medullary canal of bone (central or intermedullary) or from the bone's surface (peripheral or juxtacortical). Central lesions are classified by tissue type as conventional, clear-cell, and mesenchymal. Last, conventional lesions are subclassified by low-, medium-, or high-grade aggressiveness.[222]

Low-grade lesions resemble enchondromas cytologically, but are more aggressive radiologically and often have associated clinical complaints with no potential for metastasis. Medium-grade lesions reveal increased cellularity, local aggressiveness, and potential for metastasis. High-grade lesions are less common, have high cellularity, appear as aggressive lesions on imaging studies, and have a near-likelihood of metastasis.

More than 90% of chondrosarcomas are classified as low- or medium-grade conventional lesions. Chondrosarcomas are more common in male than female patients, at a ratio of 3:2.[195] Although presentation ranges widely, most patients are between the ages of 50 and 70 years. Peripheral chondrosarcomas tend to occur in slightly younger patients.[90]

IMAGING FINDINGS

Although chondrosarcomas may involve any bone, most are found in the pelvis, proximal femur, proximal humerus, distal femur, proximal tibia, and ribs (Figs. 13-74 to 13-79).[50,76,90,206] The radiographic appearance is varied, depending on the type of chondrosarcoma. Primary central chondrosarcomas appear most often as metaphyseal regions of bone destruction with scattered stippled calcification.[200] Endosteal cortical thinning is noted, but the cortex is aggressively destroyed only rarely. There may be a prominent lamellar periosteal reaction, but usually not one of perpendicular striations that are characteristic of osteosarcoma and Ewing's sarcoma. The more aggressive types exhibit extraosseous soft-tissue masses. Matrix calcification is characteristic but may be absent in

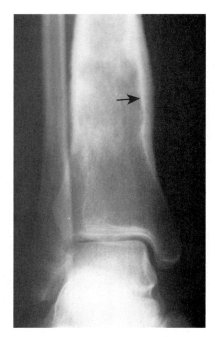

FIG. 13-76   Central chondrosarcoma of the distal tibia. Note the lack of prominent matrix calcification and the endosteal scalloping *(arrow)*, (Courtesy Steven P. Brownstein, MD, Springfield, NJ.)

up to 30% of cases. Often chondrosarcomas appear relatively nonaggressive.

On MRI examination, the low-grade lesions often appear as lobulated hyaline cartilage masses with increased signal intensity on the T2-weighted scans. High-grade lesions may demonstrate inhomogeneous increased signal intensity on the T2-weighted scans. MRI demonstrates the degree of soft-tissue involvement. CT is better to detect the presence of calcification or ossification within the matrix of the lesion.

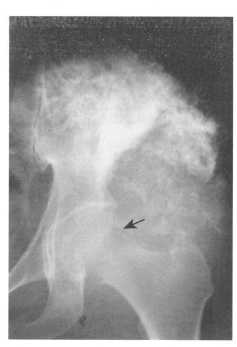

FIG. 13-77   Chondrosarcoma of the ilium with a large soft-tissue mass, stippled matrix calcification, and bone destruction *(arrow)*. (Courtesy Joseph W. Howe, Sylmar, CA.)

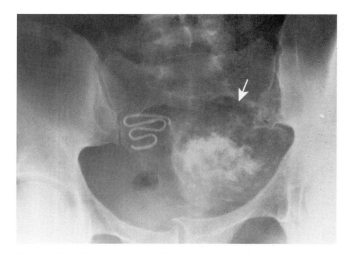

FIG. 13-78   Chondrosarcoma of the sacrum demonstrating soft-tissue mass, stippled matrix calcification, and bone destruction *(arrow)*. (Courtesy Joseph W. Howe, Sylmar, CA.)

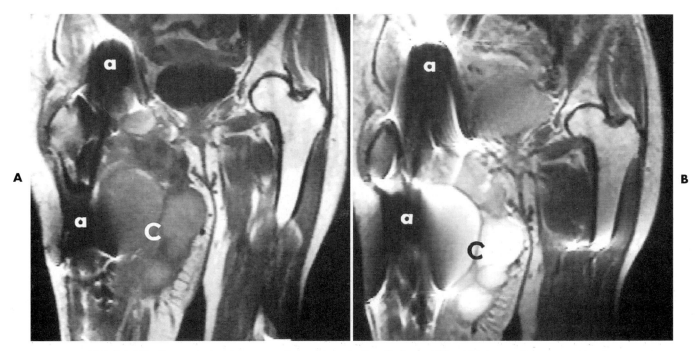

FIG. 13-79 Recurrent chondrosarcoma after surgical resection. **A,** Coronal T1-weighted magnetic resonance imaging demonstrates a lobulated mass, *C,* of low signal intensity arising from the femoral diaphysis (*a,* artifact from orthopedic hardware). **B,** The lesion, *C,* exhibits high signal intensity on a corresponding T2-weighted image (*a,* artifact from orthopedic hardware). Differential diagnosis should include consideration of other osseous and soft-tissue malignancies. (From Sartoris DJ: *Musculoskeletal imaging: the requisites,* St Louis, 1993, Mosby.)

CLINICAL COMMENTS

The most common presenting clinical complaint is progressive but not debilitating pain in the hip and buttocks of more than 3 months' duration. The pain often occurs at night and is not alleviated by rest. Aside from a slight limp and limited range of motion, the patient appears to be in excellent health. Laboratory findings typically are normal.

Resection is the preferred treatment for all chondrosarcomas. The prognosis depends on the histologic grade of the tumor and the adequacy of the resection. Irradiation and chemotherapy play minimal roles.[75,104] MRI provides the most accurate assessment of the extent of involvement and most often precedes resection.

> **KEY CONCEPTS**
> - *Chondrosarcomas are the third most common malignant primary bone tumor, arising as primary lesions or secondary to benign cartilaginous tumors (such as enchondromas and osteochondromas).*
> - *Chondrosarcomas are common in the pelvis, proximal femur, and proximal humerus.*
> - *They most often occur in patients between the ages of 50 and 70 years.*
> - *Matrix calcification is usually present and may appear nonaggressive.*

Fibrous, Histiocytic, and Fibrohistiocytic Origin

Benign

Fibrous Dysplasia

BACKGROUND

Fibrous dysplasia (FD) is a nonneoplastic disturbance of bone remodeling that is marked by inadequate maturation of osteoblasts.[148] Bone undergoing normal physiologic osteolysis becomes replaced by fibrous tissue containing small, abnormally arranged bone trabeculae. The condition may be confined to a single bone (monostotic fibrous dysplasia) or involve multiple bones (polyostotic fibrous dysplasia). These forms of the disease differ clinically, but the individual osseous lesions are pathologically

and radiographically identical. The monostotic form occurs three to four times as frequently as the polyostotic form. Approximately 3% of patients with polyostotic FD exhibit concurrent endocrinopathies, such as McCune-Albright's syndrome.

McCune-Albright's syndrome comprises a triad that includes the classic FD bony lesions in unilateral and polyostotic form, precocious puberty, and cutaneous hyperpigmentations (café-au-lait spots) located on the same side as the polyostotic lesions.[4,84,221] Mazabraud syndrome is made up of multiple fibrous and fibromyxomatous soft-tissue tumors occurring in association with polyostotic FD.[225]

FD was called osteitis fibrosa and generalized fibrocystic disease of bone in the older literature. The term *cherubism* (or *leontiasis ossea*) refers to a characteristic osseous deformity secondary to FD of the craniofacial bones. *Fibrous dysplasia protuberans* describes a rare excstotic lesion of fibrous dysplasia of small tubular bones of the hands and feet, and ribs.

FD affects men and women equally. A wide range of age is observed, affecting those from 1 to 75 years, although most cases are identified before the age of 20 years and most cases of polyostotic FD are identified before the age of 8 years.[26] The presence of concurrent endocrinopathies may lead to an earlier discovery of polyostotic FD.

IMAGING FINDINGS

FD most often occurs in the femur, tibia, craniofacial bones, pelvis, and ribs (Figs. 13-80 to 13-85).[101,107] Involvement of the pelvis typically occurs with the polyostotic form, where concurrent lesions usually are present in the femur. Spine involvement is uncommon in polyostotic FD and rare as a monostotic lesion (Fig. 13-86). Polyostotic FD has a peculiar predisposition to affect multiple bones on one side of the body.[148] The individual osseous lesions vary greatly in size, from 1 to 30 cm.

The radiographic appearance depends on the bone involved (Figs. 13-87 to 13-90). Tubular bones appear with medullary lesions that are mildly expansile, with an osteolytic or mildly sclerotic inner matrix. Mild sclerosis has been likened to the appearance of "ground glass" or "smoke" and results from the primitive and fine bone trabeculation within the lesion. The lesion also is usually marked by prominent surrounding sclerosis (rind sign). "Shepherd's crook" deformity is a lateral bowing and coxa vara deformity occurring in the proximal femur secondary to remodeling of pathologic microfracture. Skull bones appear densely sclerotic and often enlarged with FD. Involvement of the pelvis results in a distinctive bubbly appearance. MRI demonstrates low-signal-intensity medullary lesions on both T1- and T2-weighted images.

CLINICAL COMMENTS

Symptoms are more common when long tubular bones are involved; this is believed to result from microfracture. Polyostotic FD is associated with café-au-lait spots, the borders of which appear irregular ("coast of Maine") rather than smooth ("coast of California"), as occurs with spots associated with neurofibromatosis. Endocrinopathies, including McCune-Albright's syndrome (noted in the preceding), Cushing's syndrome, diabetes mellitus, acromegaly, and hyperparathyroidism are associated with polyostotic FD. Pathologic fracture is noted in up to 85% of patients with the polyostotic form of the disease.[101] Patient treatment is directed to any presenting fractures, deformity, or pain. Most lesions are small, isolated, and without associated features, requiring no treatment. Medications such as bisphosphonate (Fosamax) may be prescribed to strengthen involved bones. Malignant transformation occurs, but only rarely (<1%).

> ### KEY CONCEPTS
> - *Fibrous dysplasia is a nonneoplastic, tumorlike disturbance of bone.*
> - *The polyostotic form often is unilateral, associated with McCune-Albright's syndrome and cutaneous abnormalities.*
> - *Although a wide age range exists, the monostotic form usually occurs in patients younger than age 20 years and the polyostotic form usually occurs in patients younger than age 8 years.*
> - *Lesions of both forms appear osteolytic and expansile, most often involving the femur and tibia.*
> - *Skull lesions appear sclerotic.*

Nonossifying Fibroma and Fibrous Cortical Defect

BACKGROUND

Fibrous cortical defect (FCD) and nonossifying fibroma (NOF) are histologically identical defects of developing bone. Collectively they are called fibrous xanthomas or metaphyseal fibrous defects. They differ in age of presentation, size, frequency, and region of bone that is involved.

FCD is found on the cortical surface, and NOF is eccentrically placed within the medullary cavity (Figs. 13-91 to 13-103). Both may present as multiple lesions,[175] although multiple FCDs are more common than multiple NOFs.[105] Multiple lesions may be associated with neurofibromatosis[67] and Jaffe-Campanacci syndrome. The latter is a complex marked by café-au-lait spots, mental retardation, hypogonadism, and ocular abnormalities.[30]

FCDs are much more common than NOFs. FCDs and NOFs have been estimated to occur in 30% to 40% of children. FCDs typically are found in patients between the ages of 4 and 8 years and are twice as frequent in boys. NOFs are found in patients between the ages of 2 and 20 years, with a slight male predominance.

Jaffe-Campanacci syndrome defines multiple NOFs, café-au-lait hyperpigmentations, mental retardation, and various skeletal anomalies.[30]

IMAGING FINDINGS

FCDs and NOFs are common in the lower extremities, particularly around the knee. Most lesions are in the metaphysis, but over time may appear to migrate toward the diaphysis. There is no evidence of matrix calcification, but bone sclerosis may accompany the healing process. An FCD appears as a 1- to 3-cm round or oval geographic radiolucency eroding the cortical surface of the involved long bone.[142] It is sharply marginated by a thin rim of surrounding sclerosis. An NOF appears similarly, except it is found in the medullary cavity, more often appears multiloculated, and is larger (>3 cm) than an FCD.[47]

CLINICAL COMMENTS

Both FCDs and NOFs usually are clinically silent. They generally heal spontaneously as the peripheral rim of reactive sclerosis thickens, reducing the central radiolucent region. If large, NOFs may fracture (see Fig. 13-100), occasionally necessitating prophylactic curettage and bone grafting (see Fig. 13-103).[7]

> ### KEY CONCEPTS
> - *Fibrous cortical defects (FCDs) are common, small defects seen in patients between the ages of 4 and 8 years.*
> - *Nonossifying fibromas (NOFs) are common, larger than FCDs, and occur in patients between the ages of 2 and 20 years.*
> - *Both FCDs and NOFs usually are clinically silent, osteolytic lesions, most often found around the knee.*
> - *Both FCDs and NOFs often heal spontaneously.*

Desmoplastic Fibroma

BACKGROUND

A desmoplastic fibroma is a rare, locally aggressive solitary expression of skeletal fibromatosis. The lesion may present over a wide range of ages, from infants to senior adults, but is most typical in the second or third decade of life.

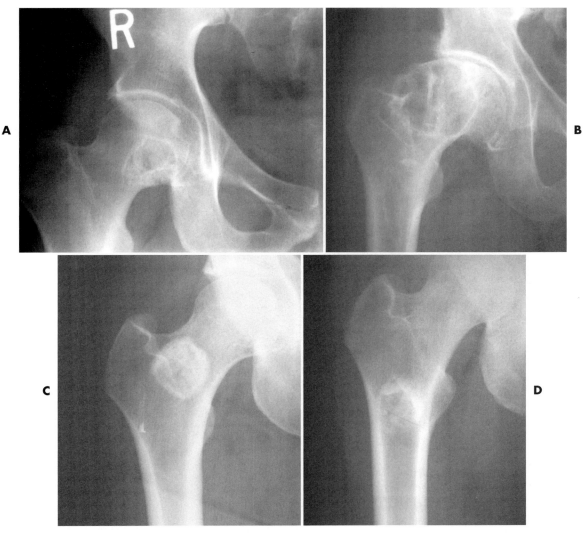

FIG. 13-80   **A** through **D,** Several cases of fibrous dysplasia of the proximal femur. The intertrochanteric region of the femur is a typical location of the disease. Note that all cases exhibit a well-defined lesion, with varying degrees of internal septation, radiodense matrix, and thickness of the surrounding rim of margination. (**A,** Courtesy Jay Brammier, Durant, IA; **D,** Courtesy William E. Litterer, Elizabeth, NJ.)

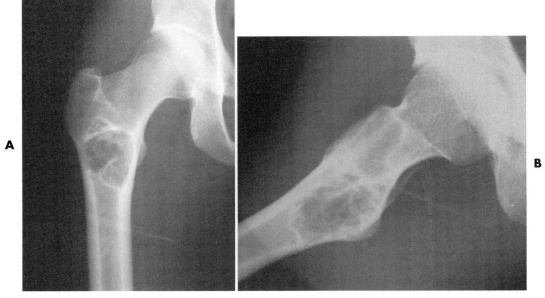

FIG. 13-81   Fibrous dysplasia of the hip, presenting on **A,** an anteroposterior and, **B,** frog-leg projection. (Courtesy Ian D. McLean, LeClaire, IA.)

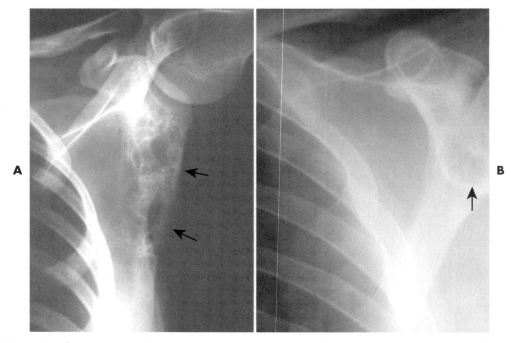

FIG. 13-82   Fibrous dysplasia of the scapula *(arrows),* appearing as, **A,** a bulbous lesion along the lateral border of the bone and, **B,** a smaller cystic defect in the subarticular region. In flat bones (i.e., scapulae and ilia), fibrous dysplasia and plasmacytomas (see Fig. 13-31) are nearly indistinguishable on plain film studies. (**B,** Courtesy Thomas Galli, Peoria, IL.)

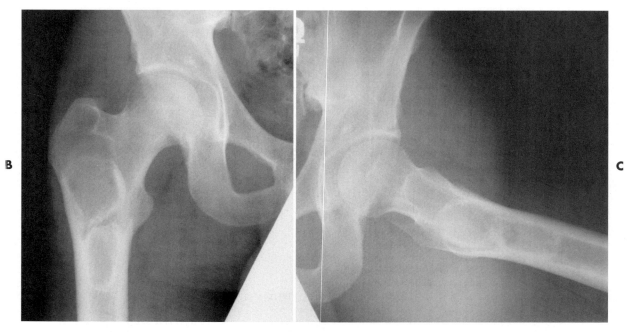

FIG. 13-83   **A** through **C,** Fibrous dysplasia of the proximal femur in a 24-year-old male patient demonstrating a hot spot on the bone scan (**A,** not shown) secondary to reactive bone sclerosis to the lesion. On these plain films, this lesion demonstrates a thick "rind" of marginal sclerosis, a feature characteristic of fibrous dysplasia. (Courtesy Ron Firth, East Moline, IL.)

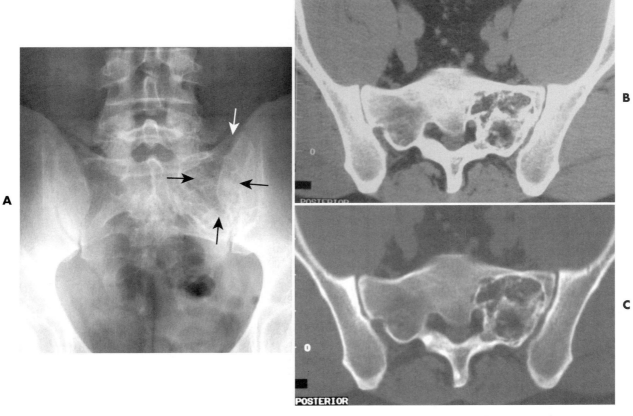

FIG. 13-84 **A,** Fibrous dysplasia of the right upper region of the sacrum noted on plain film *(arrows)* and computed tomography. **B,** Soft-tissue and, **C,** bone windows are presented.

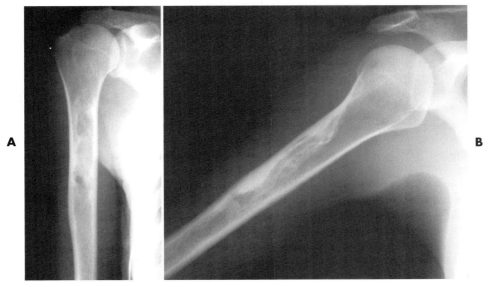

FIG. 13-85 **A** and **B,** A 32-year-old woman demonstrating fibrous dysplasia defect of the lateral margin of the proximal humerus.

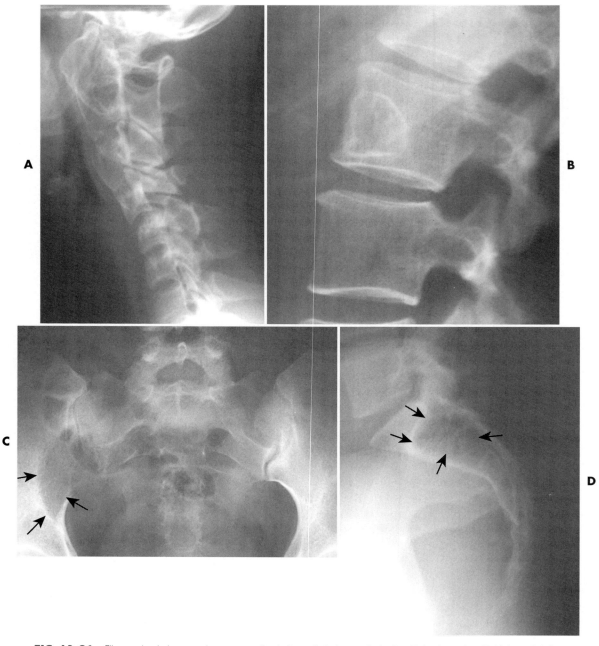

FIG. 13-86   Fibrous dysplasia appearing as expanding lesions of, **A,** the cervical spine; **B,** lumbar spine; **C,** V-shaped defect along the medial border of the ilium *(arrows);* and, **D,** faint radiolucent lesion seen on this lateral view of the sacrum *(arrows)* in different patients. (**B,** Courtesy Steven P. Brownstein, MD, Springfield, NJ; **D,** Courtesy Cheryl E. Crawford, Clarion, PA.)

IMAGING FINDINGS

The radiographic appearance denotes an expansile, radiolucent, well-defined lesion (Fig. 13-104). There may be interruption of the overlying cortex with extension into the soft tissue. The mandible and long bones usually are involved, but any bone may be affected.

CLINICAL COMMENTS

Pain and tenderness over the affected bone is most typical. Pathologic fracture may be responsible for the patient's complaint. Wide resection is the preferred method of treatment.

Malignant

Fibrosarcoma and Malignant Fibrous Histiocytoma

BACKGROUND

A fibrosarcoma is an uncommon malignant tumor derived from deep fibrous tissue. It is characterized by the presence of immature fibroblasts with variable amounts of collagen formation. Fibrosarcomas do not produce osteoid in either the primary bone lesion nor in their metastatic deposits.

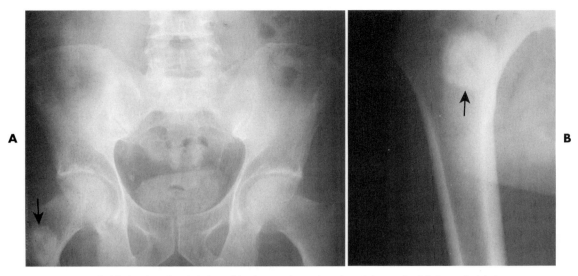

FIG. 13-87 **A,** Notice the sclerotic lesion of the intertrochanteric region of the reading left femur. **B,** It is better seen as a sclerotic lesion of fibrous dysplasia on the anteroposterior projection *(arrow).* This case illustrates the importance of not under-interpreting the periphery of the film.

A malignant fibrous tumor that contains both fibroblasts and histiocytes is termed *malignant fibrous histiocytoma* (MFH).[32,82,219,220] MFH is more commonly a lesion within soft tissue than bone. Malignant fibrous tumors arise de novo or in association with other lesions, including marrow infarct[168] previous radiation therapy, Paget's disease[43] enchondroma, chronic osteomyelitis,[48] and prosthetic replacement.[99]

Fibrosarcoma affects the sexes equally; the typical patient age is between 10 and 50 years. MFH demonstrates a 1.5:1 male predominance; the typical patient age is between 10 and 70 years.

IMAGING FINDINGS

Fifty percent of fibrosarcomas and MFHs of bone are found in the distal femur (Fig. 13-105). Other sites include the proximal tibia, humerus (Fig. 13-106), fibula, radius, and pelvis.[15,196] Any bone can be involved (Figs. 13-107 to 13-111). Up to 80% of lesions are found around the knee. Both malignant fibrous lesions appear similarly. They demonstrate geographic, moth-eaten, or permeative osteolytic destruction. Typically they are located in the metaphysis, often extending into the diaphysis. Cortical destruction, extraosseous mass, and periosteal reaction often are present.

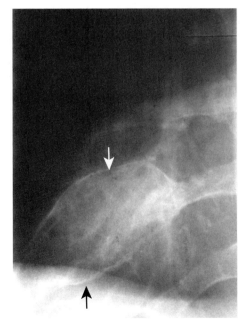

FIG. 13-88 Fibrous dysplasia of the rib. The lesion exhibits marked expansile changes *(arrows).* Other common expanding rib lesions include enchondroma, metastatic bone disease, multiple myeloma, and aneurysmal bone cyst. (Courtesy Robert C. Tatum, Davenport, IA.)

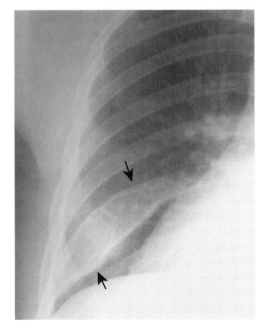

FIG. 13-89 An expansile lesion of fibrous dysplasia of the rib in a 44-year-old man *(arrows).*

PART TWO Bone, Joints, and Soft Tissues

Text continued on p. 860.

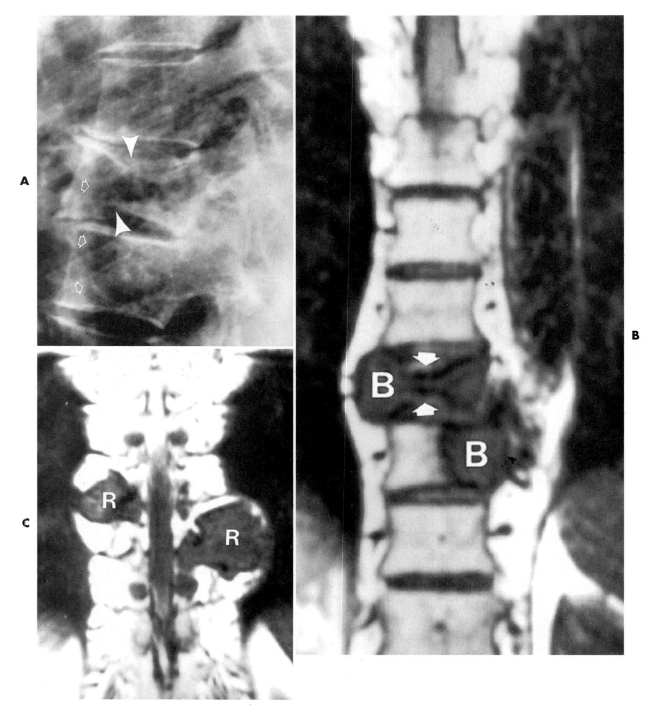

FIG. 13-90 Polyostotic fibrous dysplasia. **A,** Lateral radiograph demonstrates osteolytic involvement of two adjacent vertebral bodies *(open arrows)*, along with irregular endplate deformities *(arrowheads)*. **B** and **C,** Coronal T1-weighted magnetic resonance images reveal expansile low-signal-intensity areas within the vertebral bodies, *B,* and proximal ribs, *R.* Arrows point to the pathologic fracture. Differential diagnosis should include consideration of metastatic disease and indolent infection. (From Sartoris DJ: Musculoskeletal imaging: the requisites, St Louis, 1993, Mosby.)

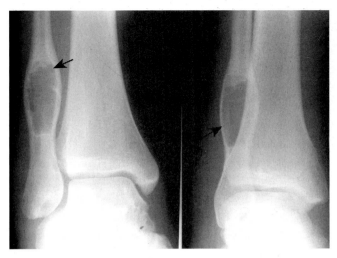

FIG. 13-91 Nonossifying fibroma appearing centrally in the diametaphyseal region of the fibula *(arrows)*. (Courtesy Ian D. McLean, LeClaire, IA.)

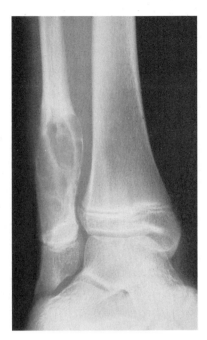

FIG. 13-92 Nonossifying fibroma of the lower fibula. (Courtesy Steven P. Brownstein, MD, Springfield, NJ.)

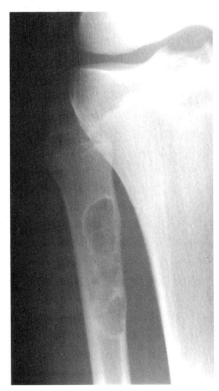

FIG. 13-93 Nonossifying fibroma of the upper fibula. (Courtesy Steven P. Brownstein, MD, Springfield, NJ.)

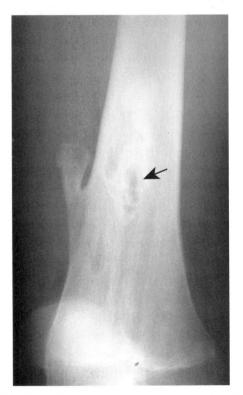

FIG. 13-94 Nonossifying fibroma of the lower femur *(arrow)* and osteochondroma, characteristically projecting away from the adjacent joint. (Courtesy Steven P. Brownstein, MD, Springfield, NJ.)

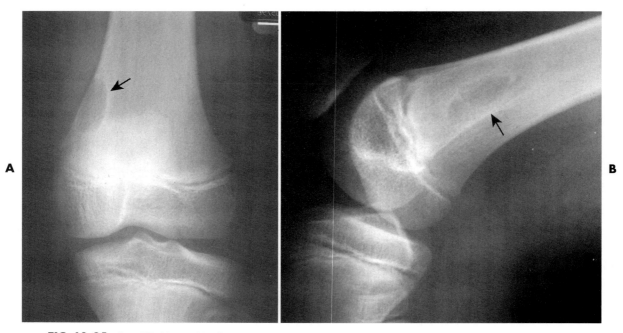

FIG. 13-95   **A** and **B,** Nonossifying fibroma of the lower femur *(arrows)*. (Courtesy Ron Firth, East Moline, IL.)

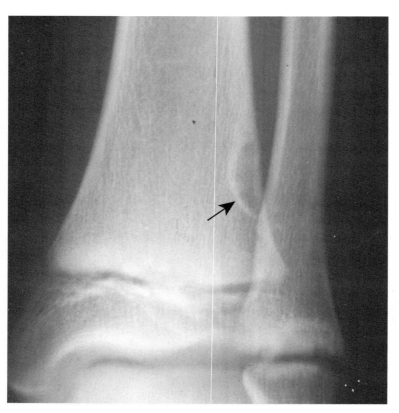

FIG. 13-96   Fibrous cortical defect presenting as a small eccentric lesion of the proximal tibia *(arrow)*.

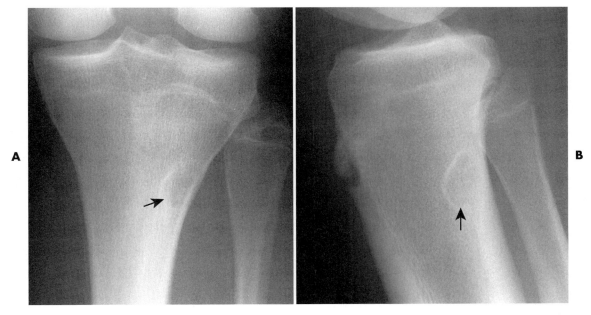

FIG. 13-97 **A** and **B,** Fibrous cortical defect of the proximal tibia *(arrows)* in a 13-year-old boy. These lesions often heal, disappearing over time. They are asymptomatic, representing no clinical concern.

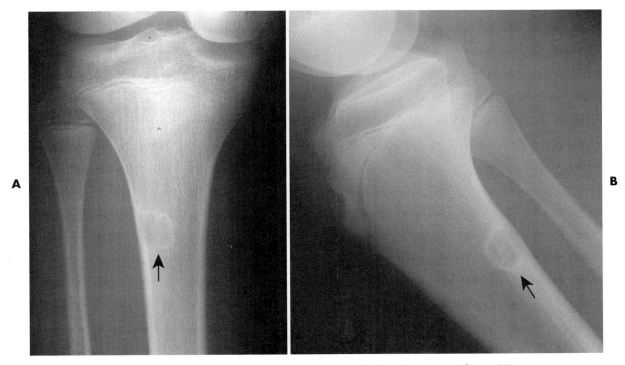

FIG. 13-98 **A** and **B,** Fibrous cortical defect of the proximal tibia *(arrows)* in a 15-year-old boy.

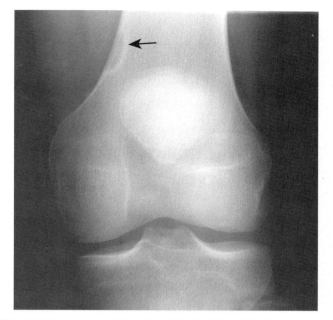

FIG. 13-99   Fibrous cortical defect of the distal femur *(arrow)*.

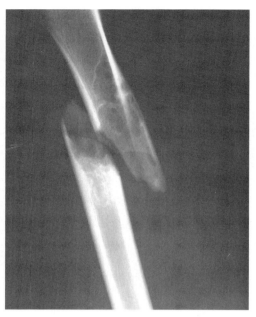

FIG. 13-100   Pathologic fracture through a nonossifying fibroma of the femur.

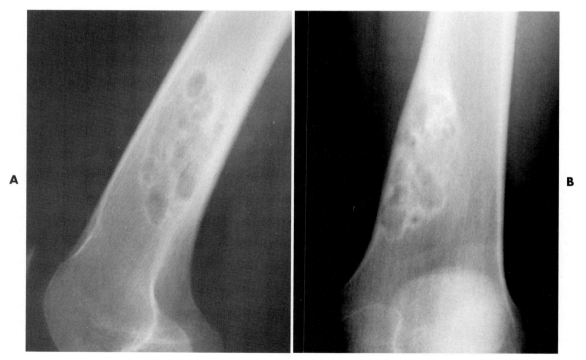

FIG. 13-101   **A** and **B,** Benign lesion eccentrically located in the distal femur consistent with either nonossifying fibroma or fibrous dysplasia.

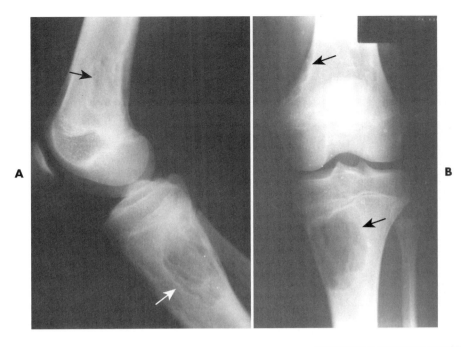

FIG. 13-102 A and **B,** Nonossifying fibroma of the distal femur and proximal tibia *(arrows).* Multiple nonossifying fibromas may occur as an isolated finding, as is the case here, or less commonly are associated with Jaffe-Campanacci syndrome or neurofibromatosis.

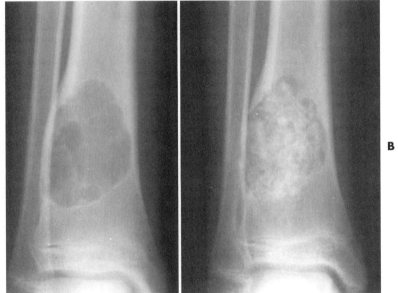

FIG. 13-103 A, Before and, **B,** after prophylactic curettage and bone grafting of a large, nonossifying fibroma of the distal tibia. (Courtesy Steven P. Brownstein, MD, Springfield, NJ.)

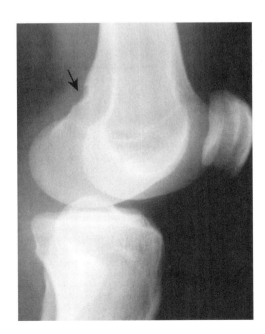

FIG. 13-104 Desmoplastic fibroma affecting the distal femur *(arrow).*

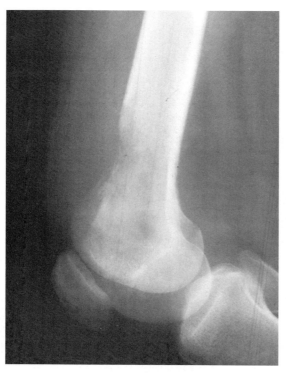

FIG. 13-105 Fibrosarcoma appearing with its most characteristic presentation of an aggressive osteolytic lesion about the knee; in this case the distal femur.

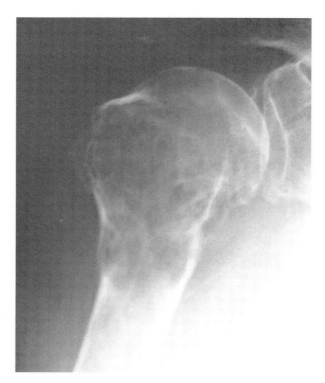

FIG. 13-106 Malignant fibrous histiocytoma with moth-eaten destruction of the proximal humerus. (Courtesy Steven P. Brownstein, MD, Springfield, NJ.)

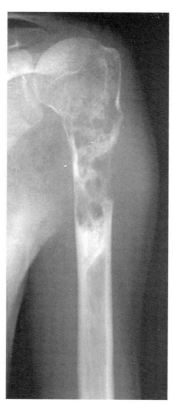

FIG. 13-107 Malignant degeneration of fibrous dysplasia to fibrosarcoma. The lesion demonstrates moth-eaten bone destruction of the proximal humerus without visible matrix calcification. (Courtesy Steven P. Brownstein, MD, Springfield, NJ.)

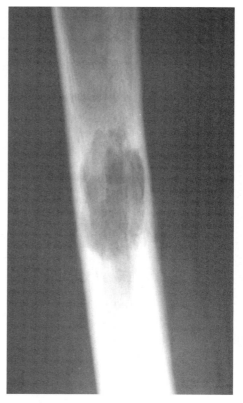

FIG. 13-108 Malignant fibrous histiocytoma presenting as central lesion with a long zone of transition between the normal bone and the lesion, and without visible matrix calcification. (Courtesy Steven P. Brownstein, MD, Springfield, NJ.)

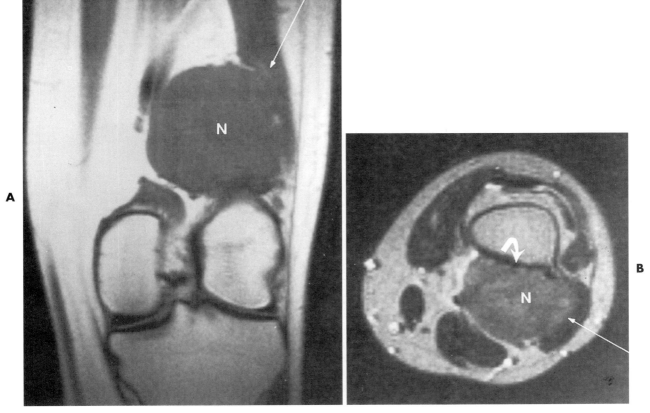

FIG. 13-109 Low-grade malignant fibrous histiocytoma. **A,** Coronal T1-weighted magnetic resonance image demonstrates a well-defined soft-tissue neoplasm, *N,* of low signal intensity superior to the femoral condyles and with displacement of the adjacent biceps femoris muscle *(arrow).* **B,** Transaxial T2-weighted image reveals intermediate signal intensity within the lesion, *N,* which has invaded the biceps femoris muscle *(arrow)* and posterior femoral cortex *(curved arrow).* Differential diagnosis should include consideration of fibrosarcoma, desmoid tumor, and other soft-tissue neoplasms of predominantly fibrous composition. (From Sartoris DJ: Musculoskeletal imaging: the requisites, St Louis, 1993, Mosby.)

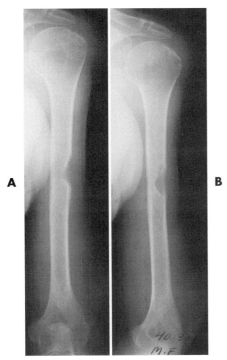

FIG. 13-110 **A** and **B,** Fibrosarcoma of the humerus appearing in a 70-year-old patient. The defect is marked by saucerization of the outer cortex of the diaphysis. (Courtesy Steven P. Brownstein, MD, Springfield, NJ.)

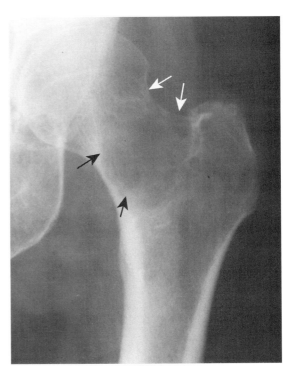

FIG. 13-111 Fibrosarcoma with permeative destruction of the femoral neck *(arrows)* and greater trochanter. (Courtesy Joseph W. Howe, Sylmar, CA.)

The tumor matrix does not exhibit calcification, although occasional bony fragments may be present. Central fibrosarcomas are more common than peripheral lesions.

CLINICAL COMMENTS

Typically patients complain of pain, tenderness, and soft-tissue swelling in the involved region. One third of patients demonstrate pathologic fracture. Fibrosarcomas and MFHs are aggressive lesions and carry poorer prognoses with soft-tissue involvement.

■ Synovial Origin

Benign

Pigmented Villonodular Synovitis

BACKGROUND

Pigmented villonodular synovitis (PVNS) is a rare, benign, inflammatory, proliferative disorder of synovium.[58] It is characterized by diffuse or localized hyperplastic outgrowth of the synovial membranes of joints, bursae, tendon sheaths, or a combination of these tissues.[18] Morphologically, the hyperplastic outgrowths may be villous, nodular, or villonodular and consist of undifferentiated connective tissue infiltrated by hemosiderin and lipid-containing macrophages. Lesions may occur as intraarticular (Fig. 13-112) or extraarticular forms, or a combination of the two. PVNS typically is monoarticular and occurs in patients between 30 and 50 years of age, without a significant sex predilection,[58] although some authorities report a slight male predominance.[91]

When PVNS involves a synovial tendon sheath, it does so as a nodular extraarticular presentation, and is termed a giant cell tumor of the tendon sheath (Fig. 13-113). However, some authorities feel it is problematic to include synovial tendon sheath lesions as PVNS.[76]

IMAGING FINDINGS

Radiographic features include soft-tissue swelling, preservation of joint space (may decrease over time), presence of well-marginated bone erosions and subchondral cysts, and absence of periarticular osteoporosis.

The spine is rarely involved.[22,55] As a tendon sheath abnormality, PVNS favors the digits. The knee is the joint most commonly involved. Other common joints include the hip, ankle, elbow, and wrist. Erosions and degenerative changes are more likely to occur in the hip and shoulder than in joints with large synovial recesses, such as the knee.

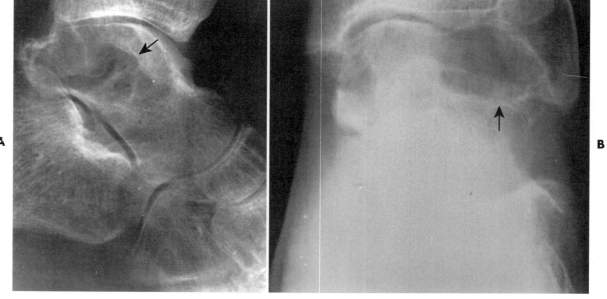

FIG. 13-112　A and **B,** Large cystic defect of the talus *(arrows)* secondary to pigmented villonodular synovitis. (Courtesy Joseph W. Howe, Sylmar, CA.)

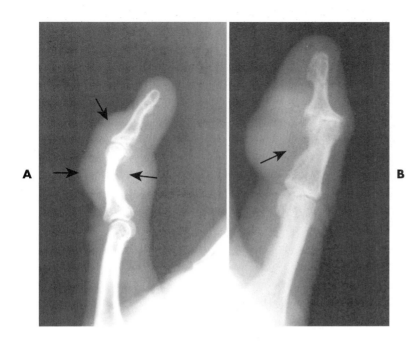

FIG. 13-113 Pigmented villonodular synovitis presenting in the tendon sheaths of, **A,** the fifth and, **B,** first digits *(arrows)* of different patients. Some authorities refer to this presentation as giant cell tumor of the tendon sheath. (**A,** Courtesy Joseph W. Howe, Sylmar, CA; **B,** Courtesy Steven P. Brownstein, MD, Springfield, NJ.)

The radiographic appearance is similar to that of noncalcified synovial chondromatosis. However, calcification is not a feature of PVNS. Another important differential is synovial sarcoma, especially if calcification is present. Other major radiographic differentials include tuberculosis, hemophilia, and juvenile rheumatoid arthritis.

PVNS has a characteristic appearance on MRI scans. PVNS is hypointense or isointense on T1-weighted images, and mixed hypointense and hyperintense on T2-weighted images (Fig. 13-114).[140] The hyperintense areas represent edema and inflamed synovium. Hemosiderin deposits account for the hypointense regions on both the T1- and T2-weighted images. Correspondingly, large effusions may appear radiodense on plain film radiographs resulting from the hemosiderin deposits.

In addition to plain film and MRI, ultrasonography, arthrography, and CT may assist in providing critical information toward the correct diagnosis when confronted with an intraarticular abnormality.[27]

CLINICAL COMMENTS

Patients with PVNS most often are accompanied by mechanical pain and limitations of motion.[32] A history of trauma is slightly more often present than not. Joint swelling and joint locking often are present. Optimal treatment is early marginal excision for the local form and total synovectomy for the diffuse form.[49,156] Although recurrence is common (approaching 30%),[29] the lesions are not malignant and radical surgical procedures are not indicated.[118]

KEY CONCEPTS

- *Pigmented villonodular synovitis (PVNS) is an uncommon, benign, inflammatory disorder of the synovial membranes of joints, bursae, and tendon sheaths.*
- *PVNS is typically monoarticular (usually involving the knee) and occurs between the ages of 30 and 50 years.*
- *Radiographic features include soft-tissue swelling, preservation of joint space (may decrease over time), presence of bone erosions and subchondral cysts, and absence of periarticular osteoporosis.*
- *Common clinical findings include mechanical pain, limitation of motion, and joint swelling.*

Synoviochondrometaplasia

BACKGROUND

Synoviochondrometaplasia synovial chondromatosis, synovial osteochondromatosis, joint chondroma is a benign disorder marked by metaplasia of hyperplastic synovium to hyaline cartilage. The hyaline cartilage calcifies or ossifies and detaches from the synovium to form loose bodies (<2 to 3 cm in diameter) within the joint, tendon sheath, or bursae in which it forms. Receiving nutrition from the surrounding synovial fluid, the loose bodies often grow.

Large weight-bearing joints are most commonly involved, but any synovial joint may be involved. The knee is the most common location, but the hip, elbow, shoulder, ankle, and other locations

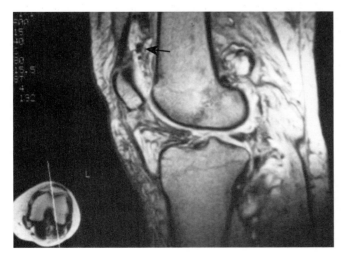

FIG. 13-114 T2-weighted magnetic resonance image of the knee revealing the characteristic mixed signal intensity with nodular low-signal foci that represent areas of hemosiderin-laden hyperplastic synovium of pigmented villonodular synovitis *(arrow).* (Courtesy Ian D. McLean, LeClaire, IA.)

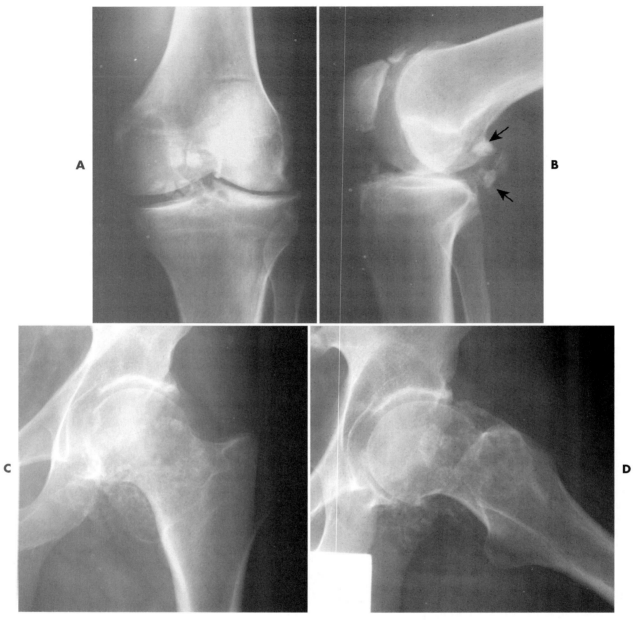

FIG. 13-115 Synoviochondrometaplasia forming many loose bodies within, **A** and **B**, the knee joint and, **C** and **D**, the hip *(arrows)* in different patients. (Courtesy Gary Longmuir, Phoenix, AZ.)

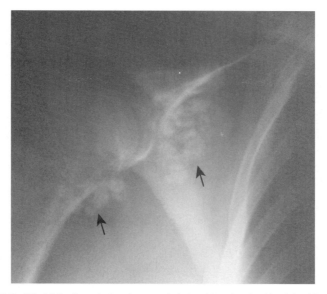

FIG. 13-116 Synoviochondrometaplasia involving the shoulder joint. Note the multiple loose bodies that define the disease *(arrows)*. At times, these loose bodies are not calcified, and therefore are not visible on radiographs. If the loose bodies are extensive and the joint capsule tight, the loose bodies may erode the adjacent bone, causing an "eaten apple core" appearance of the bone. However, this feature is not seen here. (Courtesy Ryder M. Church, Peoria, IL.)

FIG. 13-117 Synoviochrondro-metaplasia. **A,** Double-contrast arthrogram showing the granular surface of synovium anteriorly *(arrows)*. Cartilaginous bodies are poorly defined in the posterior part of the joint. **B,** Computed tomography arthrogram. Two large cartilaginous bodies outlined by contrast are seen in the olecranon fossa *(arrowheads)*. Multiple small cartilaginous bodies *(arrows)* are seen anteriorly. (From Firooznia H et al: MRI and CT of the musculoskeletal system, St Louis, 1992, Mosby.)

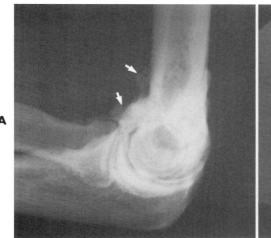

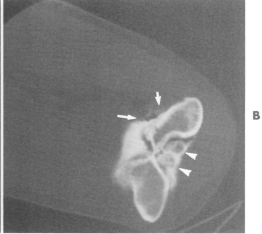

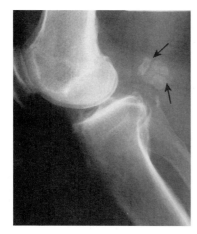

FIG. 13-118 Synoviochrondrometaplasia presenting as multiple loose bodies in the posterior aspect of the knee *(arrows)*. (Courtesy Joseph W. Howe, Sylmar, CA.)

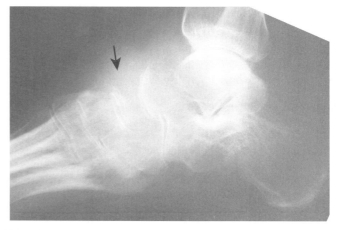

FIG. 13-119 Synovial sarcoma (synovioma) of the dorsum of the foot, causing aggressive osteolytic bone destruction with associated soft-tissue mass *(arrow)*. (Courtesy Steven P. Brownstein, MD, Springfield, NJ.)

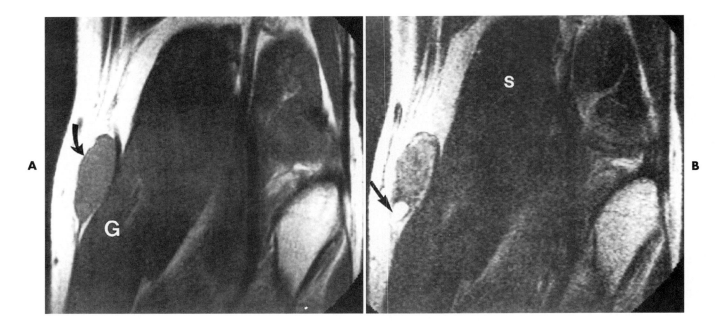

FIG. 13-120   Synovial sarcoma. **A,** Coronal T1-weighted magnetic resonance image reveals a well-defined mass of low signal intensity *(arrow)* adjacent to the medial head of the gastrocnemius muscle, G. **B,** Corresponding T2-weighted image demonstrates an inhomogeneous appearance, with high signal intensity in the inferior portion of the lesion *(arrow)* (s, semi-membranosus muscle). Differential diagnosis should include consideration of other benign and malignant soft-tissue neoplasms. (From Sartoris DJ: Musculoskeletal imaging: the requisites, St Louis, 1993, Mosby.)

are common. Occasionally the presentation is bilateral. Tendon sheath and bursae involvement are less common. Men are affected more commonly than women, and usually the disease affects young and middle-aged adults.

IMAGING FINDINGS
The radiographic appearance usually is defined by the presence of multiple radiodense loose bodies noted in the confines of the joint capsule (Figs. 13-115 to 13-118). Pressure erosions, widened joint space, and secondary degeneration may be present. Milder forms of the disease may appear similar to the radiodense debris of osteoarthritis or chondrocalcinosis of calcium pyrophosphate dihydrate (CPPD) deposition disease. Both CT and MRI are useful to define the intraarticular location.

Less commonly the loose bodies do not calcify and are not seen on the radiograph, or only a portion of them are seen radiographically. Although the loose bodies are not seen, secondary mechanical bone erosions may be visible, mimicking the appearance of pigmented villonodular synovitis and synovioma.

CLINICAL COMMENTS
Symptoms include intermittent pain, joint swelling, stiffness, and episodes of joint "locking" secondary to the internal joint mice. Limitations of movement, synovial thickening, crepitus, and palpable loose bodies are present sometimes. Although the condition is largely self-limiting and may undergo spontaneous regression, the presence of intraarticular loose bodies often produces mechanical derangement and leads to secondary degeneration of the joint. For this reason, surgical excision of the loose bodies and abnormal synovium often is recommended.

Malignant

Synoviosarcoma

BACKGROUND
Synovial sarcoma (synovioma) is an uncommon malignant soft-tissue tumor arising from the mesenchyme rather than mature synovial tissues.[33] These tumors express epithelial and supporting tissue features.[33,208] Synovial sarcoma occurs most often in patients between the ages of 15 and 40 years[5,74] and more predominantly in males.[118]

IMAGING FINDINGS
Synovial sarcomas occur more often in paraarticular regions, close to tendon sheaths, bursae, and joint capsules, in the lower extremities. They appear as soft-tissue masses with associated calcifications and bony erosions.[108,118] Common sites include the knee, hip, thigh,

ankle, elbow, wrist, hands, and feet (Figs. 13-119 and 13-120). Rare variants occur in the oral cavity, anterior abdominal wall, larynx, heart, and mediastinum.

CLINICAL COMMENTS

Pain is a very common complaint, often preceding the clinical recognition of the tumor by several years.[74] Treatment includes surgical excision with or without radiation or chemotherapy.[163]

Muscle Origin

Benign

Leiomyoma

See the abdomen section in Chapter 29.

Malignant

Leiomyosarcoma

Leiomyosarcoma of the soft tissue is rare. It is divided into four presentations: cutaneous, subcutaneous, intraabdominal, and vascular. It is most commonly present in patients over the age of 40 years; the cutaneous variety presents in young adults. Leiomyosarcoma is composed of interlacing fascicles of spindle cells with blunted (cigar-shaped) nuclei histologically. They appear as masses with irregular borders and high vascularity, blending into the collagen stroma of the involved tissue.

Leiomyosarcoma as a primary tumor of bone is extremely rare, with less than 50 documented cases. The tumor is of mesenchymal derivation predominantly of spindle cells that exhibit smooth muscle tissue. In the skeletal system, it occurs as either a primary tumor of bone, or more likely, a metastatic deposit in bone from a primary soft-tissue lesion of the uterus or gastrointestinal tract.[85] It appears as a moth-eaten destructive osteolytic lesion with an ill-defined zone of transition between the lesion and host bone. The femur and tibia are the most common bones involved. Confirmation of this lesion depends on tissue biopsy.

Rhabdomyosarcoma

Rhabdomyosarcoma is a rare tumor showing skeletal muscle differentiation. The adult variety is seen most commonly in the head and neck of middle-aged adults. It is characterized histologically by polygonal eosinophilic cells with granular cytoplasm and focal vacuolation. The fetal variety also presents in the head and neck, marked by primitive mesenchymal cells at the center of the lesion. Rhabdomyosarcoma is a rare primary lesion of bone. The radiographic presentation exhibits osteolytic destruction.

Fat Origin

Benign

Lipoma

BACKGROUND

A lipoma is a common, benign collection of mature fat cells within subcutaneous tissue, nerves, synovium, and between or within muscles. Rarely, lipomas occur as intraosseous, cortical, or parosteal lesions.[146,166,178] Soft-tissue lesions typically occur as palpable, compressive, moveable, subcutaneous masses, most often found in women. Osseous lesions usually occur during middle age, with no gender predilection.

IMAGING FINDINGS

Soft-tissue lipomas appear as radiolucent regions of fat radiodensity surrounded by the less radiolucent water density of the adjacent soft tissues (Figs. 13-121 to 13-126). Usually they involve the extremities.

Intraosseous lesions appear radiolucent, surrounded by a thin sclerotic rim of bone. Often a centrally located radiodense nidus of calcification is noted within the radiolucency (see Fig. 13-122).[39]

Osseous lesions are found predominantly in the proximal femur and calcaneus (see Fig. 13-124).

Lipomas demonstrate fat signal intensity on MRIs. The lesions are bright on T1-weighted images and bright to isointense on T2-weighted images (see Fig. 13-126). Interosseous lesions may not be well delineated on MRI because they exhibit similar signal to that of the normal bone marrow.

CLINICAL COMMENTS

Lipomas usually are asymptomatic, but localized pain, tenderness, and a soft-tissue mass can occur, often exacerbated by activity of the affected region.[141] Multiple lesions may be associated with systemic hyperlipoproteinemia.[89]

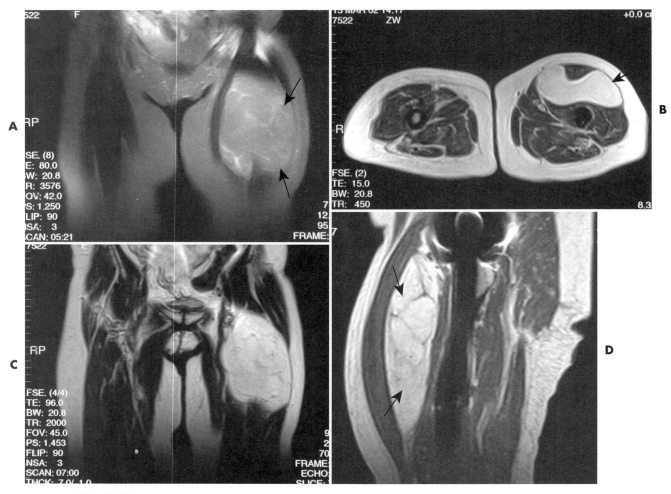

FIG. 13-121 Large intermuscular lipoma of the anterior portion of the patient's left thigh *(arrows).* The signal intensity within the lesion is homogeneous and appears with high signal intensity on, **A** and **B,** the T1- and, **C** and **D,** T2-weighted scans. Notice that the lesion is well circumscribed and without evidence of aggressive infiltration within the surrounding tissues.

Malignant

Liposarcoma

BACKGROUND

A liposarcoma is a malignant tumor of adults, usually occurring in the deep intermuscular or periarticular planes of the buttocks, thigh, calf, and retroperitoneal tissues. Liposarcoma is the second most common soft-tissue sarcoma, after MFH. Liposarcoma of bone is extremely rare. Liposarcoma usually occurs in patients between 30 and 50 years of age.

IMAGING FINDINGS

The appearance is variable, from a highly aggressive lesion with soft-tissue density to a well-defined mass often of fat radiodensity. They appear most commonly in the buttocks, thigh (Figs. 13-127 and 13-128), calf, and retroperitoneal space. Often, dystrophic calcification or ossification can be observed within the soft-tissue mass.

The MRI appearance is marked by increased signal intensity on the T2-weighted image and mixed to increased signal intensity on the T1-weighted images. Most aggressive soft-tissue lesions demonstrate a high signal intensity on the T2-weighted images, but the increased signal intensity on the T1-weighted scans is characteristic of the fatty tissues of the liposarcoma, although this appearance is not seen necessarily in all liposarcomas.

CLINICAL COMMENTS

Liposarcomas often are asymptomatic during early stages of development and therefore may be extremely large at clinical presentation. Once the lesion has been identified, surgery is indicated and accomplished through wide excision, which often is combined with chemotherapy. Recurrence and metastasis, usually to the lungs, is common.

KEY CONCEPTS

- *Liposarcoma is the second most common soft-tissue sarcoma.*
- *Common locations for liposarcoma include the buttocks, thigh, calf, and retroperitoneal tissues.*
- *Patients are usually 30 to 50 years of age.*
- *Liposarcomas are often asymptomatic initially and therefore may be large when clinically recognized.*

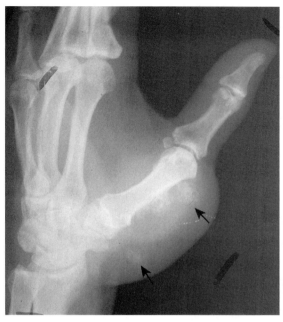

FIG. 13-122 Parosteal lipoma with several scattered foci of calcification *(arrows)*. The appearance is similar to a soft-tissue hemangioma with phleboliths. (Courtesy Steven P. Brownstein, MD, Springfield, NJ.)

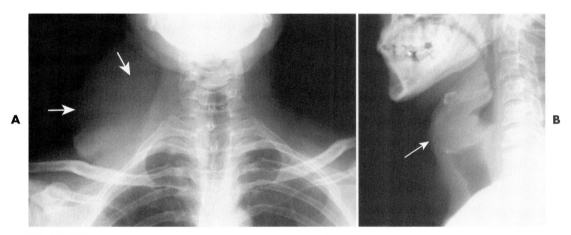

FIG. 13-123 Soft-tissue lipoma presenting as a suprascapular mass *(arrows)* on, **A,** the frontal projection and, **B,** extending as an anterior neck mass on the lateral projection *(arrow)*. (Courtesy William E. Litterer, Elizabeth, NJ.)

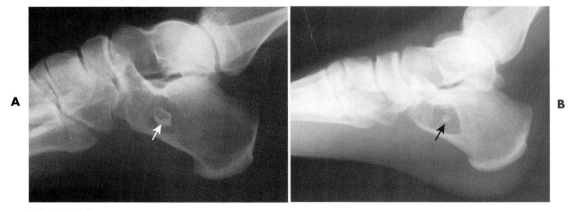

FIG. 13-124 **A** and **B,** Two cases of an interosseous lipoma of the calcaneus demonstrating a central nidus of calcification *(arrows)*. (**A,** Courtesy Steven P. Brownstein, MD, Springfield, NJ.)

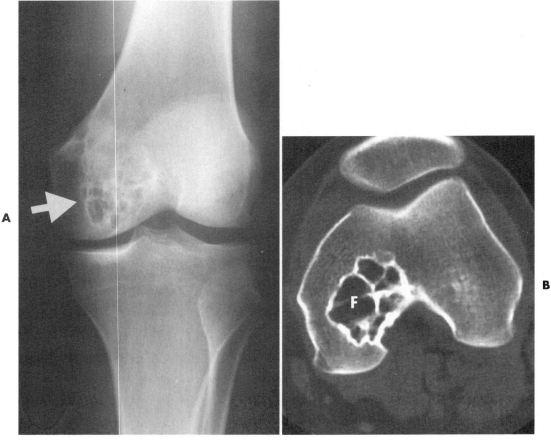

FIG. 13-125   Interosseous lipoma of the distal femur. **A,** Frontal radiograph reveals a well-defined lytic and septate lesion *(arrow)* in the epiphysis. Differential diagnosis for lytic epiphyseal lesions should include consideration of chondroblastoma, giant cell tumor, intraosseous ganglion, clear-cell chondrosarcoma, infection, and (rarely) eosinophilic granuloma. **B,** Computed tomography eliminates these possibilities by documenting low-density fat, *F,* within the lesion. (From Sartoris DJ: Musculoskeletal imaging: the requisites, St Louis, 1993, Mosby.)

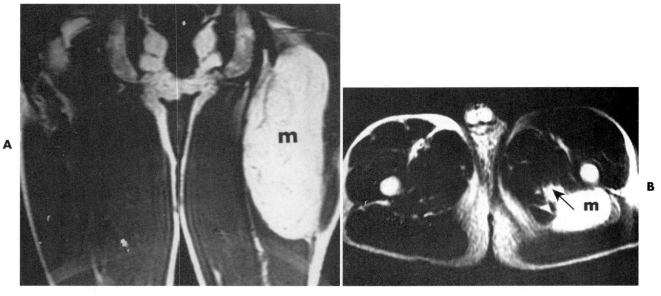

FIG. 13-126   Soft-tissue lipoma of the thigh. **A,** Coronal T1-weighted magnetic resonance imaging documents a large, relatively homogeneous fat-containing mass, *m,* in the posterior compartment. **B,** Transaxial T2-weighted image demonstrates predominant displacement of the adductor magnus muscle *(arrow)* by the mass, *m.* Differential diagnosis should include consideration of well-differentiated liposarcoma. (From Sartoris DJ: Musculoskeletal imaging: the requisites, St Louis, 1993, Mosby.)

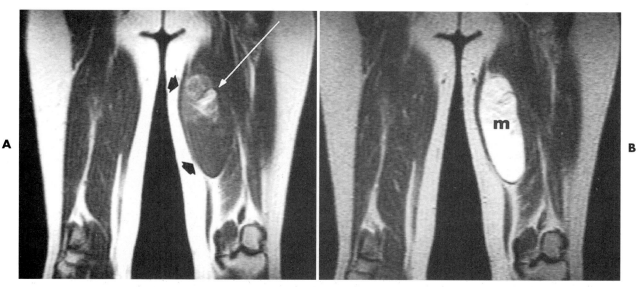

FIG. 13-127 Liposarcoma of the thigh. **A,** Coronal T1-weighted magnetic resonance imaging reveals a heterogeneous fat-containing *(white arrow)* mass *(black arrows)*, suggesting the correct diagnosis. **B,** The mass, *m*, exhibits uniformly high signal intensity on a corresponding T2-weighted image. Other fat-containing soft-tissue lesions include lipoma, macrodystrophia lipomatosa, hemangioma, and neurofibromatosis. (From Sartoris DJ: Musculoskeletal imaging: the requisites, St Louis, 1993, Mosby.)

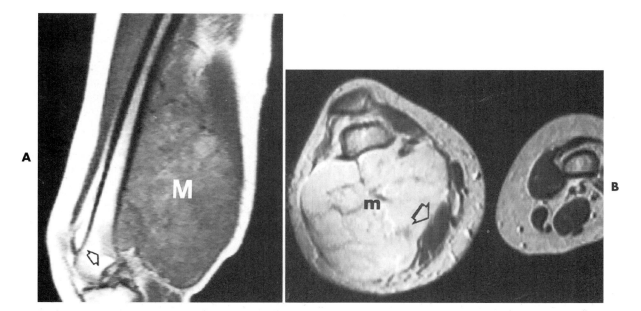

FIG. 13-128 Poorly differentiated liposarcoma of the thigh. **A,** Sagittal T1-weighted magnetic resonance image demonstrates a large inhomogeneous mass, *M*, containing only sparse fat with early invasion of the distal femur *(arrow)*. **B,** Transaxial T2-weighted image reveals predominantly high signal intensity within the mass, *m*, which has invaded and displaced the semimembranous muscle *(arrow)*. Differential diagnosis should include consideration of other soft-tissue sarcomas. (From Sartoris DJ: Musculoskeletal imaging: the requisite, St Louis, 1993, Mosby.)

Vascular Origin

Benign

Hemangioma

BACKGROUND

A hemangioma is a congenital anomaly in which a proliferation of vascular endothelium leads to a benign mass that resembles neoplastic tissue. Hemangiomas occur in bone, skin, and viscera. They are considered the most common benign tumors of the spine. In general, osseous hemangiomas are predominantly of two broad categories: capillary hemangiomas, which consist of haphazardly arranged, capillary-sized vessels, and the more common cavernous hemangiomas, which contain dilated vessels, lined with attenuated endothelial cells. Less commonly osseous hemangiomas demonstrate a histologic appearance consistent with venous soft-tissue lesions.[184]

Hemangiomas may be encountered in patients of any age, although most are recognized in the fifth decade of life with a 3:2 female-to-male predominance.[63]

IMAGING FINDINGS

More than 50% of osseous hemangiomas are in the spine (Figs. 13-129 to 13-133),[212] 20% are in the skull, and the remaining lesions are found in the ribs, patella, long bones, and short tubular bones of the hands and feet. Hemangiomas usually occur as solitary lesions.

Capillary hemangiomas appear most commonly in the frontal bone, appearing as radiating radiolucent striations from a central radiolucent focus ("sunburst appearance"). Cavernous hemangiomas are most commonly seen in the vertebral bodies of the lower thoracic and upper lumbar spine[245] and are marked by exaggerated vertical radiopaque striations of the involved vertebral body ("accordion," "corduroy cloth," or "jail bar pattern"). Cervical vertebral body lesions often exhibit a "honeycomb" appearance of coarse trabeculation. Infrequently vertebral lesions extend into the neural arch.

Contrary to most tumors, vertebral hemangiomas appear as round, well-circumscribed lesions with increased signal intensity on both T1- and T2-weighted MRI scans, reflecting their fatty and vascular stroma (Figs. 13-134 to 13-137).[196] Sometimes vertebral hemangiomas histologically exhibit less fatty stroma than usual, causing them to appear hypointense on the T1-weighted scans, but often enhancing after contrast administration.[139]

Contrary to most tumors, hemangiomas demonstrate increased signal intensity on both T1- and T2-weighted MRI.[169] Hemangiomas produce an interesting "polka-dot" pattern on the axial images of CT.

Soft-tissue hemangiomas present as soft-tissue radiodense shadows, with scattered phleboliths (Fig. 13-138).

CLINICAL COMMENTS

As evidenced by the large number of asymptomatic lesions found at autopsy (10% to 12%), most hemangiomas are unnoticed.[245] Symptoms usually are secondary to pathologic fracture, occurring in long bones. Because of the concern of pathologic fractures,

it may be prudent to avoid chiropractic spinal adjustments of grossly involved segments.

Rarely, an expanding spinal lesion may cause spinal canal stenosis.[197] MRI examination always should be considered in patients exhibiting radiographic findings of hemangioma when neurologic symptoms are present. No treatment is applied to asymptomatic lesions. The treatment for painful lesions depends on their location and degree of osseous involvement. Radiation alleviates painful lesions, although the radiographic appearance remains unchanged.[155]

KEY CONCEPTS

- *Hemangiomas are common bone lesions located in the skull (capillary) and spine (cavernous) and are clinically silent.*
- *The radiographic appearance of a spine lesion is marked by thick vertical striations.*
- *Hemangiomas exhibit increased signal intensity on both T1- and T2-weighted magnetic resonance images.*
- *Most lesions are asymptomatic and nearly incidental findings; however, pathologic fractures and expansion should be considered.*

Glomus Tumor

The glomus is an arteriovenous anastomosis present in the reticular dermis and frequently the subungual regions. The glomus tumor is a rare benign lesion of vascular channels. Glomus tumors are most common between the ages of 20 and 40 years, and usually are located in the subungual region of the fingers. Very rarely, intraosseous glomus tumors have been described, usually in the distal phalanges.[151] They present radiographically as well-defined osteolytic defects of less than 1 cm in diameter. Most often the associated symptoms are pronounced. Simple excision is curative.

Lymphangioma

Lymphangiomas are benign tumors composed of immature lymph vessels, representing hamartomatous malformations more than true tumors.[120] Lesions rarely occur after the age of 20 years. Radiographically lymphangiomas exhibit marked expansion with "sunburst" periosteal reaction. Lesions stabilize over time and generally have a good prognosis.

Malignant

Angiosarcoma

Angiosarcoma covers a wide range of malignant endothelial vascular tumors, most commonly of the dermis and subcutis regions of the head and neck, or liver and spleen.[10] They may be induced by radiation and chemical exposure.[37] Primary angiosarcoma of bone is very rare, presenting as solitary (Fig. 13-139), ill-defined lesions. They are very aggressive with early metastases, necessitating radical en bloc resection or amputation.

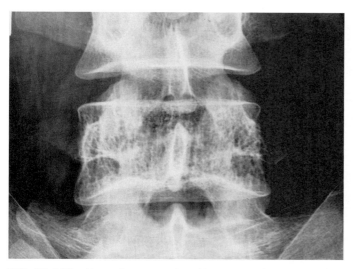

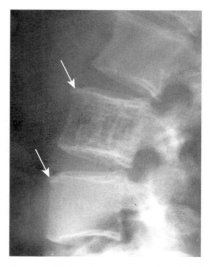

FIG. 13-129 Hemangioma presenting with a coarsened appearance of the L5 segment. (Courtesy Steven P. Brownstein, MD, Springfield, NJ.)

FIG. 13-130 Coarsened trabecular appearance characteristic of hemangioma. Notice also, the vacuum cleft phenomenon *(arrows)*.

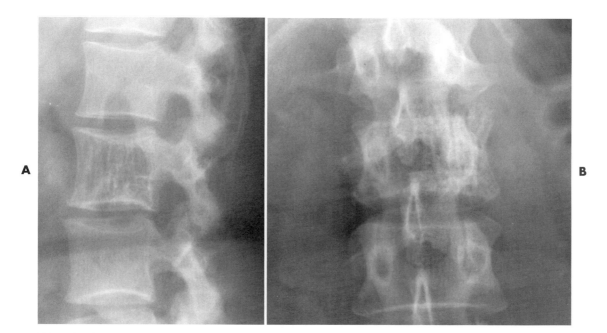

FIG. 13-131 **A,** L3 segment has prominent vertical striations, a feature known as "corduroy cloth" or "jail bar" appearance of hemangioma. **B,** Anteroposterior projection has a coarsened appearance of the trabeculation. (Courtesy Gary Longmuir, Phoenix, AZ.)

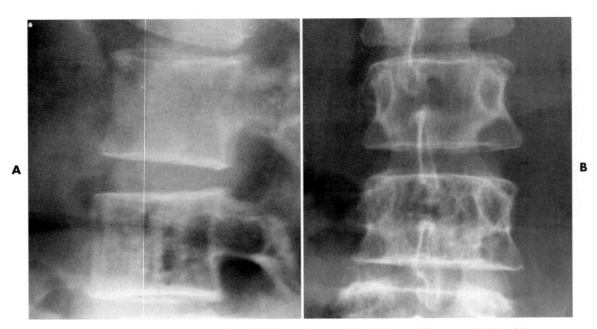

FIG. 13-132   Hemangioma presenting with, **A,** prominent vertical striations and, **B,** coarsened trabeculation.

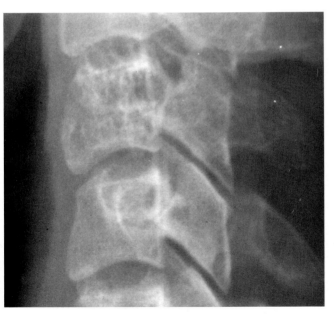

FIG. 13-133   Hemangioma of C3 noted by coarsened trabeculation. (Courtesy Steven P. Brownstein, MD, Springfield, NJ.)

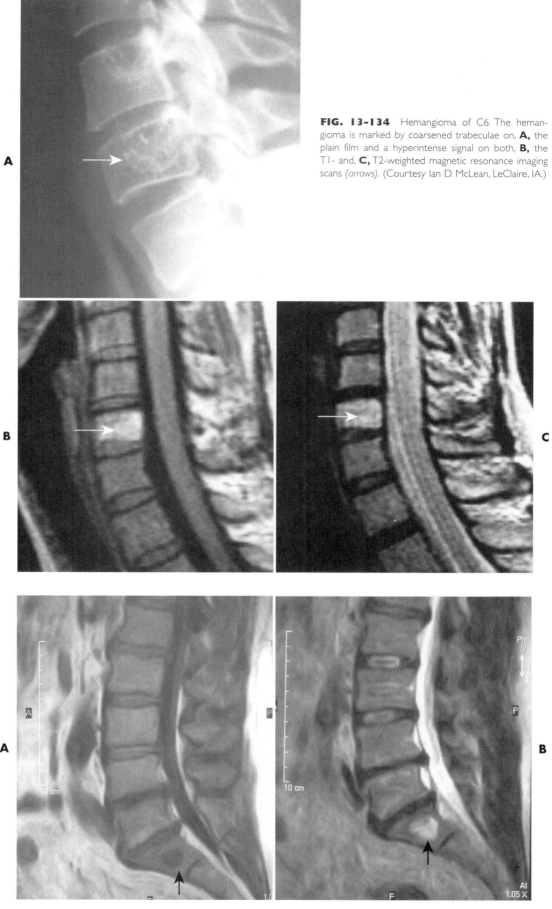

FIG. 13-134 Hemangioma of C6. The hemangioma is marked by coarsened trabeculae on, **A,** the plain film and a hyperintense signal on both, **B,** the T1- and, **C,** T2-weighted magnetic resonance imaging scans *(arrows)*. (Courtesy Ian D. McLean, LeClaire, IA.)

FIG. 13-135 Forty-five-year-old man with a hemangioma of the S1 segment appearing as a hypointense signal on, **A,** the T1-weighted magnetic resonance imaging sequence and hyperintense on, **B,** the T2-weighted image *(arrows)*.

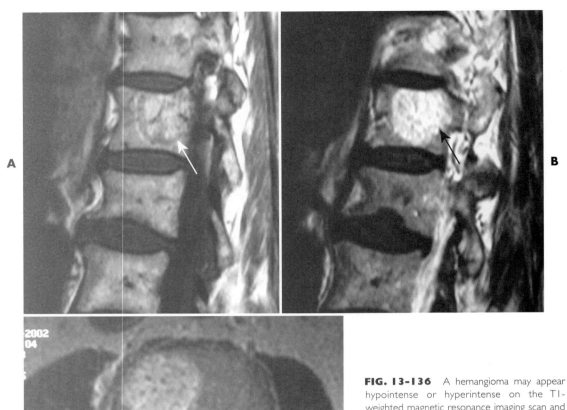

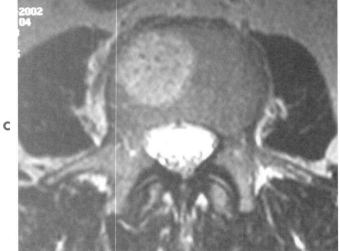

FIG. 13-136 A hemangioma may appear hypointense or hyperintense on the T1-weighted magnetic resonance imaging scan and is typically hyperintense on the T2-weighted scans, reflecting the water, fat, and blood composition of the lesions. This 104-year-old man exhibits the most typical signal present of a region of slight hyperintensity on, **A** and **C,** the T1-weighted scan that becomes more hyperintense on, **B,** the T2-weighted scan *(arrows).* (Courtesy Kevin Cunningham, Eldridge, IA.)

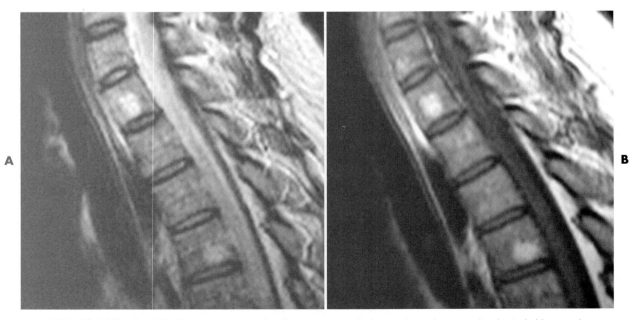

FIG. 13-137 **A** and **B,** Magnetic resonance imaging appearance of a hemangioma, demonstrating the typical increased signal intensity on both the T1- and T2-weighted scans. Two levels are involved. Hemangioma traditionally has been regarded as the most common benign tumor of the spine. With the advent of magnetic resonance imaging, hemangiomas are even more common than traditionally thought, based on plain film findings.

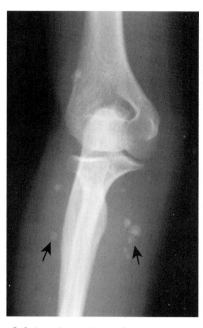

FIG. 13-138 Soft-tissue hemangioma of the elbow. Notice the small phleboliths presenting as radiodense shadows scattered throughout the soft-tissue mass (arrows).

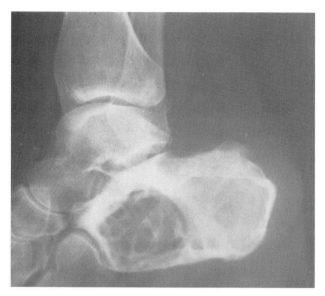

FIG. 13-139 Aggressive lesion of the calcaneus representing angiosarcoma. (Courtesy Steven P. Brownstein, MD, Springfield, NJ.)

 # Notochord Origin

Malignant

Chordoma

BACKGROUND

A chordoma is an uncommon, solitary, malignant neoplasm that develops from remnant portions of the notochord.[228] The cells of the tumor are arranged in lobules with abundant quantities of extracellular mucus. Some of the cells contain vacuoles of mucus that resemble soap bubbles, known as *physaliphorous cells*. Chordomas are slow-growing, recurring neoplasms that incapacitate by locally aggressive growth; less than 10% of cases demonstrate distal metastasis. They are the fifth most common primary malignancy of bone after multiple myeloma, osteosarcoma, chondrosarcoma, and Ewing's tumor. Parachordoma describes an extraaxial, soft-tissue tumor that is histologically similar to a chordoma.[114,207,214]

Chordomas may develop in men and women of all ages.[126] Sacrococcygeal chordomas occur most often in patients between the ages of 40 and 70 years, with greater male predominance in a ratio of 2:1. Sphenooccipital (clivus) lesions occur most often in patients between the ages of 30 and 60 years, with equal gender distribution.

IMAGING FINDINGS

In the sacrococcygeal region, 48% of chordomas arise, in the sphenoocciput 39%, and in the mobile spine less than 13%.[18] Rarely chordomas have been noted in the mandible, maxilla, and scapula. Chordomas are twice as common in the cervical spine as the other mobile spinal regions; the C2 vertebral body is the most common site.

Chordomas are midline lesions, characterized by the presence of bone destruction and a large soft-tissue mass (Figs. 13-140 and 13-141). Calcification is noted in up to 40% of lesions on plain films. Although most of the calcification is probably dystrophic tissue calcification, undoubtedly some also represent bony debris. Contrary to other neoplasms, chordomas may cross the intervertebral disc to involve adjacent segments. Vertebral lesions produce masses that expand anteriorly and posteriorly, compressing the dural sac. MRI reveals the lobulated composition of the lesion, with signal enhancement on the T2-weighted image.

CLINICAL COMMENTS

Regardless of the location, lesions may produce local pain and soft-tissue mass. Sphenooccipital chordomas may have accompanying headaches, sinus pain, and symptoms related to the eyes (diplopia is characteristic), ears, or throat.[86,169] Bowel and bladder dysfunction may accompany sacrococcygeal lesions.[1] Radiation is applied to those lesions that cannot be resected.[21,238]

KEY CONCEPTS

- *Chordomas are tumors histologically derived from the notochord.*
- *Approximately 48% of chordomas appear in the sacrococcygeal region, 39% in the sphenooccipital region, and 13% in the mobile spine (usually the C2 body).*
- *Most lesions occur in patients 30 to 70 years old.*

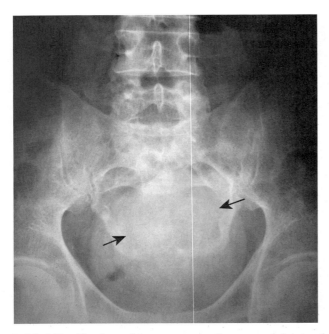

FIG. 13-140   Chordoma of the sacrum, presenting as a central destructive osteolytic lesion (*arrows*). (Courtesy Steven P. Brownstein, MD, Springfield, NJ.)

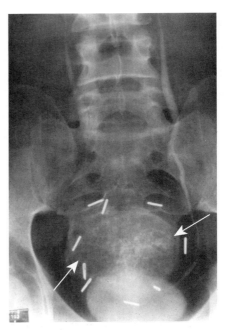

FIG. 13-141   Sacrococcygeal chordoma appearing as a midline osteolytic lesion with dystrophic calcification within the matrix (*arrows*). Surgical vascular clips and contrast from intravenous pyelogram are noted incidentally. (Courtesy Joseph W. Howe, Sylmar, CA.)

■ Miscellaneous or Unknown Origin

Benign

Aneurysmal Bone Cyst

BACKGROUND

An aneurysmal bone cyst (ABC) is a solitary, expansile, benign osteolytic lesion (Figs. 13-142 to 13-151), usually in the metaphysis of long bones. The tumor represents blood-filled spaces that are separated by fibrous tissue containing multinucleated giant cells. Its name is a misnomer; it is neither an aneurysm nor a cyst. Instead it gets its name for the markedly expansile appearance on radiographs, not for the constituents of the lesion. ABCs may appear as de novo primary lesions of bone in which no other concurrent lesion is present. Alternatively, ABCs may develop in areas of past trauma or concurrent to other tumors, a presentation called secondary ABCs. Secondary lesions account for about 30% of all cases. Most commonly, secondary ABCs are found concurrent to giant cell tumors, although fibrous dysplasia, osteoblastoma, angioma, chondroblastoma, chondromyxoid fibroma, solitary bone cyst, and osteosarcoma also are seen. Approximately 80% of patients with an ABC are younger than 20 years old.[132,210] There is no gender predilection.

IMAGING FINDINGS

The radiographic appearance is characterized by an eccentric location with cortical thinning producing a blown-out or "ballooned" contour of the host bone, geographic bone destruction with well-defined edges, and absence of periosteal reaction, visible matrix, or floating debris ("fallen fragment sign").[88,210] They appear as "bone blisters" defined by a "soap bubble" saccular protrusion of cortex filled with extravasated blood. Cortical thickening (or buttressing) is often seen at the site where the lesion expands out of the bone. ABCs range in size from 2 to 25 cm.

At times the cortical expansion may appear very thin (see Fig. 13-149) and mimic an aggressive periosteal change suggestive of a primary malignant tumor. The blown-out features usually are more pronounced in long bones. ABCs most often are eccentric in the metaphysis of long bones.[132] The spine accounts for 10% to 30% of lesions, typically found in the posterior osseous elements (see Figs. 13-142, 13-143, 13-145, 13-147, and 13-148). The pelvis accounts for half of all flat bone lesions.[132]

On MRI, ABCs appear lobulated and multiseptated with fluid levels and blood products. Fluid levels result from settling of degraded blood products within the cysts. As is generally the case with MRI scans, the fluid levels show the dependent layer with higher signal intensity than the supernatant on the T1-weighted image. Fluid levels also are seen on MRI scans of giant cell tumors and chondroblastomas. The thin, expanded, well-defined hypointense margin on T1- and T2-weighted images of the ABC may aid in differentiation.

CLINICAL COMMENTS

Most patients complain of pain, swelling, and tenderness of less than 6 months' duration.[132] Their complaint is related to the lesion itself or an associated pathologic fracture. The lesion's expansile nature may lead to stenosis of the vertebral canal or intervertebral

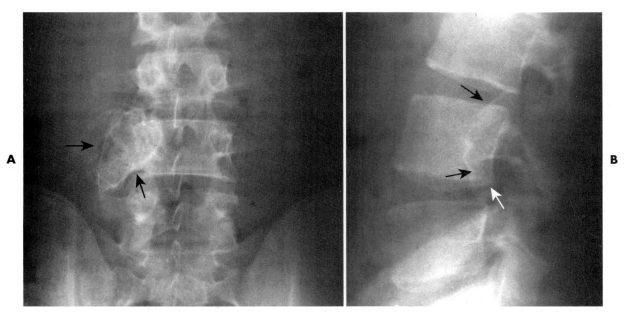

FIG. 13-142 **A** and **B,** Aneurysmal bone cyst of the transverse process of the lumbar spine *(arrows).* Expanding lesions of the neural arch are most commonly due to aneurysmal bone cysts and osteoblastomas. (Courtesy William E. Litterer, Elizabeth, NJ.)

foramen.[98] Intralesional excision with adjunctive cryosurgery is an effective method for the treatment of ABCs.[156]

KEY CONCEPTS
- *Aneurysmal bone cysts (ABCs) occur as primary or secondary (e.g., preexisting giant cell tumor) lesions.*
- *ABCs are solitary, grossly expansile, classically eccentric lesions of the metaphysis of long bones.*
- *Patients usually are younger than 20 years of age.*

Giant Cell Tumor

BACKGROUND
A giant cell tumor (GCT) is an osteolytic tumor believed to originate from undifferentiated cells within the supporting tissues of bone marrow. It is composed mostly of large mononuclear stromal cells and fewer osteoclastic-like multinucleated giant cells.[223] As a gross specimen, the tumor appears as a brown mass with dark red areas of hemorrhage.

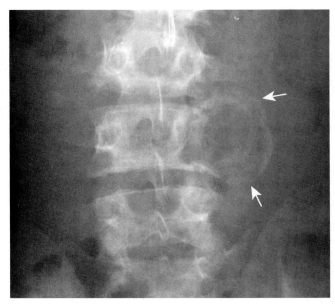

FIG. 13-143 Aneurysmal bone cyst presenting as an expansile lesion of the patient's left transverse process *(arrows).* (Courtesy Ian McLean, Davenport, IA.)

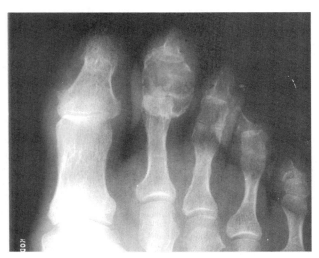

FIG. 13-144 Aneurysmal bone cyst presenting as an expanding lesion of the middle phalanx, second digit of the right foot.

PART TWO Bone, Joints, and Soft Tissues

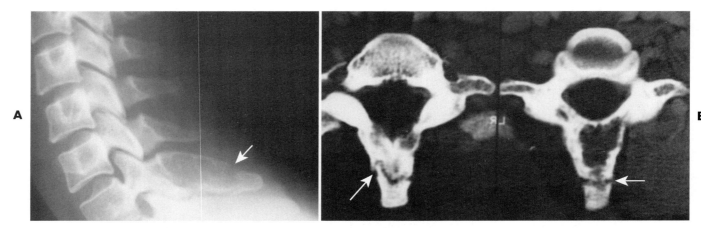

FIG. 13-145   **A,** Plain film cervical projection revealing cystic enlargement of the C7 spinous process with fracture through its distal portion *(arrow).* **B,** Computed tomogram confirming the expanded cortex consistent with aneurysmal bone cyst *(arrows).*

Approximately 18% of benign bone tumors are GCTs. Uncommonly, GCTs are associated with Paget's disease[17,187] and aneurysmal bone cysts.[158] About 5% to 10% of GCTs are malignant.[5,68] Most malignant lesions represent conventional GCTs, which transform into fibrosarcoma, or less commonly osteosarcoma, after irradiation. Few GCTs are malignant from their onset. Unlike most osseous neoplasms, GCTs demonstrate a slight female predominance.[93,159,176] GCT is rare among the skeletally immature or the elderly.[93,205] Most lesions occur in patients between the ages of 20 and 40 years. A racial predisposition has been reported, more common among the Chinese.[226]

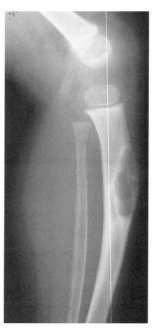

FIG. 13-146   Aneurysmal bone cyst appearing as an expanded cystic lesion of the anterior margin of the tibial diaphysis. Note the eccentric location. (Courtesy Steven P. Brownstein, MD, Springfield, NJ.)

A tumor with a similar name, giant cell reparative granuloma, occurs mostly within the craniofacial bones or small bones of the hands and feet, probably as a result of intraosseous hemorrhage occurring alone or secondary to fibrous dysplasia, hyperparathyroid bone disease, and Paget's disease.[54,56] Microscopically a giant cell reparative granuloma is nearly indistinguishable from an aneurysmal bone cyst.

IMAGING FINDINGS

Although controversial in the past, it is now generally accepted that GCTs arise within the metaphysis.[131,242] As they enlarge, 84% to 98% extend to within 1 cm of the subarticular cortex.[109,160] They appear as epiphyseal or epiphyseal-equivalent lesions in skeletally mature patients (Figs. 13-152 to 13-158). Their appearance in the metaphysis is limited to the skeletally immature and is exceptionally rare. Almost half of all GCTs are found around the knee in either the distal femur or proximal tibia (see Figs. 13-152 and 13-156).[140] In decreasing order of frequency, some other sites include distal radius (see Figs. 13-154, 13-155, and 13-157), proximal femur, distal tibia, sacrum, distal ulna, proximal fibula, and pelvis. Spinal sites above the sacrum are rare. Involvement of the short bones of the hands and feet is uncommon.

The classic radiographic description of a GCT includes an eccentric osteolytic lesion with a narrow zone of transition and without surrounding sclerosis that arises in the metaphysis and extends to the epiphyseal subarticular cortex, usually around the knee in young adults. Most lesions do not have internal septation, but occasionally lesions appear with a marked "soap bubble" appearance, especially when found in a weight-bearing location.

A minority of lesions appear locally aggressive on radiographs. These malignant lesions are suggested by the presence of cortical breakthrough and soft-tissue mass (see Figs. 13-154 and 13-155). However, radiographic features of aggressiveness do not directly correlate to histologic features of aggressiveness.

Lesions appear with mixed signal, and as a multicompartmental cystic mass, often containing blood degradation products. A hypointensive rim around the lesion on the T2-weighted image suggests a benign lesion.[6]

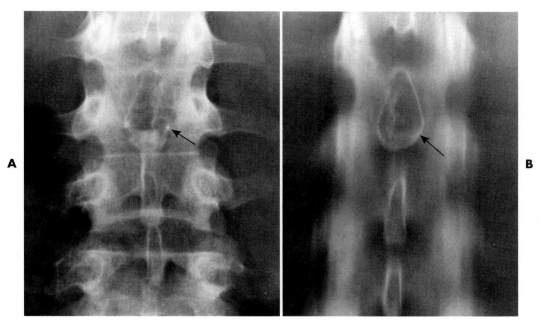

FIG. 13-147 A, Plain film and, **B,** linear tomogram of an aneurysmal bone cyst of the L3 spinous process *(arrows).*

CLINICAL COMMENTS

Patients complain of pain, limited range of motion, swelling, and tenderness. Treatment for GCT usually involves marginal or wide resection. Marginal resection is associated with a high rate of recurrence (25% to 35%),[66] whereas wide resection typically compromises the function of the affected limb. Conventional treatment involves curettage and bone grafting (Fig. 13-152). Wide resection is indicated for recurrent or malignant lesions.[66] Pulmonary metastases occurs in 1% to 2% of patients with GCT. Individual pulmonary nodules are slow growing and usually respond well to surgical excision.

> ### KEY CONCEPTS
> - *Giant cell tumor (GCT) appears as an osteolytic, nonmarginated, eccentric lesion, located in the epiphysis or metaphysis with subarticular extension.*
> - *GCT occurs in patients 20 to 40 years of age and is occasionally malignant, suggested by a painful soft-tissue mass.*
> - *Lesions are managed with curettage and bone grafting.*

Simple Bone Cyst

BACKGROUND

A simple (solitary or unicameral) bone cyst is a common, nonneoplastic, osteolytic, fluid-filled bone lesion of uncertain etiology (Figs. 13-159 to 13-169). Its development may be related to a local disturbance of venous drainage, leading to increased intraosseous pressure, bone resorption, and replacement with intracellular fluid.[38,237] Cysts have been classified as active (demonstrating continued growth) when they abut the epiphyseal plate (see Fig. 13-160), or inactive (latent) when they are separated from the plate by a length of normal cancellous bone (see Fig. 13-159). However, even cysts separated from the plate can continue to grow.[186] Growth is probably more related to the patient's age than to location within the bone.

The majority of cases are discovered in patients before the age of 20 years, with an average age of 9 years.[24] Males are more commonly affected than females at a ratio of 3:1. Lesions in the ilium and calcaneus (see Figs. 13-168 and 13-169) occur in a slightly older patient population than do lesions in long bones.

IMAGING FINDINGS

Ninety percent of simple bone cysts are found in the proximal humerus and femur, with nearly a 2:1 ratio of the former to the latter. The ilium and calcaneus[218] are involved, usually in a slightly older patient population.

Simple cysts appear as mildly expansile, well-marginated, geographic osteolytic lesions in the metaphysis, less frequently the diaphysis, or rarely the epiphysis. The cortex is thinned but remains intact.[149] The cyst's long axis parallels that of the host bone. A "fallen fragment" sign describes the appearance of bony fragments in the gravity-dependent portion of a fractured cyst and is present in up to 20% of all simple cysts.[224] A similar phenomenon occurring with an incomplete fracture is termed a "trap door" sign. A fragment may appear to float within the cyst as a "lily pad" sign. The interior of the cyst often has ridges that may anchor true fibrous septations; therefore use of the term *unicameral* (meaning monolocular, or one chamber) to describe simple bone cysts should be discouraged.

CLINICAL COMMENTS

Two thirds of patients seek clinical attention because of a pathologic fracture of the cyst.[2] Clinical signs and symptoms in those patients without fracture are uncommon, usually consisting of pain, swelling, and stiffness in adjacent joints.[172]

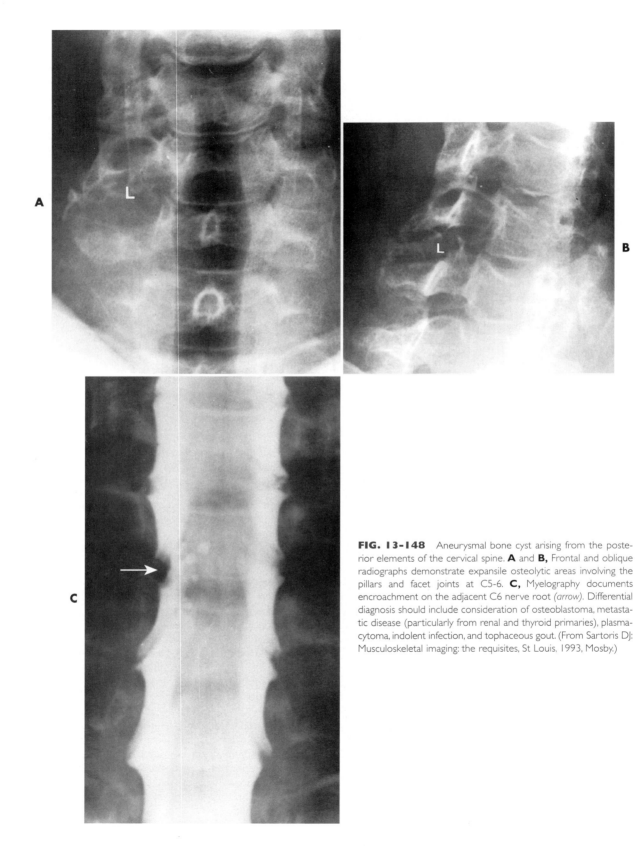

FIG. 13-148 Aneurysmal bone cyst arising from the posterior elements of the cervical spine. **A** and **B,** Frontal and oblique radiographs demonstrate expansile osteolytic areas involving the pillars and facet joints at C5-6. **C,** Myelography documents encroachment on the adjacent C6 nerve root *(arrow)*. Differential diagnosis should include consideration of osteoblastoma, metastatic disease (particularly from renal and thyroid primaries), plasmacytoma, indolent infection, and tophaceous gout. (From Sartoris DJ: Musculoskeletal imaging: the requisites, St Louis, 1993, Mosby.)

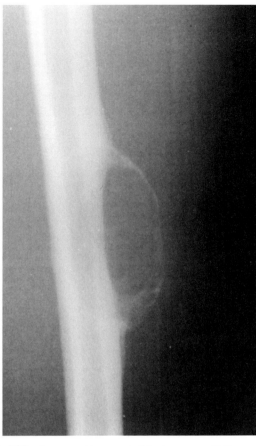

FIG. 13-149 Aneurysmal bone cyst of the humerus exhibiting an expanded and a thin cortex. The appearance has been likened to a bone blister, or the work of a glassblower. (Courtesy Joseph W. Howe, Sylmar, CA.)

Simple cysts in tubular bones often require treatment to prevent recurring pathologic fractures and possible deformity. Treatment includes curettage and grafting, excision, saucerization, and more recently, percutaneous steroid injection.[92,172,179] Recurrence rates after curettage are around 18% to 20%.[9,24]

KEY CONCEPTS

- *Simple bone cysts are common benign tumors, 90% of which are found in the proximal humerus and femur.*
- *Patients usually are younger than 20 years of age at the time of diagnosis.*
- *Lesions appear as central geographic lesions in the metaphysis, migrating to the diaphysis over time.*

Epidermoid Cyst

Epidermoid cysts are squamous cell–lined interosseous lesions. Many of the lesions are believed to be the result of an interosseous displacement of epithelial tissue as the result of puncture trauma, known as inclusion cysts. Epidermoid cysts are most commonly seen in the acral skeleton, primarily the distal aspects of the phalanges.[144] They typically occur in adults and appear as well-defined, small cysts, occasionally with slight expansion.

Developmental epidermoid cysts occur in the skull of young children as osteolytic lesions. Dermoid cysts are similar to epidermoid cysts, except the former includes dermal components, such as hair follicles, and are most common to the sacrum. Also, dermoid cysts are midline and epidermoid cysts are parasagittal or peripheral.

Interosseous Ganglion Cyst

Interosseous ganglion cysts are nonneoplastic mucoid-filled cysts of bone that are identical to their soft-tissue counterparts. It likely represents a degenerative process, with some similarity to the

FIG. 13-150 A, Aneurysmal bone cyst of the femur. Notice the scalloped bone defect along the internal margin of the femur. On this image the outer cortex of the femur is not visible. **B,** However, on the corresponding axial magnetic resonance image (MRI) a thin cortical shell (appearing as a black signal void on this MR image) is noted around the entire margin of the tumor *(arrows)*. Often aneurysmal bone cysts may be so expansile that the outer rim is difficult to see without computed tomography (CT) or MRI. CT would better demonstrate the outer cortex.

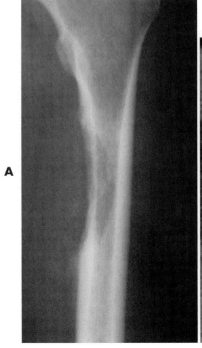

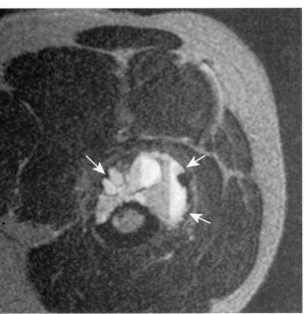

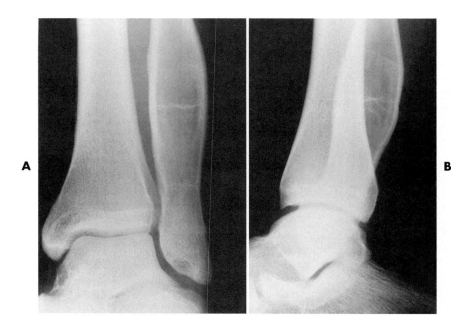

FIG. 13-151   A, Lateral and, **B,** oblique projections of the ankle demonstrating an expansile, central aneurysmal bone cyst in the distal fibula. As a central, slightly expansile lesion, this radiographic appearance appears similar to a simple bone cyst. Simple bone cysts typically present in the skeletally immature, but so do most aneurysmal bone cysts, making radiographic differentiation difficult if the presentations are similar, as they appear in this case. Although not exhibited here, aneurysmal bone cysts are usually eccentric. (Courtesy Jack C. Avalos, Davenport, IA.)

typical subchondral cysts seen with joint degeneration. The designation of interosseous ganglion should be applied when subchondral cysts are present without degeneration.[152] The lesion affects middle- to older-aged patients most commonly, without marked gender predisposition. Interosseous ganglion cysts most often occur in the subchondral bone adjacent to articular surfaces (Fig. 13-170). The most characteristic sites include the hip, knee, and ankle. They appear as well-delineated cysts of 1 to 2 cm in size. Most lesions are asymptomatic and are discovered incidentally. When pain syndromes are reported, they may be exacerbated by weight bearing.

Malignant

Adamantinoma

An adamantinoma (angioblastoma) is a rare, locally aggressive or malignant lesion composed of epithelium-like cells in dense fibrous stroma (Fig. 13-171).[112] Similar appearing lesions of the mandible or maxilla are known as ameloblastomas (see presentation in the following). Adamantinomas typically occur between the ages of 25 and 40 years and are slightly more common in females.[201]

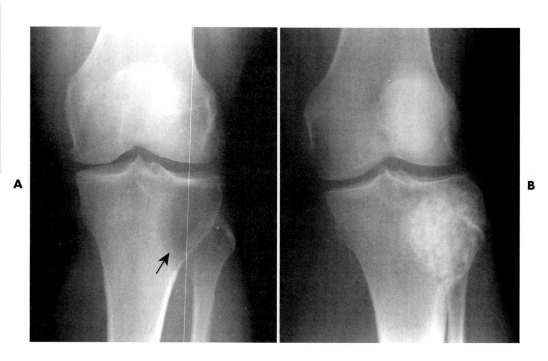

FIG. 13-152   A, Giant cell tumor presenting as a typical radiolucent, eccentric, subarticular lesion about the knee, in this case the proximal tibia *(arrow).* **B,** After curettage and bone packing, the lesion appears radiodense. (Courtesy Steven P. Brownstein, MD, Springfield, NJ.)

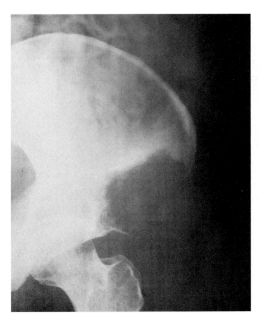

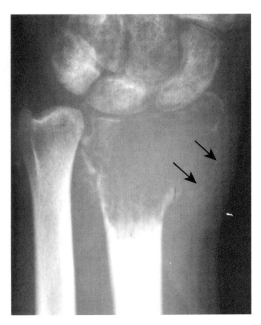

FIG. 13-153 A giant cell tumor presenting in the ilium as an aggressive lesion with cortical destruction. The lesion appears malignant. (Courtesy Steven P. Brownstein, MD, Springfield, NJ.)

FIG. 13-154 Malignant degeneration of a giant cell tumor in the distal radius. Note the cortical breakthrough and soft-tissue mass *(arrows)*. (Courtesy Steven P. Brownstein, MD, Springfield, NJ.)

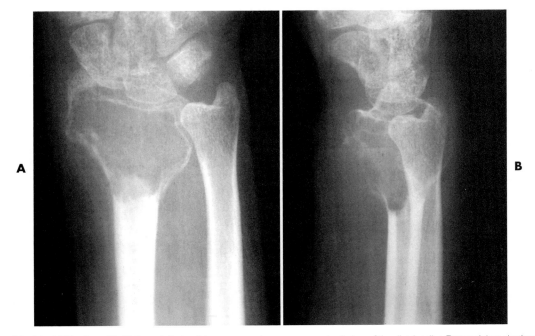

FIG. 13-155 **A** and **B,** Malignant giant cell tumor, appearing as an aggressive lesion of the distal radius. Determining whether a giant cell tumor is malignant is not definitively possible on radiographs. (Courtesy Steven P. Brownstein, MD, Springfield, NJ.)

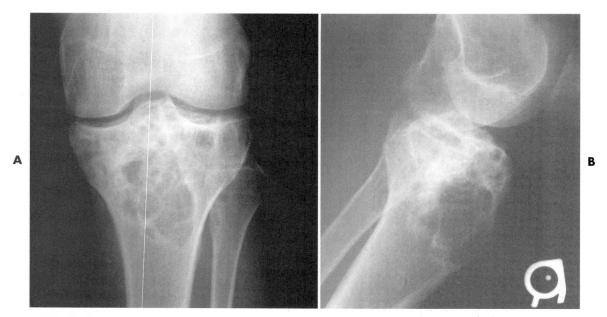

FIG. 13-156   **A** and **B,** Giant cell tumor appearing as a subarticular "soap bubble" lesion. (Courtesy Mitch Mally, Davenport, IA.)

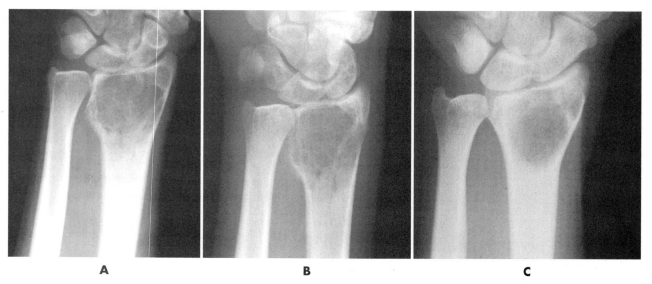

FIG. 13-157   Giant cell tumor in the distal radius. **A** through **C,** Three different patients exhibiting the common radiographic features of a subarticular, eccentric, well-defined lesion distally, poorly defined lesion proximally, and without margination. (Courtesy William E. Litterer, Elizabeth, NJ.)

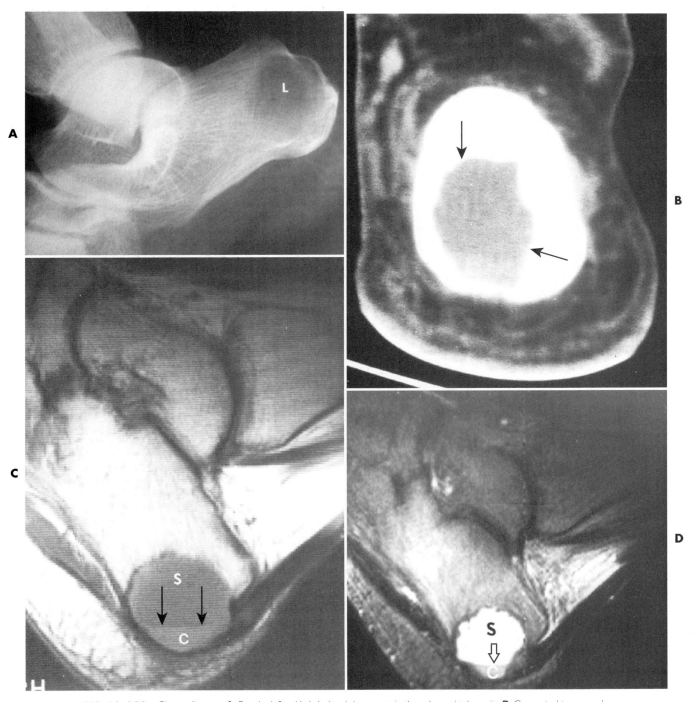

FIG. 13-158 Giant cell tumor. **A,** Poorly defined lytic lesion, *L,* is present in the calcaneal tuberosity. **B,** Computed tomography demonstrates a homogenous tissue-density process *(arrows)* without radiodense matrix. **C,** Sagittal T1-weighted magnetic resonance image reveals a fluid-fluid level *(arrows)* within the lesion, indicating a hematocrit effect (*S,* serum; *C,* cells). **D,** The finding *(arrow)* is confirmed on a sagittal T2-weighted image, in which the serum, *S,* manifests high signal intensity (*C,* cells). Fluid-fluid level indicates a blood-filled lesion, the differential diagnosis of which should include consideration of aneurysmal bone cyst, hemorrhagic metastasis, and other vascular tumors. (From Sartoris DJ: Musculoskeletal imaging: the requisites, St Louis, 1993, Mosby.)

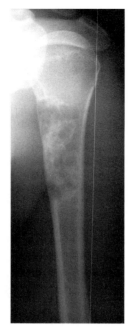

FIG. 13-159   Simple bone cyst presenting as a central lesion in the proximal humerus.

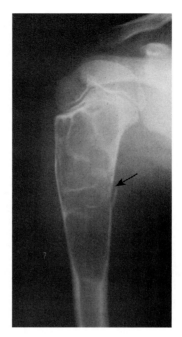

FIG. 13-160   Simple bone cyst in the proximal humerus with pathologic fracture of the thinned medial cortex *(arrow)*. (Courtesy Ian D. McLean, LeClaire, IA.)

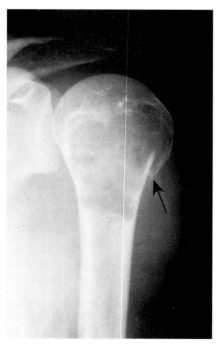

FIG. 13-161   Simple bone cyst in the proximal humerus. The thinned outer cortex of the lesion has fractured *(arrow)*. (Courtesy Steven P. Brownstein, MD, Springfield, NJ.)

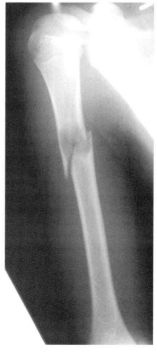

FIG. 13-162   Pathologic fracture through a central bone defect that represents a simple bone cyst. (Courtesy Steven P. Brownstein, MD, Springfield, NJ).

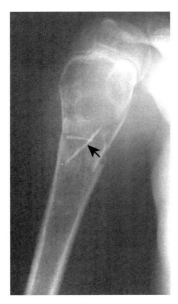

FIG. 13-163 Simple bone cyst in the proximal humerus. The lesion's internal septations are fractured, and have migrated inferiorly ("fallen fragment" sign, *arrow*). In addition, the cortex of the bone is pathologically fractured. (Courtesy Steven P. Brownstein, MD, Springfield, NJ.)

Ninety percent of lesions are found in the middle third of the tibia; less common sites include the fibula, ulna, carpals, and metacarpals. They appear as central or eccentric, slightly expansile, well-circumscribed, osteolytic lesions. Multifocal lesions are found, often as synchronous lesions of the tibia and fibula.[13]

Patients often relate a history of trauma with clinical findings of swelling, pain, and bowing deformity of the involved extremity.

A palpable mass also may be present. Lesions tend to recur after excision.

Ameloblastoma

BACKGROUND

An ameloblastoma is an extremely rare, locally aggressive, odontogenic epithelial neoplasm that histologically mimics embryonal enamel but does not form hard dental tissue. Men and women are affected equally. The average patient age is 36 years,[198] and most patients are between the ages of 30 and 50 years.

IMAGING FINDINGS

An ameloblastoma appears as a slowly growing, expansile, well-defined, radiolucent lesion occurring most commonly in the molar regions of the mandible and less commonly in the maxilla (5:1 ratio).[123,180,198] Less often ameloblastoma has a peripheral, nonosseous, mucosal location within the jaw.[8,12,181] In contrast, adamantinoma (or angioblastoma) has a similar radiographic appearance but occurs in the long bones of the skeleton, primarily the tibia.

CLINICAL COMMENTS

Lesions often are accompanied by painless swelling and a slow-growing mass in the jaw. A marked tendency exists for lesions to reoccur if inadequately excised. Radiographic unilocular lesions are treated less aggressively than multiloculated lesions.

> **KEY CONCEPTS**
> - *Ameloblastoma is a rare, radiolucent, slightly expansile lesion of the mandible.*
> - *It is usually found in patients 30 to 50 years of age.*

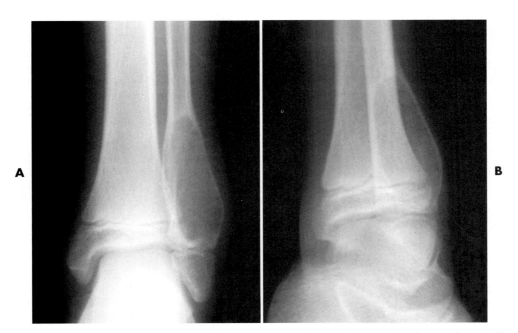

FIG. 13-164 Simple bone cyst with a characteristic appearance of a subepiphyseal, central, slightly expansile lesion. Simple bone cysts are differentiated from nonossifying fibromas, because the latter is eccentric. (Courtesy Steven P. Brownstein, MD, Springfield, NJ.)

PART TWO
Bone, Joints, and Soft Tissues

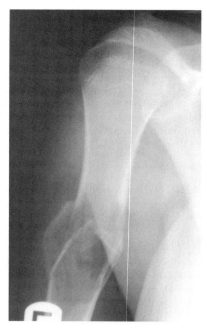

FIG. 13-165 Pathologic fracture resulting from the presence of a simple bone cyst in a 13-year-old girl who had a sudden onset of arm pain after a trivial fall.

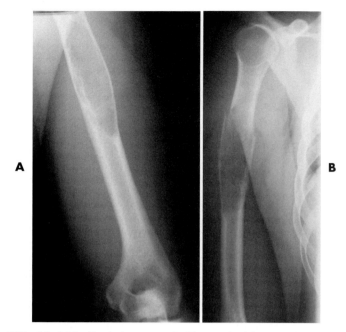

FIG. 13-166 Simple bone cyst. **A,** The proximal humerus is a typical location for a simple bone cyst. **B,** After a trivial fall, the patient suffered a pathologic fracture through the cyst. (Courtesy Gary Longmuir, Phoenix, AZ.)

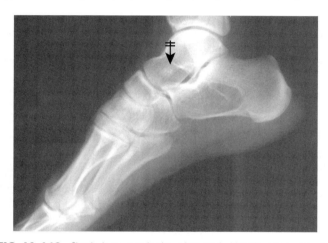

FIG. 13-168 Simple bone cyst in the calcaneus. Incidentally, a bone island is noted in the talus (crossed arrow). (Courtesy Steven P. Brownstein, MD, Springfield, NJ.)

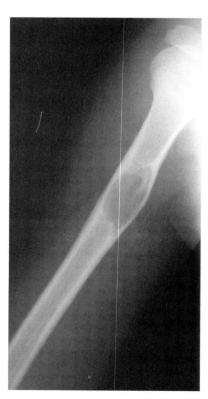

FIG. 13-167 Simple bone cyst appearing as a well-defined central lesion in the proximal humerus. (Courtesy Ian D. McLean, LeClaire, IA.)

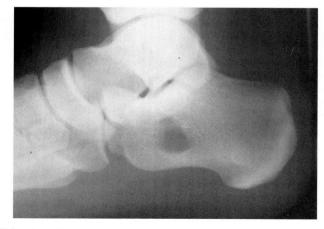

FIG. 13-169 Simple bone cyst of the calcaneus. (Courtesy Ian D. McLean, LeClaire, IA.)

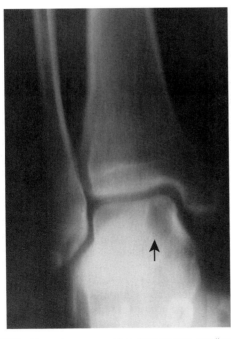

FIG. 13-170 Linear tomogram of an intraosseous ganglion of the talus (*arrow*). (Courtesy Joseph W. Howe, Sylmar, CA.)

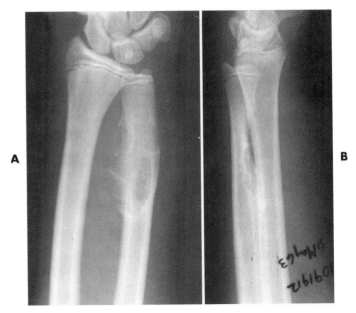

FIG. 13-171 **A** and **B,** Adamantinoma of the distal radius. (Courtesy Steven P. Brownstein, MD, Springfield, NJ.)

■ Nonneuromusculoskeletal Origin

Malignant

Metastatic Bone Disease

BACKGROUND

Dissemination. Metastatic bone disease represents osseous seeding of cells that originated from a primary malignant neoplasm. Skeletal metastases are most common from epithelial malignancies (carcinomas). Skeletal metastases from connective tissue malignancies (sarcomas) are much less common. Metastasis is the hallmark of malignancy, occurring late in the process of cancer development.

The most common mechanism of metastasis is antegrade arterial means. For metastasis to be successful, primary tumor cells must invade the extracellular tumor matrix and penetrate the arterial channels, usually through venous or lymphatic access. Continued proliferation, embolism, and extravasation from the vessel at a distal site occurs, followed by tumor cell proliferation as a first order metastasis (primary metastasis) in the new location. The first-order cells may then seed as secondary metastasis. Less commonly metastasis may occur by a retrograde venous mechanism. The most common examples of retrograde venous mechanisms are intraabdominal malignancy and increased intraabdominal pressure leading to diversion of blood flow from the systemic caval network to enter the valveless venous network of Batson connecting to the lumbar spine and seeding the vertebrae. Last, malignancies may directly extend to adjacent structures. For instance, a bronchogenic carcinoma of the lung may directly extend to the adjacent ribs, sternum, or vertebrae.

Metastasis is very common to the lungs, liver, and red marrow, traditionally explained by the rich vascularization of these structures. For instance, metastasis is common to the axial skeletal in adult patients because of the highly vascularized hemopoietic red bone marrow found in this location.[133,162] In adult patients, metastasis is less common in the extremities, containing relatively hypovascular yellow bone marrow. Moreover, skeletal metastasis is more widespread in children, commonly involving the axial and appendicular skeleton, paralleling the wider distribution of red marrow present in children.

Skeletal distribution. Ninety percent of skeletal metastasis occurs in the axial skeleton, ribs, skull, pelvis, proximal humeri, and proximal femora. Metastasis is more common in the lumbar and thoracic spine than in the cervical spine. Skeletal involvement distal to the elbows or knees, called *acral metastasis,* is unusual and when present is usually from a primary lung neoplasm.

The preferential disposition of some areas of the body to metastasis is generally explained by either specific features of the vascular architecture, traditional (mechanical model) as described above, or the affinity some malignant cells seem to exhibit toward particular antigen characteristics of selected tissues (soil and seed model).

The progression of metastasis begins with progressive displacement of the marrow elements, following the path of least resistance, gradually promoting pressure resorption of adjacent bone. In addition to direct pressure, the tumor cells stimulate host bone osteoclastic resorption through important mediators such as cytokines, interleukin-1, and interleukin-6. The elevated interosseous pressures from the resulting proliferation and resorption of bone

PART TWO Bone, Joints, and Soft Tissues

may be responsible for the bone pain experienced by the patient. Bone resorption may lead to pathologic fractures (seen in about 60% of patients with metastasis), and when advanced, elevated serum calcium levels. Pathologic fracture is less common when the metastatic deposits promote an osteoblastic response within the host bone.

Cellular origin. Skeletal metastases are much more common than primary malignant neoplasms of bone. Although deriving an accurate prevalence ratio is complicated by patient age,[87] cell type, bones involved, and other sampling factors, the overall ratio of metastatic lesions to primary bone malignancies has been reported at 25:1.[154]

Metastasis occurs in approximately 80% of patients with advanced cancer.[239] At autopsy, 70% of patients who died of carcinoma demonstrate evidence of skeletal metastasis.[117] Bone scans show abnormal uptake in up to 85% of carcinoma patients. Often the metastatic lesions are discovered before the primary lesion. For example, in one survey, less than 50% of primary lesions could be established in a group of patients with known metastasis.[216]

Not all primary malignant neoplasms have an equal propensity to metastasis to bone. Metastatic bone disease most often originates from primary lesions in the prostate, breast, kidney, thyroid, and lung. Sixty percent of metastatic bone disease in males arises from prostate neoplasms and 70% in women arises from primary neoplasms of the breast. Considering both sexes, the most common carcinoma metastasis to bone originates from the breast, prostate, lung, colon, stomach, bladder, uterus, rectum, thyroid, and kidney, in descending order. In children, metastasis is most often associated with neuroblastomas, leukemia, retinoblastoma, Ewing's tumor, osteosarcoma, and lymphoma.

Age. Although metastasis may occur at any age, the disease predominantly affects those over the age of 40 years.

Sensitivity of imaging. Diagnostic imaging is a pivotal tool in the detection, diagnosis, prognostication, and management of bone tumors. Plain film radiology is relatively insensitive to alterations of osseous density. Lesions are radiographically apparent when 30% to 50% of bone destruction is present.[36,41,71] The lack of radiographic findings early in the disease process is a reflection of the proliferating tumor's tendency to displace bone marrow as it infiltrates the bone, and the insensitivity of radiographs to exhibit early loss of bone. Only later, when more extensive osseous resorption occurs, does the bone become rarefied enough for it to be evident on plain film radiographs.

In contrast, radionuclide studies can demonstrate as little as 5% to 10% osseous change.[188] The early stages of bone resorption promote reciprocal osteoblastic activity, leading to positive findings on the bone scan. Bone scans are 50% to 80% more accurate than radiographs in detecting skeletal metastasis.[28] Although the sensitivity of radionuclide imaging is much greater during early stages of metastases, the difference in practical circumstances probably is less pronounced because most patients present with advanced disease, causing both the radionuclide imaging and plain films to be positive.[230] However, up to 40% of patients with positive bone scans have normal radiographs with early metastatic disease.[35,143]

Radionuclide imaging can demonstrate abnormal findings on average 4 months before positive findings on plain film arise.[119] Because of its sensitivity, cost-effectiveness, and ability to demonstrate the whole skeleton, a bone scan can be used to determine if skeletal metastasis exists in a patient with proven nonmusculoskeletal primary malignancy, and if metastasis is present, a bone scan can detail the extent of involvement.

Radionuclide imaging is sensitive but not specific for metastatic disease. In fact, up to 30% of solitary abnormalities detected on bone scans of patients with primary malignancy have been shown to be benign processes.[42] Often positive scans require follow-up biopsies,[40] radiographs, or other specialized imaging studies to identify the pathologic process.

In addition to their diagnostic sensitivity, a bone scan also can be used as a sign of favorable response to treatment. For instance, a "flare phenomenon" may develop, describing increased intensity and number of lesions on the bone scan over the weeks after successful therapy, which gradually decrease in uptake over the following months.

Although bone scans and plain film imaging are most popular in assessing patients for metastatic disease, CT and MRI are helpful in further delimiting the extent of involvement, especially when plain film findings are equivocal. MRI is an excellent secondary technique to bone scan when the bone scan findings are inadequate for addressing clinical questions. MRI proves sensitive and likely more specific for metastasis in certain locations of the spine than bone scans.[94] However, because of their smaller region of study and higher cost, CT and MRI are rarely the first imaging choices. CT commonly is applied to help guide the selection of biopsy samples. MRI is helpful in detailing the extent of the lesion in preparation of surgery. Whole-body MRI and 2-[fluorine 18]-fluoro-2-deoxy-D-glucose (FDG) positron emission tomography (PET) are promising techniques that demonstrate large field of view and high sensitivity. They are certain to have wider application as examination cost declines and availability broadens.

IMAGING FINDINGS

The imaging findings reflect the aggressiveness of the primary lesion. An enlarging metastatic mass of primary tumor cells elicits varying amounts of osteoclastic bone resorptive and osteoblastic bone deposition response. The location and cell type of the tumor (with varying cytokines and growth factors) dictate which of the three presentations predominates: osteolytic, osteoblastic, or mixed appearance (Figs. 13-172 to 13-200). Overall, osteolytic lesions are much more common than either osteoblastic or mixed appearances. Multiple lesions are usual; nearly 90% of metastasis patients present with multiple lesions.

Metastatic bone disease typically appears as a polyostotic moth-eaten pattern of destruction with poorly defined zones of transition surrounding the lesions. Periosteal reaction and soft-tissue masses usually are small or absent. Lesions usually begin in the medullary canal and involve the cortex secondarily. Spinal metastases may present radiographically as only an indistinct compression fracture. Metastasis has a propensity to involve the vertebrae, pelvis, and ribs. Vertebral involvement is most common in the body or pedicles. Bilateral pedicle destruction causes a "blind" vertebra (see Fig. 13-185), and unilateral destruction causes a "one-eyed" vertebra (see Fig. 13-184).

An atypical presentation of expansile, bubbly, solitary geographic lesions is associated with primary lesions of the thyroid and kidney.[64] Purely osteoblastic lesions occur most often from breast, prostate, gastrointestinal, bladder, and lung neoplasms. When involving the vertebrae, homogeneously osteoblastic metastasis is termed "ivory vertebra" (see Figs. 13-179 to 13-181). Extremities are uncommonly involved (see Fig. 13-192), especially distal to

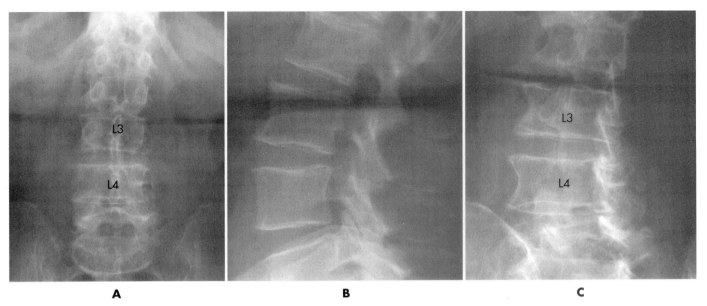

FIG. 13-172 A through **C,** Metastatic bone disease appearing with osteolytic destruction of the reading right L3 pedicle shadow and the reading left L4 pedicle shadow. **C,** L3 missing pedicle is more clearly seen on the oblique projection. (Courtesy Terence Perrault, Bridgeport, CT.)

the knees and elbows (acral metastasis). When present, lung cancer is usually the primary site of malignancy associated with metastasis of the hands and feet. Renal carcinomas also are known for their distal metastasis.

On MRI, normal bone marrow is hyperintense on T1-weighted images and hypointense on T2-weighted images. The replacement of bone marrow by the infiltrating tumor causes four abnormal appearances of the marrow, including focal lytic, focal sclerotic, diffuse homogenous, and diffuse heterogenous. Focal lytic is the

most common pattern and appears hypointense on T1-weighted images and hyperintense on T2-weighted images. Sclerotic lesions appears hypointense on both T1-weighted images and T2-weighted images. Diffuse homogeneous lesions appear hypointense on T1-weighted images, and hyperintense on T2-weighted images, and because it is diffuse, it involves multiple vertebral levels or osseous structures. The diffuse heterogenous pattern involves multiple vertebral levels or osseous structures with mixed signals on both the T1- and T2-weighted images.

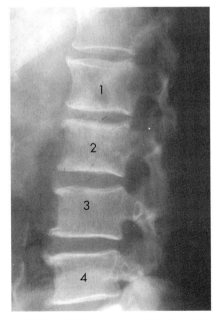

FIG. 13-173 Subtle mottled appearance of the L1 and L2 radiodensity in a patient with lumbar bone metastasis.

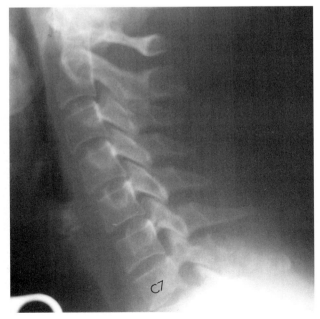

FIG. 13-174 Metastatic bone disease of the C7 spinous process. (Courtesy Gary Longmuir, Phoenix, AZ.)

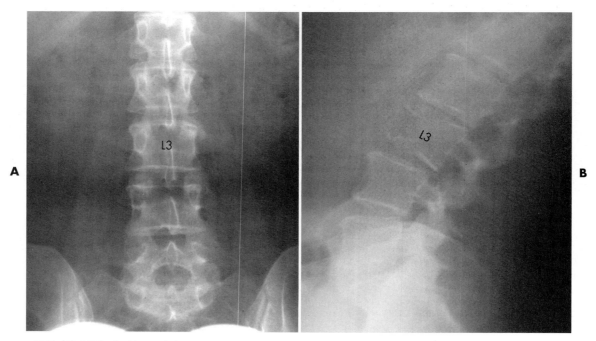

FIG. 13-175   A, Metastatic bone disease of L3 with a missing reading right pedicle shadow on the frontal projection. **B,** Vertebral body involvement seen on the lateral projection. (Courtesy Gary Longmuir, Phoenix, AZ.)

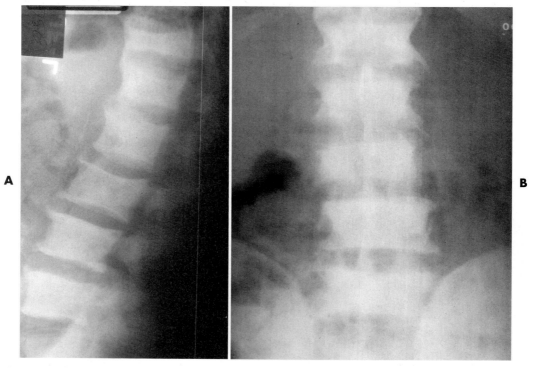

FIG. 13-176   A and **B,** Osteoblastic metastatic bone disease presenting in an 80-year-old patient with prostate cancer as a uniform increased radiodensity of the lumbar spine. (Courtesy Robin Canterbury, Davenport, IA.)

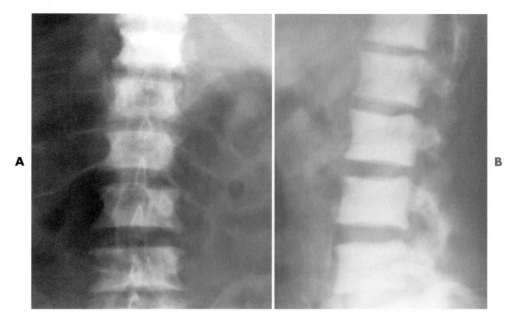

FIG. 13-177 **A** and **B,** Osteoblastic bone metastasis from a primary prostate lesion in this 73-year-old male patient. Primary malignancy of the prostate has a propensity to metastasize to the lumbar spine, and appears osteoblastic. (Courtesy Steven P. Brownstein, MD, Springfield, NJ.)

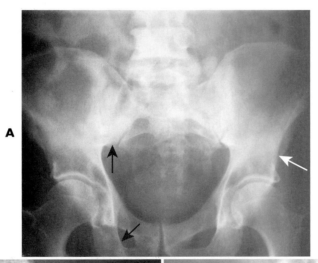

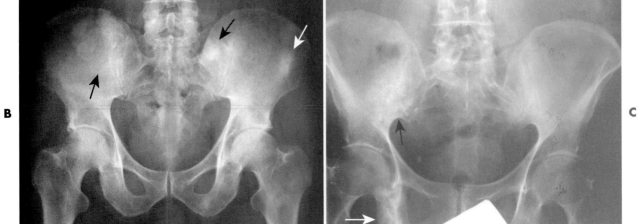

FIG. 13-178 **A** through **C,** Three cases of osteoblastic metastatic deposits involving the pelvis (arrows).

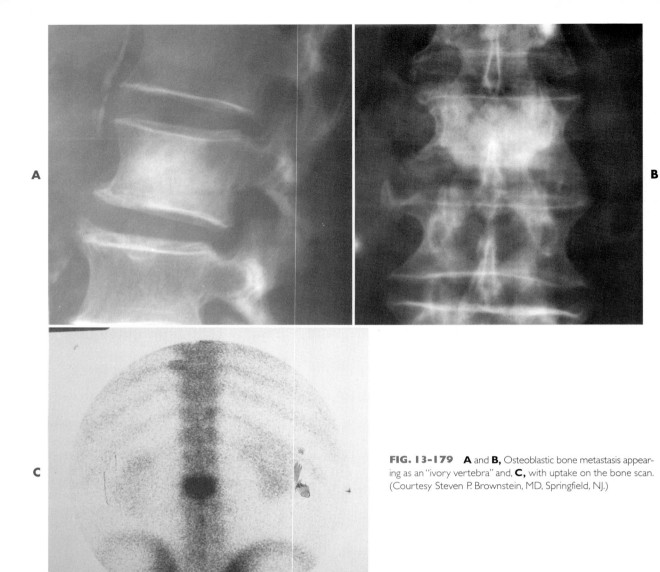

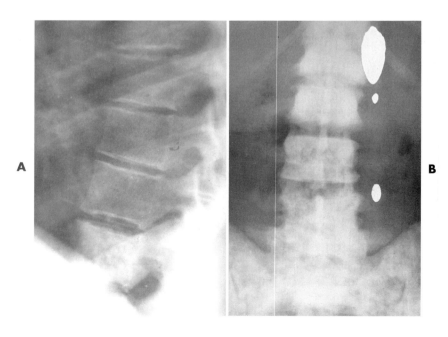

FIG. 13-179 **A** and **B,** Osteoblastic bone metastasis appearing as an "ivory vertebra" and, **C,** with uptake on the bone scan. (Courtesy Steven P. Brownstein, MD, Springfield, NJ.)

FIG. 13-180 "Ivory vertebra" manifestation of metastatic bone disease, **A,** at one level or, **B,** multiple levels as demonstrated by these two different patients. (Courtesy Steven P. Brownstein, MD, Springfield, NJ.)

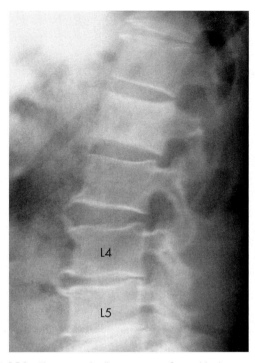

FIG. 13-181 "Ivory vertebra" appearance of osteoblastic metastatic bone disease involving L2. (Courtesy Brad Stauffer, Gretna, NE.)

CT is helpful to further delineate cortical bone involvement. On bone scintigraphy, the metastatic lesions appear as hot spots often widely scattered throughout the skeleton. In diffuse metastatic disease, the radioisotope accumulation of a bone scan may be so uniform that the pattern mimics a normal scan. This phenomenon, known as a *superscan,* is distinguished from a normal scan by a superscan's near-lack of radioisotope collection in the kidneys and bladder.

Chest radiography may reveal pulmonary abnormality in a patient in whom skeletal metastasis is suspected. The pulmonary pattern is characteristically marked by multiple nodules or masses. In addition, rib metastasis may lead to an extrapleural sign (Fig. 13-194).

CLINICAL COMMENTS

A high index of clinical suspicion for the presence of metastasis accompanies patients presenting with spinal pain who are over the age of 40, and who have a known primary malignancy. Characteristically the pain they experience is not related to trauma or appreciably affected by activity. It is commonly more severe at night, often reported to awaken the patient. Expanding osseous lesions or pathologic fractures may encroach on the spinal canal, producing neurologic signs and symptoms. Swelling, tenderness, and local pain are typical clinical findings. Anemia may present secondary to bone marrow replacement by tumor tissue.

At first, with metastases, laboratory parameters remain normal. As the disease progresses, an increased erythrocyte sedimentation rate (ESR), serum alkaline phosphatase (especially in osteoblastic lesions), and serum calcium concentration (especially in osteolytic lesions) are often found, although their absence does not exclude disease.

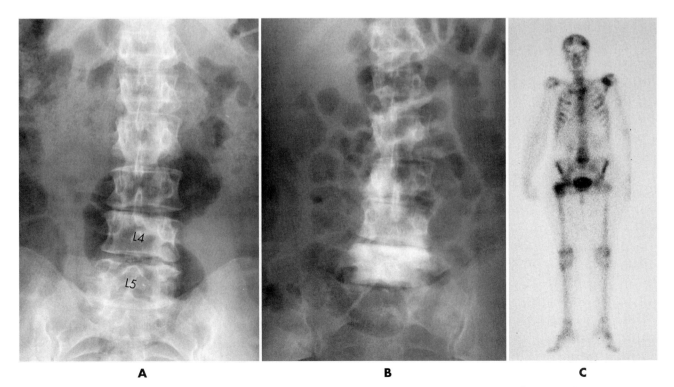

A   **B**   **C**

FIG. 13-182 **A,** Patient with breast cancer and normal-appearing anteroposterior lumbar radiograph. One year and seven months later, osteoblastic metastasis involves the lower lumbar spine on, **B,** plain film and, **C,** bone scan. The bone scan shows additional involvement in the reading left hip, right scapula, and several ribs. (Courtesy Steven P. Brownstein, MD, Springfield, NJ.)

PART TWO Bone, Joints, and Soft Tissues

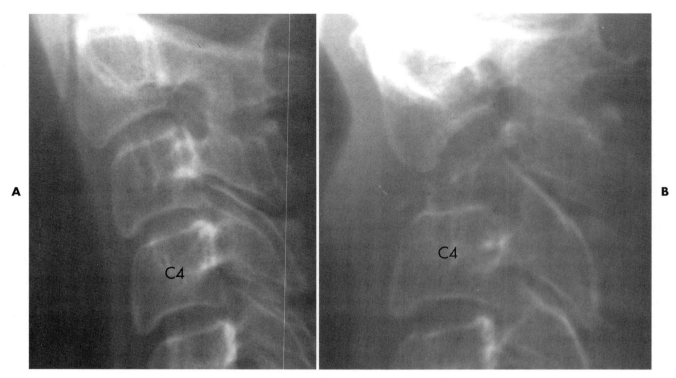

FIG. 13-183 Osteolytic metastasis to the upper cervical spine. **A,** First film appears osteopenic, but without evidence of bone destruction. **B,** Second radiograph is taken 9 months later and exhibits marked collapse of the C3 segment. (Courtesy Blair Hunt, Peoria, IL.)

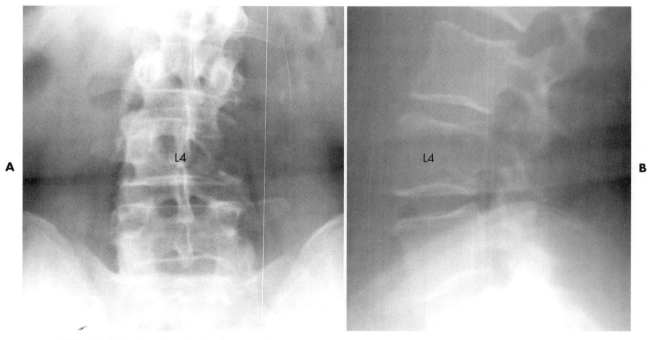

FIG. 13-184 Lumbar spine involvement with osteolytic metastasis. **A,** Frontal radiograph of this 55-year-old woman demonstrates destruction of the reading right side of the vertebral body, pedicle, and other elements of the posterior arch. **B,** Lateral radiograph appears nearly normal, with only slight reduction of the bone density of the L4 vertebral body and pedicles.

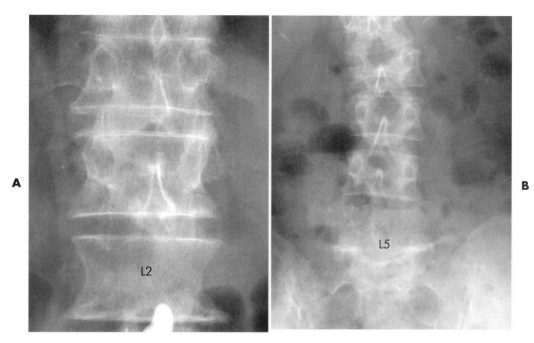

FIG. 13-185 Two cases of "blind vertebra" resulting from bilateral pedicle destruction presenting at, **A,** L2 and, **B,** L5. If the pedicles were missing on only one side, the presentation would be termed "winking owl" sign. (**A,** Courtesy Steven P. Brownstein, Springfield, NJ; **B,** Courtesy Robert C. Tatum, Davenport, IA.)

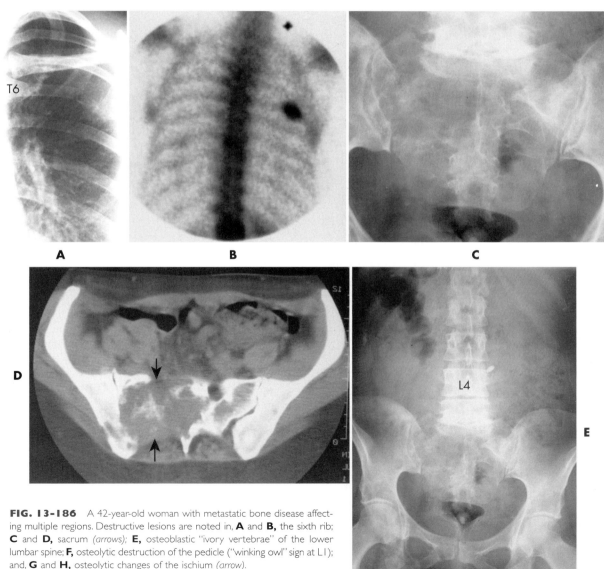

FIG. 13-186 A 42-year-old woman with metastatic bone disease affecting multiple regions. Destructive lesions are noted in, **A** and **B,** the sixth rib; **C** and **D,** sacrum *(arrows)*; **E,** osteoblastic "ivory vertebrae" of the lower lumbar spine; **F,** osteolytic destruction of the pedicle ("winking owl" sign at L1); and, **G** and **H,** osteolytic changes of the ischium *(arrow)*.

Continued

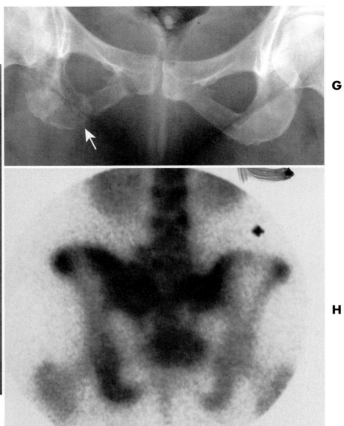

G

H

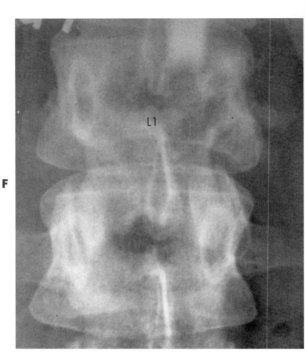

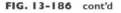

FIG. 13-186   cont'd

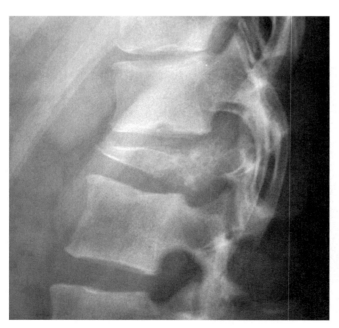

FIG. 13-187   Pathologic compression fracture secondary to osteolytic metastasis. A pathologic mechanism is suspected when the vertebra is compressed severely, as noted in this case. Metastasis, multiple myeloma, and advanced osteoporosis are the most common underlying pathologies.

Metastasis is a very grave finding, severely affecting the patient's quality of life and life expectancy. The treatment of bone metastases is often directed against the malignancy and may include systemic approaches with chemotherapy or hormonal therapy. Treatment also is directed at alleviating the patient's pain and includes radiotherapy,[127] corticosteroids, and decompressive laminectomy.[57] Also, bisphosphonate therapy can help to strengthen diseased bones to prevent fractures.

KEY CONCEPTS

- *Skeletal metastasis is approximately 25 times as common as primary malignant tumors of bone.*
- *The most common mechanism is hematogenous seeding from primary tumors; the breast gives rise to 70% of female lesions, the prostate to 60% of male lesions.*
- *Skeletal metastasis has a predilection for the axial skeleton and is rarely found distal to elbows or knees.*
- *Patients typically are older than 40 years of age.*
- *Lesions appear as areas of osteolytic destruction with no or small soft-tissue mass and periosteal reaction.*
- *Bone metastasis is clinically associated with pain, fractures, and anemia.*
- *Bone metastasis is typically incurable, representing an advanced disease state.*

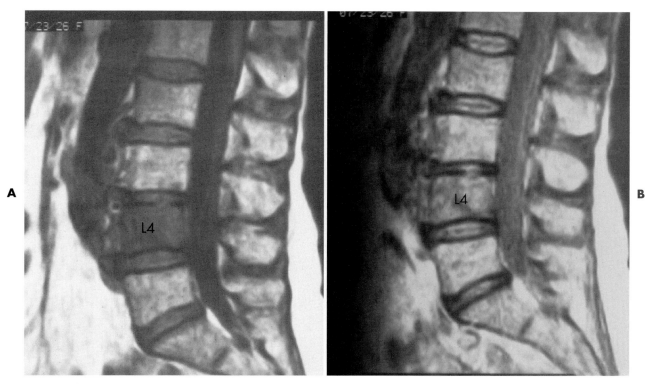

FIG. 13-188 Metastatic bone disease. **A,** T1-weighted (TR 600, TE 25) sagittal magnetic resonance image demonstrating hypointense signal from the L4 vertebral body secondary to tumor replacement of the normally bright bone marrow *(arrow)*. **B,** On the proton density (TR 2260, TE 30) sagittal magnetic resonance image, the L4 vertebra demonstrates a bright signal intensity, indicating the presence of a water-based pathology representing the tumor.

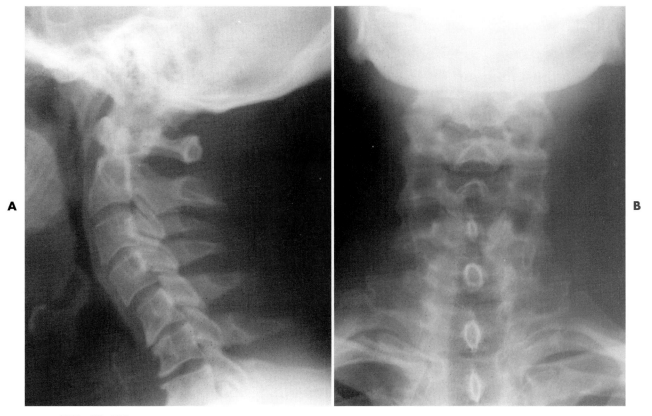

FIG. 13-189 Osteoblastic metastasis in a 63-year-old man. **A** and **B,** Initial lateral and frontal cervical projections demonstrate only kyphosis and spondylosis; the bone density is normal.

Continued

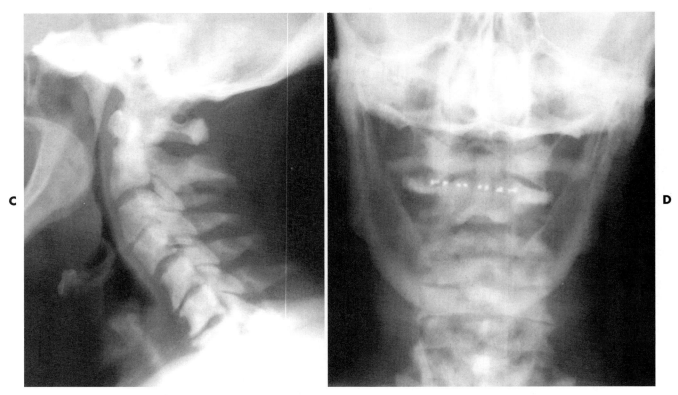

FIG. 13-189 cont'd   C and **D,** Approximately 3 years later, the same projections present a generalized increase in the bone density consistent with diffuse metastasis. (Courtesy Steven P. Brownstein, MD, Springfield, NJ.)

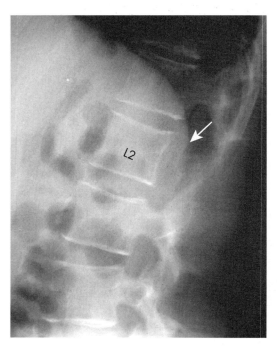

FIG. 13-190   Metastatic bone disease. Lateral lumbar radiograph of a 54-year-old woman demonstrating missing pedicles at the L2 level *(arrow).*

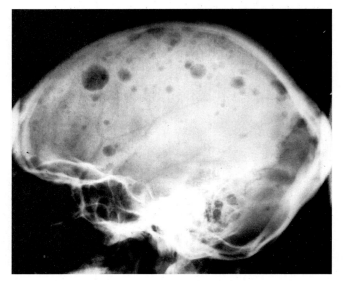

FIG. 13-191   Metastatic bone disease of the skull. Destructive defects of the skull are seen with many diseases. Typically very small permeative lesions are due to hyperparathyroidism ("salt and pepper" skull). Small "punched-out," uniform moth-eaten destruction is seen with multiple myeloma ("raindrop" skull). Metastasis causes nonuniform patterns of destruction with some small and some bigger lesions. Lastly, a larger radiolucent lesion of skull destruction is seen with Paget's disease ("osteoporosis circumscripta").

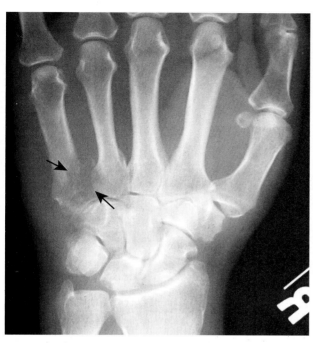

FIG. 13-192 Acral metastasis. The distal extremities, seen here in the hand *(arrows)*, are uncommon sites for metastatic bone disease. (Courtesy Steven P. Brownstein, MD, Springfield, NJ.)

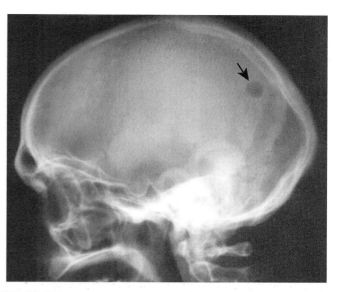

FIG. 13-193 Small singular defect of osteolytic bone metastasis to the skull *(arrow)*.

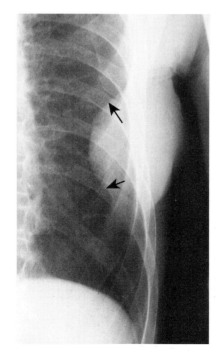

FIG. 13-194 Inward soft-tissue mass of the chest wall secondary to rib metastasis *(arrows)*. (Courtesy Steven P. Brownstein, MD, Springfield, NJ.)

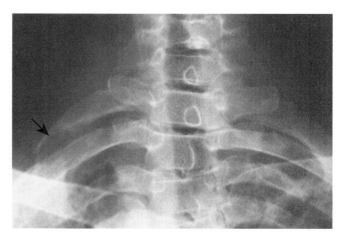

FIG. 13-195 Destruction and pathologic fracture of the first rib on the reading left *(arrow)* occurring secondary to bone metastasis. (Courtesy Steven P. Brownstein, MD, Springfield, NJ.)

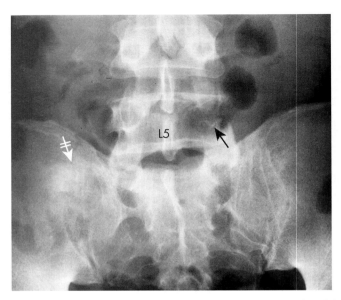

FIG. 13-196 Mixed presentation of osteolytic metastasis to the L5 pedicle ("winking owl" sign, *arrow*) and osteoblastic deposit in the ilium *(crossed arrow)*. (Courtesy Steven P. Brownstein, MD, Springfield, NJ.)

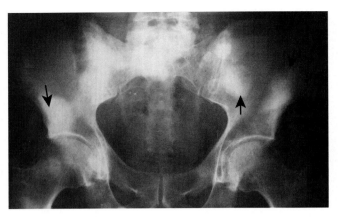

FIG. 13-197 Well-defined osteoblastic metastasis occurring throughout the pelvis *(arrows)*. (Courtesy Joseph W. Howe, Sylmar, CA.)

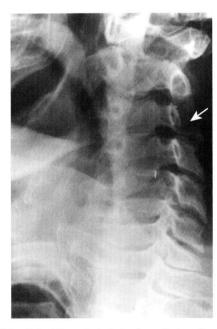

FIG. 13-199 Osteolytic metastasis to the articular pillar of C3 *(arrow)*. (Courtesy Joseph W. Howe, Sylmar, CA.)

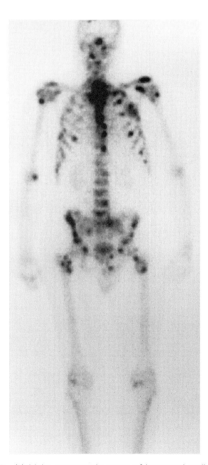

FIG. 13-198 Multiple, asymmetric areas of increased radionuclide uptake ("hot spots") widely distributed throughout the spine, ribs, skull, and pelvis. (Courtesy Ian D. McLean, LeClaire, IA.)

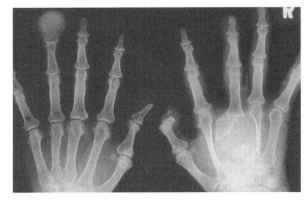

FIG. 13-200 Bone metastasis manifesting as an expansile destructive lesion of the third metacarpal of the right hand and distal phalanx of the fourth digit, left hand.

References

1. Aguilar JL et al: Difficult management of pain following sacro-coccygeal chordoma: 13 months of subarachnoid infusion, *Pain* 59:317, 1994.

2. Ahn JI, Park JS: Pathological fractures secondary to unicameral bone cysts, *Int Orthop* 18:20, 1994.

3. Albregts AE, Rapini RP: Malignancy in Maffucci's syndrome, *Dermatol Clin* 13:73, 1995.

4. Albright F et al: Syndrome characterized by osteitis fibrosa disseminata, areas of pigmentation and endocrine dysfunction, with precocious puberty in females, *N Engl J Med* 216:727, 1937.

5. Amble FR et al: Head and neck synovial cell sarcoma, *Otolaryngol Head Neck Surg* 107:631, 1992.

6. Aoki J et al: Giant cell tumors of bone containing large amounts of hemosiderin; MR pathologic correlation, *J Comput Assist Tomogr* 15:1024, 1991.

7. Arata MA, Peterson HA, Dahlin DC: Pathological fractures through nonossifying fibromas, *J Bone Joint Surg* 63A:980, 1981.

8. Baden E, Doyle JL, Petriella V: Malignant transformation of peripheral ameloblastoma, *J Oral Pathol Med* 75:214, 1993.

9. Baker DM: Benign unicameral bone cyst, *Clin Orthop* 71:140, 1970.

10. Bardwil JM et al: Angiosarcoma of the head and neck region, *Am J Surg* 116:548, 1968.

11. Bataille R, Chappard D, Klein B: Mechanisms of bone lesions in multiple myeloma, *Hematol Oncol Clin North Am* 6:285, 1992.

12. Batsakis JG, Hicks MJ, Flaitz CM: Peripheral epithelial odontogenic tumors, *Ann Otol Rhinol Laryngol* 102:322, 1993.

13. Benevenia J et al: Imaging rounds. Multifocal adamantinoma of the tibia and fibula, *Orthop Rev* 21:996, 1992.

14. Bennett MH et al: Classification of non-Hodgkin's lymphomas, *Lancet* 2:405, 1974.

15. Bertoni F et al: Primary central (medullary) fibrosarcoma of bone, *Semin Diagn Pathol* 1:185, 1984.

16. Bessler W, Grauer W, Allemann J: Case report 726. Enchondromatosis of the left femur and hemipelvis (Ollier's disease), *Skeletal Radiol* 21:201, 1992.

17. Bhambhani M et al: Giant cell tumors in mandible and spine: a rare complication of Paget's disease of bone, *Ann Rheum Dis* 51:1335, 1992.

18. Bjornsson J et al: Chordoma of the mobile spine, a clinicopathologic analysis of 40 patients, *Cancer* 71:735, 1993.

19. Blank N, Lieber A: The significance of growing bone islands, *Radiology* 85:508, 1965.

20. Bloem JL, Kroon HM: Osseous lesions, *Radiol Clin North Am* 31:261, 1993.

21. Bohm B et al: Our approach to the management of congenital presacral tumors in adults, *Int J Colorectal Dis* 8:134, 1993.

22. Borges AM, Huvos AG, Smith J: Bursa formation and synovial chondrometaplasia associated with osteochondromas, *Am J Clin Pathol* 75:648, 1981.

23. Boriani S et al: Periosteal chondroma. A review of twenty cases, *J Bone Joint Surg* 65A:205, 1983.

24. Boseker EH, Bickel WH, Dahlin DC: A clinicopathological study of simple unicameral bone cysts, *Surg Gynecol Obstet* 127:550, 1968.

25. Braunstein EM, White SJ: Non-Hodgkin lymphoma of bone, *Radiology* 135:59, 1980.

26. Brenner RJ, Hattner RS, Lilien DL: Scintigraphic features of nonosteogenic fibroma, *Radiology* 131:727, 1979.

27. Brien EW, Mirra JM, Ippolito V: Chondroblastoma arising from a nonepiphyseal site, *Skeletal Radiol* 24:220, 1995.

28. Brown ML: Bone scintigraphy in benign and malignant tumors, *Radiol Clin North Am* 31:731, 1993.

29. Burkitt DP: A sarcoma involving the jaws in African children, *Br J Surg* 46:218, 1968.

30. Campanacci M, Laus M, Boriani S: Multiple nonossifying fibromata with extraskeletal anomalies: a new syndrome? *J Bone Joint Surg* 65B:627, 1983.

31. Campanacci M: Osteofibrous dysplasia of long bones: a new clinical entity, *Ital J Orthop Traumatol* 2:221, 1976.

32. Capanna R et al: Malignant fibrous histiocytoma of bone, *Cancer* 54:177, 1984.

33. Carrillo R, Rodriguez-Peralto JL, Batsakis JG: Synovial sarcomas of the head and neck, *Ann Otol Rhinol Laryngol* 101:367, 1992.

34. Carson CP, Ackerman LV, Maltby JD: Plasma cell myeloma: clinical, pathologic and roentgenologic review of 90 cases, *Am J Clin Pathol* 25:849, 1955.

35. Charkes ND, Malmud LS, Caswell T: Preoperative bone scans: use in women with early breast cancer, *JAMA* 233:516, 1975.

36. Charkes ND, Young J, Sklaroff DM: The pathologic basis of the strontium bone scan, *JAMA* 206:2482, 1968.

37. Chen KT, Hoffman KD, Hendricks EJ: Angiosarcoma following therapeutic irradiation, *Cancer* 44:2044, 1979.

38. Chigira M et al: The aetiology and treatment of simple bone cysts, *J Bone Joint Surg* 65B:633, 1983.

39. Chow LT, Lee KC: Intraosseous lipoma. A clinicopathologic study of nine cases, *Am J Surg Pathol* 16:401, 1992.

40. Collins JC et al: Percutaneous biopsy following positive bone scans, *Radiology* 132:439, 1979.

41. Copeland MM: Metastases to bone from primary tumors in other sites, *Proc Natl Cancer Conf* 6:743, 1970.

42. Corcoran RJ et al: Solitary abnormalities in bone scans of patients with extraosseous malignancies, *Radiology* 121:663, 1976.

43. Cossetto D, Nade S, Blackwell J: Malignant fibrous histiocytoma in Paget's disease of bone: a report of seven cases, *Aust NZ J Surg* 62:52, 1992.

44. Cowan WK: Malignant change and multiple metastases in Ollier's disease, *J Clin Pathol* 18:650, 1965.

45. Craver LF: Lymphosarcoma: a review of 1269 cases, *Medicine* 40:31, 1961.

46. Crim JR et al: Case report 748: chondroblastoma of the femur with an aneurysmal bone cyst, *Skeletal Radiol* 21:403, 1992.

47. Cunningham JB, Ackerman LV: Metaphyseal fibrous defects, *J Bone Joint Surg* 38A:797, 1956.

48. Czerwinski E, Skolarczyk A, Fransik W: Malignant fibrous histiocytoma in the course of chronic osteomyelitis, *Arch Orthop Trauma Surg* 111:58, 1991.

49. Dahlin DC, Coventry MB, Scanlon PW: Ewing's sarcoma: a critical analysis of 165 cases, *J Bone Joint Surg* 43A:185, 1961.

50. Dahlin DC: Bone tumors: general aspects and data on 6,221 cases, ed 3, Springfield, IL, 1978, Charles C Thomas.

51. Dahlin DC: Giant cell tumor of bone: highlights of 407 cases, *AJR Am J Roentgenol* 144:955, 1985.

52. Damron TA, Pritchard DJ: Current combined treatment of high-grade osteosarcomas, *Oncology* 9:327, 1995.

53. Davies JA et al: Positive bone scan in a bone island, *J Bone Joint Surg* 61A:943, 1979.

54. De Smet AA, Travers H, Neff JR: Case report 207: giant cell reparative granuloma of the left femur arising in polyostotic fibrous dysplasia, *Skeletal Radiol* 8:314, 1982.

55. Dehner LP: Primitive neuroectodermal tumor and Ewing's sarcoma, *Am J Surg Pathol* 17:1, 1993.

56. Desai P, Steiner GC: Ultrastructure of brown tumor of hyperparathyroidism, *Ultrastruct Pathol* 14:505, 1990.

57. Dewald RL et al: Reconstructive spinal surgery as palliation for metastatic malignancies of the spine, *Spine* 10:21, 1985.

58. Dijkhuizen T et al: Cytogenetics as a tool in the histologic subclassification of chondrosarcomas, *Cancer Genet Cytogenet* 76:100, 1994.

59. Dimopoulos MA et al: Risk of disease progression in asymptomatic multiple myeloma, *Am J Med* 94:57, 1993.

60. Dimopoulos MA et al: Solitary plasmacytoma of bone and asymptomatic multiple myeloma, *Hematol Oncol Clin North Am* 6:359, 1992.

61. Dorfman HD, Czerniak B: Bone tumors, St Louis, 1998, Mosby.

62. Dorfman HD, Czerniak B: Bone cancer, *Cancer* 75:2003, 1995.

63. Dorfman HD, Steiner GC, Jaffe HL: Vascular tumors of bone, *Hum Pathol* 2:349, 1971.

64. Dorn W, Gladden P, Ranken EA: Regression of a renal-cell metastatic osseous lesion following treatment, *J Bone Joint Surg Am* 57:869, 1975.

65. Du YK et al: Dedifferentiated chondrosarcoma arising from osteochondromatosis. A case report, *Chang Keng I Hsueh* 14:130, 1991.

66. Duncan CP, Morton KS, Arthur JS: Giant cell tumor of bone: its aggressiveness and potential for malignant change, *Can J Surg* 26:475, 1983.

67. Durie BGM, Salmon SE, Mundy GR: Relation of osteoclast activating factor production to extent of bone disease in multiple myeloma, *Br J Haematol* 47:21, 1981.

68. Eckardt J, Grogan T: Giant cell tumor of bone, *Clin Orthop* 204:45, 1986.

69. Edeiken J: Roentgen diagnosis of diseases of bone, ed 3, Baltimore, 1981, Williams & Wilkins.

70. Edel G et al: Chondroblastoma of bone. A clinical, radiological, light and immunohistochemical study, *Pathol Anat Histopathol* 421:355, 1992.

71. Edelstyn GA, Gillespie PJ, Grebbell FS: The radiological demonstration of osseous metastases: experimental observations, *Clin Radiol* 18:158, 1967.

72. Eggli KD, Quiogue T, Moser RP: Ewing's sarcoma, *Radiol Clin North Am* 31:325, 1993.

73. El-Khoury GY, Bassett GS: Symptomatic bursa transformation with osteochondromas, *AJR Am J Roentgenol* 133:895, 1979.

74. Enterline HT: Histopathology of sarcomas, *Semin Oncol* 18:133, 1981.

75. Eriksson AL, Schiller A, Mankin HJ: The management of chondrosarcoma of bone, *Clin Orthop* 153:44, 1980.

76. Evans HL, Ayala AG, Romsdahl MM: Prognostic factors in chondrosarcoma of bone. A clinicopathologic analysis with emphasis on histologic grading, *Cancer* 40:818, 1977.

77. Eversole LR, Leiden AS, Nelson K: Ossifying fibroma: a clinicopathologic study of sixty-four cases. *Oral Surg Oral Med Oral Pathol* 60:505, 1985.

78. Ewing J: Diffuse endothelioma of bone, *Proc NY Pathol Soc* 21:17, 1921.

79. Fang Z et al: Extraskeletal osteosarcoma: a clinicopathologic study of four cases, *Jap J Clin Oncol* 25:55, 1995.

80. Fauré C et al: Multiple and large nonossifying fibromas in children with neurofibromatosis, *Ann Radiol* 29:396, 1986.

81. Feldman F, Hecht HL, Johnson AD: Chondromyxoid fibroma of bone, *Radiology* 94:249, 1970.

82. Feldman F, Lattes R: Primary malignant fibrous histiocytoma (fibrous xanthoma) of bone, *Skeletal Radiol* 1:145, 1977.

83. Ferrant A et al: Detection of skeletal involvement in Hodgkin's disease: a comparison of radiography, bone scanning, and bone marrow biopsy in 38 patients, *Cancer* 35:1346, 1975.

84. Feuillan PP: McCune-Albright's syndrome, *Curr Ther Endocrinol Metab* 5:205, 1994.

85. Fornasier VL, Paley D. Leiomyosarcoma in bone: primary or secondary? A case report and review of the literature, *Skeletal Radiol* 10:147, 1983.

86. Forsyth PA et al: Intracranial chordomas: a clinicopathological and prognostic study of 51 cases, *J Neurosurg* 78:741, 1993.

87. Francis KC, Hutter RVP: Neoplasms of the spine in the aged, *Clin Orthop* 26:54, 1963.

88. Freeby JA, Reinus WR, Wilson AJ: Quantitative analysis of the plain radiographic appearance of aneurysmal bone cysts, *Invest Radiol* 30:433, 1995.

89. Freiberg RA et al: Multiple intraosseous lipomas with type IV hyperlipoproteinemia, *J Bone Joint Surg* 56A:1729, 1974.

90. Gitelis S et al: Chondrosarcoma of bone. The experience at the Istituto Ortopedico Rizzoli, *J Bone Joint Surg* 45A:1450, 1981.

91. Giudici MA, Moser RP, Kransdorf MJ: Cartilaginous bone tumors, *Radiol Clin North Am* 31:237, 1993.

92. Goel AR et al: Unicameral bone cysts: treatment with methylprednisolone acetate injections, *J Foot Ankle Surg* 33:6, 1994.

93. Goldenberg RR, Campbell CJ, Bonfiglio M: Giant cell tumor of bone. An analysis of 218 cases, *J Bone Joint Surg* 52A:619, 1970.

94. Gosfield E, Alavi A, Kneeland B: Comparison of radionuclide bone scans and magnetic resonance imaging in detecting spinal metastases, *J Nuclear Med* 34:2191, 1993.

95. Green T et al: Multiple primary cutaneous plasmacytomas, *Arch Dermatol* 128:962, 1992.

96. Greenspan A: Bone island (enostosis): current concept: a review. *Skeletal Radiol* 24:111, 1995.

97. Grufferman S, Delzell E: Epidemiology of Hodgkin's disease, *Epidemiol Rev* 6:76, 1984.

98. Gupta VK et al: Aneurysmal bone cysts of the spine, *Surg Neurol* 42:428, 1994.

99. Haag M, Adler CP: Malignant fibrous histiocytoma in association with hip replacement, *J Bone Joint Surg* 71B:701, 1989.

100. Harned RK et al: Extracolonic manifestations of the familial adenomatous polyposis syndromes, *AJR Am J Roentgenol* 156:481, 1991.

101. Harris WH, Dudley HR, Barry RV: The natural history of fibrous dysplasia, *J Bone Joint Surg* 44A:207, 1962.

102. Harris WH, Heaney RP: Skeletal renewal and metabolic bone disease, *N Engl J Med* 280:193, 1969.

103. Harsha WN: The natural history of osteocartilaginous exostoses (osteochondroma), *Am Surg* 20:65, 1954.

104. Harwood AR, Krajbich JL, Fornasier VL: Radiotherapy of chondrosarcoma of bone, *Cancer* 45:2769, 1980.

105. Hatcher CH: The pathogenesis of localized fibrous lesions in the metaphysis of long bones, *Ann Surg* 122:1016, 1945.

106. Healy JH, Ghelman B: Osteoid osteoma and osteoblastoma: current concepts and recent advances, *Clin Orthop* 204:76-85, 1986.

107. Henry A: Monostotic fibrous dysplasia, *J Bone Joint Surg* 51B:300, 1969.

108. Horowitz AL, Resnick D, Watson RC: The roentgen features of synovial sarcomas, *Clin Radiol* 24:481, 1973.

109. Hudson TM et al: Benign exostoses and exostotic chondrosarcomas: evaluation of cartilage thickness by CT, *Radiology* 152:595, 1984.

110. Hudson TM et al: Radiology of giant-cell tumors of bone: computed tomography, arthro-tomography, and scintigraphy, *Skeletal Radiol* 11:85, 1984.

111. Hudson TM, Chew FS, Manaster BJ: Scintigraphy of benign exostoses and exostotic chondrosarcoma, *AJR Am J Roentgenol* 140:581, 1983.

112. Huvos AG et al: Telangiectatic osteogenic sarcoma: a clinicopathologic study of 124 patients, *Cancer* 49:1979, 1982.

113. Huvos AG: Bone tumors: diagnosis, treatment and prognosis, ed 2, Philadelphia, 1991, WB Saunders.

114. Ishida T et al: Parachordoma: an ultrastructural and immunohistochemical study, *Pathol Anat Histopathol* 422:239, 1993.

115. Ishida T, Dorfman HD: Plasma cell myeloma in unusually young patients: a report of two cases and review of the literature, *Skeletal Radiol* 24:47, 1995.

116. Ishida T, Kikuchi F, Machinami R: Histological grading and morphometric analysis of cartilaginous tumours, *Virchows Arch* 418A:149, 1991.

117. Jaffe HL: Tumors and tumorous conditions of the bones and joints, Philadelphia, 1958, Lea & Febiger.

118. Jong B et al: Imaging and differential diagnosis of synovial sarcoma, *J Belge Radiol* 75:335, 1992.

119. Joo KG et al: Bone scintigrams: their clinical usefulness in patients with breast carcinoma, *Oncology* 36:94, 1979.

120. Jumbelic M, Feuerstein I, Dorfman HD: Solitary intraosseous lymphangioma, *J Bone Joint Surg* 66A:1479, 1984.

121. Kaplan RP et al: Maffucci's syndrome: two case reports with a literature review, *J Am Acad Dermatol* 29:894, 1993.

122. Kattapuram SV et al: Osteoid osteoma: an unusual cause of articular pain, *Radiology* 147:383, 1983.

123. Katz JO, Underbill TE: Multilocular radiolucencies, *Dent Clin North Am* 38:63, 1994.

124. Keim HA, Reina EG: Osteoid osteoma as a cause of scoliosis, *J Bone Joint Surg* 57A:159, 1975.

125. Kempson RL: Ossifying fibroma of long bones: a light and electron microscopic study, *Arch Pathol* 82:218, 1966.

126. Keneko Y et al: Chordoma in early childhood: a clinicopathological study, *Neurosurgery* 29:442, 1991.

127. Khan FR et al: Treatment by radiotherapy of spinal cord compression due to extradural metastases, *Radiology* 89:495, 1967.

128. Kim SK, Barry WF: Bone islands, *Radiology* 90:77, 1968.

129. Kneisl JS, Simon MA; Medical management compared with operative treatment for osteoid osteoma, *J Bone Joint Surg* 74A: 179, 1992.

130. Knowles DM: Neoplastic hematopathology, Baltimore, 1992, Williams & Wilkins.

131. Kransdorf MJ et al: Giant cell tumor in skeletally immature patients, *Radiology* 184:233, 1992.

132. Kransdorf MJ, Sweet DE: Aneurysmal bone cyst: concept, controversy, clinical presentation, and imaging, *AJR Am J Roentgenol* 164:573, 1995.

133. Krishnamurthy GT et al: Distribution pattern of metastatic bone disease: a need for total body skeletal image, *JAMA* 237:2504, 1977.

134. Kroon HM, Schuurmans J: Osteoblastoma: clinical and radiologic findings in 98 new cases, *Radiology* 175:783, 1990.

135. Kyle RA: Incidence of multiple myeloma in Olmsted County, Minnesota; 1978 through 1990, with a review of the trend since 1945, *J Clin Oncol* 12:1577, 1994.

136. Kyle RA: Diagnostic criteria of multiple myeloma, *Hematol Oncol Clin North* 6A:347, 1992.

137. Kyle RA: Prognostic factors in multiple myeloma, *Stem Cells* 13:56, 1995.

138. Lange RH, Lange TA, Rao BK: Correlative radiographic, scintigraphic, and histologic evaluation of exostoses, *J Bone Joint Surg* 66A:1454, 1984.

139. Laredo JD, Reizine D, Bard M: Vertebral haemangiomas: radiologic evaluation. *Radiology* 161:183, 1986.

140. Larsson SE, Lorentzon R, Boquist L: Giant-cell tumor of bone, *J Bone Joint Surg* 57A:167, 1975.

141. Lauf E et al: Intraosseous lipoma of distal fibula. Biomechanical considerations for successful treatment, *J Am Podiatry Assoc* 74:434, 1984.

142. Laus M, Vicenzi G: Hiostiocytic fibroma of bone (a study of 170 cases), *Ital J Orthop Traumatol* 5:343, 1979.

143. Lee YTN: Bone scanning in patients with early breast carcinoma. Should it be a routine staging procedure? *Cancer* 47:486, 1981.

144. Lerner MR, Southwick WO: Keratin cysts in phalangeal bones: report of an unusual case, *J Bone Joint Surg* 50A:365, 1968.

145. Li FB et al: Rarity of Ewing's sarcoma in China, *Lancet* 1:1255, 1980.

146. Liapi-Avgeri G et al: Intraosseous lipoma. A report of three cases, *Arch Anat Cytol Pathol* 42:334, 1994.

147. Lichenstein L, Bernstein D: Unusual benign and malignant chondroid tumors of bone, *Cancer* 12:1422, 1959.

148. Lichtenstein L: Polyostotic fibrous dysplasia, *Arch Surg* 36:878, 1938.

149. Lodwick GS: Juvenile unicameral bone cyst, *AJR Am J Roentgenol* 80:495, 1958.

150. Loizaga JM: What's new in Ewing's tumor? *Pathol Res Pract* 189:616, 1993.

151. Mackenzie DH: Intraosseous glomus tumor: report of two cases, *J Bone Joint Surg* 44B:648, 1962.

152. Mainzer F, Minagi H: Intraosseous ganglion: a solitary subchondral lesion of bone, *Radiology* 94:387, 1970.

153. Malloy PC, Fishman EK, Magid D: Lymphoma of bone, muscle, and skin: CT findings, *AJR Am J Roentgenol* 159:805, 1992.

154. Manaster BJ: Handbook of skeletal radiology, ed 2, St Louis, 1997, Mosby.

155. Manning JH: Symptomatic hemangioma of the spine, *Radiology* 56:58, 1951.

156. Marcove RC et al: The treatment of aneurysmal bone cyst, *Clin Orthop* 311:157, 1995.

157. Marsh BW et al: Benign osteoblastoma: range of manifestations, *J Bone Joint Surg* 57A:1, 1975.

158. Martinez V, Sissons HA: Aneurysmal bone cyst: a review of 123 cases including primary lesions and those secondary to other bone pathology, *Cancer* 61:2291, 1988.

159. McDonald DJ et al: Giant cell tumor of bone, *J Bone Joint Surg* 68A:235, 1986.

160. McInemey DP, Middlemiss JH: Giant-cell tumor of bone, *Skeletal Radiol* 2:195, 1978.

161. McLeod RA, Dahlin DC, Beabout JW: Spectrum of osteoblastoma, *AJR Am J Roentgenol* 126:321, 1976.

162. McNeil BJ: Value of bone scanning in neoplastic disease, *Semin Nucl Med* 14:277, 1984.

163. Menendez LR, Brien E, Brien WW: Synovial sarcoma. A clinicopathologic study, *Orthop Rev* 21:465, 1992.

164. Mertens WC, Bramwell V: Osteosarcoma and other tumors of bone, *Curr Opin Oncol* 7:349, 1995.

165. Milgram JW: The origins of osteochondromas and enchondromas, *Clin Orthop* 174:264, 1983

166. Miller MD, Ragsdale BD, Sweet DE: Parosteal lipomas: a new perspective, *Pathology* 24:132, 1992.

167. Miller RW: Contrasting epidemiology of childhood osteosarcoma, Ewing's tumor and rhabdomyosarcoma, *Monogr Natl Cancer Inst* 56:9, 1981.

168. Mirra JM et al: Malignant fibrous histiocytoma and osteosarcoma in association with bone infarcts. Report of four cases, two in caisson workers, *J Bone Joint Surg* 56A:932, 1974.

169. Mizerny BR, Kost KM: Chordoma of the cranial base: the McGill experience, *J Otolaryngol* 24:14, 1995.

170. Moberg E: The natural course of osteoid osteoma, *J Bone Joint Surg* 33A:166, 1951.

171. Moore TM et al: Closed biopsy of musculoskeletal lesions, *J Bone Joint Surg* 61A:375, 1979.

172. Moreau G, Letts M: Unicameral bone cyst of the calcaneus in children, *J Pediatr Orthop* 14:101, 1994.

173. Moriwaka F, Hozen H, Nakane K: Myelopathy due to osteochondroma: MR and CT studies, *J Comput Assist Tomogr* 14:128, 1990.

174. Moser RP et al: Giant cell tumor of the upper extremity, *Radiographics* 10:83, 1990.

175. Moser RP et al: Multiple skeletal fibroxanthomas: radiologic-pathologic correlation of 72 cases, *Skeletal Radiol* 16:353, 1987.

176. Moser RP: Cartilaginous tumors of the skeleton, Philadelphia, 1990, Hanley & Belfus.

177. Moulopoulos LA et al: Extraosseous multiple myeloma: imaging features, *AJR Am J Roentgenol* 161:1083, 1993.

178. Murphey MD et al: Parosteal lipoma: MR imaging characteristics, *AJR Am J Roentgenol* 162:105, 1994.

179. Mylle J, Burssens A, Fabry G: Simple bone cysts. A review of 59 cases with special reference to their treatment, *Arch Orthop Trauma Surg* 111:297, 1992.

180. Nastri AL et al: Maxillary ameloblastoma: a retrospective study of 13 cases, *Br J Oral Maxillofac Surg* 33:28, 1995.

181. Naula JM et al: Peripheral ameloblastoma. A case report and review of the literature, *Int J Oral Maxillofac Surg* 21:40, 1992.

182. Neff JR: Nonmetastatic Ewing's sarcoma of bone: the role of surgical therapy, *Clin Orthop* 204:111, 1986.

183. Ngan H: Growing bone islands, *Clin Radiol* 23:199, 1972.

184. Niechajev IA, Stemby NH: Diagnostic accuracy and pathology of vascular tumors and tumor-like lesions, *Chir Maxillofac Plast* 7:153, 1983.

185. Nimityongskul P, Anderson LD, Dowling EA: Chondromyxoid fibroma, *Orthop Rev* 21:863, 1992.

186. Norman A, Schiffman M: Simple bone cysts: factors of age dependency, *Radiology* 124:779, 1977.

187. Nusbacher N, Sclafani SJ, Birla SR: Case report 155: polyostotic Paget's disease complicated by benign giant cell tumor of left clavicle, *Skeletal Radiol* 6:233, 1981.

188. O'Mara RE: Bone scanning in osseous metastatic disease, *JAMA* 229:1915, 1974.

189. Osborn AG: Tumors, cysts and tumor-like lesions of spine and spinal cord. In Osborn AG, editor: Diagnostic Neuroradiology, St Louis, 1994, Mosby.

190. Parham DM et al: Childhood multifocal osteosarcoma, clinicopathologic and radiologic correlates, *Cancer* 55:2653, 1985.

191. Parker BR, Marglin S, Castellino RA: Skeletal manifestations of leukemia, Hodgkin disease and non-Hodgkin lymphoma, *Semin Roentgenol* 15:302, 1980.

192. Peterson HA: Multiple hereditary osteochondromata, *Clin Orthop* 239:222, 1989.

193. Picci P et al: Giant-cell tumor of bone in skeletally immature patients, *J Bone Joint Surg* 65A:486, 1983.

194. Picci P et al: Treatment recommendations for osteosarcoma and adult soft tissue sarcomas, *Drugs* 47:82, 1994.

195. Pritchard DJ et al: Chondrosarcoma: a clinicopathologic and statistical analysis, *Cancer* 45:149, 1980.

196. Pritchard DJ et al: Fibrosarcoma of bone and soft tissues of the trunk and extremities, *Orthop Clin North Am* 8A:869, 1977.

197. Reeves DL: Vertebral hemangioma with compression of the spinal cord, *J Neurosurg* 21:710, 1964.

198. Reichart PA, Philipsen HP, Sonner S: Ameloblastoma: biological profile of 3677 cases, *Eur J Cancer B Oral Oncol* 31B:86, 1995.

199. Reinus WR, Gilula LA: Radiology of Ewing's sarcoma: intergroup Ewing's sarcoma study (IESS), *Radiographics* 4:929, 1984.

200. Reiter FB, Ackerman LV, Staple TW: Central chondrosarcoma of the appendicular skeleton, *Radiology* 105:525, 1972.

201. Resnick D: Diagnosis of bone and joint disorders, ed 4, Philadelphia, 2002, WB Saunders.

202. Rodman D, Raymond AK, Phillips WC: Case report 201: primary lymphoma of bone (PLB) left fibula, *Skeletal Radiol* 8:235, 1982.

203. Roodman GD: Osteoclast function in Paget's disease and multiple myeloma, *Bone* 17:575, 1995.

204. Rosenberg ZS et al: Osteosarcoma: subtle, rare, and misleading plain film features, *AJR Am J Roentgenol* 165:1209, 1995.

205. Ross JS et al: Vertebral hemangiomas: MR imaging, *Radiology* 165:165, 1987.

206. Sanerkin NF, Gallagher P: A review of the behavior of chondrosarcoma of bone, *J Bone Joint Surg* 61B:395, 1979.

207. Sangueza OP, White CR: Parachordoma, *Am J Dermatopathol* 16:185, 1994.

208. Santavirta S: Synovial sarcoma. A clinicopathological study of 31 cases, *Arch Orthop Trauma Surg* 111:155, 1992.

209. Saville DP: A medical option for the treatment of osteoid osteoma, *Arthritis Rheum* 23:1409, 1981.

210. Schmidt RG, Kabbani YM, Mayer DP: Aneurysmal bone cyst, *J Am Podiatr Med Assoc* 83:595, 1993.

211. Schwartz HS et al: The malignant potential of enchondromatosis, *J Bone Joint Surg* 69A:269, 1987.

212. Sherman RS, Wilner D: The roentgen diagnosis of hemangioma of bone, *AJR Am J Roentgenol* 86:1146, 1961.

213. Sherman RS, Wolfson S: Roentgen diagnosis of lymphosarcoma and reticulum cell sarcoma in infancy and childhood, *AJR Am J Roentgenol* 86:693, 1961.

214. Shin HJ et al: Parachordoma, *Ultrastruct Pathol* 18:249, 1994.

215. Sickles EA, Genant HK, Hoffer PB: Increased localization of 99mTc-pyrophosphate in a bone island: case report, *J Nucl Med* 17:113, 1976.

216. Simon MA, Bartucci EJ: The search for the primary tumor in patients with skeletal metastases of unknown origin, *Cancer* 58:1088, 1986.

217. Small IA et al: Gardner's syndrome with an unusual fibro-osseous of the mandible, *Oral Surg* 49:477, 1980.

218. Smith SB, Shane HS: Simple bone cyst of the calcaneus. A case report and literature review, *J Am Podiatr Med Assoc* 84:127, 1994.

219. Spanier SS, Enneking WF, Enrique P: Primary malignant histiocytoma of bone, *Cancer* 36:2084, 1975.

220. Spanier SS: Malignant fibrous histiocytoma of bone, *Orthop Clin North Am* 8:947, 1977.

221. Sposto MR et al: Albright's syndrome: review of the literature and case report, *J Nihon Univ School Dent* 36:283, 1994.

222. Springfield DS, Gebhardt MC, McGuire MH: Chondrosarcoma: a review, *J Bone Joint Surg* 78A:141, 1996.

223. Steiner HJ, Shosh L, Dorfman HD: Ultrastructure of giant cell tumors of bone, *Hum Pathol* 3:569, 1972.

224. Struhl A et al: Solitary (unicameral) bone cyst: the fallen fragment sign revisited, *Skeletal Radiol* 18:261, 1989.

225. Sundaram M, McDonald DJ, Merenda G: Intramuscular myxoma: a rare but important association with fibrous dysplasia of bone, *AJR Am J Roentgenol* 153:107, 1989.

226. Sung HW et al: Giant-cell tumor of bone: analysis of two hundred and eight cases in Chinese patients, *J Bone Joint Surg* 64A:755, 1982.

227. Szendroi M: New aspects in the treatment of bone sarcomas, *Acta Med Hungarica* 50:237, 1994.

228. Tashiro T et al: Intradural chordoma: case report and review of the literature, *Neuroradiology* 36:313, 1994.

229. Tertti R, Alanen A, Remes K: The value of magnetic resonance imaging in screening myeloma lesions of the lumbar spine, *Br J Haematol* 91:658, 1995.

230. Thrall JH, Ellis BI: Skeletal metastases, *Radiol Clin North Am* 25:1155, 1987.

231. Turcotte RE et al: Chondroblastoma, *Hum Pathol* 24:944, 1993.

232. Unroe BJ, Kissel CG, Rosenberg JC: Maffucci's syndrome. Review of the literature and case report, *J Am Podiatr Med Assoc* 82:532, 1992.

233. van Loon CJ et al: Aneurysmal bone cyst: long-term results and functional evaluation, *Acta Orthop Belg* 61:199, 1995.

234. Varma DG et al: MRI of extraskeletal osteosarcoma, *J Comput Assist Tomogr* 17:414, 1993.

235. Varvares MA et al: Chondroblastoma of the temporal bone. Case report and literature review, *Ann Otol Rhinol Laryngol* 101:763, 1992.

236. Vieta JO, Friedell HL, Craver LF: A survey of Hodgkin's disease and lymphosarcoma of the bone, *Radiology* 39:1, 1942.

237. Watanabe H, Arita S, Chigira M: Aetiology of a simple bone cyst. A case report, *Int Orthop* 18:16, 1994.

238. Weber AL et al: Chordomas of the skull base. Radiologic and clinical evaluation, *Neuroimaging Clin North Am* 4:515, 1994.

239. Weber MH et al: Mechanisms of tumor metastasis to bone, *Crit Rev Eukaryot Gene Expr* 10:281, 2000.

240. Wheelhouse WW, Griffin PP: Periosteal chondroma, *South Med J* 75:1003, 1982.

241. Wicklund CL et al: Natural history study of hereditary multiple exostoses, *Am J Med Genet* 55:43, 1995.

242. Willis RA: Pathology of osteoblastoma of bone, *J Bone Joint Surg* 31B:236, 1949.

243. Wiltshaw E: The natural history of extramedullary plasmacytoma and its reaction to solitary myeloma of bone and myelomatosis, *Medicine* 55:217, 1976.

244. Winkler K et al: Treatment of osteosarcoma: experience of the Cooperative Osteosarcoma Study Group (COSS), *Cancer Treat Res* 62:269, 1993.

245. Wold LE, Swee RG, Sim FH: Vascular lesions of bone, *Pathol Ann* 20:101, 1985.

246. Woods ER et al: Reactive soft tissue mass associated with osteoid osteoma: correlation of MR imaging features with pathologic findings, *Radiology* 186:221, 1993.

247. Young JW, Liebscher LA: Postirradiation osteogenic sarcoma with unilateral metastatic spread within the field of irradiation, *Skeletal Radiol* 8:279, 1982.

248. Yunis EJ: Ewing's sarcoma and related small round cell neoplasms in children, *Am J Surg Pathol* 10(suppl 1):54, 1986.

chapter 14

Endocrine, Metabolic, and Nutritional Diseases

D. ROBERT KUHN

ENDOCRINE DISORDERS
Acromegaly
Cushing Syndrome
Giantism (Gigantism)
Hyperparathyroidism
Hypoparathyroidism

Pseudohypoparathyroidism
Pseudopseudohypoparathyroidism
Hypothyroidism

METABOLIC DISORDERS
Osteoporosis

NUTRITIONAL DISORDERS
Hypervitaminosis A
Hypervitaminosis D
Osteomalacia
Rickets
Scurvy (Hypovitaminosis C)

 # Endocrine Disorders

Acromegaly

BACKGROUND

Acromegaly is marked by the oversecretion of growth hormone (somatotropin) in a skeletally mature patient. Oversecretion is caused by an adenoma in the anterior lobe of the pituitary. Anterior pituitary tumors account for about 18% of all intracranial tumors. The incidence of acromegaly is reportedly 50 to 60 cases per million and the prevalence 3 to 4 cases per million per year.[2] Acromegaly has no gender bias. If the level of growth hormone increases, it produces overgrowth of bone, particularly those bones that are formed intramembranously, principally the skull and mandible. Enlarged joint spaces and soft-tissue swelling are typical, producing enlarged hands and feet with thickening of the tongue.

Because the growth centers have not closed, increased levels of growth hormone in skeletally immature patients result in giantism.[2,68,76] Giantism patients with persistent increases in growth hormone also demonstrate acromegalic features. Complications include degenerative joint disease (DJD), increased risk for colonic polyps and colon cancers, and death caused by cardiovascular and cerebral vascular disease. Patients who exhibit diabetes mellitus or hypertension have the highest mortality rate.[2,76]

IMAGING FINDINGS

Increased disc spaces and other joint spaces are demonstrated early. This is followed by generalized osteoporosis and DJD in advanced cases. Increased anteroposterior (AP) diameter of the thorax and enlargement of the ribs at the costochondral junction is typical.[2,68,76] Sella turcica expansion (Fig. 14-1) or destruction, enlarged sinus cavities, malocclusion, and widened mandibular angle (prognathism) are common. The hands and feet exhibit thickening of the tubular bones and prominent ungual tufts (Fig. 14-2). Soft-tissue thickening may be seen at the heel pad (Fig. 14-3) measuring 20 mm or more.[2,76] Although this measure varies, the heel pad thickness should not exceed 23 mm among female and 25 mm among male patients.

CLINICAL COMMENTS

Acromegaly is a gradually progressive disorder in which the symptoms often precede diagnosis by 5 to 10 years. The classic features are a prominent forehead, malocclusion associated with a wide mandibular angle, thickening of the tongue, and large hands and feet. Soft-tissue swelling may produce neural compression in the carpal tunnel. Barrel chest, seborrhea, sweating, hypertrichosis, hyperglycemia, hypertension, and cardiomyopathy are frequently occurring features.[2,68,76] Diagnosis is accomplished by documenting excess growth hormone secretion. In cases of episodic excess of growth hormone, documentation of oral glucose administration that fails to suppress growth hormone secretion is helpful. Magnetic resonance imaging (MRI) or computed tomography (CT) documentation of pituitary hyperplasia is suggested.[2,76] Treatment revolves around removal or destruction of the pituitary tumor, reversal of hypersecretion, and maintenance of normal anterior and posterior pituitary function.[2,76]

KEY CONCEPTS

- *Acromegaly is excessive secretion of growth hormone from the anterior lobe of the pituitary gland in a skeletally mature patient.*
- *Excessive secretion of growth hormone from the anterior lobe in a skeletally immature patient results in giantism.*
- *Acromegaly leads to an elaboration of intramembranously formed bone.*
- *The disease manifests prominently in the skull, hands, feet, and chondral tissues.*
- *Thickening of the skin overlying the calcaneus can be assessed through the heel pad sign.*
- *Acromegaly is associated with diabetes mellitus, premature degenerative joint disease, increased mortality, colon cancer, hypertension, and atherosclerosis.*

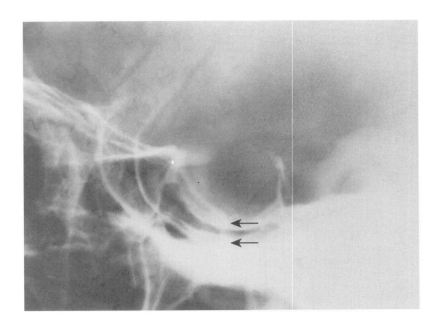

FIG. 14-1 Pituitary adenoma causing acromegaly. Expansion of the sella turcica with the "double floor sign" *(arrows)*. (From Eisenberg RL, Johnson NM: Comprehensive radiographic pathology, ed 3, St Louis, 2003, Mosby.)

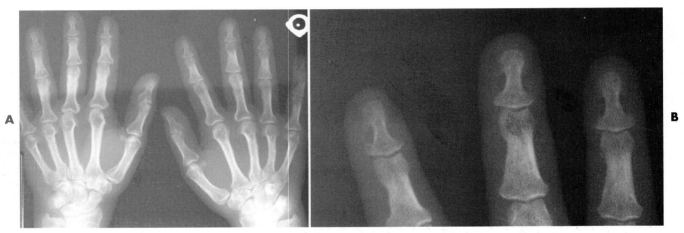

FIG. 14-2   A, Acromegaly presenting in the hands with tufting of the distal phalanges, forming spade digits. **B,** Enlarged view. (Courtesy Gary Longmuir, Phoenix, AZ.)

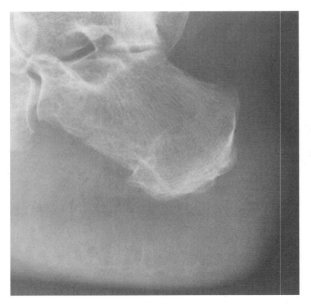

FIG. 14-3 Acromegaly. Positive heel pad sign measuring 32 mm. This value is beyond the normal upper limit of 23 mm for females and 25 mm for males. (From Eisenberg RL, Johnson NM: Comprehensive radiographic pathology, ed 3, St Louis, 2003, Mosby.)

Cushing's Syndrome

BACKGROUND

Cushing's syndrome (CS) is hyperadrenocorticism secondary to anterior lobe pituitary tumors, tumors that secrete ectopic adreno-corticotropic hormone (ACTH), adrenal cortex tumors, or as a complication of glucocorticoid therapy (Fig. 14-4). Cushing's disease adds an additional component, hypothalamic-pituitary dysfunction. The incidence of adrenal tumors in the United States is 0.5 per million people per year.[39] Pituitary tumors producing Cushing's syndrome are more frequent.[72] Women are more commonly affected, and a wide age distribution is seen.[22,34,39] Growth retardation and suppressed sexual maturation are most notable in children. Additional characteristics include rapid weight gain associated with abnormal fat distribution. A thick layer of facial fat rounds out the cheeks, producing the typical circular "moon face" appearance. In addition, a prominent fat pad is deposited over the upper thoracic spine, producing a mass called a *buffalo hump*. The abdomen typically is pendulous. Patients also may demonstrate hypertension, rapid hair growth,[19,48] muscular atrophy,[33] and striae.[39,48]

IMAGING FINDINGS

The hallmark radiographic sign is generalized osteoporosis typified by marked loss of trabecular bone and less evident loss of cortical bone. Also evident is an increased number of insufficiency fractures of the vertebrae, scapula, ribs, and pubic bones.[19,22,34,48,76] Corticosteroid therapy producing Cushing's syndrome also may lead to osteonecrosis[48,76] and insufficiency fractures.[48]

CLINICAL COMMENTS

Excessive production of cortisol is caused by ACTH hypersecretion by pituitary adenomas and occasionally ectopic ACTH-secreting tumors.

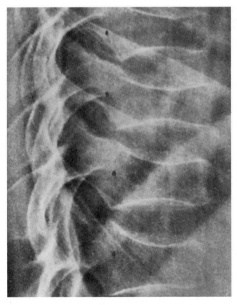

FIG. 14-4 Cushing's syndrome produced by prolonged administration of adrenocorticoids. Generalized osteopenia and bone softening produce deep endplate concavities ("codfish" vertebra) and loss of vertical height by repeated microfractures. (From Kuhn JP, Slovis T, Haller J: Caffey's pediatric diagnostic imaging, ed 10, St Louis, 2004, Mosby.)

Characteristic features. These features include facial-trunk obesity (buffalo hump, moon face), abdominal striae, growth retardation, rapid hair loss, and muscular atrophy. Generalized osteopenia, insufficiency fractures, and occasional osteonecrosis are the primary imaging findings.* Enlarged sella turcica or evidence of pituitary hypertrophy[29] may be present but is not a routine finding.[9] Plain films of the skull, chest, and abdomen often are normal. CT, MRI, and ultrasound (US) often are necessary.[9,40] Angiography and venous sampling are useful to document the hypovascularity that is typical of endocrine tumors.[40,72] Occult secretory tumors may be found with scintigraphy.[33] In cases of recurrent Cushing's disease, the treatment of choice is transsphenoidal pituitary adenectomy. Surgery is followed by irradiation (4000 to 5000 rad). Surgical success rate is 90% for skilled neurosurgeons.[38] Hypercortisolemia, external pituitary irradiation, and posttreatment hypopituitarism may increase the risk of brain infarction.[42]

KEY CONCEPTS

- *Cortisol levels are elevated secondary to glucocorticoid therapy or a pituitary or adrenal cortex tumor.*
- *The physical appearance is marked by a rounded moon face and buffalo hump fat accumulation along the upper back.*
- *Other findings include hypertension, abdominal striae, retarded growth maturation in children, inappropriate osteopenia, possibly osteonecrosis, and insufficiency fractures.*
- *Surgery and occasional use of irradiation are highly successful.*

Giantism (Gigantism)

BACKGROUND

Hypersecretion of growth hormone (GH) occurring in a skeletally immature patient produces excessive proportional bone growth, known as *giantism*. This unusual condition is produced typically by adenomas of the anterior lobe of the pituitary gland or, less commonly, by diffuse hyperplasia of acidophilic cells elsewhere. Organomegaly and commensurate hypertrophy of muscles and connective tissue are associated findings.

IMAGING FINDINGS

The hallmark imaging findings of true giantism are of proportional, yet exaggerated, skeletal growth. The bones are increased in both length and diameter.[5,17] Enlargement of the sella turcica or evidence of pressure erosion may be seen occasionally on plain film or, more reliably, with CT. MRI better demonstrates the abnormal pituitary gland. Combinations of imaging may be necessary to identify ectopic sources of GH.[77]

CLINICAL COMMENTS

Remarkable proportional growth is typical. The skeletal maturation of patients with giantism may exceed that of their age-related peers by 11 standard deviations. A case study reported a 3½-year-old boy who demonstrated a level of skeletal maturity consistent with a 10½-year-old child. At 7 years of age he was a well-proportioned boy 182 cm (6 feet, ¾ inches) tall, weighing 99.4 kg (219 lb) and wearing size 13EEE shoes.[77] Laboratory profiles include elevations of 24-hour GH secretion, paradoxic growth response to administered thyrotropin-releasing hormone (TRH), and failure to suppress serum growth hormone levels with oral

---

*References 19, 22, 23, 34, 39, 72.

glucose loading.[5,17,77] Hypercalcemia, hyperphosphaturia, and elevated levels of alkaline phosphatase are consistent findings.

Hyperparathyroidism

BACKGROUND

Hyperparathyroidism (HPT) is the condition of elevated levels of parathormone (PT), resulting from a variety of direct and indirect stimuli.[16,66,76] Excess levels of PT produce disorders of calcium, phosphate, and bone metabolism; this is the most common cause of hypercalcemia.[64,66] HPT occurs in approximately 1 in 700 persons. HPT is divided into three categories: primary, secondary, and tertiary.

Primary HPT is most commonly produced by a single adenoma (80% to 85% of cases), less commonly, parathyroid hyperplasia (10% to 15% of cases), multiple adenomas (4% to 5% of cases), and rarely secretory carcinomas (1% to 3% of cases).[23,66] Secondary HPT results from chronic renal failure in most cases (Fig. 14-5), representing an end organ dysfunction[27,32,76] PT secretion is stimulated by elevated serum levels of phosphate and reduced ionized serum calcium.[27,76] Diffuse enlargement of all parathyroid glands is typical.[23] Tertiary HPT may be described as a complication of dialysis. Parathyroid glands may act independently

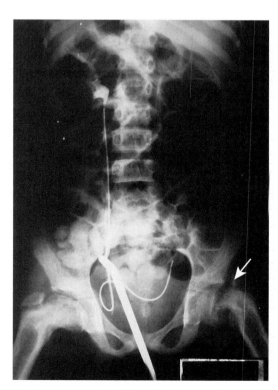

FIG. 14-5 Secondary hyperparathyroidism produced in this child by renal hypoplasia. Also note the slipped capital femoral epiphysis on the reading right (*arrow*) and coxa plana deformity of healed Legg-Calvé-Perthes disease on the reading left.

of the serum calcium levels.[27,76] In this setting, as serum phosphate levels increase, stimulus for PT secretion also increases.

PT acts predominantly on the skeleton, the kidneys and gastrointestinal tract to mobilize skeletal calcium into circulation, reducing the renal excretion of calcium and increasing gastrointestinal absorption of calcium by a diversity of metabolic actions.[23,66] Although primary HPT remains the most common form of hyperparathyroidism, secondary and tertiary HPT are increasing in frequency. This is most likely a result of an increasingly larger geriatric population, more frequent encounters with the causes of secondary and tertiary HPT, and increased longevity. Primary HPT is a disease that affects predominantly middle-age women, one half of whom are postmenopausal. The balance of the cases are equally divided between men and premenopausal women.[16,23,64] It is rare to find patients younger than 16 years of age.[66]

IMAGING FINDINGS

It is now recognized that HPT is more common than previously thought[16,23,55,64,66] and is most likely to demonstrate little or no specific signs or symptoms.[16,55,64] The insensitivity of plain film and earlier recognition of HPT by laboratory examination often produce essentially normal radiographs.[55] Bone mineral density assessments using single- or dual-energy x-ray absorptiometry or quantitative CT are more useful and should be used to investigate asymptomatic HPT.[16,55,76] Bone biopsy is definitive, but it is not used on a routine basis and is primarily a research tool.[27,64]

The radiographic analysis must answer two basic questions. First, what is the cause of the elevations of PT? Determining this establishes presurgical localization, treatment of renal disease if possible, and change in dialysis technique if necessary. Second, what is the clinical status and what skeletal and extraskeletal manifestations are present?

Follow-up examinations monitor successful treatments or identify progressive disease. Experts do not agree on which imaging strategy is best. Successful imaging often includes several complementary modalities. Because the majority of cases of primary HPT are caused by a single adenoma (80% to 85%), high-resolution ultrasound by an experienced sonographer is advocated as a first step. This study is considered safe, cost-effective, and relatively sensitive. Its value is diminished by small or ectopic lesions.[23,58,64] Scintigraphy in the form of ^{99m}Tc-sestamibi localizes parathyroid tumors normally situated and in ectopic locations. It also can determine parathyroid gland functionality.[23,58,64] MRI is indicated in cases of HPT with essentially normal parathyroid glands or persistent postsurgical elevations of PT. This clinical picture often is associated with ectopic secretory tissue.[23,58] Contrast-enhanced CT, arthrography, and selected venous sampling may be used in difficult cases or if reoperation is contemplated.[40,58,66]

The effects of HPT on the skull and extraskeletal structures are numerous. Some are classically, if not exclusively, associated with HPT. HPT effects on bone probably include a higher remodeling rate of the haversian canals. Ultimately, longitudinal defects appear in cortical bone.[27,37,55,66] Hyperthyroidism, Sudeck's atrophy, and Paget's disease may appear similarly. Cortical endosteal and trabecular resorption also occur.[27] Subperiosteal reabsorption is seen early and most often found along the radial side of the middle phalanx of the hand, particularly the second and third digits. Fine grain screens producing images with great detail[18] are necessary for early recognition of this virtually pathognomonic sign.* If progression of the

---

*References 16, 27, 32, 49, 55, 66, 76.

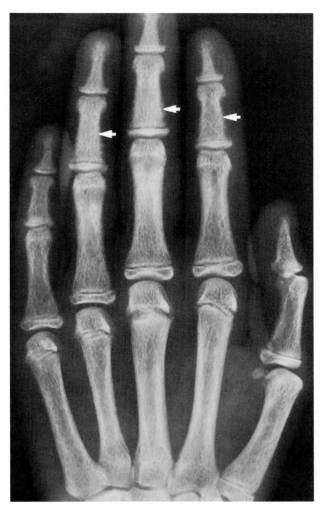

FIG. 14-6 Hyperparathyroidism. Resorption of bone from subperiosteal sites typically located along the radial side of the middle phalanges of second, third, and fourth rays *(arrows)*. This patient also demonstrates acroosteolysis of the terminal tufts. (From Eisenberg RL, Johnson NM: Comprehensive radiographic pathology, ed 3, St Louis, 2003, Mosby.)

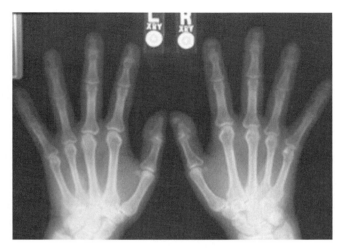

FIG. 14-7 Hyperparathyroidism. The distal phalanges of the right thumb and index finger demonstrate the classic appearance of acroosteolysis. Phalangeal and subperiosteal bone resorption are seen to a lesser degree.

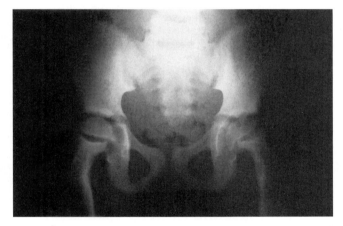

FIG. 14-8 Hyperparathyroidism. Subchondral resorption producing pseudowidening and sclerotic margins of the sacroiliac joints bilaterally. The ilia are affected to a greater extent. (Courtesy Gary M. Guebert, Maryland Heights, MO.)

PART TWO Bone, Joints, and Soft Tissues

disease occurs, ungual tufts (acroosteolysis), proximal phalanges, and metacarpals are involved (Figs. 14-6 and 14-7).[27]

Reports exist of generalized osteopenia[16] with accentuated trabeculae pattern caused by resorption of nonessential trabeculae and loss of cortical definition. The latter involves both periosteal and endosteal cortices. This produces blurring and irregular, thinned cortices with widened yet rarified medullary cavities.[27,76] Pseudowidening of the joint space may be seen as resorption of the sacroiliac (Fig. 14-8), acromioclavicular (Fig. 14-9), and pubic joint surfaces.[27,76] The upper medial surface of the humerus, tibia, calcaneus, ischial tuberosities, and the upper border of the ribs may demonstrate resorption.[27] The fine permeative destructive pattern of the skull, known as "salt-and-pepper" skull, is also typical of HPT (Fig. 14-10).[66,76] Resorption of the lamina dura surrounding the tooth socket also is seen. Administration of vitamin D and calcium leads to accelerated loss of bone mineral density in some patients, and cases of hyperphosphatemia exhibit increased incidence of soft-tissue calcification.

Osteitis fibrosa cystica, also called a *brown tumor* (Fig. 14-11), is a collection of fibrous tissue and giant cells in bone that is found in primary and secondary HPT.[9,23,66] These present as geographic lucencies. Slightly expansile, they are most commonly found in the mandible, pelvis, ribs, and femora.[22] Overall, brown tumors are seen infrequently.[64] Soft-tissue calcifications are seen in later stages of HPT (Figs. 14-12 and 14-13).[27,76] Nephrocalcinosis is still considered to be a common presenting complaint.[64] Chondrocalcinosis of menisci in the knee, as well as other sites, is seen. Secondary HPT is thought to produce more frequent soft-tissue calcifications of vascular and periarticular structures.[27,40,76] Osteosclerosis of the spine ("rugger jersey" spine) (Fig. 14-14) is a characteristic yet unusual sign.[14,76] Periarticular condensation of bone may be seen in the presence of open growth plates.[14]

CLINICAL COMMENTS

As our understanding of HPT has increased, it has become recognized that the most common presenting sign is hypercalcemia.*

---

*References 16, 23, 27, 58, 64, 66.

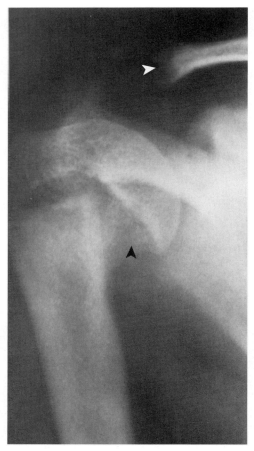

FIG. 14-9 Hyperparathyroidism. Acroosteolysis of the clavicle is common. Subperiosteal resorption of the humerus has led to slipped capital epiphysis *(arrowheads)*. (From Eisenberg RL, Johnson NM: Comprehensive radiographic pathology, ed 3, St Louis, 2003, Mosby.)

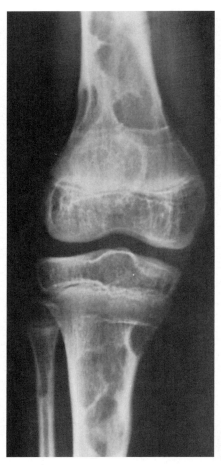

FIG. 14-11 Hyperparathyroidism. Brown tumors, collections of fibrous tissue and giant cells, producing lytic regions within the osseous structures of the knee. (From Eisenberg RL, Johnson NM: Comprehensive radiographic pathology, ed 3, St Louis, 2003, Mosby.)

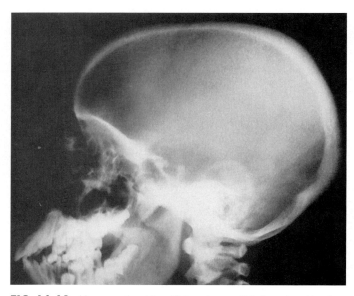

FIG. 14-10 Hyperparathyroidism. "Salt-and-pepper" skull produced by alternating zones of lucency and sclerosis. Loss of trabecular detail in the diploic space blurs the separation between inner and outer tubules. (Courtesy Gary M. Guebert, Maryland Heights, MO.)

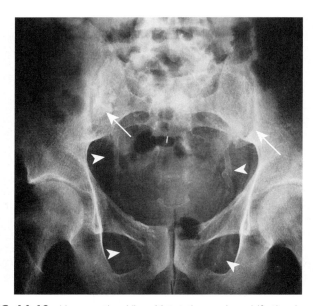

FIG. 14-12 Hyperparathyroidism. Metastatic vascular calcification is seen *(arrowheads)*. Note the pseudowidening of the sacroiliac joints *(arrows)*.

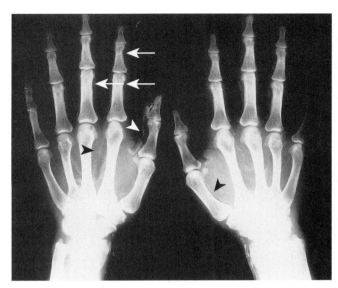

FIG. 14-13 Hyperparathyroidism. Metastatic vascular calcifications in the hand *(arrowheads)*. Note the subperiosteal resorption of bone on the radial margins of the middle phalanges *(arrows)*.

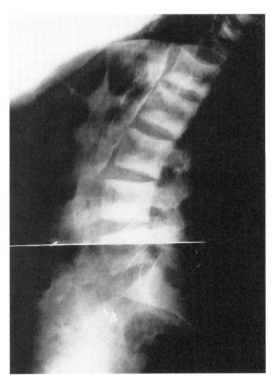

FIG. 14-14 Hyperparathyroidism. Unusual yet characteristic osteosclerosis in the spine ("rugger jersey" spine).

Hypercalcemia in the presence of elevated PT by immunoradiometric assay (IRMA) or immunochemoluminescent assay (ICMA) is a definitive diagnosis.[64] Some patients have persistent high normal levels of serum calcium. If this resulted from anything other than primary or secondary parathyroid disease, the PT levels would be low or nonexistent.[64] Otherwise a paucity of presenting features exists.[9] Silverberg and Bilezikian found that one half of

their patients were asymptomatic or demonstrated nonspecific complaints.[64] These may include depression, subjective weakness, memory and sleep abnormalities, constipation, "bone pain," loss of appetite, nausea, vomiting, or polydipsia.[58,64,66] Some report an association between childhood irradiation of the neck and primary HPT.[64] The classic features of HPT are decreased bone density, brown tumors, leontiasis ossea, renal calculi, chondrocalcinosis, and metastatic calcification. These features, although classic, are uncommon presenting features. Of these, renal calculi are the most frequent finding, occurring in 20% of all cases.[32,64]

Hypoparathyroidism

BACKGROUND

Hypocalcemia secondary to low or absent PT is the hallmark of hypoparathyroidism. Hypoparathyroidism most commonly follows thyroidectomy or radical laryngeal surgery.[17] Cases of hypoparathyroidism have followed radioactive iodine treatments for HPT.[10] Reports exist of metastases (typically breast cancer) and transient forms relating to surgical cure for hyperparathyroidism.[14] Sporadic idiopathic and familial idiopathic conditions have a more variable presentation. Familial forms may be associated with pernicious anemia and hypoadrenalism. This is characterized further by circulating antibodies to the parathyroid, thyroid, and adrenal glands, supporting the concept of an autoimmune etiology in some cases.[53] The earliest age of onset is seen in the familial form, often within the first year of life. Sporadic forms are typically found in patients 5 through 10 years old. The acquired form of hypoparathyroidism occurs later in life.

IMAGING FINDINGS

Generalized or localized sclerosis is the most common skeletal abnormality. Thickened calvarium and hypoplastic dentition, radiodense metaphyseal bands seen in the long bones, iliac crest, and vertebral margins also are potential findings. Occasionally reported are osteopenia, typically in pseudohypoparathyroidism.

Asymptomatic periarticular calcifications, particularly those involving the hips and shoulders, are not rare.[53]

CLINICAL COMMENTS

The predominant features of hypoparathyroidism evolve as a result of chronic hypoglycemia. These include tetany, epilepsy, cataracts, and papilledema with elevated intracranial pressure. Common yet not absolute features include short stature and mental impairment. Alopecia occurs in varying degrees. Underdevelopment of the dental roots is a common presenting complaint. Excessive renal reabsorption of phosphorus as a consequence of hypocalcemia is inevitable. Hypocalcemia and hyperphosphatemia combine to suppress 1,25-dihydroxy vitamin D synthesis to low levels.

Effective treatment includes calcium and vitamin D analogs. Serum calcium levels raise once the hyperphosphatemia reduces. Candidiasis of the nail beds or orogenital regions occurs in some sporadic or familial cases.[5,17]

> ### KEY CONCEPTS
> - *Low or undetectable levels of parathormone leading to chronic hypocalcemia and hyperphosphatemia define hypoparathyroidism.*
> - *Acquired forms occur later in life and may result from neck surgery (often for hyperthyroidism) after iodine treatment of breast metastasis.*
> - *Radiology features are marked by osteosclerosis, thickened calvarium, hypoplastic dentition, and periarticular calcification around the hips and shoulders.*

Pseudohypoparathyroidism

BACKGROUND

Pseudohypoparathyroidism (PHP) is an X-linked genetic disorder associated with normal or enlarged parathyroid glands and parathyroid target organ (bone, kidney) insensitivity. Often but not always a typical skeletal phenotype occurs in addition to PT resistance and is called *Albright hereditary osteodystrophy (AHO) type I*.[5,17,51,61] These skeletal changes include shortened fourth and fifth metacarpals, short stature, round face, premature hair loss, and some degree of mental impairment.[5,61,78]

IMAGING FINDINGS

It is rare to see PHP in the absence of metacarpal shortening; it most frequently affects the first, fourth, and fifth digits. Metatarsals also may be affected. A positive metacarpal sign frequently is observed.[17,51,53,78] That is, a line tangential to the heads of the fourth and fifth metacarpals should be distal to or just contact the head of the third metacarpal. Failure to do so indicates a positive metacarpal index.[51,53] However, variability in the pattern and degree of metacarpal shortening may render the metacarpal index unreliable (Fig. 14-15).[5] In addition, the metacarpals and phalanges, particularly those of the first digit, may appear wide with cup-shaped epiphyses and perpendicularly oriented exostoses.[51,78] Thickening of the skull (Fig. 14-16) and calcification of the basal ganglion (Fig. 14-17)[47] also may be present. Reports of spinal stenosis also exist.

CLINICAL COMMENTS

PHP presents with the classic phenotypic changes, and laboratory studies indicate hypocalcemia, hyperphosphatemia, and elevated PT levels. The renal and osseous PT receptors do not respond.[47,78] Treatment of PHP involves administration of vitamin D derivatives.[17] Short stature, obesity, round face, and early hair loss are typical.[1,47,51]

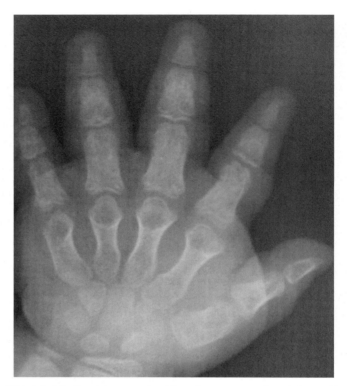

FIG. 14-15 Pseudohypoparathyroidism. Short metacarpals and short, wide phalanges are demonstrated here. The uniform shortening of all the metacarpals prevents demonstration of a positive metacarpal index. (From Taybi H: Pseudohypoparathyroidism [PH], *Semin Roentgenol* 8:214, 1973.)

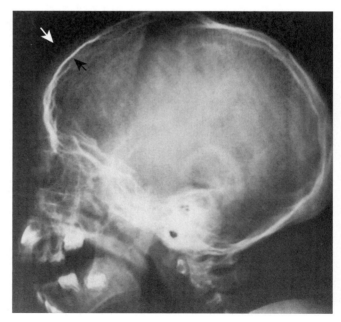

FIG. 14-16 Pseudohypoparathyroidism. A thickened skull *(arrows)* demonstrated in a short, obese 4-year-old child. (From Taybi H: Pseudohypoparathyroidism [PH], *Semin Roentgenol* 8:214, 1973.)

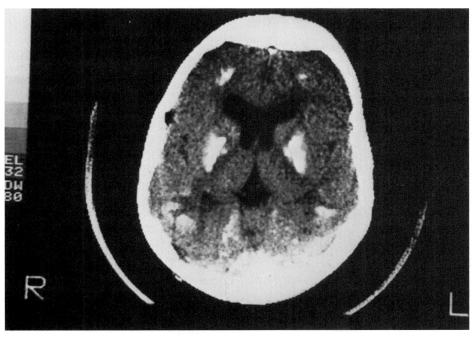

FIG. 14-17 Pseudohypoparathyroidism. Axial computed tomography demonstrates thickening of the cranial vault and several sites of intracerebral calcification. (From Taybi H, Lachman RS: Radiology of syndromes, metabolic and skeletal dysplasias, ed 4, St Louis, 1996, Mosby.)

KEY CONCEPTS

- *Pseudohypoparathyroidism represents end-organ insensitivity to parathormone; also known as Albright hereditary osteodystrophy type I, when patients exhibit a characteristic phenotype.*
- *Hypocalcemia and hyperphosphatemia occur despite elevated serum levels of parathormone.*
- *Positive metacarpal index is frequent and suggestive of the condition.*
- *The small bones of the hands and feet appear short and wide, with cup-shaped epiphyses, and exostoses perpendicular to the long axis of the bones.*
- *Those afflicted often exhibit mild mental retardation, round face, obesity, and a short stature.*

Pseudopseudohypoparathyroidism

BACKGROUND

Pseudopseudohypoparathyroidism (PPHP) is the normal calcemic form of PHP. PPHP and PHP may appear in the same family, suggesting a close genetic similarity.[1,51] These entities share common skeletal and developmental defects without the laboratory findings suggestive of hypothyroidism.[1] PPHP patients, unlike those with PHP, have a normal cyclic adenosine monophosphate (cAMP) response to parathormone in the kidney, suggesting an adequate number of membrane receptors.

IMAGING FINDINGS

The findings of PPHP are indistinguishable from PHP.[51] They share the features of short stature, metacarpal shortening (Fig. 14-18), and shortened, wide phalanges with cupped epiphyses. Exostoses may be seen.[17,51,78]

CLINICAL COMMENTS

The classic radiographic features also are seen in conjunction with obesity, round face, absent knuckles, and a prematurely receding hair line.[17,51,78] Mild mental retardation, abnormal dentition, strabismus, and impaired taste and olfaction complete the clinical picture.[53]

KEY CONCEPTS

- *Pseudopseudohypoparathyroidism is the normocalcemic form of pseudohypoparathyroidism.*
- *Skeletal and phenotypical changes are indistinguishable from pseudohypoparathyroidism, including short metacarpals, positive metacarpal index, and exostoses.*

Hypothyroidism

BACKGROUND

Hypothyroidism involves decreased levels of thyroid hormones, such as triiodothyronine (T_3) and thyroxin (T_4) in peripheral tissues. The condition results from disorders of the thyroid gland (primary) or decreased stimulating hormone secondary to disorders of the pituitary (secondary) or hypothalamus (tertiary). However, rare, peripheral resistance to the circulating hormone also may occur. A long list of primary, secondary, and tertiary causes have been identified, including dietary deficiencies, gland atrophy and inflammation, or destruction of gland tissue secondary to radioactive iodine treatments, surgery, and infiltrative disorders such as amyloidoses, metastases, and lymphoma.

Dietary deficiencies of iodine pose a significant health problem in endemic regions. Deficiency of dietary iodine represents the most common preventable cause of mental impairment. In 1991

PART TWO Bone, Joints, and Soft Tissues

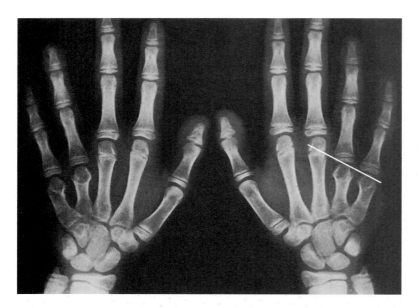

FIG. 14-18   Pseudopseudohypoparathyroidism (PPHP). A positive metacarpal index *(line)* was demonstrated by this short but normally proportioned patient with PPHP. (From Kuhn JP, Slovis T, Haller J: Caffey's pediatric diagnostic imaging, ed 10, St Louis, 2004, Mosby.)

the World Health Organization stated that 20% of the world's population was at risk.[11,35] Although endemic iodine deficiency is the most common cause of goiter and hypothyroidism worldwide, autoimmunity is the most common cause in nonendemic regions. Surgery and radioiodine treatments for thyroid toxicosis account for approximately one third of all cases of hypothyroidism.[5,11,20]

Hypothyroidism in utero produces cretins. Two types are reported: myxedematous and neurologic.[20] By contrast, juvenile myxedema occurs in children and with fewer musculoskeletal abnormalities. The pattern of involvement in the adult varies further.

IMAGING FINDINGS

The majority of radiographic abnormalities occur in younger patients who demonstrate cretinism or juvenile myxedema. Delayed osseous maturation (Fig. 14-19), persistent sutures with wormian bones, brachycephaly, and enlarged sella turcica are features commonly seen. Prognathism and hypoplasia of the sinuses may be present. Multiple epiphyseal growth centers arise, producing irregular articular surfaces. Coxa vara, coxa valga, and slipped femoral capital epiphysis all have been described.[35,53] The spine may demonstrate a bullet shape, osteoporosis, and delayed development.[20,53] The adult occasionally may demonstrate osteosclerosis secondary to a decreased rate of turnover (Fig. 14-20).

CLINICAL COMMENTS

Although regions of endemic cretinism exist, it is not a significant problem in North America. The hallmark features of juvenile myxedema include mental retardation, lethargy, constipation, large tongue, abdominal distention, hypotonia, dry hair and skin, and delayed dentition. Adults who acquire hypothyroidism are typically female with dry, coarse skin and hair, easy fatigability, lethargy, edema, hoarseness, constipation, and bradycardia. The most common neurologic complaint is carpal tunnel syndrome.

KEY CONCEPTS

- *Deficiency of thyroid hormones (triiodothyronine [T_3] and thyroxin [T_4]) produces a variable clinical picture based on the stage of development.*
- *Hypothyroidism in infants results in cretinism; in children it results in juvenile myxedema.*
- *Osseous changes are predominant in children and may include delayed ossification, persistent sutures, wormian bones, brachycephaly, prognathic jaw, enlarged or altered shape of the sella turcica secondary to pituitary hypertrophy, multiple epiphyseal growth centers, hip abnormalities, bullet-shaped vertebrae, and osteopenia.*
- *Signs and symptoms include lethargy, dry hair and skin, mental retardation, constipation, large tongue, abdominal distention, hypotonia, and delayed dentition.*

Metabolic Disorders

Osteoporosis

BACKGROUND

Osteoporosis is defined as qualitatively normal bone present in pathologically deficient quantities. Osteoporosis is the most common cause of generalized metabolic osteopenia. Osteopenia literally means "poverty of bone" and defines a generic state of less than the normal amount of bone. There are many causes of osteopenia, including tumors, metabolic conditions, disuse syndromes. Osteoporosis is a pathological state of osteopenia.

Females are affected by osteoporosis to a greater degree than males. Osteoporosis is mostly a disease of older patients; young patients are rarely affected. It is estimated that up to 20 to 25 million individuals are affected in the United States.[74] Osteoporosis is associated with 1.5 million fractures per year in the female population over 40 years of age. The United States spends in excess of 8 billion dollars per year on direct and indirect costs related to osteoporosis.

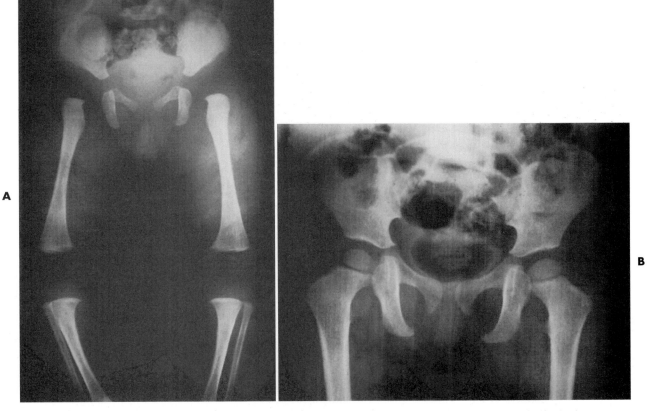

FIG. 14-19 Hypothyroidism. **A,** Delayed ossification of the acetabulum-simulated acetabular dysplasia. **B,** Ossification has progressed and no longer appears dysplastic after 30 months of thyroid medication. (From Silverman FN, Currarino G: Roentgen manifestations of hereditary metabolic diseases in childhood. *Metabolism* 9:248, 1960.)

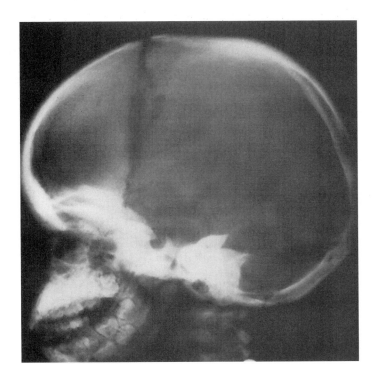

FIG. 14-20 Cretinism. The diploic space is poorly differentiated, the anterior fontanelle shows delayed closure, and the cranial sutures are wide. The pneumatization of the skull is delayed. (From Eisenberg RL, Johnson NM: Comprehensive radiographic pathology, ed 3, St Louis, 2003, Mosby.)

TABLE 14-1
Pattern of Osteoporosis

Pattern	Definition	Classic examples
Generalized	Osteoporosis affecting the majority of the skeleton	Senile osteoporosis Postmenopausal Hyperparathyroidism Cushing's disease Widespread malignant disease (e.g., metastasis, multiple myeloma)
Regionalized	Osteoporosis affecting one limb or section of the body	Disuse atrophy (immobilization) Reflex sympathetic dystrophy Transient regional osteoporosis Regional migratory osteoporosis
Localized	Focal osteoporosis in one or multiple discrete portions of bone	Lytic metastasis Osteomyelitis Inflammatory arthritides

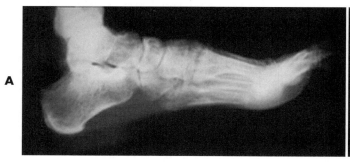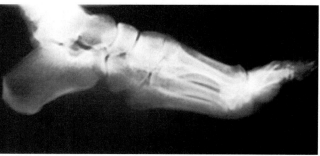

FIG. 14-21　Reflex sympathetic dystrophy. **A,** The patient's right foot demonstrates the classic regionalized pattern of osteopenia. **B,** The patient's unaffected left foot is offered for comparison. (*Note:* The left foot image has been reversed for ease of comparison.) (Courtesy M. Kathleen Kuhn, Lake St Louis, MO.)

The three major categories of osteoporosis are described:
1. Generalized; affecting the majority of the skeleton
2. Regional; affecting one limb or section of the body
3. Localized; producing focal osteopenia in one or multiple discrete portions of bone

The more common and classic causes of generalized osteoporosis such as immobilization, disuse, and transient regional osteoporosis are discussed in this section (Table 14-1). The balance of the etiologies associated with generalized osteoporosis are discussed in this chapter and elsewhere in the text. Localized osteoporosis (typically produced by neoplastic and infectious bone destruction) and periarticular osteopenia (seen in some cases of inflammatory arthritis) are discussed in their respective chapters.

Generalized osteoporosis is typically asymptomatic until a complication occurs (usually a fracture). Decreased bone mineral density (BMD) often leads to fracture.[29,43,53,59] Vertebral fractures commonly are found in the transitional spine regions. The thoracolumbar junction, lumbosacral junction, apex of the thoracic spine, proximal femur, and distal radius are the most common locations.

Regional.　Osteoporosis may be limited to a skeletal region after disuse or immobilization, reflex sympathetic dystrophy (Sudeck's atrophy) (Fig. 14-21), and as idiopathic transient presentations (transient regional osteoporosis and regional migratory osteoporosis).

The most common of these are immobilization and disuse osteoporosis. Casted fractures, central nervous system injury producing motion loss, and bone and joint inflammations[50] are the most frequent causes. These patients demonstrate a negative calcium balance. That is, skeletal loss of calcium in the urine and reduced uptake of dietary calcium occur. Variable patterns of presentation include osteopenia, spotty lucencies, bandlike zones of rarification, and cortical scalloping. These patterns may mimic aggressive osteolytic lesions at times.[53,76] The degree of BMD loss associated with disuse and immobilization may lead to further insufficiency fractures.

Transient regional osteoporosis defines a rapid onset of osteopenia in a periarticular location, which is self-limiting and spontaneously reverses without evident cause.[53,76] This disorder may take the form of transient osteoporosis of the hip or regional migratory osteoporosis.[53,76] They demonstrate similar clinical and radiologic features, prompting discussion that these disorders are related to each other, and probably related to reflex sympathetic dystrophy.[53]

Transient osteoporosis of the hip occurs in young adults. Men are more commonly affected than women (Fig. 14-22). Patients present with a painful limp and antalgic gait that predates the radiographic changes. It is well documented yet unexplained that the left hip is almost always involved in females. Full recovery is expected in 3 months to 1 year.[53,76]

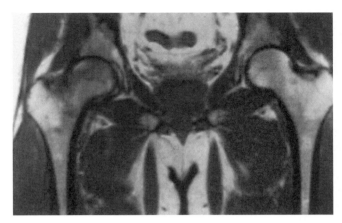

FIG. 14-22 Transient osteoporosis of the hip. Demonstration of diffuse decrease in signal intensity in the right (reading left) femur head on this T1-weighted (TR 500, TE 15) image. (From Taybi H, Lachman RS: Radiology of syndromes, metabolic and skeletal dysplasias, ed 4, St Louis, 1996, Mosby.)

Regional migratory osteoporosis, the other form of transient regional osteoporosis,[53,76] involves the hip less frequently. The knee, ankle, and foot are the typical locations.[53] Men are affected more than women.[76] Regional migratory osteoporosis presents in the fourth and fifth decades of life. The progression starts with pain and swelling, typically involving the lower extremity. Radiographic changes appear in weeks to months, then regression occurs within 9 months,[53,76] and involvement of another region may follow. Plain film demonstrates a regional pattern of profound osteopenia and rarified subchondral bone. A bone scan may be positive, and MRI demonstrates signal intensity consistent with intraosseous edema.[53,69]

IMAGING FINDINGS

Generalized osteoporosis is demonstrated on the plain film as widespread osteopenia produced by thin cortices and expanded intratrabecular spaces.[4,53,59] The relative insensitivity of plain film requires a decrease in BMD of approximately 30% to 50% before it is demonstrated on the plain films. Bone scans are invariably normal unless fracture repair is present.[29,53,76] Evaluation of BMD is most effective by single photon absorptiometry, dual photon absorptiometry, and quantitative CT. These bone mineral density studies must be age-, gender-, and race-matched to normal values.[15]

By the time osteoporosis is readily apparent on plain film, it is usually beyond the mild or moderate stage and increasingly likely that the classically associated findings are present. The spine, proximal femur, and tubular bones of the extremities display the most characteristic features of osteoporosis. First and foremost is osteopenia.[59] The remaining bone is histologically normal; it is simply rarified. The cortex is thin and porous (Figs. 14-23 and 14-24). Resorption occurs in the horizontal trabeculae, which uncover the fibers that sit predominantly along the lines of stress, thus accentuating their appearance (Figs. 14-25 and 14-26). Piezoelectric activity is thought to account for the disparate resorption rates between horizontal and vertical trabeculae.[50] Use of fine grain screens produces the best detail and demonstrates osseous structures with distinct, sharp cortical margins.[18] This is not a feature of osteomalacia, another common cause of osteopenia.

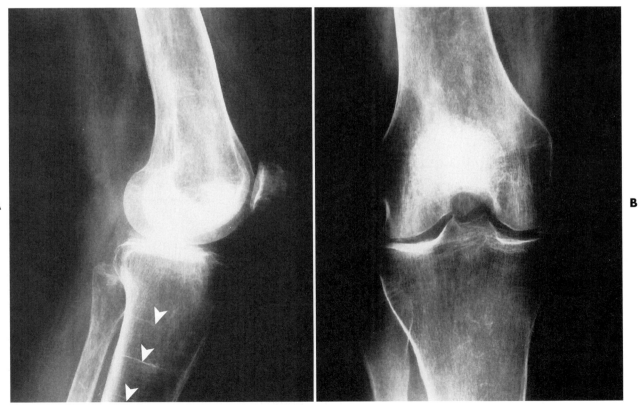

FIG. 14-23 A and **B,** Osteoporosis. Marked cortical thinning and widened medullary cavity are classic features. Note the horizontal bone bars or reinforcement lines *(arrowheads).*

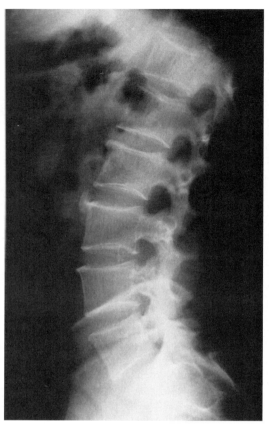

FIG. 14-24 Osteoporosis. Resorption of the horizontal trabeculae has "uncovered" the vertical fibers, accentuating their appearance.

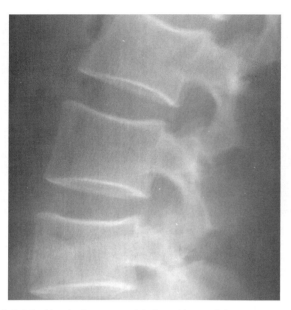

FIG. 14-25 Vertebral osteoporosis indicated by a radiolucent appearance of the vertebrae and relative highlighting of the cortices.

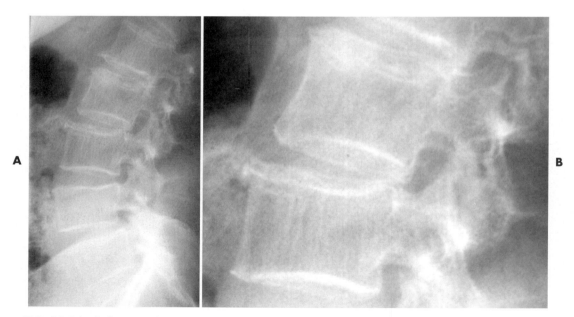

FIG. 14-26 **A,** Osteoporosis presents with vertical striations of the vertebrae, sometimes known as *pseudohemangiomas* of the vertebrae. **B,** Close-up. The two conditions can be differentiated by the number of levels involved. Hemangioma causes prominent trabeculation at one level; osteoporosis causes prominent trabeculation at all levels.

Change in the shape of a spinal segment also may indicate osteoporosis. Chronic microfractures producing bone remodeling typically are represented by the "fish" or "codfish" vertebrae.[54] This deformity is marked by deepened concavities of the vertebral endplates, without significant alteration of the anterior and posterior vertebral margins.[53,54] The expansile pressures of the intervertebral disc produces the deformity in the weakened vertebrae. On occasion, focal intrusion of nuclear material into the vertebral bodies may be seen (Schmorl's nodes). The wedge-shaped fracture[4] and vertebrae plana, or "pancake" vertebrae, are signs of abrupt osseous failure resulting from single traumatic events. In cases of severe osteoporosis, trivial trauma such as coughing and sneezing may be the proximate cause of the spinal fracture and a common cause of localized pain.

The expression of osteoporosis in the proximal femur is in the alteration of Ward's triangle.[28,53,76] Ward's triangle is bordered by three groups of trabecular fibers. The principal compressive group, secondary compressive group, and tensile group make up the boundaries of Ward's triangle (Fig. 14-27). Normally it is difficult to resolve the individual groups of fibers. These groups are readily visible as trabecular absorption progresses and Ward's triangle continues to enlarge until the secondary compression group disappears. The last fibers to resorb belong to the principal compressive group.[25,53,76] Femoral neck fracture is a common, serious, and potentially life-threatening complication of osteoporosis. The aging population in the United States guarantees that this incidence of femoral neck fracture will increase. This will continue to cost billions of dollars until proper preventive and management protocols are perfected.

CLINICAL COMMENTS

The pathogenesis of osteoporosis is unclear. Studies of the processes associated with senile and postmenopausal osteoporosis have explored theories of primary failure of bone formation, as well as excessive bone resorption, with conflicting results.

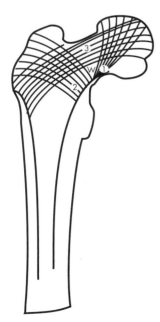

FIG. 14-27 *W,* Ward's triangle is an area in the lower femoral neck nearly devoid of trabeculae. It is surrounded by three patterns of trabeculae: *1,* Principal compressive group; *2,* secondary compressive group; and, *3,* principal tensile group.

Hormone imbalance with loss of estrogenic activity features prominently in today's preventive and therapeutic models.[29,43,53]

Other factors considered are calcium deficiency and fluctuations in gonadal and adrenocortical hormones, thyroid hormone, and growth hormone. These are known to be influential, but why and to what extent remains unclear.[53] Dietary deficiency of calcium has been strongly supported.[25,43] The type and degree of physical activity demonstrated by patients during their adolescent and young adult years certainly play a role in developing bone mineral density.[43] Men and women have a positive BMD increase until approximately 30 years of age. After 40 years of age, men and women lose BMD at a rate of 0.3% per year. This rate continues for men, unless aggravated by some other factor, through the end of their lives. As women reach menopause, the rate of decline in BMD jumps to 3% per year for approximately 8 to 10 years. Over this interval, women lose approximately 30% of their BMD.[25,43,53]

Laboratory values. Laboratory values are routinely normal with the exception of hydroxyproline found in urine. Osteoporosis most frequently comes to light as a result of some complication of the process. Typically fracture is the elucidating event. In patients with proximal femoral neck fractures, 75% to 80% have demonstrable osteoporosis at the time of injury. Femoral fractures are associated with a high mortality rate, 10% to 20% in excess of their age-matched peers. Although most patients survive the hip fracture, 20% to 30% still acquire enough disability and dependency that institutionalization occurs.[43]

Although hip fractures are the most devastating, several other sites of fracture are common. Fractures of the distal radius, foot/toe, and vertebrae, although typically cared for in nonhospital settings, still represent significant, and yet poorly elucidated, morbidity.[43] A less common but serious form of vertebral body fracture is the one associated with a retropulsion of an osseous fragment, producing cord injury.

Treatment. The burgeoning elderly population in the Unites States guarantees a dramatic rise in the number of fractures, with ever-increasing health care costs. This creates an urgent need for the adoption of adequate preventive programs. Treatment options are numerous and represent the various etiologic viewpoints. Estrogen therapy, bisphosphonate,[29,30,74] calcium, and vitamin D supplementation are potential therapeutic models. Some combination of the preceding treatments often is proposed with the additional instruction to exercise.

Exercise must produce skeletal loading to be effective. Activities such as hill walking, weightlifting, and jogging appear beneficial. These exercises should be considered by any individual under the age of 30 years who wishes to increase his or her peak BMD. Swimming has been demonstrated not to be effective for reversal or even slowing the loss of BMD. At best, this is considered a bridging activity to enhance cardiovascular fitness.

Calcitonin has demonstrated some ability to slow, if not reverse, BMD loss. Therapeutic agents may be divided into two categories. One group is aimed at slowing or minimally reversing osteoporosis. This course of action represents an interim course because these agents do not significantly reduce the patient's incidence of fracture.[29] Sodium fluoride does add new bone, but it is of poor quality. Fracture rates are decreased, yet frequent side effects and a 25% nonresponder rate continue to drive interest in other directions. Currently, biphasic treatment models are being explored and may provide significant relief. This treatment model involves the administration of bone-forming agents followed by treatment protocols in which bone conservation is promoted.[29]

KEY CONCEPTS

- Osteoporosis is characterized by decreased quantity, not quality, of bone.
- Women are affected more often than men; the incidence increases with age.
- Typically those afflicted remain asymptomatic until fractures occur.
- Hip fractures are associated with a 10% to 20% mortality rate; 20% to 30% become institutionalized as a result of their fracture.
- Radiographic appearance is noted by thin cortex with accentuated trabecular pattern.
- Osteoporotic vertebrae may appear biconcave (codfish or fish vertebrae), flat (vertebrae plana), or narrowed anteriorly (wedge fracture).

- Hydroxyproline in urine is a nonspecific sign.
- Diagnosis is achieved by bone mineral density assessments using single photon absorptiometry, dual photon absorptiometry, or quantitative computed tomography.
- Regional osteoporosis results most commonly from disuse or immobilization, injury to the central nervous system, and bone and joint inflammation.
- Transient regional osteoporosis and regional migratory osteoporosis are idiopathic, self-limiting types of regional osteoporosis; they are typically evident on plain films, and magnetic resonance imaging is particularly helpful in the diagnosis.

Nutritional Disorders

Hypervitaminosis A

BACKGROUND

Elevations of vitamin A resulting from dietary excess, common cold prophylaxis, antiacne therapies, and treatment of keratosis follicularis have been reported.[21,62,76] Hypervitaminosis A affects the central nervous system, skeleton, and integument.[8,62,76]

IMAGING FINDINGS

Painful regions that show subperiosteal cortical thickening (Fig. 14-28)[21,62,76] commonly affect the ulna (Fig. 14-29) and metacarpals. Generalized osteoporosis may be seen.

CLINICAL COMMENTS

Vitamin A administration in unknowing conjunction with medical therapy for acne and keratosis follicularis is an important and preventable cause of this entity. Self-administered, high doses of vitamin A also cause this condition.[62] Headache, blurred vision, palsies of cranial nerves, and increased intracranial pressure are presenting central nervous system complaints. Chronic toxicity may produce perioral fissures, hair loss, hair coarsening, and

desquamation of the skin of the palms and soles. Pruritus may be present.[21,62,76] Hepatosplenomegaly sometimes is observed. The liver must become saturated before toxicity is noted. Elimination of vitamin A and management of the complications of hypervitaminosis A are fundamental to the cure.[8,62,76]

KEY CONCEPTS

- Hypervitaminosis A results from iatrogenic and dietary excess intake of vitamin A, leading to liver saturation.
- Signs and symptoms include hepatosplenomegaly, blurred vision, headache, increased intracranial pressure, cranial nerve neuropathy, perioral fissures, hair loss, coarse hair, pruritus, and desquamation of palms and soles.
- Radiographic changes include solid, painful subperiosteal cortical thickening and osteoporosis.

Hypervitaminosis D

BACKGROUND

Hypervitaminosis D is a product of excessive vitamin D intake in children and adults.[7,26,31,60] Nearly 98% of the milk sold today is fortified with vitamin D. This practice began in the 1930s[7] to combat the epidemic presentation of rickets seen in many industrial cities of the United States.[52,56] The current practice is aimed at preventing the onset of rickets[7,26,31,56,63] but also to limit senile, postmenopausal, and glucocorticoid-induced osteoporosis. Vitamin D therapies also have been suggested in cases of Paget's disease and rheumatoid arthritis.[53]

Toxic levels of vitamin D have been produced by accidental overfortification,[7,26] prolonged administration of therapeutic levels of vitamin D,[24] and coincidental self-administration of vitamin D. Renal failure and thiazide diuretics lower the threshold for the expression of vitamin D toxicity.[60]

IMAGING FINDINGS

Generalized osteopenia produced by the enhanced resorption of calcium by osteoclasts is evident.[7] In skeletally immature patients, alternating bands of sclerosis and lucencies are seen in the metaphyseal regions of the tubular bones (Fig. 14-30).[53] Appositional bone thickening is produced. Metastatic calcium deposits are found in periarticular locations (Fig. 14-31), vasculature, and a variety of other organs, including the falx cerebri (Fig. 14-32) and tentorium cerebelli.[53]

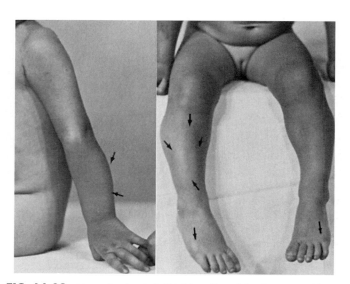

FIG. 14-28   Hypervitaminosis A. Painful swelling of the forearm and lower leg (arrows). (From Kuhn JP, Slovis T, Haller J: Caffey's pediatric diagnostic imaging, ed 10, St Louis, 2004, Mosby.)

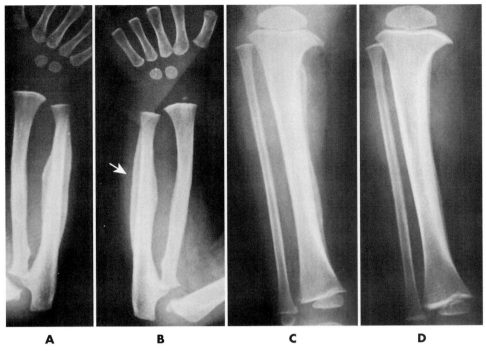

FIG. 14-29 Hypervitaminosis A. **A,** Right and, **B,** left forearms showing symmetric cortical hyperostosis (arrow). **C,** Tibial hyperostosis at the time of diagnosis of hypervitaminosis A. **D,** Five weeks after removal of dietary vitamin A. (From Kuhn JP, Slovis T, Haller J: Caffey's pediatric diagnostic imaging, ed 10, St Louis, 2004, Mosby.)

CLINICAL COMMENTS

Vitamin D toxicity can occur abruptly with high doses or in the presence of renal disease.[60] Toxic levels of vitamin D may accumulate over long periods of time.[31] The effects of hypervitaminosis D include the following: anorexia, weight loss, weakness, fatigue, disorientation, vomiting, dehydration, polyuria, constipation, and bone pain.[7,53] Laboratory findings include hypercalcemia, hypercalcuria, hematuria, albuminuria, and documentation of elevated levels of vitamin D_2 or D_3.[53]

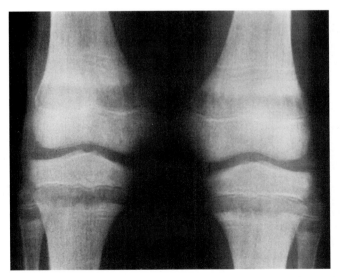

FIG. 14-30 Hypervitaminosis D. Alternating bands of sclerosis and lucency in this 9-year-old child who subsequently died of vitamin D toxicity. (From Kuhn JP, Slovis T, Haller J: Caffey's pediatric diagnostic imaging, ed 10, St Louis, 2004, Mosby.)

Osteomalacia

BACKGROUND

Osteomalacia, also called *adult rickets*,[45,69] is typified by the presence of poor bone quality. Osteomalacia is more accurately described as a group of entities that can produce similar yet nonspecific radiographic changes. The clinical and biochemical profile of osteomalacia varies. Osteomalacia often is camouflaged by the associated complaints of the various etiologic entities. Delayed or inadequate mineralization of the osteoid matrix, demonstrated by bone biopsy (the gold standard diagnostic tool), which produces bone rarefaction and osseous deformities, classically describes this lesion.[6,45] These findings and alteration of the growth plate and metaphysis represent rickets, which was discussed previously. Although several varied and distinct etiologies are able to produce osteomalacia, the majority of the cases involve abnormal calcium, vitamin D, or phosphorus metabolism (Box 14-1).[6,13,76] These are produced by dietary deficiencies, malabsorption, renal disease, and a small group of miscellaneous diseases.

IMAGING FINDINGS

Osteomalacia in adults is less severe than rickets, which appears in children.[13] Generalized osteopenia with coarse, hazy-appearing trabeculae is typical. The skeletal detail appears out of

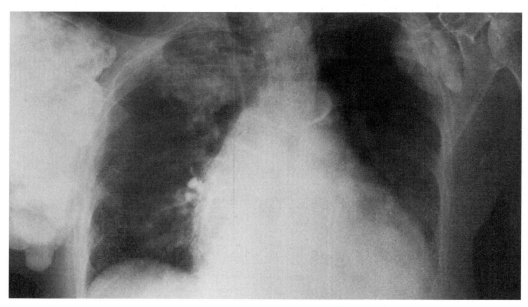

FIG. 14-31   Hypervitaminosis D. Metastatic deposits of calcium in region of the right and left shoulders. (From Eisenberg RL, Johnson NM: Comprehensive radiographic pathology, ed 3, St Louis, 2003, Mosby.)

focus (Fig. 14-33). Looser's lines or pseudofractures (focal accumulations of osteoid that occur perpendicular to and through the cortex) may be present.[13,53,76] Common sites of involvement are the femoral necks, scapulae, pelvis (Fig. 14-34), ribs, occiput, and long bones of the extremities.[5,13,45,75,76]

Other bone-softening processes also produce this feature. Bowed proximal femoral necks, "shepherd's crook" deformity, and basilar invagination are findings in Paget's disease, fibrous dysplasia, and rickets, as well as osteomalacia. The periosteal and endosteal cortical margins are blurred. Increased osteoid volumes and expanded, irregular haversian canals produce intracortical lucencies.[5,45,53]

CLINICAL COMMENTS

Common presenting complaints are bone pain with subjective or objective lower extremity weakness, waddling gait, bony tenderness, and osseous deformity. These features may suggest the diagnosis but are not exclusive to osteomalacia.[6,45,71] Biochemical analysis most often demonstrates elevated alkaline phosphatase and less often hypocalcemia and hypophosphatemia. Other features are deficiencies in the hormone vitamin D, secondary hyperparathyroidism, and elevated hydroxyproline in the urine. Osteomalacia encompasses many clinical signs and symptoms, biomechanical abnormalities, and radiographic features that are suggestive of the diagnosis; nonetheless, histologic analysis of an

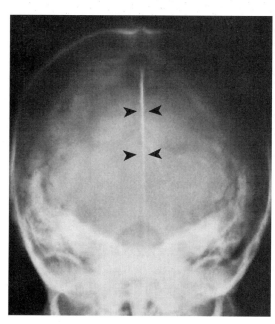

FIG. 14-32   Hypervitaminosis D. Calcification of the falx cerebri *(arrowheads)* and tentorium cerebelli are demonstrated on this Towne view. (From Kuhn JP, Slovis T, Haller J: Caffey's pediatric diagnostic imaging, ed 10, St Louis, 2004, Mosby.)

BOX 14-1
Etiologies of Osteomalacia

Dietary deficiencies
- Vitamin D
- Calcium
- Phosphate
- Dietary chelate

Malabsorption
- Gastrointestinal
- Hepatobiliary
- Pancreatic

Renal disease
- Chronic renal failure
- Renal tubular disease

Miscellaneous
- Solar irradiation deficiency
- Neoplastic invasion
- Fibrous dysplasia
- Neurofibromatosis
- Hypophosphatasia
- Medications (anticonvulsants)

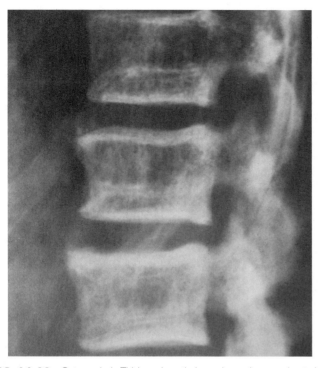

FIG. 14-33 Osteomalacia. Thickened cortical margins and coarsening trabecular patterns without overall enlargement are typical. (From Eisenberg RL, Johnson NM: Comprehensive radiographic pathology, ed 3, St Louis, 2003, Mosby.)

iliac crest bone biopsy is often relied on to definitively establish the diagnosis.[6] Attempts are being made to formulate suitable screening examinations for the diagnosis of osteomalacia; however, no procedure has garnered unequivocal support to date.[6,75]

KEY CONCEPTS

- *Osteomalacia is the lack of appropriate mineralization of normal osteoid resulting in poor bone quality in adults.*
- *Several contributing factors have been identified, including abnormal calcium, vitamin D, or phosphorus metabolism.*
- *Osteopenia is typical; shepherd's crook deformity, basilar invagination, and pseudofracture deformities are also noted.*

Rickets

BACKGROUND

More than 30 causes of rickets and osteomalacia exist.[13] Rickets is closely related to osteomalacia. Rickets demonstrates additional features of disorganized growth plates and widened epiphysis with rarefaction of the zone of provisional calcification (ZPC).[13,45,76] The most frequently encountered cases involve defects in vitamin D, calcium, or phosphate absorption or metabolism.[46]

IMAGING FINDINGS

Typically generalized osteopenia occurs.[13,45,46,76] The remaining trabeculae are coarse.[45,76] The flared metaphysis may be cupped, and the epiphysis is enlarged in all planes (Fig. 14-35). The costochondral junction is enlarged and demonstrates the "rosary bead" appearance (Fig. 14-36).[13,45,46,76] Pectus carinatum is seen with notching found at the diaphragmatic attachment sites and hyperkyphosis.[13]

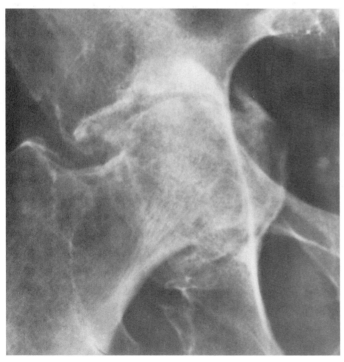

FIG. 14-34 Osteomalacia. Weak, poor-quality bone producing acetabular protrusion in this patient. (From Eisenberg RL, Johnson NM: Comprehensive radiographic pathology, ed 3, St Louis, 2003, Mosby.)

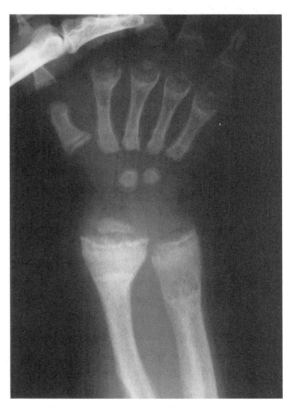

FIG. 14-35 Vitamin D–resistant rickets. The typical flaring and cupping of the metaphysis is seen. (Courtesy Gary M. Guebert, Maryland Heights, MO.)

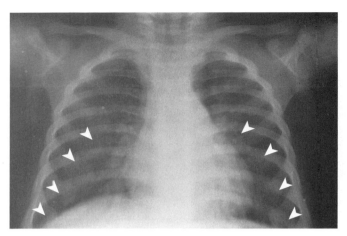

FIG. 14-36   Vitamin D–resistant rickets. Enlargement of the costochondral junction *(arrowheads)* produces the "rosary bead" chest. (Courtesy Gary M. Guebert, Maryland Heights, MO.)

As the child becomes ambulatory, bowing of the long bones is typical (Figs. 14-37 and 14-38).[46,63,70]

CLINICAL COMMENTS

Vitamin D deficiency existed in epidemic proportions in the United States until the early 1920s.[63,56] Rickets in several forms continues to plague our society, although in greatly reduced numbers.[63] High-risk populations are listed in Box 14-2.

Vitamin D–deficiency rickets is a thoroughly preventable disease.[63] Mild cases are effectively treated with standard vitamin D supplements of 400 international units per day. Other causes of rickets include renal osteodystrophy, vitamin D–resistant rickets, and renal hypophosphatemia rickets. Renal osteodystrophy produces features of hyperparathyroidism in addition to rickets (Fig. 14-39).[3] Vitamin D resistance is characterized by end-organ insensitivity to the hormone vitamin D_3 and the inability to respond to vitamin D supplementation.[24] Failure of renal resorption of phosphate-producing hypophosphatemia leads to deficient mineralization.[57] Successful treatment produces remineralization of metaphyseal bone and the ZPC returns (Fig. 14-40).

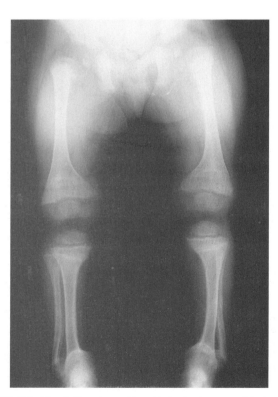

FIG. 14-37   Vitamin D–resistant rickets. Underdevelopment of the long bones and wide, irregular metaphysis are typical. The zone of provisional calcification is rarified and disorganized. The long bones are bowed. (Courtesy Gary M. Guebert, Maryland Heights, MO.)

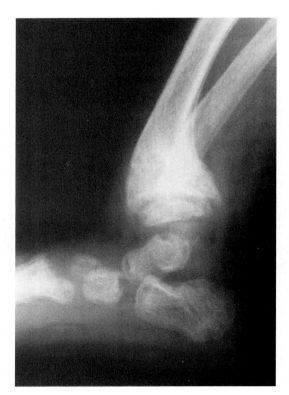

FIG. 14-38   Vitamin D–resistant rickets. The lateral view demonstrates the flared, cupped tibial metaphysis with bowing of the long bones. (Courtesy Gary M. Guebert, Maryland Heights, MO.)

- *Rickets is a lack of appropriate mineralization of normal osteoid resulting in poor bone quality in children.*
- *Radiographic changes are most marked at areas of rapid growth: wide, irregular, cupped metaphyses; wide, lucent zones of provisional calcification; and osseous deformities.*
- *Deficiencies of vitamin D, calcium, or phosphate intake or metabolism are the most frequent causes.*
- *Rickets is a largely preventable disease.*

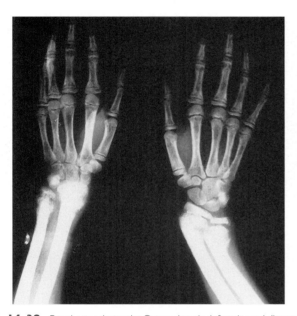

FIG. 14-39 Renal osteodystrophy. Osteosclerosis deformity and disorganization of the growth centers are demonstrated by this young patient.

Scurvy (Hypovitaminosis C)

BACKGROUND

Dietary deficiency of vitamin C for a duration of 4 months or more leads to the typical changes of scurvy. Infantile and adult forms have been identified. Infantile scurvy is infrequent and adult scurvy is rare.

IMAGING FINDINGS

Infantile scurvy leads to reduced osteoblast function, producing intraosseous collagen and a disorganized growth plate, which causes a widened metaphysis and sclerotic ZPC (Fig. 14-41). Beaklike metaphyseal outgrowths (Pelken's spurs) and a radiodense band surrounding ossification centers (Wimberger's sign of scurvy) are typical findings (Fig. 14-42). Subperiosteal hemorrhage, localized or generalized, may lift the periosteal layer (Fig. 14-43). Hemarthrosis may be found in the larger, lower joints chest. Permanent reduction in growth is infrequent.[12,53,76]

CLINICAL COMMENTS

Affected persons fall into one of several groups: infants who are fed exclusively pasteurized or boiled milk, elderly people who have chronic dietary insufficiencies, patients with malabsorption of water-soluble vitamins, and citizens of developing nations where there are widespread dietary deficiencies. Signs and symptoms include irritability, petechiae, swollen and bleeding gums, scorbutic "rosary bead" chest, periarticular swelling, and tenderness of the lower limbs. Interarticular hemorrhage may lead to infants assuming a frog-leg position to decrease the pain.[12,44]

- *Scurvy results from deficient vitamin C intake, occurring primarily in infants fed pasteurized or boiled milk.*
- *Radiographic abnormalities include growth plate abnormalities, wide metaphyses, sclerotic zones of provisional calcification, Wimberger's sign, Pelken's spurs, and periosteal lifting resulting from hemorrhage.*
- *Patients exhibit bleeding gums, irritability, "rosary bead" chest, and periarticular soft-tissue swelling.*

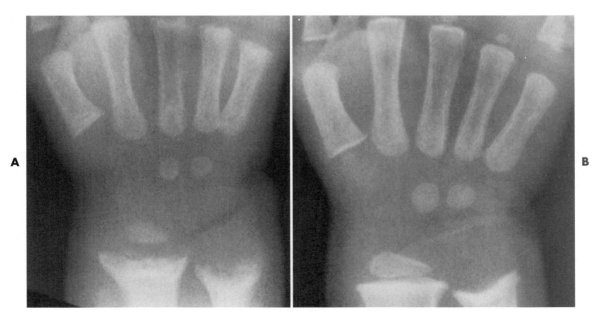

FIG. 14-40 Rickets. **A,** Pretreatment and, **B,** posttreatment radiographs demonstrate the increasing density of the zone of provisional calcification, a sign of successful treatment. (From Eisenberg RL, Johnson NM: Comprehensive radiographic pathology, ed 3, St Louis, 2003, Mosby.)

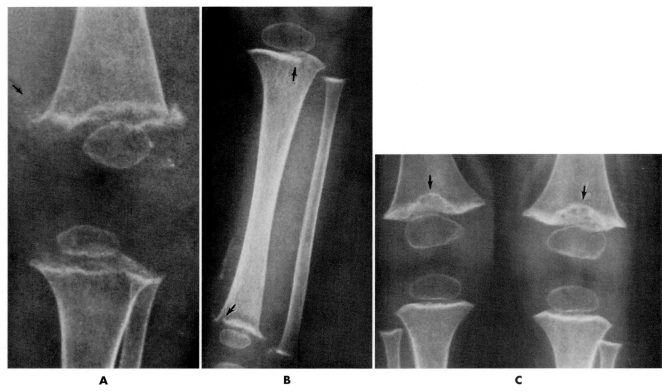

A   **B**   **C**

FIG. 14-41 Advanced scurvy with fractures of thickened, brittle zones of provisional calcification. **A,** Multiple infarctions in the provisional zone, with peripheral spurring and beginning subperiosteal ossification *(arrow)* of the terminal segment of the shaft by the externally displaced periosteum. The osteogenetic layer is lifted by hemorrhage and continues to form normal cortical bone. The bones generally are rarefied, but the provisional zones of the femur, tibia, and ulna and of the femoral and tibial ossification centers are thickened. **B,** Longitudinal fractures of provisional zones and distal ends of the tibia *(arrows).* **C,** Crumpling fractures of proximal and distal provisional zones of the ends of the femora, with incomplete cupping of ends of the shafts *(arrows).* (From Kuhn JP, Slovis T, Haller J: Caffey's pediatric diagnostic imaging, ed 10, St Louis, 2004, Mosby.)

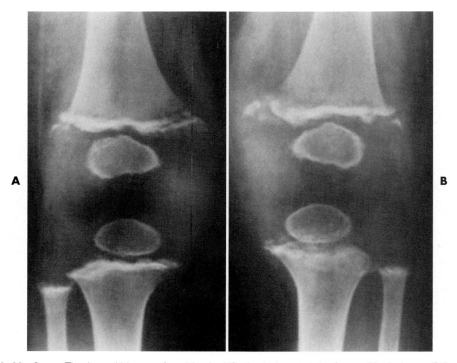

A   **B**

FIG. 14-42 Scurvy. The dense, thick zone of provisional calcification is characteristic of scurvy. Marginal spurs (Pelken's spurs) and a dense ring of sclerosis surrounding the impoverished growth center (Wimberger's sign) are present in, **A,** the right and, **B,** left knees. (From Eisenberg RL: Atlas of signs in radiology, Philadelphia, 1984, Lippincott.)

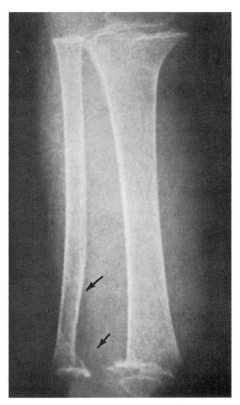

FIG. 14-43 Scurvy. The insecurely attached periosteum is easily lifted in cases of subperiosteal bleeding *(arrows)*. (From Kuhn JP, Slovis T, Haller J: Caffey's pediatric diagnostic imaging, ed 10, St Louis, 2004, Mosby.)

References

1. Ablow RC, Hsia YE, Brandt IK: Acrodysostosis coinciding with pseudohypoparathyroidism and pseudo-pseudohypoparathyroidism, *AJR Am J Roentgenol* 128:95, 1977.

2. Aron DC, Tyrrell JB, Wilson CB: Pituitary tumors: current concepts in diagnosis and management, *West J Med* 162:340, 1995.

3. Ballantyne ES, Findlay GFG: Thoracic spinal stenosis in two brothers due to vitamin D-resistant rickets, *Eur Spine J* 5:125, 1996.

4. Bauer RL: Assessing osteoporosis, *Hosp Pract* 26s:23, 1991.

5. Besser GM, Thorner MO, editors: Clinical endocrinology, ed 2, London, 1994, Wolfe.

6. Bingham CT, Fitzpatrick LA: Noninvasive testing in the diagnosis of osteomalacia, *Am J Med* 95:519, 1993.

7. Blank S et al: An outbreak of hypervitaminosis D associated with the overfortification of milk from a home-delivery dairy, *Am J Public Health* 85:656, 1995.

8. Braun L: Vitamin A excess common deficiency, requirements, metabolism, and misuse, *Pediatr Clin North Am* 9:935, 1962.

9. Buchfelder M et al: The accuracy of CT and MR evaluation of the sella turcica for detection of adrenocorticotrophic hormone-secreting adenomas in Cushing's disease, *AJNR* 14:1183, 1993.

10. Burch WM, Posillico JT: Hypoparathyroidism after I-313 therapy with subsequent return of parathyroid function, *J Clin Endocrinol Metab* 57:398, 1983.

11. Cao XY et al: Timing of a vulnerability of the brain to iodine deficiency in endemic cretinism, *N Engl J Med* 331:1739, 1994.

12. Capistol PJ et al: Scurvy, presentation of six cases, *Ann Espana Pediatr* 12:745, 1979.

13. Doppelt SH: Vitamin D, rickets and osteomalacia, *Orthop Clin North Am* 15:671, 1984.

14. Genant HK et al: Osteosclerosis in primary hyperparathyroidism, *Am J Med* 59:104, 1975.

15. Grampp S et al: Radiographic diagnosis of osteoporosis, *Radiol Clin North Am* 31:1133, 1993.

16. Grey AB et al: Effect of hormone replacement therapy on bone mineral density in postmenopausal women with mild primary hyperparathyroidism: a randomized, controlled trial, *Ann Intern Med* 125:360, 1996.

17. Grossman A, editor: Clinical endocrinology, Boston, 1992, Blackwell Scientific.

18. Guebert GM, Pirtle OL, Yochum TR: Essentials of diagnostic imaging, St Louis, 1995, Mosby.

19. Haddad G, Haddad JG, Kaplan FS: Severe symptomatic osteopenia in a man with pigmented micronodular adrenal hyperplasia, *Clin Orthop* 313:220, 1995.

20. Halpern JP et al: The neurology of endemic cretinism: a study of two endemias, *Brain* 114:825, 1991.

21. Hathcock JM et al: Evaluation of vitamin A toxicity, *Am J Clin Nutr* 52:183, 1990.

22. Hermus AR et al: Bone mineral density and bone turnover before and after surgical cure of Cushing's syndrome, *J Clin Endocrinol Metab* 80:2859, 1995.

23. Higgins CB: Roll of magnetic resonance imaging in hyperparathyroidism, *Radiol Clin North Am* 31:1017, 1993.

24. Hochberg Z et al: 1,25-dehyroxyvitamin D resistance, rickets, and alopecia, *Am J Med* 77:805, 1984.

25. Jackson DW, editor: Instructional course lectures, 1995, American Academy of Orthopedic Surgeons, 1995.

26. Jacobus CH et al: Hypervitaminosis D associated with drinking milk, *N Engl J Med* 326:1173, 1992.

27. Jensen PS, Kliger AS: Early radiographic manifestations of secondary hyperparathyroidism associated with chronic renal disease, *Radiology* 125:645, 1977.

28. Kerr R et al: Computerized tomography of proximal femoral trabecular patterns, *J Orthop Res* 4:45, 1986.

29. Kimmel DB, Slovik DM, Lane NE: Current and investigational approaches for reversing established osteoporosis, *Rheum Dis Clin North Am* 20:735, 1994.

30. Kirk JK, Spangler JG: Alendronate: a bisphosphonate for treatment of osteoporosis, *Am Fam Phys* 54:2053, 1996.

31. Kuroume T: Hypervitaminosis D after prolonged defeat with premature formula, *Pediatrics* 92:862, 1993.

32. Lee VS et al: Uremic leontiasis ossea: "big head" disease in humans? Radiologic, clinical, and pathologic features, *Radiology* 199:233, 1996.

33. Lefebvre H et al: Characterization of the somatostatin receptor subtype in a bronchial carcinoid tumor responsible for Cushing's syndrome, *J Clin Endocrinol Metab* 80:1423, 1995.

34. Leong GM et al: The effect of Cushing's disease on bone mineral density, body composition, growth, and puberty: a report of an identical adolescent twin pair, *J Clin Endocrinol Metab* 81:1905, 1996.

35. Maberly GF: Symposium: clinical nutrition in developing countries: toward the application of contemporary concepts and technology iodine deficiency disorders, *Contemp Sci Issues* 1473 (suppl), 1994.

36. Meema S, Banker MC, Meema HE: Preventive effect of estrogen on postmenopausal bone loss, *Arch Intern Med* 135:1436, 1975.

37. Meema HE, Meema S: Microradioscopic bone structure of the hand in thyrotoxicosis, renal osteodystrophy and acromegaly; clinical aspects of metabolic bone disease, *Excerpta Medica* 10:10, 1973.

38. Melby JC: Therapy of Cushing's disease: a consensus for pituitary microsurgery, *Ann Intern Med* 109:445, 1988.

39. Mendonca BB et al: Clinical, hormonal and pathological findings in a comparative study of adrenocortical neoplasms in childhood and adulthood, *J Urol* 154:2004, 1995.

40. Miller DL: Endocrine angiography and venous sampling, *Radiol Clin North Am* 31:1051, 1993.

PART TWO Bone, Joints, and Soft Tissues

41. Mimouni F: Etiology of nutritional rickets: geographic variations, *J Pediatr* 128:600, 1996.
42. Mizokami T et al: Risk factors for brain infarction in patients with Cushing's disease: case reports, *Angiology* 47:1011, 1996.
43. Nevitt MC: Epidemiology of osteoporosis, *Rheum Dis Clin North Am* 20:535, 1994.
44. Nicol M: Vitamins and immunity, *Allerg Immunol (Paris)* 25:70, 1993.
45. Nugent CA, Gall EP, Pitt MJ: Osteoporosis, osteomalacia, rickets and Paget's disease, *Prim Care* 11:353, 1984.
46. Oginni LM et al: Etiology in rickets in Nigerian children, *J Pediatr* 128:692, 1996.
47. Okada K et al: Pseudohypoparathyroidism-associated spinal stenosis, *Spine* 19:1186, 1994.
48. Ontell FK, Shelton DK: Multiple stress fractures: an unusual presentation of Cushing's disease, *West J Med* 162:364, 1995.
49. Parfitt AM: Hormonal influences on bone remodeling and bone loss: application to the management of primary hyperparathyroidism, *Ann Intern Med* 125:413, 1996.
50. Parfitt AM, Duncan H: In Rothman RH, Simeone FE, editors: Metabolic bone disease affecting the spine, Philadelphia, 1975, WB Saunders.
51. Poznanski AK et al: The pattern of shortening of the bones of the hand in PHP and PPHP: a comparison with brachydactylia E, Turner's syndrome, and acrodysostosis, *Radiology* 123:707, 1977.
52. Recker RR: Bone biopsy and histomorphometry in clinical practice, *Rheum Dis Clin North Am* 20:609, 1994.
53. Resnick D: Diagnosis of bone and joint disorders, ed 4, Philadelphia, 2002, WB Saunders.
54. Resnick DL: Fish vertebrae, *Arthritis Rheum* 25:1073, 1982.
55. Richardson ML et al: Bone mineral changes in primary hyperparathyroidism, *Skeletal Radiol* 15:85, 1986.
56. Saffran M: Rickets: return of an old disease, *J Am Podiatr Med Assoc* 85:222, 1995.
57. Saggese G et al: Long term growth hormone treatment in children with renal hypophosphatemic rickets: effects on growth, mineral metabolism, and bone density, *J Pediatr* 127:395, 1995.
58. Santos E, Higgins CB, Clark O: Clinical image: recurrent hyperparathyroidism caused by a parathyroid cystic adenoma: localization by MRI, *J Comput Assist Tomogr* 20:996, 1996.
59. Schneider R: Radiologic methods of evaluating generalized osteopenia, *Orthop Clin North Am* 15:631, 1984.
60. Schwartzman MS, Franck WA: Vitamin D toxicity complicating the treatment of senile, postmenopausal, and glucocorticoid-induced osteoporosis: four case reports and a critical commentary on the use of vitamin D in these disorders, *Am J Med* 82:224, 1987.
61. Shapira H et al: Familial Albright's hereditary osteodystrophy with hypoparathyroidism: normal structural G^5 a Gere, *J Clin Endocrinol Metab* 81:1660, 1996.
62. Sharieff GQ, Hanten K: Pseudotumor cerebri and hypercalcemia resulting from vitamin A toxicity, *Ann Emerg Med* 27:518, 1996.
63. Sills IN et al: Vitamin D deficiency rickets: reports of its demise are exaggerated, *Clin Pediatr* 33:491, 1994.
64. Silverberg SJ, Bilezikian JP: Extensive personal experience: evaluation and management of primary hyperparathyroidism, *J Clin Endocrinol Metab* 81:2036, 1996.
65. Star VL, Hochberg MC: Osteoporosis in patients with rheumatic disease, *Rheum Dis Clin North Am* 20:561, 1994.
66. Stulberg BN, Licata AA, Bauer TW, Belhobek GH: Hyperparathyroidism, hyperthyroidism, and Cushing's disease, *Orthop Clin North Am* 15:697, 1984.
67. Suarez F et al: Expression and modulation of the parathyroid hormone (PTH)/PTH-related peptide receptor messenger ribonucleic acid in skin fibroblasts from patients with type IB pseudohypoparathyroidism, *J Clin Endocrinol Metab* 80:965, 1995.
68. Subbarao K, Jacobson HG: Systemic disorders affecting the thoracic cage, *Radiol Clin North Am* 22:497, 1984.
69. Tannebaum H, Esdacle J, Rosenthall L: Joint imaging in regional migratory osteoporosis, *J Rheumatol* 7:237, 1980.
70. Taylor A, Mandel G, Norman ME: Calcium deficiency rickets in a North American child, *Clin Pediatr* 33:494, 1994.
71. Verbruggen LA, Bruyland M, Shahabpour M: Osteomalacia in a patient with anorexia nervosa, *J Rheumatol* 20:512, 1993.
72. Vincent JM et al: The radiological investigation of an occult ectopic ACTH-dependent Cushing's syndrome, *Clin Radiol* 48:11, 1993.
73. Wang LD: Preliminary study on nutrition and precancerous lesions of the esophagus in the adolescent, *Chung HUA Chung Liu Tsa Chih* 14:94, 1992.
74. Watts NB: Treatment of osteoporosis with bisphosphonates, *Rheum Dis Clin North Am* 20:717, 1994.
75. Wilton TJ et al: Screening for osteomalacia in elderly patients with femoral neck fractures, *J Bone Joint Surg Br* 69:765, 1987.
76. Yochum TR, Rowe LJ: Essentials of skeletal radiology, ed 2, Baltimore, 1996, Williams & Wilkins.
77. Zimmerman D et al: Congenital giantism due to growth hormone-releasing hormone excess and pituitary hyperplasia with adenomas transformation, *J Clin Endocrinol Metab* 76:216, 1993.
78. Zung A, Herzenberg JE, Chalew SA: Radiological case of the month: ectopic ossification and calcification in pseudohypoparathyroidism and pseudopseudohypoparathyroidism, *Arch Pediatr Adolesc Med* 150:643, 1996.

chapter 15

Miscellaneous Bone Diseases

DENNIS M. MARCHIORI

Amyloidosis
Dermatomyositis
Gaucher's Disease
Heavy Metal Poisoning
Histiocytosis
Hypertrophic Osteoarthropathy
Infantile Cortical Hyperostosis
Mastocytosis
Neurofibromatosis
Paget's Disease
Scoliosis

Amyloidosis

BACKGROUND

Amyloidosis is a rare systemic disease caused by the extracellular accumulation of insoluble amyloid proteins in various organs and tissues of the body. Although several classifications exist, the simplest divides amyloidosis into primary and secondary forms. Amyloidosis without associated antecedent or coexisting disease is primary (idiopathic). Secondary amyloidosis is associated with chronic systemic disease (e.g., rheumatoid arthritis, Crohn's disease, cystic fibrosis, chronic drug abuse), infections (e.g., familial Mediterranean fever, tuberculosis), and tumors (e.g., multiple myeloma). Usually amyloidosis is systemic; only 10% to 20% of cases demonstrate localized disease.[120] Primary amyloidosis affects men more than women and typically occurs between the ages of 40 and 80 years. The presentation of secondary amyloidosis depends on the associated underlying disorder.

IMAGING FINDINGS

Amyloidosis demonstrates a wide spectrum of imaging findings because a variety of systems, including the musculoskeletal, genitourinary, gastrointestinal, and cardiovascular systems, may be involved.[48,116]

Osteonecrosis may develop from vessel occlusion after amyloid accumulation around capillaries and endothelial cells of larger blood vessels. Other findings include osteolytic bone destruction, periarticular joint swelling, osteoporosis, pathologic vertebral fractures, joint subluxations (e.g., proximal femur and humerus), and coarse trabeculae. Calcification may be seen in the amyloid deposits.

CLINICAL COMMENTS

The clinical presentation depends on which systems are involved. Amyloid deposits in the heart produce pleural effusion and dyspnea. Gastrointestinal involvement is associated with bowel obstruction and malabsorption. Localized amyloid deposits in the upper respiratory system may cause hoarseness and dysphagia. Definitive diagnosis requires biopsy confirmation; imaging studies are nonspecific.

KEY CONCEPTS

- Amyloidosis results from localized or systemic protein deposits, known to involve a variety of systems.
- It occurs as a primary disease or secondary to multiple myeloma, rheumatoid arthritis, Crohn's disease, and other systemic disorders.
- Associated bone changes include osteonecrosis, osteolytic destruction, periarticular joint swelling, and pathologic vertebral collapse.

Dermatomyositis

BACKGROUND

Inflammatory myopathies represent a group of disorders involving chronic inflammation, weakness, and wasting of skeletal muscle tissue. Inflammatory cells surround and destroy muscle fibers by a probable autoimmune-mediated mechanism.[86] Dermatomyositis, polymyositis, juvenile myositis, and inclusion body myositis all represent inflammatory myopathies.[85]

Dermatomyositis represents chronic inflammation of the skeletal muscle and skin, affecting 5 out of every 10,000 people. It is the most easily recognized inflammatory myopathy resulting from the presence of a distinctive reddish rash occurring over the eyelids, cheeks, and nose. It occurs in all ages but is most common in adult women. Dermatomyositis is more common in children than are other myopathies. It is associated in adults with an elevated incidence of visceral carcinomas that increases with age.[6,103,104]

IMAGING FINDINGS

The presence of subcutaneous calcifications is the most striking radiographic feature of dermatomyositis. Subcutaneous calcifications appear most commonly as linear or curvilinear radiodensities around the knees, elbows, and fingers (Fig. 15-1). Widespread calcifications (calcinosis universalis) develop in a few cases, severely limiting mobility. Calcification of intramuscular septa occurs in the deep muscles of the proximal limbs.

Dermatomyositis is associated with arthritis primarily in the small joints of the hands, appearing with misalignment and juxtaarticular osteoporosis and soft-tissue swelling. Particularly characteristic is the "floppy thumb" sign, indicating subluxation of the interphalangeal joint of the first digit. A diffuse interstitial pattern is often present on the chest radiograph.

Magnetic resonance imaging (MRI) is helpful in localizing focal inflammatory myopathy, muscle atrophy, and fatty replacement of muscle.[87] MRI signal intensity correlates to the activity and distribution of the disease processes.

CLINICAL COMMENTS

Dermatomyositis often is not immediately painful; it may become noticeable only after muscle weakness and atrophy occur. The weakness may interfere with basic movements such as walking and raising arms. The diagnosis is made after an analysis of blood enzyme levels, electromyography, and muscle biopsy.

Steroids (e.g., prednisone) and immunosuppressive drugs (e.g., azathioprine) are given in an attempt to limit inflammation.[41] Passive range of motion and ice are indicated during acute exacerbations. Moderate exercise is advocated beyond the initial inflammatory stages. Muscle stretching appears to limit limb contracture.

The course of the disease is extremely variable, with some rapidly progressing to muscle wasting and weakness in just days, whereas others take years to progress to this stage. Disease complications include acute renal failure and malignancy.

KEY CONCEPTS

- *Dermatomyositis is a chronic inflammation of the skeletal muscle and skin, probably an autoimmune mechanism.*
- *Malignancy occurs with a higher incidence in adults. Dermatomyositis occurs in people of all ages but is most common in adult women.*
- *Dermatomyositis presents as a reddish rash occurring over the eyelids, cheeks, and nose.*
- *Linear or curvilinear subcutaneous calcifications may be found, primarily around the knees, elbows, and fingers.*
- *Misalignment, effusion, and osteoporosis of small joints of the hand accompany this disease.*
- *Standard treatment entails steroids, immunosuppressive drugs, passive range of motion, moderate exercise, and muscle stretching.*

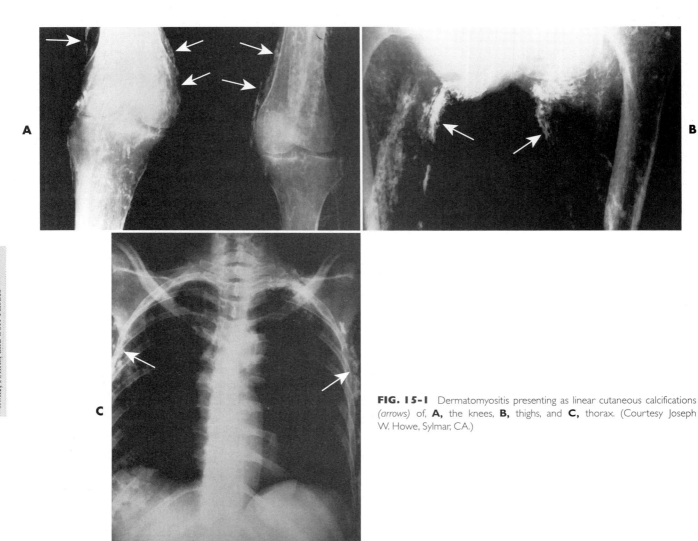

FIG. 15-1 Dermatomyositis presenting as linear cutaneous calcifications *(arrows)* of, **A,** the knees, **B,** thighs, and **C,** thorax. (Courtesy Joseph W. Howe, Sylmar, CA.)

Gaucher's Disease

BACKGROUND

Gaucher's disease is a lipid storage disorder resulting from a genetic deficiency of the enzyme glucocerebrosidase (glucosylceramidase), resulting in glucocerebroside accumulations within the cells of the reticuloendothelial system.[78] Gaucher's disease is the most common hereditary metabolic storage disorder.[15]

The disease may develop in individuals of any age, but it is more severe in children and especially infants. A higher incidence of the disease is seen in individuals who have Ashkenazi ancestry.[15]

IMAGING FINDINGS

Accumulations of glucocerebroside may suppress bone marrow activity and cause destructive bone lesions and enlargement of the liver, spleen, and lymph nodes. The distal femur may exhibit thinned cortex and bone expansion ("Erlenmeyer flask" deformity). Single or multiple osteolytic lesions may occur and mimic the presentation of an infection or neoplasm (Fig. 15-2). Osteonecrosis may result from vascular occlusion, which follows the increase in the reticulum component of bone marrow (Fig. 15-3). The femoral head, humeral head, and wrist are particularly susceptible. Similar changes may produce H-shaped vertebrae at multiple levels (Fig. 15-4). MRI is useful to assess the extent and activity of bone marrow involvement (Fig. 15-5).[10,55]

CLINICAL COMMENTS

The clinical presentation of Gaucher's disease is divided into three forms based on phenotype.[15] All three types are marked by hepatosplenomegaly and the presence of Gaucher's cells in the bone marrow. Bone changes are more apparent in the chronic forms of the disease. The disease is more severe in infants because of cerebroside accumulations in neurons. All patients are predisposed to

osteomyelitis. Intravenous infusion of glucocerebrosidase is an effective therapy but its application is limited because of its cost.[81]

KEY CONCEPTS

- *Gaucher's disease is a lipid storage disorder resulting from a genetic deficiency of the enzyme glucocerebrosidase; it is rare.*
- *Findings include anemia, hepatosplenomegaly, Erlenmeyer flask deformity, solitary or multiple osteolytic defects, osteonecrosis (usually femoral head), and H-shaped vertebrae.*

Heavy Metal Poisoning

BACKGROUND

Poisoning may develop from the injection, implantation, ingestion, or inhalation of aluminum, bismuth, copper, lead, arsenic, phosphorus, mercury, or zinc. Lead is the most prevalent heavy metal, sometimes called the "silent epidemic." Lead accumulates in the body over time, affecting multiple systems but principally the brain. Exposure is highest among occupations associated with extracting and processing lead, and among children who live in dilapidated housing whose exposure is related to the ingestion of peeling paint (Fig. 15-6). Lead-contaminated dust and soil are other potential threats of exposure for children.[74]

IMAGING FINDINGS

The most striking radiographic feature of lead, phosphorus, copper, or bismuth heavy metal poisoning is the presence of transverse radiodense lines in the metaphyses of long bones, especially around the knee.[11,128] The density of the bands is similar to that of cortical bone. Similar lines are noted with treated rickets, scurvy, and congenital syphilis, but they may also represent a normal variant. Copper, zinc, and aluminum toxicity are associated with altered bone mineralization and osteopenia.

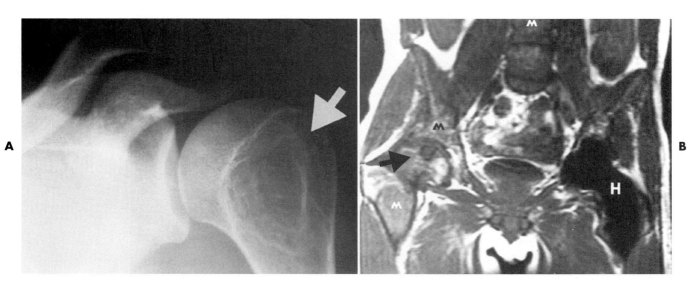

FIG. 15-2 Gaucher's disease. **A,** A lytic lesion in the proximal humerus *(arrow)* has resulted from a focal accumulation of lipid-laden cells. **B,** Coronal T1-weighted magnetic resonance imaging demonstrates diffuse low signal intensity, *M,* within the bone marrow, along with, *H,* osteonecrosis of the right femoral head *(arrow)* and contralateral hip replacement for the same process. The combination of findings is virtually diagnostic of the disease. (From Sartoris DJ: Musculoskeletal imaging: the requisites, St Louis, 1996, Mosby.)

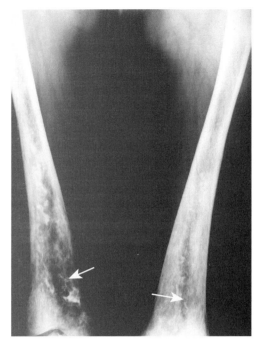

FIG. 15-3 Gaucher's disease. Marrow infarct of the distal femora appearing as serpiginous ca cifications in the distal femora *(arrows)*. (Courtesy Steven P. Brownstein, MD, Springfie d, NJ.)

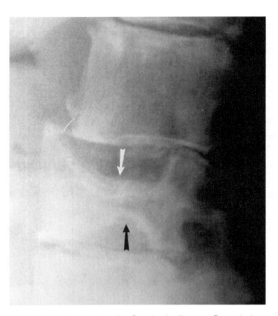

FIG. 15-4 H-shaped vertebra in Gaucher's disease. Central depression of the endplates *(arrows)* with sparing of the periphery is characteristic and occurs secondary to bone infarction. Differential diagnosis should include consideration of sickle-cell anemia and sickle-thalassemia. (From Sartoris DJ: Musculoskeletal imaging: the requisites, St Louis, 1996, Mosby.)

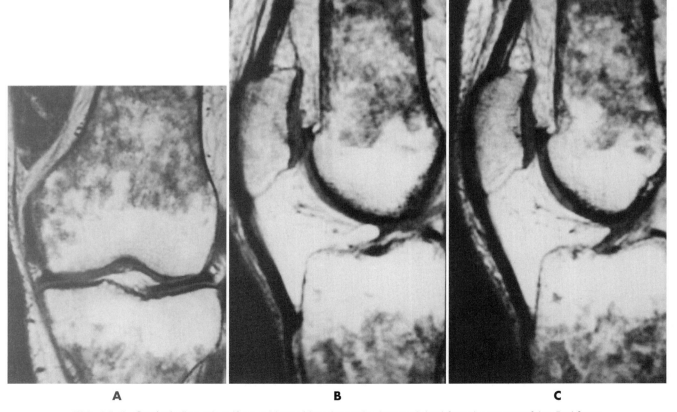

A   **B**   **C**

FIG. 15-5 Gaucher's disease in a 63-year-old man. Note the patchy decreased signal from the marrow of the distal femur and proximal tibia on, **A,** the coronal and, **B** and **C,** sagittal T1-weighted images. (From Firooznia H et al: MRI and CT of the musculoskeletal system, St Louis, 1992, Mosby.)

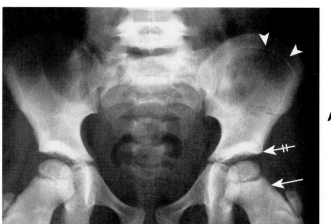

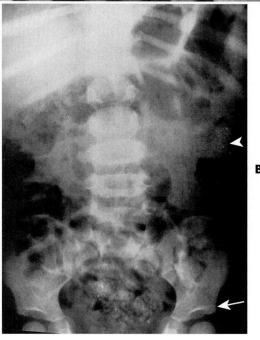

FIG. 15-6 Lead intoxication. **A,** Radiodense bands in the ilium *(arrowheads),* proximal metaphyses of the femora *(arrow),* acetabuli *(crossed arrow),* and L5 vertebra secondary to lead intoxication. **B,** Another case of lead intoxication demonstrating mild radiodense lines in the acetabuli *(arrow).* Observe the radiodense ingested lead fragments in the gastrointestinal tract of the left upper abdominal quadrant *(arrowhead).*

CLINICAL COMMENTS

Heavy metal poisoning is associated with a wide variety of nonspecific clinical findings, including anorexia, irritability, apathy, abdominal colic, vomiting, diarrhea, headaches, and convulsions. Toxic exposures damage the central nervous system, blood-forming organs, gastrointestinal tract, and other systems.[96,100]

KEY CONCEPTS

- *Lead, phosphorus, copper, and bismuth poisoning are associated with transverse, radiodense metaphyseal bands.*
- *Copper, zinc, and aluminum toxicity are associated with altered bone mineralization and osteopenia.*

Histiocytosis

BACKGROUND

Langerhans cell histiocytosis, formerly known as "histiocytosis X," is the abnormal proliferation of histiocytes resulting in focal or systemic manifestations. Although the true etiology is not known, the prevailing opinion is that Langerhans histiocytosis represents a reactive rather than a neoplastic process.[126] Recently a better understanding of the disease has resulted from advances in specialized imaging and the development of immunohistochemical, morphologic, and clinical standards of diagnosis.[38]

Langerhans cell histiocytosis describes three clinical syndromes: eosinophilic granuloma (60% to 80% of cases), Hand-Schüller-Christian disease (15% to 40% of cases), and Letterer-Siwe disease (10% of cases). Eosinophilic granuloma is the least aggressive form, usually seen in patients between the ages of 5 and 15 years.

Hand-Schüller-Christian disease is the chronic disseminated variety, characterized by multifocal bone lesions and extraskeletal involvement of the reticuloendothelial system. Typically it is seen in children between the ages of 1 and 5 years. Uncommonly (in 10% of cases) a clinical triad of exophthalmus, diabetes insipidus, and lytic skull lesions is present.

Letterer-Siwe disease represents an acute, disseminated, fulminant variety of the disease, seen in children younger than 2 years of age. Its aggressive clinical presentation may mimic leukemia. Most cases are fatal.

IMAGING FINDINGS

The osseous lesions of eosinophilic granuloma, Hand-Schüller-Christian, and Letterer-Siwe diseases are very similar. They appear as one or more medullary-based, lytic lesions with geographic destruction (Figs. 15-7 and 15-8), lobular contour, endosteal scalloping (Fig. 15-9), periosteal reaction (long bone lesions only) (Fig. 15-10), and well-defined, uneven, or beveled margins.[42] Matrix calcification and subarticular extension are not characteristic.[42] Alternatively, sclerotic lesions with or without periosteal reactions may occur.

Overall, more than 50% of osseous lesions occur in the flat bones of the skull, pelvis, and ribs; about 30% of lesions occur in long bones (Fig. 15-11).[114] Spinal involvement usually spares the vertebral arch and may lead to advanced vertebral collapse (vertebral plana). As the lesions heal, the diminished vertebral height may reconstitute (Fig. 15-12). Soft-tissue masses may occur, representing extension from adjacent bone marrow involvement.[58] Advanced bony destruction of the mandible produces an isolated, "floating" appearance of the teeth. Pulmonary manifestation of eosinophilic granuloma includes a reticulonodular pattern of the middle and upper lung zones, often progressing to honeycomb lung.

Osseous lesions occurring with Letterer-Siwe disease typically are limited to the skull, often appearing as widespread and multiple osteolytic lesions. Eosinophilic granuloma typically presents as a solitary lesion and involves the appendicular skeleton more often than Letterer-Siwe or Hand-Schüller-Christian disease. Each of the three types, especially Letterer-Siwe, may appear permeative with widespread bone destruction, mimicking findings of leukemia, Ewing's sarcoma, or infection. In general, Langerhans histiocytosis has such a variable appearance that it should be considered in every destructive bone lesion that appears in patients younger than 30 years of age.

Although radionuclide scintigraphy is more sensitive than radiographic skeletal surveys in detecting histiocytic lesions in the

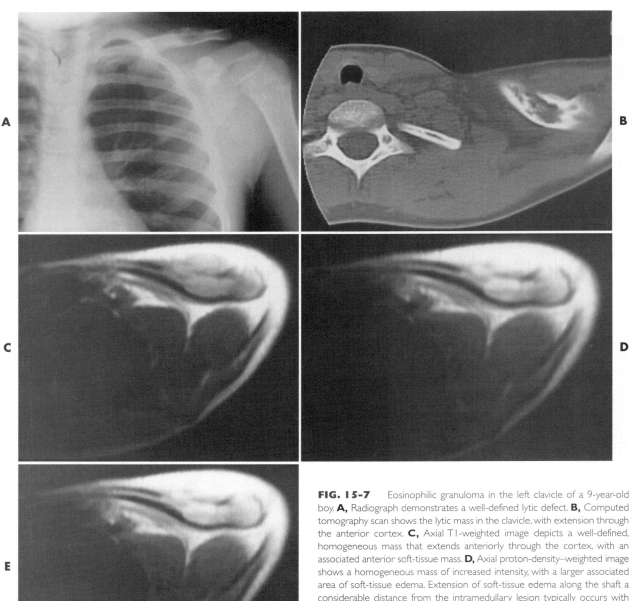

FIG. 15-7   Eosinophilic granuloma in the left clavicle of a 9-year-old boy. **A,** Radiograph demonstrates a well-defined lytic defect. **B,** Computed tomography scan shows the lytic mass in the clavicle, with extension through the anterior cortex. **C,** Axial T1-weighted image depicts a well-defined, homogeneous mass that extends anteriorly through the cortex, with an associated anterior soft-tissue mass. **D,** Axial proton-density–weighted image shows a homogeneous mass of increased intensity, with a larger associated area of soft-tissue edema. Extension of soft-tissue edema along the shaft a considerable distance from the intramedullary lesion typically occurs with eosinophilic granuloma. **E,** The lesion brightens on the T2-weighted axial image. (From Stark DD, Gradley WG: Magnetic resonance imaging, ed 3, St Louis, 1999, Mosby.)

spine, pelvis, and ribs, it is less sensitive in identifying lesions in the skull.[35]

CLINICAL COMMENTS

Pain, fever, elevated erythrocyte sedimentation rate, progressive anemia, hepatosplenomegaly, lymphadenopathy, and diabetes insipidus may be present.[33] The clinical presentation may mimic an infection. Overall, the prognosis of Langerhans cell histiocytosis is excellent in children with either localized or multifocal disease occurring in the absence of organ dysfunction, chronic disease, new-onset pituitary involvement, or long-term pulmonary fibrosis.[1,76]

Current therapeutic approaches involve chemotherapies, immunosuppressives, bone marrow transplant, and gene therapy.[1]

KEY CONCEPTS

- *Langerhans cell histiocytosis is marked by an abnormal proliferation of histiocytes.*
- *Langerhans cell histiocytosis lesions demonstrate a wide variety of osseous presentations and should be considered as a diagnostic differential in every destructive bone lesion occurring in patients younger than 30 years of age.*

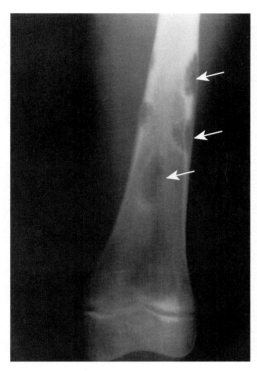

FIG. 15-8 Several well-defined osteolytic regions secondary to eosinophilic granuloma *(arrows)*. (Courtesy Joseph W. Howe, Sylmar, CA.)

- *Letterer-Siwe disease, which occurs in 10% of these cases, is the acute disseminated variety occurring in children younger than 2 years of age. Osseous lesions usually consist of multiple lytic skull lesions.*
- *Hand-Schüller-Christian disease, which occurs in 15% to 40% of these cases, is the chronic disseminated variety occurring in children between 1 and 5 years of age. Osseous lesions typically are multiple geographic osteolytic lesions, occurring in the skull, pelvis, and long bones.*
- *Eosinophilic granuloma (which occurs in 60% to 80% of cases) is the least aggressive form, usually seen in patients between the ages of 5 and 15 years. Osseous lesions usually are solitary geographic osteolytic lesions, occurring in the skull, pelvis, long bones, mandible, and spine.*

Hypertrophic Osteoarthropathy

BACKGROUND

Hypertrophic osteoarthropathy describes a primary (pachydermoperiostosis or Touraine-Solente-Golé syndrome) or secondary (Pierre-Marie-Bamberger syndrome) disorder accompanied by digital clubbing, painful swollen joints, and a symmetric, undulated, periosteal reaction.[9,72] All features of the disorder may not be present. Although the etiology remains elusive, vascular flow, vascular endothelium, and platelet-derived growth factors have all been implicated.[32,63,71] The primary form is less common (occurring in 3% to 5% of cases), has an adolescent onset and a predominance for males and blacks, and is associated with a thickened appearance of the skin of the face and scalp.

Secondary hypertrophic osteoarthropathy is associated with bronchogenic carcinoma (which occurs in up to 12% of cases),[125] pulmonary abscess, pulmonary metastasis, Hodgkin disease,[89] emphysema, cystic fibrosis, heart disease, and occasionally in other acute and chronic disorders.[21,111] Lesions of the abdominal cavity (e.g., dysentery, Crohn's disease, biliary atresia) may produce secondary hypertrophic osteoarthropathy; however, intrathoracic causes predominate, especially bronchogenic carcinoma. The age of onset is related to the underlying pathology.

IMAGING FINDINGS

The radiographic features of primary and secondary hypertropic osteoarthropathy are similar. Both are marked by periosteal reaction occurring most commonly in the tubular bones of the extremities, especially the tibia, fibula, radius, and ulna. Less commonly the wrist, ankle, and small bones of the hands and feet are involved. The periosteal reaction is nonaggressive, thick, and widespread, occurring in the diaphysis and metaphysis (Fig. 15-13). The thickness of the periosteal reaction may increase proportionally to the duration of the disease.

The differences between the primary and secondary forms are that the periosteal reaction occurring in patients with primary hypertrophic osteoarthropathy involves the epiphyses (secondary does not) and appears more "fluffy," "shaggy," or less well defined than does the reaction associated with secondary osteoarthropathy. Ligamentous calcifications and bony excrescences are features of primary hypertrophic osteoarthropathy, often involving the calcaneus, patella, and interosseous membrane between the radius and ulna.

Traditionally the diagnosis of hypertrophic osteoarthropathy has been made on plain film radiographs. However, radionuclide bone scintigraphy provides a sensitive method of detection that correlates well to the clinical presentation.[12,26]

CLINICAL COMMENTS

The clinical onset of primary hypertrophic osteoarthropathy is insidious, marked by clubbing of the distal hands and feet. The skin of the face and scalp appears thickened (pachydermia). The clinical presentation of secondary osteoarthropathy is similar but also is dependent on the underlying condition. A clinical presentation of vague bone pain and joint swelling occurs more commonly in the secondary form of the disease. The primary form usually is self-limiting after many years of involvement.

KEY CONCEPTS

- *Primary hypertrophic osteoarthropathy is marked by a solid, thick, shaggy periosteal reaction involving the epiphysis, metaphysis, and diaphysis of the tibia, fibula, radius, and ulna. Clubbing of the fingers, ligamentous calcification, and skin changes of the scalp and face are noted.*
- *Secondary hypertrophic osteoarthropathy occurs secondary to underlying disease (usually bronchogenic tumor) and demonstrates a solid, thick, well-defined periosteal reaction involving the metaphysis and diaphysis of the tibia, fibula, radius, and ulna. Clubbing of the fingers and joint swelling are common clinical features.*

PART TWO Bone, Joints, and Soft Tissues

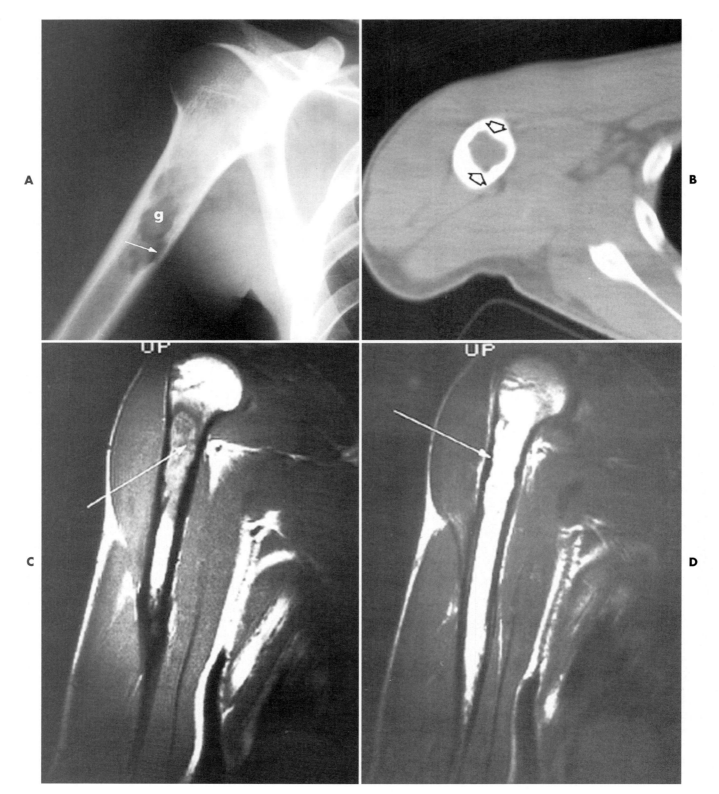

FIG. 15-9 Eosinophilic granuloma. **A,** Radiography demonstrates, *g,* a well-defined lytic lesion in the proximal humeral diaphysis with endosteal scalloping *(arrow).* **B,** Computed tomography documents endosteal erosion *(arrows)* to better advantage. **C,** Coronal T1-weighted magnetic resonance image reveals predominantly low signal intensity *(arrow)* within the lesion. **D,** The lesion exhibits high signal intensity *(arrow)* on a corresponding T2-weighted image. Differential diagnosis should include consideration of fibrous dysplasia, plasmacytoma, metastatic disease, and indolent infection. (From Sartoris DJ: *Musculoskeletal imaging: the requisites,* St Louis, 1996, Mosby.)

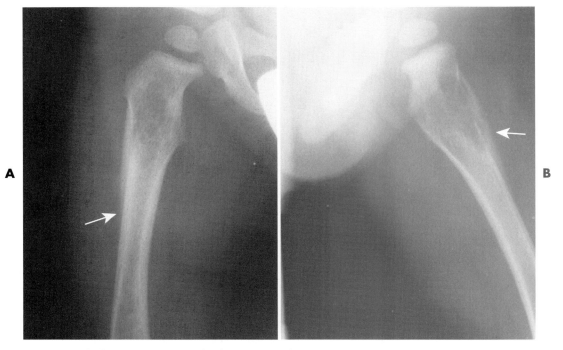

FIG. 15-10 **A,** Anteroposterior and, **B,** frog-leg projections of an aggressive osteolytic lesion in the proximal femur resulting from eosinophilic granuloma. Also noted is parallel periostitis of the lateral femur *(arrows)*. (Courtesy Joseph W. Howe, Sylmar, CA.)

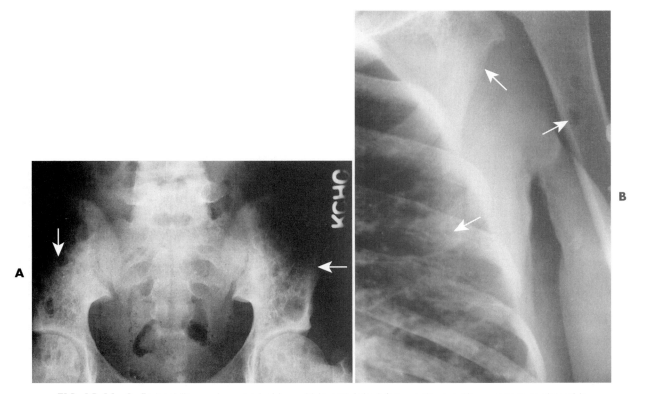

FIG. 15-11 **A,** Eosinophilic granuloma marked by multiple osteolytic defects causing a cystic appearance to the pelvis *(arrows)*. **B,** The same patient exhibits two well-defined osteolytic changes in the proximal humerus, ribs, and scapula *(arrows)*. (Courtesy Steven P. Brownstein, MD, Springfield, NJ.)

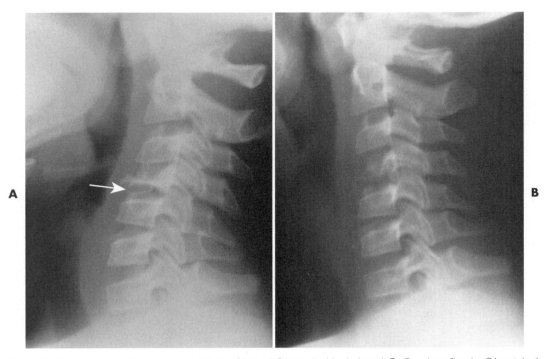

FIG. 15-12   A, Eosinophilic granuloma leading to flattened C4 vertebral body *(arrow)*. **B,** On a later film, the C4 vertebral body has partially reconstituted. (Courtesy Steven P. Brownstein, MD, Springfield, NJ.)

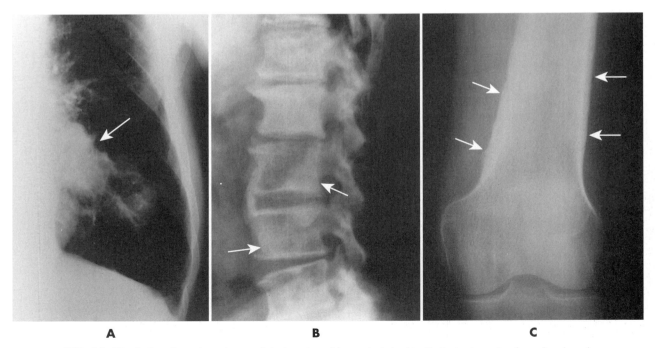

FIG. 15-13   A, Bronchogenic carcinoma of the lung *(arrow)* has metastasized to, **B,** the lumbar spine *(arrows)* and manifested with hypertrophic osteoarthropathy by producing thick periostitis along, **C,** the distal femora *(arrows)*. (Courtesy Joseph W. Howe, Sylmar, CA.)

Infantile Cortical Hyperostosis

BACKGROUND

Infantile cortical hyperostosis (Caffey's disease, Caffey's-Silverman syndrome) is an uncommon familial or sporadic syndrome marked by subperiosteal bone formation. The etiology is unknown, and it usually manifests before 6 months of age, with equal incidence in males and females.[7,45,62]

IMAGING FINDINGS

The radiographic features include a symmetric, thick periosteal reaction most commonly involving the mandible (80% of cases), clavicle, ulna, and less commonly the ribs, scapulae, calvarium, or diaphysis of tubular bones (Fig. 15-14).[45] Although the mandible is the most commonly affected bone in the sporadic form, the tibia is the predominant bone affected in patients with the familial form.[14]

Physiologic periostitis is a much more common cause of periosteal reaction in infants younger than 6 months of age. A similar appearance may occur in rickets and scurvy but rarely before 6 months of age, and each demonstrates additional metaphyseal findings. Pleural effusion may accompany rib involvement. Radionuclide scintigraphy may be useful to further delineate the extent of skeletal involvement. MRI is useful to assess the presence and extent of subperiosteal hemorrhage.[102]

CLINICAL COMMENTS

The clinical manifestation is marked by fever, hyperirritability, soft-tissue swelling over the involved bone, and often an elevated erythrocyte sedimentation rate. On palpation, the masses of involved bone and soft-tissue swelling are hard and painful. The clinical course is typically self-limiting within a few months.[14]

KEY CONCEPTS

- *Infantile cortical hyperostosis occurs before 6 months of age.*
- *Fever, hyperirritability, and painful soft-tissue swelling over affected bones are clinical symptoms.*
- *This disease most commonly involves the mandible and clavicle.*

Mastocytosis

BACKGROUND

Mastocytosis is a term used collectively to describe a heterogeneous group of disorders all characterized by an abnormal proliferation and accumulation of mast cells in various tissues and organs.[112,121] The etiology is largely unknown, but limited evidence points to an abnormality of stem cell factor receptors.[44] Mastocytosis usually is limited to the skin (90% of cases), but rarely it may become systemic, involving primarily the bone marrow and gastrointestinal tract.[30,44,49] Systemic disease usually manifests in adults, although a pediatric form of systemic disease exists.[64] Men and women are affected equally.

IMAGING FINDINGS

The radiographic appearance of systemic mastocytosis is variable. Histamine and heparin released from the mast cells may produce generalized osteopenia similar to osteoporosis.[28,59] Localized osteopenic or osteolytic defects are observed less commonly. The osteolytic lesions occur most often in the ribs, skull, and long tubular bones. Mast cell proliferation and infiltration may cause reactive sclerosis of the host bone, producing multiple osteosclerotic foci. The osteosclerotic lesions are more common in the axial skeleton and may be accompanied by thickened trabeculae. The osteolytic and osteosclerotic regions often coexist (Fig. 15-15). Radionuclide bone scintigraphy may be helpful to determine the full extent of skeletal involvement.

CLINICAL COMMENTS

Systemic mastocytosis comprises a wide spectrum of clinical features, depending on the organs involved, age of onset, and associated hematologic diseases.[44] Clinical features are related to the release of mast-cell–derived mediators (e.g., heparin, histamine, platelet-activating factor, prostaglandin, peptide leukotrienes) and include vomiting, flushing, diarrhea, hepatosplenomegaly, weight loss, and skin lesions.[91] Treatment is directed toward symptom relief and the prognosis is dependent on the extent of involvement.

KEY CONCEPTS

- *Mastocytosis involves the rare proliferation of mast cells, typically affecting adults.*
- *This disease involves general or local osteopenia, local osteosclerosis, or a mixed pattern of presentation.*
- *The clinical symptoms of mastocytosis are vomiting, flushing, weight loss, and diarrhea.*

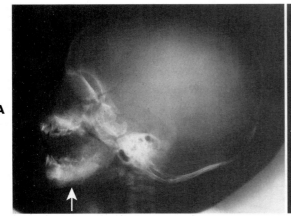
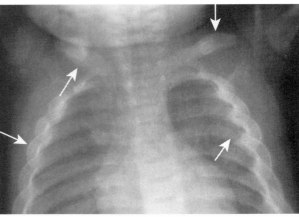

FIG. 15-14 Infantile cortical hyperostosis (Caffey's disease) presenting with bilaterally symmetric thick periostitis *(arrows)* of, **A,** the mandible clavicles and, **B,** ribs. (Courtesy Ian D. McLean, Davenport, IA.)

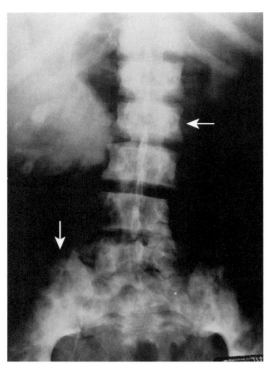

FIG. 15-15 Mastocytosis causing increased radiodensity and a mottled appearance *(arrows)* in the lumbar spine and pelvis. (Courtesy Steven P. Brownstein, MD, Springfield, NJ.)

Neurofibromatosis

BACKGROUND

Neurofibromatosis is the most common of a heterogeneous group of diseases known as *phakomatoses*. Phakomatoses are disorders of embryologic neuroectoderm tissue derivatives and are characterized by hamartomas of various tissues. Other phakomatoses include Lindau disease, Sturge-Weber syndrome, and tuberous sclerosis.

Neurofibromatosis is a genetic disorder affecting primarily the cell growth of neural tissue.[80] At least eight presentations of the disease exist; however, only two are widely recognized: neurofibromatosis type I (von Recklinghausen's disease, peripheral neurofibromatosis, or NF-1) and neurofibromatosis type II (central neurofibromatosis, or NF-2).[109] Both types have an autosomal dominant pattern of inheritance, no sexual or racial predilection, and are marked by nerve sheath tumors. Each appears to be influenced by hormones, and women may notice exacerbations during pregnancy. Other than these common points, the two types appear very different clinically and reflect defects of two different genes (chromosome 17 in NF-1 and chromosome 22 in NF-2).

Neurofibromatosis type I. NF-1 is the most common form of the disorder, affecting approximately 1 in 4000 individuals.[80] It is diagnosed when at least two of the following criteria are present:

1. Six or more cutaneous macules (café-au-lait spots), larger than 5 mm before puberty, larger than 15 mm after puberty
2. Two or more neurofibromas
3. One or more plexiform neurofibromas
4. Axillary or inguinal flecking
5. Optic gliomas
6. Two or more iris hamartomas (Lisch nodules)

7. One or more characteristic bone lesions
8. First-degree relative (parent, child, or sibling) with the disease[81]

NF-1 is associated with a variety of intracranial hamartomatous and neoplastic lesions of the white matter and globus pallidus, including optic nerve and parenchymal gliomas.[88] Those afflicted exhibit characteristic nonelevated brownish cutaneous hyperpigmentations, known as *café-au-lait spots*. The hyperpigmentations exhibit smooth margins ("coast of California"), as opposed to the jagged margins ("coast of Maine") of similar hyperpigmentations that occur with polyostotic fibrous dysplasia. Other cutaneous lesions include the presence of multiple, widely dispersed soft nodules known as *fibroma molluscum*. In addition to the intracranial and cutaneous lesions, patients with NF-1 exhibit osseous defects of the skull, spine, and extremities, which are detailed under Imaging Findings.[51]

Neurofibromatosis type II. NF-2 is a much less common form of neurofibromatosis than NF-1, affecting 1 in 50,000 individuals.[80] It is diagnosed by the presence of bilateral acoustic schwannomas or a unilateral acoustic schwannoma occurring in a patient who has a first-degree relative (parent, child, or sibling) with the disease.[80] It is common for patients to develop unilateral acoustic schwannomas unrelated to neurofibromatosis. In addition to acoustic schwannomas, patients often develop schwannomas of other cranial nerves, and solitary or multiple meningiomas.[115] In contrast to NF-1, cutaneous and osseous changes are not characteristic of NF-2.

IMAGING FINDINGS

Plain film radiography offers little in the evaluation of the intracranial manifestations of NF-1 or NF-2, although many of the skeletal changes occurring with NF-1 are clearly seen on plain film radiography. Rarely an enlarged internal acoustic or optic canal may be seen, but these osseous changes always are delineated better with computed tomography (CT). MRI offers superb imaging of intracranial and spinal lesions (Fig. 15-16). Patients with NF-1 often show hyperintense foci in the areas of brain involvement on T2-weighted images. The intensity of these areas varies over serial studies. Neurofibromas often demonstrate a characteristic pattern of peripheral hyperintensity and central hypointensity on T2-weighted images (target sign). The intracranial lesions of NF-2 (acoustic schwannomas and less frequently associated meningiomas) also are imaged best by MRI. On MRI film, schwannomas are hypointense or isointense relative to brain parenchyma on T1-weighted scans, are hyperintense on T2-weighted scans, and enhance after gadolinium.[95]

Skull. Congenital deficiency of the greater and lesser wing of the sphenoid and posterosuperior orbital wall creates a "bare orbit" appearance (Fig. 15-17). This abnormality allows the temporal lobe of the brain to directly contact the soft tissues around the eye, producing pulsatile exophthalmus.[20] Other changes include a radiolucent cranial defect at the lambdoidal suture (asterion defect) just posterior to the junction of the parietomastoid and occipitomastoid sutures (Fig. 15-18). This defect is more common on the left side and may be associated with ipsilateral hypoplasia of the mastoid. Enlargement of cranial foramen may be present, especially of the optic and internal auditory canals. Enlargement of the entire skull (macrocranium) is a common and prominent feature in up to 75% of individuals. An additional finding may be the presence of scattered calcifications over the temporal lobe similar to those that occur in the choroid plexus.[130]

Spine. The spine is affected commonly.[67,129] Kyphoscoliosis is seen in 50% of patients and is marked by a short segment; angular, progressive curvature most often occurs in the thoracic spine.

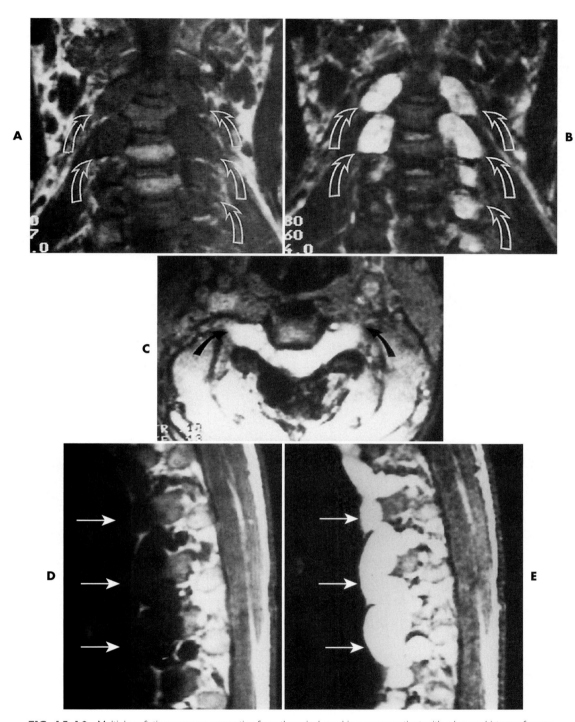

FIG. 15-16 Multiple soft-tissue masses emanating from the spinal canal in a young patient with a known history of neurofibromatosis. **A,** A T1-weighted coronal image through the cervical spine shows that the masses are both intradural and extradural *(arrows)*. **B,** A T2-weighted image through the same region demonstrates increased signal within the lesions. Some have ill-defined areas of decreased signal, characteristic of neurofibromas *(arrows)*. **C,** A 10-degree FISP gradient echo (fast imaging with steady-state precession) image shows widening of the cervical neural foramina by the high-signal lesions *(arrows)*. **D,** A T1-weighted parasagittal image through the thoracic spine reveals multiple septate cavities just lateral to the canal *(arrows)*. **E,** Homogeneously increased signal consistent with a thoracic meningocele *(arrows)*.

Continued

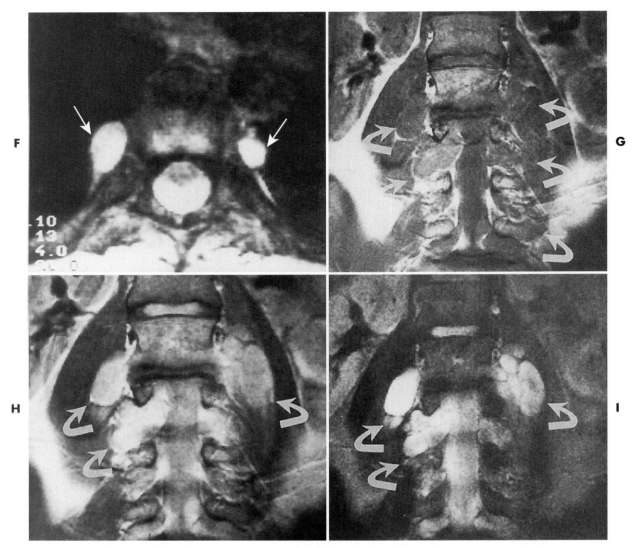

FIG. 15-16 cont'd   F, The 10-degree gradient echo axial study again shows the lateral meningocele *(arrows).* **G,** A T1-weighted coronal image through the lumbar spine demonstrates multiple intradural and extradural "dumbbell" neurofibromas that have the signal intensity of soft tissue *(arrows).* **H,** A proton-density–weighted coronal scan through the lumbar spine shows the dumbbell shape of the neurofibromas, which now are of increased signal intensity *(arrows).* **I,** A T2-weighted coronal scan through the lumbar spine reveals the high-signal neurofibromas, some of which have a lower signal intensity within *(arrows).* (From Modic et al: Magnetic resonance imaging of the spine, St Louis, 1994, Mosby.)

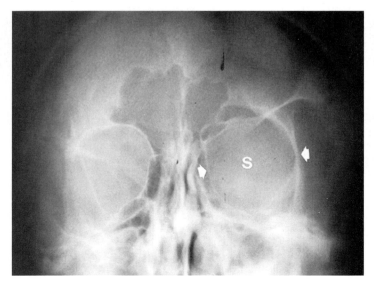

FIG. 15-17   Unilateral absence of the sphenoid wing *(s)* with orbital enlargement *(arrows)* in neurofibromatosis. The findings are virtually specific for this condition and occur secondary to mesodermal dysplasia. (From Sartoris DJ: Musculoskeletal imaging: the requisites, St Louis, 1996, Mosby.)

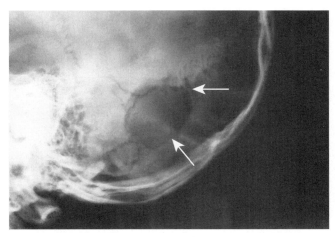

FIG. 15-18 Neurofibromatosis with lambdoidal suture (asterion) defect *(arrows).*

The kyphoscoliosis may lead to paraplegia. Scalloping of the posterocentral portion of the vertebral body is related to dural ectasia. Neurofibromas of the exiting nerve roots may cause scalloping defects of the posterior vertebral body and other borders of the corresponding intervertebral foramen (Figs. 15-19 to 15-23). Large scalloped osseous defects and paraspinal masses occur with intrathoracic meningoceles, which represent lateral protrusions of the spinal canal's meninges into the extrapleural space.

Ribs. Ribs may appear irregular, twisted, ribbonlike, or eroded. These changes are related to either adjacent intercostal neurofibromas or mesodermal dysplasia.

Extremities. Osseous dysplasia of the long bones (Fig. 15-24) manifests as bowing deformity and thin cortices, with or without pseudofractures of the convex cortex. Pseudoarthrosis of long bones results from loose periosteum and poor callus response after pathologic fracture. Bowing deformity and pseudoarthrosis most often involve the tibia. A peculiar feature of the disease is focal giantism involving a single bone or the entire extremity. Occasionally multiple cystic bone defects, thought to represent nonossifying fibromas, are encountered.

CLINICAL COMMENTS

A suspected diagnosis of NF-1 should be accompanied by a review of the patient's history for the following: psychomotor deficits, pain, vision problems, progressive neurologic deficits, and constipation.[80] A review of family history for other afflicted patients is important.

Further manifestations of NF-1 (e.g., eye, central nervous system, peripheral nervous system, bone) should be evaluated with plain film radiography, MRI, appropriate laboratory tests, and consultation with a specialist. Therapeutic options include surgical intervention, chemotherapy, and radiation therapy. All are used sparingly. The prognosis of the disease is poorly defined and may include serious complications (e.g., disfigurement, language disorders, hypertension, malignancies) in some individuals. The associated hypertension type usually is "essential," but renal artery stenosis and pheochromocytoma should be excluded. Leukemia and lymphoma are more common in children with NF-1.[113] Most patients with NF-1 have normal intelligence, although about half experience some degree of learning disability.[110]

A suspected diagnosis of NF-2 warrants a review of the patient's history for dizziness, headaches, tinnitus, loss of balance, seizures, and hearing loss.[80] Again, the family history is important, and physical examination should include a detailed neurologic assessment of the eighth cranial nerve. Audiograms and tests

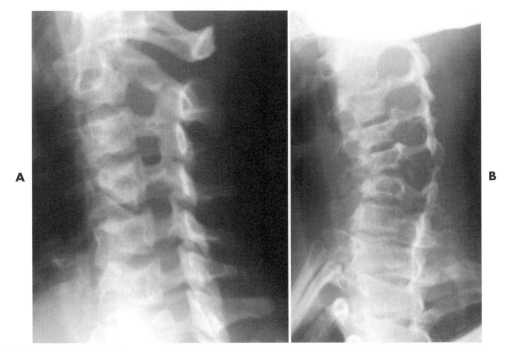

FIG. 15-19 A, Normal oblique projection demonstrating the normal appearance of the cervical intervertebral foramen. **B,** Case of neurofibromatosis presenting with enlargement of the cervical intervertebral foramen resulting from pressure erosions of the neurofibromas contained within the foramen. One or more levels of enlarged intervertebral foramen are typical of the disease.

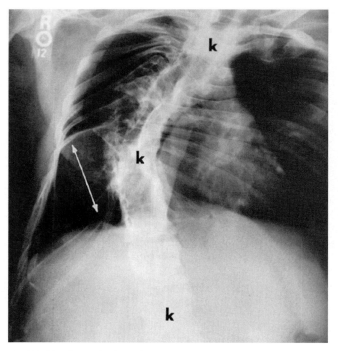

FIG. 15-20 Severe kyphoscoliosis, *k*, with associated rib deformities *(arrows)* in neurofibromatosis. Although this is the most common musculoskeletal manifestation of the disease, the differential diagnosis should include consideration of idiopathic scoliosis, Marfan's syndrome, Ehlers-Danlos syndrome, spondyloepiphyseal and spondylometaphyseal dysplasias, and a large number of other congenital malformation syndromes. (From Sartoris DJ: Musculoskeletal imaging: the requisites, St Louis, 1996, Mosby.)

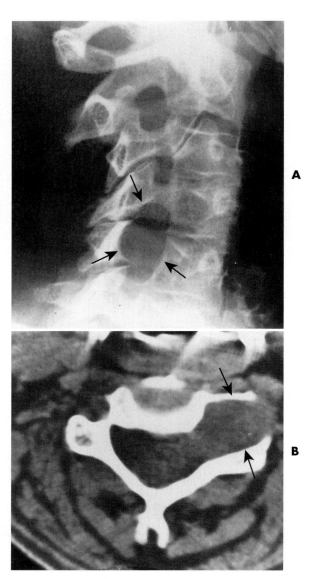

FIG. 15-21 **A,** Oblique radiograph demonstrating an enlarged C4-5 and C5-6 left intervertebral foramen with complete destruction of the C5 pedicle and posterior scalloping of the vertebral body of C4 and C5 *(arrows)* caused by, **B,** a solitary neurofibroma noted on computed tomography *(arrows)*. (Courtesy Ian D. McLean, Davenport, IA.)

of vestibular function commonly are applied. Patients often experience total loss of hearing and marked balance disturbance as the disease progresses. Therapeutics includes surgery, stereotactic radiation therapy, and hearing augmentation with mechanical aids.

KEY CONCEPTS

- *Neurofibromatosis is the most common of four diseases collectively known as phakomatoses.*
- *One of the most common genetic diseases, neurofibromatosis has no sexual or racial predilection.*
- *Two widely recognized types include neurofibromatosis type I (von Recklinghausen's disease) and neurofibromatosis type II (central neurofibromatosis).*
- *Neurofibromatosis type I manifests as changes in the nervous system (optic nerve gliomas, neurofibromas of the spinal and peripheral nerves), skin (café-au-lait spots, fibroma molluscum), and bones (erosions of vertebrae and ribs; kyphoscoliosis; dysplasia of the sphenoid, ribs, and long bones; lambdoid suture defects).*
- *Neurofibromatosis type II is marked by bilateral acoustic schwannomas, often with one or more concurrent meningiomas.*
- *Magnetic resonance imaging offers the best imaging of the intracranial- and spine-related manifestations.*

Paget's Disease

BACKGROUND

In 1877 Sir James Paget's described the condition that now bears his name. Paget's disease (also known as *osteitis deformans*) is a relatively common familial disorder of osteoclasts characterized by abnormal remodeling, hypertrophy, and structure of bone, leading to pain and deformity.[65,75]

Determining the true incidence of Paget's disease is problematic, because many limited presentations of the disease go unnoticed resulting from of a lack of symptoms.[84] Autopsy studies have estimated the incidence at 3% of those over the age of 40 years, 10% of those over 80 years, and slightly more common in men.[24,37] The incidence decreases with decreasing age. Less than 4% of patients with Paget's disease are under the age of 40 years.[5] A rare disease of similar radiographic appearance occurs in childhood and has been termed *juvenile Paget's disease*. However, this disease results from hyperphosphatasia and does not share a similar pathogenesis with Paget's disease. Paget's disease is more common in England, Australia, New Zealand, and the northern United States and is rare in Asia, Africa, and Scandinavia.[4,31,107]

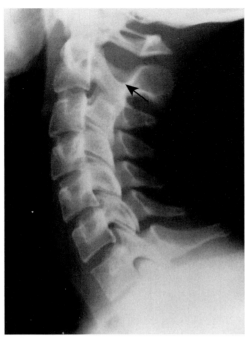

FIG. 15-22 Neurofibroma causing erosive defect of the vertebral arch of C2 *(arrow)*. (Courtesy Steven P. Brownstein, MD, Springfield, NJ.)

In Paget's disease, osteoclasts are morphologically abnormal and contain viral-like nuclear inclusions.[98] Pagetic osteoclasts are approximately five times their normal size, containing an average of 20 nuclei per cell, compared with the three or four nuclei of a normal, nonpagetic osteoclast. Although a viral etiology is widely suspected, it has not been confirmed. Osteoblasts are normal; however, the massive osteolysis propagated by the abnormal large osteoclasts leads to a matched response of bone formation.

Traditionally the pathophysiology of Paget's disease expresses as three phases of bone involvement: lytic, mixed, and blastic. At any one time, multiple phases may exist in the same patient and the rate of progression from one phase to the next is highly variable. The initial or osteolytic phase is marked by bone resorption secondary to increased osteoclastic activity. Osteoblastic activity increases in response, and the two opposing actions lead to concurrent bone formation and resorption, which characterizes the mixed phase of Paget's disease. The third or blastic phase occurs when the osteoclastic activity ceases and osteoblastic activity predominates. A quiescent period usually ensues after these actions. Pagetic bone is hypervascular (especially during the lytic phase), immature, disorganized, and structurally weak, leading to deformity and possibly pathologic fracture.

Uncommonly a locus of pagetic bone may transform into an osteosarcoma (in 50% of malignant cases), fibrosarcoma (in 25% of malignant cases), or chondrosarcoma (in 5% of malignant cases).[95] Malignant transformation (often termed the *fourth phase*) is noted in 1% to 3% of localized Paget's disease and 5% to 10% of generalized Paget's disease (Fig. 15-25).[53,95] Rarely giant cell tumors of the skull and facial bones are associated with Paget's disease.[8,13]

IMAGING FINDINGS

Paget's disease may involve any bone. It is typically localized to a bone or skeletal region and is of limited clinical consequence. Less commonly the disease is widespread, leading to extensive osseous deformity and clinical complications. Transformation from monostotic to polyostotic involvement is not inevitable.

Paget's disease has a predilection to involve the pelvis, sacrum, spine (especially lumbar), skull, and proximal femora. The characteristic radiographic features include osseous enlargement, osteosclerosis, cortical thickening, and thickened, prominent trabeculae (Figs. 15-26 through 15-35). Characteristic features occur at various skeletal regions.

Skull. The lytic phase of Paget's disease of the skull appears with a geographic destructive lesion termed *osteoporosis*

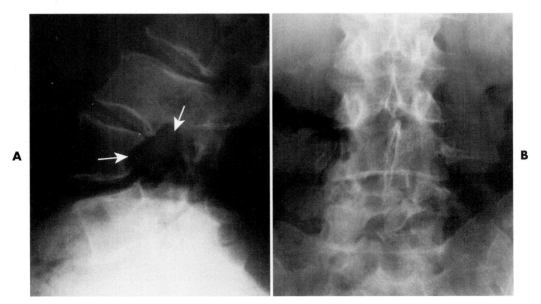

FIG. 15-23 A and **B,** Posterior vertebral scalloping, enlarged intervertebral foramen secondary to neurofibroma *(arrows).* (Courtesy Robert C. Tatum, Davenport, IA.)

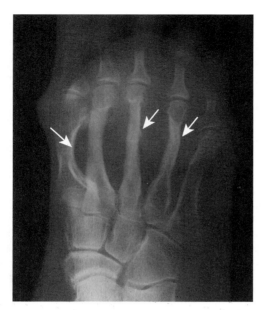

FIG. 15-24   Osseous irregularity and soft-tissue masses noted in a patient with neurofibromatosis *(arrows)*. (Courtesy Joseph W. Howe, Sylmar, CA.)

circumscripta. This lesion usually begins in the frontal or occipital regions. Mixed and blastic phases produce a "cotton wool" appearance resulting from focal osteosclerosis. Bone softening at the base of the skull often leads to basilar invagination.

Spine. Vertebral involvement is common (occurring in 75% of cases) and is marked by enlargement, endplate thickening ("picture frame"), and increased radiodensity ("ivory vertebrae") of the segments (Fig. 15-36 to 15-41). Bone softening develops biconcave vertebral body endplates. The weakened bone structure predisposes to compression fractures, although loss of vertebral height is more commonly the result of bone deformity than acute fracture.

Pelvis. Cortical thickening of the inner margin (arcuate line) of the ilium is the earliest finding of Paget's disease of the pelvis. The pelvis may appear asymmetric because of unilateral involvement with Paget's disease. Protrusio acetabuli may follow bone softening.

Extremities. Long bones are involved in about 30% of cases, most often the femur, tibia, and humerus. The hands and feet are rarely involved.[29] The earliest radiographic manifestation of long bone involvement begins as an oval, slanted, V-shaped, osteolytic defect in the subarticular region, which progresses through the length of bone ("flame," "V," "candle flame," or "blade of grass" sign) (Figs. 15-42 and 15-43). Cortical thickening often is present. Long bones exhibit bowing deformity, which occurs secondary to bone softening, often with pseudofractures fractures on the convex cortex (see Fig. 15-42). These lines are distinguished from similarly appearing transverse lucent lines (pseudofractures) occurring on the concave cortex of patient with osteomalacia, fibrous dysplasia, and other disease. Uncommonly Paget's disease may begin in the diaphysis, usually the tibia or radius.

The extent of skeletal involvement is assessed by radionuclide bone scans with follow-up radiographs of suspicious areas. Repeated bone scans may be useful to assess the patient's response to therapeutics. MRI and CT are employed to further delineate osseous or neurologic complications. The sole use of MRI to diagnose Paget's disease without the benefit of plain films may be problematic because of the variable appearance of pagetic bone on MRI scans.[95]

CLINICAL COMMENTS

Complications. The clinical features of Paget's disease vary. The localized form of the disease is typically asymptomatic and discovered incidentally.[56] Local pain (worse at night and often unrelated to activity) and tenderness over the involved bone is the

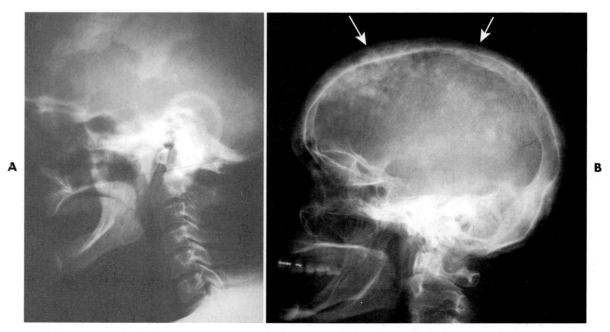

FIG. 15-25   **A** and **B,** The lytic phase of Paget's disease presents in the skull with large regions of radiolucent defect known as *osteoporosis circumscripta*. Mixed osteolytic and osteoblastic phases of Paget's disease relate a "cotton wool" appearance to the skull *(arrows)*. (Courtesy Steven P. Brownstein, MD, Springfield, NJ.)

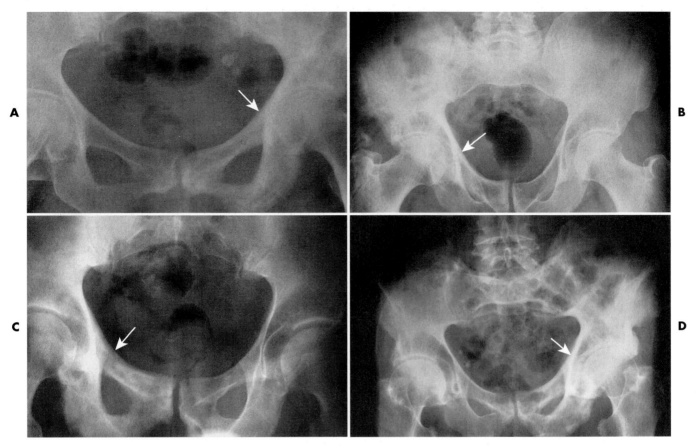

FIG. 15-26 Paget's disease is very common in the pelvis and proximal femora. **A** through **D,** In each case notice the unilateral thickening of the ridge of bone around the pelvis, especially the iliopectineal line. This is an early feature of the Pagetic involvement of the pelvis. The thickened iliopectineal line is known as a *brim sign.* (**A** and **D,** Courtesy Joseph W. Howe, Sylmar, CA; **B,** Courtesy Steven P. Brownstein, MD, Springfield, NJ.)

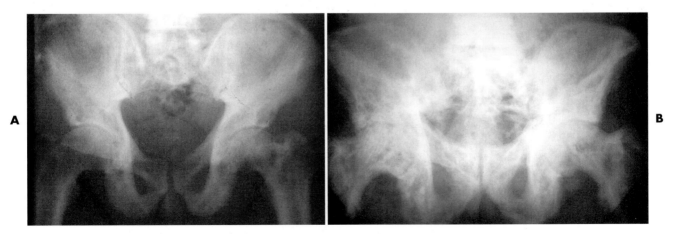

FIG. 15-27 **A** and **B,** Anteroposterior views of the pelvis in two cases demonstrate increased bone density with prominent trabeculation and gross enlargement of the bone elements. Other diseases such as metastatic bone disease cause increased bone radiodensity, but the bone enlargement and prominent trabeculation are more characteristic of Paget's disease.

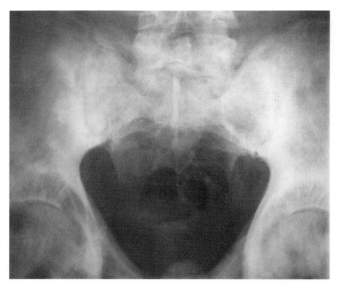

FIG. 15-28   Paget's disease involving the pelvis in a bilateral and nearly symmetric manner. Note the thickened iliopectineal lines (brim sign).

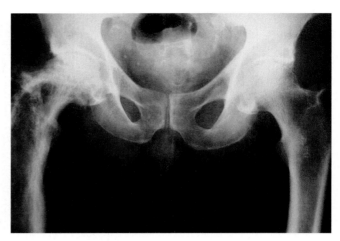

FIG. 15-29   Paget's disease isolated to the reading left proximal femur, presenting with general bone enlargement and thickening of the trabeculae and cortices of the bone. (Courtesy Jack C. Avalos, Davenport, IA.)

most common clinical complaint. Alternatively, patients with advanced disease may complain of severe pain and develop complications of the cardiovascular, skeletal, and neuromuscular systems.

High-output congestive heart failure and temperature differences are cardiovascular complications resulting from the hyperemic pagetic bone.[52] Skeletal complications include progressive osseous enlargement, bowing of long bones, degenerative joint disease, extramedullary hematopoieses, and pathologic fractures.[101] Neuromuscular complications are mainly the result of bone enlargement. Deafness may result from eighth cranial nerve compression by an enlarging temporal bone, deformity resulting from basilar impression, or enlarged dysfunctional ossicles. Pathologic fracture or enlarged vertebrae may compress the spinal cord, leading to muscle weakness, paralysis, and incontinence.

Laboratory values.   Laboratory analysis reveals elevated serum alkaline phosphatase resulting from increased bone formation and elevated urinary hydroxyproline levels secondary to bone resorption.[66] Monitoring these laboratory values may provide insight to the activity and progression of Paget's disease.[60] Serum calcium levels are usually not affected, unless pathologic fracture occurs.[60]

Treatment.   There is no cure for Paget's disease. Therapeutics are directed at alleviating pain and slowing the progression of the disease. The risk of progression and complications depends on the age of the patient, skeletal location, and aggressiveness of the Paget's disease.[75] Isolated monostotic involvement may be asymptomatic and of no consequence; however, some manifestations of the disease are marked.

Four components to the treatment regimen can be defined, including conditioning to improve muscle strength, pharmacologic therapy to stabilize bone remodeling, analgesics for pain relief, and surgical correction to address skeletal deformity. Surgical treatment may be used to stabilize pathologic fractures, osteotomies to realign the knee or other bone deformity, or joint arthroplasty for advanced joint involvement.

Pharmacology.   As part of the pharmacologic management strategy, bisphosphates and calcitonin are widely used therapeutic agents that may arrest the disease process, partially restore normal bone architecture, and alleviate pain.[92,99,106] Bisphosphates are given

for a period of 3 to 6 months and appear to offer longer-lasting benefits than can be obtained with calcitonin once treatment stops.[90,92]

Bisphosphonates bind to bone minerals acting directly to suppress the activity of osteoclasts, and indirectly by stimulating osteoblasts, which produce osteoclastic inhibitory factors. There are currently six bisphosphonates in common use: etidronate, tiludronate, alendronate, risedronate, clodronate, and pamidronate. The first four are given orally, and pamidronate intravenously. Risedronate is the newest of the group and is approximately 1000 times as potent as etidronate. Bisphosphonates (especially alendronate and clodronate) are associated with side effects of flulike gastrointestinal disturbances. Calcium and vitamin D supplements often accompany the use of these drugs. Mild forms of Paget's disease respond readily to the bisphosphonate therapy.

Calcitonin management predates the development of bisphosphonates, and is mainly used only when bisphosphonate therapy is not tolerated by the patient. Calcitonin administration involves subcutaneous injections of salmon calcitonin. Calcitonin has been shown to reduce bone turnover, speed healing of osteolytic lesions, and decrease symptoms of bone pain.

Pain management generally is accomplished with the antiosteoclastic bisphosphonates and calcitonin drugs. However, nonsteroidal antiinflammatory drugs (NSAIDs) or the newer COX-2 inhibitors also may be applied.

KEY CONCEPTS

- *Paget's disease is a relatively common familial disorder characterized by abnormal remodeling, hypertrophy, and structure of bone, leading to pain and deformity in middle-aged and older individuals.*
- *Although the bone appears thickened, it is architecturally unsound, potentially leading to bone deformity and skeletal fragility.*
- *Pathophysiology is divided into lytic, mixed, and blastic phases, replacing normal bone with immature, weak, and hypervascular bone.*
- *Sarcomatous malignant transformation is a severe but uncommon complication that may involve any bone. It is most common in the pelvis, sacrum, spine, skull, and proximal femora. Characteristic findings include osseous enlargement, osteosclerosis, cortical thickening, and thickened prominent trabeculae.*
- *Paget's disease may affect the skull (osteoporosis circumscripta, "cotton wool," basilar impression), spine ("picture frame," ivory, and biconcave*

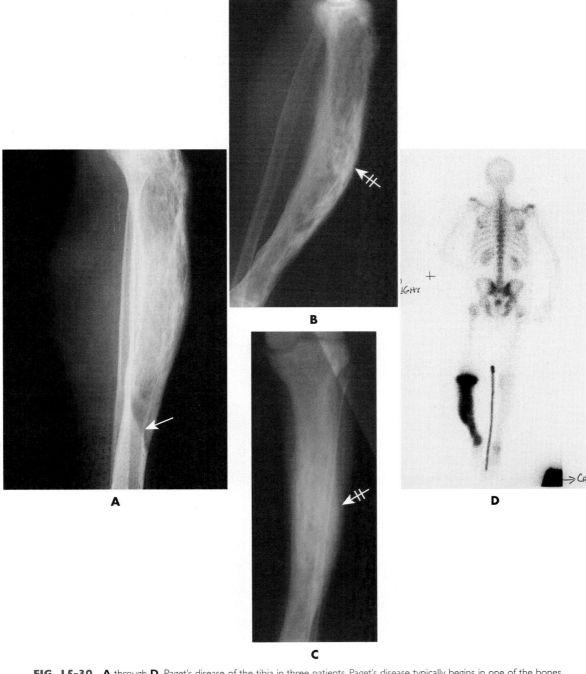

FIG. 15-30 A through **D.** Paget's disease of the tibia in three patients. Paget's disease typically begins in one of the bones and progresses as a front of osteolysis *(arrows)* ("blade of grass" sign). The cortex is thick *(crossed arrows)*, and the trabecular pattern is prominent. Each case demonstrates an anterior bowing ("saber shin") deformity. **C** and **D,** The osseous changes noted on radiographs correlate to increased metabolic activity, which can be seen on a bone scan. (Courtesy Steven P. Brownstein, MD, Springfield, NJ.)

- vertebrae, compression fractures), pelvis ("brim" sign, protrusio acetabuli), and extremities ("flame" or "blade of grass" sign, bowing, transverse fractures).
- Diagnosis is made by radionuclide bone scanning and plain film radiographs for initial assessment; magnetic resonance imaging and computed tomography are used to image complications (especially neurologic).
- The localized form is typically asymptomatic; most common clinical complaints are local pain and tenderness over involved bone.

- Related complications occur in the osseous (e.g., enlargement, deformity, spinal stenosis), cardiovascular (e.g., congestive heart failure), and neurologic (e.g., deafness, paralysis, incontinence) systems.
- Laboratory values exhibit elevated serum alkaline phosphatase, elevated urinary hydroxyproline, and normal serum calcium.
- Therapeutic agents include bisphosphonates (e.g., tiludronate, pamidronate, alendronate) and calcitonin.

Text continued on page 956

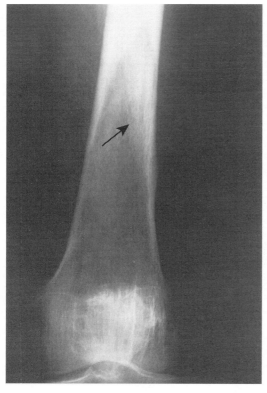

FIG. 15-31 Paget's disease of the distal femur appearing as a well-demarcated osteolytic process ("blade of grass" sign) beginning at the distal end of the femur and proceeding proximally in this case (arrow). (Courtesy Joseph W. Howe, Sylmar, CA.)

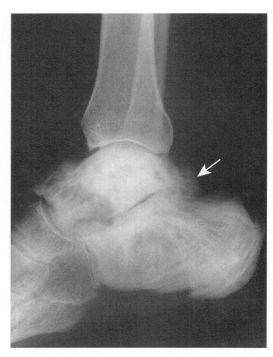

FIG. 15-32 Prominent trabeculae and bone enlargement consistent with Paget's disease of the calcaneus and navicula (arrow). (Courtesy Joseph W. Howe, Sylmar, CA.)

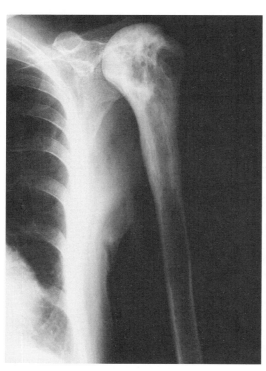

FIG. 15-33 Paget's disease of the proximal humerus marked by cortical enlargement and prominent trabeculae. (Courtesy Steven P. Brownstein, MD, Springfield, N.)

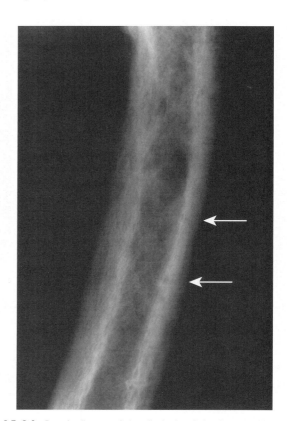

FIG. 15-34 Paget's disease of the diaphysis of the femur, exhibiting thick cortex, prominent trabecular pattern, and bowing deformity. In addition, radiolucent defects are noted in the cortex, perpendicular to the long axis of the bone (arrows), representing pseudofractures. Pseudofractures represent fibrous tissue replacement of bone and are also seen osteomalacia, fibrous dysplasia, and several other conditions. (Courtesy Joseph W. Howe, Sylmar, CA.)

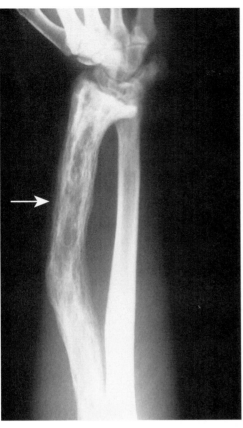

FIG. 15-35 Bone enlargement, cortical thickening, and prominent trabecular pattern *(arrow)* are noted in this radiograph of Paget's disease of the radius.

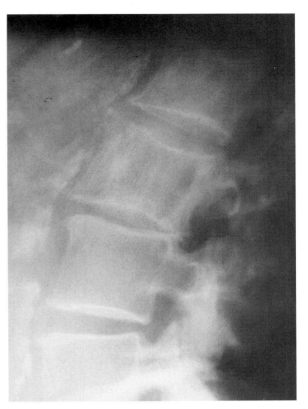

FIG. 15-37 Paget's disease noted by an enlarged, mottled appearance of the L3 segment.

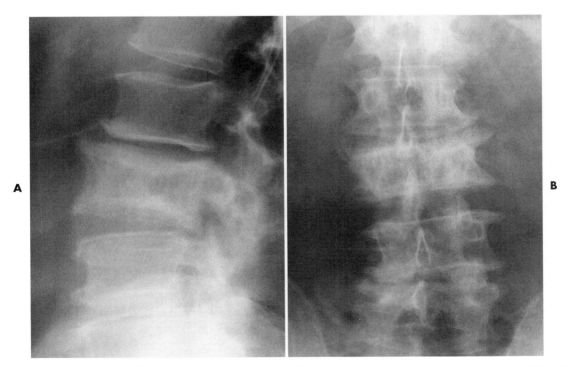

FIG. 15-36 **A** and **B,** Paget's disease of the L3 segment. The thickened cortex of the segment is called a *picture frame sign.* The segment is enlarged in the anteroposterior and lateral projection.

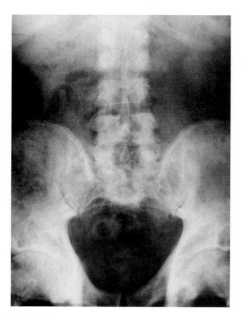

FIG. 15-38 The lumbar spine and pelvis appear radiodense. This appearance may be due to blastic metastasis, Paget's disease, and several other systemic diseases; however, the thickened cortices of the bones, prominent trabeculae, and general enlargement of the bones is most characteristic of Paget's disease.

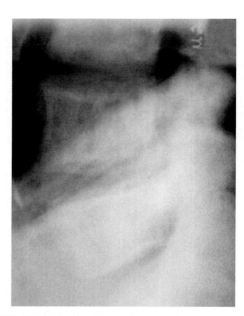

FIG. 15-39 Multiple levels of picture frame vertebrae consistent with Paget's disease. The vertebrae are enlarged with thick cortices.

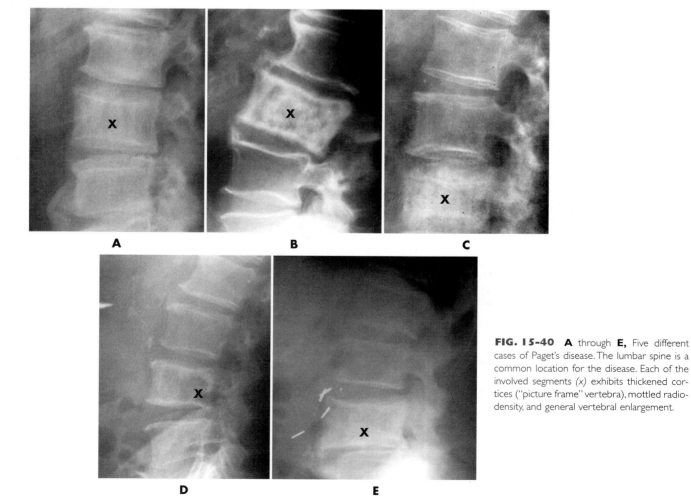

A

B

C

D

E

FIG. 15-40 A through **E,** Five different cases of Paget's disease. The lumbar spine is a common location for the disease. Each of the involved segments *(x)* exhibits thickened cortices ("picture frame" vertebra), mottled radiodensity, and general vertebral enlargement.

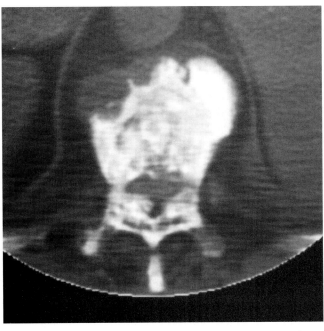

FIG. 15-41 Paget's disease. This computed tomographic image shows a radiodense "ivory vertebra" suggesting metastatic bone disease, Paget's disease, or lymphoma. Paget's disease is most likely given the mottled, enlarged appearance of the segment.

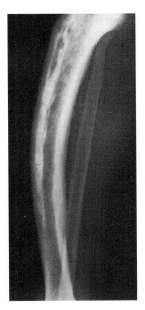

FIG. 15-42 Pagetic bone is thick, but immature and therefore mechanically weak. Bowing deformity and pathologic fractures are common complications. This lateral view of the tibia exhibits an anterior bowing secondary to extensive involvement with Paget's disease. Bowing of the anterior tibia is known as *saber shin deformity*. It is not a unique sign to Paget's disease; it is also evident in congenital syphilis and yaws. In addition, although it is not termed *saber shin deformity*, similar anterior bowing is noted in rickets.

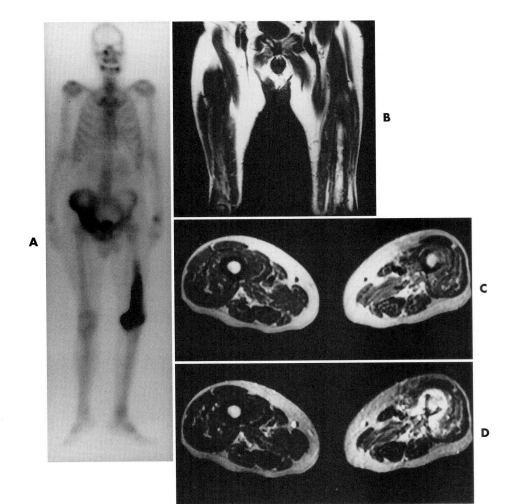

FIG. 15-43 A, Radionuclide bone scan in an 80-year-old man with known Paget's disease shows intense uptake in the distal left femur. **B,** Coronal T1-weighted (SE 1000/20) image demonstrates irregular areas of mildly decreased intensity in the distal left femur. **C** and **D,** Axial proton-density weighted (SE 2550/20) and T2-weighted (SE 2550/80) image show patchy increased intensity in the soft tissues and marrow that resembles the signal intensity of tumor or infection. The radiographs are diagnostic. (Stark DD, Gradley WG: Magnetic resonance imaging, ed 2, St Louis, 1992, Mosby.)

Scoliosis

BACKGROUND

Definition. In the purest use of the word, *scoliosis* is defined as any lateral curvature of the spine occurring in a coronal plane. However, because small lateral curvatures are nearly ubiquitous, the term *scoliosis* typically is reserved for curvatures of at least 10 degrees in magnitude (using Cobb's method). Moreover because of potential employment and medicolegal ramifications, the term *scoliosis* should be reserved for clinically significant or potentially significant presentations.

In addition to the lateral bending, the vertebrae involved in the curvature usually are rotated, giving rise to the term *rotatory scoliosis*. Kyphosis is a convex posterior curvature and lordosis a convex anterior curvature of the spine, both occurring in a sagittal plane. *Kyphoscoliosis* refers to spinal curvature, which is both convex lateral and posterior. A sharply angled kyphosis is termed a *gibbous*.

Prevalence. The frequency of scoliosis is dependent on the degree of curvature. A study in Montreal indicated a prevalence of 4.5% of curvatures greater than 5 degrees Cobb's angle.[97] Curvatures exceeding 10 degrees Cobb's angle are found in about 2% to 4% of adults in the United States.[17] Curvatures greater than 25 degrees Cobb's angle occur in 1.5 per 1000 individuals in the United States. Overall, the incidence is higher in females. Moreover, the greater the curvature is, the higher the female predilection.[94] Adolescents 9 to 15 years of age are most at risk.[94]

Classification. Scolioses are broadly divided into structural and nonstructural types. Structural scolioses (Fig. 15-44) are fixed, do not correct on side-bending radiographs, and demonstrate a rib humping on the convex side of the curvature. Nonstructural or functional scolioses lessen or disappear on lateral bending, and any rib humping disappears on forward flexion.

More than 50 conditions are associated with scoliosis. Etiologies and further classifications are listed in Fig. 15-45. In nearly 80% of cases of scoliosis, an etiology cannot be determined. Overall, these idiopathic curvatures more commonly occur in females (a 7:1 ratio of females to males). They are subdivided into infantile (0 to 3 years of age), juvenile (4 to 10 years of age), and adolescent (most common; older than 10 years of age) types based on age of onset. Research efforts are focused on growth and dysfunction of the central nervous system as a possible cause of the currently idiopathic subtype.[21,22,93,105]

Scoliosis may also result from a variety of neurogenic and myogenic causes (see Fig. 15-45). Poliomyelitis and muscular dystrophy are the most common causes, respectively. These types typically appear as long-segment, C-type configurations.

Congenital causes of scoliosis are related to abnormal vertebral formation or segmentation. The result is asymmetric anatomy leading to a lateral curvature (see Fig. 15-44). Because of the proximity of embryonic tissue, developmental defects of the skeletal system often are associated with defects of the genitourinary system. Discovery of skeletal abnormalities necessitates a review of these systems.

IMAGING FINDINGS

Radiographic assessment begins with standing anteroposterior (AP) and lateral projections of the spine, preferably each as a single full-spine projection using 14×36 inch film and cassette.[118] The radiograph should include the entire spine from occiput to sacrum. The degree of spinal curvature is quantified using the Cobb method on the anterolateral projection (Fig. 15-46). An alternative,

the Risser's-Ferguson method, is used less commonly because of its inaccuracy (Fig. 15-47). Gonadal shielding, rare earth screens, collimation, and a 72- to 84-inch focal-spot-to-film distance are effective in limiting the amount of radiation exposure. Employing a posteroanterior patient position will limit thyroid and gonadal exposure if temporal examinations are anticipated as part of long-term treatment.[57,79]

Lateral bending radiographs are useful to determine the rigidity of the spinal curvature and differentiate structural from nonstructural curvatures. Compensatory curvatures lessen or disappear on lateral bending films; structural curvatures persist.

The description of the spinal curvature should detail the following: the spinal region or levels involved (Fig. 15-48), direction of the lateral convexity, degree of curvature, vertebral end used for the measurement, and abrupt (short segment, acute) or gradual (long segment, smooth) appearance of the curvature. The most prominent curve is known as *major* or *primary,* and concurrent lesser curvatures are called *minor, secondary,* or *compensatory.*

Vertebral bodies. The vertebral bodies involved in the curvature are rotated. The rotation of each vertebra is marked by spinous process rotation opposite the curve's convexity, or, alternatively, vertebra body rotation toward the curve's convexity (Fig. 15-49). Prolonged vertebral compression on the concave side of the scoliosis leads to a wedged appearance of the vertebrae and intervertebral disc. Both are narrowed on the concave side of the scoliosis. The lateral trapezoidal configuration is particularly pronounced if the scoliosis exists in an immature skeleton. When growth plates are open, the trapezoidal shape is a manifestation of the Heuter-Volkmann principle, which states that increased pressure on the growth plate causes decreased growth and decreased pressure causes increased growth, promoting the trapezoidal appearance.

Ribs. The ribs are roughly on the concave side of the curvature. The posterior ribs on the convex side are pushed posteriorly, narrowing the width of the ipsilateral hemithorax and producing rib humping. The rib humping is more obvious on physical examination of a patient who is in the forward-bending position. On the concave side, the anterior portions of the ribs are pushed anteriorly.

Skeletal maturity. Curvatures progress more rapidly in skeletally immature patients. Radiographs offer several methods to assess the bone maturity of an individual. Radiographs of the hand can be compared with development standards, such as those listed in *Greulich and Pyle's Radiographic Atlas of Skeletal Development of the Hand and Wrist.*[47,108] A more convenient method consists of qualifying the degree of bone maturity by observing the stage of ossification of the iliac crest apophysis on the AP projection (Risser's sign) (Fig. 15-50).

If the iliac crest apophysis is completely ossified to the ilium, the patient is skeletally mature. Children who exhibit Risser's 0 and 1 are much more likely to demonstrate curvature progression than children who are Risser's 2 to 5. It takes approximately 2 to 3 years for the patient to progress from a Risser's 0 to Risser's 5. Ossification and fusion of the iliac apophysis occurs earlier and more quickly in girls, generally beginning at age 14 in girls and 15 in boys (Fig. 15-51).

The Risser's sign is a convenient method to estimate skeletal maturity because the iliac wings frequently are included on a full-length spine radiograph. Although easily obtained, the Risser's sign is not as accurate as hand and wrist radiographs and is no more accurate than the use of chronologic age alone.[68] The appearance of the vertebral body endplates provides evidence of skeletal maturity (Fig. 15-52). The endplates are completely fused and blend imperceptibly with the vertebral bodies at skeletal maturity.

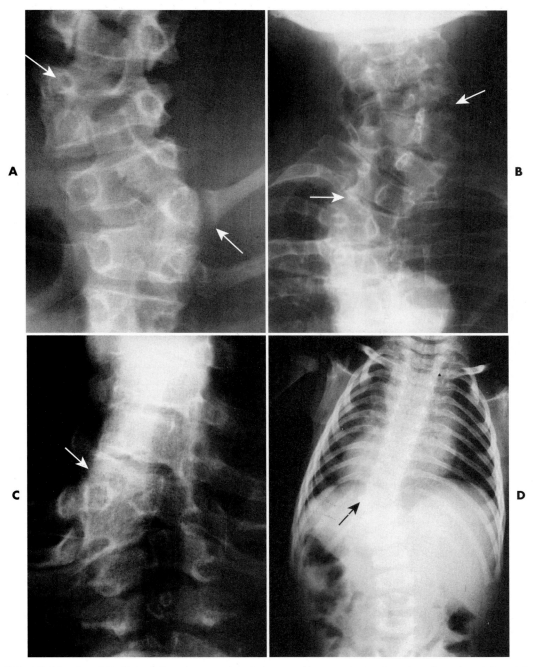

FIG. 15-44 **A** and **B,** Short, S-shaped structural scoliosis created by opposing hemivertebrae (*arrows*) and, **C** and **D,** C-shaped structural scoliosis created by the presence of a single hemivertebra (*arrows*). A second, opposing hemivertebra tends to straighten the curvature created around the first hemivertebra.

CLINICAL COMMENTS

Most curvatures are not painful, especially in young patients. Pain and deformity are the most common complaints that bring a patient to a health care provider, but typically these are expressed by middle-aged adults and are related to spinal degeneration that develops, in part, as a long-term consequence of the spinal curvature.[122]

Adolescent idiopathic scoliosis is a diagnosis of exclusion. Mainly the goal of taking the patient's history and conducting the physical examination is to exclude causes of scoliosis, such as

congenital maldevelopment (Fig. 15-53) or transient muscle spasm (Fig. 15-54). The diagnosis of adolescent idiopathic scoliosis should not be accompanied with significant pain or neurologic symptoms. The patient will likely demonstrate a family history of the disease. In fact, when both parents have scoliosis, their children's risk of developing a significant scoliosis is 50%.[69]

Screening. Most commonly scoliosis first appears during late childhood or the early teenage years. Therefore screening is targeted to children in the fifth and sixth grade. About half of the

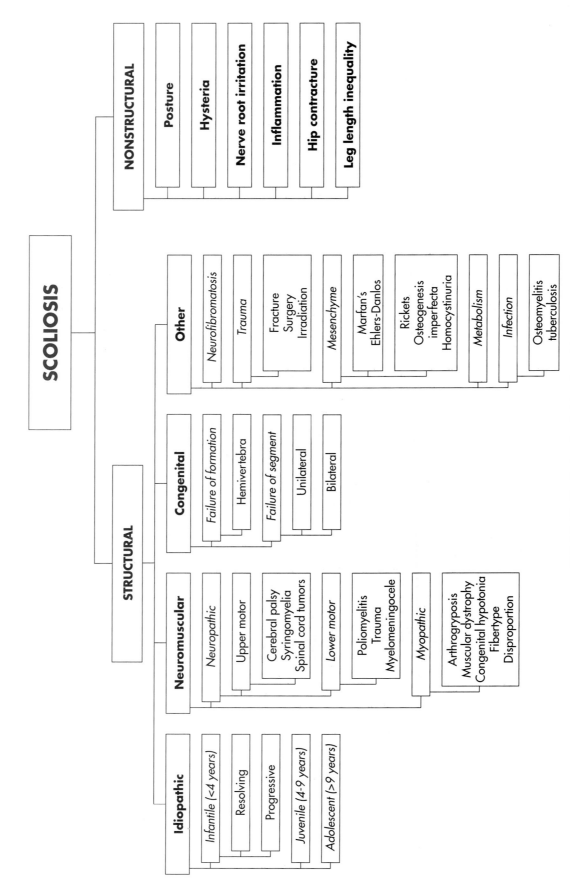

FIG. 15–45   Classification of scoliosis based on etiology.

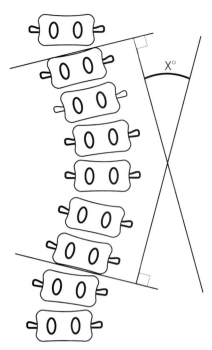

FIG. 15-46 Cobb's method of measuring scoliosis. Line segments are drawn across the superior endplate of the upper and inferior endplate of the lower vertebrae involved with the curvature. These end vertebrae are chosen using the criteria that they tilt most severely toward the scoliosis convexity. Perpendicular lines are drawn from the endplate lines, and the superior or inferior angle at their intersection (X°) is measured.

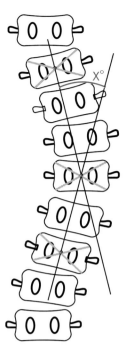

FIG. 15-47 Risser's-Ferguson method of measuring scoliosis. Line segments are drawn from the center of the upper vertebra to the center of the vertebra at the apex of the lateral curvature (apical vertebra) and from the center of the lower vertebra to the center of the apical vertebra. The next step is to measure the superior or inferior angle at the intersection of these lines (X°). This method is used less often than Cobb's method.

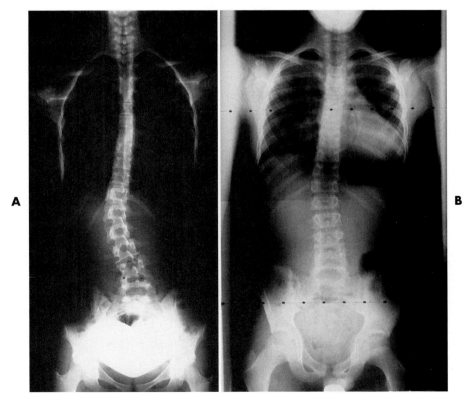

FIG. 15-48 **A** and **B,** Scoliosis evaluated on the full spine projection. Curvatures are defined by the cause, direction of the convexity, magnitude, and degree of coupled rotation of the apical segments.

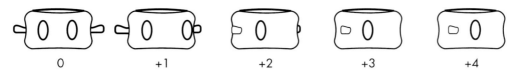

FIG. 15-49 Vertebral rotation is expressed by the pedicle appearance. The normal vertebral alignment is a Grade 0. Grade +4 indicates maximum vertebral rotation, leaving only one pedicle visible and found at the midline on the frontal projection.

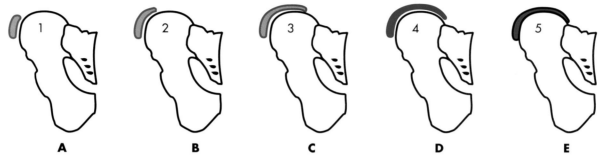

FIG. 15-50 Risser's sign. On the anteroposterior projection, the appearance of the iliac apophysis provides a stable indicator of skeletal maturity. If the apophysis is not seen, a Grade 0 is designated. **A** through **D,** The apophysis forms from the lateral aspect and progresses medially along the superior margin of the ilium (Grades 1 through 4) and, **E,** eventually fuses (Grade 5).

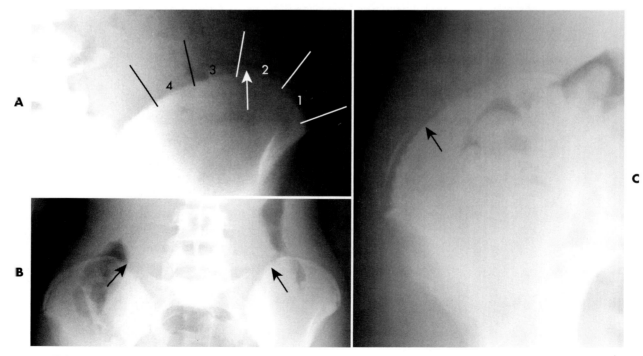

FIG. 15-51 Risser's sign in three different patients. **A,** Late Grade 2 Risser's sign in a 16-year-old girl *(arrow).* **B,** Late Grade 3 in a 17-year-old girl *(arrows).* **C,** Grade 1 Risser's sign in a 15-year-old girl *(arrow).* Adolescents usually progress from a Risser's Grade 1 to a Grade 5 in less than a 3-year period.

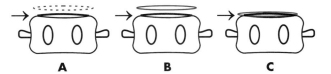

FIG. 15-52 The appearance of the vertebral endplates indicate skeletal maturation. **A,** The endplates are incompletely ossified. **B,** The endplates are ossified but now not fused to vertebra. **C,** The endplates are ossified and fused to the adjacent vertebra, indicating skeletal maturity.

schools in the United States participate in screening. Clues to the presence of curvature include a prominent scapula, high hip or shoulder, unilateral prominent chest wall or breast, and tilt of the body, including a forward lean (Fig. 15-55). During screening, the most efficient examination involves the examination of a rib hump with the Adam's test.

Adam's test is a safe and convenient screening procedure for scoliosis. Adam's test is performed by having the patient bend 90 degrees forward from a standing position in front of and facing away from the examiner. Once the patient reaches toward the floor to a horizontal position, the examiner visually scans the patient's back for asymmetry, particularly a rib hump. A rib hump noted on an Adam's test correlates to a spinal curvature of at least

10 degrees, and is an indicator of the need for more accurate radiographic evaluation of the patient.

Management. Once the diagnosis has been made, the principal concern of the clinician is to eliminate serious underlying concerns and determine the risks of progression. Seriously progressive scoliosis is related to back pain, fatigue, spinal stenosis, disfigurement, and heart and lung problems. Fortunately only about 10% of adolescent patients with scoliosis exhibit significant curvature progression that necessitates focused management.[77] The risk of progression has been estimated. Adolescent curvatures less than 30 degrees are unlikely to progress, curvatures between 30 and 50 degrees progress an average of 10 to 15 degrees over the patient's lifetime, and curvatures that measure more than 50 degrees at the time of skeletal maturity tend to progress at a rate of 1 degree per year.[77]

Adolescents and juveniles with curvatures greater than 10 degrees, but less than 20 degrees, should be closely monitored with radiographs every 3 to 6 months to determine if there is any progression.[83] Radiographs should not be taken more frequently than a 3-month interval. There is approximately 3 degrees of error associated with the Cobb's method of scoliosis measurement, and curvatures that are progressing in a skeletally immature patient typically do so at a rate slower than 1 degree per month. Therefore a progressing scoliosis needs at least 3 months to demonstrate a real change using the Cobb's method.

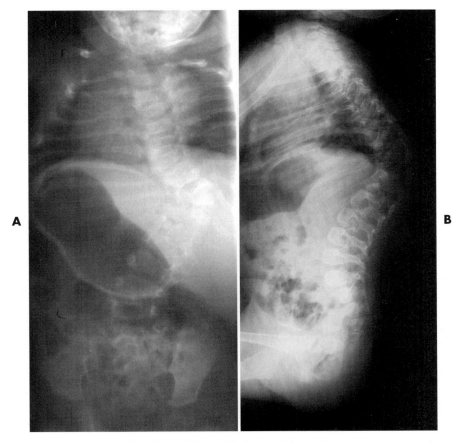

FIG. 15-53 A and **B,** A 1-year-old patient exhibiting a 75-degree left lateral thoracic curvature secondary to a thoracolumbar hemivertebra formed on the left. (Courtesy Robin Canterbury, Davenport, IA.)

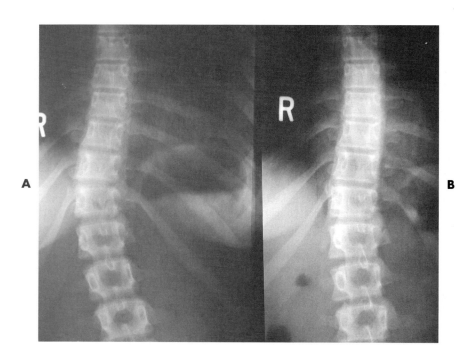

FIG. 15-54 A, Right lateral thoracolumbar curvature measuring 29 degrees from T9 to L2. **B,** A radiograph taken 2 months later demonstrates a curvature of only 11 degrees. Curvatures with such large changes in magnitude over a short period of time usually are related to muscle spasm (antalgic). (Courtesy Robert C. Tatum, Davenport, IA.)

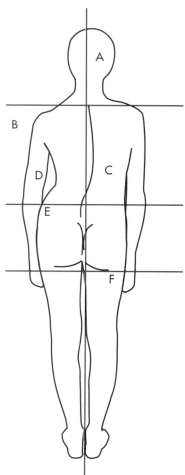

FIG. 15-55 From the posterior perspective, the physical presentation of scoliosis is marked by, *A,* a lateral head position; *B,* high shoulder; *C,* deviation of the furrow of the back; *D,* increased space between the trunk and the arm; *E,* high hip; and *F,* low gluteal fold.

Failure to recognize progression of the curve and initiate conservative treatment may delay more aggressive treatment options, possibly leading to increased deformity and complications. Positive prognostic factors for scoliosis progression include a female gender (females are 10 times more likely than males to exhibit progression), young age at time of diagnosis, pronounced vertebral rotation, early stage of skeletal maturity, early menarche, and increased magnitude of the curvature.[17,49,70,124] In general, curvatures under 30 degrees are highly unlikely to progress after skeletal maturity.

Currently scoliosis is treated by bracing, electrical stimulation, chiropractic care, surgery, or a combination of these.[127] Most curvatures can be treated nonoperatively if recognized early. Bracing is the most common conservative management.

Bracing. Bracing has a long history of use with scoliosis, dating back at least to the time of Hippocrates. Early braces were constructed of metal or plaster used merely to keep the spine straight. They were heavy, hot, and generally uncomfortable for the patient. Over time more sophisticated orthotics were developed with the inclusion of pressure pads placed to more specifically reduce the curvatures.

For decades the Milwaukee brace has been considered the gold standard in conservative scoliosis management. It is a long brace, extending from the base of the cervical spine to the pelvis. In the 1970s as research into the topic advanced, newer short torso braces were developed. As a category they are called TLSO (thoraco-lumbo-sacral-orthosis), and include the Boston brace,[39,61] Wilmington jacket,[19] Rosenberger orthosis,[43] and Miami brace.[73] These shorter braces are more comfortable than the Milwaukee brace and allow patients to completely conceal them with clothing. However, the less comfortable Milwaukee brace is not obsolete. It is still applied, especially when the curvature is high (apex of T8 or more cephalic).[18]

A brace is not an easy treatment for teenagers who may be more concerned about appearing different from their peers than they may be about their curve progression. For years, compliance has

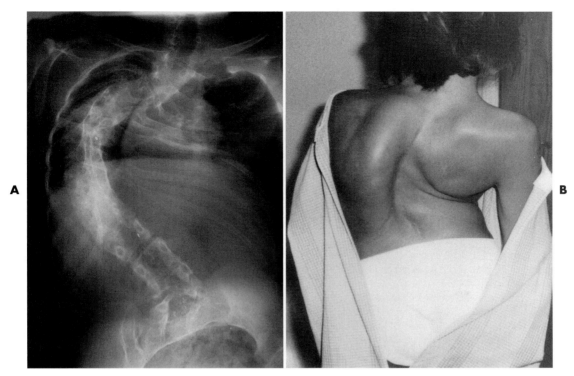

FIG.15-56 A 119-degree left lateral thoracolumbar curvature. **A,** Surgical sutures and absence of the posterior arches of the lumbar segments are noted as residua to laminectomy. **B,** Notice the high right hip, left rib humping, and high left shoulder consistent with the spinal deformity. (Courtesy Ian Shaw, Port Huron, MI.)

been a major impediment to effective management with bracing. Past research indicates that patients wore their braces for approximately 65% of the time prescribed.[34] The more comfortable and concealable torso braces have lead to increased patient compliance and hence the effectiveness of the management plan and outcomes research related to bracing.

The goal of bracing and other conservative management options is to limit progression of the curvature. Spinal curvatures generally are not related to cardiopulmonary symptoms or other serious clinical concerns until they exceed 70 degrees, so there is no immediate clinical concern for a small curvature to cause cardiopulmonary compromise. The concern is rather for possible progression of the curvature and associated cosmetic deformity. Later, as the patient ages, spinal degeneration and associated pain syndromes develop, but during youth, progression is the central clinical concern. Curvatures greater than 30 degrees nearly always progress when present in the skeletally immature,[70] and rarely progress in the skeletally mature.[124]

Braces are widely advocated to limit further progression in skeletally immature patients with flexible curvatures measuring between 20 and 40 degrees.[36,39] Bracing is more effective with smaller curvatures. Beyond 45 degrees, most applications of a brace are ineffective; therefore early detect of the curvature is paramount to a successful outcome.

Surgery. Surgery is the most aggressive management option for patients with scoliosis. Rods, hooks, and screws can be placed to reduce the scoliosis, stop further progression, stabilize the spine, and provide cosmetic improvement. In general, the magnitude of the curvature can be reduced by 50% through surgery. Surgery may be considered with curvatures that exceed 50 degrees.[83]

However, surgery is based on more than an arbitrary Cobb's measurement. Skeletal maturity, balance, age of onset, location, and size of the curve should be considered.[16,119] Spinal decompressive surgery may be performed to alleviate spinal stenosis related to the vertebral rotation (Fig. 15-56).

Although chiropractic care lacks explanatory research of its effectiveness in limiting curve progression, various descriptive reports suggest palliative relief of associated symptoms.[2,3,27,83,117] In addition, anecdotal evidences supports its use; however, more research is needed to determine chiropractic's full potential in managing patients with scoliosis.

Recent reports have indicated that left thoracic curvatures are associated with a higher incidence of neuropathology (e.g., syrinx); however, evidence of sampling bias may exist, indicating that caution should be taken so that preliminary reports are not over-interpreted.[46] Left thoracic curvatures usually are mild and benign and should be viewed as suspicious for neuropathy only if they are severe or rapidly progressive.[46]

PART TWO Bone, Joints, and Soft Tissues

KEY CONCEPTS

- *Scoliosis is lateral curvature of the spine (>10 degrees); often it is a progressive condition that can lead to significant disability.*
- *Prevalence is dependent on degree of curvature. Overall, scoliosis is more common in females. Adolescents 9 to 15 years of age are most at risk.*
- *Curvatures greater than 25 degrees Cobb's angle occur in 1.5 per 1000 individuals in the United States.*
- *Scolioses are broadly divided into nonstructural types and the more common structural type.*
- *Most structural scolioses are idiopathic and subdivided into infantile (0 to 3 years of age), juvenile (4 to 10 years of age), and adolescent*

(most common; older than 10 years of age) types, based on age of onset.

- *Radiographic assessment begins with standing frontal and lateral projections of the spine, preferably each as a single full-spine projection using 14 × 36 inch film and cassette.*
- *The degree of spine curvature is quantified using the Cobb method or less accurate Risser's-Ferguson method on the anterolateral projection.*
- *The description of the spinal curvature should include the spinal region or levels involved, the direction of the lateral convexity, degree of curvature, which end vertebrae were used for the measurement, and whether the curvature appears abrupt (short segment, acute) or gradual (long segment, smooth).*
- *The most prominent curve is known as major or primary; concurrent lesser curvatures are called minor, secondary, or compensatory.*
- *Curvatures progress more rapidly in skeletally immature patients.*
- *Pain and deformity are the most common complaints that bring a patient to a health care provider.*
- *Scoliosis is treated by bracing, electrical stimulation, surgery, chiropractic care, or a combination of all four; do not overdiagnose and unnecessarily apply premature bracing or surgery.*
- *In adolescent and juvenile patients, a curvature less than 20 degrees should be monitored every 3 to 6 months for progression. Bracing should be considered with curvatures of 20 degrees to 40 degrees. Surgery is considered when curvature is beyond 50 degrees.*
- *Prognostic factors for scoliosis progression include age at time of diagnosis vertebral rotation, stage of skeletal maturity, early or late menarche, and magnitude and pattern of curvature.*

References

1. Arceci RJ: Treatment options: commentary, *Br J Cancer* 23:58, 1994.
2. Arthur BE, Nykoliation JW, Cassidy JD: The chiropractic management of adult scoliosis: a case study, *Eur J Chiro* 34:46, 1986.
3. Barge FH: Idiopathic scoliosis, vol 3, Davenport, IA, 1986, Bawder Bros.
4. Barker DJP: The epidemiology of Paget's disease of bone, *Br Med Bull* 40:396, 1984.
5. Barry HC: Paget's disease of bone, Edinburgh, 1969, Livingstone.
6. Bernard P, Bonnetblanc JM: Dermatomyositis and malignancy, *J Invest Dermatol* 100(suppl):128, 1993.
7. Bernstein RM, Zaleske DJ: Familial aspects of Caffey's disease, *Am J Orthop* 24:777, 1995.
8. Bhambhani M et al: Giant cell tumours in mandible and spine: a rare complication of Paget's disease of bone, *Ann Rheum Dis* 51:1335, 1992.
9. Bianchi L et al: Pachydermoperiostosis: study of epidermal growth factor and steroid receptors, *Br J Dermatol* 132:128, 1995.
10. Bisagni-Faure A et al: Magnetic resonance imaging assessment of sacroiliac joint involvement in Gaucher's disease, *J Rheumatol* 19:1984, 1992.
11. Blickman JG, Wilkinson RH, Graef JW: The radiologic "lead band" revisited, *AJR: Am J Roentgenol* 146:245, 1986.
12. Boas SR et al: Hypertrophic osteoarthropathy in a child with follicular bronchiolitis, *Clin Nucl Med* 20:49, 1995.
13. Bonakdarpour A, Harwick R, Pickering J: Case report 34, *Skeletal Radiol* 2:52, 1977.
14. Borochowitz Z et al: Familial Caffey's disease and late recurrence in a child, *Clin Genet* 40:329, 1991.
15. Brady RO, Barton NW, Grabowski GA: The role of neurogenetics in Gaucher's disease, *Arch Neurol* 50:1212, 1993.
16. Bridwell KH: Surgical treatment of adolescent idiopathic scoliosis: the basics and controversies, *Spine* 19:1095, 1994.
17. Brunnel WP: The natural history of idiopathic scoliosis, *Clin Orthop* 229:20, 1988.
18. Bunch WH, Patwardhan AG: Scoliosis: making clinical decisions, St Louis, 1989, Mosby.
19. Bunnell WP, MacEwen GD, Jayakumar S: The use of plastic jackets in the non-operative treatment of idiopathic scoliosis, *J Bone Joint Surg* 62A:31, 1980.
20. Burrows EH: Orbitocranial assymmetry, *Br J Radiol* 51:610, 1978.
21. Burwell RG et al: Pathogenesis of idiopathic scoliosis, the Nottingham concept, *Acta Orthop Belg* 58(suppl 1):33, 1992.
22. Byrd JA: Current theories on the etiology of idiopathic scoliosis, *Clin Orthop* 229:114, 1988.
23. Carcassi U: History of hypertrophic osteoarthropathy (HOA), *Clin Exp Rheumatol* 10(suppl 7):3, 1992.
24. Collins DH: Paget's disease of bone-incidence and subclinical forms, *Lancet* 2:51, 1956.
25. Dahlin DC: Classification and general aspects of amyloidosis, *Med Clin North Am* 34:1107, 1950.
26. Daly BD: Thoracic metastases from nasopharyngeal carcinoma presenting as hypertrophic pulmonary osteoarthropathy: scintigraphic and CT findings, *Clin Radiol* 50:545, 1995.
27. Danbert RJ. Scoliosis: biomechanics and rationale for manipulative treatment, *J Man Physiol Ther* 12:38, 1989.
28. de Gennes C, Kuntz D, de Vernejoul MC: Bone mastocytosis. A report of nine cases with a bone histomorphometric study, *Clin Orthop* 279:281, 1992.
29. De Smet L et al: Monostotic localization of Paget's disease in the hand, *Acta Orthop Belg* 60:184, 1994.
30. Debeuckelaele S, Schoors DF, Devis G: Systemic mast cell disease: a review of the literature with special focus on the gastrointestinal manifestations, *Acta Clin Belg* 46:226, 1991.
31. Detheridge FM, Guyer PB, Barker DJP: European distribution of Paget's disease of bone, *Br Med J* 285:1005, 1982.
32. Dickinson CJ: The aetiology of clubbing and hypertrophic osteoarthropathy, *Eur J Clin Invest* 23:330, 1993.
33. DiMaggio LA, Lippes HA, Lee RV: Histiocytosis X and pregnancy, *Obstet Gynecol* 85:806, 1982.
34. DiRaimondo CV, Green NE: Brace-wear compliance in patients with adolescent idiopathic scoliosis, *J Pediatr Orthop* 8:143, 1988.
35. Dogan AS et al: Detection of bone lesions in Langerhans cell histiocytosis: complementary roles of scintigraphy and conventional radiography, *J Pediatr Hematol Oncol* 18:51, 1996.
36. Dutro CL, Keene KJ: Electrical muscle stimulation in the treatment of progressive adolescent idiopathic scoliosis: a literature review, *J Man Physiol Ther* 8:257, 1985.
37. Edeiken J, DePalma AF, Hodes PJ: Paget's disease: osteitis deformans, *Clin Orthop* 146:141, 1966.
38. Egeler RM, D'Angio GJ: Langerhans cell histiocytosis, *J Pediatr* 127:1, 1995.
39. Emans J: The Boston bracing system for idiopathic scoliosis: follow-up results in 295 patients, *Spine* 11:792, 1986.
40. Emans JB: Scoliosis: detecting the curves that mandate treatment, *J Musculoskeletal Med* 2:11, 1985.
41. Euwer RL, Sontheimer RD: Dermatologic aspects of myositis, *Curr Opin Rheumatol* 6:583, 1994.
42. Fisher AJ et al: Quantitative analysis of the plain radiographic appearance of eosinophilic granuloma, *Invest Radiol* 30:466, 1995.
43. Gavin TM, Bunch WH, Dvonch V: The Rosenberger scoliosis orthosis, *J Assoc Child Prosthet Orthot Clin* 21(3):35, 1986.
44. Genovese A et al: Clinical advances in mastocytosis, *Int J Clin Lab Res* 25:178, 1995.
45. Gentry RR et al: Infantile cortical hyperostosis of the ribs (Caffey's disease) without mandibular involvement, *Pediatr Radiol* 13:236, 1983.
46. Goldberg CJ, Dowling FE, Fogarty EE: Left thoracic scoliosis configurations. Why so different? *Spine* 19:1385, 1994.
47. Greulich WW, Pyle SI: Radiographic atlas of skeletal development of the hand and wrist, ed 2, Stanford, CA, 1959, Stanford University Press.

48. Grossman RE, Hensley GT: Bone lesions in primary amyloidosis, *AJR: Am J Roentgenol* 101:872, 1967.

49. Gruchalla RS: Mastocytosis: developments during the past decade, *Am J Med Sci* 309:328, 1995.

50. Gunnoe BA: Adolescent idiopathic scoliosis, *Orthop Rev* 19:35, 1990.

51. Gupta SK et al: Skeletal overgrowth with modelling error in neurofibromatosis, *Clin Radiol* 36:643, 1985.

52. Guyer PB: Research into Paget's disease: clues to the etiology and clinical significance, *Radiography* 48:185, 1982.

53. Hadjipavlou A et al: Malignant transformation in Paget's disease of bone, *Cancer* 70:2802, 1992.

54. Haher TR et al: Meta-analysis of surgical outcome in adolescent idiopathic scoliosis, *Spine* 20:1575, 1995.

55. Hainaux B et al: Gaucher's disease. Plain radiography, US, CT and MR diagnosis of lungs, bone and liver lesions, *Pediatr Radiol* 22:78, 1992.

56. Hamdy RC: Clinical features and pharmacologic treatment of Paget's disease, *Endocrinol Metab Clin North Am* 24:421, 1995.

57. Hellstrom G, Irstam L, Nachemson A: Reduction of radiation dose in radiologic examination of patients with scoliosis, *Spine* 8:28, 1983.

58. Henck ME et al: Extraskeletal soft tissue masses of Langerhans' cell histiocytosis, *Skeletal Radiol* 25:409, 1996.

59. Huang TY, Yam LT, Li CY: Radiological features of systemic mast-cell disease, *Br J Radiol* 60:765, 1987.

60. Hughes S, Peel-White AL, Peterson CK: Paget's disease of bone: current thinking and management, *J Man Physiol Ther* 15:242, 1992.

61. Jodoin A et al: Treatment for idiopathic scoliosis by the Boston brace system: early results, *Orthop Trans* 5:22, 1981.

62. Jones ET, Hensinger RN, Holt JF: Idiopathic cortical hyperostosis, *Clin Orthop Rel Res* 163:210, 1982.

63. Kahaleh MB: The role of vascular endothelium in fibroblast activation and tissue fibrosis, particularly in scleroderma (systemic sclerosis) and pachydermoperiostosis (primary hypertrophic osteoarthropathy), *Clin Exper Rheumatol* 10(suppl 7):51, 1992.

64. Kettelhut BV, Metcalfe DD: Pediatric mastocytosis, *Ann Allergy Asthma Immunol* 73:197, 1994.

65. Klein RM, Norman A: Diagnostic procedures for Paget's disease. Radiologic, pathologic, and laboratory testing, *Endocrinol Metab Clin North Am* 24:437, 1995.

66. Krane SM, Simon LS: Metabolic consequences of bone turnover in Paget's disease of bone, *Clin Orthop* 217:26, 1987.

67. Leeds NE, Jacobson HG: Spinal neurofibromatosis, *AJR: Am J Roentgenol* 126:617, 1976.

68. Little DG, Sussman MD: The Risser's sign: a critical analysis, *J Pediatr Orthop* 14:569, 1994.

69. Lonstein JE: Adolescent idiopathic scoliosis, *Lancet* 344:1407, 1994.

70. Lonstein JE, Carlson JM: The prediction of curve progression in untreated idiopathic scoliosis during growth, *J Bone Joint Surg* 66:1061, 1984.

71. Martinez-Lavin M: Pathogenesis of hypertrophic osteoarthropathy, *Clin Exper Rheumatol* 10:49, 1992.

72. Matucci-Cerinic M et al: The spectrum of dermatological symptoms of pachydermoperiostosis (primary hypertrophic osteoarthropathy): a genetic, cytogenetic and ultrastructural study, *Clin Exper Rheumatol* 10:45, 1992.

73. McCollough NC III et al: Miami TLSO in the management of scoliosis: preliminary results in 100 cases, *J Ped Orthop* 1:141, 1981.

74. McElvaine MD et al: Prevalence of radiographic evidence of paint chip ingestion among children with moderate to severe lead poisoning, St. Louis, 1989 through 1990, *Pediatrics* 89:740, 1992.

75. Meunier PJ, Vignot E: Therapeutic strategy in Paget's disease of bone, *Bone Suppl* 17:4895, 1995.

76. Meyer JS et al: Langerhans cell histiocytosis: presentation and evolution of radiologic findings with clinical correlation, *Radiographics* 15:1135, 1995.

77. Miller NH: Cause and natural history of adolescent idiopathic scoliosis, *Orthop Clin North Am* 30:343, 1999.

78. Morales LE: Gaucher's disease: a review, *Ann Pharmacother* 30:381, 1996.

79. Nash CL et al: Risks of exposure to x-rays in patients undergoing long term treatment for scoliosis, *J Bone Joint Surg* 61A:371, 1979.

80. National Institutes of Health Consensus Development Conference: Neurofibromatosis: conference statement, *Arch Neurol* 45:575, 1988.

81. National Institute of Health Technology Assessment Panel on Gaucher's Disease: Gaucher's disease: current issues in diagnosis and treatment, *JAMA* 275:548, 1996.

82. Neurofibromatosis: a handbook for patients, families, and healthcare professionals, New York, 1990, Thieme.

83. Nykoliation JW et al: An algorithm for the management of scoliosis, *J Man Physiol Ther* 9:1, 1986.

84. O'Doherty DP et al: Paget's disease of bone, *Curr Orthop* 3:262, 1989.

85. Oddis CV, Medsger TA: Inflammatory myopathies, *Baillieres Clin Rheumatol* 9:497, 1995.

86. Ostezan LB, Callen JP: Cutaneous manifestations of selected rheumatologic diseases, *Am Fam Physician* 53:1625, 1996.

87. Pachman LM: Juvenile dermatomyositis (JDMS): new clues to diagnosis and pathogenesis, *Clin Exper Rheumatol* 12:569, 1994.

88. Parkinson D, Hay R: Neurofibromatosis, *Surg Neurol* 25:109, 1986.

89. Peck B: Hypertrophic osteoarthropathy with Hodgkin's disease in the mediastinum, *JAMA* 238:1400, 1986.

90. Plosker GL, Goa KL: Clodronate. A review of its pharmacological properties and therapeutic efficacy in resorptive bone disease, *Drugs* 47:945, 1994.

91. Ray D, Williams G: Pathophysiological causes and clinical significance of flushing, *Br J Hosp Med* 50:594, 1993.

92. Reginster JY, Lecart MP: Efficacy and safety of drugs for Paget's disease of bone, *Bone Suppl* 17:4855, 1995.

93. Renshaw TS: Idiopathic scoliosis in children, *Curr Opin Pediatr* 5:407, 1993.

94. Renshaw TS: Screening schoolchildren for scoliosis, *Clin Orthop* 229:26, 1988.

95. Resnick D: Diagnosis of bone and joint disorders, ed 4, Philadelphia, 2002, WB Saunders.

96. Ringenberg QS et al: Hematologic effects of heavy metal poisoning, *South Med J* 81:1132, 1988.

97. Rogala EJ, Drummond OS, Gurr J: Scoliosis: incidence and natural history, *J Bone Joint Surg Am* 60:173, 1978.

98. Roodman GD: Osteoclast function in Paget's disease and multiple myeloma, *Bone Suppl* 17:575, 1995.

99. Rosen CJ, Kessenich CR: Comparative clinical pharmacology and therapeutic use of bisphosphonates in metabolic bone diseases, *Drugs* 51:537, 1996.

100. Rovira M et al: Radiological diagnosis of inorganic lead poisoning, *J Clin Gastroenterol* 11:469, 1989.

101. Ryan MD, Taylor TK: Spinal manifestations of Paget's disease, *Aust NZ J Surg* 62:33, 1992.

102. Sanders DG, Weijers RE: MRI findings in Caffey's disease, *Pediatr Radiol* 24:325, 1994.

103. Scerri L et al: Dermatomyositis associated with malignant melanoma-case report and review of the literature, *Clin Exper Dermatol* 19:523, 1994.

104. Seda H, Alarcon GS: Musculoskeletal syndromes associated with malignancies, *Curr Opin Rheumatol* 7:48, 1995.

105. Shaughnessy WJ: Management of adolescent idiopathic scoliosis, *Curr Opin Rheumatol* 5:301, 1993.

106. Singer FR, Minoofar PN: Bisphosphonates in the treatment of disorders of mineral metabolism, *Adv Endocrinol Metab* 6:259, 1995.

PART TWO Bone, Joints, and Soft Tissues

107. Sirikulchayanonta V, Naovaratanophas P, Jesdapatarakul S: Paget's disease of bone-clinico-pathology study of the first case report in Thailand, *J Med Assoc Thai* 75(suppl 1):136, 1992.

108. Skaggs DL, Bassett GS: Adolescent idiopathic scoliosis: an update, *Am Fam Physician* 53:2327, 1996.

109. Smirniotopoulos JG, Murphy FM: The phakomatoses, *AJNR* 13:725, 1992.

110. Solot CB et al: Communication disorders in children with neurofibromatosis type I. In Rubenstein AE, Korf BR, editors: Neurofibromatosis, New York, 1990, Thieme.

111. Staalman CR, Umans U: Hypertrophic osteoarthropathy in childhood malignancy, *Med Pediatr Oncol* 21:676, 1993.

112. Stein DH: Mastocytosis: a review, *Pediatr Dermatol* 3:365, 1989.

113. Stiller CA, Chessells JM, Fitchett M: Neurofibromatosis and childhood leukaemia/lymphoma: a population-based study, *Br J Cancer* 70:969, 1994.

114. Stull MA, Kransdorf MJ, Devaney KO: Langerhans cell histiocytosis of bone, *Radiographics* 12:801, 1992.

115. Stull MA et al: Magnetic resonance appearance of peripheral nerve sheath tumors, *Skeletal Radiol* 20:9, 1991.

116. Subbarano K, Jacobson HG: Amyloidosis and plasma cell dyscrasias of the musculoskeletal system, *Semin Roentgenol* 21:139, 1986.

117. Tarola GA: Manipulation for the control of back pain and curve progression in patients with skeletally mature idiopathic scoliosis: two cases, *J Man Physiol Ther* 17:253, 1994.

118. Taylor JAM: Full-spine radiography: a review, *J Man Physiol Ther* 16:460, 1993.

119. Tolo VT: Surgical treatment of adolescent idiopathic scoliosis, *Instr Course Lect* 38:143, 1989.

120. Urban BA et al: CT evaluation of amyloidosis: spectrum of disease, *Radiographics* 13:1295, 1993.

121. Valent P: Biology, classification and treatment of human mastocytosis, *Wien Klin Wochenschr* 108:385, 1996.

122. van Dam BE: Nonoperative treatment of adult scoliosis, *Orthop Clin North Am* 19:347, 1988.

123. Weinstein SL: Adolescent idiopathic scoliosis: prevalence and natural history, *Instr Course Lect* 38:115, 1989.

124. Weinstein SL, Zavala DC, Ponseti IV: Curve progression in idiopathic scoliosis, *J Bone Joint Surg* 65A:447, 1983.

125. Wierman WH, Clagett OT, McDonald JR: Articular manifestations in pulmonary disease. An analysis of their occurrence in 1024 cases in which pulmonary resection was performed, *JAMA* 155:1459, 1954.

126. Willman CL: Detection of clonal histiocytes in Langerhans cell histiocytosis: biology and clinical significance, *Br J Cancer Suppl* 23:29, 1994.

127. Winter RB: The pendulum has swung too far. Bracing for adolescent idiopathic scoliosis in the 1990s, *Orthop Clin North Am* 25:195, 1994.

128. Woolf DA et al: Lead lines in young infants with acute lead encephalopathy: a reliable diagnostic test, *J Trop Pediatr* 36:90, 1990.

129. Yaghmai I: Spine changes in neurofibromatosis, *Radiographics* 6:261, 1986.

130. Zatz LM: Atypical choroid plexus calcifications associated with neurofibromatosis, *Radiology* 91:1135, 1968.

chapter 16

Skull Patterns

DENNIS M. MARCHIORI

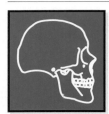

SK I | Basilar Invagination

Basilar invagination (or basilar impression) is an upward migration deformity of the base of the skull. *Platybasia* is an anthropologic term describing flattening of the skull base and should not be used synonymously with basilar invagination. The major causes of basilar invagination are summarized by the mnemonic COOP (congenital, osteogenesis imperfecta, osteomalacia, and Paget's disease).

McGregor's line is a widely used roentgenometric method to detect the presence of basilar invagination. It involves drawing a line segment from the posterior aspect of the hard palate to the inferior margin of the skull on the lateral radiograph. Basilar invagination is probable if the tip of the odontoid process is more than 8 mm above the line segment in men or 10 mm in women.

The diagnosis of basilar invagination is made with conventional radiography and is supplemented by computed tomography (CT) and magnetic resonance imaging (MRI). MRI is particularly helpful to assess possible concurrent neurologic involvement.

DISEASE	COMMENTS
More common	
Bone-softening disorders (FIG. 16-1)	Alterations of the skull base secondary to bone-softening diseases: osteogenesis imperfecta, rickets, osteomalacia, and Paget's disease.
Less common	
Congenital anomalies	Alterations of the skull base associated with atlantooccipital fusion (occipitalization or assimilation), Klippel-Feil syndrome, and stenosis of the foramen magnum.
Achondroplasia [p. 421]	Rhizomelic dysplasia resulting from a congenital defect of enchondral bone formation; characteristics include rounded lumbar "bullet-nosed" vertebrae, lumbar spine kyphosis, posterior vertebral body scalloping, increased intervertebral disc height, flattened vertebral bodies, narrowed spinal canal, and alterations of the skull base; the pelvis may appear hypoplastic; milder expressions of the disease may occur.
Arnold-Chiari malformation [p. 1395]	Malformation of the skull base with caudal displacement of the cerebellomedullary region; several levels of inferior displacement are recognized.
Cleidocranial dysplasia [p. 425]	Defect of intramembranous bone formation manifesting as osseous defects of the calvarium, clavicles, and pelvis; associated with persistence of metopic suture.
Trauma	Posttraumatic deformity from a skull fracture.

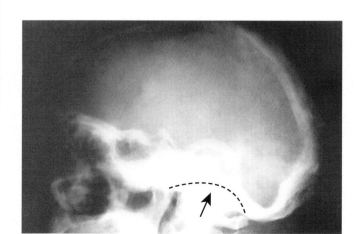

FIG. 16-1   Basilar invagination secondary to bone softening from Paget's disease of the skull *(arrow).* (Courtesy Joseph W. Howe, Sylmar, CA.)

SK2 | Button Sequestration of the Skull

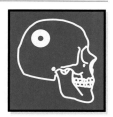

A button sequestration is a small, solitary osteolytic bone lesion that contains a central focus of calcification. Often this change represents a normal variant, particularly if it is surrounded by an osteosclerotic margin ("donut lesion"); however, aggressive pathologies should be considered.

DISEASE	COMMENTS
More common	
Eosinophilic granulomas **(FIG. 16-2)** [p. 935]	Common cause of osteolytic skull defects; the inner and outer skull tables are affected; however, the defects in the skull tables do not completely superimpose, leaving an appearance of a beveled margin.
Infection	Osteolytic defects may occur secondary to *Staphylococcus,* syphilis, or tuberculosis infections; often result from contiguous spread of scalp infection.
Bone metastasis [p. 889]	Primary carcinomas from the lung, breast, prostate, and colon commonly metastasize to the skull.
Normal variant	Radiolucent defects with central calcification and surrounding sclerosis, possibly representing normal variants; these defects are differentiated from true button sequestrations by the absence of reported pain and disability; these variants usually are discovered incidentally and are not clinically significant.
Less common	
Necrosis	Osteonecrosis resulting from irradiation, electric shock therapy, or electric burns; often a latent period of several years elapses before osteolytic lesion becomes apparent.
Postsurgical	Burr hole or shunt placement.
Primary neoplasm	Epidermoid, dermoid cyst, meningioma, and hemangiomas may cause radiolucent skull lesions.

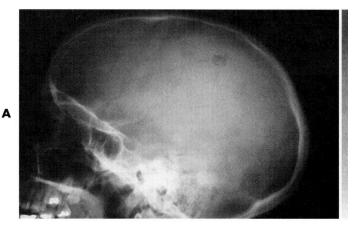
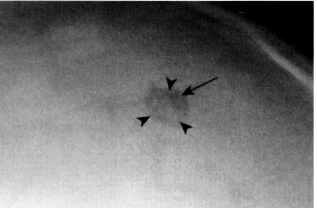

FIG. 16-2   A, Lateral skull projection and, **B,** close-up of eosinophilic granuloma, producing an osteolytic defect of the skull (*arrowheads*) with a central radiodense sequestrum (button sequestration) (*arrow*). (Courtesy Stan Higgins, Davenport, IA.)

PART TWO Bone, Joints, and Soft Tissues

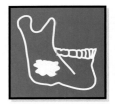

SK3 | Cystic Lesions of the Mandible

Cystic lesions of the mandible are often caused by pathologies that produce cystic lesions elsewhere in the skeleton and a variety of causes that are seen only in the mandible. Most pathologies comprising the latter group are related to pathological conditions of the teeth.

DISEASE	COMMENTS
More common *Dentigerous (follicular) cyst* **(FIG. 16-3)**	Well-circumscribed mandibular cyst that characteristically contains the crown of an unerupted tooth; this cyst is usually found in children.
Periodontal cyst	Common cyst of the jaw that develops from chronic infection; it appears as a well-defined radiolucent cyst in the periapical location and is contained within osteosclerotic margins.
Periapical granulomas	Well-circumscribed cyst in a periapical location, which may develop into periodontal cyst.
Less common *Ameloblastoma (adamantinoma)* **(FIG. 16-4)** [p. 883]	Multilocular radiolucent lesion with coarse inner trabeculation; it may grow very large, distorting the symmetry of the face. The condition usually is noted in patients older than 30 years of age.
Aneurysmal bone cyst/osteoblastomas/hemangiomas **(FIG. 16-5)**	Benign nonodontogenic tumors, including aneurysmal bone cysts, osteoblastomas, and hemangiomas, all producing osteolytic, expansile lesion of the mandible; each is much more common in other skeletal locations.
Cherubism	Bilateral, symmetric enlargement of the mandible, histologically similar to fibrous dysplasia, although the former has a familial incidence and is limited to the jaw.
Fibrous dysplasia [p. 846]	Unilateral, expansile, usually osteolytic, well-circumscribed lesions appearing locally or in association with other skeletal lesions. The osteosclerotic form of the disease is more typical of the maxilla. The craniofacial form (leontiasis ossea) of the disease is limited to the calvarium and face.
Giant cell reparative granuloma [p. 878]	Expansile osteolytic lesion of the mandible and maxilla with thin overlying cortex; this lesion is believed to represent a nontumorous reparative process.
Histiocytosis X (eosinophilic granuloma) **(FIG. 16-6)** [p. 935]	Common in the mandible; the destruction may be so advanced that the teeth appear to "float" without surrounding osseous support; Ewing's tumor, metastatic neuroblastoma, and non–Hodgkin lymphoma may produce similar appearances of "floating teeth."
Hyperparathyroidism [p. 910]	Single or multiple osteolytic lesions representing brown tumors; the lamina dura thins, as is also noted in fibrous dysplasia, Paget's disease, and osteomalacia.
Infection	Infections of the mandible and maxilla may develop from hematogenous seeding or via direct extension from dental or sinus infection; they appear as irregular osteolytic lesions, often with accompanying sequestration; trauma and local carcinoma also have been implicated.
Metastasis	Osteolytic lesions similar to those of other skeletal sites; metastasis may appear secondary to hematogenous seeding or direct extension from general nasal, oral, cutaneous, or salivary gland primary lesions.
Multiple myeloma [p. 819]	Multiple osteolytic lesions that appear well defined and of uniform size; concomitant skull changes are present nearly always.
Paget's disease [p. 946]	Diffuse osteolytic, osteosclerotic, or mixed pattern of bone disease with bilateral enlargement; concomitant skull changes nearly always occur.
Solitary bone cyst (hemorrhagic bone cyst) [p. 879]	Poorly defined irregular cyst of the mandible; this condition is seen in children; usually accompanied by a history of trauma.

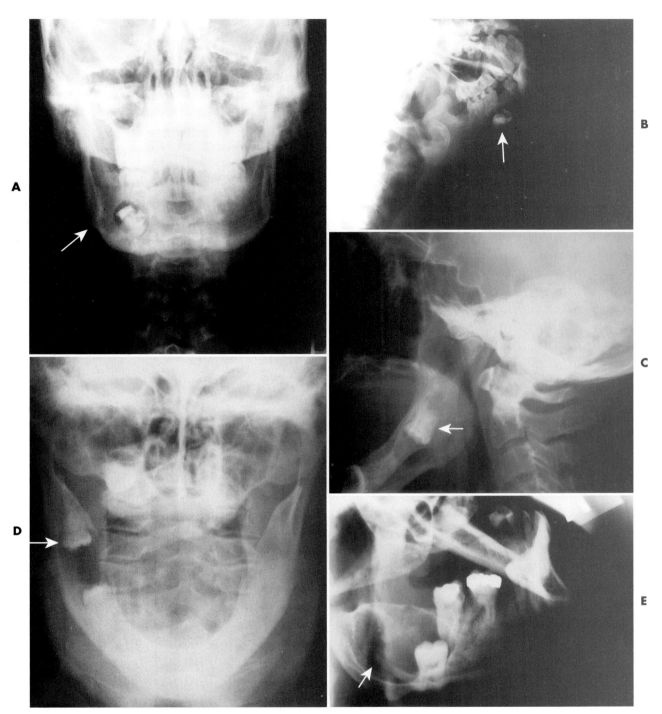

FIG. 16-3 Three patients (**A-B, C-D,** and **E**) all with a dentigerous cyst of the right ramus of the mandible. Each appears as a radiolucency with a central radiodense unerupted tooth *(arrows)*. (Courtesy Steven P. Brownstein, MD, Springfield, NJ.)

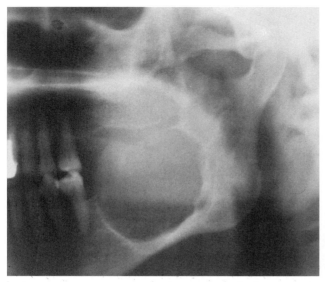

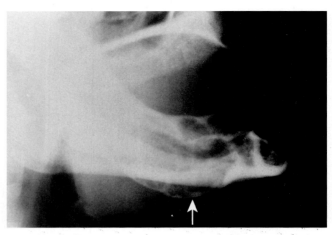

FIG. 16-5   Aneurysmal bone cyst, presenting as a cystic expansile lesion of the mandible *(arrow)*. (Courtesy William E. Litterer, Elizabeth, NJ.)

FIG. 16-4   Ameloblastoma. Oblique view of mandible reveals a large cystic lesion in body and ramus of mandible with attenuation and loss of bone superiorly. The esion has broken through upper part of mandible. (From Som PM, Curtin HD: Head and neck imaging, ed 4, St Louis, 2003, Mosby.)

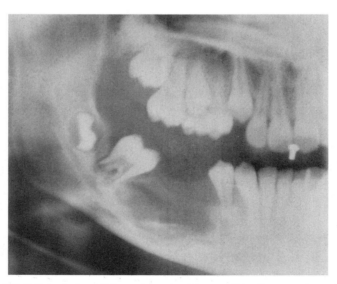

FIG. 16-6   Eosinophilic granuloma in right mandible. Panorex view of mandible reveals a lucent, irregular area that is fairly well defined in the body of the mandible between the second molar tooth and first premolar tooth. Some loss of lamina dura has occurred in the lower second molar tooth. (From Som PM, Curtin HD: Head and neck imaging, ed 4, St Louis, 2003, Mosby.)

SK4 | Diffuse Demineralization

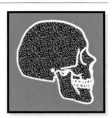

Diffuse demineralization of the skull typically is related to senile osteoporosis; however, many other conditions have classic presentations in the skull. Hyperparathyroidism mimics the radiographic appearance of osteoporosis; both appear with pure patterns of diffuse demineralization. Most of the other conditions listed in the following table produce patterns of diffuse demineralization that occur in combination with larger osteolytic lesions. For example, hemolytic anemias, leukemia, and metastatic neuroblastoma may produce a classic "hair-on-end" appearance in addition to diffuse demineralization.

DISEASE	COMMENTS
More common *Osteoporosis* [p. 451]	Appears with diffuse demineralization and is typically related to aging; less commonly, osteoporosis develops from steroid supplementation or endocrinopathy.
Less common *Anemias*	Possible diffuse osteoporosis related to marrow hyperplasia caused by sickle-cell anemia and thalassemia; other findings include a "hair-on-end" appearance involving the outer table of the calvarium.
Hyperparathyroidism **(FIG. 16-7)** [p. 910]	Granular, or "salt-and-pepper," appearance of the skull as a result of diffuse demineralization; rarely larger focal osteolytic lesions develop.
Infection [p. 785]	Diffuse presentation of infection is uncommon; in general, infections of the skull are less common in the United States than in underdeveloped countries.
Metastatic bone disease [p. 889]	Typically noted with multiple, ill-defined osteolytic lesions; this disease infrequently results in a diffuse demineralization pattern; breast, lung, and prostate origins are common in the adult; in the child, neuroblastoma and leukemia are more likely.
Multiple myeloma [p. 819]	Characterized by diffuse demineralization with focal "punched-out" lesions.
Paget's disease [p. 946]	Diffuse demineralization that may accompany the more classic presentation of large osteolytic areas of bone destruction (osteoporosis circumscripta); demineralization occurs most often in the outer table of the skull during the lytic phase of the disease.

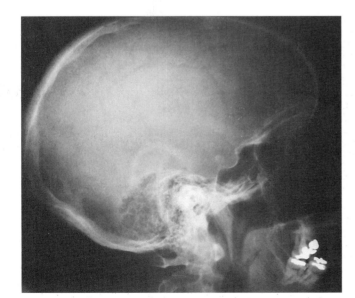

FIG. 16-7 Hyperparathyroidism. Granular deossification appearance of the calvarium, resulting in a salt-and-pepper appearance to skull. (From Deltoff MN, Kogon PL: The portable skeletal x-ray library, St Louis, 1998, Mosby.)

PART TWO Bone, Joints, and Soft Tissues

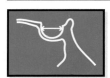

SK5 | Enlargement or Destruction of the Sella Turcica

Although variations exist, the sella turcica generally should not exceed an anteroposterior dimension of 16 mm or a vertical depth of 12 mm on the lateral skull radiograph. Also, normally the floor of the sella turcica is well defined by a single cortical line. The appearance of two cortical lines represents a "double-floor" sign, suggesting osseous erosion of the floor by an expansile mass. Hurler's disease is associated with elongation of the posterior aspect of the sella, creating a J-shaped configuration.

DISEASE	COMMENTS
More common	
Aneurysm of internal carotid vessel	Enlarged sella resulting from expanded cavernous segment of the carotid artery; linear vascular calcification often is present, projecting over the enlarged sella on a lateral radiograph.
Craniopharyngioma	Seen in children and young adults, tumor that may produce bone destruction of the sella; most lesions calcify; gliomas of the optic chiasm may cause similar changes.
Empty sella syndrome **(FIG. 16-8)** [p. 1396]	Appears as an enlarged sella without bone destruction or considerable deformity; the syndrome is believed to result from a congenital or acquired defect of the diaphragm sellae, which allows an intrasellar extension of the suprasellar arachnoid space; pulsations of the cerebrospinal fluid are thought to cause the sellar enlargement; the pituitary function typically is normal.
Pituitary tumors **(FIG. 16-9)**	Enlarged sella, uneven erosion of the floor, producing a "double-floor" appearance; pituitary tumors may be classified by size (a microadenoma is <1 cm and a macroadenoma is >1 cm in diameter) or by their appearance after staining; eosinophilic adenoma (causing acromegaly), chromophobe adenomas (causing hypopituitarism), and basophilic adenoma (causing Cushing's disease) occur.
Less common	
Chordoma [p. 875]	Blumenbach's clivus, representing the sloping surface of bone between the dorsum sellae and the foramen magnum (composed of the body of the sphenoid and pars basilaris of the occiput); the clivus is a target location for chordomas, which may secondarily involve the sella turcica from its posterior aspect; their appearance is marked by bone destruction and likely tumor matrix calcification; chordoma occurs most often in 30- to 60-year-old individuals.
Increased intracranial pressure	Associated with other conditions such as hydrocephalus, intracranial tumors, and edema; chronic increased intracranial pressure may manifest as erosion and deformity of the sella, resulting from downward pressure of an enlarged third ventricle.
Meningioma [p. 1335]	Arising from arachnoid and dura mater in the area of the diaphragma sellae, not within the pituitary fossa; meningioma appears with bone destruction and sclerosis; calcification is uncommon.

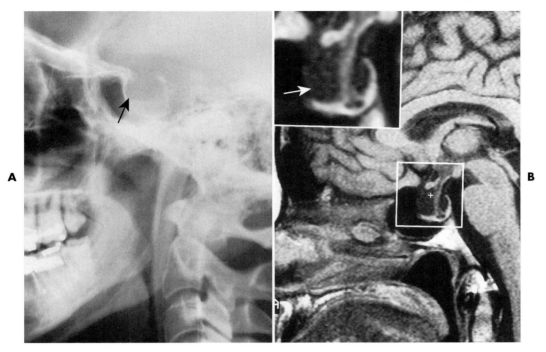

FIG. 16-8 A, The lateral cervical projection reveals an enlarged sella turcia (beyond 12 × 16 mm on the original film) with a double density of the floor of the sella *(arrow)*. **B,** The sagittal T1-weighted magnetic resonance image denotes hypointense fluid signal intensity in the sella turcica consistent with cerebrospinal fluid *(arrow)*.

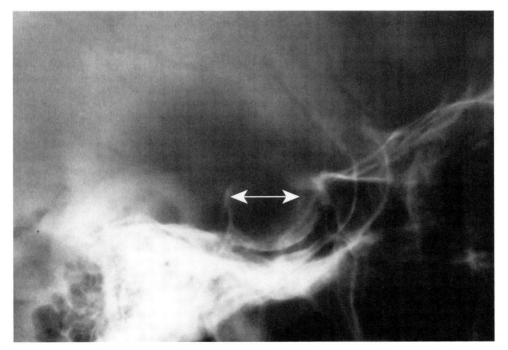

FIG. 16-9 Enlarged sella turcica *(arrow)* secondary to pituitary adenoma.

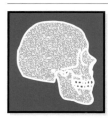

SK6 | Increased Radiodensity of the Calvarium

Increased radiodensity of the skull results from pathologic thickening of the inner, outer, or both tables of the calvarium. Generally it is difficult to determine which table is involved from plain film radiographs. At times the diploic space may be entirely obliterated by sclerosis. Increased density may be localized or generalized throughout much of the skull. Osteomas, meningiomas, and cephalohematomas usually result in localized changes. Renal osteodystrophy, fluorosis, myelosclerosis, acromegaly, hemolytic anemias, and selected congenital diseases typically produce a generalized increase in the radiodensity of the skull. Paget's disease, fibrous dysplasia, metastasis, and hyperostosis frontalis interna may occur as localized or generalized patterns.

DISEASE	COMMENTS
More common	
Fibrous dysplasia **(FIG. 16-10)** [p. 846]	Localized or generalized increased radiodensity, typically involving the skull base or facial bones; the skull is commonly involved if multiple skeletal sites are found.
Meningioma [p. 1385]	Hyperostosis of the inner table occurring over the areas of the tumor; an exaggerated appearance of the meningeal grooves and foramen spinosum is a common result.
Paget's disease [p. 946]	Thickened trabeculae leading to a localized or, more typically, generalized increased radiodensity; eventually the delineation of an inner and outer table is lost; the osteoblastic ("cotton-wool") appearance signifies an advanced stage of the disease.
Less common	
Acromegaly [p. 907]	Thickening and generalized increased radiodensity of the skull; concurrent enlargement of the jaw, sella turcica, and frontal sinuses also is noted.
Calcified cephalohematoma	Describes a localized calcific skull radiodensity or thickening that develops from a subperiosteal hematoma; the area of involvement usually is in a parietal location and is confined by suture borders; this condition often is associated with forceps delivery.
Congenital diseases **(FIG. 16-11)**	Osteopetrosis, pyknodysostosis, and Pyle disease associated with generalized increase in skull radiodensity and other skeletal changes.
Fluorosis	Generalized increase in skull radiodensity; changes are more prominent in the spine.
Hematologic anemias **(FIG. 16-12)**	Hyperplastic marrow changes associated with thalassemia, hereditary spherocytosis, and sickle-cell anemia leading to spicules of new bone growth; these spicules are oriented perpendicular to the calvarium ("hair-on-end" appearance), producing a generalized increase in the radiodensity of the skull.
Hyperostosis frontalis interna	Localized idiopathic process more common in women over the age of 40 years; it does not cross the midline and involves the inner table of the skull; hyperostosis interna generalisata describes more widespread changes of the skull.
Metastatic disease [p. 1393]	Localized or, more commonly, generalized skull involvement; this disease develops from breast or prostate carcinoma after therapy; an osteolytic presentation is more common than an osteodense presentation.
Myelosclerosis	Generalized increase in skull radiodensity; concurrent splenomegaly is usual.
Osteoma **(FIG. 16-13)**	Most common primary calvarial neoplasm; osteoma develops only in intramembranously formed bone. This disease appears as a localized region of dense cortical hyperostosis and may arise from the inner or outer skull table; it is more common in the sinuses, particularly the frontal sinus. Osteomas are to intramembranously formed bones what bone islands are to enchondrally formed bones.
Renal osteodystrophy	Generalized increase in skull radiodensity that parallels changes elsewhere in the skeleton; appearance may be similar to Paget's disease.

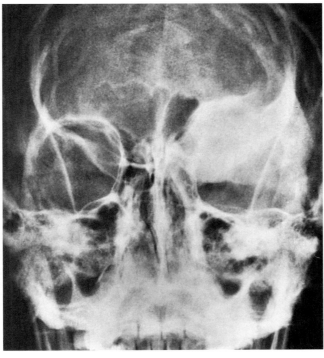

FIG. 16-10 Fibrous dysplasia of the skull on a Caldwell view shown as a very dense expansile lesion of the left frontal and zygomatic bones that has encroached on the left orbit. (From Som PM, Curtin HD: Head and neck imaging, ed 4, St Louis, 2003, Mosby.)

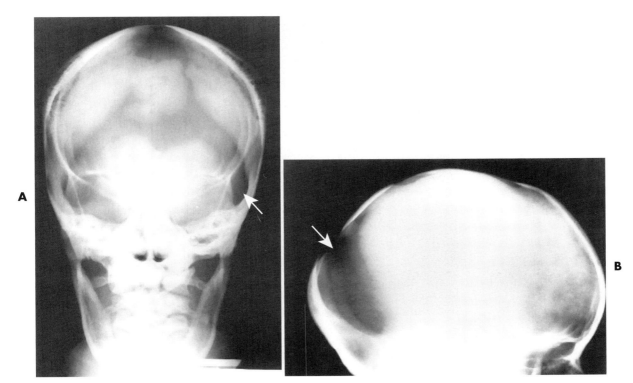

FIG. 16-11 A, Anteroposterior and, **B,** lateral projection of pyknodysostosis, demonstrating a radiodense skull and widened radiolucent sutures *(arrows)*. (Courtesy Joseph W. Howe, Sylmar, CA.)

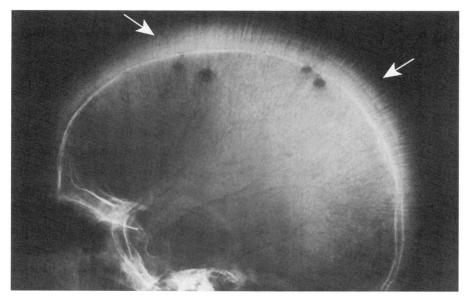

FIG. 16-12   Thalassemia (Cooley anemia), causing diffuse demineralization and "hair-on-end" appearance *(arrows)* of the anterior calvarium related to marrow hyperplasia. (Courtesy Joseph W. Howe, Sylmar, CA.)

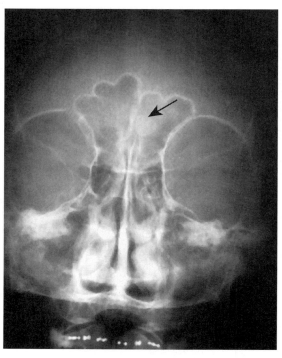

FIG. 16-13   Osteoma arising near the frontal sinus *(arrow)*. (Courtesy Steven P. Brownstein, MD, Springfield, NJ.)

SK7 | Intracranial Calcifications

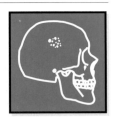

Intracranial calcifications are a common finding on plain film radiographs and even more common on CT scans of the skull. Although most represent physiologic calcifications of limited clinical significance, aggressive pathology (e.g., tumor, infection, vascular disturbance) is an important consideration in the differential diagnosis. Intracranial calcifications typically are localized; they are associated commonly with infections or tuberous sclerosis when they present with a scattered pattern.

DISEASE	COMMENTS
More common *Physiologic calcifications* **(FIG. 16-14)**	Those that involve the pineal and habenula commonly found in the midline in a frontal skull projection; physiologic calcifications of the basal ganglia and choroid plexus often are bilateral and symmetric in a frontal projection; physiologic calcification of the dura mater typically occurs along the superior sagittal sinus, falx, and tentorium; short, nearly horizontal linear calcifications located immediately posterior to the posterior clinoids in a lateral projection often are seen in the elderly and represent calcifications of the petroclinoid ligaments; physiologic calcifications are usually of no clinical significance; however, a shift in their normal location may indicate a space-occupying lesion (mass, hemorrhage, etc.); additionally, if they occur in young children, they may suggest underlying pathology; the typical age of presentation is noteworthy: pineal, older than 10 years; choroid plexus, older than 3 years; habenular, older than 10 years; petroclinoid, older than 5 years; and falx or tentorium, older than 3 years.
Less common *Tumors*	Oligodendroglioma, craniopharyngioma, ependymoma, choroid plexus papilloma, meningioma, teratoma, pinealoma, pituitary adenoma, and so on; craniopharyngiomas are more common in children; meningiomas are more common in middle-aged adults and are rare in children.
Infections	Cysticercosis, cytomegalovirus, paragonimiasis, torulosis, toxoplasmosis, tuberculomas, viral encephalitis, and so on; infections usually occur with multiple scattered foci of calcification.
Vascular	Including aneurysm, arteriosclerosis, and arteriovenous malformations (AVMs), which are common vascular causes of intracranial calcification; arteriosclerotic calcifications of the internal carotid arteries typically are seen in the parasellar region where the arteries pass through the cavernous sinuses; by contrast, an aneurysm is more often in a suprasellar location and therefore is suspected when a sellar pattern of calcification extends superiorly beyond the confines of the sella.
Basal ganglia	Pathologic basal ganglia calcification appears as bilateral, central scattered radiodensities occurring secondary to endocrine disorders (hypoparathyroidism, pseudohypoparathyroidism, pseudopseudohypoparathyroidism), infections (cytomegalovirus, toxoplasmosis, and cysticercosis), and toxic exposure (lead and carbon monoxide poisoning).
Phakomatosis **(FIG. 16-15)**	Various patterns of calcifications are produced by neurofibromatosis (meningiomas and gliomas), Sturge-Weber syndrome (parallel serpentine plaques), tuberous sclerosis (scattered nodules), and von Hippel-Lindau disease (retina and intracranial angiomas).
Trauma	Localized areas of calcification after posttraumatic hemorrhage.
Artifacts	Hair braids, toupees, barrettes, and other artifacts simulating intracranial calcifications.

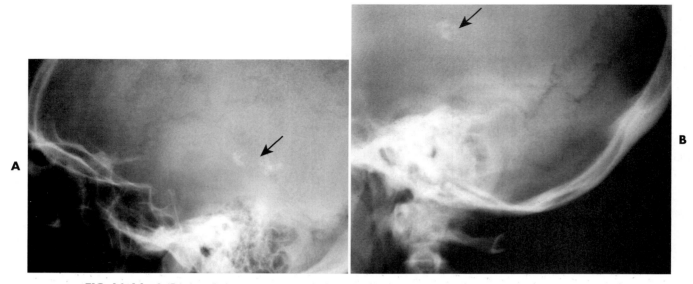

FIG. 16-14   **A,** Faintly radiodense scattered calcific foci with the choroid plexus. **B,** A small focus of calcification in the pineal gland *(arrows)*.

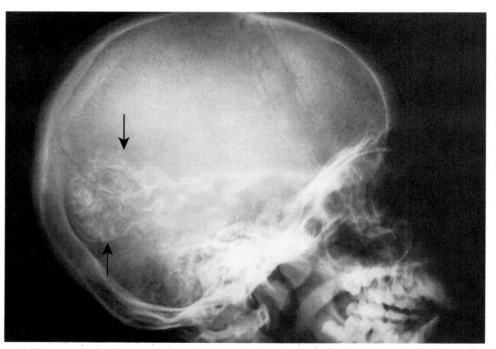

FIG. 16-15   Parallel serpentine calcifications consistent with Sturge-Weber syndrome *(arrows)*.

SK8 | Mass in the Paranasal Sinuses

The paranasal sinuses comprise the paired frontal, ethmoid, sphenoid, and maxillary sinuses. Alteration in the normally radiolucent appearance of the sinus suggests the presence of pathology. Aggressive pathology within the sinuses may have serious complications because of the sinuses' anatomic proximity to the brain and eye. Multiple radiographic projections and possibly CT are needed to evaluate all of the paranasal sinuses.

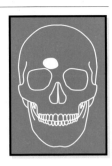

DISEASE	COMMENTS
More common	
Fracture	Paranasal sinus opacification resulting from recent trauma and hemorrhage or, less often, old fracture and residual bone deformity.
Infection	Typically follows dental or sinus infection; the appearance of thick mucosa with bone demineralization and destruction is suggestive; osteomyelitis involving the calvarium above the frontal sinus has been called *Pott's puffy tumor.*
Mucocele	Radiodense accumulation of mucous secretions secondary to obstruction of the involved sinus ostium; obstruction usually is the result of swollen mucosa, thick secretions, or both; mucoceles may completely opacify the sinus; most mucoceles are found in the frontal sinuses, followed by ethmoid sinuses; an infected mucocele is known as a *pyocele.*
Mucus retention cyst/serous cyst **(FIG. 16-16)**	Smooth, rounded, radiodense mass representing a plugged and consequentially expanded sinus mucous gland; the floor of the maxillary sinus most commonly is involved; the serous cyst is radiographically identical to the mucus retention cyst, representing fluid accumulation between submucosal layers; both cysts are related to chronic sinusitis.
Sinusitis (acute or chronic) **(FIG. 16-17)**	Opacification, mucosal thickening, and regional bone demineralization; an air-fluid level is characteristic; sinusitis occurs secondary to acute sinus infection; the maxillary sinuses are most commonly involved with acute or chronic sinusitis; sphenoid sinuses are least involved.
Less common	
Benign tumors **(FIG. 16-18)**	Masses of varying radiodensity, ranging from the very radiodense osteomas to the more radiolucent lipomas; others include chondroma, dermoid, and hemangioma, and lesions extending from the maxilla and mandible.
Fibrous dysplasia/Paget's disease	Paranasal sinus opacification related to Paget's disease or fibrous dysplasia involving the adjacent bone; leontiasis ossea is the bilateral enlargement and distortion of the facial bones secondary to fibrous dysplasia.
Malignant tumors	Characterized by a soft-tissue mass and bone destruction; squamous cell carcinomas are the most common; others include lymphoma, extramedullary plasmacytoma, adenoid cystic carcinomas (cylindromas), and mixed salivary tumors; the maxillary sinus is involved most commonly.
Polypoid rhinosinusitis	Complication of allergies, tobacco, and chronic nasal or paranasal sinusitis manifesting as multiple polypoid enlargements and degeneration of the mucosa.
Wegener granulomatosus	Autoimmune necrotizing granulomatosus usually affecting pulmonary, renal, and sinus tissues; sinus mucosal thickening with regional bone destruction is common; involvement of the mastoid sinus is characteristic.

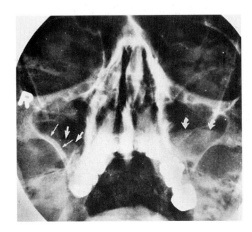

FIG. 16-16 Waters view shows a large "flat" retention cyst *(curved arrows)* in the left antrum. This can simulate an air-fluid level if careful attention is not paid to its slightly convex upper surface. The mucosa has thickened slightly in the right antrum *(thin arrows)*, and another small retention cyst is present in the lower right maxillary sinus *(arrows)*. (From Som PM, Curtin HD: Head and neck imaging, ed 4, St Louis, 2003, Mosby.)

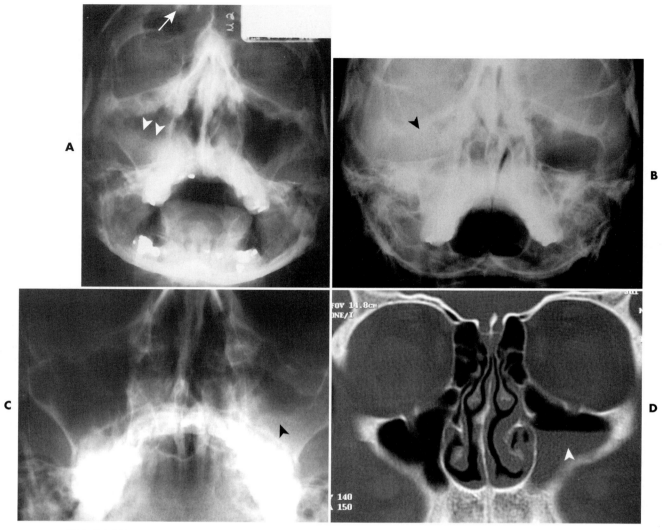

FIG. 16-17 Three cases (**A, B,** and **C-D**) of sinus opacification associated with sinusitis *(arrowheads)*. (**A,** Courtesy Ian D. McLean, Davenport, IA; **C** and **D,** Courtesy Sean Mathers, Pittsburgh, PA.)

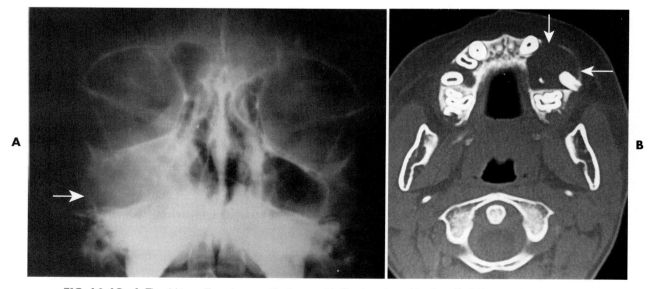

FIG. 16-18 **A,** The right maxillary sinus opacification on plain film *(arrow)*, resulting from, **B,** fluid accumulations related to a dentigerous cyst of the maxilla, seen on computed tomography *(arrows)*.

SK9 | Multiple Wormian Bones

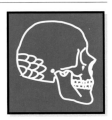

Wormian bones are intrastructural islands of bone occurring in the lambdoid, posterior sagittal, and tympanosquamosal sutures. Their appearance often is a variant of normal, particularly when found in a child younger than the age of 6 months. Wormian bones have been associated with a number of pathologic conditions. Many of the conditions are described by the mnemonic *PORK CHOPS* (pyknodysostosis, osteogenesis imperfecta, rickets in healing phase, kinky hair syndrome, cleidocranial dysplasia, hypothyroidism [and hypophosphatasia], otopalatodigital syndrome, primary acroosteolysis [and pachydermoperiostosis], Down syndrome).

DISEASE	**COMMENTS**
More common	
Variant	Wormian bones may present as a variant of normal, without associated features.
Cleidocranial dysplasia **(FIG. 16-19)** [p. 425]	Defect of intramembranous bone formation largely involving the calvarium, clavicles, and pelvis; this disease is associated with persistence of the metopic suture.
Osteogenesis imperfecta [p. 451]	Defect of connective tissue formation; characteristics include blue sclera, brittle bones, multiple fractures, and delayed closure of sutures.
Less common	
Hypoparathyroidism/hypophosphatasia [p. 913]	Metabolic disturbances resulting from low levels of parathormone or alkaline phosphatase, respectively; both are associated with delayed closure of sutures.
Pyknodysostosis [p. 456]	Rare syndrome of bone dysplasia marked by short stature, mandibular hypoplasia, and a failure of sutures to close.
Rickets [p. 925]	Defect of calcification resulting from deficiency of vitamin D (dietary or poor metabolism) associated with altered skull shape and delayed closure of sutures.

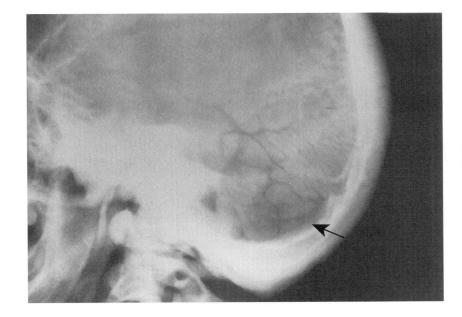

FIG. 16-19 Cleidocranial dysostosis with multiple wormian bones *(arrow)*. (Courtesy Joseph W. Howe, Sylmar, CA.)

PART TWO Bone, Joints, and Soft Tissues

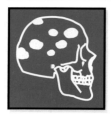

SK10 | Osteolytic Defects of the Skull

The calvarium (or skull cap) is composed of a central, marrow-filled diploic space sandwiched between inner and outer cortical tables of bone. Osteolytic lesions of the skull may involve primarily either the inner or outer skull tables or may arise from the diploic space, progressively involving both the inner and outer layers equally.

Osteolytic defects of the skull may be solitary or multiple. A solitary lesion with surrounding osteosclerotic border is known as a *donut lesion;* one with a central nidus of calcification is known as a *button sequestration* and is detailed in pattern SK2.

Osteolytic defects of the skull are described by the mnemonic *HELP ME* (hemangioma, epidermoid/dermoid, leptomeningeal cyst [and lambdoidal suture defect], Paget's disease [osteoporosis circumscripta], postsurgical, metastasis, and eosinophilic granuloma/encephalocele).

DISEASE	COMMENTS
SOLITARY	
More common	
Donut lesion	Defect with surrounding sclerosis of variable thickness; these defects are of no clinical significance.
Parietal foramina	Bilateral, symmetric lucent defects in the posterior region of the parietal bones; these defects are of no clinical significance.
Metastasis **(FIG. 16-20)** [p. 1393]	Usually occur in patients older than 40 years of age; typically patients have a history of primary malignancy; breast carcinoma is a particularly common source of skull metastasis; lesions usually are multiple.
Hemangioma **(FIG. 16-21)**	Benign solitary osteolytic lesion that demonstrates characteristic "honeycomb" or "spoke-wheel" trabecular patterns; histologically these are the same as those lesions occurring in the vertebrae.
Infection [p. 785]	Acute infection resulting in irregular, poorly defined osteolytic margins that have a tendency to coalesce; often develops secondary to contiguous spread from paranasal or middle ear infections.
Less common	
Encephalocele	Rare, representing a herniation of brain substance through a congenital defect in the skull.
Histiocytosis X [p. 935]	Abnormal proliferation of histiocytes that encompasses several clinical entities, all of unknown origin; few bone changes are noted with Letterer-Siwe disease; Hand-Schüller-Christian disease may demonstrate bone lesions of the calvarium, skull base, and mandible; eosinophilic granuloma represents the most common and proliferative form of the disease; it is marked by osteolytic skeletal defects, most prominent in the skull; bone lesion resulting from histiocytosis X involves the inner and outer tables of the skull; the lesions do not completely superimpose, forming a characteristic "beveled-edge" appearance; although lesions are usually solitary, multiple lesions often occur.
Lambdoid suture	Wide appearance of the lambdoidal suture often seen in neurofibromatosis.
Necrosis	Radiation, electric shock therapy, or electric burns.
Postsurgical	Burr holes or shunt placement.
Primary malignancy **(FIG. 16-22)**	Malignancies of the scalp, bone, orbit, dura, and brain.
Epidermoid, dermoid	Benign tumors presenting with well-defined radiolucent defects, often with osteosclerotic borders; they form from tissues that become trapped in the diploic space secondary to a defect in the formation of the neural tube; dermoids usually are located in the midline and form from ectodermal and mesodermal tissue; epidermoids form from ectodermal tissue.
Leptomeningeal cyst	Describes an entrapment of the arachnoid dura between the margins of an existing skull fracture; the continuous pulsations of the cerebrospinal fluid cause erosions of the skull, giving a "growing" nature to the fracture.
MULTIPLE	
More common	
Hyperparathyroidism [p. 910]	Classic appearance of demineralization and fine granular or "salt-and-pepper" appearance to the skull; less commonly, larger osteolytic skull defects appear.
Metastasis **(FIGS. 16-23 and 16-24)** [p. 1393]	Multiple osteolytic defects of varying sizes; most patients have metastasis elsewhere in the skeleton. Resulting from an increased blood supply, the calvarium is more commonly involved than the skull base. Patients are usually older than 40 years of age; breast and lung primaries are most common in adults; neuroblastoma and leukemia are most common in children.

DISEASE	COMMENTS
Multiple myeloma **(FIG. 16-25)** [p. 819]	Characteristic presentation of demineralization with multiple, well-defined osteolytic defects of generally uniform size (ranging from 0.5 to 4 cm); the lesions appear as "punch-out" defects without osteosclerotic borders.
Pacchionian bodies (arachnoid granulations or villi)	Fingerlike extensions of the arachnoid mater into the dural venous sinus; extensions exert pressure on the thinned dura mater, forming pit or erosion defects of the supraadjacent inner table of the skull; defects are located within several centimeters of the sagittal sinus and are of no clinical significance.
Paget's disease **(FIG. 16-26)** [p. 946]	Single or multiple osteolytic areas occurring with the osteolytic phase of Paget's disease, known as *osteoporosis circumscripta;* usually begins in the frontal or occipital regions and progresses as a wave of osteoporosis; the osteolytic areas are well demarcated, often bilateral, involving the outer table more than the inner table of the skull; more common among patients older than 40 years of age.
Less common *Radiation*	Mixed osteosclerotic and osteolytic pattern of bone disease with widely scattered irregular defects usually presenting a year after irradiation.
Cushing's syndrome [p. 909]	Demineralization and fine granular osteolytic defects similar in appearance to hyperparathyroidism.
Fibrous dysplasia **(FIG. 16-27)** [p. 846]	Single or multiple defects, usually appearing with a mixed osteosclerotic and osteolytic pattern in the calvarium.
Histiocytosis X **(FIG. 16-28)** [p. 935]	Abnormal proliferation of histiocytes that encompasses several clinical entities, all of unknown origin; few bone changes are noted with Letterer-Siwe disease; Hand-Schüller-Christian disease may demonstrate bone lesions of the calvarium, skull base, and mandible. Eosinophilic granuloma represents the most common and proliferative form of the disease. It is marked by osteolytic skeletal defects, most prominent in the skull. Bone lesion resulting from histiocytosis X involves the inner and outer tables of the skull. The lesions do not completely superimpose, relating a characteristic "beveled-edge" appearance. Although lesions usually are solitary, multiple lesions often occur.
Neurofibromatosis [p. 942]	Single or multiple defects in the occipital and temporal bone, more commonly involving the greater wing of the sphenoid.

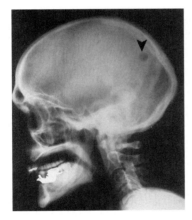

FIG. 16-20 Metastatic disease presenting with one prominent osteolytic defect *(arrowhead).* (Courtesy Ian D. McLean, Davenport, IA.)

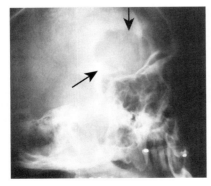

FIG. 16-22 Osteolytic defect of the skull *(arrows)* secondary to squamous cell carcinoma of the orbit. (Courtesy Steven P. Brownstein, MD, Springfield, NJ.)

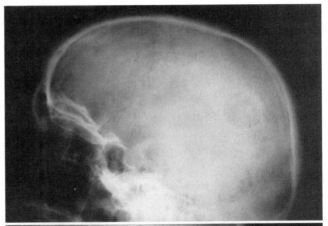

A

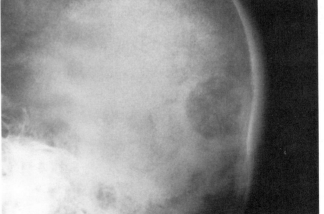

B

FIG. 16-21 **A,** Lateral skull and, **B,** close-up view of a hemangioma exhibiting the typical radiolucent defect with internal radiodense striations.

PART TWO Bone, Joints, and Soft Tissues

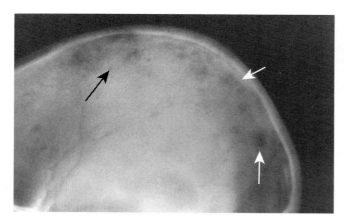

FIG. 16-23 Metastatic bone disease of the skull with multiple well-defined osteolytic defects *(arrows)*. This appearance is also strongly suggestive of multiple myeloma. (Courtesy Joseph W. Howe, Sylmar, CA.)

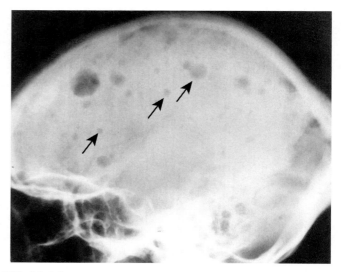

FIG. 16-24 Metastatic bone disease appearing as multiple osteolytic defects *(arrows)*. Metastatic lesions are often larger than depicted in this case. (Courtesy Ian D. McLean, Davenport, IA.)

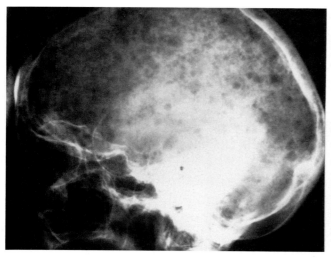

FIG. 16-25 Multiple "punch-out" osteolytic lesions of consistent size, characteristic of multiple myeloma of the skull.

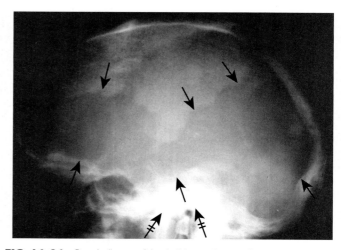

FIG. 16-26 Paget's disease of the skull. Large circumscribed regions of osteolysis (osteoporosis circumscripta) *(arrows)*, with basilar impression *(crossed arrows)*.

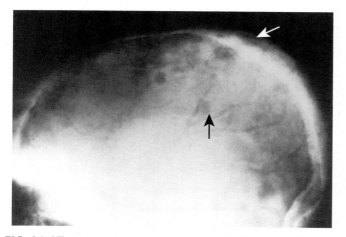

FIG. 16-27 Mixed pattern of bone sclerosis with focal osteolytic regions *(arrows)* secondary to fibrous dysplasia of the calvarium. (Courtesy Joseph W. Howe, Sylmar, CA.)

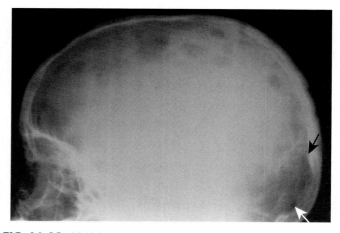

FIG. 16-28 Multiple osteolytic regions of bone destruction. In the occipital region the area of bone destruction of the inner and outer table are not identical. The lack of overlap produces a "beveled-edge" appearance, characteristic of histiocytosis X *(arrows)*. (Courtesy Joseph W. Howe, Sylmar, CA.)

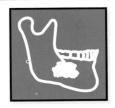

SK11 Radiodense Mandible Lesions

Osteosclerotic lesions of the mandible may appear solitary, multiple, or generalized throughout the bone. The appearance often changes over time. Many diseases originally appear as radiolucent osteolytic bone lesions and become osteosclerotic over time.

DISEASE	COMMENTS
More common *Cementinoma/cementoma*	Tumor of mesodermal origin, most often involving the anterior portion of the mandible; this disease is more common among women 30 to 40 years of age; lesions may appear solitary or multiple; in its initial stages the lesion appears as a radiolucent cyst and becomes radiodense in the late stages, having an appearance of a mass within a cyst.
Odontoma **(FIG. 16-29)**	Radiodense mass with two appearances; a complex odontoma represents a single mass of maldeveloped solid dental tissues (e.g., enamel, dentin, pulp) that appear radiographically as an amorphous radiodense mass; the second type—compound odontomas—are similar, but they may contain discernible, poorly developed, misshapen teeth.
Sclerosing infection	Infection of the jaw typically secondary to trauma or a dental or sinus infection; the appearance may originally be osteolytic, later forming a sequestrum and becoming osteosclerotic.
Less common *Fibrous dysplasia* [p. 846]	Usually osteolytic; however, fibrous dysplasia may present as solitary or multiple radiodense lesions with an occasionally expansile appearance; less commonly a mixed osteolytic-osteosclerotic pattern occurs.
Infantile cortical hyperostosis (Caffey's disease) **(FIG. 16-30)** [p. 941]	Bilateral, symmetric thickening of the mandible resulting from intramembranous new bone formation; although other skeletal sites are involved (e.g., clavicle), the mandible is the most common location; clinical findings include hard, tender soft-tissue enlargement over involved region; this disease occurs before 5 months of age.
Osteosarcoma/chondrosarcoma	Similar appearance to that of lesions elsewhere in the skeleton; mandibular lesions are less common and typically follow lesions at other skeletal sites.
Torus palatinus/torus mandibularis	(Torus palatinus) exostoses arising from the median suture of the hard palate; (torus mandibularis) bone projections from the internal, anterior portion of the mandible are similar to that of torus palatinus; both are typically bilateral and symmetric.
Paget's disease [p. 946]	Appears as a radiodense, bilateral, symmetric, enlarged appearance of bone during its blastic phase; the mandible is more commonly involved than the maxilla.

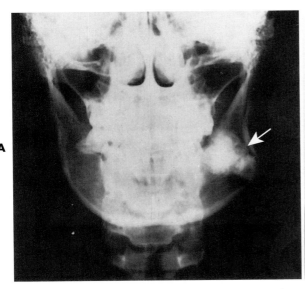

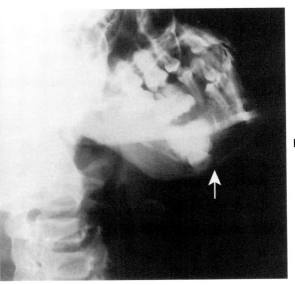

A

B

FIG. 16-29 A and **B,** Odontoma appearing as a radiopaque mass of the left ramus of the mandible *(arrows).* (Courtesy Steven P. Brownstein, MD, Springfield, NJ.)

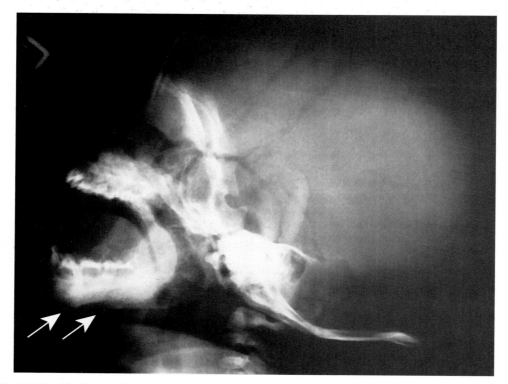

FIG. 16-30   Infantile cortical hyperostosis. Note thick and radiodense jaw *(arrows)*. (Courtesy William E. Litterer, Elizabeth, NJ.)

Suggested Readings

Burgener FA, Kormano M: Differential diagnosis in conventional radiology, ed 2, New York, 1991, Thieme.

Chapman S, Nakielny R: Aids to radiological differential diagnosis, ed 4, Philadelphia, 2003, WB Saunders.

Dahnert W: Radiology review manual, Baltimore, 1991, Williams & Wilkins.

Dolan KD Cervicobasilar relationships, *Radiol Clin North Am* 15(2):155, 1977.

Eisenberg R: An atlas of differential diagnosis, ed 2, Gaithersburg, MD, 1992, Aspen.

Jacobson HG: Dense bone-too much bone: radiographical considerations and differential diagnosis, *Skeletal Radiol* 13:1, 1985.

Keller JD: Basics of head and neck film interpretation, Boston, 1990, Little, Brown.

Ravin CE, Cooper C, Leder RA: Review of radiology, Philadelphia, 1994, WB Saunders.

Reeder MM, Bradley WG: Reeder and Felson's gamuts in radiology, ed 3, New York, 1993, Springer-Verlag.

Taybi H, Lachman RS: Radiology of syndromes, metabolic disorders, and skeletal dysplasias, ed 4, St Louis, 1996, Mosby.

Teodori JB, Painter MJ: Basilar impression in children, *Pediatrics* 74(6), 1997.

Unger JM: Head and neck imaging, New York, 1987, Churchill Livingstone.

Weissleder R, Wittenberg J, Harisinghani MG: Primer of diagnostic imaging, ed 3, St Louis, 2003, Mosby.

chapter 17

Spine Patterns

DENNIS M. MARCHIORI

SP1 Altered Vertebral Shape

Altered vertebral shape typically results from congenital conditions. Although a vertebra's appearance may be altered in a myriad of ways, the following table includes some of the more commonly encountered alterations. Vertebral collapse and vertebral expansion are larger topics and therefore are discussed separately in this chapter.

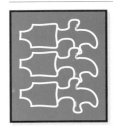

SP1a | Beaked or Hooked Vertebrae

DISEASE	COMMENTS
More common *Achondroplasia* [p. 421]	Congenital defect of endochondral bone formation, producing characteristic rounded lumbar "bullet-nosed" vertebrae, lumbar kyphosis, posterior scalloping of the vertebrae, increased intervertebral disc height, flattened vertebral bodies, and narrowed spinal canal; the pelvis may appear hypoplastic; milder forms of the disease may occur.
Mucopolysaccharidoses [p. 444]	A group of lysosomal storage diseases marked by a common disorder in mucopolysaccharide metabolism, evidenced by various mucopolysaccharides excreted in the urine; these substances collect in connective tissue, resulting in bone, cartilage, and connective tissue defects; characteristics are platyspondyly with dwarfism, kyphosis, and alterations in the appearance of the vertebrae; mucopolysaccharidosis I (Hurler's syndrome) is associated with oval, posteriorly scalloped, anterior inferiorly beaked vertebrae; mucopolysaccharidosis IV (Morquio's syndrome) is associated with flattened, anterior centrally beaked vertebrae.
Normal variant	Slightly beaked vertebrae, most often occurring in the thoracic spine; the vertebral defect usually appears more wedged than beaked; the vertebral body may appear anteriorly beaked before ossification of the ring epiphyses; these steplike defects contain the cartilage growth centers of the vertebral endplate; as ossification proceeds, a focus of bone fills the radiolucent defect (6 to 12 years of age), fusing to the vertebral body at 20 to 25 years of age.
Less common *Diastrophic dysplasia* [p. 429]	Autosomal, recessive, rhizomelic dwarfism secondary to a cartilage disorder; it is characterized by multiple skeletal disorders, including progressive kyphoscoliosis, anteriorly deformed vertebrae, hypoplastic first metacarpal, clubfoot, and deformed flattened epiphyses.
Neurofibromatosis *(von Recklinghausen's disease)* [p. 942]	Congenital disturbance of mesodermal and neuroectodermal tissue development, appearing clinically with cutaneous markings, bone deformity, and neurofibromas; spinal changes include posterior vertebral scalloping, enlarged intervertebral foramina, kyphoscoliosis, and anteriorly beaked or wedged vertebrae.
Cretinism [p. 915]	Congenital hypothyroidism with delayed appearance of ossification centers, skeletal underdevelopment, wormian bones, and poorly developed sinuses; sail-like or tonguelike vertebrae and kyphosis at the thoracolumbar junction are common; changes may regress in adulthood.

SP1b | Biconcave Vertebrae

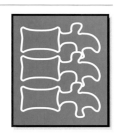

DISEASE	COMMENTS
More common	
Metastatic bone disease [p. 889]	Metastatic bone deposition and subsequent tumor growth may weaken the vertebrae promoting endplate impaction, producing a biconcave deformity; metastasis typically occurs in patients over the age of 40 years and is more common in those with a personal history of primary malignancy.
Notochordal persistence **(FIG. 17-1)**	Nonfocal, congenital, smooth, inward deformity of all or part of the superior, inferior, or both vertebral endplates; this type of deformity is less focal and involves more of the endplate than Schmorl's nodes.
Osteopenia (metabolic disorders)	Deformity from decreased bone mass secondary to rickets, osteomalacia, steroid therapy, hyperparathyroidism, malnutrition, senile osteoporosis, immobilization, or postmenopausal bone alterations.
Schmorl's nodes [p. 456]	Prolapse of the nucleus pulposus into the vertebrae, producing abrupt, inward deformities of a focal area of the endplate; both endplates and multiple vertebrae may be involved.
Less common	
Gaucher's disease [p. 933]	Genetic deficiency of glucocerebroside, with clinical findings of hepatosplenomegaly, osteopenia, osteonecrosis, focal osteolytic bone changes; biconcave vertebrae is a less common feature of the disease.
Homocystinuria **(FIG. 17-2)** [p. 438]	Genetic disorder causing defect in collagen metabolism. Its presentation is similar to Marfan's disease; vertebrae appear osteopenic and biconcave or flattened.
Renal osteodystrophy [p. 910]	Secondary to renal glomerular disease; vertebral changes present with osteosclerosis ("rugger jersey") and, less commonly, a biconcave appearance.
Sickle-cell anemia **(FIG. 17-3)** [p. 771]	Genetic abnormality in which red blood cells assume a sickled configuration in low oxygen tension; the sickled cells may occlude small vessels with resulting ischemia; skeletal changes include osteopenia, coarse trabeculae, biconcave (more precisely, steplike or H-shaped) vertebrae, and dactylitis.

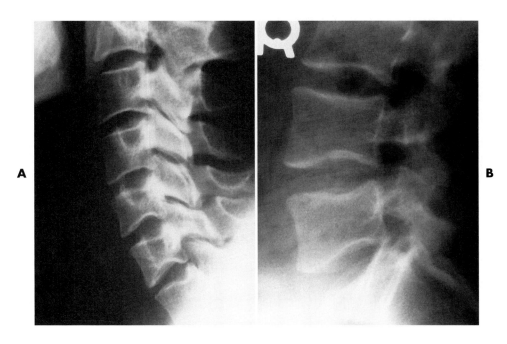

A

B

FIG. 17-1 Biconcave appearance of, **A,** the cervical and, **B,** lumbar vertebrae in different patients' notochordal persistency (or nuclear impression).

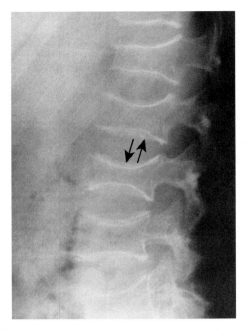

FIG. 17-2 Homocystinuria presenting with osteoporosis and biconcave vertebrae *(arrows)*. (Courtesy Steven P. Brownstein, MD, Springfield, NJ.)

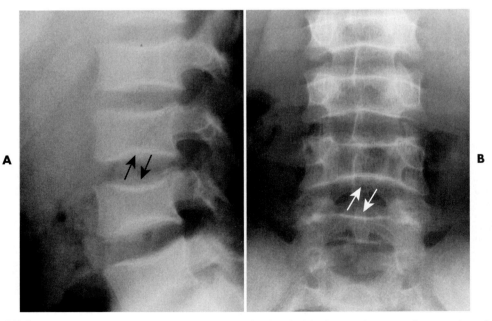

FIG. 17-3 **A** and **B,** Sickle cell anemia causing biconcave deformity of the lumbar vertebrae secondary to underperfusion of the center of the vertebrae in two patients *(arrows)*.

SP1c | Blocked Vertebrae

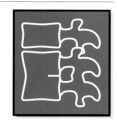

DISEASE	COMMENTS
Congenital *Isolated anomalies* **(FIG. 17-4)**	Congenital failure of segmentation; presentation varies from slight hypoplasia of intervertebral disc space to complete fusion of adjacent vertebral bodies and neural arches; interbody fusion and neural arch fusion are most common in the lumbar spine but frequently occur in the thoracic and cervical regions as well; the sagittal diameter of the vertebrae is decreased with an inward concavity of the anterior body margins at the site of segmentation failure; fusion of posterior elements and under-development of the intervertebral disc space is common and used to differentiate congenital from acquired etiology.
Klippel-Feil syndrome **(FIGS. 17-5 and 17-6)** [p. 439]	Congenital failure of segmentation occurring at multiple levels; associated radiographic findings may include Sprengel's deformity (elevation and medial rotation of the scapula), syndactyly, platybasia, and renal anomalies; patients usually demonstrate a clinical triad of a short neck, restricted cervical motion, and low posterior hairline.
Acquired *Ankylosing spondylitis* [p. 739]	Acquired interbody fusion, seronegative spondyloarthropathy characterized by involvement in the sacroiliac joints and spine; the vertebrae appear square with ossification of the annulus fibrosus; disc height maintained; the disease has a strong male predominance and always involves the sacroiliac joints.
Infections	Acquired interbody fusion secondary to pyogenic (e.g., *Staphylococcus*) or tuberculosis infections; disc height usually is decreased or absent.
Rheumatoid arthritis **(FIGS. 17-7 and 17-8)** [p. 472]	Chronic inflammatory arthritide that may demonstrate acquired interbody fusion; occurs more commonly with juvenile than adult rheumatoid presentations; the spinous processes do not fuse, but the remaining vertebral arches may fuse, particularly in the juvenile form.
Surgical fusion	Acquired interbody fusion resulting from surgery; multiple levels may be involved; posterior joints typically are spared, intervertebral disc spaces are not visible; vertebral bodies may have a thick, square appearance, resulting from surgically placed paraspinal layers of bone as part of the fusion surgery.
Trauma	Acquired interbody fusion from bone remodeling after severe trauma.

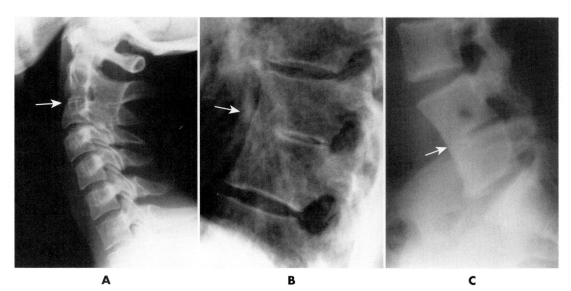

A   B   C

FIG. 17-4 A, Cervical; **B,** thoracic; and **C,** lumbar congenital blocked vertebrae. All three patients exhibit hypoplasia of the intervertebral disc *(arrows).*

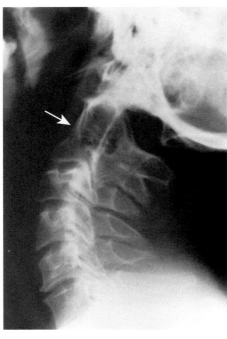

FIG. 17-5 Klippel-Feil syndrome characterized by the multiple blocked segments in the cervical spine. The occipitoatlantal space is nonexistent because of occipitalization of atlas, and the C2 and C3 levels are fused across the vertebral bodies and neural arches *(arrow)*. (Courtesy Joseph W. Howe, Sylmar, CA.)

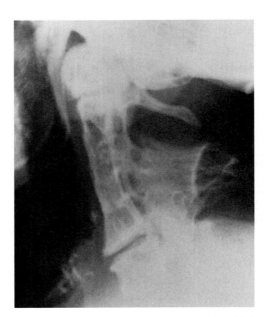

FIG. 17-6 Multiple congenital blocked segments of Klippel-Feil syndrome. Fusion is noted across the disc spaces and the vertebral arches. (Courtesy Joseph W. Howe, Sylmar, CA.)

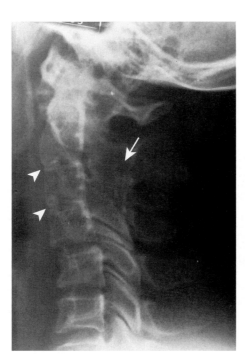

FIG. 17-7 Juvenile rheumatoid arthritis demonstrating fusion across the posterior joints of C2-4 *(arrow)* and underdevelopment of the vertebral bodies and disc spaces *(arrowheads)*. (Courtesy Joseph W. Howe, Sylmar, CA.)

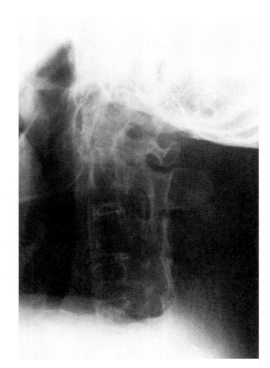

FIG. 17-8 Rheumatoid arthritis with multiple levels of disc and posterior joint fusion, appearing as blocked segments. (Courtesy Joseph W. Howe, Sylmar, CA.)

SPId | Wide Enlarged Vertebrae

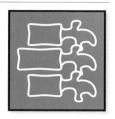

DISEASE	**COMMENTS**
Acromegaly [p. 907]	Pituitary eosinophilic adenoma that produces excess somatotropin, leading to increased levels of growth hormone; the disorder is marked by progressive enlargement of the hands, feet, head, jaw, and abdominal organs; vertebrae are enlarged with posterior body scalloping; patients may have diabetes mellitus.
Expansile bone lesions **(FIGS. 17-9 through 17-11)**	Examples of expansile lesions known to develop in the vertebrae: giant cell tumor, hemangioma, aneurysmal bone cyst, osteoblastoma, Paget's disease, hydatid cyst, eosinophilic granuloma, fibrous dysplasia, chordoma, metastasis, osteosarcoma, chondrosarcoma, and angiosarcoma.
Paget's disease **(FIG. 17-12)** [p. 946]	A generalized skeletal disease in which bone formation and resorption are both increased, leading to abnormally thick and soft bones with disorganized "mosaic" trabeculae; skull, pelvis, and vertebrae are common sites of involvement; vertebrae appear enlarged with thick cortices ("picture-framed" vertebrae).

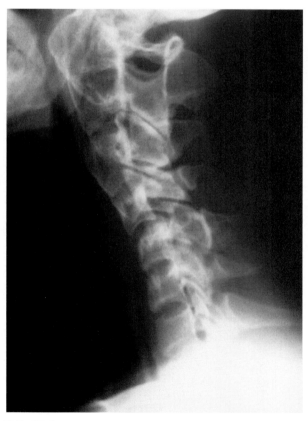

FIG. 17-9   Fibrous dysplasia causing expansile lesions of C2 and C3.

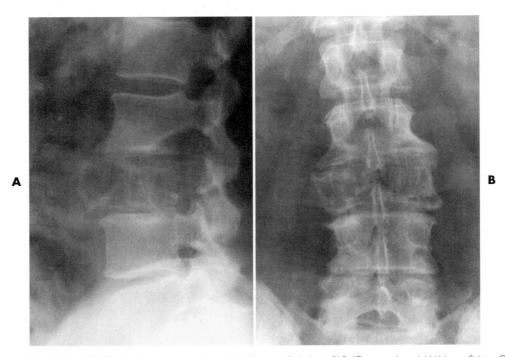

FIG. 17-10   A and **B,** Giant cell tumor appearing as a cystic expansile lesion of L3. (Courtesy Joseph W. Howe, Sylmar, CA.)

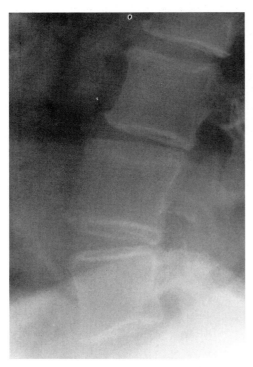

FIG. 17-11 Hemangioma of L4 presenting as an expansile body lesion. (Courtesy Joseph W. Howe, Sylmar, CA.)

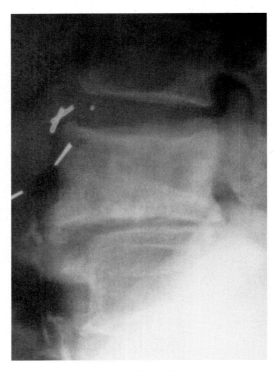

FIG. 17-12 Marked enlargement of the L3 vertebra secondary to Paget's disease.

SP1e | Tall Enlarged Vertebrae

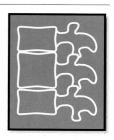

DISEASE	COMMENTS
Blocked vertebrae [p. 439]	Associated with congenital or acquired etiologies, may appear as a single "tall" vertebra; a congenital etiology is indicated when the posterior arches are fused.
Gibbus formation	A gibbus formation, often developed from tuberculosis discitis in a child, may be associated with altered compressive forces on the vertebra, causing the lower segment of the gibbus to appear with increased vertical height along its posterior margin.
Marfan's syndrome (arachnodactyly) [p. 441]	Congenital disturbance of collagen formation primarily expressed as defects of the skeleton and heart valves; skeletal changes include "tall" vertebrae, posterior vertebral scalloping, wide spinal canal, scoliosis, and a long, slender appearance of the metatarsals, metacarpals, phalanges, and long narrow bones (dolichostenomelia).

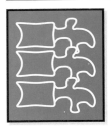

SP1f | Anterior Scalloped Vertebrae

DISEASE	COMMENTS
Aortic aneurysms **(FIGS. 17-13 and 17-14)** [p. 1155]	Because of proximity, may cause erosions along the anterior left side of the vertebrae, which are sometimes termed *Oppenheimer's erosions*; although not always present, the majority of cases also demonstrate calcification of the dilated vessel walls; the intervertebral disc is not involved.
Lymphadenopathy	Enlarged lymph nodes resulting from lymphoma, inflammatory lymphadenopathy, or metastatic lymphadenopathy may cause pressure erosions on the anterior surfaces of the vertebrae, primarily the lumbar vertebrae.
Normal variant	Mild in concavity; multiple levels are common; variants are most often seen in the lower thoracic and upper lumbar spine.
Tuberculosis [p. 779]	Common to find infectious erosions of the vertebral margins with paraspinal masses and involvement of the intervertebral disc.

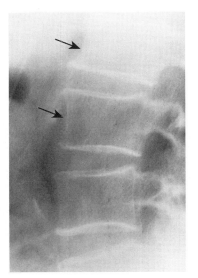

FIG. 17-13 Lateral lumbar radiograph with an increased anterior concavity of the upper lumbar vertebrae *(arrows)*, which was thought to represent pressure erosions from an aneurysm later diagnosed in this patient. (Courtesy Joseph W. Howe, Sylmar, CA.)

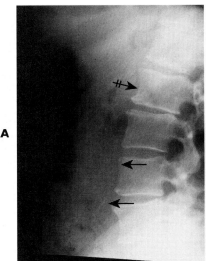 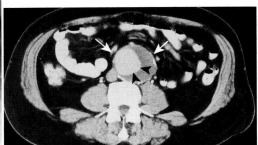

FIG. 17-14 Lateral lumbar radiographs with, **A,** vascular calcification in the posterior wall of the abdominal aorta and, **B,** poor visualization of the anterior wall. There is an exaggerated anterior concavity of the L2 vertebral body, suspicious for erosion secondary to the aneurysm *(crossed arrow).* The contrast-enhanced computed tomography scan demonstrates an aneurysm of the abdominal aorta *(arrows).* The central, more radiodense region (where the arrowheads are pointing) corresponds to the region of blood flow; the less radiodense outer region (space where the arrowheads are located) denotes lack of contrast corresponding to clotted blood.

SP1g | Posterior Scalloped Vertebrae

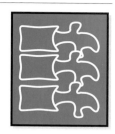

DISEASE	COMMENTS
Achondroplasia [p. 421]	Congenital defect of endochondral bone formation resulting in the following spinal changes: posterior scalloping of the vertebrae, increased intervertebral disc height, flattened vertebral bodies, narrow spinal canal, lumbar kyphosis, "bullet-shaped" lumbar vertebrae; the pelvis may appear hypoplastic; milder forms of the disease may occur.
Acromegaly [p. 907]	Excess levels of growth hormone resulting from a pituitary eosinophilic adenoma overproducing soma-totropin; the disorder is marked by progressive enlargement of the hands, feet, head, jaw, and abdominal organs; vertebrae are enlarged with posterior scalloping; patients may have diabetes mellitus.
Congenital syndromes **(FIGS. 17-15 and 17-16)**	Arachnodactyly (see previous Enlarged Vertebrae discussion), mucopolysaccharidosis syndromes (e.g., Hurler's, Hunter's, Morquio's), Marfan's syndrome, Ehlers-Danlos syndrome, and others.
Increased intraspinal pressure	Increased intraspinal pressure from an ependymoma or communicating hydrocephalus may cause adjacent bone erosions.
Neurofibromatosis *(von Recklinghausen's disease)* [p. 942]	Congenital disturbance of mesodermal and neuroectodermal tissues, appearing clinically with cutaneous markings, bone deformity, and neurofibromas; selected skeletal changes include kyphoscoliosis, enlarged intervertebral foramina, posterior vertebral body scalloping from dural ectasia or neurofibroma, and bowing deformity of the lower extremities.
Tumors	Bone erosion from adjacent spinal canal tumors (e.g., meningioma, ependymoma, lipoma, neurofibroma).

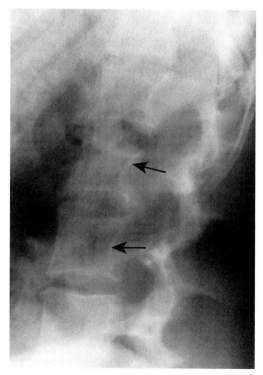

FIG. 17-15 Posterior body scalloping secondary to dural ectasia of unknown etiology *(arrows)*. (Courtesy Joseph W. Howe, Sylmar, CA.)

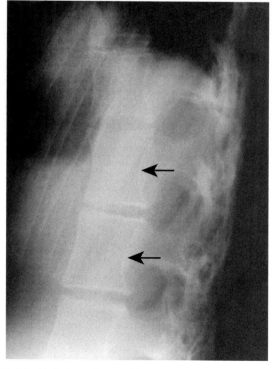

FIG. 17-16 Marfan's syndrome with prominent scalloping of the posterior vertebral bodies *(arrows)*.

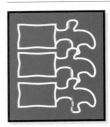

SPIh | Square Vertebrae

DISEASE	COMMENTS
Inflammatory arthropathies (FIG. 17-17)	Square vertebrae is one of the earliest findings of ankylosing spondylitis; square vertebrae also may be a feature of psoriatic arthritis, Reiter's syndrome, and rheumatoid arthritis (usually juvenile); the seronegative inflammatory arthropathies usually involve the sacroiliac joints.
Paget's disease [p. 946]	A generalized skeletal disease in which bone formation and resorption are both increased, leading to abnormally thick, soft bones with disorganized "mosaic" trabeculae; skull, pelvis, and vertebrae are common sites of involvement; vertebrae usually appear enlarged and square with thick cortices ("picture-framed" vertebrae).

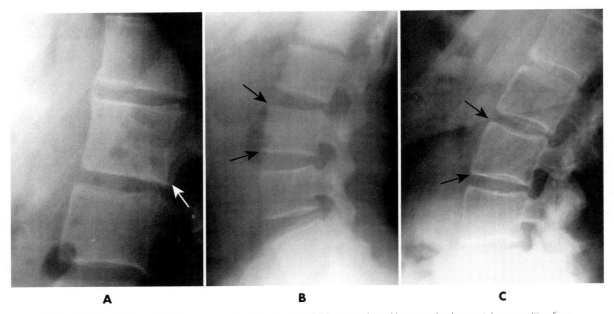

A **B** **C**

FIG. 17-17 **A** through **C,** Three cases of ankylosing spondylitis presenting with square lumbar vertebrae resulting from corner erosion and proliferation *(arrows).* (**A** and **B,** Courtesy Joseph W. Howe, Sylmar, CA.)

SPIi | Wedged Vertebrae

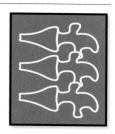

DISEASE	**COMMENTS**
Congenital syndromes	Possible causes of wedged congenital vertebrae and other characteristic alterations; syndromes include achondroplasia, hypothyroidism, and mucopolysaccharidoses; usually multiple levels are involved.
Hemivertebrae **(FIG. 17-18)**	Focal vertebral hypoplasia, resulting in a lateral, anterior, or posterior wedged hemivertebra at one or multiple levels; lateral hemivertebrae produce scoliosis; posterior hemivertebrae are commonly posteriorly displaced up to 3 mm and produce a kyphosis.
Infections **(FIG. 17-19)**	Tuberculosis and pyogenic infections (e.g., *Staphylococcus*); clues to an infection include involvement of intervertebral disc space, paraspinal masses and calcifications, cortical demineralization, and angular kyphosis.
Normal variant	Slightly wedged vertebrae may occur as normal variants, usually in the thoracolumbar region.
Scheuermann's disease [p. 456]	Posttraumatic defect of vertebral endplate maturation presenting during adolescence with three or more levels of wedged vertebrae, narrowed anterior disc space, multiple Schmorl's nodes, and vertebral endplate irregularity; the disease usually develops in the middle and lower thoracic spine.
Trauma **(FIGS. 17-20 and 17-21)**	Compression fracture leading to wedged configuration; endplate defects, cortical offset of anterior body margin ("step defect"), horizontal zone of bone impaction within vertebrae (zone of condensation), and history of trauma are clues to traumatic etiology.

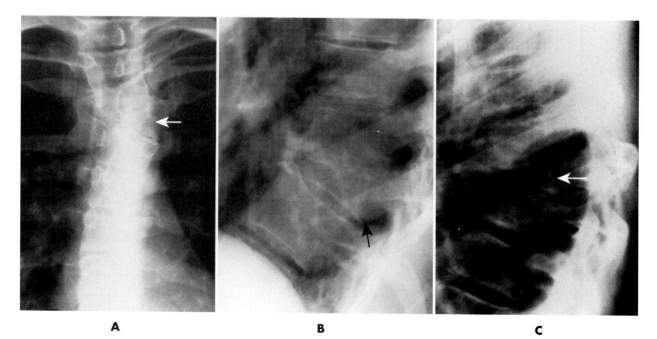

A   **B**   **C**

FIG. 17-18   **A,** Lateral; **B,** dorsal; and, **C,** thoracic hemivertebrae *(arrows).* (**A** and **B,** Courtesy Joseph W. Howe, Sylmar, CA.)

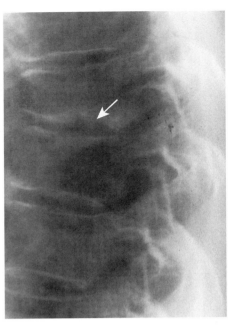

FIG. 17-19 Infection leading to the trapezoidal shape of a middle thoracic vertebra with destructive endplate changes and narrowing of the intervertebral disc space (*arrow*). (Courtesy Joseph W. Howe, Sylmar, CA.)

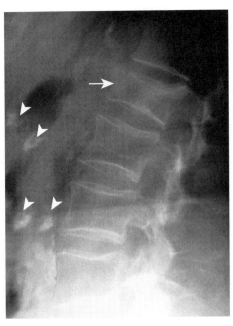

FIG. 17-20 Compression fracture in the upper lumbar spine (*arrow*) and multiple levels of costal cartilage calcification (*arrowheads*). (Courtesy Steven P. Brownstein, MD, Springfield, NJ.)

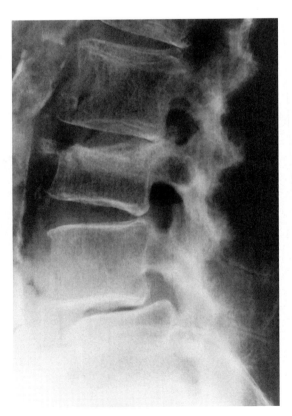

FIG. 17-21 Compression fracture and resulting wedged vertebral configuration. In addition, a Grade I degenerative spondylolisthesis of L4 on L5 is present with degenerative vacuum phenomena at L4. Calcification of the abdominal aorta anterior to the spine also can be seen.

SP2 | Atlantoaxial Subluxation

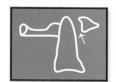

The normal measurement of the atlantodental interval (ADI) is less than or equal to 5 mm in children and 3 mm in adults. A measurement beyond these limits suggests instability of the atlantoaxial articulation. Instability results from compromise of the transverse atlantal ligament or C2 odontoid process. Because the joint is most stressed during flexion, forward flexion radiographs provide a more specific measure of ADI enlargement than neutral lateral radiographs. If the anterior tubercle or odontoid process does not represent fixed, clearly defined points of mensuration, atlantoaxial instability can be assessed by choosing another point on the atlas and axis, such as the distance between the posterior surface of the odontoid and the anterior surface of the posterior tubercle of the atlas (this space is known as the *posterior atlantodental interval* or *PADI*).

DISEASE	COMMENTS
Congenital conditions	Occipitalization of atlas, Down syndrome (20% of cases), Morquio's syndrome, and spondyloepiphyseal dysplasia; these are associated with atlantoaxial subluxation secondary to absence or attenuation of the transverse atlantal ligament, occurring as an isolated anomaly or in association with other defects.
Inflammatory spondyloarthropathy **(FIG. 17-22)**	Condition that includes rheumatoid (adult and juvenile types) arthritis, ankylosing spondylitis, psoriatic arthritis, Reiter's syndrome, and systemic lupus erythematosus; these are associated with synovitis, ligament attenuation, and odontoid erosions, which may lead to instability of the atlantoaxial articulation; rheumatoid arthritis is the most common inflammatory arthropathy to involve the atlantodental joint.
Marfan's syndrome [p. 441]	Genetic disorder of connective development that leads to ocular, cardiovascular, and musculoskeletal abnormalities; joint instability follows ligamentous laxity.
Odontoid anomalies [p. 309]	Aplasia, hypoplasia, or malunion of the odontoid process may lead to instability.
Regional infections	Include retropharyngeal abscesses, otitis media, mastoiditis, cervical adenitis, parotitis, and alveolar abscesses.
Trauma	Instability resulting from fracture or torn ligaments.

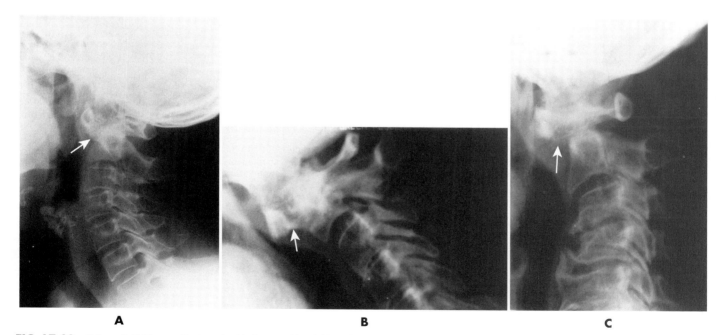

A   B   C

FIG. 17-22 **A** through **C,** Three patients, each with rheumatoid arthritis and an increased atlantodental space *(arrows).* (Courtesy Joseph W. Howe, Sylmar, CA.)

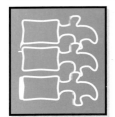

SP3 | Bony Outgrowths of the Spine

Most bony outgrowths of the spine represent osteophytes, related to degenerative arthropathy of the intervertebral disc spaces or posterior joints. An appearance of multilevel, flowing, thick, mostly anterior paravertebral outgrowths is characteristic of diffuse idiopathic skeletal hyperostosis (DISH). Large, coarse, incompletely bridging paravertebral outgrowths are associated with Reiter's syndrome and psoriatic arthropathy. In contrast delicate, thin, completely bridging outgrowths (marginal syndesmophytes) are characteristic of ankylosing spondylitis. As the terms are generally used, osteophytes denote a degenerative etiology and syndesmophytes an inflammatory etiology. Because the condition is classified as idiopathic, the bony outgrowths of DISH are neither osteophytes nor syndesmophytes; rather, exostasis or another generic term is used to describe the changes.

DISEASE	COMMENTS
More common	
Ankylosing spondylitis **(FIG. 17-23)** [p. 492]	Seronegative spondyloarthropathy characterized by arthritis targeted to the sacroiliac joints and spine; bilateral, symmetric, thin intervertebral connections, known as syndesmophytes, are prominent features, representing ossification of the outermost lamellae of the annulus fibrosis; posterior joint fusion is common; collectively, multiple levels produce a "bamboo spine" appearance; in addition, the anterior body margins appear straight or square.
Diffuse idiopathic skeletal hyperostosis **(FIG. 17-24)** [p. 583]	Idiopathic disease marked by thick, flowing anterior longitudinal ligament ossifications along the anterior and lateral body margins; diffuse idiopathic skeletal hyperostosis (DISH) is most common in the thoracolumbar region.
Reiter's syndrome and psoriatic arthropathy **(FIGS. 17-25 and 17-26)** [p. 510]	Inflammatory arthropathies associated with paravertebral ossifications incompletely bridging the intervertebral disc spaces; usual to the thoracolumbar spine; the paravertebral ossifications are typically thick, but uncommonly may appear thin; the latter appearance is identical to those of ankylosing spondylitis.
Spondylosis deformans (degenerative disc disease) **(FIG. 17-27)** [p. 578]	Degenerative disease involving principally the outer portions of the intervertebral disc, appearing as curved ("claw") or horizontal ("traction") vertebral osteophytes, with or without other findings of degenerative disc disease (e.g., endplate osteosclerosis and irregularity, narrowed disc space, misalignment). Osteophytes form in response to increased tension at the Sharpey's fibers, anchoring the outer annulus into the cortical bone of the adjacent endplate. Degenerative osteophytes are moderately thick (thicker than ankylosing spondylitis, thinner than DISH) and typically incompletely bridge the intervertebral disc space.
Less common	
Acromegaly [p. 907]	Excess levels of growth hormone resulting from a pituitary eosinophilic adenoma overproducing somatotropin; the disorder is marked by progressive enlargement of the hands, feet, head, jaw, and abdominal organs. Vertebrae are enlarged with posterior scalloping and new bone growth along the anterior body margins.
Fluorosis	Chronic fluoride intoxication associated with osteophytosis and vertebral hyperostosis with calcification of the paraspinal ligaments; vertebrae have increased radiodensity; fluorosis is most marked in the innominates and lumbar spine.
Hypoparathyroidism [p. 913]	Inadequate parathormone from undersecretion or surgical removal of the gland; skeletal changes include increased or decreased radiodensity, thickened calvarium, premature fusion of ossification centers, and ossification of the paraspinal ligaments.
Neuropathic spine [p. 584]	Primarily caused by diabetes mellitus, syringomyelia, and tabes dorsalis; the radiographic appearance is marked by loss of intervertebral disc height, increased bone radiodensity, misalignment, fragmentation, and prominent osteophytosis.
Ochronosis	Inherited disorder of excessive homogentisic acid production and subsequent accumulation within connective tissues; the spine is affected by multiple levels of intervertebral disc calcification and massive osteophytosis and ankylosis, especially in the elderly.
Trauma	May cause bony outgrowths from degenerative joint changes or dystrophic tissue calcifications.

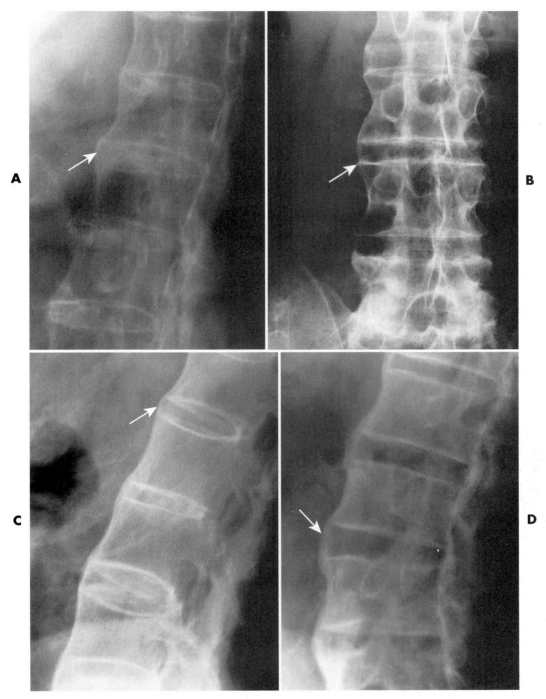

FIG. 17-23 **A** through **D,** Thin, bridging syndesmophytes characteristic of ankylosing spondylitis in four patients *(arrows).* (**A** and **C,** Courtesy Joseph W. Howe, Sylmar, CA.)

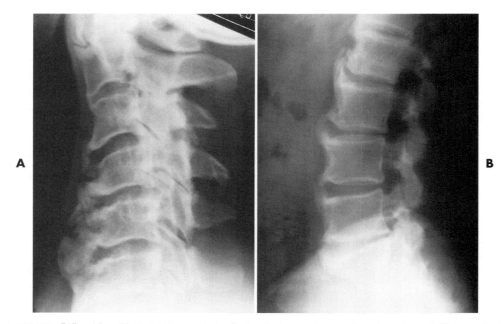

FIG. 17-24 Diffuse idiopathic skeletal hyperostosis affecting, **A,** the cervical and, **B,** lumbar spines of different patients.

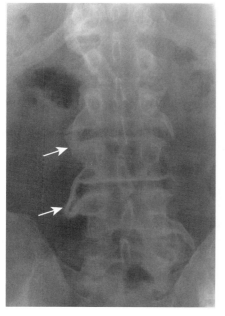

FIG. 17-25 Reiter's disease with prominent syndesmophytes at multiple lumbar levels *(arrows)*. (Courtesy Joseph W. Howe, Sylmar, CA.)

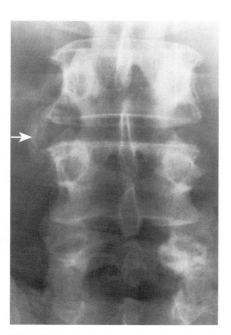

FIG. 17-26 Psoriatic spondyloarthropathy with characteristic thick syndesmophytes incompletely bridging the disc space *(arrow)*. (Courtesy Joseph W. Howe, Sylmar, CA.)

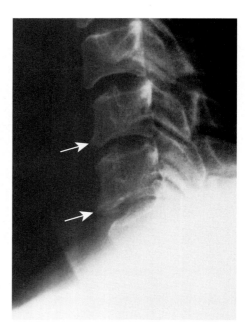

FIG. 17-27 Degenerative osteophytes projecting from the anterior vertebral body margins *(arrows)*.

SP4 | Calcification of the Intervertebral Disc

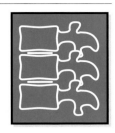

Calcification of the intervertebral disc is noted by increased radiopacity within the normally radiolucent disc space. The appearance represents dystrophic calcification of the nucleus pulposus or surrounding annulus. The appearance usually is stable, with the notable exception of idiopathic juvenile disc calcification, which disappears by adulthood.

DISEASE	COMMENTS
More common	
Blocked segmentation **(FIG. 17-28)** [p. 439]	Dystrophic disc calcification occurring with congenital block segmentation, Klippel-Feil syndrome, myositis ossificans progressiva, and surgical fusion; it is probably related to a loss or reduction of intersegmental motion with consequential nutritional deprivation of tissue.
Degenerative spondylosis [p. 578]	Common findings of degenerative arthropathy of the intervertebral disc: vertebral marginal osteophytosis, vertebral endplate sclerosis, Schmorl's nodes, disc vacuum phenomena, and narrowing of the disc space; another finding, particularly in the elderly, includes calcification of the posterior portion of the nucleus pulposus.
Idiopathic **(FIGS. 17-29 and 17-30)**	Includes childhood and adult forms; the childhood variety is transient (usually of the cervical spine), restricted to the nucleus pulposus (often at only one level), and commonly associated with clinical symptoms; the adult variety is asymptomatic, persistent, and probably related to degeneration.
Posttraumatic	Potential of developing one or more levels of disc calcification if spine has been injured previously; patients with poliomyelitis may have disc calcification, which is believed to result from trauma caused by lack of muscular support.
Less common	
Ankylosing spondylitis [p. 492]	Seronegative spondyloarthropathy characterized by involvement in the sacroiliac joints and spine; single or multiple levels of disc calcification may be seen, usually concurrent with facet ankylosis and syndesmophytes at the same level.
Crystal deposition disease (chondrocalcinosis) [p. 518]	Calcium pyrophosphate dihydrate (CPPD) deposition disease, presenting with crystal-induced synovitis (pseudogout) and cartilage calcification (chondrocalcinosis); spine involvement appears with calcification of the annulus fibrosis, reduction of the disc space, and sclerotic vertebral body margins; CPPD more commonly involves the extremities.
Hemochromatosis [p. 521]	A disorder of iron metabolism leading to hemosiderin deposits in the viscera and connective tissues; calcification of the nucleus pulposus and annulus fibrosus may occur.
Hyperparathyroidism [p. 910]	Overproduction of parathormone from primary or secondary disorders of the parathyroid glands; the disease is marked by osteopenia, osteosclerosis, bone resorption, and soft-tissue and vascular calcification; both the nucleus pulposus and annulus fibrosis may become calcified; specifically, the central regions of the vertebral bodies appear osteopenic with characteristic homogeneous radiodense bands traversing horizontally at each end of the vertebra ("rugger jersey" spine).
Ochronosis **(FIG. 17-31)**	Inherited disorder of excessive homogentisic acid production and subsequent accumulation within connective tissues; degeneration of the cartilage results; multiple levels of disc calcification essentially are pathognomonic; the disease typically develops in elderly people and may be accompanied by advanced degenerative disease of the spine.
Sequestered disc prolapse	May have dystrophic calcification in displaced portions of the intervertebral disc; more common in posterior fragments.

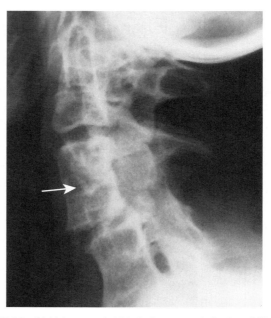

FIG. 17-28   Multiple congenital blocked segments indicative of Klippel-Feil syndrome. There appears to be a focus of intervertebral disc calcification at the C3 disc space *(arrow)*.

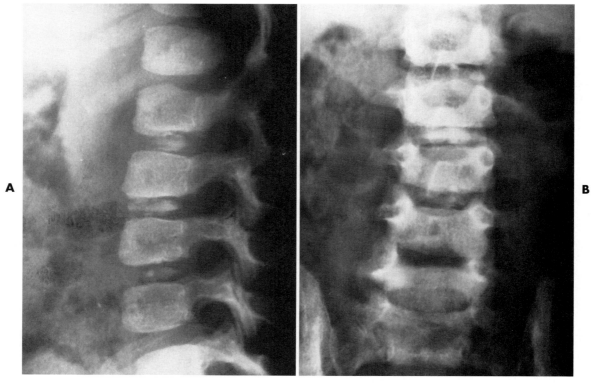

FIG. 17-29   **A** and **B,** Multiple levels of idiopathic lumbar intervertebral disc calcification. (Courtesy Steven P. Brownstein, MD, Springfield, NJ.)

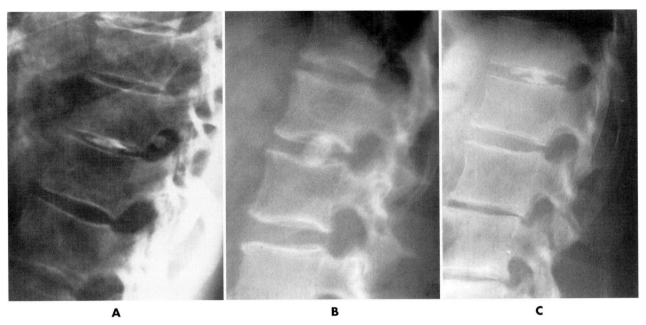

A   **B**   **C**

FIG. 17-30 **A** through **C,** Idiopathic disc calcification in three patients who do not demonstrate degenerative changes at the level of calcification. (Courtesy Joseph W. Howe, Sylmar, CA.)

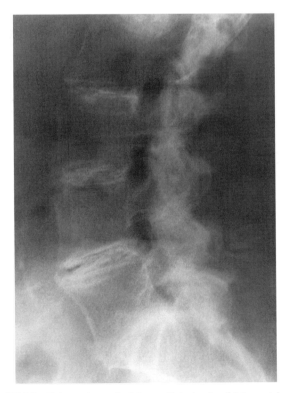

FIG. 17-31 Ochronosis marked by multiple levels of intervertebral disc calcification. In addition, advanced posterior joint arthrosis is indicated by the radiodense and irregular appearance. (Courtesy Joseph W. Howe, Sylmar, CA.)

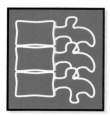

SP5 | Narrow Intervertebral Disc Height

Narrowing of the intervertebral disc spaces in the adult patient typically is related to degenerative disc disease. Degenerative narrowing of the disc usually is accompanied by other degenerative findings (e.g., osteophytes, subchondral sclerosis, joint misalignment) and in its advanced stages involves multiple levels and the posterior joints. Grossly advanced degenerative spinal changes may result from neuropathy. Infections represent more serious causes of a narrowed disc space, presenting with bone destruction, paraspinal mass, and less prominent degenerative findings. In particular, intradiscal vacuum phenomena are not seen with infection and may help in differentiating degeneration from infection. The following lists causes of narrowed intervertebral disc spaces at one or more levels.

DISEASE	COMMENTS
More common *Hypoplastic disc (developmental)* **(FIG. 17-32)**	Congenital underdevelopment of the intervertebral disc seen as an isolated anomaly at the L5 level, in conjunction with congenital block segmentation at practically any level (most common at C5-6 and C2-3), or in the thoracic and lumbar spine associated with Scheuermann's disease.
Inflammatory arthritides	Seropositive (e.g., rheumatoid arthritis) or seronegative (e.g., ankylosing spondylitis) inflammatory arthritide involving the spine, which manifests with osteoporosis, osteosclerosis of the vertebral body margins, and concurrent involvement of the posterior joints; reduction of the disc spaces is uncommon, with the exception of rheumatoid arthritis (usually juvenile) in the cervical spine; ankylosing spondylitis has a propensity to involve the sacroiliac joints, and rheumatoid arthritis to involve the metacarpophalangeal joints.
Infections **(FIGS. 17-33 through 17-35)**	Spinal infections secondary to various causative agents (e.g., pyogenic, tuberculosis, brucellosis, typhoid infections) producing bone destruction, indistinct cortical margins, intervertebral disc space narrowing, and paraspinal mass; usually involve only one level, not multiple levels as occurs with a degenerative etiology.
Intervertebral osteochondrosis *(degenerative disc disease)* **(FIG. 17-36)** [p. 578]	Degenerative disease involving principally the inner portions of the intervertebral disc (nucleus pulposus and cartilaginous endplate), typically presenting with other degenerative findings: osteophytes, misalignment, vacuum phenomena, endplate osteosclerosis, and irregularity.
Less common *Neuropathic spine* [p. 584]	Primary causes: diabetes mellitus, syringomyelia, and tabes dorsalis; the radiographic appearance is marked by loss of intervertebral disc height, increased bone radiodensity, misalignment, fragmentation, and prominent osteophytosis; the changes are more advanced than those of age-related degeneration.
Ochronosis	Inherited disorder of excessive homogentisic acid production and subsequent accumulation within connective tissues; the spine is affected by multiple levels of intervertebral disc calcification and massive osteophytosis and ankylosis, especially in elderly people.
Calcium pyrophosphate dihydrate deposition disease (chondrocalcinosis) [p. 518]	Calcium pyrophosphate dihydrate (CPPD) deposition disease, presenting with crystal-induced synovitis (pseudogout) and cartilage calcification (chondrocalcinosis); spine involvement appears with calcification of the annulus fibrosis, reduction of the disc space, and sclerotic vertebral body margins; extremities are much more commonly involved than the spine.

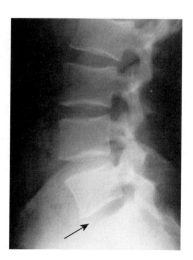

FIG. 17-32 The L5 disc space is slightly decreased *(arrow)*; however, because no other signs of degeneration are present (e.g., osteophytes, vacuum phenomena), the narrowing of the L5 disc is more likely representative of disc hypoplasia. Disc hypoplasia is a common cause of a narrow disc space at the L5 level and is particularly suggested by an L5 disc space that appears narrow in a younger patient who is not likely to exhibit degeneration.

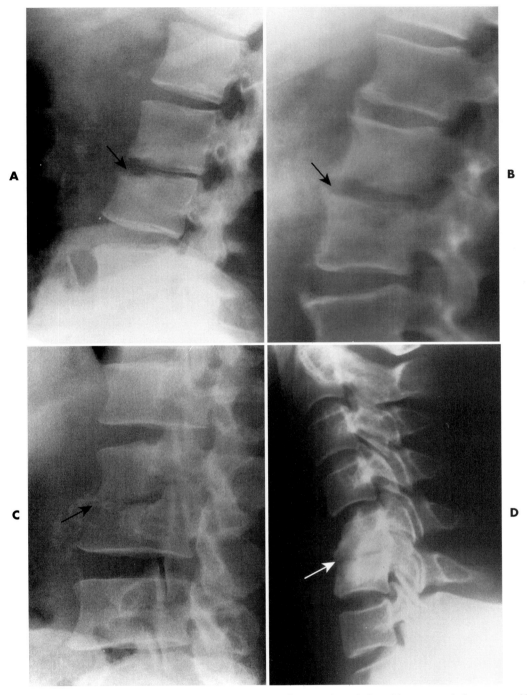

FIG. 17-33 **A** through **D,** Intervertebral disc infections in different patients indicated by narrowed disc spaces with accompanying endplate destruction *(arrows).* (Courtesy Joseph W. Howe, Sylmar, CA.)

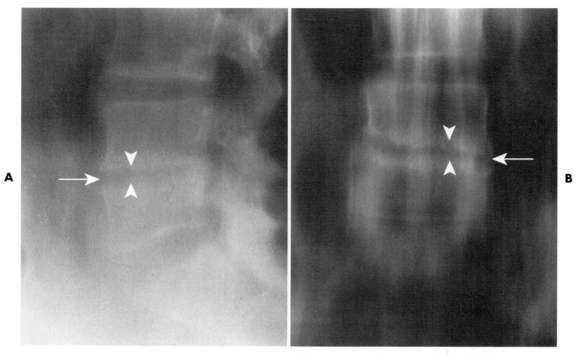

FIG. 17-34 Lumbar intervertebral disc infection seen on, **A,** a lateral radiograph and, **B,** an anteroposterior linear tomogram. Both studies demonstrate a narrowed L4 intervertebral disc space *(arrows)* with endplate irregularity following bone destruction *(arrowheads).*

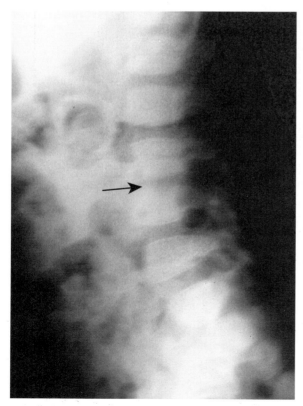

FIG. 17-35 Child with reduction of the L3 intervertebral disc space secondary to infective discitis *(arrow).*

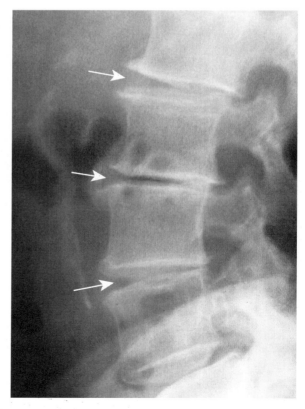

FIG. 17-36 Degenerative narrowing of the intervertebral disc space *(arrows).*

SP6 | Osteolytic Lesions of the Spine

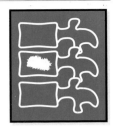

This pattern encompasses solitary and multiple osteolytic lesions of the spine and sacrum. A lesion may involve the vertebral body, neural arch, or appendages of the segments. The list of differentials is long but can be functionally abbreviated by noting the area of the vertebrae that is involved primarily.

Lesions that more commonly involve the vertebral body include chordoma, aneurysmal bone cyst, leukemia, lymphoma, hemangioma, hydatid cyst, osteoblastoma, multiple myeloma, metastasis, and eosinophilic granuloma. A helpful mnemonic for these lesions is *CALL HOME*. Each often appears as an osteolytic lesion.

Lesions primarily seen in the neural arch and transverse processes include giant cell tumor, osteoblastoma, aneurysmal bone cyst, plasmacytoma, and eosinophilic granuloma. A helpful mnemonic for these lesions is *GO APE*. Most of these lesions also appear expansile.

The conditions that most often involve the sacrum include giant cell tumor, aneurysmal bone cyst, plasmacytoma, chordoma, chondrosarcoma, and hemophilic pseudotumor. If multiple vertebrae are involved, the list can be abbreviated to metastasis, myeloma, lymphoma, Paget's disease, angiosarcoma, and eosinophilic granuloma. Regardless of their location in the vertebrae, lesions most noted for their expansile tendencies include aneurysmal bone cysts, hemangioma, and osteoblastoma. Any expanding spinal lesions may encroach on the neural canal. Specialized imaging may be needed to assess the canal and assist in definitive diagnosis.

DISEASE	COMMENTS
More common	
Fibrous dysplasia **(FIGS. 17-37 and 17-38)** [p. 846]	Nonneoplastic disturbance of bone maintenance; spine involvement is uncommon; it may have a nonhomogeneous "ground glass" appearance.
Hemangioma [p. 870]	Common congenital proliferation of vascular endothelium that leads to a benign osteolytic appearance, commonly with characteristic vertical struts ("jail bar" vertebrae); most occur in the vertebral bodies.
Infections **(FIGS. 17-39 and 17-40)**	Spinal infections secondary to various causative agents (e.g., pyogenic, tuberculosis, brucellosis, typhoid infections), producing bone destruction, indistinct cortical margins, intervertebral disc space narrowing, and paraspinal mass.
Metastatic bone disease **(FIG. 17-41)** [p. 889]	Bone metastasis is common to the spine and other portions of the axial skeleton; it rarely involves the skeleton distal to the elbows or knees (acral metastasis). It is usually polyostotic with a moth-eaten pattern of osteolytic bone destruction and poorly defined zones of transition. Periosteal reaction and soft-tissue masses typically are small or absent. Metastasis usually develops in patients over the age of 40 years; neuroblastoma, retinoblastoma, rhabdomyosarcoma, and Ewing's tumors are common causes of metastasis among infants and children.
Multiple myelomas/plasmacytomas [p. 819]	Malignant proliferations of plasma cells developing in predominantly the red marrow of various bones; the skull, vertebral bodies, ribs, and proximal humeri and femora are most commonly involved.
Paget's disease **(FIG. 17-42)** [p. 946]	Chronic skeletal disease of aberrant bone remodeling, marked by bone enlargement, softening, and rarely sarcomatous changes. The lumbar spine is one of the most common areas of involvement, appearing with enlarged and thickened vertebral cortices that form radiodense bands around the perimeter of the vertebra (known as "picture frame"); less commonly Paget's disease appears predominantly as a solitary osteolytic or sclerotic lesion of the vertebral body.
Less common	
Aneurysmal bone cysts **(FIG. 17-43)** [p. 876]	Solitary, benign osteolytic lesions that expand within a long bone or a vertebra (10% to 30%), are associated with local pain and tenderness, and usually develop before age 20 years.
Angiosarcoma	A rare, malignant, expansile neoplasm occurring most often in the breast and skin, with only 10% occurring in the spine (mostly lumbar).
Chordomas **(FIG. 17-44)** [p. 875]	Rare, low-grade malignancies arising from notochord remnants; only 13% arise in the spine (above sacrum), usually at C2; appearance may include body collapse and anterior vertebral mass; tumor may cross the intervertebral disc space.
Eosinophilic granuloma **(FIG. 17-45)** [p. 935]	Proliferation of eosinophils seen most commonly in children and young adults, with spine involvement in less than 10% of cases; it may appear with advanced body collapse "vertebra plana" and at multiple levels.

DISEASE	COMMENTS
Giant cell tumors **(FIG. 17-46)** [p. 878]	Occasionally malignant, well-defined, osteolytic lesions of bone; spine involvement (above sacrum) is rare.
Hydatid (Echinococcus) *cysts* **(FIG. 17-47)** [p. 1310]	Cysts that may be formed in bone (but usually are formed in the liver) by the larval stage of *Echinococcus;* they appear as slow-growing, destructive lesions surrounded by sclerotic borders and are mostly limited to endemic areas.
Lymphoma [p. 1203]	Primary and secondary (from systemic non–Hodgkin's lymphoma and Hodgkin's disease) lymphoma of bone that appears as permeative radiolucent lesions of the lower extremities, pelvis, and spine; less commonly the lesions appear with dense vertebral sclerosis.
Osteoblastomas **(FIG. 17-48)** [p. 809]	Benign bone lesions that have a propensity to involve the neural arches of the spine; they may be expansile or appear as a radiodense lesion with a central nidus.

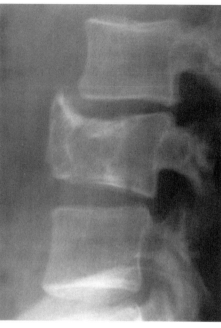

FIG. 17-37   Cystic expansile lesion resulting from fibrous dysplasia of the L3 vertebral body. (Courtesy Joseph W. Howe, Sylmar, CA.)

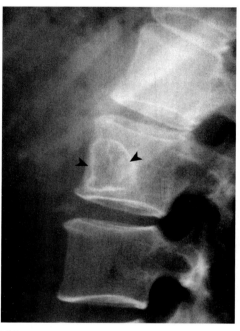

FIG. 17-38   Fibrous dysplasia appearing as a well-marginated *(arrowheads)* osteolytic lesion of the vertebral body. The matrix of the lesion is not radiolucent, but it appears "smoky" or similar to ground glass. (Courtesy Steven P. Brownstein, MD, Springfield, NJ.)

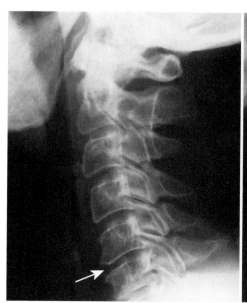

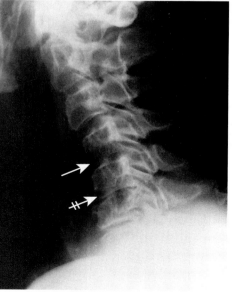

FIG. 17-39   **A,** Initial cervical radiograph of a patient with neck pain reveals only moderated disc degeneration at C5 *(arrow)* and reduced cervical curvature. **B,** One month later, the kyphotic cervical spine exhibits osteolytic bone destruction of the C4 vertebral body *(arrow)* and more advanced disc space narrowing at C5 *(crossed arrow)* consistent with multiple levels of infection. (Courtesy Steven P. Brownstein, MD, Springfield, NJ.)

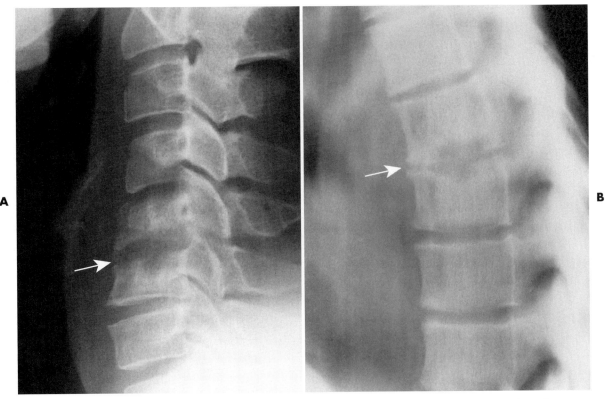

FIG. 17-40 Two patients exhibit narrowed intervertebral disc spaces and osteolytic endplate changes *(arrows)* consistent with infection in, **A,** the cervical and, **B,** thoracic spine. (Courtesy Steven P. Brownstein, MD, Springfield, NJ.)

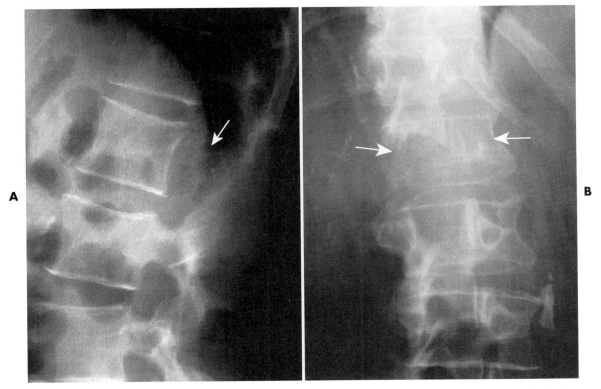

FIG. 17-41 **A,** Lateral and, **B,** anteroposterior lumbar projections revealing osteolytic destruction of the vertebral arch of L1 *(arrows)* secondary to bone metastasis.

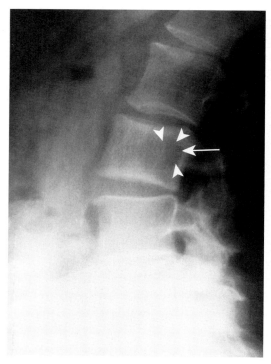

FIG. 17–42 Osteolytic appearance of the center of the L4 vertebral body (*arrowheads*) secondary to Paget's disease. The L4 vertebral body appears enlarged (*arrow*), and the cortices are thick.

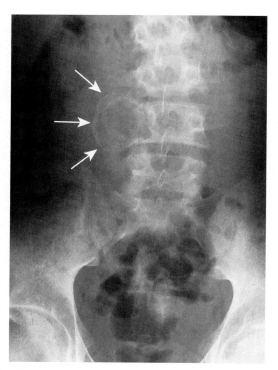

FIG. 17–43 Aneurysmal bone cyst involving the right transverse process of L4 (*arrows*).

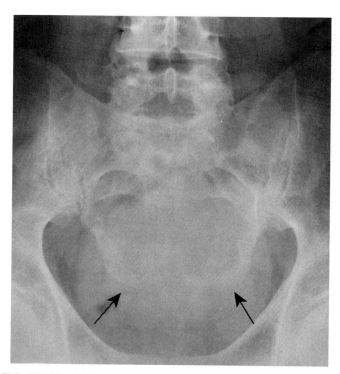

FIG. 17-44 Midline osteolytic sacrococcygeal chordoma (*arrows*). (Courtesy Steven P. Brownstein, MD, Springfield, NJ.)

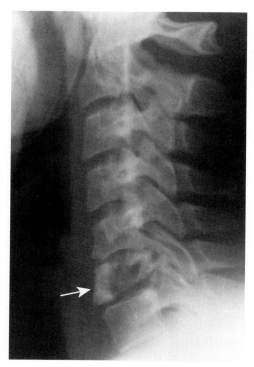

FIG. 17-45 Osteolytic defect of the C6 vertebral body secondary to eosinophilic granuloma (*arrow*). (Courtesy Joseph W. Howe, Sylmar, CA.)

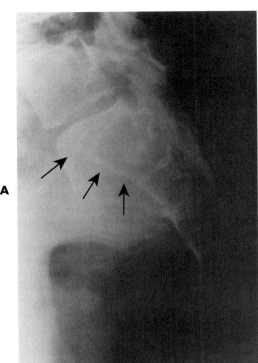

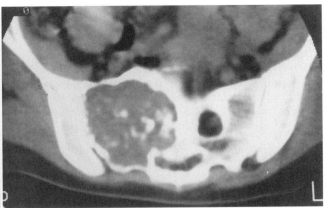

FIG. 17-46 Giant cell tumor appearing on, **A,** plain film *(arrows)* and, **B,** computed tomogram as a cystic lesion of the sacrum. (Courtesy Joseph W. Howe, Sylmar, CA.)

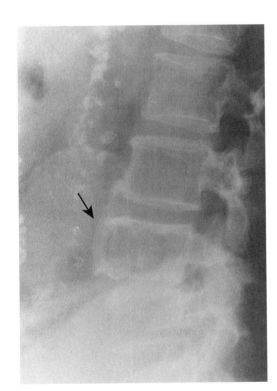

FIG. 17-47 Hydatid cyst causing an expansile osteolytic lesion of the L4 vertebral body *(arrow)*. (Courtesy Joseph W. Howe, Sylmar, CA.)

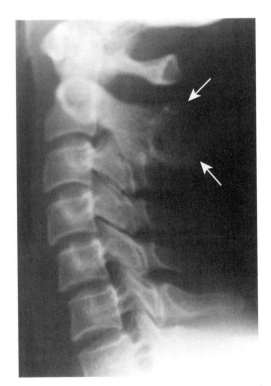

FIG. 17-48 Expansile lesion of the C2 spinous process consistent with osteoblastoma *(arrows)*. An aneurysmal bone cyst may have an identical appearance. (Courtesy Joseph W. Howe, Sylmar, CA.)

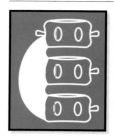

SP7 | Paraspinal Mass

Paraspinal masses often result from infections, particularly tuberculosis in countries where it is prevalent. A tumor mass is probably the most important differential to exclude in most patients. Tumors in the pediatric age group include neuroenteric cysts, histiocytosis X, leukemia, neuroblastomas, and tumors of the kidney. In adults, neurofibromas, metastasis, and myeloma should be excluded. A paraspinal mass of traumatic etiology should have associated features of fracture and are historically indicated. Aneurysms are common in elderly patients.

DISEASE	COMMENTS
More common	
Aortic aneurysms **(FIGS. 17-49 and 17-50)** [p. 1155]	Circumscribed dilations of the aorta secondary to atherosclerosis, trauma, syphilis, and so on; the dilated segments may produce elongated paraspinal masses in the thoracic or lumbar regions; often in the lumbar region an abdominal aortic aneurysm demonstrates thin, curvilinear calcification of the vessel's walls in the region of L2 to L4; with increasing age, uncoiling of the aortic arch occurs, and the resulting tortuosity of the descending aorta may mimic an aneurysm. Thoracic aneurysms may occur along the right margin of the middle thoracic spine (ascending aorta), left margin of the upper thoracic spine (arch of the aorta), or left margin of the lower thoracic spine (descending portion of the thoracic aorta).
Hiatal hernia [p. 1297]	Herniation of part or all of the stomach through the esophageal hiatus of the diaphragm, possibly appearing as a largely left-sided paraspinal mass near the level of the diaphragm with an air-fluid level.
Infections	Infectious spondylitis (tuberculosis, sarcoid, fungal, brucella, salmonella, and others) with associated paraspinal abscess; osteolytic vertebral changes and narrowed disc spaces accompany findings.
Trauma	May produce a focal paraspinal mass (e.g., a hematoma forming from spinal fractures or direct soft-tissue injury); a history of trauma and possible evidence of fracture are clues.
Less common	
Achalasia	Esophageal motility disorder marked by failure of the lower esophageal sphincter to relax, resulting in dilatation of the upper third of the esophagus; the distended esophagus produces a paraspinal mass in the middle to upper thoracic spine in the frontal projection; an air-fluid level may be appreciated.
Expansile spine lesions **(FIG. 17-51)**	Expansile lesions of the vertebrae (e.g., osteoblastoma, osteochondroma, aneurysmal bone cyst).
Extramedullary hematopoiesis	Vertebral bone marrow extrusion seen with the congenital anemias (e.g., thalassemia), producing smooth-appearing paravertebral masses in the posterior mediastinum and often associated with splenomegaly.
Lymphadenopathy	Because of their paraspinal location, enlargement of the lymph nodes from tumor (e.g., metastasis, lymphoma), infection (e.g., granuloma), or other etiologies may produce paraspinal masses.
Neurogenic tumors **(FIG. 17-52)**	Include neurofibroma, neurilemoma, ganglioneuroma, and neuroblastoma; because of the proximity of the intervertebral foramina and chain ganglia, they may produce a paraspinal mass.

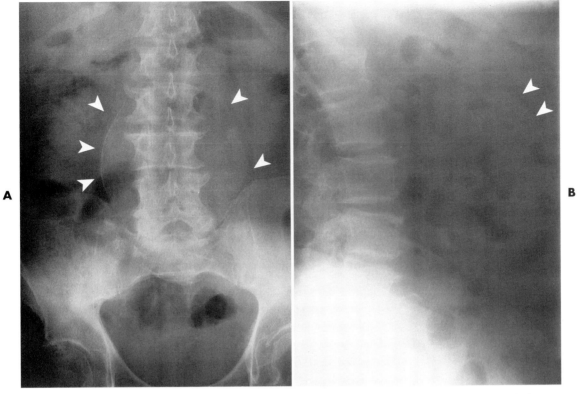

FIG. 17-49 **A,** Anteroposterior and, **B,** lateral lumbar projections demonstrating, **A,** a paraspinal and, **B,** prespinal mass, resulting from, **A,** a large abdominal aortic aneurysm with calcification of the outer wall *(arrowheads).* (**A,** Courtesy Joseph W. Howe, Sylmar, CA.)

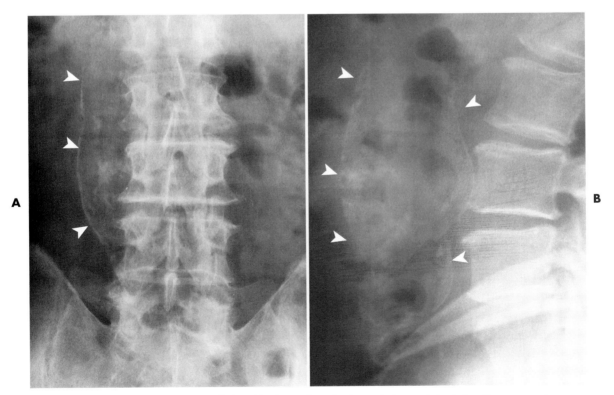

FIG. 17-50 **A,** Anteroposterior and, **B,** lateral lumbar radiographs demonstrating an abdominal aortic aneurysm demarcated by the calcified curvilinear lines representing the anterior and posterior walls of the vessels *(arrowheads).* (Courtesy Robert C. Tatum, Davenport, IA.)

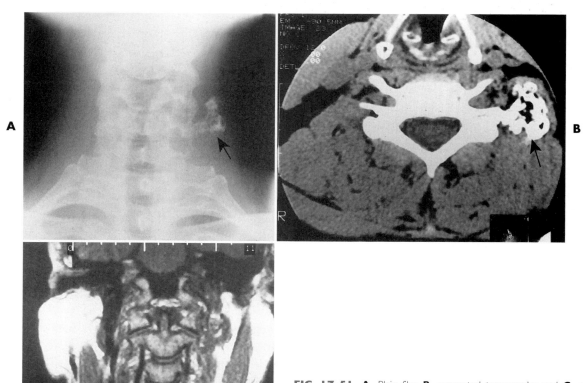

FIG. 17-51 A, Plain film; **B,** computed tomography; and **C,** magnetic resonance imaging of an osteochondroma extending laterally from the spine as a left paraspinal mass *(arrows)*. (Courtesy Ian D. McLean, Davenport, IA.)

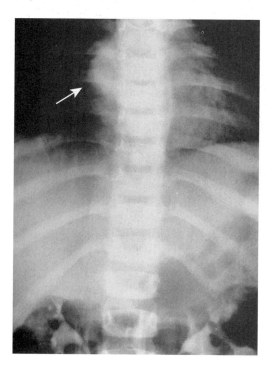

FIG. 17-52 Neuroblastoma presenting as a paraspinal mass *(arrow)*. It is not certain whether this is a primary intrathoracic lesion or metastatic lesion from the abdomen. (Courtesy Steven P. Brownstein, MD, Springfield, NJ.)

SP8 | Radiodense "Ivory" Vertebrae

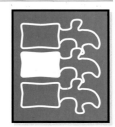

This pattern includes the appearance of a radiodense ("ivory") vertebra at one or more levels. If the entire spine is involved, the list of causes under the pattern of generalized increased bone density may be more applicable. The most common causes of an ivory vertebra are osteoblastic metastasis, Paget's disease, and lymphoma. Other less common conditions are included in the following table to provide a more comprehensive differential list of causes.

Some of the conditions listed in the table may appear as foci of vertebral sclerosis instead of the more uniform radiodense appearance of an ivory vertebra. Conditions associated with foci of vertebral sclerosis include bone islands, fractures, osteoblastic metastases, sclerosing spondylosis, lymphomas, chronic osteomyelitis, and osteoid osteomas.

DISEASE	COMMENTS
More common *Lymphoma* **(FIG. 17-53)** [p. 1203]	Malignancy of the lymphocytes arising in the spleen, lymph nodes, and other lymphoid tissues; sclerotic vertebral lesions are more typical of Hodgkin disease; involved vertebrae are not enlarged but may exhibit concavity of the anterior body margin secondary to erosions from enlarged prevertebral lymph nodes.
Osteoblastic metastases **(FIGS. 17-54 through 17-57)** [p. 809]	Secondary to hematogenous metastases, are most commonly a result of breast or prostate primary malignancies, and exist at one or multiple levels; patients are usually over the age of 40 years; typically the size and shape of the vertebrae remain normal.
Paget's disease **(FIG. 17-58)** [p. 946]	Chronic skeletal disease of aberrant bone remodeling, marked by bone enlargement, softening, and (rarely) sarcomatous changes. The lumbar spine is one of the most common areas; single or multiple vertebrae may be involved, typically appearing enlarged, with thick cortices ("picture frame"); alternatively, it may present as a densely sclerotic or osteolytic lesion of the vertebrae; the disc space is uninvolved.
Less common *Fluorosis*	Chronic fluoride intoxication associated with osteophytosis and vertebral hyperostosis with calcification of the paraspinal ligaments; vertebrae have increased radiodensity; fluorosis is most marked in the innominates and lumbar spine.
Fractures	Compression or healing vertebral fractures, usually appearing as focal areas of increased radiodensity, that typically do not appear uniformly dense enough to be mistaken for true ivory vertebrae.
Infections	Chronic sclerosing infections seen with tuberculosis, syphilis, brucellosis, and typhoid; bone destruction and disc space narrowing are typical.
Myelofibrosis **(FIG. 17-59)**	Extensive and progressive bone marrow fibrosis of unknown etiology occurring in hematopoietic bones (vertebrae, pelvis, ribs, and long bones); involved areas appear osteoporotic first, later becoming patchy, then homogeneously dense; splenic enlargement also noted.
Osteopetrosis (Albers-Schünberg's disease) [p. 451]	Hereditary failure of calcified cartilage resorption that interferes with the development of mature bone; the appearance is marked by sclerotic, fragile bones; vertebrae may appear "doubled" by smaller "endobones" within their bodies; well-defined transverse radiodense bands characteristically are found subjacent to the endplates; multiple levels are involved.

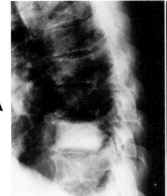
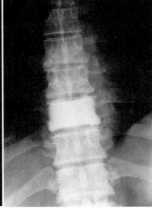

A   **B**

FIG. 17-53 A and **B,** Lymphoma presenting as an ivory vertebra. (Courtesy Steven P. Brownstein, MD, Springfield, NJ.)

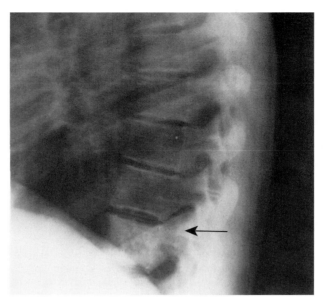

FIG. 17-54 Ivory vertebra from osteoblastic spinal metastasis *(arrow).* (Courtesy Ian D. McLean, Davenport, IA.)

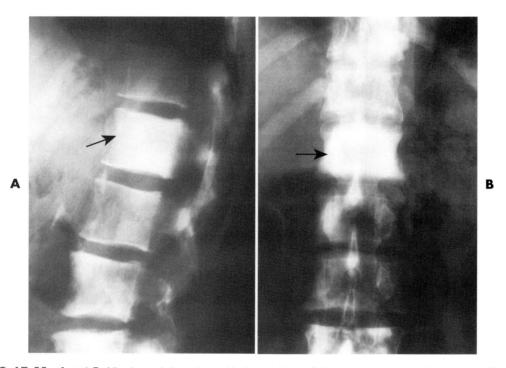

FIG. 17-55 **A** and **B,** Mixed osteolytic and osteoblastic metastasis of the lumbar spine presenting as several ivory vertebrae. The increased density of the L1 vertebrae is most notable *(arrows).* (Courtesy Joseph W. Howe, Sylmar, CA.)

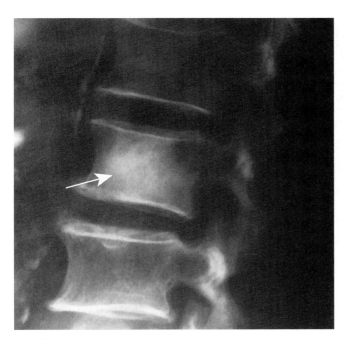

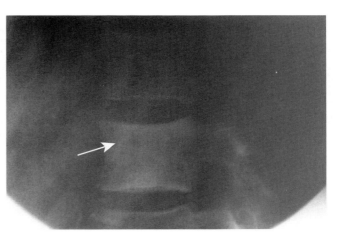

FIG. 17-57 Lateral lumbar projection demonstrating an early ivory vertebra secondary to osteoblastic metastasis *(arrow)*. (Courtesy Steven P. Brownstein, MD, Springfield, NJ.)

FIG. 17-56 Lateral lumbar spine demonstrating an early ivory vertebra appearance resulting from blastic metastatic bone disease affecting the L3 segment *(arrow)*. (Courtesy Steven P. Brownstein, MD, Springfield, NJ.)

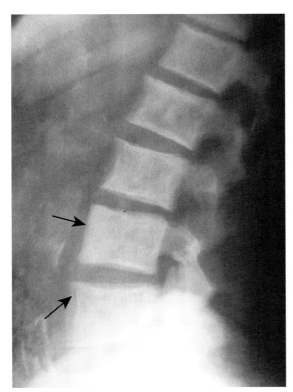

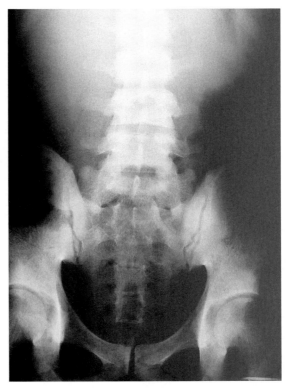

FIG. 17-58 Radiodense appearance of the lower lumbar vertebrae occurring as a result of Paget's disease. In addition, the L4 and especially L5 vertebrae are enlarged *(arrows)*.

FIG. 17-59 Myelofibrosis producing radiodense vertebrae and pelvis. (Courtesy Steven P. Brownstein, MD, Springfield, NJ.)

PART TWO
Bone, Joints, and Soft Tissues

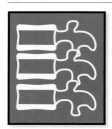

SP9 | Radiodense Vertebral Stripes

The appearance of radiodense vertebral stripes that are clearly defined and located immediately below the vertebral endplates is most closely associated with osteopetrosis. Less well-defined stripes of similar location are suggestive of hyperparathyroidism. Trauma and hypercorticism may be associated with more centrally located stripes. Other causes of dense vertebral stripes include spondylosclerosis, which has concurrent degenerative findings, and Paget's disease, which is systemic and usually has some degree of vertebral enlargement.

DISEASE	COMMENTS
More common *Hyperparathyroidism* **(FIG. 17-60)** [p. 1393]	Overproduction of parathormone, resulting from primary or secondary disorders of the parathyroid glands; the disease is marked by osteopenia, osteosclerosis, bone resorption, and soft-tissue and vascular calcification; specifically, vertebrae appear osteopenic, with characteristic homogeneous radiodense bands traversing horizontally at each end of the vertebrae ("rugger jersey" spine). The vertebral stripes of hyperparathyroidism (HPT) are less well defined than those of osteopetrosis ("sandwich vertebrae").
Osteopetrosis (Albers-Schönberg's disease) **(FIGS. 17-61 and 17-62)** [p. 451]	Hereditary failure of calcified cartilage resorption that interferes with the development of mature bone; the appearance is marked by sclerotic, fragile bones; vertebrae may appear "doubled" by smaller "endobones" within their bodies; well-defined transverse radiodense bands characteristically are found subjacent to the endplates ("sandwich vertebrae").
Sclerosing spondylosis	Degenerative disc disease that may produce a prominent subchondral sclerosis of the subjacent vertebra ("hemispheric spondylosclerosis") and is most common in the lower lumbar levels. In contrast to the "rugger jersey" appearance of HPT and the "sandwich vertebrae" appearance of osteopetrosis, sclerosing spondylosis involves the inferior and superior endplates adjacent to the degenerative disc, not necessarily the superior and inferior endplates of the same vertebrae.
Less common *Compression fractures*	Fracture manifesting as decreased vertical height of the vertebra (generally <2 mm); recent fractures may demonstrate a horizontal radiodense zone of condensation just below the endplate and sometimes a cortical offset "step defect" along the anterior body margin. Compression fractures are often found at the L1, L2, and T12 levels.
Hypercorticism	Excess levels of corticosteroids (e.g., Cushing's disease, steroid therapy); hypercorticism is associated with osteopenia, avascular necrosis, pathologic fractures; repeated microfractures of the vertebral endplate may produce horizontal, poorly defined zones of increased radiodensity in the subjacent bone.
Paget's disease [p. 946]	Chronic skeletal disease of aberrant bone remodeling, marked by bone enlargement, softening, and rarely sarcomatous changes; the lumbar spine is one of the most common areas of involvement; the enlarged and thickened vertebral cortices appear as radiodense bands around the perimeter of the vertebra ("picture frame").

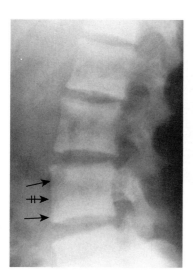

FIG. 17-60 Hyperparathyroidism. Radiodense horizontal bands *(arrows)* adjacent to the vertebral endplates create a radiolucent horizontal band across the middle of the vertebrae *(crossed arrow)*. (Courtesy Joseph W. Howe, Sylmar, CA.)

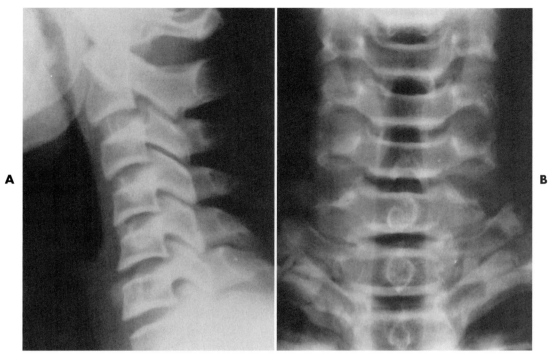

FIG. 17-61 **A** and **B,** Osteopetrosis appearing with radiodense stripes along the vertebral endplates throughout the cervical spine.

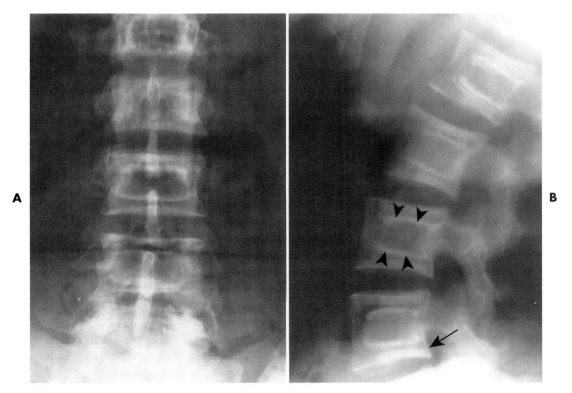

FIG. 17-62 **A,** Anteroposterior and, **B,** lateral lumbar projections demonstrating radiodense endplate stripes *(arrow)* and "bone-within-a-bone" appearance *(arrowheads)* of osteopetrosis. (Courtesy Joseph W. Howe, Sylmar, CA.)

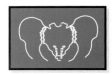

SP10 | Sacroiliac Joint Disease

The sacroiliac joint comprises a lower synovial portion and an upper ligamentous portion. Some diseases demonstrate predisposition to a specific area of the joint. For example, DISH affects the upper portion of the joint, whereas ankylosing spondylitis first affects the lower portion.

In general, sacroiliitis is initially assessed on plain film radiographs. The standard antero-posterior radiograph is most often taken. Additional radiographic projections are helpful to further assess the sacroiliac joint, such as a posteroanterior bilateral view of the sacroiliac joints or unilateral anteroposterior projections of each joint. The radiographic appearance of sacroili-itis is marked by marginal erosions, subchondral sclerosis, loss of cortical joint margins, widened joint space with possible eventual fusion, osteoporosis, and a gradual return to normal bone density. Often changes are better seen on the iliac side when the lower two thirds, or syn-ovial, portion of the sacroiliac joint is affected. Radionuclide bone scintigraphy, computed tomography, and magnetic resonance imaging augment the plain film radiographs if findings are equivocal or if infection or other serious progressive arthropathy is suspected.

Although some variation is expected, each of the diseases and conditions listed in the table below exhibits a typical presentation in the sacroiliac joints that is either bilateral symmetric, bilateral asymmetric, or unilateral. The certainty of the presentation is expressed by denoting a usual presentation with (+++), a common presentation with (++), and a rare presentation with (+).

DISEASE	COMMENTS
Typically bilateral symmetric presentation *Ankylosing spondylitis* **(FIGS. 17-63 and 17-64)** [p. 739]	Seronegative spondyloarthropathy characterized by involvement in the sacroiliac joints and spine; the vertebrae appear square with ossification of the annulus fibrosus and paraspinal ligaments; fusion of the posterior joints is typical, and the proximal joint of the limbs are involved; sacroiliac distribution is bilateral symmetric (+++);* sacroiliitis is virtually always present; the disease has a male predomi-nance; onset is between 15 and 35 years of age.
Diffuse idiopathic skeletal hyperostosis [p. 583]	Generalized articular disorder characterized by prolific hypertrophic ligamentous ossifications, espe-cially the anterior longitudinal ligament of the spine; less commonly the sacroiliac joints are involved, usually in a bilateral symmetric (+++) distribution of sacroiliitis that is marked by fusion at the upper and lower margins of the joint after more advanced spinal changes.
Inflammatory bowel disease	Includes Crohn's disease, ulcerative colitis, and Whipple's disease, which are sometimes accompanied by inflammatory arthropathy, especially of the sacroiliac joints; the bilateral symmetric (+++) distri-bution is indistinguishable from ankylosing spondylitis.
Osteitis condensans ilia **(FIG. 17-65)**	Bilateral symmetric (+++) triangular osteosclerosis of the iliac bones immediately adjacent to the lower, anterior portion of the sacroiliac joint; joint space appears normal; this condition represents a common variant seen among women of childbearing age, or stress reaction of multiparous women.
Paraplegia	Paralysis of both lower extremities and, generally, the lower trunk; sacroiliitis with a bilateral sym-metric (+++) distribution appears as joint space widening and osteoporosis.
Typically bilateral asymmetric presentation *Hyperparathyroidism* [p. 910]	Overproductive parathyroid glands, resulting from primary or secondary causes; the disease is marked by osteopenia, osteosclerosis, bone resorption, and soft-tissue and vascular calcification; vertebrae have characteristic homogeneous radiodense bands traversing horizontally at each end of the verte-brae ("rugger jersey" spine); uncommon cause of sacroiliitis with a bilateral symmetric (++) or bilat-eral asymmetric (++) distribution, noted by limited subchondral bone resorption, causing apparent widened joint space.
Psoriatic arthritis **(FIG. 17-66)** [p. 505]	Common skin disease with an associated inflammatory arthropathy; sacroiliitis is common, and distri-bution may be unilateral (+), bilateral asymmetric (+++), or bilateral symmetric (++).
Reiter's syndrome **(FIG. 17-67)** [p. 510]	Encompasses triad of urethritis, conjunctivitis, and polyarthritis following sexually transmitted disease or dysentery; sacroiliitis is common and distribution may be unilateral (+), bilateral asymmetric (+++), or bilateral symmetric (++).

*Sacroiliac distribution: (+++), usual; (++), common; (+) rare.

DISEASE

Rheumatoid arthritis
[p. 472]

Typically unilateral presentation
Gout
[p. 514]

Infections

Osteoarthritis
[p. 469]

COMMENTS

Systemic connective tissue disorder characterized by inflammatory arthropathy most pronounced in the hands and feet; sacroiliitis is rare, but when present it is marked by mild loss of joint space and (less commonly) erosion; distribution is bilateral asymmetric (+++), bilateral symmetric (++), or unilateral (+) sacroiliac.

Primarily a disorder of purine metabolism that causes crystal deposits, resulting in synovial pannus, arthropathy, and large well-defined bony marginal erosions; infrequent cause of sacroiliitis of a unilateral (++), bilateral asymmetric (++), or bilateral symmetric (++) distribution.

Suppurative or tuberculosis infections of the sacroiliac joint or surrounding bone; involvement is unilateral (+++); fever and other signs of infection are helpful for differentiation when present; intravenous drug abusers are prone to *Pseudomonas* species infections, which target the "s joints" (spine, sacroiliac, symphysis pubis, and sternoclavicular).

Degenerative joint changes that usually develop after 40 years of age; precocious degeneration may follow biomechanical or traumatic stresses; characteristics include smooth, sclerotic joint margins with anterior osteophytes and joint space narrowing; distribution is unilateral (+++) or bilateral asymmetric (++).

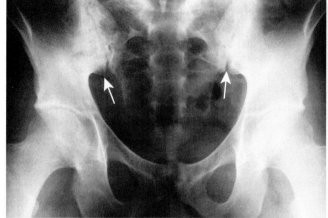

A

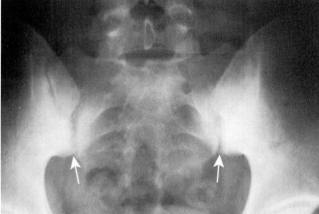

B

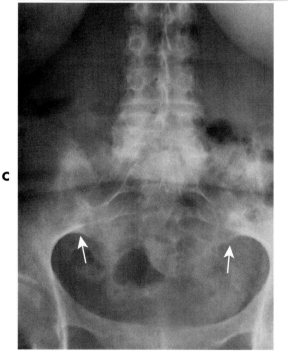

C

FIG. 17-63 **A** through **C,** Three different patients with early ankylosing spondylitis, who all demonstrate bilateral symmetric sacroiliitis *(arrows).* (**A,** Courtesy Jack C. Avalos, Davenport, IA.)

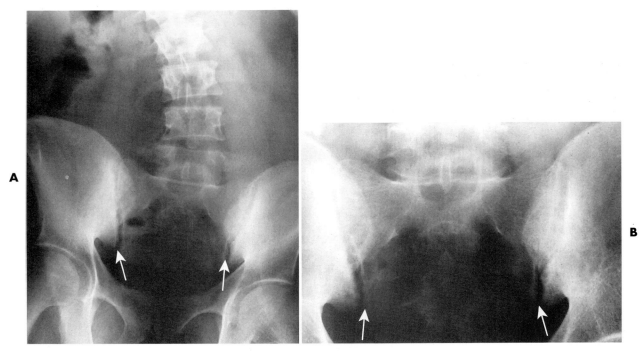

FIG. 17-64　A and **B,** Bilateral sacroiliitis in a patient with ankylosing spondylitis *(arrows).*

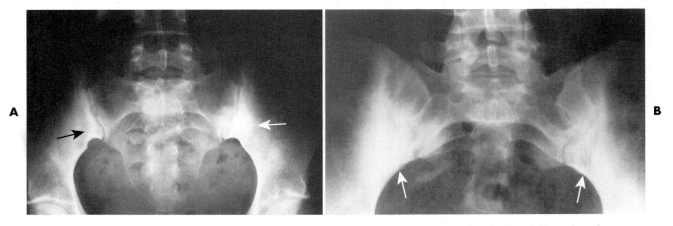

FIG. 17-65　A and **B,** Two cases of osteitis condensans ilia appearing with bilateral, triangular-shaped iliac region of osteosclerosis adjacent to the low margin of the sacroiliac joint *(arrows).* This stress reaction of bone may appear similar to ankylosing spondylitis on the iliac side of the joint. (**A,** Courtesy Joseph W. Howe, Sylmar, CA.)

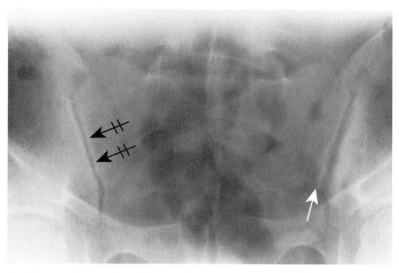

FIG. 17-66 Psoriatic sacroiliitis appearing with osteosclerosis and erosions of the left joint margins *(arrow)* and only slight osteosclerosis on the right *(crossed arrows)*. (Courtesy Joseph W. Howe, Sylmar, CA.)

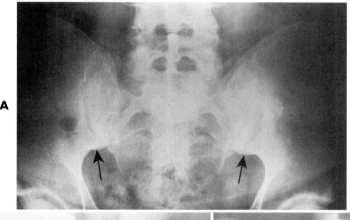

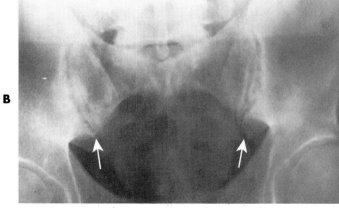

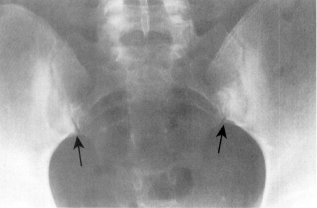

FIG. 17-67 Sacroiliitis secondary to Reiter's syndrome with, **A** and **B,** bilateral asymmetric and, **C,** nearly bilateral symmetric patterns *(arrows)*. (Courtesy Joseph W. Howe, Sylmar, CA.)

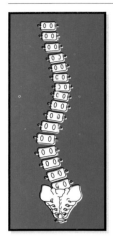

SP11 | Scoliosis

Scoliosis is a lateral curvature of the spine, usually implying a curvature of more than 15 degrees. The degree of curvature is quantified on a full-spine frontal projection, using Cobb's method of assessment. Progression is assessed by periodic reevaluations. The majority of scoliosis cases that present before skeletal maturity are idiopathic in nature. By contrast, those that present after skeletal maturity typically are related to degeneration, osteoporosis, or iatrogenic causes (e.g., following extensive decompressive surgery for spinal stenosis). The following table lists causes of scoliosis for all age groups.

DISEASE	COMMENTS
More common *Congenital spinal anomaly* **(FIG. 17-68)**	Spinal curvatures that result from structural changes of the spine such as congenital blocked vertebrae, Klippel-Feil syndrome, hemivertebrae, dysraphism, osseous bridging vertebral bars, and others; a short segment of the spine typically is involved.
Degenerative diseases	Degeneration is the most common cause of scoliosis, presenting in patient past the age of skeletal maturity; scoliosis may be related to advanced degeneration of the intervertebral disc and posterior joints of the spine, particularly if the degenerative changes are asymmetric.
Idiopathic **(FIG. 17-69)**	Unknown. The most common type of scoliosis presenting before skeletal maturity, much more common in girls.
Leg length deficiencies	Secondary to amputation, chiropractic subluxation, pelvic unleveling, and foot deformity.
Spasms	Lateral deviation resulting from such phenomena as asymmetric muscle spasm in response to spinal injury, retroperitoneal or abdominal abscess, hemorrhage, or ureteral or renal calculi.
Less common *Chest wall abnormalities*	Related to asymmetric chest wall, rib anomalies, Sprengel's deformity, or postsurgical deformities (e.g., thoracoplasty, pneumonectomy).
Congenital syndromes	Occurring with achondroplasia, cretinism, mucopolysaccharidoses, neurofibromatosis, osteogenesis imperfecta, Marfan's syndrome, homocystinuria, and others.
Iatrogenic	Typically related to extensive surgical procedures that significantly alter the spine's structural integrity (e.g., extensive decompressive laminectomy performed for spinal canal stenosis).
Infections	Examples of spinal infections: tuberculosis, pyogenic infections, brucellosis; these infections may cause focal spinal curvature secondary to bone destruction; a sharply angled kyphosis (gibbus) deformity is characteristic.
Neuromuscular disorders	Most common: poliomyelitis; others include cerebral palsy, muscular dystrophy, Friedreich ataxia, Charcot's-Marie-Tooth atrophy, and syringomyelia.
Osteoid osteoma [p. 809]	Most common neoplasm causing scoliosis; osteoid osteomas affect the vertebral arch; a painful scoliosis with sclerotic pedicle shadow on the concave side is the classic presentation; often the tumor is radiographically occult, requiring a bone scintigraphy or computed tomography scan to detect and confirm the diagnosis.
Osteoporosis [p. 916]	Reduction in the quantity of bone that occurs most often in postmenopausal women and elderly men; sparse, thin trabeculae are present, as well as thinning (but no destruction) of cortex; smooth indentations of endplates centrally in the region of the nucleus pulposus are noted, as well as solitary or multiple level vertebral collapse; it is more typical in the lumbar and thoracic regions; severe demineralization may result in bone deformity and related mild scoliosis.
Radiation	In a growing spine, may cause asymmetric arrest of growth centers with resulting lateral curvature; involvement in the lumbar spine is most often in relation to treatment for Wilms' tumor and neuroblastoma; the convexity of the lateral curvature is opposite the side of irradiation.
Trauma	Fracture or dislocation involving the spine resulting in structural deformity; in particular, fractures of the transverse processes at multiple levels are associated with scoliosis—convex to the same side.

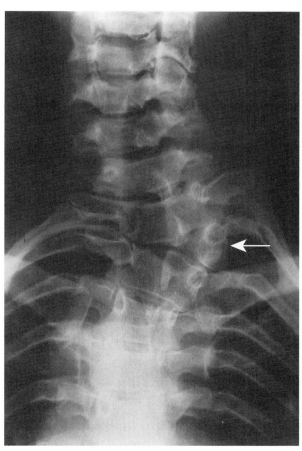

FIG. 17-68 Structural left lateral cervicothoracic scoliosis secondary to a hemivertebra interposed between the first and second thoracic segments *(arrow)*. (Courtesy Joseph W. Howe, Sylmar, CA.)

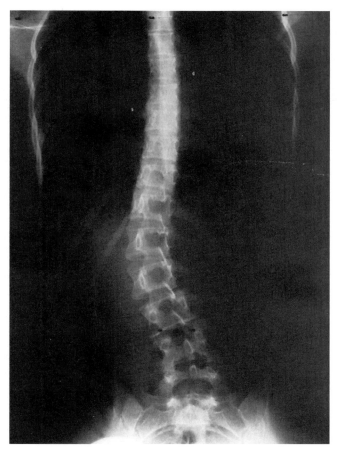

FIG. 17-69 Idiopathic right lateral lumbar scoliosis.

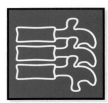

SP12 | Diminished Vertebral Height (Collapsed Vertebra)

Vertebral collapse is marked by a decrease of the normal vertical dimension of the vertebral body, often accompanied by an expansion of the horizontal dimension of the body. If the anterior vertebral body is more involved than the posterior margin, the appearance may resemble a "wedged" vertebra, and the differential list found in the first pattern (SP1i) of this chapter may be more helpful. A collapsed vertebra is not necessarily wedged. Collapse secondary to fracture may lead to posterior migration and encroachment of bone fragments on the spinal canal, leading to serious neurologic complications. In addition, changes in the vertebra's structure may have accompanying biomechanical consequences.

Most conditions known to cause a solitary vertebral collapse also cause multiple levels of vertebral collapse. Contrary to this general statement, benign bone tumors, chordomas, and traumatic ischemic necrosis virtually always involve only one level, and Scheuermann's disease and sickle-cell anemia typically involve multiple levels.

Advanced vertebral collapse, in which the vertebral body appears as a thin wafer disc, is termed *vertebra plana* and is characteristic of eosinophilic granuloma.

DISEASE	COMMENTS
More common *Fractures*	Usually involve only the anterior vertebral body height, creating a "wedged" vertebra appearance; it is more common for pathologic fractures (those resulting from tumor, infection, or other causes) to also involve the posterior margin of the vertebra, which is a rare feature of fractures with purely traumatic etiologies; fractures may occur at one or several levels.
Infections	Chronic sclerosing infections (e.g., tuberculosis, syphilis, brucellosis, fungus, typhus) and pyogenic infections; bone destruction and disc space narrowing are typical, distinguishing infection from metastasis and myeloma; solitary or multiple-level vertebral collapse occurs; involvement is typically localized to a level and not generalized throughout the spine; areas of cortical demineralization and destruction develop; a paraspinal mass may develop.
Metastases **(FIGS. 17-70 and 17-71)** [p. 1393]	Osteolytic metastases occurs most commonly from primary metastases of the lung and breast; patients are usually over the age of 40 years; involvement of the pedicles and other areas of the neural arch is common and distinguishes metastasis from multiple myeloma, which does not demonstrate this tendency; solitary or multiple-level vertebral collapse occurs; the intervertebral disc space remains uninvolved, differentiating metastasis from infection.
Multiple myelomas/plasmacytomas **(FIG. 17-72)** [p. 819]	Malignant proliferation of plasma cells occurring in predominantly the red marrow of various bones; the skull, vertebral bodies, ribs, proximal humerus, and femur most commonly are involved; osteolytic lesions simulate metastatic disease, without tendency to involve vertebral arch, which is common in metastasis; osteopenia and solitary or multiple-level vertebral collapse simulating osteoporosis occur.
Normal variant	Mild anterior wedged configuration of vertebral body that occurs at one or several levels; the posterior vertebral body margin typically is not involved, which gives it more of a "wedged" appearance; it is common in the middle cervical spine and thoracolumbar junction.
Osteoporosis [p. 916]	Reduction in the quantity of bone that occurs most often in postmenopausal women and elderly men; sparse, thin trabeculae, as well as thinning (but no destruction) of cortex are noted; there are smooth indentations of endplates centrally, in the region of the nucleus pulposus; solitary or multiple-level vertebral collapse occurs; the condition is more typical in the lumbar and thoracic regions.
Scheuermann's disease [p. 456]	Posttraumatic defect in endplate maturation presenting during adolescence with multiple levels of anteriorly wedged vertebrae, narrowed anterior disc space, multiple Schmorl's nodes, and vertebral endplate irregularity; the disease is usually seen in the middle and lower thoracic spine; the anteriorly wedged vertebrae produce a kyphosis.
Less common *Benign bone tumors*	Giant cell bone tumors, hemangiomas, aneurysmal bone cysts, and other benign bone tumors; may present with loss of vertebral body height secondary to pathologic fracture.
Chordoma [p. 875]	A rare, low-grade malignancy arising from notochord remnants; only 13% arise in the spine (above the sacrum), usually at C2; appearance may include body collapse and anterior vertebral mass; tumor may cross the intervertebral disc space; there is solitary vertebral collapse.

DISEASE	COMMENTS
Dwarfing syndromes **(FIG. 17-73)**	Advanced flattened deformity of multiple vertebral levels, known as *platyspondyly;* associated with Morquio's syndrome, spondyloepiphyseal dysplasia, thanatophoric dysplasia, and other dwarfing dysplasias.
Eosinophilic granuloma **(FIG. 17-74)** [p. 935]	Proliferation of eosinophils seen most commonly in children and young adults; spine involvement in less than 10%; may appear with advanced body collapse "vertebra plana" or "coin vertebra" and involve one or multiple levels; the disease usually develops in children younger than 10 years of age.
Hydatid (Echinococcus) *cysts* [p. 1310]	Cysts that may be formed in bone (usually formed in the liver) by the larval stage of *Echinococcus;* such a cyst appears as a slow-growing, destructive lesion surrounded by sclerotic borders; they may cause solitary or multiple level vertebral collapse.
Hypercorticism	Excess levels of corticosteroids (e.g., Cushing's disease, steroid therapy); hypercorticism is associated with osteopenia, avascular necrosis, pathologic fractures; repeated microfractures of the vertebral endplate may produce horizontal, poorly defined zones of increased radiodensity in the subjacent bone; solitary or multiple-level vertebral collapse occurs.
Hyperparathyroidism [p. 910]	Overproductive parathyroid glands, resulting from primary or secondary causes; the disease is marked by osteopenia, osteosclerosis, bone resorption, and soft-tissue and vascular calcification; specifically, vertebrae appear osteopenic with characteristic homogeneous radiodense bands traversing horizontally at each end of the vertebrae ("rugger jersey" spine); solitary or multiple-level vertebral collapse occurs; the appearance may simulate osteoporosis, presenting with concave endplate deformities and marked demineralization.
Ischemic necrosis (Kümmell disease)	Controversial condition believed to represent delayed posttraumatic vertebral collapse related to ischemic necrosis of the vertebral body; presence of an intravertebral vacuum phenomenon is characteristic; solitary vertebral collapse occurs.
Lymphoma [p. 1203]	Primary and secondary (systemic non–Hodgkin lymphoma and Hodgkin disease) lymphoma of bone appears as permeative radiolucent lesions of the lower extremities, pelvis, and spine; less commonly the lesions appear as dense vertebral sclerosis; solitary or multiple-level vertebral collapse may occur.
Neuropathic spine [p. 584]	Primarily caused by diabetes mellitus, syringomyelia, congenital indifference to pain, and tabes dorsalisopathy; the radiographic appearance is marked by loss of intervertebral disc height, increased bone radiodensity, misalignment, fragmentation, and prominent osteophytosis; solitary or multiple-level vertebral collapse may occur.
Osteogenesis imperfecta [p. 451]	Inherited abnormal fragility and plasticity of bone, marked by recurring fractures following minimal trauma; other findings include ligamentous laxity, long bone deformity, blue sclerae, osteopenia, and otosclerosis; severe (congenita) and more mild forms (tarda) exist; multiple levels of wedged or completely narrowed vertebrae with biconcave endplates develop.
Osteomalacia [p. 923]	Inadequate mineralization of bone, characterized by gradual softening and deformity, which develops secondary to lack of vitamin D or renal tubular dysfunction; more common in women than in men, osteomalacia often begins during pregnancy; the smooth concave deformity of the vertebral endplates simulate osteoporosis; solitary or multiple-level vertebral collapse occurs.
Paget's disease [p. 946]	A generalized skeletal disease in which bone deposition and resorption are both increased, leading to abnormal thick and soft bones with disorganized, "mosaic" trabeculae; skull, pelvis, and vertebrae are common sites of involvement; vertebrae appear enlarged with thick cortices, "picture-framed" vertebrae; concave endplate deformity involving one or more levels may occur but is not typical.
Sickle-cell anemia **(FIG. 17-75)** [p. 771]	Genetic abnormality in which red blood cells assume a sickled configuration in low oxygen tension; the sickled cells may occlude small vessels with resulting ischemia; skeletal changes include osteopenia, coarse trabeculae, dactylitis, and biconcave (more precisely, steplike or H-shaped) central endplate deformity occurring at multiple levels.

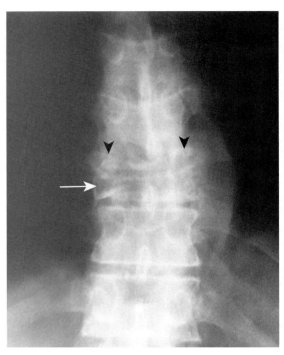

FIG. 17-70   Anteroposterior thoracic projection demonstrating vertebral collapse of T10 *(arrow).* The interpedicular distance is increased, and the pedicles are poorly seen *(arrowheads).*

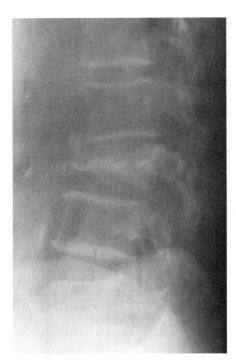

FIG. 17-71   Lateral lumbar projection revealing pathologic collapse secondary to metastasis involving the L3 segment. The anterior and posterior vertebral body heights are decreased, a characteristic of pathologic collapse. In addition, the anteroposterior width of the vertebra has increased, causing potential narrowing of the spinal canal. (Courtesy Joseph W. Howe, Sylmar, CA.)

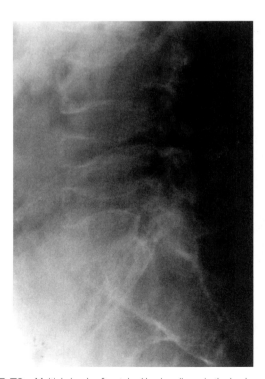

FIG. 17-72   Multiple levels of vertebral body collapse in the lumbar spine secondary to advanced multiple myeloma. The collapsed vertebrae exhibit decreased anterior and posterior vertebral body heights, a characteristic of pathologic collapse. As in this case, multiple myeloma may produce decreased bone density, mimicking senile osteoporosis. (Courtesy Joseph W. Howe, Sylmar, CA.)

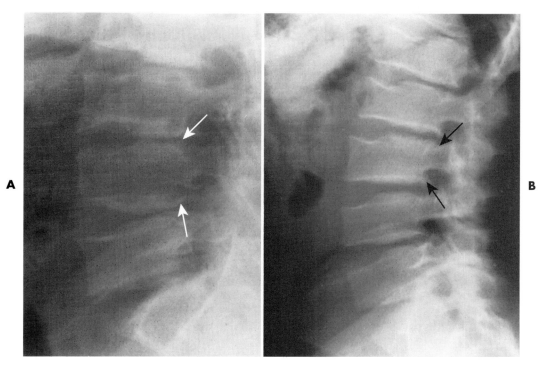

FIG. 17-73 A and **B,** Two cases of spondyloepiphyseal dysplasia appearing with decreased vertical body height and characteristic appearance of the vertebral endplates *(arrows).* (**A,** Courtesy Joseph W. Howe, Sylmar, CA.)

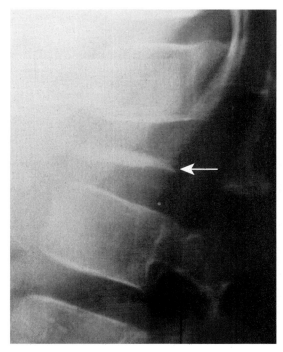

FIG. 17-74 Vertebra plana defect resulting from eosinophilic granuloma of the vertebral body *(arrow).*

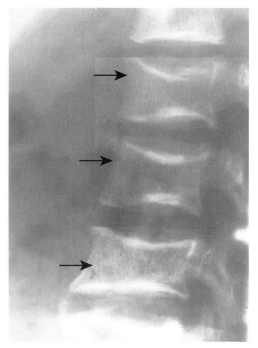

FIG. 17-75 Sickle cell anemia presenting with biconcave or H-shaped lumbar vertebrae. The segments are deceased in vertical height *(arrows).* (Courtesy Joseph W. Howe, Sylmar, CA.)

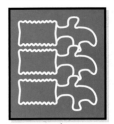

SP13 | Vertebral Endplate Alterations

Some of the more common endplate alterations include zones of increased osteosclerosis, irregularity, steplike defects, and fragmentation. One or multiple spinal levels may be involved. Often other osseous changes are present, which suggest a specific disease.

DISEASE	COMMENTS
More common *Limbus bone* **(FIG. 17-76)**	Designates a small, well-corticated fragment of bone at the edge or fringe of a vertebra that develops from interosseous herniation of the nucleus pulposus between the vertebral centra and endplate, prohibiting fusion of secondary growth center to the vertebral centra; it is differentiated from fracture fragment by its well-corticated margin, lack of displacement, presence in the lumbar region, and absence of serious trauma history.
Normal growth centers **(FIG. 17-77)**	In the lateral projection, steplike defects are seen at the vertebral endplate margins (more prominent anteriorly); these defects contain the cartilage growth centers of the vertebral endplate; as ossification proceeds, a focus of bone fills the radiolucent defect (6 to 12 years of age), fusing to the vertebral body at 20 to 25 years of age.
Nuclear impressions (notochordal persistence) **(FIG. 17-78)**	Nonfocal, congenital, smooth, inward deformity of all or part of the superior, inferior, or both vertebral endplates; in the frontal projection the defect has a "double-hump" or "cupid's bow" appearance.
Osteoporosis [p. 916]	Reduction in the quantity of bone that occurs most often in postmenopausal women and elderly men; sparse, thin trabeculae, as well as thinning (but no destruction) of cortex are noted; there are smooth indentations of endplates centrally, in the region of the nucleus pulposus; bone sclerosis along endplates and solitary or multiple-level vertebral collapse occur; the disease is more typical in the lumbar and thoracic regions.
Scheurmann's disease **(FIG. 17-79)** [p. 456]	Posttraumatic defect in endplate maturation presenting during adolescence with multiple levels of anteriorly wedged vertebrae, narrowed anterior disc space, multiple Schmorl's nodes, and vertebral endplate irregularity; usually it is seen in the middle and lower thoracic spine; the anteriorly wedged vertebrae produce a kyphosis.
Schmorl's nodes **(FIG. 17-80)**	Prolapse of the nucleus pulposus into the vertebra producing abrupt, inward deformities of a focal area of the endplate, usually with notable surrounding sclerosis; both endplates and multiple vertebrae may be involved; multiple Schmorl's nodes are encountered in Scheuermann's disease.
Less common *Hyperparathyroidism* [p. 910]	Overproduction of parathyroid glands, resulting from primary or secondary causes; the disease is marked by osteopenia, osteosclerosis, bone resorption, and soft-tissue and vascular calcification; specifically, vertebrae appear osteopenic with characteristic homogeneous, radiodense bands traversing horizontally at each end of the vertebrae ("rugger jersey" spine).
Osteopetrosis (Albers-Schönberg's disease) **(FIGS. 17-81 and 17-82)** [p. 451]	Hereditary failure of calcified cartilage resorption, which interferes with the development of mature bone; the appearance is marked by sclerotic, fragile bones; vertebrae may appear "doubled" by smaller "endobones" within their bodies; well-defined, transverse, radiodense bands characteristically are found subjacent to the endplates.
Radiation **(FIGS. 17-83 and 17-84)**	In the growing spine, may arrest the growth of the vertebra through endplate necrosis, producing short vertebrae with irregular endplates, involvement of the lumbar spine is most often in relation to treatment for Wilms' tumor and neuroblastoma; if the radiation is applied asymmetrically, scoliosis may develop with a convexity of the lateral curvature opposite the side of irradiation.
Sickle-cell anemia **(FIG. 17-85)** [p. 771]	Genetic abnormality in which red blood cells assume a sickled configuration in low oxygen tension; the sickled cells may occlude small vessels with resulting ischemia; skeletal changes include osteopenia, coarse trabeculae, biconcave (more precisely steplike or H-shaped) vertebrae, and dactylitis.

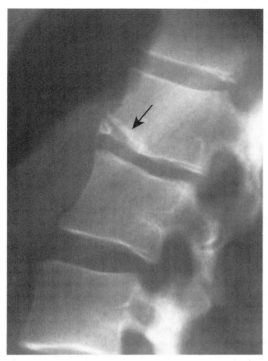

FIG. 17-76 Limbus bone with a characteristic, well-marginated appearance located at anterior inferior corner of the L2 vertebra. In contrast, a teardrop fracture is not well-marginated, does not exhibit a sclerotic band on the vertebra *(arrow)*, and is usually displaced from the vertebra.

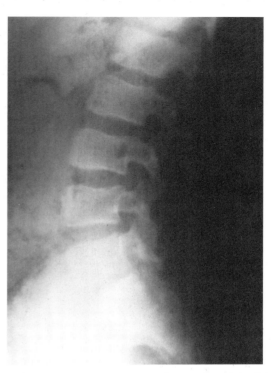

FIG. 17-77 Lateral lumbar projection demonstrating mild inward defects of the endplates with central radiodensity. This is a normal developmental appearance.

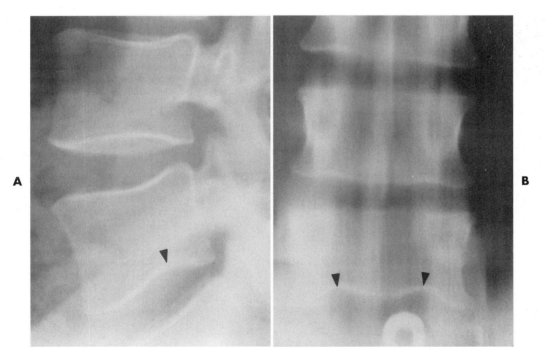

FIG. 17-78 **A,** Lateral plain film and, **B,** anteroposterior linear tomogram radiograph demonstrating notochordal persistency *(arrowheads)*. (Courtesy Steven P. Brownstein, MD, Springfield, NJ.)

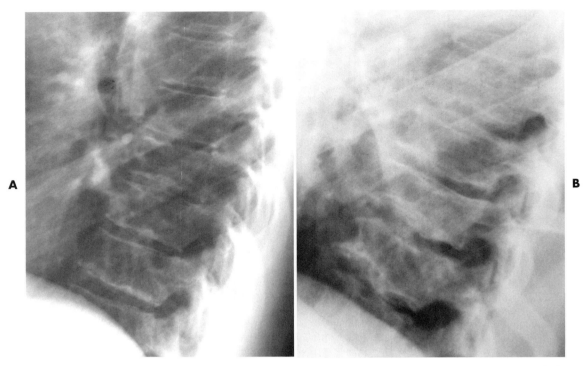

FIG. 17-79 A and **B,** Scheuermann's disease indicated by multiple levels of endplate irregularity and anterior vertebral wedging in the thoracolumbar spine.

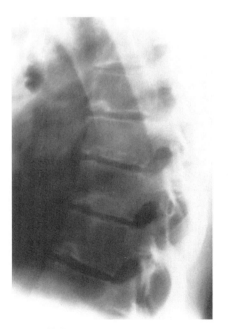

FIG. 17-80 Deformity of the vertebral endplates caused by multiple Schmorl's nodes.

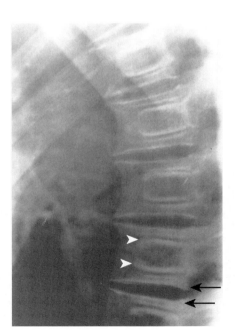

FIG. 17-81 Osteopetrosis appearing with characteristic endobone shadows in each of the thoracic vertebrae *(arrowheads)*. In addition, radiodense endplate stripes are noted *(arrows)*. The endplate stripes are not a prominent feature in this case.

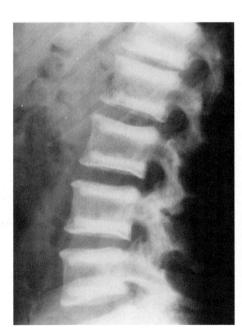

FIG. 17-82 Osteopetrosis producing radiodense stripes along the vertebral endplates throughout the lumbar spine.

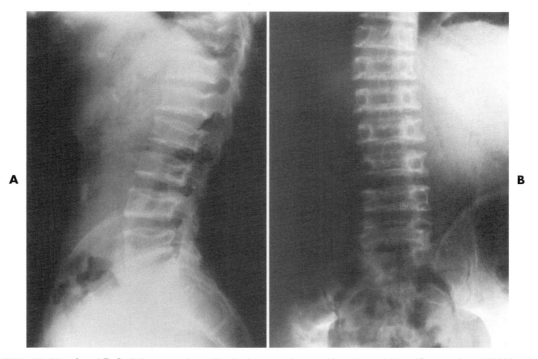

FIG. 17-83 **A** and **B,** Radiation necrosis resulting in short vertebrae and irregular endplates. (Courtesy Joseph W. Howe, Sylmar, CA.)

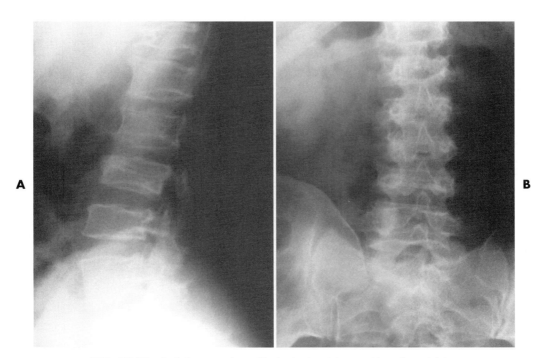

FIG. 17-84 Radiation necrosis resulting in short vertebrae and irregular endplates.

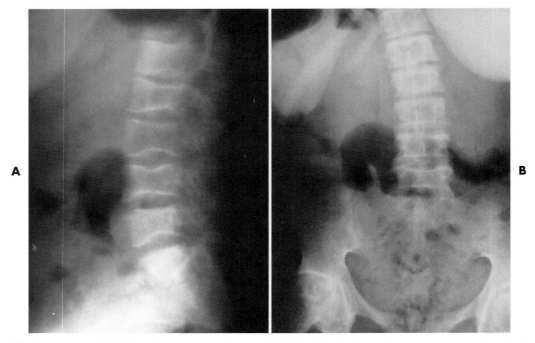

FIG. 17-85 **A** and **B,** Sickle-cell anemia causing biconcave deformity of the lumbar vertebrae secondary to underperfusion of the center of the vertebrae.

Suggested Readings

Aliabadi P, Nikpoor N: Imaging evaluation of sacroiliitis, *Rheum Dis Clin North Am* 17(3):809, 1991.

Burgener FA, Kormano M: Differential diagnosis in conventional radiology, ed 2, New York, 1991, Thieme.

Chapman S, Nakielny R: Aids to radiological differential diagnosis, ed 4, Philadelphia, 2003, WB Saunders.

Dahnert W: Radiology review manual, Baltimore, 1991, Williams & Wilkins.

Dolan KD: Cervicobasilar relationships, *Radiol Clin North Am* 15(2):155, 1977.

Eisenberg RL: An atlas of differential diagnosis, ed 2, Gaithersburg, MD, 1992, Aspen.

Herman TE, McAlister WH: Inherited diseases of bone density in children, *Radiol Clin North Am* 29(1):149, 1991.

Jacobson HG: Dense bone—too much bone: radiographical considerations and differential diagnosis, *Skeletal Radiol* 13:1, 1985.

Jacobson HG, Edeiken J: Radiology of disorders of the sacroiliac joints, *JAMA* 253(19):2863, 1985.

Ravin CE, Cooper C, Leder RA: Review of radiology, Philadelphia, 1994, WB Saunders.

Reeder MM, Bradley WG: Reeder and Felson's gamuts in radiology, ed 3, New York, 1993, Springer-Verlag.

Weinberger A, Myers AR: Intervertebral disc calcification in adults: a review, *Semin Arthritis Rheum* 8(1):69, 1978.

Weissleder R, Wittenberg J, Harisinghani MG: Primer of diagnostic imaging, ed 3, St Louis, 2003 Mosby.

Extremity Patterns

DENNIS M. MARCHIORI

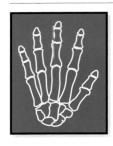

EX I | Acroosteolysis

Acroosteolysis represents bone resorption of the distal phalanges of the hands and feet. A wide range of congenital and acquired etiologies is responsible. Swelling or atrophy of the overlying soft tissues also may be present.

DISEASE	COMMENTS
More common	
Hyperparathyroidism (FIG. 18-1) [p. 910]	Overproduction of parathormone resulting from primary or secondary factors affecting the parathyroid glands. The disease is marked by osteopenia, osteosclerosis, bone resorption, and soft-tissue and vascular calcification. Vertebrae appear osteopenic with characteristic, homogeneous, radiodense bands traversing horizontally at each end of the vertebrae ("rugger jersey" spine); resorption of the distal tufts and radial side of the digits is characteristic.
Neurotrophic disease [p. 584]	Bone resorption secondary to diabetes, leprosy, tabes dorsalis, syringomyelia, meningomyelocele, and congenital indifference to pain.
Psoriatic arthritis [p. 505]	Arthritis occurring in fewer than 7% of patients with psoriasis; this condition involves the carpal, interphalangeal (distal interphalangeal common), and less commonly the sacroiliac joints. The digits are marked by nail pitting, swelling of the soft tissues, and less commonly erosions of the distal tufts, which relate a tapered appearance of the distal phalanges.
Scleroderma (progressive systemic sclerosis) (FIG. 18-2) [p. 487]	Disease of small vessels and organ fibrosus; the soft tissues of the hands and feet undergo atrophy and calcification in addition to resorption of distal phalanges.
Thermal injury (FIG. 18-3)	Resorption of the distal phalanges secondary to burns or frostbite injury; characteristically the thumb is spared in frostbite injury as the individual makes a fist around the thumb, protecting it from low temperatures.
Less common	
Arteriosclerosis obliterans	Arteriosclerosis producing narrowing and occlusion of the arterial lumen; the resulting ischemia causes bone resorption.
Lesch-Nyhan syndrome	Disorder characterized by hyperuricemia and uric acid urolithiasis, mental retardation, spastic cerebral palsy, and biting (self-mutilation) of fingers and lips.
Pyknodysostosis (FIG. 18-4) [p. 456]	Hereditary sclerosing dysplasia of bone, marked by short stature, dense bones (often with transverse fractures), hypoplastic angle of mandible, wormian bones, delayed closure of the fontanelles, and hypoplasia of the terminal phalanges.
Raynaud disease	Spasms of the digital arteries leading to distal tuft resorption, blanching, and pain in the hands; condition is associated with scleroderma.
Sarcoidosis (FIG. 18-5) [p. 1218]	Systemic granulomatous disease most pronounced in the lungs; less commonly the disease involves arthritis or acroosteolysis of the hand with coarsened trabeculae and well-defined osteolytic lesions.
Vinyl chloride exposure	Systemic toxicant, abbreviated VC, which is particularly noxious to endothelium and is used for polyvinyl chloride (PVC) synthesis. Occupational exposure is associated with acroosteolysis and neuritis; the acroosteolysis presents as transverse, bandlike radiolucent defects of the distal phalanges, usually the thumb.

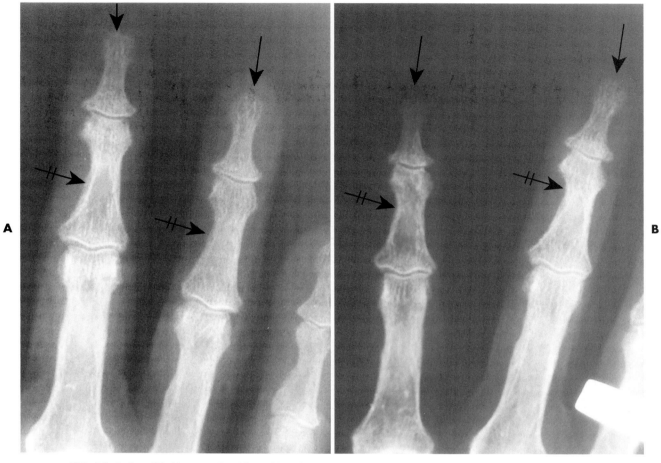

FIG. 18-1 A and **B,** Hyperparathyroidism with mild resorption of the distal tufts *(arrows)* and along the radial side of the middle phalanx of the second and third digits *(crossed arrows).* (Courtesy Joseph W. Howe, Sylmar, CA.)

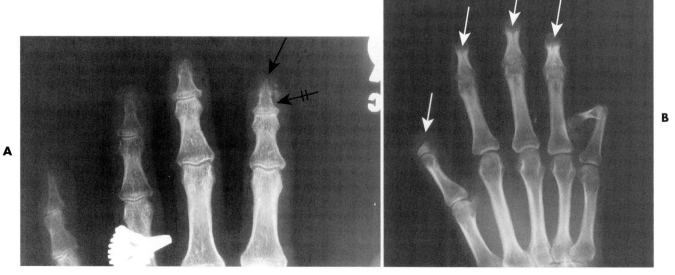

FIG. 18-2 A and **B,** Different patients with scleroderma presenting as acroosteolysis *(arrows).* The first cases exhibits soft-tissue calcification *(crossed arrow).* (Courtesy Joseph W. Howe, Sylmar, CA.)

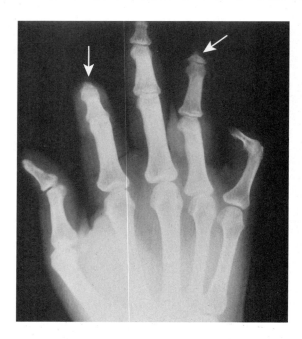

FIG. 18-3 Acroosteolysis *(arrows)* secondary to frostbite. (Courtesy Steven P. Brownstein, MD, Springfield, NJ.)

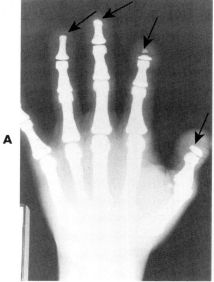

A

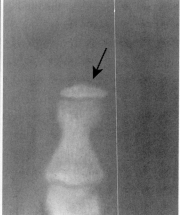

B

FIG. 18-4 Pyknodysostosis presenting, **A,** with increased radiodensity and acroosteolysis and, **B,** acroosteolysis alone in a second case *(arrows).*

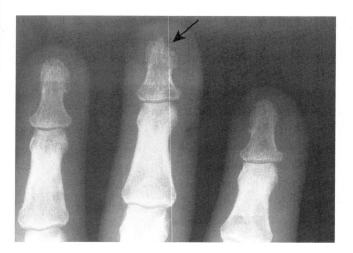

FIG. 18-5 Sarcoidosis causing acroosteolysis *(arrow).* Sarcoidosis is an uncommon cause of acroosteolysis. (Courtesy Joseph W. Howe, Sylmar, CA.)

EX2 | Calcified Intraarticular Loose Bodies

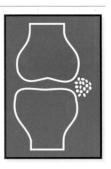

Loose intraarticular bodies typically are found in the large weight-bearing joints (e.g., knees). Degenerative disease probably represents the most common etiology. Noncalcified intraarticular bodies are not visible on plain film radiographs and necessitate specialized imaging to detect their presence. Symptoms are variable, ranging from acute joint locking to asymptomatic states.

DISEASE	COMMENTS
More common *Degenerative joint disease* [p. 525]	Very common, progressive, noninflammatory disorder involving the large weight-bearing joints and smaller joints of the hand. The radiographic appearance is characterized by joint subluxation, articular deformity, nonuniform reduction in joint space, marginal osteophytes, subchondral sclerosis, subchondral bone cysts, and intraarticular loose bodies. The knee is most commonly involved; this disease usually is seen in elderly patients.
Trauma	Single or multiple loose bodies representing bone, ligament, or meniscal fragments arising from trauma. Fragments may not be calcified, and therefore are not visible with plain film radiography.
Less common *Neuropathic (Charcot's) joint* [p. 584]	Destructive arthropathy secondary to altered joint sensory innervation, resulting in either unchecked repetitive injury as a result of absence of pain or loss of trophic influences of innervations with local hyperemia and bone resorption. Varieties are atrophic and hypertrophic; hypertrophic changes include premature and advanced degeneration marked by dislocation, destruction, intraarticular loose bodies (debris), and disorganization; the knee, hip, ankle, and lumbar spine are commonly affected.
Osteochondrosis dissecans [p. 734]	Complete or incomplete separation of a portion of the joint cartilage and subjacent bone from a traumatic or osteonecrotic etiology. Occurs adolescence; the knee usually is involved, classically the lateral aspect of the medial condyle; fragments that do not reunite exist as intraarticular loose bodies.
Synovial osteochondromatosis **(FIGS. 18-6 and 18-7)** [p. 862]	Nonneoplastic hypertropic metaplasia of synovial tissue, producing multiple cartilage nodules, which eventually may ossify; nodules detach to become loose bodies in the joint, bursal, and tendon sheath spaces. This condition may be asymptomatic or produce acute pain with joint locking; in adults, the knee, hip, ankle, and elbow are most commonly affected.

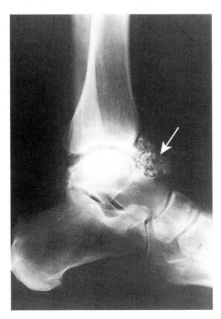

FIG. 18-6 Synovial osteochondromatosis of the ankle, demonstrating calcified loose bodies *(arrow)*. (Courtesy Joseph W. Howe, Sylmar, CA.)

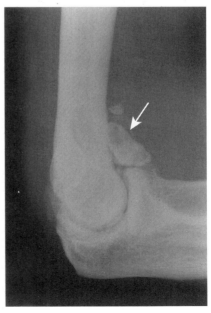

FIG. 18-7 Synovial osteochondromatosis of the elbow *(arrow)*. (Courtesy Joseph W. Howe, Sylmar, CA.)

PART TWO Bone, Joints, and Soft Tissues

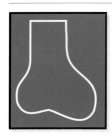

EX3 | Change in Size and Shape of Epiphyses

Alterations in the size and shape of epiphyses are related to traumatic, congenital, and metabolic disturbance of bone growth, or they may represent normal variants of bone growth and development. Joint effusion or bleeding may cause overgrowth, as is the case in juvenile rheumatoid arthritis and hemophilia. A long list of eponyms is applied to irregularity of the epiphysis associated with avascular necrosis.

DISEASE	COMMENTS
More common *Avascular necrosis* **(FIGS. 18-8 through 18-12)** [p. 755]	Etiologies related to vascular insufficiency (e.g., sickle-cell disease, steroid therapy, trauma, alcoholism); necrosis gives the epiphyses a fragmented, radiodense, thin, and small appearance. Proximal femoral epiphysis is most common; weight bearing, joint effusion, and decreased range of motion cause pain.
Trauma	Traumatic separation or changes in the size and shape of the epiphysis; including battered child syndrome.
Less common *Achondroplasia* [p. 421]	Congenital defect of enchondral bone formation, producing characteristic rounded lumbar "bullet-nosed" vertebrae, lumbar kyphosis, posterior scalloping of the vertebrae, increased intervertebral disc height, flattened vertebral bodies, and narrowed spinal canal; the pelvis may appear hypoplastic; epiphyses may appear "cone-shaped"; cone-shaped epiphyses also are seen with sickle-cell disease, various congenital dysplasias, and as a normal variant.
Congenital syndromes **(FIG. 18-13)**	Chondrodysplasia punctata (Conradi's disease), multiple epiphyseal dysplasia (Fairbank-Ribbing disease), Down syndrome, and other congenital syndromes associated with irregularity, fragmentation, and stippling of multiple epiphyses.
Cretinism [p. 915]	Juvenile hypothyroidism during the first year of life resulting from thymic agenesis or low maternal iodine intake during pregnancy. Patients exhibit delayed skeletal and mental development result; epiphyses appear stippled during infancy and fragmented during childhood; cone-shaped epiphyses may develop. The proximal femoral epiphyses are most commonly involved.
Hemophilia [p. 768]	Inherited X-linked defect of blood coagulation marked by a permanent tendency toward hemorrhages. Hemarthrosis is associated with red, swollen joints, osteoporosis, precocious degeneration, and an enlargement of the epiphyses; knee, ankle, and elbow are most common; rarely, osteolytic expansile bone lesions (hemophilic pseudotumors) develop.
Juvenile rheumatoid arthritis [p. 482]	Chronic arthritis beginning in childhood (before 16 years of age), manifesting as one of several clinical types; characteristic large, overgrown, "ballooned" epiphyses, osteoporosis, joint fusion, periostitis, and gracile long bones are secondary to hyperemia.
Normal variant	May be represented by symmetric, fragmented, or irregular appearance of the epiphysis; these variants may mimic osteonecrosis.
Rickets **(FIG. 18-14)** [p. 925]	Infantile or juvenile osteomalacia secondary to vitamin D deficiency, characterized clinically by irritability, listlessness, and generalized muscle weakness. An overproduction and deficient calcification of osteoid tissue results in disturbances of bone growth with resulting deformity. Fractures are common; epiphyses may appear indistinct, epiphyseal plates are wide, and metaphyses appear frayed.
Scurvy (Barlow's disease) **(FIG. 18-15)** [p. 927]	Defective osteogenesis occurs secondary to abnormal collagen from vitamin C deficiency, beginning between 6 to 14 months of age. The disease is marked clinically by irritability, bleeding gums, tendency toward hemorrhage, and tenderness and weakness of lower limbs; epiphyses appear radiolucent with surrounding sclerotic rim (Wimberger's sign or ring epiphyses).

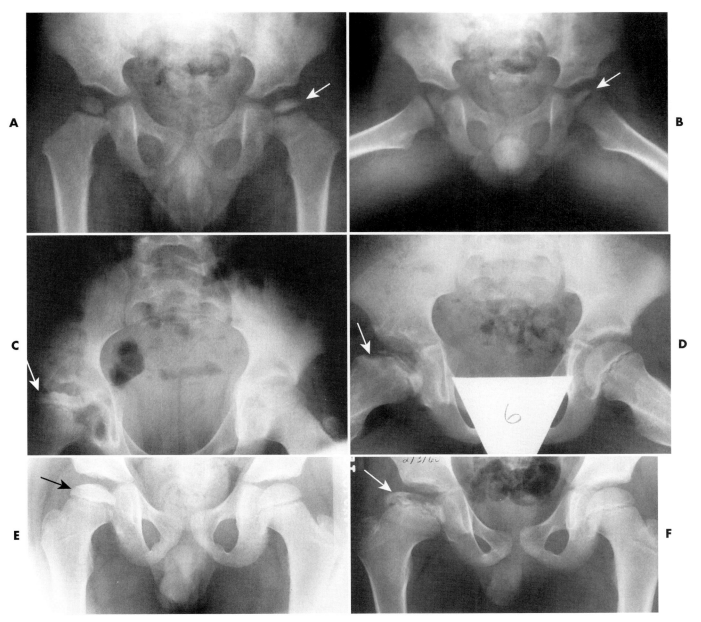

FIG. 18-8 Three cases of Legg-Calvé-Perthes (LCP) disease. **A,** Anteroposterior and, **B,** frog-leg pelvic projection of a child with a left proximal femoral epiphysis *(arrows)*, which appears small and dense consistent with LCP. Second case with, **C,** anteroposterior and, **D,** frog-leg projection of a patient with similar findings of a small, fragmented, dense right epiphysis *(arrows)*. The third case exhibits progressive changes of fragmentation, increased density, and diminution occurring, **E,** initially and, **F,** 2 years after the initial film *(arrows)*. (**C** and **D,** Courtesy Jack C. Avalos, Davenport, IA; **E** and **F,** Courtesy Joseph W. Howe, Sylmar, CA.)

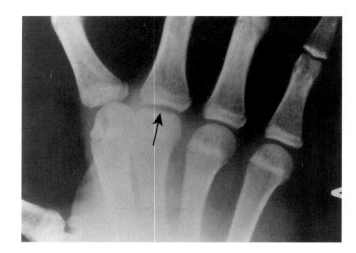

FIG. 18-9 Mauclaire disease, presenting as avascular necrosis of the third metacarpal head *(arrow)*. (Courtesy Joseph W. Howe, Sylmar, CA.)

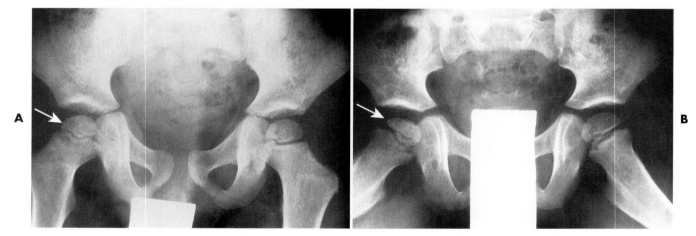

FIG. 18-10 Legg-Calvé-Perthes disease presenting with proximal femoral epiphyses that appear nearly normal, **A,** on the anteroposterior radiography and, **B,** with loss of vertical height of the proximal femoral epiphysis on the frog-leg projection *(arrows)*. (Courtesy Robert C. Tatum, Davenport, IA.)

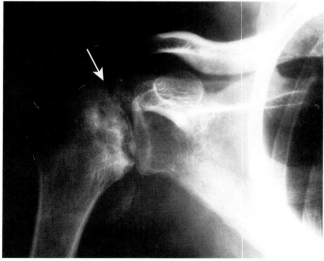

FIG. 18-11 Avascular necrosis of the humeral head (Hass disease) *(arrow)*. (Courtesy Steven P. Brownstein, MD, Springfield, NJ.)

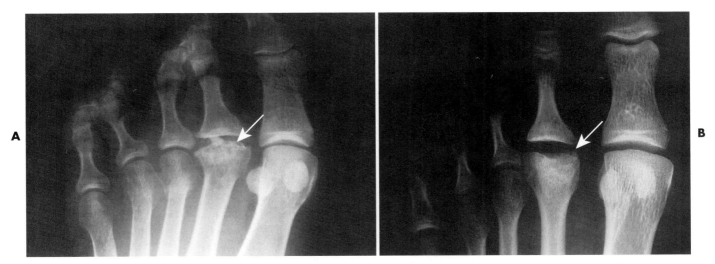

FIG. 18-12 **A** and **B,** Two patients with flattened deformity of the metatarsal head consistent with avascular necrosis (Freiberg disease) *(arrows).*

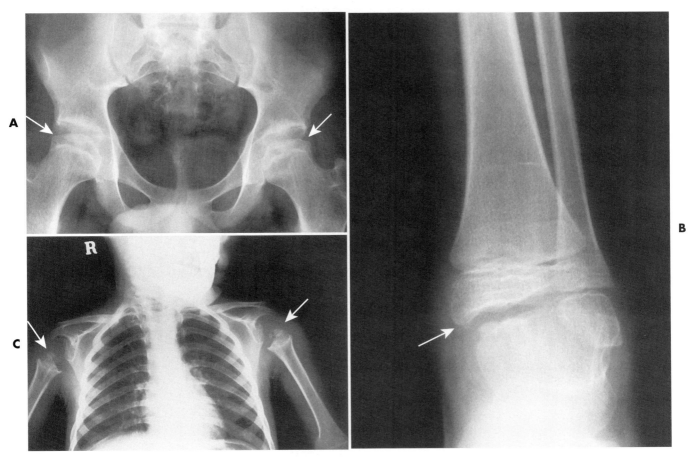

FIG. 18-13 Multiple epiphyseal dysplasia, resulting in irregular-appearing epiphyses, **A,** of the proximal femora and, **B,** distal tibia *(arrows).* **C,** Another patient with irregularity of the proximal humeri *(arrows).* (**A** and **B,** Courtesy Jack C. Avalos, Davenport, IA; **C,** Courtesy Joseph W. Howe, Sylmar, CA.)

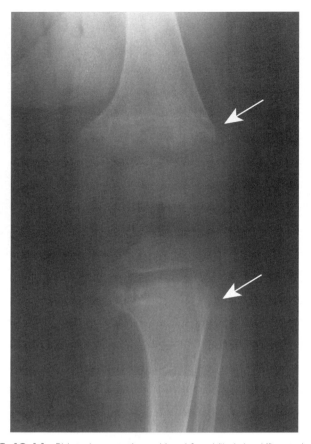

FIG. 18-14   Rickets demonstrating a widened, frayed ("paintbrush") metaphyses *(arrows)* with an indistinct epiphysis. (Courtesy Joseph W. Howe, Sylmar, CA.)

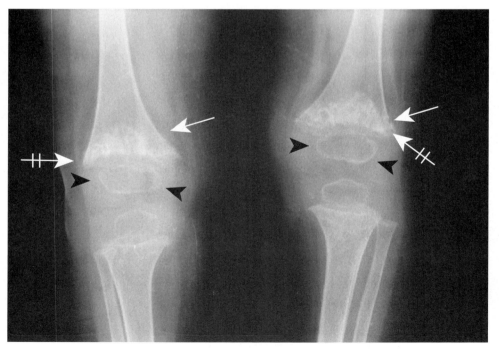

FIG. 18-15   Scurvy appearing with bilateral radiolucent epiphyses, which are outlined by a surrounding radiodense rim *(arrowheads)*. Radiolucent metaphyseal bands *(arrows)* and radiodense zone of provisional calcification *(crossed arrows)* are evident. (Courtesy Steven P. Brownstein, MD, Springfield, NJ.)

EX4 | Cystic Lesions of Extremities and Ribs

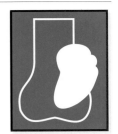

This pattern lists lesions occurring mostly in the epiphyses and metaphyses of long bones that appear as solitary or, less commonly, multiple well-defined holes in the bone. The age of presentation, host bone, presence of calcification, and symptoms are useful discriminators for the list of lesions. The popular mnemonic *FEGNOMASHIC* includes many of this list: fibrous dysplasia, enchondroma (and eosinophilic granuloma), giant cell tumor, nonossifying fibroma, osteoblastoma, metastatic disease (and multiple myeloma/plasmacytoma), aneurysmal bone cyst, simple bone cyst, hyperparathyroidism (and hemophilic pseudotumors) infection, and chondroblastoma (and chondromyxoid fibroma).

The full list may be modified if the presentation is of multiple lesions or is epiphyseal in location. A presentation of multiple lesions suggests the following etiologies: infection, fibrous dysplasia, metastasis, multiple myeloma, subchondral cysts, hyperparathyroidism, enchondromatosis, and eosinophilic granuloma. An epiphyseal location suggests infection, giant cell tumor, chondroblastoma, subchondral cyst, pigmented villonodular synovitis, and interosseous ganglion. Cystic bone lesions occurring in patients younger than 30 years of age most often result from eosinophilic granuloma, aneurysmal bone cyst, simple bone cyst, chondroblastoma, and nonossifying fibroma/fibrous cortical defect.

The mnemonic *FAME* describes cystic rib lesions: fibrous dysplasia, aneurysmal bone cyst, metastatic disease (and multiple myeloma), and enchondroma.

DISEASE	COMMENTS
More common	
Enchondroma **(FIG. 18-16)** [p. 828]	Solitary or multiple benign cystic cartilage lesion, appearing most often in the small bones of the hands and feet; stippled cartilage matrix is seen typically; no periostitis or pain is present unless fractured.
Fibrous cortical defect/nonossifying fibroma **(FIGS. 18-17 and 18-18)** [p. 847]	Very common, benign asymptomatic cystic bone lesions seen before the age of 30 years; marked by a thin sclerotic border without matrix calcification; common in the lower extremities, particularly around the knee.
Fibrous dysplasia **(FIGS. 18-19 and 18-20)** [p. 846]	Disturbance of bone maintenance in which bone is replaced by abnormal proliferation of fibrous tissue, possibly involving one or multiple bones. The matrix often has a characteristic "ground glass" radiodensity; lesions may be surrounded by a thick rind of bone sclerosis; most common locations are femur, ribs, tibia, craniofacial bones, and pelvis; lesion should not be painful.
Infection **(FIG. 18-21)**	May occur at practically any location during any age; if found in a subarticular location, the joint is often involved with effusion. Soft-tissue mass and central bone sequestrum often are present; appearance varies from cystic to sclerotic; alternatively, infections may present as aggressive bone lesions.
Metastatic disease **(FIG. 18-22)** [p. 1393]	Common cause of one or more osteolytic bone lesions in patients over the age of 40 years; atypical presentations of expansile, bubbly, solitary geographic lesions are associated with primary lesions of the thyroid and kidney; purely blastic lesions occur most often from breast, prostate, gastrointestinal, bladder, and lung neoplasms.
Simple (solitary) bone cyst **(FIGS. 18-23 and 18-24)** [p. 879]	Fluid-filled cyst of uncertain etiology; the majority of cases are discovered before the age of 20 years; 90% of simple bone cysts are found in the proximal humerus and femur. Bone cysts appear as mildly expansile, well-marginated, geographic lytic lesions in the metaphysis, less frequently in the diaphysis, or rarely in the epiphysis; fracture causes pain, otherwise, it is usually painless.
Subchondral bone cyst **(FIGS. 18-25 and 18-26)**	Related to arthritic or synovial disorder (osteoarthritis, gout, calcium pyrophosphate deposition disease, rheumatoid arthritis, hemophilia, intraosseous ganglion, amyloidosis, and avascular necrosis). This well-defined cyst is located in the epiphysis subjacent to the articular cortex.
Less common	
Adamantinoma [p. 883]	Also known as *angioblastoma*, a rare, locally aggressive or malignant lesion composed of epithelium-like cells in dense fibrous stroma; 90% are found in the middle third of the tibia. Lesions appear as central or eccentric, slightly expansile, well-circumscribed, osteolytic lesions.
Aneurysmal bone cyst [p. 876]	Solitary, benign, osteolytic lesion of bone, characterized by cortical expansion, usually found in patients younger than 20 years of age; this bone cyst most commonly presents as an eccentric lesion in the metaphyses of long bones; typically it causes pain.

DISEASE	COMMENTS
Chondroblastoma [p. 829]	Rare, benign bone tumor arising in the secondary growth centers of long bones; usually in patients younger than 25 years of age; 50% demonstrate matrix calcification and a rim of surrounding sclerosis.
Chondromyxoid fibroma [p. 832]	Rare, benign bone tumor of mixed histology, arising most commonly in the proximal tibia and fibula; usually in patients younger than 30 years of age, they appear as noncalcified lytic lesions.
Eosinophilic granuloma [p. 935]	Proliferation of eosinophils seen most commonly in children and young adults; spine involvement is present in less than 10% of patients; advanced body collapse ("vertebra plana") and multiple levels may accompany the condition. Long bone involvement typically occurs in the diaphysis; patients younger than 30 years of age almost exclusively represent the population affected by this disease; it may be present with solitary or multiple lesions.
Giant cell tumor **(FIG. 18-27)** [p. 878]	Sometimes malignant cystic lesion of bone; subarticular, eccentric (early), sharply defined lesion appears without surrounding sclerosis; most commonly found around the knee; tumor occurs between 20 and 40 years of age.
Hydatid (Echinococcus) *cyst* [p. 1310]	Cyst that may be formed in bone (usually formed in the liver) by the larval stage of *Echinococcus*. It appears as a slow-growing, destructive lesion surrounded by sclerotic borders; it is primarily limited to endemic areas.
Hyperparathyroidism [p. 910]	Overproduction of parathyroid glands because of primary or secondary causes; the disease is marked by osteopenia, osteosclerosis, bone resorption, and soft-tissue and vascular calcification; vertebrae have characteristic homogeneous radiodense bands traversing horizontally at each endplate ("rugger jersey" spine). Subchondral bone resorption occurs, particularly at the radial aspects of the middle phalanges; lytic or sclerotic cystic bone lesion (brown tumors) may be present.
Intraosseous lipoma **(FIG. 18-28)** [p. 866]	Intraosseous collections of fat appearing as a radiolucent lesion surrounded by a thin sclerotic rim of bone, often with a centrally located radiodense nidus. The proximal femoral and calcaneal epiphyses predominantly house the lipoma; it typically presents as an asymptomatic lesion during middle age.
Multiple myeloma/plasmacytoma **(FIG. 18-29)** [p. 819]	Malignant proliferation of plasma cells, occurring predominantly in the red marrow of various bones; the skull, vertebral bodies, ribs, and proximal humerus and femur are involved most commonly. Single or multiple osteolytic lesions simulate metastatic disease, without tendency to involve vertebral arch, as is common in metastasis; osteopenia and solitary or multiple levels of vertebral collapse together simulate osteoporosis; it rarely occurs before 30 years of age.
Osteoblastoma [p. 809]	Histologically similar to osteoid osteoma, but different in radiographic appearance; osteoblastomas appear as medium-sized (≥1.5 cm), geographic, expansile, generally nonaggressive, eccentric medullary lesions. Most commonly located in the posterior elements of the spine, and less frequently in the proximal femur, tibia, talus, ribs, and hands; they usually appear before 25 years of age.
Pigmented villonodular synovitis **(FIG. 18-30)** [p. 801]	Chronic condition marked by diffuse hyperplastic outgrowths of a joint's synovial membrane; osteolytic appearance may result from pressure erosions of bone if joint capsule is tight. Usually pigmented villonodular synovitis (PVNS) occurs before 40 years of age, although wide age range is possible; the most common locations are the knee, hip, ankle, elbow, and shoulder.

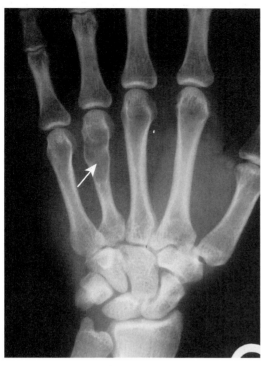

FIG. 18-16   Enchondroma of the distal fourth metacarpal *(arrow)*.

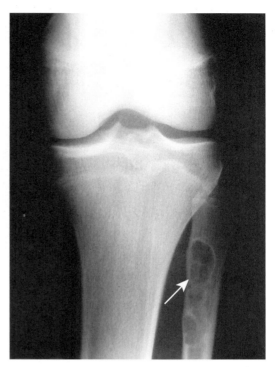

FIG. 18-17   Nonossifying fibroma of the proximal fibula *(arrow)*. (Courtesy Steven P. Brownstein, MD, Springfield, NJ.)

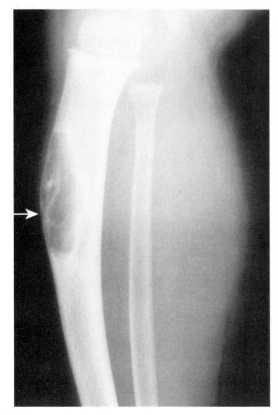

FIG. 18-18   Nonossifying fibroma of the proximal tibia *(arrow)*. (Courtesy Steven P. Brownstein, MD, Springfield, NJ.)

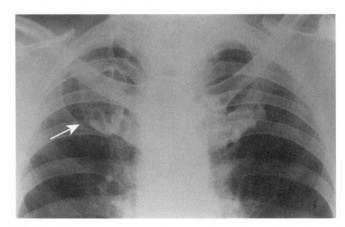

FIG. 18-19   Fibrous dysplasia causing a cystic lesion of the right first rib *(arrow)*. (Courtesy Joseph W. Howe, Sylmar, CA.)

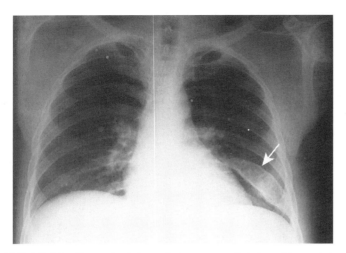

FIG. 18-20   Fibrous dysplasia, producing an expansile lesion of the posterior portion of the left eighth rib *(arrow)*.

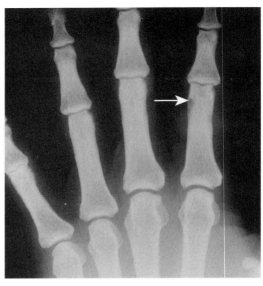

FIG. 18-21   Well-defined, seemingly relatively nonaggressive infection of the distal portion of the proximal phalanx of the second digit secondary to a puncture wound *(arrow)*. (Courtesy Steven P. Brownstein, MD, Springfield, NJ.)

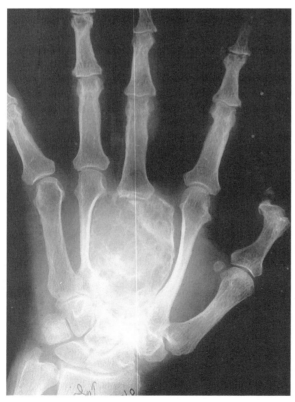

FIG. 18-22   Expansile lesion of the third metacarpal, representing metastatic bone disease secondary to primary thyroid malignancy. (Courtesy Steven P. Brownstein, MD, Springfield, NJ.)

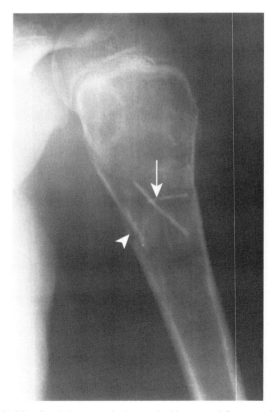

FIG. 18-23   Simple bone cyst in the proximal humerus. A fragmented septum is noted obliquely oriented and inferiorly displaced ("fallen fragment" sign) in the large radiolucent lesion *(arrow)*. Fracture of the thinned cortex is noted on the medial side of the humerus *(arrowhead)*. (Courtesy Steven P. Brownstein, MD, Springfield, NJ.)

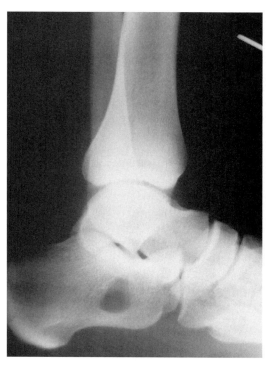

FIG. 18-24 Simple bone cyst of the calcaneus. A similar appearance may occur with interosseous lipoma or giant cell tumor. (Courtesy Steven P. Brownstein, MD, Springfield, NJ.)

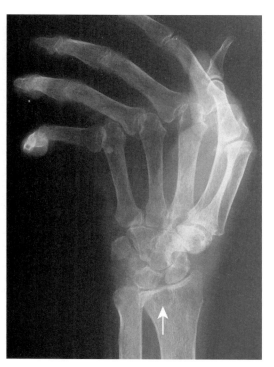

FIG. 18-25 Subchondral cyst in the radius *(arrow)* of a patient with advanced rheumatoid arthritis. (Courtesy Jack C. Avalos, Davenport, IA)

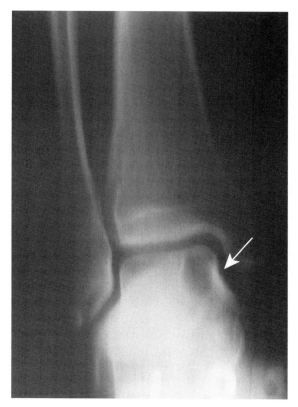

FIG. 18-26 Linear tomogram of an intraosseous ganglion of the talus *(arrow)*. (Courtesy Joseph W. Howe. Sylmar, CA.)

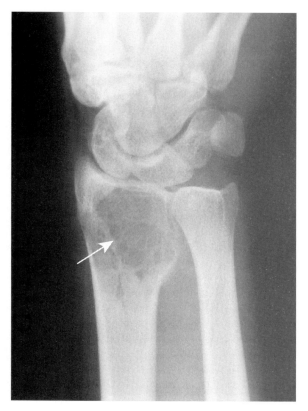

FIG. 18-27 Giant cell tumor of the distal radius. The lesion presents the characteristic osteolytic, well-defined, subarticular, and eccentric appearance *(arrow)*. (Courtesy William E. Litterer, Elizabeth, NJ.)

PART TWO
Bone, Joints, and Soft Tissues

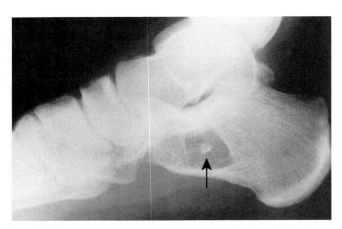

FIG. 18-28 Interosseous lipoma appearing as a cystic lesion in the calcaneus with a central nidus of calcification *(arrow)*. (Courtesy Steven P. Brownstein, MD, Springfield, NJ.)

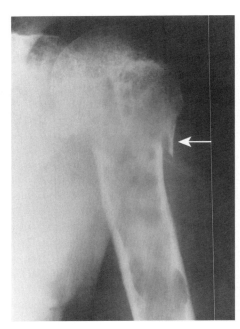

FIG. 18-29 Multiple myeloma presenting with multiple osteolytic lesions in the proximal humerus. The larger cystic lesion of the surgical neck is fractured *(arrow)*. (Courtesy Joseph W. Howe, Sylmar, CA.)

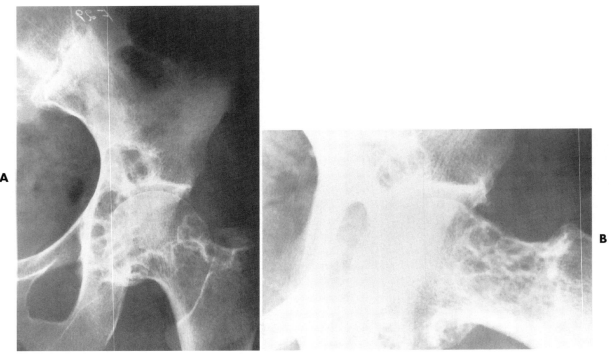

FIG. 18-30 Pigmented villonodular synovitis of the hip, causing cystic bone erosions of the femoral neck ("apple core" deformity) and the surrounding acetabulum. The bone erosions are secondary to the proliferation of the synovium. (Courtesy Joseph W. Howe, Sylmar, CA.)

EX5 | Aggressive Osteolytic Lesions of Extremities and Ribs

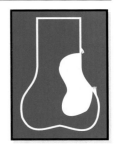

The following diseases produce usually ill-defined osteolytic lesions of bone, most characteristically of the long bones. They arise from permeative or moth-eaten patterns of bone destruction, which may coalesce over time. Radiographic findings of ill-defined bone destruction suggest aggressive pathology. The majority of these patterns represent malignant bone or marrow tumors. Patients usually complain of pain and soft-tissue mass over the involved bone.

Malignant bone tumors with marked periosteal reaction include Burkitt's lymphoma, Ewing's tumor, osteosarcoma, neuroblastoma metastasis, and leukemia presenting in a child. Tumors that arise in the midshaft of long bones and contain cells with round nuclei are known as *round cell lesions*. Round cell lesions are listed by the mnemonic *LEMON:* leukemia (and lymphoma), eosinophilic granuloma (and Ewing's tumor), multiple myeloma, osteomyelitis (mimics tumor), and neuroblastoma metastasis.

DISEASE	COMMENTS
More common *Infection* **(FIG. 18-31)**	Infection resulting from broad spectrum causative organisms involving bone by hematogenous spread, contiguous involvement, or direct implantation. Bones with rich marrow supply are frequently involved (e.g., metaphyses of long bones, spine, and ribs). Bone findings begin as subtle areas of destruction; subperiosteal extension causes thick, laminated periosteal response, which encases (involucrum) the infection; disruption of the blood supply may produce osteonecrotic bone fragments (sequestrum) within the lesion.
Metastasis **(FIGS. 18-32 to 18-34)** [p. 1393]	Bone metastasis is common to the spine and rarely involves the skeleton distal to the elbows or knees (acral metastasis). Typically appears as a polyostotic, moth-eaten pattern of osteolytic bone destruction with poorly defined zones of transition; periosteal reaction and soft-tissue masses typically are small or absent; usually occurs in patients older than 40 years of age.
Multiple myeloma/plasmacytoma **(FIGS. 18-35 and 18-36)** [p. 819]	Malignant proliferation of plasma cells occurring predominantly in the red marrow of various bones; the skull, vertebral bodies, ribs, and proximal humerus and femurs are most commonly involved. Single or multiple osteolytic lesions simulate metastatic disease but typically do not involve vertebral arch, as is demonstrated by metastasis. Osteopenia and solitary or multiple-level vertebral collapse may simulate osteoporosis; these diseases rarely occur before 30 years of age.
Less common *Central chondrosarcoma* [p. 844]	Aggressive malignant tumor of cartilage arising within the medullary canal of patients usually between the ages of 40 and 70 years; lesions are found in the pelvis, proximal femur, proximal humerus, distal femur, proximal tibia, and ribs. Chondrosarcoma appears most often as metaphyseal regions of bone destruction with scattered stippled matrix calcification with endosteal cortical scalloping, but the cortex is destroyed only rarely.
Eosinophilic granuloma **(FIG. 18-37)** [p. 935]	Abnormal proliferation of eosinophils seen most commonly in children and young adults; lytic skull and long bone defects mark this condition. The spine is involved in less than 10% of patients and appears as advanced body collapse ("vertebra plana"), possibly at multiple levels; long bone involvement typically occurs in the diaphysis appearing as solitary, or less commonly, multiple osteolytic defects. Almost exclusively, patients younger than 30 years of age exhibit this disease.
Ewing's sarcoma **(FIG. 18-38)** [p. 822]	Highly malignant primary bone tumor occurring mostly in children and teenagers; may occur in any bone of the body, although the majority of cases present in the pelvis and long bones of the lower extremities. A diaphyseal location is classic, but the metadiaphysis is more often involved. Lesion is marked by permeative lytic bone destruction, cortical erosion (saucerization), laminated or "onion skin" periosteal reaction, and large soft-tissue mass.
Fibrosarcoma/malignant fibrous histiocytoma **(FIGS. 18-39 and 18-40)** [p. 850]	Uncommon malignant tumors that involve fibrous tissues; most lesions are found around the knee and appear as osteolytic lesions with geographic, moth-eaten, or permeative bone destruction. Typically tumors are located in the metaphysis; cortical destruction, extraosseous mass, and aggressive periosteal reaction often are present; the tumor matrix does not exhibit calcification, although occasional bony fragments may be present.

DISEASE	COMMENTS
Leukemic [p. 770]	Proliferation of abnormal leukocytes within hemopoietic tissues and other organs. A variety of types exist, based on cell type and duration from onset to death; the most common, leukemia of bone, is typically acute lymphoblastic. Skeletal manifestations include diffuse demineralization, osteolytic defects, smooth periosteal reaction, and radiolucent metaphyseal bands, which become dense after chemotherapy.
Lymphoma **(FIG. 18–41)** [p. 1203]	Primary and secondary (systemic non–Hodgkin lymphoma and Hodgkin disease) lymphoma of bone, appearing as permeative radiolucent lesions of the lower extremities, pelvis, and spine; occurs over wide range of ages.
Osteosarcoma **(FIG. 18-42)** [p. 813]	Highly aggressive, malignant tumor of bone-forming cells most commonly arising in the metaphysis of long bones, usually around the knee. People 10 to 25 years of age are affected primarily; lesions appear as lytic or blastic areas of bone destruction with a surrounding cloudlike density of tumor matrix and aggressive periosteal reaction ("sunburst").

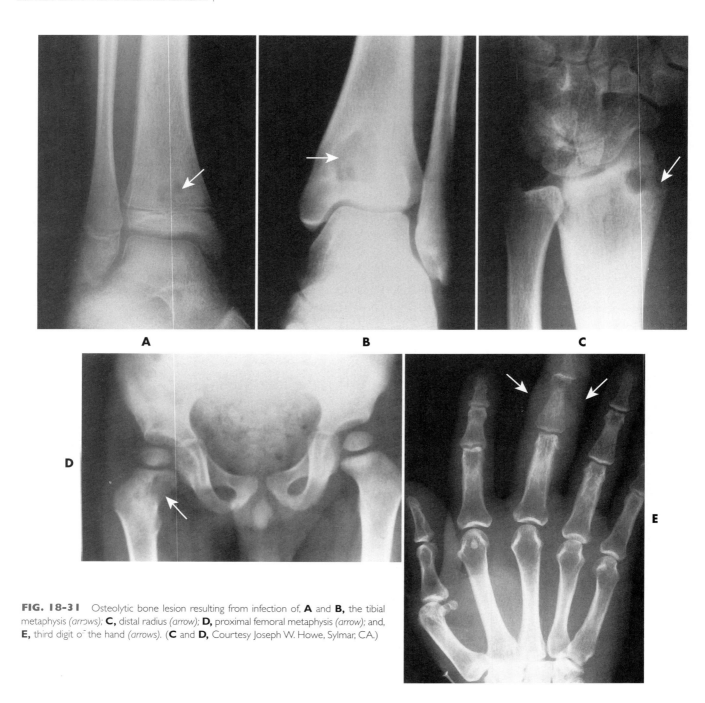

FIG. 18-31 Osteolytic bone lesion resulting from infection of, **A** and **B,** the tibial metaphysis *(arrows);* **C,** distal radius *(arrow);* **D,** proximal femoral metaphysis *(arrow);* and, **E,** third digit of the hand *(arrows).* (**C** and **D,** Courtesy Joseph W. Howe, Sylmar, CA.)

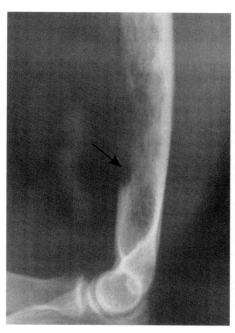

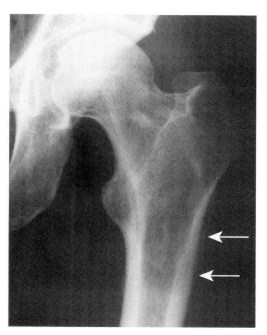

FIG. 18-32 Metastatic bone disease producing osteolytic bone destruction of the anterior, distal portion of the humerus (*arrow*). (Courtesy Joseph W. Howe, Sylmar, CA.)

FIG. 18-33 Permeative osteolytic bone destruction of the proximal femur resulting from metastatic bone disease (*arrows*). Lymphoma may present with a similar appearance. (Courtesy Joseph W. Howe, Sylmar, CA.)

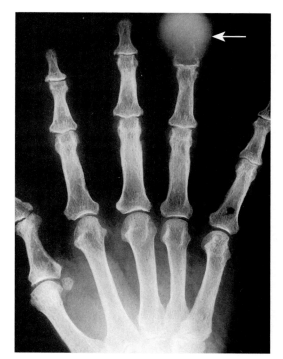

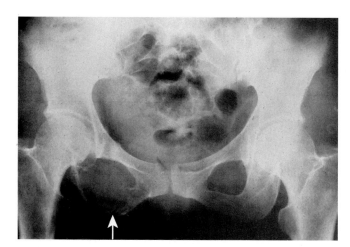

FIG. 18-34 Metastatic disease causing an aggressive lesion of the distal phalanx of the fourth digit of the left hand (*arrow*).

FIG. 18-35 Osteolytic destruction of the ischial tuberosity (*arrow*) secondary to multiple myeloma. (Courtesy Steven P. Brownstein, MD, Springfield, NJ.)

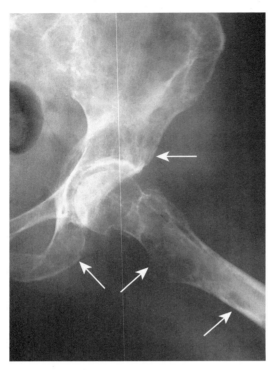

FIG. 18-36   Multiple myeloma producing multiple punched-out osteolytic lesions of the innominate and proximal femur *(arrows)*. (Courtesy Steven P. Brownstein, MD, Springfield, NJ.)

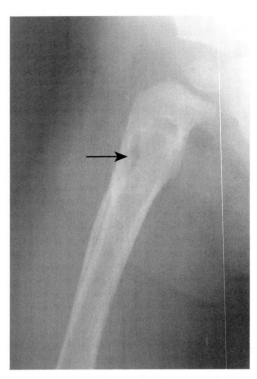

FIG. 18-37   Eosinophilic granuloma presenting as an osteolytic defect in the proximal femur *(arrow)*. (Courtesy Joseph W. Howe, Sylmar, CA.)

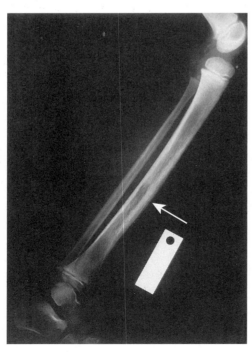

FIG. 18-38   Ewing's sarcoma representing a poorly defined osteolytic lesion of the tibial diaphysis *(arrow)*. (Courtesy Ian D. McLean, Davenport, IA.)

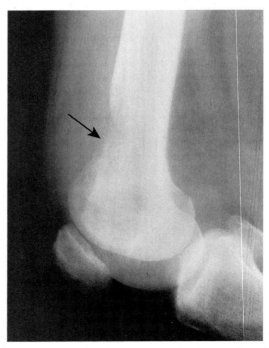

FIG. 18-39   Fibrosarcoma of the distal femur, demonstrating permeative bone destruction with no matrix calcification *(arrow)*. (Courtesy Steven P. Brownstein, MD, Springfield, NJ.)

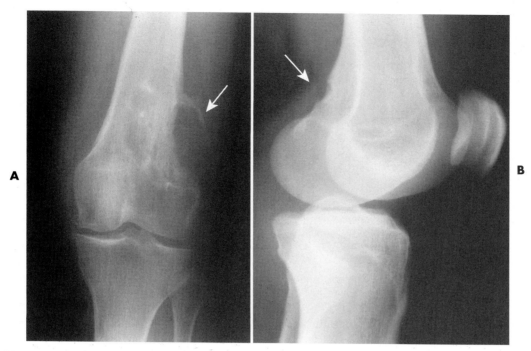

FIG. 18-40 Desmoplastic fibroma. **A,** Desmoplastic fibromas *(arrow)* represent rare benign lesions that are histologically identical to the nontumorous alteration of the periosteum known as, **B,** *juxtacortical desmoids (arrow).* As in this case, desmoplastic fibromas often appear as osteolytic lesions with prominent trabeculation. Often the lesions are difficult to differentiate from fibrosarcomas. (**A,** Courtesy Joseph W. Howe, Sylmar, CA; **B,** Courtesy Steven P. Brownstein, MD, Springfield, NJ.)

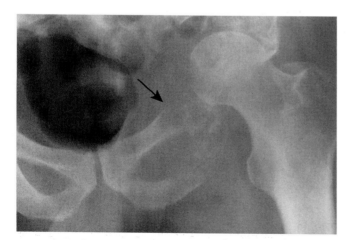

FIG. 18-41 Primary lymphoma of bone causing permeative destruction of the ischium *(arrow).* (Courtesy Joseph W. Howe, Sylmar, CA.)

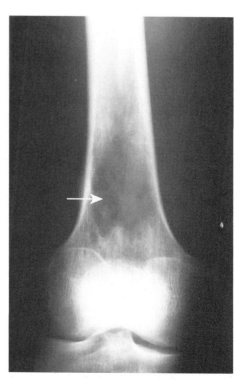

FIG. 18-42 Osteosarcoma of the distal femur, demonstrating an aggressive, purely osteolytic lesion of the distal femur *(arrow).* No periosteal reaction is demonstrated in this single view. Approximately 25% of osteosarcomas are osteolytic, 25% osteoblastic, and 50% mixed. (Courtesy Steven P. Brownstein, MD, Springfield, NJ.)

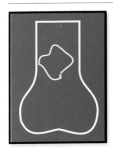

EX6 | Osteosclerotic Bone Lesions

This pattern describes solitary or multiple osteosclerotic bone lesions in the extremities. Many of the diseases listed also occur in the spine, making the pattern functional for osteosclerotic spinal lesions as well. Asymptomatic solitary osteosclerotic lesions usually represent bone islands or entities of limited consequence. In general, multiple presentations in patients over the age of 40 years are suggestive of metastatic disease.

DISEASE	COMMENTS
More common *Bone infarct/epiphyseal avascular necrosis* **(FIGS. 18-43 and 18-44)** [p. 755]	Healed bone infarcts usually appear as serpiginous calcifications in the metadiaphysis of long bones. Epiphyseal avascular necrosis is characterized by sclerosis, cystic formations, and flattening or diminution of the involved epiphysis; both conditions most often follow trauma, irradiation, corticosteroid use, and so on.
Bone island/osteopoikilosis/osteomas **(FIG. 18-45)** [p. 807]	Benign, common, solitary (bone island) or less common, multiple (osteopoikilosis) foci of compact, nontrabeculated bone occurring in the extremities and less commonly the spine. Similar formations in the skull and facial bones are known as *osteomas,* often occurring around the paranasal sinuses.
Fibrous dysplasia [p. 846]	Nonneoplastic disturbance of bone maintenance; femur, tibia, craniofacial bones, and pelvis are the most common sites. Fibrous dysplasia usually appears as an osteolytic lesion with mild sclerosis within, but rarely may present as densely sclerotic lesions; usually it is solitary.
Fracture	Radiodense appearance secondary to callus around healing fractures or stress fractures that often emerge in predictable locations; both usually are solitary lesions.
Metastasis [p. 1393]	Bone metastasis is common to the spine and rarely involves the skeleton distal to the elbows or knees (known as *acral metastasis*). Osteosclerotic lesions are less common than osteolytic lesions, usually related to primary malignancy of the breast, prostate, gastrointestinal system, bladder, or lung and usually found in patients over the age of 40 years; soft-tissue masses typically are small or absent; lesions may be solitary or multiple.
Paget's disease **(FIG. 18-46)** [p 946]	Chronic skeletal disease of aberrant bone remodeling, marked by bone enlargement, softening, and rarely sarcomatous changes. The pelvis, proximal femora, and lumbar spine are common areas; single or multiple osteosclerotic lesions are marked by bone enlargement, cortical thickening, and prominent trabeculae affecting middle-aged people.
Primary bone tumors (benign) **(FIGS. 18-47 and 18-48)**	Primary benign (osteoid osteoma, enchondromas, and osteochondroma) and malignant tumors (osteosarcoma, rarely multiple myeloma, and Ewing's sarcoma), possibly producing osteosclerotic lesions.
Less common *Healing bone lesions*	Osteolytic bone lesions may become sclerotic spontaneously or after treatment (e.g., radiation therapy).
Melorheostosis **(FIG. 18-49)** [p. 444]	Begins as a region of linear hyperostosis at the proximal end of a tubular bone and progresses distally to involve both sides of the cortex; one or more bones may be involved.
Sclerosing osteomyelitis	Usually related to clinical symptoms; Garré sclerosing osteomyelitis, Brodie's abscess, and chronic osteomyelitis may produce osteosclerotic bone lesions.

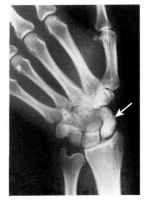

FIG. 18-43 The lunate appears osteosclerotic secondary to avascular necrosis *(arrow).* (Courtesy Joseph W. Howe, Sylmar, CA.)

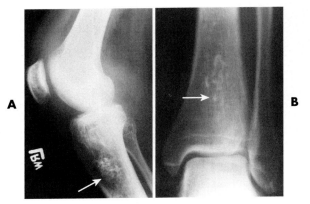

FIG. 18-44 Different patients with stippled calcification within the medullary cavity of, **A,** proximal and, **B,** distal tibia *(arrows).* The appearance is consistent with medullary infarct or enchondroma. (Courtesy Joseph W. Howe, Sylmar, CA.)

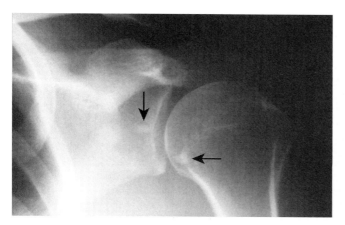

FIG. 18-45 Several bone islands in the scapula and proximal humerus *(arrows).* (Courtesy Arthur W. Holmes, Foley, AL.)

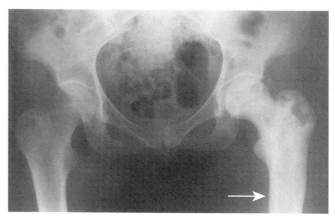

FIG. 18-46 Paget's disease. The proximal left femur appears osteosclerotic and enlarged with thick cortex *(arrow).*

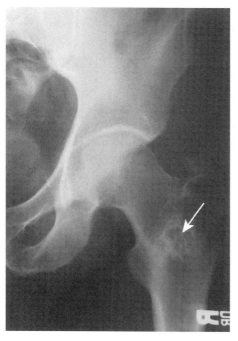

FIG. 18-47 Fibrous dysplasia presenting as a radiodense lesion of the intertrochanteric region of the left proximal femur *(arrow).* (Courtesy Steven P. Brownstein, MD, Springfield, NJ.)

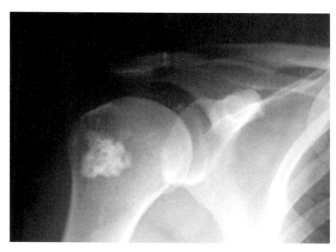

FIG. 18-48 Enchondroma presenting as a sclerotic radiodense shadow of the proximal humerus.

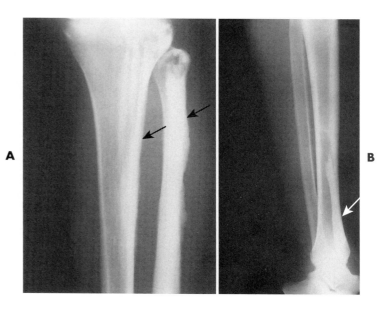

FIG. 18-49 **A** and **B,** Melorheostosis in two patients. In both patients, thick endosteal osteosclerosis is noted *(arrows).* (**A,** Courtesy Joseph W. Howe, Sylmar, CA; **B,** Courtesy Steven P. Brownstein, MD, Springfield, NJ.)

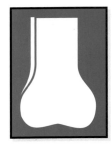

EX7 Periosteal Reactions

Periosteal irritation occurs as a result of a wide variety of etiologies, ranging from fractures to malignant tumors. The radiographic appearance of the periosteum correlates to the aggressiveness and chronicity of the underlying lesion. Aggressive lesions (e.g., malignant bone tumors) disrupt the periosteum before bone deposition and periosteal consolidation can occur, resulting in a disrupted, spiculated, amorphous, or laminated appearance of the periosteum.

A less aggressive, benign appearance of the periosteum occurs when the underlying pathology is slowly progressive (e.g., benign bone tumors) and allows the periosteum to consolidate. Benign periosteal reaction is marked by a thick, wavy, and uniformly dense appearance. Although some benign processes may cause aggressive periosteal changes, aggressive lesions are rarely associated with a benign periosteal appearance. The periosteal reaction may be localized to a bone or appear generalized to a limb or the entire skeleton.

EX7a Localized Periosteal Reactions

DISEASE	COMMENTS
More common *Fracture*	Traumatic or stress fractures; more generalized appearance occurs with battered child syndrome.
Infection **(FIGS. 18-50 and 18-51)**	Solid, thick, laminated periosteal reaction resulting from subperiosteal extension of infection; resulting development of involucrum surrounds central necrotic sequestrum of bone.
Malignant bone tumor **(FIGS. 18-52 and 18-53)**	Solid, laminated, spiculated, or amorphous appearance usually associated with either osteosarcoma or Ewing's sarcoma; multiple sites of involvement suggest leukemia or metastasis from neuroblastoma.
Subperiosteal hemorrhage **(FIG. 18-54)**	Solid, thick, laminated periosteal reaction resulting from subperiosteal hemorrhage; it is related to trauma, hemophilia, or scurvy.
Less common *Arthritis*	Solid or laminated periosteal reaction associated with juvenile rheumatoid arthritis and Reiter's syndrome. Periosteal response may appear localized or generalized.
Benign bone tumor **(FIG. 18-55)**	Solid, thick (e.g., osteoid osteoma) or thin (e.g., aneurysmal bone cyst) periosteal reaction associated with benign bone lesion.
Eosinophilic granuloma **(FIG. 18-56)** [⊃. 935]	Abnormal proliferation of histiocytes marked by osteolytic skull and long bone defects that exhibit a characteristic, beveled edge; solid or laminated periosteal reaction may be localized or generalized.

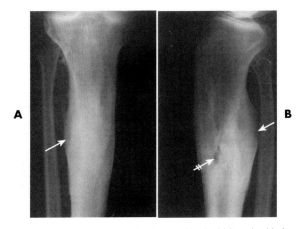

FIG. 18-50 A and **B,** Bone infection resulting in thick periostitis *(arrows)* and central radiolucent nidus *(crossed arrow).* (Courtesy Joseph W. Howe, Sylmar, CA.)

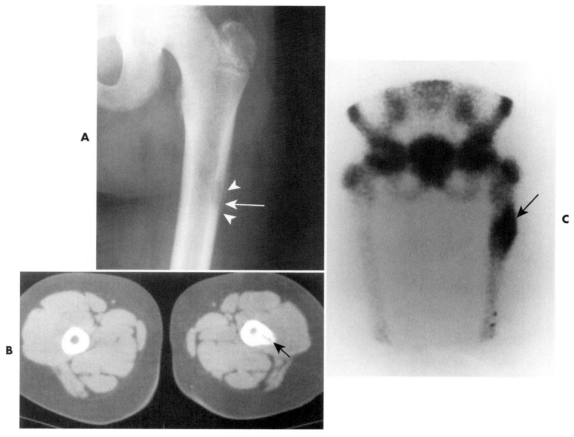

FIG. 18-51 **A,** Infection appearing with a focal region of the osteolysis *(arrow)* with benign periosteal reaction *(arrowheads)*. The infection demonstrates, **B,** a cortical channel *(arrow)* on computed tomography and, **C,** uptake on the radionuclide scan *(arrow)*. (Courtesy Joseph W. Howe, Sylmar, CA.)

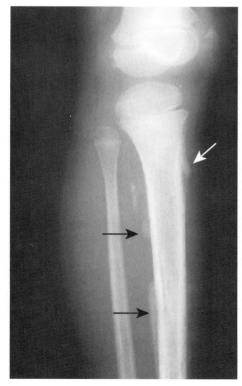

FIG. 18-52 Thick but aggressive periostitis *(arrows)* associated with infection or tumor in the proximal tibia.

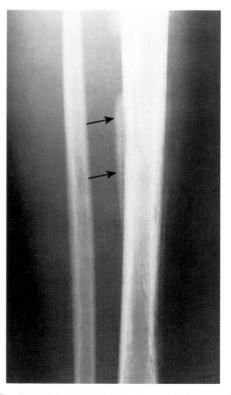

FIG. 18-53 Aggressive periostitis *(arrows)* associated with metastasis from neuroblastoma. (Courtesy Joseph W. Howe, Sylmar, CA.)

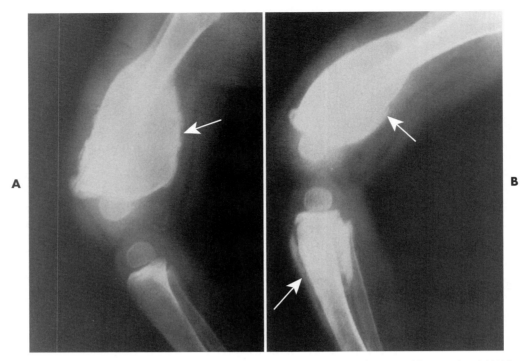

FIG. 18-54 **A** and **B,** Bilateral subperiosteal hemorrhage *(arrows)* in a patient with scurvy. (Courtesy Joseph W. Howe, Sylmar, CA.)

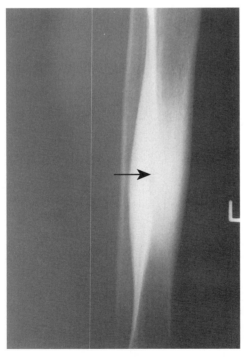

FIG. 18-55 Osteoid osteoma in the tibial diaphysis with surrounding sclerosis. New periosteal bone formation causes the localized increase in bone density. There is a subtle radiolucent nidus in the center of the sclerosis *(arrow).* (Courtesy Joseph W. Howe, Sylmar, CA.)

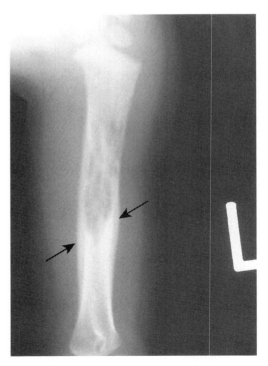

FIG. 18-56 Eosinophilic granuloma appearing as an aggressive diaphyseal lesion of the humerus with solid periosteal reaction along the medial and lateral cortices *(arrows).*

EX7b | Generalized Periosteal Reactions

DISEASE	COMMENTS
More common *Vascular stasis*	Localized or generalized solid periosteal reaction; most often the long bones of the lower extremity are involved; vascular calcification and phleboliths may be present.
Less common *Congenital syphilis* **(FIG. 18-57)** [p. 777]	Acute or chronic infectious disease caused by *Treponema pallidum* via direct contact, usually through sexual intercourse. Congenital syphilis is acquired by the fetus in utero; generalized or localized diaphyseal and metaphyseal solid periosteal reaction, osteolysis, striped metaphyseal bands (radiolucent and dense), and hepatosplenomegaly are characteristic findings of congenital syphilis.
Fluorosis **(FIG. 18-58)**	Chronic fluoride intoxication associated with osteophytosis, vertebral hyperostosis leading to increased radiodensity, and calcification of the paraspinal ligaments; vertebrae have increased radiodensity; fluorosis is marked in the innominates and lumbar spine; solid, symmetric periosteal reaction is most prominent in the tubular bones.
Gaucher's disease [p. 933]	Genetic deficiency of glucocerebroside, presenting with clinical findings of hepatosplenomegaly, osteopenia, osteonecrosis, and focal osteolytic bone changes; biconcave vertebrae is a less common feature of the disease; long tubular bones may exhibit generalized solid periosteal reaction.
Hypertrophic osteoarthropathy **(FIG. 18-59)** [p. 937]	Primary (e.g., pachydermoperiostosis or Touraine-Solente-Golé syndrome) or secondary (e.g., Pierre-Marie-Bamberger syndrome) disorder that presents clinically with digital clubbing, painful and swollen joints, and symmetric undulated periosteal reaction; diaphyses of tubular bones are involved, most commonly the long bones of the arms and legs; the thickness of the periosteal reaction depends on the duration of the disease: the more chronic, the thicker the changes; secondary hypertrophic osteoarthropathy occurs in bronchogenic carcinoma (up to 10%), pulmonary abscess, pulmonary metastasis, Hodgkin disease, cystic fibrosis, heart disease, and occasionally in other acute and chronic disorders; primary hypertrophic osteoarthropathy is less common; onset occurs during adolescence and causes thickened appearance of face and scalp, and may involve the epiphyses.
Hypervitaminosis A [p. 922]	Condition resulting from the ingestion of an excessive amount of vitamin A. Alopecia, pruritus, dermatitis, and a yellow hue to the skin are noted clinically. Radiographically patient may demonstrate a solid periosteal reaction involves that long tubular bones.
Infantile cortical hyperostosis (Caffey's disease) **(FIG. 18-60)** [p. 941]	Rare disease marked by irritability, fever, swelling of the soft tissues, and palpable soft-tissue masses over affected bones. Periosteal new bone formation occurs over many bones, especially the mandible, clavicles, and shafts of long bones (usually ulna). Although the periosteal reaction usually is generalized, a localized appearance can occur. The disease typically is present before 6 months of age, disappearing during childhood.
Sickle-cell disease [p. 771]	Disease characterized by altered shape and plasticity of red blood cells under low oxygen tension, causing vascular occlusion, infarct, and necrosis. Predisposition to *Salmonella osteomyelitis;* generalized or localized, solid, thick, undulated periosteal reaction and osteosclerosis develop in response to diaphyseal bone infarct. Dactylitis (hand-foot syndrome) occurs in children with sickle-cell disease, marked by periosteal reaction and soft-tissue swelling of the short tubular bones, mimicking osteomyelitis.
Thyroid acropachy	Rare complication of hyperparathyroidism therapy; asymmetric, thick, spiculated periosteal reaction occurs in the small tubular bones of the hands and, less commonly, the feet, with a predilection to the radial side. Soft-tissue swelling and digital clubbing occur. The disease can present at any age and has an equal sex incidence. Patients usually are hypothyroid or euthyroid when symptoms arise.
Tuberous sclerosis (Bourneville disease)	Multisystem, neuroectodermal disorder characterized by the triad of seizures, mental retardation, and skin nodules of the face. Cerebral and retinal lesions and intracranial calcifications occur. Multifocal areas of osteosclerosis are best seen in the skull and vertebrae. Cortical thickening manifests in long, tubular bones; irregular solid metacarpal periosteal reaction occurs.

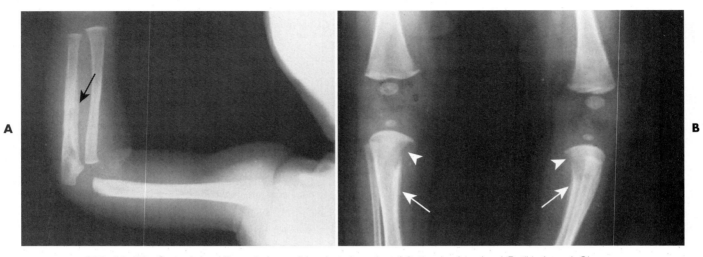

FIG. 18-57   Congenital syphilis producing a solid periosteal reaction of, **A,** the ulna *(arrow)* and, **B,** tibia *(arrows)*. Observe the characteristic bilateral destruction of the medial proximal tibia *(arrowheads)*, known as *Wimberger's sign*. (Courtesy Steven P. Brownstein, MD, Springfield, NJ.)

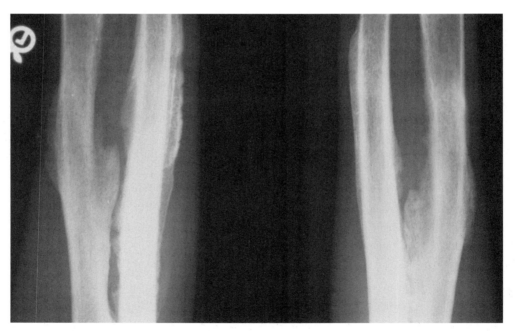

FIG. 18-58   Thick periostitis along the diaphysis of the radius secondary to fluorosis. (Courtesy Steven P. Brownstein, MD, Springfield, NJ.)

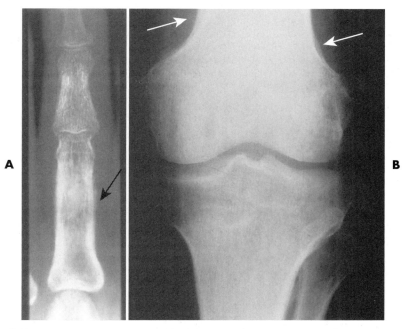

FIG. 18-59 **A,** Hypertrophic osteoarthropathy manifesting in one patient with periostitis of the small bones of the hand *(arrow).* **B,** In a different patient, hypertrophic osteoarthropathy manifests as periostitis, seen as a thick, radiodense band parallel to the cortex in the distal femur *(arrows).* (**A,** Courtesy Joseph W. Howe, Sylmar, CA; **B,** Courtesy Steven P. Brownstein, MD, Springfield, NJ.)

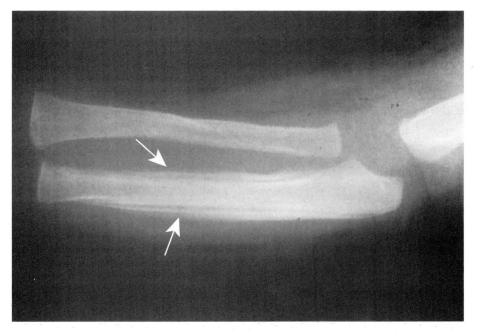

FIG. 18-60 Infantile cortical hyperostosis presenting as thick periostitis along the ulna *(arrows).* (Courtesy William E. Litterer, Elizabeth, NJ.)

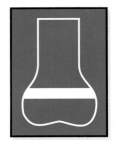

EX8 | Radiodense Metaphyseal Bands

Transverse radiodense metaphyseal bands describe zones of osteosclerosis across the metaphyses of long bones. The appearance may represent a normal variant of growth in children younger than 3 years of age. Other etiologies are described by the mnemonic *Heavy cretins shift scurrilously through rickety systems*. This mnemonic describes the following list of conditions: heavy metal poisoning, cretinism, syphilis, scurvy (congenital), rickets, and systemic illness (e.g., leukemia).

DISEASE	COMMENTS
More common *Normal variant*	Dense metaphyseal band found in long bones of children younger than 3 years of age; alternatively, multiple, fine, dense bands can occur, representing persistence of calcified cartilage (growth arrest lines).
Rickets (healing) **(FIG. 18-61)** [p. 925]	Infantile or juvenile osteomalacia secondary to vitamin D deficiency, characterized clinically by irritability, listlessness, and generalized muscle weakness. An overproduction and deficient calcification of osteoid tissue results in disturbances of bone growth with resulting deformity. Fractures are common; epiphyses may appear indistinct with irregular and wide epiphyseal plates. With successful therapy the zone of provisional calcification is reinstated and is radiographically visible as a dense metaphyseal band.
Scurvy (Barlow's disease) [p. 927]	Defective osteogenesis secondary to abnormal collagen from vitamin C deficiency. Onset occurs between 6 and 14 months of age; irritability, bleeding gums, tendency toward hemorrhage, and tenderness and weakness of lower limbs are clinical manifestations. Epiphyses appear radiolucent with surrounding sclerotic rim (Wimberger's sign or ring epiphyses); dense metaphyseal band represents zone of provisional calcification; this zone may remain after healing.
Trauma	Radiodense metaphyseal bands related to current fracture (particularly stress type), or remodeling residuum of past fracture.
Less common *Congenital syphilis* [p. 777]	Acute or chronic infectious disease caused by *Treponema pallidum*. Direct contact usually occurs via sexual intercourse. Congenital syphilis is acquired by the fetus in utero. Generalized or localized diaphyseal and metaphyseal solid periosteal reaction, osteolysis, striped metaphyseal bands (dense and radiolucent), and hepatosplenomegaly are characteristic findings of congenital syphilis.
Lead poisoning **(FIG. 18-62)** [p. 933]	Inhalation or ingestion of lead, causing wide metaphyses with dense transverse bands in the metaphyses of growing bones. Multiple bands suggest repeat episodes of toxicity; physiologic bands may be differentiated by the involvement of other bones around the joint (e.g., fibula and tibia).
Leukemia [p. 770]	Proliferation of abnormal leukocytes within hemopoietic tissues and other organs. There are several types of the disease, based on cell type and duration from onset to death. Leukemia of bone typically is acute lymphoblastic; skeletal manifestations include diffuse demineralization, osteolytic defects, smooth periosteal reaction, and radiolucent metaphyseal bands that become dense after chemotherapy.
Osteopetrosis (Albers-Schönberg's disease) [p. 451]	Hereditary failure of calcified cartilage resorption that interferes with the development of mature bone. The appearance is marked by sclerotic, fragile bones; vertebrae may appear "doubled" by smaller "endobones" within their bodies; well-defined transverse radiodense bands characteristically are found subjacent to the vertebral endplates and in the metaphyses of long bones.

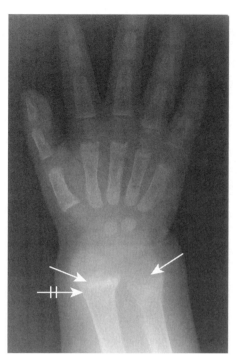

FIG. 18-61 Rickets demonstrating a widened, frayed ("paintbrush") appearance to the metaphyses *(arrows)* with indistinct epiphyses. A radiodense zone stretches across the metaphysis, indicating reconstitution of the provisional zone of calcification and the beginning stages of healing *(crossed arrow)*. (Courtesy Joseph W. Howe, Sylmar, CA.)

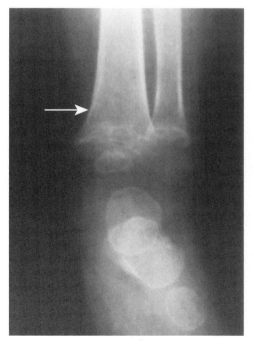

FIG. 18-62 Radiodense metaphyseal bands *(arrow)* secondary to lead intoxication. (Courtesy Joseph W. Howe, Sylmar, CA.)

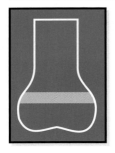

EX9 | Radiolucent Metaphyseal Bands

Radiolucent metaphyseal bands are zones of decreased bone density extending perpendicularly to the long axis of the bone. They are found at the ends of long bones. Their causes are non-specific, representing disorganized bone growth, infection, trauma, and others.

DISEASE	**COMMENTS**
More common *Congenital syphilis* [p. 777]	Acute or chronic infectious disease caused by *Treponema pallidum* via direct contact, usually through sexual intercourse. Congenital syphilis is acquired by the fetus in utero. Generalized or localized diaphyseal and metaphyseal solid periosteal reaction, osteolysis, striped metaphyseal bands (radiolucent and dense), and hepatosplenomegaly are characteristic findings of congenital syphilis.
Leukemia [p. 770]	Proliferation of abnormal leukocytes within hemopoietic tissues and other organs. Several types are noted, based on cell type and duration from onset to death. Leukemia of bone is typically acute lymphoblastic. Skeletal manifestations include diffuse demineralization, osteolytic defects, smooth periosteal reaction, and radiolucent metaphyseal bands, which become dense after chemotherapy.
Metastatic neuroblastoma	Highly malignant tumor of immature nerve cells arising in a retroperitoneal (usually adrenal) or mediastinal location. Tumor usually develops before the age of 5 years; metastases to the liver, lungs, lymph nodes, cranial cavity, and skeleton are common. Skull metastases are characteristic, appearing as wide sutures with bone spicules of the surrounding bone. Extremity involvement resembles leukemia with radiolucent metaphyseal bands.
Normal variant	Radiolucent metaphyseal bands seen as a normal variant in neonates.
Scurvy (Barlow's disease) **(FIG. 18-63)** [p. 927]	Defective osteogenesis secondary to abnormal collagen from vitamin C deficiency, occurring between 6 to 14 months of age. Irritability, bleeding gums, tendency toward hemorrhage, and tenderness and weakness of lower limbs are clinical manifestations. Epiphyses appear radiolucent with surrounding sclerotic rim (Wimberger's sign or ring epiphyses). Radiolucent metaphyseal bands (scorbutic or Trümmerfeld zone) represent disorganized osteoid.
Systemic illness	Serious childhood illnesses may interfere with normal bone development and cause radiolucent metaphyseal bands.
Trauma	Radiolucent metaphyseal band after traumatic fracture or battered child syndrome.

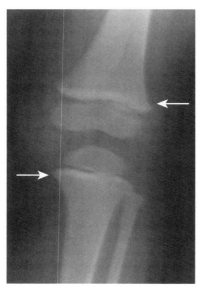

FIG. 18-63   Scurvy presenting with radiolucent metaphyseal bands *(arrows)* of the distal fibula and tibia, representing disorganized osteoid material (Trümmerfeld zone). (Courtesy Joseph W. Howe, Sylmar, CA.)

Suggested Readings

Brant WE, Helms CA: Fundamentals of diagnostic radiology, Baltimore, 1994, Williams & Wilkins.

Burgener FA, Kormano M: Differential diagnosis in conventional radiology, ed 2, New York, 1991, Thieme.

Chapman S, Nakielny R: Aids to radiological differential diagnosis, ed 4, Philadelphia, 2003, WB Saunders.

Dahnert W: Radiology review manual, Baltimore, 1991, Williams & Wilkins.

Eisenberg RL: An atlas of differential diagnosis, ed 2, Gaithersburg, MD, 1992, Aspen.

Forrester DM, Brown JC, Nesson JW: The radiology of joint disease, ed 2, Philadelphia, 1978, WB Saunders.

Ravin CE, Cooper C, Leder RA: Review of radiology, Philadelphia, 1994, WB Saunders.

Reeder MM, Bradley WG: Reeder and Felson's gamuts in radiology, ed 3, New York, 1993, Springer-Verlag.

Weissleder R, Wittenberg J, Harisinghani MG: Primer of diagnostic imaging, ed 3, St Louis, 2003, Mosby.

chapter 19

General Skeletal Patterns

DENNIS M. MARCHIORI

PART TWO Bone, Joints, and Soft Tissues

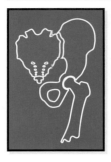

GN I | Acetabular Protrusion

Protrusio acetabuli exists if, in a frontal projection of the pelvis, the dome of the acetabulum extends medially beyond a line segment drawn from the pelvic border of the ilium to the medial border of the body of the ischium (Köhler's line). It occurs most frequently secondary to rheumatoid arthritis and Paget's disease, or as a primary anomaly (Otto pelvis).

DISEASE	COMMENTS
Bone softening **(FIG. 19-1)**	Bone deformity resulting from congenital (osteogenesis imperfecta) or acquired bone-softening diseases (e.g., Paget's disease, rickets, osteomalacia, osteoporosis).
Inflammatory arthritides	Most commonly associated with advanced rheumatoid arthritis of the hip; associated findings include osteopenia, uniform loss of joint space, bilateral distribution, nonproliferative joint margins; less commonly associated with rheumatoid variants (e.g., ankylosing spondylitis, psoriatic arthritis, Reiter's syndrome, inflammatory bowel disease).
Miscellaneous disorders	Bone deformity resulting from posttraumatic remodeling, tumor, and infection.
Normal variant **(FIG. 19-2)**	May include medial protrusion of the femoral head in children.
Osteoarthritis **(FIG. 19-3)** [p. 525]	Usually less advanced degree of protrusion; patients manifest with a unilateral distribution of proliferative joint changes marked by nonuniform reduction of joint space. Osteoarthrosis occurs secondary to trauma, hemophilia, ochronosis, and so on. In distinction to its listing here, osteoarthritis typically reduces the weight-bearing superior joint space, not the medial.
Otto pelvis **(FIG. 19-4)**	Primary protrusio acetabuli; Otto pelvis usually is bilateral and exhibits a female predominance.

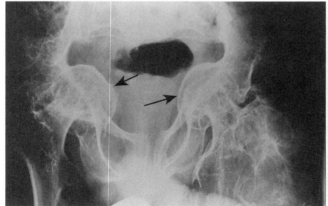
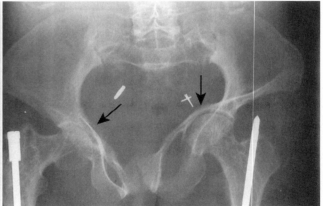

FIG. 19-1   **A** and **B,** Two cases of acetabular protrusion *(arrows)* developing in patients with osteogenesis imperfecta. (Courtesy Joseph W. Howe, Sylmar, CA.)

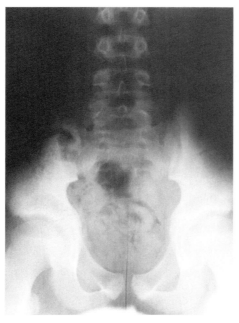

FIG. 19-2 Bilateral protrusio acetabuli presenting as a normal developmental variant. (Courtesy Lawrence J. Shell, Sandwich, MA.)

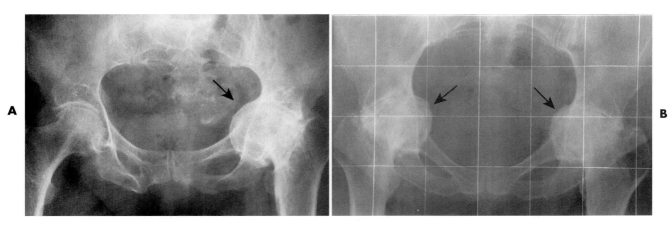

FIG. 19-3 **A,** Unilateral and, **B,** bilateral protrusio acetabuli secondary to degeneration *(arrows)*.

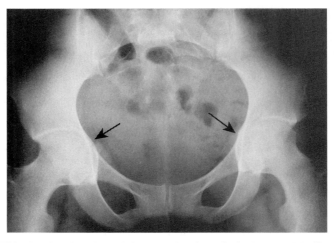

FIG. 19-4 Bilateral acetabular protrusion *(arrows)* of unknown origin (Otto pelvis).

GN2 | Arthritides

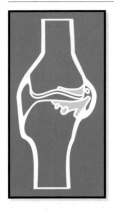

Many disorders result in joint pathology. Arthritides are broadly divided into two groups: those affecting one joint and those affecting multiple joints (polyarthritis). Polyarthritis can be further divided into inflammatory, degenerative, and metabolic subcategories. Knowledge of the overall prevalence, skeletal target locations, and demography of those affected helps to narrow the long list of etiologies.

Types of arthritis occurring more commonly among men include ankylosing spondylitis, gout, hemophilia, ochronosis, and Reiter's syndrome. Common monoarticular arthritides include secondary osteoarthritis (e.g., trauma, avascular necrosis, mechanical stress), gout, and infection. Suppurative arthropathy and rheumatoid arthritis are commonly associated with surrounding osteoporosis. Behçet syndrome, dermatomyositis, Jaccoud's arthritis, and Sjögren syndrome characteristically produce transient arthritis, which remisses without residual bone deformity. Joint effusions are pronounced with gout, infection, hemorrhage, and rheumatoid arthritis.

DISEASE	COMMENTS
Inflammatory (seropositive) *Jaccoud's arthritis* [p. 491]	Uncommon, nondestructive arthritis marked by reversible joint derangements, soft-tissue swelling, and pain, classically after an episode of rheumatic fever; Jaccoud's arthritis resembles rheumatoid arthritis and affects the joints of the hands and feet.
Rheumatoid arthritis, adult **(FIGS. 19-5 and 19-6)** [p. 472]	Systemic connective tissue disorder that targets synovial tissues; juxtaarticular osteoporosis, soft-tissue nodules, symmetric reduction of joint space, marginal erosions, subchondral cysts, symmetric distribution, and rarely joint ankylosis are characteristic; most commonly the hands and feet are involved, particularly the intercarpal, metacarpophalangeal, and proximal interphalangeal joints, and counterparts in the foot; rheumatoid arthritis occurs most commonly in middle-aged women.
Rheumatoid arthritis, juvenile **(FIG. 19-7)** [p. 472]	Chronic arthritis beginning in childhood (before 16 years of age), manifesting as one of several clinical types; monoarticular distribution is more common than occurs in adult rheumatoid arthritis; target areas include cervical spine, hands, feet, and knees; joint fusion, periostitis, and growth abnormalities are characteristic.
Scleroderma (progressive systemic sclerosis) [p. 487]	Disease of small vessels and organ fibrosis; symptoms include atrophy and systemic dystrophic calcifications of the soft tissues of the hands and feet with resorption of distal phalanges; limited soft-tissue swelling, juxtaarticular osteoporosis, marginal erosions, and other similar findings to rheumatoid arthritis occurring in the hands.
Systemic lupus erythematosus **(FIG. 19-8)** [p. 486]	Systemic inflammatory connective tissue disease marked by fever, weakness, erythematous skin lesions on the face, and arthritis most visible in the hands as reversible subluxations and dislocations of the digits, predominantly the metacarpophalangeal joints.
Inflammatory (seronegative) *Ankylosing spondylitis* [p. 739]	Seronegative spondyloarthropathy characterized by arthritis targeted to the sacroiliac joints and spine; bilateral, symmetric, thin intervertebral connections known as *syndesmophytes* are a prominent feature, representing ossification of the outermost lamellae of the annulus fibrosis; collectively multiple levels produce a "bamboo spine" appearance; in addition, the anterior body margins appear straight or square.
Psoriatic arthritis **(FIGS. 19-9 and 19-10)** [p. 505]	Arthritis occurs in fewer than 7% of patients with psoriasis; patients experience symptoms in the carpal, interphalangeal, and less commonly the sacroiliac joints; the digits are marked by nail pitting, swelling of the soft tissues, and erosions of the distal tufts, relating a tapered appearance of the distal phalanges.
Reiter's syndrome **(FIG. 19-11)** [p. 510]	Describes triad of urethritis, conjunctivitis, and polyarthritis; men, especially those between the ages of 20 and 40 years, contract this condition much more frequently than women; arthritis is targeted to the sacroiliac joints and lower extremities, especially the foot; erosions at the calcaneal insertions of the plantar and Achilles tendons are characteristic.
Metabolic/Endocrine *Acromegaly* [p. 907]	Excess levels of growth hormone result from a pituitary eosinophilic adenoma that is overproducing somatotropin; this condition is marked by progressive enlargement of the hands, feet, head, jaw, and abdominal organs, in addition to enlarged vertebrae with posterior scalloping and new bone growth along the anterior body margins; arthritis is targeted to the metacarpophalangeal and hip joints.

DISEASE	COMMENTS
Chondrocalcinosis **(FIG. 19-12)** [p. 518]	Radiographically evident cartilage calcification relating to calcium pyrophosphate dihydrate crystal or other crystal deposition disease; chondrocalcinosis is associated with arthritis targeted to the wrist, knees, elbows, hips, and shoulders.
Gout [p. 514]	Primarily a disorder of purine metabolism with crystal deposits causing synovial pannus, arthropathy, and large, well-defined, bony marginal erosions; infrequently patients demonstrate sacroiliitis and systemic dystrophic calcifications; typical sites include first metatarsophalangeal joint, insertion of the Achilles tendon, and olecranon bursa.
Hemochromatosis **(FIG. 19-13)** [p. 521]	Disorder of iron metabolism resulting from excessive absorption of ingested or injected iron; disorder is accompanied by cirrhosis of the liver, diabetes, bronze skin pigmentation, generalized osteoporosis, and arthropathy secondary to iron deposits in synovium; the arthritis is targeted to the metacarpophalangeal and interphalangeal joints of the hands; women are protected by menstruation.
Multicentric reticulohistiocytosis **(FIG. 19-14)**	Rare disorder marked by cutaneous and joint deposits of histiocytes containing glycolipids; the interphalangeal joints of the hands and feet manifest well-defined marginal erosions; shortening of the fingers often results.
Ochronosis	Inherited disorder of excessive homogentisic acid production and subsequent accumulation within connective tissues; the spine is affected by multiple levels of intervertebral disc calcification and massive osteophytosis and ankylosis, especially in elderly people; osteoporosis occurs in adjacent vertebrae; advanced degenerative joint disease may develop in the large proximal joints of the extremities (e.g., hip, knee, and shoulder).
Degenerative *Erosive osteoarthritis* [p. 469]	Seronegative inflammatory variant of osteoarthritis particularly common in 40- to 50-year-old women; proliferative joint changes, central joint erosions, and painful, swollen joints occur; arthritis is targeted to the distal interphalangeal joints of the hands.
Osteoarthritis [p. 469]	Common, noninflammatory, degenerative joint disease with clinical presentation of pain, stiffness, and crepitus; characteristic radiographic features include bilateral asymmetric distribution, nonuniform reduction of joint space, sclerosis of subarticular bone, marginal osteophytosis, joint malalignment, subchondral cysts, and others; primary osteoarthritis is seen with increasing age and mostly affects weight-bearing joints (e.g., knees, hips, spine) and hands (e.g., distal interphalangeal, first tarsophalangeal, and first carpometacarpal joints); degeneration also occurs secondary to trauma or osteonecrosis.
Miscellaneous *Hemophilia* [p. 768]	Inherited X-linked defect of blood coagulation, marked by a permanent tendency toward hemorrhages; hemarthrosis is associated with red, swollen joints, precocious degenerative arthritis, and an enlargement of the epiphyses; knees, ankles, and elbows are affected most commonly; expansile bone lesions (hemophilic pseudotumors) develop rarely; arthritis is targeted to the knees, elbows, and ankles.
Infection **(FIGS. 19-15 through 19-18)** [p. 785]	Suppurative or tuberculosis infections marked by soft-tissue swelling, juxtaarticular osteoporosis, joint space narrowing, and bone destruction; radiographic findings follow clinical presentation of pain and soft-tissue swelling by 8 to 10 days; infection may affect any joint, most commonly the hip, knee, or spine.
Neuropathic (Charcot's) joints [p. 584]	Destructive arthropathy secondary to altered joint sensory innervation, resulting in either unchecked repetitive injury ensuing from absence of pain or loss of trophic influences of innervations with local hyperemia and bone resorption; atrophic and hypertrophic varieties exist; hypertrophic changes include premature and advanced degeneration, marked by dislocation, destruction, intraarticular loose bodies (debris), and disorganization; this type of arthropathy is common in the knee, hip, ankle, and lumbar spine; etiologies include diabetes, syphilis, syringomyelia, and alcoholism.
Pigmented villonodular synovitis [p. 801]	Chronic condition marked by diffuse hyperplastic outgrowths of a joint's synovial membrane; osteolytic appearance results from pressure erosion of adjoining bone; wide age range is possible, although pigmented villonodular synovitis usually occurs before 40 years of age; no juxtaarticular osteoporosis or loss of joint space exists; the most common locations are the knee, hip, ankle, elbow, and shoulder.
Sarcoidosis **(FIG. 19-19)** [p. 1218]	Systemic granulomatous disease most pronounced in the lungs; less commonly the disease involves arthritis of the hand with coarsened trabeculae and well-defined osteolytic lesions.
Others	Transient and episodic arthritis associated with Sjögren syndrome, dermatomyositis, relapsing polychondritis, Behçet syndrome, and so on; patterns of involvement vary.

PART TWO Bone, Joints, and Soft Tissues

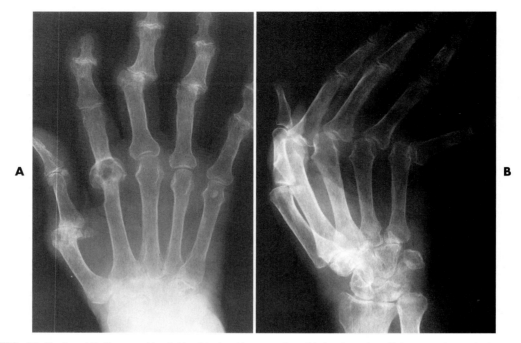

FIG. 19-5 A and **B,** Rheumatoid arthritis of the hand in two patients. Notice the reduced joint spaces, juxtaarticular osteoporosis, and misalignment of the involved joints. (**A,** Courtesy Joseph W. Howe, Sylmar, CA.)

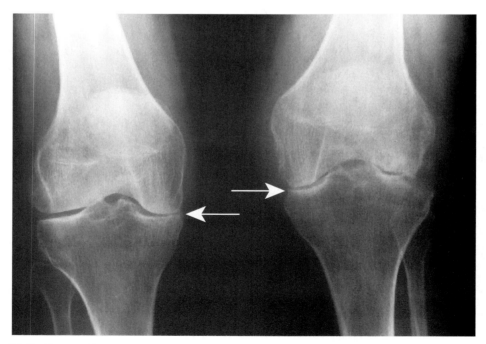

FIG. 19-6   Rheumatoid arthritis of the knees marked by nonproliferative loss of joint space *(arrows)*. (Courtesy Steven P. Brownstein, MD, Springfield, NJ.)

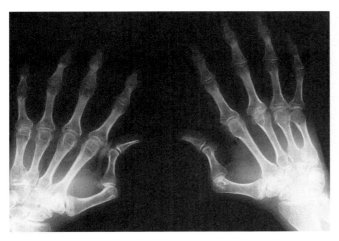

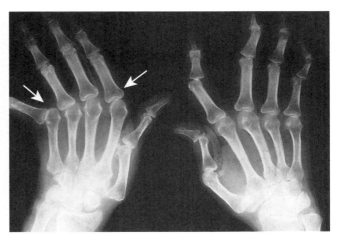

FIG. 19-7 Juvenile rheumatoid arthritis manifesting in the hands with osteoporosis, underdevelopment of the small tubular bones, and arthritis targeted to the wrist. (Courtesy Jack C. Avalos, Davenport, IA.)

FIG. 19-8 Systemic lupus erythematosus of the hands, marked by multiple bilateral, reversible subluxations of the hands (arrows). (Courtesy Steven P. Brownstein, MD, Springfield, NJ.)

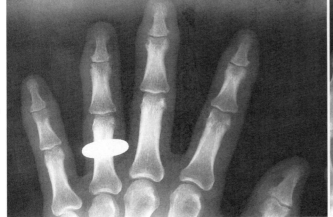

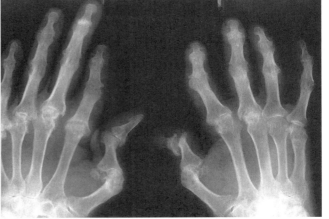

FIG. 19-9 **A,** Early and, **B,** late psoriatic arthropathy of the hands. The changes are marked by lack of osteoporosis, soft-tissue swelling, central articular erosions, proliferative marginal changes, and a pattern of distribution that is more prominent across all joints in the same digit (ray pattern) than in the same joint across different digits. **A,** A wedding band is noted incidentally on the fourth digit. (Courtesy Steven P. Brownstein, MD, Springfield, NJ.)

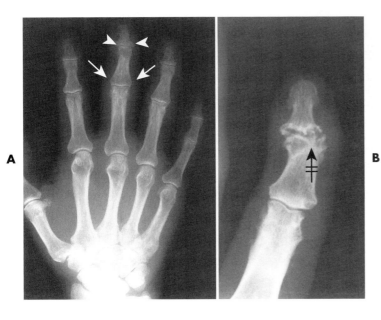

FIG. 19-10 **A** and **B,** Psoriatic arthropathy of the hands in different patients who exhibit soft-tissue hypertrophy (arrows), central erosions (crossed arrow), and proliferative changes on the joint margins (arrowheads). (Courtesy Joseph W. Howe, Sylmar, CA.)

PART TWO Bone, Joints, and Soft Tissues

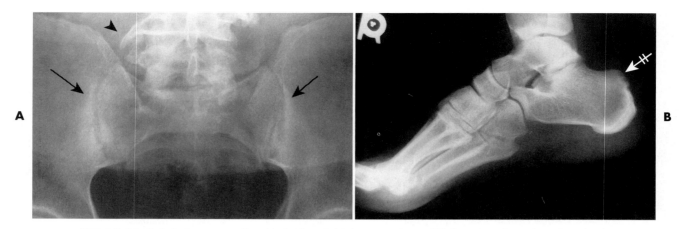

FIG. 19-11   Reiter's disease, presenting with, **A,** bilateral, slightly asymmetric sacroiliitis *(arrows)*, syndesmophytes *(arrowhead)*, and, **B,** erosions at the insertion of the calcaneal (Achilles) tendon *(crossed arrow)* in a different patient. (**A,** Courtesy Joseph W. Howe, Sylmar, CA; **B,** Courtesy Arthur W. Holmes, Foley, AL.)

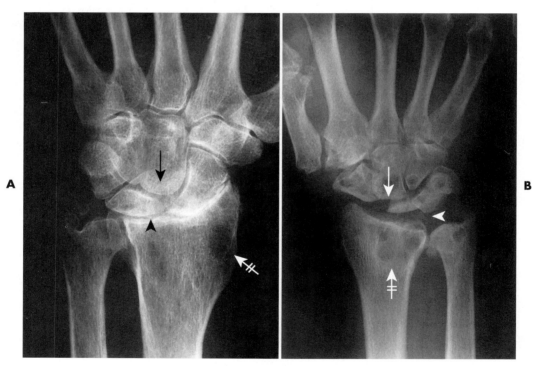

FIG. 19-12   Calcium pyrophosphate dihydrate deposition disease of the wrist in two different patients. **A** and **B,** Both radiographs exhibit scapholunate advanced collapse deformity of the capitate toward the radius *(arrows)*, degeneration subchondral cysts *(crossed arrows)*, and chondrocalcinosis *(arrowheads)*. **B,** In addition, this radiograph exhibits a radiodense appearance of the lunate consistent with lunate avascular necrosis (Keinböck disease). (**B,** Courtesy Joseph W. Howe, Sylmar, CA.)

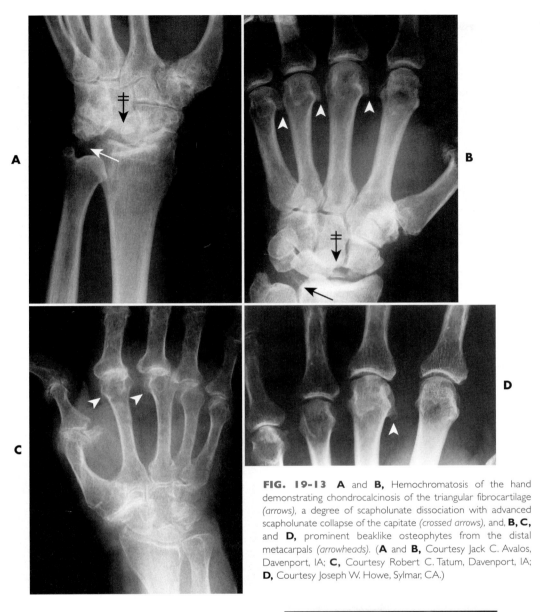

FIG. 19-13 **A** and **B,** Hemochromatosis of the hand demonstrating chondrocalcinosis of the triangular fibrocartilage *(arrows),* a degree of scapholunate dissociation with advanced scapholunate collapse of the capitate *(crossed arrows),* and, **B, C,** and **D,** prominent beaklike osteophytes from the distal metacarpals *(arrowheads).* (**A** and **B,** Courtesy Jack C. Avalos, Davenport, IA; **C,** Courtesy Robert C. Tatum, Davenport, IA; **D,** Courtesy Joseph W. Howe, Sylmar, CA.)

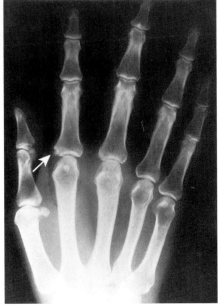

FIG. 19-14   Multicentric reticulohistiocytosis appearing with a well-defined marginal erosion of the proximal phalanges of the second digit (arrow). (Courtesy Joseph W. Howe, Sylmar, CA.)

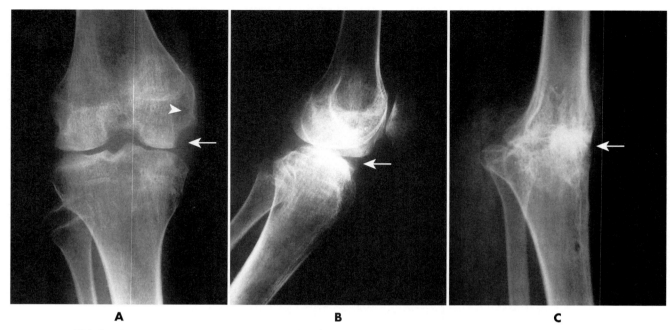

FIG. 19-15 Tuberculosis of the knee. **A** and **B,** Initial plain films demonstrate a reduced joint space *(arrows)* and a focus of osteolysis *(arrowhead).* **C,** The lateral knee projection taken 14 months later demonstrates ankylosis *(arrow).* (Courtesy Steven P. Brownstein, MD, Springfield, NJ.)

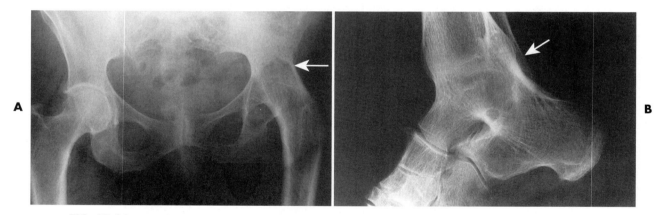

FIG. 19-16 Healed infections resulting in, **A,** fusion of the left hip joint *(arrow)* and, **B,** tibiotalar joint *(arrow).* (Courtesy Joseph W. Howe, Sylmar, CA.)

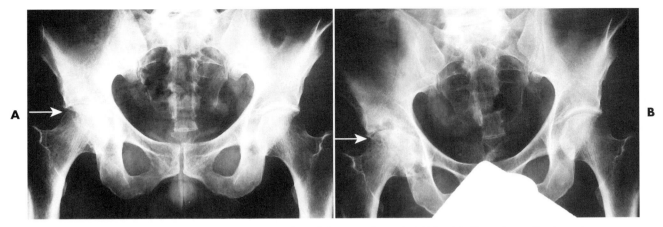

FIG. 19-17 Infection of the right hip marked by loss of joint space, **A,** on the initial and, **B,** 5 months postfilm *(arrows)*.

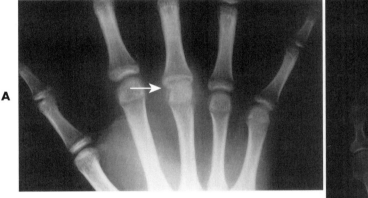

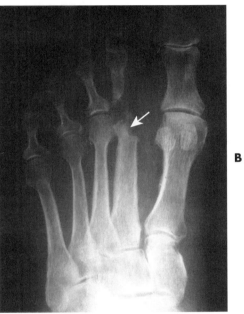

FIG. 19-18 Joint infections, **A,** of the third metacarpophalangeal joint and, **B,** second metatarsophalangeal joint. All are marked by decreased joint spaces *(arrows)* and bone destruction often involving both sides of the joint. (**A,** Courtesy Joseph W. Howe, Sylmar, CA.)

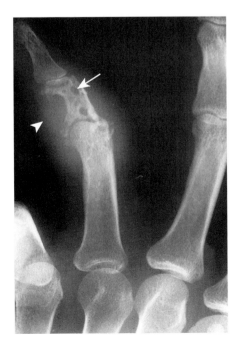

FIG. 19-19 Sarcoidosis causing multiple well-defined osteolytic defects in the middle phalanx *(arrow)* with soft-tissue swelling *(arrowhead)*. (Courtesy Steven P. Brownstein, MD, Springfield, NJ.)

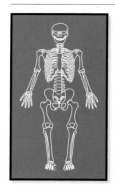

GN3 | Dwarfism

Dwarfism is the condition of being undersized. This condition may result from a variety of disorders affecting the growth and development of the tissues. Skeletal dysplasias result in dwarfism because of abnormal tissue development. Skeletal dysplasias are classified according to whether they predominantly affect the proximal or distal long bones of the limb. Rhizomelic (*rhiza-,* meaning "root," and *-melia,* meaning "limb") dysplasias affect the femur and humerus more predominantly than the tibia or radius. Mesomelic (*meso-,* meaning "middle") dysplasia describes shortening of the distal long bones (tibia, ulna, and radius), or middle of the limb in relation to the proximal limb (humerus or femur). Acromelic (*acro-,* meaning "extreme") dysplasia is a growth disturbance involving the distal portions of the limbs (hands and feet). Micromelic dysplasia involves both the proximal and distal portions of the extremity. Short spine dysplasias cause dwarfism without involving the limbs.

DISEASE	COMMENTS
More common	
Achondroplasia **(FIG. 19-20)** [p. 421]	Rhizomelic dysplasia resulting from congenital defect of enchondral bone formation; characteristics include rounded lumbar "bullet-nosed" vertebrae, lumbar kyphosis, posterior scalloping of the vertebrae, increased intervertebral disc height, flattened vertebral bodies, and narrowed spinal canal; the pelvis may appear hypoplastic; milder forms of the disease may occur.
Less common *Asphyxiating thoracic dysplasia (Jeune syndrome)* **(FIG. 19-21)**	Mild micromelic dysplasia marked by small thorax; small, flared iliac bones; and shortening of the humerus, femur (rhizomelia), and distal phalanges (acromelia).
Chondrodysplasia punctata	Autosomal dominant (nonrhizomelic) and recessive (rhizomelic) dysplasia; the nonrhizomelic form (Conradi-Hünermann's disease) demonstrates tracheal underdevelopment and mild stippled epiphyses; the rarer rhizomelic form is characterized by marked limb shortening, severe punctate calcifications (stippled) epiphyses, metaphyseal splaying, and congenital cataracts.
Cretinism [p. 915]	Hypothyroid dwarfism from delayed appearance and maturation of skeletal growth centers; stunted mental development occurs; disease appears during the first years of life and results from thymic agenesis or inadequate maternal intake of iodine during pregnancy; wormian bones and poorly developed sinuses are characteristic; sail-like or tonguelike vertebrae and kyphosis at the thoracolumbar junction are common; changes may regress in adulthood.
Diastrophic dysplasia [p. 429]	Short spine dysplasia characterized by scoliosis, hypoplastic first metacarpal "hitchhiker thumb," abnormal interphalangeal joints, cleft palate, and clubbed feet.
Dyschondrosteosis (Leri-Weill syndrome) **(FIG. 19-22)**	Mesomelic dysplasia with long-bone shortening of the upper limbs, producing bilateral Madelung's deformities, which are marked by short radii, dorsal ulnar subluxations, and carpal wedging between the radius and ulna; elbow and distal radius dislocations result.
Mucopolysaccharidosis [p. 578]	Group of lysosomal storage diseases marked by a common disorder in mucopolysaccharide metabolism, evidenced by various mucopolysaccharides excreted in the urine; these substances collect in connective tissue, resulting in bone, cartilage, and connective tissue defects; platyspondyly with dwarfism, kyphosis, and alterations in the appearance of the vertebrae are characteristic; mucopolysaccharidosis I (Hurler's syndrome) is associated with oval, posteriorly scalloped, anterior-inferiorly beaked vertebrae; mucopolysaccharidosis IV (Morquio's syndrome) is associated with flattened, anterior-centrally beaked vertebrae.
Osteogenesis imperfecta [p. 451]	Connective tissue disorder of immature collagen, marked by micromelic dwarfism, which is characterized by bone fragility and deformity, abnormal teeth, ligament laxity, and otosclerosis; it occurs with variable severity.
Spondyloepiphyseal dysplasia	Short spine dysplasia presenting in dominant and recessive forms, marked by both platyspondyly and short trunk dwarfism.
Thanatophoric dysplasia	Severe micromelic dysplasia marked by large head with prominent frontal bone, platyspondyly, short ribs, and curved long bones with bulbous ends ("telephone receiver" long bones).
Turner's syndrome [p. 459]	Chromosomal anomaly (XO syndrome) marked by absent secondary sex characteristics and presenting clinically with dwarfism, webbed neck, mental deficiency, valgus of elbows, pigeon chest, widely spaced nipples, infantile sexual development, and amenorrhea.

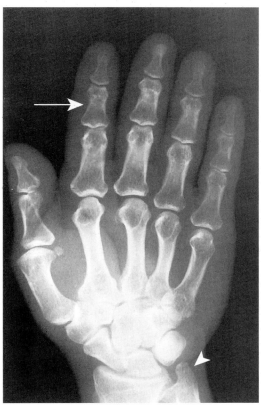

FIG. 19-20 Achondroplasia presenting as short tubular bones *(arrow)* with elongation of the ulnar styloid *(arrowhead)*. (Courtesy Joseph W. Howe, Sylmar, CA.)

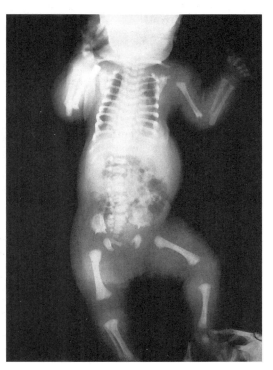

FIG. 19-21 Dwarfism related to asphyxiating thoracic dysplasia (Jeune syndrome). (Courtesy Steven P. Brownstein, MD, Springfield, NJ.)

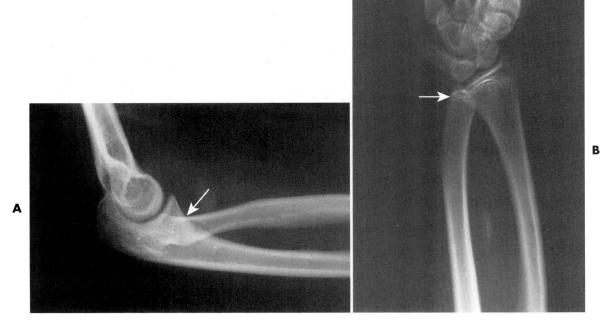

FIG. 19-22 **A** and **B,** Dyschondrosteosis exhibiting a short, bowed radius, short ulna, and dislocations *(arrows)*. (Courtesy Joseph W. Howe, Sylmar, CA.)

GN4 | Generalized Osteoporosis

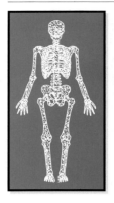

Osteoporosis is a disease of bones marked by decreased bone mass and density. The remaining bone is normal in calcification and histology. The resulting skeletal weakness increases the risk of fracture, particularly of vertebrae, wrists, and hips. Laboratory values are normal. Osteoporosis may occur as a primary, age-related phenomenon or appear secondary to an underlying condition. The term *osteopenia* describes decreased mineralization of bone, without implying causality.

Several noninvasive methods are available to evaluate bone density. These vary widely in cost, availability, and radiation dose. Dual-energy x-ray absorptiometry (DEXA) offers the greatest reliability, safety, precision, and convenience. Standard radiographs of the spine are the most widely available measure of osteoporosis; however, they are insensitive to early changes.

DISEASE	COMMENTS
More common *Drug-induced (iatrogenic)*	Large doses of steroids, heparin, vitamin A, and various chemotherapies.
Endocrine disorders **(FIG. 19-23)**	Adrenocortical abnormality (e.g., Cushing's syndrome, Addison's disease), hypogonadism (e.g., menopause, oophorectomy, prepubertal castration), thyroid abnormalities (e.g., hyperthyroidism, hypothyroidism, cretinism), pancreatic abnormality (e.g., cystic fibrosis), and pituitary abnormality (e.g., acromegaly, hypopituitarism).
Nutritional disorders	Protein deficiency (e.g., malnutrition, nephrosis, diabetes mellitus), vitamin C deficiency (e.g., scurvy), and intestinal malabsorption (e.g., sprue, scleroderma, Crohn's disease).
Senile (primary) osteoporosis **(FIG. 19-24)** [p. 916]	Common age-related decrease in bone quantity; trabecular bone is resorbed more rapidly than cortical bone; the spine, proximal femur, and distal radius are the most advanced sites; complicating fractures are common causes of morbidity; women and whites are most commonly affected; rate of bone loss may be modified by therapy.
Less common *Anemia* **(FIG. 19-25)**	Sickle-cell anemia, thalassemia, spherocytosis, severe iron deficiency, all causing thin cortices secondary to bone marrow hyperplasia.
Collagen disease	Osteoporosis possibly resulting from lupus erythematosus, scleroderma, dermatomyositis, rheumatoid arthritis, and ankylosing spondylitis.
Congenital syndrome **(FIG. 19-26)**	Homocystinuria (see later entry), mucopolysaccharidosis, osteogenesis imperfecta, pseudohypoparathyroidism, pseudopseudohypoparathyroidism, Ehlers-Danlos syndrome, and others.
Hemochromatosis [p. 521]	Disorder of iron metabolism resulting from excessive absorption of ingested or injected iron; characteristics include cirrhosis of the liver, diabetes, bronze skin pigmentation, arthropathy secondary to iron deposits in synovium, and generalized osteoporosis; women are protected by menstruation.
Hemophilia [p. 768]	Inherited X-linked defect of blood coagulation marked by a permanent tendency toward hemorrhages; hemarthrosis is associated with red, swollen joints, precocious degeneration, and an enlargement of the epiphyses; knees, ankles, and elbows are affected most commonly; rarely, expansile bone lesions (hemophilic pseudotumors) develop; advanced osteoporosis occurs.
Homocystinuria **(FIG. 19-27)** [p. 438]	Hereditary error of amino acid (methionine) metabolism leading to homocystine excretion in urine. The condition results in defects of the collagen structure and clinical features of ligamentous laxity, mental retardation, tendency to form blood clots, downward dislocation of lens, sparse blond hair, thromboembolic episodes, and osteoporosis.
Idiopathic juvenile osteoporosis	Rare, usually transient, onset of osteoporosis and pain in children.
Mastocytosis (systemic) [p. 941]	Abnormal proliferation of mast cells in multiple organ systems, usually seen in adults; skeletal involvement includes scattered, fairly well-defined sclerotic foci occasionally with diffuse involvement; regions of bone rarefaction typically are present also; diffuse osteopenia similar to osteoporosis is possible.
Neoplastic disorders	Common manifestation of multiple myeloma, metastatic bone disease, and acute leukemia secondary to neoplastic bone marrow infiltrates.
Neuromuscular diseases *and dystrophies* **(FIG. 19-28)**	Reduced muscular tone and lack of weight-bearing posture associated with cerebral palsy, spinal cord disorder, muscular dystrophy, and immobilization.

DISEASE	COMMENTS
Ochronosis	Inherited disorder of excessive homogentisic acid production and subsequent accumulation within connective tissues; the spine is affected by multiple levels of intervertebral disc calcification and massive osteophytosis and ankylosis, especially in the elderly; osteoporosis occurs in adjacent vertebrae; advanced degenerative joint disease may develop in the large proximal joints of the extremities (e.g., hip, knee, and shoulder).
Renal disease	Nephrosis, tubular acidosis, oxalosis, renal osteodystrophy.

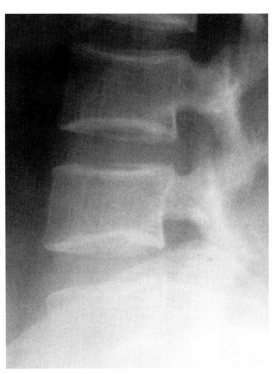

FIG. 19-23 Osteoporosis secondary to Cushing's disease.

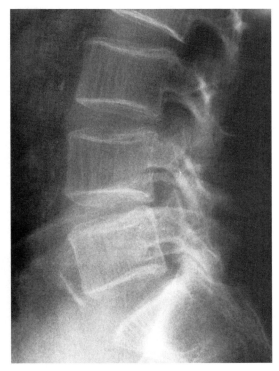

FIG. 19-24 Senile osteoporosis with prominent vertical trabecular pattern. (Courtesy Steven P. Brownstein, MD, Springfield, NJ.)

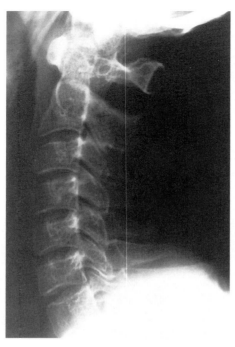

FIG. 19-25 Lateral cervical spine projection demonstrating the coarse trabecular and osteopenic pattern consistent with thalassemia (Cooley anemia). (Courtesy Joseph W. Howe, Sylmar, CA.)

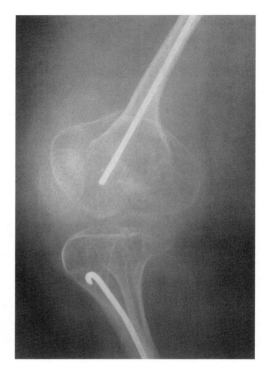

FIG. 19-26 Advanced osteopenia with bowing deformity and gracile cortices secondary to osteogenesis imperfecta. (Courtesy Joseph W. Howe, Sylmar, CA.)

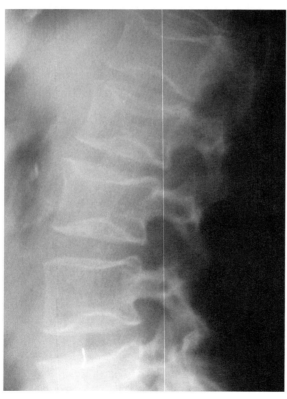

FIG. 19-27 Hcmocystinuria presenting with generalized osteoporosis of the lumbar spine with secondary concave endplate deformity.

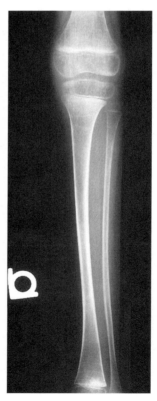

FIG. 19-28 Cerebral palsy patient with osteoporosis of the lower extremities marked by thin cortex and decreased radiopacity.

GN5 | Generalized Osteosclerosis

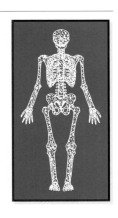

Generalized osteosclerosis describes skeletal-wide changes of increased bone density. Generalized osteosclerosis incorporates the causes of other patterns of increased bone density of the spine and extremities. Disorders that more characteristically cause focal osteosclerotic lesions include bone islands, bone infarcts, avascular necrosis, enchondroma (in a long bone), fibrous dysplasia, healed fractures, healing nonossifying fibroma, osteitis condensans ilia or pubis, osteomas, osteomyelitis, osteosarcomas, and Paget's disease.

DISEASE	COMMENTS
More common *Osteoblastic metastasis* **(FIGS. 19-29 to 19-31)** [p. 889]	Especially from breast and prostate primary lesions; typically patients are older than 40 years of age, often with a history of known malignancy; generalized osteosclerosis is less common than a presentation of multiple focal areas of osteosclerosis.
Paget's disease **(FIG. 19-32)** [p. 946]	Chronic skeletal disease of aberrant bone remodeling; one or more bones are affected; characteristics include bone enlargement, softening, and rarely sarcomatous changes; the lumbar spine is one of the most common areas of involvement; the enlarged and thickened vertebral cortices appear as radiodense bands around the perimeter of the vertebra (known as "picture frame"); less commonly the disease appears predominantly as a solitary lytic or sclerotic lesion of the vertebral body; generalized osteosclerosis may be a feature of widespread skeletal involvement.
Renal osteodystrophy [p. 910]	Secondary to renal glomerular disease; vertebral changes occur with horizontal sclerotic bands ("rugger jersey" spine) and less commonly a biconcave appearance.
Less common *Fibrous dysplasia (polyostotic)* [p. 846]	Disturbance of bone maintenance, in which bone is replaced by abnormal proliferation of fibrous tissue; the disturbance may involve one (monostotic) or multiple (polyostotic) bones; most common locations are femur, ribs, tibia, craniofacial bones, and pelvis; lesions should not be painful, unless dysplasia is widespread with bowing deformity and pathologic fractures; lesions of the medullary cavity may have radiolucent, "ground glass," or radiodense appearance.
Fluorosis **(FIG. 19-33)**	Chronic fluoride intoxication associated with enthesopathies, osteophytosis, vertebral hyperostosis with calcification of the paraspinal ligaments; solid, symmetric periosteal reaction is most prominent in the tubular bones; generalized osteosclerosis is more prominent in the axial skeleton.
Heavy metal intoxication **(FIG. 19-34)** [p. 933]	Osteosclerosis related to lead, phosphorus, bismuth, or cadmium poisoning; similar findings may occur after thorotrast injections (thorium dioxide in dextran).
Hyperphosphatasia **(FIG. 19-35)** [p. 946]	Also known as *juvenile Paget's disease;* this rare disorder of infants and children results from chronically elevated alkaline phosphatase levels; characteristics are generalized cortical thickening, bone deformity, short stature, and increased bone density.
Mastocytosis (systemic) [p. 941]	Abnormal proliferation of mast cells in multiple organ systems; primarily adults are affected; skeletal involvement includes scattered, fairly well-defined sclerotic foci occasionally with diffuse involvement; regions of bone rarefaction typically also are present.
Myelofibrosis	Extensive and progressive bone marrow fibrosis of unknown etiology occurring in hematopoietic bones (vertebrae, pelvis, ribs, and long bones); involved areas appear first osteoporotic, later becoming patchy, then homogeneously dense.
Osteopetrosis (Albers-Schönberg's disease) **(FIG. 19-36)** [p. 451]	Hereditary failure of calcified cartilage resorption, which interferes with the development of mature bone; the appearance is marked by sclerotic, fragile bones; vertebrae may appear "doubled" by smaller "endobones" within their bodies; well-defined, transverse radiodense bands characteristically are found subjacent to the endplates.
Sickle-cell disease [p. 771]	Occurs almost exclusively in blacks; characterized by altered shape and plasticity of red blood cells under low oxygen tension, causing vascular occlusion, infarct, and necrosis; patient is predisposed to *Salmonella* osteomyelitis; generalized or localized, solid, thick, undulated periosteal reaction and osteosclerosis develop in response to diaphyseal bone infarct; dactylitis (hand-foot syndrome) occurs in children with sickle-cell disease, marked by periosteal reaction and soft-tissue swelling of the short tubular bones, mimicking osteomyelitis.
Pyknodysostosis **(FIG. 19-37)** [p. 456]	Hereditary sclerosing dysplasia of bone marked by short stature, dense bones (often with transverse fractures), hypoplastic angle of the mandible, wormian bones, delayed closure of the fontanelles, and hypoplasia of the terminal phalanges.

DISEASE	COMMENTS
Tuberous sclerosis (Bourneville disease) **(FIG. 19-38)**	Multisystem, neuroectodermal disorder characterized by the triad of seizures, mental retardation, and skin nodules of the face; cerebral and retinal lesions result, as well as intracranial calcifications, multifocal areas of osteosclerosis (best seen in the skull and vertebrae), cortical thickening in long, tubular bones, and irregular, solid metacarpal periosteal reaction.

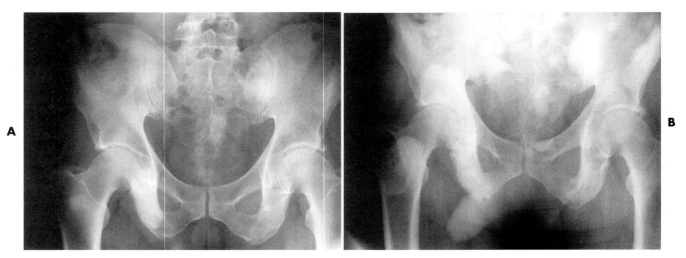

FIG. 19-29 **A,** Osteoblastic metastasis most predominantly involving the right ischium and intertrochanteric region of the femur. **B,** Increased metastasis occurs in all regions after approximately 1 year. (Courtesy Joseph W. Howe, Sylmar, CA.)

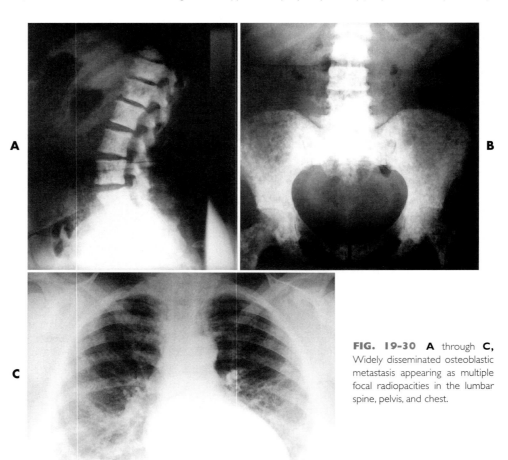

FIG. 19-30 A through **C,** Widely disseminated osteoblastic metastasis appearing as multiple focal radiopacities in the lumbar spine, pelvis, and chest.

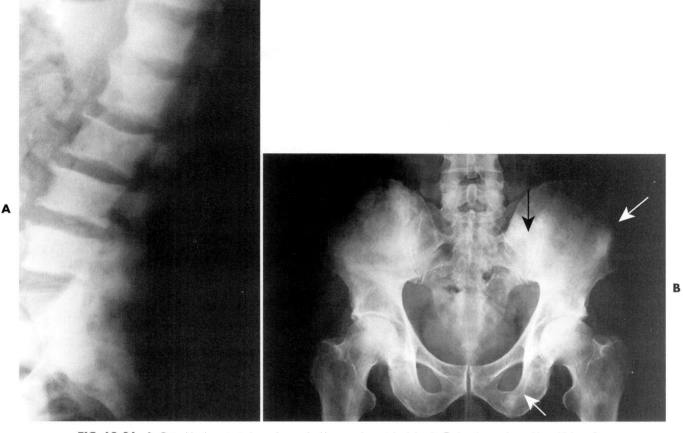

FIG. 19-31   A, Osteoblastic metastasis causing marked increase in vertebral density. **B,** Another patient with multiple radiodense regions of the pelvis secondary to osteoblastic metastasis *(arrows)*. (Courtesy Ian D. McLean, Davenport, IA.)

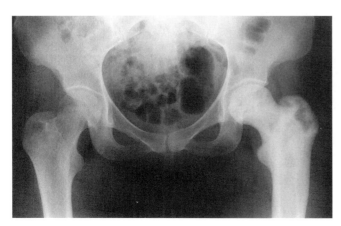

FIG. 19-32   The left femur is larger and more radiodense than the right femur secondary to Paget's disease. (Courtesy Joseph W. Howe, Sylmar, CA.)

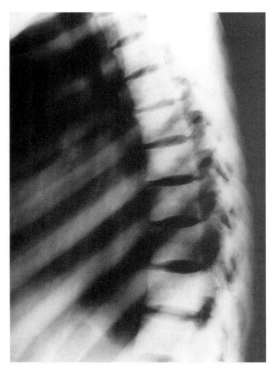

FIG. 19-33   Increased radiodense appearance of the thoracic vertebrae and ribs resulting from fluorosis. (Courtesy Steven P. Brownstein, MD, Springfield, NJ.)

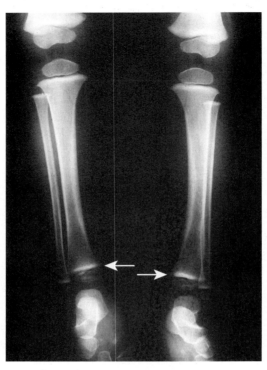

FIG. 19-34 Radiodense appearance of the tibia and fibula with metaphyseal band *(arrows)* secondary to lead intoxication. (Courtesy Steven P. Brownstein, MD, Springfield, NJ.)

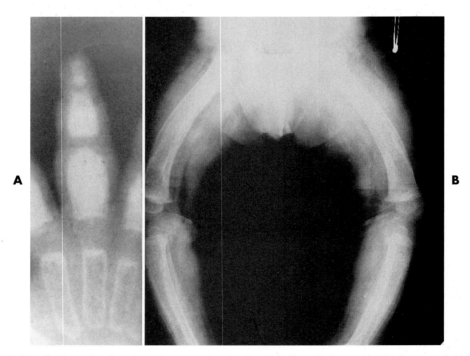

FIG. 19-35 **A,** Hyperphosphatasia causing osteosclerosis of a child's finger. **B,** A second child demonstrating increased radiodensity and thickened cortices in the lower extremities. (**A,** Courtesy Joseph W. Howe, Sylmar, CA; **B,** Courtesy Steven P. Brownstein, MD, Springfield, NJ.)

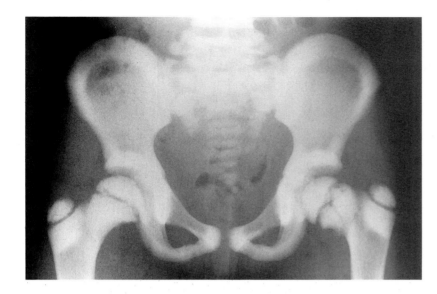

FIG. 19-36 Osteopetrosis appearing as generalized osteosclerosis of the pelvis, femora, and lumbar spine. (Courtesy Joseph W. Howe, Sylmar, CA.)

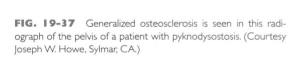

FIG. 19-37 Generalized osteosclerosis is seen in this radiograph of the pelvis of a patient with pyknodysostosis. (Courtesy Joseph W. Howe, Sylmar, CA.)

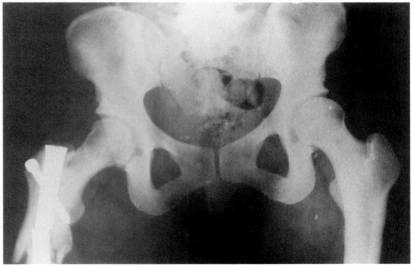

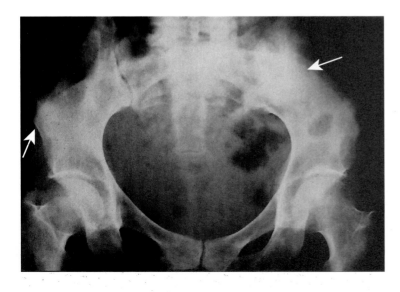

FIG. 19-38 Radiograph of a patient with tuberous sclerosis, which demonstrates multiple regions of increased bone density scattered throughout the pelvis (arrows).

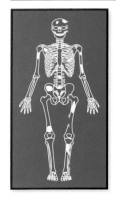

GN6 | Polyostotic Bone Lesions

Imaging studies that indicate the presence of multiple lesions substantially narrow the differential list of conditions causing a bone lesion. The skeletal location and patient age further narrow the list. Bone islands, fibrocytic lesions (e.g., fibrous dysplasia, fibrous cortical defect/nonossifying fibroma), and metastases represent some of the more common conditions listed in the following table.

DISEASE	COMMENTS
More common *Fibrous cortical defect/nonossifying fibroma* [p. 847]	Very common, benign, asymptomatic cystic bone lesions seen in patients younger than 30 years of age; a thin sclerotic border without matrix calcification marks this defect; the lower extremities, particularly around the knee, are affected commonly; multiple defects/fibromas are possible.
Fibrous dysplasia (polyostotic) [p. 846]	Disturbance of bone maintenance in which bone is replaced by abnormal proliferation of fibrous tissue; this condition may involve one (monostotic) or multiple (polyostotic) bones; the matrix often has a characteristic "ground glass" radiodensity; lesions may be surrounded by a thick rind of bone sclerosis; most common locations are femur, ribs, tibia, craniofacial bones, and pelvis; lesion should not be painful.
Fractures	Traumatic or stress fractures occurring at all ages; often seen in infants and children who are victims of battered child syndrome.
Hemangiomas [p. 870]	Common congenital proliferation of vascular endothelium leading to a benign osteolytic appearance; capillary (usually in the spine) and cavernous (usually in the calvarium) types occur; multiple lesions may be present.
Hyperparathyroidism [p. 910]	Overproduction of parathyroid glands resulting from primary or secondary causes; the disease is marked by osteopenia, osteosclerosis, bone resorption, and soft-tissue and vascular calcification; vertebrae have characteristic homogeneous radiodense bands traversing horizontally at each end of the vertebrae ("rugger jersey" spine); subchondral bone resorption occurs, particularly at the radial aspects of the middle phalanges of the second and third digits; one or more osteolytic or sclerotic cystic bone lesions (brown tumors) may be present.
Infection **(FIG. 19-39)**	May occur at practically any location during any age; if found in a subarticular location, the joint often is involved with effusion; soft-tissue mass and central bone sequestrum frequently are present; appearance varies from cystic to sclerotic; single or multiple lesions may occur.
Metastases **(FIGS. 19-40 and 19-41)** [p. 1393]	Common to the spine, rarely involve the skeleton distal to the elbows or knees (acral metastasis); metastasis typically appears as a polyostotic, moth-eaten pattern of osteolytic bone destruction with poorly defined zones of transition; it alternatively presents as predominantly mixed or purely blastic patterns; periosteal reaction and soft-tissue masses typically are small or absent; this condition usually occurs in patients over the age of 40 years; neuroblastoma, retinoblastoma, rhabdomyosarcoma, and Ewing's tumor are common causes of metastasis among infants and children.
Multiple myeloma **(FIG. 19-42)** [p. 819]	Malignant proliferation of plasma cells occurring predominantly in the red marrow of various bones; the skull, vertebral bodies, ribs, and proximal humerus and femurs are involved most commonly; single or multiple osteolytic lesions simulate metastatic disease, without tendency to involve vertebral arch, as is demonstrated by metastasis; osteopenia and solitary or multiple-level vertebral collapse simulate osteoporosis; multiple myeloma rarely occurs before 30 years of age.
Osteonecrosis [p. 755]	Multiple areas of bone and marrow necrosis related to trauma, sickle-cell disease, alcoholism, corticosteroids, and others; this disease appears as one or more regions of altered density and structure of bone.
Paget's disease [p. 946]	Chronic skeletal disease of aberrant bone remodeling, involving one or more bones; characteristics include bone enlargement, softening, and rarely sarcomatous changes; the lumbar spine is one of the most common areas of involvement; the enlarged and thickened vertebral cortices appear as radiodense bands around the perimeter of the vertebra (similar to a picture frame); less commonly it appears as a solitary lytic or sclerotic lesion of the vertebral body; generalized osteosclerosis may be a feature of widespread skeletal involvement.

DISEASE	COMMENTS
Subchondral cysts	Related to arthritic or synovial disorder (osteoarthritis, gout, calcium pyrophosphate deposition disease, rheumatoid arthritis, hemophilia, intraosseous ganglion, amyloidosis, and avascular necrosis); this solitary or multiple, well-defined cyst is located in the epiphysis subjacent to the articular cortex; usually occurs in adults.
Less common *Anemias* **(FIG. 19-43)**	Multiple osseous lesions associated with hemolytic anemias, including sickle-cell disease, thalassemia, and hereditary spherocytosis.
Enchondromatosis (Ollier's disease) **(FIG. 19-44)** [p. 828]	Childhood presentation of multiple benign cystic cartilage lesions, most often in the small bones of the hands and feet; stippled matrix calcification is typical; 30% of cases exhibit malignant transformation; Ollier's disease with multiple soft-tissue hemangiomas is termed *Maffucci's syndrome* and may have an even higher malignant transformation rate.
Eosinophilic granuloma [p. 935]	Proliferation of eosinophils seen most commonly in children and young adults; spine involvement occurs in less than 10%; this condition may appear with advanced body collapse ("vertebra plana") possibly at multiple levels; long bone involvement typically occurs in the diaphysis; patients are almost exclusively younger than 30 years of age; solitary or multiple lesions may occur.
Hemophilia [p. 768]	Inherited X-linked defect of blood coagulation, marked by a permanent tendency toward hemorrhages; hemarthrosis is associated with red, swollen joints, precocious degeneration, and an enlargement of the epiphyses; knees, ankles, and elbows are affected most commonly; rarely, expansile bone lesions (hemophilic pseudotumors) develop; advanced osteoporosis occurs.
Hereditary multiple exostosis **(FIG. 19-45)** [p. 834]	Describes the inherited condition of multiple osteochondromas involving growth deformity; the hips, knees, and forearms most frequently are involved; patients typically are younger than 20 years of age at time of diagnosis.
Hydatid (Echinococcus) *disease* [p. 1310]	Cysts that may be formed in bone (usually formed in the liver) by the larval stage of *Echinococcus;* cysts appear as slow-growing, destructive lesions surrounded by sclerotic borders; multiple lesions may appear; this occurs in endemic geographic areas.
Infantile cortical hyperostosis (Caffey's disease) [p. 941]	Rare disease marked by irritability, fever, swelling of the soft tissues, and palpable soft-tissue masses over affected bones; periosteal new bone formation occurs over many bones, especially the mandible and clavicles and the shafts of long bones (usually the ulna); although the periosteal reaction usually is generalized, a localized appearance can occur; this condition usually is present before 6 months of age and disappears during childhood; periosteal reaction also may be localized.
Leukemia [p. 770]	Proliferation of abnormal leukocytes within hemopoietic tissues and other organs; variety of types is based on cell type and duration from onset to death; leukemia of bone typically is acute lymphoblastic; skeletal manifestations include diffuse demineralization, osteolytic defects, smooth periosteal reaction, and radiolucent metaphyseal bands, which become dense after chemotherapy; leukemia occurs in infants and children.
Lymphoma [p. 1203]	Primary and secondary (systemic non–Hodgkin lymphoma and Hodgkin disease) lymphoma of bone, appearing as permeative radiolucent lesions of the lower extremities, pelvis, and spine; lymphoma occurs over wide range of ages.
Mastocytosis (systemic) [p. 941]	Abnormal proliferation of mast cells in multiple organ systems; most patients are adult age; skeletal involvement includes scattered, fairly well-defined sclerotic foci occasionally with diffuse involvement; regions of bone rarefaction typically also are present.
Neurofibromatosis (von Recklinghausen's disease) [p. 942]	Congenital disturbance of mesodermal and neuroectodermal tissue development, appearing clinically with cutaneous markings, bone deformity, and neurofibromas; spinal changes include posterior vertebral scalloping, enlarged intervertebral foramina, kyphoscoliosis, and anteriorly wedged vertebrae.
Syphilis [p. 777]	Acute or chronic infectious disease caused by *Treponema pallidum.* Direct contact transmits this disease, usually through sexual intercourse; congenital syphilis is acquired by the fetus in utero. Generalized or localized diaphyseal and metaphyseal solid periosteal reaction, osteolysis, striped metaphyseal bands (lucent and dense), and hepatosplenomegaly are characteristic findings of congenital syphilis. Acquired syphilis is marked by ill-defined osteolytic lesions in the skull, spine, and long bones secondary to gumma formation; both congenital and acquired types are marked by multiple foci of osteomyelitis.

PART TWO Bone, Joints, and Soft Tissues

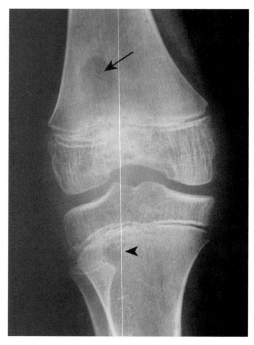

FIG. 19-39　Brodie's abscess infection noted in the distal femur *(arrow)* with a second lesion noted in the proximal tibia *(arrowhead).* (Courtesy Steven P. Brownstein, MD, Springfield, NJ.)

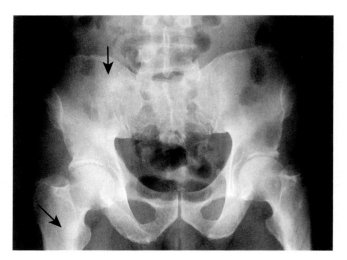

FIG. 19-40　Multiple radiodense regions of the femoral, lumbar vertebrae, and pelvis secondary to osteoblastic metastasis *(arrows).* (Courtesy Steven P. Brownstein, MD, Springfield, NJ.)

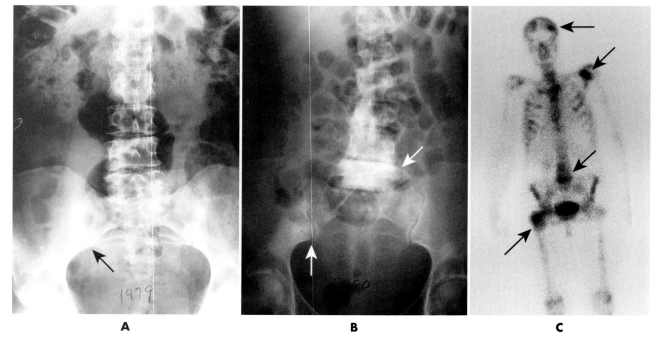

A　　　　　　　　　　**B**　　　　　　　　　　**C**

FIG. 19-41　**A,** Initial radiograph demonstrating slight osteosclerosis of the medial right ilium *(arrow).* **B,** One year later L5 vertebral osteosclerosis also is noted *(arrows).* **C,** Radionuclide bone scan performed around the time of the second radiograph reveals further metastatic involvement of the skull, ribs, and extremities *(arrows).* (Courtesy Steven P. Brownstein, MD, Springfield, NJ.)

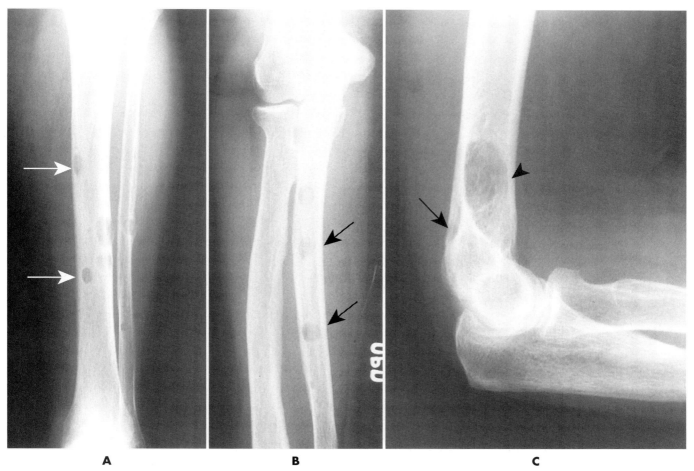

A   **B**   **C**

FIG. 19-42   Multiple myeloma involving, **A,** the tibia and fibula; **B,** ulna, and, **C,** humerus with osteolytic lesions of consistent size and appearance *(arrows).* The larger and more central radiolucent defect of the distal humerus (**C,** *arrowhead*) represents the pseudocyst appearance of the epicondyle and does not represent an osteolytic bone lesion. (Courtesy Joseph W. Howe, Sylmar, CA.)

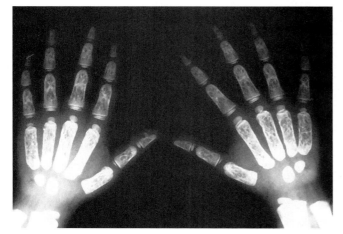

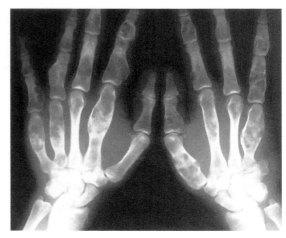

FIG. 19-43   Bilateral thin cortices and prominent coarsened trabecular pattern, characteristic of thalassemia. (Courtesy Steven P. Brownstein, MD, Springfield, NJ.)

FIG. 19-44   Bilateral cystic bone lesions, characteristic of multiple enchondromatosis or Ollier's disease.

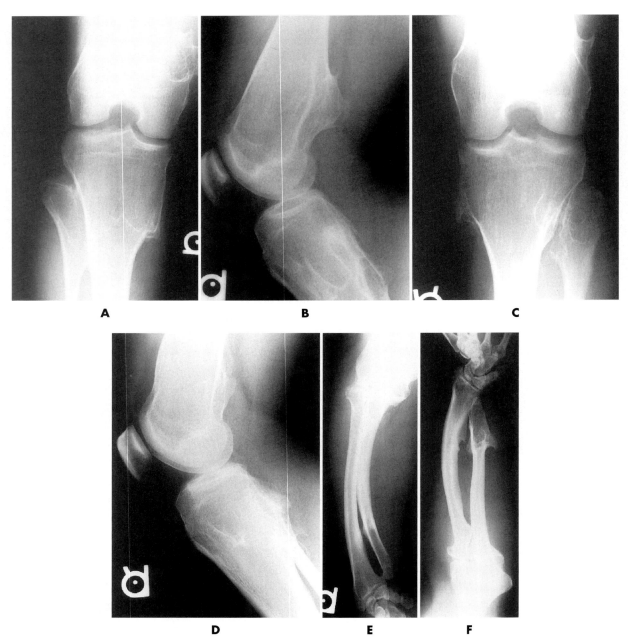

FIG. 19-45 **A** through **D,** Multiple osteochondromas leading to bone deformity about the knees bilaterally. **E** and **F,** This patient also exhibits the characteristic "bayonet" deformity of the forearms.

GN7 | Soft-Tissue Calcification and Ossification

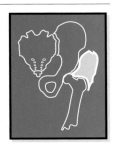

Soft-tissue calcification describes a process in which tissue becomes hardened by deposition of calcium salts, which normally occurs only in bone and teeth. Soft-tissue calcification can be classified as dystrophic, metastatic, or idiopathic.

Dystrophic calcification occurs in devitalized tissue as a result of tissue damage, degeneration, or necrosis. Associated conditions include Ehlers-Danlos syndrome, arteriosclerosis obliterans, and crystal deposition disease. Some authors describe age-related dystrophic calcification as physiologic calcification (e.g., costal cartilages).

Metastatic calcification occurs as a result of abnormal serum calcium or phosphorus levels in trophic tissues. Conditions associated with metastatic calcifications include hyperparathyroidism, selected neoplasms, milk-alkali syndrome, hypervitaminosis D, and tumoral calcinosis.

Idiopathic calcinosis is unrelated to degeneration or serum calcium and phosphorus levels. Associated conditions include calcinosis universalis and calcinosis circumscripta.

Calcification is termed *ossification* if the calcified structure appears as a bone with cortex and possibly trabeculae. Nearly all disorders that cause calcification may ossify secondarily.

Vascular wall calcification is a common finding in the large arteries of the abdomen and pelvis. Etiologies of vascular calcifications include arteriosclerosis, diabetes, hemangiomas, hyperparathyroidism, Mönckeberg medial wall sclerosis, and thrombus.

Phleboliths represent dystrophic calcification of thrombi within a vein ($\approx$0.5 cm in diameter). Phleboliths are common, usually homogeneously dense, and particularly common in the perirectal veins of the lower pelvis.

Lymph node calcifications, usually resulting from tuberculosis or histoplasmosis infection, appear as thin, curvilinear ("eggshell") segments or mottled dense nodules in characteristic locations (e.g., cervical chain, axillary).

GN7a | Soft-Tissue Calcification

DISEASE	COMMENTS
Dystrophic or metastatic	
More common	
Calcific bursitis and tendinitis **(FIGS. 19-46 and 19-47)**	Dystrophic calcification after degenerative, inflammatory, tumorous, or necrotic processes in tendons and bursae, often resulting in pain and limitation of joint motion; this condition is common in the supraspinatus tendon, and subacromial and trochanteric bursa.
Chondrocalcinosis **(FIG. 19-48)** [p. 518]	Radiographically evident cartilage calcification relating to calcium pyrophosphate dihydrate or other crystal deposition disease; it may lead to symptoms of joint pain and advanced arthropathy.
Fracture	Localized dystrophic soft-tissue calcifications occurring in damaged tissues and regions of hemorrhage.
Gout **(FIG. 19-49)** [p. 514]	Disorder of purine metabolism with crystal deposits causing synovial pannus, arthropathy, and large, well-defined bony marginal erosions; infrequent sacroiliitis and systemic dystrophic calcifications occur; classic sites include the first metatarsophalangeal joint, insertion of the Achilles tendon, and the olecranon bursa.

DISEASE	COMMENTS
Hyperparathyroidism [p. 910]	Overproduction of parathyroid glands resulting from primary or secondary causes; the disease is marked by osteopenia, osteosclerosis, bone resorption, and widespread metastatic soft-tissue and vascular calcification; vertebrae appear osteopenic with characteristic homogeneous, radiodense bands traversing horizontally at each end of the vertebrae ("rugger jersey" spine); bone resorption is located predominantly at the radial aspect of the middle phalanges of the second and third digits.
Infections	Soft-tissue and lymph node calcifications along the spine or roots of the limbs secondary to infections of tuberculosis, histoplasmosis, and so on.
Injection granuloma	Localized postinflammatory dystrophic focus of soft-tissue calcification after injection (e.g., bismuth, antibiotics, insulin, quinine) or inoculation (e.g., *Bacillus* Calmette-Guerin vaccine); this disease is most commonly seen in the buttocks.
Scleroderma (progressive systemic sclerosis) **(FIGS. 19-50 and 19-51)** [p. 487]	Disease of small vessels and organ fibrosis; atrophy and calcifications of the soft tissues of the hands and feet occur with resorption of distal phalanges.
Less common *Dermatomyositis* **(FIG. 19-52)** [p. 490]	Progressive disorder of muscular weakness and atrophy, occurring in children and adults; characteristics include linear and confluent systemic dystrophic soft-tissue calcifications.
Hypervitaminosis D [p. 922]	Condition resulting from the ingestion of an excessive amount of vitamin D; symptoms include nausea, anorexia, drowsiness, headaches, polyuria, and polydipsia; bone deossification (parathormone-like effects) and extensive periarticular metastatic soft-tissue calcification are characteristic.
Idiopathic (nondystrophic, nonmetastatic etiologies) *Parasites*	Systemic dystrophic calcifications of various configurations occurring secondary to parasitic infections (e.g., cysticercosis, guinea worm, trichinosis).
Soft-tissue tumors **(FIG. 19-53)**	Benign (e.g., leiomyoma, lipoma, fibroma, hemangioma) and malignant (e.g., leiomyosarcoma, liposarcoma, fibrosarcoma) calcified soft-tissue masses; synovial sarcomas (synoviomas) are aggressive malignant tumors of the bursa, joint capsule, or tendon.
Tumoral calcinosis **(FIGS. 19-54 and 19-55)**	Large, progressively enlarging, nodular, juxtaarticular soft-tissue calcifications of unknown etiology common in the hips, shoulders, wrists, and ankles; primarily otherwise healthy young individuals 5 to 25 years old are affected; disease is more common among blacks; this condition tends to recur after surgical removal.

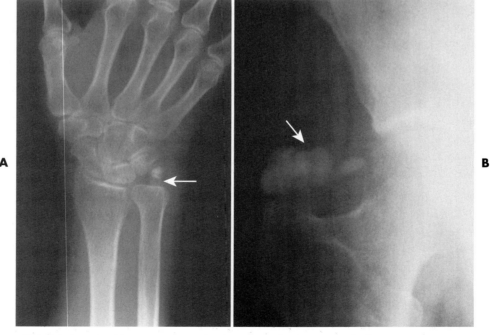

FIG. 19-46   Calcification (*arrows*) in, **A,** the triangular fibrocartilage and, **B,** supratrochanteric bursae.

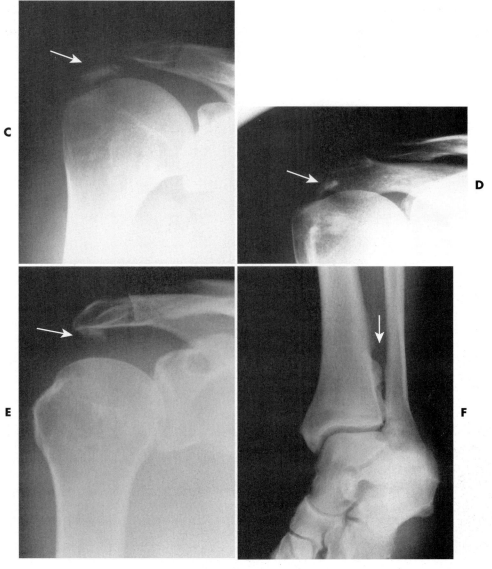

FIG. 19-46 cont'd Calcification *(arrows)* in, **C** through **E,** the supraspinatus tendons and, **F,** interosseous ligament. The calcification represents postinflammatory dystrophic hydroxyapatite deposition disease, and signifies degeneration. (**A,** Courtesy Joseph W. Howe, Sylmar, CA.)

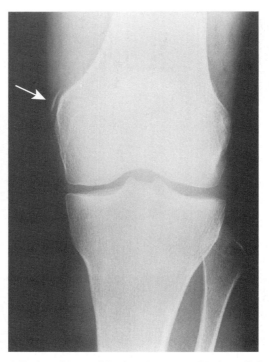

FIG. 19-47   Dystrophic calcification of the medial collateral ligament of the knee (Pellegrini-Stieda disease) *(arrow)*.

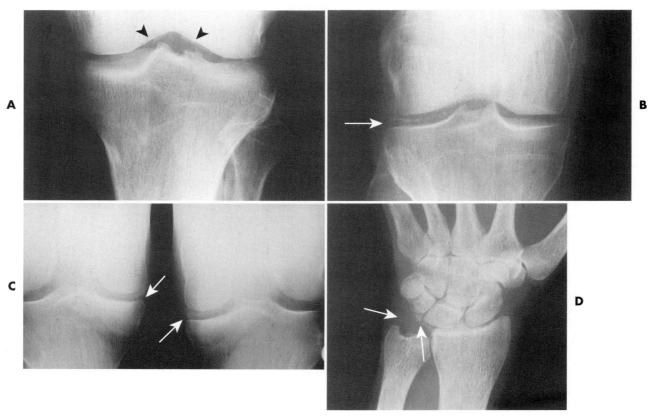

FIG. 19-48   Chondrocalcinosis resulting in calcium pyrophosphate dihydrate deposition disease. **A** through **C,** Disorder presents commonly in the knee paralleling the articular surface in the articular cartilage *(arrowheads)* or more centrally located in the menisci *(arrows).* **D,** Triangular fibrocartilage of the wrist is involved *(arrows).* (**A,** Courtesy Joseph W. Howe, Sylmar, CA.)

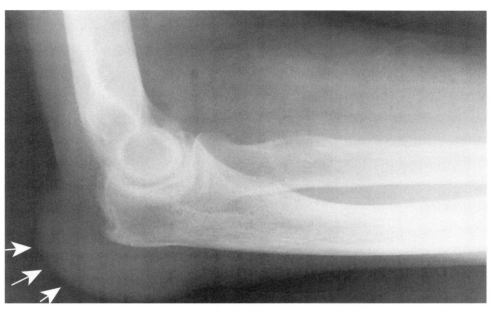

FIG. 19-49 Gout presenting with soft-tissue masses about the elbow *(arrows)*. (Courtesy Joseph W. Howe, Sylmar, CA.)

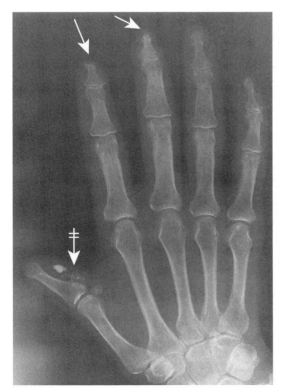

FIG. 19-50 Scleroderma with a characteristic presentation of acroosteolysis *(arrows)* and soft-tissue calcifications *(crossed arrow)*. (Courtesy Joseph W. Howe, Sylmar, CA.)

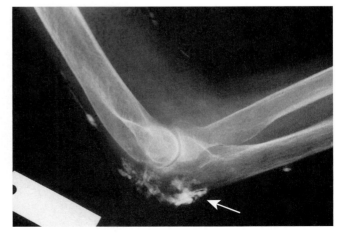

FIG. 19-51 Scleroderma with soft-tissue calcification around the elbow *(arrow)*. (Courtesy Steven P. Brownstein, MD, Springfield, NJ.)

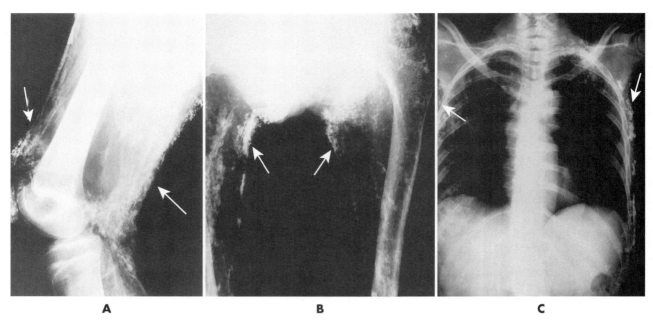

FIG. 19-52 Dermatomyositis of, **A,** the knee; **B,** thighs; and, **C,** chest in different patients. All demonstrate linear cutaneous calcifications characteristic of the disease (arrows). (**A,** Courtesy Joseph W. Howe, Sylmar, CA; **B** and **C,** Courtesy Steven P. Brownstein, MD, Springfield, NJ.)

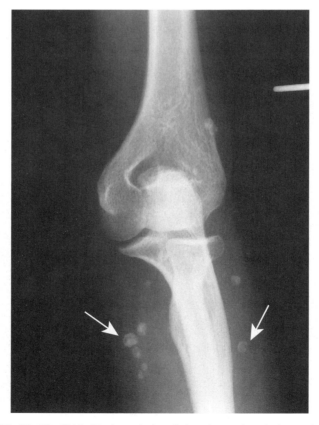

FIG. 19-53 Phleboliths (arrows) of a soft-tissue hemangioma in the proximal forearm. (Courtesy Steven P. Brownstein, MD, Springfield, NJ.)

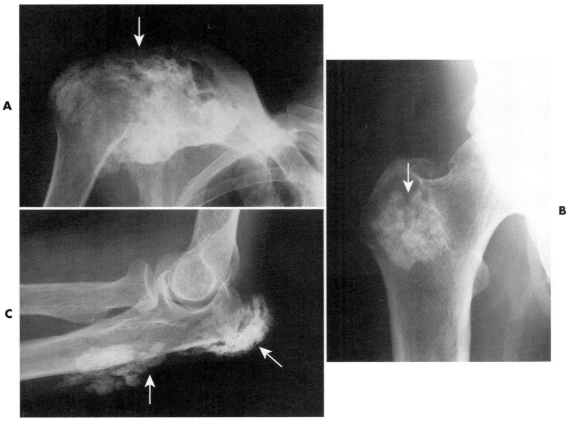

FIG. 19-54 Tumoral calcinosis of, **A,** the shoulder; **B,** hip; and **C,** elbow *(arrows)*. (Courtesy Jack C. Avalos, Davenport, IA.)

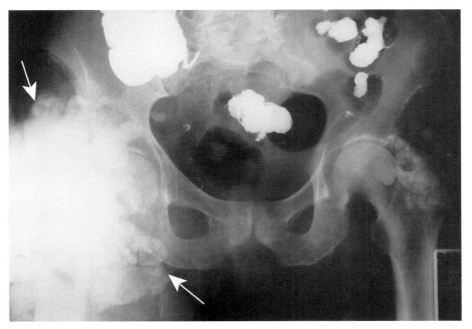

FIG. 19-55 Large, radiodense, soft-tissue masses of tumoral calcinosis *(arrows)*. (Courtesy Steven P. Brownstein, MD, Springfield, NJ.)

GN7b | Soft-Tissue Ossification

DISEASE	COMMENTS
More common *Degenerative*	Intraarticular ossification of degenerative debris usually related to trauma.
Myositis ossificans [p. 733]	Self-limiting disorder of soft-tissue metaplasia to bone usually related to trauma; in early stage, it may be difficult to distinguish from primary bone tumor; a systemic, inherited, progressive form also exists.
Less common *Burns*	Severely burned and damaged tissue may ossify.
Osteosarcoma [p. 813]	Extraosseous and parosteal osteosarcomas representing aggressive primary malignancies of bone; they arise in middle-aged patients, a group older than those affected with conventional osteosarcomas; lesions appear as radiodense masses.
Prolonged immobilization	Paraplegia and other neuropathic conditions with development of ossification or calcifications in muscles, tendons, and ligaments.
Surgical scar	Linear ossific or calcific densities in the location of past surgical sites.
Synovial osteochondromatosis [p. 862]	Nonneoplastic hypertropic metaplasia of synovial tissue, producing multiple cartilage nodules; nodules detach to become loose bodies in the joint, bursal, and tendon sheath spaces and become radiographically discernible after calcification or ossification; this condition may be asymptomatic or produce acute pain with joint locking and effusion; it occurs in adults, most commonly in the knees, hips, ankles, and elbows.

Suggested Readings

Bernstein ML, Neal DC: Oral lesion in a patient with calcinosis and arthritis: case report and differential diagnosis, *J Oral Pathol* 14(1):8, 1985.

Black AS, Kanat IO: A review of soft tissue calcifications, *J Foot Surg* 24(4):243, 1985.

Brant WE: Fundamentals of diagnostic radiology, Baltimore, 1994, Williams & Wilkins.

Burgener FA, Kormano M: Differential diagnosis in conventional radiology, ed 2, New York, 1991, Thieme.

Chapman S, Nakielny R: Aids to radiological differential diagnosis, ed 4, Philadelphia, 2003, WB Saunders.

Dahnert W: Radiology review manual, Baltimore, 1991, Williams & Wilkins.

Eisenberg RL: An atlas of differential diagnosis, ed 2, Gaithersburg, MD, 1992, Aspen.

Forrester DM, Brown JC, Nesson JW: The radiology of joint disease, ed 2, Philadelphia, 1978, WB Saunders.

Ravin CE, Cooper C, Leder RA: Review of radiology, Philadelphia, 1994, WB Saunders.

Reeder MM, Bradley WG: Reeder and Felson's gamuts in radiology, ed 3, New York, 1993, Springer-Verlag.

Weissleder R, Wittenberg J, Harisinghani MG: Primer of diagnostic imaging, ed 3, St Louis, 2003, Mosby.

chapter 20

Magnetic Resonance Imaging Patterns

IAN D. MCLEAN

General Indications for Magnetic Resonance Imaging Examination

Magnetic resonance imaging (MRI) is the most tissue-sensitive, noninvasive imaging modality that can be used to evaluate the extraordinarily wide range of diseases affecting the neuromusculoskeletal system. It is arguably the modality of choice for the detection of osteonecrosis, occult fractures, and soft-tissue neoplasms, and in the assessment of many soft-tissue structures of the musculoskeletal system. In many instances, MRI has replaced more invasive imaging techniques such as arthrography, myelography, and discography.

However, conventional radiography remains an important initial imaging tool. Plain film radiography provides valuable information in the evaluation of common bone and joint pathologies. Conventional radiographic techniques can be more specific than MRI in the diagnosis of many bone lesions, especially bone tumors, which often produce predictable bone changes and periosteal reactions. Consequently, plain film radiographic examinations complement the MRI examination and usually should precede it.

Critically, however, MRI has major advantages over conventional radiographic studies and even computed tomography (CT). These advantages include its ability to yield high tissue contrast, image in multiple planes, and represent a large field of view, all without radiation exposure. Consequently, MRI is helpful in the evaluation of a wide range of conditions of the neuromusculoskeletal system, including traumatic muscle and tendon injuries, hematomas, infections, masses, and internal injuries to joints, including meniscal and cruciate ligament tears and brain and spinal cord pathology.

The cost of MRI is relatively high; however, an MRI examination usually yields an accurate diagnosis of the patient's condition. Furthermore, in some instances it may preclude the need for redundant multiple examinations that may be less sensitive and specific and possibly more invasive than the MRI examination. For instance, MRI should be the primary imaging procedure in the evaluation of the spine in most clinical circumstances, particularly in the presence of neurologic symptoms. Therefore MRI represents a critically needed diagnostic tool for chiropractors, given that diagnosis of the disorders of the spine represents a daily challenge.

The following tables illustrate some of the more common pathologies encountered in imaging the spine and extremities for musculoskeletal complaints.

MRI | Spine

DISEASE	COMMENTS
Vertebral body *Yellow bone marrow* **(FIG. 20-1)**	Adult bone marrow (fatty) is normally signal hyperintense on T1-weighted and, to lesser extent, on T2-weighted sequences. Radiation therapy can also result in increased hyperintensity of the bone marrow, especially on T1-weighted sequences. Marrow appears black (low signal) focally with a bone island and metastasis, and diffusely with mastocystosis, hemosiderosis, myelofibrosis, osteopetrosis.
Red bone marrow	Typical in the pediatric skeleton with abundant hematopoietic tissue. Also occurs in adult marrow reconversion seen in conditions with increased RBC demand, anemias, and bone marrow–replacing pathologies.
Infection **(FIG. 20-2)**	Very sensitive diagnosis of infection provided by MRI when it is used in conjunction with the clinical presentation, radiographic findings, and radionuclide studies; MRI examinations reveal joint effusions on the T2-weighted images with juxtaarticular bone marrow edema and abnormal signal within the adjacent soft tissues, along with bone destruction.
Metastasis, multiple myeloma **(FIG. 20-3)**	MRI is sensitive to metastatic involvement of bone marrow. The typical MRI feature of spinal vertebral body metastasis is deformity (vertebral collapse) with low signal intensity on the T1-weighted sequences and high signal intensity on the T2-weighted sequences, often involving multiple segments. The MRI examination also can evaluate extension into the adjacent paraspinal tissues inclusive of the spinal canal. Other bone marrow–replacing disorders inclusive of multiple myeloma and lymphoma look similar.
Vertebral body compression fractures	Differentiation of osteoporosis and malignant collapse at times may be difficult; old or healed fractures show preservation of the normal marrow signal, and if the fracture is chronic, a band of low signal is evident paralleling the endplate on T2-weighted images; fresh fracture creates nonhomogeneous bone marrow changes, reflective of hemorrhage; by contrast, tumor replacement of marrow tends to create homogeneous signal changes within the vertebral bodies; multiple levels of vertebral body marrow abnormalities with fracture are typical for metastatic disease. CT findings of an osteoporotic vertebral body fracture can be applied to MRI and include cortical fractures without bone destruction, retropulsion of bone fragments, intravertebral vacuum phenomenon, and thin, diffuse paraspinal soft-tissue mass; CT findings of collapse secondary to malignancy include destruction of the anterolateral or posterior cortical bone of the vertebral body; characteristics include destruction of the vertebral body, destruction of a pedicle, and focal soft-tissue or epidural mass.
Hemangioma **(FIG. 20-4)**	Typically hyperintense on both T1-weighted (contributions from fat and vascular components) and T2-weighted (contributions from fluid or blood sequences). The signal hyperintensity on T1-weighted sequences allows discrimination from more aggressive bone marrow–replacing pathologies inclusive of metastasis and myeloma. The absence of cortical destruction also assists in differentiation. Correlation with the conventional radiographs or CT may reveal the typical features of accentuated vertical trabeculation.
Osteochondroma **(FIG. 20-5)**	Depending on the bone tumor and the matrix formation, most tumors that involve the bone marrow are signal hypointense on T1-weighted images and hyperintense on T2-weighted images. As with conventional radiography the diagnosis of bone tumors is dependent on the appearance and location. Some tumors such as osteochondroma have a characteristic appearance that is easily recognized on x-ray and MRI.
Soft-tissue tumors and masses **(FIG. 20-6)**	For normal or equivocal initial radiographs, MRI is useful for further evaluation of the presence of a serious underlying pathology such as tumor or infection; MRI is sensitive in detecting bone abnormalities; criteria to distinguish tumor or metastasis from infection are the same as in conventional radiography, but this pattern can be recognized at a far earlier stage on an MR image; in the spine, when only a single body is involved, it is difficult to distinguish infection from tumor if the differentiation is based purely on the MR images; the plain film criteria of endplate destruction and disc involvement are typical of infection rather than metastasis; extension of destruction into the posterior elements of a vertebra is more typical of metastatic disease; signal changes of infection frequently are equal to cerebrospinal fluid, whereas metastatic bone disease appears more hypointense; soft-tissue involvement of infection tends to be ill defined as opposed to the soft-tissue involvement of tumor, which often is more sharply defined; in general the signal changes within the vertebral bodies are nonspecific, and sometimes differentiation of benign from malignant lesions is difficult; however,

DISEASE	COMMENTS
Soft-tissue tumors and masses cont'd	certain masses have typical MRI characteristics allowing for confident diagnosis; in general, "white lesions are 'right' on T1-weighted images" and "white lesions are 'wrong' on T2-weighted images." For example, a vertebral fat deposit that is of limited clinical significance appears as high signal intensity on T1-weighted scans and lower signal intensity on T2-weighted scans. By contrast, metastatic bone disease, which is highly clinically significant, likely demonstrates high signal intensity on T2-weighted images.
Intervertebral disc *Anular rents*	Hyperintense focal lesions involving the posterior annular fibers (high intensity zone) on T2-weighted or gradient echo–weighted images.
Disc bulge	Diffuse contour alteration of disc space.
Disc protrusion	Relatively central, broad-based, not large, sometimes described as a *subligamentous herniation*.
Disc extrusion **(FIG. 20-7)**	Transligamentous extrusion of the disc material through the posterior longitudinal ligament.
Disc sequestration	Transligamentous disc herniation without communication (migration) to the parent disc.
Vertebral (Modic) endplate changes *Type I* **(FIG. 20-8, A and B)**	Represents edema or granulation tissue; appears hypointense on T1-weighted images and hyperintense on T2-weighted images.
Type II **(FIG. 20-8, C)**	Represents fat tissue phase; appears hyperintense on T1-weighted images and mildly hyperintense on T2-weighted images.
Type III	Represents bone sclerosis and appears hypointense on T1- and T2-weighted images.
Spinal canal **(FIGS. 20-9 to 20-14)**	MRI is excellent for imaging the spinal canal; abnormalities such as dural ectasia, multiple sclerosis, tethered cord syndrome, ligamentum flavum calcification, and syringomyelia are noted readily.

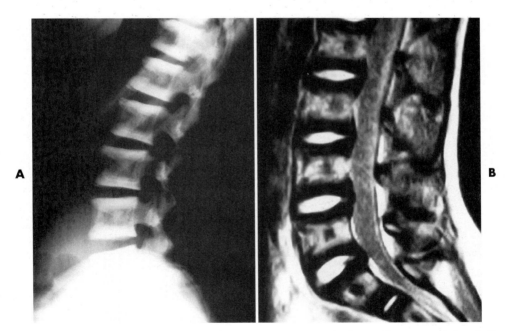

FIG. 20-1 Osteopetrosis on, **A,** plain film and, **B,** sagittal spin-density–weighted magnetic resonance image. **A,** Densely sclerotic vertebral bands that parallel the endplates appear markedly hypointense on, **B,** the magnetic resonance image.

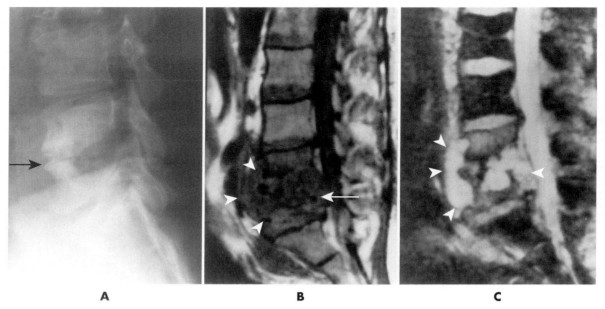

A   **B**   **C**

FIG. 20-2   A, Infection of the L4 intervertebral disc, presenting with decreased disc space on the plain film *(arrow).*
B, A large soft-tissue mass *(arrowheads)* and hypointense signal of the infection *(arrow)* is noted on the T1-weighted magnetic
resonance image. **C,** These regions become hyperintense on the T2-weighted magnetic resonance image *(arrowheads).*

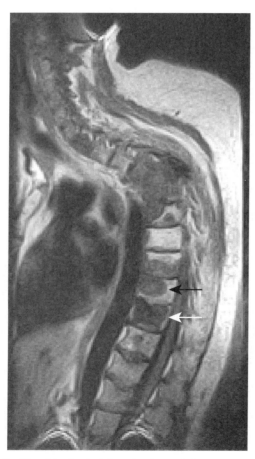

FIG. 20-3   T1-weighted sagittal, thoracic spine study showing foci of decreased
signal intensity *(arrows)* representing metastatic disease replacing the normally
high signal intensity bone marrow fat.

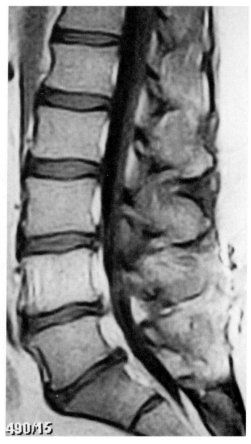

FIG. 20-4   Hemangioma at L4 with diffuse increase in signal intensity involving
the vertebral body. Close inspection shows accentuated vertical trabeculation
that correlates to the characteristic radiographic findings.

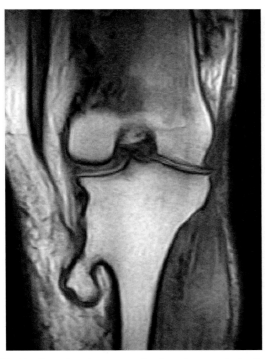

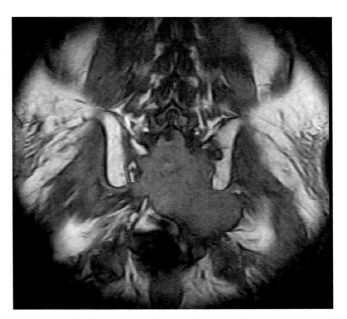

FIG. 20-6 Chordoma presenting as a T1-weighted hypointense expansile lesion involving the sacrum. This lesion would appear hyperintense on a T2-weighted image.

FIG. 20-5 Osteochondroma extending from the metaphysis of the tibia.

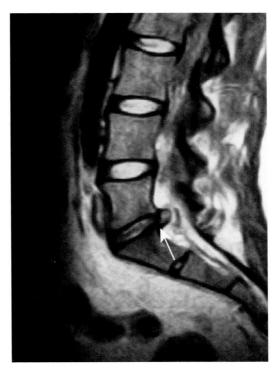

FIG. 20-7 Sagittal T2-weighted lumbar intervertebral disc extrusion at the L5 level *(arrow).*

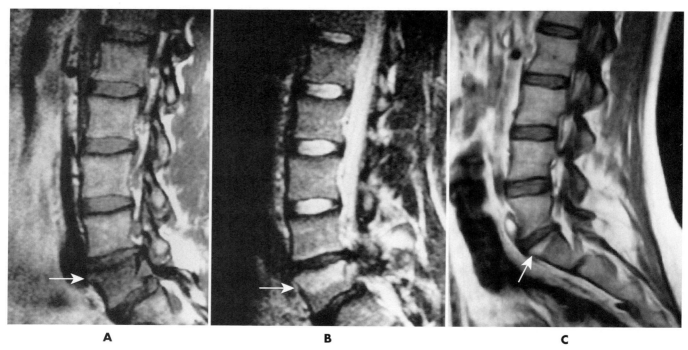

A   B   C

FIG. 20-8   Modic type I endplate changes consistent with inflammatory vertebral marrow alterations. Notably, **A,** the hypointense regions on the T1-weighted image appear, **B,** hyperintense on the T2-weighted image *(arrows).* **C,** Modic type II endplate changes consistent with fat marrow changes. The imaging findings denote focal signal hyperintensity on the sagittal T1-weighted magnetic resonance lumbar scan *(arrow).*

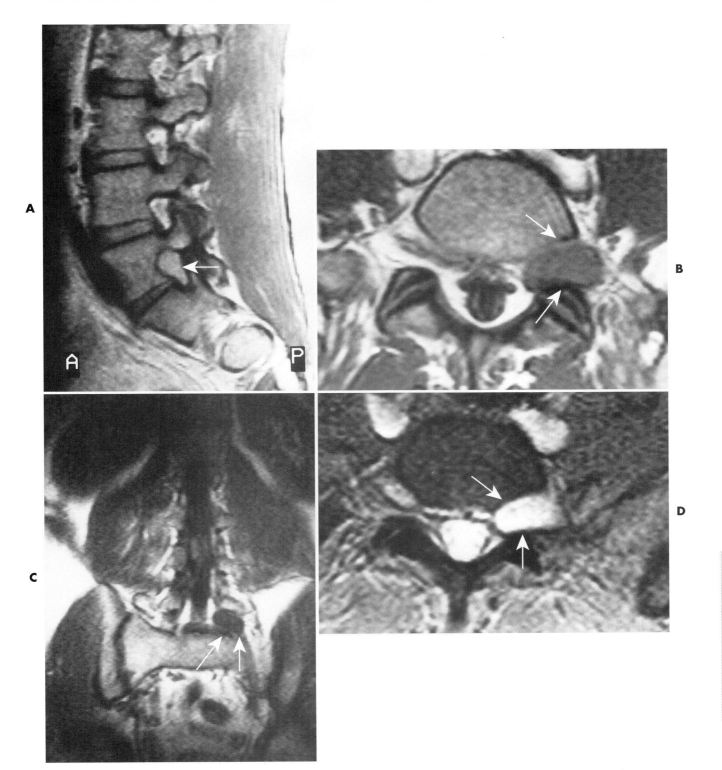

FIG. 20-9 Neurofibroma presenting as a mass in the intervertebral foramen *(arrows)* on, **A,** sagittal; **B,** axial; **C,** and coronal magnetic resonance images. **D,** Mass becomes hyperintense on T2-weighted images *(arrows)*.

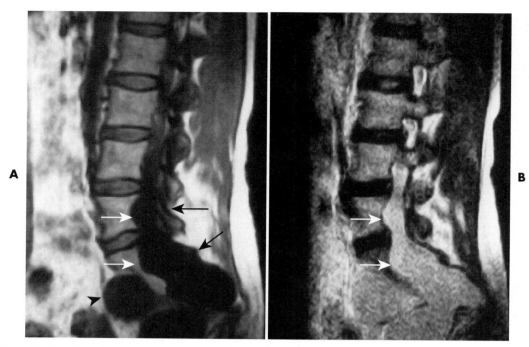

FIG. 20-10   Neurofibromatosis with dural ectasia noted as cerebrospinal fluid–filled saccular redundancy of the dura *(arrows)* with ventral meningocele *(arrowhead)* appearing, **A,** hypointense on T1-weighted images and, **B,** hyperintense on T2-weighted images *(arrows).*

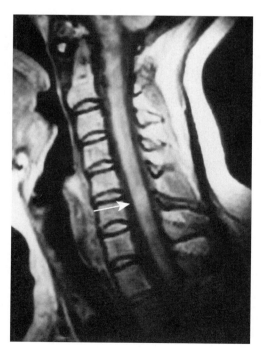

FIG. 20-11   Demyelinated, hyperintense plaque *(arrow)* of multiple sclerosis on this sagittal T1-weighted cervical magnetic resonance image without contrast.

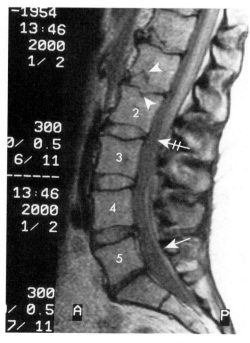

FIG. 20-12   Tethered cord syndrome. Sagittal T1-weighted magnetic resonance image demonstrating fat infiltrate of the filum terminale *(arrow).* The spinal cord termination is at the L2-L3 intervertebral disc space *(crossed arrow),* which is lower than the normal L1-L2 level of termination. Schmorl's nodes *(arrowheads)* of the upper lumbar spine and advanced degenerative disc disease at the L4 and L5 levels also are noted.

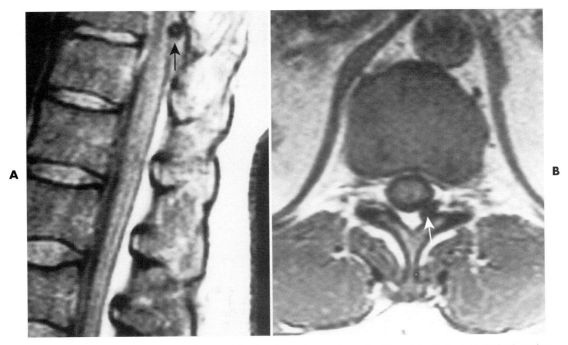

FIG. 20-13 **A** and **B,** Ligamentum flavum calcification *(arrows)* appearing as focal hypointensity in the vertebral canal at the thoracolumbar junction.

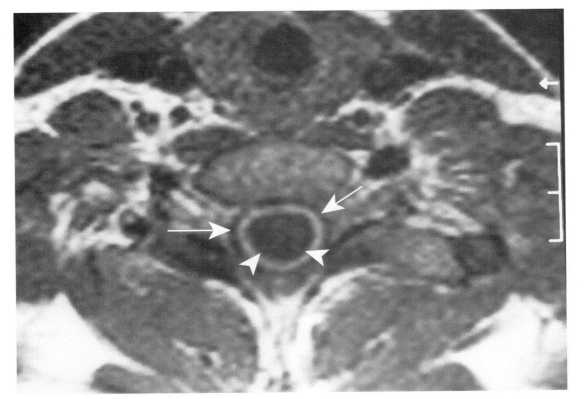

FIG. 20-14 Syringomyelia presenting as a cavity in the center of the hyperintense spinal cord *(arrows)* filled with hypointense cerebrospinal fluid *(arrowheads)* on this axial T1-weighted image.

MR2 Joints

Many causes of joint pain are well portrayed with MRI. Tissue contrast with MRI is high, and early changes in marrow, subchondral bone, and cartilage can be evaluated, including arthritis, trauma, infection, and neoplasia. MRI should be considered when a need exists to evaluate internal joint derangement and juxtaarticular pathology or if there is a poor response to conservative management.

MR2a | Shoulder

DISEASE	COMMENTS
Biceps tendon abnormalities **(FIG. 20-15)**	Rupture or dislocation is suggested when the biceps tendon is not visible in its expected location; fluid also may be observed within the biceps tendon sheath.
Glenoid labral tears **(FIG. 20-16)**	Sequelae of anterior shoulder dislocation with involvement of the anterior labrum (Bankart lesion); osseous fractures of the underlying glenoid margin may accompany labral tear. Superior labral anteroposterior lesions are specific labral pathologies involving the superior labrum from antero-posterior lesion, representing injury of the biceps labral complex inclusive of "bucket handle" tearing.
Rotator cuff tear **(FIGS. 20-17 and 20-18)**	Complete tear revealing a T2-weighted signal hyperintensity extending through the rotator cuff; the supraspinatus musculotendinous junction retracts and fluid accumulates in the subacromial bursa; secondary signs include loss of the subdeltoid fat, atrophy of the supraspinatus muscle, and cystic changes of the humeral head (principally at the site of the supraspinatus tendon insertion). Partial tears can involve the bursal surface, articular surface, or interstitium and require differentiation from tendinopathy and calcific tendinitis.
Subacromial impingement	Compression of the supraspinatus tendon and subacromial bursa between the humeral head and cora-coacromial arch; conventional radiographic examination may reveal a hooked acromion impinging on the region of the supraspinatus (subacromial space <7 mm) that can be confirmed on MRI examination; also evidence of subacromial spurs and acromioclavicular joint degeneration; MRI evaluation reveals additional findings of supraspinatus tendinopathy.
Subscapularis tear **(FIG. 20-19)**	Subscapularis muscle tendon tears can occur secondary to both anterior and posterior shoulder dislocations and along with injuries to other components of the rotator cuff. Disruption of the subscapularis with high-intensity (T2-weighted) signal within the defect represents the most outstanding MRI finding. Capsular injury also may be seen. Avulsion of the lesser tuberosity may be evident both on x-ray and MRI examinations when seen in conjunction with previous posterior shoulder dislocation. Bankart and reversed Bankart lesions may be evident as well.

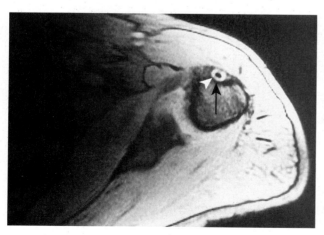

FIG. 20-15 Bicipital tendinitis noted by a hyperintense effusion *(arrow)*, surrounding the central hypointense biceps tendon *(arrowhead)* within the bicipital groove on this T2-weighted axial magnetic resonance image.

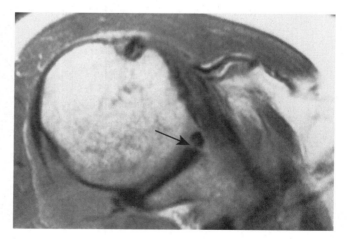

FIG. 20-16 Bucket handle tear of the glenoid labrum. Larger bucket handle-type tears can be seen as areas of linear high signal intensity within the labrum on multiple images *(arrow)*. (From Stark DD, Gradley WG: *Magnetic resonance imaging,* ed 2, St Louis, 1992, Mosby.)

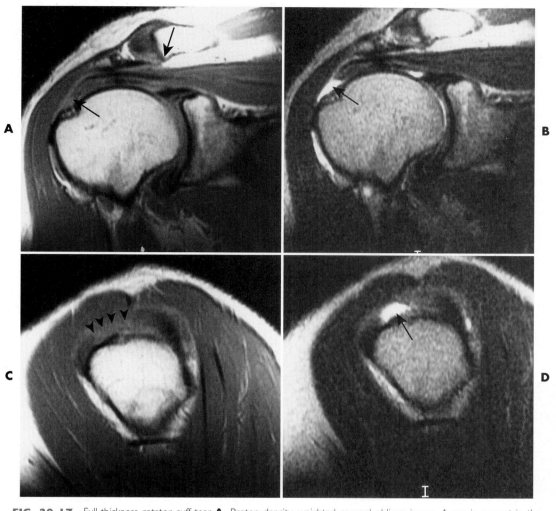

FIG. 20-17 Full-thickness rotator cuff tear. **A,** Proton density–weighted coronal oblique image. A gap is present in the supraspinatus tendon near its insertion site *(arrow)*. Some proliferative changes affect the acromioclavicular joint, including a small, downward-pointing spur *(small arrow)*. **B,** T2-weighted²⁵⁰⁰/⁷⁰ coronal oblique image. The tendon gap is bright *(arrow)* and is most likely filled with fluid. No intact tendon exists above or below the abnormal area. **C,** Proton density–weighted²⁵⁰⁰/⁷⁰ sagittal oblique image. Anterosuperiorly the normal dark band of the rotator cuff is interrupted by a fuzzy area of relatively increased signal *(arrowheads)*. **D,** T2-weighted²⁵⁰⁰/⁷⁰ sagittal oblique image. The anterior part of this area becomes very bright *(arrow)*. The remainder brightens only slightly. Often a tear is adjacent to or surrounded by an area of tendinopathy. (From Haaga JR: Computed tomography and magnetic resonance imaging of the whole body, St Louis, 1994, Mosby.)

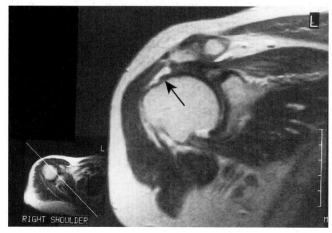

FIG. 20-18 Full-thickness tear of the supraspinatus with the tendon gap filled with fluid on this T1-weighted coronal magnetic resonance image *(arrow)*.

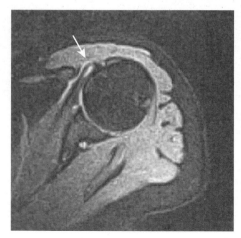

FIG. 20-19 Focal increase in signal intensity representing tear involving the expected position of the subscapularis tendon at the lesser tuberosity of the humerus *(arrow)*.

MR2b | Wrist

The multiplanar imaging potential of MRI is advantageous in evaluating the complex anatomy of the wrist, an area that is often difficult to visualize with conventional imaging techniques.

DISEASE	COMMENTS
Scapholunate ligament tear **(FIG. 20-20)**	Ligamentous disruption between the scaphoid and lunate with resulting disassociation; radiographic features include rotatory subluxation of the scaphoid (signet ring) and scaphoid-lunate diastases ("Terry Thomas"). These features are confirmed by MRI with the additional findings of partial or complete tear of the scapholunate ligament complex (dorsal, volar, intrinsic components). Chronic scaphoid-lunate disassociation may result in scaphoid-lunate advanced collapse in which there is chronic scaphoid-lunate diastasis with proximal migration of the capitate.
Triangular fibrocartilage tear	Evidenced as direct extension of fluid across the triangular fibrocartilage.
Carpal tunnel syndrome **(FIG. 20-21)**	Compression of the median nerve with flattening, swelling, and increased signal intensity; palmar bowing of the transverse ligament occurs.
Osteonecrosis of the scaphoid and lunate **(FIG. 20-22, A through C)**	Typically low signal intensity within the bone marrow on T1-weighted images with regions of increased signal intensity on T2-weighted images; the T2-weighted appearance is thought to represent hemorrhage or edema.

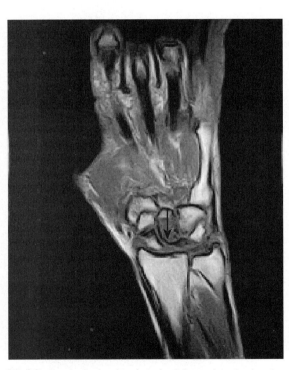

FIG. 20-20 Proximal migration (*arrow*) of the capitate in chronic scapholunate diastases.

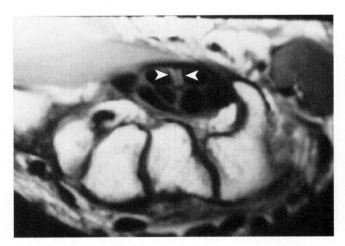

FIG. 20-21 Axial T1-weighted magnetic resonance scan of the wrist, demonstrating alteration of the normally oval median nerve width (*arrowheads*), suggesting compression within the carpal tunnel.

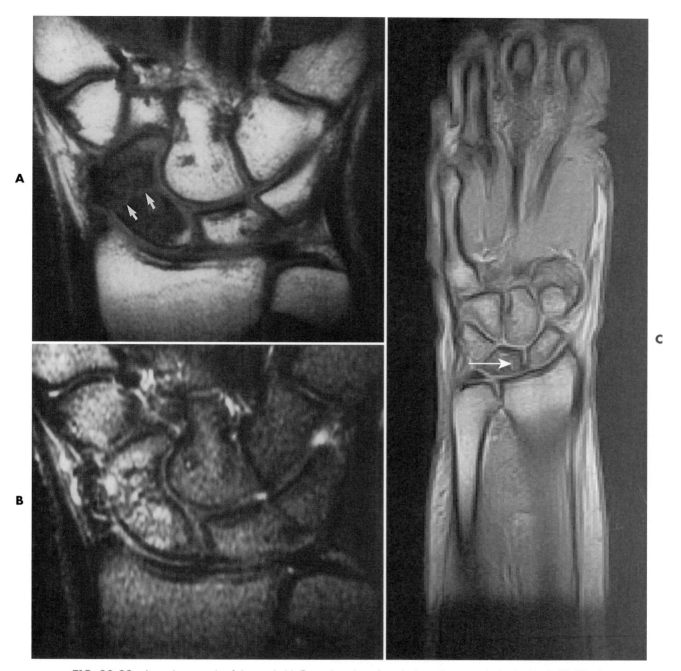

FIG. 20-22 Avascular necrosis of the scaphoid. Coronal sections through the wrist were obtained with, **A,** TR/TE of 500/20 and, **B,** TR/TE of 200/80. **A,** A fracture of the scaphoid is present (*arrows*). A diffuse loss of the normally high signal intensity of the bone marrow is seen on the T1-weighted image, and mottled high and low signal intensity is seen on the T2-weighted image. **C,** Alteration of signal intensity consistent with lunate avascular necrosis (*arrow*). (**A** and **B,** From Stark DD, Gradley WG: Magnetic resonance imaging, ed 2, St Louis, 1992, Mosby.)

MR2c | Hip

DISEASE	COMMENTS
Legg-Calvé-Perthes disease	Idiopathic osteonecrosis of the femoral head in children, usually between 4 and 8 years of age; characteristic radiographic findings include increase in density of the femoral head, subchondral collapse, flattening, and diffuse sclerosis of an irregularly ossified femoral capital epiphysis.
Osteonecrosis **(FIGS. 20-23 and 20-24)**	Condition that results from ischemic death of the cellular aspects of bone marrow and bone; MRI is optimal for use in patients with normal or equivocal conventional radiographs after clinical complaint of the hip; radiography is comparatively insensitive in the early diagnosis of osteonecrosis. The classic radiographic findings become obvious when stages of bone repair or collapse become evident; radionuclide bone scintigraphy is sensitive but lacks specificity, consequently MRI detects early osteonecrosis and differentiates osteonecrosis from other bone pathology. Characteristic features of osteonecrosis of the hip include a circumscribed ovoid- or crescent-shaped rim of low signal on T1-weighted scans occurring in a subchondral location with a band of increased signal on the T2-weighted scan corresponding to the interface of repair between ischemic bone and hypervascular granulation tissue ("double line" sign); joint effusions along with the presence of a diffuse signal abnormality of the head and neck also are observed.
Transient osteoporosis of the hip	Condition of unknown etiology; it may be related to regional migratory osteoporosis and reflex sympathetic dystrophy; conventional radiographs often are normal; MRI reveals a diffuse loss of normal bone marrow fat signal on T1-weighted images, with hyperintense signal on T2-weighted images representing bone marrow edema; condition tends to resolve spontaneously in 6 to 12 months.

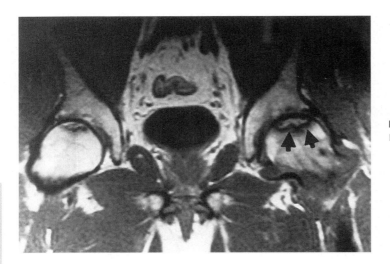

FIG. 20-23   T1-weighted coronal section demonstrating bilateral femoral head avascular necrosis, more advanced on the patient's left *(arrows)*.

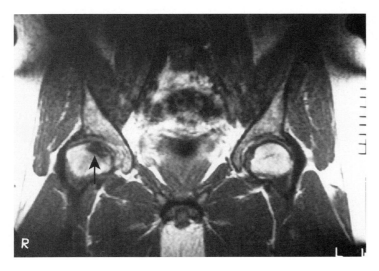

FIG. 20-24   T1-weighted coronal section demonstrating a hypointense focus in the right femoral head, consistent with avascular necrosis *(arrow)*.

MR2d | Knee

DISEASE	COMMENTS
Anterior cruciate injuries **(FIG. 20-25)**	Midsubstance discontinuity, abnormal angulation of the course of the anterior cruciate, abnormal cruciate buckling, increased curvature of the posterior cruciate ligament (PCL), anterior tibial subluxation, thinning of the fibers of the anterior cruciate ligament (ACL), hematomas about the intact fibers of the ACL, and increased signal intensity within the ACL but with intact fibers.
Posterior cruciate ligament injuries **(FIG. 20-26)**	Midsubstance discontinuity of the ligament with avulsion occurring at the tibial insertion; isolated posterior cruciate ligament tears are uncommon, and associated injuries to the ACL or the menisci should be sought.
Chondromalacia patellae	MRI studies showing early cartilage thinning or erosion of the cartilaginous surface along with focal regions of edema and later marked hypointensity (sclerosis) on T1- and T2-weighted images of the subchondral bone.
Collateral ligament injuries **(FIG. 20-27)**	T2-weighted images demonstrating edema and hemorrhage surrounding the usually low signal intensity fibers of the ligament; complete tears are seen as a loss of continuity of the ligament fibers.
Meniscal tears **(FIGS. 20-28 and 20-29)**	Three grades of abnormal signal intensity associated with abnormal menisci: Grade I represents globular foci of abnormal signal correlating with mucinous degeneration (the signal does not extend to the meniscal articular surface); Grade II represents a linear, horizontal region of increased signal intensity that does not extend to the articular surface; Grades I and II are arthroscopically normal; Grade III represents an abnormal signal intensity (often linear) that extends to an articular surface.
Bucket handle tear **(FIG. 20-30)**	A vertical tear of the meniscus with displacement of the medial component into the intercondylar notch ("fragment-in-notch" sign); truncation of the normal triangular appearance of the meniscus also is a good diagnostic clue ("absent bow tie" sign); the fragment may parallel the PCL on sagittal sequences, creating the "double PCL sign."
Popliteal (Baker's) cyst **(FIG. 20-31)**	Distention of the gastrocnemius/semimembranosus bursa with extension to the joint space. High signal intensity (T2-weighted) mass posterior to the medial femoral condyles, interposed between the tendons of the medial gastrocnemius and semimembranosus.
Plica **(FIG. 20-32)**	Represents incomplete resorption of the synovial membrane that compartmentalizes the knee during embryologic development; three plica are most common: the suprapatellar, medial patellar, and infrapatellar; may thicken and cause knee pain; the medial plica presents as a low signal linear structure on the medial aspect of the knee joint capsule.
Osteochondritis dissecans	Low signal intensity, subchondral foci involving the non–weight-bearing lateral surface of the medial femoral condyle on both T1- and T2-weighted images; in situ bone and cartilage fragment with or without evidence of displacement or migration.
Bone infarct **(FIG. 20-33)**	Serpiginous defect involving the subchondral marrow; commonly presents with a "double line sign" of decreased signal intensity periphery with an adjacent increased signal intensity inner border; more common within the metaphysis.
Patellar subluxation	Triad of patellar bone bruise, femoral bone bruise, and associated tearing of the medial retinacular attachments; patellar subluxation may involve a large effusion; this condition is associated with hypoplastic lateral femoral condyle, genu valgum, abnormal lateral insertion of the patellar tendon, and patella alta.
Patella tendon tear **(FIG. 20-34)**	Disruption with high-intensity T2-weighted, low-intensity T1-weighted gap most commonly adjacent to the inferior pole of the patella involving the proximal one third of the tendon; avulsion involving the inferior pole of the patellar also may be evident.

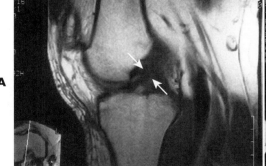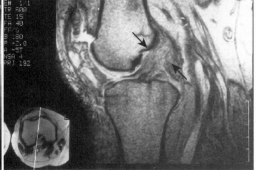

FIG. 20-25   **A** and **B,** Anterior cruciate ligament tear noted by the interruption of the normally hypointense ligament band with surrounding hemorrhage and edema present on the sagittal T1- and T2-weighted magnetic resonance images *(arrows).*

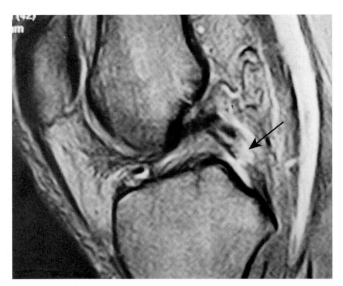

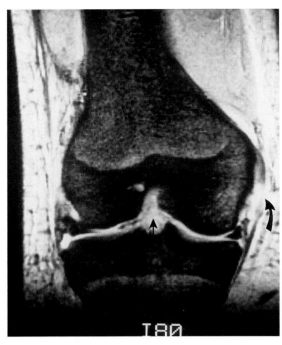

FIG. 20-26 Disruption of the proximal component of the posterior cruciate ligament tear. Sagittal T2-weighted image shows hyperintense hemorrhage and edema replacing the region of a complete tear *(arrow)*.

FIG. 20-27 Medial collateral ligament tear, Grade III. Coronal gradient echo image shows complete disruption of the medial collateral ligament *(curved arrow)*. In addition a normal anterior cruciate ligament is not seen at the intercondylar region and therefore is torn *(small arrow)*. (From Haaga JR: Computed tomography and magnetic resonance imaging of the whole body, St Louis, 1994, Mosby.)

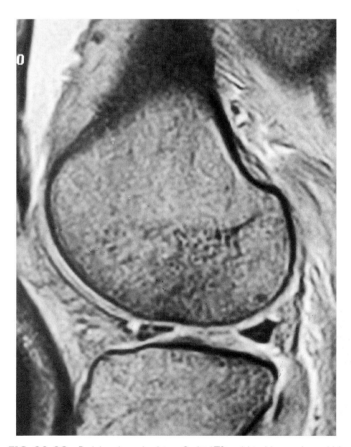

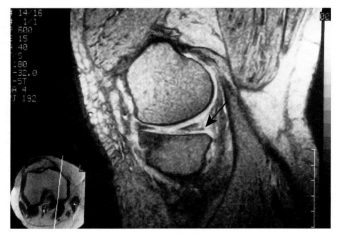

FIG. 20-28 Peripheral meniscal tear. Sagittal T2-weighted image shows high signal intensity at the periphery of the anterior horn of the medial meniscus.

FIG. 20-29 Hyperintense tear of the posterior horn of the lateral meniscus *(arrow)*.

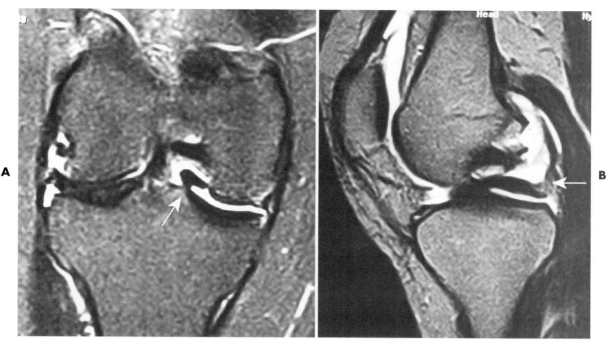

FIG. 20-30 A, Bucket handle tear with the displaced fragment evident within the intercondylar notch *(arrow)* on the coronal sequence and, **B,** paralleling the posterior cruciate ligament on the sagittal image *(arrow).*

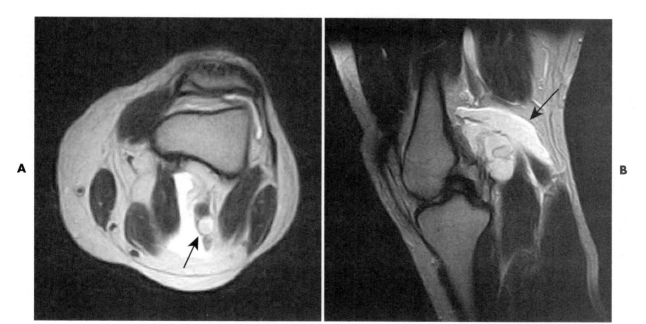

FIG. 20-31 A and **B,** Popliteal cyst with a T2-weighted signal hyperintense collection within the gastrocnemius/semi-membranosus bursa *(arrows).*

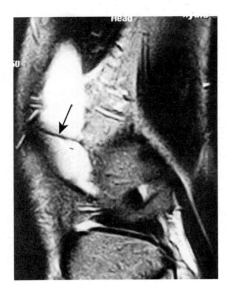

FIG. 20-32 Signal hypointense plica dividing the medial knee joint compartment *(arrow)*.

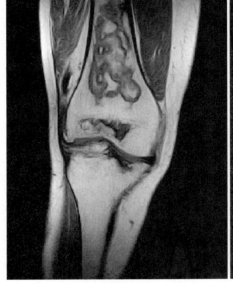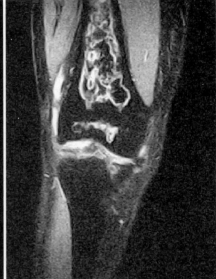

FIG. 20-33 **A** and **B,** Serpiginous defect involving the bone marrow with characteristic "double line" appearance.

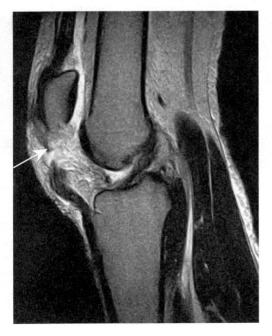

FIG. 20-34 Complete disruption of the patella tendon exhibiting amorphous increase in signal intensity *(arrow)*.

MR2e | Ankle

DISEASE	COMMENTS
Tendon ruptures	Most commonly affecting the Achilles tenden and tibialis posterior; the peroneus brevis and longus also are affected frequently.
Transchondral injuries	Including osteochondral fractures, osteochondritis dissecans, and talar dome fractures, which usually are found to involve either the medial or lateral talar dome with extension into both the articular cartilage and subchondral bone; characteristics include associated focal cartilaginous signal alteration and joint effusion.

MR3 | General Skeletal

DISEASE	COMMENTS
Bone marrow disorders **(FIGS. 20-35 and 20-36)**	Healthy bone marrow of adults is composed of predominantly fat with characteristic high signal intensity on T1-weighted images. Disease processes that replace bone marrow, including fluid, blood, pus, or calcification, cause an abnormal MRI bone marrow signal; consequently, MRI is exquisitely sensitive to such diseases as osteonecrosis, primary and secondary tumors, infection, systemic bone marrow diseases, and trauma. The signal characteristics of the medullary space also depend on the age of the patient, the quantity of cancellous bone, and the ratios of red and yellow marrow; in children and young adults, high signal intensity of yellow marrow is observed in the femoral epiphyses, in contrast with the intermediate signal intensity of the hematopoietic marrow in the metaphysis and pelvis. With aging, fatty marrow gradually replaces hematopoietic marrow and the MRI signal changes to the characteristic high signal intensity on T1-weighted images; MRI provides critical diagnostic information on bone marrow disorders; bone marrow processes include age-related marrow conversion and reconversion, hematologic disorders, neoplasia processes, ischemic disorders, infection, and metabolic bone disorders.
Bone bruises **(FIG. 20-37)**	Representative of microfracture of the cancellous bone with hemorrhage and edema involving the medullary spaces; usually secondary to an impaction injury; expected appearance of a diffuse low T1-weighted and high T2-weighted signal intensity; conspicuity is increased on short tau inversion recovery (STIR) sequences; in the knee these are commonly associated with anterior and posterior cruciate ligament injuries and medial collateral ligament injuries.
Fractures **(FIGS. 20-38 to 20-40)**	MRI is sensitive in the diagnosis of acute and stress fractures and should be used when conventional radiographs show no abnormalities or only questionable findings; the typical findings of fatigue fractures include linear regions of decreased signal intensity on T1-weighted images with associated edematous changes of low signal intensity on T1-weighted images and high signal intensity on T2-weighted images within the marrow; importantly, stress fractures may be bilateral.
Joint effusions **(FIG. 20-41)**	Low signal intensity on T1-weighted images and high signal intensity on T2-weighted scans; a characteristic "saddlebag" look appears on the coronal images within the suprapatellar bursa.
Osteoarthritis	Characteristic features include osteophytes, loss of joint space, and subchondral cysts.
Pigmented villonodular synovitis	Monoarticular synovial proliferative disorder presenting as soft-tissue masses about the joint; MRI findings consist of mixed signal intensity changes; the T2-weighted images show foci of decreased signal intensity consistent with hemosiderin deposition in addition to areas of increased signal intensity in the adjacent synovial fluid.
Rheumatoid arthritis	Multicompartmental disease with subchondral and marginal erosions with diffuse loss of cartilage; moderate joint effusions with popliteal cysts about the knee are common, best demonstrated on the T2-weighted images; thickening of the synovium is a relatively consistent feature of inflammatory joint disease; MRI examination of rheumatoid joints also helps to exclude osteonecrosis as a complication of steroid therapy.
Synovial osteochondromatosis	Joint effusions and multiple filling effect shown on MRI within the effusions that represent osteocartilaginous loose bodies; calcified cartilaginous bodies may be seen on conventional radiographs; however, calcification is not apparent in approximately one third of cases.

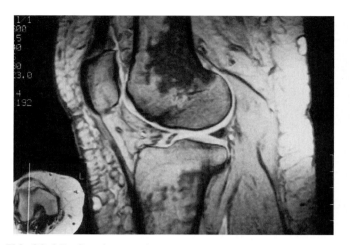

FIG. 20-35 Conspicuous red marrow reconversion in a long-term smoker. Most notable are the focal regions of hypointense hemopoietic marrow within the normal hyperintense adult yellow marrow, yielding a heterogeneous marrow signal pattern.

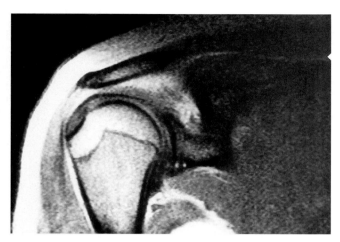

FIG. 20-36 Coronal T1-weighted magnetic resonance scan of the proximal humerus, denoting normal bone marrow contrast of the epiphyses and the signal hypointense hemopoietic metaphysis in a young patient.

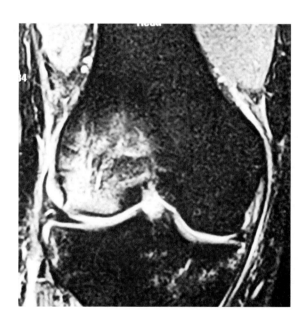

FIG. 20-37 Diffuse increase in marrow signal intensity involving the lateral femoral condyle, representing bone bruise well demonstrated on this short tau inversion recovery (STIR) sequence.

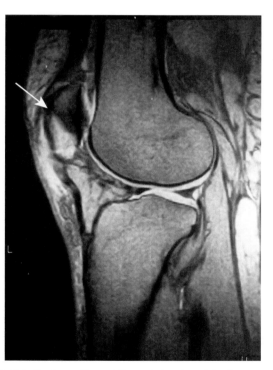

FIG. 20-38 Fracture of the patella, producing altered signal pattern appearing as a hypointense signal in the upper pole and hyperintense signal in the lower pole (arrow).

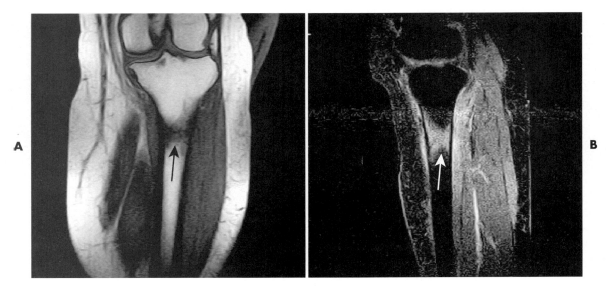

FIG. 20-39 **A** and **B,** Stress fracture involving the proximal diaphysis of the tibia with linear T1-weighted signal hypo-intensity and hyperintensity on the short tau inversion recovery (STIR) sequence *(arrows).*

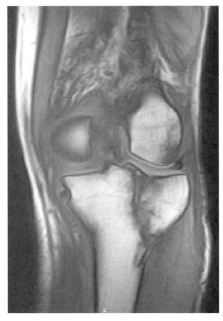

FIG. 20-40 Fracture involving the tibial plateau with extension into the articular surface. Bone edema and hemorrhage are evident as diffuse hypointense signal changes at the fracture margins.

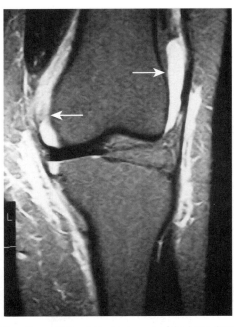

FIG. 20-41 Coronal T2-weighted sequence of the knee, showing a homogeneous posttraumatic collection of fluid-producing joint effusion *(arrows).*

Suggested Readings

Gosfield E, Alavi A, Kneeland B: Comparison of radionuclide bone scans and magnetic resonance imaging in detecting spinal metastases, *J Nucl Med* 34:2191, 1993.

Gundry CR, Fritts HM: Magnetic resonance imaging of the musculoskeletal system, part 8, the spine, section 1, *Clin Orthop Rel Res* 338:275, 1997.

Haaga JR: Computed tomography and magnetic resonance imaging of the whole body, ed 3, St Louis, 1994, Mosby.

Kneeland JB: Magnetic resonance imaging of the musculoskeletal system, part 1, Fundamental principles, *Clin Orthop Rel Res* 321:274, 1995.

Mitchell DG et al: Femoral head avascular necrosis: correlation with MR imaging, radiographic staging, radionuclide imaging, and clinical features, *Radiology* 162:709, 1987.

Pomeranz SJ: Pitfalls and variations in neuro-orthopedics, Cincinnati, 1995, MRI-EFI Publications.

Runge VM: Magnetic resonance imaging of the spine, Philadelphia, 1995, JB Lippincott.

Stoller DW, Tirman PF, Bredella MA: Diagnostic imaging orthopedics, Salt Lake City, 2004, AMIRSYS.

Chest

chapter 21

Introduction to Chest Radiography

DENNIS M. MARCHIORI

Chest Radiography
Anatomy
Radiographic Signs
Pattern Recognition

Chest Radiography

Radiographic examination of the chest plays an important role in the diagnosis and management of pulmonary disease. Chest radiographs account for the majority of radiographs taken each year by the medical profession. Chest radiography plays a less dominant but no less important clinical role in chiropractic practice. Although limitations exist, when combined with a thorough history and physical examination, chest radiography offers a sensitive method for detecting serious pathology of the thorax.

The standard radiographic examination of the chest consists of a posteroanterior (PA) and right or left lateral projection (Figs. 21-1 and 21-2). Oblique, lateral decubitus, and apical lordotic views are some of the more helpful accessory projections that may augment the standard views (Figs. 21-3 and 21-4). The lateral projection adds little as a screening procedure in the younger patient.[14] Consequently, the PA projection alone generally is accepted as adequate screening of the thorax in young individuals who are without symptoms directly referable to the chest. All patients older than 40 years of age or patients of any age who exhibit clinical findings directly referable to the chest should have both a PA and lateral projection radiograph taken during routine evaluation.

Because the side of the body closest to the film is demonstrated with better detail and much of the left lung is obscured by the heart in the frontal projection, the left side of the body is customarily positioned next to the film in the lateral projection.[5] However, if pathology is known or suspected on the right, then the right side of the patient is placed next to the film to exhibit the area of concern with better detail.

Chest radiography employs high peak kilovoltage (110 to 150 kVp) exposures during full patient inspiratory effort, with a film-focal distance of 72 inches. In the frontal projection, rotation is present if the clavicles are not equidistant from the patient's midline. Although individual preferences exist, generally a properly exposed chest radiograph should barely outline the thoracic spine through the heart shadow. The radiograph should display the entire thorax and particularly the costophrenic angles on the film. Good patient inspiratory result is noted by observing the posterior portions of the first 10 ribs (or anterior portions of the first 7 ribs) above the right hemidiaphragm. The right hemidiaphragm is used as a reference for the reason that the position of the left hemidiaphragm is more variable because of the subjacent gastric air bubble. Diagnostic purposes sometimes warrant taking films during patient expiration. For instance, if a "check-valve" bronchial obstruction is present, the involved lung demonstrates a pathologic state in which it remains well inflated on an expiration film.

The criteria for ordering chest films vary and often are individualized at the personal, departmental, or institutional level. Some of the more common indications include chronic cough; hemoptysis; expectoration; shortness of breath; cyanosis; clubbing of the fingers; and pain in the chest, thoracic spine, or upper extremities. Routine chest radiographs in an otherwise healthy patient population are discouraged. However, when these baseline films are available, they offer valuable comparative studies for equivocal radiographic findings on subsequent studies. Often patients exhibit residue of an old or inactive disease, such as healed granulomas, chronic obstructive pulmonary disease (COPD), and pulmonary scarring. Frequently the availability of old films for comparison may eliminate the need for continued evaluation, limiting further cost and patient exposure. Likewise, practitioners should apply serial radiographs cautiously to follow a disease process, and then only at large enough intervals that overirradiation does not become an issue.

Many times it is necessary to augment the information gathered from the chest radiographs with other imaging modalities to more completely evaluate the patient. Fluoroscopy is an often overlooked but valuable procedure for localizing pulmonary nodules and evaluating diaphragmatic movement. Computed tomography (CT) probably is the most useful additional procedure and has all but replaced conventional tomography. CT is particularly advantageous when shadows of the chest wall, pleura, lung, hilum, or mediastinum should be better visualized when partially obstructed by overlying densities. CT is most widely used to delineate and assess neoplastic disease.

Magnetic resonance imaging (MRI) is used most often to distinguish pathology of the hilar and mediastinal lymph nodes from adjacent vascular anatomy. It has a particular advantage over CT for distinguishing mediastinal lymph node involvement from vascular masses, because flowing blood has no signal on MRI and therefore appears black, readily distinguishing vessels from the high signal intensity of the lymph nodes. The ventilation and perfusion scans of lung scintigraphy are valuable in the diagnosis of pulmonary embolism, although the more invasive pulmonary

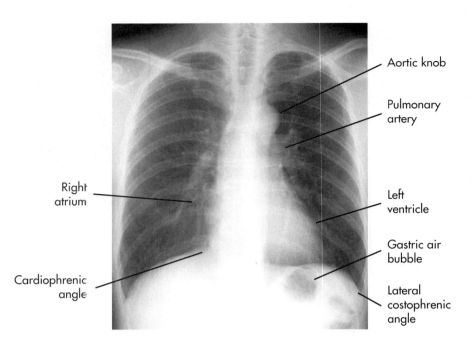

FIG. 21-1 Normal posteroanterior chest.

Aortic knob

Pulmonary artery

Right atrium

Left ventricle

Gastric air bubble

Cardiophrenic angle

Lateral costophrenic angle

angiography remains the imaging standard for questionable scan results.

Although imaging examinations are valuable in the study of intrathoracic disease, they do not supplant the importance of a thorough physical examination and history. In addition, blood tests, diagnostic skin tests, sputum cultures, biopsy, and especially bronchoscopy each has the ability to add a unique information perspective to the diagnostic case. The clinician is cautioned to be cognizant of the limitations of imaging and the unique benefits provided by other diagnostic studies.

Anatomy

Selected normal structures on PA and lateral chest radiographs are identified in the normal anatomy chapter of this book (see Chapter 6). Some common variants and misinterpretations are presented in Figures 21-5 to 21-10. The bony thorax consists of 12 thoracic vertebrae, 12 pairs of ribs with costal cartilages, and the sternum. The scapulae and clavicles are superimposed over the thorax on the PA chest radiograph. Individual muscles of the thorax generally are not discernible on radiographs. However, absence of large muscles,

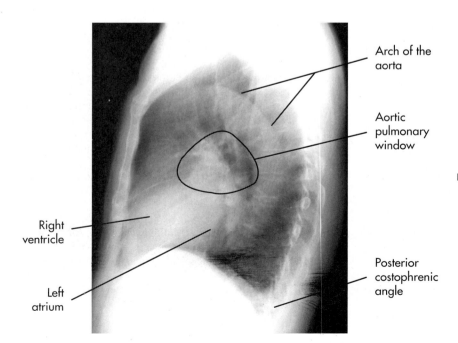

FIG. 21-2 Normal lateral chest.

Arch of the aorta

Aortic pulmonary window

Right ventricle

Left atrium

Posterior costophrenic angle

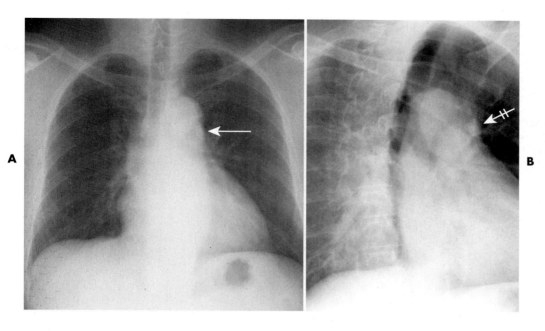

A

B

FIG. 21-3 By providing another angle to the anatomy, oblique views may present a clearer view of pulmonary, rib, or mediastinal lesions. **A,** There is a small radiodense lesion overlying the shadow of the descending aorta *(arrow)* on the posteroanterior chest film. **B,** Oblique projection casts the radiodense shadow of interest laterally *(crossed arrow),* allowing it to be more easily seen and, in this case, confirmed as a granuloma given the homogenous calcification.

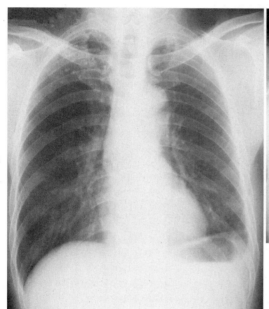

A

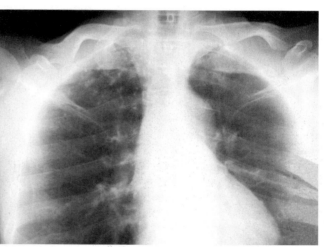

B

FIG. 21-4 Apical lordotic view reduces the interpretation distraction caused by the overlying ribs and clavicle on the anatomy of the lung apices. In this case, the small tuberculosis granulomas seen on, **A,** the posteroanterior projection are more clearly demonstrated on, **B,** the apical lordotic view. (Courtesy John A.M. Taylor, Seneca Falls, NY.)

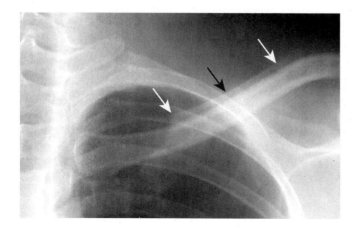

FIG. 21-5 Skin overlying the clavicle (companion shadow) causes a parallel density that should not be confused with a periosteal reaction *(arrows).*

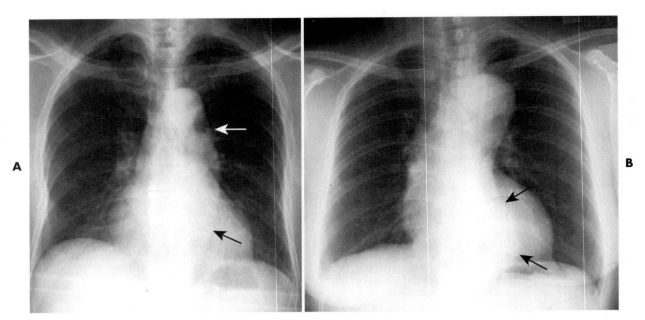

FIG. 21-6 **A** and **B,** With advancing age, supportive tissue laxity and increased thoracic kyphosis lead to an unwinding (alternatively described as unfolding or uncoiling) of the arch of the aorta. As a result, the thoracic aorta appears lengthened and more lateral than usual *(arrows)*. The appearance must be differentiated from an aneurysm or other mediastinal lesion. A tortuous aorta maintains the size of the vessel; therefore both the medial and lateral walls of the vessel deviate laterally together. By contrast, an aneurysm exhibits less deviation of the medial wall, defining the expanded vessel. Computed tomography may be needed to better define the appearance to exclude aneurysm.

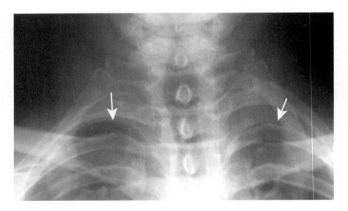

FIG. 21-7 Sickle-shaped, concave inferior soft-tissue shadows along the upper margins of the thoracic cavity usually represent normal brachiocephalic vessels. They may be unilateral or bilateral, and often are asymmetric *(arrows)*. For any apical shadow, prime consideration should be given to excluding a Pancoast lesion or mesothelioma. At times a similar but more focused appearance is caused by the subcostal muscles.

FIG. 21-8 Dextrocardia describes an anomalous presentation of a left-sided heart. It is usually found with reversal of other organ systems, a condition called *situs inversus*. Situs inversus may present as an isolated finding or as part of a larger syndrome, such as Kartagener syndrome. Kartagener syndrome describes the clinical triad of chronic sinusitis, bronchiectasis, and situs inversus. Deafness, infertility, and other clinical outcomes also are associated with the ciliary defects that mark this autosomal recessive syndrome.

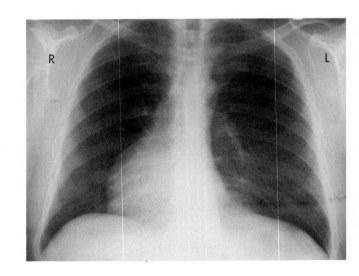

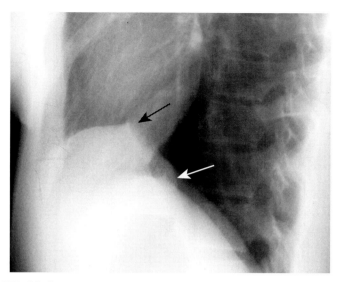

FIG. 21-9 A tent or nipple configuration of the diaphragm correlates to the attachment of the inferior pulmonary ligaments (arrows).

such as the pectorals, appears as a region of decreased density. The intercostal arteries, veins, and nerves pass along the inferior border of the ribs; enlargements of these structures may cause a characteristic erosion deformity of the inferior rib margin.

The thoracic cavity is divided into two pleural cavities surrounding a centrally located mediastinum (Fig. 21-11). The mediastinum is divided into four anatomic (superior, anterior, middle, and posterior) or three radiographic (anterior, middle, and posterior) areas, as depicted in Figure 21-12. The heart, great vessels, esophagus, thymus, and lymph tissues are all important structures contained within the mediastinum.

Visceral pleurae cover the lungs and line the pulmonary fissures; parietal pleurae line the inside of the pleural cavities. The largely potential pleural space created by these membranes may become enlarged by fluid accumulating in response to disease, known as *pleural effusion*. Visceral pleurae also line the pulmonary fissures. The right oblique and transverse fissures separate the right lung into three lobes (upper, middle, and inferior), and a left oblique fissure separates the left lung into two lobes (upper and lower) (Figs. 21-13 and 21-14).

Accessory lung fissures are noted occasionally. Inferior accessory lung fissures are the most common in autopsy studies but are difficult to recognize on radiographs. The rarer azygous fissures actually are more commonly seen on radiographs. About 1% of patients demonstrate an azygous fissure. The azygous fissure is created by the downward migration of the azygous vein, taking with it a portion of the apical parietal and visceral pleurae of the right upper lobe. It appears as a right-sided, thin, curvilinear structure of several centimeters, which ends inferiorly as a teardrop-shaped radiopacity, representing the invaginated azygous vein (Figs. 21-15 and 21-16). Azygous fissures are normal variants of no clinical significance. The portion of the right upper lobe that is medial to the fissure is termed an *azygous lobe*.

The lower trachea divides into two primary (main) bronchi, one directed to each lung. In addition, each lung is supplied by two pulmonary veins, a single pulmonary artery, a bronchial artery,

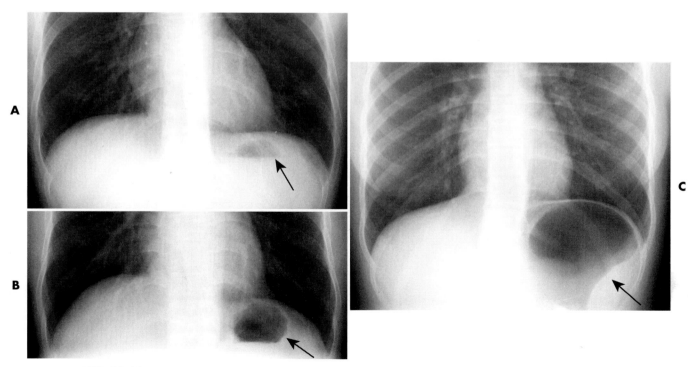

FIG. 21-10 Gastric air bubble. The gastric air bubble (or magenblase) is located subadjacent to the left hemidiaphragm. It normally exhibits, **A,** a flattened hemispheric shape but can enlarge, **B,** slightly or, **C,** extensively in relation to ingestion, especially of carbonated beverages (arrows). The location of the gastric air bubble is more critical than its size. For instance, the air bubble is displaced superiorly with a hiatal hernia or may displace medially with splenic enlargement.

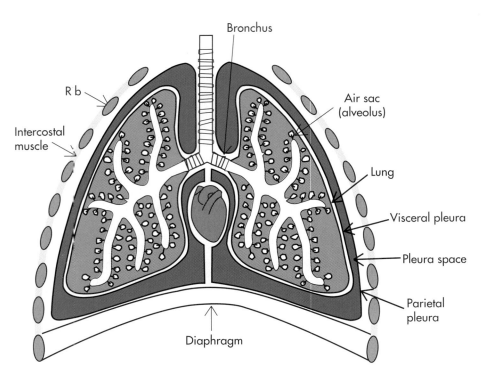

Bronchus

R b

Intercostal muscle

Air sac (alveolus)

Lung

Visceral pleura

Pleura space

Parietal pleura

Diaphragm

FIG. 21-11   The thoracic cavity consists of two pleural cavities and an interposed mediastinum.

and multiple nerves and lymph vessels. These structures enter the lung through the hilum (root of the lung). The hila are important areas to interpret. Serious pathology such as metastasis, lymphoma, and bronchogenic carcinoma has a propensity to involve these areas, as well as vascular disease such as pulmonary embolism. The left hilum typically is 1 to 3 cm higher than the right. Atelectasis or mass may distort this normal configuration. Each hilum should exhibit a branching pattern, appearing similar to a sideways tree. Lymphadenopathy may cause the hilum to appear more similar to a sideways shrub than a tree. In the lateral view, the right hilum is anterior to the left.

The arteries and bronchi follow a similar branching pattern within the lung, whereas the veins have an individual path. Reflecting gravitational forces, perfusion is greatest in the lower regions of the lung in the upright patient. This, coupled with the fact that the lung's base is thicker in an anteroposterior (AP) dimension than at its apex, accounts for the more prominent appearance of normal vascular markings in the lower regions of the lung.ˉ Increased perfusion also results in more blood-borne infections, metastasis, and pulmonary emboli occurring in the lower lung regions. Contrary to perfusion, ventilation is fairly uniform throughout the lung. Stable ventilation and relatively

FIG. 21-12   Mediastinal divisions. **I,** Anatomic divisions of the mediastinum include: *A,* Anterior; *B,* middle; *C,* posterior; and, *D,* superior. **II,** Roentgenometric divisions of the mediastinum include: *A,* Anterior; *B,* middle; and, *C,* posterior.

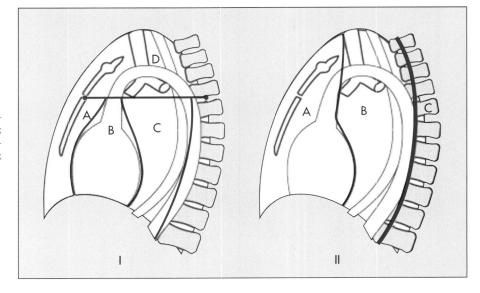

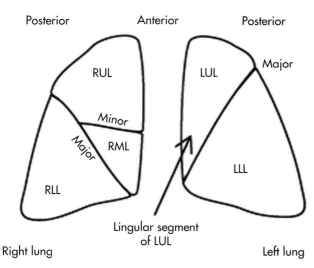

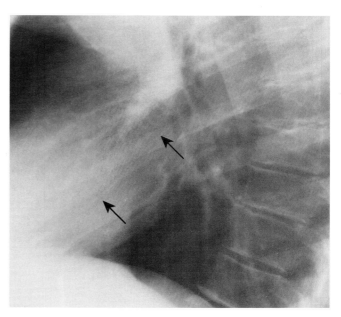

FIG. 21-13 The right lung is divided into three lobes. The right major (or oblique) fissure separates the right lower lobe *(RLL)* from the right middle lobe *(RML)*. The minor (or horizontal) fissure separates the RML from the right upper lobe *(RUL)*. The left major fissure separates the left upper lobe *(LUL)* from the left lower lobe *(LLL)*. The lingular segment of the left upper lobe is homologous to the right middle lobe. A left minor fissure is not found normally. The drawing above depicts each lung in its lateral view.

FIG. 21-14 The major and minor fissures usually are difficult to see. When present, they appear as very fine radiodense lines *(arrows)*. A portion of the major fissure is seen on this lateral chest view.

lower perfusion results in a higher Po₂ in the upper lung segments, possibly contributing to the predilection of tuberculosis reinfections in the upper regions of the lung.

AIRWAY

Each primary bronchus divides into secondary or lobar bronchi (two in the left lung and three in the right lung). The secondary bronchi further divide into tertiary or segmental bronchi, each supplying specific sectors of lung, termed *bronchopulmonary segments* (Fig. 21-17). The bronchial branching varies, but typically

8 to 25 generations of divisions exist.[8] Bronchial branching ends with the terminal or lobular bronchioles.

AIR-SPACE

The pulmonary region distal to the respiratory bronchiole is termed an *acinus* or *primary lobule*, representing the basic functional unit of respiration (Fig. 21-18). The aggregation of four to five primary lobules constitutes a secondary lobule. Secondary lobules are 1 to 2 cm in diameter and are separated from one another by connective tissue layers known as *interlobular septa*. Accessory pathways of communication exist between adjacent alveoli (pores of Kohn) and alveoli and distal bronchioles (canals of Lambert). Accessory communications influence the spread of disease through lung parenchyma.

Pulmonary lobules contain respiratory bronchioles, alveolar ducts, and alveolar sacs. The alveolar ducts and sacs are lined with

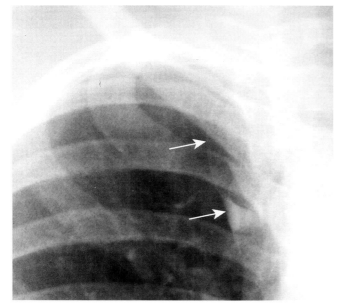

FIG. 21-15 Azygous fissure presenting as a curvilinear radiopaque line in the apex of the right upper lobe ending in a teardrop-shaped radiodensity *(arrows)*. (Courtesy C. Robert Tatum, Davenport, IA.)

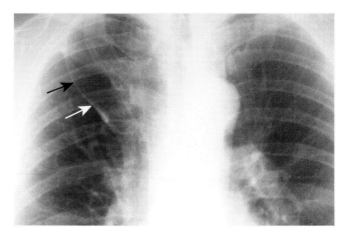

FIG. 21-16 Azygous fissure. This particular example is slightly more lateral than is typical *(arrows)*.

PART THREE Chest

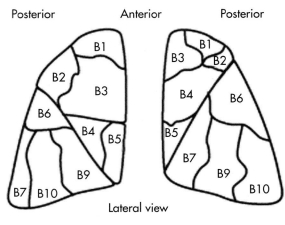

Posterior   Anterior   Posterior

Lateral view

Right lung   Left lung

Superior lobe

B1   Apical segment
B2   Posterior segment
B3   Anterior segment
B4   Lateral segment
B5   Medial segment

Inferior lobe

B6   Superior segment
B7   Posterior basal segment
B8   Anterior basal segment
B9   Medial basal segment
B10 Lateral basal segment

FIG. 21-17   The lung tissue distal to a tertiary bronchus is termed a *bronchopulmonary segment*. The segmental anatomy of the lung is important and relates to the localization and pathophysiology of lung disease. The divisions of the right and left lung with their corresponding Boyden number are presented. There is some variation in the division of bronchopulmonary segments. For instance, the apicoposterior segment of the left upper lobe and anteromedial basal segment of the left lower lobe may present together as one segment or separate into individual segments. The drawing above depicts the lateral view of each lung.

cup-shaped alveoli, functionally representing the area of gas exchange. Two types of epithelial cells, or pneumonocytes, line the alveoli. The type I pneumonocytes comprise 95% of the cell population. They are squamous cells, which lack the ability of mitosis. The second cell type, type II pneumonocytes, are cuboidal cells responsible for maintaining type I pneumonocytes and producing surfactant (a substance that reduces alveoli surface tension, maintaining an open alveolar sac).

Radiographically, the normally radiolucent lung tissue becomes radiopaque if the air within the acini is replaced by pathology of water density (e.g., blood, edema, exudate, tumor cells, proteins). The resulting radiopaque regions may be completely opaque if the alveolar filling is extensive (homogeneous or complete consolidation) or appears patchy and poorly defined if the alveolar filling is incomplete (heterogeneous or incomplete consolidation). Therefore consolidation is loss of air (replacement of air) in the alveolar space without overall loss in lung volume.

INTERSTITIUM

The interstitium, also termed *interstitial space,* provides a supporting framework for the delicate alveolar sacs. The interstitium comprises three freely communicating compartments: axial, parenchymal, and peripheral.[1] The axial (or peribronchovascular) space surrounds the primary bronchi and pulmonary artery as they enter the lung. The axial interstitium follows the bronchial and arterial branching, eventually becoming continuous with the interlobular septa, which separate adjacent secondary lobules. The parenchymal or alveolar interstitium provides delicate fibers to support the intralobular air-exchanging portion of the lung. The space between the visceral pleura and the lung parenchyma is

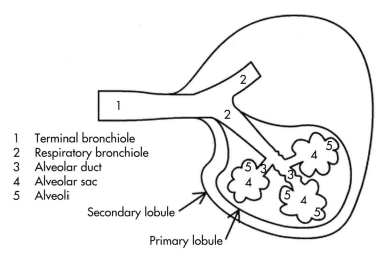

1   Terminal bronchiole
2   Respiratory bronchiole
3   Alveolar duct
4   Alveolar sac
5   Alveoli

Secondary lobule

Primary lobule

FIG. 21-18   The secondary lobule is the smallest structural segment of the lung that is enveloped within a connective tissue septum. Primary lobules (or acini) are within the secondary lobules and represent the pulmonary tissue distal to the respiratory bronchiole. The primary lobule is the basic functional unit of respiration, consisting of an alveolar duct, alveolar sac, and alveoli. Alveoli are cup-shaped structures formed within the alveolar sac. The primary lobule is the air-space of the lung. Disease processes that occupy a significant amount of the air-space of the lung appear cloudy and ill defined on the radiograph.

termed the *peripheral* (or *subpleural*) *interstitium* and sends strong supporting fibers to the parenchyma.

An explanation of the arrangement between the capillary and alveolus within the parenchymal interstitium is necessary to fully understand the radiographic appearance of interstitial and air-space patterns of lung disease. The cell junctions of the portion of the capillary walls that are in contact with alveoli are tight, maintaining the relative "dryness" of the alveoli by limiting fluid movement from the capillaries to the alveoli. In contrast, the capillary cell junctions are relatively loose where the capillary is not in contact with the alveoli. This allows a slow "drip" of fluid into the surrounding parenchymal interstitium (the space that separates the capillary from neighboring alveoli). Under normal circumstances, fluid entering the interstitium is balanced by the fluid reabsorbed into lymphatics. Because parenchymal interstitium does not contain lymphatics, the excessive fluid flows to the lymphatics of the adjacent axial and subpleural interstitium.

Normally the interstitium is not seen on radiographs. However, alterations in the amount of fluid entering the interstitium, impairment in the lymphatic clearing mechanism, or alterations in permeability of the capillary walls result in excessive fluid accumulation and distention of the interstitium, producing radiographic linear shadows. Moreover, the interstitium may become visible on the radiographs if it is distended by space-occupying lesions (e.g., blood, edema, pus, tumor) or thickened in response to such disorders as connective tissue disorders. Distention of the axial interstitium appears as peribronchial cuffing and perihilar haze; parenchymal interstitium relates a "ground glass" appearance, and the peripheral interstitium appears as thick pleura.

Radiographic Signs

Signs are useful clues to the presence of specific disease presentations. There are many radiographs signs related to chest radiography. Selected signs are presented in the following text.

AIR-BRONCHOGRAM SIGN

Intrapulmonary airways are not well seen on radiographs unless they appear on end. The thin air tubes are surrounded by the air-filled lung parenchyma and therefore are not well seen because of the lack of contrast. However, if the lung parenchyma is filled with pathology of water density, and the airways are not involved, they appear as lucent tubes traversing the region of lung consolidation. The presence of this sign is indicative of air-space pathology, usually pneumonia or pulmonary edema. Air-alveologram describes a similar concept of an air-filled lobule surrounded by consolidated parenchyma.

AIR CRESCENT SIGN

The air-crescent sign is a radiolucent defect at the periphery of a lung mass or spherical region of lung consolidation. The crescent represents a region of necrotizing cavitation or region around complicating pneumonia, commonly a fungal infection.

CERVICOTHORACIC SIGN

The cervicothoracic sign is based on the observation that an intrathoracic soft-tissue lesion is typically surrounded by air, hence its borders are well delineated. If the lesion extended into the soft tissues of the neck, that portion of the lesion's border would not be seen because it is continuous with the soft-tissue density (known as a *cervicothoracic sign*) (Fig. 21-19). Also, sometimes the sign is used to describe an apical location of a lesion. The apical segments of the upper lobes extend superior to the clavicles; therefore radiographic

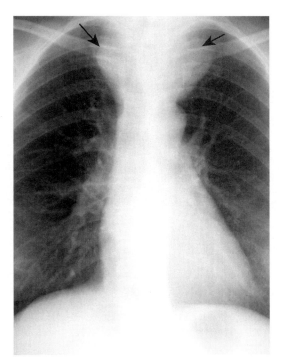

FIG. 21-19 Substernal thyroid presenting with a cervicothoracic sign. The superior edge of the mediastinal mass ends abruptly at the level of the clavicles (*arrows*). This appearance indicates that the mass is continuous with the anterior soft tissues of the neck (in this case a substernal thyroid) and not located in the pulmonary tissues. (Courtesy John A.M. Taylor, Seneca Falls, NY.)

shadows extending above the clavicle shadows are located posteriorly. Anterior structures entering the neck (e.g., brachiocephalic artery) are not seen above the clavicle shadows and appear cut off at the level of the clavicles. This is also the case for mediastinal lesions. For example, a mediastinal soft-tissue lesion that appears to extend superiorly above the clavicles must be retrotracheal and posteriorly situated. Conversely, a lesion effacing along its superior margin and not extending above the clavicles must be located anteriorly.

EXTRAPLEURAL SIGN

As lesions originating from the chest wall extend into the lung field, their extrapleural location is indicated by sloping, tapered superior and inferior margins denoting the inward deviation of the pleura. A completely intrapulmonary lesion would lack the tapered pleural tails (Fig. 21-20). An extrapleural lesion is characterized by a peripheral location, concave edges, and indistinct outer margin. Extrapleural signs are common with rib metastasis or fracture.

FALLEN LUNG SIGN

Fallen lung sign describes an inferior displacement of the lung, suggesting a fractured bronchus.

FIGURE 3 SIGN

A "3" configuration develops along the outer contour of the proximal descending aorta with coarctation of the aorta.

FLAT WAIST SIGN

The flat waist sign refers to a flattened appearance of the aortic knob and pulmonary trunk occurring as a result of left lower lobe collapse.

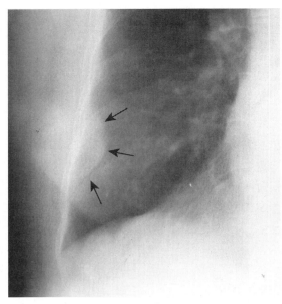

FIG. 21-20 Extrapleural sign denotes the appearance of a convex expansion into the lung field from the chest wall. It is marked by tapering margins, simulating the appearance of something shoved under a rug (arrows).

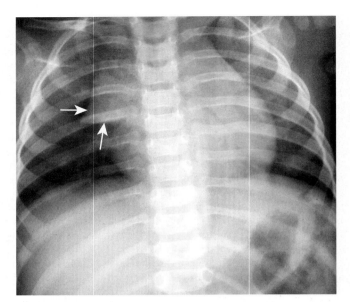

FIG. 21-21 Sail sign denotes the right lower margin of the thymus in infants (arrows).

GLOVED FINGER SIGN

Bronchial impaction appears as a longitudinal radiodensity. Impaction is seen in asthmatics and allergic bronchopulmonary aspergillosis.

HILUM OVERLAY SIGN

The hilum overlay sign is used to distinguish a true hilar lesion from a pulmonary lesion located in front of or behind the hilum, appearing as a hilar lesion on the PA radiograph. Normally the pulmonary artery of the hilum is well defined. The pulmonary artery is poorly defined if a true hilar mass is present (e.g., lymphadenopathy). A hilum overlay sign is present when the apparent hilar mass continues to reveal a well-defined pulmonary artery, indicating that the lesion is superimposed.

"S" SIGN OF GOLDEN

Collapse of the right upper lobe promotes a superior migration of the horizontal fissure. The medial portion of the displaced fissure may be bulged inferiorly by a hilar mass, causing the fissure to have a slanted and reversed "S" configuration.

SAIL SIGN

The thymus enlarges during the first few months of life. The right lobe of the enlarged thymus may project laterally along the superior right margin of the mediastinum. The appearance has been likened to a ship's sail (Fig. 21-21).

SILHOUETTE SIGN

The silhouette sign was popularized by Felson,[4] who summarized the concept as follows: "An intrathoracic lesion touching a border of the heart, aorta, or diaphragm will obliterate that border on the roentgenogram. An intrathoracic lesion not anatomically contiguous with a border of one of these structures will not obliterate that border." Loss of the anatomic border is described as a positive silhouette sign.[3] Obscuring lesions may be large or small, positioned within or outside of the lung (Fig. 21-22).

Structures are visualized on the radiograph because they are contiguous with another structure of different density. For instance, the right heart border is seen because it is contiguous with the air-filled right middle lobe. If pathology of similar density to that of the heart filled the right middle lobe, the right heart border would be lost, creating a positive silhouette sign. Absence of anatomic borders aids in localizing lesions within the chest. In general, the left heart border is adjacent to the lingula of the left upper lobe, the right heart border is adjacent to the right middle lobe, the diaphragm is adjacent to the inferior lobes, the ascending aorta is next to the anterior segment of the right upper lobe, and the aortic arch is next to the apical segment of the left upper lobe. Loss of these borders suggests adjacent pathology.

Pattern Recognition

Generally it is more efficient to group abnormal radiographic findings into "patterns of disease" than to describe or conclude on each finding individually. The concept of grouping radiographic findings into patterns of chest disease has been advocated by other authors* and certainly predates this publication.

The radiographic appearance of parenchymal disease of the lung is commonly dichotomized into air-space and interstitial patterns (Figs. 21-23 and 21-24). *Air-space, alveolar,* and *consolidation* are all terms used to describe the poorly marginated parenchymal opacities that follow space-taking lesions within the alveolar sacs. The opacities have a tendency to coalesce and most commonly are segmental or lobar in distribution. Air-alveolograms and air-bronchograms are characteristic, appearing respectively as radiolucent spheres or tubes within the consolidated lung. Diffuse interstitial disease appears as linear, reticular, nodular, or reticulonodular patterns of pulmonary disease. A reticular pattern appears as a "net" overlying the lung. The net may be fine or coarse, as in

---

*References 4, 5, 7, 10–13, 15.

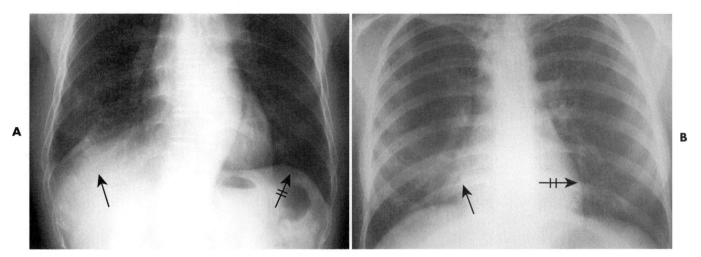

FIG. 21-22 The silhouette sign is used to localize air-space disease in the lung. **A,** Notice that the superior margin of the patient's right (reading left) hemidiaphragm is not clearly demarcated *(arrow),* as it is on the contralateral side *(crossed arrow).* This is a positive silhouette sign because the hemidiaphragm's silhouette is obscured by adjacent air-space disease (in this case, pneumonia of the right lower lobe). **B,** Second example with pneumonia of the right middle lobe *(arrow).* Because the right middle lobe is in contact with the right heart border, the heart border is not seen when the air of the right middle lobe becomes replaced with pneumonia (compare with the normal appearance of the left heart border *(crossed arrow).* In other words, the heart border typically is seen clearly because it is surrounded by air within the right middle lobe on the right and lingula of the left upper lobe on the left. If the air density of either region is replaced (e.g., by pneumonia), the border of the heart is obscured.

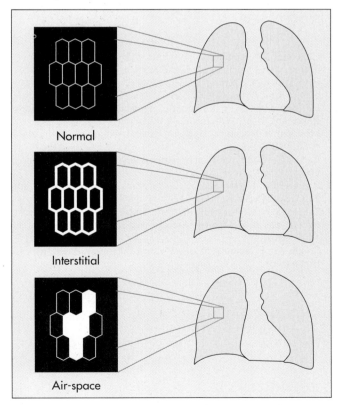

FIG. 21-23 Disease of the lung parenchyma can be categorized as air-space or interstitial. Air-space disease describes the presence of water-based pathology (e.g., tumor, infection, hemorrhage, edema) within the alveolar sacs, causing consolidation. An interstitial pattern of lung disease results from thickening of the connective tissues of the lung (e.g., rheumatoid arthritis) or water-based pathology within the interstitial space (e.g., Kerley's lines of pulmonary edema), causing a thickened linear or "honeycomb" appearance.

"honeycomb" lung, which represents end-stage lung fibrosis. Small, well-circumscribed, homogenous nodules occur alone or may accompany the linear shadows; the latter presentation denotes a reticulonodular pattern.

Although patterns of lung disease are largely descriptive in nature, some degree of radiologic–pathologic correlation exists. In other words, it is possible to anatomically localize pathology to either an interstitial or air-space location based on the radiographic appearance.[8] For instance, a poorly defined region of incomplete consolidation in the peripheral lung field is consistent with an air-space pattern of disease. This is not solely a descriptive "tag"; the appearance most often correlates to pathology within the "air-space" of the lung. Unfortunately, this is not always the case. The alveolar stages of sarcoidosis appear as fluffy, ill-defined, air-space filling of the lung, but they actually represent granulomatous deposits within the interstitium, not the air-space of the lung.

A more accurate assessment of the underlying pulmonary disease is obtained when the radiographic patterns are combined with clinical information. The pattern's chronicity, complexity, severity, and correlation to clinical findings aid in determining the significance and lead to a narrowed list of possibilities. At the very least they suggest which follow-up examination should be applied to provide the missing information.

The chest section continues the general theme of this book. Radiographic abnormalities are grouped into common radiographic patterns. Each pattern lists diseases that are commonly associated with the radiographic appearance and provides short descriptions of each listing to aid in differential diagnosis between listings. The second portion of the chest section comprises chapters presenting detailed descriptions of some of the more commonly encountered disease entities that are listed with each pattern.

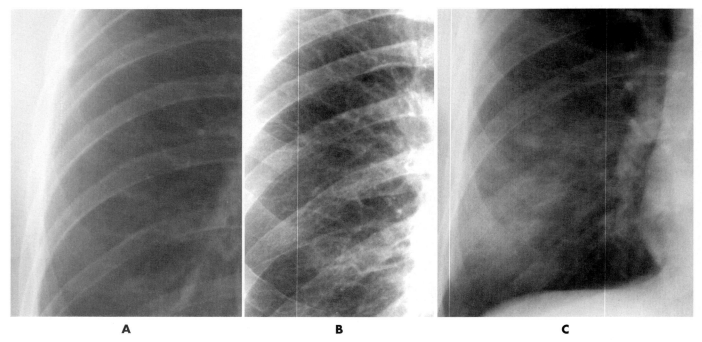

A   **B**   **C**

FIG. 21-24 A, Normally the pulmonary tissue is radiolucent with interspersed radiodense bronchovascular markings. Disease of the lung parenchyma can be broadly divided into, **B** that affecting the interstitial connective tissue, producing a thickened linear appearance, and, **C,** that affecting the air-space of the lung, yielding a hazy, cloudy, diffusely radiodense appearance.

References

1. Bachofen H, Bachofen M, Weibel ER: Ultrastructural aspects of pulmonary edema, *J Thorac Imaging* 3:1, 1988.
2. Burgener FA, Kormano M: Differential diagnosis in conventional radiology, New York, 1991, Thomas.
3. Felson B, Felson H: Localization of intrathoracic lesions by means of the posteroanterior roentgenogram, the silhouette sign, *Radiology* 55:363, 1955.
4. Felson B: A new look at pattern recognition of diffuse pulmonary diseases, *AJR Am J Roentgenol* 133:183, 1979.
5. Felson B: Chest roentgenology, Philadelphia, 1973, WB Saunders.
6. Felson B: The roentgen diagnosis of disseminated pulmonary alveolar diseases, *Semin Roentgenol* 2:3, 1967.
7. Fraser RG, Pare JAP: Tables of differential diagnosis and decision trees. In Fraser RG, Pare JAP, editors: Diagnosis of diseases of the chest, ed 2, Philadelphia, 1979, WB Saunders.
8. Genereux GP: Pattern recognition in diffuse lung disease: a review of theory and practice, *Med Radiog Photog* 61:2, 1985.
9. Horsfield K, Cumming G: Morphology of the bronchial tree in man, *J Appl Physiol* 24:373, 1968.
10. Lillington GA: A diagnostic approach to chest diseases, Baltimore, 1987, Williams & Wilkins.
11. Meschan I: Roentgen signs in clinical diagnosis, Philadelphia, 1956, WB Saunders.
12. Reed JC: Chest radiology: patterns and differential diagnosis, Chicago, 1981, Year Book.
13. Reeder MM: Reeder and Felson's gamuts in radiology, New York, 1993, Springer-Verlag.
14. Sagel SS et al: Efficacy of routine screening and lateral chest radiographs in a hospital-based population, *N Engl J Med* 291:1001, 1974.
15. Simon G: Principles of chest x-ray diagnosis, London, 1956, Butterworth.

chapter 22

Diseases of the Airways

DENNIS M. MARCHIORI

Atelectasis
Bronchial Asthma
Bronchiectasis
Bronchopulmonary Sequestration
Congenital Bronchogenic Cysts
Emphysema

Atelectasis

BACKGROUND

General. Atelectasis is defined as incomplete air filling and underexpansion of pulmonary tissue. It should be distinguished from consolidation, which also represents incomplete air filling of the lung. However, in consolidation, the missing air is replaced by blood, edema, pus, or another space-occupying substance, whereas missing air of an atelectatic region is not replaced, resulting in segmental collapse. Atelectasis may involve the entire lung or appear localized to a lobe, segment, or subsegment of the lung. It is not a disease itself, but rather a radiographic sign suggesting the presence of another pathology. Based on the underlying mechanism, atelectasis is divided into five categories: obstructive, passive, compressive, adhesive, and cicatrization.

Obstructive atelectasis. The first and most common type of atelectasis is termed obstructive or resorptive atelectasis. It is caused by intrinsic or extrinsic obstruction of an airway by such phenomena as neoplasm, infection, foreign body, and heavy secretions.[2,6] Over time, air distal to the airway obstruction is resorbed and not replaced, leading to an airless, radiolucent, collapsed portion of lung tissue (Figs. 22-1 through 22-6). Often the lung distal to bronchial obstruction exhibits increased radiopacity correlating to replacement of the alveolar air with inflammatory transudate, exudate, or other substance. Less commonly, a check-valve or obstruction develops, creating a hyperlucent, overinflated portion of lung tissue.

A check-valve mechanism involves accumulation of air distal to an airway obstruction. Airways dilate during inhalation, permitting air to pass by a partial bronchial obstruction. Airways constrict tightly around an obstruction during exhalation, effectively limiting the expiration of air distal to the obstruction. With each breathing cycle, more air is "pumped" into the overinflated lung tissue distal to the obstruction. Check-valve obstructions in a small airway are of limited clinical significance; however, they may result in respiratory distress when present in a large airway.

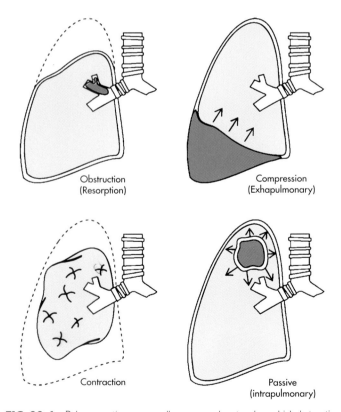

FIG. 22-1 Pulmonary tissue may collapse secondary to a bronchial obstruction (obstructive), expanding intrapleural lesion (passive), expanding intrapulmonary lesion (compressive), and scarring contracture of the lung tissue (cicatrization). A fifth type, adhesive, is less common and presents in infants with hyaline membrane disease.

1143

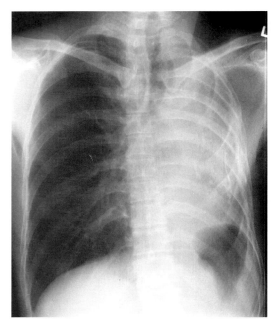

FIG. 22-2 Collapse of the patient's left lung with proximal shift of the patient's left hemidiaphragm, heart, and trachea. (Courtesy John A.M. Taylor, Seneca Falls, NY.)

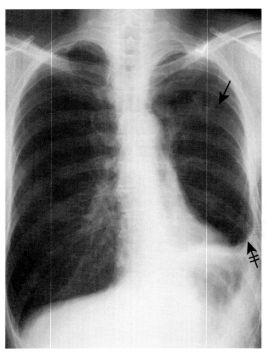

FIG. 22-3 A 53-year-old male patient with a fracture of the left sixth rib *(arrow)*. The elevated left hemidiaphragm suggests volume loss of the left lung. Also, blunting of the lateral costophrenic angle denotes pleural effusion *(crossed arrow)*. (Courtesy John A.M. Taylor, Seneca Falls, NY.)

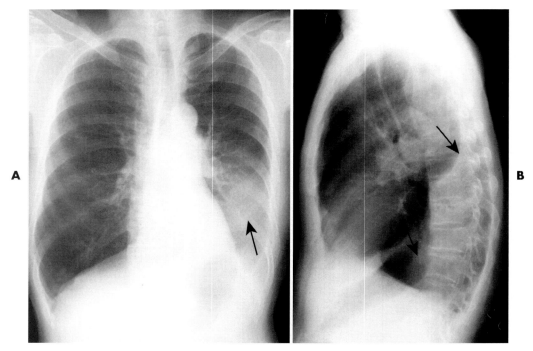

FIG. 22-4 **A,** Atelectasis of the left lower lobe presenting as a hazy radiodense shadow in the left lower margin of the lung field *(arrow)* and, **B,** posterior shift of the oblique fissure *(arrows)*. (Courtesy John A.M. Taylor, Seneca Falls, NY.)

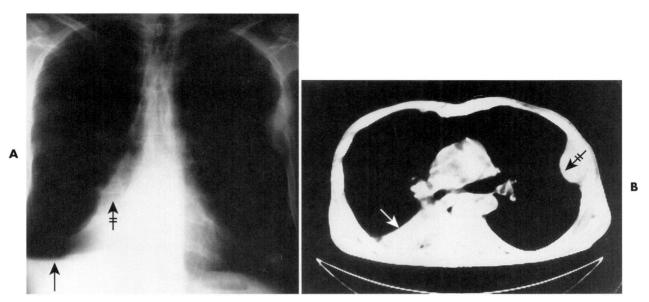

FIG. 22-5 Obstructive atelectasis of the right middle and lower lobe. **A,** The plain film radiograph demonstrates an elevated right hemidiaphragm *(arrow)* and loss of the silhouette of the right heart border *(crossed arrow).* **B,** Computed tomography reveals an airless lung mass in the right costal angle *(arrow)* and left rib mass, representing costal metastasis *(crossed arrow).*

Passive atelectasis. Passive (relaxation) atelectasis is the second type of atelectasis and results from the presence of a space-occupying lesion external to the lung. Pleural fluid (blood, exudate, transudate, and chyle) or air may accumulate to such an extent that the adjacent lung is "pushed" aside, resulting in partial or complete pulmonary collapse. Diaphragmatic elevation or herniation of abdominal viscera also may compress the lung. The amount of collapse is proportional to the size of the space-taking lesion.

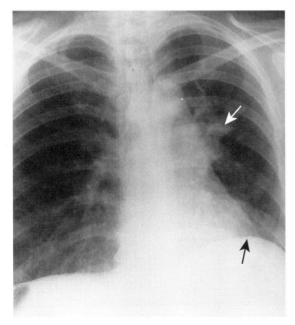

FIG. 22-6 Tracheal carcinoma with left hilar mass *(white arrow)* and partial obstructive atelectasis of the left lung and elevation of the left hemidiaphragm *(black arrow).* (Courtesy Steven P. Brownstein, MD, Springfield, NJ.)

Compressive atelectasis. Compressive atelectasis is a form of passive atelectasis in which the space-taking lesion is located within the involved lung. Large bullae, neoplasms, abscesses, and other large lesions may result in compressive atelectasis of adjacent lung tissue.

Adhesive atelectasis. Adhesive atelectasis refers to the non-obstructive, noncompressive pulmonary collapse secondary to decreased surfactant production by the type II pneumonocytes.[31] Pneumonocyte damage results from genetic defects, general anesthesia, ischemia, or radiation damage. Adhesive atelectasis is seen in neonates afflicted with hyaline membrane disease.

Cicatrization atelectasis. Finally, cicatrization atelectasis represents scarring and contracture of pulmonary tissue after infection, pneumoconioses, scleroderma, radiation, idiopathic pulmonary fibrosis, and so on. This condition may appear localized (tuberculosis in the lung apices) or generalized (interstitial pulmonary fibrosis).

IMAGING FINDINGS

The presence of atelectasis is suggested by direct and indirect radiographic signs (Box 22-1). Displacements of intralobar fissures are the most reliable findings. The radiographic appearance differs based on the degree of lung involvement, location, and type of atelectasis (Table 22-1). Combined lobar collapse may complicate the radiographic appearance.[16] Rounded atelectasis is a form of peripheral pulmonary collapse that must be differentiated from similarly appearing neoplastic masses.[20,32]

CLINICAL COMMENTS

Whenever atelectasis is noted, it should prompt a vigorous search for a cause. Although several mechanisms of collapse have been identified, obstruction of the airway resulting from neoplasm is a common cause of lobar or segmental atelectasis that should direct patient management.

BOX 22-1
Direct and Indirect Signs of Lobar Atelectasis

Direct signs
Displacement of interlobular fissures
Increased radiopacity*

Indirect signs
Elevation of the diaphragm
Mediastinal displacement
Hilar displacement
Overinflation of remaining normal lung
Approximation of pulmonary vessels
Approximation of ribs

*Some sources consider increased radiopacity an indirect sign of atelectasis.

KEY CONCEPTS
- *Atelectasis is a sign of underlying disease process, defined as incomplete inflation of the lung.*
- *The five categories of atelectasis are obstructive, compressive, passive, adhesive, and cicatrization. Obstructive is the most common.*
- *The radiographic appearance depends on the location and extent of collapse; findings include loss of pulmonary volume, increased radiopacity, and distorted anatomic structures.*

Bronchial Asthma

BACKGROUND
Bronchial asthma is characterized by widespread, episodic, reversible narrowing of the airways resulting from smooth muscle spasm, mucosal edema, or excess mucus in the lumen of the bronchi and bronchioles. A wide variety of inciting factors have been identified, including the following: exercise, infection, pharmaceuticals, and hypersensitivity to known allergens, such as pollen, animal fur, and fungi.

IMAGING FINDINGS
Early in the disease process no imaging findings are evident between acute episodes of the disease. However, radiographs taken at the time of an acute attack demonstrate increased radiolucency secondary to general lung overinflation and depression of the diaphragm.[21,23] Patients who suffer from chronic asthma attacks may demonstrate increased prominence of the central interstitial markings and, when projected on end, bronchial wall thickening greater than 1 mm.[13,18] The radiographic findings may be complicated by the presence of infection or mucous plugs resulting in atelectasis[5] (Fig. 22-7) or consolidation.[3]

CLINICAL COMMENTS
Asthma attacks are characterized by wheezing, prolonged expiration phases of respiration, dyspnea, and cough.[1] Asthma may be complicated by pneumonia, pneumomediastinum, pneumothorax, emphysema, and mucous plugs in the airway.

KEY CONCEPTS
- *Asthma is a common condition marked by well-defined clinical symptoms.*
- *The radiographic appearance varies from normal to increased radiolucency of lung fields secondary to overinflation.*
- *The chronicity, nature of the attacks, and presence of complicating infection influence the radiographic appearance.*

TABLE 22-1
Radiographic Appearance of Atelectasis

Atelectasis	Imaging findings
Lung	Opacification of the entire hemithorax, compensatory shift of the mediastinum with overinflation and herniation of opposite lung toward collapsed lung side
Lobe*	
Right upper lobe	Radiodense lobe displaced superomedially, superiorly displaced diaphragm, oblique and horizontal fissures; can see the characteristic reversed "S-shape of Golden sign"[10] when a central mass is found in combination with the displaced horizontal fissure
Right middle lobe	Best demonstrated on the lateral projection, where the minor and major fissure approximate one another, bordering a thin, oblique-to-horizontal density; loss of silhouette of the left heart border on the frontal projection; on frontal projection, lordotic projection best for visualizing a wedge-shaped density with base adjacent to heart border
Right lower lobe	Radiodense lobe displaced posteromedially with posterior displacement of oblique fissure noted on lateral projection
Left upper lobe	Radiodense lobe displaced anterolaterally with overinflation of lower lobe occasionally located between collapsed upper lobe and mediastinum, "Luftsichel" sign[35]
Left lower lobe	Radiodense lobe displaced posteromedially, often obstructed by heart shadow; posterior displacement of the oblique fissure on the lateral projection
Segment	Increased radiodensity and volume loss that correspond to region collapsed and appear less marked than lobe involvement
Subsegment	Also known as *platelike, discoid,* or *linear atelectasis;* represents peripheral atelectasis of small areas of pulmonary tissue appearing as 2 to 10 cm horizontal linear density in the lower lung field
Round (folded lung)	Rare form of atelectasis associated with asbestosis-related pleural disease, in which the involved lung appears as a round mass (2 to 7 cm) in the lower lung

*Multiple lobes may be collapsed, yielding a combination of findings.

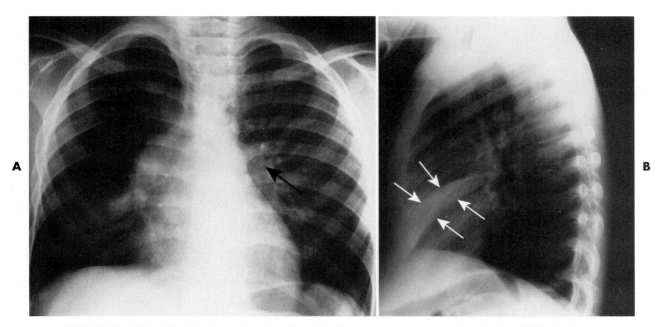

FIG. 22-7 Right middle lobe obstructive atelectasis resulting from a mucous plug in an asthmatic patient. **A,** The right heart border is poorly demarcated because it is in contact with the collapsed lobe (arrow). **B,** The collapsed lobe appears as a triangular density with the apex anchored at the hilum in the lateral projection (arrows). (Courtesy Steven P. Brownstein, MD, Springfield, NJ.)

Bronchiectasis

BACKGROUND

Bronchiectasis is chronic, irreversible dilation of bronchi or bronchioles that occurs as a sequela of inflammatory disease,[11,12] obstruction, or congenital alteration in either the smooth muscle or cartilage of an airway. The disease may be localized (e.g., tuberculosis) or generalized (e.g., cystic fibrosis) and predominates in the lower lobes. Based on the macroscopic appearance, cylindrical, varicose, and saccular forms of the disease have been described (Table 22-2).[25]

TABLE 22-2 Types of Bronchiectasis	
Type	**Macroscopic and high-resolution computed tomography appearance**
Cylindrical (tubular)	Mild form, mild bronchial dilatation ("tram lines," "signet ring"), normal branching of tracheobronchial tree
Varicose	Moderate bronchial dilatation with intervening constrictions producing a "beaded" appearance, reduced branching of tracheobronchial tree
Saccular (cystic)	Severe form, grossly dilatated bronchi ("string of cysts"), greatly reduced branching of tracheobronchial tree, reduced functional lung parenchyma

IMAGING FINDINGS

Imaging findings include alterations in lung volume and thickened bronchial walls, which appear as linear or cystic radiopacities as depicted in Figures 22-8 and 22-9.[11] The computed tomography (CT) and bronchography appearance is more specific and may be characteristic of a morphologic type (Table 22-2).

CLINICAL COMMENTS

Patients with localized bronchiectasis may have little or no pulmonary impairment. The patient may exhibit shortness of breath and wheezing in the more generalized form. The most common associated clinical finding is a chronic cough with purulent expectorant. Often hemoptysis and clubbing of the fingers are present.[7]

KEY CONCEPTS

- Bronchiectasis is chronic dilation of the airways secondary to infection, obstruction, or congenital structural defects.
- Bronchiectasis may be categorized into cylindrical, varicose, and saccular types.
- Each type is associated with alterations of bronchial branching and linear or cystic radiodensities.
- The radiographic appearance is nonspecific. Characteristic findings are seen with high-resolution computed tomography and bronchography.

Bronchopulmonary Sequestration

BACKGROUND

Bronchopulmonary sequestration represents congenital malformation of the foregut, resulting in a portion of lung that is not connected to the tracheobronchial tree (Fig. 22-10).[8] The sequestered segment of lung retains its embryonic systemic blood supply and may be found within (intralobar) or, less commonly, outside (extralobar) of the lung's pleural envelope.[27]

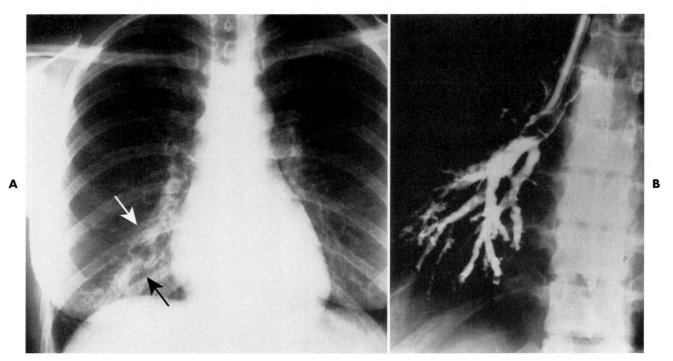

FIG. 22-8 A, Bronchiectasis appearing as prominent, thick bronchial markings in the right paracardiac region of the lung *(arrows)*. **B,** Bronchogram demonstrating ectasia and irregularity of the bronchi.

IMAGING FINDINGS

An extralobar sequestration appears as a dense mass located immediately above or within the left hemidiaphragm in 90% of cases. Less frequent locations include mediastinum, pericardial, and retroperitoneal spaces. By contrast, 60% of intralobar sequestrations are found on the right and may appear dense or cystic if infection has formed communication with the bronchial tree.[19]

Intralobar lesions rarely are found in the upper regions of the lung.[14]

CLINICAL COMMENTS

Extralobar sequestered regions of lung are asymptomatic, incidental findings. Intralobar types often represent areas of recurrent infection.

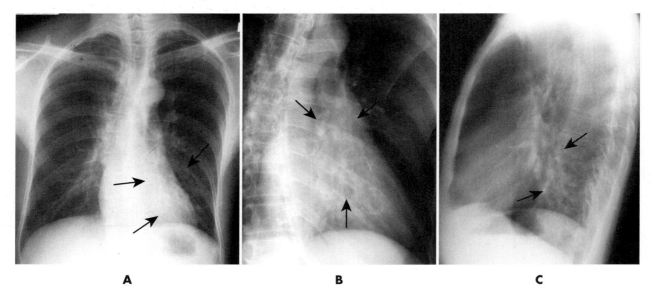

FIG. 22-9 A through **C,** Bronchiectasis exhibits a thickened, radiodense appearance of the normal bronchial pattern. In this 45-year-old male patient. The appearance is noted in the lower medial region of the patient's left (reading right) field *(arrows).* (**A** through **C,** Courtesy John A.M. Taylor, Seneca Falls, NY.)

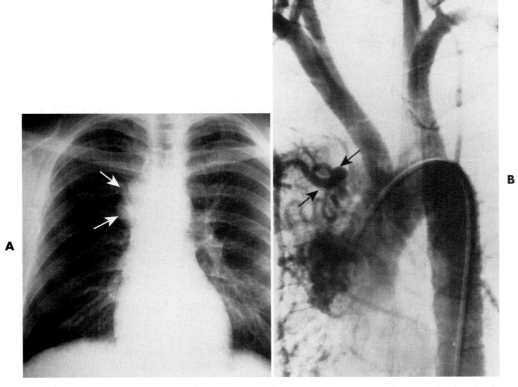

FIG. 22-10   A, Extralobar pulmonary sequestration appearing as a solid mass in the right paratracheal region *(arrows).* **B**, The angiogram demonstrates an anomalous systemic blood supply to the sequestration *(arrows).* (Courtesy Steven P. Brownstein, MD, Springfield, NJ.)

KEY CONCEPTS

- *Bronchopulmonary sequestration results in a nonfunctioning segment of lung not connected to the bronchopulmonary tree.*
- *Intralobar location is more common than extralobar, and it may represent an area of recurrent infection.*
- *Extralobar location is an incidental finding.*

Congenital Bronchogenic Cysts

BACKGROUND

Bronchogenic cysts represent anomalous outpouching of the primitive foregut. The outpouchings become separated from the tracheobronchial tree, but unlike bronchopulmonary sequestrations do not undergo further tissue development. Bronchogenic cysts do not communicate with the tracheobronchial tree. The mediastinum contains 80%, and 20% are in a pulmonary, hilar,[24,30] or ectopic location.[22]

IMAGING FINDINGS

The radiographic appearance is that of a well-defined mass in the mediastinum, hilum, or lung (Fig. 22-11). Bronchogenic cysts are typically in close proximity to the large airways. An air-filled cystic appearance may follow infection and result in communication between the cyst and tracheobronchial tree. The cyst's thin wall aids in its differentiation from an abscess. Calcification is unusual.

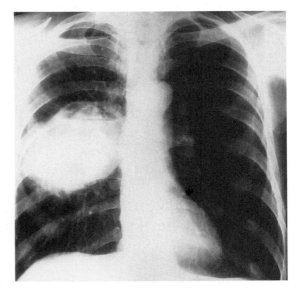

FIG. 22-11   Fluid-filled bronchogenic cyst. (Courtesy Steven P. Brownstein, MD, Springfield, NJ.)

CLINICAL COMMENTS

Infants may exhibit respiratory distress secondary to extrinsic airway obstruction.[9] Typically they are asymptomatic in the adult.[15]

Emphysema

BACKGROUND

Emphysema is defined as chronic dilatation of the air space distal to a terminal bronchiole, an area known as a *secondary lobule*. The acinar walls are destroyed, leading to large aggregate air spaces, effectively decreasing the number of acini. Little or no evidence of fibrosis is present.[29] In Table 22-3, emphysema is classified into structural types based on the portion of the acinus most affected. Several types may coexist in the same patient.

Bullae are a prominent feature of emphysema. Bullae represent parenchymal collections of air resulting from advanced tissue destruction and are associated with emphysema, Marfan's syndrome, Ehlers-Danlos syndrome, human immunodeficiency virus infection, intravenous drug use, and others. Typically they are in a subpleural location and vary from a few centimeters to a lobe or larger in size. Many use the term *bleb* interchangeably with bulla; however, *bleb* should be reserved for much smaller interstitial collections of air, typically in a peripheral, subpleural location. Bullous emphysema describes the condition of patients with emphysema in whom bullae are a prominent feature of the radiographic presentation. Spontaneous pneumothorax may result from ruptured blebs and bullae.

TABLE 22-3
Structural Types of Emphysema

Type	Comments
Centrilobular	Upper lobes, patchy distribution, associated with chronic bronchitis and smoking, involves center of pulmonary acinus
Panacinar	Lower lobes, homogenous distribution, associated with alpha 1-antitrypsin deficiency and smoking, involves all of pulmonary acinus
Distal acinar (paraseptal)	Along septal lines, peripheral distribution, associated with smoking, involves distal portion of acinus
Irregular (paracicatricial)	No consistent distribution, associated with lung fibrosis, irregular involvement of the acinus

IMAGING FINDINGS

The most prominent radiographic findings result from lung overinflation, which manifests as increased pulmonary radiolucency and a bilaterally flat, depressed hemidiaphragm (below the anterior portion of the seventh rib or the posterior portion of the tenth rib),[17,34] increased retrosternal space (>4.5 cm on the lateral film measured from a point 3 cm below the sternal angle),[28] accentuated kyphosis, and increased intercostal spaces (Figs. 22-12 through 22-16). The number of vessels is decreased in emphysemic tissue. The central pulmonary arteries are more prominent and appear truncated peripherally. Increased prominence of the interstitial markings often is present.[4,33] Bullae may appear as

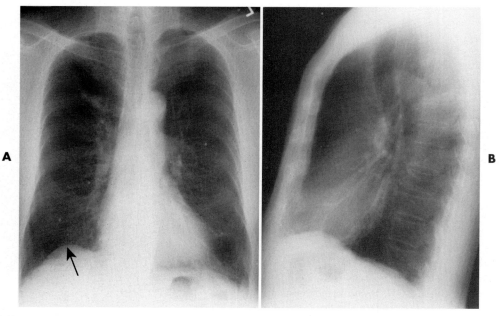

FIG. 22-12   A and **B,** Emphysema marked by hyperinflation, oligemic upper lung fields, prominent truncated pulmonary arteries, enlarged retrosternal clear space, obtuse sternodiaphragmatic angle, and depressed and flattened hemidiaphragms. Incidentally, partial congenital eventration of the right hemidiaphragm is noted *(arrow).* (Courtesy John A.M. Taylor, Seneca Falls, NY.)

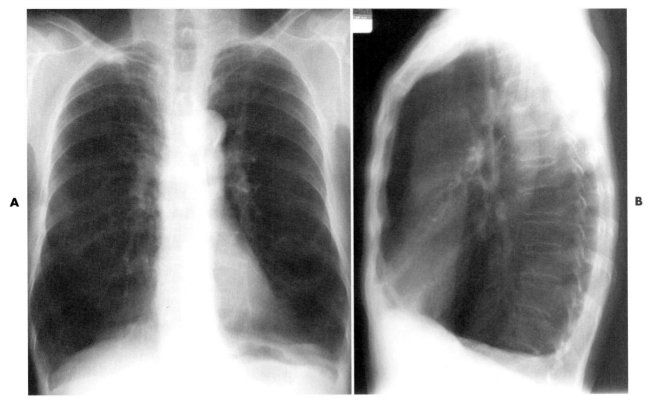

FIG. 22-13 **A** and **B,** The characteristic features of emphysema are noted in this case, including flat, depressed hemidiaphragms, thin heart shadow, prominent hilar vasculature, more radiolucent lung fields, wide intercostal spaces, and an increased retrosternal clear space. (Courtesy John A.M. Taylor, Seneca Falls, NY.)

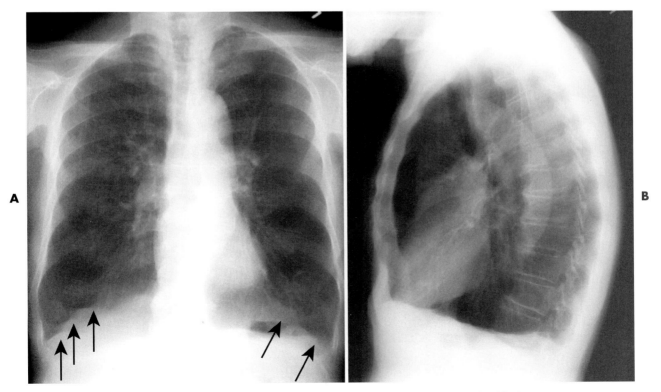

FIG. 22-14 **A** and **B,** An 83-year-old male patient with emphysema. At times, the depressed hemidiaphragm may appear rippled or scalloped in the posteroanterior view as in this case (arrows). (Courtesy John A.M. Taylor, Seneca Falls, NY.)

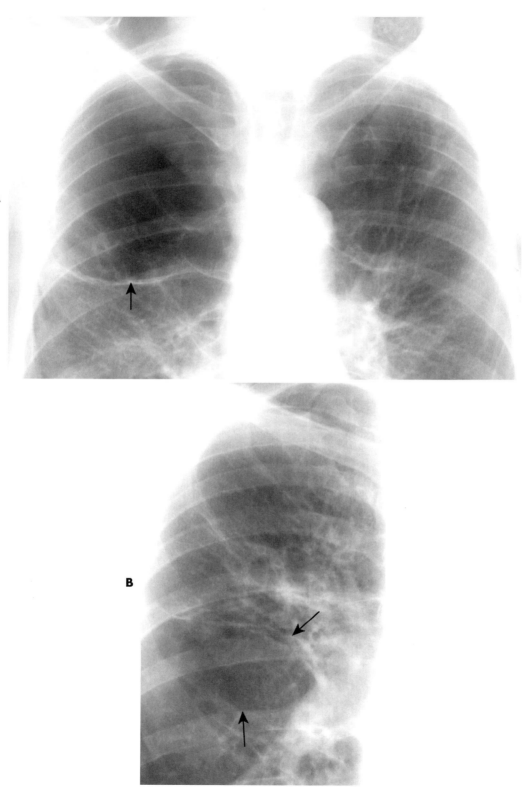

FIG. 22-15   A and **B,** Two cases of men in their early sixties. Both patients exhibit extensive bullae formation within the apices of the lungs. The bullae appear as thin-walled air sacs within the lung *(arrow)*. Small bullae formations are difficult to see on radiographs. In some patients, bullae may be surgically resected in an attempt to improve pulmonary function.

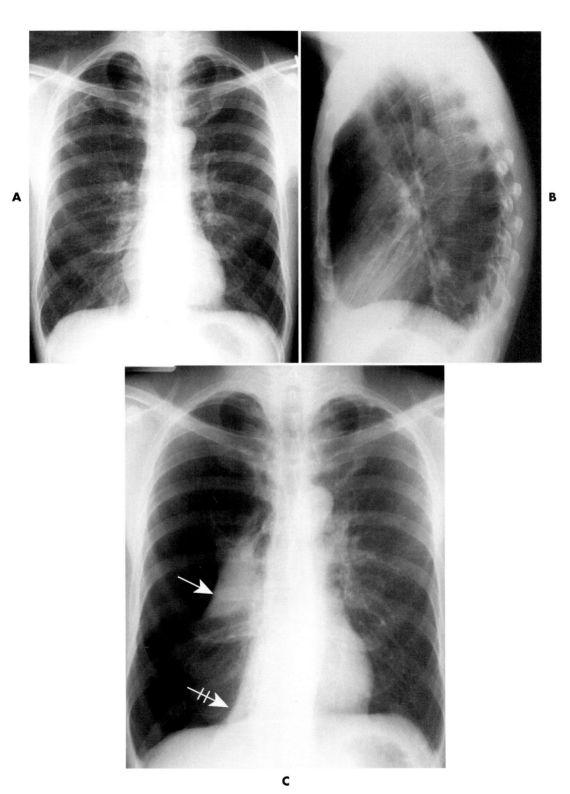

FIG. 22-16 **A** and **B,** This 49-year-old male patient demonstrates the characteristic radiographic signs of emphysema, including flattened low hemidiaphragms, thin heart shadow, and prominent hilar vasculature. **C,** Bullae are not seen directly, but a ruptured bulla is the believed mechanism for the collapsed right upper and middle lobes *(arrow)* and right lower lobe *(crossed arrow)*.

radiolucent air sacs in the periphery of the apex or base of the lungs. Only moderate to severe forms of emphysema are detectable on plain film radiography.[26,33] CT may identify early manifestations of the disease.

CLINICAL COMMENTS

Emphysema is characterized by breathlessness on exertion, secondary to reduced surface area for gas exchange. The presence of a productive cough is related to chronic bronchitis, which often accompanies emphysema. Patients may exhibit a "barrel chest" appearance physically, caused by the collapse of small airways with trapping of alveolar gas during expiration, which in turn causes the chest to be held in the position of inspiration with prolonged expiration effort and increased residual volume. Most patients relate a history of cigarette smoking.

KEY CONCEPTS

- *Emphysema results in overinflation of the distal air spaces of the lung.*
- *Emphysema may be divided into the following categories: centrilobular, panacinar distal acinar, and irregular types.*
- *Radiographic findings include hyperinflation, interstitial changes, vascular changes, and possibly bullae.*

References

1. American Thoracic Society: Definitions and classifications of chronic bronchitis, asthma and pulmonary emphysema, *Am Rev Resp Dis* 85:762, 1962.
2. Barbato A et al: Use of fiberoptic bronchoscopy in asthmatic children with lung collapse, *Pediatr Med Chir* 17:253, 1995.
3. Blair DN, Coppage L, Shaw C: Medical imaging in asthma, *J Thorac Imag* 1:23, 1986.
4. Boushy SF et al: Lung recoil pressure, airway resistance, and forced flows related to morphologic emphysema, *Am Rev Respir Dis* 104:551, 1971.
5. Brashear RE, Meyer SC, Manion MW: Unilateral atelectasis in asthma, *Chest* 63:847, 1973.
6. Brooks-Brunn JA: Postoperative atelectasis and pneumonia: risk factors, *Am J Crit Care* 4:340, 1995.
7. Clark NS: Bronchiectasis in childhood, *Br Med J* 1:80, 1963.
8. De Parades CG et al: Pulmonary sequestrations in infants and children: a 20 year experience and review of the literature, *J Pediatr Surg* 5:136, 1970.
9. Eraklis AJ, Griscom NT, McGovern JB: Bronchogenic cysts of the mediastinum in infancy, *N Engl J Med* 281:1150, 1969.
10. Golden R: The effect of bronchostenosis upon the roentgen-ray shadows in carcinoma of the bronchus, *AJR Am J Roentgenol* 13:21, 1925.
11. Gudbjerg CE: Roentgenologic diagnosis of bronchiectasis, *Acta Radiol* 143:209, 1955.
12. Heard BE et al: The morphology of emphysema, chronic bronchitis, and bronchiectasis: definition, nomenclature, and classification, *J Clin Pathol* 32:882, 1979.
13. Hodson CJ, Trickey SE: Bronchial wall thickening in asthma, *Clin Radiol* 11:183, 1960.
14. Hoeffel JC, Bernard C: Pulmonary sequestration of the upper lobe in children, *Radiology* 160:513, 1986.
15. Kirwan WO, Walbaum PR, McCormack RJM: Cystic intrathoracic derivatives of the foregut and their complications, *Thorax* 8:424, 1973.
16. Lee KS et al: Combined lobar atelectasis of the right lung: imaging findings, *AJR Am J Roentgenol* 163:43, 1994.
17. Lennon EA, Simon G: The height of the diaphragm in the chest radiograph of normal adults, *Br J Radiol* 38:937, 1965.
18. Lynch DA et al: Uncomplicated asthma in adults: comparison of CT appearance of the lungs in asthmatic and healthy subjects, *Radiology* 188:829, 1993.
19. Niaidich DP et al: Intra-lobar pulmonary sequestration, MR evaluation, *J Comput Assist Tomogr* 11:531, 1987.
20. Ohri SK, Townsend ER: Folded lung: a masquerader of malignancy, *Scand J Thorac Cardiovasc Surg* 26:213, 1992.
21. Petheram IS, Kerr IH, Collins JV: Value of chest radiographs in severe acute asthma, *Clin Radiol* 32:281, 1981.
22. Ramenofsky ML, Leape Ll, McCauley RGK: Bronchogenic cyst, *J Pediatr Surg* 14:219, 1979.
23. Rebuck AS: Radiological aspects of severe asthma, *Aust Radiol* 4:264, 1970.
24. Reed JC, Sobonya RE: Morphologic analysis of foregut cysts in the thorax, *AJR Am J Roentgenol* 120:851, 1974.
25. Reid LM: Correlation of certain bronchographic abnormalities seen in chronic bronchitis with the pathological changes, *Thorax* 10:199, 1955.
26. Sanders C: The radiographic diagnosis of emphysema, *Radiol Clin North Am* 29:1019, 1991.
27. Savic B et al: Lung sequestration: report of seven cases and review of 540 published cases, *Thorax* 34:96, 1979.
28. Simon G et al: Relation between abnormalities in the chest radiograph and changes in pulmonary function in chronic bronchitis and emphysema, *Thorax* 28:15, 1973.
29. Snider GL et al: The definition of emphysema: report of a National Heart, Lung, and Blood Institute, Division of Lung Diseases workshop, *Am Rev Respir Dis* 132:182, 1985.
30. St-Georges R et al: Clinical spectrum of bronchogenic cysts of the mediastinum and lung in the adult, *Ann Thorac Surg* 52:6, 1991.
31. Sutnick AI, Soloff LA: Atelectasis with pneumonia. A pathophysiologic study, *Ann Intern Med* 60:39, 1964.
32. Szydlowski GW et al: Rounded atelectasis: a pulmonary pseudotumor, *Ann Thoracic Surg* 53:817, 1992.
33. Thurlbeck WM et al: Chronic obstructive lung disease: a comparison between clinical, roentgenologic, functional and morphologic criteria in chronic bronchitis, emphysema, asthma and bronchiectasis, *Medicine* 49:82, 1970.
34. Thurlbeck WM, Simon G: Radiographic appearance of the chest in emphysema, *AJR Am J Roentgenol* 130:429, 1978.
35. Webber M, Davies P: The Luftsichel: an old sign in upper lobe collapse, *Clin Radiol* 32:271, 1981.

chapter 23

Circulation and the Heart

DENNIS M. MARCHIORI

Acquired Valvular Heart Disease　　**Congestive Heart Failure**
Aortic Aneurysms　　　　　　　　　**Pleural Effusion**
Coarctation of the Aorta　　　　　　**Pulmonary Edema**
Congenital Heart Disease　　　　　　**Pulmonary Thromboembolism**

Acquired Valvular Heart Disease

BACKGROUND

Acquired valvular heart disease is caused by rheumatic heart disease,[31] arteriosclerosis,[9] hypertension, or congenital heart defects. The mitral and aortic valves usually are involved.

IMAGING FINDINGS

Chest radiographs of patients with valvular heart disease typically demonstrate changes in the size of the cardiac shadow, alterations in the size and configuration of specific heart chambers, and alterations in pulmonary vascularity (Figs. 23-1 and 23-2). Valvular calcification also may be present, suggesting mitral and aortic stenosis of the involved value. Specific radiographic findings are listed in Table 23-1. Magnetic resonance imaging (MRI) may be helpful in providing anatomic and functional information about patients with valvular heart disease.[8,17]

CLINICAL COMMENTS

The diagnosis of valvular heart disease is made based on the patient's clinical history, a physical examination, electrocardiography, chest radiography, and echocardiography.[45] In the past, acquired valvular disease most often was caused by rheumatic fever. This is still the case in underdeveloped countries, but other causes predominate today in developed countries.

> **KEY CONCEPTS**
> - *Acquired valvular heart disease presents with a variety of symptoms and findings that vary according to the specific valve involved.*
> - *Radiographic changes in the size of the heart and specific chamber, along with the degree of pulmonary blood flow and presence of calcification, aid in locating the valve involved.*

Aortic Aneurysms

BACKGROUND

Aneurysms are circumscribed dilations of an arterial wall. Saccular aneurysms involve part of the circumference of the vessel, whereas fusiform aneurysms involve the entire circumference. If all three arterial layers (the tunica intima, media, and adventitia) are affected, the aneurysm is called a *true aneurysm*. False aneurysms disrupt arterial walls but are contained by the surrounding connective tissue. A number of conditions, including atherosclerosis, syphilis, mycoses, posttraumatic conditions, congenital conditions, cystic media necrosis, and arteritis, have been named as possible causes of aneurysms (Table 23-2; Figs. 23-3 through 23-7). Atherosclerosis is the most common cause and usually involves the descending aorta.

Aortic dissection occurs when a hematoma in the middle to outer third of the aortic wall longitudinally separates the aortic wall proximally and distally. Hematomas often develop as a result of a vasa vasorum hemorrhage, which is seen in patients with hypertension. The tunica intima may rupture and reconnect the hematoma with its aortic lumen, creating a "double barrel" aorta. A number of classification schemes have been developed to describe the nature and region of aortic involvement (e.g., DeBakey, Stanford).

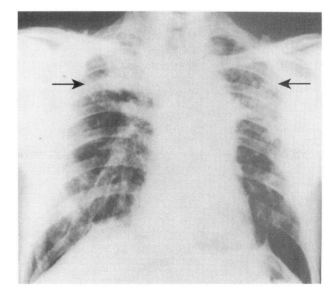

FIG. 23-1　Raised pulmonary venous pressures in a patient with mitral stenosis. Note that the vessels in the third and fourth interspace *(arrows)* are large compared with equivalent vessels in the lower zones of the lung. (From Armstong P et al: Imaging of diseases of the chest, ed 2, St Louis, 1995, Mosby.)

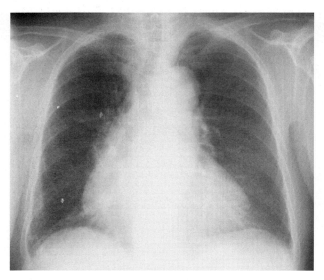

FIG. 23-2   Marked enlargement of the right atrium consistent with tricuspid valve disease in this 86-year-old man. (Courtesy John A.M. Taylor, Seneca Falls, NY.)

IMAGING FINDINGS

The radiographic features of an aneurysm are limited to contour changes in the frontal and lateral projections. Although it does not indicate the presence of an aneurysm, vessel calcification provides a means of visualizing distortions of the vessel's wall. Aortic dissection is suggested by mediastinal widening, cardiomegaly, pleural effusion, and (in rare cases) medial displacement of the

TABLE 23-1
Radiographic Appearance of Acquired Valvular Heart Disease

Condition	Radiographic appearance
Mitral stenosis	Large left atrium, right ventricle, and pulmonary trunk; long, straight left heart border; cephalization of pulmonary blood flow; narrowed retrosternal clear space and occasional calcification
Mitral insufficiency	Large left atrium and left ventricle, pulmonary edema in severe cases
Mitral prolapse (floppy mitral valve syndrome)	Normal (unless regurgitation develops)
Aortic stenosis	Large left ventricle, prominent ascending arch, small aortic knob, valve calcification
Aortic insufficiency	Large left ventricle, prominent aortic knob
Tricuspid stenosis	Large right atrium
Tricuspid insufficiency	Large right atrium and right ventricle, dilated superior vena cava and dilated azygous vein
Pulmonary stenosis	Large left pulmonary artery, increased left lung vascularity, and large right ventricle
Pulmonary insufficiency	Large right ventricle

TABLE 23-2
Types of Aneurysms

Type	Comments
Cystic media necrosis–related	An aneurysm seen in patients with Marfan's syndrome, Ehlers-Danlos syndrome, and other diseases in which collagen production is altered; commonly involves the ascending aorta or sinus of Valsalva
Atherosclerotic	An aneurysm in which the vasa vasorum is impaired; often demonstrates calcification; commonly affects the aortic arch or descending aorta
Congenital	An aneurysm involving a congenital discontinuity of arterial wall; commonly involves the sinus of Valsalva
Arteries-related	An aneurysm seen in patients with Takayasu's disease and other diseases involving intimal proliferation and fibrosis; most often affects the ascending aorta
Mycotic	A saccular aneurysm caused by infection; does not result in calcification
Posttraumatic	An aneurysm involving a vessel tear; common near the ligamentum arteriosum; has a poor prognosis
Syphilitic	An aneurysm in which the vasa vasorum has been impaired by *Treponema* organisms; most commonly affects the ascending aorta and aortic arch

calcified plaque more than 1 cm inward from the outer vessel wall of the descending aorta (which is called the *calcification sign*).[10,11] MRI and computed tomography (CT) provide the best initial and follow-up evaluations of the aorta.[27,56] Angiography may be used preoperatively to better define the vessel.

CLINICAL COMMENTS

The clinical presentation of an aneurysm depends on its size and location; the majority are asymptomatic.[41] Compression of the vena cava (vena cava syndrome), stridor, hoarseness (caused by laryngeal nerve compression), dysphagia, and sternal chest pain may develop in patients who have a large aneurysm mass.

The risk of rupture is related to the size of the aneurysm. Aneurysms of the aortic arch or descending aorta that have a diameter of less than 5 cm rarely rupture. Those exceeding 6 cm have a significant risk of rupturing; 40% of those greater than 10 cm rupture. A patient with a rapidly expanding aneurysm of any size has a poor prognosis.[41]

KEY CONCEPTS

- *Aneurysms are localized dilations of all (true aneurysms) or some (false aneurysms) of the arterial wall layers and involve part (saccular aneurysms) or all (fusiform aneurysms) of the vessel's circumference.*
- *Although many have no clinical symptoms, large aneurysms are significant and life-threatening.*

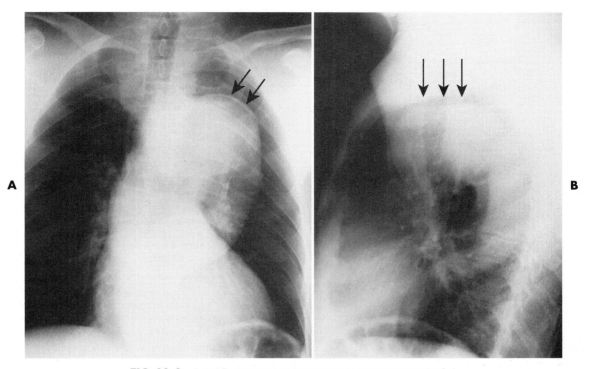

FIG. 23-3 **A** and **B,** Arteriosclerotic aneurysm in the aortic arch *(arrows).*

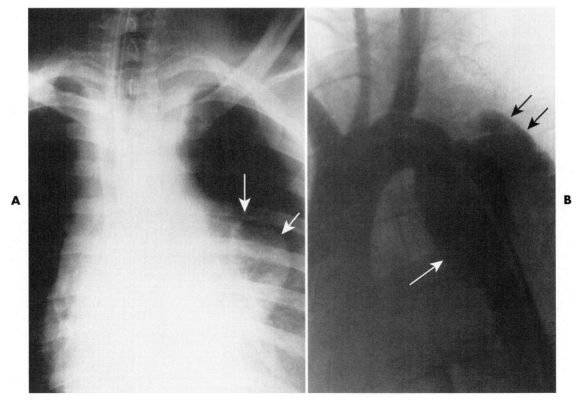

FIG. 23-4 **A,** Plain film and, **B,** angiogram of 21-year-old car accident victim with a traumatic tear of the proximal descending aorta *(arrows).* (Courtesy Steven P. Brownstein, MD, Springfield, NJ.)

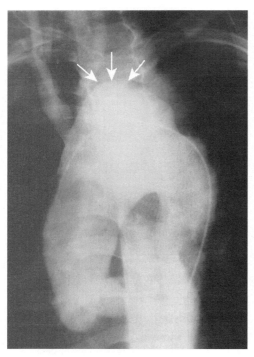

FIG. 23-5 Angiogram showing an aneurysm in the aortic arch *(arrows)*. (Courtesy Steven P. Brownstein, MD, Springfield, NJ.)

Coarctation of the Aorta

BACKGROUND

Juxtaductal, or adult type, coarctation of the aorta is a discrete narrowing of the aortic isthmus (the region between the arch and descending aorta) distal to the origin of the left subclavian artery and near the ductus or ligamentum arteriosus.[46] Tubular hypoplasia, or infantile-type coarctation of the aorta, is less common and involves narrowing of a segment of the transverse aortic arch. Coarctation is more common in males and often develops in conjunction with other cardiovascular defects, particularly when it is found in infants.

Although the aorta is narrowed, the collateral circulation typically prevents hypoperfusion of the trunk and lower extremities. In one such collateral path, blood from the subclavian arteries (before the coarctation has developed) enters the internal mammary arteries. It flows to the anterior intercostals and across the intercostal anastomoses, reversing the normal blood flow of the posterior intercostals and causing it to enter the aorta distal to the coarctation that developed. The hypertrophy of the intercostal arteries causes characteristic inferior rib notching.

Pseudocoarctation is kinking of the aorta that commonly is seen secondary to arteriosclerosis in elderly patients.

IMAGING FINDINGS

Imaging features of infants with coarctation of the aorta may include cardiomegaly and possibly increased pulmonary vascular markings. In children and adults a characteristic inward deformity of the proximal descending aorta may be present with bulging of the vessel immediately above and below (the "figure 3" sign). This sign is seen uncommonly on images of infants because the aortic arch is difficult to observe. Although not pathognomonic for coarctation, bilateral inferior rib notching is common at the posterior angles of the third through ninth ribs (Fig. 23-8). Rib notching is not seen in the infant. MRI is the modality of choice for further assessment.

CLINICAL COMMENTS

Most symptomatic infants with coarctation of the aorta have concurrent cardiovascular abnormalities (e.g., aortic stenosis, patent ductus arteriosus, ventricular septal defect).[42] Associated cardiac anomalies are uncommon in adults. A blood pressure difference of 20 mm Hg between the arms and legs is strongly indicative of coarctation.[33,42] Treatment involves surgical correction of the deformity.[25]

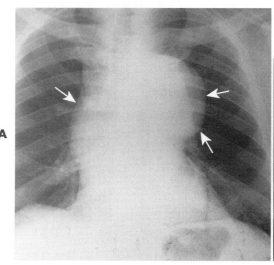
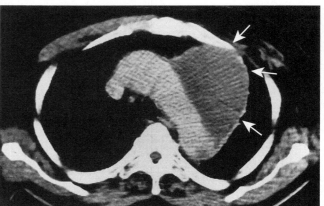

FIG. 23-6 **A,** Plain film and, **B,** computed tomography scan demonstrating an aneurysm in the aortic arch *(arrows)*.

Congenital Heart Disease

BACKGROUND

Congenital heart disease (Table 23-3) encompasses a wide variety of defects that appear at birth as either isolated anomalies or part of larger complexes. Patients with congenital heart disease are categorized based on the presence or absence of cyanosis. Further subdivisions can be made based on the heart size and pulmonary vascularity.

IMAGING FINDINGS

Plain film radiography is used to evaluate pulmonary vascularity, heart size, and configuration of the great vessels (Fig. 23-9).[15,50] Echocardiography, angiocardiography, and MRI are all useful imaging modalities for evaluating congenital heart defects.[13,55]

CLINICAL COMMENTS

Although congenital heart disease can be so severe that an affected unborn fetus cannot survive, also it can be largely asymptomatic. Many infants with the condition seem to be healthy immediately after birth, but their condition changes as the ductus arteriosus closes and adult circulation begins. Some congenital heart diseases may not appear until adulthood (e.g., floppy mitral valve syndrome).

Clinical findings are often nonspecific.[35] Cyanosis, indicated by clubbing of the fingers and toes, hypertrophic osteoarthropathy,

and polycythemia, is a prominent feature of many forms of the disease. Congestive heart failure, impaired growth and development, and pulmonary vascular disease also may be found.[21]

Congestive Heart Failure

BACKGROUND

Four factors are involved in heart functioning: preload (the end-diastolic volume), afterload (the ejection resistance), myocardium contractility, and heart rate. Disturbance of one or several of these factors results in heart failure, the mechanical inability of the heart to circulate an adequate supply of blood. In rare cases the four cardiac factors may appear normal, but the heart still cannot meet the tissues' increased metabolic and flow needs; this is called *high-output heart failure* and is seen in patients with conditions such as Paget's disease and severe anemia.

Forward heart failure refers to the inability of the heart to pump an adequate volume of blood. Symptoms of this condition are related to underperfusion of vital organs (e.g., the brain, leading to fatigue; skeletal muscle, leading to weakness). Backward heart failure refers to the inability of the heart to pump blood that enters it through the venous system. Backward failure results in increased venous pressure and produces transudate in the tissues. During left-sided heart failure, blood is not expelled from the left side of the heart at the same rate as it is on the right, and as a consequence

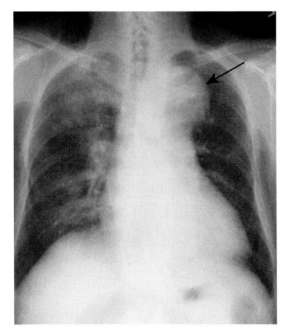

FIG. 23-7 An 86-year-old man with an enlarged aortic knob *(arrow)* that is suspicious of aneurysm. Computed tomography is indicated as follow-up. In addition, pneumonia is seen as an air-space pattern in the middle right (reading left) lung field. (Courtesy John A.M. Taylor, Seneca Falls, NY.)

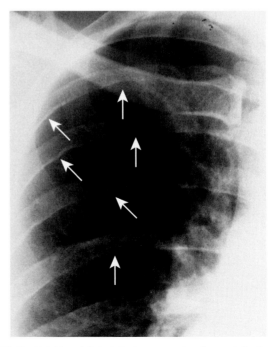

FIG. 23-8 Notching defect at the lower margin of several ribs in a patient with coarctation of the aorta *(arrows).* (Courtesy Steven P. Brownstein, MD, Springfield, NJ.)

TABLE 23-3

Summary of Common Congenital Heart Diseases

Defect	Physical appearance*	Pulmonary vascularity†	Frequency‡	Comments
Ventricular septal defect (VSD)	A	↑	25%	A defect that is usually in the fibrous portion of the septum; second most common congenital heart defect (with bicuspid aortic valve defect being the most common); asymptomatic if small[30]
Atrial septal defect (ASD)	A	↑	—	Defect of the ostium secundum; most common congenital defect recognized in adults; often asymptomatic
Patent ductus arteriosus	A	↑	15%	Defect in which the ductus arteriosus fails soon after birth, resulting in aortic/pulmonary artery shunt
Coarctation of the aorta	A	=	12%	Localized or generalized stenosis of aortic isthmus; results in a large heart in infants and rib notching in adults[25,43]
Aortic stenosis	A	=	10%	Valvular or vessel stenosis; usually asymptomatic; in severe cases in infants, results in congestive heart failure
Pulmonary stenosis	A	=	10%	Valvular or vessel stenosis; usually asymptomatic; results in loud systolic murmur and poststenotic dilation of pulmonary trunk
Tetralogy of Fallot	C	↓	10%	(1) Obstructed pulmonary outflow tract, (2) ventricular septal defect, (3) right ventricular hypertrophy, (4) aorta overriding interventricular septum[18] (in addition, normal heart size); most common congenital heart defect with cyanosis after 1 year of age
Pentalogy of Fallot	C	↓	—	Defect comprising the tetralogy of Fallot and an ASD; increased heart size
Ebstein anomaly	C	↓	—	Defect in which a caudally displaced tricuspid valve creates an enlarged right atrium and small right ventricle; increased heart size
Tricuspid atresia	C	↓	2%	Absence of tricuspid valve and presence of ASD; increased heart size
Total anomalous pulmonary venous return (TAPVR)	C	↑	—	Aberrant communication between pulmonary and systemic veins; an ASD is needed for the defect to be compatible with life; "figure 8" or "snowman" configuration of heart shadow
Truncus arteriosus	C	↑	—	Defect in which a failure of septation forces the pulmonary, systemic, and cardiac arteries to share a single cardiac outlet
Transposition of great vessels	C	↑	10%	Defect in which the aorta arises from the right ventricle and the pulmonary trunk arises from the left ventricle; most common cause of neonatal cyanosis; results in a wide heart shadow[55]
Double outlet right ventricle	C	↑	—	Defect in which the aorta and pulmonary trunk arise from the right ventricle; VSD present
Single ventricle	C	↑	—	Defect in which the ventricular septum is absent and associated defects of the atrioventricular valves are present

*A, Acyanotic; C, cyanotic.
†↑, Increased; ↓, decreased: =, normal.
‡Frequency of congenital heart disease cases in children.

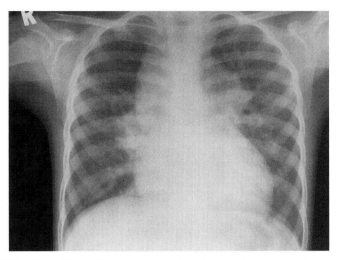

FIG. 23-9 "Figure 8," or "snowman," configuration of total anomalous pulmonary venous return. (Courtesy Steven P. Brownstein, MD, Springfield, NJ.)

the blood backs up and "congests" the pulmonary tissues.[6,36] During right-sided heart failure, blood accumulates on the venous side of the major circulation pathways but typically spares the lungs. Right-sided heart failure usually is caused by left-sided heart failure.

These types of heart failure are not mutually exclusive, but rather are useful categories for conceptualizing the cause and expected dynamics of heart failure.

IMAGING FINDINGS

The radiographic features of patients with congestive heart failure are summarized in Table 23-4. One or more chambers of the heart usually are enlarged, and signs of pulmonary congestion and edema often are present (Figs. 23-10 and 23-11). Pleural effusion is found frequently[29] and may be bilateral or predominantly right-sided. The radiographic findings change as time passes. Patients with isolated right-sided heart failure may exhibit few pulmonary findings.

CLINICAL COMMENTS

Although symptoms and physical findings are helpful in diagnosing congestive heart failure, they have limited sensitivity and specificity.[26] Common clinical findings include shortness of breath (which often worsens with activity), a chronic and nonproductive cough, nocturia, pulmonary rales, pitting edema, an enlarged and tender liver, and engorged neck veins. The prevalence of congestive heart failure increases with age.[2,23,53] The majority of the patients have irreversible heart damage and a poor prognosis. Drugs combined with modifications in diet and activity are part of most treatment programs.

KEY CONCEPTS

- *Heart failure is the mechanical inability of the heart to circulate an adequate volume of blood because of a disturbance in one or more of the cardiac factors needed for proper functioning.*
- *Chest radiographs provide important information about the size and shape of the heart and congestion of pulmonary tissues.*

TABLE 23-4
Radiographic Appearance of Congestive Heart Failure

Finding	Appearance
Enlarged heart shadow	Suggested if the widest transverse dimension of the cardiac shadow in the frontal projection is more than one half the internal dimension of the hemithorax (spinous process to body wall)
Left ventricular enlargement	In the frontal projection, an enlarged left lower heart border. In the lateral projection, an enlarged posteroinferior heart border (more than 2 cm posterior to the inferior vena cava shadow)
Left atrial enlargement	In frontal projection, appears more than 7 cm inferolaterally from center of left bronchus (may form right heart border if massive enlargement present)
Cephalization of blood flow	Increased vascular markings in the superior lung fields
Enlarged superior vena cava and azygous vein	Enlarged right mediastinal border
Perivascular cuffing Peribronchial cuffing	Hazy, blurred pulmonary vessels Thick, "donut," or on-end appearance of bronchial walls
Kerley's lines (A, B, C, etc.)	Interstitial accumulation of fluid
Thickening of interlobar fissures	Fluid accumulation in fissures
Pleural effusion	Transudate accumulation in the pleural space, common
Pulmonary edema	Perihilar edema accumulations appearing as "bat-wing," "butterfly," or "perihilar haze"

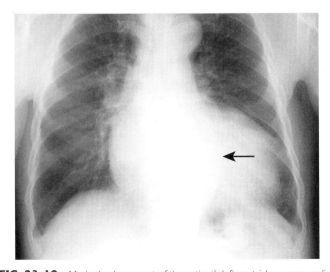

FIG. 23-10 Marked enlargement of the patient's left ventricle corresponding to congestive heart failure. Currently the lungs fields appear clear of excess fluid. Age-related tortuosity accounts for the lateral deviation of the descending thoracic aorta (arrow). (Courtesy John A.M. Taylor, Seneca Falls, NY.)

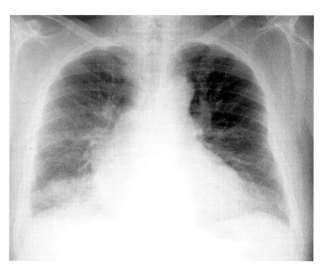

FIG. 23-11   Congestive heart failure in a 65-year-old man. The heart is enlarged and there is a hazy appearance of the perihilar regions consistent with pulmonary edema. (Courtesy John A.M. Taylor, Seneca Falls, NY.)

Pleural Effusion

BACKGROUND

Normally little more than a potential space exists between the visceral and parietal pleurae, containing less than 2 ml of fluid. Pleural effusion is the presence of a larger collection of transudate, exudate, blood, or chyle in this pleural space. More specific terms, such as hydrothorax, hemothorax, or chylothorax, are used if the fluid content is known. The composition of the fluid cannot be determined by its radiographic appearance.

Pleural effusion typically is secondary to diseases of the mediastinum, lungs, or chest wall. Radiographs often provide additional characteristics of a chest disease that may be associated with effusion. Large effusions may obscure part of the lung in some radiographs; therefore CT is needed to visualize much of the parenchyma.

IMAGING FINDINGS

Pleural fluid can be free or loculated by surrounding fibrosus. Free pleural fluid occupies the most gravity-dependent portion of the lung, making first the posterior costophrenic angle and then the lateral costophrenic angle appear blunted (Figs. 23-12 through 23-17).[14] Capillary pressure may draw the effusion upward along the body wall, creating a meniscus sign. Loculated fluid in an interlobar fissure may appear as a mass ("pseudotumor") that characteristically shrinks and disappears ("vanishing" or "phantom" tumor) as its fluid is absorbed (Fig. 23-18).[22] Loculated effusion is more common in the right lung[12] and typically affects the minor fissures.[22] A pseudotumor can be correctly identified by the way its characteristic tapered margins enter into the fissure.

Occasionally, fluid occupies a subpulmonary location, a condition that mimics an elevated hemidiaphragm. Subpulmonic effusion is more common on the right.[39] Left-sided subpulmonic effusion is more easily recognized because the increased distance (>1 cm) between the gastric air bubble and the top of the subpulmonary fluid presents as an easily recognizable finding. Regardless of the side of the body affected, the pseudodiaphragm created by the top of the subpulmonic fluid appears more lateral than the true dome of the hemidiaphragm.[3]

A lateral decubitus projection (with the affected side placed down) can help the clinician distinguish between pleural effusion and an elevated diaphragm (see Fig. 23-12). Free effusion moves to the most gravity-dependent position and spreads out laterally on the dependent side. Lateral decubitus projections provide a more sensitive evaluation of early effusions.[52] Massive effusion may opacify the hemithorax and shift the mediastinum toward the contralateral side.

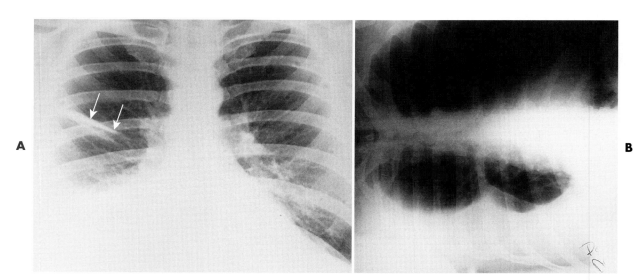

A   B

FIG. 23-12   **A,** Posteroanterior projection demonstrating right-sided pleural effusion in the lower pleural space and loculated pleural effusion in the lateral portion of the horizontal fissure presenting as a linear radiodense shadow in the middle right lung field *(arrows)*. **B,** Lateral decubitus projection in which fluid from the effusion spills laterally, creating a fluid level along the right side of the chest wall. (Courtesy Steven P. Brownstein, MD, Springfield, NJ.)

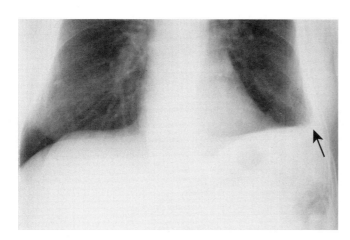

FIG. 23-13 A 56-year-old male cancer patient with excess fluid in the pleural space. The fluid has accumulated in the left (reading right) lateral costophrenic angle *(arrow)* on this upright posteroanterior chest film. (Courtesy John A.M. Taylor, Seneca Falls, NY.)

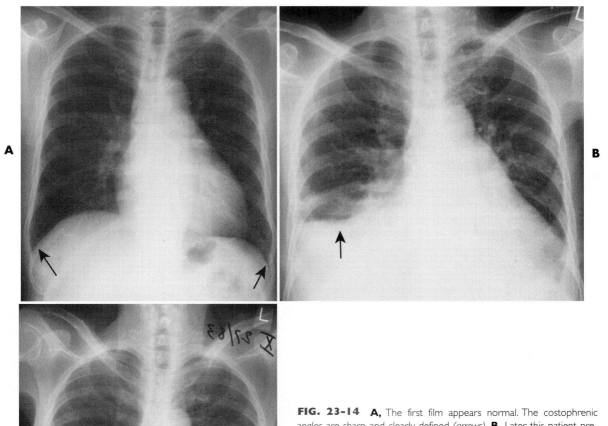

FIG. 23-14 **A,** The first film appears normal. The costophrenic angles are sharp and clearly defined *(arrows)*. **B,** Later this patient presented with pneumonia and fluid accumulation that filled the lateral costophrenic space and the subpulmonic space, mimicking a high diaphragm *(arrow)*. **C,** A third film taken 5 months after the second film demonstrates only slight blunting *(arrow)*. Most of the fluid has cleared. (Courtesy John A.M. Taylor, Seneca Falls, NY.)

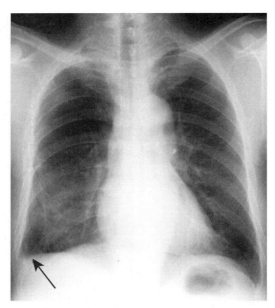

FIG. 23-15 Subtle blunting of the patient's right costophrenic angle *(arrow)* consistent with pleural effusion.

CLINICAL COMMENTS

Pleural effusion is a nonspecific indication of some other underlying problem, such as a neoplasm, trauma, embolism, or pulmonary edema. The observation of pleural effusion should prompt a thorough review of the patient's history and concurrent radiographic findings for a cause. Often a pleural tap is necessary to rule out certain significant pathologic factors.

The symptoms of patients with pleural effusion often include well-localized pleuritic pain that typically is described as "stabbing" and may be aggravated by actions such as coughing, inhaling deeply, or sneezing. Severe dyspnea also may develop, necessitating

thoracocentesis. Although physical examinations cannot reliably detect small effusions, large effusions may cause certain areas to produce dull or flat sounds during percussion.

Pulmonary Edema

BACKGROUND

Pulmonary edema is excess fluid accumulation in the extravascular lung space. The most common cause of increased fluid accumulation is elevated venous and capillary pressures caused by left-sided heart disease. The increased capillary pressure forces excessive amounts of fluid from vessels to the interstitial spaces. Normally the lymphatics drain excess fluid from the interstitial spaces and transport it back to the systemic circulation. However, interstitial fluid accumulations can become excessive and overwhelm the draining ability of the lymphatics, leading to a breakdown of the tight junctions between adjacent alveolar cells. Consequently, fluid may force its way into the air space of the lungs and accumulate.

Other factors leading to excessive extravascular fluid accumulations include those that increase capillary wall permeability (e.g., noxious substances, high altitude, pancreatitis), cause fluid overload syndromes (e.g., excessive intravenous fluid administration, renal failure), or cause obstruction of the lymphatic vessels (e.g., neoplasms, neurogenic factors).[1,48] (See Chapter 27, pattern CS-12, for a more complete list of causes.)

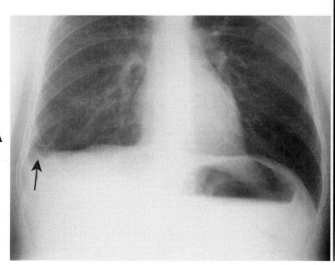

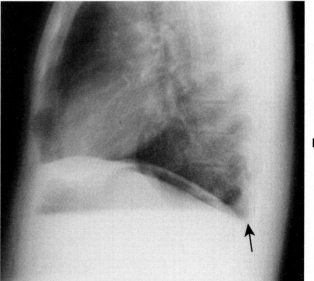

FIG. 23-16 **A** and **B,** Pleural effusion accumulated in the patient's right and posterior costophrenic angles *(arrows)*. (Courtesy John A.M. Taylor, Seneca Falls, N.Y.)

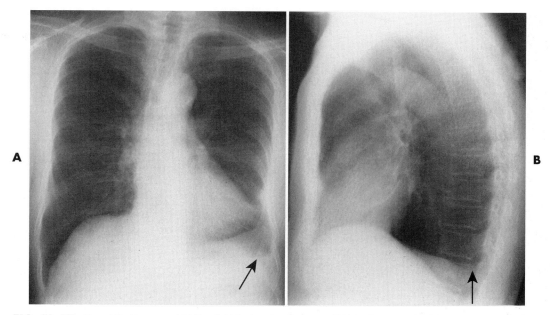

FIG. 23-17 **A** and **B,** On an upright film, fluid in the pleural space will blunt the normally sharp lateral and posterior costophrenic angles. The blunting sometimes is called a *meniscus sign.* If the fluid is free to move, it will accumulate to a greater extent in the lower posterior costophrenic angle *(arrows).* Fluid in the pleural space is not a specific finding. It may occur from trauma, heart failure, pulmonary embolism, or general inflammation. (Courtesy John A.M. Taylor, Seneca Falls, NY.)

IMAGING FINDINGS

The radiographic appearance of pulmonary edema is largely based on whether the fluid accumulation is in the interstitial or alveolar spaces (Box 23-1 and Figs. 23-19 through 23-22). Interstitial edema precedes alveolar edema, although they can be present concurrently. Identifying the cause of pulmonary edema from the radiographic appearance alone is difficult, but classic appearances of several causes have been identified.

- Cardiac failure presents with a cephalic redistribution of pulmonary blood flow that results in prominent vascular markings in the upper lung zone. An enlarged heart shadow and pleural effusion also are present and often are more prominent on the right side of the patient.[37,57]
- Features of pulmonary edema caused by renal failure may include heart enlargement, normal pulmonary vascular distribution, and symmetric, bilateral perihilar opacities.
- Pulmonary edema caused by increased vascular permeability is associated typically with a widespread pattern of alveolar filling and a normal-sized heart shadow and vascular distribution.

CLINICAL COMMENTS

Acute pulmonary edema presents with characteristic symptoms that include severe dyspnea; tachypnea; pink, frothy sputum; diaphoresis; and cyanosis. Examination of the lungs reveals rales and wheezing.

KEY CONCEPTS

- *Pulmonary edema represents increased extravascular fluid accumulations because of hydrostatic, permeability, or lymphatic factors.*
- *The radiographic appearance changes rapidly; it is generally seen as an interstitial or air-space pattern depending, on the location of the excess fluid.*

Pulmonary Thromboembolism

BACKGROUND

Pulmonary emboli arise from thrombi in the venous circulation, tumors in the venous system, or nonvenous sources such as amniotic fluid, bone marrow, or air. Most pulmonary emboli originate from clots in the deep veins of the lower extremities. Predisposing clinical factors for the formation of deep venous thrombi include prolonged standing, obesity, prolonged bed rest, surgery, stroke, congestive heart disease, and fractures of large bones.

Pulmonary emboli become lodged in the pulmonary trunk, pulmonary arteries, or arterial tree. Emboli may have both hemodynamic (e.g., obstructive) and physiologic (e.g., vasoconstrictive) effects on blood flow. (The effects of vasoconstriction probably are less clinically significant.)[45]

Most pulmonary emboli resolve, restoring pulmonary arterial flow.[5,16,32] Embolism results in pulmonary infarction in up to 15% of patients,[34] typically involving the lower lobes. It appears as pleural-based triangular radiopacities resulting from alveolar filling with edema and hemorrhage.

IMAGING FINDINGS

Although many radiographic findings have been associated with pulmonary embolism, none are specific for or highly sensitive to the disease.[4,19] The pulmonary arteries may appear enlarged (>16 mm). Oligemia distal to the site of arterial obstruction may appear radiolucent (Westermark's sign) in patients who have a pulmonary embolism but no infarct. A triangular, pleural-based radiopacity is seen in patients with a pulmonary embolism and infarct. This radiographic feature, called *Hampton's hump,* is an accumulation of blood and edema in the alveolar space of a lung infarct. Over a period of months, the periphery of the hump "melts away," resolving completely or remaining as a small, horizontal, linear tissue scar.

The combination of ventilation and perfusion (V/Q) radionuclide imaging demonstrates the air distribution and blood flow to

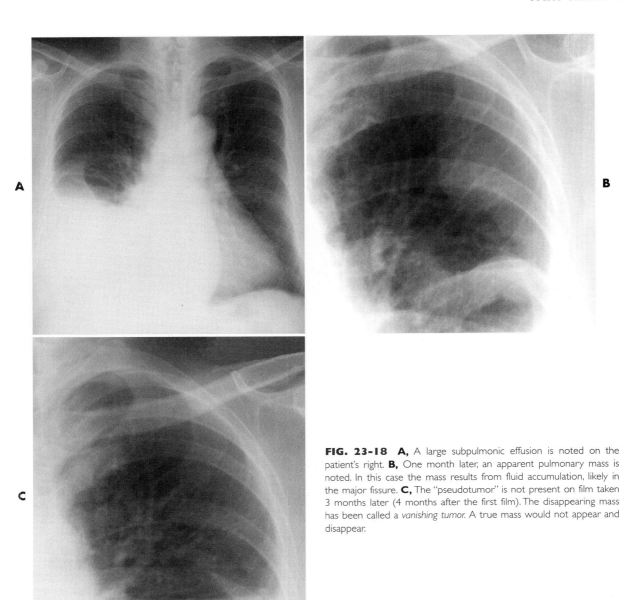

FIG. 23-18 A, A large subpulmonic effusion is noted on the patient's right. **B,** One month later, an apparent pulmonary mass is noted. In this case the mass results from fluid accumulation, likely in the major fissure. **C,** The "pseudotumor" is not present on film taken 3 months later (4 months after the first film). The disappearing mass has been called a *vanishing tumor.* A true mass would not appear and disappear.

FIG. 23-19 Pulmonary edema appears with an air-space pattern of disease proximally and an interstitial pattern of disease laterally, reflecting the difference in venous pressure (higher proximally).

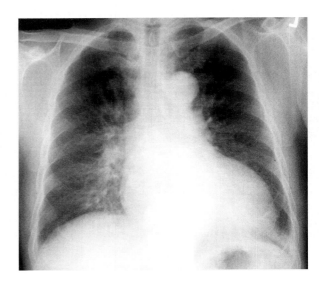

BOX 23-1
Radiographic Appearance of Pulmonary Edema

Interstitial pattern

Septal lines

Kerley's A lines: Thin, 5- to 10-cm lines seen in the upper lung fields representing distention of the interlobular septa, suggesting acute disease.

Kerley's B lines: Dense, 1- to 2-cm horizontal lines perpendicular to the pleura of the lower lung representing distention of the subpleural interlobular septa.

Kerley's C lines: Thin lines that radiate peripherally from the hilum, relating a diffuse reticular pattern.

Hilar haze

A loss of definition of the large pulmonary vessels.

Subpleural edema[20,41]

Fluid accumulations immediately beneath the visceral pleura. Appears as linear thickening, thick fissures if interlobular visceral pleura is involved.

Peribronchovascular blurring and cuffing[7]

Loss of definition of the bronchi and vessels because of surrounding fluid accumulations.

Apical cap

Fluid accumulations at the apex of the pleura.

Alveolar pattern

Bilateral hilar densities[24]

"Butterfly," "sunburst," "bat's wing" or "fan-shaped" radiopacities extending from the hila bilaterally. The opacification may be partial (appearing patchy and mottled) or complete (appearing homogeneously radiodense).

Air-bronchogram

A radiolucent transverse shadow representing an air-filled bronchus contrasted by surrounding fluid-filled air spaces.

Transient

Typically, air-space patterns of pulmonary edema change rapidly over time.

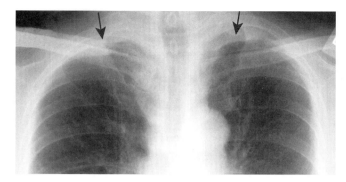

FIG. 23-20 Bilaterally apical capping is noted in this case as thickened appearance of the superior pleura. This feature may be seen with edema, as in this case, tumor, or generally any condition that inflames the pleura *(arrows)*.

the lung. Radionuclide imaging is an important imaging modality for use in patients who already show clinical or radiographic evidence indicative of a pulmonary embolism.

CLINICAL COMMENTS

The clinical presentation of a pulmonary embolism depends largely on the size of the embolus and the patient's health status. Up to 80% of patients with a known embolism do not exhibit significant clinical symptoms.[47] However, pulmonary emboli are a major cause of death for up to 15% of adults in acute care hospital settings. When present, clinical manifestations are diffuse, poorly defined, and nonspecific,[49] causing many cases to go unnoticed.[43] Common clinical findings include chest pain, dyspnea, cough, hemoptysis, rales, tachypnea, and fever.

KEY CONCEPTS

- *Pulmonary emboli arise from deep venous thrombi, bone marrow, amniotic fluid, air, and other sources. They are more common in the lower portions of the lungs.*

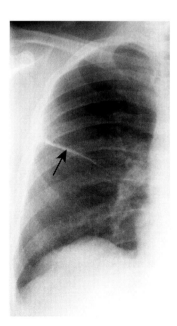

FIG. 23-21 During episodes of fluid overload (e.g., congestive heart failure, renal failure, drug overdose), fluid may become loculated in the fissures, appearing as a radiodense linear shadow in the lung field *(arrow)*. Subsegmental atelectasis has a similar appearance, but is not as rapidly transient as a fluid accumulation.

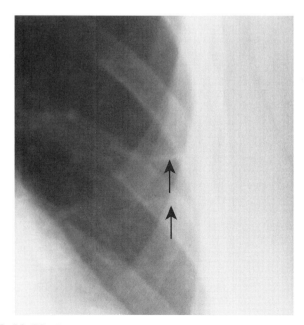

FIG. 23-22 Distention of the subpleural interstitial space appearing as two horizontal, 1cm-long radiodense lines perpendicular to the visceral pleura in the lower periphery of the lung field; these lines are known as *Kerley's B-lines (arrows)*.

Continued

- *Of the patients who develop a pulmonary embolism, 15% also develop a pulmonary infarct, which often is indicated radiographically by a triangular, pleural-based, radiodense region.*
- *Although many patients remain asymptomatic, complaints of dyspnea, cough, hemoptysis, and chest pain are suggestive of a pulmonary embolism.*
- *Ventilation and perfusion (V/Q) radionuclide scanning is helpful in diagnosing patients in whom clinical suspicion of pulmonary embolism is high.*

Acknowledgment

Special thanks to James C. Reed for his contribution as a reviewer of this material.

References

1. Aryre SM: Mechanisms and consequences of pulmonary edema, *Am Heart J* 103:97, 1982.
2. Besse S et al: Is the senescent heart overloaded and already failing? *Cardiovasc Drugs Ther* 8:581, 1994.
3. Bryk D: Infrapulmonary effusion: effect of expiration on the pseudodiaphragmatic contour, *Radiology* 120:33, 1976.
4. Buckner CB, Walker CW, Purnell GL: Pulmonary embolism: chest radiographic abnormalities, *J Thoracic Imag* 4:23, 1989.
5. Dalen JE et al: Pulmonary angiography in acute pulmonary embolism: indications, techniques, and results in 367 patients, *Am Heart J* 81:175, 1971.
6. Dhalla NS et al: Pathophysiology of cardiac dysfunction in congestive heart failure, *Can J Cardiol* 9:873, 1993.
7. Don C, Johnson R: The nature and significance of peribronchial cuffing in pulmonary edema, *Radiology* 125:577, 1977.
8. Duerinckx AJ, Higgins CB: Valvular heart disease, *Radiol Clin North Am* 32:613, 1994.
9. Duncan AK et al: Cardiovascular disease in elderly patients, *Mayo Clin Proc* 71:184, 1996.
10. Earnest F, Muhm JR, Sheedy PF: Roentgenographic findings in thoracic aortic dissection, *Mayo Clin Proc* 54:43, 1979.
11. Eyler WR, Clark MD: Dissecting aneurysms of the aorta. Roentgen manifestations including a comparison with other types of aneurysms, *Radiology* 85:1047, 1965.
12. Feder EH, Wilk SP: Localized interlobar effusion in heart failure: phantom lung tumor, *Dis Chest* 30:289, 1956.
13. Fellows KE et al: Evaluation of congenital heart disease with MR imaging: current and coming attractions *AJR Am J Roentgenol* 159:925, 1992.
14. Fleischner FG: Atypical arrangement of free pleural effusion, *Radiol Clin North Am* 1:347, 1963.
15. Foster E: Congenital heart disease in adults, *West J Med* 163:492, 1995.
16. Fred HL et al: Rapid resolution of pulmonary thromboemboli in man, *JAMA* 196:1137, 1966.
17. Globits S, Higgins CB: Assessment of valvular heart disease by magnetic resonance imaging, *Am Heart J* 129:369, 1995.
18. Greenberg SB, Faerber EN, Balsara RK: Tetralogy of Fallot: diagnostic imaging after palliative and corrective surgery, *J Thorac Imag* 10:26, 1995.
19. Greenspan RH et al: Accuracy of the chest radiograph in diagnosis of pulmonary embolism, *Invest Radiol* 17:539, 1982.
20. Harrison MO, Conte P, Heitzman ER: Radiological detection of clinically occult cardiac failure following myocardial infarction, *Br J Radiol* 44:265, 1971.
21. Higgins IT: The epidemiology of congenital heart disease, *J Chronic Dis* 18:699, 1965.
22. Higgins JA et al: Loculated interlobar pleural effusion due to congestive heart failure, *Arch Intern Med* 96:180, 1955.
23. Hixon ME: Aging and heart failure, *Prog Cardiovasc Nurs* 9:4, 1994.
24. Hodsun CJ: Pulmonary edema and bat-wing shadows, *J Fac Radiol* 1:176, 1950.
25. Hougen TJ, Sell JE: Recent advances in the diagnosis and treatment of coarctation of the aorta, *Curr Opin Cardiol* 10:524, 1995.
26. Jimenez MQ: Ten common congenital cardiac defects, *Pediatrician* 10:3, 1981.
27. Karon BL: Diagnosis and outpatient management of congestive heart failure, *Mayo Clin Proc* 70:1080, 1995.
28. Kersting-Sommerhoff BA et al: Aortic dissection: sensitivity and specificity of MRI imaging, *Radiology* 166:651, 1988.
29. Maher GG, Berger HW: Massive pleural effusion: malignant and nonmalignant causes in 46 patients, *Am Rev Respir Dis* 105:458, 1972.
30. Mahoney LT: Acyanotic congenital heart disease. Atrial and ventricular septal defects, atrioventricular canal, patent ductus arteriosus, pulmonic stenosis, *Cardiol Clin* 11:603, 1993.
31. Majeed HA et al: Acute rheumatic fever and the evolution of rheumatic heart disease: a prospective 12 year follow-up report, *J Clin Epidemiol* 45:871, 1992.
33. Mathur VS et al: Pulmonary angiography one to seven days after experimental pulmonary embolism, *Invest Radiol* 2:304, 1967.
34. McNamara DG: Coarctation of the aorta: difficulties in clinical recognition, *Heart Dis Stroke* 1:202, 1992.
35. Moser KM: Pulmonary embolism: state of the art, *Am Rev Respir Dis* 115:829, 1977.
36. Moss AJ: Clues in diagnosing congenital heart disease, *West J Med* 156:392, 1992.
37. Navas JP, Martinez-Maldonado M: Pathophysiology of edema in congestive heart failure, *Heart Dis Stroke* 2:325, 1993.
38. Nessa CB, Rigler LG: The roentgenological manifestations of pulmonary edema, *Radiology* 37:35, 1941.
39. Ober WB, Moore TE: Congenital cardiac malformations in the neonatal period. An autopsy study, *N Engl J Med* 253:271, 1955.
40. Petersen JA: Recognition of infrapulmonary pleural effusion, *Radiology* 74:34, 1960.
41. Pistolesi M, Giuntini C: Assessment of extravascular lung water, *Radiol Clin North Am* 16:551, 1978.
42. Posniak HV, Demus TC, Marsan RE: Computed tomography of the normal aorta and thoracic aneurysms, *Semin Roentgenol* 24:7, 1989.
43. Rao PS: Coarctation of the aorta, *Semin Nephrol* 15:87, 1995.
44. Rosenow EC, Osmundson PJ, Brown ML: Pulmonary embolism: subject review. *Mayo Clin Proc* 56:161, 1981.
45. Ruttley MS: The chest radiograph in adult heart valve disease, *J Heart Valve Dis* 2:205, 1993.
46. Sabiston DC: Pathophysiology, diagnosis, and management of pulmonary embolism, *Am J Surg* 138:384, 1979.
47. Shinebourne EA, Elseed AM: Relations between fetal blood flow patterns, coarctation of the aorta and pulmonary blood flow, *Br Heart J* 36:492, 1974.
48. Spittell JA: Pulmonary thromboembolism-some editorial comments, *Dis Chest* 54:401, 1968.
49. Staub NC: Pulmonary edema due to increased microvascular permeability to fluid protein, *Annu Rev Med* 32:291, 1981.
50. Stein PD, Saltzman HA, Weg JG: Clinical characteristics of patients with acute pulmonary embolism, *Am J Cardiol* 68:1723, 1991.
51. Steiner RM et al: Congenital heart disease in the adult patient: the value of plain film chest radiology, *J Thorac Imag* 10:1, 1995.
52. Storstein O: Congenital cardiac disease. An analysis of 1,000 consecutive cases, *Acta Med Scand* 176:195, 1964.
53. Vix VA: Roentgenographic recognition of pleural effusion, *JAMA* 229:695, 1974.
54. Walker JE: Congestive heart failure in the elderly, *Conn Med* 7:293, 1993.
55. Webb GD et al: Transposition complexes, *Cardiol Clin* 11:651, 1993.
56. Wexler L, Higgins CB: The use of magnetic resonance imaging in adult congenital heart disease, *Am J Card Imag* 9:15, 1995.
57. Wolff DA et al: Aortic dissection: Atypical patterns seen at MR imaging, *Radiology* 181:489, 1991.
58. Youngberg AS: Unilateral diffuse lung opacity, *Radiology* 123:277, 1977.

chapter 24

Pulmonary Infections

DENNIS M. MARCHIORI

Empyema
Lung Abscess
Pneumonia
Tuberculosis

Empyema

BACKGROUND

Empyema is an intrapleural infection that is distinguished from simple parapneumonic effusions on the basis of positive cultures. The most likely infectious agents are tuberculosis or *Staphylococcus*, although many others have been identified. Often other radiographic evidence accompanies empyema, including pneumonia, surgery, trauma, and abdominal infections.[2,20]

IMAGING FINDINGS

The radiographic appearance varies from a slight chest wall mass producing an inward deformity and pleural effusion to the presence of a massive radiopacity obscuring most of the hemithorax. The infective process may become extensive, encasing the lung. Computed tomography (CT) is instrumental in determining if the infection is largely pleural or pulmonary (Fig. 24-1).

CLINICAL COMMENTS

Fever, chills, chest pain, and other clinical findings consistent with infection typically are present. Thoracentesis may be necessary to establish the causative agent.[4] Most lung abscesses respond to appropriate antimicrobial therapy, with only about 10% requiring external drainage or surgical therapy.[39]

KEY CONCEPTS

- *Empyema most often develops from pulmonary infection.*
- *Empyema is distinguished from pleural effusion by the presence of a positive culture.*

Lung Abscess

BACKGROUND

A lung abscess is a localized suppurative process marked by tissue necrosis. It most commonly results from aspiration and bronchogenic spread of foreign material or infectious debris secondary to oropharyngeal surgery, sinobronchial infections, dental sepsis,

and so on. Aspiration is common among patients who have a suppression of the cough reflex from any of a variety of reasons, including alcoholism, coma, general anesthesia, and narcotic use. Antecedent bacterial pneumonias (commonly *Staphylococcus aureus* and *Klebsiella pneumoniae*) may result in abscess formation.

IMAGING FINDINGS

When secondary to aspiration, the most gravity-dependent portions of the lung are typically involved; namely, the posterior segment of the upper lobes during an upright posture and the superior segments of the lower lobes during a supine posture. Lesions typically begin as areas of spherical consolidation. If the cavity forms a communication with the adjacent airways, the cavity's fluid is replaced by air (Fig. 24-2), creating an air-fluid level within the once radiopaque cavity.

CLINICAL COMMENTS

The clinical presentation is characterized by cough, fever, and abundant amounts of foul-smelling, purulent, or sanguineous sputum. Chest pain and weight loss are common. Complications result if the infection extends into the pleural space. The radiographic appearance of a lung abscess should alert the interpreter of the radiograph to the possibility of bronchogenic carcinoma, which may arise in long-standing abscesses and empyemas.

KEY CONCEPTS

- *Lung abscesses are aggressive infections of the lung often secondary to aspiration of infectious debris.*
- *Cavitation follows a communication with the adjacent airway.*

Pneumonia

BACKGROUND

Pneumonia represents inflammation of the alveolar parenchyma of the lung from a variety of causes (e.g., infections, inhalation of chemicals, and trauma to the chest wall). Unless otherwise stated, the common usage of the term *pneumonia* implies an

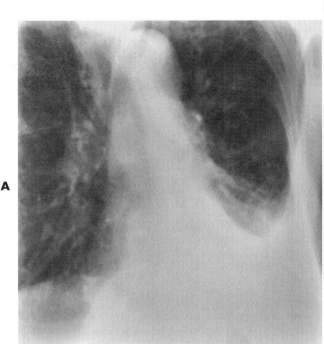

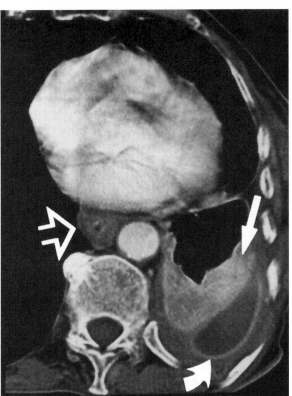

FIG. 24-1 **A,** Chest radiograph shows consolidation and volume loss of the left lower lobe. An associated left pleural effusion is evident. **B,** Contrast-enhanced computed tomography shows consolidation of a portion of the left lower lobe *(straight arrow)*. This is aspiration pneumonia. This patient had an esophageal hiatal hernia that resulted in a Barrett's esophagus. Note the thickened esophageal wall *(open arrow)*. Gastroesophageal reflux results in aspiration pneumonia. The aspiration pneumonia is complicated by a parapneumonic effusion that became infected; therefore an empyema *(curved arrow)*. (From Swenson SJ: Radiology of thoracic diseases: a teaching file, St Louis, 1993, Mosby.)

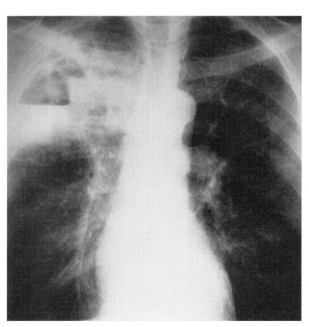

FIG. 24-2 Pneumonia and pulmonary abscess within the right upper lobe. (Courtesy Steven P. Brownstein, MD, Springfield, NJ.)

infectious etiology. Pneumonias are classified by their causative organism (e.g., virus, bacteria, mycoplasma, yeasts, or fungi), radiographic appearance (lobar, lobular or bronchostitial, interstitial, and spherical or round), or etiology (community-acquired, nosocomial, immunosuppressed, or aspiration).

Infections are transmitted to the lung parenchyma by one or more of the following pathways: direct extension, hematogenous spread, inhalation of airborne agents, and aspiration of gastric or nasopharyngeal organisms. The characteristics of selected pneumonias are presented in Table 24-1.

IMAGING FINDINGS

Chest radiography remains the primary tool to establish the presence and extent of pneumonia. Although it should be emphasized that the lack of radiographic evidence does not exclude pneumonia, neither does the presence of consolidation exclusively indicate the presence of pneumonia. It is imperative that clinical findings be correlated to the radiographic appearance.

Although large areas of crossover exist, several radiographic patterns of lung infection have been identified (Table 24-2). However, except for a few classic presentations (Table 24-3), the radiographic appearance of most lung infections is so general that radiographs offer little help in isolating a particular causative agent.[36]

TABLE 24-1
Characteristics of Selected Pneumonias

Causative agent	Comments
Bacterial (gram-positive)	
Streptococcus pneumoniae (*S. pneumoniae,* pneumococci)	Most common bacterial community-acquired agent[35] and common hospital-acquired pneumonia; it occurs at any age; prototype lobar pneumonia appears as homogenous consolidation;[16] children often demonstrate spherical pattern
Streptococcus pyogenes (*S. pyogenes*)	Seen rarely today, although common in early 1900s; appears as homogenous consolidation, typically of lower lobes; often it is accompanied by large pleural effusion and empyema[5]
Staphylococcus aureus (S. aureus)	Commonly results from aspiration of gastric contents; patchy segmental consolidation; cavitation, pneumatoceles, pleural effusion, and empyema are common
Anthrax *(Bacillus anthracis)*	Uncommon in the United States, typically acquired in the Middle East from contact with infected goats; it produces patchy consolidation of the lower lungs with occasional mediastinal widening because of lymphadenopathy[38]
Bacterial (gram-negative)	
Klebsiella pneumoniae (*K. pneumoniae,* Friedländer's disease)	Typically affects individuals with chronic debilitating disease or alcoholism; it appears as homogenous nonsegmental consolidation, often rapidly progressing to involve the entire lobe;[17] regions of lung involvement may appear expanded[14,21]
Legionella pneumophila (*L. pneumophila*)	Found in aquatic environments (humidifiers, water towers, reservoirs, etc.); radiographic appearance begins as patchy peripheral densities, rapidly progressing to involve the entire lobe;[12] pleural effusion often is noted
Pertussis *(Bordetella [Haemophilus] pertussis)*	Marked by streaking peribronchial consolidation in one or more lobes;[3,4] a tendency exists to involve the right lung to a greater extent
Haemophilus influenzae (*H. influenzae*)	Common in patients with chronic obstructive pulmonary disease,[6] alcoholism, and diabetes mellitus, as well as children;[37] it exhibits a lower lobe bronchopneumonia pattern; *H. influenzae* is often concomitant with empyema, meningitis, or epiglottitis
Pseudomonas aeruginosa (*P. aeruginosa*)	Common in hospitalized ventilated patients with lowered immunity; it appears as extensive, bilateral, ill-defined opacities in the lower lobes, often with small pleural effusion[22] and abscess formation
Mycobacterial	
Mycobacterium tuberculosis (*M. tuberculosis*)	Distribution largely impacted by social and economic factors; few patients demonstrate signs or symptoms with primary infection; secondary infections are marked by clinical symptoms and radiographic changes in the lung parenchyma, tracheobronchial tree, and hilar and mediastinal lymph nodes
Mycoplasmal	
Mycoplasma pneumoniae (*M. pneumoniae*)	Exhibits bacterial and viral characteristics; this type generally is recognized as the most common nonbacterial cause of pneumonia;[15] it appears similar to viral pneumonias with primarily an interstitial pattern in the early stages of the disease,[9] possibly progressing to an air-space pattern
Viral	
Influenza (Groups A, B, and C)	Usually confined to the upper respiratory tract, rarely produces pneumonia; when present appears as patchy, bilateral lower lobe consolidation; localized consolidation occurs less commonly
Varicella-zoster	Affects immunosuppressed patients or may complicate lymphoma; the radiographic appearance of acute disease appears as patchy diffuse air-space consolidation;[34] a less common presentation consists of multiple 5- to 10-mm diffusely scattered bilateral radiopacities that have a tendency to calcify[8]
Fungal	
Actinomyces israelii (A. israelii)	Represents normal inhabitant of oropharynx; infection results when organism reaches devitalized tissue and proliferates; mandibular infection may complicate dental extractions; pulmonary infection develops from direct extension or aspiration of infectious debris; it appears as peripheral lower lobe air-space consolidation
Histoplasma capsulatum (*H. capsulatum*)	Endemic to the Mississippi, Ohio, and St. Lawrence River valleys and Puerto Rico; the majority of infections are asymptomatic with a past presence suggested by multiple scattered discrete calcific densities with (or without) accompanying calcified hilar and mediastinal lymph nodes; chronic involvement of the mediastinum may lead to fibrosing mediastinitis

Continued

TABLE 24-1 cont'd
Characteristics of Selected Pneumonias

Causative agent	Comments
Fungal—cont'd	
Coccidioides immitis (C. immitis)	Endemic to the southwest United States (San Joaquin Valley); infected individuals may describe arthralgias and erythema nodosum (valley fever); imaging findings include well-defined segmental radiopacities that typically resolve over time; mediastinal and hilar lymphadenopathy may be present; the chronic progressive form of the disease is similar to postprimary tuberculosis or histoplasmosis
Aspergillus fumigatus (A. fumigatus)	Presents as aspergilloma ("fungal ball" or "mycetoma"), representing a mass in a preexisting pulmonary cavity; more invasive varieties of parenchymal infection are seen in the immunocompromised patient[41]
Blastomyces dermatitidis (B. dermatitidis)	Chronic systemic infection that appears as nonsegmental homogenous consolidation with a tendency to involve the upper lobes of the lung; less commonly it presents as single or multiple mass lesions[19]
Cryptococcus neoformans (C. neoformans; formerly *Torula histolytica)*	Worldwide distribution; infection results from inhalation of contaminated dust; a wide variety of radiographic presentations exists; it is associated with lymphomas, steroid therapy, and acquired immunodeficiency syndrome (AIDS); meningitis and encephalitis represent the most serious complications; the most common radiographic appearance is a single well-defined nodule or mass,[18] less commonly a region of consolidation[13]
Parasitic	
Pneumocystis carinii (P. carinii)	Significant pneumonia among immunocompromised patients (e.g., AIDS and organ transplant patients), demonstrates bilateral perihilar fine, "ground-glass" radiographic appearance;[30] it may progress to air-space consolidation pattern; pleural effusion and lymphadenopathy are uncommon
*Echinococcus granulosus (E. granulosis—*infection called hydatid disease)	Tapeworm whose definitive host is dogs and intermediate host is sheep; when humans become the accidental intermediate host, disease results; pulmonary involvement is marked by a well-defined, three-layered pulmonary mass[7] or cyst, most often in the lower lobes; rupture of the cyst may produce a radiodense air shadow ("crescent" sign) or noticeable floating debris on the internal fluid of the cyst ("water lily" sign)

TABLE 24-2
Radiographic Appearance of Pneumonia

Radiographic type	Radiographic appearance
Broncho (lobular) pneumonia	Represents the most common pneumonic pattern, in which inflammatory exudate involves some and spares some of the parenchymal tissue along a large airway; it appears as fluffy, patchy, multifocal densities tracking along a large airway; because the airways are affected, there may be volume loss, and air-bronchograms are uncommon; common agents include *S. aureus, H. influenza,* gram-negative bacteria
Lobar pneumonia	Inflammatory exudate beginning in the periphery of the lung and spreading circumferentially through pores of Kohn and canals of Lambert to involve adjacent lung tissue, involving the entire bronchopulmonary segment and eventually lobe; the region of pneumonia appears homogenously radiodense; because the airways are not involved, volume loss is rare and air bronchograms are common; common agents include *S. pneumoniae, K. pneumoniae,* and *S. aureus*
Interstitial pneumonia	Localized or generalized thickening of the interstitium producing peribronchial or reticulonodular radiographic patterns; typically it is caused by viral or mycoplasma infections
Aspiration pneumonia	Bilateral, poorly defined consolidation in gravity-dependent portions of the lung

TABLE 24-3
Classic Radiographic Presentations of Pneumonia

Radiographic appearance	Organisms
Consolidation of all or nearly all of a lobe	Bacteria
Consolidation with cavitation or pneumatoceles	*Staphylococcus aureus*
Consolidation with expansion of the lobe	*Klebsiella pneumoniae* (see Fig. 24-15)
Spherical (nodular) pneumonia	Pneumococcal,[33] *Legionella micdadei*,[31] and Q fever[28]
Localized or widespread reticulonodular pattern	Viruses[10] or mycoplasma
Miliary nodules	Tuberculosis, fungi, or varicella-zoster
Patchy upper lobe consolidations	Tuberculosis, histoplasmosis, blastomycosis, cryptococcosis, etc.
Large pleural effusions	*S. aureus* and *Streptococcus pyogenes*

The essential radiographic finding of pneumonia is partial or complete lung consolidation, often with associated pleural effusion, a silhouette sign, air-bronchogram, lung cavitation, and empyema (Figs. 24-3 through 24-17). Selected causative agents and their radiographic appearances are presented in Table 24-1.

CLINICAL COMMENTS

Pneumonia is the most life-threatening infectious disease.[32] Its clinical importance depends on the causative organism involved, the patient's age, and any predisposing illness. Mortality is higher for individuals with a preexisting condition or otherwise healthy children and elderly patients. Clinical findings of pneumonia typically precede radiographic evidence. Further clinical findings resolve before imaging findings of pneumonia resolve. Serial films may help in assessing treatments. However, given the often low correlation between imaging findings and patient symptoms, it is difficult to support frequent radiographs used to follow the course of pneumonias in the general population.

Most pneumonias resolve within 4 weeks in otherwise healthy individuals. Those who remain unresponsive to conservative measures or exhibit common reoccurrence suggest misdiagnosis or the presence of an underlying condition.[40]

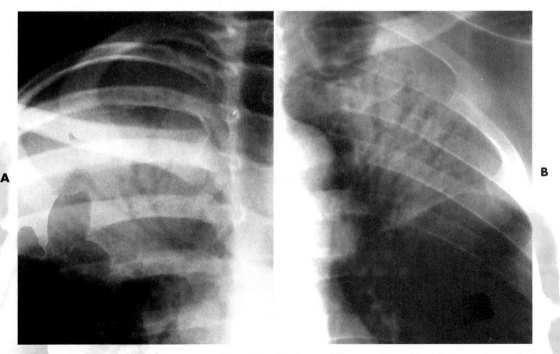

FIG. 24-3 In different patients, **A,** the upper lobe of the right lung and, **B,** upper lobe of the left lung are incompletely consolidated by water-based pathology, namely, pneumonia. Tubular radiolucent shadows are noted traversing the region of consolidation, forming an air-bronchogram sign. The air-bronchogram is seen with an air-space pattern of parenchymal involvement. Normally the air-filled bronchi are adjacent to air-filled alveolar sacs. If the surrounding alveolar sacs become filled with a water-based pathology (e.g., pneumonia), the bronchi become contrasted and are visible as radiolucent tubular shadows, hence an air-bronchogram. (Courtesy Steven P. Brownstein, MD, Springfield, NJ.)

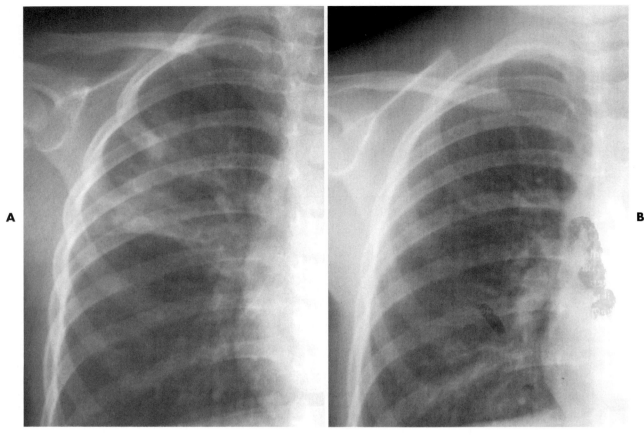

FIG. 24-4 A, The right upper lobe of this 4-year-old girl has an ill-defined cloudy radiodense appearance consistent with pneumonia. **B,** The appearance cleared 3 weeks later. Pneumonia is transient over a several-week period in otherwise healthy individuals. (Courtesy John A.M. Taylor, Seneca Falls, NY.)

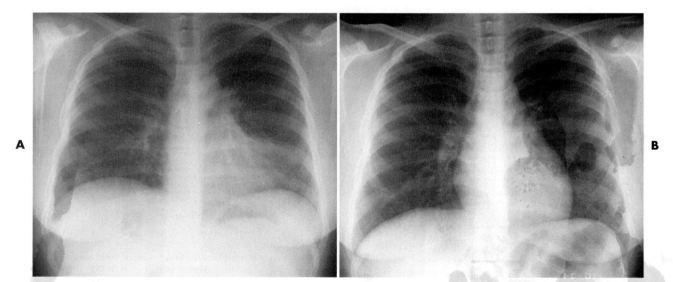

FIG. 24-5 A, A lingular pneumonia is present in this 14-year-old girl. The lingular location can be confirmed in this posteroanterior projection by the lack of a visualized complete left heart border (positive silhouette sign). **B,** In 3 weeks, the left heart border is seen, and the pneumonia has cleared.

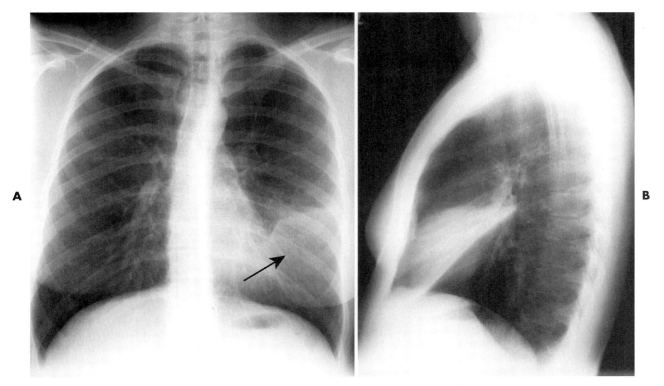

FIG. 24-6 **A,** Left heart border cannot be followed along its entire length. The apex of the heart does not demonstrate a definite border *(arrow)* with the adjacent pulmonary tissue (positive silhouette sign resulting from an absence of a clear silhouette of the heart). The lack of a clear border is caused by pathologic filling of the alveolar sacs with a water-based pathology, most typically pneumonia. Because the lingular segment of the left upper lobe is in direct contact with the apex of the heart, the interpreter can assume that the lingular segment is involved when the heart apex is not clearly demarcated. **B,** Involvement of the lingular segment can be confirmed by the wedge-shaped radiodense shadow seen in the lateral projection and correlating to the pathologic filling of the lingular segment with a water density. (Courtesy John A.M. Taylor, Seneca Falls, NY.)

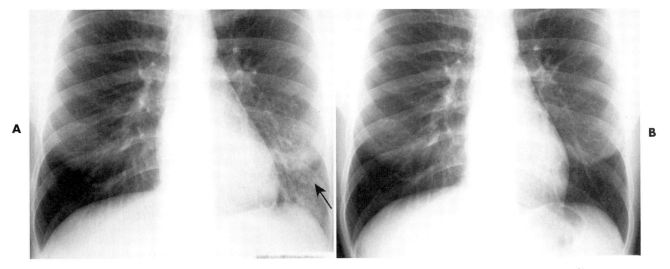

FIG. 24-7 The heart shadow is typically obscured by pneumonia of the lingula of the left upper lobe. Involvement of lung tissue anterior or posterior to the lingula does not obscure the left heart border. In this case, the hazy radiodense shadow over the patient's left (reading right) lower lung field *(arrow)* correlates to the left lower lobe because, **A,** the heart shadow remains as well visualized on the active film as it does on, **B,** a film taken 1 month later after the pneumonia has resolved. (Courtesy John A.M. Taylor, Seneca Falls, NY.)

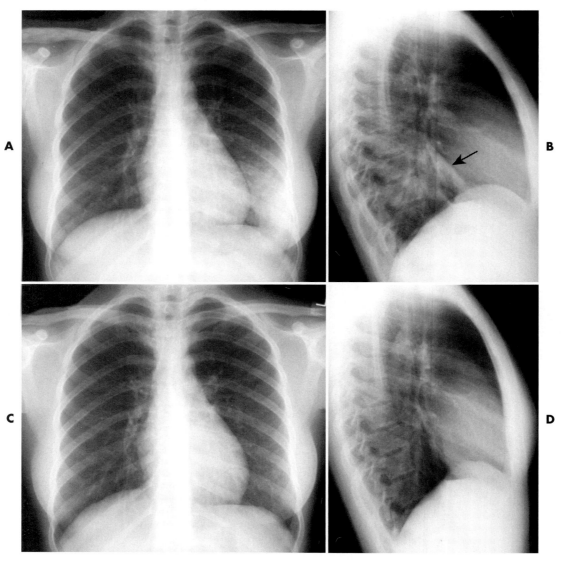

FIG. 24-8   Nineteen-year-old woman with pneumonia of her left lower lung. **A,** Heart border is well delineated, establishing a nonlingula location for the pneumonia. That is, because the cloudy region of air-space disease is seen in the lower lung field, it must be in either the lingula of the left upper lobe or some portion of the left lower lobe. The left lower lobe location is more likely in this case because of the finding of a clear heart silhouette (absence of silhouette sign) present on the posteroanterior radiograph. **B,** Lateral film confirms an air-space pattern of disease that has a smooth anterior margin *(arrow)* corresponding to the major fissure and a lower lobe location. Smooth borders of pathology usually are caused by anatomic structures, such as fissures. **C** and **D,** Films taken 1 month later reveal a normal appearance, indicating that the pneumonia has cleared. (Courtesy John A.M. Taylor, Seneca Falls, NY.)

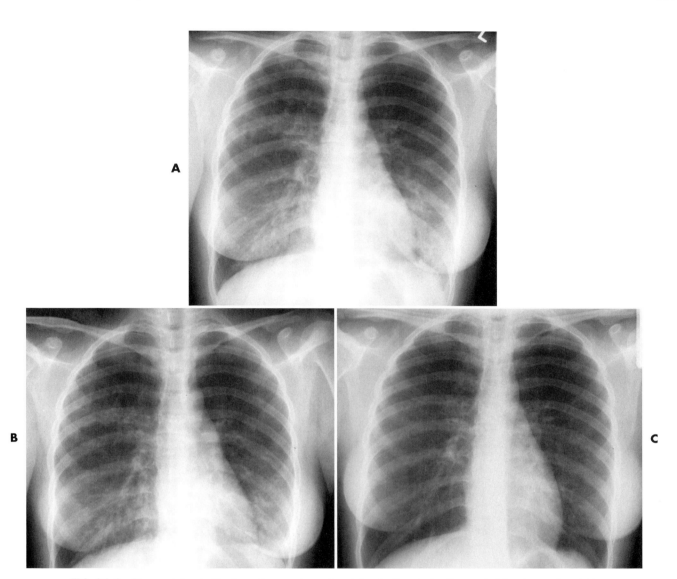

FIG. 24-9 Pneumonia is noted for its rapid progression and resolution in otherwise healthy people. It is not generally a stable radiographic feature. A timeframe of a few weeks produces notable changes. **A,** In this 23-year-old woman, a bilateral presentation of pneumonia of the right and left lower lobes is noted. **B,** Incomplete consolidation begins to resolve 3 days later and, **C,** is nearly completely resolved 9 days later (12 days from the first film, **A**). (Courtesy John A.M. Taylor, Seneca Falls, NY.)

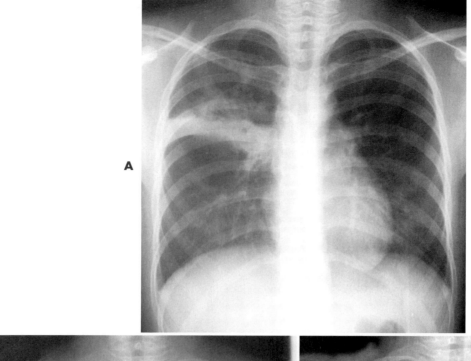

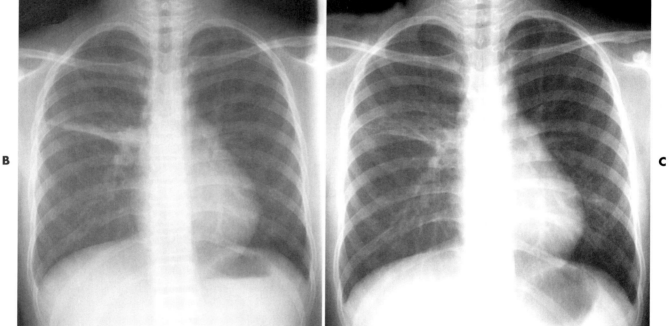

FIG. 24-10 A, Initial film; **B,** 13 days later; and, **C,** 5 days later (18 days after the first film, **A**) exhibit a resolving pneumonia of the right upper lobe. The right upper lobe location is suggested by the smooth lower border of the consolidation. Smooth borders typically are anatomic; in this case the smooth border corresponds to the minor fissure. (Courtesy John A.M. Taylor, Seneca Falls, NY.)

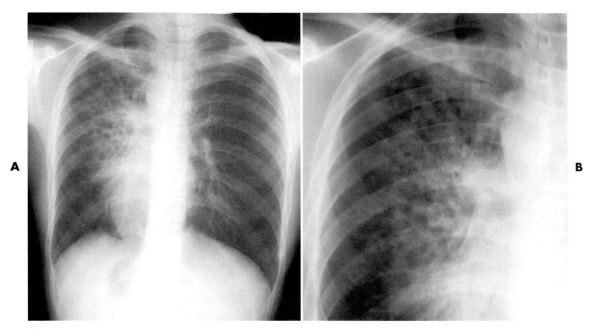

FIG. 24-11 Although there is much crossover, pneumonias can be divided by their radiographic appearance, as described in Table 24-2. **A** and **B**, In this case, a bronchopneumonia pattern is exhibited resulting from the patchy radiodense shadow around the proximal large airways. (Courtesy John A.M. Taylor, Seneca Falls, NY.)

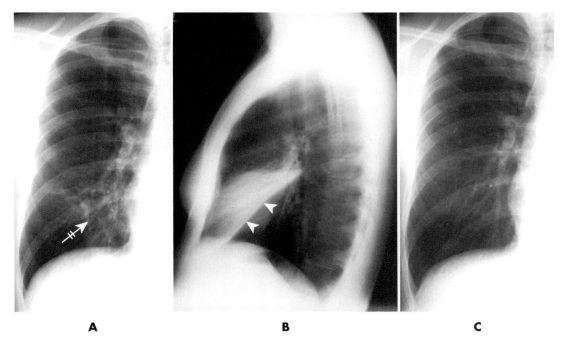

FIG. 24-12 Pneumonia of the right middle lobe. **A,** Although there is only slight abnormality on the posteroanterior (PA) projection *(crossed arrow)*, **B,** the lateral projection exhibits consolidation of the lung tissue immediately anterior to the lower portion of the major fissure *(arrowheads)*. This location corresponds to either the right middle lobe or the lingula of the left upper lobe. The right middle lobe location is confirmed by the appearance on the PA film (**A,** *crossed arrow*). **C,** Three weeks later, the region of the right middle lobe appears clearer and offers a comparison to see the abnormal heavy and thick bronchovascular pattern present on, **A,** the first film. (Courtesy John A.M. Taylor, Seneca Falls, NY.)

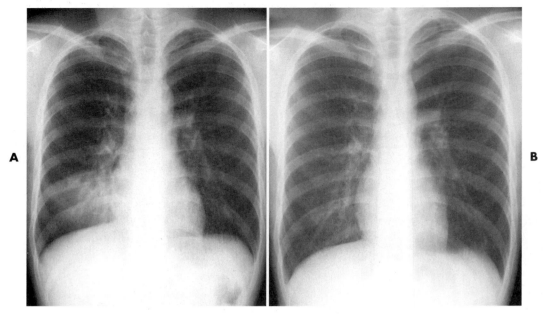

FIG. 24–13 Silhouette sign. **A,** Right lateral margin of the heart of this 17-year-old male patient is not clearly seen on the posteroanterior projection but is clear on, **B,** a follow-up film taken 3 weeks later. Obstruction of the right heart border corresponds to the right middle lobe. (Courtesy John A.M. Taylor, Seneca Falls, NY.)

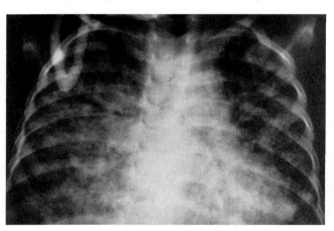

FIG. 24–14 Bilateral consolidating pulmonary radiodense areas in a 15-month-old boy with primary invasive aspergillosis. (Courtesy Steven P. Brownstein, MD, Springfield, NJ.)

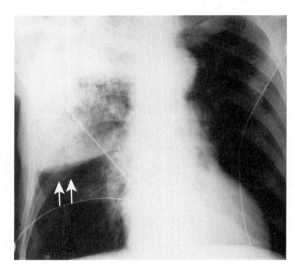

FIG. 24–15 Inferiorly bulging right horizontal fissure secondary to *Klebsiella pneumoniae* within right upper lobe *(arrows)*. (Courtesy Steven P. Brownstein, MD, Springfield, NJ.)

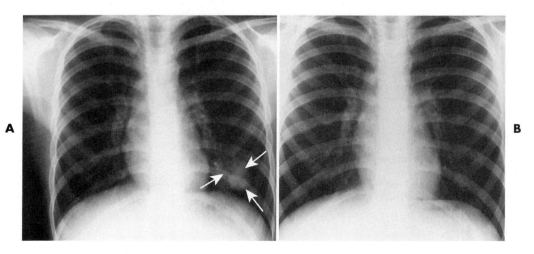

FIG. 24–16 Round pneumonia located adjacent to the left heart border *(arrows)*, **A,** before and, **B,** after antibiotic therapy. (Courtesy Steven P. Brownstein, MD, Springfield, NJ.)

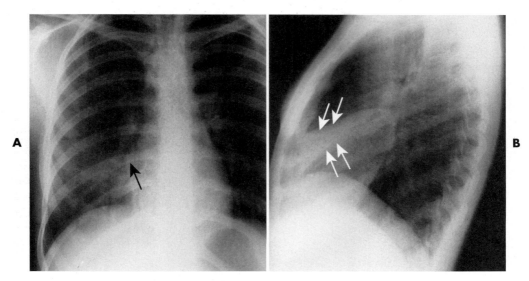

FIG. 24-17 Pneumonia of right middle lobe. **A,** Posteroanterior projection with absence of a clearly demarcated right heart border resulting from contact of the fluid-filled right middle lobe (silhouette sign) *(arrow).* **B,** Lateral projection demonstrating a wedge-shaped consolidated right middle lobe with the apex of the consolidated segment directed toward the hilum *(arrows).* (Courtesy Steven P. Brownstein, MD, Springfield, NJ.)

KEY CONCEPTS

- *Pneumonia is a commonly encountered clinical entity.*
- *It is classified by causative organism (e.g., virus, bacteria, mycoplasma, yeasts, and fungi), radiographic appearance (lobar, lobular or broncho, interstitial, and spherical or round) or etiology (community-acquired, nosocomial, immunosuppressed, or aspiration).*
- *Radiographic findings typically are marked by partial or complete lung consolidation.*
- *Most pneumonias resolve within 4 weeks in otherwise healthy individuals; children, elderly people, and patients with comorbidity should be monitored more closely.*

Tuberculosis

BACKGROUND

Pulmonary tuberculosis (TB) is a chronic granulomatous disease characterized pathologically by caseating granulomas or pneumonia.[23] Although widespread at the turn of the century, tuberculosis has declined markedly throughout most of the past century in developed countries. However, in recent years a slight increase has been noted.[29] This is related to higher incidence among the homeless, prisoners, elderly people in nursing homes, intravenous drug users, and acquired immunodeficiency syndrome (AIDS) patients.[1,11]

For the most part, tuberculosis infections result from inhalation of *Mycobacterium tuberculosis* sputum droplets produced by coughing of infected persons. The pathogen is disseminated by homogenous, bronchogenic, and lymphangitic mechanisms. Pulmonary infections are classified into primary and secondary (postprimary or reinfection) types based on clinical and radiographic criteria. Primary infection represents the first recorded exposure to the pathogen, in which no immunity exists. Secondary infections occur in subsequent exposures in which some degree of immunity is present.

Classically, primary tuberculosis is a childhood disorder, and because of the lack of clinical symptoms, the infection often goes unnoticed. An inflammatory focus develops if the immune response is overcome by the inhaled bacilli. The surrounding tissue response to the acute tuberculous infection results in caseous necrosis and fibrosus. The area may undergo dystrophic calcification and granuloma (tuberculoma) formation, in which the active disease and containment of the disease are balanced. Postprimary infection occurs in adults as either a reactivation of a primary infection or may represent a slow continuation of the active state of a primary infection with no intervening indolent stage.[25]

IMAGING FINDINGS

Chest radiography remains the mainstay in the radiologic evaluation of suspected or proven pulmonary TB (Figs. 24-18 through 24-28).[27] Because TB often passes unrecognized, radiographs are not always available during the initial exposure. Lymphadenopathy, with or without parenchymal consolidation, is the hallmark imaging finding of primary tuberculosis.[26] Hilar lymphadenopathy represents lymphangitic spread from the parenchymal lesion. Alternatively, no radiographic evidence of infection may

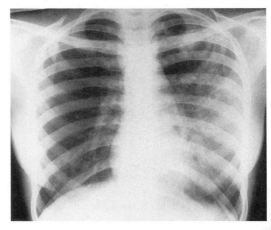

FIG. 24-18 Primary tuberculosis presenting as incomplete pulmonary consolidation in the middle left lung field. (Courtesy Steven P. Brownstein, MD, Springfield, NJ.)

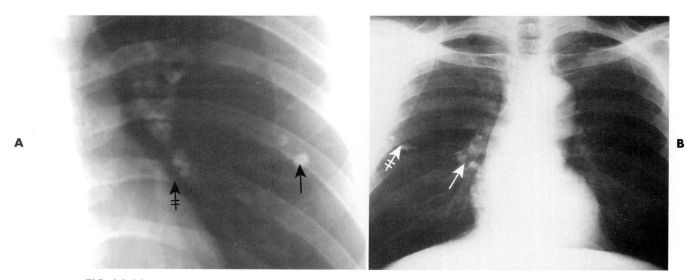

FIG. 24-19 A and **B,** Different patients, both demonstrating a Ranke complex. Ranke complex describes a paired hilar *(crossed arrow)* lymph node calcification and peripheral *(arrow)* parenchymal granuloma that are residual to the primary tuberculosis infection.

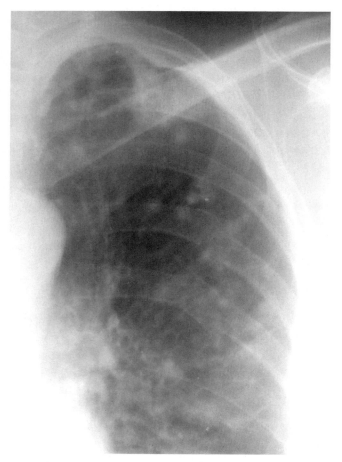

FIG. 24-20 Multiple small radiodense nodules consistent with granulomas in a 42-year-old man. The central "target" calcifications are more typical of histoplasmosis than tuberculosis. (Courtesy John A.M. Taylor, Seneca Falls, NY.)

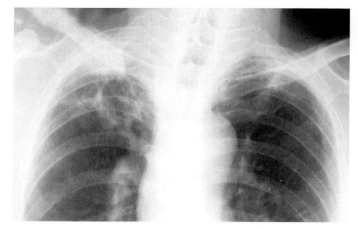

FIG. 24-21 The lung apices exhibit irregular coarse linear shadowing implying fibrosis, and consistent with secondary tuberculosis in this 64-year-old woman. (Courtesy John A.M. Taylor, Seneca Falls, NY.)

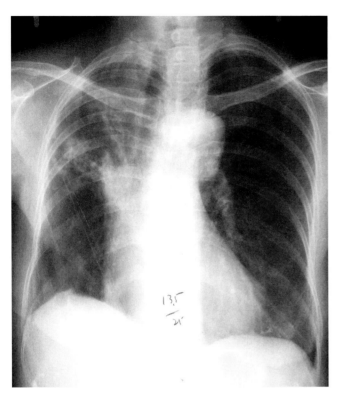

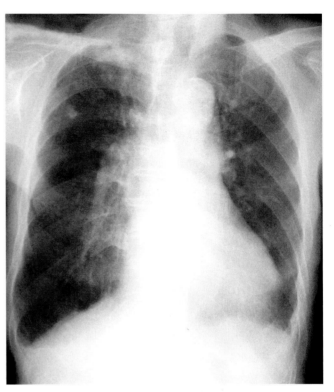

FIG. 24-22 Secondary tuberculosis in a 75-year-old woman. The patient's right lung is more involved, with evidence of volume loss indicated by the superior shift of the horizontal fissure, hilum, and hemidiaphragm. In addition, apical strandlike coarsening is noted bilaterally, but more advanced on the patient's right side. (Courtesy John A.M. Taylor, Seneca Falls, NY.)

FIG. 24-23 Secondary tuberculosis. The right hilum is enlarged, suggesting lymphadenopathy, and multiple granulomas are noted in the lung apices in this 88-year-old patient. (Courtesy John A.M. Taylor, Seneca Falls, NY.)

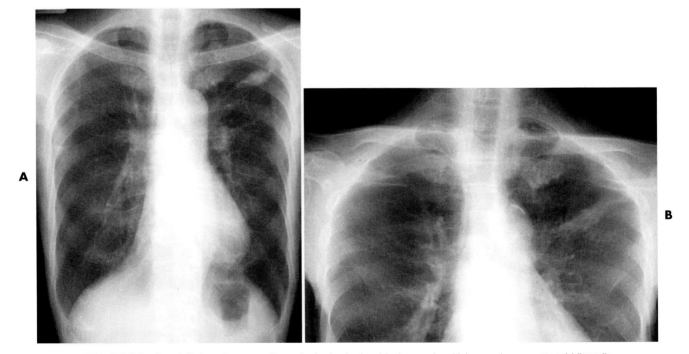

FIG. 24-24 **A** and **B,** Irregular coarse linear shadowing in the right lung and multiple granulomas scattered bilaterally consistent with tuberculosis in this 54-year-old man. (Courtesy John A.M. Taylor, Seneca Falls, NY.)

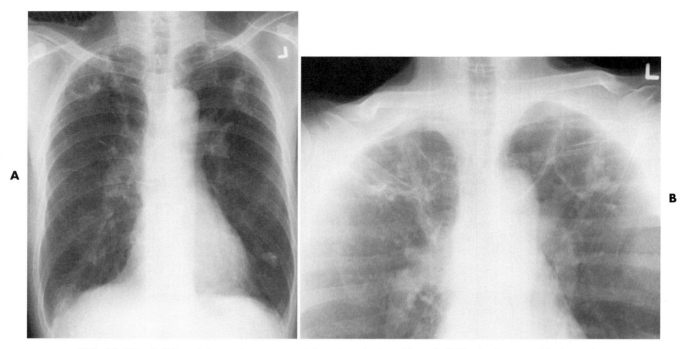

FIG. 24-25   A, Tuberculosis granulomas scattered throughout the lungs bilaterally. **B,** The involvement of the lung apices is seen more clearly on the apical lordotic projection. (Courtesy John A.M. Taylor, Seneca Falls, NY.)

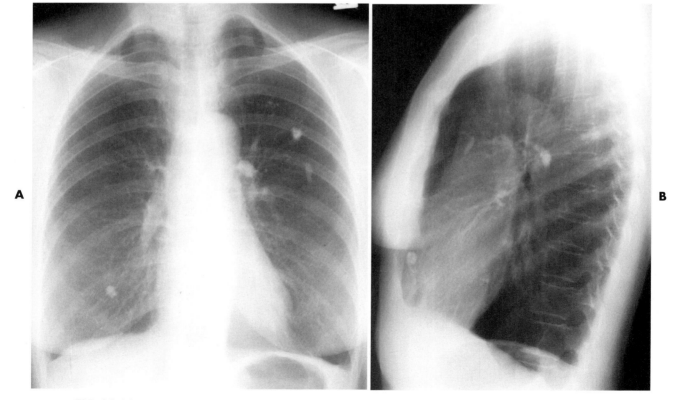

FIG. 24-26   A and **B,** Several densely calcified pulmonary granulomas in this 54-year-old man. Granulomas represent pulmonary scars that develop from past infections with a granulomatous agent, such as tuberculosis, coccidiomycosis, or histoplasmosis. Over time the pulmonary scar undergoes dystrophic calcification. The calcification is an important radiographic finding because it helps in differentiating a benign nodular presentation from something more sinister (e.g., bronchogenic carcinoma). (Courtesy John A.M. Taylor, Seneca Falls, NY.)

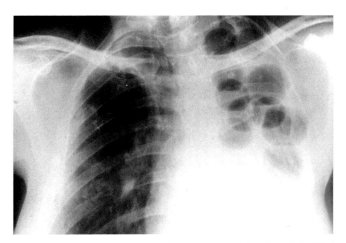

FIG. 24-27 Oblique radiographs of a patient treated for tuberculosis (TB) by stripping the parietal pleura from the chest wall and packing the space with inert Lucite balls, known as *plombage*. TB thrives best in a high-oxygen level environment. Plombage was a twentieth-century method of treating TB by means of iatrogenic atelectasis to reduce the air in the lung, thereby limiting the growth and progression of TB. Antibiotic therapy has replaced most surgical treatments for TB.

be present.[26] The right side is more commonly involved, and no predilection for the upper or lower lobes exists.

The imaging findings typically resolve completely in otherwise healthy individuals. Occasionally a characteristic primary complex (Ranke complex) provides residual evidence of a primary infection, as seen in Figure 24-19. A Ranke complex is the combination of a calcified region of parenchymal involvement (known as a *Ghon tubercle*) and corresponding hilar lymph node calcification.

Reinfection tuberculosis produces a progressive infection with predilection of the posterior and apical segments of the upper lobes and, like primary infections, is more common on the right.

Lymphadenopathy is a less common manifestation than in the primary form of the disease. Parenchymal involvement appears as subsegmental, poorly defined, incomplete consolidations, which have a tendency to coalesce into strandlike radiopacities (see Figs. 24-21 and 24-22). The presence of cavitation indicates reinfection TB and suggests that the disease is active.

Calcified hilar lymph nodes may erode adjacent airways to become broncholiths, which may lead to obstructive atelectasis. Also, bronchogenic spread of TB may produce a widespread lung infection. Hematogenous spread of TB results in discrete miliary nodules widely scattered throughout both lungs, as well as systemic foci of disease. Pleural effusion may occur in response to primary or postprimary infections and is more common when parenchymal involvement is present.

CLINICAL COMMENTS

Predisposing conditions for primary infection include alcoholism, corticosteroids, and diabetes mellitus. Symptoms of cough and productive sputum are rarely present. As with other infections the presence of a single opacity without a confirmed history of TB is presumed to be a solitary pulmonary nodule or "coin lesion" of undetermined etiology. Postprimary infections are more likely associated with symptoms. Typically the patient exhibits cough, night sweats, weight loss, and pleuritic chest pain. Hematogenous spread of TB is an uncommon but serious problem resulting in multiple systemic sites of infection, and necessitating immediate attention.

KEY CONCEPTS

- *Persons at risk for tuberculosis infection include the homeless, prisoners, elderly people in nursing homes, intravenous drug users, and acquired immunodeficiency syndrome (AIDS) patients.*
- *Infections are classified into primary and secondary (postprimary or reinfection) types based on clinical and radiographic criteria.*
- *Primary findings present with no or limited imaging findings; secondary infections exhibit predilection for the upper lung regions and appear as lung scarring and possible cavity formations.*

PART THREE Chest

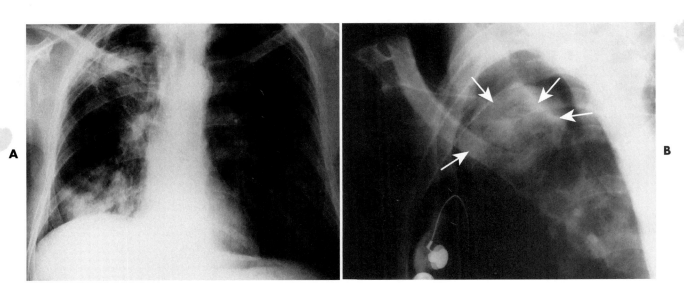

FIG. 24-28 Right lung field demonstrates hazy increased radiodensity consistent with pneumonia. **A,** Lung contracture has caused volume loss, indicated by the slight elevation of the patient's right hemidiaphragm. **B,** Close-up of an oblique view demonstrates an aspergillosis fungal ball within a tuberculosis cavity *(arrows)*. (Courtesy Steven P. Brownstein, MD, Springfield, NJ.)

References

1. Agrons GA, Markowitz RI, Kramer SS: Pulmonary tuberculosis in children, *Semin Roentgenol* 28:58, 1993.

2. Alfageme I et al: Empyema of the thorax in adults: etiology, microbiologic findings, and management, *Chest* 103:839, 1993.

3. Barnhard HJ, Kniker WT: Roentgenologic findings in pertussis with particular emphasis on the "shaggy heart" sign, *AJR Am J Roentgenol* 4:445, 1960.

4. Bartlett JG: Anaerobic bacterial pneumonitis, *Am Rev Respir Dis* 119:19, 1979.

5. Basiliere JL, Bistrong HW, Spence WF: Streptococcal pneumonia: recent outbreaks in military recruit populations, *Am J Med* 44:580, 1968.

6. Bates JH: The role of infection during exacerbations of chronic bronchitis, *Ann Intern Med* 97:130, 1982.

7. Beggs I: The radiology of hydatid disease, *AJR Am J Roentgenol* 145:639, 1985.

8. Brunton FJ, Moore ME: A survey of pulmonary calcification following adult chicken-pox, *Br J Radiol* 42:256, 1969.

9. Cameron DC, Borthwick RN, Philip T: The radiographic patterns of acute *Mycoplasma* pneumonitis, *Clin Radiol* 28:173, 1977.

10. Conte P, Heitzman EK, Markarian B: Viral pneumonia: roentgen pathological correlations, *Radiology* 95:267, 1970.

11. Couser JI, Glassroth J: Tuberculosis: an epidemic in older adults, *Clin Chest Med* 14:491, 1993.

12. Fairbank JT, Patel MM, Dietrich PA: Legionnaire's disease, *J Thorac Imag* 6:6, 1991.

13. Feigin DS: Pulmonary cryptococcosis: radiologic-pathologic correlation of its three forms, *AJR Am J Roentgenol* 141:1263, 1983.

14. Felson LB, Rosenberg LS, Hamburger M: Roentgen findings in acute Friedländer's pneumonia, *Radiology* 53:559, 1949.

15. Foy HM et al: Radiographic study of *Mycoplasma pneumoniae* pneumonia, *Am Rev Respir Dis* 108:469, 1973.

16. Fraser RG, Wortzman G: Acute pneumococcal lobar pneumonia: the significance of nonsegmental distribution, *J Can Assoc Radiol* 3:37, 1959.

17. Frommhold W, Lagemann K, Wolf KJ: Die akute Klehsiellenpneumonie, *Fortschr Geb Romtgellstr* 121:25, 1974.

18. Gordonson J et al: Pulmonary cryptococcosis, *Radiology* 112:557, 1974.

19. Halvorsen RA et al: Pulmonary blastomycosis: radiologic manifestations, *Radiology* 150:1, 1984.

20. Hanna JW, Reed JC, Choplin RH: Pleural infections: clinicoradiologic review, *J Thorac Imag* 6:68, 1991.

21. Holmes RB: Friedlander's pneumonia, *AJR Am J Roentgenol* 75:728, 1956.

22. Iannini PB, Claffey T, Quintiliani R: Bacteremic *Pseudomonas* pneumonia, *JAMA* 230:558, 1974.

23. Im JG et al: CT—pathology correlation of pulmonary tuberculosis, *Crit Rev Diagn Imag* 36:227, 1995.

24. Krysl J et al: Radiologic features of pulmonary tuberculosis: an assessment of 188 cases, *J Can Assoc Radiol* J 45:101, 1994.

25. Lee KS et al: Adult-onset pulmonary tuberculosis: findings on chest radiographs and CT scans, *AJR Am J Roentgenol* 160:753, 1993.

26. Leung AN et al: Primary tuberculosis in childhood: radiographic manifestations, *Radiology* 182:87, 1992.

27. McAdams HP, Erasmus J, Winter JA: Radiologic manifestations of pulmonary tuberculosis, *Radiol Clin North Am* 33:655, 1995.

28. Millar JK: The chest film findings in Q fever: a series of 35 cases, *Clin Radiol* 29:371, 1978.

29. Nainar HS: Tuberculosis: revisited, *ASDC J Dent Child* 59:450, 1992.

30. Peters SG, Prakash UB: Pneumocystis carinii pneumonia. Review of 53 cases, *Am J Med* 82:73, 1987.

31. Pope TL et al: Pittsburgh pneumonia 3 agent: chest film manifestations, *AJR Am J Roentgenol* 138:237, 1983.

32. Putnam JS, Tuazon CU: Symposium on infectious lung diseases: foreword, *Med Clin North Am* 64:317, 1980.

33. Rose RW, Ward BH: Spherical pneumonias in children simulating pulmonary and mediastinal masses, *Radiology* 106:179, 1973.

34. Sargent EN, Carson MJ, Reilly ED: Roentgenographic manifestations of varicella pneumonia with postmortem correlation, *AJR Am J Roentgenol* 98:305, 1966.

35. Smith CB, Overall IC: Clinical and epidemiologic clues to the diagnosis of respiratory infections, *Radiol Clin North Am* 11:261, 1973.

36. Tew J, Calenoff L, Berlin BS: Bacterial or nonbacterial pneumonia: accuracy of radiographic diagnosis, *Radiology* 124:607, 1977.

37. Trollfors B et al: Incidence, predisposing factors and manifestations of invasive *Haemophilus influenzae* infections in adults, *Eur J Clin Microbiol* 3:180, 1984.

38. Vessal K et al: Radiological changes in inhalational anthrax: a report of radiological and pathological correlation in two cases, *Clin Radiol* 25:471, 1975.

39. Wiedemann HP, Rice TW: Lung abscesses and empyema, *Semin Thorac Cardiovasc Surg* 7:119, 1995.

40. Winterbauer RH, Bedon GA, Ball WC Jr: Recurrent pneumonia: predisposing illness and clinical patterns in 158 patients, *Ann Intern Med* 70:689, 1969.

41. Young RC et al: *Aspergillosis:* the spectrum of the disease in 98 patients, *Medicine* 49:47, 1970.

chapter 25

Thoracic Neoplasms

DENNIS M. MARCHIORI

Bronchial Carcinoid Tumors
Bronchogenic Carcinoma
Hamartoma
Lymphoma

Metastatic Lung Disease
Pleural Mesothelioma
Teratomas
Thymic Masses

Bronchial Carcinoid Tumors

BACKGROUND

Bronchial carcinoid tumors are uncommon pulmonary tumors, formerly termed *bronchial adenomas*. The term adenoma to describe these lesions is a misnomer resulting from their locally invasive nature, tendency for recurrence, and occasional metastasis to extrapulmonary tissues. They typically occur in patients at least 40 years of age but represent the most common primary lung tumors in patients under the age of 16 years. These tumors arise from neuroectodermal cells[49,68] and are hormonally active, known to produce symptoms similar to Cushing's disease.[22,25] Overall, 75% arise in the lobar bronchi, 10% in the mainstem bronchi, and 15% in the periphery of the lung.[18] Ninety percent of bronchial carcinoids are well-differentiated lesions. Atypical carcinoids are less common but exhibit a higher malignancy rate than well-differentiated lesions.

IMAGING FINDINGS

Often a solitary nodule can be seen on plain films. This is more likely if the lesion is peripherally located. Bronchial carcinoids commonly are discovered by recognizing associated findings of bronchial obstruction. If the airway obstruction is partial, a check-valve obstruction may result in overexpansion of the distal air-space. Atelectasis results if obstruction is complete. Recurrent pneumonia, bronchiectasis, and calcification of the lesion also may occur.[6] Computed tomography (CT) is helpful in confirming suspected lesions (Fig. 25-1).

CLINICAL COMMENTS

Because bronchial carcinoid tumors commonly are centrally located in the lobar divisions of bronchi, they often present with findings related to bronchial obstruction (recurrent atelectasis and pneumonia). Clinical findings of hemoptysis, wheezing, cough, and atypical asthma may be noted. A small percentage of patients remain asymptomatic. Resection is typical, with a 5-year survival rate of 95%. The prognosis is usually excellent and is more specifically determined when the pathologic grade and stage of the tumor are known.

KEY CONCEPTS

- Bronchial carcinoid tumors are low-grade malignancies most commonly arising in the lobar bronchi.
- Well-differentiated carcinoid tumors represent almost 90% of all bronchial carcinoids.
- Lesions may be seen directly on radiographs or often are found by recognizing concurrent findings of airway obstruction. Resection usually is associated with an excellent prognosis.

Bronchogenic Carcinoma

BACKGROUND

Risk factors. Bronchogenic carcinoma (lung cancer) was a relatively uncommon tumor at the beginning of the century. It has grown to become the leading cause of cancer-related deaths among men and women. Lung cancer accounts for approximately 20% of cancer deaths among men and 10% among women, replacing breast cancer as the most common cause of cancer death among women.[44] Cancer rates correlate positively with population density, chronic lung disease, urbanization, industrialization, cigarette smoking, and carcinogenic inhalants (e.g., asbestos, nickel, uranium, chromates).[21,69] Genetic factors seem to play a role in the development of lung cancer, but the influence is confounded by environmental factors such as cigarette smoking.

Cigarette smoking is the most common important risk factor for developing lung cancer, with approximately 90% of lung cancer worldwide attributed to cigarette smoking. Its development is related to both the duration and dose of cigarette smoking, with risk of lung cancer death reported in the realm of 12 to 20 times that of nonsmokers. Although rates of smoking among men appear to have leveled off, smoking among women has increased[7] and is likely to be responsible for the contemporary increase in lung cancer rates among women. The risks of smoking may be compounded when other risks are present. For instance, asbestos exposure alone relates approximately five times the baseline risk for developing lung cancer; however, the combination of work-related asbestos exposure and cigarette smoking is associated with a 50 to 100 times baseline risk, a synergistic risk that far exceeds the risk derived by simply adding the risks of the individual factors.

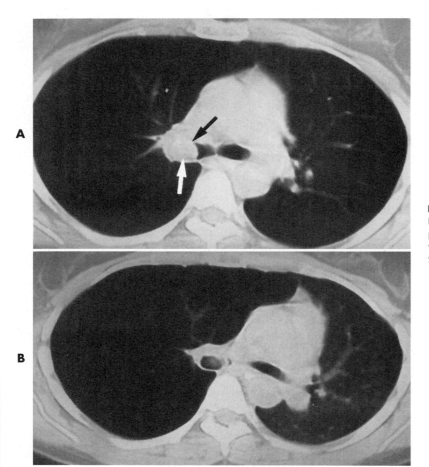

FIG. 25-1 A, Computed tomography (CT) shows an endobronchial tumor in the right mainstem bronchus *(arrows)*. **B,** CT performed after exhalation shows a significant mediastinal shift to the patient's left as a result of air trapping on the right. (From Swenson SJ: Radiology of thoracic diseases: a teaching file, St Louis, 1993, Mosby.)

Categorization. Bronchogenic carcinomas develop from the airways, not the lung parenchyma. Parenchymal neoplasms are represented by leiomyomas, fibromas, chondromas, and other mesenchymal derivatives.[60] Bronchogenic tumors are divided into four groups, based on histology: squamous cell (epidermoid) carcinoma, adenocarcinoma, large cell carcinoma, and small (oat) cell carcinoma (Table 25-1).[33,51] Bronchoalveolar carcinoma is a subtype of the adenocarcinoma cell type.[14]

Often lesions are divided by location into central (near the hilum) or peripheral (lateral to the hilum) location (Figs. 25-2 through 25-11). Peripheral lesions appear as masses (>3 cm diameter) or nodules (≤3 cm diameter)[26] in the lateral lung field arising from the third or fourth order bronchi and beyond. Central lesions arise from the mainstem, lobar, or segmental bronchi and appear as hilar enlargements or present with secondary findings related to airway obstruction. Approximately 60% of lesions are central and 40% are peripheral.[4] Sixty percent of lesions (peripheral and central) are right sided. Similarly, 60% of peripheral lesions are in the upper lung (Fig. 25-12), 30% in the lower, and the remaining 10% in the middle and lingual segments. The average age of patients with recently recognized lung cancer is 53 years, with 80% of lesions developing between 40 and 70 years.[66]

IMAGING FINDINGS

The radiographic features of a nodule or mass are important to the clinical management of the patient. When considered with the patient age, the growth rate, calcification, size, and location of the lesion are significant indicators of a benign versus malignant lesion (Fig. 25-13). Associated bone destruction is a strong indicator of malignancy (Figs. 25-14 and 25-15).

Location. Central tumors demonstrate radiographic changes related to airway obstruction. Airway obstruction leads to volume changes presenting as atelectasis or overinflation (if a check-valve mechanism develops), both of which may displace the mediastinum, heart shadow, diaphragm, or other anatomic borders. A consolidated radiographic pattern may result from postobstructive pneumonitis, which refers to marked retention of lung secretions in the alveolar spaces secondary to airway obstruction.[9]

An enlarged hilum is a common finding of central tumors.[56] The enlarged hilum represents the tumor mass itself or associated lymph node involvement. A classic radiographic appearance, known as the S-sign of Golden, develops when the hilar mass is found with concurrent radiopacity of the right upper lobe secondary to either atelectasis or postobstructive pneumonitis resulting from airway obstruction. The inferior border of the parenchymal radiopacity appears as a smooth, reversed S-shape. The radiographic appearance appears S-shaped when present on the patient's left side.

Pancoast (superior sulcus) tumors are defined as dense, homogenous masses with smooth borders located in the lung apex (Figs. 25-16 to 25-18). Lesions often demonstrate adjacent rib or vertebral destruction (see Fig. 25-15). Most Pancoast tumors are

TABLE 25-1
Radiographic Appearance of Bronchogenic Carcinoma Types

Type	Radiographic appearance*
Squamous cell (epidermoid) carcinoma	Most often a central lesion with locally invasive hilar and mediastinal involvement, often presenting as lobar collapse; peripheral presentation appears as nodule, mass, or cavity
Adenocarcinoma	Most common cell type, nearly always presents as peripheral mass; smaller in size than large cell type
Alveolar cell carcinoma (bronchoalveolar cell carcinoma)	Subtype of adenocarcinoma, most commonly presents as a nodule, but is more noted for its presentation of diffuse or localized air-space disease pattern
Small (oat) cell carcinoma	Classically presents as a hilar or mediastinal metastasis, whereas the primary tumor remains occult; it is the most aggressive cell type, having the worst prognosis; central involvement may lead to atelectasis or superior vena cava syndrome
Large cell carcinoma	Like adenocarcinoma, presents in a peripheral location, but is most often larger in size than adenocarcinoma cell type

*Considerable crossover exists in radiographic appearance, making distinction among types difficult.

caused by squamous cell carcinomas, although other types of bronchogenic tumors may be responsible. Alternatively, Pancoast tumors may appear with little more than subtle pleural thickening.

Size. Peripheral lesions often present as only a spherical radiopacity.[10] Lesions present in variable sizes, but they are difficult to detect on plain films if less than 1 cm in diameter.[28,42] The average diameter at the time of discovery is 5 cm.[66] Lesions greater than 3 cm in diameter are malignant 85% of the time.[53] Most solitary pulmonary nodules (lesions ≤3 cm in diameter) are indeterminate at the time of discovery. Further procedures (CT, biopsy, and thoracotomy) are necessary to reach a definitive diagnosis.[30]

Nipple shadows, moles, and other body wall lesions may mimic pulmonary nodules, particularly in the periphery of the lung (Figs. 25-19 through 25-22). Repeating the radiograph with metallic markers over the area in question is a simple method to exclude such body wall lesions (Fig. 25-23).

Borders. The appearance of the outer border of the lesion has been emphasized in the past. Circumferential strandlike radiopacities radiating from the outer border of the tumor (corona radiata) have been described[71] as characteristic but not specific to bronchogenic tumor.[35] The irregular outer border is believed to represent tissue fibrosis or radial spread of the tumor. A lobulated appearance of the outer border, representing areas of rapid growth, is found in 50% of peripheral tumors. Cavitation has been described in 16% of peripheral lesions,[66] most often seen in the squamous cell type.

Calcification. Calcification of bronchogenic tumors rarely is demonstrated on plain film studies. CT demonstrates calcification in 6% to 7% of lesions.[45,73] As depicted in Figure 25-24, certain patterns of calcification strongly suggest a benign etiology. Central, laminated, or total homogeneous calcification is typical of granulomas. A "comma-shaped" or "popcorn" calcification pattern suggests a hamartoma. Eccentric calcification is associated with bronchogenic carcinoma, representing calcium produced by the tumor, dystrophic calcification of ischemic tissue, or a granuloma that has

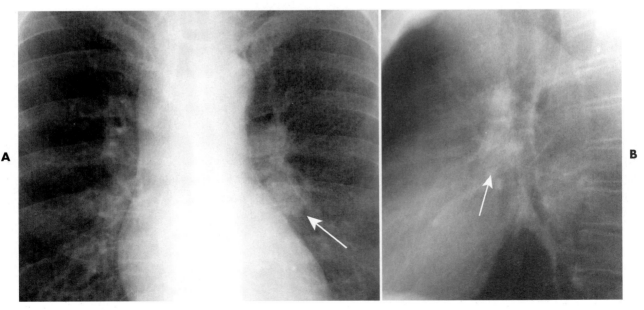

FIG. 25-2 **A** and **B,** Central bronchogenic carcinoma of the patient's left hilum *(arrows)* in a 59-year-old male patient. (Courtesy John A.M. Taylor, Seneca Falls, NY.)

Text continued on p. 1199.

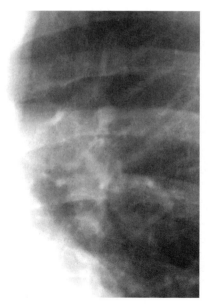

FIG. 25-3 Bronchogenic carcinoma presenting as an enlarged hilum. Normally the hila are well defined and exhibit a branching pattern that is absent in this examp e.

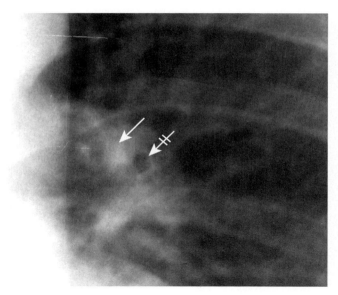

FIG. 25-5 At times a large hilar vessel may be confused with a pulmonary nodule. One clue to differentiation is provided by the observation that pulmonary vessels and bronchi follow a similar branching pattern. Therefore if a radiodense ring shadow accompanies the suspicious homogeneous radiodense shadow, the apparent nodule is likely a vessel, not a true pulmonary nodule. This finding of a radiodense circle *(arrow)* next to a radiodense ring (with radiolucent center) *(crossed arrow)* is known as a *monocle sign.*

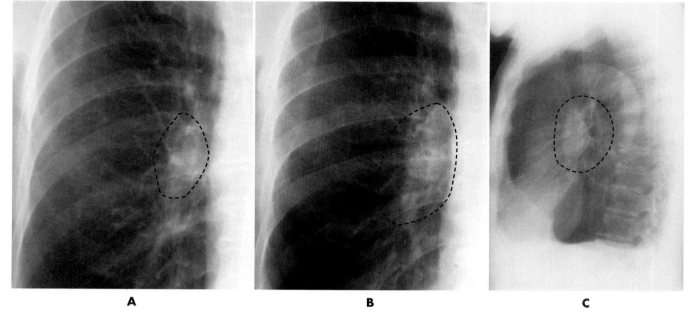

A   **B**   **C**

FIG. 25-4 Bronchogenic carcinoma enlarging the hilum. **A,** First film exhibiting an abnormal bulky appearance of the hilum. **B,** Second film taken 4 months later revealing that the lesion has grown. **C,** Lesion in the right hilum, as noted by its appearance anterior to the bronchi in the aortic pulmonary window of the lateral projection. (Courtesy John A.M. Taylor, Seneca Falls, NY.)

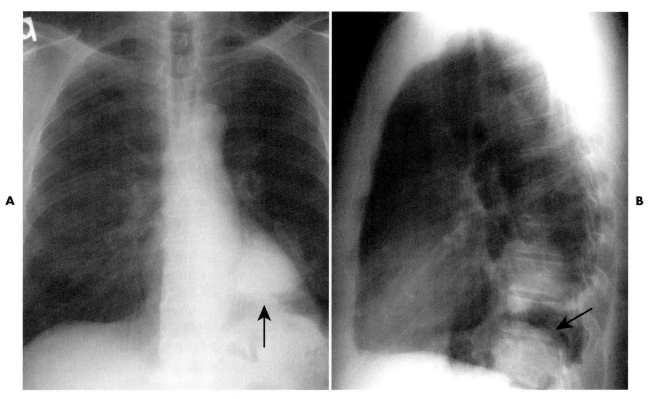

FIG. 25-6 Large malignant mass presenting behind the heart shadow *(arrows).* **A,** Pulmonary lesions presenting behind and in front of the heart are missed easily. **B,** Care should be taken to look closely through the heart shadow and augment this difficult-to-interpret area with the addition of a lateral view. (Courtesy Gary Longmuir, Phoenix, AZ.)

PART THREE
Chest

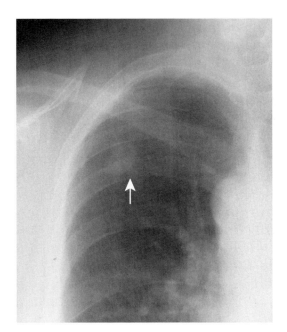

FIG. 25-7 Bronchogenic carcinoma presenting as a solitary pulmonary nodule without evidence of calcification *(arrow)* in a 56-year-old man. The lack of calcification necessitates further evaluation to exclude malignancy in middle-aged and older patients. (Courtesy John A.M. Taylor, Seneca Falls, NY.)

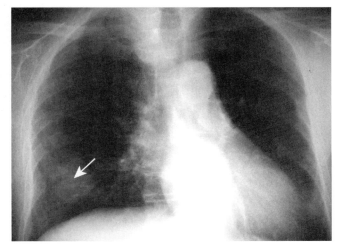

FIG. 25-8 Large malignant mass in the patient's lower right lung *(arrow).*

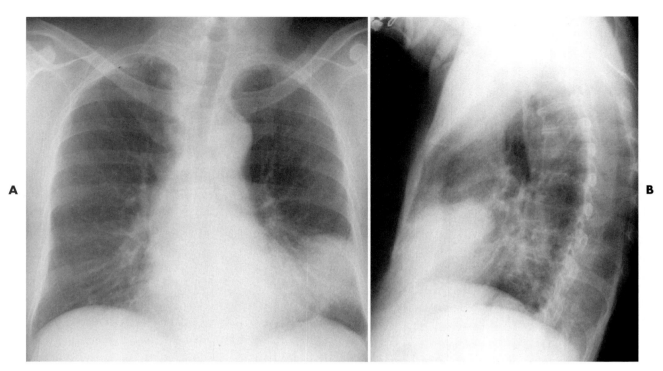

FIG. 25-9 **A** and **B,** Bronchogenic carcinoma in a 70-year-old male patient. The lesion presented as a large noncalcified mass. The larger a lesion, the more likely it is malignant. (Courtesy John A.M. Taylor, Seneca Falls, NY.)

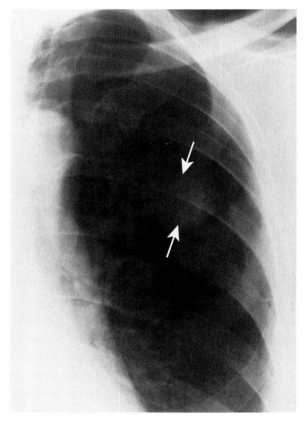

FIG. 25-10 Squamous cell bronchogenic carcinoma presenting as a noncalcified solitary pulmonary nodule at the level of the posterior angle of the sixth left rib (arrows). (Courtesy Steven P. Brownstein, MD, Springfield, NJ.)

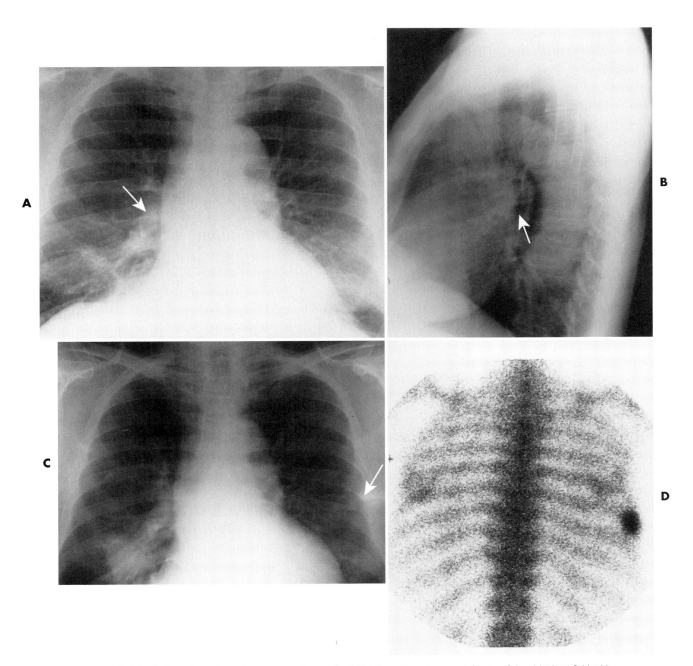

FIG. 25-11 **A,** Bronchogenic carcinoma presenting on the initial film with pulmonary infiltrate of the right lung field with enlargement of the right hilum *(arrow)*. **B,** Lateral projection revealing radiodense region in the aortic pulmonary window corresponding to the right hilum *(arrow)*. **C,** Thirteen months later the pulmonary infiltrate has consolidated into a mass. Also of interest is an unrelated fracture of the lateral margin of the seventh left rib *(arrow)*. **D,** Radionuclide bone scan demonstrating radionuclide uptake at the fracture site. (Courtesy Steven P. Brownstein, MD, Springfield, NJ.)

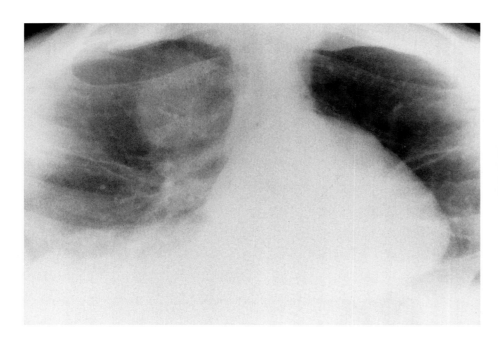

FIG. 25-12 Apical lordotic projection demonstrating noncalcific mass in the right lung apex, consistent with bronchogenic carcinoma. (Courtesy Steven P. Brownstein, MD, Springfield, NJ.)

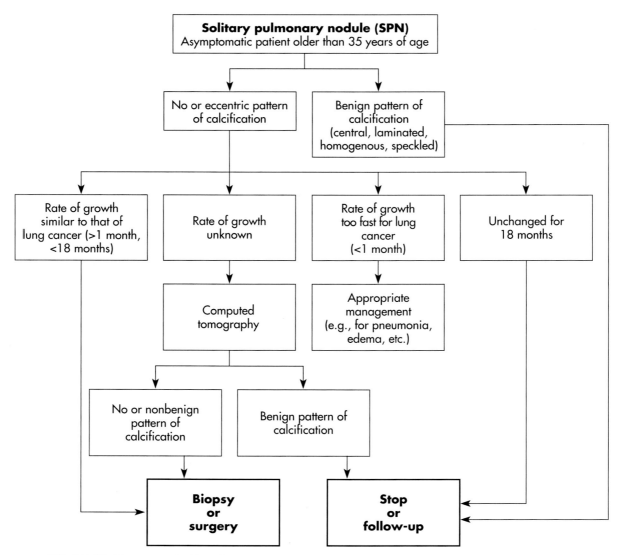

FIG. 25-13 Management algorithm of solitary pulmonary nodules of patients in cancer age group, based on imaging findings.

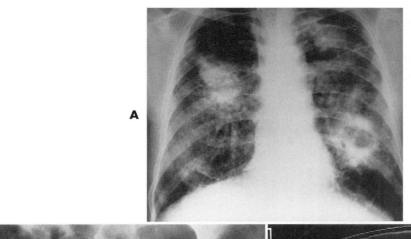

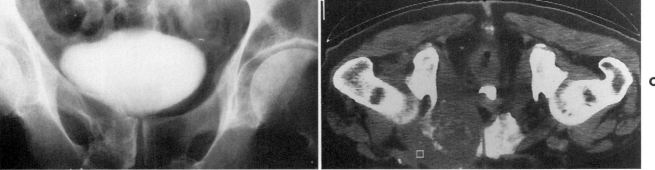

FIG. 25-14 A, Cavitating squamous cell carcinoma of the left lower lung field in a patient with progressive massive fibrosis noted by the bilateral, asymmetric radiodensities in the lung fields. **B,** Plain film radiograph and, **C,** computed tomography scan reveal lytic bone destruction of the right pubis resulting from metastasis of the lung carcinoma. (Courtesy Steven P. Brownstein, MD, Springfield, NJ.)

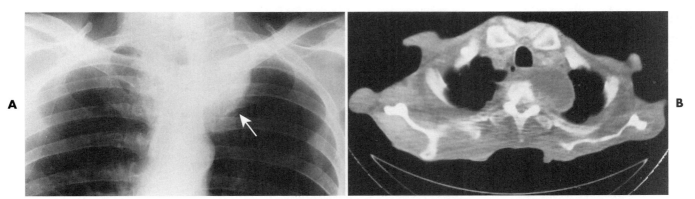

FIG. 25-15 A, Bronchogenic carcinoma within the medial portion of the patient's left lung apex (Pancoast tumor) *(arrow).* **B,** Computed tomography reveals the tumor mass with associated vertebral body destruction. (Courtesy Steven P. Brownstein, MD, Springfield, NJ.)

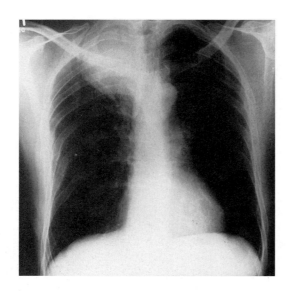

FIG. 25-16 Bronchogenic carcinoma presenting as a right apical mass.

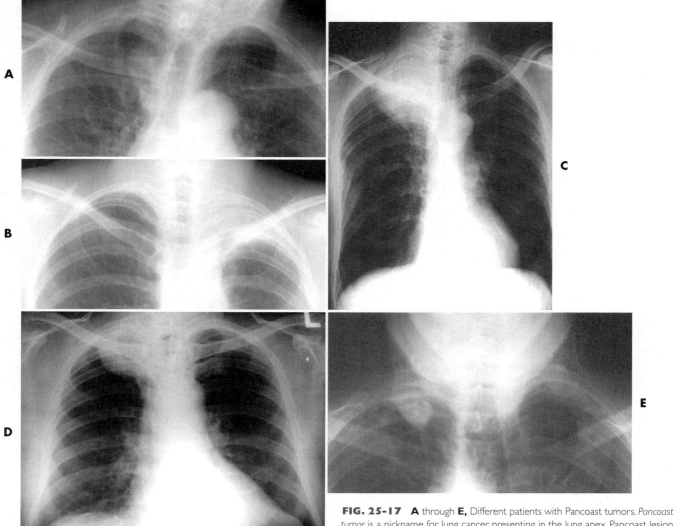

FIG. 25-17 **A** through **E,** Different patients with Pancoast tumors. *Pancoast tumor* is a nickname for lung cancer presenting in the lung apex. Pancoast lesion may present clinically with Horner syndrome, upper extremity neurovascular compromise, and rib destruction. (**A** and **B,** Courtesy John A.M. Taylor, Seneca Falls, NY; **C** and **D,** Courtesy Steven P. Brownstein, MD, Springfield, NJ.)

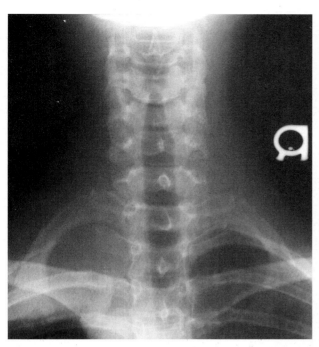

FIG. 25-18 Care should be taken not to underinterpret the apices of the lungs on an anteroposterior lower cervical radiograph. As seen here in the patient's left lung apex, Pancoast tumors are common serious pathologies that may present in this radiographic view. (Courtesy Gary Longmuir, Phoenix, AZ.)

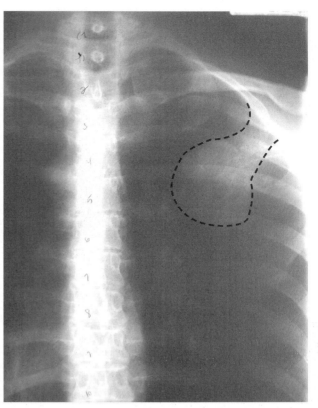

FIG. 25-19 Apparent pulmonary mass that latter studies confirmed was a benign lesion of the rib, likely an osteochondroma. (Courtesy C. Robert Tatum, Davenport, IA.)

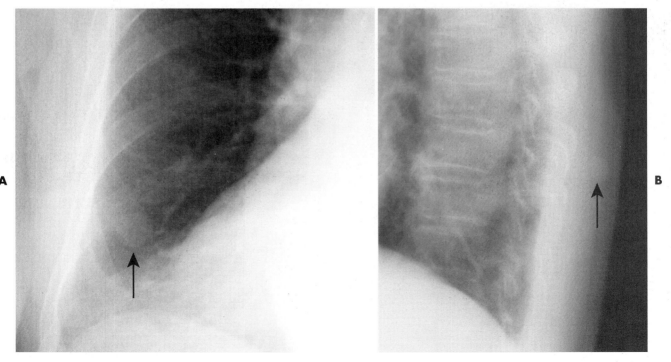

FIG. 25-20 **A,** The small radiodense shadow appears to be in a pulmonary location. **B,** However, the lateral view and patient examination confirm it as large a mole *(arrows)*. (Courtesy John A.M. Taylor, Seneca Falls, NY.)

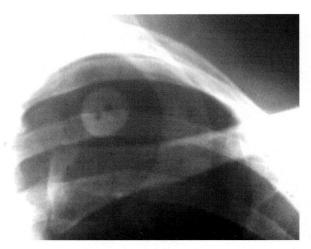

FIG. 25-21 A button mimics a solitary pulmonary nodule. In this case the two holes in the center of the shadow readily confirm it as a clothing artifact.

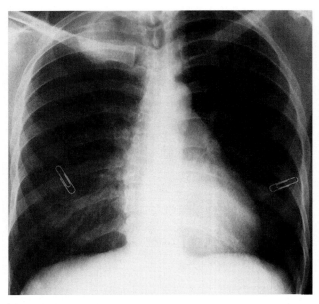

FIG. 25-23 Paper clips confirming that nipple shadows represent bilateral symmetric pulmonary nodules. In addition, a bronchogenic carcinoma is in the apex of the patient's right lung (Pancoast tumor) causing the radiodense shadow above the patient's right clavicle. (Courtesy Steven P. Brownstein, MD, Springfield, NJ.)

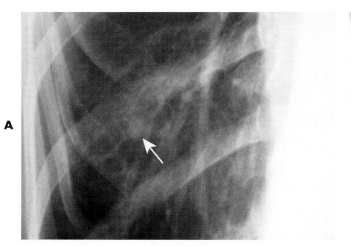

FIG. 25-22 At times, **A,** a male or, **B,** female patient's nipple (arrows) may be confused as a solitary pulmonary nodule. The nipple often appears more well defined laterally from better air contrast when the medial side of the nipple is pushed against its adjacent soft tissue as a result of placing the anterior chest wall against the grid cabinet during the posteroanterior chest patient setup. Also, the nipple shadow often is bilateral and generally is found in an expected anatomic location relative to the breast shadow that also may be seen on the film. If differentiation between the nipple shadow and pulmonary nodule cannot be made, a metallic marker is placed over the nipple and the chest x-ray is repeated (see Fig. 25-23).

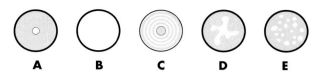

FIG. 25-24 Benign patterns of nodule calcification. **A,** Central; **B,** homogenous (total); **C,** laminated; **D,** amorphous; and **E,** speckled.

been engulfed by the growing tumor mass. Patients who demonstrate masses and nodules with no calcification or calcification only in the periphery of the lesions should be studied vigorously for the possibility of malignancy (Figs. 25-25 through 25-31).

Growth rate. It has been estimated that on average bronchogenic tumors double in volume every 1 to 18 months (see Fig. 25-11).[27,34] Doubling in volume is equal to a 25% increase in diameter. Lesions that double in size more rapidly or slowly than normal suggest another cause (e.g., infection, edema). Lesions known to be stable over a 2-year period can be assumed to be benign (Fig. 25-32).

Growth rate most often is assessed by comparing the appearance of a lesion with its appearance on earlier radiographs of the same patient that may be available. If the past radiographs reveal a stable lesion, no further workup may be necessary. However, if past studies do not reveal the lesion, or if the lesion appears to have grown, further workup is necessary to exclude aggressive pathology.

CLINICAL COMMENTS

Twenty-five percent of lung cancer patients are asymptomatic at the time of diagnosis.[58] When clinical findings are present, they are nonspecific and of little diagnostic value. When carcinoma is still confined to the lung, clinical findings of cough, wheezing, and hemoptysis are common clinical manifestations. Mediastinal involvement is suggested with hoarseness, chest pain, brachial plexus neuropathy, Horner syndrome, superior vena cava obstruction, and dysphagia. Recurrent, unresolving, or persistent (unchanged over 2 weeks) patterns of pneumonia suggest underlying airway obstruction.

Because of their anatomic location, Pancoast tumors are often associated with clinical findings of Horner syndrome (ptosis, miosis, anidrosis, and enophthalmos) and brachial plexus neuropathy.

Treatments for lung cancer are disappointing, with a 5-year survival rate of less than 10%[55] to 13%.[23] The poor prognosis results in part from the advanced stage of the disease at the time of initial recognition. The tumor is in its later stages by the time clinical symptoms are noted.[70] The formation of lung tumors predates their initial identification by 8 to 17 years.[53] Peripheral lesions have a slightly better prognosis, caused by the more diverse surgical techniques available to these lesions when compared with central lesions. A preventive approach to the disease is crucial because 90% of cases are related to smoking.[50]

Patients with a solitary pulmonary nodule on the chest radiograph should be vigorously investigated for the possibility of malignancy. The patient's age, size and borders of the lesion, presence of calcification, and growth over time (evaluated by previous radiographs) may be helpful in determining malignancy.

KEY CONCEPTS

- *The majority of lung cancers appear as either a solitary parenchymal nodule/mass or a hilar mass that demonstrates progressive growth with time.*
- *Plain film radiology may reveal the tumors themselves or, as is often the case with central lesions, abnormalities related to bronchial obstruction by the tumor (e.g., postobstructive pneumonitis or obstructive emphysema).*
- *A lesion's size, pattern of calcification, borders, and growth over time are helpful criteria in differentiating a benign versus malignant etiology.*

Hamartoma

BACKGROUND

Hamartomas are focal tissue malformations representing faulty tissue development at the organ level. Lung hamartomas are composed of fibrous, cartilaginous, muscle, fatty, and epithelial tissues

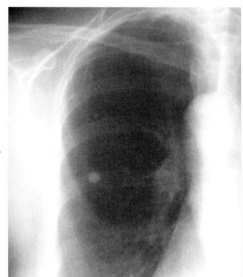

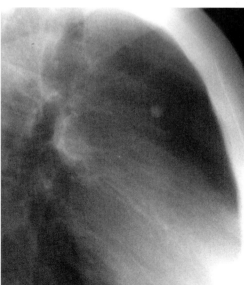

FIG. 25-25 A and **B,** Isolated small densely calcified nodule consistent with a benign etiology. (Courtesy Julie-Marthe Grenier, Davenport, IA.)

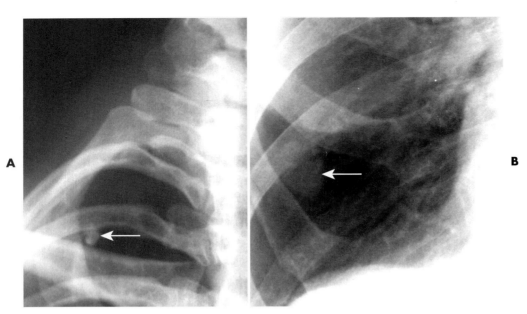

FIG. 25-26 **A,** Small completely calcified granuloma *(arrow)*. **B,** In contrast, the lack of any visible calcification in the second nodule *(arrow)* warrants further investigation to excluded malignancy. The absence or presence of calcification is a strong determinant of whether the lesion is benign or malignant.

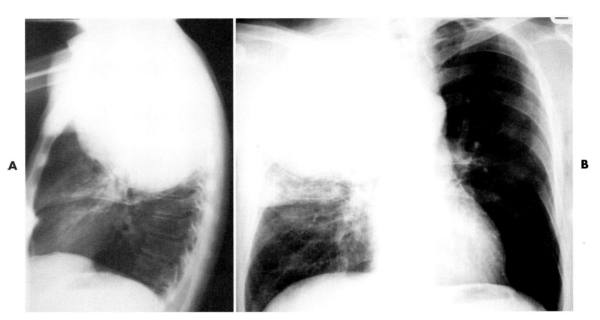

FIG. 25-27 **A** and **B,** Oat cell carcinoma presenting as a huge pulmonary mass.

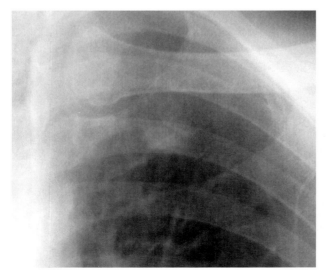

FIG. 25-28 Pulmonary nodule with added radiodensity from superimposed ribs. This nodule is not calcified and is suspicious of malignancy. The degree of radiodensity that is present is caused by the overlying osseous structures of the anterior margin of the first rib and the posterior margin of the fourth rib. One should not attribute the additive density of overlying structures to calcification of the nodule, and consequently, by mistake, interpret a malignant lesion as benign.

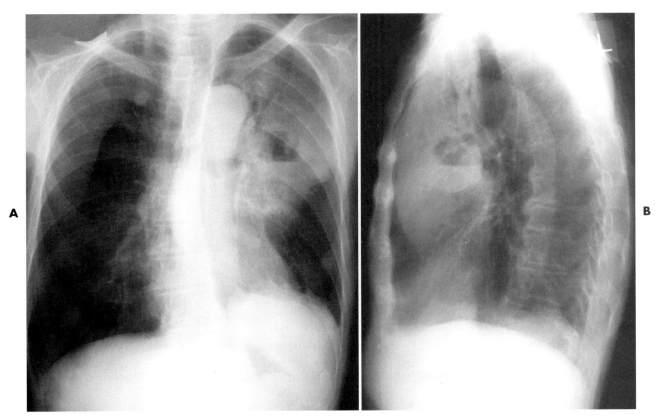

FIG. 25-29 A and **B,** An 87-year-old man presenting with cavitating bronchogenic carcinoma. (Courtesy John A.M. Taylor, Seneca Falls, NY.)

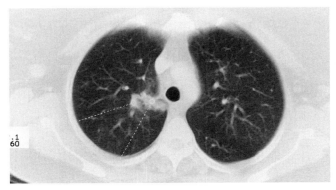

FIG. 25-30 Computed tomography (CT) of an enlarged right hilum. Because of its greater accuracy, CT is indicated as follow-up to an abnormal feature noted or suspected on plain film studies.

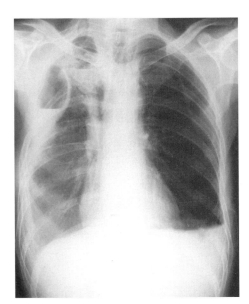

FIG. 25-31 Malignant cavitating lesion in the periphery of the patient's right lung. (Courtesy John A.M. Taylor, Seneca Falls, NY.)

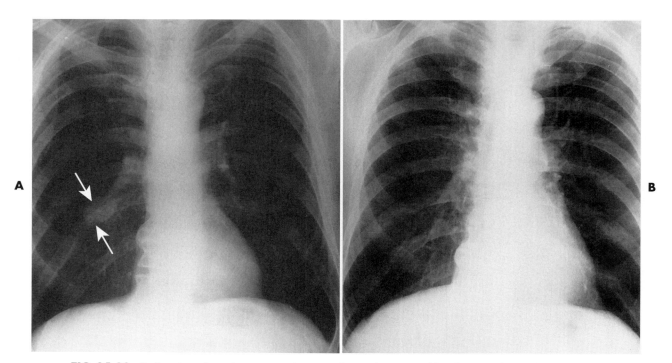

FIG. 25-32 A, Bronchogenic carcinoma presenting as a solitary pulmonary nodule adjacent to the anterior end of the fifth right rib *(arrows)*. **B,** Radiograph of the same patient 8 years earlier without the tumor nodule. (Courtesy Steven P. Brownstein, MD, Springfield, NJ.)

normally found in lung, but the quantity, proportions, and arrangement of the tissues are abnormal.

Hamartomas represent the most common type of benign lung tumor, representing 5% of all solitary pulmonary nodules.[5] The average age at discovery is 58 years, with a range of 14 to 76 years reported.[32]

IMAGING FINDINGS

Hamartomas grow at the same rate as their parent organ, and therefore do not exhibit neoplastic pressure erosion of adjacent tissues.

Hamartomas typically are peripheral, presenting as well-defined pulmonary nodules.[5] Peripheral lesions are distributed equally among the lobes. Hamartomas may appear large (Fig. 25-33)[17] but typically are less than 4 cm in diameter; an average diameter of 2.2 cm has been reported.[32] Typically calcification is demonstrated in 25%[5] to 30% of patients, with rates as high as 75% reported.[61] When present, the pattern of calcification often has a pathognomonic "popcorn" or "comma-shaped" appearance. Approximately 8% of hamartomas are in an endobronchial location,[52] possibly leading to airway obstruction.

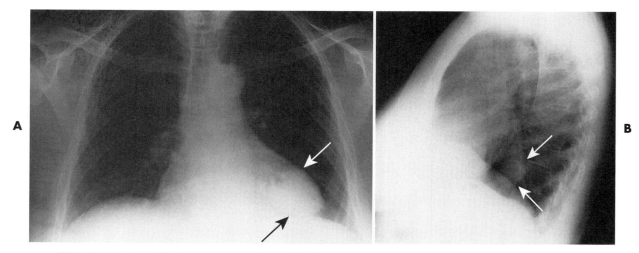

FIG. 25-33 Noncalcific hamartoma presenting as, **A,** pulmonary mass overlying the apex of the heart shadow in the frontal projection *(arrows)* and, **B,** in the retrocardiac clear space in the lateral projection *(arrows)*. (Courtesy Steven P. Brownstein, MD, Springfield, NJ.)

CLINICAL COMMENTS

Most lesions are asymptomatic clinically, although hemoptysis, cough, and chest pain are present occasionally. Surgical resection is considered for expanding lesions found in young and middle-aged patients and in those with clinical symptoms.

Lymphoma

BACKGROUND

Lymphomas are malignant tumors composed of lymphocytes and less commonly histiocytes that arise in the lymph nodes, spleen, or other sites of lymphoid tissue elsewhere in the body. Lymphomas are classified by cell type, degrees of differentiation, and nodular or diffuse pattern of distribution. Hodgkin disease (HD) is a distinctive form of lymphoma, separated from the larger spectrum of non–Hodgkin lymphoma (NHL) on the basis of a characteristic appearance of cellular morphology (Reed-Sternberg cells). When disseminated, lymphomas, especially the lymphocytic type, may invade the peripheral blood and manifest as leukemia.

HD has a bimodal age distribution, 15 to 34 years and over 45 years. It has a propensity toward involvement of the mediastinum, hilum, or lung parenchyma. Intrathoracic disease is more common in HD than NHL.[24] HD involves the mediastinum in 67% to 87% of cases.[11,24]

NHL is seen in patients 30 to 70 years of age. Thoracic involvement is seen in less than half of patients. Pulmonary involvement is much less common than lymphadenopathy of the hilum or mediastinum.

IMAGING FINDINGS

Moderate to extensive adenopathy is demonstrated easily with conventional radiographs; CT is more sensitive to early or more subtle presentations. Both HD and NHL demonstrate hilar and mediastinal lymph node enlargement.

Mediastinal lymph nodes from the thoracic inlet to the diaphragm may be involved. Involvement may be extensive, exhibiting huge conglomerate masses, or more subtle limited nodal masses. The pattern of involvement is contiguous for HD in the mediastinum, spreading from one node to another. In contrast, adenopathy resulting from NHL may be noncontiguous. Rarely is hilar involvement noted without concurrent involvement of the mediastinum (Figs. 25-34 through 25-36). Typically lymphoma spreads from mediastinal or hilum involvement along the bronchovascular lymphatics to involve the pulmonary tissue.

Pulmonary parenchymal involvement with HD usually is associated with hilar and mediastinal nodal disease;[24,39] the pulmonary tissues are virtually never involved alone. This is not the case for NHL, in which the pattern is more unpredictable and pulmonary involvement may be seen without hilar or mediastinal adenopathy.

Parenchymal involvement typically is nodular, sometimes demonstrating poorly defined borders. The appearance may be similar to metastatic lung disease. An interstitial pulmonary pattern is rare. Patterns of consolidation and atelectasis of a lobe or segment often are seen. This results from either extrinsic bronchial compression by enlarged lymph nodes or endobronchial tumors.[59,62]

Pleural effusions are noted in 7% to 10% of cases.[24] Solid pleural[62] and pericardial masses are seen less often. Chest wall lesions most often are anterior, resulting from direct extension of anterior mediastinal disease. Occasionally posterior nodes invade adjacent vertebrae or the spinal canal.

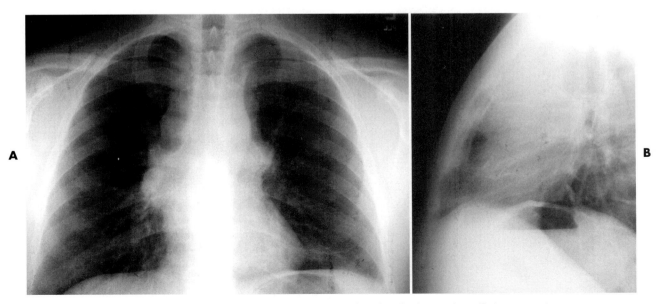

FIG. 25-34 **A** and **B,** Hodgkin lymphoma presenting with an enlarged mediastinum and opacified retrosternal space.

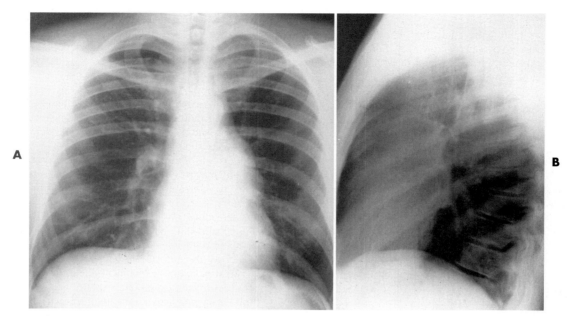

FIG. 25-35 A, Wide mediastinum and, **B,** opacified retrosternal space in a patient with non–Hodgkin lymphoma. (Courtesy Michael Whitehead, Kansas City, MO.)

CLINICAL COMMENTS

The clinical presentation of lymphoma is variable. Both HD and NHL may present with either an indolent or rapidly progressing course. Indolent disease presents with painless lymphadenopathy, whereas the progressive course is marked by constitutional symptoms such as fever, drenching night sweats, or weight loss. Once the pathologic diagnosis is established, the patient should be evaluated to determine the extent of disease. Staging determines whether regional therapy, such as surgery or radiation therapy, is appropriate or if the disease must be approached in a systemic fashion with chemotherapy.

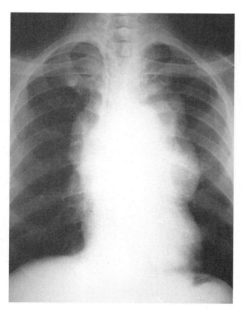

FIG. 25-36 Lymphoma with marked widening of the mediastinum.

KEY CONCEPTS

- *Lymphoma is separated into Hodgkin and non–Hodgkin types. Each type is further classified by cell type, degrees of differentiation, and nodular or diffuse pattern of distribution.*
- *Both Hodgkin disease and non–Hodgkin lymphoma are marked by hilar and mediastinal lymphadenopathy; parenchymal involvement is less common.*
- *Both Hodgkin disease and non–Hodgkin lymphoma may demonstrate a clinically indolent or rapidly progressing course.*

Metastatic Lung Disease

BACKGROUND

The lungs are a common location for metastasis, reflecting their rich vascularity and central location in the vascular system.[15,63] At autopsy, 30% to 50% of cancer patients have pulmonary metastasis. Both carcinomas and sarcomas arising anywhere in the body may spread to the lungs via the blood, lymphatics, or direct extension of a contiguous lesion.

Most lung metastases are blood-borne arising from mesenchymal tumors, melanomas, sarcomas, and primary renal and thyroid tumors. Lymphangitic carcinomatosis refers to pulmonary dissemination and tumor growth in the lymphatics, most commonly related to primaries of the stomach, pancreas, prostate, and breast.[37] Growth of contiguous tumors of the lungs occurs most often with esophageal and thyroid carcinomas[67] and mediastinal lymphomas.

IMAGING FINDINGS

Blood-borne metastasis typically presents as multiple well-defined nodules ranging from 1 to 5 cm in size located in the peripheral lung fields (Figs. 25-37 through 25-42).[16,19,54] Nodules tend to

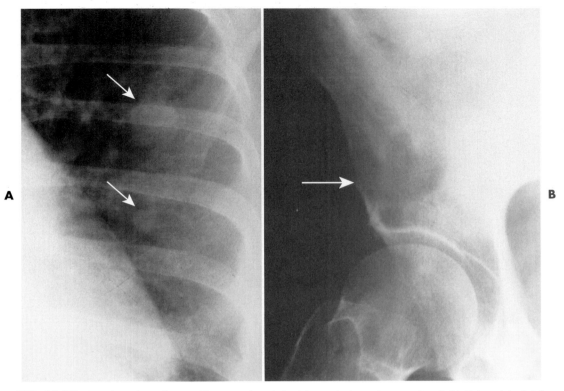

FIG. 25-37 Bronchogenic carcinoma with metastasis to skeletal sites and other pulmonary sites. **A,** Multiple nodules in left lung *(arrows)*. **B,** Osteolytic bone destruction in right supraacetabular region *(arrow)*. (Courtesy Steven P. Brownstein, MD, Springfield, NJ.)

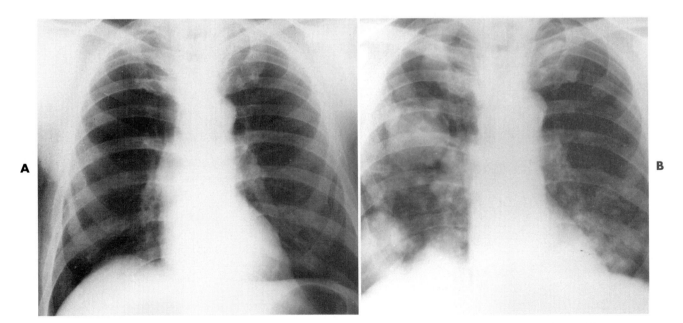

FIG. 25-38 Pulmonary metastasis developing from adenocarcinoma of the colon. **A,** Initial film with no abnormalities. **B,** Film taken 16 months later, demonstrating multiple bilateral masses and nodules characteristic of pulmonary metastasis. (Courtesy Steven P. Brownstein, MD, Springfield, NJ.)

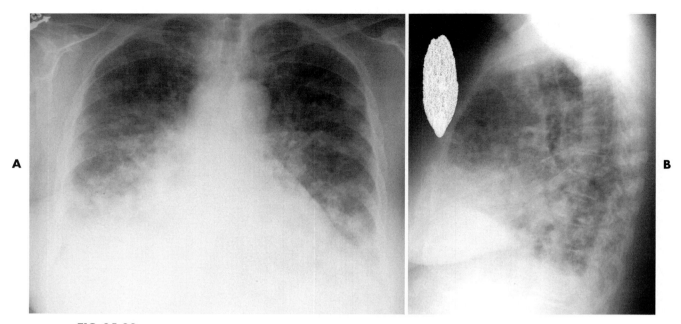

FIG. 25-39   A and **B,** Advanced pulmonary metastasis presenting with multiple masses and nodules in this patient with a history of breast cancer. (Courtesy John A.M. Taylor, Seneca Falls, NY.)

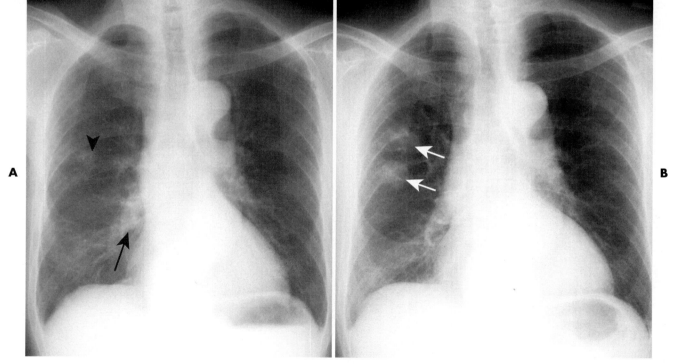

FIG. 25-40   A, Seventy-six-year-old male cancer patient demonstrating an enlarged left hilum *(arrow)* and faint pulmonary nodule *(arrowhead).* **B,** Second film taken 9 months later, demonstrating a second pulmonary nodule with the first *(arrows).* Multiple pathologic findings strongly indicate metastasis, as seen in this case. (Courtesy John A.M. Taylor, Seneca Falls, NY.)

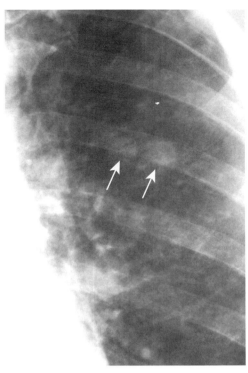

FIG. 25-41 Faint noncalcified radiodense nodules consistent with pulmonary metastasis (*arrows*). (Courtesy Blair Hunt, Peoria, IL.)

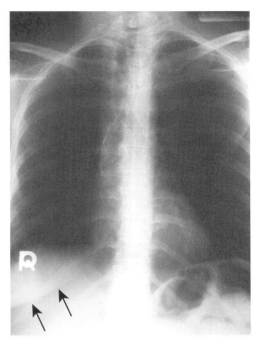

FIG. 25-42 This radiograph of a 45-year-old woman exhibits only the patient's right breast (*arrows*). A left breast shadow is not seen. A missing breast shadow suggests a past malignant history and should prompt the interpreter to examine the film closely for any signs of bone or pulmonary metastasis. (Courtesy Brian Frank, Sunnyland, IL.)

involve the basal portions of lungs, possibly related to preferential blood flow.[16] Larger lesions are termed *cannonball metastasis*. Lymphangitic spread of metastasis presents with Kerley's lines, discrete nodules, and linear shadows, denoting a reticulonodular interstitial pattern of pulmonary disease.

The pattern typically is bilateral. A unilateral solitary presentation suggests a primary lesion, such as bronchogenic carcinoma. Radiographs of other skeletal sites may reveal bone destruction, as in Figure 25-37. Abnormal radiographic findings may occur less than 2 years after normal radiographic studies (Fig. 25-38). Cavitation is present in 6% to 7%,[20] and is more common with squamous cell carcinoma than adenocarcinomas. The uterus, cervix, colon, head, and neck are common sites of origin.[12]

Calcification is unusual unless the metastasis is from osteosarcoma or chondrosarcoma. The higher-contrast resolution and fewer blind spots make CT the most sensitive imaging technique for detecting pulmonary metastasis.

Pleural effusion is a common manifestation accompanying lung metastasis or may signify pleural metastasis. It most often accompanies carcinoma of the lung, breast, stomach, and pancreas.[1,13,46]

CLINICAL COMMENTS

Pulmonary metastases are a devastating complication for the cancer patient. Their presence usually signals a lethal outcome. Often no signs or symptoms are present at the time of discovery, and although helpful when known, a reported history of primary tumor elsewhere in the body may not exist. Pleural involvement may cause dyspnea on exertion. The disease is mostly limited to those over the age of 50 years.

> **KEY CONCEPTS**
> - *The lungs are common recipients of metastatic disease.*
> - *Hematogenous metastasis results in multiple well-delineated peripheral nodules; lymphangitic metastasis appears as an interstitial pattern resulting from engorgement of the axial interstitial space; and direct extension most often results from tumors of the esophagus and mediastinal lymphoma.*
> - *Pleural effusion is common.*

Pleural Mesothelioma

BACKGROUND

Primary tumors of the pleura are much less common than metastatic pleural disease, which typically arises from breast or lung primary tumors. Mesotheliomas are the most common primary tumors of the pleura,[3,31] arising from either the visceral or parietal pleura.[38] Two forms are recognized: localized benign (pleural fibroma) and diffuse malignant. The localized form, typically seen in patients 45 to 65 years of age, is rare and not related to asbestos exposure. It arises most often from the visceral pleura and frequently is not recognized until it becomes large.

The malignant variety is recognized in patients 40 to 70 years of age and is more common in men. It is caused primarily by asbestos exposure, with the duration and intensity of exposure relating to the risk of developing the disease.[2] The lifetime risk of developing mesothelioma with heavily exposed individuals is approximately 10%. The incidence is rising because the disease's 15-year latent period is resulting in current cases that are attributed to past asbestos exposure.

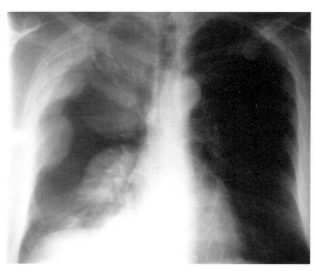

FIG. 25-43 Malignant mesothelioma involving the right lung. (Courtesy Steven P. Brownstein, MD, Springfield, NJ.)

IMAGING FINDINGS

The localized form appears as a solitary mass in the lung periphery,[57] or occasionally in the lung fissure. It may be attached to the pleura by a pedicle. Calcification and accompanying pleural effusion are rare.

Malignant mesotheliomas begin as nodules on the visceral or parietal pleura that progress widely through the pleural space and form a thick rind encasing and constricting the lung. A shift of the mediastinum toward the involved side is seen in advanced cases. The radiographic appearance is that of multiple areas of pleural thickening or pleural masses with or without pleural effusion (Fig. 25-43). The main differential diagnostic considerations are metastatic tumor and lymphoma.

CLINICAL COMMENTS

Unless large, the benign localized form typically is clinically silent. The diffuse malignant variety may demonstrate presenting complaints of chest pain, shortness of breath, cough, weight loss, fever, and recurrent pleural effusions.[2]

> **KEY CONCEPTS**
> - *Localized benign (pleural fibroma) and diffuse malignant forms are recognized.*
> - *The malignant variety is closely related to asbestos exposure.*
> - *The benign localized form is typically clinically silent the diffuse malignant variety is associated most often with clinical symptoms.*

Teratomas

BACKGROUND

Teratomas are neoplasms composed of multiple tissues derived from all three germ cell layers, including tissues not normally found in the lung.[41] Within the mass, it is not uncommon to find such elements as skin, teeth, hair, muscle, bone, cartilage, and fat. The thorax represents the third most common site for teratomas, following gonadal and sacrococcygeal locations. Nearly all intrathorax lesions are mediastinal, accounting for 10% of mediastinal tumors.[72] Grossly they appear as benign cystic or solid malignant lesions.[29,40]

IMAGING FINDINGS

Teratomas are anterior mediastinal lesions most frequently arising near the junction of the heart and great vessels (Fig. 25-44). Benign lesions are well defined; malignant lesions appear lobulated and often asymmetric. Peripheral calcification may be noted, similar to thymomas. On average they are larger than thymomas. Intrapulmonary locations are described rarely.[48]

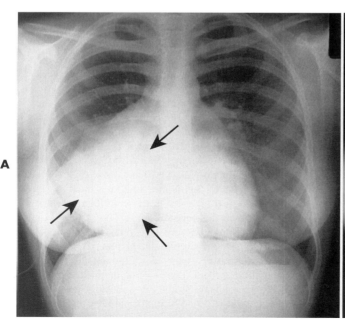 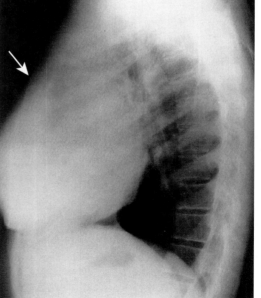

FIG. 25-44 **A** and **B,** Large teratoma in the anterior portion of the mediastinum (*arrows*).

CLINICAL COMMENTS

Teratomas usually produce no symptoms, although large lesions may cause shortness of breath and coughing. Some patients relate a feeling of fullness or pain in the retrosternal area. Those lesions presenting later in life are malignant more often than those presenting in younger individuals. Malignant teratomas usually are highly aggressive lesions, often resulting in patient death within a short period after diagnosis.

KEY CONCEPTS

- *Teratomas are lesions containing tissue from all three germ cell layers.*
- *They are found most commonly in the anterior mediastinum, although an intrapulmonary location has been identified.*
- *Most are benign and produce few symptoms; the less common malignant variety is highly aggressive.*

Thymic Masses

BACKGROUND

Thymomas may be benign or malignant. Appearing most commonly in middle-aged patients, thymomas represent 10%[47] of anterior mediastinal lesions and follow lymphoma as the second most common primary tumor to affect the mediastinum.[36] Thymolipomas are uncommon anterior mediastinal tumors consisting of an admixture of fat and thymic epithelial and lymphoid tissue of unknown etiology.[65] Thymic cysts are uncommon, accounting for less than 3% of anterior mediastinal lesions. Thymic hyperplasia also is rare overall, but it represents the most common anterior mass among infants and children.

IMAGING FINDINGS

All the lesions present as anterior mediastinal masses (Figs. 25-45 and 25-46). Typically thymomas are located near the junction of the heart and great vessels and are 5 to 10 cm in diameter. If large they may displace the heart or great vessels posteriorly. Thymolipomas extend inferiorly from the base of the heart, creating an enlarged appearance of the heart shadow.

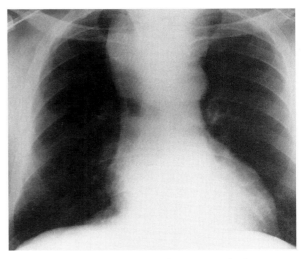

FIG. 25-45 Substernal thyroid presenting as a mass in the upper anterior mediastinum. (Courtesy Steven P. Brownstein, MD, Springfield, NJ.)

CLINICAL COMMENTS

Patients with thymomas typically experience symptoms related to either pressure from an anterior mediastinal mass, producing cough, chest pain, and shortness of breath;[43] or myasthenia gravis, which is noted in 35% of patients with thymomas.[8,72] Thymolipomas cause few symptoms and typically are discovered incidentally.

KEY CONCEPTS

- *Tumors, cysts, and hyperplasia of the thymus are common anterior mediastinal lesions.*
- *Clinical symptoms typically depend on the size of the mass.*
- *Clinical data and radiographic appearance may assist in differentiating various thymic lesions.*

PART THREE Chest

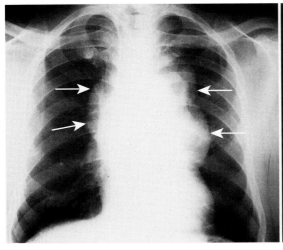
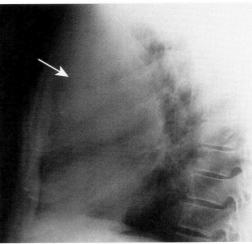

FIG. 25-46 **A** and **B,** Thymoma presenting as a solid mass in the anterior portion of the mediastinum (*arrows*). (Courtesy Steven P. Brownstein, MD, Springfield, NJ.)

References

1. Anderson CB, Philpott GW, Ferguson TB: The treatment of malignant pleural effusions, *Cancer* 33:916, 1974.
2. Antman C: Malignant mesothelioma, *N Engl J Med* 303:200, 1981.
3. Antman KH: Natural history and epidemiology of malignant mesothelioma, *Chest* 103(suppl 4):373, 1993.
4. Auerbach O, Garfinkel L: The changing pattern of lung carcinoma, *Cancer* 68:1973, 1991.
5. Bateson EM: An analysis of 155 solitary lung lesions illustrating the differential diagnosis of mixed tumors of the lung, *Clin Radiol* 16:51, 1965.
6. Bateson EM, Whimster WF, Woo-Ming M: Ossified bronchial adenoma, *Br J Radiol* 43:570, 1970.
7. Beamis JR, Stein A, Andrews JL: Epidemiology of lung cancer, *Med Clin North Am* 59:315, 1975.
8. Benjamin SP et al: Critical review: "primary tumors of the mediastinum." *Chest* 62:297, 1972.
9. Burke M, Fraser R: Obstructive pneumonitis: a pathologic and pathogenetic reappraisal, *Radiology* 166:699, 1988.
10. Byrd RB et al: The roentgenographic appearance of squamous cell carcinoma of the bronchus, *Mayo Clin Proc* 43, 1968.
11. Castellino RA et al: Hodgkin's disease: contributions of chest CT in the initial staging evaluation, *Radiology* 160:603, 1986.
12. Chaudhuri MR: Cavitary pulmonary metastases, *Thorax* 25:375, 1970.
13. Chernow B, Sahn SA: Carcinomatous involvement of the pleura, *Am J Med* 63:695, 1977.
14. Clayton F: The spectrum and significance of bronchoalveolar carcinoma, *Pathol Annu* 23(part 2):361, 1988.
15. Coppage L, Shaw C, Curtis AM: Metastatic disease to the chest in patients with extrathoracic malignancy, *J Thorac Imag* 2:24, 1987.
16. Crow J, Slavin G, Kreel L: Pulmonary metastasis: a pathologic and radiologic study, *Cancer* 47:2595, 1981.
17. Darke CS et al: The bronchial circulation in a case of giant hamartoma of the lung, *Br J Radiol* 45:147, 1972.
18. Davila DG et al: Bronchial carcinoid tumors, *Mayo Clin Proc* 68:795, 1993.
19. Davis SD: CT evaluation for pulmonary metastases in patients with extrathoracic malignancy, *Radiology* 180:1, 1991.
20. Dodd GD, Buyle JS: Excavating pulmonary metastases, *AJR Am J Roentgenol* 85:277, 1961.
21. Doll R: The age distribution of cancer; implications for models of carcinogenesis, *J Roy Stat Soc Series A*, 133 (part 2):66, 1971.
22. Doppman JL et al: Ectopic adrenocorticotrophic hormone syndrome: localization studies in 28 patients, *Radiology* 172:115, 1989.
23. Epstein DM: The role of radiologic screening in lung cancer, *Radiol Clin North Am* 28:489, 1990.
24. Filly R, Blank N, Castellino RA: Radiographic distribution of intrathoracic disease in previously untreated patients with Hodgkin's disease and non-Hodgkin's lymphoma, *Radiology* 120:277, 1976.
25. Findling JW, Tyrell B: Occult ectopic secretion of corticotropin, *Arch Intern Med* 146:929, 1986.
26. Fleischner Society: Glossary of terms for thoracic radiology: recommendations of the nomenclature committee of the Fleischner Society, *AJR Am J Roentgenol,* 143:509, 1984.
27. Geddes DM: The natural history of lung cancer: a review based on rates of tumor growth, *Br J Dis Chest* 73:1, 1979.
28. Goldmeier E: Limits of visibility of bronchogenic carcinoma, *Am Rev Respir Dis* 91:232, 1955.
29. Gonzales-Crussi F: Extragonadal teratomas. In: Atlas of Tumor Pathology, Washington, DC, 1982, Armed Forces Institute of Pathology.
30. Gurney JW: Determining the likelihood of malignancy in solitary pulmonary nodules with bayesian analysis, *Radiology* 186:405, 1993.
31. Hammar SP: The pathology of benign and malignant pleural disease, *Chest Surg Clin North Am* 4:405, 1994.
32. Hansen CP et al: Pulmonary hamartoma, *J Thorac Cardiovasc Surg* 104:674, 1992.
33. Haque AK: Pathology of carcinoma of lung: an update on current concepts, *J Thorac Imag* 7:9, 1991.
34. Hayabuchi N, Russell WJ, Murakami J: Slow-growing lung cancer in a fixed population sample: radiologic assessments, *Lancet* 52:1098, 1983.
35. Heitzman ER et al: Pathways of tumor spread through the lung: radiologic correlations with anatomy and pathology, *Radiology* 144:3, 1982.
36. Ingels GW et al: Malignant schwannomas of the mediastinum, *Cancer* 27:1190, 1971.
37. Janower ML, Blennerhassett JB: Lymphangitic spread of metastatic cancer to the lung: a radiologic-pathologic classification, *Radiology* 101:267, 1971.
38. Kannerstein M et al: Asbestosis and mesothelioma, *Pathol Annu* 13(part 1):81, 1978.
39. Kaplan HS: Contiguity and progression in Hodgkin's disease, *Cancer Res* 31:1811, 1971.
40. Keslar PJ, Buck JL, Suarez ES: Germ cell tumors of the sacrococcygeal region: radiologic-pathologic correlation, *Radiographics* 14:607, 1994.
41. Kountakis SE et al: Teratomas of the head and neck, *Am J Otolaryngol* 15:292, 1994.
42. Kundel HL: Predictive value and threshold detectability of lung tumors, *Radiology* 139:25, 1981.
43. Lewis JE et al: Thymoma. A clinicopathologic review, *Cancer* 60:2727, 1987.
44. Loeb LA et al: Smoking and lung cancer: an overview, *Cancer Res* 44:5942, 1984.
45. Mahoney MC et al: CT demonstration of calcification in carcinoma of the lung, *AJR Am J Roentgenol* 154:255, 1990.
46. Matthay RA et al: Malignancies metastatic to the pleura, *Invest Radiol* 25:601, 1990.
47. Meza MP, Benson M, Slovis TL: Imaging of mediastinal masses in children, *Radiol Clin North Am* 31, 1993.
48. Morgan DE et al: Intrapulmonary teratoma: a case report and review of the literature, *J Thorac Imag* 7:70, 1992.
49. Muller NL, Miller RR: Neuroendocrine carcinomas of the lung, *Semin Roentgenol* 25:96, 1990.
50. Petty TL: What to do when an x-ray film suggests lung cancer, *Postgrad Med J* 89:101, 1991.
51. Pietra GG: The pathology of carcinoma of the lung, *Semin Roentgenol* 25:25, 1990.
52. Poirier TJ, Van Ordstrand HS: Pulmonary chondromatous hamartoma: report of seventeen cases and review of the literature, *Chest* 59:50, 1971.
53. Pugatch RD: Radiologic evaluation in chest malignancies: a review of imaging modalities, *Chest* 107(suppl):294, 1995.
54. Remy-Jardin M et al: Pulmonary nodules detection with thick-section spiral CT versus conventional CT, *Radiology* 187:513, 1993.
55. Ries LG, Pollack ES, Young JL: Cancer patient survival: surveillance, epidemiology, and end results program, 1973–79, *J Natl Cancer Inst* 70:693, 1983.
56. Rigler LG: The roentgen signs of carcinoma of the lung, *AJR Am J Roentgenol* 74:415, 1955.
57. Robinson LA, Reilly RB: Localized pleural mesothelioma. The clinical spectrum, *Chest* 106:1611, 1994.
58. Rosenow EC, Carr DT: Bronchogenic carcinoma, *Cancer J Clin* 29:233, 1979.
59. Samuels ML et al: Endobronchial malignant lymphoma: report of five cases in adults, *AJR Am J Roentgenol* 85:87, 1961.
60. Sargent EN, Barnes RA, Schwinn CP: Multiple pulmonary fibroleiomyomatous hamartomas, *AJR Am J Roentgenol* 110:694, 1970.

61. Shin MS, McElvein RB, Ho KJ: Radiographic evidence of calcification in pulmonary hamartomas, *J Natl Med Assoc* 84:329, 1992.

62. Stolberg HO et al: Hodgkin's disease of the lung: roentgenologic-pathologic correlation, *AJR Am J Roentgenol* 92:96, 1964.

63. Suster S, Moran CA: Unusual manifestations of metastatic tumors to the lungs, *Semin Diagn Pathol* 12:193, 1995.

64. Suzuki Y: Diagnostic criteria for human diffuse malignant mesothelioma, *Acta Pathol Jpn* 42:767, 1992.

65. Teplick JG, Nedwich A, Haskin ME: Roentgenographic features of thymolipoma, *AJR Am J Roentgenol* 117:873, 1973.

66. Theros EG: Varying manifestations of peripheral pulmonary neoplasms: a radiologic-pathologic correlative study, *AJR Am J Roentgenol* 128:893, 1977.

67. Tsumori T et al: Clinicopathologic study of thyroid carcinoma infiltrating the trachea, *Cancer* 56:2843, 1985.

68. Warren WH, Gould VE, Faber LP: Neuroendocrine neoplasms: a clinicopathologic update, *J Thorac Cardiovasc Surg* 98:321, 1989.

69. Weiss W: Cigarette smoke as a carcinogen, *Am Rev Respir Dis* 108:364, 1973.

70. Weiss W: Tumor doubling time and survival in men with bronchogenic carcinoma, *Chest* 65:3, 1974.

71. Wenckebach KF: The radiology of the chest, *Arch Roentgen Ray* 18:169, 1913.

72. Wychulis AR et al: Surgical treatment of mediastinal tumors, *J Thorac Cardiovasc Surg* 62:379, 1971.

73. Zwirewich CV et al: Solitary pulmonary nodule: high-resolution CT and radiologic-pathologic correlation, *Radiology* 179:469, 1991.

chapter 26

Miscellaneous Chest Diseases

DENNIS M. MARCHIORI

**Adult Respiratory Distress
  Syndrome**
Extrinsic Allergic Alveolitis
Pneumoconioses
Pneumothorax
Sarcoidosis

Adult Respiratory Distress Syndrome

BACKGROUND

Adult respiratory distress syndrome (ARDS) is a condition in which the pulmonary system is affected as a result of more generalized, multiorgan capillary damage.[14] The pathogenic sequence appears to be related to inappropriate activation of the complement cascade,[32,18] resulting in increased capillary permeability and pulmonary edema. Eventually fluid spills into the alveolar spaces, leading to hemorrhaging, reduced surfactant levels, and a resultant smaller functional area for gas exchange. A wide range of factors and conditions is associated with the development of ARDS (Box 26-1).

IMAGING FINDINGS

No changes are detectable radiographically during the initial stage of ARDS unless it is caused by pneumonia, aspiration, or another pulmonary condition, in which case the pulmonary findings of the

concurrent disease may be noted. The latter stages of the disease are marked by alveolar filling. Patchy areas of incomplete lung consolidation are noted at first (Fig. 26-1), which eventually become more uniform, generalized, and homogenous. The radiographically detectable features gradually resolve during the ensuing weeks. Pleural effusion is rare.

CLINICAL COMMENTS

ARDS is characterized by rapidly progressing respiratory distress.[2,12] Alveolar filling is followed by acute respiratory failure that necessitates mechanical ventilation and oxygen administration. The eventual clinical outcome depends heavily on whether the patient develops

---

BOX 26-1

Partial List of Factors Associated with Adult Respiratory Distress Syndrome[2,26,31]

- Amniotic fluid embolism
- Arterial embolism
- Aspiration
- Drug abuse
- Eclampsia
- Fat embolism
- Fractures
- Heat stroke
- High-altitude pulmonary edema
- Pancreatitis
- Pulmonary contusions
- Radiation pneumonitis
- Shock
- Smoke inhalation
- Transplantation

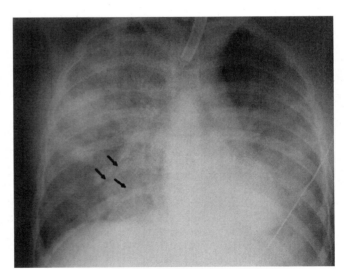

FIG. 26-1 Diffuse pulmonary consolidations with air bronchograms (arrows) are the result of adult respiratory distress syndrome after viral pneumonia. This appearance is radiologically indistinguishable from pulmonary alveolar edema and diffuse pneumonia. (From Reed JC: Chest radiology: plain film patterns and differential diagnoses, ed 5, St Louis, 2003, Mosby.)

a nosocomial infection, hemorrhage, sepsis, lung barotrauma, or another major complication.[18]

Extrinsic Allergic Alveolitis

BACKGROUND

Extrinsic allergic alveolitis (EAA), also known as *hypersensitivity pneumonitis,* is a nonatopic, nonasthmatic allergic lung disease. EAA manifests as an occupational lung disease caused by the inhalation of organic dusts, which produces granulomatous and interstitial lung changes. Several etiologic agents are listed in Table 26-1.

IMAGING FINDINGS

The radiographic presentation of EAA is the same regardless of the type of organic dust inhaled,[43] but it varies according to the intensity of the exposure.[30] The early stages of EAA usually are characterized by reversible, multiple, small (1- to 3-mm), nodular radiodensities that are scattered bilaterally throughout the lung zones; although it is less common, the lung apices may be spared (Fig. 26-2).* Repeated exposures may result in a chronic interstitial (honeycomb) pattern[3,42] with upper lobe predominance.

CLINICAL COMMENTS

Acute EAA is characterized by the sudden onset of malaise, chills, fever, cough, dyspnea, and nausea within hours after exposure to the offending agent. Subacute and chronic forms are characterized by a persistent cough and slowly progressing dyspnea, anorexia, and weight loss. The patient's history of exposure preceding the clinical symptoms is important for a proper diagnosis.

Pneumoconioses

BACKGROUND

Pneumoconioses are a group of diseases caused by inhalation of inorganic dust and its accumulation in the lung.[30] The dust deposits cause a nonneoplastic lung reaction that is often seen on radiographs. Asbestos, silicon, and coal dust incite a fibrogenic tissue reaction throughout the lung. Tin, barium, iron, and other inert particles do not incite fibrogenic changes but do cause particle-laden macrophages to accumulate in the lung.[4] These reactions are called

---

*References 10, 15, 31, 42, 43.

TABLE 26-1

Selected Provocative Agents of Extrinsic Allergic Alveolitis

Disease	Provocative agent
Bagassosis	Moldy sugar cane
Bird fancier's lung	Avian excreta
Farmer's lung	Moldy hay
Humidifier lung	Contamination from humidifying, heating, and air conditioning systems
Malt worker's lung	Moldy malt
Maple bark stripper's lung	Moldy maple bark
Mushroom worker's lung	Mushroom spores
Sequoiosis	Redwood dust
Suberosis	Moldy cork dust

benign pneumoconioses (even though their radiographic appearance can be dramatic) because they are less aggressive.

IMAGING FINDINGS

The chest radiograph is the primary means of determining the presence and extent of pneumoconiosis.[45] The International Labour Office (ILO) has established a classification system for the radiographic appearance of pneumoconioses[20,39] that focuses on the size and shape of the lung nodules. The classification also includes a detailed categorization of pleural thickening.

The radiographic appearance of pneumoconiosis depends on the type and amount of dust inhaled and individual immunologic lung reactions (Table 26-2).[5,22] In general nonfibrogenic pneumoconioses show nodular opacities. A fibrogenic lung response is associated with lymphadenopathy; interstitial parenchymal patterns; and pleural thickening, calcification (Figs. 26-3 through 26-5), and effusion.

CLINICAL COMMENTS

Radiographic and clinical findings often are not consistent. Extensive changes may be seen in radiographs of relatively asymptomatic patients. Dyspnea and rales are present occasionally. The treatment is supportive.

Pneumothorax

BACKGROUND

A pneumothorax is a collection of air in the pleural space that has a spontaneous or traumatic etiology. A traumatic pneumothorax results from blunt or penetrating injuries and is often iatrogenic.

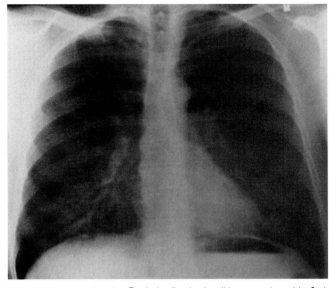
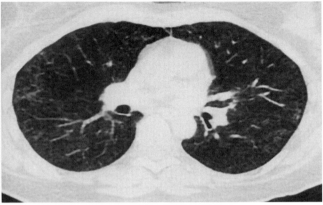

FIG. 26-2 Extrinsic allergic alveolitis presenting with, **A,** bilateral diffuse infiltrate and, **B,** small pulmonary nodules on a computed tomogram after exposure to pigeon droppings. (From Swensen SJ: Radiology of thoracic diseases: a teaching file, St Louis, 1993, Mosby.)

TABLE 26-2
Selected Pneumoconioses

Condition and causative agent	Comments
Nonfibrogenic (benign)	
Stannosis: tin	Stannosis is caused by deposits of tin in the lung that lead to formation of opaque nodules.
Baritosis: barium	Baritosis is caused by inhalation of barium sulfate, which produces small, rounded opacities that exceed the attenuation of calcium.
Siderosis: iron	Siderosis develops in workers who inhale fumes containing iron oxide particles, which produce scattered radiopacities in the lung fields.
Fibrogenic	
Asbestosis: asbestos	Construction workers, insulation workers, pipe fitters, ship builders, and asbestos miners may be exposed to asbestos fibers of varying levels of pathogenicity (e.g., crocidolite > amosite > anthophyllite > chrysotile), causing interstitial lung disease (asbestosis), pleural thickening (asbestos-related pleural disease), and malignancies. Asbestosis appears as linear radiopacities in the lung bases progressing to the apex. Asbestos-related pleural disease may be focal (plaques) or diffuse and usually appears in a posterolateral location. It is assumed to be the result of asbestos fibers that have pierced the visceral pleura.[29] Asbestos exposure increases the risk of developing mesothelioma[1,7] and lung cancer.[6,23]
Silicosis: silicon dioxide	Silicosis results from exposure to silicon dioxide,[40] which is abundant in the earth's crust and commonly encountered in mining, quarrying, sandblasting, and ceramic work. Small, radiopaque nodules are seen throughout the perihilar and apical regions. The nodules coalesce to form large (>2 cm) conglomerate masses that progressively migrate toward the hilum in a bilateral but asymmetric pattern known as progressive massive fibrosus (PMF). Occasionally hilar lymphadenopathy with possible peripheral "eggshell" calcifications of the hilar lymph nodes is present.
Coal worker's pneumoconiosis (CWP): coal	Coal miners are almost the only individuals who inhale enough carbon-containing inorganic material to cause a reaction. Carbon deposits in the lung form coal dust macules that are seen as round, 1- to 5-mm nodules scattered throughout the upper lung fields.[33] This feature is the hallmark of simple CWP and is radiographically indistinguishable from silicosis. Complicated CWP develops when the simple pattern is complicated by the formation of PMF similar to that seen in silicosis. Caplan syndrome is CWP in patients who also have rheumatoid arthritis; Erasmus syndrome is CWP in patients who also have progressive systemic sclerosis.

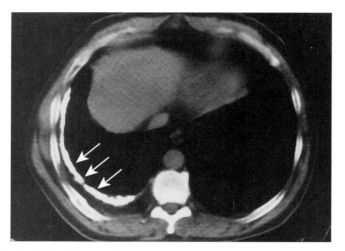

FIG. 26-3 Computed tomogram demonstrating calcific asbestosis-related pleural plaques in the right posterior region *(arrows)*. (Courtesy Steven P. Brownstein, MD, Springfield, NJ.)

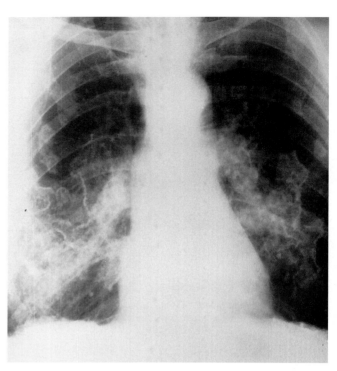

FIG. 26-4 Asbestosis with calcific pleural plaques and an interstitial parenchymal pattern.

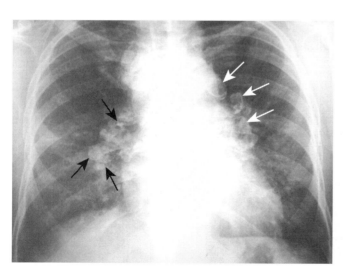

FIG. 26-5 Rim "eggshell" calcifications of the lymph nodes seen in silicosis *(arrows)*. In addition to silicosis, eggshell hilar lymph node calcification is also noted in coal worker's pneumoconiosis, sarcoidosis, treated Hodgkin lymphoma, scleroderma, amyloidosis, histoplasmosis, and blastomycosis.

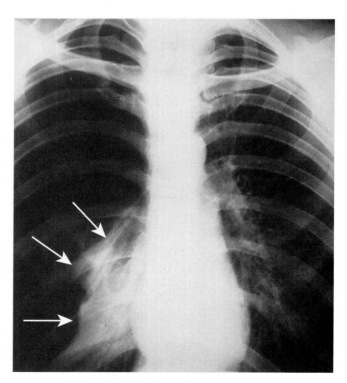

FIG. 26-6 Atelectasis of right lung with tension pneumothorax maintaining the midline position of the mediastinum and heart. The collapsed lung remains as a radiodense mass along the right heart border *(arrows)*. (Courtesy Steven P. Brownstein, MD, Springfield, NJ.)

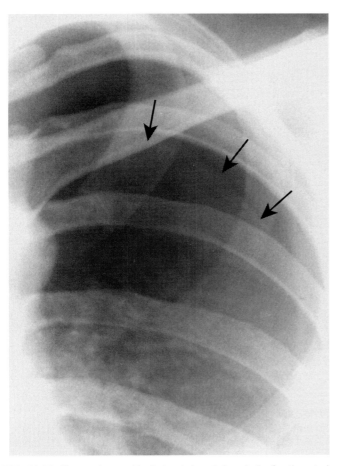

FIG. 26-7 Pneumothorax with displaced visceral pleura in the fourth posterior rib interspace *(arrows)*.

A pneumothorax is caused by rupturing of the parietal or visceral pleura, which permits air from outside the body or in the lung to collect in the pleural space.

A spontaneous pneumothorax has primary and secondary forms. The primary form most often develops in young or middle-aged men.[35] A primary spontaneous pneumothorax is thought to result from rupturing of subpleural air collections that are known as *blebs*.[25] A spontaneous pneumothorax also may be secondary to chest diseases that produce cysts and cavities in the lung, such as chronic obstructive pulmonary disease,[26] cystic fibrosis, Ehlers-Danlos syndrome,[9] histiocytosis X, and Marfan's syndrome.[19]

Tension pneumothoraces develop in a small percentage of patients. Their etiology probably involves a pleural "flap" defect. In a patient with a flap defect, the flap opens during inspiration and allows air to enter the pleural space; the flap closes during expiration and traps the air in the space. Each respiratory cycle pumps air into the overexpanded pleural space. Tension pneumothoraces may become large and lead to atelectasis (Fig. 26-6), impairing venous return to the heart and displacing the mediastinum and hemidiaphragm.

IMAGING FINDINGS

On a chest radiograph of a patient in the upright position, trapped air in the pleural space usually appears as a crescent-shaped radiolucent shadow between the lung and chest wall in the upper chest (Figs. 26-7 through 26-9). The absence of lung markings indicates that the air is extrapulmonary. The subjacent visceral pleura is contrasted by air on both sides and is seen as a thin, curvilinear, radiodense line. A pneumothorax is difficult to detect on radiographs taken with the patient in the supine position.[41] Suspected pneumothorax may be seen more easily on radiographs of patients in a state of full expiration. Full expiration decreases the radiolucent

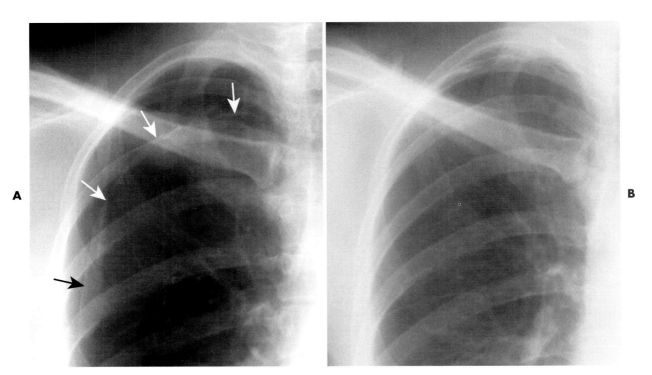

A   **B**

FIG. 26-8 **A,** The pleural space is expanded, and the displaced visceral pleural appears as a fine sickle-shaped radiodense shadow *(arrows)*. There are no bronchovascular markings in the apex of the lung, denoting the air with the expanded pleural space that defines pneumothorax. **B,** A second film taken 1 month later shows a resolution of the pneumothorax. (Courtesy John A.M. Taylor, Seneca Falls, NY.)

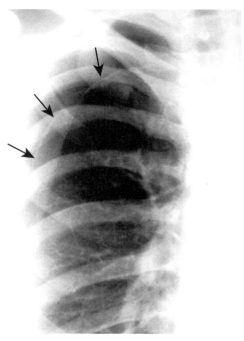

FIG. 26-9 Pneumothorax with characteristic linear density in the right upper lung field representing the displaced visceral pleura *(arrows)*.

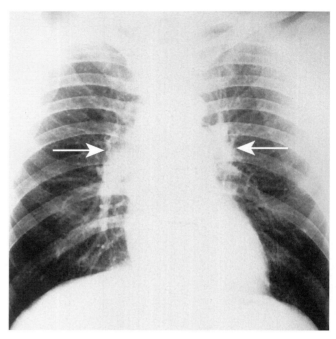

FIG. 26-10 Bilateral enlargement of the hila, consistent with early stage 1 sarcoidosis *(arrows)*. (Courtesy Steven P. Brownstein, MD, Springfield, NJ.)

appearance of the lung, leading to greater contrast between the lung and pleural air of the pneumothorax.

CLINICAL COMMENTS

Pneumothoraces typically present with a sudden onset of ipsilateral chest pain and dyspnea. A tension pneumothorax is characterized by tachypnea, tachycardia, cyanosis, and hypotension. A tension pneumothorax is a medical emergency that requires immediate action to alleviate the progressive lung collapse.

KEY CONCEPTS

- *A pneumothorax is classified as either traumatic or spontaneous based on its etiology.*
- *The spontaneous variety is further subdivided into primary and secondary types based on the presence of underlying disease.*
- *A radiograph of the patient in the upright position is helpful for recognizing pneumothorax.*
- *Tension pneumothoraces are uncommon, but when they develop they require immediate medical attention to alleviate the intrathoracic pressure and halt progressive lung collapse.*

Sarcoidosis

BACKGROUND

Sarcoidosis is a multisystem disease of unknown etiology that is characterized by the formation of noncaseating epithelioid granulomas. Intrathoracic involvement occurs in nearly all patients. Sarcoidosis typically presents between the ages of 20 and 40 years, is more common in women, and is 10 to 20 times more common in blacks.*

---

*References 13, 17, 21, 24, 28, 38.

IMAGING FINDINGS

Sarcoidosis is staged according to its radiographic appearance.[11] Stage 0 has no radiographic changes present. Stage 1 is characterized by the formation of extensive bilateral hilar, paratracheal, tracheobronchial, and azygous lymphadenopathy (Fig. 26-10). In stage 2, radiography shows bilateral hilar adenopathy with parenchymal radiopacities, usually in a diffuse nodular or reticulonodular pattern. The presence of parenchymal opacities with no associated hilar lymphadenopathy defines stage 3 (Fig. 26-11). Radiographs of patients in stage 4 show pulmonary fibrosis without concurrent lymphadenopathy or parenchymal opacities. Patients may not necessarily progress sequentially through all four stages.

Endobronchial involvement is common, and physiologic evidence of airway obstruction may be present in up to 63% of patients.[8] Lobar atelectasis may develop in rare cases as a result of endobronchial obstruction or extrinsic bronchial compression by adjacent adenopathy.[37] Pleural effusion and "eggshell" calcifications of the hilar lymphadenopathy occasionally are present.

In addition to the intrathoracic changes, about 15% of patients with sarcoidosis develop lacelike or honeycombed osteolytic bone lesions predominantly in the small tubular bones of the hands. Arthritis is an uncommon finding. The majority of patients with bone involvement also have skin lesions and intrathoracic involvement.

CLINICAL COMMENTS

Patients with sarcoidosis usually are initially asymptomatic, but up to 50% may develop pulmonary symptoms, including a nonproductive cough, dyspnea, chest pain, and hemoptysis. Extrathoracic manifestations of the disease include osteolytic bone lesions, hepatosplenomegaly, erythema nodosum, and cutaneous granulomas.

Sarcoidosis is considered as a diagnosis only after neoplastic and infectious diseases with similar radiographic presentations have

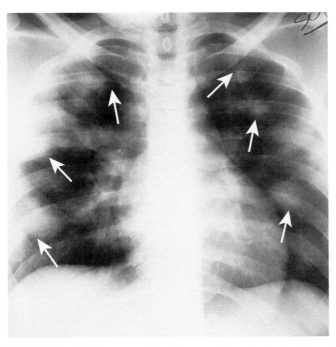

FIG. 26-11 Multiple mass and nodule presentation of alveolar (stage 3) sarcoidosis. (Courtesy Steven P. Brownstein, MD, Springfield, NJ.)

been considered. Definitive diagnosis is aided by biopsy or the less accurate Kveim skin test.[34] Spontaneous regression of the thoracic sarcoidosis occurs in 80% of cases, with the remainder progressing to extensive tissue fibrosis and the end stages of lung disease.

KEY CONCEPTS

- *Sarcoidosis is a condition of unknown etiology characterized by noncaseating granulomatous deposits in multiple organ systems.*
- *The thorax is the most common site of involvement.*
- *The radiographic appearance of sarcoidosis is typically characterized by small or massive bilateral hilar lymphadenopathy.*

References

1. Andersen HA, Lilis R, Daum SM: Household-contact asbestos neoplastic risk, *Ann NY Acad Sci* 271:310, 1976.
2. Balk R, Bone RC: The adult respiratory distress syndrome, *Med Clin North Am* 67:685, 1983.
3. Braun SR et al: Farmer's lung disease: long-term clinical and physiologic outcome, *Am Rev Respir Dis* 119:185, 1979.
4. Brooks SM: An approach to patients suspected of having an occupational pulmonary disease, *Clin Chest Med* 2:271, 1981.
5. Burrell R: Immunological aspects of coal workers' pneumoconiosis, *Ann NY Acad Sci* 200:94, 1972.
6. Casey KR, Rom WN, Moatamed F: Asbestos-related diseases, *Clin Chest Med* 2:179, 1981.
7. Chen W, Mattet NK: Malignant mesothelioma with minimal asbestos exposure, *Hum Pathol* 9:253, 1978.
8. Cieslicki J, Zych D, Zielinski J: Airway obstructions in patients with sarcoidosis, *Sarcoidosis* 8:42, 1991.
9. Clark JG, Kuhn C, Uitto J: Lung collagen in type IV Ehlers-Danlos syndrome: ultrastructural and biochemical studies, *Am Rev Respir Dis* 122:971, 1980.
10. Cook PG, Wells IP, McGavin CR: The distribution of pulmonary shadowing in farmer's lung, *Clin Radiol* 39:21, 1988.
11. DeRemee RA: The roentgenographic staging of sarcoidosis, *Chest* 83:128, 1983.
12. Divertie MB: The adult respiratory distress syndrome: subject review, *Mayo Clin Proc* 57:371, 1982.
13. Edmondstone WM, Wilson AG: Sarcoidosis in Caucasians, blacks and Asians in London, *Br J Dis Chest* 79:27, 1985.
14. Effros RM, Mason GR: An end to "ARDS," *Chest* 89:162, 1986.
15. Emanuel UA et al: Farmer's lung: clinical, pathologic and immunologic study of twenty-four patients, *Am J Med* 37:392, 1964.
16. Epler GR: Clinical overview of occupational lung disease, *Radiol Clin North Am* 30:1121, 1992.
17. Freundlich LM et al: Sarcoidosis: typical and atypical thoracic manifestations and complications, *Clin Radiol* 21:376, 1970.
18. Greene R: Adult respiratory distress syndrome: acute alveolar damage, *Radiology* 163:57, 1987.
19. Hall JR et al: Pneumothorax in the Marfan's syndrome: prevalence and therapy, *Ann Thorac Surg* 37:500, 1984.
20. International Labour Office: Guidelines for the use of ILO international classification of radiographs of pneumoconioses, Geneva, 1980, International Labour Office.
21. Israel HL, Sones M: Sarcoidosis: clinical observation on one hundred sixty cases, *Arch Intern Med* 102:766, 1958.
22. Jacobsen M: New data on the relationship between simple pneumoconiosis and exposure to coal mine dust, *Chest* 78:408, 1980.
23. Kipen HM et al: Pulmonary fibrosis in asbestos insulation workers with lung cancer: a radiologic and histopathological evaluation, *Br J Ind Med* 44:96, 1987.
24. Kirks DR, Greenspau RH: Sarcoid, *Radiol Clin North Am* 11:279, 1973.
25. Kjaergaard H: Spontaneous pneumothorax in the apparently healthy, *Acta Med Scand* 43(suppl):1, 1932.
26. Light RW: Management of spontaneous pneumothorax, *Am Rev Respir Dis* 148:245, 1993.
27. Matthay MA: Pathophysiology of pulmonary edema, *Clin Chest* 6:301, 1985.
28. Mayock RL et al: Manifestations of sarcoidosis: analysis of 145 patients, with a review of nine series selected from the literature, *Am J Med* 35:67, 1963.
29. McLoud TC: Conventional radiography in the diagnosis of asbestosis-related disease, *Radiol Clin North Am* 30:1177, 1992.
30. McLoud TC: Occupational lung disease, *Radiol Clin North Am* 29:931, 1991.
31. Mindell HJ: Roentgen findings in farmer's lung, *Radiology* 97:341, 1970.
32. Morgan PW, Goodman LR: Pulmonary edema and adult respiratory distress syndrome, *Radiol Clin North Am* 29:943, 1991.
33. Morgan WKC, Lapp NL: Respiratory disease in coal miners, *Am Rev Respir Dis* 113:531, 1976.
34. Munro CS, Mitchell DN: The Kveim response: still useful, still a puzzle, *Thorax* 42:321, 1987.
35. Primrose WR: Spontaneous pneumothorax: a retrospective review of aetiology, pathogenesis and management, *Scott Med J* 29:15, 1984.
36. Reynold HY: Hypersensitivity pneumonitis, *Clin Chest Med* 3:503, 1982.
37. Rockoff SD, Rohatgi PK: Unusual manifestations of thoracic sarcoidosis, *AJR Am J Roentgenol* 144:513, 1985.
38. Romer FK: Presentation of sarcoidosis and outcome of pulmonary changes, *Danish Med Bull* 29:27, 1982.
39. Shipley RT: The 1980 ILO classification of radiographs of the pneumoconioses, *Radiol Clin North Am* 30:1135, 1992.
40. Stark P, Jacobsen F, Shaffer K: Standard imaging in silicosis and coal worker's pneumoconiosis, *Radiol Clin North Am* 30:1147, 1992.

41. Tocino IM, Miller MH, Fairfax WR: Distribution of pneumothorax in the supine and semirecumbent critically ill patient, *AJR Am J Roentgenol* 144:901, 1985.

42. Uargreave F et al: The radiological appearances of allergic alveolitis due to bird sensitivity (bird fancier's lung), *Clin Radiol* 23:1, 1972.

43. Unger GF et al: A radiologic approach to hypersensitivity pneumonias, *Radiol Clin North Am* 11:339, 1973.

44. Unger J, Fink JN, Unger GF: Pigeon breeder's disease: a review of the roentgenographic pulmonary findings, *AJR Am J Roentgenol* 90:683, 1968.

45. Wagner GR, Attfield MD, Parker JE: Chest radiography in dust-exposed miners: promise and problems, potential and imperfections, *Occup Med* 8:127, 1993.

Chest Patterns

DENNIS M. MARCHIORI

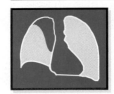

CS I | Atelectasis

Atelectasis is defined as incomplete air filling and underexpansion of the lung. It may involve the entire lung or appear localized to a lobe, segment, or subsegment. The collapsed lung may displace the diaphragm, fissures, hila, mediastinum, or other anatomic borders. Regions of increased radiopacity and approximation of vascular markings, ribs, or other structures are apparent occasionally. Atelectasis is always secondary to underlying pathology; therefore its presence should prompt a vigorous search for a cause. Although several mechanisms of collapse have been identified, obstruction of the airway is the most common.

DISEASE	COMMENTS
Adhesive (adhesion of the alveolar interior walls)	
Hyaline membrane disease	Decreased surfactant production in the neonate.
Postoperative	Tissue adhesions related to cardiac or thoracic surgery.
Cicatrizing (scarring, fibrosus, and contraction of lung interstitium)	
Connective tissue disease	Widely disseminated radiopacities resulting from tissue fibrosus related to rheumatoid arthritis, scleroderma, idiopathic pulmonary fibrosis, and so on.
Infections **(FIG. 27-1)** [p. 1147]	Scattered linear and circular radiopacities in the upper lung fields correlating to a history of granulomatous infections (e.g., tuberculosis, histoplasmosis, coccidioidomycosis); lesions have a tendency to form irregular thick-walled cavities.
Radiation	Nonanatomic regions of involvement that correlate to history and site of past therapeutic radiation exposure.
Compressive (intrapulmonary lesions compressing normal lung tissue)	
Bullous emphysema [p. 1150]	Large, thin-walled air sacs associated with emphysema and typically found in the upper lung; these sacs may compress adjacent normal lung tissue.
Pulmonary mass	Space-occupying mass lesion within the lung (e.g., neoplasms, sarcoidosis).
Obstructive (intrinsic or extrinsic airway obstruction)	
Broncholithiasis	Occurs occasionally when a radiodense, calcified lymph node from prior granulomatous infection erodes through the bronchial wall and obstructs the lumen of the airway.
Foreign bodies	Seen in infants, children (e.g., marble, peanut), and adults (e.g., dentures, tooth fragments after trauma, nails or screws held in mouth, meat) after aspiration of a foreign body; usually a characteristic history exists; occasionally patients exhibit an asymptomatic period of hours to days after incident.
Mucus plugs	Most often associated with asthma, chronic bronchitis, surgery, and neurologic suppression of cough reflex.
Tumors **(FIG. 27-2)** [p. 1187]	Bronchogenic carcinoma is a common cause of obstruction in patients over the age of 50 years; these patients may exhibit concurrent enlargement of the involved hilum or mediastinum. Bronchial carcinoid tumors are more common in younger patients.
Passive (extrapulmonary lesions compressing normal lung tissue)	
Body wall lesions	Expansile rib lesions, pleural-based disease, and intercostal soft-tissue lesions.
Pleural space filling	Space-occupying lesions in the pleural space (e.g., edema, chyle, hemorrhage, air).
Subsegmental, platelike, discoid (linear radiopacity in periphery of lung) **(FIG. 27-3)**	
Hospitalization	Resulting from hypoventilation because of painful breathing, anesthesia, pleural effusion, pneumonia, and so on.
Pulmonary embolism [p. 1165]	Commonly involves collapse as a nonspecific finding of acute pulmonary embolism, often associated with pleural effusion; when the collapse occurs in the late manifestations of the disease, it represents pulmonary scar formations.

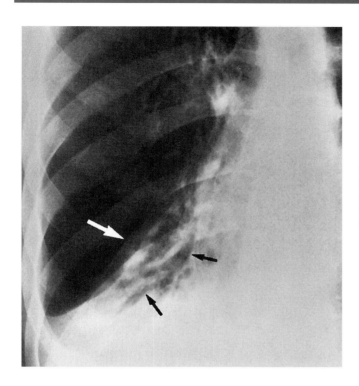

FIG. 27-1 Right lower lobe collapse caused by destruction and fibrosis from past infection. Air in dilated bronchi *(black arrows)* is an important clue to fibrosis and resulting bronchiectasis as the cause of the collapsed lobe. White arrow points to displaced major fissure. (From Armstrong P et al: Imaging of diseases of the chest, ed 3, St Louis, 2000, Mosby.)

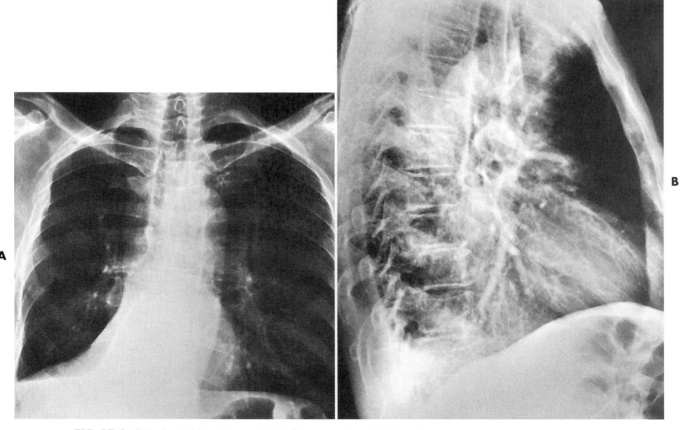

FIG. 27-2 Right lower lobe collapse resulting from bronchial carcinoma. Although the obstructing bronchial lesion is not seen, metastatic bone disease is present in the right eighth rib, and there are multiple old fractures of the right ribs. **A,** Posteroanterior radiograph. **B,** Lateral radiograph.

Continued

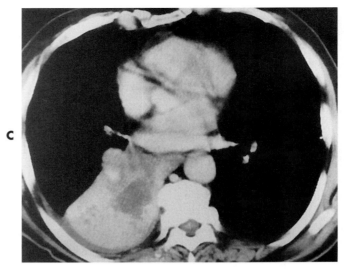

FIG. 27-2 cont'd   **C,** Computed tomography scan in a different patient with right lower lobe collapse. (From the Armstrong P et al: Imaging of diseases of the chest, ed 3, St Louis, 2000, Mosby.)

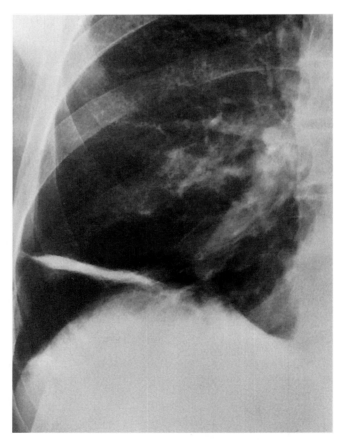

FIG. 27-3   Discoid atelectasis showing a typical bandlike shadow. (From Armstrong P et al: Imaging of diseases of the chest, ed 3, St Louis, 2000, Mosby.)

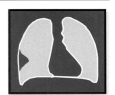

CS2 | Chest Wall and Pleural-Based Lesions

Chest wall and pleural-based lesions often are marked by a characteristic radiographic appearance of a radiopaque convexity extending inward, toward the lung, with sloping superior and inferior tails. The outer border of the lesion is incompletely defined, confirming an extrapulmonary location. A variety of etiologies are responsible, including infections, primary neoplasms, metastasis, and trauma.

DISEASE	COMMENTS
Abscess [p. 1376]	Most commonly results from *Staphylococcus* infection, tuberculosis, and actinomycosis; associated characteristics include rib involvement, pulmonary infiltrate, pleural effusion, and a painful, red, subcutaneous mass.
Hematoma	Suggested by the presence of pleural effusion, history of trauma, evidence of trauma (e.g., rib fracture), or hemoptysis; retrosternal hematomas occasionally are seen in the lateral projection on those patients experiencing automobile accidents, in which the steering wheel inflicts blunt trauma to the chest.
Pleural fluid [p. 1162]	Free or loculated transudate, exudate, blood, chyle, etc., presenting as a well-defined density in the pleural space.
Rib fracture	Secondary to blunt or penetrating trauma to normal ribs or less forceful trauma to ribs affected by pathology (e.g., tumor or infection). Fracture occurs as a thin, vertical radiolucent line with offset of rib cortices, often best seen on an oblique projection; acute fracture warrants a careful search for associated hemothorax or pneumothorax.
Rib tumors **(FIG. 27-4)**	Most common benign tumors: osteochondromas, followed by enchondromas and osteoblastomas; metastatic bone disease, chondrosarcoma, and multiple myeloma produce multiple lytic regions; nonneoplastic lesions such as fibrous dysplasia commonly involve the ribs.
Skin lesions	Soft-tissue densities (e.g., nipples, moles, neurofibromas) typically appear with incomplete borders because of region of contact with the skin. Examination of the skin surface or repeat radiographs using a radiopaque marker confirms questionable lesions.
Soft-tissue benign tumor	Variety of tissue types, appearing as a smooth protruding mass from body wall into lung field; lipomas are most common and may present as intrathoracic or extrathoracic lesions.
Soft-tissue malignant tumor	Often visible, painful mass with associated bone destruction; the most common malignant soft-tissue neoplasms of the chest wall in adults are fibrosarcoma and liposarcoma; metastasis, mesotheliomas, and bronchogenic (Pancoast) tumors may involve the pleura; a past history of radiation therapy is a risk factor.

PART THREE Chest

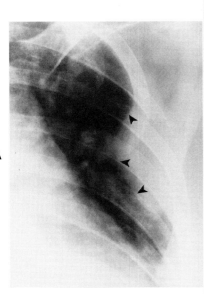

A

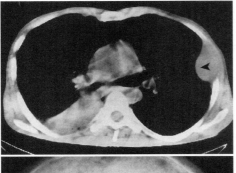

B

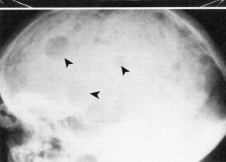

C

FIG. 27-4 Multiple myeloma of the rib appearing as an extrapleural lesion *(arrowheads)* and pathologic rib fracture. **A,** Peripheral pulmonary radiopacity extending inward from a broad-based chest wall origin (extrapleural sign). **B,** The appearance is better demarcated on computed tomography scans *(arrowhead)*. **C,** Involvement of the skull also is noted in this patient *(arrowheads)*. (Courtesy Steven P. Brownstein, MD, Springfield, NJ.)

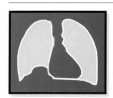

CS3 | Diaphragmatic Abnormalities

The right hemidiaphragm typically is one intercostal space higher than the left. With proper inspiratory effort, the right hemidiaphram should be below the level of the posterior portion of the tenth rib or the anterior portion of the seventh rib. The position of the left hemidiaphram is more variable than that of the right because of the subjacent gastric air bubble. Unilateral or bilateral changes of the diaphragm's position may suggest underlying pathology of the thorax or abdomen.

CS3a | Depressed Diaphragm

DISEASE	COMMENTS
Increased pulmonary volume **(FIG. 27-5)**	Unilateral lung overinflation resulting from a large bulla, a pulmonary cyst, or in response to a contralateral small lung; chronic bilateral overinflation results from diffuse obstructive emphysema or is transient with asthma and expiratory air trapping because of bronchial obstruction.
Large pleural effusion [p. 1162]	Difficult to detect because the fluid obliterates the diaphragm contour; the position of the gastric air bubble indicates the position of the left hemidiaphragm.
Pneumothorax [p. 1214]	Other radiographic findings of pneumothorax: absence of interstitial and bronchovascular lung markings and the characteristic, thin, radiodense line represents visceral pleura; if large, the pneumothorax may invert the dome of the diaphragm.

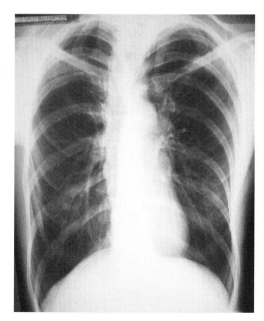

FIG. 27-5 Emphysema demonstrated by hyperlucent, overexpanded lung fields, prominent truncated pulmonary arteries, and flattened hemidiaphragms.

CS3b | Elevated Diaphragm

DISEASE	COMMENTS
Congenital eventration (FIGS. 27-6 and 27-7)	Represents an elevated segment of the diaphragm, resulting from congenital absence or weakness of a portion of the diaphragmatic musculature; this condition results in poor contractility and inability to resist infradiaphragmatic visceral pressure; total hemidiaphragm eventration is more common on the left; partial hemidiaphragm eventration is more common on the right and usually involves the antero-medial segment.
Diaphragm splinting	Lack of diaphragm excursion in response to pain, fracture, infection, and so on.
Diaphragmatic hernia	Most commonly the esophageal hiatal hernia presents as a centrally located air-fluid level behind the heart shadow in the frontal projection; an esophagram is confirmatory; Bochdalek's hernias typically appear as posterolateral masses above the left hemidiaphragm and represent herniations of retroperitoneal contents; Morgagni's hernias typically appear as anteromedial right-sided masses in the cardiophrenic angles.
Intraabdominal mass (FIG. 27-8)	Unilateral elevation resulting from renal, hepatic, or splenic abscess, tumor, cyst, or gas distention of the bowel, stomach, or peritoneal cavity; bilateral elevation results from pregnancy, obesity, and ascites.
Phrenic nerve paralysis	Reduces the contractility of hemidiaphragm by damage to the phrenic nerve (surgical transection, pressure from hilar mass, poliomyelitis, and Erb's palsy); the affected diaphragm exhibits paradoxic motion under fluoroscopic observation by ascending rather than descending movement during inspiration (positive sniff test).
Poor inspiratory result	*Inspiratory effort* is defined as the patient's compliance with inspiratory instructions during the radiographic exposure. *Inspiratory result* is a general term encompassing both inspiratory effort and mechanical obstacles to full inspiration, such as obesity, pregnancy, and ascites.
Reduced pulmonary volume	Loss of lung volume resulting from congenital hypoplasia, pneumonectomy, atelectasis, and other diseases.
Ruptured diaphragm (FIG. 27-9)	Significant blunt, crushing, or penetrating thoracoabdominal trauma possibly causing abdominal contents to herniate into the thoracic cavity; the rupture is nearly always left-sided because the liver dissipates traumatic forces on the right; a ruptured diaphragm appears as a gas-filled bowel or stomach seen in the left lower lung field.
Subpulmonary effusion [p. 1165]	Pleural fluid under the lung possibly simulating elevation of the diaphragm; commonly the pseudodiaphragm, or dome of the fluid, appears more lateral than its normal position; lateral decubitus projections may aid in differentiating subpulmonary effusion from an elevated diaphragm.

PART THREE Chest

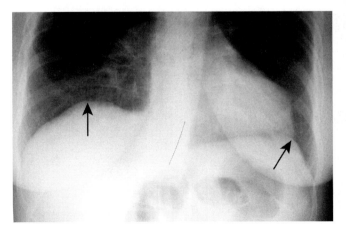

FIG. 27-6 Bilateral partial congenital eventration of the diaphragm *(arrows)*.

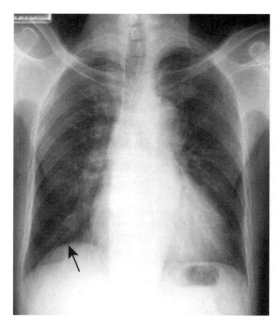

FIG. 27-7 Unilateral presentation of partial congenital eventration of the diaphragm *(arrow)*.

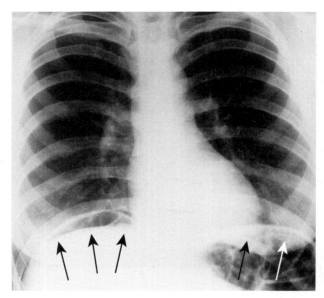

FIG. 27-8 Radiolucent, sickle-shaped air shadows subjacent to the right and left hemidiaphragm secondary to perforated ulcer *(arrows)*. (Courtesy Steven P. Brownstein, MD, Springfield, NJ.)

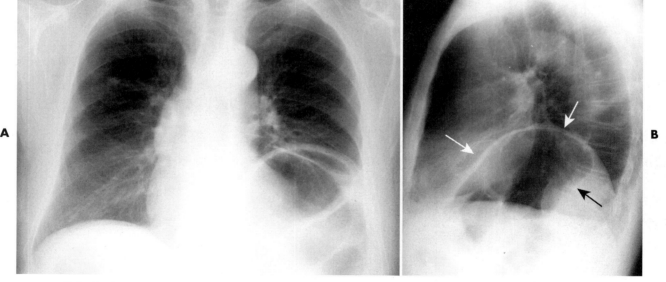

FIG. 27-9 **A,** Posteroanterior and, **B,** lateral projections demonstrating traumatic rupture of the left hemidiaphragm with herniation of an air-filled portion of the stomach into the thoracic cavity *(arrows)*. As a result, there is a gastric air-fluid level. (Courtesy John A.M. Taylor, Seneca Falls, NY.)

cs4 | Diffuse Alveolar (Air-Space) Disease

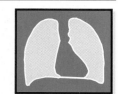

Diffuse alveolar disease comprises bilateral, widely disseminated opacifications that may appear very dense (homogenous consolidation) and correlate to complete filling of the alveolar space. Alternatively, a patchy and fluffy appearance (heterogeneous consolidation) denotes incomplete filling of the alveolar space.

The opacifications of lung vary in size and exhibit a tendency toward coalescence. Within the regions of opacification, characteristic tubular radiolucent shadows are seen occasionally, representing air-filled bronchi transversing water-filled parenchyma (air-bronchogram sign).

The diseases are divided into acute and chronic forms based on history and serial radiography. Although an exact timeline is difficult to develop, patterns that remain largely unchanged for several weeks or months are chronic.

DISEASE	COMMENTS
Acute diffuse alveolar disease *Adult respiratory distress syndrome* [p. 1213]	Increased capillary permeability resulting from a wide variety of systemic and pulmonary insults (e.g., drug abuse, fractures, smoke inhalation, shock), causing excessive fluid accumulation in the alveolar spaces.
Near-drowning **(FIG. 27-10)**	May be prevented by laryngeal spasm; otherwise fluid may enter the lung from drowning or submersion events.
Pneumonia [p. 1169]	Related to aggressive infections of the lung; patients typically are extremely ill, exhibiting fever, productive cough, difficulty breathing, and malaise; although many organisms may be associated with this presentation, gram-negative infections are notorious for producing this appearance.
Pulmonary edema **(FIG. 27-11)** [p. 1164]	Accumulates within the interstitium during the early stages; the resulting linear densities are termed *Kerley's lines* and are subdivided by position within the lung; lymphatic drainage is overwhelmed as fluid accumulates, and edema spills over to the alveolar lumen, relating an alveolar pattern; the appearance may be "cloudlike," diffusely involving the lung fields bilaterally; as pulmonary edema progresses, the alveolar pattern is seen centrally with interstitial extensions to the periphery.
Pulmonary hemorrhage	Associated with anticoagulant therapy, pulmonary contusion, or less commonly Goodpasture's syndrome; hemoptysis and patient history are indicative.
Chronic diffuse alveolar disease *Alveolar proteinosis* **(FIG. 27-12)**	Bilateral confluent radiopacities, less commonly diffuse nodular pattern; appearance may be transient, and there are surprisingly few associated clinical symptoms apart from dyspnea.
Radiation pneumonitis	Diffuse pulmonary damage with accompanying history of therapeutic radiation.

PART THREE Chest

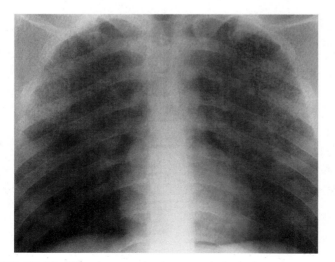

FIG. 27-10 Bilateral, symmetric, air-space radiodense shadows in a near-drowning victim. (Courtesy Steven P. Brownstein, MD, Springfield, NJ.)

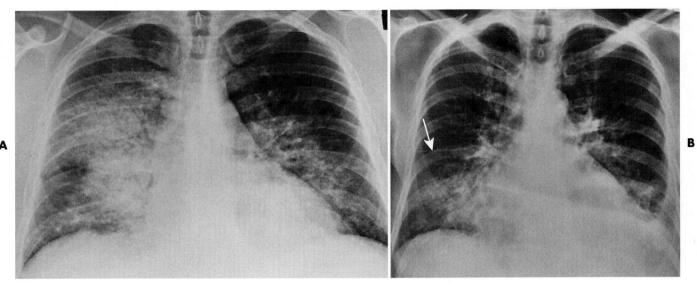

FIG. 27-11 Cardiogenic alveolar edema. **A,** Butterfly pattern. **B,** Bibasilar edema in a different patient showing septal lines and a left pleural effusion. Note also the bronchial wall thickening and thickening of the minor fissure *(arrow)*. (From Armstrong P et al: Imaging of diseases of the chest, ed 3, St Louis, 2000, Mosby.)

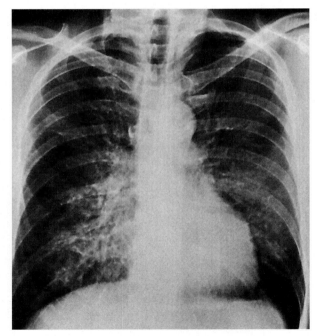

FIG. 27-12 "Bat's wing" shadowing in alveolar proteinosis. (From Armstrong P et al: Imaging of diseases of the chest, ed 3, St Louis, 2000, Mosby.)

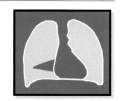

CS5 | Localized Alveolar (Air-Space) Disease

Solitary or multiple localized alveolar disease is marked by extensive filling of the alveolar spaces with space-occupying lesions (e.g., blood, edema, pus, protein, cells), relating a complete (homogenous) or partial (heterogeneous) consolidation or opacification of a segment, lobe, or entire lung.

This pattern differs from the previous pattern of diffuse alveolar pattern because the involved pulmonary region is localized, unilateral, and peripherally well defined. However, similar to the previous pattern of lung disease, it may be separated into acute and chronic presentation based on the patient's history and available serial radiographs. Although an exact timeline is difficult to develop, patterns that remain largely unchanged for several weeks or months are chronic.

DISEASE	COMMENTS
Acute localized alveolar disease *Bronchioloalveolar (alveolar cell) carcinoma* **(FIG. 27-13)** [p. 1187]	May appear as well-defined consolidation similar to pneumonia; however, it does not respond to appropriate management of pneumonia.
Pulmonary contusion	Appearance corresponding to alveolar collections of edema and atelectasis of the lung in response to bronchial obstruction; the obstruction may develop slowly (e.g., bronchogenic carcinoma, bronchial carcinoid tumors) or rapidly (e.g., foreign body, mucus plug).
Obstructive pneumonitis	Consolidation of lung parenchyma (lung, lobe, or segment) resulting from filling of the normally air-filled alveolar sacs with exudate and inflammatory cells of similar radiopacity to water. Causative agents include bacteria, fungi, and viruses; clinical features of malaise, fever, and purulent expectorant typically accompany the radiographic findings; the consolidated area becomes patchy and fades to normal after successful treatment.
Pneumonia **(FIG. 27-14)** [p. 1169]	Transient densely radiopaque or incompletely consolidated patchy regions that extend from the body wall and represent blood and edema in the alveolar sacs; history of blunt trauma to the chest and presence of rib fractures are strongly indicative.
Chronic localized alveolar disease *Atelectasis* [p. 1143]	Incomplete inflation of a lung (or segment) possibly appearing as a region of increased radiopacity resulting from increased lung density; concurrent finding of incomplete inflation (hilar, diaphragm, or mediastinum displacement) and clinical absence of fever and purulent cough distinguish atelectasis from pneumonia.
Lymphoma [p. 1203]	Appearance of radiopacities that represent pulmonary infiltrate of neoplasm or superimposed infection secondary to immunosuppression after treatment; often lymphoma presents with mediastinal widening; pulmonary involvement occurs as a result of direct lymphatic extension from the mediastinum.
Pulmonary infarct **(FIG. 27-15)** [p. 1181]	Radiopaque parenchymal density (classically pleural-based triangular appearance with apex toward hilum) located most commonly in the peripheral lower lung field. Over time the lesions tend to resolve from the periphery, inward to the center, preserving the radiopacity's triangular configuration ("melting" sign).
Radiation pneumonitis	Patchy, irregular areas of incomplete consolidation resulting from tissue "weeping" and edema produced from tissue irradiation; a history of radiation is suggestive; the location corresponds to the radiation port.
Sarcoidosis [p. 1218]	Patchy, irregular, radiopaque areas representing noncaseating, granulomatous deposits in the interstitium; it appears as an alveolar pattern; parenchymal involvement only is an uncommon presentation of the disease; more commonly, findings include concurrent enlarged hilar lymph nodes or adenopathy that precedes the pulmonary disease; sarcoidosis is more common in blacks and women.
Tuberculosis [p. 779]	Transmitted by repeated contacts with infected individuals through inhalation; tuberculosis is not easily contracted in immunocompetent individuals; consequently, the immunocompromised and those of low socioeconomic scale (e.g., acquired immunodeficiency syndrome [AIDS] patients, alcoholics, elderly people, homeless persons) are vulnerable. The radiographic features of the primary infection include consolidation with pleural effusion; any lung segment may be involved and the findings typically resolve without complication; reactivation infections typically involve the upper lobes, often with scarring and a tendency toward cavitation.

PART THREE
Chest

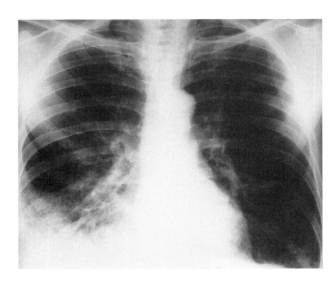

FIG. 27-13 Localized pattern of bronchioloalveolar carcinoma appearing as air-space consolidation in the right lower lung. (Courtesy Steven P. Brownstein, MD, Springfield, NJ.)

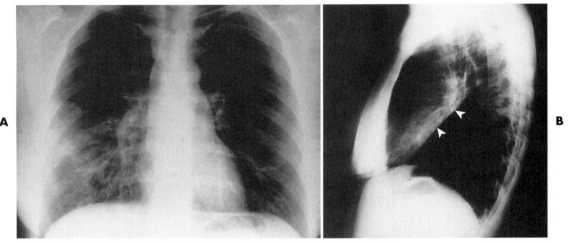

FIG. 27-14 **A,** Posteroanterior chest radiograph demonstrating partial consolidation of the lateral portion of the right middle lobe. **B,** The partially consolidated segment is noted as a radiodense zone anterior to the oblique fissure *(arrowheads)* on the overexposed lateral projection.

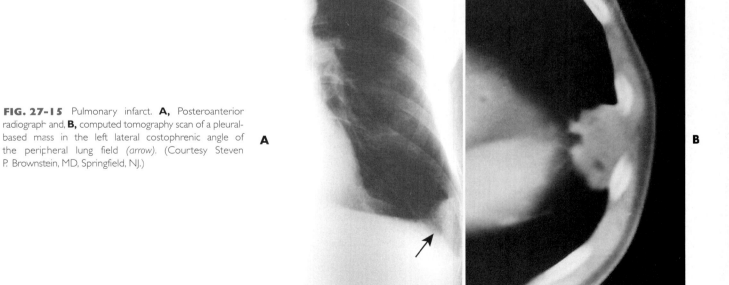

FIG. 27-15 Pulmonary infarct. **A,** Posteroanterior radiograph and, **B,** computed tomography scan of a pleural-based mass in the left lateral costophrenic angle of the peripheral lung field *(arrow).* (Courtesy Steven P. Brownstein, MD, Springfield, NJ.)

CS6 | Diffuse Interstitial Disease

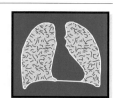

Diffuse interstitial disease describes a general radiographic pattern that can be more specifically separated into miliary, nodular, reticular, reticulonodular, and honeycomb patterns. These patterns represent disease in the interstitium, although often air-space (alveolar) disease is concurrently present, making the radiographic appearance confusing to the observer.

In its uncomplicated presentation, interstitial disease is marked by well-defined linear or nodular radiopacities widely disseminated throughout the lung fields, usually in a bilateral, symmetric distribution.

Similar to those of an alveolar pattern, the causes of an interstitial radiographic pattern can be divided into acute and chronic, based on history and, in the case of chronicity, serial studies. Although an exact timeline is difficult to develop, patterns that remain largely unchanged for several weeks or months are chronic.

DISEASE	COMMENTS
Acute diffuse interstitial disease *Infection* [p. 1169]	Appearance resulting from inflammation and thickening of interstitial spaces often appearing as reticulonodular opacities; an interstitial pattern is an uncommon presentation of pneumonia, seen most commonly with viral or mycoplasmic agents; the appearance typically is more prominent in the lower lung regions with accompanying clinical findings suggestive of infection.
Pulmonary edema [p. 1164]	Pulmonary edema accumulates within the interstitium during the initial stages; the resulting linear densities are termed *Kerley's lines* and are subdivided by position within the lung; as fluid accumulates, lymphatic drainage is overwhelmed, and edema spills over to the alveolar lumen, relating an alveolar pattern. As pulmonary edema progresses, the alveolar pattern is seen centrally with interstitial extensions at the periphery.
Chronic diffuse interstitial disease *Connective tissue disorders*	Group of systemic disorders causing chronic interstitial patterns that are more pronounced in the lower lung fields; examples include rheumatoid arthritis, dermatomyositis, systemic lupus erythematosus, and scleroderma.
Cystic fibrosis **(FIG. 27-16)**	Coarse interstitial pattern with mixed areas of consolidation, atelectasis, and peribronchial thickening; cystic fibrosis is seen in patients younger than 30 years of age.
Histiocytosis X (Langerhans cell histiocytosis)	Coarse interstitial appearance more common in the upper lung fields; radiographic changes are often seen in the absence of clinical findings.
Idiopathic interstitial fibrosis **(FIG. 27-17)**	Describes a group of conditions of unknown origin associated with a chronic interstitial pattern predominantly in the lower peripheral lung regions; the initial presentation is that of diffuse, thin linear densities that progress to thickened cystic "end-stage" or "honeycomb" lung disease; symptoms include dyspnea and cough.
Lymphangitic metastasis	Lymph dissemination of primary malignancy (most commonly breast, stomach, thyroid, or lung) through pulmonary tissue; it is more prominent in the lower lung field, commonly associated with hilar enlargement, unilateral presentation, and history of primary malignancy.
Pneumoconioses [p. 1214]	Chronic inhalation of inorganic dust particles (e.g., asbestos, silicon, iron, tin, barium) is associated with interstitial patterns and varying degrees of clinical complaints. Involvement by silicosis is noted more commonly in the upper lung fields, whereas asbestosis has a lower lobe distribution; a history of exposure is usual.
Sarcoidosis **(FIG. 27-18)** [p. 1218]	Marked by a progression of radiographic appearances from hilar and mediastinal lymphadenopathy to an interstitial pattern. It is characterized by a disparity between the advanced radiographic presentation and mild patient symptoms; it is seen more commonly in blacks and women.

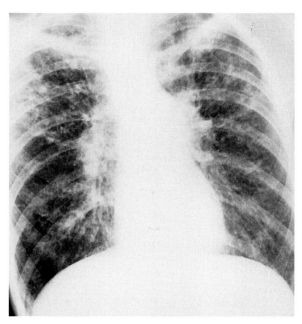

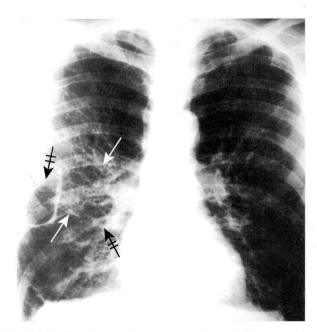

FIG. 27-16 Generalized multiple linear and cystic radiodensities scattered bilaterally through the lung fields indicative of cystic fibrosis. (Courtesy Steven P. Brownstein, MD, Springfield, NJ.)

FIG. 27-17 Chronic obstructive pulmonary disease relating linear and cystic radiodense shadows characteristic of an interstitial pattern of parenchymal disease *(arrows)*. Cyst formation is noted also *(crossed arrows)*.

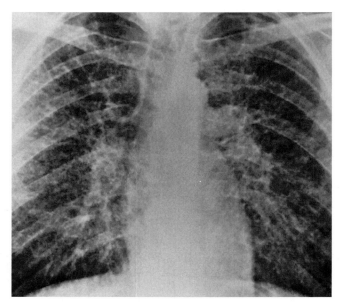

FIG. 27-18 Parenchymal sarcoidosis. Note mild adenopathy and mild hilar elevation. Parenchymal shadowing is reticulonodular with pronounced linear elements that suggest development of scarring. Uniformity of changes in all zones is unusual. (From Armstrong P et al: Imaging of diseases of the chest, ed 3, St Louis, 2000, Mosby.)

CS7 | Enlarged Hilum

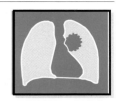

The hilum is the root of the lung, representing the connection between the lung and mediastinum. Anatomically it is a conduit for the primary bronchi, pulmonary artery, bronchial artery, two pulmonary veins, and lymphatics. On the radiograph, the hilum appears as the radiopacity at the central, medial portion of the lung. Alterations in the size, configuration, or density of the hilum may indicate a disease process of one of these elements entering the lung.

Minor changes in size are difficult to differentiate from variants of normal. Abnormalities are detected best by comparing questionable appearances with the contralateral hilum or old radiographs. An enlarged or altered hilum may occur alone or in combination with other imaging findings (e.g., parenchymal disease, pleural effusion, mediastinal involvement). In the frontal projection, the normal pulmonary artery alone measures around 16 mm in diameter.

DISEASE	COMMENTS
Airway	
Bronchogenic carcinoma **(FIG. 27-19)** [p. 1149]	Represents the most common cause of unilateral hilar enlargement in the adult patient; the tumor arises in the large bronchi and extends to the surrounding lymph nodes, which account for much of the mass seen; obstructive pneumonitis and atelectasis may be the first signs of disease.
Bronchial carcinoid tumors [p. 1187]	Arise in the central bronchi and are recognized by the appearance of hilar mass or secondary findings of bronchial obstruction, including obstructive pneumonitis and atelectasis.
Lymph nodes *Infectious adenopathy*	Tuberculosis, coccidioidomycosis, and histoplasmosis may present as a bilateral or unilateral hilar mass; the involved nodes generally calcify over time and may be associated with unilateral parenchymal disease; more aggressive infections also cause hilar enlargement but typically are dominated by their parenchymal patterns.
Leukemia	Bilateral, symmetric enlargement of hila and mediastinum commonly seen in adults with chronic lymphocytic leukemia, but rarely seen in childhood leukemias. Pleural effusion and parenchymal involvement are common and must be differentiated from opportunistic infections and drug reactions.
Lymphoma **(FIG. 27-20)** [p. 1203]	Characteristic bilateral enlargement for Hodgkin and non–Hodgkin types; mediastinal involvement (especially anterior) and pleural effusion are common; patient also may exhibit peripheral lymphadenopathy and splenomegaly and symptoms of weakness and fever.
Metastatic adenopathy [p. 1393]	Unilateral or bilateral involvement, commonly with accompanying wide mediastinum and sometimes with interstitial pattern resulting from lymphangitic spread.
Sarcoidosis **(FIGS. 27-21 and 27-22)** [p. 1218]	Common early manifestation is bilateral hilar enlargement from large, well-defined "potato nodes." These nodes may regress spontaneously, or the disease may progress to further stages of parenchymal involvement; mediastinal involvement is common and enlarged right paratracheal nodes are characteristic.
Vessels *Pulmonary artery aneurysm* **(FIGS. 27-23 and 27-24)**	Rare, usually secondary to pulmonary hypertension or infection (e.g., mycotic and bacterial endocarditis).
Pulmonary artery hypertension	Bilateral enlargement of the central pulmonary vessels, which taper peripherally, relating a truncated appearance. In addition, the patient may exhibit cardiomegaly, suggesting a cardiogenic origin of hypertension.
Pulmonary embolism [p. 1165]	Bilateral or unilateral pulmonary artery enlargement resulting from massive central or multiple peripheral emboli.

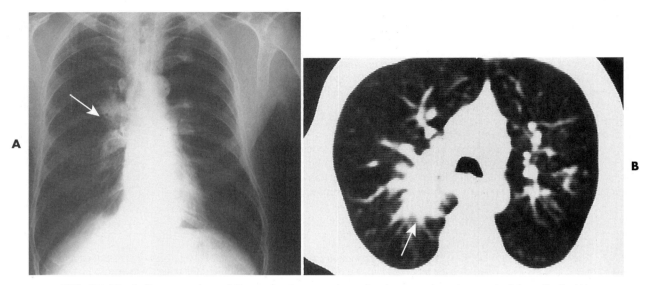

FIG. 27-19 **A,** Posteroanterior and, **B,** computed tomography studies demonstrating enlargement of the patient's right hilum secondary to bronchogenic carcinoma *(arrows)*. (Courtesy Steven P. Brownstein, MD, Springfield, NJ.)

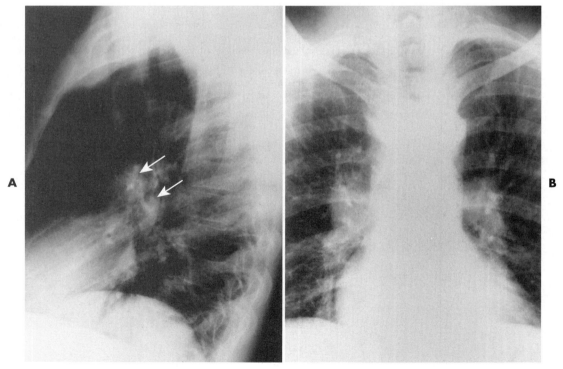

FIG. 27-20 **A** and **B,** Bilateral hilar enlargement secondary to lymphoma *(arrows)*. (Courtesy Steven P. Brownstein, MD, Springfield, NJ.)

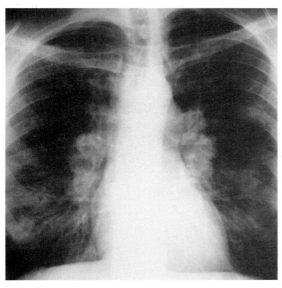

FIG. 27-21 Bilateral hilum enlargement and linear pulmonary radiopacities consistent with stage 2 sarcoidosis. (Courtesy Steven P. Brownstein, MD, Springfield, NJ.)

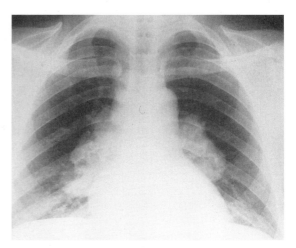

FIG. 27-22 Bilateral hilar adenopathy without parenchymal abnormality consistent with stage I sarcoidosis. (Courtesy Steven P. Brownstein, MD, Springfield, NJ.)

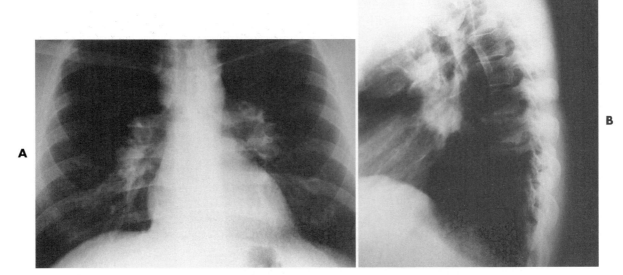

FIG. 27-23 **A** and **B,** Stage I sarcoidosis presenting with bilateral, symmetric hilar adenopathy. (Courtesy Robert C. Tatum, Davenport, IA.)

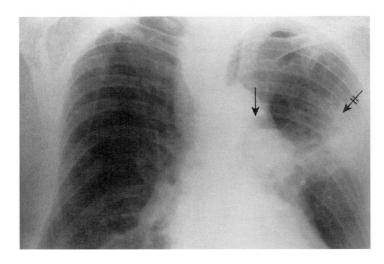

FIG. 27-24 Enlarged left hilum *(arrow)* resulting from pulmonary artery aneurysm with pneumonitis producing the parenchymal air-space pattern in the periphery of the middle left lung field *(crossed arrow)*. (Courtesy Steven P. Brownstein, MD, Springfield, NJ.)

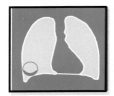

cs8 | Focal Radiolucent Lesions

Holes in the lung are broadly divided into cysts and cavities on the basis of appearance and etiology. Cysts are thin-walled (1- to 3-mm) circular defects of lung appearing alone or in groups. Cavities are defined as areas of radiolucency that represent areas of tissue necrosis and clearing within areas of parenchymal opacification. The radiolucency is surrounded by the remaining opacification, creating a surrounding rim of more than 3 mm. Cavities also appear alone or in groups. The presence of a cavity suggests a more aggressive pathology than can be inferred from the presence of a cyst.

cs8a | Cavities

DISEASE	COMMENTS
Infections **(FIGS. 27-25 and 27-26)**	Common for cavitation to become a chronic development among the granulomatous diseases; tuberculosis is the most widely recognized of these diseases and usually involves the lung apices with associated pulmonary findings. Cavitation in the presence of clinical symptoms (e.g., fever, elevated white blood cell counts, and positive sputum and cultures) strongly suggests an infection from pyogenic agents; these cavitations are called *abscesses*.
Neoplasms **(FIG. 27-27)**	Thick-walled cavities with irregular, lobulated inner margins; they most often occur with bronchogenic carcinomas (especially squamous cell type), lymphoma, and metastasis from various origins.
Septic embolism **(FIG. 27-28)**	Typically multiple in the lower lung regions resulting from shower of emboli; related to right-sided bacterial endocarditis or history of intravenous drug abuse.
Wegener's granulomatosis **(FIG. 27-29)**	Common for cavitation to develop within the multiple granulomatous lesions of Wegener's granulomatosus; often the kidney and nasal cavity are involved concurrently; cavities may regress with treatment.

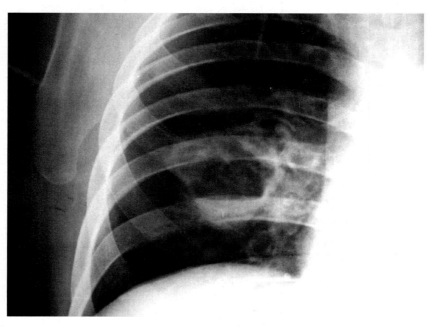

FIG. 27-25 Staphylococcal infection with cavity in right middle lung field. (Courtesy Steven P. Brownstein, MD, Springfield, NJ.)

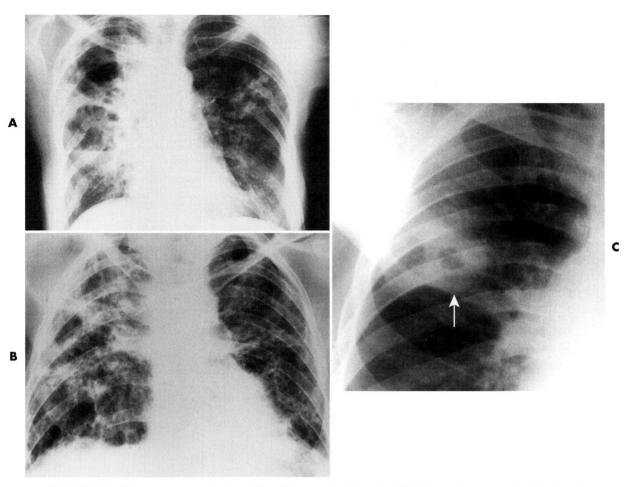

FIG. 27-26 Different patients with, **A** and **B,** multiple and, **C,** solitary *(arrow)* infectious pulmonary cavities. Associated volume loss of right lung is marked by the elevated right hemidiaphragm in **A** and **B.**

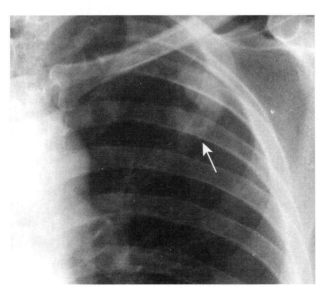

FIG. 27-27 Cavitating squamous cell bronchogenic carcinoma located in the periphery of the left upper lobe *(arrow).* (Courtesy Steven P. Brownstein, MD, Springfield, NJ.)

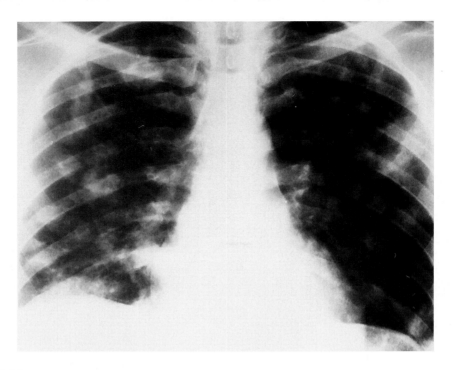

FIG. 27-28 Septic emboli presenting as multiple bilateral pulmonary nodules. (Courtesy Steven P. Brownstein, MD, Springfield, NJ.)

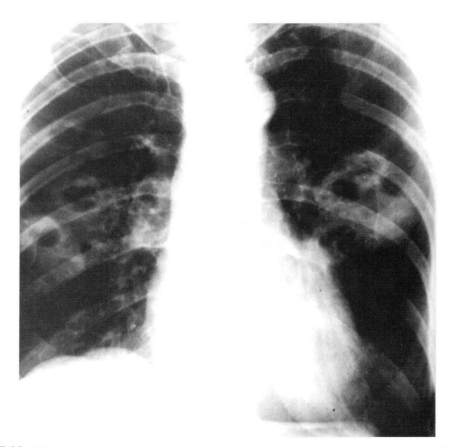

FIG. 27-29 Wegener's granulomatosis, appearing with bilateral cavitating nodules in the central regions of the lungs. (Courtesy Steven P. Brownstein, MD, Springfield, NJ.)

CS8b | Cysts

DISEASE	COMMENTS
Bronchogenic cyst [p. 1149]	Appear as solitary, moderately large lesions within the lung or mediastinum; most begin as radiopaque, fluid-filled lesions and become air-filled cysts only after connection to an airway is established.
Bulla/bleb	Thin-walled cysts in the upper lung fields of various sizes; associated with emphysema and recurrent pneumothorax; although some authorities use the terms bulla and bleb interchangeably, others use bleb to represent a smaller lesion of subpleural location.
Cystic fibrosis	Multiple, ringlike shadows associated with an interstitial pattern; they may be filled with fluid.
Hydatid cyst (*Echinococcus granulosus*)	Typically in the lower lobe; if ruptured, debris may appear floating on the internal fluid ("water lily" sign).
Pneumatocele (FIG. 27-30)	Small cyst resulting from a check-valve obstruction of an airway, usually secondary to *Staphylococcus* infection in children.
Rheumatoid arthritis (FIG. 27-31)	Single or multiple, thin- or thick-walled peripheral subpleural defects that may be associated with pleural effusion; lesions typically demonstrate smooth inner walls that may regress with remission of the disease.
Traumatic lung cyst	Development of single or multiple peripheral subpleural cysts after pulmonary trauma.

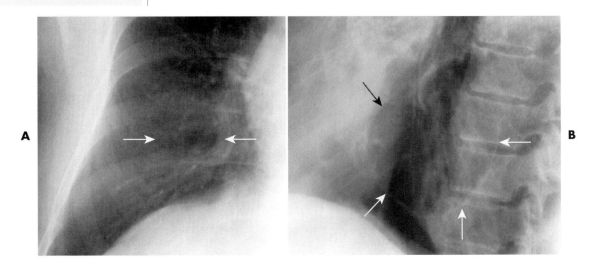

FIG. 27-30 **A** and **B,** Pneumatocele presenting as a faint cystic defect *(arrows)* in this 80-year-old man. (Courtesy John A.M. Taylor, Seneca Falls, NY.)

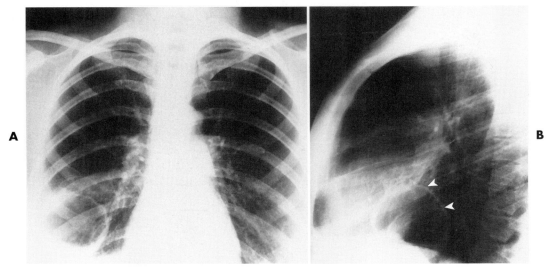

FIG. 27-31 **A** and **B,** Rheumatoid cyst within the lower right lobe *(arrowheads).* (Courtesy Steven P. Brownstein, MD, Springfield, NJ.)

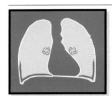

cs9 | Intrathoracic Calcifications

hest radiographs commonly demonstrate calcification within the thorax. Most often calcifications are dystrophic, occurring in degenerated or necrotic tissue. Physiologic age-related calcification often is present in the costal cartilages. Calcification within masses of the parenchyma and mediastinum is important clinically, often helping to establish the etiology of the lesion.

cs9a | Cardiovascular Calcifications

DISEASE	COMMENTS
Aortic calcification	Linear calcification of the aortic wall, consistent in location with the path of the vessel, most often resulting from atherosclerosis; dilation of the vessel may indicate aneurysm.
Aortic annulus or valve calcification	Annular calcification is typically more pronounced than that of the valve, often secondary to rheumatic valve disease.
Coronary artery calcification	Best demonstrated in the lateral projection; typically involves the left circumflex artery.
Mitral annulus or valve calcification	Dense, curved, calcified band secondary to rheumatic valve disease.
Myocardial calcification	Secondary to infarct, tumor, aneurysm, trauma, and so on.
Pericardial calcification (FIG. 27-32)	Calcification most often associated with pericardial infection.

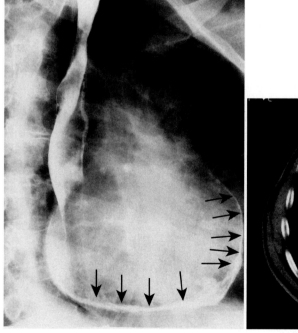
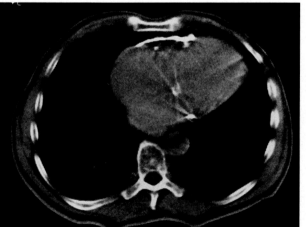

FIG. 27-32 A, Plain film demonstrating calcification of the pericardium *(arrows)* and barium in the esophagus. **B,** Computed tomography scan demonstrating calcification of the anterior pericardium. (Courtesy Steven P. Brownstein, MD, Springfield, NJ.)

CS9b | Hilar/Mediastinal Calcifications

DISEASE	COMMENTS
Granuloma (FIG. 27-33)	Central focal or widespread calcification of involved lymph nodes occasionally associated with a calcified parenchymal nodule (Ghon's lesion); this is associated with histoplasmosis, tuberculosis, and coccidioidomycosis infections.
Calcification secondary to radiation therapy	May result in the presence of multiple calcifications of irradiated lymph nodes.
Silicosis	Ring or "eggshell" calcification of the periphery of involved lymph nodes; a similar appearance is noted in sarcoidosis and irradiated nodes with Hodgkin disease.
Teratoma	Indicated by peripheral calcification, anterior mediastinal location, and the presence of rudimentary dental elements.
Thyroid calcification	Peripheral calcification, most often present in the upper anterior mediastinum.
Tracheobronchial cartilage calcification	Physiologic calcification of the tracheal rings occasionally noted in elderly patients.

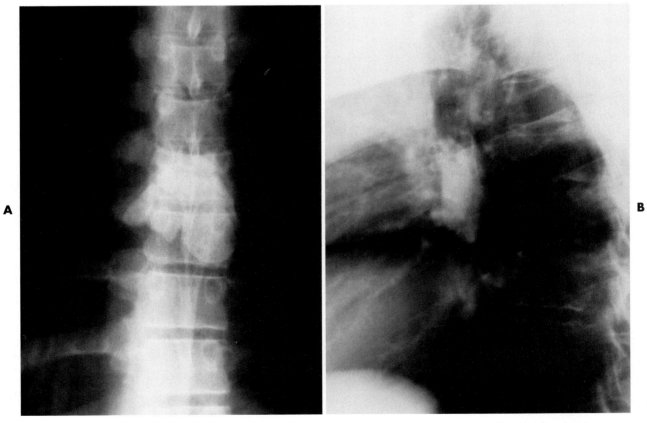

FIG. 27-33 A, Frontal and, **B,** lateral chest radiographs demonstrating calcification of the subcarinal lymph nodes secondary to past granulomatous infection in two patients.

CS9c | Lung Parenchymal Calcifications

DISEASE	COMMENTS
Fungal ball	Scattered calcification within the mass.
Granuloma	Probably the most common intrathoracic calcification; the presence of calcification in a benign pattern and stability of size over time help differentiate from other, more aggressive lesions; often granuloma is associated with other sites of calcification in the lymph nodes or spleen, secondary to histoplasmosis, tuberculosis, and coccidioidomycosis infections.
Hamartoma [p. 1202]	Benign, focal lung malformation with a "popcorn" or "comma-shaped" pattern of calcification.
Metastasis [p. 1393]	Calcification of multiple widespread nodules resulting from osteosarcoma or chondrosarcoma.
Pneumoconioses [p. 1214]	Silicosis demonstrating multiple small densities of calcification scattered throughout the parenchyma with associated "eggshell" calcification of the hilar lymph nodes; asbestosis is associated with pleural plaquelike calcification near the diaphragm.
Varicella (chickenpox)	Small, discrete calcifications scattered throughout lower lung fields after varicella infection; typically no lymph node involvement.

CS9d | Pleural Calcifications

DISEASE	COMMENTS
Empyema **(FIG. 27-34)** [p. 1169]	Unilateral board sheet or multiple smaller regions of calcification commonly in a posterolateral location similar to traumatic hemothorax; a history positive for infection and negative for trauma may differentiate between the two entities.
Hemothorax	Unilateral broad sheet or multiple smaller regions of calcification accompanying history of trauma; most commonly occurs in a posterolateral location.
Pneumoconioses [p. 1214]	Asbestos-related pleural disease resulting in bilateral calcified pleural plaques, most commonly appearing parallel to the diaphragm; a similar presentation is seen in talcosis.

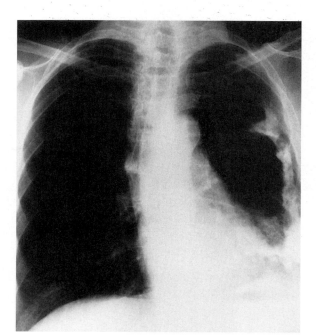

FIG. 27-34 Hemothorax with thick pleural calcifications and left lung atelectasis, causing a shift of the heart shadow to the left.

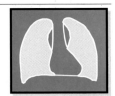

CS10 | Mediastinal Lesions

The mediastinum is the central portion of the thorax. It can be subdivided into anterior and middle parts by an imaginary line drawn posterior to the heart shadow on the lateral projection (see Chapter 21). A second line constructed 1 cm posterior to the anterior thoracic vertebral body margins, drawn parallel to the thoracic spine, separates the middle and posterior parts. This method of subdivision, known as the *roentgen divisions,* is employed commonly by radiologists and surgeons.

The roentgen divisions differ from the traditional anatomic divisions, which subdivide the mediastinum into anterior, middle, and posterior parts by constructing lines along the anterior and posterior margins of the cardiac shadow. Using the anatomic approach, a third line extends horizontally from the sternal angle to the T4 intervertebral disc space, creating a superior part of the mediastinum above the line. The roentgen divisions extend to the thoracic inlet, eliminating the superior mediastinal subdivision.

Mediastinal lesions may appear as radiodensities of various sizes and shapes. If possible there should be an attempt to localize lesions to a division by the radiographic appearance on multiple projections.

CS10a | Anterior Mediastinum

DISEASE	COMMENTS
Ascending aortic aneurysm [p. 1156]	Fusiform or saccular in configuration it appears as radiopacity continuous with the aortic shadow, seen anteriorly on the lateral projection and to the patient's right on the frontal projection; ascending aortic aneurysm may be atherosclerotic, luetic, mycotic, or traumatic in origin.
Lipoma **(FIG. 27-35)**	Localized fat accumulation often occurring around the heart.
Lymphoma **(FIG. 27-36)** [p. 1203]	Follows cardiomegaly as the second most common cause of mediastinal enlargement; accompanying hilar masses are common; although both Hodgkin disease and non–Hodgkin lymphoma may occur, the former presents more commonly as an anterior mediastinal mass.
Morgagni's hernia	Most often in a right posterolateral location, often occurs with a gas-filled loop representing a herniated bowel; opaque mass correlates with herniation of abdominal omentum or liver; it appears in middle-aged patients and usually is small.
Pericardial cyst	Asymptomatic mass in right anterior costophrenic angle, less often left-sided; pericardial cyst appears as a dense, radiopaque, rounded, well-circumscribed mass.
Substernal thyroid **(FIG. 27-37)**	Smooth, often lobulated mass, which has a propensity to calcify, located at the superior region of the neck. More commonly it projects to the patient's right and may deviate the tracheal air shadow on frontal projection.
Teratoma **(FIG. 27-38)** [p. 1392]	Appears as mass, often with calcification, teeth, or fat contained within lesion; dense lobulated lesions may be malignant.
Thymic masses [p. 1209]	Thymic masses including hyperplasia, cysts, and tumors of the gland; the most common is thymoma, which represents a large, smooth mass often associated with myasthenia gravis.

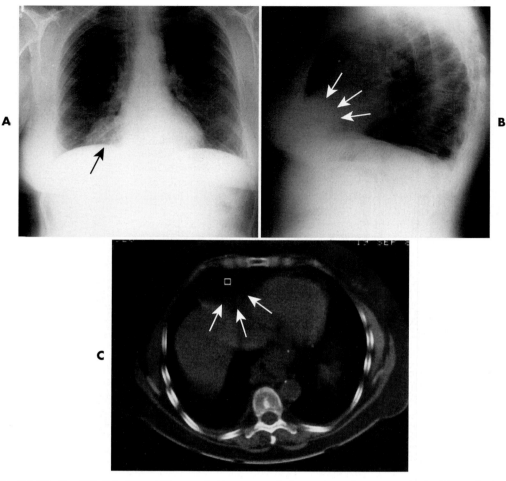

FIG. 27-35 **A** and **B,** Plain film and, **C,** computed tomogram of a lipoma presenting as a mass in the right cardiophrenic angle *(arrows).*

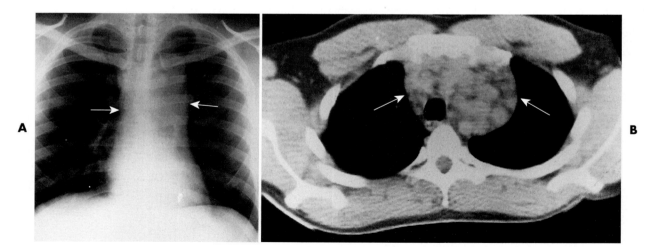

FIG. 27-36 Lymphoma appearing on, **A,** the posteroanterior radiograph and, **B,** computed tomography scan as wide anterior and middle mediastinal compartments *(arrows).*

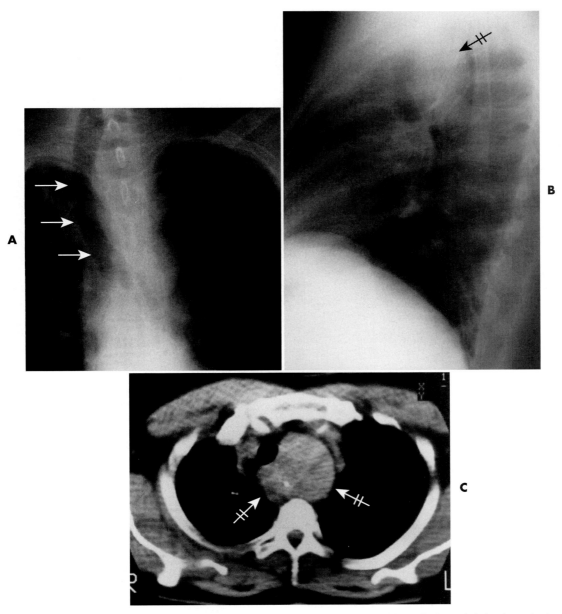

FIG. 27-37   Substernal thyroid *(crossed arrows)* presenting as a mass in the upper middle mediastinum, deviating the tracheal air shadow to the right *(arrows)* on, **A** and **B**, the posteroanterior radiograph and, **C**, computed tomography scan. (Courtesy Steven P. Brownstein, MD, Springfield, NJ.)

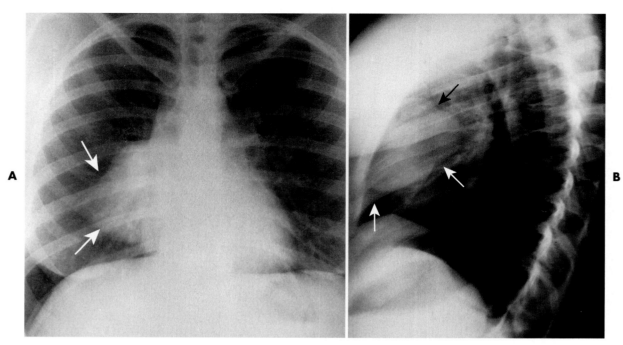

FIG. 27-38 **A** and **B,** Large teratoma in the anterior portion of the mediastinum *(arrows).*

CS10b | Middle Mediastinum

DISEASE	COMMENTS
Aortic aneurysm [p. 1155]	Atherosclerotic, mycotic, luetic, and traumatic etiologies; it may obliterate the aortic window in the lateral projection and project to either the left or right side in the frontal projection; position and contour are consistent with the vessel's path; hemorrhage causes symmetric massive enlargement of the superior mediastinum.
Bronchogenic cyst [p. 1149]	Round, well-defined fluid-filled cyst usually located just inferior and to the right of the carina; the cyst may become air-filled after communication with the tracheobronchial tree.
Esophageal neoplasm (FIG. 27-39)	Occasionally large enough to be seen on the radiograph, appearing as a smooth, rounded mass demonstrated best on an esophagram.
Hiatal hernia	Retrocardiac mass of variable size appearing solid or containing an air-fluid level positioned immediately above the diaphragm; in the frontal projection the density can be seen through the cardiac shadow; an esophagram is diagnostic.
Lymph node enlargement	Enlargement secondary to neoplasm (metastasis and lymphoma), granulomatous infection (tuberculosis, histoplasmosis, and coccidioidomycosis), pneumoconiosis (silicosis and asbestosis), and sarcoidosis.
Mediastinal lipomatosis (FIG. 27-40)	Fat deposits resulting in diffuse enlargement of the mediastinum; the condition is associated with hyperadrenocorticism, diabetes, obesity, and so on.
Pneumomediastinum (mediastinal emphysema)	Air within the mediastinum, typically secondary to blunt or penetrating trauma.

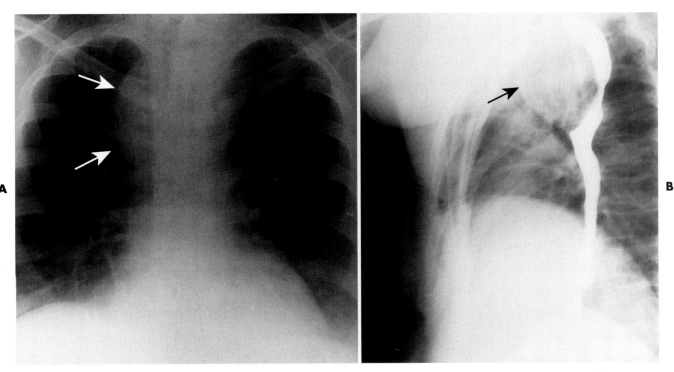

FIG. 27-39 **A,** Posteroanterior radiograph and, **B,** lateral projection of esophagram revealing a solid middle mediastinal mass of undetermined etiology *(arrows)*. On the esophagram, the column of barium is posteriorly distended around the mass. (Courtesy Steven P. Brownstein, MD, Springfield, NJ.)

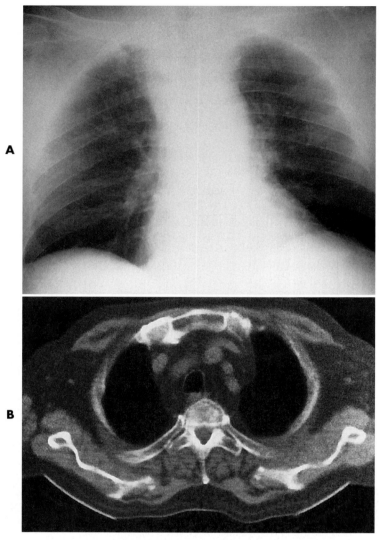

FIG. 27-40 Lipomediastinum. **A,** Posteroanterior radiograph and, **B,** computed tomography scan show a widened mediastinum and thoracic inlet secondary to fatty infiltrate. (Courtesy Steven P. Brownstein, MD, Springfield, NJ.)

CSI0c Posterior Mediastinum

DISEASE	**COMMENTS**
Aneurysm of descending aorta [p. 1156]	Mass on the left side of the patient's mediastinum that appears continuous with the vascular shadow of the aorta; it may calcify and erode vertebral bodies.
Bochdalek's hernia	Radiodense retrocardiac mass nearly always on the left.
Extramedullary hematopoiesis	Vertebral bone marrow extrusion seen with the congenital anemias (e.g., thalassemia), producing smooth-appearing paravertebral masses in the posterior mediastinum. Often it is accompanied by splenomegaly.
Neurogenic neoplasm **(FIGS. 27-41 AND 27-42)**	Unilateral and paravertebral well-circumscribed mass, often representing neurofibroma and neurolemmoma in adult, or neuroblastoma and ganglioneuromas in children. Rib or vertebral erosions may accompany this disease.
Spinal neoplasm **(FIG. 27-43)**	Bony destruction resulting from osteochondroma, aneurysmal bone cyst, osteogenic sarcoma, metastasis, and so on. Soft-tissue paravertebral mass is uncommon.

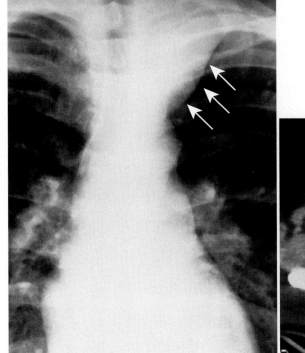
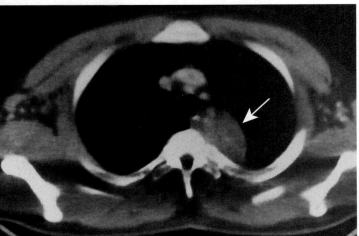

FIG. 27-41 **A** and **B,** Ganglioneuroma presenting as a posterior mediastinal mass *(arrows).* (Courtesy Steven P. Brownstein, MD, Springfield, NJ.)

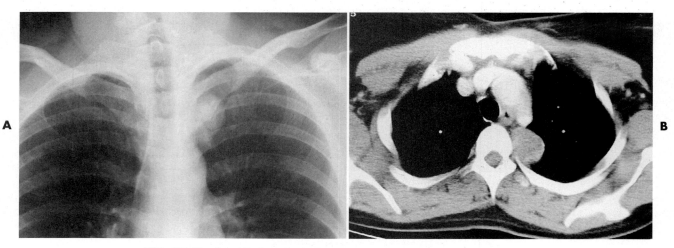

FIG. 27-42   A and **B,** Posterior mediastinal lesion consistent with a neurogenic tumor.

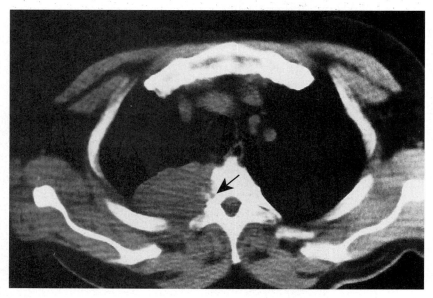

FIG. 27-43   Computed tomography scan demonstrating bronchogenic tumor mass with associated destruction of the adjacent rib and vertebral body *(arrow)*. (Courtesy Steven P. Brownstein, MD, Springfield, NJ.)

CS II | Pleural Effusion

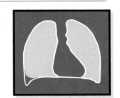

Pleural effusion describes larger collections of transudate, exudate, blood, or chyle in the pleural space. Radiographic findings vary from blunting of the costophrenic angles with mild effusion to opacification of the hemithorax with shifting the mediastinum with massive fluid accumulations. Pleural effusion is a nonspecific sign of underlying neoplasm, trauma, embolism, pulmonary edema, or other disease. The presence of pleural effusion should prompt a thorough search for concurrent disease.

DISEASE	COMMENTS
Abdominal diseases	Effusion often accompanies subphrenic abscesses, acute pancreatitis, and hepatitis.
Chylothorax	Accumulations of chyle from ruptured thoracic duct secondary to trauma or neoplasm.
Collagen diseases	Small, bilateral pleural effusions may accompany rheumatoid arthritis, systemic lupus erythematosus, Sjögren syndrome, mixed connective tissue diseases, and dermatomyositis.
Congestive heart failure [p. 1159]	Represents the most common cause of transudate effusion; resulting effusion is bilateral most often, but if unilateral it occurs most commonly on the right side; congestive heart failure is accompanied by findings of an enlarged heart shadow, cephalization of pulmonary vascularity, and pulmonary edema.
Empyema [p. 1169]	Purulent effusions often result from the spread of infection from contiguous lung structures.
Malignancies	Pleural effusion frequently accompanying primary and metastatic lesions of the pleura or adjacent tissues; malignant effusions typically are massive and rapidly reoccur after aspiration; examples include bronchogenic carcinoma, lymphoma, mesothelioma, and multiple myeloma.
Pneumonia [p. 1169]	Small unilateral effusion often accompanying radiographic findings of pneumonia; effusion occurs more commonly with bacterial agents.
Pulmonary infarct [p. 1181]	Typically small or moderate effusions; they are nonprogressive and may represent the only radiographic findings of a pulmonary infarct; pulmonary infarct is commonly accompanied by localized pleuritic pain or chest wall discomfort.
Renal diseases	Effusions of varying degrees produced by neoplasms, infections, and failure of the renal system.
Trauma	Chest wall trauma or surgical procedures; these may cause blood or edema accumulations in the pleural space.
Tuberculosis **(FIG. 27-44)** [p. 779]	Effusion is a common early manifestation of primary intrathoracic tuberculosis and often is the only radiographic finding; effusions typically are unilateral and small.

PART THREE
Chest

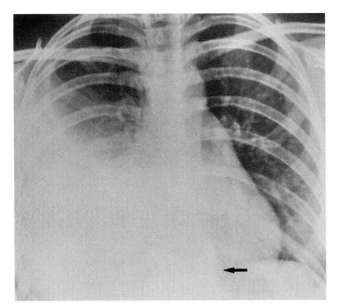

FIG. 27-44 Pleural effusion. Right-sided opacity has the classic feature of free pleural effusion in an erect patient. Opacity is homogeneous, occupies the inferior part of chest, and has concave upper margins that extend higher laterally than medially. The medial to lateral limb of meniscus exhibits characteristic haziness without a clear upper border. At first glance, a shadow low and to the left *(arrow)* resembles a displaced azygoesophageal recess, as sometimes occurs with pleural effusion. However, its configuration is not quite as expected, and it was found to result from tuberculosis paravertebral abscess of the effusion. (From Armstrong P et al: Imaging of diseases of the chest, ed 3, St Louis, 2000, Mosby.)

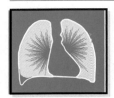

CS12 | Pulmonary Edema

Pulmonary edema represents fluid accumulation in the lungs from increased capillary permeability, increased hydrostatic capillary pressure, or blockage of lymphatic canals. Excessive fluid accumulates in the interstitium, overwhelms the lymphatics, and spills over to the air-space of the lung. The resultant appearance is one of confluent radiopaque perihilar densities with peripheral irregular linear shadows. A symmetric, bilateral pattern has been called *bat-wing consolidation* or *perihilar haze*. Changes in patient position or blood flow (such as are seen in patients with emphysema) may alter the fluid distribution and radiographic appearance. The appearance reflects a combination of interstitial and alveolar patterns.

DISEASE	COMMENTS
Adult respiratory distress syndrome (FIG. 27-45) [p. 1213]	Hemorrhagic pulmonary edema resulting from a variety of toxic substances ingested, inhaled, or aspirated; findings are related to alterations in capillary permeability and develop 2 to 36 hours after the exposure; this clinical feature helps to differentiate adult respiratory distress syndrome from other causes of pulmonary edema.
Aspiration pneumonia [p. 1172]	Bilateral, often asymmetric pattern resulting from aspiration of vomitus related to anesthesia, alcohol abuse, seizures, coma, or neurologic disturbance of the swallowing reflex.
Cardiogenic (FIG. 27-46)	Represents the most common cause of pulmonary edema. Results from hydrostatic factors typically secondary to mitral valve disease or left heart failure. Although cardiomegaly is common, it does not always indicate cardiogenic disease (e.g., chronic renal failure), nor does its absence rule out cardiogenic disease (e.g., heart arrhythmia); patients may demonstrate dyspnea, orthopnea, and pink frothy sputum. Pleural effusions are common.
Extrinsic allergic alveolitis [p. 1214]	Hypersensitivity pneumonitis resulting from inhalation of antigenic organic dusts; a wide variety of agents have been identified, such as moldy hay (farmer's lung) and avian excreta (bird fancier's lung).
Fat embolism	Occurs 12 to 36 hours after trauma, usually a fracture in lower limbs, which releases fatty marrow embolism into the circulation.
Near-drowning	Indicated by a history of fresh or saltwater near-drowning; edema results from asphyxia secondary to laryngeal spasm and aspiration of water.
Nephrogenic	Occurs secondary to glomerulonephritis and chronic renal failure; heart shadow may be enlarged.
Neurogenic (FIG. 27-47)	Observed in individuals with seizures, head trauma, and increased intracranial pressure; atypical distributions of pulmonary edema have been reported; the heart shadow is normal unless concurrent heart disease is present.

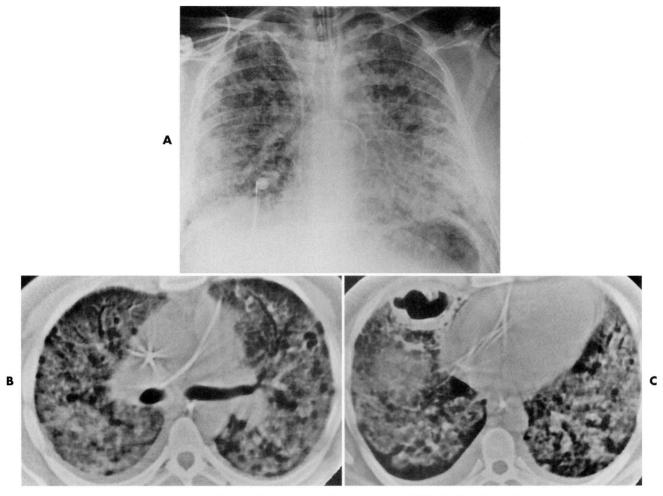

FIG. 27-45 Lung abscess complicating adult respiratory distress syndrome (ARDS). **A,** Plain chest radiograph shows features of ARDS, but a complicating pneumonia with abscess formation is difficult to recognize. **B,** Computed tomographic (CT) scan shows widespread but patchy distribution of the air-space shadows. **C,** CT section at a lower level shows a large abscess in the middle lobe. Sputum cultures revealed mixed gram-positive and gram-negative bacteria. (From Armstrong P et al: Imaging of diseases of the chest, ed 3, St Louis, 2000, Mosby.)

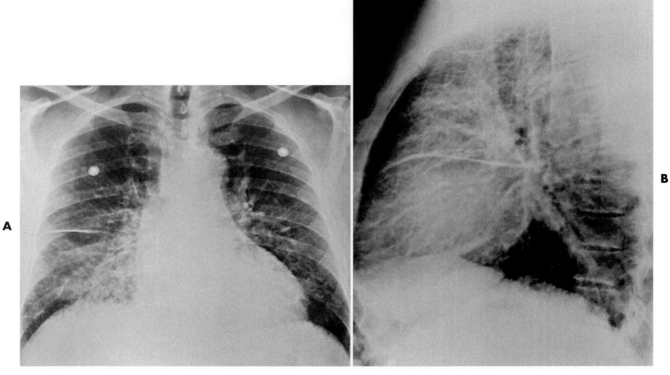

FIG. 27-46 Cardiogenic pulmonary edema after myocardial infarction in a 52-year-old man, illustrating widespread fissural thickening and lack of clarity of the intrapulmonary vessels and septal lines. Frank alveolar edema is evident in the right lower zone. The fissural thickening caused by subpleural edema is particularly striking. **A,** Frontal view. **B,** Lateral view. (From Armstrong P et al: Imaging of diseases of the chest, ed 3, St Louis, 2000, Mosby.)

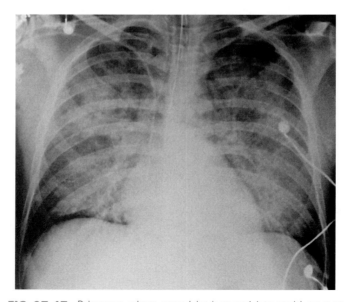

FIG. 27-47 Pulmonary edema caused by increased intracranial pressure after a subarachnoid hemorrhage caused by a ruptured aneurysm. (From Armstrong P et al: Imaging of diseases of the chest, ed 3, St Louis, 2000, Mosby.)

CS13 | Solitary Pulmonary Nodule and Mass

Well-circumscribed pulmonary radiopacities of 3 cm or less in diameter are nodules; those greater than 3 cm are masses. The presentation of a mass is more serious than a nodule; the larger the lesion, the more likely that it is malignant. Although multiple etiologies have been identified, the differential diagnosis often is between granuloma and malignancy. The growth rate of the lesion, age of patient, presence of calcification, and associated clinical presentation are valuable clues to determine its etiology. Although any calcification is strong evidence against malignancy, periphery calcification may exist in malignant lesions. Central, stippled, laminated, and complete patterns of calcification more accurately indicate a benign etiology. Early detection of pulmonary nodules and masses is directly related to a successful patient outcome.

DISEASE	COMMENTS
Abscess [p. 1376]	Pulmonary abscesses begin as solid radiopacities that cavitate and then appear as poorly circumscribed masses. Most often they are associated with clinical findings consistent with infection.
Arteriovenous malformation (FIG. 27-48)	Congenital defect of capillaries that results in an abnormal vascular communication between a pulmonary artery and vein. Arteriovenous malformations typically are located in the medial portion of the lower lobes; they appear as dense bands extending from the lesion to the hilum, representing a feeding artery and draining vein ("rabbit ear" sign).
Bronchial carcinoid tumors [p. 1187]	Low-grade malignancies most commonly arising from the lobar bronchi, often presenting with radiographic findings of airway obstruction.
Bronchogenic carcinoma (FIG. 27-49) [p. 1187]	May exhibit fuzzy or lobulated borders, classically never with a laminated, central, or completely calcified pattern, although it may demonstrate focus of peripheral calcification. Serial chest films demonstrate increased growth rate over time. Bronchogenic carcinoma is seen more commonly in those over 35 years of age; it may present with a history of chronic cough and hemoptysis.
Bronchogenic cyst [p. 1149]	Sharply defined mass in the lower lung fields representing a fluid-filled cyst; it may appear air filled if a communication with an adjacent airway is established.
Chest wall lesion (FIG. 27-50)	Moles, nipples, cutaneous neurofibromas, and other skin lesions may mimic pulmonary lesions. Reevaluation with the use of metallic markers is helpful in determining if the location is extrathoracic. Rib lesions also may appear as pulmonary masses.
Granulomas	Most common cause of solitary pulmonary nodules; represents nearly 90% of lesions in patients younger than 35 years of age; granulomas are associated with tuberculosis, histoplasmosis, and coccidioidomycosis infections; typically no or little change in size is noted on serial films.
Hamartoma [p. 1202]	Most common benign lung tumor; commonly calcified (characteristic popcornlike pattern); usually no clinical symptoms emerge, and the growth rate is slow.
Intralobar sequestration [p. 1147]	Sharply defined mass of variable shape in the lower lung field, representing poorly developed pulmonary tissue; lesions are most commonly left-sided, appearing in contact with the diaphragm.
Metastasis [p. 1393]	May uncharacteristically present as a solitary nodule or mass; calcification is rare, but when present it usually indicates a primary bone tumor.
Progressive massive fibrosus	Large, bilateral, slightly asymmetric masses in the upper portion of the lungs; the lesions begin peripherally and can be seen to migrate toward the hila on serial chest films. The presence of progressive massive fibrosus is related to silicosis or coal worker's pneumoconiosis.

PART THREE Chest

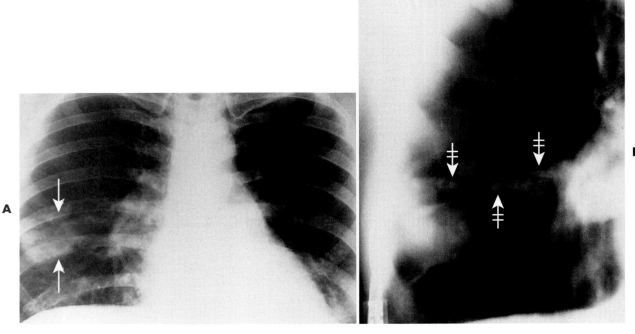

FIG. 27-48 Pulmonary arteriovenous malformation. **A,** Peripheral mass *(arrows)* formed from a communication between, **B,** the large artery and vein *(crossed arrows),* which extend from the hilum. Linear tomogram demonstrating the large artery and vein as cords connecting the hilum to the peripheral mass. (Courtesy Steven P. Brownstein, MD, Springfield, NJ.)

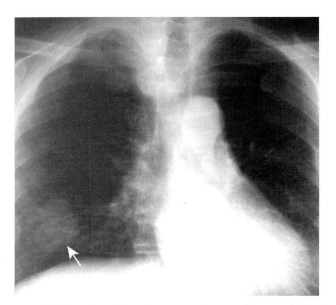

FIG. 27-49 Bronchogenic carcinoma presenting as a solitary mass in the right lower lung field *(arrow).* (Courtesy Steven P. Brownstein, MD, Springfield, NJ.)

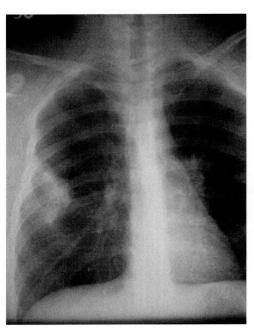

FIG. 27-50 Osteochondroma of the right side that appears as a pulmonary mass *(arrow).*

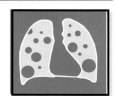

CS14 | Multiple Nodules and Masses

A multiple nodule or mass presentation is strongly suggestive of metastatic lung disease, particularly if a primary tumor already has been established in the patient's history. The primary tumor may originate from any organ system, with the notable exception of the central nervous system, from which tumors rarely metastasize to the lungs. Although most primary tumors appear as solitary lesions, lymphoma and alveolar cell carcinoma are exceptions, often presenting as multiple lesions.

Pneumonia is the most common cause of noncircumscribed lesions, appearing as fluffy, poorly defined, inhomogeneous consolidation, strongly indicative of alveolar filling (see pattern CS4). The presence of multiple, discrete, calcified nodules suggests granulomatous disease, in particular, coccidioidomycosis, histoplasmosis, and tuberculosis. Thromboemboli may cause ill-defined regions of pulmonary infarct (usually in the lower lung fields adjoining the pleural surface).

DISEASE	COMMENTS
Alveolar cell carcinoma	Subtype of pulmonary adenocarcinoma; it appears as single or multiple poorly defined regions, often resembling pneumonia or other alveolar disease pattern.
Granuloma	Well-defined, small lesions related to tuberculosis, histoplasmosis, and coccidioidomycosis infections; calcification is common.
Lymphoma [p. 1203]	More often in the lower lung regions, appearing as radiopacities with irregular borders; it may be associated with hilar or mediastinal enlargement.
Metastasis (FIG. 27-51) [p. 1393]	Multiple lesions of small (miliary) or large (cannonball) size, more often in the lower lobes; calcification is rare, but when seen is highly suggestive of primary bone tumor (osteosarcoma); cavitation is associated with metastasis from squamous cell neoplasms.
Rheumatoid arthritis	Small, well-defined lesions occurring in peripheral subpleural locations; cavitation is common; the lesions regress with remission of the arthritis.
Sarcoidosis [p. 1218]	Less common presentation of the disease; sarcoidosis usually is associated with hilar or mediastinal lymphadenopathy; sarcoidosis is more common in blacks and women.
Wegener's granulomatosis (FIG. 27-52)	Widely scattered irregular nodules mostly in the lower lung regions; nodules have a tendency to cavitate, producing shaggy inner margins.

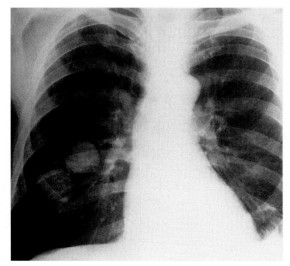

FIG. 27-51   Multiple small masses in the lower lung field, representing pulmonary metastasis from a primary carcinoma of the colon. (Courtesy Steven P. Brownstein, MD, Springfield, NJ.)

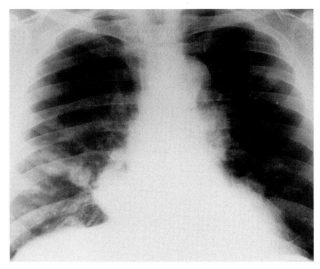

FIG. 27-52   Wegener's granulomatosis occurring with scattered bilateral pulmonary nodules, most notably in the right lower lung field. (Courtesy Steven P. Brownstein, MD, Springfield, NJ.)

Suggested Readings

Burgener FA, Kormano M: Differential diagnosis in conventional radiology, New York, 1991, Thieme.

Dahnert W: Radiology review manual, Baltimore, 1991, Williams & Wilkins.

Eisenberg RL: An atlas of differential diagnosis, ed 2, Gaithersburg, MD, 1992, Aspen.

Felson B: A new look at pattern recognition of diffuse pulmonary diseases, *AJR Am J Roentgenol* 133:183, 1979.

Fraser RG, Pare JAP: Tables of differential diagnosis and decision trees. In Fraser RG, Pare JAP: Diagnosis of Diseases of the Chest, ed 2, Philadelphia, 1979, WB Saunders.

Genereux GP: Pattern recognition in diffuse lung disease: a review of theory and practice, *Med Radiog Photog* 61:2, 1985.

Goodman LR: Felson's principles of chest roentgenology, ed 2, Philadelphia, 1999, WB Saunders.

Lillington GA: A diagnostic approach to chest diseases, Baltimore, 1987, Williams & Wilkins.

Meschan I: Roentgen signs in clinical diagnosis, Philadelphia, 1956, WB Saunders.

Ravin CE, Cooper C, Leder RA: Review of radiology, Philadelphia, 1994, WB Saunders.

Reed JC: Chest radiology: patterns and differential diagnoses, Chicago, 1981, Year Book.

Reeder MM, Bradley WG: Reeder and Felson's gamuts in radiology, ed 3, New York, 1993, Springer-Verlag.

Simon G: Principles of chest x-ray diagnosis, London, 1956, Butterworth.

Weissleder R, Wittenberg J, Harisinghani MG: Primer of diagnostic imaging, ed 3, St Louis, 2003, Mosby.

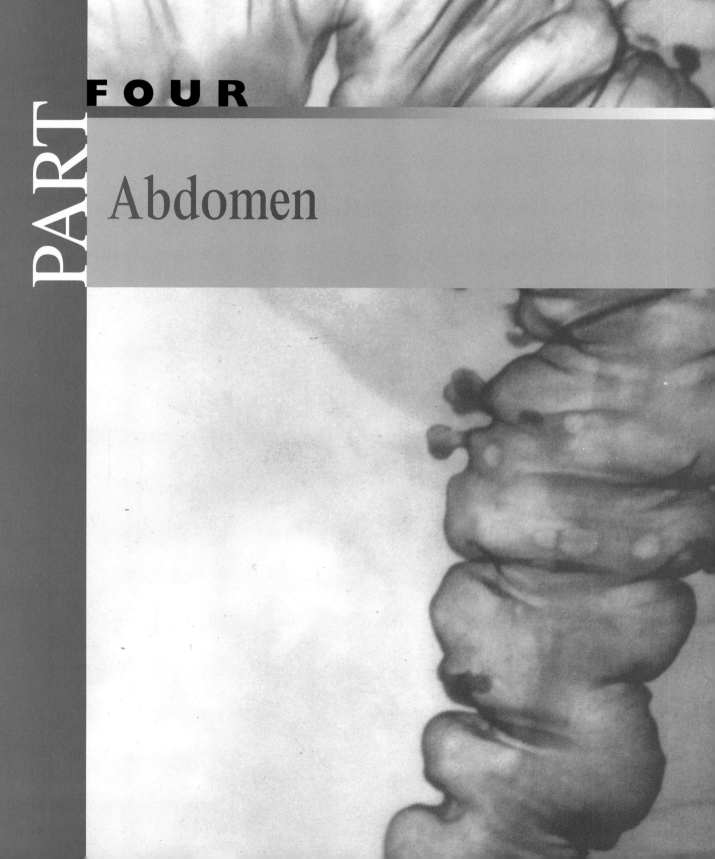

PART FOUR

Abdomen

chapter 28

Introduction to Abdomen Radiography

BEVERLY L. HARGER

LISA E. HOFFMAN

RICHARD ARKLESS

Plain Film Anatomy
Diagnostic Procedures

As an initial imaging procedure, plain film radiography of the abdomen can be useful in evaluating serious and even life-threatening conditions. Even though it may not reveal abnormalities shown by diagnostic ultrasonography and computed tomography (CT), this imaging modality can be a cost-effective method for use in diagnosing and managing abdominal pathosis. The recognition of key diagnostic features (seen incidentally on spine radiographs or noted on abdomen views used in the initial investigation of abdominal complaints) on plain film can be critical to patient management.

LIMITATIONS

A caveat to keep in mind is that the diagnostic yield of plain film of the abdomen is low in the absence of signs and symptoms; therefore an abdomen radiograph usually is not recommended as a survey tool. Box 28-1 lists many conditions for which plain film radiographs are not indicated because roentgenographic findings rarely occur.

INDICATIONS

Common conditions for which abdominal plain films may be of value, especially if the patient presents with moderate to severe pain or if significant abdominal tenderness is present, are listed in Box 28-2. Other indications for plain film radiography of the abdomen include trauma, abdominal distention or pain, vomiting, diarrhea, and constipation (Box 28-3).

TECHNICAL CONSIDERATIONS

When clinically indicated, obtaining a single radiograph showing a recumbent anteroposterior (AP) view of the abdomen is the first step. Upright or decubitus views may add valuable information about gas and fluid patterns, free air, abnormal calcifications, masses, and abnormal organs. Oblique views may aid in further localizing abnormal findings. The entire abdomen should be visualized from the hemidiaphragms to the pubic symphysis.

An upright, posteroanterior (PA) view of the chest may reveal valuable information about the presence of infiltrates in the lung bases, pleural fluid, or free peritoneal air that could explain the abdominal symptoms. Without the aid of contrast, abdominal contents generally are seen only if they contain gas or are surrounded by fat.

Before selecting the kilovolt peak (kVp), the patient's size and clinical problem should be considered. Although a high peak kilovoltage is correlated with a low x-ray dose, the higher the peak kilovoltage, the less is the contrast. Often a peak kilovoltage of 80 to 90 kV is optimal, depending on what type of x-ray generator is being used (e.g., single phase, three-phase, high frequency). To minimize motion artifact, lower the exposure time and use a higher milliamperage (mA) setting.

BOX 28-1

Limitations of Abdominal Plain Film

Conditions in which diagnosis is rarely aided by abdominal plain films
Gastrointestinal bleeding
Hepatobiliary disease other than calcified gallstones
Acute cholecystitis, better diagnosed by ultrasonography or technetium-99m cholescintigraphy
Cholangitis
Acute hepatitis
Liver masses except when intrahepatic calcifications or hepatosplenomegaly is present
Acute pancreatitis
Ulcers
Inflammatory bowel diseases
Pyelonephritis

Modified from Baker SR, Kyunghee CC: The abdominal plain film with correlative imaging, ed 2, Stamford, CT, 1999, Appleton & Lange.

BOX 28-2

Indications for Abdominal Plain Films

Conditions that may be diagnosed with plain film radiography

Perforated viscus
Intestinal obstruction
Adynamic ileus
Abdominal abscess
Bowel infarction
Fat versus ascitic fluid in obese patients
Emphysematous cholecystitis and colitis
Gallstone ileus
Urinary tract calculi
Abdominal aortic aneurysm
Preliminary films for contrast studies of urinary tract

Modified from Baker SR, Kyunghee CC: The abdominal plain film with correlative imaging, ed 2, Stamford, CT, 1999, Appleton & Lange.

BOX 28-3

Indications for Abdominal Films in the Adult Patient

Abdominal pain is moderate to severe
Abdominal pain is of any severity accompanied by significant abdominal tenderness

OTHER DIAGNOSTIC PROCEDURES

Complete evaluation of abdominal pathosis usually requires additional imaging, which may include barium-filled bowel or intravenous contrast studies, ultrasonography, CT, magnetic resonance imaging (MRI), angiography, and nuclear medicine (Table 28-1). Some portions of the gastrointestinal (GI) tract can be visualized directly via fiberoptic scoping. Because the uterus is within the primary beam for abdominal imaging, pregnancy should be ruled out before conducting any imaging study that uses x-rays or radioactive material. Alternative imaging such as ultrasound should be considered if a patient is pregnant.

OTHER CLINICAL CONSIDERATIONS

When evaluating patients with musculoskeletal pain, it is imperative that the clinician be aware that many organ diseases refer pain. The more common sites of pain referral are listed in Table 28-2.

Plain Film Anatomy

GENERAL

Interpretation of abdominal radiographs is aided by knowledge of basic anatomic relationships. The location and relative mobility of abdominal organs are important factors in the evaluation of radiographic signs (Fig. 28-1). Whether a viscus is solid or hollow also can be important. Gas in the stomach, portions of the small bowel, and most of the colon and rectum usually makes identification of these structures possible. Fat surrounding the renal capsules, along the psoas muscle edges, and abutting the inferior aspect of the liver aids in their visualization.

Retroperitoneal structures are relatively fixed in position, which increases their potential for traumatic injury, among other factors.

Consistently retroperitoneal structures include the kidneys and adrenal glands, third portion of the duodenum, ascending and descending portions of the colon, psoas muscles, pancreas, and abdominal aorta. Fascial planes provide channels for the spread of fluids, cells, and pathogens. Processes affecting the psoas muscle may follow the fascial sheath as far as the lesser trochanter of the femur.

Intraperitoneal structures can be categorized by their location within conceptual quadrants of the abdomen. The liver location is fixed in the right upper quadrant (RUQ). The liver shadow generally is well outlined inferiorly by intraperitoneal fat. Basic guidelines indicate that the liver should have a homogenous density and should not extend below the level of the iliac crest (although some normal anatomic variants do this) or past the midline. The lower liver margin may be delineated by gas in the adjacent small and large bowel. Although the gallbladder almost always is in the RUQ, closely opposed to the anteroinferior aspect of the liver, it is mobile in some patients and may be found in any quadrant. Much of the ascending colon is found in the RUQ. The transverse colon is mobile and its position may vary greatly, from running crosswise in the upper abdomen to dipping well into the pelvic area.

STOMACH

Most of the stomach is located in the left upper quadrant (LUQ), although its distal part does cross the midline into the RUQ and may extend ptotically into the lower abdomen. The stomach is identified on plain film by the gas it contains, especially the magenblase (stomach bubble) seen superiorly in the fundus on upright views (although gas may be seen throughout the stomach on supine views). The stomach is relatively fixed proximally at the gastroesophageal junction, with the remainder of the stomach being relatively mobile. A spatial relationship of the stomach with the transverse colon exists from attachment of the gastrocolic ligament. If distention or displacement affects one, the other's position is affected as well.

SMALL BOWEL

The duodenum is primarily a fixed retroperitoneal structure, making it more vulnerable to injury in cases of blunt abdominal trauma. Although the duodenal bulb frequently contains some air, contrast material such as barium generally is necessary to visualize the duodenum adequately. The descending, or second, portion of the duodenum is associated closely with the head of the pancreas and is the emptying site of the pancreatic and common bile ducts. Processes affecting these structures may be identified by secondary changes involving the duodenum.

The jejunum often does not contain enough gas to serve any diagnostic purpose for plain film radiography and requires contrast material for optimal visualization. Mucosal folds tend to be fine and "feathery." This portion of the small bowel is mobile; its mesenteric attachment to the posterior abdominal wall may serve as an axis for torsion.

The ileum also has the potential to be mobile, except when it is obstructed, involved with infiltrating diseases, or paralyzed. Like other portions of the small bowel, the ileum usually contains too little gas to be used for diagnostic purposes on plain film radiography except when obstructed or paralyzed. Differentiation between the jejunum and ileum can be difficult. The distal end of the ileum is connected to the colon at the ileocecal junction. Several diseases, including Crohn's disease and tuberculosis, tend to develop in this region.

TABLE 28-1
Diagnostic Procedures Used for Abdominal Imaging

Imaging modality	Technology	Advantages	Limitations
Ultrasound	Uses a combined transducer and receiver head to produce images based on the difference in tissue impedance or echogenicity to sound waves.	Noninvasive and has no notable risks or side effects; No ionizing radiation; Equipment purchase and maintenance is relatively low; Highly available; Examination time is relatively short; Capable of imaging most abdominal organs (except gas-filled bowel); Capable of identifying and measuring masses; Can determine the internal architecture of most masses (cystic, solid, complex); Can provide significant information about blood flow in masses or organs; Dynamic study allowing the investigator to pursue further questions that may arise as information is obtained.	Diagnostic ultrasound is highly operator dependent; Cannot image gas-filled bowel; Detail hampered in obese patients.
Computed tomography (CT)	Relies on contrast between radiographic densities as plain film does. It produces significantly greater resolution by using thin, fan-shaped beam and computer analysis to produce images of thin "slices" of anatomy.	Provides significantly greater detail than either plain film or ultrasound of the abdomen; Most organ architecture is well represented; Addition of contrast material to the vessels, renal collecting system, bowel, or other hollow structures provides better differentiation of those tissues from surrounding structures; Addition of intravenous contrast agents can provide information about the functional activity of masses and structures.	Uses ionizing radiation, so care must be taken to keep dosages down, especially in children; Availability may be an issue; Technology is reducing examination time, but time may still be somewhat prohibitive for seriously ill or uncooperative patients.
Magnetic resonance imaging (MRI)	MRI uses magnetic resonance technology to differentiate tissues by their cellular and extracellular contents. This provides important anatomic and functional information. The addition of intravenous contrast materials can provide further information about tissue metabolism.	Provides diagnostic information about solid, immobile organs such as the liver and kidney parenchyma.	Presence of gas in the bowel limits the usefulness of MRI in the abdomen; The mobility of abdominal contents also degrades MR images; Less available than CT.
Plain film with contrast	The use of barium- or iodine-based contrast agents greatly improves the value of radiography in evaluating the abdomen. Contrast agent is administered to fill a hollow structure such as the gastrointestinal (GI) tract (e.g., barium swallow, upper GI with small bowel follow-through, barium enema);	Lumen of structures can be evaluated for filling defects, mass effects, and irregularity of the lumen wall such as ulceration; Timed studies using contrast agents can give functional information regarding the motility of the bowel, contractibility, distensibility, and the ability of the kidney to concentrate urine.	Three-dimensional information is not available as it is with CT; Limited detail is provided regarding filling defects, mass effects, and constrictions.

TABLE 28-1 cont'd
Diagnostic Procedures Used for Abdominal Imaging

Imaging modality	Technology	Advantages	Limitations
Pain film with contrast—cont'd	the collecting system of the kidneys (intravenous pyelogram, retrograde pyelogram); the uterine body and fallopian tubes (hysterosalpingogram). Video fluoroscopy may be used to allow more complete and specific evaluation.		
Fiber optic exams	Fiber optics may be used to directly evaluate the lumen of accessible areas of the GI tract such as the esophagus, stomach, and colon, as well as the bladder and uterine cavity.	Direct visualization provides information about the lumen of hollow structures such as filling defects, constrictions, and mass effects; Direct observation also can detail subtle changes in the tissue lining the lumen that may not be available through other indirect studies.	Wireless endoscopy (a swallowable camera with transmitter) is still in the early stages of introduction to the field of diagnostic imaging.

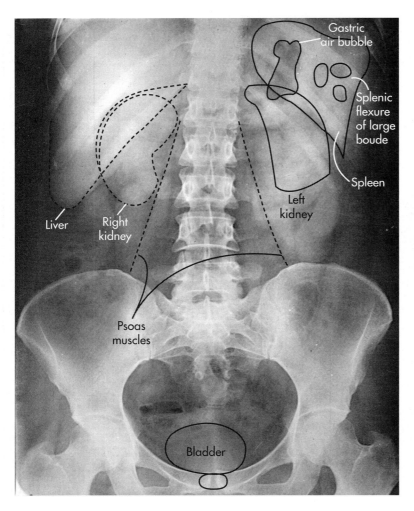

FIG. 28-1 Normal radiographic anatomy of the abdomen. (From Ballinger PW: Merrill's atlas of radiographic positioning and radiologic procedures, vol 2, ed 8, St Louis, 1995, Mosby.)

TABLE 28-2
Musculoskeletal Pain Referral Sites Associated with Organ Disease

Diseased organ or disease process	Site of pain referral
Aorta	Lumbar spine
Colon	Midlumbar spine
Gallbladder	Inferior scapula, interscapular, right shoulder
Gynecologic disorders	Lumbar spine; rarely above L4, pelvis
Kidneys, ureters	Groin, flank
Pancreas	Lower thoracic spine
Peptic ulcer	Midthoracic spine, heart area
Rectum	Sacral region
	Left lumbar paraspinal region
Sigmoid colon	Sacral region

LARGE BOWEL

The colon is relatively well visualized because of its gas content, but it still requires contrast material for an adequate evaluation. The large bowel is recognized easily by haustral, or semilunar mucosal, folds that are much further apart than the closely packed small bowel folds. The cecum usually is found in the right lower quadrant (RLQ), even though it is not a fixed retroperitoneal structure. It can be mobile in some patients, sometimes even undergoing volvulus. The contents of the cecum are mostly fluid with small gas bubbles interspersed, as opposed to the distal colon that has solid lumps of stool. This collection of small gas bubbles typically allows identification of the cecum. This appearance may produce a confusing mottled density over the right ilium. The ascending and descending portions of the colon are found retroperitoneally in the right and left lateral regions of the abdomen, respectively. The sigmoid colon is freely movable and usually is seen in the middle or left lower region of the abdomen, although occasionally it rises all the way up to the stomach. The rectum is relatively fixed and often contains gas and formed stool. Gas outlining the posterior wall of the rectum can be used on lateral spinal radiographs to measure the presacral space. The distance from the anterior cortex of the sacrum to the posterior margin of the rectum (presacral space) should not exceed 2 cm in the adult patient, with the exception of an extremely obese patient. Ascites, blood, or an inflammatory or neoplastic mass may increase the quantity of soft tissues in this space.

APPENDIX

The vermiform appendix generally is filled with gas only under pathologic conditions. It is mobile and may even be retrocecal. The appendix may not fill during contrast studies; therefore diagnostic ultrasound may be useful in cases of suspected appendicitis, although CT has been shown to be more sensitive and accurate.

LIVER

The liver is seen as a relatively homogeneous density in the RUQ. The inferior and lateral margins usually are defined by thin linings of intraperitoneal fat. The hepatic flexure of the colon also may aid in localizing liver margins. Gas overlying the liver shadow should be considered a possible abnormality and be carefully evaluated, although occasionally normal bowel is found between the liver and diaphragm.

GALLBLADDER

The gallbladder is associated closely with the anteroinferior aspect of the liver, although in some patients it can occupy an area deep inside the liver or be mobile and seem unrelated to the lower liver edge. This is one of the more common sites of abnormal abdomen calcifications (gallstones), even though only a modest percentage of gallstones are calcified.

PANCREAS

The pancreas is one of the more difficult organs to visualize. The head of the pancreas lies in the duodenal sweep, with the tail extending posteriorly and to the left. CT with contrast in the adjacent bowel generally provides the best images of the pancreas, but in some cases meticulous ultrasonography may be all that is needed. Endoscopic retrograde cholangiopancreatography (ERCP) provides images of the ductal system, but is an invasive and expensive examination. Chronic pancreatitis may show stippled calcifications.

SPLEEN

The spleen is located in the LUQ, lateral and somewhat posterior to the stomach. The lower pole of the spleen may be seen when contrasted with intraperitoneal fat. Images of the spleen may be obtained with CT or diagnostic ultrasound. Gas shadows overlying the spleen should be considered possible pathosis and evaluated further. In certain areas of the country, prior histoplasmosis can produce multiple small clinically unimportant calcifications. Histoplasmosis is endemic to the Ohio, upper Mississippi, Missouri, and St. Lawrence river valleys.

KIDNEYS

The kidneys are outlined by pericapsular fat, and their profiles are seen in many patients. Failure to visualize the renal outline is not necessarily abnormal. The kidneys are retroperitoneal and therefore relatively fixed. Regardless, a few centimeters of excursion normally are seen between images of the upright and recumbent or between inspiration and expiration views. During respiration or with the patient upright, the right kidney occasionally drops into the bony pelvis and presents clinically with a pelvic mass. The normal renal shadow spans two to three vertebral body heights. The kidneys are located at approximately the L1 to L3 levels, with the left positioned slightly more cephalad than the right. The normal axis of the kidney extends from a medial position of the superior pole to a more lateral position caudally.

ADRENALS

The adrenal glands are bilateral, V-shaped organs seen superior and somewhat anterior to the superior poles of the kidneys; they are not identified on plain film radiographs. Cross-sectional imaging modalities such as CT or MRI (or occasionally ultrasound) are necessary to evaluate the adrenal glands adequately.

URETERS

The ureters are not seen on plain film radiographs and can be difficult to visualize completely even with the use of intravenous contrast material that is excreted by the kidneys, because peristaltic waves transiently empty them of contrast material. They extend from their junction with the renal pelvis anteriorly along the psoas muscles to their posterior junction with the bladder. Few pathoses primarily affect the ureters, but they are the sites of most symptomatic calculi. Three common sites for calculi to lodge are the sites of anatomic ureter narrowing: where they exit the renal pelvis, at the point where they cross the iliac crest, and at the ureter's junction with the bladder. Clinical symptoms, especially pain in the kidney or groin area, typically develop as a calculus passes along a ureter. Microscopic (or macroscopic) hematuria is present around 95% of the time. It must be remembered that if a small blood clot is passed (e.g., from a kidney cancer), it may present with signs and symptoms mimicking a stone.

BLADDER

Often the bladder is seen as a water density immediately superior to the pubic symphysis. In females the uterus may lay against the superior aspect of the bladder, causing an indentation. Other indentations may be fluid-filled or partially gas-filled loops of bowel.

UTERUS

The uterus is located in the pelvic bowl between the bladder and rectum and is only seen on plain films if it indents the bladder, is grossly enlarged, or contains calcifications of uterine fibroids.

OVARIES

The ovaries are considered to be contents of the pelvic bowl, but their exact location can vary significantly. Large benign or malignant ovarian tumors may extend well into the abdomen unless containing fat or calcium in a tumor; the ovaries are not seen on plain films.

VAS DEFERENS

The vas deferens is not visualized on plain film radiographs unless calcified, which is seen in diabetic patients.

PROSTATE

The prostate gland lies just above the pubic symphysis and normally is not seen on plain film radiographs unless it has calcifications from prior inflammation. Prostate enlargement may be shown by displacement of the bladder and its ureter insertions superiorly after intravenous contrast is given.

BLOOD VESSELS

The abdominal aorta runs along the left anterolateral aspect of the lumbar spine and bifurcates into common iliac arteries at approximately the L4-5 level. Calcification within the walls is more common in elderly persons; younger people with calcification often have a history of smoking or significant predisposing pathology such as aortitis. Ultrasound is the imaging modality of choice for evaluating aortic diameter and searching for aneurysms, occlusion, or stenosis. CT (especially after a rapid bolus of contrast) or MRI may reveal valuable information (e.g., concerning a leaking aneurysm and whether renal arteries are involved). Search for aortic calcium on plain radiographs, because they may reveal a life-threatening aneurysm.

The common iliac arteries branch from the aortic bifurcation and extend downward and outward to the groin. Like the aorta, they are common sites of calcification. The inferior vena cava runs parallel to the right side of the abdominal aorta. Calcification in the walls of abdominal venous structures is rare. Ultrasound can be used to determine the presence of blood clots, extension of kidney or other cancers, and obstructions.

Diagnostic Procedures

Abdominal pathoses are diagnosed using the patient's history, physical examination findings, and laboratory investigations. Although not always necessary, diagnostic imaging sometimes adds an integral part of the evaluation of abdominal disease and abnormality.

Some common conditions and the procedures that may be used to diagnose, evaluate, or follow their disease progress are organized according to the target organ they affect in Tables 28-4 through 28-12; however, some conditions that are not organ-specific are listed in Table 28-3. All listed modalities may not be necessary in each case, and some uncomplicated conditions require no imaging studies whatsoever.

STOMACH

Endoscopic evaluation, passing a thin fiberoptic tube through the esophagus, is often the first procedure selected in the diagnosis of many conditions affecting the gastroesophageal junction or stomach. This procedure provides direct visualization of the gastric mucosa, allowing for detection of damaged mucosa. Endoscopy is

---

TABLE 28-3

Diagnostic Imaging Procedures Applied to Non–Organ-Specific Conditions

Suspected condition	Diagnostic procedure
Abdominal abscess	Computed tomography (CT), abdomen and pelvis with intravenous contrast* Ultrasound Plain film radiography Nuclear medicine Magnetic resonance imaging (MRI)
Abdominal mass, palpable	CT Ultrasound MRI
Abdominal trauma (blunt)	Plain film radiography, upright chest, supine, abdomen, and upright or decubitus abdomen* CT of abdomen and pelvis is first choice in severe trauma Ultrasound
Ascites	Ultrasound* CT Laparoscopy
Diarrhea (acute)	Sigmoidoscopy
Diarrhea (chronic)	Radiography, abdomen Upper GI barium study with small bowel follow-through CT, abdomen and pelvis Sigmoidoscopy
Dyspepsia	Upper gastrointestinal (UGI)* study Endoscopy Ultrasound (gallbladder and pancreas) Echocardiogram to rule out heart attack
Nausea and vomiting	Plain film radiography, upright and recumbent abdomen Ultrasound, CT (for hepatic origin) UGI barium study

*Usual first imaging modality.

TABLE 28-4
Diagnostic Imaging Procedures Applied to Selected Conditions of the Stomach

Suspected condition	Diagnostic procedure
Dyspepsia	Endoscopy Upper gastrointestinal (UGI) barium study* Ultrasound (when gallbladder or pancreas disease is suspected)
Gastric tumor	Endoscopy* UGI barium study Endoscopic ultrasound
Gastritis	Endoscopy* UGI barium study
Gastroesophageal reflux disease, esophagitis, dysphagia	Barium swallow* Endoscopy
Peptic ulcer	Endoscopy UGI barium study*
Ulcer perforation	Plain film radiography, upright or decubitus abdomen UGI study with water-soluble contrast

*Usual first imaging study.

TABLE 28-5
Diagnostic Imaging Procedures Applied to Selected Conditions of the Small Bowel

Suspected condition	Diagnostic procedure
Small bowel obstruction	Plain film radiography, supine and upright abdomen* (for identification of complications) Barium small bowel follow-through Computed tomography (CT) of abdomen and pelvis
Crohn's disease	Barium small bowel follow-through* CT Small bowel enteroclysis Magnetic resonance enteroclysis Barium enema Colonoscopy
Small bowel tumors (rare)	Barium small bowel follow-through Small bowel enteroclysis CT, abdomen and pelvis

*Usual first imaging modality.

TABLE 28-6
Diagnostic Imaging Procedures Applied to Selected Conditions of the Large Bowel

Suspected condition	Diagnostic procedure
Colitis, antibiotic associated	Plain film radiography, abdomen* Contrast enema Sigmoidoscopy
Colorectal cancer	Colonoscopy Barium enema Computed tomography (CT), abdomen and pelvis Radiography, chest (for metastases)
Constipation, colon obstruction	Plain film radiography, supine and upright abdomen films* Barium enema Colonoscopy, sigmoidoscopy
Crohn's disease	Upper gastrointestinal (GI) scan with small bowel follow-through* Barium enema Colonoscopy CT
Diverticulitis	Plain film radiography, abdomen Sigmoidoscopy Barium enema CT, abdomen and pelvis Nuclear medicine (for occult bleeding)
GI bleeding Lower, acute Upper, acute Occult	Sigmoidoscopy, colonoscopy Barium enema Occasional angiography Endoscopy Upper GI barium study Upper GI and barium enema* Colonoscopy and endoscopy
Irritable bowel syndrome	Barium enema* Sigmoidoscopy, colonoscopy
Polyps	Barium enema, especially double contrast Sigmoidoscopy, colonoscopy
Ulcerative colitis	Sigmoidoscopy Plain film radiography, abdomen (for identification of complications)

*Usual first imaging modality.

TABLE 28-7
Diagnostic Imaging Procedures Applied to the Gallbladder

Suspected condition	Diagnostic procedure
Cholecystitis, cholelithiasis	Ultrasound* Oral cholecystography Percutaneous transhepatic cholangiography Computed tomography, abdomen and pelvis

*Usual first imaging modality.

valuable for monitoring and endoscopic removal of lesions as well. Other than endoscopic methods, mucosal detail is best provided by barium contrast studies. Barium contrast studies also may reveal mass effects, ulcers, tumors, scars, strictures, swollen folds, and motility disorders. CT with diluted barium contrast may be necessary for processes that do not alter the lumen. The degree of contraction of the stomach at the time of CT imaging may alter its appearance markedly; therefore conclusions often cannot be drawn from a single image.

Table 28-4 lists some common conditions affecting the gastroesophageal junction and stomach and the most frequently diagnostic procedures utilized.

TABLE 28-8
Diagnostic Imaging Procedures Applied to the Liver

Suspected condition	Diagnostic procedure
Cirrhosis	Ultrasound Computed tomography (CT) Plain film radiography (may show enlargement) Magnetic resonance imaging (MRI)
Hemochromatosis	MRI, CT (not diagnostic alone)
Hepatic abscess	Ultrasound* CT MRI Radiography, chest
Hepatic tumor	CT* MRI Arteriography
Jaundice	Ultrasound* CT MRI Endoscopic retrograde cholangiopancreatography (ERCP) Percutaneous transhepatic cholangiography (PTHC)

*Usual first imaging modality.

TABLE 28-9
Diagnostic Imaging Procedures Applied to the Pancreas

Suspected condition	Diagnostic procedure
Pancreatic tumors	Computed tomography (CT)* Magnetic resonance imaging (MRI) Endoscopic retrograde cholangiopancreatography (ERCP)
Pancreatitis, acute or chronic	CT* Plain film radiography (often nondiagnostic) ERCP (chronic)

*Usual first imaging modality.

SMALL BOWEL

In contrast to the assessment of the esophagus, stomach, and colon, in which endoscopy has taken the forefront over barium x-rays, imaging of the small intestine continues to be an unsolved diagnostic problem despite the technical advances in medicine. Wireless endoscopy (a swallowable camera with transmitter) is still in the early stages of introduction to the field of diagnostic imaging. Orally ingested barium often is necessary for evaluation of the small bowel. Enteroclysis is another method is which the

TABLE 28-10
Diagnostic Imaging Procedures Applied to the Kidneys and Bladder

Suspected condition	Diagnostic procedure
Bladder cancer	Intravenous urography* Computed tomography (CT) Magnetic resonance imaging (MRI) Cystoscopy, cystourethroscopy (this may be the procedure of choice)
Renal calculi	Plain film radiography, abdomen (kidney, ureter, and bladder) Ultrasound Intravenous pyelogram (IVP) with tomograms
Renal function abnormalities	Radionuclide studies Ultrasound IVP, CT (not performed if blood urea nitrogen or creatinine are too high or rising) MRI Arteriography, renal venography
Renal tumors	Ultrasound* IVP CT (second choice) MRI

*Usual first imaging modality.

TABLE 28-11

Diagnostic Imaging Procedures Applied to the Gynecologic Conditions

Suspected condition	Diagnostic procedure
Cervical cancer	Computed tomography (CT) Magnetic resonance imaging 　(MRI) (for staging)
Dysmenorrhea, secondary	Ultrasound* Laparoscopy MRI Hysteroscopy Hysterogram
Endometrial carcinoma	Intravenous urography (IVU) Cystoscopy Sigmoidoscopy Ultrasound (can be procedure of 　choice) MRI (can be useful) Chest radiography to 　determine extent
Endometriosis	Ultrasound MRI Barium enema Laparoscopy
Infertility	Hysterosalpingography* Laparoscopy
Ovarian tumors	Ultrasound* CT, abdomen and pelvis Laparoscopy Plain film radiography, chest 　(to check for metastasis)
Pelvic inflammatory 　disease	Ultrasound* Hysterosalpingogram
Uterine bleeding, 　abnormal	Ultrasound* MRI Hysteroscopy Hysterosalpingogram
Uterine fibroids	Ultrasound* MRI Hysteroscopy, hysterography

*Usual first imaging modality.

TABLE 28-12

Diagnostic Imaging Procedures Applied to the Prostate and Scrotum

Suspected condition	Diagnostic procedure
Prostate mass/enlargement	Intravenous urography* Ultrasound Magnetic resonance imaging
Scrotal tumors	Ultrasound* Computed tomography

*Usual first imaging modality.

diseases. More recently MRI enteroclysis has emerged as a diagnostic procedure for detecting inflammatory or neoplastic diseases and small bowel obstruction.

LARGE BOWEL

A useful procedure for examination of the colon is the single- or double-contrast barium enema. This procedure is indicated for the detection of several conditions (Table 28-6). Proper colon preparation is essential to achieve a colon free of fecal material. For a single-contrast examination, a low-density barium suspension is administered rectally. Double-contrast examination uses a high-density barium suspension and air that are administered under fluoroscopic control to achieve adequate coating and distention of the colon. Special CT techniques can be used to search for premalignant polyps, but there is controversy concerning its value, especially in lesions smaller than 1 cm.

APPENDIX

Ultrasound and especially CT are the primary diagnostic procedures used in the diagnosis of appendicitis, the most common disease affecting the appendix, although a wide range of other uncommon conditions, infectious and neoplastic, may involve the appendix as well.

GALLBLADDER

Ultrasonography usually provides adequate information for diagnosing gallbladder pathoses such as gallstones and cholecystitis (Table 28-7) and should be the imaging procedure of choice. In cases requiring contrast for visualization, endoscopic retrograde cholangiopancreatography (ERCP) or percutaneous transhepatic cholangiography (PTHC) is often used. Laparoscopic cholecystectomy may be indicated when the patient presents with acute RUQ pain and has gallstones.

LIVER

Several conditions, which are listed in Table 28-8, may target the liver. CT can be valuable for evaluating most liver pathoses; however, diagnostic ultrasound is extremely useful in evaluating the liver and gallbladder and should be the primary study used in evaluation. Occasionally nuclear medicine or MRI examinations can reveal even more information.

PANCREAS

The advent of dual-phase helical CT (hCT) has improved the staging performance of CT in pancreatic cancer (a disease that is usually not detected until late and has a dismal prognosis), and the ability to

entire length of the small bowel is examined. In this procedure, a tube is inserted into the patient's nose and through the stomach into the small intestine. A barium suspension is then administered through the tube. Films are taken as the barium passes through the small intestine. Clinical applications of both these procedures include the detection of gastrointestinal bleeding, small bowel obstruction, Crohn's disease, nonspecific abdominal pain, and chronic diarrhea and small bowel tumors (Table 28-5).

Complementary to these procedures is CT for the detection of mural and extramural lesions and the assessment of exocentric manifestations of inflammatory or neoplastic small intestinal detect metastatic extension of disease (Table 28-9). Endoscopic ultrasound originally was conceived for the detection of early pancreatic cancer and continues to have a role in the evaluation of small pancreatic tumors not seen by with other imaging modalities and those in which hCT is equivocal for vascular invasion.

KIDNEYS AND BLADDER

Until recently, intravenous pyelogram (IVP) was the procedure of choice for renal evaluation, but this is being replaced by CT in searching for tumors, stones, and complications of infections. Ultrasound and nuclear medicine studies can be useful in renal evaluation but have limited application in ureter and bladder evaluation (Table 28-10).

The mucosal surface of the bladder is best defined with contrast material, although even moderate-sized tumors may not be seen on

an intravenous urogram (IVU). Although CT and MRI are better ways to evaluate abnormalities, the most definitive way to search for potentially serious abnormalities is still cystoscopy.

UTERUS AND OVARIES

The best way to evaluate the uterus with imaging studies is by ultrasound, although for certain problems CT (or MRI) can be helpful (Table 28-11). Ultrasound is the most useful technique for locating and evaluating ovaries. CT or MRI occasionally may be necessary to clarify abnormalities.

PROSTATE

Transrectal ultrasound provides the best imaging of the prostate, with CT or MRI sometimes used to evaluate the full extent of lesions and spread of cancers (Table 28-12).

chapter 29

Genitourinary Diseases

BEVERLY L. HARGER
LISA E. HOFFMAN
RICHARD ARKLESS

Portions of the genitourinary system are readily visible on plain film radiographs, which may aid in the localization of abnormal densities. This is a common site for concretions and some calcifying masses. Table 29-1 lists the common appearance of the genitourinary system and some of the abnormal findings that may be visible on plain film.

Angiomyolipoma (Hamartoma)

BACKGROUND

Angiomyolipoma (AML) is the most common benign renal neoplasm diagnosed radiologically. It is a hamartomatous tumor containing varying amounts of fat, smooth muscle, and vascular tissues, and it may range in size from a few millimeters to more than 20 cm.[21] AMLs are found in young adults to elderly patients and are four and a half times more common in women.[10,21] Multiple, bilateral, small AMLs that may be symptomatic are found in up to 80% of patients with tuberous sclerosis, an uncommon heritable condition.[10,13,21] However, most angiomyolipomas arise sporadically.

IMAGING FINDINGS

The radiolucent fatty tissue of these tumors is seldom appreciated on plain film radiographs. The AML may be revealed by its mass effect after contrast injection on an intravenous pyelogram but cannot be differentiated from other masses. Attenuation of the collecting system with displacement and focal dilation of the calyces may be visible.[21]

A renal tumor containing fat density tissue is essentially diagnostic for AML. Unenhanced computed tomography (CT) scans, use of small areas for attenuation measurements, and use of thin sections may be necessary to detect small amounts of fat.[3,12,21]

Sonography characteristically shows a very hyperechoic lesion compared with adjacent renal parenchyma.* The high fat content, heterogeneous cellular architecture, and presence of multiple vessels all contribute to the marked echogenicity, but still this lesion cannot accurately be separated from renal cell carcinoma on ultrasound; therefore CT is necessary.[14,21]

CLINICAL COMMENTS

Angiomyolipomas generally are asymptomatic and usually are identified during evaluation for unrelated genitourinary conditions. Flank pain, hematuria, and palpable mass are classic symptoms and usually are seen in otherwise healthy patients with isolated, unilateral lesions.[21] Parenchymal, subcapsular, or perirenal hemorrhage may lead to hypotension.[21]

Embolization or partial excision is usual for large or symptomatic lesions. Overall, treatment for AMLs is usually conservative with follow-up alone being sufficient for most small, asymptomatic tumors.[10,21]

KEY CONCEPTS

- *Angiomyolipoma is the most common radiologically diagnosed benign renal neoplasm.*
- *Classic symptoms, when present, are flank pain, hematuria, and palpable mass.*
- *Fatty attenuation seen on computed tomography is virtually diagnostic for angiomyolipoma.*

Bladder Calculi

BACKGROUND

Ninety-eight percent of bladder calculi identified in the United States occur in elderly men.[16] The instigating factor in their formation usually is urinary retention with high residual urine. Superimposed infections add to susceptibility. The presence of bladder stones is associated with an increased incidence of carcinoma.[16]

IMAGING FINDINGS

Bladder calculi often are nonopaque or only faintly opaque, allowing them to be frequently overlooked. Fecal material and gas in the rectosigmoid colon and the sacrum itself also overlie the area and may further obscure them. Bladder calculi usually are located centrally in the pelvis (Fig. 29-1). Those that are found more laterally may lie in a bladder diverticulum.[16]

---

*References 6, 7, 14, 21, 26, 27.

TABLE 29-1
Genitourinary Plain Film Organ Appearance

Organ	Plain film visibility	Plain film location	Retroperitoneal versus intraperitoneal	Fixed versus mobile	Appearance specifics	Plain film abnormalities
Kidneys	Surrounding pericapsular fat	T12 to L2 level, right slightly lower than left	Retroperitoneal	Fixed; some translation with upright posture or inspiration	Height = 2 to 2.5 vertebral bodies plus intervertebral disc (IVD); long axis oriented superomedial to inferolateral	Lobulated contour; enlargement; ectopic; abnormal axis; nephrolith
Adrenals	None	Adjacent to body margins of T12 or L1	Retroperitoneal	Fixed	None	Calcifications (masslike or cystic)
Ureters	None	Along anterior aspect of psoas muscle to posterosuperior bladder	Intraperitoneal	Fixed	None	Nephrolith
Bladder	Domed water density	Midline in pelvic bowl	Intraperitoneal	Fixed	Inferior margin less than 1 cm above pubic symphysis; superior margin may be indented by uterus	May appear as mass, may become distended (e.g., neurogenic bladder); superiorly displaced by enlarged prostate
Prostate	None	Midline at pubic symphysis	Intraperitoneal	Fixed	None	Calcifications
Uterus	None	Midline, pelvic bowl	Intraperitoneal	Fixed	None	Calcifications (fibroids)
Ovaries	None	Variable	Intraperitoneal	Somewhat mobile	None	Calcifications (dermoid cyst)

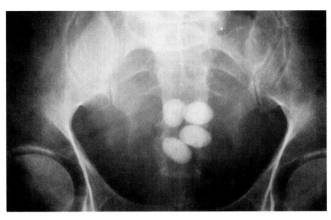

FIG. 29-1 Multiple bladder calculi. Four oval radiopaque bladder stones are visible centrally in the pelvis. Most bladder calculi are round or oval but they may be amorphous, laminated, or even spiculated.

KEY CONCEPTS
- Urinary retention with high residual urine is a common cause for formation.
- It may be difficult to detect on plain radiographs.
- Bladder calculi usually lie centrally in the pelvis on plain radiographs.
- The incidence of carcinoma of the bladder increases in the presence of stones.

Nephroblastoma (Wilms' Tumor)

BACKGROUND

Nephroblastoma (Wilms' tumor) is the most common abdominal malignancy in childhood.[8,13] Overall, leukemia-lymphoma, brain tumors (astrocytoma and medulloblastoma), and neuroblastoma have a higher incidence in pediatric populations when other sites of the body are also considered.[19] The highest incidence occurs in 3- and 4-year-old individuals, with 80% of Wilms' tumors occurring in individuals 1 to 5 years old.[2,5,19]

IMAGING FINDINGS

Wilms' tumor appears radiographically as a complex renal mass (Fig. 29-2). Approximately 5% to 10% of these lesions show areas of calcification, but calcium, when seen in a mass in this area, is much more likely to be in a neuroblastoma of the adrenal or other similar tissue.[19] Intravenous pyelogram shows either a displaced or a nonfunctioning kidney. Ultrasound typically reveals a well-defined tumor, often surrounded by a hyperechoic halo of compressed normal renal tissue.[13,17] Noncontrast CT usually reveals a large intrarenal mass of lower attenuation than the adjacent

CLINICAL COMMENTS

Bladder calculi may abrade and irritate the mucosa and predispose to infection. Bladder infections are more difficult to treat when calculi are present. Ureteral or bladder outlet obstruction may also be present.[16] Approximately 15% of patients with gout, as well as hyperuricemic patients, produce uric acid stones.[16]

Standard treatment of bladder stones consists of endoscopic visualization and fragmentation by electrohydraulic probe.[31] Massive calculi may require open surgery.[31]

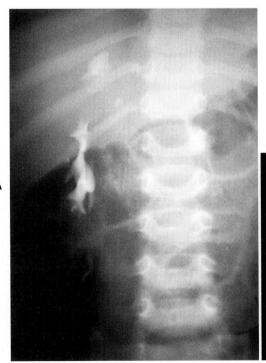
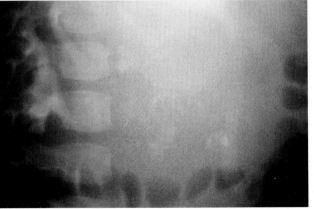

FIG. 29-2 Nephroblastoma (Wilms' tumor). **A,** Intravenous urogram anteroposterior projections show diffuse amorphous calcification of a large right upper quadrant mass in a pediatric patient. **B,** Intravenous urogram lateral view of this same patient demonstrates the retroperitoneal location of this mass. Nephroblastoma is the most common abdominal malignancy of children, with 80% occurring between 1 and 5 years of age.

normal kidney. Cystic spaces or areas of tumor necrosis appearing as inhomogeneous, low-density areas are seen in most tumors.[13]

CLINICAL COMMENTS

Patients with Wilms' tumor present with an abdominal mass in more than 90% of cases.[13] Approximately 50% of patients experience hypertension or fever. Hematuria is relatively uncommon.[13,19] No male or female predominance is noted.[13] Up to 30% with the rare condition of aniridia (congenital absence of the iris) develop nephroblastoma.[19] Four to five percent of cases show bilateral tumors.[19]

> ### KEY CONCEPTS
> - *Wilms' tumor is the most common abdominal malignancy of children.*
> - *Abdominal mass is the most common clinical presentation.*
> - *Radiographically, Wilms' tumor is seen as a complex renal mass; 5% to 10% have internal calcification.*

Nephrocalcinosis

BACKGROUND

Based on its location, calcification in the kidney can be classified broadly into two categories: calcification within the pyelocalyceal lumina or nephrolithiasis, and intraparenchymal calcification or nephrocalcinosis. Nephrocalcinosis also can be categorized with respect to its predominant location. A limited group of diseases, cortical nephrocalcinosis, may produce calcification confined to, or predominantly located in, the renal cortex. Other conditions, such as medullary nephrocalcinosis, spare the cortex and cause calcium salt deposition in the medulla, interstitium, or lumina of the nephrons.

IMAGING FINDINGS

Radiographically cortical nephrocalcinosis can be differentiated from the medullary variety by the peripheral location of the calcification (Fig. 29-3). Medullary calcification is typically that of bilateral, diffuse, fan-shaped clusters of stippled calcifications, primarily in the renal pyramids (Fig. 29-4).

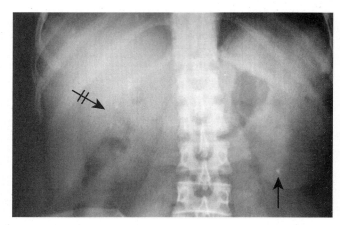

FIG. 29-3　Nephrocalcinosis. Cortical *(arrow)* and medullary *(crossed arrow)* nephrocalcinosis.

CLINICAL COMMENTS

The two most common etiologies of cortical nephrocalcinosis are acute cortical necrosis and chronic glomerulonephritis, although radiographically evident calcification is rare in both conditions. Persons on chronic dialysis may have similar calcifications.

Roughly 40% of cases of medullary nephrocalcinosis are attributable to primary hyperparathyroidism, another 20% to renal tubular acidosis, and the remaining 40% divided among many other causes.

> ### KEY CONCEPTS
> - *Renal intraparenchymal calcification is known as nephrocalcinosis.*
> - *Two categories of nephrocalcinosis are cortical and medullary.*
> - *Peripheral location is seen with cortical nephrocalcinosis.*
> - *Cortical nephrocalcinosis is rare.*
> - *Bilateral, diffuse, fan-shaped clusters of stippled calcifications typically are seen with medullary nephrocalcinosis.*
> - *Primary hyperparathyroidism and renal tubular acidosis are the most common causes of medullary nephrocalcinosis.*

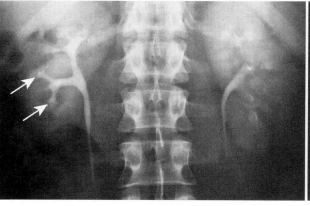
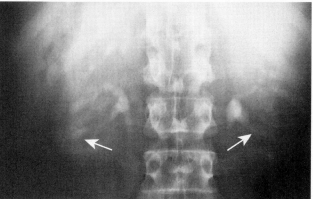

FIG. 29-4　Medullary sponge kidney. **A,** Faint calculi are seen in the renal pyramids *(arrows)*. Medullary sponge kidney is characterized by ectatic collecting ducts and associated small cysts communicating with these ducts. **B,** Renal tubular acidosis. This parenchymal renal calcification results from renal tubular acidosis. The calcifications occur within the tubules surrounding the calyces *(arrows)*.

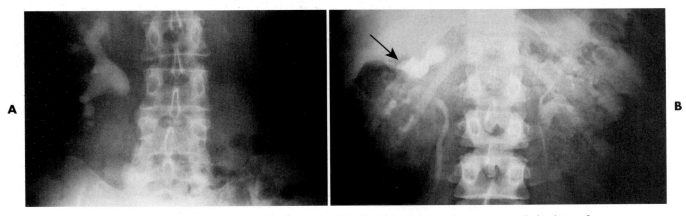

FIG. 29-5 Staghorn calculus in two different patients. **A,** Plain film of the abdomen demonstrates a calculus that conforms to the shape of the calyces, infundibulum, and pelvis. **B,** Intravenous pyelogram showing bilateral duplication of the collecting systems with a staghorn calculus obstructing the upper collecting system on the right *(arrow)*.

Nephrolithiasis (Renal Calculi)

BACKGROUND

Nephrocalcinosis is calcification in renal parenchyma, whereas nephrolithiasis is concretion calcification in the luminal portion of the urinary tract (Fig. 29-5). The composition of renal stones varies with geography. In the United States, approximately 75% of renal stones are calcium oxalate. The remaining 25% of renal calculi are noncalcareous and are composed of uric acid, struvite, or cystine.

IMAGING FINDINGS

Ultrasonographically, most stones larger than a few millimeters show shadowing. However, ultrasound is not the procedure of choice in diagnosis because too many false-negative studies exist. In intravenous pyelography, the radiolucent stones can be difficult to differentiate from blood clots or sloughed tissue. (All of these can obstruct drainage from the kidney.) With CT, all stones are denser than unenhanced renal parenchyma and urine.

Segments of the urinary tract proximal to the stone may show varying degrees of dilation depending on the degree and chronicity of occlusion created by the stone (Fig. 29-6). Not all dilated drainage systems are from stones and other intrinsic filling defects; crossing bands of vessels or congenital narrowing can give the same appearance on intravenous pyelograms. Up to 90% of renal calculi are opaque enough to be seen on plain film radiographs.

CLINICAL COMMENTS

Low urine volume and stasis contribute to formation of both calcareous and noncalcareous stones by increasing the urinary concentration of stone-forming constituents.

Renal calculi in the ureters cause renal colic, which has a dramatic clinical presentation, often with severe flank pain. Stones remaining in the renal pelvis may lead to obstruction. If they pass into the bladder, on unusual occasions, they may act as the nidus of a bladder calculus.

KEY CONCEPTS

- *Nephrolithiasis is produced in conditions causing urinary stasis or providing a nidus for stone formation.*
- *Symptoms usually are produced by obstruction.*
- *Nearly 90% are opaque enough to be seen on plain film radiographs.*

Ovarian Dermoid Cysts

BACKGROUND

Approximately 80% of ovarian tumors are benign. Most are discovered in women of reproductive age. In patients between 20 and 45 years old, approximately 30% to 50% of benign ovarian neoplasms are mature teratomas (dermoid cysts). Dermoid cysts represent only 10% of benign tumors in patients over 45 years;[23] however, malignancy can never be ruled out without complete tissue diagnosis.

IMAGING FINDINGS

The radiographic image of teratomas is influenced by the presence of tissues from all three germ layers. Characteristic densities

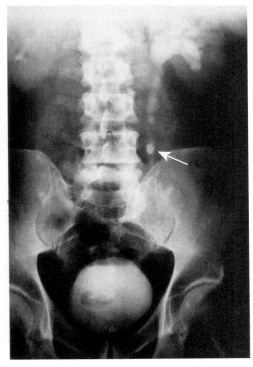

FIG. 29-6 Nephrolithiasis. Ureteral stone *(arrow)* with associated proximal ureter dilation and hydronephrosis.

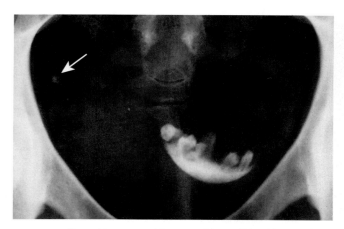

FIG. 29-7   Dermoid cyst containing a partial mandible with multiple well-formed teeth. The speck of calcification on the opposite side most likely represents another dermoid cyst *(arrow)*.

frequently aiding in the diagnosis of these tumors include fat and teeth (Figs. 29-7 and 29-8). Both fat and calcium result in high-level reflective echoes on ultrasound, creating a relatively high degree of specificity for this imaging modality. Calcium also results in acoustic shadowing. Cystic-type calcification is seen in the walls of about 10% of cystic teratomas. High signal foci on T1-weighted MRIs reflect the characteristic fat content.

CLINICAL COMMENTS

Dermoid cysts usually are found incidentally in young women. Although usually asymptomatic, they are prone to torsion, perforation, and infection (often salmonella). The complication rate for dermoid cysts is high compared with other ovarian tumors. Sudden rupture can result in chemical peritonitis and shock.[23] Benign teratomas usually are surgically removed to avoid these complications. Up to 25% of dermoid cysts are bilateral. Malignant transformation is rare, but it cannot be excluded by imaging studies alone.[11]

Other Ovarian Lesions

BACKGROUND

Approximately 80% of ovarian neoplasms are benign, and the majority occur in patients of reproductive age.[23] Approximately one half to two thirds of lesions considered suspicious based on ultrasound, physical examination, and laboratory findings are determined to be benign (Fig. 29-9).

Ovarian cancers are more common in perimenopausal and postmenopausal women (Figs. 29-10 and 29-11). The odds of an ovarian lesion being malignant increase to one in three for patients over the age of 45. Only 10% of benign tumors are seen in patients over 45 years old. The most common malignant ovarian tumors are adenocarcinoma, serous or mucinous cystadenocarcinoma, and endometrioid carcinoma.[23]

IMAGING FINDINGS

Ultrasound is used extensively as the initial imaging modality for evaluation of the adnexa.[23,28] Ultrasound findings usually are adequate to differentiate functional cysts, dermoids, some endometriomas, ectopic pregnancies, and more complex masses that require additional evaluation. The usefulness of ultrasound is limited by obesity, the presence of gas and bone in the area of concern, and the experience of the operator.[28] Transvaginal ultrasound offers better spatial resolution than transabdominal, but it has a more limited field of view.[25,28]

CT is appropriate for identifying fat or calcium within lesions and is recommended for staging ovarian carcinoma.[23] Magnetic

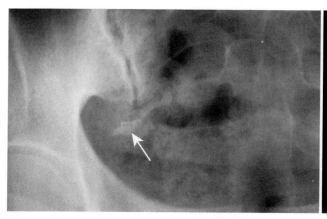

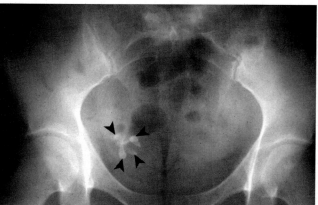

FIG. 29-8   **A,** Single well-formed tooth in the pelvis indicative of a dermoid cyst *(arrow)*. The wall of the cyst is not visible in either case. **B,** Second case demonstrating several well-formed teeth in the reading left of the patient's pelvis *(arrowheads)*. (**B,** Courtesy Gary Longmuir, Phoenix, AZ.)

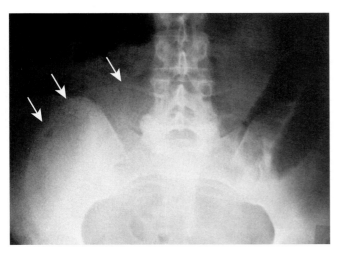

FIG. 29-9 Cystadenoma of the ovary. An extremely large cystadenoma is occupying the majority of the pelvis *(arrows)*.

resonance imaging (MRI) is capable of distinguishing adnexal from uterine masses, as well as identifying fat or hemorrhage within lesions. MRI is useful in identifying metastatic lesions.[23,25]

Irregular walls, thick septations and papillary projections are characteristic of malignant lesions.[23] Other findings suggestive of malignancy include large size, complex architecture, solid components, and cystic lesions that fail to resolve on serial ultrasound examinations.[25] Solid portions of the lesion typically enhance and may show signs of necrosis.

No demonstrable difference in sensitivity or specificity in the detection of malignancy has been reported between MRI and CT, but MRI with contrast does provide better detail of the internal architecture of lesions.[23] CT has been recommended as the preferred modality for staging to assist in surgical and chemotherapeutic planning.[23]

CLINICAL COMMENTS

Nonneoplastic cysts or functional cysts rarely cause symptoms unless they become large, rupture, or hemorrhage. Malignancies of

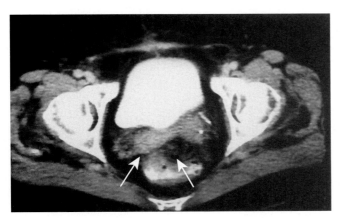

FIG. 29-10 Ovarian carcinoma. Computed tomography examination reveals an adnexal mass that was proven to be an ovarian carcinoma *(arrows)*.

the ovaries are notorious for their presentation of minimal symptoms such as abdominal distention.[23]

Pheochromocytoma

BACKGROUND

Pheochromocytoma is a rare, potentially life-threatening neoplasm characterized by its marked production of catecholamines. Approximately 85% to 95% occur in the adrenal medulla. The remainder occur in parts of the sympathetic nervous system in other abdominal locations, the thorax, or the neck, and are called *paragangliomas*. Most cases occur sporadically, but in 10% an association is seen with other neuroectodermal disorders such as simple familial pheochromocytoma, von Recklinghausen's neurofibromatosis, multiple endocrine neoplasm (MEN) type II syndromes, Sturge-Weber syndrome, and von Hippel-Lindau disease.[4,18,29]

IMAGING FINDINGS

The role of diagnostic imaging is to localize the tumor. CT is 85% to 95% accurate in detecting adrenal masses larger than 1 cm in diameter, but it cannot accurately differentiate between pheochromocytoma and other adrenal masses such as adenomas or metastasis (see Fig. 32-45). Nuclear medicine scanning with metaiodobenzylguanidine (MIBG) specifically localizes adrenergic tissue and is recommended if CT is negative with the appropriate clinical and laboratory findings.[29] MRI is less sensitive than CT, but it may differentiate pheochromocytoma from other adrenal tumors by its marked enhancement on T2-weighted images.[18,29] These tumors tend to be encapsulated and highly vascular. Larger tumors often contain hemorrhagic and necrotic areas. Diffuse or nodular adrenal hyperplasia often is seen before or with development of pheochromocytoma.[29]

CLINICAL COMMENTS

The presenting signs and symptoms of pheochromocytoma reflect the tumor's marked production of catecholamines (epinephrine and norepinephrine). Adrenocorticotropic hormone (ACTH) and other renal and vasoactive hormones may be produced as well. The hallmark symptom is sustained or paroxysmal hypertension. Abnormalities of glucose regulation also occur.[29] The classic clinical triad of headache, sweating, and palpitations occurs only in approximately 40% of patients.[18] Laboratory detection of serum or urinary catecholamines and their metabolites provides the diagnosis. Surgery is the only effective treatment.

Identification of malignant pheochromocytoma cannot be made on the basis of clinical presentation, biochemical assay, or histologic evaluation. Surgical identification of local tissue invasion or the presence of metastasis or recurrence after resec-tion indicates malignancy. Approximately 10% prove to be malignant.[4,18,29]

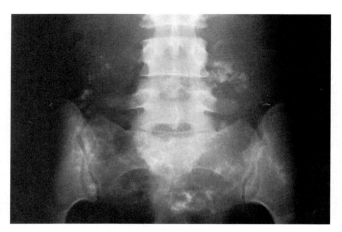

FIG. 29-11 Calcification in a hemangiopericytoma of the ovary. This represents a rare primary tumor of the ovary. This pattern of calcification is similar to the psammomatous calcifications associated with ovarian malignancy.

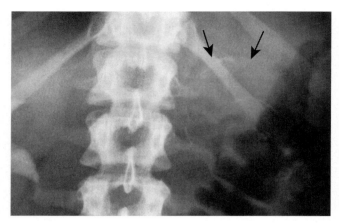

FIG. 29-12 Renal cell carcinoma. Calcification is present within the wall of a renal mass simulating a cyst but proved at biopsy to be a renal cell carcinoma (arrows).

KEY CONCEPTS

- *Pheochromocytoma is a rare tumor characterized by marked production of catecholamines.*
- *Catecholamines primarily affecting blood pressure and glucose regulation produce presenting symptoms.*
- *Pheochromocytoma is occasionally associated with genetic neuroectodermal syndromes.*
- *Computed tomography and metaiodobenzylguanidine scans localize the tumor for surgical resection.*

Renal Cell Carcinoma

BACKGROUND

Renal cell carcinoma accounts for 80% to 90% of primary malignant renal neoplasms and approximately 3% of all malignancies in the adult population. The median age at diagnosis is 57 years, although renal cell carcinoma may occur at any age.[2,20] Renal cell carcinoma is about twice as common in men as in women. Most of these tumors occur sporadically and the etiology is unknown.[20]

IMAGING FINDINGS

Radiologic identification of a renal mass requires differentiation of renal cell carcinoma from simple cyst, abscess, hematoma, lymphoma, renal metastasis, oncocytoma, or angiomyolipoma.[24]

Several excretory urography findings may suggest renal cell carcinoma, although this procedure cannot fully characterize a renal mass. Calcification occurs in approximately 13% of renal cell carcinomas, and it is usually amorphous and centrally located.[9,20] The calcification may simulate a calcified simple cyst and appear as a peripheral or central curvilinear or annular calcification (Figs. 29-12 and 29-13).[1,20,30]

Size, vascularity, and the extent of necrosis or cystic change affect the CT appearance. On unenhanced CT scans the neoplasm may appear hypodense, isodense, or hyperdense as compared with the normal renal parenchyma (Fig. 29-14).[20,32] Tumor calcification is readily identified and characterized on CT. On ultrasound, the mass appears solid with or without cystic components to its walls. Any cystic component is not as thin as a pencil line, as is typical of a benign cyst.

Unenhanced MRI spin-echo (SE) sequences vary based on the homogeneity of the lesion. Signal intensity of renal cell carcinoma is comparable to normal renal parenchyma on both T1- and T2-weighted images. Areas of hemorrhage and necrosis result in a heterogeneous appearance on unenhanced images.[15,20] Unenhanced SE images detect only 63% of tumors less than 3 cm in diameter.[15,20] MRI is somewhat limited in usefulness in evaluating renal masses because of the difficulty of appreciating calcification on almost any MRI pulse sequence.

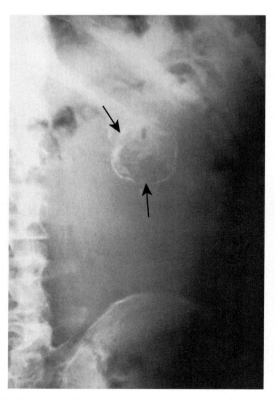

FIG. 29-13 Renal cell carcinoma. Mottled calcification within a renal cell carcinoma (arrows).

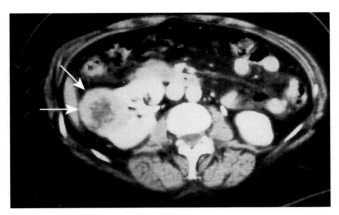

FIG. 29-14 Computed tomography of renal cell carcinoma *(arrows)*.

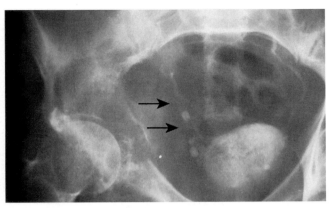

FIG. 29-15 Renal cell metastasis. Osteolytic metastasis. Osteolytic destructive lesions of left ilium and superior pubic rami, acetabulum, and ischium. *Note:* Phleboliths are displaced toward midline *(arrows)*.

CLINICAL COMMENTS

Renal cell carcinoma produces signs and symptoms in as few as 5% of patients. Metastatic spread is present at initial presentation in up to 45% of patients (Fig. 29-15). Classic presenting symptoms include flank pain sometimes because of a subcapsular bleed, flank mass, and hematuria.[22]

KEY CONCEPTS

- *Renal cell carcinoma accounts for 80% to 90% of primary malignant renal neoplasms.*
- *Radiologic identification of a renal mass requires differentiation from simple cyst, abscess, hematoma, lymphoma, renal metastasis, oncocytoma, or angiomyolipoma.*
- *Classic presenting symptoms include flank pain, flank mass, and hematuria, but patients often have only some or none of these findings.*

Uterine Fibroma (Leiomyoma)

BACKGROUND

Leiomyomas are seen in approximately 40% of women over 35 years of age and are the most common benign uterine tumor. They can be intramural, subserosal, or submucosal. Sometimes they are associated with infertility. Subserosal and submucosal types may be pedunculated, and the uterus may be deformed by these tumors. A unique characteristic of leiomyomas is their ability to detach from the uterus and develop a new blood supply from another organ. Tumor growth is affected primarily by estrogen. Estrogen levels increased by pregnancy or oral contraceptives can lead to tumor growth. Growth ceases after menopause without estrogen replacement therapy.[11]

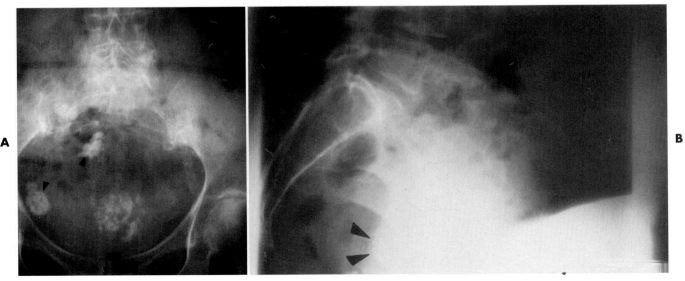

FIG. 29-16 **A** and **B,** Multiple uterine leiomyomas presenting with characteristic stippled or whorled calcific appearance *(arrowheads)*.

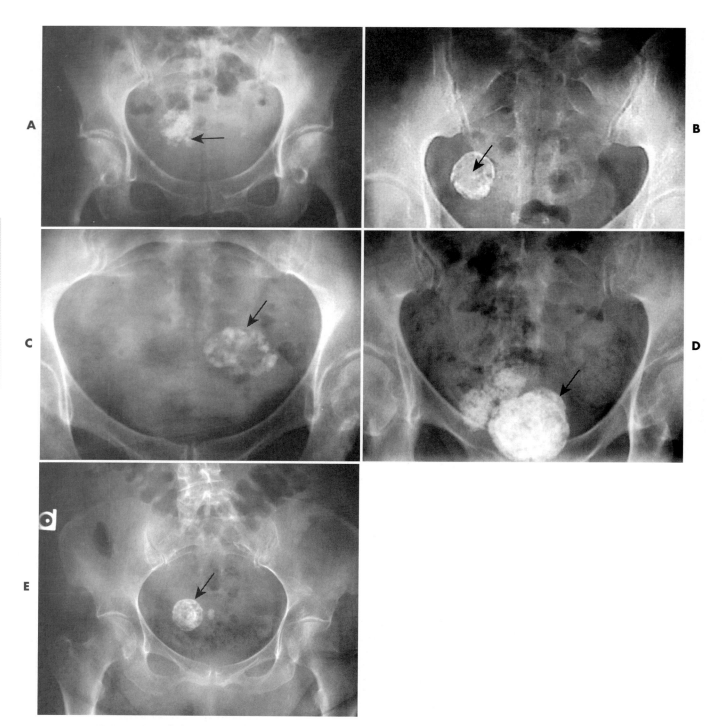

FIG. 29-17 **A** through **E,** Uterine leiomyoma in different patients *(arrows)*. Notice the typical stippled calcification of a uterine fibroid; several cases exhibit calcification of the outer wall of the lesion.

IMAGING FINDINGS

Most uterine fibroids are identified either by pelvic examination, by palpation of a uterine enlargement or mass, or by discovering them on plain x-ray examination done for other purposes (by seeing either a mass or calcifications). Pelvic ultrasound is the most useful tool for evaluating these masses. The appearance of leiomyomas may vary, but common findings include general enlargement of the uterus (longer than 10 cm and wider than 5 cm), focal bulges in the uterine contour, and areas of inhomogeneous mural echoes.[11] Acoustic shadowing usually occurs when calcifications are present. However, obviously tissue diagnosis cannot be definitively made with ultrasound alone.

Plain radiographs or computed tomographs may reveal "popcornlike" or "cauliflower-like" mass-type calcifications, which develop in necrotic areas of leiomyomas (Figs. 29-16 through 29-21).

Leiomyomas without areas of degeneration produce an MRI signal isointense with myometrium on T1-weighted images and hypointense on T2-weighted images. Degeneration of leiomyomas produces heterogenicity of signal and a wide range of intensities.[11] Again, diagnosis cannot be 100% definitive with imaging studies alone.

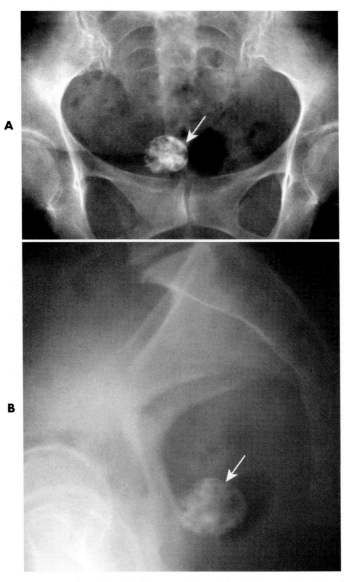

FIG. 29-18 A small uterine leiomyoma is noted in, **A,** the central portion of the pelvis and, **B,** anterior to the sacrum in the lateral projection *(arrows).*

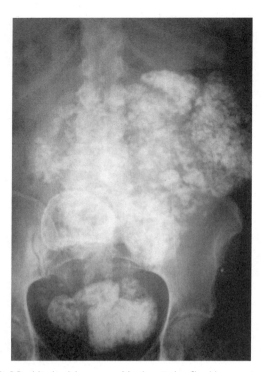

FIG. 29-19   Uterine leiomyomas. Massive uterine fibroids are extending out of the pelvis in this patient.

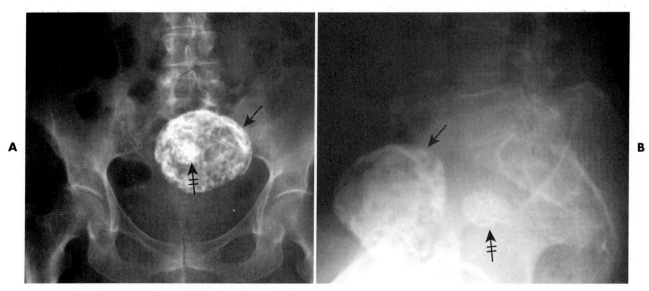

FIG. 29-20   **A,** Superimposed uterine leiomyomas *(arrow* and *crossed arrow)* on the anteroposterior projection and, **B,** seen as two bodies *(arrow* and *crossed arrow)* in the lateral projection.

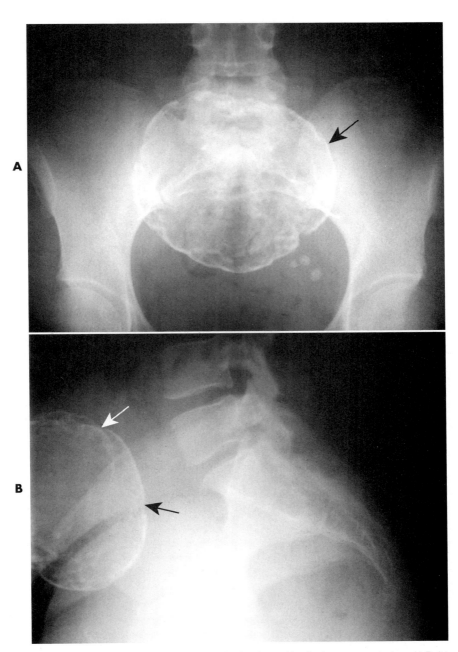

FIG. 29-21 Large leiomyoma appearing with cystic calcification *(arrows)* in, **A,** the anteroposterior and, **B,** lateral projection. (Courtesy Randy Hurt, Rock Island, IL.)

CLINICAL COMMENTS

More than 50% of uterine fibroids are asymptomatic and are not a health concern for women. Abnormal bleeding presenting as heavier and longer menses is the most common chronic symptom. Acute degeneration occurs in approximately one third of cases. Infertility is an occasional result. Symptoms secondary to pressure on adjacent abdominal contents and an increase in abdominal girth may occur as the tumor increases in size. Malignant degeneration occurs in less than 3% of cases of leiomyoma.[11]

KEY CONCEPTS

- *Leiomyoma is the most common benign uterine tumor; it occurs in approximately 40% of women over 35 years of age.*
- *Tumor growth is affected by estrogen.*
- *Most uterine fibroids are identified first by pelvic examination or on x-ray alone for other reasons.*
- *More than 50% are asymptomatic.*
- *"Popcornlike" or "cauliflower-like" mass calcification may be seen on plain film.*

References

1. Arkless R: Cyst-like calcification in renal cell carcinomas, *Clin Radiol* 17:397, 1966.
2. Bennington JL, Beckwith JB: Tumors of the kidney, renal pelvis and ureter. In: Atlas of Tumor Pathology, Washington, DC, 1975, Armed Forces Institute of Pathology.
3. Bosniak MA et al: CT diagnosis of renal angiomyolipoma: the importance of detecting small amounts of fat, *AJR Am J Roentgenol* 151:497, 1988.
4. Bravo EL: Evolving concepts in the pathophysiology, diagnosis, and treatment of pheochromocytoma, *Endocr Rev* 15:356, 1994.
5. Breslow N et al: Age distribution of Wilms' tumor study, *Cancer Res* 48:1653, 1988.
6. Bret PM et al: Small, asymptomatic angiomyolipomas of the kidney, *Radiology* 154:7, 1985.
7. Charboneau JW et al: Spectrum of sonographic findings in 125 renal masses other than benign simple cyst, *AJR Am J Roentgenol* 140:87, 1983.
8. Cris WM, Kun LE: Common solid tumors of childhood, *N Engl J Med* 324:461, 1991.
9. Daniel WW et al: Calcified renal masses: a review of ten years' experience at the Mayo Clinic, *Radiology* 103:503, 1972.
10. Earthman WJ, Mazer MJ, Winfield AC: Angiomyolipomas in tuberous sclerosis: subselective embolotherapy with alcohol, with long-term follow-up study, *Radiology* 160:437, 1986.
11. Hall DA, Hann LE: Gynecologic radiology: benign disorders. In Taveras JM, Ferrucci JR, editors: Radiology-Diagnosis-Imaging-intervention, vol 4, Philadelphia, 1996, Lippincott-Raven.
12. Hansen GC et al: Computed tomography diagnosis of renal angiomyolipoma, *Radiology* 128:789, 1978.
13. Hartman DS: Pediatric renal tumors. In Taveras JM, Ferrucci JR, editors: Radiology-Diagnosis-Imaging-Intervention, vol 4, Philadelphia, 1996, Lippincott-Raven.
14. Hartman DS et al: Angiomyolipoma: ultrasonic-pathologic correlation, *Radiology* 139:451, 1981.
15. Hricak H et al: Detection and staging of renal neoplasms: a reassessment of MR imaging, *Radiology* 166:643, 1988.
16. Imray TJ, Kaplan P: Lower urinary tract infections and calculi in the adult, *Semin Roentgenol* 18: 267, 1983.
17. Jaffe MH et al: Wilms' tumor: ultrasonic features, pathologic correlation, and diagnostic pitfalls, *Radiology* 140:147, 1981.
18. Kazantsev GB, Prinz RA: Functioning tumors of the adrenal gland, *Compr Ther* 19:232, 1993.
19. Kissane JM, Dehner LP: Renal tumors and tumor-like lesions in pediatric patients, *Pediatr Nephrol* 6:365, 1992.
20. Levine E: Renal cell carcinoma: clinical aspects, imaging diagnosis, and staging, *Semin Roentgenol* 30:128, 1995.
21. Meilstrup JW et al: Other renal tumors, *Semin Roentgenol* 30:168, 1995.
22. Mevorach RA et al: Renal cell carcinoma: incidental diagnosis and natural history: review of 235 cases, *Urology* 39:519, 1992.
23. Occhipinti KA, Frankel SD, Hricak H: The ovary, *Radiol Clin North Am* 31:1115, 1993.
24. O'Toole KM, Brown M, Hoffmann P: Pathology of benign and malignant kidney tumors, *Urol Clin North Am* 20:193, 1993.
25. Outwater EK, Dunton CJ: Imaging of the ovary and adnexa: clinical issues and applications of MR imaging, *Radiology* 194:1, 1995.
26. Raghavendra BN, Bosniak MA, Megibow AJ: Small angiomyolipoma of the kidney: sonographic-CT evaluation, *AJR Am J Roentgenol* 141:575, 1983.
27. Scheible W et al: Lipomatous tumors of the kidney and adrenal: apparent echographic specificity, *Radiology* 129:153, 1978.
28. Scott LM, McCarthy SM: Imaging of ovarian masses: magnetic resonance imaging, *Clin Obstet Gynecol* 34:443, 1991.
29. Werbel SS, Ober KP: Pheochromocytoma: update on diagnosis, localization, and management, *Med Clin North Am* 79:131, 1995.
30. Weyman PJ et al: CT of calcified renal masses, *AJR Am J Roentgenol* 138:1095, 1982.
31. Wickman JEA: Treatment of urinary tract stones, *BMJ* 307:1414, 1993.
32. Zagoria RJ et al: CT features of renal cell carcinoma with emphasis on relation to tumor size, *Invest Radiol* 25:261, 1990.

chapter 30

Gastrointestinal Diseases

BEVERLY L. HARGER
LISA E. HOFFMAN
RICHARD ARKLESS

Radiographic Anatomy of the Gastrointestinal Tract

A thorough understanding of the normal plain film appearance of the gastrointestinal tract is critical when evaluating for the presence of serious conditions that may affect this system. For example, swallowed air within the stomach has a different appearance than gas within the small bowel or colon. Table 30-1 reviews the plain film appearance of the gastrointestinal tract.

Cholelithiasis (Gallstones)

BACKGROUND

The incidence of gallstones in patients in the United States approaches 20% of men and 35% of women by the age of 75 years;[24] thus, gallstones exhibit a greater prevalence in women and in older age groups. Obesity and certain diseases also are associated with the development of gallstones (Table 30-2).

IMAGING FINDINGS

Ultrasonography generally is the preferred imaging modality for evaluating patients for possible gallstones or biliary duct obstruction. Gallstones produce hyperechoic foci with acoustic shadowing, and mobility of the stone usually is apparent (Fig. 30-1).[5,15] The patient should fast for 4 or more hours because these stones can be missed in a contracted gallbladder.[25]

These stones may be imaged incidentally on plain film radiographs even in asymptomatic patients, but only 10% to 15% of them contain enough calcium to be visible (Figs. 30-2 through 30-4).[11,31] Oral cholecystography (OCG) requires the patient to take an oral contrast agent, which is absorbed from the bowel, excreted by the liver, and concentrated in the gallbladder (except when the gallbladder cystic duct is blocked or sometimes when the gallbladder is inflamed). The gallbladder also is not seen in cases of a lack of absorption or significant liver damage.

OCG does demonstrate most gallstones, but since the development of ultrasound to accomplish this task, it is thought by some to be most useful for providing information about the functional status of the gallbladder (see Fig. 30-3).[7] However, the clinical usefulness of this is still controversial.

Uncommonly, the noncontrasted gallbladder forms a radiodense "milk of calcium" bile that mimics the gallbladder's appearance during OCG (Fig. 30-5). This phenomenon is thought to develop from chronic obstruction of the cystic duct by one or more gallstones in patients with chronic cholecystitis. The duct obstruction leads to decreased gland function, bile stasis, and radiographic visible accumulations of a radiodense calcium carbonate in viscous intraluminal bile. Review of the patient's history to exclude any recent intake of contrast material (oral or intravenous) must be accomplished before the milk of calcium bile diagnosis can be made. On radiographs, the fluid is found in the gravity-dependent portion of the gallbladder. The ultrasound appearance is not consistent because the composition of the milk of calcium bile varies from a semisolid to fluid suspension.

"Porcelain gallbladder" describes extensive calcification of the wall of the gallbladder; also known as calcifying cholecystitis or cholecystopathic chronica calcarea (Figs. 30-6 and 30-7). Specifically the term refers to the blue-greenish discoloration and brittle condition of the gallbladder observed at surgery. A porcelain gallbladder typically is found incidentally on plain film studies. Patients generally are asymptomatic and more commonly are women (5:1 ratio). Concurrent gallstones are usual. A porcelain gallbladder is associated with higher incidence of adenocarcinoma of the gallbladder, typically warranting prophylactic excision.

CLINICAL COMMENTS

Cholelithiasis usually is discovered incidentally during other studies. In the first 5 years after diagnosis, only approximately 10% of patients experience symptoms resulting from gallstones.[31] Right upper quadrant pain is the most commonly reported symptom.[31] The pain usually is steady, lasting for several hours. Radiation to the lower abdomen, back, or tip of the right scapula is not uncommon; vomiting may occur.[5]

Complications seen with gallstone disease include cholecystitis, choledocholithiasis, pancreatitis (migration of a stone to the

PART FOUR
Abdomen

TABLE 30-1
Gastrointestinal Tract Plain Film Organ Appearance

Organ	Visibility	Location	Retroperitoneal versus intraperitoneal	Fixed versus mobile	Appearance specifics	Plain film abnormalities
Esophagus	Air occasionally visible in cervical region	Anterior and left of spine from laryngopharynx to diaphragm	Not applicable	Fixed	None on plain film	Abnormalities including dilation or neoplasm may present as posterior mediastinal mass (hiatal hernia)
Stomach	Air in fundus on upright with inferior fluid level, spreads to body of stomach and may outline rugae on supine image	Magenblase immediately inferior to left lung base on upright image; should not extend to midline or lateral body	Intraperitoneal	Fixed proximal and distal; mobile body	None on plain film	Displacement of magenblase laterally suggests hepatomegaly
Duodenum	Occasional air in bulb	Right upper quadrant medially	Retroperitoneal (most)	Fixed	None	None
Small bowel	Occasional small segment air-filled	Most of abdomen; jejunum primarily left upper quadrant and middle lower ileum	Intraperitoneal	Mobile	Small, thin mucosal folds	Long segments air-filled; dilated air-filled (>3 cm)
Cecum	Fluid feces and gas bubbles mixed	Right lower quadrant	Intraperitoneal	Mobile, usually right lower quadrant location	None	Distention (>10 cm risk of rupture); volvulus ("coffee bean" sign)
Appendix	May be visible gas in appendix	Considerable variation, although usually in right lower quadrant	Intraperitoneal	Can move with the cecum	None	Normal or may show slight distention of adjacent ileum; possible appendicolith
Ascending and descending colon	Visible gas in haustra	Ascending along right flank; descending along left flank	Retroperitoneal	Fixed	Widely spaced, thick mucosal folds Lateral margin of both should be within 2 to 3 mm of adjacent flank stripe (fat plane medial to abdominal muscle wall). Splenic flexure should be most superior portion of colon.	Dilation

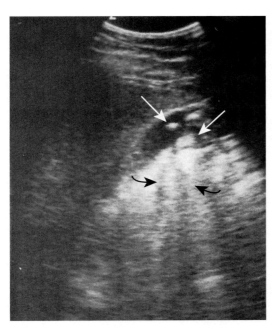

FIG. 30-1 Choleliths. Ultrasound image shows multiple echogenic foci within the gallbladder lumen *(arrows)* with posterior acoustic shadowing *(curved arrows)*. (Courtesy John A.M. Taylor, Seneca Falls, NY.)

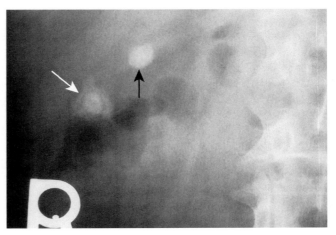

FIG. 30-2 Choleliths. Two laminated and faceted calculi in the gallbladder characteristic of concretion calcifications *(arrows)*.

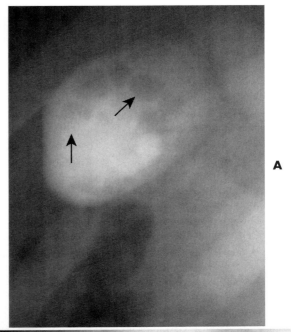

A

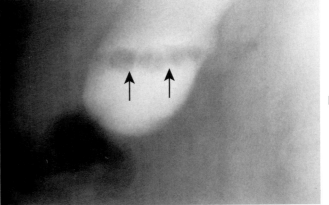

B

FIG. 30-3 Oral cholecystographic appearance of gallstones. **A,** Oral cholecystogram with the patient in the recumbent position demonstrates several nonopaque stones within the gallbladder *(arrows)*. **B,** With the patient in the upright position, the stones float just above the fundus *(arrows)*. (Courtesy John A.M. Taylor, Seneca Falls, NY.)

TABLE 30-2
Associated Factors for Gallstone Formation

Associated factors	Comments
Obesity	Rapid weight loss resulting in increased risk of symptomatic gallstone formation
Increasing age	Associated with increased cholesterol secretion
Northern European ethnic group	Associated with increased cholesterol secretion
Estrogen replacement therapy and oral-contraceptive use	Increases biliary output of cholesterol and also reduces synthesis of bile acid in women
Pregnancy	Associated with increased risk of gallstones and symptomatic gallbladder disease
Sickle-cell anemia or other hemolytic conditions	Hemolysis increases bilirubin excretion
Crohn's disease	Disease of the terminal ileum causing disruption of bile acid reabsorption

From Johnston DE, Kaplan MM: Pathogenesis and treatment of gallstones, *N Engl J Med* 328:412, 1993; Liddle RA, Goldstein RB, Saxton J: Gallstone formation during weight-reduction dieting, *Arch Intern Med* 149:1750, 1989; Tait N, Little JM: The treatment of gallstones, *BMJ* 311:99, 1995.

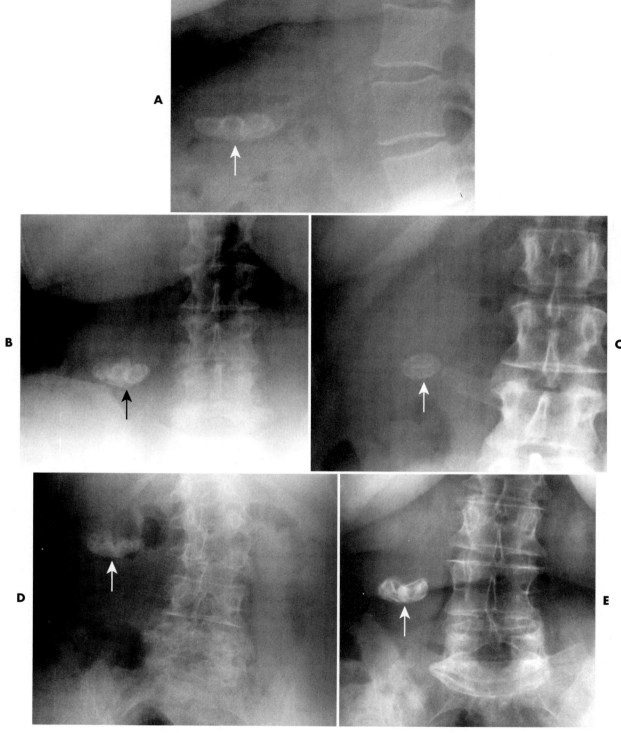

FIG. 30-4 Gallstones appearing as radiodense calculi of the right upper abdominal quadrant on, **A,** an anteroposterior and, **B,** lateral lumbar projection; and, **C** through **E,** in three other patients (arrows).

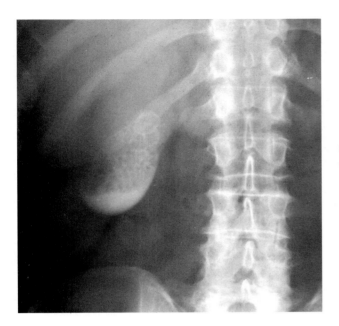

FIG. 30-5 Milk of calcium bile. Multiple gallstones are noted in the lower portion of the gallbladder. The stones are contrasted by an opaque fluid of calcium carbonate, known as *milk of calcium bile.* (Courtesy Ian D. McLean, LeClaire, IA.)

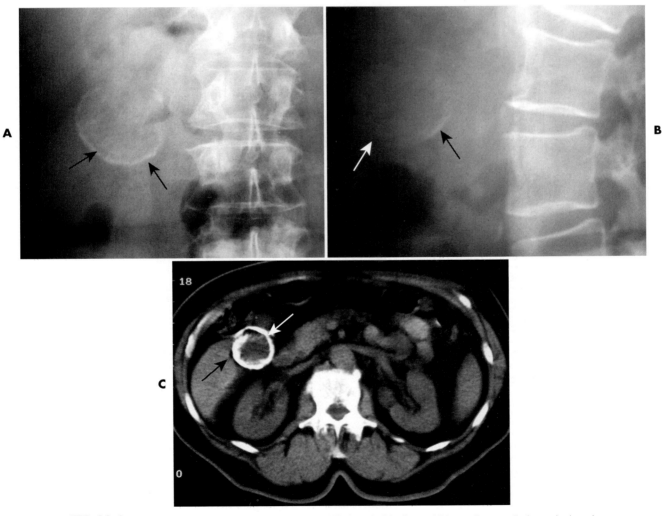

FIG. 30-6 Porcelain gallbladder. **A,** Anteroposterior and, **B,** lateral plain films exhibit curvilinear radiodense shadows in the right upper abdominal quadrant that correspond to partial calcification of the wall of the gallbladder. **C,** On computed tomography without contrast, the circumference of the gallbladder is calcified. Gallstones are not present *(arrows).* (Courtesy Kevin Paustian, Durant, IA.)

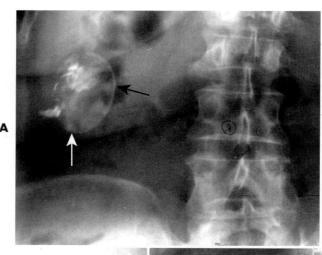

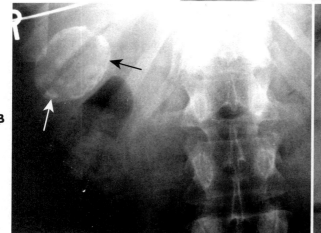

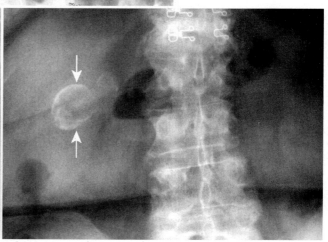

FIG. 30-7   A through **C,** Porcelain gallbladder in several patients *(arrows).* The finding of a porcelain gallbladder typically warrants surgical excision because of the approximately 20% associated increased risk of developing gallbladder carcinoma.

TABLE 30-3
Complications Associated with Gallstones

Complications	Comments
Acute cholecystitis	May remit temporarily, but sometimes progresses to gangrene and perforation
Choledocholithiasis	Gallstones obstructing the common bile duct
Cholangitis	Infection of the bile ducts following obstruction possible
Acute pancreatitis	Probably secondary to transient obstruction of the main pancreatic duct
Gallstone ileus	Follows perforation of the duodenum or bowel by gallstone; classic plain film triad: small bowel obstruction, biliary tract air, and an opaque concretion in the small bowel

From Johnston DE, Kaplan MM: Pathogenesis and treatment of gallstones, *N Engl J Med* 328:412, 1993.

distal common duct where the pancreatic duct enters), cholangitis, stone perforation of the duodenum or colon, and gallstone ileus (Table 30-3).[2,3,5,19,31] Symptomatic gallbladder disease may require surgical intervention if nonsurgical techniques such as lithotripsy (using strong ultrasound waves to break up the stone) are ineffective, unsuitable, or unavailable.[31]

KEY CONCEPTS
- *The prevalence of cholelithiasis increases with age.*
- *It is more common in women.*
- *Obesity is a risk factor.*
- *Symptoms vary and clinical correlation is required.*
- *Plain film radiography plays a minor role.*

Colon Polyps

BACKGROUND

Colon polyps are found in up to 12% of the population.[33] The adenomatous polyp is considered the precursor to colorectal cancer.[16] Therefore detection of colonic polyps is extremely important. The incidence of malignancy increases with increased size of the polyp

TABLE 30-4
Incidence of Malignancy in Relation to Polyp Size

5 mm or less	5 mm to 10 mm	10 mm to 20 mm	More than 20 mm
<0.5%	1% to 2.5%	10%	46%

From Thoeni RFL, Bischof TP: Colonic polyps. In Traveras JM, Ferrucci JT, editors: Radiology Diagnosis-Imaging-Intervention, vol 4, Philadelphia, 1996, Lippincott-Raven.

(Table 30-4). Most polyp development is incidental, but polyps also appear as part of familial polyposis syndromes (not common). Table 30-5 reviews the characteristics of several polyposis conditions.

IMAGING FINDINGS

Barium examination and endoscopy are the most important methods for detecting polyps.[32] Polyps appear as discrete masses, sessile or pedunculated, which protrude into the lumen of the gut (Figs. 30-8 through 30-10). Recent investigations report up to 98% accuracy in identification of polyps by double-contrast barium enema. Older studies report less accuracy, but the accuracy depends on the meticulousness and quality of the exam. Lesions smaller than 1 cm in diameter are more difficult to detect.

In general the inner margin of a polyp appears sharper than the outer margin because it is an intraluminal mass surrounded by barium. On occasion a diverticulum coated with barium and filled with air can mimic a polyp on one or more x-rays, but with meticulous evaluation it should not be misdiagnosed.

TABLE 30-5
Review of Polyposis Conditions

Complications	Comments
Nonfamilial adeonomatous polyps	Present in 30% of adults over 50 years of age; malignancy correlates with polyp size, villous features, and degree of dysplasia
Familial adenomatous polyposis	Autosomal dominant; it begins to appear between ages of 10 and 35 years; colon cancer usually occurs by age 50
Gardner syndrome	Variant of familial adenomatous polyposis; it is characterized by extraintestinal osteomas, fibromas, and desmoid tumors
Familial juvenile polyposis	Autosomal dominant; most common—colon
Peutz-Jehgers syndrome	Autosomal dominant; mucocutaneous pigmented macules appear on lips, buccal mucosa, and skin; 50% of patients develop malignancies in gastrointestinal and nonintestinal organs
Turcot syndrome	Autosomal recessive; central nervous system neoplasm

From Jones B, Braver JM: Essentials of gastrointestinal radiology, Philadelphia, 1982, WB Saunders.

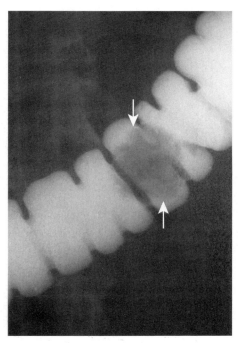

FIG. 30-8 Sessile polyp. Filling defect of a sessile-based polyp is well demonstrated *(arrows)*.

CLINICAL COMMENTS

Most patients with multiple small polyps or even small carcinomas have no overt symptoms. Chronic occult blood loss from polyps may lead to iron deficiency. Occasionally, symptoms from large polyps are related to complications such as intussusception or colonic obstruction.[32] Polyps measuring 1 cm or larger definitely should be removed and histologically examined, although some experts believe even smaller ones should be removed also.

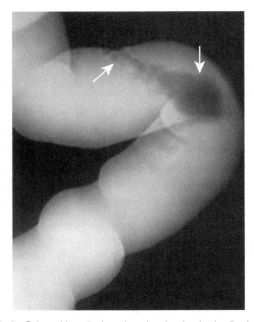

FIG. 30-9 Polyp with stalk. A pedunculated polyp is visualized within this contrast-filled bowel *(arrows)*.

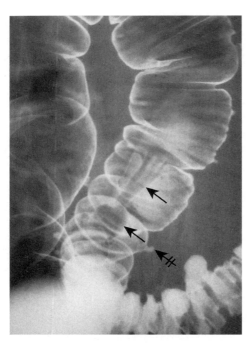

FIG. 30-10   Polyp with stalk. Double-contrast (air and barium) study reveals a pedunculated polyp (*arrows*). Diverticulae are seen with this study also (*crossed arrow*).

TABLE 30-6
High-Risk Groups for Colorectal Carcinoma

Risk factors	Comments
Familial polyposis	100% risk of cancer if untreated
Gardner's syndrome	Characterized by precancerous colorectal polyps; associated with osteomas, fibromas, soft-tissue desmoids, and lipomas
Ulcerative colitis	Patients with long-standing and extensive ulcerative colitis at high risk
Crohn's disease	Risk not as high as for those with ulcerative colitis
Family history	Positive family history for colorectal cancer or polyps
Hereditary cancer of multiple anatomic sites	Autosomal dominant syndrome, such as breast, endometrium, ovary, and colon

From Realini JP: Screening for colorectal cancer: issues for primary care physicians, *Prim Care* 15:63, 1988.

KEY CONCEPTS

- *Colonoscopy and barium enema are two possibly equal modalities in evaluating the colon for polyps.*
- *Adenomatous polyps may be a precursor to colon cancer.*
- *The incidence of malignancy increases with increased size of the polyp.*

Colorectal Carcinoma

BACKGROUND

Colorectal cancer is second only to lung cancer in men and breast and lung cancer in women as a cause of death.[38] The incidence of colorectal cancer increases after 35 to 45 years of age; however, high-risk persons (Table 30-6) develop colorectal cancer at a much younger age.[26,34] Most colorectal cancers are thought to arise from malignant transformation of an adenomatous polyp.[34]

IMAGING FINDINGS

Colorectal cancer may produce changes that are imaged as infiltration, mucosal destruction, and masses (Fig. 30-11). Colonoscopy demonstrates these changes and is the preferred diagnostic procedure when patient history is suggestive of colon cancer or barium enema has demonstrated abnormalities consistent with colon cancer. Any large, broad-based polyp with an irregular surface is highly suggestive of carcinoma.[29] The classic appearance on barium enema is the annular "napkin ring" or "apple core" lesion produced by an infiltrating tumor, which causes narrowing of the lumen, thickening of the wall, and rigidity. However, this is an advanced stage tumor; obviously cancer is best discovered when much smaller. Mucosal destruction and overhanging edges also are components of this appearance.

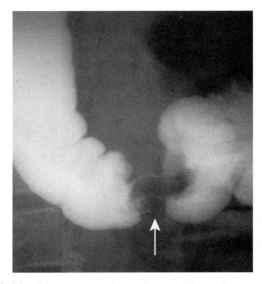

FIG. 30-11   Colon carcinoma. An annular constricting carcinoma can be seen as a narrowed segment of bowel with a markedly narrowed lumen, abrupt transition, and overhanging edges known as "napkin ring" or "apple core" lesion (*arrow*).

CLINICAL COMMENTS

Clinical features do not consistently reflect tumor size; therefore large carcinomas may remain clinically silent. However, patients presenting with rectal bleeding or hemoccult-positive stools must be evaluated for colorectal cancer.[18,29,35] In individuals older than 40 years of age, a change in bowel habits or particularly constipation, weight loss, and unexplained anemia are other clinical features that suggest possible colorectal cancer.[290]

KEY CONCEPTS

- *Colorectal cancer is suspected in any patient over 40 years of age with change in bowel habits, weight loss, and unexplained anemia.*
- *Characteristic findings on barium enema include narrowing of bowel lumen, thickening of bowel wall, and rigidity.*
- *Colonoscopy with biopsy establishes diagnosis.*

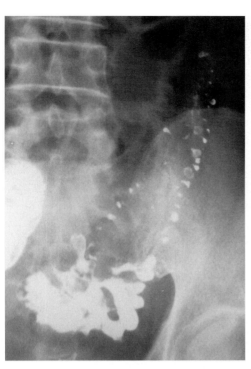

FIG. 30-16 Diverticulosis. Postevacuation study demonstrates diverticulae. (Courtesy John A.M. Taylor, Seneca Falls, NY.)

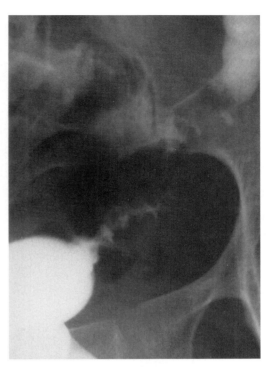

FIG. 30-17 Diverticulitis. Contrast enema depicts spasm of a portion of the sigmoid colon. This finding is indicative of diverticular disease but not diagnostic for diverticulitis.

Hiatal Hernia

BACKGROUND

Hiatal hernia is the most common diagnostic entity identified on radiographic examination of the upper gastrointestinal tract. The sliding or axial hiatal hernia, in which the esophagogastric junction and a portion of the gastric fundus herniates into the chest, comprises more than 95% of hiatal hernias.[1] At least 10% of the adult North American population have a sliding hiatal hernia, but with Valsalva's maneuver one can demonstrate at least a tiny hiatal hernia in many, if not most, people.[1] The paraesophageal type, in which the junction remains fixed below the diaphragmatic hiatus but a portion of the gastric fundus herniates into the chest alongside the lower esophagus, represents about 1% of all hiatal hernias.[6] A mixed type represents the third type of hiatal hernia. Presence or absence of this hernia is not nearly as important as presence or absence of gastroesophageal reflux, which can occur even in the absence of a hernia and may not occur even with a large hernia.

IMAGING FINDINGS

Identification of the esophagogastric junction at least 2 cm above the diaphragm, usually seen with the aid of barium contrast, is needed. Identification of a mucosal web is helpful but often is not present. A soft-tissue mass or air-fluid level in the posterior mediastinum on a plain film chest radiograph may indicate hiatal hernia (Figs. 30-19 through 30-21). Use of barium esophagram allows differentiation from other posterior mediastinal masses (see Fig. 30-20).

CLINICAL COMMENTS

Hiatal hernias are common and the associated symptoms of reflux are usually their only clinical significance. Endoscopic evidence of reflux esophagitis is absent in most patients with hiatal hernia.[22,31] However, hiatal hernia can be imaged in 90% of patients with gastroesophageal reflux disease.[22] The more severe forms of reflux esophagitis are less common in patients without hiatal hernia, but normal esophagogastric junction does not rule out reflux esophagitis.[22] A rare but potentially life-threatening complication of massive hiatal hernia is volvulus of the stomach ("upside-down stomach") with strangulation.[8]

KEY CONCEPTS

- *Hiatal hernia commonly occurs in adults.*
- *The presence or absence of hiatal hernia poorly predicts presence of gastroesophageal reflux disease.*
- *Most are sliding (axial) hernias.*
- *Volvulus of stomach with strangulation can be life threatening with massive hiatal hernia.*

Pancreatic Lithiasis

BACKGROUND

Relative obstruction of the pancreatic ductal system is the likely underlying mechanism for pancreatic calculus development.[20,28] The calculi primarily represent calcified masses of inspissated secretions.[20,28] A history of high alcohol intake is elicited in nearly 90% of patients with pancreatic calculi.[27] Table 30-8 lists other conditions that may lead to pancreatic calculus formation.

IMAGING FINDINGS

Pancreatic calculi secondary to alcoholic pancreatitis usually appear as small, irregular concretions, commonly numerous and scattered throughout the gland. These concretions are seen on the

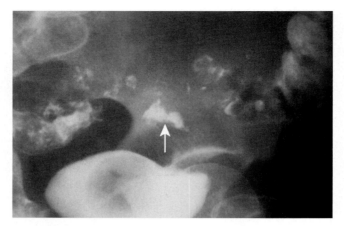

FIG. 30-18   Diverticulitis. Extravasation of contrast material is noted *(arrow)*. A specific diagnosis of perforated diverticulitis can be made with this finding.

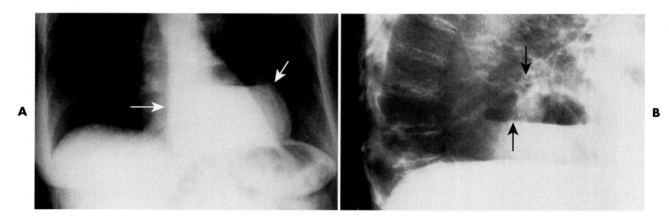

FIG. 30-19   Hiatal hernia. **A,** Posteroanterior projection. A mass with an air-fluid level within can be seen behind the heart *(arrows)*. **B,** Lateral view of hiatal hernia *(arrows)*.

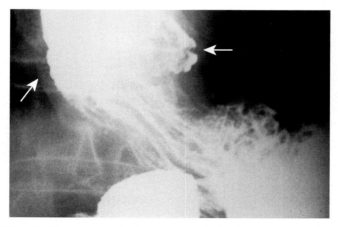

FIG. 30-20   Hiatal hernia. Upper gastrointestinal study demonstrates a sliding hiatal hernia *(arrows)*.

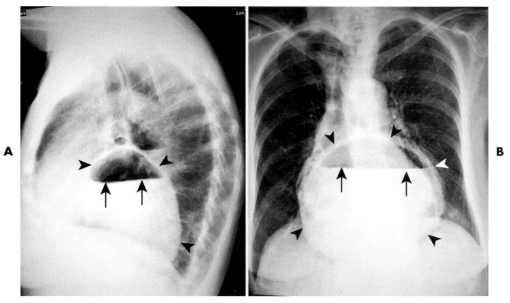

FIG. 30-21 **A** and **B,** Large hiatal hernia *(arrowheads).* The gastric air bubble *(small arrows)* is outlined by arrows. (Courtesy Ian D. McLean, LeClaire, IA.)

TABLE 30-8
Conditions That May Lead to Pancreatic Calcification

Condition	Pattern	Comments
Alcoholic pancreatitis	Small concretions widely scattered throughout gland	Usually develops after 5 to 10 years of pain
Pseudocysts	Widely scattered or rim calcification usually in or near pancreas	Up to 20% of cases exhibit calcification similar to chronic pancreatitis
Pancreatic cancer	Diffusely present throughout gland; however, most pancreatic cancers do not calcify	Higher incidence of pancreatic cancer in patients with chronic pancreatitis
Hyperparathyroidism	Pancreatic and renal calcification	Pancreatitis occurs as a complication of hyperparathyroidism in 10% of cases
Cystadenoma or cystadenocarcinoma	Sunburst pattern—pathognomonic, but not common	Tumor calcification in 10% of patients

From Ring EJ, Ferrucci JT, Short WF: Differential diagnosis of pancreatic calcification, *AJR Am J Roentgenol* 117:446, 1973.

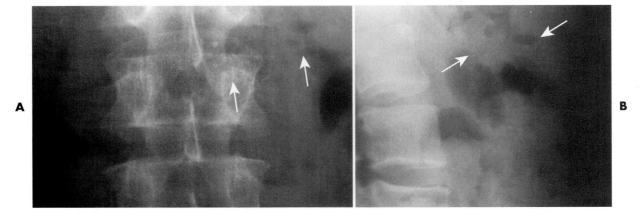

FIG. 30-22 Pancreatic lithiasis. **A,** Anteroposterior projection demonstrates faint discrete calculi superimposed over and near the L2 vertebral body *(arrows).* **B,** Lateral view reveals multiple, tiny, dense, discrete opacities typical of pancreatic lithiasis *(arrows).*

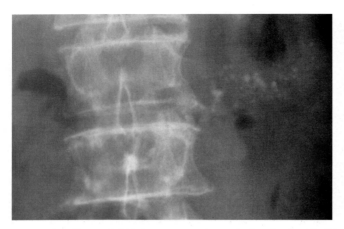

FIG. 30-23   Pancreatic lithiasis, anteroposterior projection. On the right side the stippled opacities are close to the midline, but on the left the calcification extends far peripherally, conforming to the shape of the pancreas. (Courtesy Cynthia Peterson, Toronto, Ontario, Canada.)

abdominal films at the level of L1-2 and conform to the shape of the pancreas. On the right side, the densities are close to the midline, but on the left the calcifications may extend far peripherally (Figs. 30-22 and 30-23). In approximately 25% of cases the calcifications are seen in only the head or tail of the pancreas.[27]

CLINICAL COMMENTS

Patients with pancreatic calcifications secondary to alcoholic pancreatitis usually have a 5- to 10-year history of episodic abdominal pain.[27]

Peptic Ulcer Disease

BACKGROUND

Peptic ulcer disease is the result of erosion of the gastric or duodenal mucosa. Although the etiology of peptic ulcer disease can be complex, the presence of *Helicobacter pylori* bacteria in the stomach is thought to be a major factor.[4] *Helicobacter pylori* infection is identified in more than 90% of patients with duodenal ulcers and more than 80% of patients with gastric ulcers.[4] The vast majority of peptic ulcers are benign. Ninety-five percent occur in the duodenum with virtually no association with malignancy.[12] Only 5% of gastric ulcers are associated with malignancies.[12]

IMAGING FINDINGS

Although debate continues regarding the best imaging method, double-contrast studies have shown a sensitivity of 95% for lesions identified by endoscopy.[30]

Small gastric ulcers produce a defect that is filled by barium or air. This niche is persistent in multiple images and usually projects beyond the gastric mucosa margin. Slight notching (incisura) may be visible along the wall opposite the ulcer. The edematous collar of tissue around the ulcer becomes visible as gastric distention from

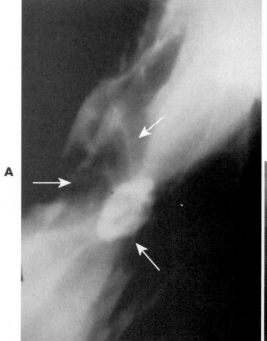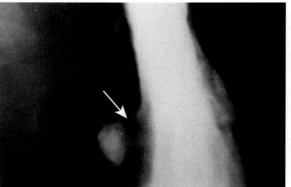

FIG. 30-24   Benign gastric ulcer. **A,** View of the ulcer end on shows that the mucosal folds are thin and regular and extend up to the margin of the ulcer crater *(arrows)*. **B,** Tangential view demonstrating the ulcer collar *(arrow)*. Moderately edematous tissue at the ulcer mouth produces a lucent mound when seen in profile. A large ulcer is seen along the lesser curvature of the stomach. Notice that the ulcer projects beyond the normal expected lesser curvature, a sign suggesting benignancy.

TABLE 30-9
Roentgen Findings of Benign Gastric Ulcers

Roentgen findings	Comments
Radiation of folds	Gastric folds connecting to the ulcer crater
Crater beyond lumen	When viewed in profile, a benign ulcer typically penetrating beyond the expected margin of the lumen
Hampton's line	A thin (1 to 2 mm), lucent line occasionally visible crossing the base of the ulcer
Ulcer collar	Moderately edematous tissue at the ulcer mouth producing a lucent band when seen in profile
Ulcer mound	Lucent mound produced by a large amount of edema surrounding an ulcer, especially when seen in profile; it indicates some retraction from prior scarring
Incisura	Indrawing of the wall opposite the ulcer is a sign of a benign ulcer
Peristalsis	Peristalsis continuing normally through the region of the ulcer; area should be pliable

From Wolf BS: Observations of roentgen features of benign and malignant gastric ulcers, *Semin Roentgenol* 6:140, 1971; Zboralske FF, Stargardter FL, Harell GS: Profile roentgenographic features of benign greater curvature ulcers, *Radiology* 127:63, 1978.

barium or air decreases (Fig. 30-24).[30] When the ulcer crater is seen on profile, a 1-mm thin lucent line traversing the orifice of the ulcer crater, known as the *Hampton line,* may be seen. Table 30-9 identifies the criteria for benign gastric ulcers.

Imaging of the duodenal ulcers does not differ significantly from gastric ulcers. A constant, reproducible collection of barium must be seen, and folds radiating to the crater are characteristic.[12] Duodenal bulb is deformed more often by changes from prior ulcers than is the stomach.[12] The so-called cloverleaf deformity is one created by marked contraction of tissues toward the site of a present or prior ulcer (Fig. 30-25).

CLINICAL COMMENTS

Epigastric pain (dyspepsia) is present in 90% of patients.[9] The more common pain pattern includes increased pain between meals and at night. Ulcer penetration or perforation should be suspected if pain becomes constant or radiates to the back or shoulders. Most patients experience symptomatic periods lasting up to several weeks with intervening pain-free months to years.[9] Gastric outlet obstruction (or gastric malignancy) should be suspected if significant vomiting or weight loss is noted.[12]

KEY CONCEPTS

- *Epigastric pain occurs in 90% of patients with peptic ulcer disease.*
- *Duodenal ulcers are virtually never malignant.*
- *5% of gastric ulcers occur in malignancies.*
- *Upper gastrointestinal study is the procedure of choice for diagnosis of duodenal and gastric ulcers.*

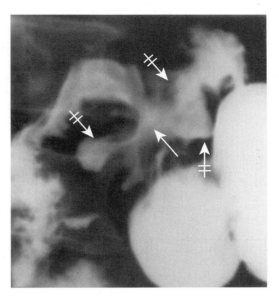

FIG. 30-25 Duodenal ulcer. A small ulcer *(arrow)* is seen in the central portion of the bulb. Note the radiating folds *(crossed arrows)* and bulbar deformity associated with the ulcer.

Ulcerative Colitis

BACKGROUND

Ulcerative colitis is an idiopathic inflammatory condition affecting the mucosal surface of the colon and resulting in diffuse friability and erosions with bleeding. This disease involves only the rectosigmoid region in roughly half of patients.[34] In approximately 30% of patients, ulcerative colitis extends to the splenic flexure and in less than 20% it extends more proximally.[34] Alternating episodes of exacerbations and remissions characterize this process.[34]

IMAGING FINDINGS

Plain radiographs of the abdomen are used to identify significant colonic dilation (>6.5 cm) associated with toxic megacolon (a serious and potentially life-threatening condition) in patients with severe colitis.[34] Barium enema may reveal variable loss of the haustra pattern, a coarse granular appearance of the mucosa, collar button ulcerations, pseudopolyps, decreased rectal distensibility,

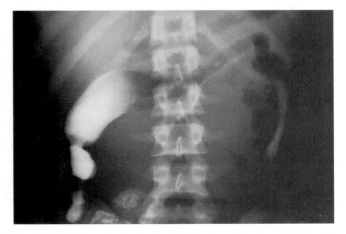

FIG. 30-26 Chronic ulcerative colitis. The colon is shortened, tubular, lacks haustra, and is narrow. (Courtesy John A.M. Taylor, Seneca Falls, NY.)

TABLE 30-10
Complications of Ulcerative Colitis

Complications	Comments
Colorectal cancer	Occurs in approximately 3% of patients
Complications involving bone	Nondeforming migratory polyarthritis of large joints, sacroiliitis and ankylosing spondylitis, osteonecrosis in patients receiving steroids
Hepatobiliary abnormalities	Fatty liver; hepatitis; cirrhosis; ascending cholangitis; portal hypertension
Gallbladder abnormalities	Increased incidence of cholelithiasis, sclerosing cholangitis
Toxic dilatation	Diameter of transverse colon exceeding 6.5 cm

From Kirsner JB: Inflammatory bowel disease part I: nature and pathogenesis, *Disease-a-Month* 37:605, 1991.

and frequent shortening of the colon (Fig. 30-26).[13] As opposed to Crohn's disease, the colon is involved continuously without skip areas; also, no strictures, fistulae, or fissures are present, unlike with Crohn's disease.

CLINICAL COMMENTS

In contrast to Crohn's disease, bloody diarrhea is the hallmark finding in patients with ulcerative colitis.[34] Other symptoms include abdominal cramping, rectal urgency, anorexia, and weight loss.[13] Secondary colon cancer becomes an increasingly significant concern the longer the disease is present. Complications of ulcerative colitis are listed in Table 30-10.[14]

KEY CONCEPTS

- *Bloody diarrhea is the hallmark of ulcerative colitis.*
- *About one half of patients have disease limited to the rectosigmoid region.*
- *Plain films are obtained to look for toxic megacolon.*
- *Barium enema reveals distinctive findings, including a loss of haustra pattern and coarse, granular appearance of the mucosa.*

References

1. Aronson MR, Szucs RA, Turner MA: Gastrointestinal tract abnormalities related to diaphragmatic disorders, *Postgrad Radiol* 16:3, 1996.
2. Ashur H et al: Calcified gallbladder, *Arch Surg* 113:594, 1978.
3. Aucott JN et al: Management of gallstones in diabetic patients, *Arch Intern Med* 153:1053, 1993.
4. Brooks MJ, Maxson CJ, Rubin W: The infectious etiology of peptic ulcer disease: diagnosis and implications for therapy, *Prim Care* 23:443, 1996.
5. Cohen SM, Kurtz AB: Biliary sonography, *Radiol Clin North Am* 29:1171, 1991.
6. Dodds WJ: Esophagus and esophagogastric region including diaphragm. In Margulis AR, Burhenne HJ, editors: Alimentary Tract Radiology, St Louis, 1989, Mosby.
7. Gelfand DW et al: Oral cholecystography vs gallbladder sonography: a prospective, blinded reappraisal, *AJR Am J Roentgenol* 151:69, 1988.
8. Gerson DE, Lewicki AM: Intrathoracic stomach: when does it obstruct? *Radiology* 171:385, 1989.
9. Glick SN: Duodenal ulcer, *Radiol Clin North Am* 32:1259, 1994.
10. Homer MJ, Danford RO: Acute diverticulitis in the young adult, *Radiology* 125:623, 1977.
11. Johnston DE, Kaplan MM: Pathogenesis and treatment of gallstones, *N Engl J Med* 328:412, 1993.
12. Jones B, Braver JM: Essentials of gastrointestinal radiology, Philadelphia, 1982, WB Saunders.
13. Kirsner JB: Inflammatory bowel disease part I: nature and pathogenesis, *Disease-a-Month* 37:605, 1991.
14. Kirsner JB: Inflammatory bowel disease part II: clinical and therapeutic aspects, *Disease-a-Month* 37:669, 1991.
15. Laing FC: Ultrasound diagnosis of choledocholithiasis, *Semin Ultrasound CT MR* 8:103, 1987.
16. Levine MS et al: Atypical hyperplastic polyps at double-contrast barium enema examination, *Radiology* 175:691, 1990.
17. Liddle RA, Goldstein RB, Saxton J: Gallstone formation during weight-reduction dieting, *Arch Intern Med* 149:1750, 1989.
18. Mandel JS et al: Reducing mortality from colorectal cancer by screening for fecal occult blood, *N Engl J Med* 328:1365, 1993.
19. Milner LR: Cancer of the gallbladder: its relationship to gallstones, *Am J Gastroenterol* 39:480, 1963.
20. Minagi H, Margolia FR: Pancreatic calcifications, *Am J Gastoenterol* 57:139, 1972.
21. Norman DC, Yoshikawa TT: Intra-abdominal infections: diagnosis and treatment in the elderly patient, *Gerontology* 30:327, 1984.
22. Ott DJ: The esophagus: diaphragmatic hernias. In Traveras JM, Ferrucci JT, editors: Radiology Diagnosis-Imaging-Intervention, vol 4, Philadelphia, 1996, Lippincott-Raven.
23. Painter NS: Diverticular disease of the colon: a disease of Western civilization, *BMJ* 2:450, 1971.
24. Ranshohoff DF, Gracie WA: Treatment of gallstones, *Ann Intern Med* 119:606, 1993.
25. Raptopoulos V et al: Comparison of real-time and gray scale static ultrasonic cholecystography, *Radiology* 140:153, 1981.
26. Realini JP: Screening for colorectal cancer: issues for primary care physicians, *Prim Care* 15:63, 1988.
27. Ring EJ, Ferrucci JT, Short WF: Differential diagnosis of pancreatic calcification, *AJR Am J Roentgenol* 117:446, 1973.
28. Sarles H, Sahel J: Pathology of chronic calcifying pancreatitis, *Am J Gastroenterol* 66:117, 1976.
29. Skucas J, Gasparaitis AE: Colon cancer. In Traveras JM, Ferrucci JT, editors: Radiology Diagnosis-Imaging-Intervention, vol 4, Philadelphia, 1996, Lippincott-Raven.
30. Stevenson GW: Gastric ulcers. In Traveras JM, Ferrucci JT, editors: Radiology Diagnosis-Imaging-Intervention, vol 4, Philadelphia, 1996, Lippincott-Raven.
31. Tait N, Little JM: The treatment of gallstones, *BMJ* 311:99, 1995.
32. Thoeni RFL, Bischof TP: Colonic polyps. In Traveras JM, Ferrucci JT, editors: Radiology Diagnosis-Imaging-Intervention, vol 4, Philadelphia, 1996, Lippincott-Raven.
33. Thoeni RFL, Menuck L: Comparison of barium enema and colonoscopy in the detection of small colonic polyps, *Radiology* 124:631, 1977.
34. Tierney LM Jr, McPhee SJ, Papadakis MA, editors: The alimentary tract. In Current Medical Diagnosis and Treatment 1997, ed 36, Stanford, CT, 1997, Appleton & Lange.
35. Toribara NW, Sleisenger MH: Screening for colorectal cancer, *N Engl J Med* 332:861, 1995.
36. Williams I, Fleischchner FG: Diverticular disease of the colon. In Margulis AR, Burhenne HJ, editors: Alimentary Tract Roentgenology, ed 2, St Louis, 1973, Mosby.
37. Wilson JM: Diverticular disease of the colon, *Prim Care* 15:111, 1988.
38. Wingo PA, Tong T, Bolden S: Cancer statistics 1995, *CA Cancer J Clin* 45:8, 1995.
39. Wolf BS: Observations of roentgen features of benign and malignant gastric ulcers, *Semin Roentgenol* 6:140, 1971.
40. Zboralske FF, Stargardter FL, Harell GS: Profile roentgenographic features of benign greater curvature ulcers, *Radiology* 127:63, 1978.

chapter 31

Miscellaneous Abdomen Diseases

BEVERLY L. HARGER
LISA E. HOFFMAN
RICHARD ARKLESS

Abdominal Aortic Aneurysm
Acute Abdomen
Hydatid Disease

Abdominal Aortic Aneurysm

DEFINITION

Focal dilation of the infrarenal abdominal aorta of at least 150% of the normal diameter (range 1.4 to 3.0 cm, average 2.0 cm) is the usual definition of an aneurysm.[18] Therefore aortic dilation above 3 cm indicates a possible aneurysm. Some sources state that 4.0 cm is clearly diagnostic.[18,10] Consultation with an experienced surgeon is indicated when it reaches a diameter of 5.0 cm (some say 5.5 cm).

INCIDENCE

Abdominal aortic aneurysm (AAA) affects approximately 2% to 8% of the population over 60 years of age.[18] Incidence increases rapidly in men after age 55 and in women after age 70. Overall incidence and deaths resulting from AAA are more common in men.[6,14] In one screening study of nearly 30,000 65-year-old men, the prevalence of AAA (confirmed by at least two ultrasound studies) was 5% and 80% of AAAs detected were smaller than 4.0 cm.[11]

RUPTURE (RATES AND MORTALITY)

Each year in the United States more than 15,000 deaths, many of which are preventable, are attributed to abdominal aortic aneurysm.[4] Natural history of most aneurysms is one of gradual enlargement; growth rates have been estimated to average 0.2 cm/year for aneurysms under 4 cm and 0.5 cm/year for those over 6 cm.[18] Although impossible to predict for a given individual, the risk of AAA rupture increases with larger initial aneurysm diameter, hypertension, and chronic obstructive pulmonary disease (COPD). Expansion rates of AAAs for men 65 years of age are listed in Table 31-1.[11] Rupture of AAA is considered essentially inevitable if the patient lives long enough.[14] Once rupture occurs, massive intraabdominal bleeding usually occurs and usually is fatal, with a mortality rate of 80% to 90%, unless prompt surgery can be performed.[4,18] A relatively low risk of rupture is seen for asymptomatic, slow-growing AAA under 6 cm. Table 31-2 lists the estimated annual rates of rupture related to AAA.[9,18]

RISK FACTORS

The underlying cause of AAA is multifactorial, including such factors as smoking, hypertension, and processes that result in an inflammation that may lead to dilatation and subsequent plaque deposition.[7] Other uncommon possible causes include infection, inflammatory disease, increased protease activity within the arterial wall, genetically regulated defects in collagen and fibrillin, and mechanical factors.[7] An individual's risk is increased twelve-fold if a first-degree relative has an AAA.[6] In addition to family history of aneurysms, increasing age and male gender are established risk factors. Understanding the established as well as possible risk factors assists the clinician in determining an index of suspicion for the presence of AAA (Table 31-3). AAA is best repaired as an elective, not emergency, procedure.

IMAGING FINDINGS

Ultrasonography (US) reaches almost 100% accuracy[18] in detecting AAA, making it ideal for screening, diagnosis, and follow-up studies in suspected cases.[3] Obesity and excessive bowel gas may interfere with US imaging.[14] Approximately 50% of AAAs may be seen as cystlike calcifications on plain film radiography resulting from the calcium content of atherosclerotic plaques (Figs. 31-1 through 31-9).[14]

Computed tomography (CT) provides better anatomic detail, especially regarding the aneurysm's relationship to the renal arteries, which is very important information for surgical planning (see Fig. 31-3). Magnetic resonance imaging (MRI) demonstrates excellent anatomic detail and sizing of aneurysms but provides no

TABLE 31-1

Expansion Rate of Abdominal Aortic Aneurysm Based on Initial Size

Initial size measured on ultrasound	Expansion rate per year
2.6–2.9 cm	0.09 cm
3.0–3.4 cm	0.16 cm
3.5–3.9 cm	0.32 cm

TABLE 31-2

Estimated Annual Rates of Rupture Related to Abdominal Aortic Aneurysm Size

Size of abdominal aortic aneurysm	Annual rate of rupture
4.0–4.9 cm	1%
5.0–5.9 cm	3%
6.0–6.9 cm	9%
≥7.0 cm	25%

distinct advantage and is more expensive than CT. Aortography often is ordered for surgical planning, although it is not appropriate for diagnosis.[14] It may significantly underestimate the width of the aneurysm because large areas of thrombus can fill an aneurysm and aortography shows only the residual central canal (which can resemble a normal-sized aorta).

Diagnosis is made by US for the majority of patients, and preoperative planning is based on aortography. US (which is faster and less expensive than other methods) and CT are ways to follow up nonsurgical cases in which the diameter is less than 5 cm, although some surgeons feel this is too large a dividing point.[14]

SCREENING FOR ABDOMINAL AORTIC ANEURYSM

Most AAA are asymptomatic and are discovered on routine physical examination or via imaging for other complaints.[16] A pulsatile abdominal mass may be palpated, although the aorta in a thin person with an accentuated lower lumbar lordosis can feel spuriously aneurysmal. Also, the larger the aneurysm, the less likely it is that pulsations will be felt. Obesity limits the effectiveness of abdominal palpation for the detection of AAA.[4,10] A caveat is that physical examination should not be relied on to rule out the

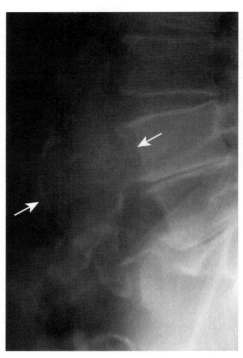

FIG. 31-1   Abdominal aortic aneurysm. Lateral view demonstrates a calcified wall of a fusiform abdominal aorta (arrows). Plain film visualization is possible because of the calcium content of atherosclerotic plaques. Most abdominal aortic aneurysms occur between the renal artery and iliac bifurcation.

presence of AAA in cases with clinical suspicion.[10] Abdominal examination plays a complementary rather than competitive role to US in the detection of AAA.[19]

Conclusive evidence that screening is cost-effective and significantly reduces overall mortality in older patients is still unavailable; however, a selective screening program may be useful in white

TABLE 31-3

Risk Factors for Developing Abdominal Aortic Aneurysm

Established risk factors	Comments
Increasing age	Most studies focus on ages 65–80
Male gender	More frequent and at an earlier age than in females. The male to female ratio for death from abdominal aortic aneurysm (AAA) is 11:1 between ages 60 and 64 and narrows to 3:1 between 85 and 90
Family history of aneurysm	Increases individual's risk twice, especially first-degree male relative
Possible risk factors	**Comments**
Tobacco use	Long-term smoking increases individual's risk five times over the baseline
Systemic atherosclerosis disease	Including peripheral arterial disease, cerebrovascular disease, history of coronary artery bypass, history of myocardial infarct have modest correlation; less association with smaller AAA than with larger AAAs
Chronic obstructive pulmonary disease	Difficult to establish as an independent risk factor
Hypertension	Weak correlation
Hypercholesterolemia	Weak correlation, specifically related to hypertriglyceridemia
Caucasian race	AAAs are uncommon in African Americans, Asians, and Hispanics

From Ebaugh JL, Garcia ND, Matsumura JS: Screening and surveillance for abdominal aortic aneurysms: who needs it and when, *Semin Vasc Surg* 14(3):193, 2001; Lederle FA, Simel DL: Does this patient have abdominal aortic aneurysm? *JAMA* 281:17, 1999; U.S. Preventive Services Task Force: Guide to clinical preventive services, ed 2, Washington, DC, 1996, U.S. Department of Health and Human Services, Office of Disease Prevention and Health Promotion.

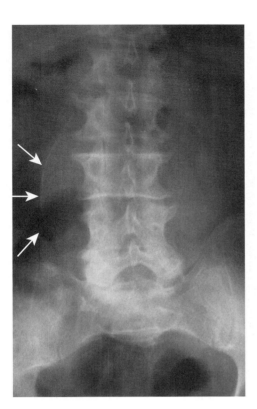

FIG. 31-2 Abdominal aortic aneurysm presenting in an anteroposterior lumbar projection. Note the characteristic thin rim of curvilinear calcification *(arrows)*. The location to the right of the spine indicates an extremely large aneurysm. (Courtesy Cynthia Peterson, Toronto, Ontario, Canada.)

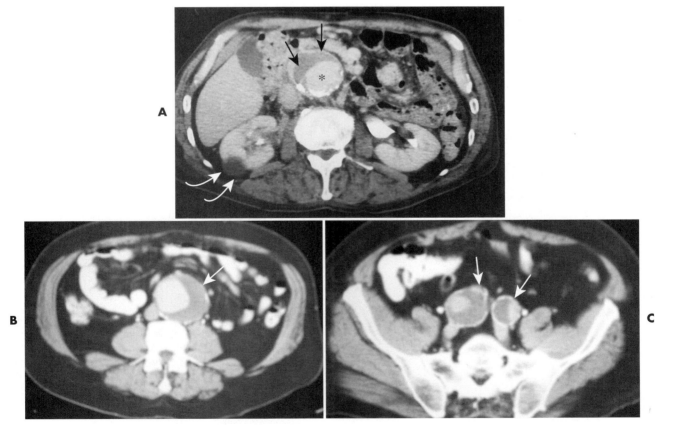

FIG. 31-3 **A,** Abdominal aortic aneurysm: computed tomography with intravenous contrast. This scan shows a large, partially calcified abdominal aortic aneurysm anterior to the spine. Within the aneurysm is a region of increased density *(asterisk)* that corresponds to the functional lumen of the aneurysm; the remaining low-attenuated region represents a large thrombus *(arrows)*. Note the renal cyst *(curved arrows)*. **B** and **C,** Same imaging methods applied to a different patient reveal abdominal aortic and iliac aneurysms *(arrows)*. (**B** and **C,** Courtesy Julie-Marthe Grenier, Davenport, IA.)

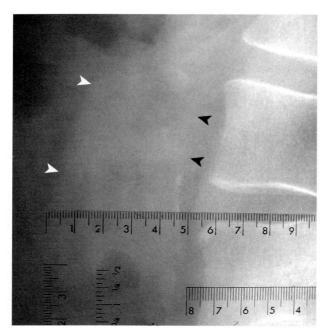

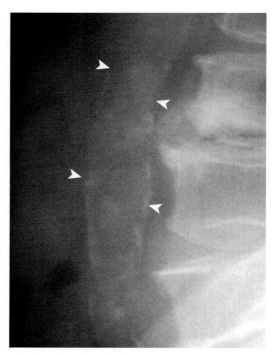

FIG. 31-4 Abdominal aortic aneurysm measuring 4.7 cm on the lateral 40-inch focal film distance lateral lumbar projection. Any measure larger than 3.0 cm is suspicious of aneurysm, and values over 4.0 cm warrant further investigation with ultrasound. In this case, the ultrasound examination validated the presence of aneurysm. Note the faint linear radiodensity of the anteroposterior margin of the vessel *(arrowheads)*. Interpreters are cautioned not to assume that wall calcification is requisite to aneurysm formation. Any suggestive linear shadows, as seen in this case, warrant consideration for an ultrasound examination.

FIG. 31-5 Aorta is calcified, but not enlarged *(arrowheads)*. No evidence of aneurysm is present in this case. The sole finding of vascular wall calcification of the abdominal aorta does not warrant further investigation.

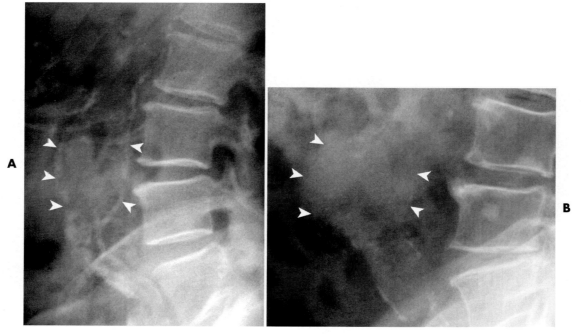

FIG. 31-6 **A** and **B,** Two cases of an expanded aorta *(arrowheads)* consistent with aneurysm.

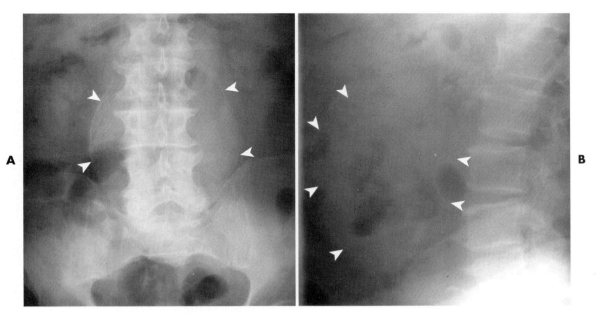

FIG. 31-7 A 12.5-cm aneurysm seen in prominently in, **A,** the anteroposterior projection and, **B,** only faintly in the lateral projection (*arrowheads*). (Courtesy Robert C. Tatum, Davenport, IA.)

PART FOUR
Abdomen

men over the age of 60, especially those with a history of smoking; patients with aneurysms of the popliteal or femoral arteries; or patients who have a first-degree relative with an AAA.[4,14]

MANAGEMENT

Leakage, rapid expansion, or rupture may produce mild to severe flank, back, abdominal, testicular, or groin pain. Hypovolemic

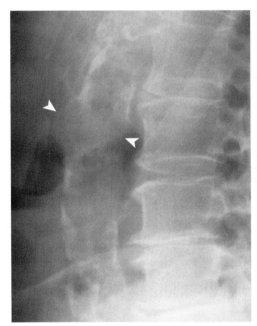

FIG. 31-8 A 74-year-old man exhibiting prominent calcification of the anterior and posterior walls of the abdominal aorta. A focal dilation of 4.7 cm is noted (*arrowheads*), consistent with aneurysm. In addition to the overall size of the vessel, aneurysms often exhibit a focal bulge, disrupting the parallel continuity of the walls of the vessel. For instance, the focal nature of the budge seen in this case would represent a concern for aneurysm, regardless of its size.

shock may follow rupture. The death rate increases twelve-fold in patients experiencing rupture versus patients undergoing elective surgery. Surgical repair is recommended for all symptomatic or ruptured AAAs, and for asymptomatic AAAs measuring over 5 cm, unless strong contraindications to surgery are identified.[3] Surgery is not commonly recommended for AAAs measuring less than 4 cm.[3] Those measuring 4 to 5 cm represent a gray area, in which case the risk of surgery is weighed against the risk of rupture.[3,6] All saccular AAAs should be treated because of an increased risk of rupture.

> ### KEY CONCEPTS
> - *The incidence of abdominal aortic aneurysms (AAAs) increases in men after age 55 and in women after age 70.*
> - *Risk is increased in patients with a first-degree relative who has AAA, patients with a history of smoking, patients with hypertension, and patients with a connective tissue disease.*
> - *Most patients are asymptomatic.*
> - *Fifty percent of AAAs can be seen on plain film.*
> - *Ultrasound is a sensitive and specific modality for detection of AAA.*

Acute Abdomen

BACKGROUND

Plain film radiography typically follows history and physical examination in the evaluation of the acute abdomen. Nevertheless, plain film findings are interpreted most often as nonspecific or normal in these cases. Sensitivity is extremely low for common causes such as appendicitis, pyelonephritis, pancreatitis, and diverticulitis.[12] CT often is the first choice in imaging modalities in the evaluation of patients with acute abdominal pain.[15] Abdominal and pelvic CT is rapidly developing as the most appropriate imaging modality. Improvements in resolution, reduced acquisition time, and other technical improvements are leading to increased applicability of multislice CT in the evaluation of acute abdominal disease.[8]

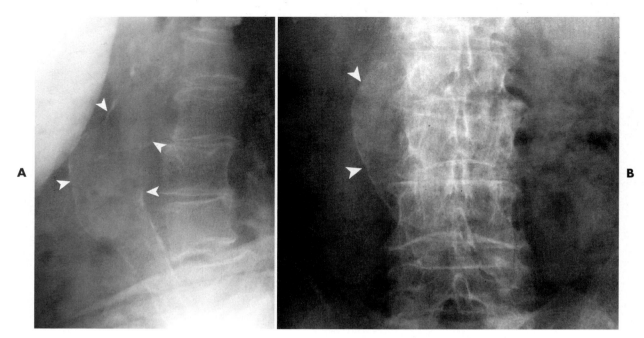

FIG. 31-9 **A** and **B,** Aneurysm of the abdominal aorta presenting in an 87-year-old man. Largest visible diameter of the vessel measures 5.8 cm *(arrowheads).*

US may be a useful tool in acute situations because of its accessibility.[18] MRI often is used as a second modality in problematic cases. Its lack of ionizing radiation can be of importance in some cases.[13] Nuclear medicine is indicated typically for the localization of acute gastrointestinal (GI) bleeding.[20] Plain film radiographs can aid in diagnosis by revealing the configuration of intestinal gas and the presence and location of tubes and surgical artifacts. Plain film can provide significant information in the evaluation of obstruction or adynamic ileus.[15]

IMAGING FINDINGS AND CLINICAL COMMENTS

Appendicitis is the most common cause of acute abdominal pain, and CT frequently provides a specific diagnosis (Box 31-1).[12] Some of the more common diagnoses presenting with acute abdominal pain are listed in Table 31-4. Other conditions that may present with acute abdominal pain and that can be diagnosed with CT include Crohn's disease, epiploic appendagitis, infectious ileitis, mesenteric adenitis, omental infarction, Meckel's diverticulitis, cholecystitis, ureteral stone, aortic aneurysm, large and small bowel volvulus, intussusception, diverticulitis, ruptured ovarian cyst, perforated ulcer, various types of hernias, and intestinal ischemia.[12]

Historically, diagnostic imaging has not been a significant tool in the diagnosis of acute appendicitis, but the classic diagnostic signs and symptoms are not always present. This has produced a high rate of false-positive diagnoses, particularly in young women who have acute gynecologic conditions. CT and US significantly reduce this rate. Sensitivity of CT in the diagnosis of acute appendicitis is reported to be in the 90% to 96% range. CT also is reasonably accurate in differentiating competing diagnoses. US has a sensitivity rate reported to be near 75% (although probably considerably lower than that in most centers) but does not expose the patient to ionizing radiation.[12]

US is the preferred imaging modality in suspected acute gallbladder pathosis, and hepatobiliary scintography is helpful in

---

BOX 31-1

Computed Tomographic Features of
Acute Appendicitis

Appendiceal diameter >6 mm with periappendiceal inflammation
Nonopacification of appendix with oral or rectal contrast material
  with periappendiceal inflammation
Presence of an appendicolith

TABLE 31-4
Acute Abdominal Pain

Diagnosis	Percent of 10,682 patients
Appendicitis	28
Cholecystitis	9.7
Small bowel obstruction	4.1
Gynecologic disorders	4
Pancreatitis	2.9
Renal colic	2.9
Peptic ulcer disease	2.5
Cancer	1.5
Diverticular disease	1.5
Other conditions	9
No specific diagnosis	34

From De Dombal FT: Diagnosis of acute abdominal pain, ed 2, New York, 1991, Churchill Livingstone.

problem cases. CT is seldom needed here unless there is the clinical question of another possible abnormality.[1] CT provides more information about the abdomen in general and may be more likely to provide the diagnostic information for a wider range of differential diagnoses. CT can accurately assess complications of many pathologies, thus providing significant management information.[1]

The classic triad of radiographic findings (small bowel obstruction, large gallstone, and pneumobilia) is a rare condition that is present in 30% to 35% of cases of gallstones ileus. CT is more sensitive to these findings and more accurate in determining the site of obstruction.[1]

GI perforation may follow blunt, penetrating, or iatrogenic trauma, inflammatory conditions such as Crohn's disease, ruptured stomach or bowel ulcer, clostridium colon infection, diverticulitis, or invasive neoplasm (Table 31-5). CT and luminal water-soluble contrast agents are the preferred imaging modalities for demonstrating perforation. CT best demonstrates extraluminal air, fluid, or abscess and can delineate extraluminal changes secondary to the perforation. Contrast GI studies often best determine the site of perforation and can provide information regarding the etiology. Plain film radiographs may demonstrate free intraperitoneal gas but are inferior to both CT and contrast studies in the evaluation of the cause of the perforation.[15]

Adynamic ileus is a significant clinical concern, and the underlying cause must be determined. Clinically it can suggest bowel obstruction but results from immotility rather than mechanical obstruction. The radiographic appearance of mechanical obstruction, especially partial obstruction, and adynamic ileus can be similar, with both presenting dilated, fluid-filled loops of bowel. However, in obstruction the dilated loops show a hairpinlike appearance, as opposed to the flaccid loops of bowel seen with "paralyzed" (adynamic) bowel in adynamic ileus. The presence of "thumbprinting" (thickening of mucosal folds) can indicate bowel infarction in cases of obstruction. Both entities can result in bowel rupture. Table 31-6 displays some of the differentiating factors

TABLE 31-5
Sites and Causes of Perforation

Location of perforation	Causes
Esophagus	Boerhaave syndrome
	Mallory-Weiss tears
	Sudden increase in intraabdominal pressure
Stomach	Ulcers
	Postsurgical leaks
Small bowel	Ischemia
	Blunt trauma
	Inflammatory conditions such as Crohn's disease and diverticulitis
	Perforating tumors
	Postsurgical complications
Colon	Diverticulitis
	Carcinoma
	Volvulus
	Barium enema complication
	Colonoscopy complication
Biliary tree	Trauma
	Cholecystitis
	Surgery
	Endoscopic retrograde cholangiopancreatography
	Percutaneous transhepatic cholangiography

From Rubesin GE, Levine MS: Radiologic diagnosis of gastrointestinal perforation, *Radiol Clin North Am* 41:1095, 2003.

TABLE 31-6
Differentiating Adynamic Ileus and Mechanical Obstruction

Finding	Adynamic ileus	Mechanical obstruction
Clinical signs/symptoms	Minimal tenderness Distention Nausea, vomiting Decreased bowel sounds Tympany	Vomiting Cramping pain Tenderness Late in obstruction the bowel may become adynamic
Radiographic signs	Gas-filled, dilated loops of both large and small bowel; "sentinel loop" is limited to a smaller segment, often a single loop, of bowel with localized cause	Dilated loops of small bowel, often with fluid levels Decreased air in colon
Causes	Postsurgical complication Peritonitis Electrolyte imbalance Severe systemic illness Acute pancreatitis Ruptured viscus Hemorrhage Acute appendicitis Trauma Some medications	Adhesions Hernias Crohn's disease Volvulus Gallstone ileus Radiation enteritis Bowel wall hematoma Neoplasm

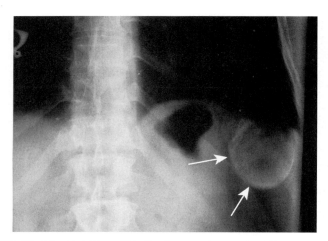

FIG. 31-10　Hydatid cyst. Plain film demonstrates a cystic calcified abdominal mass in the left upper quadrant *(arrows)*, proved to be a hydatid cyst of the spleen.

between these two diagnoses. Plain film radiographs can confirm and monitor adynamic ileus but may not be able to rule out obstruction. Obstruction is evaluated best with intraluminal contrast studies.

KEY CONCEPTS

- *Plain film findings most often are nonspecific or normal.*
- *Computed tomography (CT) often is the first choice imaging modality, except in gallbladder and female reproductive organ diseases.*
- *Appendicitis is the most common cause of acute abdomen.*
- *CT and ultrasonography should be considered, especially if a woman presents with an acute abdomen.*

Hydatid Disease

BACKGROUND

Hydatid cysts represent infestation by the *Echinococcus granulosus* or *Echinococcus multilocularis* (tapeworm) parasite. Sheep,

cattle, hogs, and deer are the common intermediate hosts for *E. granulosus;* dogs often play an important role in transmitting this parasite to humans. Rodents are the primary intermediate host for *E. multilocularis.*[5] Hydatid cysts are slow growing and may affect the liver, lungs, muscle, bone, kidney, and brain. *Echinococcus* infestation is most common in ranching areas of Australia, South America, and Mediterranean countries. The disease is rare in North America but occasionally is seen in sheepherders of Basque descent in California and Idaho and sheep ranchers in Utah, New Mexico, and Arizona. It is seen more often in immigrants who bring the disease with them. Cases in Alaska have been linked to caribou.[5]

IMAGING FINDINGS

Hydatid cysts may be seen involving the liver, peritoneum, kidney, spleen, or bladder on abdominal imaging. The liver is involved frequently; multiple cysts occur in about 20% of cases.[5] These cysts average 5 cm in diameter but may grow to 50 cm. Cystic calcification may be seen on plain film (Figs. 31-10 through 31-13). CT shows well-defined round masses with or without internal septations. The cyst wall and septations are visible with contrast. Frequently US demonstrates a complex heterogeneous mass. Well-defined anechoic cysts are another common presentation. Identification of "daughter cysts" within a cyst is pathognomonic but rare.[17]

CLINICAL COMMENTS

Most hydatid cysts are asymptomatic when discovered. Symptoms are produced most commonly by mass effect or are a result of leakage or rupture of the cyst. Eosinophilia may result from allergic reaction to slow leaks. Anaphylaxis and death can result from acute rupture.[5] The only treatment is surgical excision, which is recommended for liver cysts over 5 cm and all pulmonary cysts. Cysts located in nonvital areas may be monitored.[5] Aspiration is contraindicated because of the potentially life-threatening allergic reaction to leakage.[5]

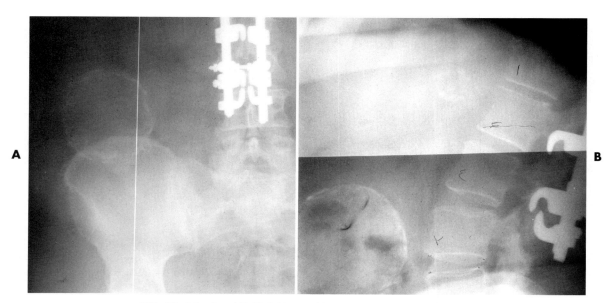

FIG. 31-11　**A** and **B,** Hydatid cyst of the right lower abdominal quadrant.

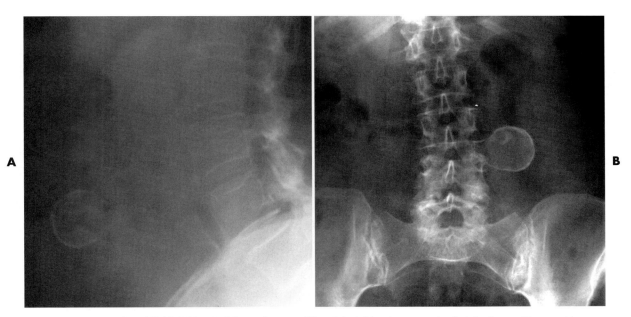

FIG. 31-12 **A** and **B,** Hydatid cyst of the peritoneum. Although hydatid cysts commonly affect the liver and lung, a wide range of tissues and organs may be involved. (Courtesy Gary Longmuir, Phoenix, AZ.)

KEY CONCEPTS

- *Sheep, cows, and pigs are intermediate hosts with dogs providing a route to humans.*
- *Most cysts are asymptomatic; mass effect, leakage, or rupture produces symptoms.*
- *Cystic calcification may be seen.*
- *Aspiration is contraindicated because of potential anaphylactic response to rupture.*

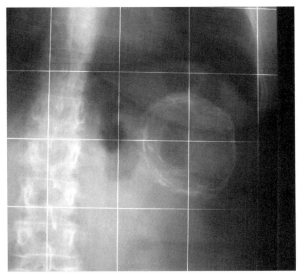

FIG. 31-13 Large hydatid cyst of the spleen.

References

1. Bennett GL, Balthazar EJ: Ultrasound and CT evaluation of emergent gallbladder pathology, *Radiol Clin North Am* 41:1203, 2003.
2. De Dombal FT: Diagnosis of acute abdominal pain, ed 2, New York, 1991, Churchill Livingstone.
3. Desforges JF: Abdominal aortic aneurysm, *N Engl J Med* 328:1167, 1993.
4. Ebaugh JL, Garcia ND, Matsumura JS: Screening and surveillance for abdominal aortic aneurysms: who needs it and when, *Semin Vasc Surg* 14(3):193, 2001.
5. Elliot DL et al: Pet-associated illness, *N Engl J Med* 313:985, 1985.
6. Fine LG: Abdominal aortic aneurysm: grand round, *Lancet* 341:215, 1993.
7. Gorski Y, Ricotta JJ: Weighing risks in abdominal aortic aneurysm, *Postgrad Med* 10692:69, 1999.
8. Kundra V, Silverman PM: Impact of multislice CT on imaging of acute abdominal disease, *Radiol Clin North Am* 41:1083, 2003.
9. Law MR, Morris J, Wald NJ: Screening for abdominal aortic aneurysms, *J Med Screening* 1:110, 1994.
10. Lederle FA, Simel DL: Does this patient have abdominal aortic aneurysm? *JAMA* 281:17, 1999.
11. McCarthy R et al: Recommendations for screening intervals for small aortic aneurysms, *Br J Surg* 90:821, 2003.
12. Macari M, Balthazar EJ: The acute right lower quadrant: CT evaluation, *Radiol Clin North Am* 41:1117, 2003.
13. Pedrosa I, Forsky NM: MR imaging in abdominal emergencies, *Radiol Clin North Am* 41:1243, 2003.
14. Rose WW III, Ernst CB: Abdominal aortic aneurysm, *Compr Ther* 21:339, 1995.
15. Rubesin GE, Levine MS: Radiologic diagnosis of gastrointestinal perforation, *Radiol Clin North Am* 41:1095, 2003.

16. Tierney LM, Messina LM: Blood vessels and lymphatics. In Tierney LM, McFhee SJ, Papadakis MA, editors: Current Medical Diagnosis and Treatment, ed 36, Stamford, CT, 1997, Appleton & Lange.

17. Tierney LM, Messina LM: Infectious diseases: protozoal & helminthic. In Tierney LM, McPhee SJ, Papdakis MA, editors: Current Medical Diagnosis and Treatment, ed 36, Stamford, CT, 1997, Appleton & Lange.

18. U.S. Preventive Services Task Force: Guide to clinical preventive services, ed 2, Washington, DC, 1996, U.S. Department of Health and Human Services, Office of Disease Prevention and Health Promotion.

19. Venkatasubramaniam AK et al: The value of abdominal examination in the diagnosis of abdominal aortic aneurysm, *Eur J Vasc Endovasc Surg* 24:56, 2004.

20. Zuckier LS, Freeman LM: Selective role of nuclear medicine in evaluating the acute abdomen, *Radiol Clin North Am* 41:1275, 2003.

chapter 32

Abdomen Patterns

BEVERLY L. HARGER
LISA E. HOFFMAN
RICHARD ARKLESS

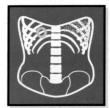

AB 1 | Abdominal Calcifications

Numerous pathologic processes in the abdomen may cause soft-tissue calcification. A pattern approach that evaluates the morphologic features, location, and mobility of an abnormal opacity often provides sufficient information for a definitive diagnosis or at least narrows the etiologic considerations to a few possibilities.[3] Almost all abdominal calcifications fall into four major morphologic categories. Each one of the four categories possesses characteristic roentgen features based on shape, border sharpness, marginal continuity, and internal architecture.[3] The four morphologic categories are concretions, conduit wall calcification, cystic calcification, and solid mass calcification (Table 32-1).[3] A concretion represents calcification within the lumen of a vessel or hollow viscera. The most common of these are listed in Table 32-2. Concretions typically do not pass through vascular or visceral walls; therefore they seldom are seen outside their expected locations. Calcification with the wall of fluid-containing hollow tubes (e.g., parts of the urinary tract, the pancreatic ducts, vas deferens, biliary ductal system, and arteries and veins) is known as *conduit wall pattern*. Calcification within the wall of a hollow mass is characteristic of the cystic morphologic category. Lastly, the solid mass calcification can be found anywhere within the abdomen and may be central or peripheral, adjacent to or within organs, or in the intraperitoneal or retroperitoneal spaces.

Several limitations of classification according to radiographic morphology exist. When a calcification is small, it is difficult to categorize. Furthermore, faint calcification cannot be classified if no information about margins or internal matrix can be ascertained.[3]

The following is a brief presentation of each of the four major morphologic categories (AB1a through AB1d) with the most common etiologic considerations.

TABLE 32-1
Comparison of Roentgen Features of Abdominal Calcifications

Morphology	Shape	Border	Margin	Internal appearance
Concretion (stone)	Varied (round or oval, faceted); occasional unique shape such as star-shaped bladder calculi or "staghorn" calculus	Sharp, clearly defined; may occasionally have irregular bulges	Continuous; if outer perimeter is incomplete, it is unlikely a stone	Varied Multiple laminations (unequivocal indication of concretion) Homogenously dense Single central lucency Outer margin is dense and continuous with lucent internal appearance
Conduit	Tubular, tracklike appearance when viewed in profile; ringlike appearance when viewed en face	May be indistinct	Discontinuous, irregular	None; presence of internal radiopacity suggests another morphologic category
Cystic	Round or oval; may be compressed on one side; shape depends on location	Smooth, curvilinear rim of opacification	Rim calcification may be continuous or interrupted; short arcs may be only visibly calcified portion	Surfaces with extensive calcium deposition that are not tangential to x-ray beam may simulate internal matrix (masslike) calcification; interior calcifications less dense than marginal calcifications
Mass	Varied	Irregular calcified border; occasionally, the border is more densely calcified than interior resembling cyst	Interrupted; margins typically appear notched or slightly angulated	Extensive interior calcification; mottled densities with scattered radiolucencies; flocculent calcification superimposed on lucent background

From Baker SR: The abdominal plain film, ed 1, Norwalk, CT, 1990, Appleton & Lange.

TABLE 32-2
Sites of Concretions

Site	Comments
Pelvic veins (phleboliths)	Represent calcification within preexisting venous thrombi; typical appearance is round opacity with a central or slightly eccentric single lucency
Gallbladder (choleliths)	Circumferential laminations are encountered frequently
Urinary tract (nephroliths)	Ureteral calculi are often angular; bladder stones are most often smooth and laminated; renal calculus occupying the pelvicaliceal system may have an appearance of a "staghorn" distinguishing it from other abdominal radiopacities
Prostate	Predominantly within elderly men
Appendix (appendicolith, fecalith)	Usually encountered in younger patients; appendicoliths often are laminated; essentially considered a surgical indicator
Pancreas	Typically present as discrete opacities that cross the midline at the level of the L1-2 vertebral bodies; discrete opacities present in head of pancreas alone (25% of cases)

ABIa | Concretions

A concretion (also called a *stone* or *calculus*) is a calcified mass that forms in a tubular or hollow structure such as the lumen of a vessel or hollow viscus. A fairly constant appearance of concretions is a sharp, clearly defined external margin that almost always is continuous.[3] This continuity may help differentiate a concretion in a hollow viscus (e.g., renal pelvis, gallbladder, urinary bladder) from a calcified cyst. Discontinuity of the outer margin makes a diagnosis of a stone unlikely. The internal architecture of concretions may vary in appearance. Concretions may have concentric laminations, contain a slightly eccentric area of lucency, or be homogenously dense. On occasion a concretion's outer margin is dense and continuous with a lucent internal appearance. Generally concretions are seen in association with anatomic structures and do not pass through the vascular or visceral wall. Concretions appearing outside of common, expected anatomic locations are unusual.

CONCRETION	COMMENTS
Appendicolith (FIG. 32-1)	Frequently associated with current or future appendiceal perforation, especially in children;[18] it is seen most commonly in the right lower quadrant but location may vary.
Cholelithiasis (FIG. 32-2) [p. 1287]	Ten to fifteen percent are calcified and therefore visible on plain film;[30,62] cholelithiasis occurs more frequently in elderly and obese people, predominantly in women;[30] typically cholelithiasis occurs in the right upper quadrant, but location may vary.
Pancreatic calculi (FIG. 32-3)	Most commonly associated with chronic pancreatitis secondary to alcoholism;[61] the typical appearance is multiple, tiny, dense, discrete opacities that cross the midline at the level of L1-2.
Phleboliths (FIG. 32-4)	Most commonly encountered calcification in pelvis;[3] they are frequently multiple and bilateral; sometimes a concentric or slightly eccentric interior lucency occurs; they can be confused with urinary tract stones; should not appear midline; collections of phleboliths outside the area of the pelvic bowl veins may indicate the presence of a soft-tissue hemangioma.
Prostatic calculi (FIG. 32-5)	Multiple concretions of varied sizes clustered behind pubic symphysis in men usually more than 40 years of age;[3] this condition results from prior prostatitis; prostatic calculi often are asymptomatic.
Urinary tract calculi (FIGS. 32-6 TO 32-8)	May be seen in the renal calyces or pelvis, ureters, and bladder; they are uncommon in the urethra;[52] sometimes urinary tract calculi are associated with conditions producing hypercalcemia or hypercalciuria.[3]

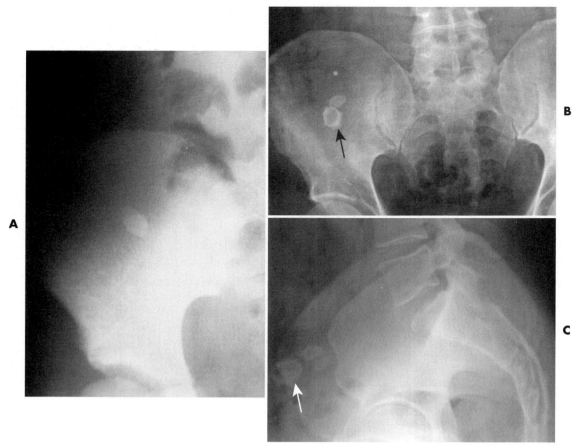

FIG. 32-1   Appendicoliths. **A,** Concretion in the right lower quadrant in a child. Appendicolith may indicate appendicitis with perforation and abscess. Notice the sharp, continuous external margin characteristic of a concretion. The concretion in this case is uniformly dense. **B** and **C,** Large concretion of the right lower abdominal quadrant consistent with appendicolith *(arrows)* in a second patient. (**B** and **C,** Courtesy C. Robert Tatum, Davenport, IA.)

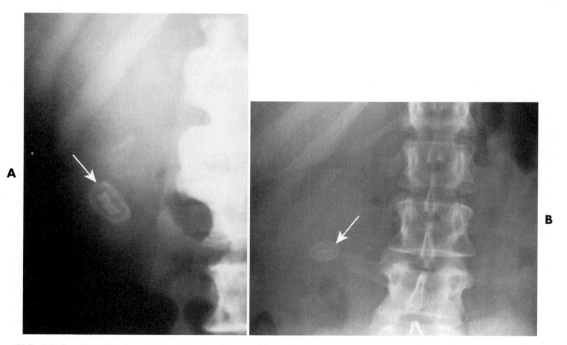

FIG. 32-2   Cholelith. **A** and **B,** Laminated gallstone with continuous outer margin typical of a concretion *(arrow)* in different patients. (**A,** Courtesy John A.M. Taylor, Seneca Falls, NY.)

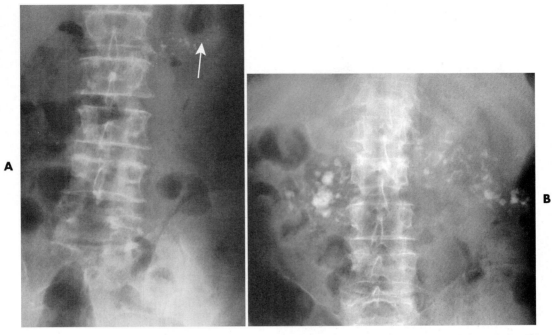

FIG. 32-3 A and **B,** Two patients with pancreatic calculi and chronic pancreatitis in a patient suffering from alcoholism. This is the typical appearance of numerous dense, discrete opacities that cross the midline at the level of L1-2 *(arrow)*. The normal pancreas is not visible on abdominal plain films.

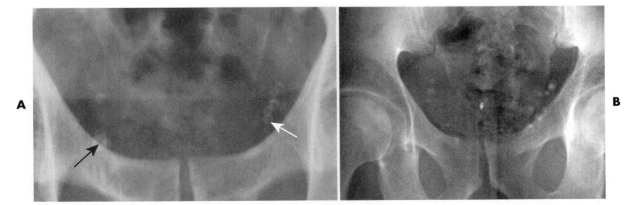

FIG. 32-4 A and **B,** Numerous phleboliths in two patients. Phleboliths frequently are multiple and bilateral, and they are asymptomatic. They are inconsequential concretions of thrombi attached to the walls of veins. Observe the concentric interior lucency of the phleboliths *(arrows)*. These should not be confused with ureteral stones or calcifications of a pelvic mass.

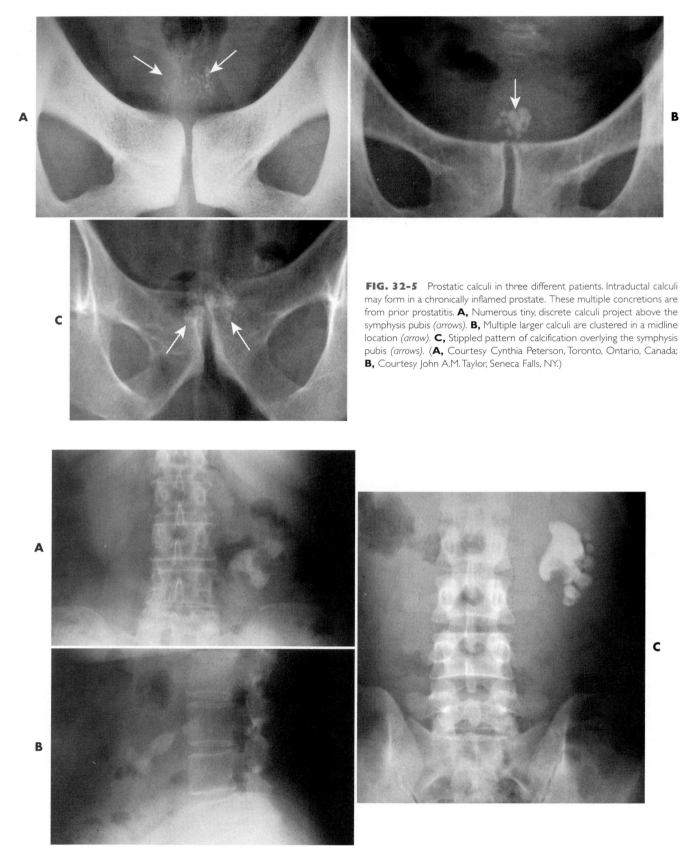

FIG. 32-5 Prostatic calculi in three different patients. Intraductal calculi may form in a chronically inflamed prostate. These multiple concretions are from prior prostatitis. **A,** Numerous tiny, discrete calculi project above the symphysis pubis *(arrows).* **B,** Multiple larger calculi are clustered in a midline location *(arrow).* **C,** Stippled pattern of calcification overlying the symphysis pubis *(arrows).* (**A,** Courtesy Cynthia Peterson, Toronto, Ontario, Canada; **B,** Courtesy John A.M. Taylor, Seneca Falls, N.Y.)

FIG. 32-6 Staghorn calculi. **A,** Anteroposterior projection shows a concretion taking the shape of the pelvicaliceal system (staghorn calculus). **B,** Lateral view. Superimposition of the concretion over the vertebral body indicates the retroperitoneal location. **C,** Second patient with staghorn calculus. (**A** and **B,** Courtesy Cynthia Peterson, Toronto, Ontario, Canada.)

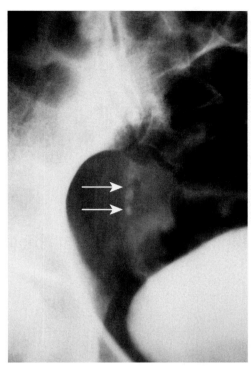

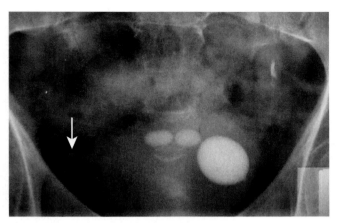

FIG. 32-8 Bladder calculi. Three homogeneously dense bladder stones with a continuous rim of calcification typical of concretions. Incidentally noted is a phlebolith with the diagnostic concentric lucency that should not be mistaken for a ureteral stone (arrow).

FIG. 32-7 Ureteral stones. Intravenous urogram demonstrates multiple small opacities located within the lower segment of the ureter (arrows).

ABIb | Conduit Wall Calcification

Conduits are channels or tubular structures through which fluids are conducted.[3] Conduit wall calcifications are confined to only the tubular walls, which are seen radiographically as parallel, linear opacities or, when seen on end, as ringlike calcifications.[3] Therefore any internal radiopacity indicates another class of calcification.

The calcification in conduit walls is not homogeneous. The most common site is in the walls of arteries, where one sees interrupted but basically linear calcifications.[3] This feature helps differentiate them from concretions, which usually have a continuous calcified external margin. The calcification also can outline a vessel's branching pattern.[3]

LOCATION	COMMENTS
Aorta and iliac arteries **(FIG. 32-9)**	Occurs mostly as a result of atherosclerosis; patients younger than 40 years of age are rarely affected; this may be associated with smoking or diabetes; patients can be hypertensive or have coronary artery disease.
Renal arteries	Arise from abdominal aorta at or near L1 and usually extend laterally or infralaterally; calcification occurs primarily as a consequence of atherosclerosis or diabetes;[2,59] this often is accompanied by aortic calcification.
Splenic artery **(FIG. 32-10)**	Frequently calcifies and has a characteristic serpentine course in the left upper quadrant.
Iliac veins and inferior vena cava	Veins not subjected to either high pressure or pulsatile flow and are relatively protected from the risk of intimal layer damage (see Figs. 32-4 and 32-68).[3]
Gallbladder wall **(FIG. 32-11)**	Also known as *porcelain gallbladder*, can resemble a large gallstone; a significant percentage of these patients also develop gallbladder cancer, usually adenocarcinoma.* Typically prophylactic surgery is indicated.
Vas deferens **(FIG. 32-12)**	Most often in diabetic patients, rarely secondary to infection;[11,23,35] most often it is bilateral, curved, symmetric, and parallel to the pubic rami.

*References 5, 10, 17, 33, 44, 51

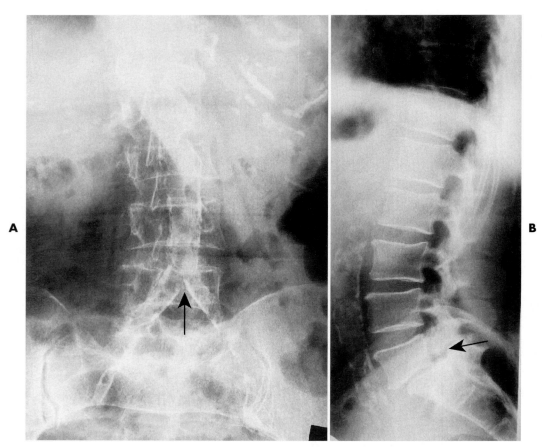

FIG. 32-9 Abdominal aorta and iliac arteries calcification. **A,** Anteroposterior projection. Tubular appearance characteristic of conduit wall calcification. The aortic bifurcation is seen clearly *(arrow)*. **B,** Lateral view. Notice that the anterior and posterior walls are parallel and the abdominal aorta diameter does not exceed 3.5 cm. Aneurysm should be suspected if the diameter of the abdominal aorta exceeds 3.5 cm. A spondylolytic spondylolisthesis of L5 also is visible *(arrow)*. (Courtesy John A.M. Taylor, Seneca Falls, NY.)

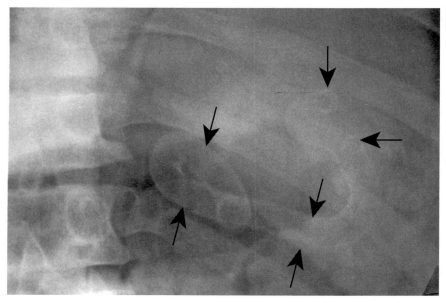

FIG. 32-10 Splenic artery calcification. A convoluted and tubular appearance is typical of the splenic artery *(arrows)*.

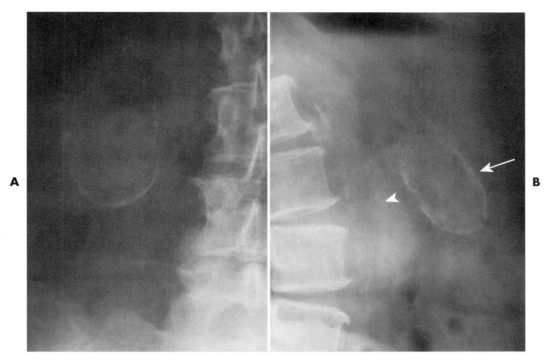

FIG. 32-11 Calcification within the wall of the gallbladder. **A,** Anteroposterior projection. Calcification within the wall of the gallbladder mimics a cyst. This condition is important to recognize, because adenocarcinoma is a common complication. **B,** Lateral view confirms the intraperitoneal location *(arrow)*. Conduit calcification of the abdominal aorta also is visible *(arrowhead)*. (Courtesy John A.M. Taylor, Seneca Falls, NY.)

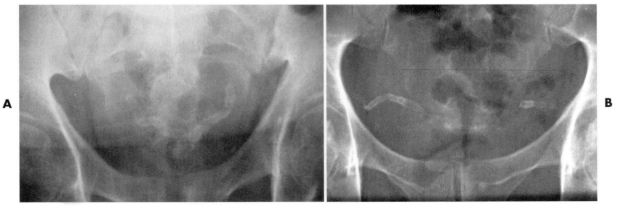

FIG. 32-12 Vas deferens calcification. **A** and **B,** Two cases of tramlike calcification paralleling the superior pubic rami are typical of vas deferens calcification. Location helps differentiate this from arterial calcification.

AB1c | Cystic Calcifications

Calcium deposition in the wall of an abnormal fluid-filled structure defines cystic calcification.[3] Calcium around the surface of a tumor occasionally mimics this appearance. Examples of cystic calcification include epithelial-lined cysts, pseudocysts that have fibrous integument, and arterial aneurysms. Calcification shows up as a smooth, curvilinear rim of opacity.[3] This rimlike appearance usually is larger than that of conduit wall calcification; however, calcification may be interrupted in spots in both types, appearing as an incomplete circle. Single, incomplete calcified margins likely represent a cystic density, in contrast to a concretion, in which one should expect a continuous margin of calcification.[3] The external border of the cyst usually is smooth, whereas the internal aspect is irregular, reflecting the interface with the contained fluid.[3] In contrast to a solid mass type of pattern, the outer margin of a cystic structure usually exhibits a relatively well-defined margin. Adjacent organs or vessels may be displaced or distorted by either solid masses or cystic structures.

CYST	COMMENTS
Left upper quadrant (above L3) *Spleen* **(FIG. 32-13)**	Two thirds of splenic cysts caused by *Echinococcus granulosis* (rare in the United States);[60] other possibilities include hemorrhagic and serous cysts, usually secondary to trauma;[13] cystic changes may be secondary to subcapsular hematoma and metastatic mucinous adenocarcinoma of the ovary;[47] occasionally an aneurysm of splenic artery may mimic a cyst; see also the Renal and Adrenal sections that follow.
Right upper quadrant (above L3) *Liver*	Rare hepatic cysts except those associated with *Echinococcus granulosis;* occasionally gallbladder carcinoma calcification can reside high and inside the liver.[7,21]
Right or left upper quadrant *Renal* **(FIG. 32-14)**	Benign and malignant neoplasms of the kidney and renal cysts; renal cysts are more common with advancing age, but usually they do not calcify;[31,34,50] renal artery aneurysm and subcapsular hematoma also may present as cystic calcifications.
Adrenal **(FIG. 32-15)**	Infrequent; pseudocysts are the most common cysts to calcify;[46] calcified cystic pheochromocytomas and other benign and malignant tumors are rare.[20,54,68]
Midabdomen *Pancreas*	Rare calcification of the wall of a pancreatic pseudocyst;[36] cystic calcifications may be seen in benign and malignant tumors.[19]
Right lower quadrant (below L3) *Appendix*	Mucocele calcification rarely appears as a calcified cyst; it occurs primarily in middle-aged persons and is slightly more common in men.[14]
Left lower quadrant (below L3)	Least likely of the abdominal regions to contain calcific densities; when present, they are likely to be ureteral stones, vascular densities, and leiomyomas; cystic calcifications are especially rare.
Pelvic bowl *Bladder*	Schistosomiasis of the bladder, worldwide, is the most common cause of mural calcification and is seen as a thin, continuous curvilinear calcification of cyst type; it is rare in the United States.[65]
Ovary	Most common ovarian lesion: cystic teratoma (dermoid cyst);[67] about 10% of cystic teratomas show calcification of cyst type;[12,67] benign cystadenomas and cystadenocarcinomas may appear as curvilinear calcifications of cystic type;[45] any cystic calcification in this area must be considered a possible malignancy unless proved otherwise.
Any location *Mesentery and omentum*	Cysts resulting from inflammation, trauma, or congenital rests;[3] they can move on sequential films; they are located anterior to pancreas, kidney, spleen, and adrenal glands.
Cystic calcifications that cross midline *Aorta* **(FIG. 32-16)**	Abdominal aortic aneurysm: most common abnormality with the radiographic appearance of the cystic calcification in this location.[3]

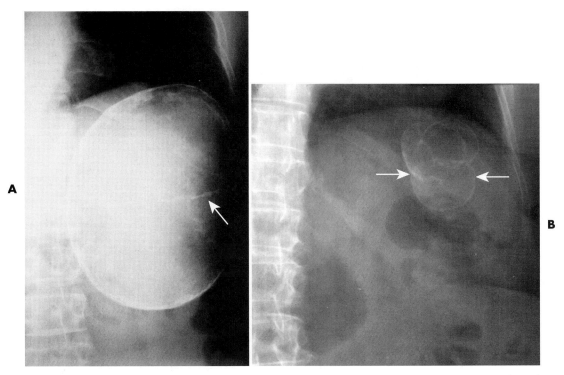

FIG. 32-13 Calcified splenic cyst. **A,** Observe the smooth, curvilinear rim of opacity in the wall of the cyst; although continuous in this case, most cysts have an interrupted rim of calcification. A central, horizontal line of calcification indicates septation *(arrow)*. **B,** Another patient demonstrates a smaller splenic cyst *(arrows)*. (**B,** Courtesy Gary Longmuir, Phoenix, AZ.)

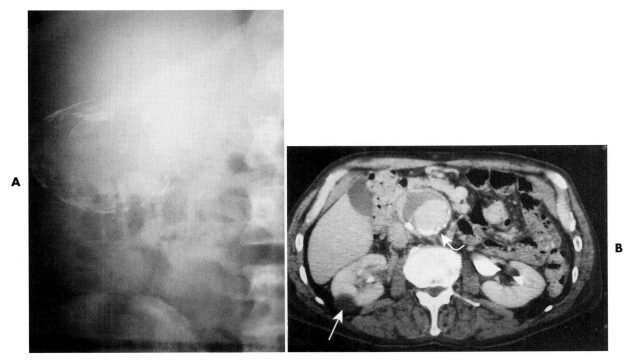

FIG. 32-14 **A,** Renal cell carcinoma. This cystic lesion proved to be a malignant neoplasm of the kidney. Note the rim calcification characteristic of a cyst. **B,** Computed tomography scan of a noncalcified benign renal cyst *(arrow)*, which would not be visible on plain film. Note the calcification in the wall of an abdominal aortic aneurysm *(curved arrow)*.

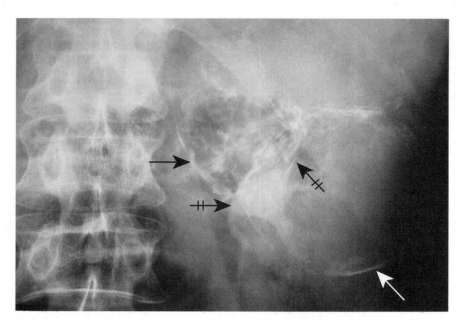

FIG. 32-15 Massive adrenal cyst with septations. This massive lesion proved to be adrenal carcinoma *(arrows)*. Contrast opacification of the pelvicaliceal system and proximal ureter is noted *(crossed arrows)*.

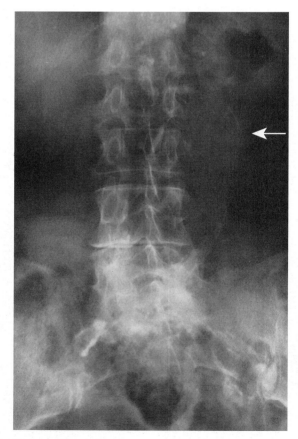

FIG. 32-16 Abdominal aortic aneurysm. Curvilinear calcification of the wall of an abdominal aortic aneurysm presenting as a cystic calcification *(arrow)*.

AB1d Solid Mass Calcification

This category comprises the most diverse presentation of the four. Irregularly calcified borders and complex internal architecture are characteristic of solid mass calcification.[3] Prominent but irregular and inhomogeneous calcification in the more central portion of the mass and discontinuity of the outer border are encountered frequently.[3]

MASS	COMMENTS
Left upper quadrant *Spleen* **(FIG. 32-17)**	Splenic densities most often resulting from calcium deposition in granulomas, often from histoplasmosis if multiple or occasionally from tuberculosis.[22,58] Frequently they have the morphologic appearance of concretions.
Right upper quadrant *Liver*	Most common universal cause of solid calcifications: tuberculosis and histoplasmosis;[1,16] calcified metastases (usually from colon and ovary) and benign neoplasms, such as cavernous hemangioma, may cause solid calcifications.[40]
Right or left upper quadrant *Adrenal* **(FIG. 32-18)**	In the adult, a normal-sized adrenal gland with calcification may be seen secondary to tuberculosis, Addison's disease, and old neonatal hemorrhage; solid adrenal calcification in an enlarged gland may result from cortical carcinoma; adenomas rarely calcify.[6]
Renal **(FIG. 32-19)**	Hypernephromas make up 90% of all solid mass type of calcification involving the kidney;[15] among inflammatory diseases, tuberculosis most frequently shows calcification;[64] solid mass calcification can occur in other primary malignancies, metastases (rare), and hamartomas.[53]
Midabdomen *Pancreas* **(FIG. 32-20)**	Pancreatic cystadenoma and cystadenocarcinoma solid mass calcification varying from a large stellate to closely aggregated solid masses to scattered clumps.[28,48]
Pelvic bowl *Bladder*	Detectable calcifications seen in only 0.5% of bladder tumors;[43] bladder calcification is rare with urinary tuberculosis;[27] schistosomiasis can calcify but is rare in the United States.
Uterine **(FIG. 32-21)**	Coarse, granular calcifications resembling popcorn or cauliflower developing within necrotic areas of uterine leiomyoma (common) and leiomyosarcoma (rare).[56]
Ovary	Two thirds of all ovarian malignancies: papillary serous cystadenocarcinomas that may calcify at the primary site and in metastatic deposits;[8,63] the calcification, known as *psammomatous* calcification, can vary from a flocculent, sharply demarcated focus to a less well-defined density and sometimes are found throughout the abdomen.
Any location *Intestinal tract*	Adenocarcinomas or colloid carcinomas of the intestinal tract with characteristically mottled, speckled, or granular pattern calcification; however, calcified small bowel tumors rarely are seen on x-rays; when seen, carcinoid tumors are more common.[32]
Subcutaneous **(FIG. 32-22)**	Extensive calcification resulting from scleroderma, dermatomyositis, and subcutaneous fat necrosis; this calcification can project over the abdomen and seem to be intraabdominal.[26]
Lymph node **(FIG. 32-23; SEE ALSO FIG. 32-28, A)**	Mesenteric lymph nodes: most common abdominal nodes to calcify;[57] they are one of the more common types of abdominal calcifications seen; healed tuberculosis is sometimes the cause of these calcifications, with exposure usually occurring several decades previously.[57]
Peritoneal	Psammomatous calcifications appearing within ovarian cystadenocarcinoma and its peritoneal implants; they may be widespread.[63]
Scars **(FIG. 32-24)**	Occasionally peculiar-shaped calcifications, often located in the abdominal wall.

PART FOUR Abdomen

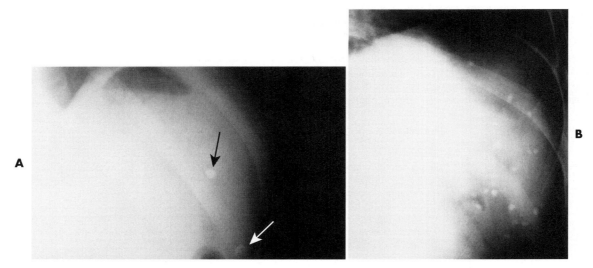

FIG. 32-17   Splenic mass calcifications in two different patients. **A,** Splenic granulomas are seen as solid mass calcification in the left upper quadrant *(arrows)*. **B,** Multiple calcified granulomas. These are most often from histoplasmosis.

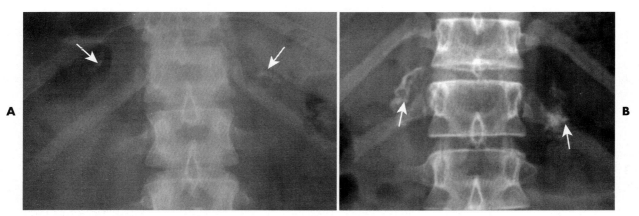

FIG. 32-18   **A** and **B,** Bilateral adrenal gland calcification in two cases. The size and location of the adrenal glands are visible because of calcification *(arrows)*. These normal-sized adrenal glands show calcification most likely secondary to tuberculosis, Addison's disease, or old neonatal hemorrhage.

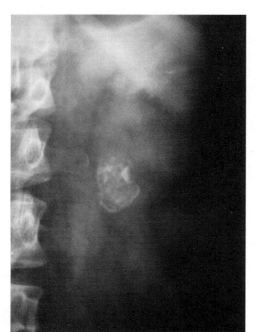

FIG. 32-19   Solid mass calcification. This was proved to be renal mass calcification from tuberculosis. Solid calcifications share the common feature of a nongeometric inner architecture and irregular, often incomplete margins.

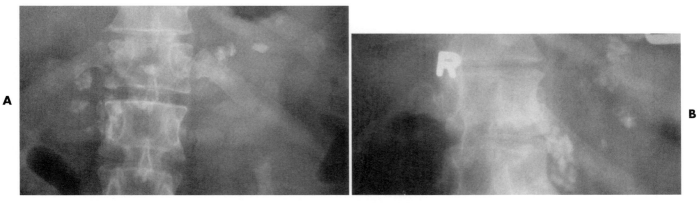

FIG. 32-20 Solid mass calcification of the pancreas. **A,** Anteroposterior projection. Notice that the calcifications are close to the midline on the right and extend far to the periphery to the left. **B,** Right anterior oblique view. These scattered clumps of calcification of the pancreas may indicate benign or malignant lesions. Pancreatic lithiasis associated with pancreatitis typically present as small, discrete opacities (concretions).

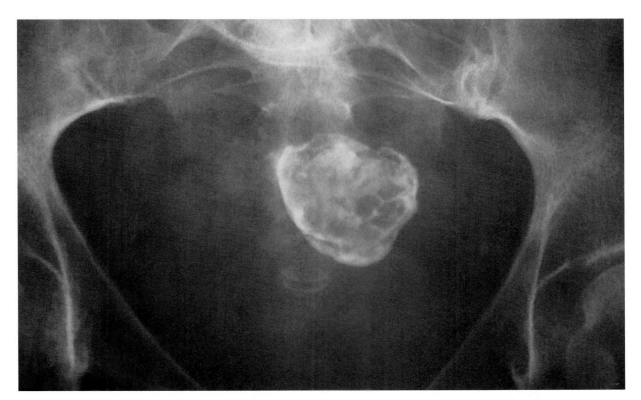

FIG. 32-21 Uterine leiomyoma. Mass calcification associated with uterine leiomyoma is very common. Location and pattern of calcification are helpful in determining the diagnosis.

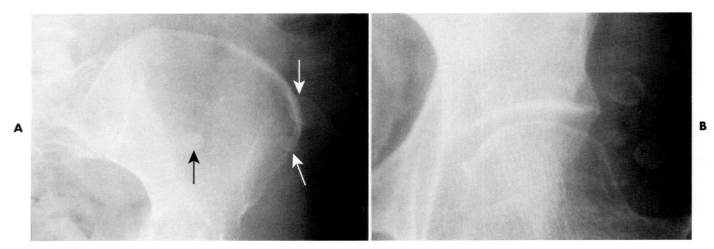

FIG. 32-22   Subcutaneous fat necrosis with calcium in two patients. **A,** Subcutaneous fat necrosis after injections can produce calcification that can project over the abdomen and seem as if it is intraabdominal *(arrows)*. **B,** Close-up view. (Courtesy John A.M. Taylor, Seneca Falls, NY.)

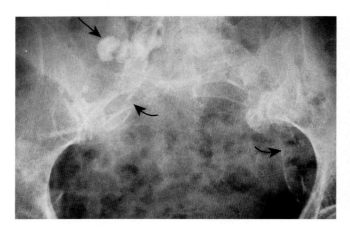

FIG. 32-23   Calcified mesenteric nodes. Mesenteric nodes are the most common abdominal nodes to calcify and present as mass calcification *(arrow)*. Observe the conduit pattern of arterial calcification *(curved arrows)*.

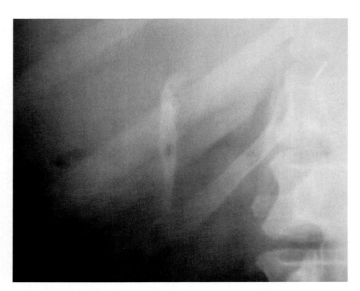

FIG. 32-24   Abdominal scar. Scars may give a peculiar pattern of calcification on occasion. Perpendicular views may indicate their surface location.

AB2 | Pneumoperitoneum

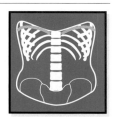

There are numerous sources of free air in the peritoneal cavity. In some patients this is a benign, inconsequential finding, but in others it indicates such grave conditions as perforation of a hollow viscus.

AB2a | Most Common Causes of Pneumoperitoneum

DISEASE	COMMENTS
Recent laparotomy	Usually present for 3 to 7 days after laparotomy, occasionally longer;[55] the volume of air decreases daily; faster resorption is seen in young adults.[25]
Trauma	Can be secondary to diagnostic studies such as peritoneoscopy and culdoscopy or from perforation during double-contrast barium enema or with colonoscopy; pneumoperitoneum may occur after severe external trauma.
Spontaneous	Most common cause: perforation of gastric or duodenal ulcer; rarely, air enters peritoneum via uterus and fallopian tubes (from puberty on).

AB2b | Plain Film Technique for Detection of Pneumoperitoneum

A complete series to detect free air includes erect and decubitus abdomen and upright posteroanterior chest views.[42] This approach occasionally requires up to 30 minutes to allow air to migrate between views, although larger amounts migrate faster and smaller amounts usually do not need more than a few minutes to migrate.

PROJECTION	COMMENTS
Left lateral decubitus	Should be performed first;[43] patient is placed in left lateral decubitus position for 10 or 20 minutes (if the condition affecting the patient permits); lower right lung field is included in the film; chest technique is used.[42]
Upright view **(FIG. 32-25)**	Patient placed in sitting or standing position for a few minutes, 5 to 10 minutes if possible; film is centered at thoracolumbar junction area.[42]
Supine film	May be only film taken in acutely ill patients; however, smaller amounts of air usually are not seen; one must be familiar with these subtle signs of pneumoperitoneum on the supine film if the condition is to be recognized.[42]

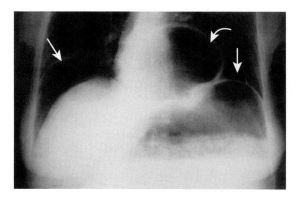

FIG. 32-25 Free air in abdomen. Air beneath both hemidiaphragms is seen in this upright view of the lower thorax and upper abdomen *(arrows)*. A large hiatal hernia is demonstrated as a mass with an air-fluid level superimposed over the cardiac silhouette *(curved arrow)*.

AB2c | Signs of Pneumoperitoneum on Supine Abdominal Films

The complete series for detection of intraperitoneal gas may not be possible, such as with debilitated patients and for those who suffer from acute abdominal pain. In such cases, recognition of free air on the supine radiograph is essential, realizing that smaller amounts (which can be just as ominous) cannot be seen.

SIGN	COMMENTS
Gas-relief or double-wall sign (FIG. 32-26)	Intraluminal and extraluminal air outlining both surfaces of the bowel wall; usually, at least 1 L of gas is necessary to demonstrate this sign.[9]
Falciform ligament sign	Falciform ligament: lies just to the right and parallel to the spine at the inferior aspect of the liver; the sign may appear as a linear density when surrounded by air.[24]
Urachus sign	Triangular soft-tissue density with its base at the urinary bladder seen in the midline below the umbilicus; urachus represents a remnant of the fetal allantois and may have its own peritoneal reflection to contrast pneumoperitoneum.[29]
Inverted V sign	Visualization of the lateral umbilical ligaments.[66]
Football sign	Large amounts of air forming a dome over free intraperitoneal fluid in the central part of the abdomen; this has an ellipsoidal shape, resembling a football; the football sign is seen most frequently in children.[3]
Morison's pouch sign	A triangular gas density projected over the superior margin of the right kidney, representing air trapped dorsally under the liver.[41]
Parahepatic air	Air may be trapped under the tip of the right lobe of the liver, presenting as an oblique, linear gas density.[39]
Triangle sign	A triangular collection of free air contrasted between three loops of bowel.[39]
Air in the fissure for ligamentum teres	Air possibly confined to the fissure for the ligamentum teres; this appears as a vertically directed area of hyperlucency in the right upper quadrant.[9]

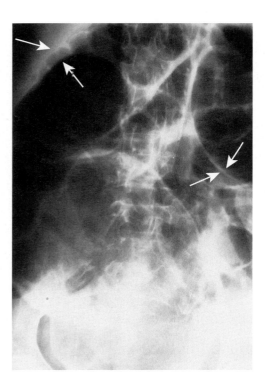

FIG. 32-26 Gas-relief sign (double-wall sign). Massive pneumoperitoneum from rupture of a duodenal ulcer allows clear demarcation of the inner and outer walls of many intestinal loops (arrows).

AB2d | Pseudopneumoperitoneum

Many processes may stimulate free air in the peritoneal cavity (pseudopneumoperitoneum).

DISEASE	COMMENTS
Double-wall finding	Two closely estimated gas-filled bowel loops, one of which may mimic free air.
Chilaiditi's syndrome (FIG. 32-27)	Gas-filled intestine between liver and diaphragm; intestine is examined for haustra and continuity with other bowel loops.
Subdiaphragmatic fat	Fat in the posterior pararenal space may extend between the diaphragm and peritoneum; its appearance as a thin black stripe can mimic free subdiaphragmatic air.
Extraperitoneal air	Streaky or bubbly air collections that do not change on decubitus views; if abutting the diaphragm this structure appears too thick; it is also seen at the edge of the abdomen in the abdominal wall.
Situs inversus	Stomach bubble appearing under right diaphragm resembling free air; however, the usual position of the stomach is devoid of gas, being occupied by the liver.

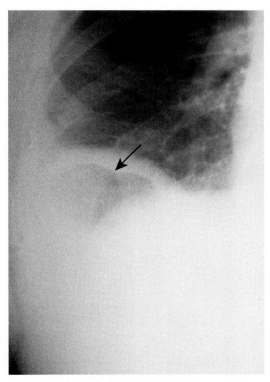

FIG. 32-27 Chilaiditi's syndrome. Anteroposterior projection of the upper abdomen reveals the colon interposed between the liver and the diaphragm. Cirrhosis and ascites predispose to Chilaiditi's syndrome. Demonstration of haustra *(arrow)* helps differentiate this from pneumoperitoneum.

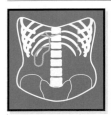

AB3 | Abnormal Localized Intraperitoneal Gas Collections

Besides free air in the peritoneal cavity, localized intraperitoneal gas collections also may be seen in the biliary ducts, gallbladder, portal veins, renal pelvis, urinary bladder, abscess, and pancreatic pseudocyst.[3]

LOCATION	COMMENTS
Gas in the biliary tract (pneumobilia) **(FIG. 32-28)**	Often a result of surgery on Oddi's sphincter during stone removal for the common duct; this surgery often allows gas to subsequently occupy the biliary tree for years; a fistula secondary to erosion of a gallstone into the intestine is the most common nonsurgical cause of pneumobilia;[4] sometimes the gallstones can be seen obstructing a loop of small bowel.
Gas in the gallbladder (emphysematous cholecystitis)	Emphysematous cholecystitis, of infectious etiology, resulting in gas either in the lumen or the wall of the gallbladder; the fatality rate is 15%, independent of patient's age.[38]
Gas in the portal vein system	May present with multiple tubular lucencies that extend to the periphery of the liver; usually this results from bowel wall necrosis or infection; therefore the mortality of these patients can be as high as 75%.[37]
Small bubbles in an abscess **(FIG. 32-29)**	Bubbly gas seen within some abscesses; often a history exists of diabetes, pancreatitis, or recent surgery; CT scan with oral contrast is the best imaging modality to differentiate abscess from bowel gas.

PART FOUR Abdomen

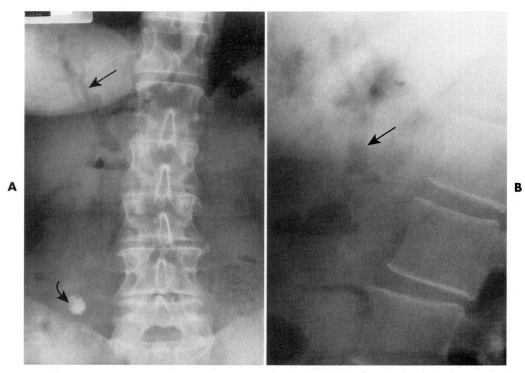

A   **B**

FIG. 32-28   Pneumobilia secondary to surgical creation of a fistula between the bile duct and duodenum (choledochoduodenostomy). **A,** Anteroposterior projection shows branched, tubular areas of lucency in the central portion of the liver characteristic of gas in the biliary tree *(arrow).* Incidentally noted is calcification of a lymph node in the right lower quadrant *(curved arrow).* **B,** Lateral view demonstrates air within the biliary duct *(arrow).* (Courtesy Cynthia Peterson, Toronto, Ontario, Canada.)

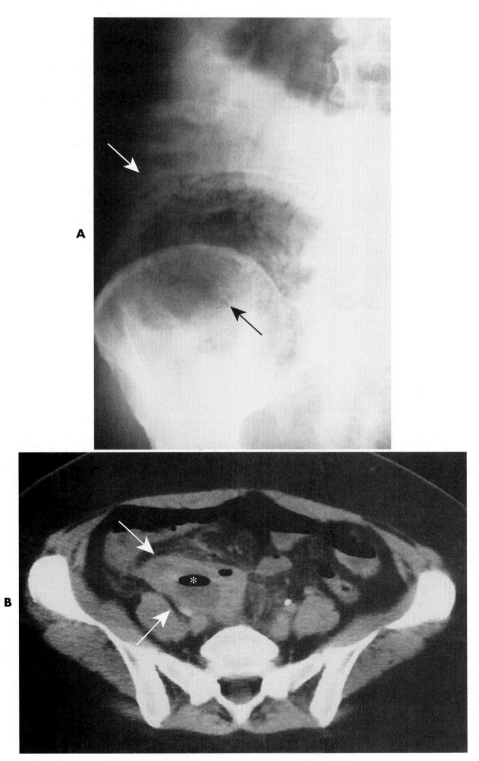

FIG. 32-29 **A,** Abnormal intraperitoneal gas collection. Bubbly gas within an abscess can be seen in this patient who recently had abdominal surgery *(arrows)*. **B,** Appendiceal abscess *(arrows)* containing air *(asterisk)*. Computed tomography scan is the best imaging modality to differentiate abscess from bowel gas.

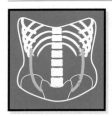

AB4 | Pneumoretroperitoneum

Pneumoperitoneum also may be simulated by air in the retroperitoneal space and its lateral and anterior continuations on supine films. Retroperitoneal and intraperitoneal air may exist simultaneously, producing even more confusing signs. The markedly different etiology, clinical course, and treatment of pneumoperitoneum and pneumoretroperitoneum make differentiation of the two crucial to patient evaluation.[3] Pneumoretroperitoneum is uncommon. The most common causes follow.

ETIOLOGY	COMMENTS
Trauma	Commonly trauma from penetrating wounds, after surgery, after diagnostic procedures such as barium enema or endoscopy, and perforation by pelvic fracture fragments.[3]
Spontaneous colon perforation	Frequently caused by perforation of colonic diverticula or carcinoma in the ascending or descending colon (which are retroperitoneal); rupture of the sigmoid colon within or posterior to the peritoneal cavity secondary to volvulus also may be a cause.[3]
Extension from pneumomediastinum	Various posterior and midline openings in the diaphragm providing a route for communication of free air in the mediastinum with the retroperitoneal space.[3]
Gas-containing retroperitoneal abscess **(FIG. 32-30)**	Infection by gas-forming organisms occurring in any retroperitoneal compartment; communication from the perirenal space may occur inferiorly to the anterior and posterior pararenal spaces;[3] this type may be caused by a recent back or kidney surgery, pancreatitis, or penetrating injury.

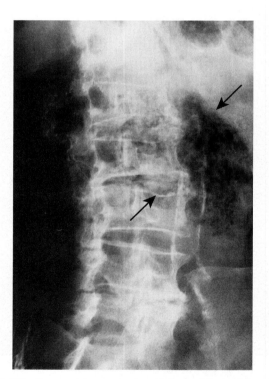

FIG. 32-30   Gas-containing retroperitoneal abscess. Infection by gas-forming organisms may occur in any retroperitoneal compartment, and on plain film the abscess may be seen as an extraluminal collection of gas *(arrows)*.

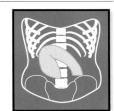

AB5 | Abnormal Bowel Gas Resulting from Obstruction

Identification of bowel obstruction on plain film can be difficult. The hallmark findings involve the small bowel. Prominent valvulae conniventes can be identified by their contrast against the gas in the lumen. Several adjacent or continuous distended loops usually are identified. The overall appearance of these tubular lucencies is affected by the site, duration, and degree of obstruction. Measuring the relative amounts of gas and liquid within the occluded segment also helps determine the radiographic presentation. Often the distended bowel loop in obstruction has a "tight" or hairpin appearance, rather than the flaccid appearance of inflamed or paralyzed bowel.

The stomach can be altered drastically in caliber and volume. The appearance of the stomach can be misleading because stomach contents can vary depending on what was ingested recently, whether the patient recently vomited or had fluid aspirated through a stomach tube, and whether stomach emptying is rapid or slow.

The colon presents with a variety of normal configurations. Obstruction also has a variety of presentations determined by the site and duration of blockage, liquid versus solid versus gaseous nature of the luminal contents, competency of the ileocecal valve, and possible concomitant dilatation of small loops. Typically dilatation of the lumen proximal to the obstructed point is seen with mechanical obstruction.[3]

Intestinal dilatation is noted secondary to many diseases. Diseases or injuries that directly or reflexively affect bowel motility or transport may lead to this appearance. Signs of nonobstructive dilatation include diffuse, symmetric, predominantly gaseous distention of the bowel in a patient who has few symptoms. A point of abrupt disruption usually is not identified with nonobstructive dilatation. Differentiation of mechanical from functional obstruction may require an oral barium study of the stomach, small bowel follow-through, and barium enema of the colon. Possible causes include reaction to medications such as narcotics, peritonitis, recent enemas, and (rarely) diseases such as scleroderma.

SITE	COMMENTS
Gastric obstruction	Occlusion of the gastric outlet sometimes caused by a chronic ulcer scar or antral carcinoma; a dilated, fluid-filled stomach may be imaged as a large water or gas density mass displacing the transverse colon downward.[3]
Small bowel obstruction (FIGS. 32-31 AND 32-32)	Identified by distention of small bowel, which normally should not exceed 3 cm in diameter; adhesions from prior surgery is the most common cause, but external and internal hernias, masses, and volvulus also can cause obstruction.[3]
Large bowel obstruction (FIGS. 32-33 AND 32-34)	The diameter of the colon, with the exception of the cecum, is normally less than 6 cm; the cecum can be somewhat larger safely, sometimes up to 8 cm; the most common cause is a distal obstruction either from colon cancer or diverticulitis, but other causes to be considered are cecal volvulus, obstruction distally by peritoneal metastases (especially ovarian cancer), pressure from a massively distended bladder or other large pelvic mass, and adhesions.[3]

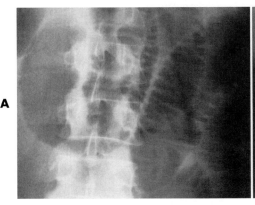
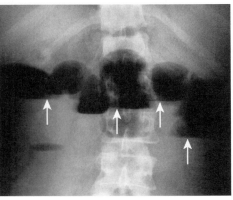

FIG. 32-31   Small bowel obstruction. **A,** Supine film demonstrates dilated small bowel in the abdomen. Note that the mucosal folds of the small bowel are much narrower than the haustral folds of the colon. **B,** Upright view shows multiple air-fluid levels *(arrows)*.

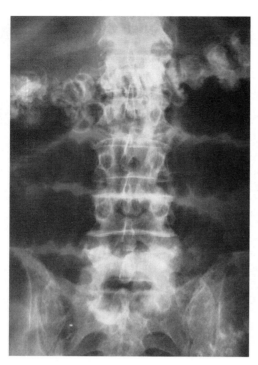

FIG. 32-32 Small bowel obstruction. Supine film reveals dilated small bowel loops greater than 3 cm diameter. Most small bowel obstructions are caused by postoperative adhesions.

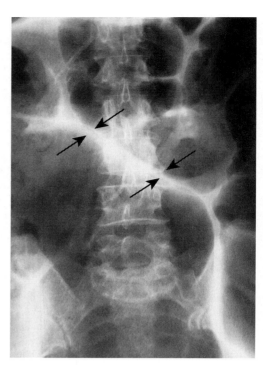

FIG. 32-33 Sigmoid volvulus. Recumbent plain film of the abdomen shows the massively dilated "inverted U" of gas-filled colon pointing toward the right upper quadrant. Opposed inner walls of the sigmoid colon form a dense white line *(arrows)*. This finding should not be confused with the double-wall sign of pneumoperitoneum.

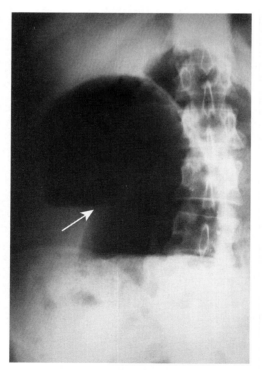

FIG. 32-34 Cecal volvulus. Erect film reveals a dilated cecum with a single air-fluid level. Ileocecal valve *(arrow)* produces a soft-tissue indentation so that the gas-filled cecum has the appearance of a coffee bean or kidney.

AB6 | Ascites

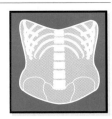

The importance of plain abdomen films in the evaluation of ascites has diminished in recent years with the introduction of ultrasound and computed tomography (CT) (Fig. 32-35). Most plain radiographic signs have limited reliability because usually large amounts of fluid must be present for identification, whereas CT and ultrasonography can accurately detect small amounts.

SIGN	COMMENTS
Loss of hepatic angle (inferior lateral tip of liver) **(FIG. 32-36, A)**	Normally the liver is contrasted by the adjacent fat; one pitfall is that adhesions may slow the flow of fluid along the right paracolic gutter, thereby preserving the hepatic angle.
Widening of paracolic gutter	Large effusions increasing the distance, which is normally 2 to 3 mm, between the flank stripe and gas in the ascending or descending colon; supine films are more likely to show this if obtained on inspiration.
Dog ears **(FIG. 32-36, B)**	Pelvic accumulation of ascites; peritoneal fluid may accumulate as symmetric bulges above the bladder resembling the contour of dog ears; smaller amounts of fluid can be seen here; upright abdomen film is best.
Ground glass sign	Ascites sometimes extensive enough to produce this overall increase in density; in such cases, other imaging and physical examination findings normally are present.

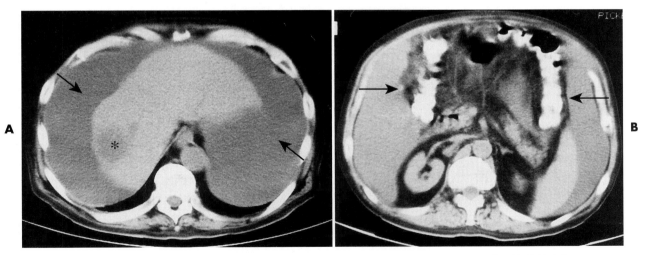

FIG. 32-35   Ascites. Ultrasound and computed tomography (CT) may detect small amounts of ascitic fluid. A larger amount of fluid, more than 500 ml, is necessary to detect ascites on plain films. **A,** CT scan shows the presence of a fluid-filled peritoneum *(arrows).* A lesion within the liver is also visible *(asterisk).* **B,** Centralization of bowel loops is occurring *(arrows)* because of the large amount of fluid in the paracolic gutters.

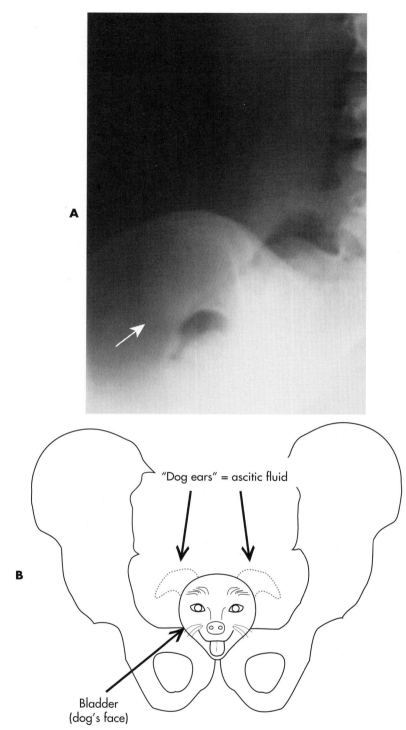

FIG. 32-36   Ascites. **A,** Normal liver edge is visible in this patient *(arrow)*. With ascites, the normal liver edge may be obscured. **B,** Symmetric bulges above the bladder resembling the contour of dog ears represent intraperitoneal fluid accumulation in the pouch of Douglas with central indentation from the bladder or rectum.

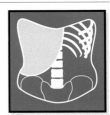

AB7 | Enlarged Organ Shadows

Radiographic evidence of enlarged organs generally comprises the recognition of displacement of adjacent structures. Mobile structures (e.g., the stomach, transverse and sigmoid colon, small bowel, urinary bladder) can be pushed easily by enlarging masses. Adjacent normal structures move as they accommodate themselves to the growth of the organ. The direction of this movement is particularly useful in the localization of small to moderate-sized masses. The kidneys also may be displaced, especially with retroperitoneal masses such as tumors or aortic aneurysm.

AB7a | Hepatomegaly

The liver fills the right upper abdomen and extends transversely from the right lateral abdominal wall to the left of the midline. On the right side the liver extends sagittally from the diaphragm to about the inferior costal margin. The usual causes of generalized hepatomegaly are fatty infiltration, congestive heart failure, primary neoplasms, leukemia, lymphoma, abscesses, hepatitis, metastases, and cystic or storage disease.

STRUCTURE DISPLACED WITH HEPATOMEGALY	DIRECTION OF DISPLACEMENT
Hepatic flexure, anterior liver	Pushed inferiorly.
Proximal transverse colon, anterior liver (FIG. 32-37)	Displaced below right renal shadow.
Hepatic shadow, anterior liver	Displaced across right psoas margin.
Right kidney, posterior liver (SEE FIG. 32-37)	Displaced inferiorly.
Stomach, left lobe of liver	Displaced laterally; depressed lesser curvature.
Right hemidiaphragm	Elevated.

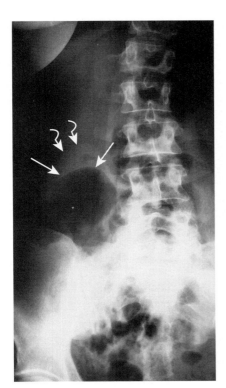

FIG. 32-37 Hepatomegaly. Proximal transverse colon and hepatic flexure *(arrows)* are displaced below the right renal shadow *(curved arrows)*. Right kidney is displaced downward as well.

AB7b | Gallbladder Enlargement

The gallbladder usually lies in a fossa on the anteroinferior surface of the right liver lobe and cannot be identified when normal. It is situated cephalad and slightly dorsal to the right transverse colon and anteriorly and slightly lateral to the descending duodenum. Gallbladder enlargement may be secondary to hydrops, acute cholecystitis, carcinoma of the gallbladder, or acute obstruction (Courvoisier's gallbladder).

STRUCTURE DISPLACED WITH GALLBLADDER ENLARGEMENT	DIRECTION OF DISPLACEMENT
Proximal transverse colon	Depressed inferiorly.
Hepatic flexure	Pushed inferiorly.
Duodenal loop	Pushed medially.

AB7c | Spleen Enlargement

The spleen usually is about 10 cm in length, although up to 13 cm is considered normal. It lies in the posterior left upper abdomen. Causes of splenomegaly include leukemia, lymphoma, infection, storage diseases, portal hypertension from hepatitis or cirrhosis, and hematologic abnormalities.

STRUCTURE DISPLACED WITH SPLEEN ENLARGEMENT	DIRECTION OF DISPLACEMENT
Splenic flexure (FIGS. 32-38 AND 32-40)	Depressed inferiorly.
Left kidney	Displaced inferiorly.
Greater curvature of stomach	Lateral impression.
Gastric lumen (FIGS. 32-39 AND 32-40)	Displaced medially.
Left hemidiaphragm	Rarely elevated except when spleen is huge.

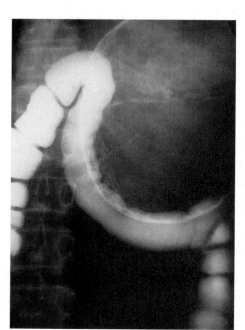

FIG. 32-38   Splenomegaly from a calcified posttraumatic cyst. Inferior displacement of the distal transverse colon and splenic flexure is seen.

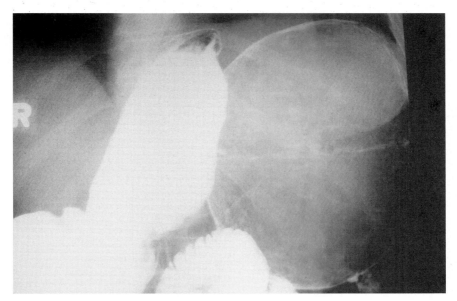

FIG. 32-39 Splenomegaly. Displacement of stomach medially is noted from a large calcified splenic cyst.

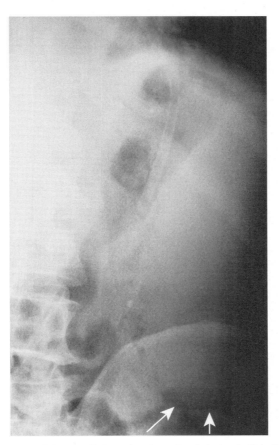

FIG. 32-40 Splenomegaly from chronic myelocytic leukemia. Plain film find-ings of splenomegaly include medial displacement of the stomach (with nasogas-tric tube) and inferior tip of the spleen projected over the iliac wing *(arrows)*. Downward depression of the splenic flexure also is observed.

AB7d | Gastric Distention

The stomach and first portion of the duodenum occupy the anterior left upper quadrant. The stomach is distensible and may vary widely in size and shape.

STRUCTURE DISPLACED WITH GASTRIC DISTENTION	DIRECTION OF DISPLACEMENT
Transverse colon	Depressed inferiorly.
Small bowel	Depressed inferiorly.

AB7e | Right Kidney Enlargement

Renal lesions are the largest group of retroperitoneal masses identified on abdominal plain film radiographs after abdominal aortic aneurysms.

STRUCTURE DISPLACED WITH RIGHT KIDNEY ENLARGEMENT	DIRECTION OF DISPLACEMENT
Proximal transverse colon (lower pole enlargement)	Elevated.
Proximal transverse colon (upper pole enlargement)	Usually not displaced.
Ascending colon or hepatic flexure	Displaced anteriorly and laterally or medially.
Descending duodenum	Indented or displaced medially and anteriorly.

AB7f | Left Kidney Enlargement

Renal lesions are the largest group of retroperitoneal masses identified on abdominal plain film radiographs after abdominal aortic aneurysms.

STRUCTURE DISPLACED WITH LEFT KIDNEY ENLARGEMENT	DIRECTION OF DISPLACEMENT
Transverse colon (FIG. 32-41)	Displaced inferiorly.
Descending colon (SEE FIG. 32-41)	Pushed laterally.
Duodenal-jejunal junction	Displaced anteriorly and medially.
Posterior gastric wall	Indented.

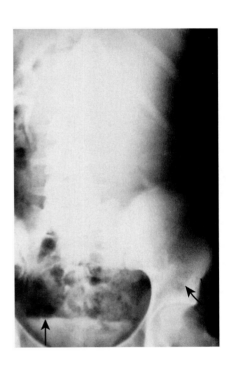

FIG. 32-41 Left kidney enlargement. Transverse colon is displaced inferiorly *(arrow)*, and distal colon is pushed laterally *(curved arrow)*.

AB7g | Adrenal Enlargement

The adrenal gland rests on the superior medial border of the adjacent kidney, with the right gland more caudally situated than the left. Normally the adrenal glands are not longer than 3 cm or wider than 2.5 cm. Common adrenal masses include congenital or posttraumatic cysts, neuroblastoma, pheochromocytoma, adenoma, and carcinoma (primary or metastatic). Smaller masses are not seen on plain films unless they are calcified or contain fat.

STRUCTURE DISPLACED WITH ADRENAL ENLARGEMENT	DIRECTION OF DISPLACEMENT
Subjacent kidney	Elevated but rarely affected.

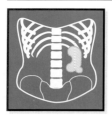

AB8 | Abdominal Masses

With the expanding role of advance imaging modalities, the abdominal radiograph often is useful as a guide to further studies. Abdominal and pelvic masses are recognized by both direct and indirect signs. The direct signs include visualization of the actual mass or an alteration in the size, contour, or density of an abdominal or pelvic organ, or identifying gas, fat, or calcium in them. The indirect signs are displacement of normal structures and obliteration of normal fat lines of the organ interfaces with adjacent fat.

One can narrow the diagnostic possibilities by determining if the mass is intraperitoneal or extraperitoneal. The lateral radiograph may be a useful supplement to the routine study if displacement of the retroperitoneal segments of the intestinal tract can be seen. A retroperitoneal mass can cause anterior displacement of the kidneys, ureters, duodenum, or vertical colon segments. However, if a mass is retroperitoneal and anterior to the kidneys, the kidneys are displaced posteriorly. Intraperitoneal masses are more mobile, and changes in position may be seen on sequential films. Fat can surround extraperitoneal masses and provide a sharp outline. This is rarely true of intraperitoneal masses.

AB8a | True Abdominal Masses

MASS	COMMENTS
Right upper quadrant (above L3) *Liver, right lobe* **(FIG. 32-42)**	Usual causes of generalized hepatomegaly: fatty infiltration, congestive heart failure, primary neoplasms, leukemia, lymphoma, abscesses, hepatitis, metastases, and cystic or storage disease.
Gallbladder	Most common causes: hydrops, acute cholecystitis, carcinoma of gallbladder, and a Courvoisier's gallbladder.
Duodenum/gastric antrum **(FIG. 32-43)**	Large mass produced by gastric leiomyoma or leiomyosarcoma; adenocarcinoma rarely displaces structures but may cause obstruction of the gastric outlet.
Left upper quadrant (above L3) *Liver, left lobe*	Focal masses caused by congenital or acquired cystic lesions, as well as benign or malignant neoplasms; these masses also may involve the right lobe of the liver.
Spleen **(FIG. 32-44)**	Most common causes for enlargement: traumatic or spontaneous hemorrhage, portal hypertension, infiltrative diseases, sickle-cell anemia, malaria, septicemia, and kala-azar.
Right or left upper quadrant (above L3) *Adrenal* **(FIG. 32-45)**	Most common adrenal mass: adenoma; these may be found as a normal variant, but they are usually only a few centimeters in size and therefore are not seen on plain x-rays; plain film identifiable lesions are uncommon but include congenital or posttraumatic cysts, neuroblastoma, pheochromocytoma, adenoma, and carcinoma (metastatic, especially from the lung, and primary).
Kidney **(FIG. 32-46)**	Cystic masses, including polycystic disease, multicystic kidney, simple renal cyst (found in up to 10% of older patients, but often small), inflammatory cyst, and pancreatic pseudocyst (in alcoholics); solid masses include pseudotumor, Wilms' tumor, renal cell carcinoma, and metastases.
Pancreas **(FIG. 32-47)**	With the exception of a pseudocyst, pancreatic masses rarely reach sufficient size to be identified on abdominal radiographs.
Right lower quadrant (below L3) *Appendix* **(FIG. 32-48)**	Appendiceal abscess common; the usual periappendiceal abscess indents the tip of the cecum and displaces local loops of ileum away from the abscess.
Cecum	Cecal carcinoma sometimes appearing as a mass or obstruction of the appendix, resulting in acute appendicitis; sometimes it can be seen as a filling defect in a gas-filled cecum.

MASS	COMMENTS
Left lower quadrant (below L3) *Rectosigmoid colon*	Common inflammatory mass produced by diverticulitis with abscess; this mass most frequently involves the descending and sigmoid portions of the colon, but usually it is too small to show up on plain films; colon carcinoma occurs most commonly in the rectosigmoid but also does not commonly present as a radiographically visible mass, except when outlined by bowel gas in a dilated loop.
Midline *Abdominal aorta* **(FIG. 32-49)**	Aneurysm possibly presenting as an abdominal mass; ultrasound is the procedure of choice in determining the presence, size, and extent of an abdominal aortic aneurysm.
Any location *Colon* **(FIG. 32-50)**	Inflammatory masses possibly resulting from diverticulitis, granulomatous colitis, amebiasis, and tuberculosis; colon carcinoma seldom presents as a mass; herniation of peritoneal structures, most occurring in the groin, may present as a palpatory mass.
Small bowel mesentery **(FIG. 32-51)**	Masses arising in the small bowel mesentery, most commonly inflammatory, from regional enteritis; mesenteric cysts also can occur and can be quite large; curvilinear calcifications may be seen in the cyst wall.
Small bowel	Jejunal or ileal masses classified as congenital, inflammatory, or neoplastic; except for the rare duplication of this area, they usually are not seen as masses on radiographs; volvulus of the bowel (especially in children) and dilated fluid-filled small bowel secondary to distal obstruction from regional enteritis (especially in young adults) both should be considerations.
Pelvic *Prostate* **(FIG. 32-52)**	Elevated base of bladder, possible result of enlarged prostate; benign prostatic hypertrophy may appear as a soft-tissue mass behind the symphysis pubis; prostatic carcinoma is more irregular but cannot be differentiated from the more common benign prostatic hypertrophy.
Uterus	Enlargement most commonly caused by pregnancy; other causes include pregnancy complications (including molar pregnancy), benign neoplasm (leiomyoma), and malignancy; the uterus can become large in a child if there is no exit point for uterine blood and debris.
Ovaries **(FIGS. 32-53 TO 32-55)**	Approximately 20% of ovarian tumors are dermoid cysts; these can be large, and sometimes fat or teeth can be seen within them;[3] other common ovarian masses include follicular cysts, corpus luteum cysts, serous or mucinous cystadenomas, and cystadenocarcinomas; endometriosis can cause cystic or solid ovarian enlargement, as can tuboovarian abscesses (both are somewhat common).
Bladder **(FIG. 32-56)**	Commonly carcinoma and leiomyosarcoma; they cannot be seen on plain radiographs unless they become large; contrast material in the bladder is needed to see them; a large bladder diverticulum may stimulate pelvic fluid or a pelvic mass.
Congenital lesions	Including urachal cyst, mesenteric cyst, pelvic kidney, and choledochal cyst.

PART FOUR Abdomen

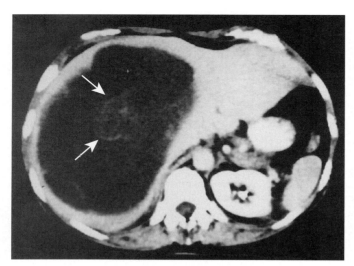

FIG. 32-42 Hepatic mass. Enhanced computed tomography scan demonstrates a large cystic-appearing lesion occupying the right lobe of the liver. Subtle areas of higher density *(arrows)* indicate that this is not a simple cyst. A malignant lesion that has undergone massive necrosis must be considered.

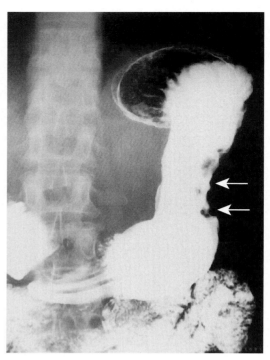

FIG. 32-43 Gastric carcinoma. Barium study reveals an infiltrating mass producing an irregular narrowing with nodularity of the mucosa of the greater curvature of the stomach *(arrows)*.

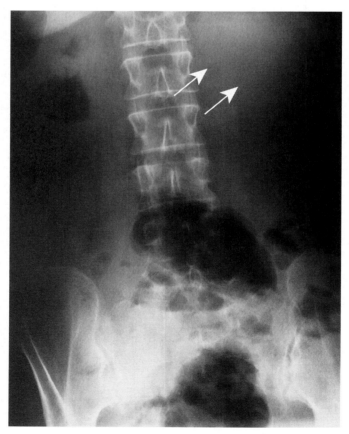

FIG. 32-44 Splenomegaly. Plain film demonstrates marked splenic enlargement with the inferior tip of the spleen extending a significant distance below the twelfth rib *(arrows)*.

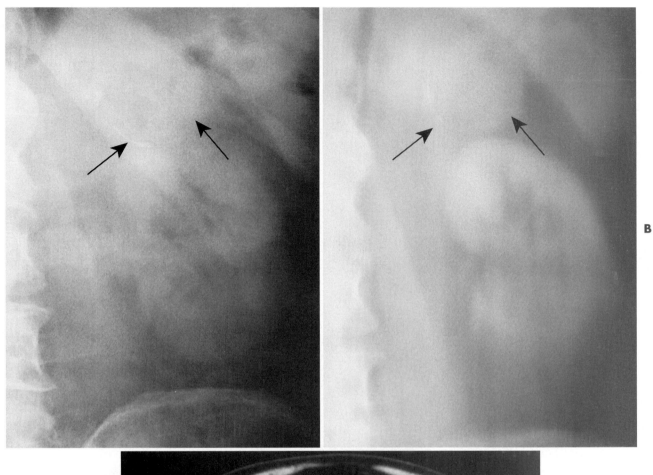

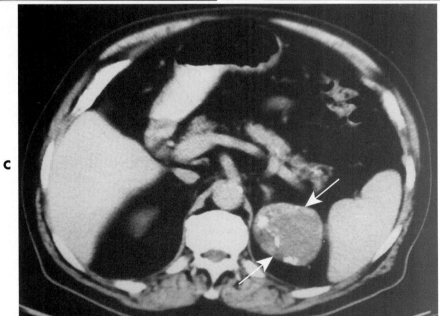

FIG. 32-45 Adrenal carcinoma. **A,** Plain film demonstrates a faint calcified mass with a cystic pattern of calcification (*arrows*). **B,** Conventional tomography confirms the suprarenal location of this mass (*arrows*). **C,** Computed tomography shows a large adrenal mass with rim calcification (*arrows*).

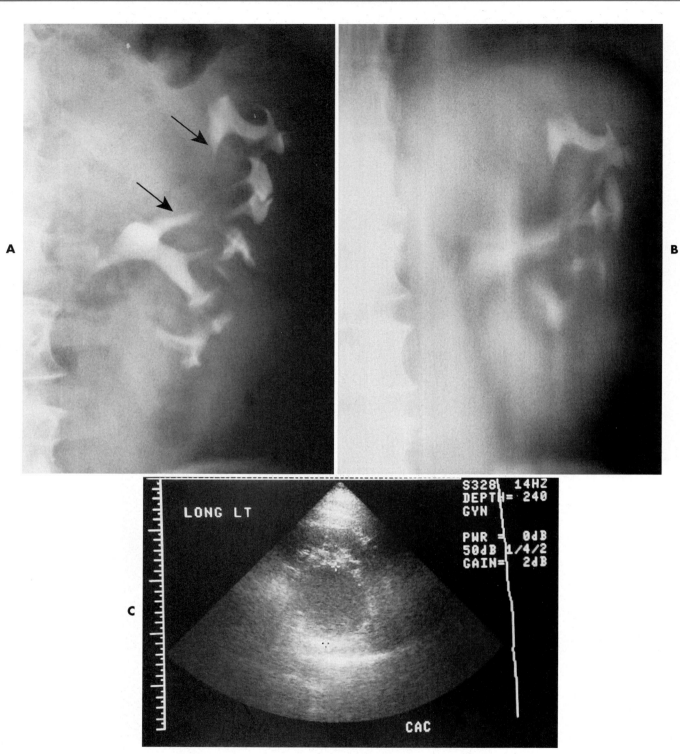

FIG. 32-46   Renal cyst in a 64-year-old man with chief complaint of hematuria. **A,** Three-hour postinjection intravenous urogram (IVU). Note the displacement and stretching of the upper and middle calyces of the left kidney around a mass *(arrows),* which proved at ultrasonography to be a cyst. **B,** Conventional tomography reveals similar findings as the IVU. **C,** Sonography shows an echolucent (black) round mass characteristic of a fluid-filled cyst (margins noted by cursors). Ultrasound usually can differentiate between a fluid-filled cyst and a solid renal tumor.

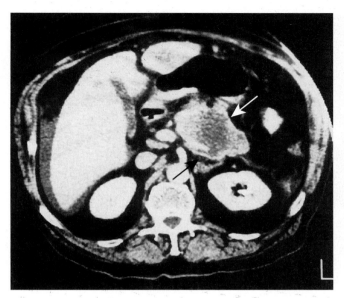

FIG. 32-47   Carcinoma of the pancreas. This mass was not visible on abdominal radiographs. Computed tomography scan demonstrates a pancreatic mass with a central zone of decreased attenuation *(arrows)*.

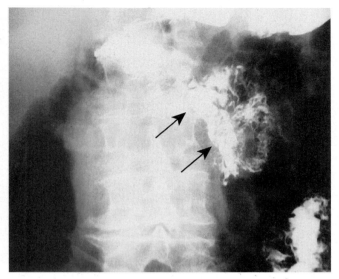

FIG. 32-49   Huge noncalcified abdominal aneurysm. Upper gastrointestinal study demonstrates displacement of the duodenum *(arrows)* from the large abdominal aneurysm.

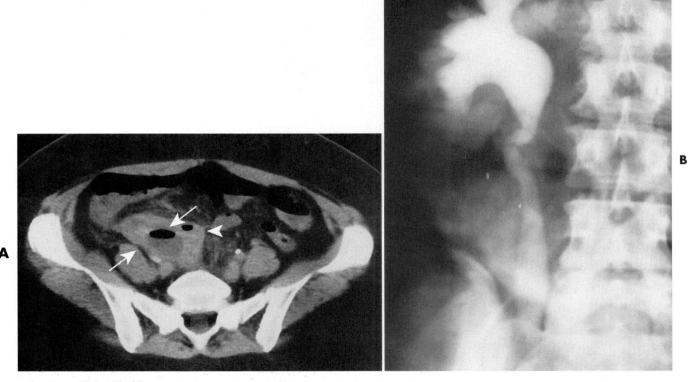

FIG. 32-48   Appendiceal abscess. **A,** Enhanced computed tomography demonstrates an air-containing abdominal mass *(arrows)* within the right lower quadrant. The left ureter *(arrowhead)* is visible, and the right ureter is obscured by the mass. **B,** Intravenous urography shows dilation of the pelvicaliceal system and ureter from obstruction secondary to this appendiceal abscess.

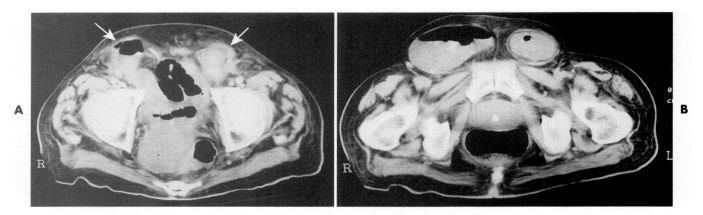

FIG. 32-50   Inguinal hernias: Computed tomographic appearance. **A,** The peritoneal sac containing bowel loops is seen protruding through both inguinal canals *(arrows)*. **B,** The same patient showing right and left well-defined groin masses produced by bowel loops.

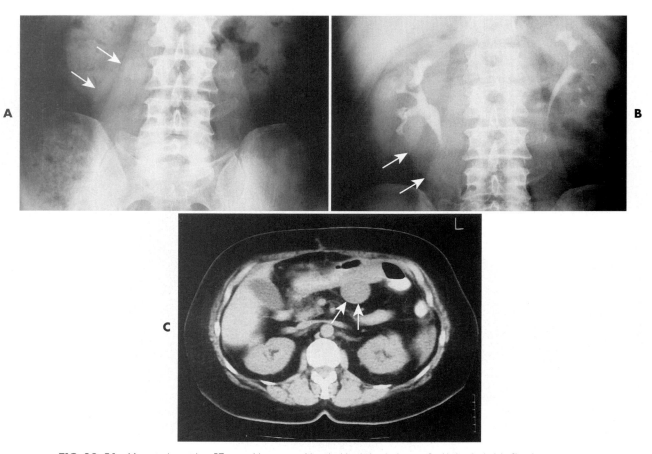

FIG. 32-51   Mesenteric cyst in a 57-year-old woman with palpable abdominal mass. **A,** Abdominal plain film demonstrates a large mass *(arrows)*. **B,** Intravenous urography shows that the mass does not involve the kidneys. The margin of the mass has changed position with the patient now recumbent *(arrows)*. **C,** Computed tomography of a different patient. This mesenteric cyst would not be visible on plain films *(arrows)*.

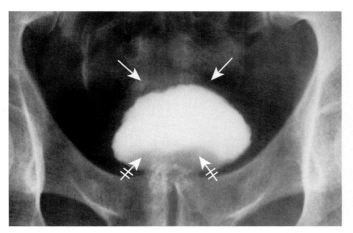

FIG. 32-52 Enlarged prostate. An enlarged prostate elevates the base of this contrast-filled bladder *(crossed arrows)*. Also, numerous calculi clustered over the symphysis pubis are seen, which are characteristic of prostatic concretions. Note the thickened bladder wall from the increased contractions necessary to overcome urethral constrictions by the enlarged prostate *(arrows)*. (Courtesy John A.M. Taylor, Seneca Falls, N.Y.)

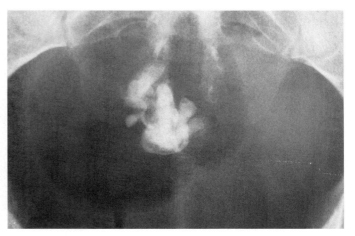

FIG. 32-53 Dermoid cyst. Radiolucent mass containing several teeth, characteristic of a dermoid cyst.

PART FOUR
Abdomen

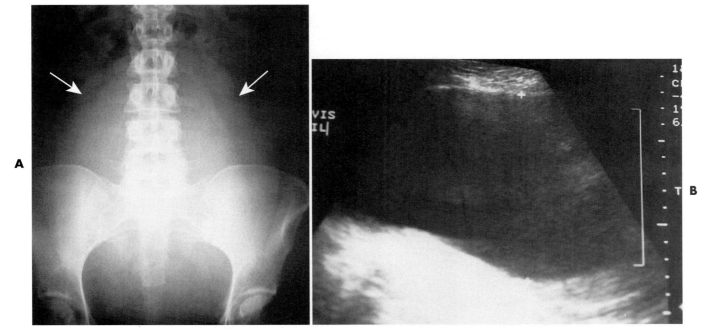

FIG. 32-54 Huge cystadenoma in a 36-year-old woman reporting a feeling of fullness in her abdomen for 6 weeks. **A,** Plain film of the abdomen demonstrates a huge soft-tissue mass extending out of pelvis to the level of L2 *(arrows)*. **B,** Ultrasound shows an echolucent mass typical of a fluid-filled cyst. Cursors delineate walls of the lesion.

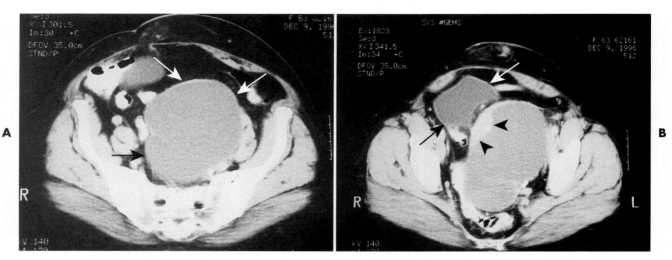

FIG. 32-55 Endometrioma. **A,** Computed tomography demonstrates a large soft-tissue mass in the pelvis of lower attenuation than muscle *(arrows)*. **B,** A more caudal section shows the urinary bladder *(arrows)* displaced to the right by the lesion. A thickened area in the wall of this lesion also is seen *(arrowheads)*.

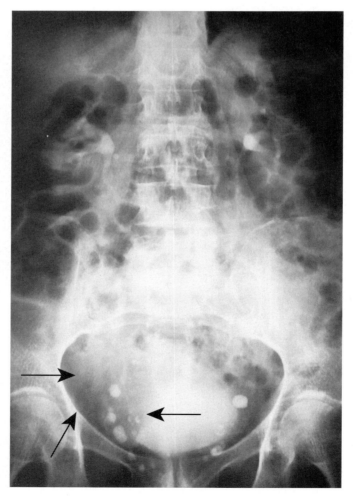

FIG. 32-56 Bladder carcinoma. Intravenous urography demonstrates a mass creating a filling defect of the bladder *(arrows)*.

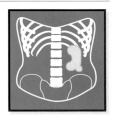

AB8b | Pseudomasses

On occasion, a fluid-containing viscus or a normal solid organ may simulate an abdominal mass. The more common pseudomasses are listed in the following.

STRUCTURE	COMMENTS
Stomach **(FIG. 32-57)**	Dilated, fluid-filled stomach projecting as a smooth homogeneous left upper quadrant mass.
Dilated urinary bladder **(FIG. 32-58)**	Dilated bladder appearing as a smooth, round mass in the lower midline pelvis; occasionally with chronic obstruction it can fill much of the abdomen.
Dilated bowel loops	In intestinal obstruction a dilated, fluid-filled loop of bowel may simulate an abdominal mass.
Ectopic kidney and anomalies **(FIG. 32-59)**	Pelvic kidney and other renal anomalies appearing as an abdominal or pelvic mass.

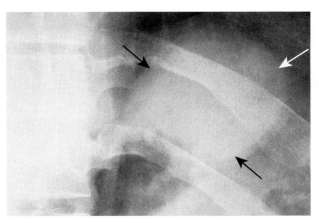

FIG. 32-57 Fluid-filled stomach in the left upper quadrant simulating a mass *(arrows)*.

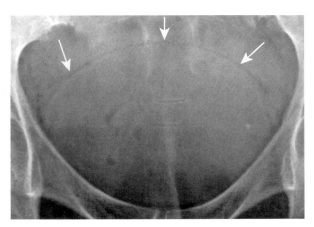

FIG. 32-58 Fluid-filled bladder may simulate a pelvic mass *(arrows)*. Note the rim of pelvic fat that defines the margin.

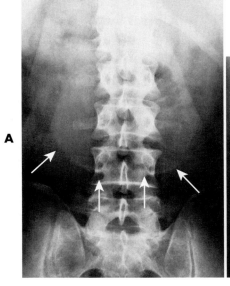

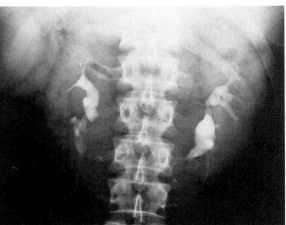

FIG. 32-59 Anomalous, conjoined horseshoe kidneys. **A,** Plain film findings simulate an abdominal mass *(arrows)*. **B,** On this intravenous pyelogram, the inferior aspects of the right and left kidneys are joined, a characteristic of horseshoe kidneys.

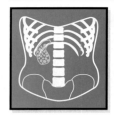

AB9 | Diseases of the Gallbladder

The gallbladder can change its volume and configuration rapidly. Nevertheless, its location next to the liver and its lack of adjacent, contrasting fat makes it rarely identifiable on plain radiograph.

DISEASE	COMMENTS
Acute cholecystitis	Most frequently caused by obstruction of the cystic duct by a gallstone;[49] gallbladder distention (hydrops) may result, a round to oval right upper quadrant (RUQ) mass may be seen.
Cholelithiasis **(FIGS. 32-60 AND 32-61)** [p. 1287]	Gallstones containing enough radiodense material to be visible on plain films in only 10% to 15% of patients;[30,62] however, most stones can be easily demonstrated with ultrasound.
Milk of calcium **(FIG. 32-62)**	Numerous, minute, calcific stones are in suspension in bile; an upright or lateral decubitus film frequently produces a fluid level with the heavier calculi in the dependent portion and a layer of bile above.
Calcification of wall **(FIG. 32-63)**	Also known as *porcelain gallbladder;* affected individuals usually are asymptomatic; five times as many women as men are affected;[5] the frequency of gallbladder carcinoma increases, so prophylactic cholecystectomy generally is performed.
Gallbladder carcinoma	Uncommon; this neoplasm rarely calcifies.
Gallstone ileus **(FIG. 32-64)**	Obstruction of the intestine by a gallstone that has eroded through the gallbladder and is in the small bowel; the typical patient is an obese, elderly woman, often diabetic, who complains of vague and poorly localized symptoms; classic plain film triad is small-bowel obstruction, biliary tract air, and an opaque concretion in the small bowel.
Emphysematous cholecystitis	Acute infection of the gallbladder caused by gas-forming organisms; air resulting from perforation is five times more common than routine acute cholecystitis; gas fills the lumen first, then the gas infiltrates the gallbladder wall; air within the gallbladder is a serious sign indicating advanced gallbladder disease.

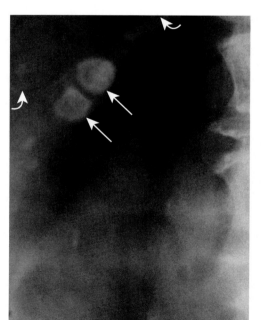

FIG. 32-60   Calcified gallstones *(arrows)* and costal cartilage calcification *(curved arrows).*

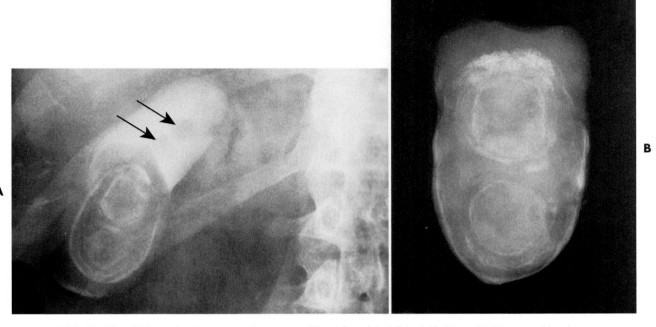

A

B

FIG. 32-61 **A,** This oral cholecystogram shows a large filling defect of the inferior half of the gallbladder created by a large partially calcified stone with two stones within it. *Note:* Two nonopaque stones create filling defects of upper half of gallbladder *(arrows).* **B,** Surgical specimen.

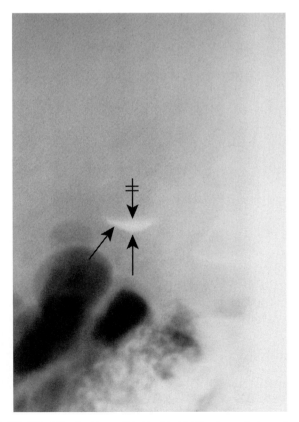

FIG. 32-62 Milk of calcium gallbladder. Upright film demonstrates radiopaque substance that layers dependently within the fundus of the gallbladder *(arrows).* Horizontal cephalad surface on the upright film indicates a fluid *(crossed arrow).* This most likely is calcium carbonate material.

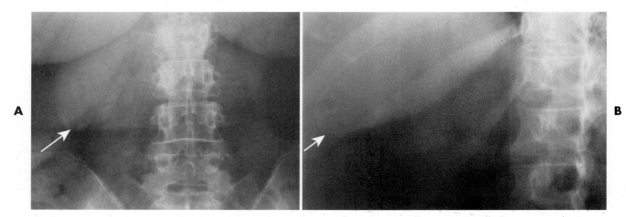

FIG. 32-63   Porcelain gallbladder. **A,** Anteroposterior plain film shows a cystlike calcification of the gallbladder *(arrow).* **B,** Calcifications of the gallbladder move further away from the spine during the right posterior oblique view *(arrow).* (Courtesy Cynthia Peterson, Toronto, Ontario, Canada.)

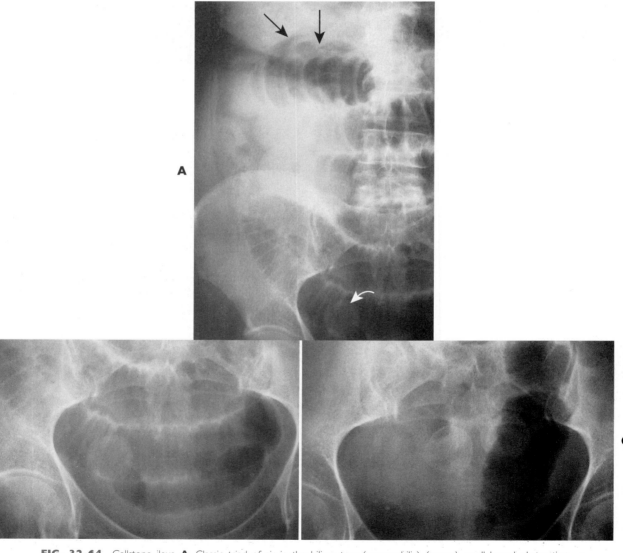

FIG. 32-64   Gallstone ileus. **A,** Classic triad of air in the biliary tree (pneumobilia) *(arrows),* small bowel obstruction evidenced by the dilated, gas-filled loops, and an ectopic gallstone *(curved arrow)* is virtually diagnostic of gallstone ileus. Observe the gallstone remaining within the right upper quadrant. **B,** Close-up view of the ectopic gallstone and small bowel obstruction. **C,** Second opaque gallstone that has eroded into the gastrointestinal tract. These gallstones often create a mechanical obstruction.

AB10 | Vascular Calcifications

This is a common finding in middle-aged and elderly patients. Typically, linear and parallel calcifications are seen along the path of the major arteries.

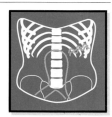

VASCULAR STRUCTURE	COMMENTS
Aorta (FIG. 32-65)	Frequently calcification in the walls of the aorta is observed in radiographs of middle-aged and elderly patients; similar calcifications also can be seen in young persons, especially those suffering from diabetes.
Iliac artery (FIG. 32-66)	Fragmentary calcification of an iliac artery just below the sacroiliac joint can be mistaken for a ureteral calculus.
Splenic artery (FIG. 32-67)	Located in the left upper quadrant; can be recognized by its extreme tortuosity.
Renal artery	Occasionally calcifies.
Celiac and superior mesenteric arteries	Occasionally can be seen coming off a calcified aorta on a lateral spine film that includes the L1 and L3 areas.
Phlebolith (FIG. 32-68)	Common in the pelvic veins; have no clinical significance; usually they are round, 1- to 5-mm calcifications; may have a lucent center; easily confused with a ureteral stone.
Portal vein	Rare imaging finding; almost always occur in patients with portal hypertension or thrombosis.
Lymph nodes (SEE FIG. 32-23)	(Mesenteric or paravascular) may be affected by granulomatous diseases, especially histoplasmosis or tuberculosis, with subsequent calcification; rarely other entities such as lymphoma or sarcoid occur.

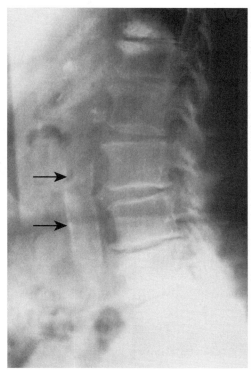

FIG. 32-65 Aorta calcification (arrows).

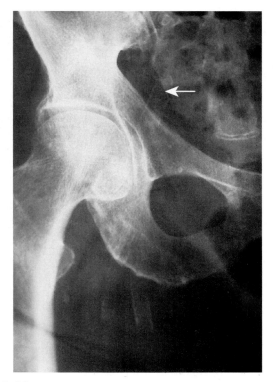

FIG. 32-66 Iliac artery calcification (arrow).

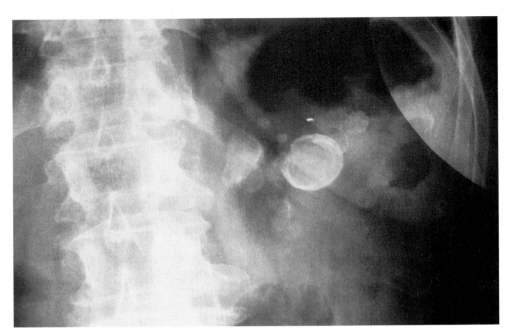

FIG. 32-67 Splenic artery calcification. Multiple ringlike calcifications represent portions of the tortuous splenic artery projected on end. The largest ring indicates aneurysmal dilation.

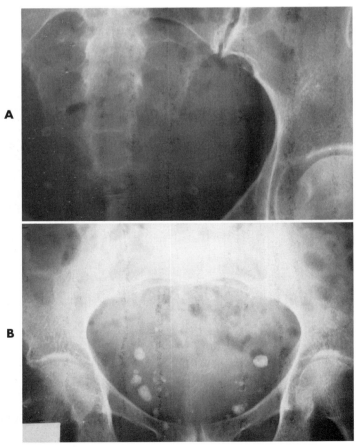

FIG. 32-68 Phleboliths in two different patients. **A,** Multiple small, round calcifications with a central lucency, which should not be confused with urinary tract calculi. **B,** Larger phleboliths found in a pattern consistent with pelvic veins.

AB11 Miscellaneous Radiopacities and Abdomen Artifacts

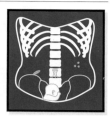

A variety of miscellaneous radiographic densities can simulate calcification on abdominal radiographs (Figs. 32-69 through 32-79).

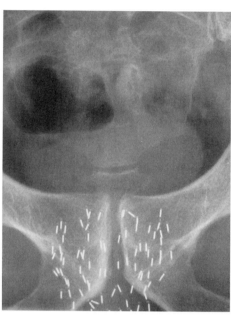

FIG. 32-69 Treatment for prostate carcinoma. Multiple metallic implants that contain radioactive material have been injected into the prostate gland.

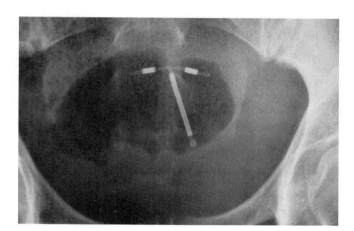

FIG. 32-70 Intrauterine device. T-shaped metal and plastic density in the region of the uterus. Note the eyelet in the caudal end for the removal.

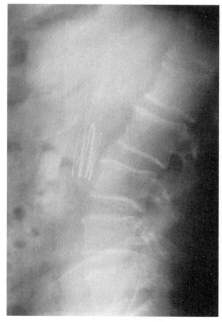

FIG. 32-71 Thrombi filter. Basketlike devices may be placed in the inferior vena cava of patients with a propensity to produce thromboemboli. (Courtesy Cynthia Peterson, Toronto, Ontario, Canada.)

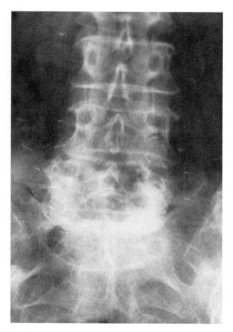

FIG. 32-72 Acupuncture needles. Hari, a Japanese form of acupuncture, consists of placement of many gold needles into the subcutaneous tissues. They are cut off at the skin surface and remain in place permanently.

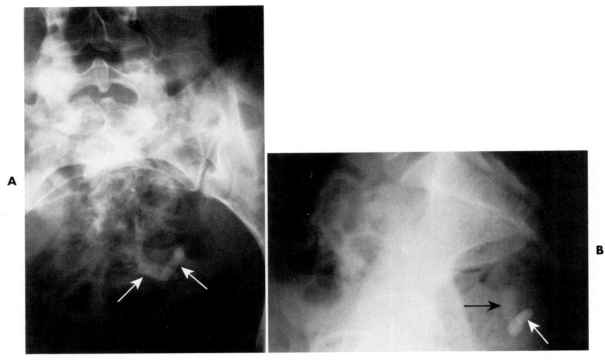

FIG. 32-73 Ingested tablets. Undigested tablets may mimic abdominal calcifications. **A,** Anteroposterior projection *(arrows).* **B,** Lateral view *(arrows).*

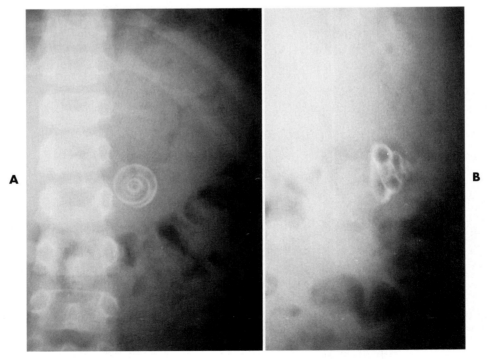

FIG. 32-74 Ingested snail shell. The characteristic spiral makes this unusual diagnosis obvious. **A,** Anteroposterior projection. **B,** Lateral view.

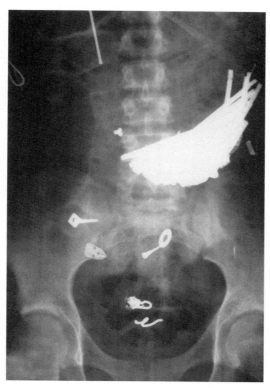

FIG. 32-75 Ingested metallic objects. Metallic foreign bodies are seen throughout the gastrointestinal tract.

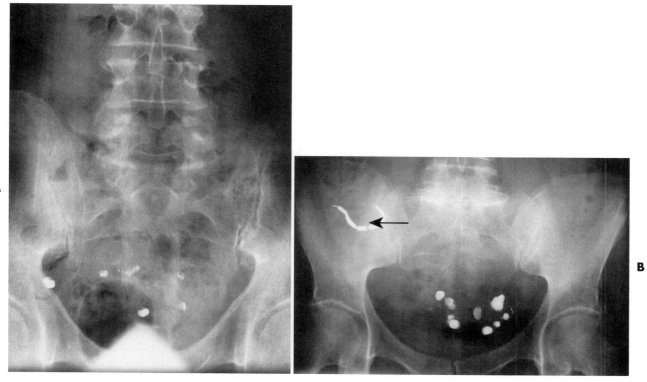

FIG. 32-76 **A,** Barium retained in diverticula after barium enema. Note their dense, homogeneous metallic opacification that can usually be distinguished from calcifications. Most diverticula occur in the sigmoid. **B,** Barium retained in appendix *(arrow)* and diverticula. Barium is present in multiple, left-sided diverticula and the appendix. (**A,** Courtesy John A.M. Taylor, Seneca Falls, NY; **B,** Courtesy Cynthia Peterson, Toronto, Ontario, Canada.)

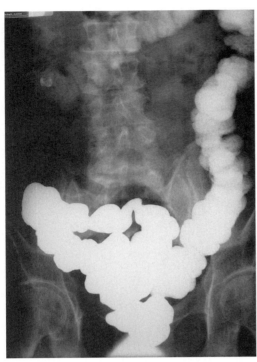

FIG. 32-77 Impaction of ingested barium occurred in the colon because of dehydration of retained barium by the colonic mucosa. (Courtesy Cynthia Peterson, Boumermouth Toronto, Ontario, Canada.)

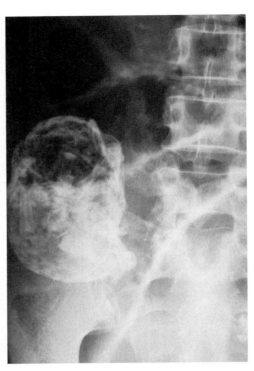

FIG. 32-78 Lithopedion.

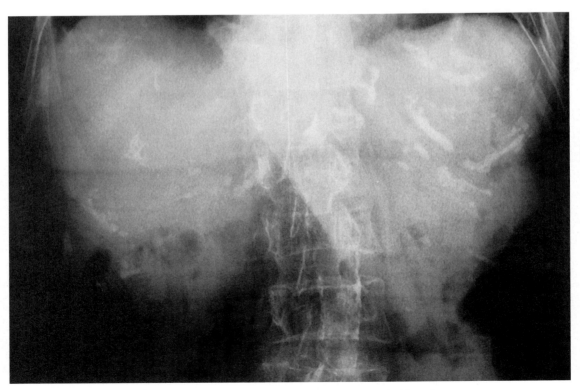

FIG. 32-79 Costal cartilage calcification of the lower ribs bilaterally.

References

1. Astley R, Harrison N: Miliary calcification of the liver: report of a case, *Br J Radiol* 22:723, 1949.
2. Azimi T, Cameron DD: Calcification of the intrarenal branches of the renal arteries, *Clin Radiol* 28:217, 1977.
3. Baker SR: The abdominal plain film, ed 1, Norwalk, CT, 1990, Appleton & Lange.
4. Balthazar EJ, Gurkin S: Cholecystenteric fistulas: significance and radiographic diagnosis, *Am J Gastroenterol* 65:168, 1976.
5. Berk RN, Armbuster TG, Saltzstein SL: Carcinoma in the porcelain gallbladder, *Radiology* 106:29, 1973.
6. Boise CL, Sears WN: Calcification in adrenal neoplasms, *Radiology* 56:731, 1951.
7. Caplan LN, Simon M: Non-parasitic cysts of the liver, *AJR Am J Roentgenol* 96:421, 1966.
8. Castro JR, Klein EW: The incidence and appearance of roentgenologically visible psammomatous calcification of papillary cystadenocarcinoma of the ovaries, *AJR Am J Roentgenol* 88:886, 1962.
9. Cho KC, Baker SR: Air in the fissure for the ligamentum teres: new sign of intraperitoneal air on plain radiographs, *Radiology* 178:489, 1991.
10. Cornell CM, Clarke R: Vicarious calcification involving the gallbladder, *Ann Surg* 149:267, 1959.
11. Culver GJ, Tannenhaus J: Calcification of the vas deferens: its relation to diabetes mellitus and arteriosclerosis, *N Engl J Med* 245:321, 1951.
12. Cusmano JV: Dermoid cysts of the ovary: roentgen features, *Radiology* 66:719, 1956.
13. Dachman AH et al: Non-parasitic splenic cysts: a report of 52 cases with radiologic-pathologic correlation, *AJR Am J Roentgenol* 147:537, 1986.
14. Dachman AH, Lichtenstein JE, Friedman AC: Review: mucocele of the appendix and pseudomyxoma peritonei, *AJR Am J Roentgenol* 144:923, 1985.
15. Daniel WW Jr et al: Calcified renal masses: a review of ten years' experience at the Mayo Clinic, *Radiology* 103:503, 1972.
16. Darlak JR, Moskowitz M, Kattan KE: Calcifications in the liver, *Radiol Clin North Am* 18:209, 1981.
17. Etala E: Cancer de la vesicula biliar, *Prensa Med Argent* 49:2283, 1962.
18. Fagenberg D: Fecaliths of the appendix, incidence of significance, *AJR Am J Roentgenol* 89:572, 1963.
19. Friedman AC, Lichtenstein JE, Dachman AH: Cystic neoplasms of the pancreas, *Radiology* 149:45, 1983.
20. Grainger RG, Lloyed GAS, Williams JL: Eggshell calcification: a sign of phaeochromocytoma, *Clin Radiol* 18:282, 1967.
21. Gonzalez LR et al: Radiologic aspects of hepatic echinococcosis, *Radiology* 130:21, 1979.
22. Gray EF: Calcifications of the spleen, *AJR Am J Roentgenol* 61:336, 1944.
23. Hafiz A, Melnick JC: Calcification of the vas deferens, *J Can Assoc Radiol* 19:56, 1968.
24. Han SY: Variations in falciform ligament with pneumoperitoneum, *J Can Assoc Radiol* 31:171, 1980.
25. Harrison I, Litwer H, Gerwig WH: Studies on the incidence and duration of post-operative pneumoperitoneum, *Ann Surg* 145:591, 1957.
26. Hilbrish TF, Bartler FC: Roentgen findings in abnormal deposition of calcium in tissues, *AJR Am J Roentgenol* 87:1128, 1962.
27. Holman CC: Urinary tuberculosis with extensive calcification of the bladder, *Br J Surg* 40:90, 1952.
28. Imhof H, Frank P: Pancreatic calcification in malignant islet cell tumors, *Radiology* 122:333, 1977.
29. Jelasco DV, Schultz EH: The urachus: an aid to the diagnosis of pneumoperitoneum, *Radiology* 92:295, 1969.
30. Johnston DE, Kaplan MM: Pathogenesis and treatment of gallstones, *N Engl J Med* 328:412, 1993.
31. Jonutis AJ, Davidson AJ, Redman HC: Curvilinear calcifications in four uncommon benign renal lesions, *Clin Radiol* 24:468, 1973.
32. Kaude JV: Calcification in carcinoid tumors, *N Engl J Med* 289:921, 1973.
33. Kazmierski RH: Primary adenocarcinoma of gallbladder with intramural calcification, *Am J Surg* 82:248, 1951.
34. Kikkawa K, Lasser ER: Ringlike or rimlike calcifications in renal cell carcinoma, *AJR Am J Roentgenol* 107:737, 1969.
35. King JC Jr, Rosenbaum HD: Calcification of the vasa deferentia in nondiabetics, *Radiology* 100:603, 1971.
36. Komaki S, Clark JM: Pancreatic pseudocyst: a review of 17 cases with emphasis on radiologic findings, *AJR Am J Roentgenol* 122:385, 1974.
37. Liebman PR et al: Hepatic-portal venous gas in adults: etiology, pathophysiology, and clinical significance, *Ann Surg* 107:281, 1978.
38. Mentzer RM et al: A comparative appraisal of emphysematous cholecystitis, *Am J Surg* 129:10, 1973.
39. Menuck L, Siemers PT: Pneumoperitoneum: importance of right upper quadrant features, *AJR Am J Roentgenol* 127:753, 1976.
40. Miele AJ, Edmonds HW: Calcified liver metastases: a specific roentgen diagnostic sign, *Radiology* 80:779, 1963.
41. Miller RE: Perforated viscus in infants: a new roentgen sign, *Radiology* 74:65, 1960.
42. Miller RE: The technical approach to the acute abdomen, *Semin Roentgenol* 8:267, 1973.
43. Miller SW, Pfister RC: Calcification in uroepithelial tumors of the bladder: report of 5 cases and survey of the literature, *AJR Am J Roentgenol* 121:827, 1974.
44. Milner LR: Cancer of the gallbladder. Its relationship to gallstones, *Am J Gastroenterol* 39:480, 1963.
45. Moncada R, Cooper RA, Garces M: Calcified metastases from malignant ovarian neoplasm: review of the literature, *Radiology* 113:31, 1974.
46. Parker JM: Calcified cyst of the adrenal gland, *Mil Med* 138:791, 1970.
47. Papavasiliou CG: Calcification in secondary tumors of the spleen, *Acta Radiol* 51:278, 1959.
48. Parientes RA et al: Cystadenoma of the pancreas: diagnosis by computed tomography, *J Comput Asst Tomogr* 4:364, 1980.
49. Phemister DB, Rewbridge AG, Rudisill H Jr: Calcium carbonate gallstone following cystic duct obstruction, *Ann Surg* 94:493, 1931.
50. Phillips TL, Chin FG, Palubinskas AJ: Calcification in renal masses: an eleven-year survey, *Radiology* 80:786, 1963.
51. Polk HC Jr: Carcinoma and the calcified gallbladder, *Gastroenterology* 50:582, 1966.
52. Roth CS, Bowyer BA, Berquist TH: Utility of the plain film abdominal radiograph for diagnosing ureteral calculi, *Ann Emerg Med* 14:311, 1985.
53. Salik JO, Abeshouse BS: Calcification, ossification and cartilage formation in the kidney, *AJR Am J Roentgenol* 88:125, 1962.
54. Samuel E: Calcification in suprarenal neoplasms, *Br J Radiol* 21:139, 1948.
55. Samuel E et al: Radiology of the post-operative abdomen, *Clin Radiol* 14:133, 1963.
56. Schabel SI, Burgener FA, Reynolds J: Radiographic manifestations of malignant mixed uterine tumors, *J Can Assoc Radiol* 26:176, 1975.
57. Schechter S: Calcified mesenteric lymph nodes: their incidence and significance in routine roentgen examination of the gastrointestinal tract, *Radiology* 27:485, 1936.
58. Schwarz J et al: The relationship of splenic calcifications to histoplasmosis, *N Engl J Med* 252:887, 1955.
59. Sheshanarayana KN, Keats TS: Intrarenal arterial calcifications: roentgen appearance and significant, *Radiology* 95:145, 1970.
60. Soler-Bechara J, Soscia JL: Calcified echinococcus (hydatid) cyst of the spleen, *JAMA* 187:62, 1964.

61. Steer ML et al: Chronic pancreatitis, *N Engl J Med* 332:1492, 1995.
62. Tait N, Little JM: The treatment of gallstones, *BMJ* 311:99, 1995.
63. Teplick JG, Haskins ME, Alavi A: Calcified intraperitoneal metastases from ovarian carcinoma, *AJR Am J Roentgenol* 127:1003, 1976.
64. Tonkin AK, Witten DM: Genitourinary tuberculosis, *Semin Roentgenol* 14:305, 1979.
65. Umerah BC: The less familiar manifestations of schistosomiasis of the urinary tract, *Br J Surg* 50:105, 1977.
66. Weiner CI, Diaconis JN, Dennis JM: The inverted V: a new sign of pneumoperitoneum, *Radiology* 107:47, 1973.
67. Wollin E, Ozonoff MB: Dermoid development of teeth in an ovarian teratoma, *N Engl J Med* 265:890, 1961.
68. Wood JC: A calcified adrenal tumor, *Br J Radiol* 25:222, 1952.

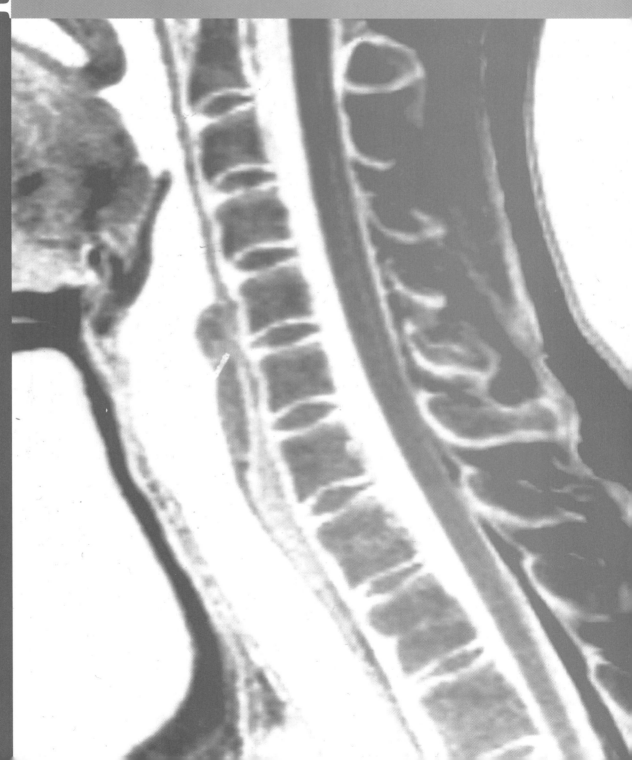

Brain and Spinal Cord

chapter 33

Brain and Spinal Cord

RAY N. CONLEY
GARY A. LONGMUIR

Trauma

BACKGROUND

Trauma to the head accounts for more deaths and disability in the United States than any other neurologic disorder among individuals under the age of 50.[185,304] More than 50,000 people die each year because of brain trauma, about one third of all injury deaths, with approximately 11,000 new cases of spinal cord injury reported during the same time.[56,59,151,185] Motor vehicle accidents cause approximately half of the traumatic brain injuries in the United States, with falls and firearms responsible for most of the remaining cases.[151,304] Traumatic brain injury (TBI) is a cause of long-term disability that annually affects an estimated 70,000 to 90,000 people.[56] Public health efforts to prevent the occurrence and mitigate the consequences of TBI have received increased attention in recent years because of the serious outcome and large number of people affected. Alcohol is often a precipitating factor in these injuries.[59,67] The clinical assessment of the posttraumatic patient is discussed with emphasis on appropriate diagnostic imaging.

IMAGING FINDINGS

Spinal trauma. It is appropriate to initially evaluate the posttraumatic patient with plain films. Radiographic examination of the cervical region should include anteroposterior (AP) open mouth, AP lower cervical, neutral lateral cervical, and possibly oblique cervical and flexion-extension projections, depending on patient presentation. If the C7 vertebral body and posterior arch structures are not well demonstrated in the routine examination, overexposed lateral cervicothoracic spot or swim lateral cervicothoracic spot radiographs are recommended. Visualization of the C7 level is extremely important because posterior arch and vertebral body fractures often are overlooked because of summation of shoulder structures. Passive flexion lateral cervical and extension lateral cervical radiographs are particularly helpful for evaluation of intersegmental stability.

Radiographic or clinical assessment may provide justification for more specialized imaging. If fracture is suspected, a three-view cervical series with computed tomography (CT) is prudent. CT is superior to oblique projections and other plain film views to demonstrate the osseous anatomy of the vertebral arch. Axial imaging often allows visualization of fractures that are not discernible on routine radiography. In addition, CT examination may render a more detailed understanding of the extent of fracture deformity previously detected in a routine radiographic examination. CT permits visualization of the central canal, including retropulsed fracture fragments and stenosis caused by misalignment. Occasionally a nuclear bone scan or single photon emission computed tomography (SPECT) might be advantageous in those patients who exhibit clinical findings suggestive of an occult posterior arch fracture. These are frequently not well demonstrated with plain films or CT because of the orientation of the fracture. Fractures in a horizontal plane may not be visible in axial imaging, although reformatting in the coronal, oblique, and sagittal planes may be beneficial. Reformatted CT images also may be useful in determining a treatment plan for complex fractures.[190,199]

If sufficient clinical indications exist, a magnetic resonance imaging (MRI) scan may be necessary to demonstrate the ligaments, intervertebral discs, and soft tissues within the spinal canal or intervertebral foramina. MRI is the preferred examination in patients with spinal cord edema, hematoma, or transection. Space-occupying lesions that may cause mass effect on the spinal cord or nerve roots are well perceived. Late effects of trauma to the spinal cord are best examined by MRI, including gliosis, myelomalacia, and syringomyelia.[192]

Examination of the thoracic and lumbar regions should proceed in the same manner as in the cervical spine with initial plain film radiography, including at least AP and lateral projections. One should demonstrate the thoracolumbar junction, because this transitional region is a common area for fracture. Lumbar oblique projections may be added, particularly for evaluation of the posterior arch anatomy. Tilting up lumbosacral spot (L5-S1 AP or Hibb's projection) and lateral lumbosacral spot radiography may help to better visualize the lumbosacral junction. Special imaging should be performed if indicated by clinical or plain radiographic findings. Lumbar or thoracic trauma may result in different neurologic findings than in the cervical region. For instance, the cauda equina and conus medullaris syndromes are indigenous to the lumbar region, whereas quadriplegia is caused by a cervical spine injury. These patients should be imaged appropriately according to their individual clinical findings.[134,275]

Brain and skull trauma. Patients with head trauma constitute a large percentage of cases referred for neuroimaging.

Imaging of hyperacute trauma (<24 hours) to the skull and brain should begin with MRI or CT, particularly in a patient with neurologic deficit, because the diagnostic yield of plain film radiography does not warrant its use. In the first 24 hours after trauma, CT is the imaging modality of choice rather than MRI. Emergency equipment is more easily used with CT rather than MRI because of the incompatibility of equipment with a strong magnetic field. However, recent advances have resulted in the commercial introduction of more MRI–compatible patient stabilization equipment.[171,229,304]

Attenuation of blood in CT scans is dependent on its constituent components because serum is less dense than protein and red blood cells. Therefore serum displays less attenuation than brain tissue, whereas the other products of hemorrhage and hematoma exhibit greater attenuation than the brain. Assessment of fractures and penetrating injuries is easily accomplished with CT in most cases and is fast, reliable, and easily accessible in most communities (Fig. 33-1, *A* to *C*). CT is compatible with

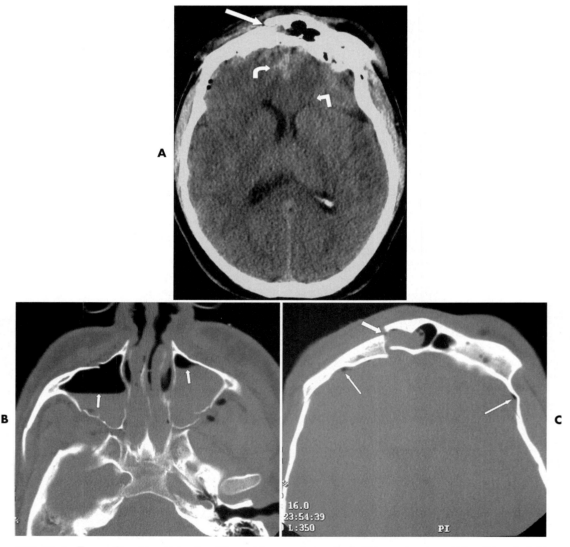

FIG. 33-1   Trauma. Closed head injury in a 48-year-old man as the result of a high-speed motor vehicle collision. **A,** Axial noncontrast soft-tissue window computed tomography image shows an oblique fracture line through the right frontal sinus *(large arrow),* bilateral frontal lobe hemorrhagic contusions with associated edema *(curved arrow),* and blunting of the anterior horn of the left lateral ventricle *(angled arrow).* **B,** Axial bone window images demonstrate a comminuted nasal fracture and extensive fractures of both maxillary sinuses with air-fluid levels *(arrows).* **C,** Axial bone window image of the frontal bone illustrates a displaced fracture through the right frontal sinus *(large arrow).* This introduces free air into the cranial vault *(small arrows)* and puts the patient at risk for meningeal infection.

patient stabilization devices and monitoring equipment.[53] Posttraumatic CT protocol should include 5- to 10-mm thick contiguous axial images from the skull base to the vertex with bone, brain, and subdural windows or level settings. Limitations resulting from beam hardening artifact should be taken into consideration, particularly in the frontal, parietal, occipital, and cerebellar regions. In those patients who require assessment of vascular injury, magnetic resonance angiography (MRA), duplex or transcranial ultrasound, CT with contrast, or conventional catheter angiography is used.[43,93,171,276]

MRI is superior to CT in the demonstration of blood products in the acute, subacute, and chronic posttraumatic patient, as well as nonhemorrhagic lesions such as diffuse axonal injury, cortical contusions, white matter shear injury, and brainstem lesions. Within the past 10 years, recognition of a deoxyhemoglobin rim in hyperacute injuries has made MRI a reasonable alternative to CT.[22] In addition, MRI is better at visualization of hemorrhages within the brain parenchyma and subcortical gray matter.[93,267] MRI provides direct multiplanar acquisitions in the axial, sagittal, or coronal planes and permits excellent soft-tissue contrast. In imaging hemorrhage or hematoma in the brain, the MRI signal is dependent not only on the length of time that the blood has been present, but also on the strength of the magnet. Familiarity with the MRI system is essential in determining the signal characteristics to be expected in the various time stages after trauma.[23,216,275]

Blood products are predominantly oxyhemoglobin with a deoxyhemoglobin rim in the hyperacute stage after trauma (<24 hours). Deoxyhemoglobin is more prevalent in the acute stage (24 to 72 hours), whereas methemoglobin predominates in the subacute/late phase (72 hours to 2 weeks). Methemoglobin remains in the central portion of the lesion, whereas hemosiderin surrounds the periphery after 2 weeks. Eventually hemosiderin deposition dominates the blood products in the late chronic stage with low signal characteristics on both T1- and T2-weighted images (Table 33-1).*

CLINICAL COMMENTS

The most common head injuries result from blunt or nonpenetrating trauma. These injuries frequently induce a temporary or longer loss of consciousness, and the brain may suffer gross damage in spite of the absence of skull fracture or penetrating injury. Skull fractures may serve to indicate the presence of significant trauma; however, the presence or absence of a skull fracture cannot be used to predict the presence or severity of intracranial injury.

Trauma to the head and spine often requires emergency evaluation and treatment performed by an emergency team at the site of injury. It is essential that the injury not be compounded by excessive movement immediately after trauma. The cervical spine must be stabilized before transport. If time allows, a cursory physical and neurologic assessment of the patient is recommended. Evaluating the ABCs (airway, breathing, and circulation) is suggested, and the Glasgow coma scale (GCS) is used to assess posttraumatic brain injury. The outcome of the GCS and severity and type of trauma are good predictors of mortality.[284] Spinal cord injury may mask injuries below the level of the trauma, particularly in the abdominal region.[59] Before the arrival of emergency medical transportation, a physician may administer cardiopulmonary resuscitation (CPR), treatment for shock, or other life-sustaining procedures, always avoiding further spinal cord injury. State Good Samaritan laws should be understood before initiating care. Even if a Good

---

*References 9, 22, 53, 134, 267, 275.

TABLE 33-1
Blood Products

Time following trauma	Hemoglobin/hemosiderin	Magnetic resonance imaging signal characteristics
Hyperacute (<24 hours)	Oxyhemoglobin-deoxyhemoglobin rim	Intermediate T1, high T2, low T2 rim
Acute (24–72 hours)	Deoxyhemoglobin	Intermediate T1, low T2
Subacute early (3–7 days)	Early, intracellular methemoglobin	High T1, low T2
Subacute late (1–2 weeks)	Later, extracellular methemoglobin	High T1, high T2
Chronic early (>2 weeks)	Extracellular methemoglobin with a hemosiderin rim	High central signal in both T1 and T2, low signal rim
Chronic late (>2 months)	Hemosiderin predominates late	Low T1, low T2

Samaritan law is in place, some jurisdictions consider it "gross negligence" to provide care at a level beyond which a person is trained.

KEY CONCEPTS

- *In spinal trauma, radiographs should be accomplished first with good visualization of C7, the thoracolumbar junction, and the lumbosacral junction.*
- *Radiography or clinical findings may suggest the need for special imaging.*
- *Computed tomography (CT) is particularly useful in evaluation of possible posterior arch fractures.*
- *Magnetic resonance imaging (MRI) is helpful in assessing the soft tissues, ligaments, discs, spinal canal, and intervertebral foramina.*
- *With skull trauma, CT or MRI should be done first; plain film generally is inadequate for patient evaluation.*

Specific Selected Injuries

Acute Cortical Contusion

BACKGROUND

By design the skull is a rigid shell that protects the brain from direct injury. The inner table of the vault has roughened edges, ridges and bony prominences along the floor of the anterior fossa, sphenoid wings, and petrous pyramids that can contuse the brain surface during the compressive force of a traumatic event.

Cortical contusions or bruises may occur by direct trauma (coup) or by the brain rebounding and striking the skull (contrecoup) because of acceleration and deceleration.[201,259] A vascular injury must be present for bruising to occur. Parenchymal lesions are found on the surface of the brain in the form of microhemorrhage with edema. Cortical contusions typically are multiple and measure approximately 2 to 4 cm in diameter. Thirty to fifty percent of these lesions are hemorrhagic.[56] Cellular disruption is associated with the release of vasoactive substances. The resulting vascular permeability to serum proteins facilitates a progressive increase of interstitial fluid. Over a short period of time, blood and edematous fluid advance within the white matter and into the subdural and subarachnoid spaces, producing a mass effect on adjacent anatomic structures and positive neurologic findings. Approximately 50% to 75% of cortical contusions involve the frontal and temporal lobes, especially the lateral aspects of both lobes and inferior surface of the frontal lobe.[56] The falx, tentorium, and cranial fossae are especially vulnerable areas.[201,218] Gliding and shearing injuries often are bilateral with tearing of the parasagittal venous structures.[218,249]

IMAGING FINDINGS

CT usually is employed for initial evaluation of hyperacute cortical contusion because it is fast, reliable, and readily available. Recognition of hyperacute cortical injury is dependent on increased attenuation in the region of the contusion. However, CT has a tendency to underestimate the size of these lesions soon after injury because of isoattenuation with edema and surrounding brain tissue. Repeat scanning often allows complete visualization of original foci and recognition of other sites of involvement. CT also produces beam-hardening artifacts that hamper imaging of more peripheral parenchymal cortical tissue adjacent to the skull.[321]

MRI typically demonstrates contusion in the hyperacute stage, particularly if gradient echo and fluid-attenuated inversion recovery (FLAIR) protocols are used.[201,250,251] MRI is particularly sensitive to surrounding edema and peripheral cortical foci that may be overlooked on CT. However, many facilities are not equipped with MRI–compatible emergency equipment. In addition, claustrophobia, sedation to reduce motion, and large body habitus must be taken into consideration if MRI is performed instead of CT. MRI is ideal for evaluation of cortical contusions in later stages when emergency equipment is no longer needed.[23,201] The signal intensity of cortical contusion is similar to other blood products produced by trauma (see Table 33-1). Cortical contusion often is associated with other intracranial lesions, such as subdural hematoma (Fig. 33-2, *A* to *C*). SPECT scans are being used occasionally for diagnosis of cortical contusion. SPECT scanning also has been used in a monitoring role to follow patients with traumatic brain injury.[155]

CLINICAL COMMENTS

Focal neurologic deficits are late-appearing clinical findings. Confusion, focal cerebral dysfunction, seizures, and personality changes are seen more frequently early in cases of cortical contusion.

> **KEY CONCEPTS**
> - *Trauma may be coup or contrecoup and result in bleeding into the brain.*
> - *Computed tomography (CT) or magnetic resonance imaging (MRI) may be performed in the hyperacute stage depending on facilities.*
> - *MRI is better than CT after 24 hours.*

Acute Epidural Hematoma

BACKGROUND

Epidural hematomas may occur within the spine or skull when blood accumulates between the dura and surrounding bone. If the arteries are torn because of a severe shear trauma that separates the dura from the bone, blood may accumulate rapidly in the potential space created by this injury. If there is venous compromise, a slower, more chronic pattern may result. The middle meningeal artery is involved most often after skull trauma, although the ethmoidal artery or sinuses (superior sagittal, transverse, or sigmoidal) may be traumatized depending on the exact site of trauma. A small percentage of epidural hematomas are bilateral (<10%), whereas the great majority exhibit skull fractures (>90%). The calvarial periosteum (dura layer) is bound down at the suture margins, creating an anatomic boundary to hemorrhage.[169,218]

There are numerous causes for spinal epidural bleeding other than high-impact trauma. Spinal epidural hematoma often occurs in conjunction with disc herniation because of involvement of the epidural venous plexus and may be responsible for neural effacement. MRI signal characteristics of disc versus blood must be thoroughly explored, because a space-occupying lesion caused by blood resolves much more quickly than disc debris. This characteristic may clarify the rapid resolution of "sequestered" disc herniations that are in reality spinal epidural hematomas.[105]

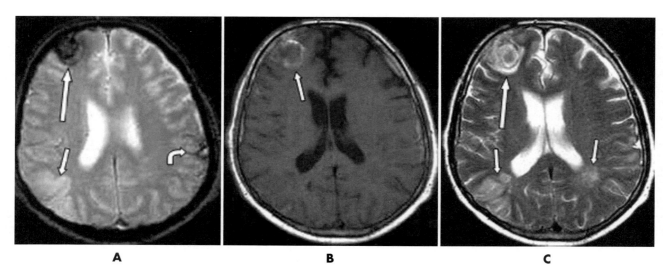

A	**B**	**C**

FIG. 33-2   Cortical contusion. **A,** Right frontal and left parietal cortical contusions are apparent *(long arrow, curved arrow)* in the gradient recall axial acquisition with an area of cortical edema in the right posterior parietal region *(short arrow)*. **B,** Peripheral enhancement is visualized in the right frontal contusion in the postcontrast T1-weighted axial image *(arrow)*. **C,** The T2-weighted axial image demonstrates heterogenous increase in signal at the right frontal cortical contusion with increased signal in areas of edema adjacent to the posterior parietal region and posterior to the posterior horn of the left lateral ventricle. A subdural hematoma is discernible incidentally anteriorly on the left side *(arrows)*. (Courtesy Bryan K. Hosler, Cincinnati, OH.)

In addition, thrombolysis, anticoagulation therapy, lumbar puncture, spinal epidural injections, hypertension, and blood dyscrasias may result in spinal epidural hematoma with compromise of neural structures caused by mass effect. These conditions produce symptoms similar to disc herniation, including back pain, numbness or paresthesias, lower extremity weakness, and incontinence (both urinary and fecal).[169]

IMAGING FINDINGS

Imaging of both intracranial and spinal epidural hematomas usually begins with CT, although MRI also is diagnostic in the stable patient or in facilities that are equipped with MRI–compatible emergency and stabilization equipment. MRI is particularly useful in evaluation of spinal epidural hematoma and its consequences with surrounding neural structures. In the brain, considerable midline shift, large hematoma volume, signs of active bleeding (mixed density clot on CT), and the presence of other associated lesions are suggestive of a poor prognosis after skull trauma. These imaging findings are correlated with clinical signs such as age, coma, papillary abnormalities, and GCS or motor score to help determine an outcome.[218,230,258,295] The hematoma typically is lentiform shaped and hyperdense on CT, although less dense areas occur in regions where there is serum or recent bleeding. The area of hematoma usually is homogeneously hyperdense 72 hours after cessation of bleeding. Signal characteristics in MRI scans are typical of other forms of hematoma (see Table 33-1).

CLINICAL COMMENTS

A transient loss of consciousness may occur with intervals of mental lucidity. Palsy of cranial nerve III may be present and is a sign of cerebral herniation. Somnolence, sleepiness, or unnatural drowsiness 24 to 96 hours after injury constitutes a medical emergency.

KEY CONCEPTS

- *Hematomas occur in the epidural space of the brain or spine.*
- *Computed tomography or magnetic resonance imaging scans are used rather than plain film radiography.*
- *Imaging findings should be correlated with clinical signs.*

Acute Subdural Hematoma

BACKGROUND

Subdural hematomas are caused more frequently by venous rather than arterial damage and are often self-limiting because of the slow bleeding process. However, if the hematoma is large, mass effect may take place, shifting cerebral structures and causing edema in the parenchyma of the brain, resulting in a poor clinical outcome. Subdural hematomas arise deep to the dura but external to the arachnoid membrane, and the untreated hematoma may become subacute or chronic. Acute subdural hematoma is more common in older age groups because the veins are less resilient and more easily damaged. Patients taking anticoagulants and alcoholic patients are also prone to acute subdural hematoma.[152,249,304,311]

IMAGING FINDINGS

MRI is more accurate than CT in assessing the size of a subdural hematoma and its effect on surrounding parenchymal tissue (Fig. 33-3).[249] Nonetheless, CT frequently is the imaging modality used because of accessibility, rapid acquisition, and compatibility with emergency equipment. On CT scans, increased density is visualized along the inner table of the skull, most commonly in the

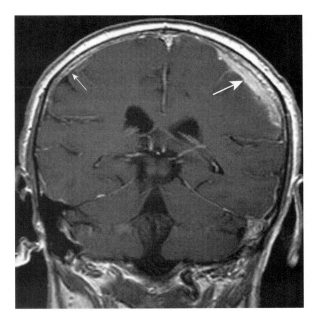

FIG. 33-3 Subdural hematoma. Large subdural hematoma *(large arrow)* present on the left side of the Gd-DTPA–enhanced T1-weighted coronal acquisition. Smaller subdural hematoma apparent on the right side *(small arrows)*. (Courtesy Bryan K. Hosler, Cincinnati, OH.)

parietal region. Small hematomas may be difficult to visualize, and adjustment of the window level or width between usual bone and soft-tissue windows may be necessary. Edema is not as easily perceived with CT as MRI. False-negative CT findings may occur as the result of a high-convexity lesion, beam-hardening artifact, or volume averaging with the high density of calvarium obscuring flat "en plaque" hematomas. Approximately 38% of small subdural hematomas are missed on CT.[56] Cerebral edema should be suspected and MRI accomplished if midline shift has occurred.[93,171,190,249,275] A blood-fluid level is appreciated occasionally.

KEY CONCEPTS

- *Acute subdural hematomas are usually caused by damage to the veins and are often slow to develop.*
- *Hematomas are more common in older patients and in those who are alcoholics or taking anticoagulants.*
- *Magnetic resonance imaging may be better for small bleeds adjacent to bone and for visualization of surrounding edema.*

Acute Subarachnoid Hemorrhage

BACKGROUND

Extravasation of blood deep to the arachnoid and above the pia mater is defined as subarachnoid hematoma and most frequently is caused by trauma, although often this type of hematoma is caused by vascular compromise, particularly aneurysm and arteriovenous malformation. Laceration of the microvessels in the superficial portion of the subarachnoid space causes subarachnoid hemorrhage. Posttraumatic subarachnoid hemorrhage may be benign. However, a communicating hydrocephalus may develop because of obstruction of the arachnoid villi or a noncommunicating hydrocephalus because there is a blood barrier for cerebrospinal fluid (CSF) flow through the third or fourth ventricle. Vasospasm and subsequent cerebral ischemia is another complication of traumatic subarachnoid hemorrhage.[43,59,323] Clinical prognosis is dependent on the volume of blood in the subarachnoid space.

IMAGING FINDINGS

CT is an extremely sensitive test for subarachnoid hemorrhage, particularly in the first 12 hours, although 1 hour is necessary for enough clot retraction to take place for sufficient protein concentration to become hyperdense. Within the past 10 years, it has become possible to demonstrate parenchymal and subarachnoid hemorrhage on MRI with confidence. Studies have shown that FLAIR MRI sequences allow visualization of acute subarachnoid hemorrhage better than CT or other MRI pulse sequences, particularly in the posterior fossa because of beam-hardening artifacts in CT.[22,46,102,212,272] Recognition of the deoxyhemoglobin border surrounding areas of oxyhemoglobin in T2-weighted MRI acquisitions also has made it possible to image blood products in the hyperacute patient.[22] Thin slice CT must be performed to recognize small bleeds; blood may be isodense with brain tissue if the hematocrit levels are below 30.[243,265] An extremely small percentage of patients have false-negative CT or MRI scans. Lumbar puncture is indicated in those patients who exhibit symptoms of subarachnoid hemorrhage who have a negative CT or MRI examination.[296] It must be remembered that lumbar punctures often are falsely negative in the first 12 hours after injury.[71,243,265]

KEY CONCEPTS

- *Posttraumatic subarachnoid hematoma may be benign but may be associated with hydrocephalus- or vasospasm-induced ischemia.*
- *Magnetic resonance imaging (MRI) or computed tomography (CT) scans are used and are extremely sensitive.*
- *If clinical findings suggest a subarachnoid hemorrhage, a lumbar puncture should be performed, even though MRI and CT scans are negative.*

Vascular Injury

BACKGROUND

Blunt trauma to the internal carotid, middle cerebral, and anterior cerebral arteries is more commonly the cause of brain ischemia than injuries to other arteries. The external carotid, vertebral, and subclavian arteries are not common sites of injury; posttraumatic brain ischemia and penetrating injuries cause most damage to these arteries. Fractures at the base of the skull and mandible frequently are encountered with traumatic carotid injuries.[44,67,92,323]

With relatively minor trauma, disruption of the vascular intima leads to a hemodynamic situation ideal for platelet deposition and thrombus formation. The thrombus eventually may occlude the entire vascular lumen, resulting in cerebral ischemia and infarction. In addition, traumatic disturbance of atherosclerotic plaque may give rise to an embolus.

Higher-force trauma may lead to more complete tearing of the intima, resulting in dissecting aneurysm as pulsatile high-pressure blood forces its way between the intima and media.[88,323] Dissecting extracranial aneurysms are most commonly found in the cervical portion of the internal carotid as it enters the skull, whereas intracranial aneurysms most frequently occur at branches of the middle cerebral artery. Turbulence may cause the aneurysm to enlarge with thrombus formation and possible distal embolization.[88]

IMAGING FINDINGS

Vascular injuries may be examined by MRA, catheter angiography, duplex ultrasound, transcranial Doppler ultrasound, and SPECT.[155,234,267,274,278] MRA is noninvasive and presents a viable alternative to conventional catheter angiography. Reconstruction of thin slice two- or three-dimensional time-of-flight axial images using "flow phenomena" allows visualization of the vessel with an angiographic appearance. Phase contrast studies provide information about volume and velocity of blood flow. The key finding in MRA of an intimal tear with dissection is demonstration of the intimal flap that separates the true from the false lumen of the vessel. The lumen may be narrowed with increased signal within the entirety of the lumen or in the periluminal region.* Catheter angiography reveals an irregular narrowing of the vessel or the classic "string sign," and the intimal flap also may be visualized. Total occlusion from hematoma or thrombus causes interruption of signal on MRA and flow void on angiography.[90,321] Duplex and transcranial ultrasound rapidly is becoming more popular because it is fast, inexpensive, sensitive, and noninvasive.[274,278]

KEY CONCEPTS

- *Trauma to the head or neck may cause arterial thrombus or dissecting aneurysm.*
- *Magnetic resonance angiography (MRA) is noninvasive, and new protocols have made MRA a feasible alternative to catheter angiography.*
- *Advances in duplex and transcranial diagnostic ultrasound have made these modalities an alternative to catheter angiography.*

Traumatic Pseudoaneurysms

BACKGROUND

A pseudoaneurysm or "false" aneurysm is created by rupture of all three arterial walls (intima, media, and adventitia), although egress of blood flow from the vessel is contained initially by surrounding fibrous tissue in the adventitia. These lesions may extravasate blood into the surrounding tissues, which may gradually or abruptly increase in size, resulting in pressure on surrounding structures. Pseudoaneurysm of the vertebral artery is usually observed at the C1-2 level. Rupture or distal embolization may take place.[276] Catheterization (particularly in patients undergoing anticoagulant therapy or antiplatelet medication), rotational trauma, and infection may be causative factors for pseudoaneurysm.[6,116,136] Treatment includes duplex-guided compression (peripheral extracranial vessels), thrombin injection, and surgical repair.[37]

IMAGING FINDINGS

Duplex and transcranial Doppler ultrasonography are becoming increasingly more reliable in early diagnosis of traumatic pseudoaneurysms. Various bone windows are being used for transcranial Doppler. For example, the temporal bone is thin and can be used as a window to reveal segments of the middle cerebral, internal carotid, anterior cerebral, and anterior communicating arteries. The ophthalmic artery is visible through the orbital window and the basilar artery by the suboccipital approach.[143,234,239]

---

*References 210, 216, 218, 233, 275, 316.

The ability of transcranial Doppler ultrasound and phase contrast MRI to measure volume and velocity of blood flow is particularly useful. However, patients undergoing surgery should have MRA or catheter angiography. MRA is a practical alternative to catheter angiography when patients are allergic to contrast dye, have renal insufficiency, or desire a noninvasive examination.[275] Accuracy for carotid stenosis is virtually assured if MRA and ultrasound findings correlate. Nonetheless, if there is no correlation between MRA and ultrasound, conventional angiography should be done, if possible.[77,78]

PART FIVE
Brain and Spinal Cord

Vascular Disorders

Specific Selected Conditions

Stroke

BACKGROUND

Disruption of the local blood supply to the brain produces ischemia and eventual infarction of brain parenchyma. Large infarctions may be associated with marked cerebral edema resulting in gross shifting of midline structures, herniation, and death caused by brainstem compression. Stroke is the third most common cause of death and the primary cause of severe disability in the United States. It is the second leading cause of death in patients over 75 years of age.[56] Stroke may result from ischemia or hemorrhage. The majority (80%) of cases result from ischemia because of extracranial embolus or intracranial thrombosis. Hemorrhagic strokes may be secondary to brain neoplasia, arteriovenous malformation, subarachnoid cyst, and anticoagulant therapy. A sudden loss of circulation to the brain results in infarction and loss of neurologic function. The site of occlusion and size of infarction control the subsequent clinical outcome.

Symptoms include nausea, vomiting, headache, vertigo, aphasia, visual disturbances, diplopia, and neurologic deficit such as sudden-onset paresis, hypesthesia, or ataxia. Risk factors include high blood cholesterol, advanced age, smoking, hypertension, atherosclerosis, and cardiac disease.[7,15]

IMAGING FINDINGS

Diffusion-weighted imaging (DWI) and apparent diffusion coefficient (ADC) make clinically relevant information available about presence, age, and location of lesions minutes after onset of ischemia that is not appreciated on conventional MRI examinations or CT (Fig. 33-4, *A* and *B*).[250,251,317] DWI relies on the differences of tissue water diffusion properties for visualization of lesional tissue. Increase in signal is directly proportional to increased water diffusion on DWI examinations. Both conventional MRI and DWI have been shown to be considerably more accurate than CT in characterization and demonstration of acute cerebral infarct.[156,294,317] Functional MRI (fMRI) permits early evaluation of stroke. The patient is instructed to perform a task during an fMRI examination. The metabolism in the brain accelerates in the area used to

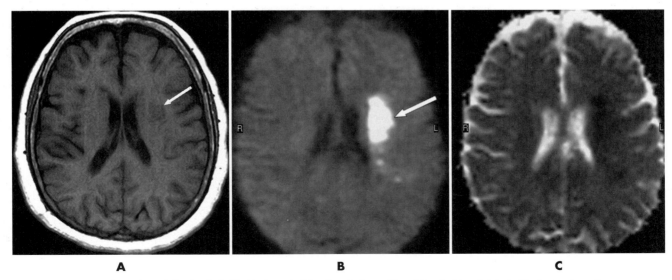

A   **B**   **C**

FIG. 33-4 Acute infarction. Left-sided brain acute infarction. **A,** Area of hypointensity *(arrow)* detected in the basal ganglia adjacent to the left lateral ventricle in the postcontrast T1-weighted axial image. Lesion does not enhance with gadolinium-diethylene-triamine-pentaacetic acid (Gd-DTPA) administration. **B,** Diffusion-weighted imaging demonstrates increased signal *(arrow).* **C,** Decreased signal in the apparent diffusion coefficient image typical of an acute infarction.

accomplish this task, altering MRI signal. fMRI is particularly useful in mapping brain tissue for surgery or radiation therapy.

Another relatively new technology, diffusion tensor imaging (DTI), uses gradients not only in the *x, y,* and *z* planes, but also in six noncollinear directions simultaneously; therefore both the direction and magnitude of water diffusion in space can be measured independently of patient or white matter fiber orientation. In DTI, an echo planar technique is used that allows determination of the structural integrity of white matter fibers by a method called *anisotropy.* Anisotropy is the diffusion of water or a metabolite in a specific direction. DTI uses the fact that myelin is a barrier to diffusion of water molecules to allow assessment of the integrity of white matter fibers on a microscopic scale.*

Transcranial Doppler is useful in evaluating the vertebrobasilar, middle cerebral, internal carotid, anterior cerebral, and anterior communicating arteries.[143,234,239] Angiography usually is not needed unless endovascular treatment is intended.

CLINICAL COMMENTS

Death during hospitalization occurs in approximately 25% of stroke patients. Patients with an alteration in consciousness, gaze preference, and dense hemiplegia have a 40% mortality rate. Survival with varying degrees of neurologic deficit occurs in 75% of patients. Forty percent of stroke patients can expect a good functional recovery. Indications for cerebrovascular testing include transient ischemic attack (TIA), progressive carotid arterial disease with 95% to 98% stenosis, and the presence of cardiogenic cerebral emboli.[56]

> ### KEY CONCEPTS
> - *Stroke is caused by interruption of normal blood flow to brain parenchyma.*
> - *Stroke may lead to severe neurologic deficit or death.*
> - *Diffusion-weighted and diffusion tensor magnetic resonance imaging allow early evaluation of stroke patients.*
> - *Transcranial Doppler diagnostic ultrasound may be useful in certain types of stroke.*

Nontraumatic Subarachnoid Hemorrhage

BACKGROUND

Approximately one third of all patients diagnosed with subarachnoid hemorrhage (SAH) have a demonstrable neurologic deficit. Forty to fifty percent of patients with SAH die within the first month. Saccular aneurysms often rupture spontaneously and account for two thirds of all nontraumatic SAH, resulting in more than 18,000 deaths per year. The remaining cases of SAH are caused by arteriovenous malformation, mycotic aneurysm, cortical thrombosis, angioma, and various other invasive neoplasia. Discrete and episodic bleeding from the wall of a saccular aneurysm, known as a "warning leak," may precede complete rupture.[96,128,209] Severe headache, often described by the patient as "the worst headache ever," is a common complaint with SAH. These headaches typically are new to the patient with abrupt onset. Meningeal irritation caused by the hemorrhage is likely to produce nuchal rigidity or other signs of meningeal irritation (Brudzinski's or Kernig's sign). Other patient complaints include nausea, vomiting, neck pain, seizure, cranial neuropathy, visual disturbances, paresis, loss of consciousness, and coma. A high percentage of SAH patients

undergo complications that include rebleeding and vasospasm. Eighty-five percent of all saccular intracranial aneurysms are found in the anterior cerebral circulation and occur at arterial junctions and branches.*

IMAGING FINDINGS

CT is sensitive for the first 24 hours after a SAH. The longer CT is delayed, the less sensitive the test becomes. In addition, it is necessary that the hemoglobin count exceed 10 g/dl or blood will be isodense to the surrounding brain tissue on CT. The bleeding event requires at least 1 hour for clot and protein concentration to be sufficiently dense to be visible on CT scans.[243,265] Catheter angiography is used to localize aneurysms and define their shape before surgery. MRA is sensitive for aneurysms exceeding 3 mm in diameter; this size is constantly decreasing as MRA becomes more sensitive (Fig. 33-5, *A* and *B*). MRI also is sensitive in SAH in both the hyperacute and subsequent stages, particularly if FLAIR, DWI, and DTI sequences are employed.[†] Lumbar puncture is positive in most cases when there is a "warning leak" or SAH, although blood is not found in the CSF until 12 hours after the onset of bleeding. Care also must be taken to exclude traumatic lumbar puncture as a cause for blood in the CSF. Lumbar puncture should not be performed if there are imaging findings suggestive of increased intracranial pressure or mass effect because of the possibility of brainstem herniation.[48,71,243,265]

> ### KEY CONCEPTS
> - *Most nontraumatic subarachnoid hemorrhage is related to aneurysmal rupture.*
> - *Severe headache is usually present.*
> - *Magnetic resonance angiography, magnetic resonance imaging, computed tomography, and lumbar puncture are diagnostic methods useful in the evaluation of subarachnoid hemorrhage.*

Vascular Malformation

BACKGROUND

Arteriovenous malformation (AVM), cavernous hemangioma, venous angioma, and capillary telangiectasia are common forms of vascular malformation. The latter two are of little clinical significance because they are relatively benign and rarely symptomatic. AVMs may be found in the brain or spine, but are much more common in the brain. The tangled masses of arteries and veins that make up an AVM communicate with one another without normal capillary function. Neural parenchyma lies between the vessels in an intracranial AVM. Blood is shunted directly between the arterial and venous systems in the AVM, resulting in an increased venous pressure that helps to facilitate hemorrhage. Although the great majority of patients with AVMs are asymptomatic, approximately 12% of patients with AVMs present with severe headaches, seizures, and progressive neurologic deficit. Aneurysms are present in more than 5% of individuals with AVM, usually in the arteries feeding the AVM. AVM should be considered in the differential diagnosis if there is a high clinical suspicion of intracranial hemorrhage. This is particularly important in young patients. Spinal AVM may present with weakness, numbness, or motor dysfunction in the extremities that may lead to paresis. Bladder and bowel dysfunction are also a consequence of spinal AVM. Treatment is surgical.[97,232,270]

---

*References 3, 17, 156, 162, 176, 294.

---

*References 15, 47, 170, 188, 209, 252.
†References 22, 46, 102, 157, 212, 272.

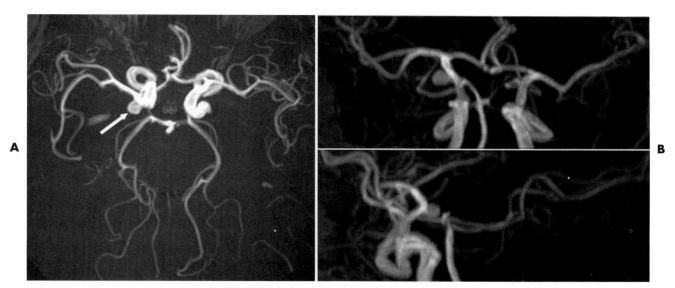

FIG. 33-5 Saccular aneurysm. **A** and **B,** Magnetic resonance angiography (MRA) of the circle of Willis illustrates a saccular aneurysm on the right side (arrow). MRA is noninvasive and may be accomplished without contrast. (Courtesy Bryan K. Hosler, Cincinnati, OH.)

Cavernous hemangiomas are also known as *cavernous angiomas* and *cavernomas*. They were previously considered angiographically occult or cryptic vascular malformations because they were not readily discernible on catheter angiography. Cavernous hemangiomas are endothelial-lined sinusoidal spaces and are slow flow lesions rather than rapid shunts. Brain tissue is not interposed between the abnormal vessels as it is in the AVM. Less than 25% of cavernomas are asymptomatic. They often bleed and may cause seizures or neurologic deficit. Hemangiomas may be seen in the spinal cord but are uncommon. The treatment of intracerebral and spinal cord hemangiomas is surgical or stereotactic radiosurgery.[97,189,232]

IMAGING FINDINGS

Often CT is used early in the diagnosis of AVM. However, non-hemorrhagic AVMs often are isodense to surrounding brain matter and overlooked on CT. Only 20% to 30% of AVMs calcify and are visible on CT. The high sensitivity of MRI to flow void makes MRI the most accurate modality for imaging of AVM. A diagnosis of AVM is established by the demonstration of multiple tortuous areas of flow void on MRI. Hemosiderin deposition secondary to hemorrhage produces a characteristic low signal, particularly on gradient echo acquisitions. In addition, high signal areas on T2-weighted images are suggestive of ischemia. Multiple serpiginous, irregular tubular structures are the hallmark of AVM in the spinal cord. Supplying arteries, lesional matrix, and venous drainage are discernible on digital subtraction catheter angiography, as well as those small aneurysms that may not be visible on MRA. Angiography usually is performed before surgery.[97,113,232]

CT is fast and widely available. For these reasons CT is useful for early diagnostic workup of cavernous hemangiomas in emergent situations. However, MRI and MRA should be considered the imaging modalities of choice because they provide considerably more information about anatomy and pathophysiology than CT. Cavernous hemangiomas are not visible on conventional angiography and CT may not demonstrate all lesions. Edema is identified easily on MRI with high signal intensity on T2-weighted acquisitions. Repeated bleeds cause deposition of hemosiderin that produces a characteristic low signal ring appearance on MRI. Gradient echo MRI sequences are particularly well suited for the discovery and evaluation of small hemangiomas due to the sensitivity of gradient echo imaging to magnetic susceptibility artifact produced by hemosiderin.[24,113]

KEY CONCEPTS

- *Arteriovenous malformations and cavernous hemangiomas are the most clinically important of the vascular malformations.*
- *Magnetic resonance imaging and magnetic resonance angiography are highly sensitive for vascular malformation and should be used if an emergent situation allows.*
- *Digital subtraction angiography is useful in visualization of small aneurysms, feeding arteries, arteriovenous malformation matrix, and draining veins in arteriovenous malformations and is usually performed before surgery.*
- *Cavernous hemangiomas are not demonstrated on digital subtraction angiography.*

Infectious and Inflammatory Processes of the Central Nervous System

BACKGROUND

The brain, spinal cord, and their associated membranes comprise the central nervous system (CNS). Life-threatening infections may ensue if bacteria, viruses, fungi, protozoa, or parasites enter the CNS. The meninges (meningitis), brain (encephalitis, abscess), epidural region (epidural abscess), and spine (discitis, epidural abscess) are common locations for infection. Brain infections most commonly arise from infections at contiguous sites. The ear, mastoid processes, mouth, and sinuses are frequent primary sites. CNS infections also may appear because of hematogenous spread from remote extracranial sites of infection or through direct penetrating injury.[279,286] Spinal infections are the result of hematogenous spread, penetrating injury, or iatrogenic causes, including injections or surgery. However, more than 25% of patients with spinal infections display no perceivable primary infection.[63,194,225]

Neck pain and stiffness, fever, vomiting, seizures, sensitivity to light, headache, weakness, and neurologic deficit are common symptoms. Signs of meningeal irritation include spinal and nuchal rigidity, Kernig's sign, and Brudzinski's sign, although these signs are not reliable indicators of infection. Numerous variable pathogens are responsible for CNS infection. Unusual pathogens and other concurrent infections should be considered in immunocompromised patients. Aggressive early treatment of CNS infections with oral or intravenous antibiotics is crucial. However, surgical intervention is necessary in some cases.[38] Antibiotic-resistant organisms have made treatment difficult or impossible in many instances.[194,225]

Specific Selected Conditions

Abscess

BACKGROUND

Brain abscesses are not common but may cause severe symptoms, depending on the location and size of the abscess and the presence of surrounding inflammation. The location of the abscess may suggest its etiology. For example, those abscesses stemming from hematogenous dissemination may be multiple and vascular in distribution, whereas those resulting from sinusitis tend to be singular and located in the frontal lobe. CNS abscess is characterized initially by the presence of necrotic tissue surrounded by inflamed brain cells. Suppuration ensues, and mature abscesses are encapsulated pus-filled sacs. Less well-capsulated abscesses are prone to metastasis within the brain, producing multiple sites that usually are monomicrobial. Mass effect from the abscess and inflammation surrounding the abscess causes the brain to swell, permanently damaging adjacent brain tissue. Bacteria are the most common pathogens responsible for brain abscess, although fungi also may cause abscesses.[70,225,231,308]

IMAGING FINDINGS

Fatalities have fallen by 90% since CT and MRI have been employed in the diagnosis of brain abscess.[26,186,308] MRI has proved to be more sensitive and specific in the diagnosis and follow-up of brain abscess than CT.[306] CT imaging findings are poor indicators of clinical progress, and CT scans tend to underestimate the number of lesions. Ring enhancement on contrast CT may be helpful in diagnosis, although a similar enhancement can be visualized in granulomas, tumors, and resolving hematomas. MRI with contrast (Gd-DTPA) allows better visualization in the initial stages of abscess formation and produces more complete imaging of the central necrotic tissue, surrounding rim, and edema with earlier detection of small satellite lesions than CT (Fig. 33-6, *A* and *B*). For this reason, an MRI scan should be performed even if the CT scan is normal when clinical evidence of infection exists. This is particularly important if the patient is immunosuppressed.[26,308] DWI appears to be a sensitive method in diagnosis of abscess and can help to differentiate necrotic-cystic tumors from abscesses. It should be noted that DWI is not specific for abscess. Treatment with steroids

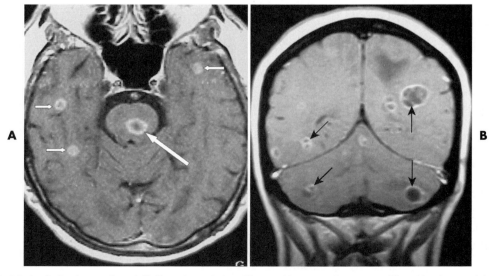

FIG. 33-6 Brain abscess. **A** and **B,** Toxoplasmosis in a 51-year-old woman. Postcontrast T1-weighted coronal images illustrates peripheral enhancement of multiple abscesses in both cerebral hemispheres and the cerebellum (*arrows*).

may impair the visualization of lesions on imaging by reducing mass effect and edema. Gallium, thallous chloride, and technetium SPECT imaging may allow discrimination between abscess and primary or metastatic brain neoplasias.[279,291]

CLINICAL COMMENTS

Symptoms include headache, nausea, vomiting, fever, altered mentation, seizures, paresis, and focal neurologic deficit; none are pathognomonic of abscess. Clinical signs are those of increased intracranial pressure and are dependent on the site of the lesion. A cerebral lesion causes different symptoms than a cerebellar abscess.[26] Complete blood count and blood cultures may be suggestive of infection and the electroencephalogram, positive (although not specific) in those cases of focal neurologic deficit or seizure. A biopsy using stereotactic CT or MRI permits accurate needle placement.[168] The biopsy specimen then is cultured and an appropriate antibiotic regimen is established. A developing cerebral abscess is a medical emergency, and larger lesions (>2.5 cm) should be excised or stereotactically aspirated.[260] Many abscesses can be avoided with the early successful treatment of the primary site of infection. Lumbar puncture should not be employed because of the possibility of transtentorial herniation. CSF assay is within normal limits in an unruptured abscess.[26,70,98]

> ### KEY CONCEPTS
> - *Although uncommon, abscess may have serious clinical consequences.*
> - *Magnetic resonance imaging is the modality of choice for evaluation of abscess.*
> - *Clinical signs and symptoms are suggestive of a central nervous system lesion but not specific for abscess.*

Meningeal Infections

BACKGROUND

Infection of the inner two membranes (leptomeninges) covering the brain and spinal cord may result in meningitis. Spread can be hematogenous or secondary to sinus and ear infections. The blood–brain barrier effectively isolates the infection from the immune system. Untreated pyogenic (bacterial) meningitis may cause death or lifelong disability. Bacterial meningitis presents the most serious clinical implications, causing 2000 deaths in the United States annually. The most common bacteria responsible are *Streptococcus pneumoniae, Neisseria meningitides, Staphylococcus,* and *Haemophilus* influenza type B bacteria (Hib). Cerebral infarcts, brain edema, paresis, seizures, hearing loss, blindness, and coma are common complications of pyogenic meningitis. In addition to bacteria, fungi and viruses may seed the leptomeninges with tuberculosis and sarcoidosis, affecting the pia mater and arachnoid. Fungal infections often are serious and usually require hospitalization. Viral meningitis is not typically fulminant and usually has a better clinical outcome that may be treated successfully with home care.[8,126,291]

IMAGING FINDINGS

MRI is more sensitive than CT in the imaging of meningitis. Contrast MRI with gadolinium (Gd-DTPA) characteristically results in diffuse enhancement of the subarachnoid space. This is not completely specific for infection; diseases such as sarcoidosis, neoplasia, or parasitic disease also may cause leptomeningeal enhancement. MRI without contrast may allow the visualization of cortical edema, distention of the subarachnoid space, and obliteration of the cisterns.[291] Inversion recovery MRI sequences are particularly sensitive

to subarachnoid exudate. MRI also is adept at imaging the primary site of infection or pathology resulting from complications such as hydrocephalus, infarction, cerebritis, and empyema.[135,282]

CLINICAL COMMENTS

The symptoms of meningitis are nonspecific and include headache, confusion, fever, stiff neck, nausea, vomiting, photophobia, diarrhea, seizures, and coma. Clinical signs include nuchal and spinal rigidity, Kernig's sign, unilateral or bilateral Babinski's sign, and Brudzinski's sign. Petechial or purpuric skin rash may be associated with meningococcal meningitis or septicemia. Intracranial pressure may occur along with rapidly falling blood pressure, causing septic shock. In addition, systemic complications, acute cortical stroke secondary to vasospasm, and massive brain infarction may lead to death.[75]

Lumbar puncture should be performed if the patient demonstrates a clinical presentation or imaging findings suggestive of meningitis. Imaging must be performed before lumbar puncture to exclude mass effect or increased intracranial pressure that may lead to herniation of the brainstem.[48] Lumbar puncture with analysis and culture of CSF should be not only diagnostic of bacterial meningitis, but a culture is essential in selecting the most effective treatment program. Septicemia is an occasional consequence of meningitis, and mortality is twice as high in cases with septicemia as with meningitis only. Early treatment with intravenous antibiotics is essential in bacterial meningitis.[8,126]

> ### KEY CONCEPTS
> - *Infection of the pia mater or arachnoid causes meningitis, an extremely severe disorder.*
> - *Magnetic resonance imaging is the most sensitive imaging examination for meningitis.*
> - *Lumbar puncture should be performed for definitive diagnosis and to establish the most effective antibiotic treatment.*

Encephalitis

BACKGROUND

Encephalitis is distinct from meningitis in that encephalitis results from inflammation of the brain parenchyma rather than the leptomeninges. However, the two often coexist, which is reflected in imaging examinations. Encephalitis is responsible for approximately 1400 deaths annually in the United States.[48] Acute encephalitis is associated more frequently with herpes simplex virus type 1 or an arbovirus than any other viral pathogen. If the infection involves the spinal cord and the brain, this is known as *encephalomyelitis.* Cerebritis implies a fulminant pyogenic bacterial infection that often leads to abscess formation and is not considered encephalitis. Untreated herpes simplex encephalitis has a mortality rate exceeding 50%. The mortality rate is highest in very young and elderly patients.[65,75,160]

IMAGING FINDINGS

MRI is considerably more sensitive than CT in its ability to image encephalitis. Approximately 40% of the acute encephalitic lesions caused by herpes simplex are not evident on CT. Comparatively MRI has been shown to demonstrate 94% of similar lesions.[48,194] If clinical indications exist, an MRI scan should be performed even if CT is negative. Mass effect, edema, and hemorrhage are visualized in the inferior frontal and temporal lobes that may be initially unilateral with eventual spread to both sides as the disease progresses.

Focal abnormalities in the basal ganglia, cerebral cortex, and substantia nigra often are discernible on MRI examination. Blood–brain barrier abnormalities are best imaged with MRI, particularly postcontrast.[48,65,150]

CLINICAL COMMENTS

Symptoms are not specific for encephalitis and include sudden fever, headache, myalgia, vomiting, photophobia, stiff neck and back, confusion, drowsiness, clumsiness, unsteady gait, and irritability. Symptoms that require emergency treatment include stupor, seizure, muscle weakness, paresis, sudden severe dementia, memory loss, impaired judgment, and coma. The GCS should be used to evaluate the level of consciousness and the GCS may be beneficial in formulating a prognosis and treatment plan. Metabolic disease, immunosuppression, medication, or illicit drug use may be indicators of etiology. Lumbar puncture may be diagnostic if increased intracranial pressure or mass effect that may lead to brainstem herniation already has been excluded by advanced imaging.[48] Definitive diagnosis requires brain biopsy that exhibits a 96% sensitivity and 100% specificity. Differential considerations include a low-grade glioma, infarction, and abscess. Antiviral drugs (especially adenine arabinoside) are helpful in herpes simplex and varicella-zoster encephalitis.* The mortality rate approximates 70%.[56]

> **KEY CONCEPTS**
> - Acute encephalitis usually results from a virus.
> - Magnetic resonance imaging is extremely sensitive and should be ordered, if available.
> - Symptoms and signs are nonspecific.
> - Brain biopsy is used for definitive diagnosis.

Epidural Abscess

BACKGROUND

An epidural abscess is a pyogenic, necrotic focus of infection superficial to the dura mater and deep to the dermal bone of the cranium or spinal canal. Most cases of intracranial epidural abscess (IEA) are secondary to direct extension from a local paranasal sinus infection, sinusitis, otitis media, mastoiditis, or dental abscess. Generalized septicemia also is a recognized cause of IEA that is often associated with pulmonary infection. Common examples include bronchiectasis, empyema, pneumonia, and bronchopleural fistula formation. IEA occasionally may be iatrogenic secondary to cranial surgery. Up to one fourth of cases of IEA are cryptogenic. Patients with a history of corticosteroids use, immunosuppressive drug therapy, and congenital or acquired immunologic deficiency are at greatest risk for IEA.

Hematogenous spread is implicated in approximately two thirds of all cases of spinal epidural abscess (SEA). The skin and supporting soft-tissue infections are the most common sources of primary infection. Direct extension of infection also has been described in association with spinal osteomyelitis, retropharyngeal abscess, perinephritic abscess, and psoas abscess. An iatrogenic SEA can occur as a complication to the administration of epidural anesthesia, lumbar puncture, and spinal epidural injection. Penetrating injuries are rarely implicated in cases of SEA. Anaerobic varieties of *Streptococcus* are the common causative

---

*References 48, 65, 75, 235, 309, 310.

organisms of IEA. Other pathogens include *Bacteroides* and *Staphylococcus*. *Staphylococcus* is the most common pathogen involved in SEA.[182,225,315]

IMAGING FINDINGS

MRI scans are ideal for use in the diagnosis of both intracranial and spinal epidural abscess. Gadolinium-enhanced MRI is not only useful to demonstrate the abscess formation, but also to identify the primary site of infection. Vertebral osteomyelitis, psoas abscess, and sinusitis are readily visualized on MRI scans. The detection of these conditions should stimulate an imaging search to exclude IEA or SEA if clinical indications are present. CT with contrast is not as sensitive or specific and should be used only if MRI is not available. Plain radiographs are useful only if adjunctive disease is advanced.

Upon use of noncontrast MRI, the abscess appears as an epidural mass that is low signal on T1-weighted images and high signal on T2-weighted acquisitions. The contrasted mass may reveal diffusely homogeneous or slightly heterogenous enhancement. In later stages, enhancement may be limited to a thick rim surrounding the mass (Fig. 33-7, *A* and *B*). CT with intravenous contrast is useful in the evaluation of associated osseous involvement; however, the use of intrathecal contrast with CT may be contraindicated due to the risk of dissemination of infection.[218,275,306]

CLINICAL COMMENTS

An insidious onset of headache (over a period of several weeks or months) may be the only presenting complaint with IEA. A persistent fever also may be present. Nausea, vomiting, neck stiffness, focal neurologic deficit, seizure, or paresis may develop as the subdural space becomes occupied by subdural empyema. Regional signs and symptoms of a primary infection often accompany intracranial epidural abscess. Early diagnosis is essential to preclude the spread of infection to the leptomeninges or brain parenchyma.

SEA may have a similar clinical presentation to that of disc herniation. Back pain, radiculopathy, paresthesias, and cauda equina syndrome are common complaints. A febrile episode may or may not precede these complaints. Acute onset usually results from hematogenous dissemination and a more insidious onset as a result of direct extension from contiguous infection.[75,207,263,315]

> **KEY CONCEPTS**
> - Intracranial epidural abscess (IEA) usually is caused by spread of infection from adjacent sites.
> - Spinal epidural abscess (SEA) is most often caused by hematogenous spread.
> - Magnetic resonance imaging is more sensitive and specific than other modalities in the diagnosis of both IEA and SEA.
> - Symptoms are not pathognomonic of either IEA or SEA, but should suggest appropriate imaging.

Spinal Infections

BACKGROUND

Spinal infections may involve the osseous structures (osteomyelitis), intervertebral discs (discitis), or contents of the spinal canal (epidural abscess, meningitis). Meningitis and spinal epidural abscess have been discussed previously. This section emphasizes osteomyelitis and discitis.

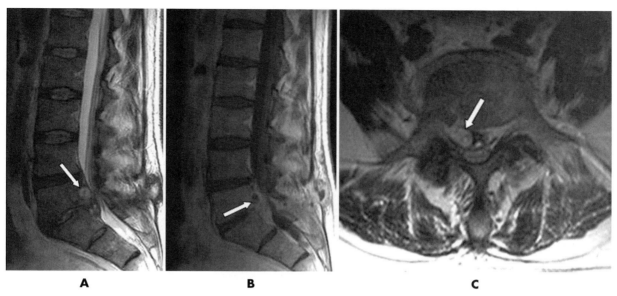

FIG. 33-7 Epidural abscess. The patient presented with severe low back pain 2 weeks after discectomy. **A,** Rounded area of intermediate signal in the T2-weighted sagittal acquisition detected posterior to the L5 vertebral body *(arrow).* **B,** Peripheral enhancement demonstrated in the postcontrast T1-weighted sagittal image *(arrow).* **C,** Abscess visualized on the right side in the axial image *(arrow).* High-grade central canal stenosis present on the right side. (Courtesy Bryan K. Hosler, Cincinnati, OH.)

Although spinal infections are somewhat uncommon, it is extremely important to recognize them to minimize their potential for devastating long-term effects. Discitis and osteomyelitis typically coexist. Hematogenous osteomyelitis usually is caused by the seeding of bone from a remote site of infection. Primary infective sources commonly include the urinary tract, respiratory tract, and skin. Spread from infected tissues to contiguous structures, open trauma, or postoperative complications are other causes of spinal osteomyelitis.[85,144] Immunocompromise and intravenous drug use are precipitating factors in the development of spinal osteomyelitis. The most common organism causing vertebral osteomyelitis among newborns, children, and adults is *Staphylococcus aureus.* The vertebral body is richly nourished by vascular structures (both arterial and venous) and is involved in approximately 95% of cases of pyogenic vertebral osteomyelitis. Posterior arch structures are infected in only 5% of all cases.[213,299] Osteomyelitis of the vascular vertebral bodies precedes discitis with the spread of infection from the osseous structures to the sparsely vascularized discs. Discitis is more prominent in males and is most commonly found, in descending order of frequency, involving the lumbar, cervical, and thoracic spine.[99,121,193]

IMAGING FINDINGS

Plain film radiography may be positive in the later stages of both spinal osteomyelitis and discitis. Findings include decreased disc space height and destruction of the subjacent cortical margins. CT is more sensitive to the early detection of spinal infection than plain film radiography. In the presence of contrast enhancement, CT may be useful in the assessment of contiguous soft-tissue involvement. For early diagnosis, the imaging modalities of choice are MRI and nuclear scanning. Radionuclide scans utilizing technetium 99 m and gallium 67 demonstrate uptake soon after the onset of symptoms. Nuclear imaging is sensitive; however, not as specific as MRI. MRI scans are useful not only for the early

detection of early osteomyelitis and discitis, but also for contiguous soft-tissue involvement and spinal epidural abscess (Fig. 33-8, *A* and *B*). Typically, the infected vertebral structures demonstrate a low signal on T1-weighted images and a higher signal than the normal osseous structures on T2-weighted acquisitions. Similarly the infected disc has a slightly lower signal on T1-weighted images and signal is considerably increased in T2 weighting. Gadolinium contrast administration results in easily recognizable enhancement of the infected intervertebral disc and vertebral body.*

CLINICAL COMMENTS

Insidious onset of back pain and minor paraspinal muscle spasm are the most common presenting complaints associated with spinal infection. The pain initially is localized to the area of infection, becoming progressively more intense with consequential limitation of motion. Regional edema, erythema, and tenderness with warmth on palpation commonly are associated clinical findings. Eventually complete bed rest and analgesics do not diminish the patient's pain. Fever is present in approximately 50% of presenting cases, and leukocytosis may be absent or minimal. Neurologic findings are not present until late in the disease, often secondary to vertebral collapse or the intraspinal mass effect of an epidural abscess. Mass effect has the ability to compress neural structures. Epidural abscess also may lead to infarction of the spinal cord. A rapidly deteriorating neurologic deficit ensues, advancing possibly to paralysis. Erythrocyte sedimentation rate (ESR) and C-reactive protein (CRP) are nonspecific blood chemistry findings associated with inflammation. However, the possibility of infectious spondylodiscitis should be entertained if these tests are positive in a patient presenting with back pain. Although a blood culture is positive in only 33% to 50% of cases, it is still prudent to perform a

---

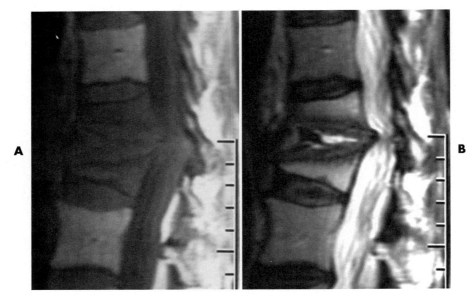

FIG. 33-8 Spinal infection. **A** and **B,** Kyphotic deformity present at the thoracolumbar junction. High signal is identified within the L1-2 disc in the T2-weighted images with destruction of the adjacent vertebral bodies consistent with discitis and osteomyelitis. Retropulsion of bone and extension of infection into the spinal canal is discernible. (Courtesy Bryan K. Hosler, Cincinnati, OH.)

culture before antibiotic therapy is attempted. In addition, CT-guided needle biopsy with tissue culture is indicated despite a positive return in approximately 50% of cases.[144] Surgical biopsy with débridement must be considered if the infection does not respond to intravenous antibiotic therapy, if needle aspiration biopsy does not yield an appropriate culture, if vertebral collapse occurs, or if there is neurologic compromise.[106,121,144,213,299]

> **KEY CONCEPTS**
> - *Spinal osteomyelitis and discitis commonly coexist.*
> - *Nuclear scans are sensitive.*
> - *Magnetic resonance imaging scans are both sensitive and specific.*
> - *Insidious onset of localized back pain with minor paraspinal muscle spasm is the most common presenting complaint.*

◼ Noninfectious Inflammatory Conditions

Multiple Sclerosis

BACKGROUND

Multiple sclerosis (MS) is the most common demyelinating disease of the central nervous system. More than 350,000 patients suffer from MS in the United States alone. The disease characteristically begins in early adulthood and is slightly more common in females. Approximately 70% of cases of MS undergo progressive exacerbation and remission of symptoms (relapsing-remitting type), whereas the remaining 30% are classified as chronic progressive.[161] It has been theorized that the etiology of MS is autoimmune, viral, genetic, or a combination of these. Evidence at this time is inconclusive, and the cause of MS still must be considered idiopathic. Environmental factors also appear to have an impact on MS, because the incidence of the disease increases in direct proportion to the distance from the equator.[64,82,287,307]

A fatty substance known as *myelin* insulates the neural axons, promoting the virtually instantaneous transfer of neural signals. Neural conduction may be diminished or blocked completely if myelin is damaged. The primary pathologic processes of MS involve the demyelinization and inflammation of axons and the plaquing of white matter parenchyma. Plaques may be found anywhere in the white matter but are most frequent in the periventricular region of the cerebrum, brainstem, optic nerves, basal ganglia, and spinal cord. The prognosis is unpredictable. Onset at an early age, female gender, infrequent exacerbation with long remission, and a small amount of plaque visible on imaging appear to predict a relatively benign course.[82,133,161]

IMAGING FINDINGS

The early diagnosis of MS requires acute clinical awareness on the part of the physician. MRI is the preferred imaging modality for MS and is not only considered diagnostic but also predictive. The presence of three or more plaques in T2-weighted MR imaging is indicative that the patient will develop clinically definitive MS within 7 to 10 years. The presence of plaque is sensitive in 80% of patients who develop MS. Fifty percent of patients with MRI findings of MS are clinically definitive within 2 years.[11,161,165] Increased signal in the periventricular white matter in T2-weighted images is highly suggestive of MS. Enhancement with a gadolinium contrast is characteristic of inflammation or an active lesion (Fig. 33-9, *A* and *B*). In approximately 20% of patients with MS, CNS lesions are confined exclusively to the spinal cord.[82]

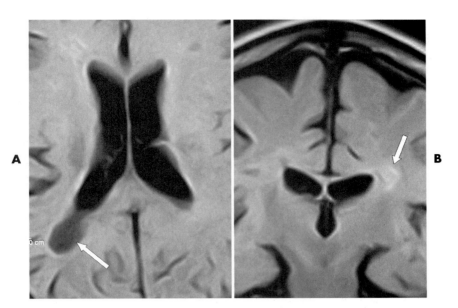

FIG. 33-9   Multiple sclerosis. Multiple sclerosis in a 49-year-old female patient presenting with tingling in the right arm and ataxia. **A,** Postinfusion T1-weighted axial acquisition displays an area of low signal *(arrow)* in the posterior right periventricular white matter. **B,** Peripheral enhancement is discernible in the lesion adjacent to the posterior horn of the right lateral ventricle in the axial image *(arrow)*. Contrast enhancement is detected in a lesion adjacent to the left lateral ventricle visualized in the coronal image. Area without enhancement represents an old or quiescent lesion.

MS plaques are isointense to hypointense on unenhanced T1-weighted MR images. T2-weighted and inversion recovery acquisitions reveal increased signal in MS plaques.[11] The recent advent of techniques using diffusion-weighted MRI or magnetization transfer permits earlier diagnosis of MS. These techniques take advantage of local tissue perfusion. Inflammation within the myelin sheath becomes evident before the formation of plaque and disruption of the blood–brain barrier. The size of MS plaques may be underestimated by as much as 250% on T2-weighted images compared with DWI.[165,177,314]

CLINICAL COMMENTS

The clinical diagnosis of multiple sclerosis often is extremely difficult, because of a frequently variable and conflicting patient presentation. Symptoms include weakness, paresis, and tremor of one or more extremities. Muscle atrophy and spasticity may be present with dysfunctional movement. Numbness, paresthesias, and visual disturbances are common. Incoordination, myasthenia, changes in mentation, and altered speech with facial and extremity pain can occur with frequency in MS. Charcot's triad of signs is intention tremor, nystagmus, and scanning speech (INS). The Schumacher criteria for MS consists of: (a) CNS dysfunction, (b) involvement of two or more parts of the CNS, (c) predominant white matter involvement, (d) two or more episodes lasting greater than 24 hours less than 1 month apart, (e) slow stepwise progression of signs and symptoms, and (f) onset at 10 to 50 years of age. The hallmark of MS is inconsistency in time and space. For example, a patient may present with speech difficulties and weakness of one of the extremities followed by a period of remission. On exacerbation, the patient may complain of spasticity of a different extremity with visual disturbances. Diagnosis is dependent upon the recognition of this extremely variable pattern and the judicious pursuit of appropriate laboratory testing and MRI.[82,133] Rudick red flags suggest a diagnosis other than MS: (a) absence of visual disturbances,

(b) no clinical remission, (c) totally localized disease, (d) no sensory findings, (e) no bladder involvement, and (f) no CSF abnormality. Laboratory tests include lumbar puncture and evoked potentials. Oligoclonal banding and immunoglobulin G (IgG) index in the CSF are positive in approximately 90% of MS cases. Evoked potentials make use of slowed conduction in demyelinated neural structures to permit the assessment of subclinical MS. However, evoked potentials are of no value in patients with known lesions.[217]

> ### KEY CONCEPTS
> - *Multiple sclerosis is a demyelinating disease of the central nervous system.*
> - *Magnetic resonance imaging is the preferred imaging modality in the diagnosis of multiple sclerosis.*
> - *The pattern of symptoms in multiple sclerosis is extremely variable, often characterized by relapses and remissions.*
> - *Lumbar puncture is specific and sensitive for multiple sclerosis.*

Sarcoidosis

BACKGROUND

Sarcoidosis is typically a multisystemic noncaseating epithelioid granulomatous disease process of unknown etiology. Although hilar and paratracheal lymphadenopathy are common, involvement of the lung parenchyma also may occur. Often the symptoms are less severe than the extent of chest involvement seem to suggest. Sarcoidosis of the CNS is localized to the leptomeninges with extended involvement of the brain parenchyma through the Virchow-Robin spaces. Neurosarcoidosis is found at autopsy in less than 10% of patients with sarcoidosis. The mortality rate in neurosarcoidosis is approximately 10%, double that found in sarcoidosis.[52,61,208,215,256]

IMAGING FINDINGS

Contrast-enhanced MRI is the preferred modality of investigation for neurosarcoidosis. Typically, the lesions are isointense to gray matter in unenhanced T1-weighted images and isointense or slightly hyperintense in T2-weighted acquisitions. Multiple white matter lesions are detected in 43% of cases.[319] Leptomeningeal enhancement takes place with the administration of gadolinium contrast. However, other diseases may simulate neurosarcoidosis, particularly infectious meningitis and meningioma. Hypermetabolism and hypometabolism in lesional tissue are discernible with positron emission tomography (PET) scans and may be beneficial in establishing a final diagnosis.[68] Spinal involvement usually is limited to the extramedullary portion of the cervical region; however, inflammation and enlargement of the cord could suggest an intramedullary neoplasm. Lesions also may occur within the thoracic and lumbar spinal canal.[224] Atrophy of the spinal cord may be demonstrated in late-stage neurosarcoidosis. A nuclear scan with gallium 67 citrate may prove informative in equivocal cases.[130,269,303]

CLINICAL COMMENTS

Neurologic manifestations of neurosarcoidosis are nonspecific and may include headache, paresis, paresthesias, dizziness, seizures, altered mentation, and visual disturbances.[61] Often the symptoms of sarcoidosis in the chest and various organs overshadow the neurologic component until late in the disease process. Hydrocephalus is the most common finding associated with sarcoidosis of the CNS and usually is the result of arachnoiditis and adhesion formation.[56] The greatest challenge for the clinician is to recognize the neurologic signs and symptoms of neurosarcoidosis in a patient with diffuse sarcoidosis in other organ systems. Definitive diagnosis is made by lymph node or skin lesion biopsy. The Kveim-Siltzbach skin test for sarcoidosis is considerably less sensitive.

> ### KEY CONCEPTS
> - *Neurosarcoidosis is an uncommon manifestation of sarcoidosis.*
> - *Gadolinium contrast-enhanced magnetic resonance imaging is the most sensitive and specific imaging modality available at this time.*
> - *Biopsy is necessary for definitive diagnosis.*

Tumors of the Central Nervous System

BACKGROUND

Tumors of the CNS are primary or metastatic in etiology. Primary tumors make up slightly less than one half of all CNS neoplasia. Neoplasms that are found within the brain parenchyma or spinal cord are intraaxial. Tumors that are located within the spinal canal or cranium but outside parenchymal tissue are extraaxial. Both intraaxial and extraaxial tumors may be primary or metastatic. Primary CNS tumors are classified by cell type (Table 33-2). Ninety-five percent of CNS neoplasia may be categorized as metastases, gliomas, meningiomas, pituitary adenomas, and acoustic neuromas.[146] Gliomas comprise approximately 60% of all primary brain tumors with meningiomas making up an additional 20%. The majority of brain tumors in children are found below the tentorium with more than 60% above the tentorium in adults. A familial history of cancer is present in 16% of patients with CNS neoplasia. Each year in the United States, more than 35,000 people develop primary or metastatic brain tumors.* Metastatic CNS

TABLE 33-2	Primary Central Nervous System Tumor Classifications

Gliomas	Nonglial tumors
Pilocytic astrocytoma	Meningioma
Subependymal astrocytoma	Neurofibroma/schwannoma
Fibrillary astrocytoma: low-grade diffuse	Pituitary adenoma: micro, macro
Oligodendroglioma	Medulloblastoma: primary neuro-ectodermal tumor
Ependymoma: myxopapillary	Lymphoma
Ependymoma: anaplastic	Craniopharyngioma
Mixed astrocytoma	Germ cell: germinoma, teratoma, choriocarcinoma, embryonal carcinoma
Anaplastic astrocytoma	Choroid plexus: papilloma, carcinoma
Glioblastoma multiforme	Pineal: pineocytoma, pineoblastoma
	Hemangioblastoma

involvement is somewhat more common than primary CNS neoplasia. Primary tumors in the breast, lung, kidney, thyroid, prostate, and skin metastasize frequently to the CNS.[62]

Tumors arising from the spinal cord, spinal nerve roots, and dura are uncommon compared with primary brain tumors. Spinal neoplasms are divided into three distinct groups, based on their location. These are extradural, intradural extramedullary, and intradural intramedullary lesions. The cell types of primary spinal tumors are essentially the same as those found in the brain. Ependymomas are the most common intrinsic primary spinal cord tumor, and along with astrocytomas, together comprise more than 75% of all primary spinal cord tumors. Approximately 15% to 20% of CNS tumors occur in the spine, although less than 5% are intramedullary. The spinal cord is a rare location for metastasis.[94] Less than 5% of metastatic spinal tumors are intradural, and less than 1% are intramedullary. The most common primary intradural extramedullary lesions are meningiomas and neurofibromas. Extradural lesions include osseous metastasis and benign bone lesions such as hemangioma, osteoid osteoma, aneurysmal bone cyst, and osteoblastoma.[†]

IMAGING FINDINGS

Multiplanar gadolinium-enhanced MRI is ideally suited for the detection and localization of CNS tumors. MRI is the preferred modality because of its ability to depict not only small solid and cystic neoplasia, but also adjunct findings such as edema, infarction, hemorrhage, and necrosis. Unenhanced MRI is sensitive to the discovery of CNS lesions. Typically neoplasms are isointense or hypointense to brain tissue in T1-weighted images and hyperintense in T2 weighting. This pattern is nonspecific for tumors and is seen in other lesions, particularly infarction. The blood–brain barrier effectively blocks contrast material from entering the

---

*References 60, 101, 122, 175, 178, 191, 301, 313.

†References 30, 74, 86, 112, 117, 164, 191, 218.

normal CNS; however, the neovascularity of most neoplasia facilitates the intake of contrast and permits enhancement. Gadolinium-enhanced MRI allows differentiation from infarction because infarcted tissue does not enhance.[36,114,120,204,275] MRI of spinal cord neoplasia frequently discloses cord enlargement and syrinx formation. CT is complementary to MRI in the evaluation of neoplastic calcification and the assessment of osseous lesions. CT and MRI are used in guidance for stereotactic biopsy.[168,218] MR spectroscopy is being used in clinical settings to determine the cell type of tumors.[120]

PET uses a low dose of a radioactive glucose (fluorodeoxyglucose) or 11C-methionine to evaluate the metabolic activity, perfusion, electrical activity, and neurochemistry of neoplastic tissue with respect to the surrounding structures. Aggressive tumors exhibit a high metabolic rate and benign lesions a lower rate. These differences are important in the staging of tumors and the formulation of a treatment plan. PET scans are also used to monitor the effects of tumor treatment and to distinguish neoplastic recurrence from radionecrosis.[68] Fusion technology is accomplished by overlaying PET scans with a modality that permits better resolution. For instance, PET and MRI scans may be used with one another, or PET and CT joined to make an image with both anatomic and functional characteristics.

CLINICAL COMMENTS

Symptoms of brain neoplasia are nonspecific. Insidious onset of "new or different" headache, disturbed mentation, altered personality, behavioral disorders, seizures, paresis, nausea, vomiting, and altered gait are common. Typically the onset of headache or cognitive impairment in patients with brain tumors is measured in weeks or months. Headaches are particularly suggestive of CNS neoplasia when combined with focal neurologic deficit or seizures.

A primary headache is a clinical entity that presents as the primary disorder and not as a symptom of another underlying and potentially catastrophic condition. The three most common examples of primary headaches are: (a) migraine headache, (b) tension headache, and (c) cluster headache. Secondary headaches are clinical entities that present as symptoms of some other underlying condition. Some secondary headaches are associated with benign or self-limiting conditions. Common examples of primary causes of secondary headaches include neoplasm, meningitis, subarachnoid hemorrhage, subdural hematoma, and temporal arteritis.

There is consensus in the literature that the presence of cognitive changes may be caused by a potentially catastrophic underlying problem. Chronic subdural hematoma often simulates a primary brain neoplasm, and these are likely to be clinically indistinguishable. Because both conditions are common to the elderly patient population, the taking of a patient history and the reliability of patient reported symptoms (both of primary importance) can make the task of differentiation even more difficult. The most frequent signs associated with brain tumors are cognitive in nature. These include confusion, lapses of memory, emotional lability, and depressive changes. Headaches associated with tumor most likely present in the range of several weeks to months in duration before examination. These headaches often are progressive in nature, and virtually any accompanying neurologic signs or combination of signs is possible. These vary depending on the location, size, and doubling time of the lesion. Vomiting in the absence of nausea often occurs with tumor headache and is a useful clinical indicator. Seizures, particularly when occurring for the first time, in an adult patient are a useful predictor of brain neoplasm. Funduscopic examination may yield papilledema associated with an increase of intracranial pressure. Although this is clinically significant, increased intracranial pressure is not unique to brain tumors. A recent change in the pain pattern of a chronic headache patient may herald the onset of an underlying problem, and it must be understood that patients with primary headaches are not statistically immune from becoming tumor headache patients. Brain tumors as the cause of headaches are not common clinical entities. Advanced imaging (to include high-field magnetic resonance imaging) has limited utility when applied as a screening technique to headache patients for the detection of neoplastic disease.

Neurologic manifestations of CNS tumors are produced by mass effect, infiltration of brain parenchyma, and the disruption of CSF flow. Both the tumor and surrounding edema contribute to the mass effect. Tumor replacement of parenchymal tissue degrades neurologic function. Occlusion of CSF through the foramina (Monro, Sylvius) or third and fourth ventricles may lead to hydrocephalus.[84,178,203,271]

Symptoms in patients with spinal neoplasia commonly are caused by cord and nerve root compression rather than parenchymal infiltration. Extradural tumors are much more common than intrinsic cord tumors. For these reasons, insidious onset of back pain and extremity symptoms (e.g., pain, weakness, numbness, paresthesias) are frequent clinical manifestations. Cauda equina syndrome also can be a presenting condition. Chronic back pain is typical of the primary glial cell spinal cord tumors. The ependymomas and astrocytomas found in the spinal cord usually are slow growing and relatively benign in nature.[74,86,112,117,164]

DIFFERENTIAL DIAGNOSIS

The differential diagnosis of CNS tumors is based on the location of the lesion, age and sex of the patient, presence of calcification, necrosis or hemorrhage, and enhancement pattern. For example, meningiomas are located adjacent to the dura in which they arise, increase in frequency with age, exhibit a female predominance, and do not calcify. In contrast, ependymomas typically arise from the ependymal surface of the fourth ventricle of pediatric patients and frequently calcify. Meningiomas typically enhance homogeneously or display ring enhancement. The enhancement pattern of ependymomas often is heterogeneous because of the varying presence of hemorrhage, necrosis, and calcification. Chronic subdural hematoma (CSH), by definition, constitutes a low-pressure (venous) intracranial lesion with accumulated blood dispersed throughout the subdural space. Generalized symptoms of increased intracranial pressure are common to both CSH and brain neoplasm. The slowly expanding, space-occupying nature of both intracranial entities lends itself to a methodical and thorough (e.g., nonemergency) evaluation. It is essential that the syndrome be recognized and referred for investigation. Differential characteristics are discussed in the individual tumor sections. Stereotactic biopsy is used for tissue cell diagnosis, staging, and treatment planning.

KEY CONCEPTS

- *Metastatic tumors are slightly more common than primary neoplasia in the brain and considerably more prevalent in the spine.*
- *Gadolinium-enhanced magnetic resonance imaging is the modality of choice for imaging central nervous system (CNS) tumors.*
- *Symptoms of CNS tumors are nonspecific and may mimic other neurologic disorders.*
- *Computed tomography or magnetic resonance imaging–guided stereotactic biopsy is utilized for definitive tissue cell diagnosis, staging, and treatment planning.*

Primary Tumors

Glioma

BACKGROUND

Gliomas are the most common of the primary brain tumors. The astrocytomas are the most prevalent of these. More than 10,000 CNS gliomas are diagnosed in the United States each year. Glial tumors not only include astrocytomas but also ependymomas, oligodendrogliomas, and mixed astrocytomas (see Table 33-2).

Numerous grading systems have been devised for astrocytomas that are confusing to clinicians, pathologists, and radiologists.[35,57,58,142,220] In general, these systems separate the low-grade or benign astrocytomas from the high-grade anaplastic or malignant tumors. The grading system developed by the World Health Organization (WHO) is the most commonly used.[145] Astrocytomas are graded I through IV. Pilocytic and giant cell astrocytomas are included in Grade I, whereas fibrillary, protoplasmic and gemistocytic astrocytomas are considered Grade II lesions. Anaplastic astrocytomas exhibit malignant characteristics and are designated Grade III. The most aggressively invasive (Grade IV) of the astrocytomas is the glioblastoma multiforme (glioblastoma), and recently has been considered a separate lesion.[35]

Cellularity, pleomorphism, anaplasia, nuclear atypia, mitoses, vascular proliferation, and necrosis are used in grading astrocytomas.[13,27,29,33,35] A wide range of these factors is present in astrocytomas with gradually greater amounts of anaplasia and necrosis culminating in the glioblastoma multiforme, considered the most malignant of the glial tumors. Glioblastoma multiforme displays frequent mitoses, endothelial proliferation, and necrosis with abnormal neovascularity.[12,13] Gliomas rarely metastasize, although glioblastoma multiforme may be multicentric. There is a tendency for glial growth along white matter tracts and for gliomas to increase in grade over time. Mixed astrocytomas are relatively common and are a low-grade combination of astrocytes and oligodendroglial cells.[14,49]

Intracranial ependymomas are most frequently found in the roof of the fourth ventricle and have a predilection for children. Spinal ependymomas typically are intramedullary or extend from the conus, cauda equina, or filum terminale. Spinal ependymomas occur most frequently in adult patients, whereas spinal astrocytomas are more common among children. Intracranial ependymomas account for less than 10% of all CNS tumors. Spinal ependymomas are the most common of the intramedullary neoplasms but are decidedly less common than intracranial ependymomas.[28]

Oligodendrogliomas account for less than 5% of all primary CNS tumors. These lesions are slow growing and common to the cerebral hemispheres. Oligodendrogliomas are most frequently diagnosed in the fourth decade of life.[111,242]

IMAGING FINDINGS

MRI, CT, and PET scans are complementary in the diagnosis of gliomas. MRI, both with and without contrast, is the imaging modality of choice. CT sometimes is useful in demonstrating calcifications within the matrix of low-grade gliomas. Ependymomas and oligodendrogliomas are the most likely of the gliomas to exhibit calcification. On unenhanced MRI, gliomas are typically low signal or isointense with brain tissue on T1-weighted images and high signal on T2-weighted images. Gadolinium contrast enhancement is moderately intense with anaplastic, malignant

lesions and less intense within low-grade gliomas. Diminished intensity of tumor enhancement is observed with steroid therapy, and areas of necrosis do not enhance. Ring enhancement is frequent, particularly in high-grade gliomas (Figs. 33-10 and 33-11).[12,29] DWI is used effectively in the characterization of necrotic, cystic, and edematous tumoral regions. DWI is of value in differentiating low-grade from high-grade gliomas.[40,72,280,289] Cell types, fiber structure, and vascularity of glial tumors can be accurately predicted using DTI.[18,149,174] fMRI is used to evaluate the effect surgical excision has on neural structures.[238,253] PET scans are useful for the evaluation and long-term monitoring of low-grade gliomas. PET scans quantify the uptake of fluorodeoxyglucose or 11C-methionine to demonstrate functional alteration in the blood–brain barrier or the presence of endothelial proliferation.[68,118] Fusion technology permits PET or SPECT scans to be used with CT or MRI. Fusion of PET or SPECT scans with one of the other higher-resolution modalities results in anatomic detail with functional information.[124,255]

Oligodendrogliomas are uncommon tumors and characteristically are found in the cerebral hemispheres. On T1-weighted MRI acquisitions these lesions are low signal or appear as a combination of isointense and low signal. T2-weighted MR images present with high signal intensity. Heterogeneity on contrast administration occurs because of a tendency for this tumor to calcify.[34,111] DWI, DTI, and fMRI are used to assist with both diagnosis and surgical planning.*

Intracranial ependymomas typically are infratentorial and arise in the ependymal lining of the ventricles, with a predilection for the fourth ventricle. Intracranial ependymomas have a tendency to extend into the foramina of Luschka and Magendie. Intracranial or spinal ependymomas may be isointense with the spinal cord, low signal, or high signal in T1-weighted images. Ependymomas uniformly increase in signal in T2-weighted acquisitions. Spinal ependymomas enlarge the cord and exhibit a more central location than spinal astrocytomas. Both intracranial and spinal ependymomas may enhance homogeneously ($\approx$50%) or heterogenously on MRI after injection of gadolinium. Contrast heterogeneity can be associated with calcification, methemoglobin, necrosis, or neovascularity (Fig. 33-12, A through D).[147,181,244] Adjacent cysts, edema, and hemorrhage are commonly detected, often at the superior or inferior pole of the tumor.[45,148,200,281] DWI, DTI, and fMRI are employed in the diagnosis and treatment stages, as in previously discussed neoplastic processes.

CLINICAL COMMENTS

The symptoms associated with a glioma are dependent on the location and size of the tumor mass. Behavioral and personality changes with headaches, altered cognition, seizures, nausea, vomiting, motor impairment, or sensory disturbances should alert the clinician to the possibility of an intracranial tumor.[84,178,203,271] Spinal cord gliomas usually are ependymomas or astrocytomas and enlarge slowly with an insidious onset of symptoms. The symptoms of a spinal cord glioma usually are related to the level of neoplastic involvement with motor and sensory impairment at the appropriate neural distribution. The slow onset of localized back pain is a common chief complaint.† Pilocytic astrocytomas and

---

*References 18, 40, 72, 149, 174, 238, 253, 280, 289.
†References 27, 29, 74, 86, 112, 117, 164.

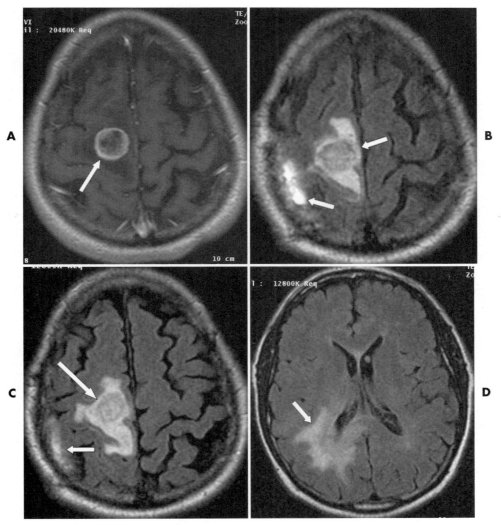

FIG. 33-10 Grade IV astrocytoma (glioblastoma multiforme) in a 62-year-old man. **A,** Postcontrast T1-weighted axial image details peripheral enhancement of a right-sided mass *(arrow)* adjacent to the falx with surrounding edema (low signal) and obliteration of the central and postcentral sulci. **B** and **C,** Contiguous axial diffusion-weighted images obtained 1 month later reveals the necrotic center, whereas the tumor appears isointense to surrounding vasogenic edema *(large arrow)*. High-signal sanguineous surgical changes are seen in the right temporoparietal region *(small arrows)*. **D,** Involvement of the right parietal lobe *(arrow)*, occipital horn of the lateral ventricle, and adjacent occipital cortex.

ependymomas are found most commonly in children and young adults. Glioblastoma multiforme is more common to older patients (mean age, 53 years).[29] Imaging always should be performed if there are symptoms suggestive of a CNS tumor. Definitive diagnosis usually is accomplished by means of stereotactic biopsy.

KEY CONCEPTS

- *Astrocytomas are the most common glial cell tumor.*
- *Magnetic resonance imaging, computed tomography, and positron emission tomography scans are complementary imaging devices.*
- *Symptoms are not pathognomonic of glioma.*
- *Biopsy is necessary for definitive diagnosis.*

Meningioma

Meningiomas comprise slightly less than 20% of all primary intracranial neoplasms and are the most common extraaxial tumor. They arise from the meningothelial cells concentrated in the arachnoid villi that penetrate dura mater and are found uncommonly in the spine. Meningiomas are most commonly located at the periphery of the brain with dural attachment. Invasion of the brain parenchyma is uncommon. Intraosseous and intraventricular meningiomas are infrequent but have been described in the literature.[31,154] Meningiomas are typically indolent and more common among females. The more aggressive meningiomas exhibit a male predominance. Most meningiomas are diagnosed in young and middle-aged adults and are rare in children.[39,55,107,154] An association with neurofibromatosis has been noted.

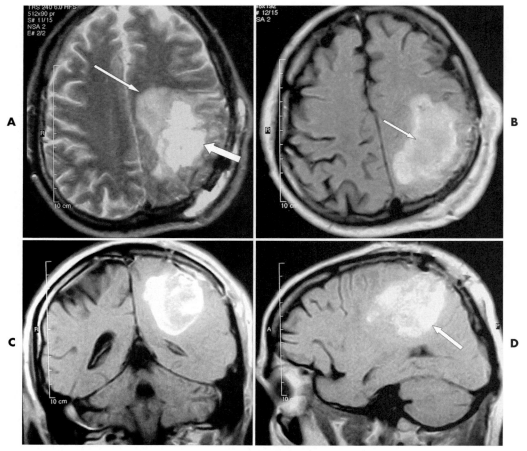

FIG. 33-11 Glioblastoma multiforme. Recurrent glioblastoma multiforme in a 65-year-old man. **A,** Axial T2-weighted; **B,** postcontrast T1-weighted axial; **C,** coronal; and **D,** sagittal sequences reveal necrosis within the tumor matrix and edema extending into the white matter of the centrum semiovale *(arrows)*. Slight deflection of the falx cerebri is apparent with distortion of the left lateral ventricle. Surgical residuals are visible in the left posterolateral skull.

IMAGING FINDINGS

MRI is the preferred imaging modality for demonstrating a meningioma and defining its relationship with the dura. Typically unenhanced T1-weighted MR acquisitions reveal the signal to be isointense with or slightly lower than the surrounding brain tissue. T2-weighted MR images display increased signal within the matrix of the meningioma. Intense gadolinium contrast enhancement occurs homogeneously in approximately 85% of cases of meningioma (Fig. 33-13, *A* to *C*). MRA demonstrates vascular effacement, encasement, or deflection secondary to the tumor mass. The morphology of the tumor is significant concerning recurrence. A round-shaped meningioma is less likely to recur than an irregular, lobulated, or "mushroomed" meningioma. The dural tail is a thickened contrast-enhanced collar adjacent to the meningioma that is present in more than 50% of cases.* DWI, DTI, fMRI, PET, and fusion technologies are used in diagnosis and treatment planning.[†] CT is complementary and is useful in demonstrating tumoral calcification and osseous involvement.[218]

CLINICAL COMMENTS

Meningiomas are slow growing and usually asymptomatic unless critical neural structures are compressed. Frequently they are large when first diagnosed. Three distinct types have been recognized:

(a) globular meningioma, a compact rounded mass with invagination of brain parenchyma (generally flat at the base with contact at the falx, tentorium, or basal dura); (b) meningioma-en-plaque that, because of a pronounced hyperostosis of adjacent bone particularly along the skull base, renders detection difficult; and (c) multicentric meningioma, which presents clinically at an earlier stage and has a tendency to localize within a single hemicranium. CSF seeding of this type is exceptional. Seizures, focal neurologic deficits, headaches, altered behavior, and disturbed mentation are frequent symptoms. Clinical signs are the result of compressed parenchymal or vascular tissue, increased intracranial pressure, and cranial nerve involvement. As always, clinical signs and symptoms should alert the clinician to the possibility of an intracranial mass. Appropriate imaging then should be performed as clinically indicated with stereotactic biopsy and excision.

KEY CONCEPTS

- *Meningiomas are found at the periphery of the brain and do not infiltrate brain parenchyma.*
- *Magnetic resonance imaging is the modality of choice to image the meningioma.*
- *Computed tomography is employed to detect calcification and related osseous alterations.*
- *Signs and symptoms are not specific for meningioma. Imaging and biopsy are necessary for diagnosis.*

*References 31, 19, 125, 179, 275, 322.
[†]References 18, 40, 72, 149, 174, 238, 253, 280, 289.

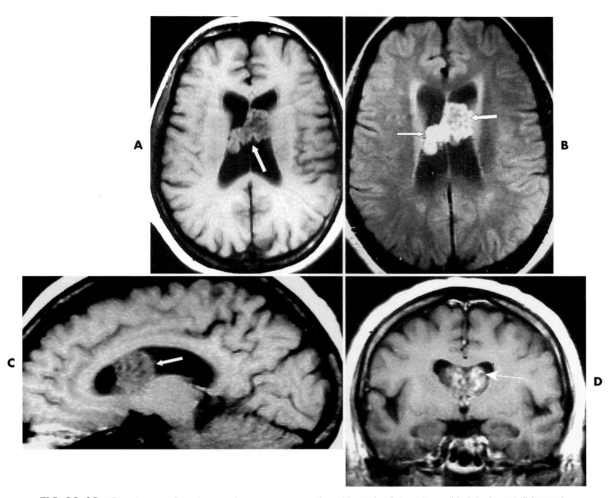

FIG. 33-12 Ependymoma. Ependymoma in a woman presenting with ptosis of the right eyelid, diplopia, and slight ataxia. **A** through **D,** Precontrast and postcontrast T1-weighted images reveal a heterogenous signal intraventricular mass in the body of both lateral ventricles extending inferiorly near the foramen of Monro (arrows). (Courtesy Steven P. Brownstein, MD, Springfield, NJ.)

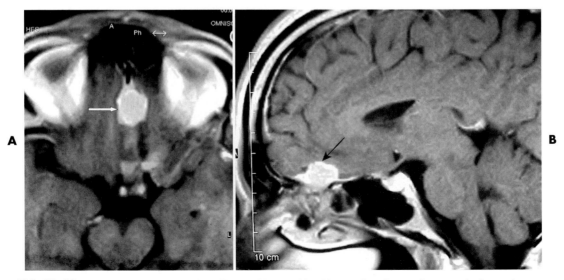

FIG. 33-13 Meningioma. Meningioma in a 35-year-old man with a history of craniotomy for removal of an optic nerve meningioma 11 years before this examination. **A,** Postcontrast T1-weighted axial, and, **B,** sagittal acquisitions reveal enhancement of the tumor matrix in the left olfactory groove (arrow). Minor ring enhancement is discernible, and a dural tail is demonstrated in the sagittal image (arrow).

Neurofibroma or Schwannoma

BACKGROUND

Schwannomas are primary neoplasms that arise in the Schwann cells of the myelin sheath, surrounding the axons of peripheral nerves. Schwannomas consist of nerve sheath cells (Schwann cells) and do not infiltrate nerve fibers. Acoustic neuroma is the most common intracranial schwannoma, followed by the less frequently seen trigeminal neuroma. Spinal schwannomas are more commonly found in the lumbar spine than in the thoracic or cervical regions. Neurofibromas are heterogenous tumors that display fewer Schwann cells and more collagen and reticulin than schwannomas. Unlike schwannomas, neurofibromas invade the neural structures and divide fibers. The majority of neurofibromas are singular, whereas plexiform neurofibromas are associated with neurofibromatosis. Neurofibromas have the capacity to erode intervertebral foramina and extend through the neuroforamina. Both neurofibromas and schwannomas can undergo malignant degeneration. Neurofibromatosis type I (NF-1, von Recklinghausen's disease) is characterized by the presence of numerous neurofibromas. Approximately 10% of plexiform neurofibromas associated with NF-1 undergo malignant degeneration.[187] Both NF-1 and neurofibromatosis type II (NF-2) are multisystem genetic disorders. NF-2 exhibits multiple schwannomas, meningiomas, and ependymomas that rarely undergo malignant degeneration. In addition, bilateral vestibular schwannomas and gliomas commonly are encountered in NF-2. Both NF-1 and NF-2 develop multiple subcutaneous nodules that may be difficult to distinguish clinically.* Patients with schwannomatosis develop numerous schwannomas, but do not produce vestibular tumors, meningiomas, neurofibromas, gliomas, or ependymomas.

IMAGING FINDINGS

Gadolinium-enhanced MRI is the imaging modality of choice for the investigation of neurofibromas, schwannomas, and neurofibromatosis. These lesions are typically isointense with muscle on T1-weighted acquisitions, increased signal on T2-weighted images,

*References 4, 5, 16, 104, 129, 273.

and enhance on contrast administration (Fig. 33-14, *A* to *C*). Homogenous signal is common with benign tumors and heterogenous signal with malignant degeneration, although this is not an extremely reliable differential finding.[187] Paravertebral neurofibromas are found at multiple spinal levels. Tumors that erode the neuroforamina and occupy both sides of the neural foramen are called "dumbbell" neurofibromas (Fig. 33-15, *A* to *C*). CT may be useful to demonstrate osseous erosions. Contrast-enhanced computed tomography (CECT) typically displays a uniformly enhanced tumor matrix.[115,277,298] Fluorodeoxyglucose positron emission tomography (FDG PET) has proven to be beneficial in the detection of plexiform neurofibromas in NF-1. FDG PET also is useful in differentiating malignant from benign neurofibromas.[79]

CLINICAL FINDINGS

Symptoms generally are dependent on the size and distribution of tumors. Vestibular schwannomas (acoustic neuromas) often are small at the onset of symptoms because of their location. As the name implies, these tumors involve the eighth cranial nerve and produce hearing loss, tinnitus, and impaired balance.[4] Singular spinal tumors grow slowly and are often large when discovered. Osseous abnormalities are common in NF-1 and include scoliosis, congenital pseudarthrosis, and sphenoid bone dysplasia. Lateral thoracic meningocele is an uncommon complication of NF-1. Café-au-lait macules, freckling in the axillary or inguinal regions, Lisch nodules, and a positive familial history are helpful in the diagnosis of NF-1.[104] Cutaneous features are found less frequently in NF-2 and schwannomatosis than in NF-1.[223] The presenting complaints in NF-2 often involve hearing loss, tinnitus, and disturbed balance resulting from bilateral involvement. Patients with schwannomatosis present most frequently with localized pain.

KEY CONCEPTS

- *Histologically dissimilar tumors are found in schwannoma, neurofibroma, neurofibromatosis type I tumors, neurofibromatosis type II tumors, and schwannomatosis.*
- *Magnetic resonance imaging is the investigational tool of choice.*
- *Symptoms are dependent on the type of tumor, size, and location.*

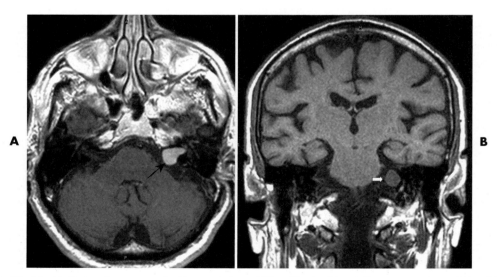

FIG. 33-14   Vestibular schwannoma. **A,** Contrast-enhanced T1-weighted axial, and, **B,** contrast enhanced T1-weighted coronal acquisitions illustrate a vestibular schwannoma (acoustic neuroma). Lesion is slightly lower signal than white matter before contrast administration and enhances after the administration *(arrow)* of Gd-DTPA.

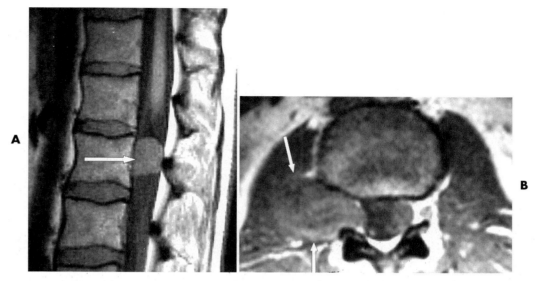

FIG. 33-15 Neurofibrosarcoma. Neurofibrosarcoma incidentally discovered in a 34-year-old man who presented with low back pain and bilateral radiculopathy. Disc herniations were identified at L4-5 and L5-S1 and surgically repaired. Lesion is well demonstrated in, **A,** T1-weighted sagittal and, **B,** axial images existing within the thecal sac and extending through the intervertebral foramen to reside in the soft tissues lateral to the spine (dumbbell lesion) *(arrows)*. Tumor was surgically excised successfully.

Pituitary Adenomas

BACKGROUND

Pituitary adenomas arise from the epithelial cells of the adenohypophysis (anterior lobe) and comprise approximately 10% of all intracranial tumors. Females are affected much more commonly than males and the peak incidence is between 20 and 60 years of age. Small adenomas (<10 mm) are more common and designated as *microadenomas*. Larger tumors (>10 mm) are called *macroadenomas*. Pituitary adenomas may be solitary or part of a syndrome such as multiple endocrine neoplasia, McCune-Albright's syndrome, and Carney complex. These lesions are classified as benign tumors, although the clinical consequences may be devastating.[202]

IMAGING FINDINGS

Contrast-enhanced MRI is the preferred imaging examination for investigation of pituitary adenomas. These lesions are typically low signal on T1-weighted images and high signal on T2-weighted images. Homogeneous or heterogenous enhancement ensues with contrast administration (Fig. 33-16, *A* to *C*). However, the normal pituitary also enhances, and delayed images are essential because the tumor continues to enhance, whereas the contrast dissipates from the gland itself. Lesions may be confined to the sella turcica or erode the sella turcica and adjacent osseous structures, extending into the brain parenchyma. Larger neoplasms tend to produce greater morbidity and mortality. Intraoperative MRI (iMRI) is used successfully for assessment of complete surgical resection of adenomas during transsphenoidal microsurgery.[19,109,184,241,318]

CLINICAL COMMENTS

Symptoms in pituitary adenoma are dependent on the particular cell type and mass effect. Somatotrophs and gonadotrophs are the most likely to be affected. Corticotrophs and thyrotrophs are less sensitive. Acromegaly is a product of excessive growth hormone, whereas testicular enlargement or ovarian hyperstimulation may occur because of excess gonadotrophic hormone. Insufficient gonadotrophic hormone resulting from mass effect may result in hypogonadism.[66,183] Hyperprolactinemia may develop because of hormonal production by a prolactinoma. Cushing's syndrome and hyperthyroidism are infrequent consequences of pituitary adenoma. Recent advances in immunocytochemical biology and radioimmunoassay permit detailed analysis of these neoplasias.[202] Surgery is the best option, even in small microadenomas.

> **KEY CONCEPTS**
> - *Pituitary adenomas may be designated as microadenomas or macroadenomas, depending on size.*
> - *Magnetic resonance imaging is extremely dependable in the investigation of pituitary microadenomas and macroadenomas.*
> - *Clinical findings are the result of the type of hormone produced and the mass effect of the adenoma.*

Medulloblastoma

BACKGROUND

Medulloblastoma accounts for 2% to 6% of all intracranial gliomas and is the most common malignant posterior fossa tumor of childhood. It accounts for 15% to 20% of all pediatric intracranial tumors.[56] There are approximately 350 new cases per year in the United States. A slight male predominance exists. Medulloblastoma originally was classified as a glial lesion, but is now considered a primary neuroectodermal tumor (PNET).

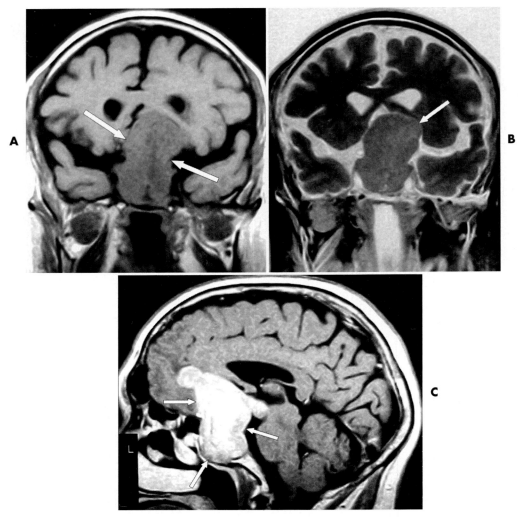

FIG. 33-16 Pituitary macroadenoma. Large pituitary macroadenoma in a 65-year-old man. **A,** T1-weighted coronal; **B,** T1-weighted inverted gray-scale; and, **C,** postcontrast sagittal T1-weighted sequences demonstrate contrast enhancement of a lesion that has eroded the sella turcica and clivus and extends superiorly into the brain parenchyma at the midline (arrows).

Most arise from the floor of the fourth ventricle and the vermis cerebelli of younger children and the hemispheres of the cerebellum in older children, often creating hydrocephalus secondary to CSF obstruction. Medulloblastoma commonly presents with the signs and symptoms of increased intracranial pressure related to hydrocephaly. Drop metastasis and leptomeningeal metastasis occur in a small percentage of cases.[81,240]

IMAGING FINDINGS
Gd-DTPA enhanced MRI is the preferred imaging study in the diagnosis of medulloblastoma (Fig. 33-17, *A* and *B*). Enhancement is typically homogeneous in children. Cysts, necrosis, hemorrhage, and calcifications are atypical. A surrounding zone of edema is frequent and is best appreciated by T2-weighted or FLAIR images. Spinal MRI is imperative if medulloblastoma is diagnosed in the brain because of the possibility of drop metastasis. Unlike CT, MRI is not susceptible to the osseous artifacts found in the posterior fossa.[167,218,275]

CLINICAL COMMENTS
The symptoms of medulloblastoma often are related to obstructive hydrocephalus. Altered behavior, malaise, vomiting, headache, and ataxia are frequent clinical findings among patients with medulloblastoma. Increased head circumference may be the only sign in infants. Papilledema is the most frequent physical finding. Torticollis is present occasionally if there is involvement of the fourth cranial nerve or herniation of the cerebellar tonsils into the foramen magnum. Obstructive hydrocephalus is an absolute contraindication to lumbar puncture.[81,240]

KEY CONCEPTS
- *Medulloblastoma is an uncommon tumor but is the most common posterior fossa neoplasia in children.*
- *Contrast-enhanced magnetic resonance imaging is the diagnostic imaging modality of choice.*
- *Signs and symptoms of obstructive hydrocephalus often dominate the clinical picture.*

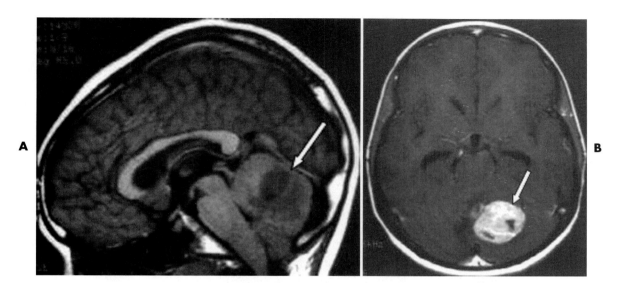

FIG. 33-17 Medulloblastoma. **A,** Unenhanced T1-weighted sagittal, and, **B,** postcontrast T1-weighted axial acquisitions demonstrate low signal in the left cerebellar hemisphere before contrast. **B,** Slightly inhomogeneous enhancement occurs on contrast administration (arrows). (Courtesy Stephen Pomeranz, Cincinnati, OH.)

Lymphoma

BACKGROUND

The incidence of primary CNS lymphoma has increased dramatically with the spread of autoimmune disease and the use of immunosuppressive drugs in chemotherapy and organ transplantation surgery. Primary brain lymphoma currently comprises greater than 7% of the primary brain tumors and is more common than secondary brain lymphoma. Primary brain lymphoma is found in approximately 2% of patients with acquired immunodeficiency syndrome (AIDS). CNS lymphoma is more common in male patients, and the peak incidence occurs in the fifth and sixth decades of life.[51,80,261]

IMAGING FINDINGS

Gd-DTPA–enhanced MRI is the imaging modality of choice to demonstrate CNS lymphoma. The most common site of involvement is the basal ganglia. Leptomeningeal involvement is less frequent. Typically the tumor is isointense to brain parenchyma or low signal on T1-weighted acquisitions and isointense or high signal on T2-weighted images. Tumor enhancement is diffuse and intense with ring enhancement, particularly among AIDS patients. Surrounding edema is found in a small percentage of lesions (Fig. 33-18, *A* through *D*). Leptomeningeal extension occurs and enhances with contrast MRI. DWI, DTI, and fMRI may be of benefit. PET scans, SPECT scans, and hybrid or fusion imaging may add information, particularly about tumoral staging, treatment, and prognosis.[18,40,174,289] Spontaneous regression of CNS lymphoma occurs with some frequency.[25]

CLINICAL COMMENTS

Clinical signs and symptoms are not specific to CNS lymphoma. Symptoms are similar to other CNS neoplasia and include headache, nausea, vomiting, paresis, behavioral disturbances, and altered personality. However, as is so frequently the case, the patient's history often is the most important step in formulating a correct diagnosis. Appropriate imaging should be performed if the symptoms are consistent with a CNS lesion and the patient has a history of immunosuppressive disease or therapy. Stereotactic biopsy is used to provide definitive diagnosis.[80]

> ### KEY CONCEPTS
> - *The incidence of lymphoma has increased significantly related to patients with immunosuppressive diseases, therapy resulting in immunosuppression, and organ transplant surgery.*
> - *Contrast-enhanced magnetic resonance imaging is the imaging modality of choice.*
> - *The patient's history of immunosuppressive disease or therapy is essential to the diagnosis of central nervous system lymphoma.*

Craniopharyngioma

BACKGROUND

The embryonal anatomic precursor to the adenohypophysis is Rathke's cleft. The craniopharyngioma evolves from epithelial cells within Rathke's cleft. The adenohypophysis and infundibulum migrate along the craniopharyngeal duct during embryonal development, and a craniopharyngioma may emanate in any location along this duct. Hence, common locations for craniopharyngioma are the suprasellar cistern, third ventricle, within the sella turcica, or the immediate region of the sella turcica. Hydrocephalus is a frequent complication resulting from the potentially obstructive location of these lesions. Craniopharyngioma is found most frequently in the pediatric population, comprising less than 5% of all brain tumors. No significant gender or race predominance exists.[245,302]

IMAGING FINDINGS

Craniopharyngioma is a slow-growing neoplasia that exhibits cysts and calcification in more than 60% of cases.[302,320] It comprises 4% of all intracranial neoplasms and make up 7% of all intracranial childhood tumors. These tumors are the most common suprasellar

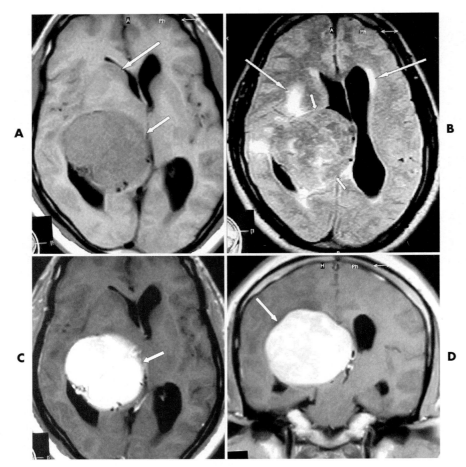

FIG. 33–18   Lymphoma. Lymphoma in a 47-year-old male AIDS patient. Precontrast and postcontrast T1-weighted sagittal and axial, postcontrast coronal, and inversion recovery axial acquisitions demonstrate a large right cerebral mass with its epicenter in the periventricular region. Lesion is slightly hypointense to the white matter in, **A,** the unenhanced T1-weighted image with, **C** and **D,** heterogenous enhancement in the postcontrast T1-weighted sequences *(arrows).* **B,** Inversion recovery acquisition permits visualization of edema adjacent to the left lateral ventricle and the brain parenchyma anterior, lateral, and posterior to the lymphoma *(arrows).* Midline shift to the left side is evident with effacement of the posterior body and horn of the right lateral ventricle.

mass of childhood.[56] MRI and CT are complementary imaging modalities. MRI with and without Gd-DTPA contrast is exceptional in the detection and characterization of the size, location, and matrix (cystic/solid) of the tumor. The solid portion of a craniopharyngioma enhances because of disruption of the blood–brain barrier by neovascularity. Cystic lesions within the tumor matrix do not enhance because of their avascular morphology.[266] CT excels in the demonstration of calcification.[108] The characteristic parasellar location in a pediatric patient exhibiting a solid tumor matrix, cysts, and calcification suggests the diagnosis.

CLINICAL COMMENTS

Symptoms in patients with craniopharyngioma range from nonspecific headaches, nausea, vomiting, and fatigue to more specific endocrine and visual disturbances related to the location of the lesion. Endocrine disturbances include delayed growth, obesity, premature or precocious puberty, and diabetes insipidus. Craniopharyngioma involving the optic tract may lead to visual defects such as bitemporal hemianopsia, amblyopia, scotoma, and blindness. Behavioral and personality alteration with disturbed mentation also are symptoms of craniopharyngioma. Hydrocephalus with increased intracranial pressure often leads to papilledema. Imaging findings and stereotactic biopsy are diagnostic.[87,245]

KEY CONCEPTS

- *Craniopharyngioma is found along the embryonal remnants of Rathke's cleft.*
- *Magnetic resonance imaging and computed tomography demonstration of a parasellar tumor in a pediatric patient with cysts and calcification is highly suggestive of craniopharyngioma.*
- *Endocrine disturbances, visual defects, and signs of increased intracranial pressure should trigger appropriate imaging.*

Teratoma

BACKGROUND

Tumors of the germinal epithelium are much more common than those composed of interstitial cells. Because germinal cells are capable of differentiating to almost any type of cell, many of these tumors contain multiple tissues, including hair, teeth, skin, muscle, and placental and endocrine tissue all found together in the same tumorous mass called a teratoma.[32,110] Intracranial teratomas are rare, comprising less than 1% of all CNS tumors; however, they are the most common brain tumor of the newborn. The pineal region is the most common site of intracranial involvement. Ovarian and sacrococcygeal teratomas are much more common than teratomas of the brain and exhibit a strong female predilection. The majority of brain teratomas are found among the male fetal or pediatric population. Intrauterine and early neonatal mortality is common.[50]

IMAGING FINDINGS

Transcranial ultrasound is the imaging modality of choice to help exclude a fetal or early neonatal teratoma.[166,172] The typical teratoma appears as a large solid or cystic mass. Associated congenital defects occur with great frequency. MRI, CT, and FDG PET scans are useful in the diagnosis and detection of reoccurrence of surgically excised lesions. MR spectroscopy is sensitive to high lipid levels, suggesting a malignant teratoma.[257] Calcification and cyst formation are frequent.[2]

CLINICAL COMMENTS

There is a high mortality rate associated with teratomas, both in utero and among neonates. Macrocephaly often makes cesarean delivery a necessity. Increased intracranial pressure resulting from hydrocephalus causes papilledema, visual disturbances, and headaches. Diabetes insipidus is a common complication. Stereotactic biopsy is used for definitive diagnosis. Treatment typically is surgical for accessible tumors, although pediatric patients younger than 3 years of age commonly are treated with chemotherapy.[2,32,50,110]

> ### KEY CONCEPTS
> - *Brain teratoma is rare. Sacrococcygeal and ovarian teratoma is much more frequent.*
> - *Ultrasound, magnetic resonance imaging, computed tomography, and positron emission tomography scans are useful imaging modalities.*
> - *Patients with brain teratomas often die before or shortly after birth.*
> - *Symptoms are often those of increased intracranial pressure resulting from hydrocephalus.*

Secondary Tumors

Metastasis

BACKGROUND

Metastasis to the brain is the most common intracranial neoplasm encountered in adult patients and makes up 40% of all intracranial tumors.[56] Tumors of the lung, breast, skin (melanoma), kidney, thyroid, and colon are the most frequent primary malignancies that metastasize to the brain. Hematogenous metastasis is the most common method of dissemination. More than one half of all metastatic brain tumors are multiple.

Metastasis to the spinal cord is uncommon, although the spine is the most common site of osseous metastasis. Spinal metastasis typically is hematogenous in etiology. Dissemination via Batson's venous plexus occurs with great frequency, particularly with carcinoma of the prostate. Lesions that metastasize to the spine frequently are primary malignancies of the lung (although squamous cell carcinoma metastasis is rare) breast, colon, and prostate. Brain metastasis from sarcomas is exceptionally rare. Approximately 70% of metastatic lesions are found in the thoracic spine, although more than 50% of metastatic tumors exhibit multiple levels of involvement.[173,290] *Drop metastasis* is the term used to describe the aqueous cerebrospinal seeding of primary brain tumors, particularly medulloblastoma and ependymoma (Fig. 33-19). An extramedullary intradural location is typical for drop metastasis.

IMAGING FINDINGS

Contrast-enhanced MRI is the preferred imaging modality in the diagnosis of brain and spinal metastatic disease. CT and radionuclide scans may be informative, particularly in cases involving osseous structures. A history of primary malignancy and multiple masses in the brain or spinal structures is highly suggestive of metastatic disease. Solitary lesions occur in approximately one third of cases, with multiple lesions in the other two thirds.[56] In the brain, T1-weighted MR images demonstrate tumors that typically are isointense with the parenchyma, but enhance intensely with contrast administration, often exhibiting ring enhancement (Fig. 33-20, *A* to *C*). Areas that do not enhance are indicative of tissue necrosis or cyst formation. Tumors are increased in signal on T2-weighted images (Fig. 33-21, *A* to *C*). FLAIR images are useful in the visualization of vasogenic edema. If hemorrhage is present, signal intensity is dependent on the age of the hemorrhage (see Table 33-1). DWI is particularly effective in characterization of areas of necrosis, cyst formation, and edema.[40,72,280,289]

Plain film radiography may be of benefit in the evaluation of a patient with osseous metastatic disease, although this has been largely supplanted by MRI, CT, and nuclear scans. Metastatic tumors to bone structures typically exhibit low signal on T1-weighted acquisitions and high signal on T2-weighted images. Gd-DTPA enhancement is intense. CT is useful in the assessment of osseous lesions but is inferior to MRI in the demonstration of soft-tissue involvement. Radionuclide scans are sensitive; however, they are nonspecific for metastatic disease.*

CLINICAL COMMENTS

Symptoms of metastasis to the brain are not pathognomonic and include headaches, nausea, vomiting, altered mentation, paresis, visual and speech disturbances, seizures, and ataxia.[140] The symptoms are dependent on the size and location of the metastatic deposits. The cerebral hemispheres are involved 57% of the time, whereas the cerebellum and brainstem are involved approximately 29% and 32%, respectively.[56] Symptoms in patients with spinal metastasis often are the result of compression of neural structures from mass effect or pathologic fracture. The majority of patients with spinal metastatic disease present with localized back pain and radicular symptoms. Sensory and motor complaints are common, and 50% of patients present with bladder and bowel dysfunction.[290]

> ### KEY CONCEPTS
> - *Metastasis to the brain and osseous structures of the spine is common.*
> - *Metastasis to the spinal cord is rare.*
> - *Gadolinium-DTPA–enhanced magnetic resonance imaging is the imaging modality of choice.*
> - *Signs and symptoms of metastasis to the brain and spine are not specific. The history of a primary malignancy and neurologic symptoms should stimulate imaging.*

*References 123, 141, 173, 222, 290.

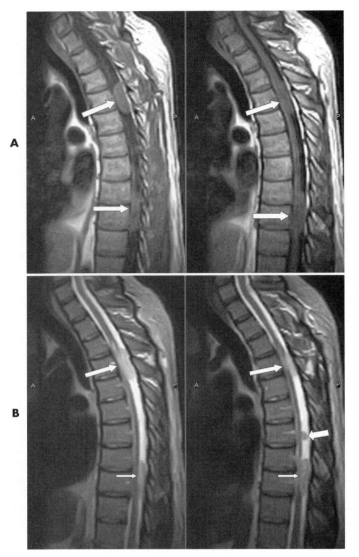

FIG. 33-19 Drop metastasis. **A,** Sagittal T1, and, **B,** T2-weighted sequences illustrate multiple intradural tumors in the thoracic spine resulting from drop metastasis (arrows). These lesions are isointense with the spinal cord in the T1-weighted images and slightly higher signal intensity than the spinal cord in the T2-weighted acquisitions.

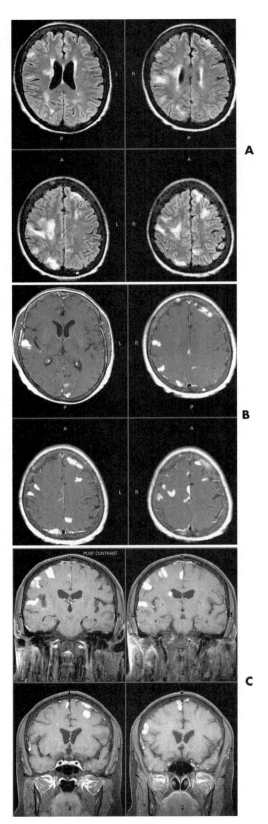

FIG. 33-20 Metastasis. Numerous enhancing metastatic nodules are visible in, **A** and **B,** the postcontrast T1-weighted axial and, **C,** coronal images. Gd-DTPA is essential in the evaluation of small lesions.

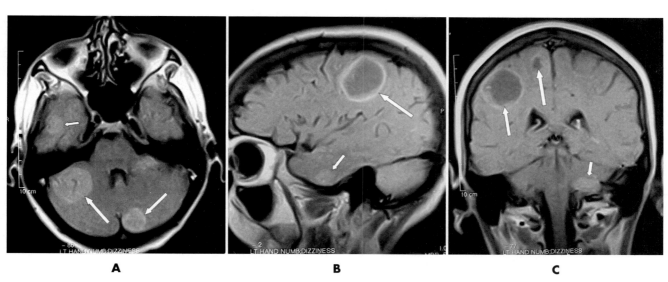

A   **B**   **C**

FIG. 33-21 Metastasis. Metastatic carcinoma in a 62-year-old woman with a history of lung carcinoma treated with chemotherapy and radiation therapy. Postcontrast T1-weighted, **A,** axial; **B,** sagittal; and, **C,** coronal acquisitions reveal multiple lesions in both the cerebrum and cerebellum (*arrows*). Peripheral enhancement is evident in a large lesion in the right parietal region.

■ Miscellaneous Selected Conditions

Arnold-Chiari Malformation

BACKGROUND

A Chiari malformation is the herniation of the cerebellar tonsils into the cervical spinal canal through the foramen magnum. Normally the cerebellar tonsils should lie no more than 3 mm below the foramen magnum. Extension below the foramen between of 3 and 5 mm is considered borderline. Chiari malformations larger than 5 mm but smaller than 10 mm are symptomatic in approximately 70% of patients. However, symptoms are invariably present in those patients with Chiari malformations greater than 12 mm.[73,195] The cerebellar tonsils ascend somewhat with increasing age, and tonsillar ectopia of greater than 5 mm may not be as clinically significant in a pediatric patient as with a geriatric patient.

Chiari malformations have been divided into four types (I, II, III, and IV). Chiari I refers to a wedge- or peg-shaped inferior displacement of the cerebellar tonsils more than 3 mm through the foramen magnum with crowding of the craniocervical junction. Basilar invagination is a frequent accompanying feature (25%). Chiari I also has been associated with occipitalization, Klippel-Feil syndrome, hydromyelia, and diminished size of the fourth ventricle.[1,198] In addition to tonsillar ectopia, Chiari II malformations display cephalocaudad elongation of the fourth ventricle with transverse narrowing and a decreased AP dimension. Hydrocephalus, syringohydromyelia, and lumbar meningoencephalocele are common to a majority of patients with Chiari II (Fig. 33-22). The posterior petrous ridge and clivus may be concave in appearance. Attenuation of the clivus can occur, and has been described. Chiari II has also been associated with lacunar skull (Lückenschädel) and a kinking of the medulla.[127] Chiari III malformation is characterized by herniation of the cerebellum through the foramen magnum, often associated with an ununited neural arch in the cervical spine, possibly leading to an encephalocele. Chiari IV malformation is a severe form of cerebellar hypoplasia without the characteristic tonsillar ectopia. It may not represent a true Chiari-type malformation.[211]

IMAGING FINDINGS

MRI is the preferred imaging modality for the evaluation of all forms of Chiari malformation. Direct multidirectional MR acquisitions are ideal for demonstration of the relationship of the cerebellar tonsils to the foramen magnum and for the exclusion of ventricular abnormality, syrinx formation, hydrocephalus, and medullary kink. Cervical encephalocele and cerebellar hypoplasia are readily evaluated with MRI.[1,73,195,275] Osseous abnormalities often can be depicted with plain film radiography or CT. Diagnostic ultrasound and transcranial ultrasound may be informative, particularly in the immediate neonatal period.[127]

CLINICAL COMMENTS

Common complaints associated with Chiari I malformation are pain, weakness, paresthesias of the upper extremities, and headaches. Clinical signs include urinary incontinence and sensory loss. Chiari II syndrome exhibits different symptoms between infants and children. Respiratory distress and impaired swallowing occurs frequently among infants. Infants may commonly present with pain, weakness, or spasticity in the extremities and nystagmus. Childhood signs and symptoms include nystagmus, syncope, upper extremity weakness, paresis, pneumonia (caused by aspiration), and exaggerated deep tendon reflexes. Chiari III and IV malformations have a high incidence of infant mortality.[127]

KEY CONCEPTS

- *Chiari I, II, and III malformations display inferior displacement of the cerebellar tonsils through the foramen magnum. Associated abnormalities determine the clinical degree and severity.*
- *Magnetic resonance imaging is preferred for demonstration of the placement of cerebellar tonsils and related abnormalities.*
- *Signs and symptoms are dependent on the degree of displacement of the cerebellar tonsils and associated disorders.*

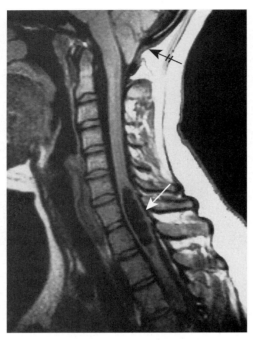

FIG. 33-22 Chiari malformation. T1-weighted sagittal acquisition demonstrates extension of the cerebellar tonsils well below the foramen magnum (crossed arrow). Syrinx within the spinal cord has signal intensity isointense to the cerebrospinal fluid (arrow). Note the enlargement of the spinal cord in the area of the syrinx. (Courtesy Ian D. McLean, Davenport, IA.)

Empty Sella Syndrome

BACKGROUND

Empty sella is a disorder involving the presence of CSF within the cavity of the sella turcica, the saddle-shaped structure that houses the pituitary gland. Empty sella syndrome describes the presence of accompanying symptoms and occurs as a primary or secondary condition. Primary empty sella syndrome likely develops from a defect in the diaphragma sella, allowing CSF to enter the sella, compress the pituitary gland, and potentially increase the size of the sella turcica cavity. Primary empty sella is associated with obesity, past pregnancy, and high blood pressure in women. Secondary empty sella describes a space void created when the pituitary gland shrinks as a result of radiation therapy, injury, surgery, and so on. The smaller pituitary gland may appear necrotic.

IMAGING FINDINGS

On a lateral radiograph, the sella turcica typically measures about 8 mm horizontally and 6 mm vertically. Dimensions larger than 16 mm horizontally or 12 mm vertically, are considered abnormal, warranting further investigation with MRI. MRI may detail an enlarged sella or presence of CSF within the sella as high signal intensity on the T2-weighted images, and possibly reveal deformity in the normal lobular shape of the pituitary gland (see Fig. 16-8).

CLINICAL COMMENTS

An enlarged sella turcica is a significant finding, suggesting the presence of a pituitary neoplasm, empty sella syndrome, extrapituitary neoplasm, or possibly a normal variant of the patient's anatomy. An empty sella can be completely asymptomatic. However, commonly reported clinical symptoms include nontraumatic CSF fluid rhinorrhea, irregular menstruation, fatigue, visual disturbances, headaches, and pituitary hyposecretion or hypersecretion. Treatment entails

supporting the patient and addressing any associated endocrine dysfunction present. Surgery may be warranted.

> **KEY CONCEPTS**
> - *Empty sella is the presence of cerebrospinal fluid within an enlarged sella turcica. Empty sella syndrome designates the presence of related symptoms.*

Syringohydromyelia

BACKGROUND

Syringohydromyelia (syrinx) is the term for a fluid-filled cavity within the spinal canal and spinal cord. Hydromyelia refers to cavitation with fluid in the central canal, whereas syringomyelia is reserved for cavitary fluid within the spinal cord. There are numerous causes for this cavitation, including trauma, tumor, infection, arachnoiditis, and idiopathic or congenital conditions, including Chiari malformation.*

IMAGING FINDINGS

The advent of MRI has made the diagnosis of syrinx considerably easier. As a result, the incidence of diagnosed syringes has increased immensely. Fluid within the spinal cord is typically isointense with CSF (low signal T1, high signal T2). A "bull's-eye" or "target" pattern is frequently discernible in axial acquisitions when a central intramedullary syrinx is present. The central portion (syrinx) is isointense with CSF, the transitional section represents the spinal cord, and surrounding CSF makes up the periphery (Fig. 33-23). The spinal cord often is enlarged in the area of the syrinx, and the cavity may appear multiloculated.[254,275] Phase contrast MRI permits demonstration of pulsatile fluid flow within the cavity and differentiates a syrinx from myelomalacia.[226]

CLINICAL COMMENTS

The signs and symptoms of syringohydromyelia are dependent on the level and extent of involvement. Stiffness and weakness of the lower

---

*References 132, 196, 197, 254, 283, 288.

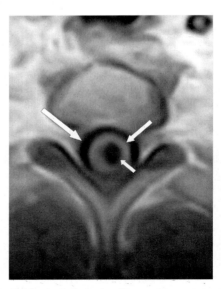

FIG. 33-23 Syringomyelia. Syrinx in a 22-year-old man presenting with complaints of cervical and left arm pain. Postcontrast T1-weighted axial sequence demonstrates the typical "bull's-eye" pattern. Central low signal represents the syrinx (small arrow) and the intermediate signal is the spinal cord (medium arrow). Low signal surrounding the spinal cord is cerebrospinal fluid (large arrow). Chiari malformation is associated (not shown).

extremities with loss of grip strength is the most common complaint. Pain, muscular atrophy, and sensory loss are found in approximately 50% of patients with syringohydromyelia. Nystagmus, dysphagia, and neurotrophic arthropathy are encountered infrequently.[247]

KEY CONCEPTS

- *Syringohydromyelia is a fluid-filled cavitation in the central canal and spinal cord.*
- *Magnetic resonance imaging is superior to other modalities in the diagnosis of syringohydromyelia.*
- *Signs and symptoms are variable and dependent upon the size and location of the cavity.*

Tarlov or Arachnoid Cyst

A Tarlov cyst is a dilatation of the subarachnoid space surrounding a spinal nerve root and is incidentally found in approximately 5% of patients undergoing a lumbosacral MRI examination. Approximately 80% are asymptomatic with no demonstrable need for care. Patients who do exhibit symptoms complain of low back pain, radicular pain, and incontinence. These symptoms must be differentiated from those symptoms caused by disc herniation. Tarlov cysts communicate with the thecal sac and thus are isointense with CSF on MR images (Fig. 33-24, *A* to *D*). Tarlov cysts are most frequently found at the S2 level, and bone erosion is a common feature of large

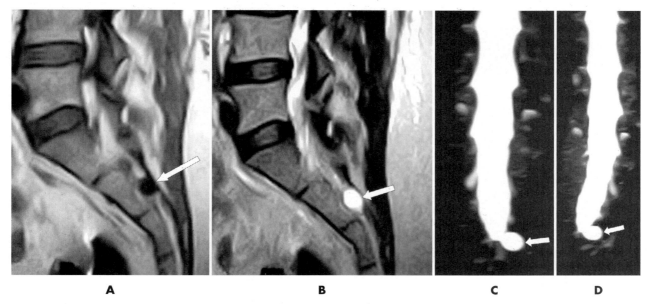

FIG. 33-24 Tarlov cyst. Small Tarlov cyst visualized at the S2 level that is isointense with cerebrospinal fluid in, **A,** the T1-, and, **B,** T2-weighted sagittal images *(arrows)*. **C,** Coronal, and, **D,** oblique magnetic resonance imaging myelography demonstrates the communication between the thecal sac and the Tarlov cyst *(arrows)*.

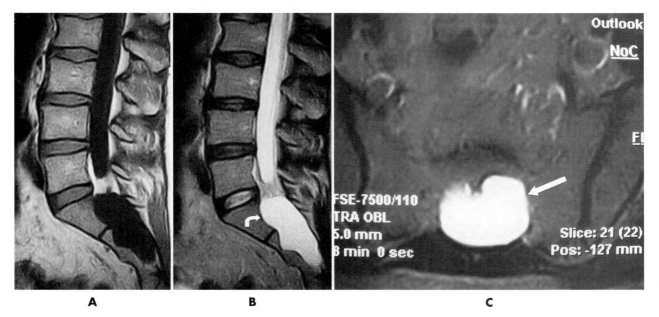

FIG. 33-25 Large Tarlov cyst. Large Tarlov cyst in a 48-year-old man, extending from the left S2 nerve root and approximately 2.2 × 7 × 4 cm. Significant bony remodeling of the sacrum secondary to mass effect *(curved arrow)*. Matrix of the lesion is isointense to the cerebrospinal fluid in, **A,** the T1-weighted sagittal, **B;** T2-weighted sagittal; and, **C,** axial T2-weighted images *(straight arrow)*.

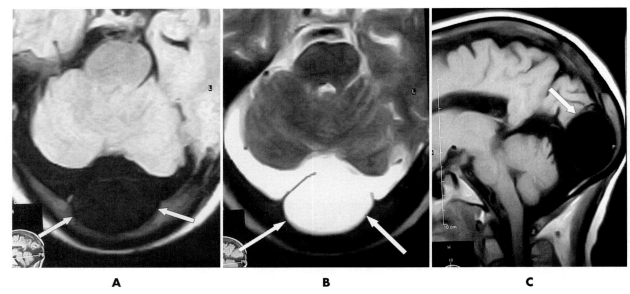

A   **B**   **C**

FIG. 33-26   Arachnoid cyst. Large arachnoid cyst with a prominent cisterna magna in a 60-year-old woman presenting with headaches, dizziness, and nausea. **A,** T1-weighted sagittal; **B,** axial; and, **C,** T2-weighted axial acquisitions demonstrate low signal in the T1-weighted images and high signal in the T2-weighted images, isointense with cerebrospinal fluid *(arrows)*.

cysts (Fig. 33-25, *A* to *C*). Trauma and increased hydrostatic pressure have been implicated in the formation of Tarlov cysts. Surgical treatment in large (>1.5 cm) symptomatic cysts may relieve symptoms.[300]

An arachnoid cyst contains CSF and does not communicate with the ventricular system. These cysts occur most frequently in the middle cranial fossa and are more common on the left side, although subdural or epidural spinal cysts may ensue. The most common spinal location is posterior to the spinal cord in the thoracic region, but arachnoid cysts are also found in the lumbar and cervical regions. The majority result from a developmental anomaly, although they may be infrequently found with neoplasms and adhesions secondary to hemorrhage, surgery, or leptomeningitis. Arachnoid cysts are easily demonstrated with MRI (Fig. 33-26, *A* to *C*). Arachnoid cysts typically are asymptomatic. Headaches, seizures, localized bulging of the cranium, and focal neurologic deficits are infrequent clinical manifestations. Surgical treatment consists of constructing a CSF shunt from the cyst to the peritoneum.[41,139,300]

KEY CONCEPTS

- *Tarlov cysts are the result of dilatation of the subarachnoid space surrounding a nerve root.*
- *The majority of Tarlov and arachnoid cysts are asymptomatic.*
- *Tarlov and arachnoid cysts are filled with cerebrospinal fluid (CSF) and are isointense with CSF on magnetic resonance imaging.*

References

1. Aboulezz AO et al: Position of cerebellar tonsils in the normal population and in patients with Chiari malformation: a quantitative approach with MR imaging, *J Comput Assist Tomogr* 9(6):1033, 1985.
2. Adkins SE et al: Teratomas and other germ cell tumors, *eMedicine* 2003, *http://www.emedicine.com/ped/topic3023.htm.*
3. Albers GW et al: Yield of diffusion-weighted MRI for detection of potentially relevant findings in stroke patients, *Neurology* 54(8): 1562, 2000.
4. Allcutt DA et al: Acoustic schwannomas in children, *Neurosurgery* 29(1):14, 1991.
5. Antinheimo J et al: Population-based analysis of sporadic and type 2 neurofibromatosis-associated meningiomas and schwannomas, *Neurology* 54(1):71, 2000.
6. Aoki H et al: Vertebral artery pseudoaneurysm: a rare complication of internal jugular vein catheterization, *Anesth Analg* 75:296, 1992.
7. Arnold JL et al: Stroke, ischemic, *eMedicine* 2003, *http://www.emedicine.com/ped/topic3023.htm.*
8. Ashwal S: Neurologic evaluation of the patient with acute bacterial meningitis, *Neurol Clin* 13(3):549, 1995.
9. Atlas SW, Thulborn KR: MR detection of hyperacute parenchymal hemorrhage of the brain, *AJNR* 19(8):1471, 1998.
10. Atlas SW: Magnetic resonance imaging of intracranial aneurysms, *Neuroimaging Clin North Am* 7(4):709, 1997.
11. Barclay L: MRI allows earlier diagnosis, treatment of multiple sclerosis: *Neurology* 61:602, 2003.
12. Barker FG 2nd et al: Necrosis as a prognostic factor in glioblastoma multiforme, *Cancer* 77(6):1161, 1996.
13. Barker FG 2nd et al: Radiation response and survival time in patients with glioblastoma multiforme, *J Neurosurg* 84(3): 442, 1996.
14. Barnard RO, Geddes JF: The incidence of multifocal cerebral gliomas. A histologic study of large hemisphere sections, *Cancer* 60(7):1519, 1987.
15. Barsan WG, Kothari R: Emergency medicine concepts and practices, *Stroke* 3:2184, 1998.
16. Baser ME et al: Neurofibromatosis 2, *Curr Opin Neurol* 16(1): 27, 2003.
17. Basser PJ, Mattiello J, LeBihan D: MR diffusion tensor spectroscopy and imaging, *Biophys J* 66(1):259, 1994.
18. Beppu T, Inoue T: Measurement of fractional anisotropy using diffusion tensor MRI in supratentorial astrocytic tumors, *J Neurooncol* 63(2):109, 2003.
19. Bohinski RJ et al: Intraoperative magnetic resonance imaging to determine the extent of resection of pituitary macroadenomas during transsphenoidal microsurgery, *Neurosurgery* 49(5): 1133, 2001.
20. Boutin RD, Brossmann J, Sartoris DJ: Update on imaging of orthopedic infections, *Orthop Clin North Am* 29(1):41, 1998.

21. Bozbuga M et al: Posterior fossa epidural hematomas: observations on a series of 73 cases, *Neurosurg Rev* 22(1):34, 1999.

22. Bradley WG, Schmidt PG: Effect of methemoglobin formation on the MR appearance of subarachnoid hemorrhage, *Radiology* 156:99, 1985.

23. Bradley WG: MR appearance of hemorrhage in the brain, *Radiology* 189:15, 1993.

24. Brant WE, Helms CA: Fundamentals in diagnostic radiology, ed 2, Baltimore, 1999, Williams & Wilkins.

25. Bromberg JE, Siemers MD, Taphoorn MJ: Is a "vanishing tumor" always a lymphoma? *Neurology* 59(5):762, 2002.

26. Brook I et al: Brain abscess, *eMedicine* 2002, *http://www.emedicine.com/ped/topic3023.htm*.

27. Bruce J et al: Glioblastoma multiforme, *eMedicine* 2001, *http://www.emedicine.com/ped/topic3023.htm*.

28. Bruce J et al: Ependymoma, *eMedicine* 2002, *http://www.emedicine.com/ped/topic3023.htm*.

29. Bruce J et al: Astrocytoma, *eMedicine* 2001, *http://www.emedicine.com/ped/topic3023.htm*.

30. Bruner JM: Neuropathology of malignant gliomas, *Semin Oncol* 21(2):126, 1994.

31. Buetow MP, Buetow PC, Smirniotopoulos JG: Typical, atypical and misleading features in meningioma, *Radiographics* 11(6):1087, 1991.

32. Buetow PC, Smirniotopoulos JG, Done S: Congenital brain tumors: a review of 45 cases, *AJR Am J Roentgenol* 155:587, 1990.

33. Burger PC, Green SB: Patient age, histologic features, and length of survival in patients with glioblastoma multiforme, *Cancer* 59(9):1617, 1987.

34. Burger PC et al: Clinicopathologic correlations in the oligodendroglioma, *Cancer* 59(7):1345, 1987.

35. Burger PC et al: Glioblastoma multiforme and anaplastic astrocytoma. Pathologic criteria and prognostic implications, *Cancer* 56:1106, 1985.

36. Byrne TN: Imaging of gliomas, *Semin Oncol* 21(2):162, 1994.

37. Calvin EB, Stanley JC: Current therapy in vascular surgery, St Louis, 1995, Mosby.

38. Carragee EJ: Pyogenic vertebral osteomyelitis, *J Bone Joint Surg Am* 79:874, 1997.

39. Castillo GC et al: Brain meningioma, *eMedicine* 2004, *http://www.emedicine.com/ped/topic3023.htm*.

40. Castillo M et al: Apparent diffusion coefficients in the evaluation of high-grade cerebral gliomas, *AJN* 22:60, 2001.

41. Cayli SR: Arachnoid cyst with spontaneous rupture into the subdural space, *Br J Neurosurg* 14(6):568, 2000.

42. Cerreta E: The role of magnetic resonance imaging studies in multiple sclerosis, *J Neurosci Nurs* 30(5):290, 1998.

43. Chesnut RM: The management of severe traumatic brain injury, *Emerg Med Clin North Am* 15(3):581, 1997.

44. Cheung DS: Evidence based emergency medicine: evaluation and diagnostic testing, *Emerg Med Clin North Am* 17:9, 1999.

45. Choi JY et al: Intracranial and spinal ependymomas: review of MR images in 61 patients, *Korean J Radiol* 3(4):219, 2002.

46. Chrysikopoulos H et al: Acute subarachnoid haemorrhage: detection with magnetic resonance imaging, *BJR* 69(823):601, 1996.

47. Clare CE, Barrow DL: Infectious intracranial aneurysms, *Neurosurg Clin North Am* 3(3):551, 1992.

48. Clifford DB: Neurologic opportunistic infections, *Curr Opin Neurol* 8:175, 1995.

49. Coffey RJ, Lunsford LD, Taylor FH: Survival after stereotactic biopsy of malignant gliomas, *Neurosurgery* 22(3):465, 1988.

50. Comiter CV et al: Prognostic features of teratomas with malignant transformation: a clinicopathological study of 21 cases, *J Urol* 159(3):859, 1998.

51. Cordoliani YS: Primary cerebral lymphoma in patients with AIDS: MR findings—17 cases, *AJR Am J Roentgenol* 159:841, 1992.

52. Cotran RS, Kumar V, Collins T: Robbins: pathologic basis of disease, ed 6, Philadelphia, 1999, WB Saunders.

53. Cox LA: The shaken baby syndrome: diagnosis using CT and MRI, *Radiol Technol* 67:513, 1996.

54. Daemerel PH et al: MRI of herpes simplex encephalitis, *Neuroradiology* 34(6):490, 1992.

55. Daffner RH, Yakuis R, Maroon JC: Intraosseous meningioma, *Skeletal Radiol* 27(2):108, 1998.

56. Dähnert W: Radiology review manual, Baltimore, 1991, Williams & Wilkins.

57. Daumas-Duport C et al: Grading of astrocytomas, a simple and reproducible method, *Cancer* 62:2152, 1988.

58. Daumas-Duport C, Scheithauer BW, Kelly PJ: A histologic and cytologic method for the spatial definition of gliomas, *Mayo Clin Proc* 62:435, 1987.

59. Dawodu ST et al: Traumatic brain injury: definition, epidemiology, pathophysiology, *eMedicine* 2003, *http://www.emedicine.com/ped/topic3023.htm*.

60. DeAngelis LM: Brain tumors, *N Engl J Med* 344(2):114, 2001.

61. DeBarge LR, Sheppard J: Sarcoidosis, *eMedicine* 2001, *http://www.emedicine.com/ped/topic3023.htm*.

62. Delattre JY, Krol G, Thaler HT: Distribution of brain metastases, *Arch Neurol* 45:741, 1988.

63. Desprechins B, Stadnik T, Koerts G: Use of diffusion-weighted MR imaging in differential diagnosis between intracranial necrotic tumors and cerebral abscesses, *AJNR* 20:1252, 1999.

64. DeStefano F et al: Multiple sclerosis, *N Engl J Med* 344:381, 2001.

65. Dichgans M et al: Bacterial meningitis in adults: demonstration of inner ear involvement using high-resolution MRI, *Neurology* 52(5):1003, 1999.

66. Diez JJ, Iglesias P: Current management of acromegaly, *Exp Opin Pharmacother* 1(5):991, 2000.

67. Dikmen SS et al: Alcohol use before and after traumatic head injury, *Ann Emerg Med* 26:167, 1995.

68. Dubey N et al: Role of fluorodeoxyglucose positron emission tomography in the diagnosis of neurosarcoidosis, *J Neurol Sci* 15;205(1):77, 2002.

69. Duffy GP: Lumbar puncture in spontaneous subarachnoid hemorrhage, *BMJ* 285:1163, 1982.

70. Duma CM, Kondziolka D, Lunsford LD: Image-guided stereotactic management of non-AIDS-related cerebral infection, *Neurosurg Clin North Am* 2:291, 1992.

71. Edlow JA, Caplan LR: Avoiding the pitfalls in the diagnosis of subarachnoid hemorrhage, *N Engl J Med* 342(1):29, 2000.

72. Eis M et al: Quantitative diffusion MR imaging of cerebral tumor and edema, *Acta Neurochir* 60:344, 1999.

73. Elster AD, Chen MY: Chiari I malformations: clinical and radiologic reappraisal, *Radiology* 183(2):347, 1992.

74. Epstein F, Farmer JP, Freed D: Adult intramedullary astrocytomas of the spinal cord, *J Neurosurg* 77:355, 1992.

75. Ericsson M, Algers G, Schliamser SE: Spinal epidural abscesses in adults: review and report of iatrogenic cases, *Scand J Infect Dis* 22(3):249, 1990.

76. Ernoehazy W et al: Brain abscess, *eMedicine* 2003, *http://www.emedicine.com/ped/topic3023.htm*.

77. Eton D, Weaver FA: A multi-specialty approach to diagnosis and management, *Landes Biosci* 27, 1998.

78. Eugene JR et al: Carotid occlusive disease: primary care of patients with or without symptoms, *Geriatrics* 54:24, 1999.

79. Ferner RE et al: Evaluation of (18)fluorodeoxyglucose positron emission tomography ((18)FDG PET) in the detection of malignant peripheral nerve sheath tumors arising from within plexiform neurofibromas in neurofibromatosis 1, *J Neurol Neurosurg Psychiatry* 68(3):353, 2000.

80. Fertikh D et al: Brain lymphoma, *eMedicine* 2003, *http://www.emedicine.com/ped/topic3023.htm*.

81. Fertikh D et al: Medulloblastoma, *eMedicine* 2002, *http://www.emedicine.com/ped/topic3023.htm.*

82. Fertikh D et al: Multiple sclerosis, spine, *eMedicine* 2002, *http://www.emedicine.com/ped/topic3023.htm.*

83. Filippi M: Enhanced magnetic resonance imaging in multiple sclerosis, *Mult Scler* 6(5):320, 2000.

84. Forsyth PA, Posner JB: Headaches in patients with brain tumors: a study of 111 patients, *Neurology* 43:1678, 1993.

85. Fouquet B, Goupille P, Jattiot F: Discitis after lumbar disc surgery, features of "aseptic" and "septic" forms, *Spine* 17(3): 356, 1992.

86. Francavilla TL et al: Intramedullary spinal cord tumors, *eMedicine* 2002, *http://www.emedicine.com/ped/topic3023.htm.*

87. Frank F et al: Stereotactic management of craniopharyngiomas, *Stereotact Funct Neurosurg* 65(1–4):176, 1995.

88. Friedman AH: Traumatic injury of neck and intracranial vessels, *Cont Neurol* 12:26, 1990.

89. Frishberg BM: The utility of neuroimaging in the evaluation of headache in patients with normal neurologic examinations, *Neurology* 44:1191, 1994.

90. Gean AD: Imaging of head trauma, New York, 1994, Raven Press.

91. Gennarelli TA, Thibault LE: Biomechanics of acute subdural hematoma, *J Trauma* 22:680, 1982.

92. Gennarelli TA: Mechanisms of brain injury, *J Emerg Med* 11:5, 1993.

93. Gentry LR: Imaging of closed head injury, *Radiology* 191(1): 1, 1994.

94. Ghosh S et al: Drop Metastasis from sinonasal undifferentiated carcinoma. Clinical implications, *Spine* 26(13):1486, 2001.

95. Giles GM, Clark-Wilson J: Brain injury rehabilitation: a neurofunctional approach, San Diego, 1993, Singular.

96. Gillingham FJ: The management of ruptured intracranial aneurysm, *Ann Roy Coll Surg (England)* 23:89, 1958.

97. Gillingham FJ: The management of ruptured intracranial aneurysm, *Scott Med J* 12:377, 1967.

98. Goldberg AN, Oroszlam G, Anderson T: Complications of frontal sinusitis and their management, *Otolaryngol Clin North Am* 34:211, 2001.

99. Gotway MB, Marder SR, Hanks DK: Thoracic complications of illicit drug use: an organ system approach, *Radiographics* 22:119, 2002.

100. Gouliamos A et al: Magnetic resonance angiography compared with intra-arterial digital subtraction angiography in patients with subarachnoid hemorrhage, *Neuroradiology* 35(1):46, 1992.

101. Greig NH et al: Increasing annual incidence of primary malignant brain tumors in the elderly, *J Natl Cancer Inst* 82:1621, 1990.

102. Griffiths PD et al: Multimodality MR imaging depiction of hemodynamic changes and cerebral ischemia in subarachnoid hemorrhage, *AJNR* 22(9):1690, 2001.

103. Grossman RI, Yousem DM: Neuroradiology: the requisites, St Louis, 1994, Mosby.

104. Grostern RJ et al: Neurofibromatosis-1, *eMedicine* 2001, *http://www.emedicine.com/ped/topic3023.htm.*

105. Gundry CR, Heithoff KB: Epidural hematoma of the lumbar spine: 18 surgically confirmed cases, *Radiology* 187:427, 1993.

106. Haas DW, McAndrew MP: Bacterial osteomyelitis in adults: evolving considerations in diagnosis and treatment, *Am J Med* 101(5):550, 1996.

107. Haddad G et al: Meningioma, *eMedicine* 2002, *http://www.emedicine.com/ped/topic3023.htm.*

108. Hald JK, Edevik OP, Skalpe IO: Craniopharyngioma identification by CT and MR imaging at 1.5 T, *Acta Radiol* 36(2):142, 1995.

109. Hald JK et al: MR imaging of pituitary macroadenomas before and after transsphenoidal surgery, *Acta Radiol* 33(5):396, 1992.

110. Hamilton C et al: Teratoma, cystic, *eMedicine* 2002, *http://www.emedicine.com/ped/topic3023.htm.*

111. Hariharan S et al: Oligodendroglioma, *eMedicine* 2002, *http://www.emedicine.com/ped/topic3023.htm.*

112. Harrop JS et al: Spinal tumors, *eMedicine* 2001, *http://www.emedicine.com/ped/topic3023.htm.*

113. Hasso AN, Bell SA, Tadmor R: Intracranial vascular tumors, *Neuroimaging Clin North Am* 4:849, 1994.

114. Healy ME et al: Increased detection of intracranial metastases with intravenous Gd-DTPA, *Radiology* 165:619, 1987.

115. Hems TE, Burge PD, Wilson DJ: The role of magnetic resonance imaging in the management of peripheral nerve tumours, *J Hand Surg (Br)* 22(1):57, 1997.

116. Henriksen SD et al: Pseudoaneurysm of a lateral internal carotid artery in the middle ear, *Int J Pediatr Otorhinolaryngol* 52: 163, 2000.

117. Henson JW: Spinal cord gliomas, *Curr Opin Neurol* 14(6):679, 2001.

118. Herholz K et al: 11C-methionine PET for differential diagnosis of low-grade gliomas, *Neurology* 50(5):1316, 1998.

119. Hodgson TJ, Kingsley DP, Moseley IF: The role of imaging in the follow up of meningiomas, *J Neurol Neurosurg Psychiatry* 59(5):545, 1995.

120. Horska A et al: Proton magnetic resonance spectroscopy of choroid plexus tumors in children, *J MRI* 14(1):78, 2001.

121. Houten JK, Cooper PR: Pyogenic osteomyelitis of the spine, *Contemp Neurosurg* 22:6:1, 2000.

122. Huff JS et al: Brain neoplasms, *eMedicine* 2003, *http://www.emedicine.com/ped/topic3023.htm.*

123. Husband DJ, Grant KA, Romaniuk CS: MRI in the diagnosis and treatment of suspected malignant spinal cord compression, *Br J Radiol* 74(886):977, 2001.

124. Hustinx R, Alavi A: SPECT and PET imaging of brain tumors, *Neuroimaging Clin North Am* 9(4):751, 1999.

125. Ikushima I et al: Dynamic MRI of meningiomas and schwannomas: is differential diagnosis possible? *Neuroradiology* 39(9): 633, 1997.

126. Incesu L et al: Bacterial meningitis, *eMedicine* 2003, *http://www.emedicine.com/ped/topic3023.htm.*

127. Incesu L et al: Chiari II malformation, *eMedicine* 2002, *http://www.emedicine.com/ped/topic3023.htm.*

128. Jakobsson KE et al: Warning leak and management outcome in aneurysmal subarachnoid hemorrhage, *J Neurosurg* 85(6): 995, 1996.

129. Jayaraman M et al: Schwannoma, cranial nerve, *eMedicine* 2002, *http://www.emedicine.com/ped/topic3023.htm.*

130. Junger SS et al: Intramedullary spinal sarcoidosis: clinical and magnetic resonance imaging characteristics, *Neurology* 43: 333, 1993.

131. Kaiser S, Jorulf H, Hirsch G: Clinical value of imaging techniques in childhood osteomyelitis, *Acta Radiol* 39(5):523, 1998.

132. Kakar A, Madan VS, Prakash V: Syringomyelia—a complication of meningitis: case report, *Spinal Cord* 35(1):629, 1997.

133. Kandel ER et al: Principles of neural science, ed 4, New York, 2000, McGraw-Hill.

134. Kaplan PA et al: Musculoskeletal MRI, Philadelphia, 2001, WB Saunders.

135. Kaplan SL: Clinical presentations, diagnosis, and prognostic factors of bacterial meningitis, *Infect Dis Clin North Am* 13(3): 579, 1999.

136. Kapral MK, Bondy SJ: Cervical manipulation and risk of stroke. *Can Med Assoc J* 165:907, 2001.

137. Kazzi AA et al: Subarachnoid hemorrhage, *eMedicine* 2003, *http://www.emedicine.com/ped/topic3023.htm.*

138. Keogh AJ, Vhora S: The usefulness of magnetic resonance angiography in surgery for intracranial aneurysms that have bled, *Surg Neurol* 50(2):122, 1998.

139. Khan AN et al: Arachnoid cyst, *eMedicine* 2002, *http://www.emedicine.com/ped/topic3023.htm.*

140. Kholsa A et al: Brain, metastases, *eMedicine* 2001, *http://www.emedicine.com/ped/topic3023.htm.*

141. Kim JK et al: Diagnosis of vertebral metastasis, epidural metastasis and malignant spinal cord compression: are T1 weighted sagittal images sufficient? *J MRI* 18(7):819, 2000.

142. Kim TS et al: Correlates of survival and the Daumas-Duport grading system for astrocytomas, *J Neurosurg* 74:27, 1991.

143. Kimura K, Hirano H, Uchinom T: Random diagnosis of MCA occlusion with TCD, *Am J Neuroradiol* 17:895, 1996.

144. King R et al: Osteomyelitis, *eMedicine* 2002, *http://www.emedicine.com/ped/topic3023.htm.*

145. Kleihues P, Burger PC, Cavenee WK: Glioblastoma. In: WHO Classification: Pathology and Genetics of Tumors of the Nervous System, ed 1, Lyon, France, 1997, International Agency for Research on Cancers.

146. Kleihues P et al: Histological typing of tumours of the central nervous system, ed 2, Berlin, 1993, Springer-Verlag.

147. Klein W et al: Brain ependymoma, *eMedicine* 2004, *http://www.emedicine.com/ped/topic3023.htm.*

148. Koeller KK, Rosenblum RS, Morrison AL: Neoplasms of the spinal cord and filum terminale: radiologic-pathologic correlation, *Radiographics* 20(6):1721, 2000.

149. Kono K et al: The role of diffusion weighted imaging in patients with brain tumors, *AJNR* 22(6):1013, 2001.

150. Koskiniemi M, Vaheri A, Taskinen E: Cerebrospinal fluid alterations in herpes simplex virus encephalitis, *Rev Infect Dis* 6:608, 1984.

151. Kraus JF, McArthur DL: Epidemiologic aspects of brain injury, *Neurol Clin* 14(2):435, 1996.

152. Kraus JF et al: Blood alcohol tests, prevalence of involvement, and outcomes following brain injury, *Am J Public Health* 79:294, 1989.

153. Kremer S et al: Dynamic contrast-enhanced MRI: differentiating melanoma and renal carcinoma metastases from high-grade astrocytomas and other metastases, *Neuroradiology* 45(1):44, 2003.

154. Kuratsu J, Kochi M, Ushio Y: Incidence and clinical features of asymptomatic meningiomas, *J Neurosurg* 92(5):766, 2000.

155. Laatsch L et al: Incorporation of SPECT imaging in a longitudinal cognitive rehabilitation therapy programme, *Brain Inj* 13(8):555, 1999.

156. Lansberg MG et al: Comparison of diffusion-weighted MRI and CT in acute stroke, *Neurology* 54(8):1557, 2000.

157. Lanzino G et al: Intracranial dissecting aneurysm causing subarachnoid hemorrhage: the role of computerized tomographic angiography and magnetic resonance angiography, *Surg Neurol* 48(5):477, 1997.

158. Lasner TM, Raps EC: Clinical evaluation and management of aneurysmal subarachnoid hemorrhage, *Neuroimaging Clin North Am* 7(4):669, 1997.

159. Latchaw RE, Silva P, Falcone SF: The role of CT following aneurysmal rupture, *Neuroimag Clin North Am* 7(4):693, 1997.

160. Lazoff M et al: Encephalitis, *eMedicine* 2002, *http://www.emedicine.com/ped/topic3023.htm.*

161. Lazoff M et al: Multiple sclerosis, *eMedicine* 2001, *http://www.emedicine.com/ped/topic3023.htm.*

162. Le Bihan D et al: Diffusion tensor imaging: concepts and applications, *J MRI* 13(4):534, 2001.

163. Ledermann HP et al: Pitfalls and limitations of magnetic resonance imaging in chronic posttraumatic osteomyelitis, *Eur Radiol* 10(11):1815, 2000.

164. Lee M et al: Nonneoplastic intramedullary spinal cord lesions mimicking tumors, *Neurosurgery* 43:788, 1998.

165. Lee MA et al: defining multiple sclerosis disease activity by using MRI T2-weighted difference imaging, *Brain* 121:2095, 1998.

166. Lee S, Cho JY, Song MJ: Prenatal ultrasound findings of fetal neoplasms, *Korean J Radiol* 3(1):64, 2002.

167. Levy RA et al: Desmoplastic medulloblastoma: MR findings, *AJNR* 18(7):1364, 1997.

168. Levy RM: Brain abscess and subdural empyema, *Curr Opin Neurol* 3:223, 1994.

169. Liebeskind D et al: Epidural hematoma, *eMedicine* 2003, *http://www.emedicine.com/ped/topic3023.htm.*

170. Liedo A et al: Acute headache of recent onset and subarachnoid hemorrhage: A prospective study, *Headache* 34(4):172, 1994.

171. Link TM et al: Substantial head trauma: value of routine CT examination of the cervicocranium, *Radiology* 196:741, 1995.

172. Lipman SP et al: Fetal intracranial teratoma; US diagnosis of three cases and a review of the literature, *Radiology* 157:191, 1985.

173. Loughrey GJ et al: Magnetic resonance imaging in the management of suspected spinal canal disease in patients with known malignancy, *Clin Radiol* 55(11):849, 2000.

174. Lu S et al: Peritumoral diffusion tensor imaging of high-grade gliomas and metastatic brain tumors, *AJNR* 24(5):937, 2003.

175. Lubin E, Sullivan PR, DeAngelis LM: Brain tumors, *N Engl J Med* 344:1478, 2001.

176. Lutsep HL et al: Clinical utility of diffusion-weighted magnetic resonance imaging in the assessment of ischemic stroke, *Ann Neurol* 41(5):574, 1997.

177. Lycklama G et al: Spinal-cord MRI in multiple sclerosis, *Lancet Neurol* 2(9):555, 2003.

178. Mahaley MS Jr et al: National survey of patterns of care for brain-tumor patients, *J Neurosurg* 71:826, 1989.

179. Maiuri F et al: Intracranial meningiomas: correlations between MR imaging and histology, *Eur J Radiol* 31(1):69, 1999.

180. Maiuri F, Iaconetta G, Gallicchio B: Spondylodiscitis. Clinical and magnetic resonance diagnosis, *Spine* 22(15):1741, 1997.

181. Maldjian JA, Patel RS: Cerebral neoplasms in adults, *Neuroimaging Clin North Am* 11:547, 2001.

182. Mandell GL et al: Principles and practices of infectious diseases, ed 5, New York, 2000, Churchill Livingstone.

183. Manieri C, DiBisceglie D, Razzore P: Gonadotroph cell pituitary adenomas in males, *Panminerva Med* 42(4):237, 2000.

184. Martin CH, Schwartz R, Jolesz F: Transsphenoidal resection of pituitary adenomas in an intraoperative MRI unit, *Pituitary* 2(2):155, 1999.

185. Masson F, Thicoipe M, Aye P: Epidemiology of severe brain injuries: a prospective population-based study, *J Trauma* 51(3):481, 2001.

186. Mathisen GE, Johnson JP: Brain abscess, *Clin Infect Dis* 25:763, 1997.

187. Mautner VF et al: Malignant peripheral nerve sheath tumors in neurofibromatosis type 1: MRI supports the diagnosis of malignant plexiform neurofibroma, *Neuroradiology* 45(9):618, 2003.

188. Mayer PL et al: Misdiagnosis of symptomatic cerebral aneurysm: prevalence and correlation with outcome at four institutions, *Stroke* 27:1558, 1996.

189. McCormick WF: The pathology of vascular ("arteriovenous") malformations, *J Neurosurg* 24(4):807, 1966.

190. McCort JJ: Caring for the major trauma victim: the role for radiology, *Radiology* 163:1, 1987.

191. McDonald DR: Low-grade gliomas, mixed gliomas, and oligodendrogliomas, *Semin Oncol* 21(2):236, 1994.

192. McDonald JW, Sadowsky C: Spinal-cord injury, *Lancet* 359(9304):417, 2002.

193. McHenry MC, Easley KA, Locker GA: Vertebral osteomyelitis: long-term outcome for 253 patients from 7 Cleveland-area hospitals, *Clin Infect Dis* 34(10):1342, 2002.

194. McKendall RR, Sadiqu SA, Calverley JR: Unusual manifestations of Epstein-Barr virus encephalomyelitis, *Infection* 19:54, 1991.

195. Meadows J et al: Asymptomatic Chiari malformations identified on magnetic resonance imaging, *J Neurosurg* 2(6):920, 2000.

196. Michals EA, Ramsey RG: Syringomyelia, *Orthop Nurs* 15(5):33, 1996.

197. Milhorat TH et al: Intramedullary pressure in syringomyelia: clinical and pathophysiological correlates of syrinx distension, *Neurosurgery* 41(5):1102, 1997.

198. Milhorat TH et al: Chiari I malformation redefined: clinical and radiographic findings for 364 symptomatic patients, *Neurosurgery* 44(5):1005, 1999.

199. Mirvis SE et al: Traumatic aortic injury: diagnosis with contrast-enhanced thoracic CT-five-year experience at a major trauma center, *Radiology* 200:413, 1996.

200. Miyazawa N et al: MRI at 1.5 T of intramedullary ependymoma and classification of pattern of contrast enhancement, *Neuroradiology* 42(11):828, 2000.

201. Morales D et al: Brain, contusion, *eMedicine* 2003, *http://www.emedicine.com/ped/topic3023.htm.*

202. Mulinda JR et al: Pituitary macroadenoma, *eMedicine* 2003, *http://www.emedicine.com/ped/topic3023.htm.*

203. Murray K, Kun L, Cox J: Primary malignant lymphoma of the central nervous system, *J Neurosurg* 65:600, 1986.

204. Murtagh R, Linden C: Neuroimaging of intracranial meningiomas, *Neurosurg Clin North Am* 5(2):217, 1994.

205. Nadalo LA et al: Brain abscess, *eMedicine* 2003, *http://www.emedicine.com/ped/topic3023.htm.*

206. Nakasu S, Nakasu Y, Nakajima M: Preoperative identification of meningiomas that are highly likely to recur, *J Neurosurg* 90(3):455, 1999.

207. Nathoo N, Nadvi SS, van Dellen JR: Cranial extradural empyema in the era of computed tomography: a review of 82 cases, *Neurosurgery* 44(4):748, 1999.

208. Newman LS, Rose CS, Maier LA: Sarcoidosis, *N Engl J Med* 336:1224, 1997.

209. Newton T et al: Subarachnoid hemorrhage, *eMedicine* 2002, *http://www.emedicine.com/ped/topic3023.htm.*

210. Nguyen Bui L et al: Magnetic resonance angiography of cervicocranial dissection, *Stroke* 24(1):126, 1993.

211. Nishikawa M et al: Pathogenesis of Chiari malformation: a morphometric study of the posterior cranial fossa, *J Neurosurg* 86(1):40, 1997.

212. Noguchi K et al: Acute subarachnoid hemorrhage: MR imaging with fluid-attenuated inversion recovery pulse sequences, *Radiology* 196:773, 1995.

213. Nolla JM, Ariza J, Gomez-Vaquero C: Spontaneous pyogenic vertebral osteomyelitis in nondrug users, *Semin Arthritis Rheum* 31(4):271, 2002.

214. Noseworthy JH et al: Multiple sclerosis, *N Engl J Med* 343(13):938, 2000.

215. Nowak DA, Widenka DC: Neurosarcoidosis: a review of its intracranial manifestation, *J Neurol* 248(5):363, 2001.

216. Ogawa T et al: Comparative study of magnetic resonance and CT scan imaging of cases of severe head injury, *Acta Neurochir Suppl (Wien)* 55:8, 1992.

217. Olek MJ: Multiple sclerosis, *Best Pract Med* 2002.

218. Osborne AG: Diagnostic neuroradiology, St Louis, 1994, Mosby.

219. Pahapill PA, Lownie SP: Conservative treatment of acute spontaneous spinal epidural hematoma, *Can J Neurol Sci* 25(2):159, 1998.

220. Patchell RA, Posner JB: Neurologic complications of systemic cancer, *Neurol Clin* 3:729, 1985.

221. Pattison J: Cavernous angiomas of the brain, *Eurorad Online* 2002.

222. Perrin RG: Metastatic tumors of the axial spine, *Curr Opin Oncol* 4(3):525, 1992.

223. Pletcher BA et al: Neurofibromatosis, type 2, *eMedicine* 2002, *http://www.emedicine.com/ped/topic3023.htm.*

224. Prelog K, Blome S, Dennis C: Neurosarcoidosis of the conus medullaris and cauda equina, *Austral Radiol* 47(3):295, 2003.

225. Pruitt AA: Infections of the nervous system, *Neurol Clin* 16:2, 1998.

226. Quencer RM, Post MJ, Hinks RS: Cine MR in the evaluation of normal and abnormal CSF flow: intracranial and intraspinal studies, *Neuroradiology* 32(5):371, 1990.

227. Ramsey RG: Neuroradiology, Philadelphia, 1994, WB Saunders.

228. Rana S et al: Diffusion-weighted imaging and apparent diffusion coefficient maps in a case of intracerebral abscess with ventricular extension, *AJNR* 23(1):109, 2002.

229. Rhea JT, Rao PM, Novelline RA: Helical CT and three-dimensional CT of facial and orbital injury, *Radiol Clin North Am* 37:489, 1999.

230. Rivas JJ et al: Extradural hematoma: analysis of factors influencing the courses of 161 patients, *Neurosurgery* 23(1):44, 1988.

231. Roberta L, DeBiasi RL, Tyler KL: Polymerase chain reaction in the diagnosis and management of central nervous system infections, *Arch Neurol* 56:1215, 1999.

232. Robinson JR, Awad IA, Little JR: Natural history of the cavernous angiomas, *J Neurosurg* 75(5):709, 1991.

233. Rollins N et al: Idiopathic ischemic cerebral infarction in childhood: depiction of arterial abnormalities by MR angiography and catheter angiography, *AJNR* 21:549, 2000.

234. Rommer B et al: Transcranial Doppler sonography, angiography and SPECT measurement in traumatic carotid artery dissection, *Acta Neurol* 126:185, 1994.

235. Roos KL: Encephalitis, *Neurol Clin* 17(4):813, 1999.

236. Rordorf G et al: Diffusion- and perfusion-weighted imaging in vasospasm after subarachnoid hemorrhage, *Stroke* 30(3): 599, 1999.

237. Rosenblum ML, Joff JT, Norman D: Decreased mortality from brain abscesses since advent of computerized tomography, *J Neurosurg* 49:658, 1978.

238. Roux FE et al: Methodological and technical issues for integrating functional magnetic resonance imaging data in a neuronavigational system, *Neurosurgery* 49(5):1145, 2001.

239. Rumack CM, Wilson SR, Charboneau WJ: Diagnostic ultrasound, ed 2, Philadelphia, 1998, Mosby.

240. Rutka JT: Medulloblastoma, *Clin Neurosurg* 44:571, 1997.

241. Sakamoto Y et al: Normal and abnormal pituitary glands: gadopentetate dimeglumine enhanced MR imaging, *Radiology* 178:441, 1997.

242. Sakata K et al: Supratentorial astrocytomas and oligodendrogliomas treated in the MRI era, *Jpn J Clin Oncol* 31(6): 240, 2001.

243. Sames TA et al: Sensitivity of new-generation computed tomography in subarachnoid hemorrhage, *Acad Emerg Med* 3(1):16, 1996.

244. Sanford RA, Gajjar A: Ependymomas, *Clin Neurosurg* 44:559, 1997.

245. Sanford RA, Mulhbauer MS: Craniopharyngioma in children, *Neurol Clin* 9:453, 1991.

246. Santiago Restrepo C, Gimenez CR, McCarthy K: Imaging of osteomyelitis and musculoskeletal soft tissue infections: current concepts, *Rheum Dis Clin North Am* 29(1):89, 2003.

247. Saremi F et al: Syringohydromyelia, *eMedicine* 2003, *http://www.emedicine.com/ped/topic3023.htm.*

248. Sawin PD, Loftus CM: Diagnosis of spontaneous subarachnoid hemorrhage, *Am Fam Phys* 55(1):145, 1997.

249. Scaletta T et al: Subdural hematoma, *eMedicine* 2002, *http://www.emedicine.com/ped/topic3023.htm.*

250. Schellinger PD et al: Stroke MRI in intracerebral hemorrhage: is there a perihemorrhagic penumbra? *Stroke* 34:1674, 2003.

251. Schellinger PD et al: A standardized MRI stroke protocol: comparison with CT in hyperacute intracerebral hemorrhage, *Stroke* 30:765, 1999.

252. Schievink WI: Intracranial aneurysms, *N Engl J Med* 336(1):28, 1997.

253. Schiffbauer H et al: Functional activity within brain tumors: a magnetic source imaging study, *Neurosurgery* 49(6):1313, 2001.

254. Schwartz ED et al: Posttraumatic syringomyelia: pathogenesis, imaging, and treatment, *AJR Am J Roentgenol* 173(2):487, 1999.

255. Scott AM et al: Clinical applications of fusion imaging in oncology, *Nucl Med Biol* 21(5):775, 1994.

256. Scott TF: Neurosarcoidosis: progress and clinical aspects, *Neurology* 43:8, 1993.

257. Seong WC et al: In-vivo proton magnetic resonance spectroscopy in adnexal lesions, *Korean J Radiol* 3(2):105, 2002.

258. Servadei F: Prognostic factors in severely head injured adult patients with epidural haematomas, *Acta Neurochir (Wien)* 139(4):273, 1997.

259. Sganzerla EP, Tomei G, Rampini P: A peculiar intracerebral hemorrhage: the gliding contusion, its relationship to diffuse brain damage, *Neurosurg Rev* 12(Suppl 1):215, 1989.

260. Shahzadi S, Lozano AM, Bernstein M: Stereotactic management of bacterial brain abscesses, *Can J Neurol Sci* 23:34, 1996.

261. Sheikh B, Siqueira E: Primary lymphoma of the central nervous system, *Br J Neurosurg* 8(4):427, 1994.

262. Shih TT, Huang KM, Hou SM: Early diagnosis of single segment vertebral osteomyelitis: MR pattern and its characteristics, *Clin Imag* 23(3):159, 1999.

263. Shukla PC et al: Intracranial epidural abscess, *eMedicine* 2002, *http://www.emedicine.com/ped/topic3023.htm*.

264. Siddiqi NH: Chiari I malformation, *eMedicine* 2002, *http://www.emedicine.com/ped/topic3023.htm*.

265. Sidman R, Connolly E, Lemke T: Subarachnoid hemorrhage diagnosis: lumbar puncture is still needed when the computed tomography scan is normal, *Acad Emerg Med* 3(9):827, 1996.

266. Skjodt K, Loft Edal A, Nepper-Rasmussen HJ: Rathke's cleft cyst. Two cases with uncommon MR signals, *Acta Radiol* 37(4):596, 1996.

267. Sklar EM et al: Magnetic resonance applications in cerebral injury, *Radiol Clin North Am* 30:353, 1992.

268. Sloan MA et al: Sensitivity and specificity of transcranial Doppler ultrasonography in the diagnosis of vasospasm following subarachnoid hemorrhage, *Neurology* 39:1514, 1989.

269. Smith JK, Matheus MG, Castillo M: Imaging manifestations of neurosarcoidosis, *AJR Am J Roentgenol* 182(2):289, 2004.

270. Smith M et al: Intracranial arteriovenous malformation, *eMedicine* 2002, *http://www.emedicine.com/ped/topic3023.htm*.

271. Snyder H, Robinson K, Shah D: Signs and symptoms of patients with brain tumors presenting to the emergency department, *J Emerg Med* 11(3):253, 1993.

272. Soong JC et al: FLAIR should be more sensitive than CT for the detection of acute subarachnoid hemorrhage, *Radiology* 209:471, 1998.

273. Sorensen SA, Mulvihill JJ, Nielsen A: Long-term follow-up of von Recklinghausen's neurofibromatosis. Survival and malignant neoplasms, *N Engl J Med* 314(16):1010, 1986.

274. Srinivasan J, Newell DW, Sturzenegger M: Transcranial Doppler in the evaluation of internal carotid artery dissection, *Stroke* 27(7):1226, 1996.

275. Stark DD, Bradley WG: Magnetic resonance imaging, ed 2, St Louis, 1999, Mosby.

276. Strandness ED: Duplex scanning in vascular disorders, Philadelphia, 2002, Lippincott Williams & Wilkins.

277. Stull MA et al: Magnetic resonance appearance of peripheral nerve sheath tumors, *Skeletal Radiol* 20(1):9, 1991.

278. Sturzenegger M, Mattle H, Rivoir A: Ultrasound findings in carotid artery dissection: analysis of 43 patients, *Neurology* 45:691, 1995.

279. Su TM et al: Streptococcal brain abscess: analysis of clinical features in 20 patients, *Surg Neurol* 56(3):189, 2001.

280. Sugahara T et al: Usefulness of diffusion-weighted MRI with echo-planar technique in the evaluation of cellularity in gliomas, *J MRI* 9:53, 1999.

281. Sun B et al: MRI features of intramedullary spinal cord ependymomas, *J Neuroimag* 13(4):346, 2003.

282. Sze G, Ziaema RD: Magnetic resonance imaging of infections and inflammatory diseases, *Radiol Clin North Am* 26:839, 1988.

283. Tamaki N, Nagashima T: Hemodynamics of syringomyelia, *Rinsho Shinkeigaku* 35(12):1398, 1995.

284. Teasdale G, Jennett B: Assessment of coma and impaired consciousness: a practical scale, *Lancet* 2:81, 1984.

285. Tehranzadeh J, Wang F, Mesgarzadeh M: Magnetic resonance imaging of osteomyelitis, *Crit Rev Diagn Imag* 33(6):495, 1992.

286. Teixeira J et al: Diffusion imaging in pediatric central nervous system infections, *Neuroradiology* 43(12):1031, 2001.

287. Thompson AJ et al: Primary progressive MS, *Brain* 120:1085, 1997.

288. Tiamkao S et al: Syringomyelia as a complication of tuberculous meningitis, *J Med Assoc Thai* 84(1):125, 2001.

289. Tien RD et al: MR imaging of high-grade cerebral gliomas: value of diffusion-weighted echoplanar pulse sequences, *AJR Am J Roentgenol* 162(3):671, 1994.

290. Tse V et al: Metastatic disease to the spine and related structures, *eMedicine* 2003, *http://www.emedicine.com/ped/topic3023.htm*.

291. Tung GA, Evangelista P: Is markedly decreased water diffusion specific for brain abscess? *AJR Am J Roentgenol* 177:709, 2001.

292. Tunkel AR: Brain abscess, *Curr Treatment Options Infect Dis* 2:449, 2000.

293. Turpin S, Lambert R: Role of scintigraphy in musculoskeletal and spinal infections, *Radiol Clin North Am* 39(2):169, 2001.

294. Urresta FL, Medina DA, Gaviria M: Diffusion MRI studies in vascular cognitive impairment and dementia, *Rev Bras Psiquiatr* 25:3, 2003.

295. Valadka AB, Narayan RK: Injury to the cranium, *Trauma* 3:267, 1996.

296. Van der Wee N et al: Detection of subarachnoid haemorrhage on early CT: is lumbar puncture still needed after negative scan? *J Neurol Neurosurg Psychiatry* 58:357, 1995.

297. Van Tassel P, Cure JK: Nonneoplastic intracranial cysts and cystic lesions, *Semin Ultrasound CT MR* 16(3):186, 1995.

298. Verstraete KL et al: Nerve sheath tumors: evaluation with CT and MR imaging, *J Belge Radiol* 75(4):311, 1992.

299. Vinas FC et al: Spinal infections, *eMedicine* 2003, *http://www.emedicine.com/ped/topic3023.htm*.

300. Voyadzis JM, Bhargava P, Henderson FC: Tarlov cysts: a study of 10 cases with review of the literature, *J Neurosurg* 95(1 Suppl):25, 2001.

301. Walker AE, Robins M, Weinfeld FD: Epidemiology of brain tumors: the national survey of intracranial neoplasms, *Neurology* 35:219, 1985.

302. Wasserman JR et al: Craniopharyngioma, *eMedicine* 2001, *http://www.emedicine.com/ped/topic3023.htm*.

303. Waubant E et al: MRI of intramedullary sarcoidosis: follow-up of a case, *Neuroradiology* 39:357, 1997.

304. Waxweiler RJ et al: Monitoring the impact of traumatic brain injury: a review and update, *J Neurotrauma* 12:509, 1995.

305. Weaver JP, Fisher M: Subarachnoid hemorrhage: an update of pathogenesis, diagnosis and management, *J Neurol Sci* 125(2):119, 1994.

306. Weingarten K et al: Subdural and epidural empyemas: MR imaging, *AJR Am J Roentgenol* 152(3):615, 1989.

307. Weinshenker BG: The natural history of multiple sclerosis, *Neurol Clin* 13:119, 1995.

308. Whelan MA, Hilal SK: Computed tomography as a guide in the diagnosis and follow-up of brain abscesses, *Radiology* 135(3):663, 1980.

309. Whitley RJ, Gnann JW: Viral encephalitis: familiar infections and emerging pathogens, *Lancet* 359:507, 2002.

310. Whitley RJ et al: Herpes simplex encephalitis. Clinical assessment, *JAMA* 247:317, 1982.

311. Wilberger JE: Contemporary treatment paradigms in head injury, *Clin Neurosurg* 46:143, 2000.

312. Winchell RJ, Hoyt DB, Simons RK: Use of computed tomography of the head in the hypotensive blunt-trauma patient, *Ann Emerg Med* 25:737, 1995.

313. Wingos PA, Tong T, Bolden S: Cancer statistics 1995, *CA Cancer J Clin* 45:8, 1995.

314. Wuerfel J et al: Changes in cerebral perfusion precede plaque formation in multiple sclerosis: a longitudinal perfusion MRI study, *Brain* 127:111, 2004.

315. Yadavalli GK et al: Epidural abscess, *eMedicine* 2002, *http://www.emedicine.com/ped/topic3023.htm.*

316. Yamada I, Suzuki S, Matsushima Y: Moyamoya disease: comparison of assessment with MR angiography and MR imaging versus conventional angiography, *Radiology* 196:211, 1995.

317. Yoneda Y et al: Diffusion-weighted magnetic resonance imaging: detection of ischemic injury 39 minutes after onset in a stroke patient, *Ann Neurol* 45(6):794, 1999.

318. Yuh WTC et al: Sequential MR enhancement patterns in normal pituitary gland and in pituitary adenoma, *AJNR* 15:101, 1994.

319. Zajicek JP et al: Central nervous system sarcoidosis—diagnosis and management, *QJM* 92(2):103, 1999.

320. Zhang YQ, Wang CC, Ma ZY: Pediatric craniopharyngiomas: clinicomorphological study of 189 cases, *Pediatr Neurosurg,* 36(2):80, 2002.

321. Zimmerman RA, Gibby WA, Carmody RF: Neuroimaging: clinical and physical principles, New York, 2001, Springer-Verlag.

322. Zimmerman RD et al: Magnetic resonance imaging of meningiomas, *AJNR* 6(2):149, 1985.

323. Zink BJ: Traumatic brain injury, *Emerg Med Clin North Am* 14(1):115, 1996.

Glossary

a-, an- a prefix meaning without or lack of.

ab-, abs- a prefix meaning away, departure, or draw away from (e.g., away from the median axis of the body).

abscess a circumscribed collection of pus that results from acute or chronic localized infection secondary to tissue necrosis.

acanthion the center point at the base of the anterior nasal spine.

accessory supplementary, auxiliary, or additional to some major structure.

acid phosphatase an enzyme that is found in many tissues, including the liver, bone marrow, red blood cells, and most notably the prostate gland. It is most useful clinically to diagnose prostatic carcinoma and monitor the effectiveness of treatments for this disease. Levels increase as the carcinoma metastasizes beyond the prostate capsule. Normal levels in the adult patient are 0.11 to 0.6 U/L.

acute sudden, brief, short-term onset; running a short, often severe course.

ad- a prefix meaning toward (e.g., toward the median axis of the body).

adenocarcinoma any one of a large group of malignant epithelial cell tumors of glands or glandlike tissues.

ALARA principle the use of ionizing radiation in diagnostic imaging should be as low as reasonably achievable.

aliasing artifact an artifact in magnetic resonance images caused by inadequate sampling. It most often occurs when the field of view is smaller than the part being imaged, and protons outside the field of view are excited. The artifact appears to be a portion of the anatomy outside the field of view being folded into the image (e.g., wraparound).

alkaline phosphatase a nearly ubiquitous enzyme found in highest concentrations in the kidneys, liver, intestine, teeth, and bone. Levels are elevated in patients who have liver and bone abnormalities. Normal levels in the adult are 42 to 128 U/L.

Andersson lesion an irregularly shaped vertebral endplate found in patients who have ankylosing spondylitis who have sustained fractures of ankylosed segments and resultant intersegmental hypermobility.

anemia any condition in which the hemoglobin in 100 ml of blood, number of red blood cells per cubic millimeter of blood, and volume of packed red blood cells per 100 ml of blood are less than normal. Anemia results from blood loss, decreased red blood cell production, or increased red blood cell destruction. Clinical manifestations include pallor of the skin and mucous membranes, shortness of breath, exertional dyspnea, dizziness, palpitations, headaches, soft systolic murmurs, and lethargy.

angiography radiography of the heart, arteries (arteriogram), or veins (venogram) using a radiopaque contrast agent.

ankylosis an abnormal bony or fibrous union across a joint; joint immobility.

anomaly a deviation from average or normal; usually pertains to a structure.

apophysis a nonpathologic outgrowth or projection, usually of bone; commonly functions as an attachment site for ligaments and tendons on nonarticular bone surfaces. It does not contribute to bone length.

arachnodactyly a congenital condition characterized by long, slender, spiderlike fingers and, in some cases, toes; characteristic of Marfan's syndrome.

Arnold-Chiari malformation congenital inferior displacement of the brainstem and lower cerebellum through the foramen magnum into the cervical vertebral canal. The defect may be associated with spina bifida and meningoceles in the upper cervical spine and lower occiput. The degree of displacement and associated defects are staged together into four types (type I–IV).

arteriosclerosis hardening of the arteries. Three types are generally recognized: atherosclerosis, Mönckeberg's arteriosclerosis, and arteriolosclerosis.

arthritis mutilans a form of advanced, severe, and destructive arthritis marked by osteolysis and pronounced changes of the joint's surfaces; usually develops in the hands and feet of patients who have chronic rheumatoid arthritis.

arthrodesis surgical stiffening or fixation of a joint.

arthrography radiography in which the introduction of air or contrast medium into a joint is used to enhance visibility of the joint's anatomy.

asterion defect a radiolucent defect of the skull found adjacent to the lambdoidal suture and just posterior to the parietomastoid and occipitomastoid sutures.

atrophy a wasting, or diminution in size, of tissues, organs, or the entire body.

axial (transverse) plane the plane located at right angles to both the sagittal and coronal planes. The axial plane divides a standing patient into upper and lower sections.

Baastrup (kissing spines) syndrome a syndrome characterized by sclerosis and interspinous pseudoarthrosis caused by approximation of spinous processes; often develops in patients who have excessive lordosis.

Baker's cyst a large collection of synovial fluid in a synovial-lined sac, which extends into the popliteal space between the medial gastrocnemius tendon and semimembranosus tendon; associated with rheumatoid arthritis.

balanitis xerotica obliterans a chronic skin disease characterized by inflammation of the glans penis and white indurated area around the meatus.

balanorrhagia a condition characterized by inflammation of the glans penis and discharge of a large amount of pus from the penis.

1405

bamboo spine (poker spine) a term used to describe the appearance of syndesmophytes and ankylosis of multiple contiguous vertebrae in patients who have ankylosing spondylitis.

Bankart lesion avulsion of a fragment of cartilage or bone from the anterior glenoid rim. Bankart lesions are associated with recurrent anterior shoulder dislocations.

bare area a region of intraarticular bone that is not covered by articular cartilage or a joint capsule; a common nidus for rheumatoid arthritis bone involvement.

bare orbit a region that develops as a result of agenesis or hypoplasia of the posterior wall of the orbit; develops in patients who have neurofibromatosis.

barium (Ba) a chemical element with an atomic weight of 137.327 and atomic number of 56; belongs to the alkaline earth metals. Barium sulfate ($BaSO_4$) is used as a contrast medium in radiography because of its high radiopacity.

barium enema a rectal infusion of barium sulfate; a radiopaque contrast medium used for imaging studies of the gastrointestinal tract.

barium meal ingestion of barium sulfate, a radiopaque contrast medium used for imaging studies of the gastrointestinal tract.

basion the midpoint on anterior margin of the foramen magnum of the occipital bone, opposite the opisthion.

Bence Jones proteins lightweight, unusually thermosoluble immunoglobulins that are made by the plasma cells of patients who have multiple myelomas. They are rapidly filtered from the blood by the kidneys; therefore they are best detected in the urine. Normally no Bence Jones proteins are present in urine.

benign mild in character (e.g., a mild illness); nonmalignant (e.g., a nonmalignant tumor).

berry aneurysm a small (usually <2 cm in diameter) saccular aneurysm resembling a berry; most often develops at vessel junctions of the circle of Willis. Frequent rupture leads to subarachnoid hemorrhage.

blade-of-grass (candle flame) sign V-shaped radiolucent defect caused by the osteolytic progression of Paget's disease moving through the tibia.

Bo the symbol used to designate the main magnetic field of a magnetic resonance imaging system; expressed in tesla (T).

bolus a round mass, especially one of masticated food; a dose of intravenous medication delivered all at once.

bone window a computed tomographic image at a window level and width that emphasize bone anatomy and make it easy to distinguish between cortical and cancellous bone. Soft tissues appear dark gray.

Boston brace a brace worn over the lower trunk used to decrease lordosis and increase pelvic flexion. The brace is worn by individuals with spondylolisthesis who still want to maintain motion.

boutonnière deformity also called the buttonhole defect; proximal interphalangeal joint flexion and concurrent distal interphalangeal joint hyperextension; a result of rupture of the extensor hood at the proximal interphalangeal joint—proximal phalanx head protrudes through the resulting defect.

bowline of Brailsford (inverted Napoleon's hat sign, Gendarme's cap) the inferiorly bowed radiodense line created by the anterior vertebral body of L5 on a frontal radiographic projection of a patient with spondylolisthesis.

brim sign cortical thickening along the pelvic brim or iliopectineal line secondary to Paget's disease.

brown tumor (osteoclastoma) a mass of fibrous tissue containing hemosiderin-pigmented macrophages and multinucleated giant cells that develop in patients who have hyperparathyroidism and replace bone; appear as small, slightly expansile, radiolucent lesions mimicking a destructive process.

Bucky the moveable housing of the film and grid used in plain film radiography.

buffalo hump an accumulation of fat seen posteriorly above the upper thoracic vertebrae; associated with Cushing's disease or prolonged use of glucosteroids.

Bywater-Dixon syndesmophyte a nonmarginal, incompletely bridging syndesmophyte that does not appear to attach to either a superior or inferior vertebra; develops in some patients who have Reiter's syndrome or psoriatic arthritis.

cachexia a physical state characterized by weight loss, emaciation, and weakness; caused by malnutrition or the poor health associated with serious illnesses.

café-au-lait spots light to dark brown cutaneous hyperpigmentations that develop normally or are cutaneous manifestations of neurofibromatosis and fibrous dysplasia.

calcitonin a peptide hormone that is an antagonist to parathormone (PTH); increases calcium and phosphate deposition in bone and lowers serum calcium levels by reversing parathormone effects on bone, the kidneys, and the intestine.

calculus a concretion formed in any part of the body; usually composed of the salts of inorganic or organic acids or of cholesterol; often found in the biliary and urinary tracts.

cancer a general term indicating the presence of a malignant growth or tumor, especially a carcinoma.

canthus angle of the eye; point at which the eyelids meet.

Caplan syndrome intrapulmonary nodules that develop in coal workers who have pneumoconiosis with rheumatoid arthritis.

carcinoma any one of the various types of malignant tumors originating from epithelial tissue.

cardiac gating a process used to reduce the number of cardiac-cycle–related motion artifacts on magnetic resonance imaging scans. The patient's heart rate is synchronized to the magnetic resonance imaging signal acquisition.

central ray the center of the x-ray beam, which is approximated by the cross marks of the light localizer.

centric pertaining to the center.

Charcot's joint the classic term for a joint with neuropathic joint disease, especially when the disease is caused by tabes dorsalis (tabetic neurosyphilis).

chemical shift artifact an artifact on magnetic resonance imaging scans that is found at fat–water tissue interfaces along the frequency encoding the axis; develops because of the similar Larmor frequencies of fat and water tissues.

Chopart's (transverse tarsal) joint the synovial joint between the talus and navicular bones medially and the calcaneus and navicular bones laterally.

chronic continuing for a prolonged period of time; long-term, protracted course of disease, often of low intensity.

cicatrix scar; contracted fibrous tissue.

Clutton's joint a joint, especially the knee, with bilateral arthrosis secondary to syphilis.

coalition a fibrous or osseous union between two or more bones.

codfish vertebra an exaggerated biconcave endplate deformity associated with advanced osteopenia.

Codman's sign, triangle, angle (periosteal cuff) a subperiosteal extension of a lesion causing subperiosteal new bone growth and elevation of the free margin of the disrupted periosteum at the interface of normal bone and a growing bone tumor.

cold spots (photopenia) a term used in scintigraphy to describe areas of decreased gamma emission caused by a lack of radioisotope absorption.

collimator an apparatus placed on the front of the x-ray tube to limit the field of exposure.

complete blood count (CBC) the number of red and white blood cells per cubic millimeter of blood.

concretion the aggregation or formation of a solid, stony mass by succeeding layers of mineral salts surrounding a foreign body.

coniosis a disease or morbid condition caused by dust.

consolidation a disease process marked by solidification of a normally porous tissue into a firm, dense mass; often applied to lung tissue infections.

contralateral related to the opposite side.

core decompression a surgical procedure used to treat avascular necrosis of the femoral head. A core of bone marrow is removed to reduce intraosseous pressure and facilitate revascularization of the head.

coronal plane the vertical plane located at right angles to the sagittal plane. The coronal plane divides a standing patient into front and back sections.

cotton's-wool skull an osteosclerotic skull with fuzzy, poorly defined edges that develop during the osteoblastic phase of Paget's disease.

coxa the hip or hip joint.

craniosynostosis premature skull ossification and suture fusion.

C-reactive protein (CRP) test a nonspecific test that detects acute inflammatory conditions such as bacterial infections or rheumatoid arthritis. The test is sensitive but not specific. It is thought to be more sensitive and responsive than the erythrocyte sedimentation rate (ESR).

crepitus crackling, fine bubbling sound produced by bone or irregular cartilage surfaces rubbing together.

dagger sign the appearance of ossified interspinous and supraspinatus ligaments in the midline of the lumbar radiograph of some patients who have ankylosing spondylitis.

deciduous temporary; that which falls off or is shed.

decubitus lying down.

dextro- a prefix meaning right.

diploë the central layer of cancellous osseous tissue in the space between the inner and outer tables of the skull.

dissecting aneurysm splitting or dissection of an arterial wall by a localized extravasation of blood from the true lumen of the vessel—longitudinal dissection between the outer and middle layers of the vessel creates a second lumen (double barrel lumen); most often occurs in the aorta and often ruptures through the outer wall.

distal away from (e.g., away from the body or the origin or beginning of some part of the body).

diverticulitis inflammation of a diverticulum.

diverticulosis the presence of multiple diverticula (abnormal).

diverticulum a blind sac or pouch extending from a main cavity or lumen.

dolicho- a prefix meaning long.

dolichostenomelia long, narrow limbs characteristic of patients who have Marfan's syndrome.

dorsal the back (e.g., the back of the body or a structure); opposite of ventral.

dys- a prefix meaning difficult or painful, abnormal or impairment; opposite of eu-.

dysplasia abnormal development of an organ or tissue.

dyspnea difficult or impaired breathing.

dysraphism incomplete closure of a raphe; dorsal fusion defect of the neural tube.

dysuria difficult or painful urination.

eburnation (subchondral sclerosis) increased radiodensity of the subarticular bone; caused by degeneration and increased mechanical forces applied to the bone that make it dense and smooth like ivory.

ec- a prefix meaning out or outside of.

eccentric off center, away from midline; opposite of concentric.

echo time (TE) one half the time interval between successive 90- and 180-degree pulses in a spin-echo magnetic resonance imaging sequence—the primary determinant of differences in contrast of T2-weighted images.

ecto- a prefix meaning outside, external, or without.

-ectomy a suffix meaning surgical removal.

edema abnormal accumulation of fluid in tissues or body spaces.

effusion escape of fluid from vessels into tissues or body spaces.

elephantiasis a chronic condition in which the affected body part becomes enlarged and overlying skin thickens, resembling an elephant's hide.

elephantiasis neuromatosa a large soft-tissue mass that causes the overlying skin to appear undulated; seen in patients who have neurofibromatosis.

em-, en- a prefix meaning in or enclosed by.

emaciation a wasted appearance associated with a chronic disease state.

embolism obstruction of a blood vessel by an embolus.

embolus a detached thrombus, air bubble, fatty fragment, or other obstructive plug that is carried by the bloodstream and lodges in small vessels.

emphysema a lung condition characterized by increased air space size distal to the terminal bronchiole, with destructive changes in the alveolar walls and reduction in the number.

empty vertebra a horizontal radiolucent lumbar vertebra defect seen on frontal radiographic projections; results from a horizontal fracture through both pedicles and transverse processes.

empyema accumulation of pus in a body cavity.

endo- a prefix meaning within.

endoscopy examination of the interior of a canal or hollow viscus with a fiberoptic scope.

enteritis inflammation of the intestines, especially the small intestines.

enthesis the insertion site of tendons and ligaments into bone, specifically the zone in which tendon and ligament fibers blend with the periosteum of bone.

enthesopathy a disease process occurring at the insertion site of tendons and ligaments into bones.

epi-, ep- a prefix meaning on, upon, over, or on the outside of.

epidural hematoma an intracranial hemorrhage that results in a collection of blood outside the dura mater of the brain and spinal cord.

epiphysial plate the cartilage plate between the metaphysis and the epiphysis of an immature bone; the site of lengthening bone growth.

epiphysis the end of a bone; develops from a center of ossification distinct from that of the bone's shaft; develops before mature bone is separated from the shaft by a cartilage plate.

Erlenmeyer flask deformity a splayed deformity caused by failure of metaphyseal modeling.

erythema an abnormal state of skin redness associated with inflammation and vasodilatation.

erythrocyte sedimentation rate (ESR) test a nonspecific test for inflammatory, neoplastic, necrotic, or infectious diseases. The test measures the amount (millimeters) of red blood cells that settle in saline in 1 hour. The C-reactive protein test may be helpful if the ESR test results are equivocal.

etiology the science of causation.

eu- a prefix meaning well or normal; opposite of dys-.

eventration protrusion of the intestine or omentum from the abdomen.

eventration of the diaphragm elevation of half or part of the diaphragm. The elevated portion is usually atrophic, abnormally thin, or poorly innervated.

evert to turn outward.

ex- a prefix meaning out, out of, or away from; outside of.

exostosis a cartilage-capped bony outgrowth from a bone.

extravasation the escape of material from a space or compartment into surrounding tissues.

exudate any proteinaceous fluid that has exuded from injured or inflamed tissues or vessels.

fabella a sesamoid bone within the tendon of the lateral head of the gastrocnemius.

facet tropism a condition in which the zygapophyseal joint planes of the spine are oriented asymmetrically; one joint plane is sagittal and the other is coronal.

Faraday shield an electrical conductor such as copper mesh or an aluminum sheet that is used to block out electromagnetic radiation. Most magnetic resonance imaging rooms are surrounded by a Faraday shield to keep extraneous radio waves from entering the room.

Felty syndrome rheumatoid arthritis with leukopenia and splenomegaly.

fibroma a benign fibrous neoplasm.

fibroma molluscum multiple, soft, nonpainful, cutaneous nodules; the cutaneous manifestation of neurofibromatosis.

fibrosis the proliferation of fibrous material in any organ or tissue.

field of view the anatomy contained within the area imaged.

fissure a narrow cleft, furrow, or slit.

fistula an abnormal passage leading from one hollow organ to another.

flaccid without firmness or tone.

FLASH fast low angle shot; magnetic resonance imaging gradient echo protocol in which a short repetition and echo time with a flip angle of less than 90 degrees are used. As the flip angle moves toward 0 degrees, the resulting image appears more T2 weighted. The gradient echo protocol is a way to quickly obtain images that appear T2 weighted. Gradient images also show joints well, but their major disadvantage is that they do not show bone marrow well.

flip angle the angle of hydrogen atom deflection resulting from the atoms' equilibrium orientation after an applied radiofrequency pulse.

flocculent the appearance of fluid containing soft flakes or shreds that resemble tufts of cotton's or wool.

focal giantism enlargement of the skin and underlying bone; seen in patients who have neurofibromatosis.

focal plane the plane of tissue in maximum focus on a tomogram.

focal plane level the distance from the tabletop to the focal plane.

fossa a pit, cavity, or depression; usually longitudinal in shape.

fovea a pit or cup-shaped depression.

frog-leg projection a frontal projection of the hip in which the femur is flexed and externally rotated.

functional scoliosis a nonstructural lateral curvature that is compensatory or positional.

fusiform aneurysm an elongated, spindle-shaped, progressive dilation of a vessel.

gadolinium (Gd) a rare earth metallic element with an atomic number of 64 and an atomic weight of 157.25. Its paramagnetic properties make it a widely used contrast medium in magnetic resonance imaging.

gallium-67 (^{67}Ga) citrate a cyclotron-produced radionuclide (the ^{67}Ga citrate salt) used as a radiotracer to localize tumor and inflammation.

gamma camera a scintigraphic camera that uses gamma emissions emanating from the patient to produce an image.

gangrene tissue necrosis caused by an insufficient blood supply to an organ or tissue.

Gardner syndrome a syndrome characterized by a triad comprising multiple osteomas, colonic polyposis, and soft-tissue fibromas.

Garré's osteomyelitis a chronic, low-grade form of osteomyelitis that appears densely sclerotic and is associated with proliferative periostitis.

gavage feeding by a stomach tube.

geode a large, subarticular, degenerative cyst.

giant bone island a bone island greater than 1 cm in diameter.

gibbus an acute or sharply angled kyphosis.

glioma a malignant tumor in the supporting or connective tissues of the central nervous system.

gradient echo sequence any one of a number of magnetic resonance imaging pulse sequences that lack the 180-degree radiofrequency refocusing pulse used in the more commonly used spin-echo sequence. Examples include fast field echo (FFE), fast imaging with steady-state precession (FISP), and gradient recalled acquisition in the steady state (GRASS).

gradient magnetic coils coils used to produce a magnetic field gradient that allows "slicing" of the patient's anatomy into sagittal, coronal, or transverse planes. During the examination, these coils switch on and off rapidly, which produces the characteristic and sometimes quite loud tapping noise associated with the magnetic resonance imaging scan.

gravid pregnant.

grid a plate consisting of a series of lead strips that is placed on the front of the Bucky between the patient and the radiographic film. A grid increases film quality by reducing the scatter radiation that reaches the film.

Guillain-Barré syndrome acute idiopathic peripheral polyneuritis that develops 1 to 3 weeks after a mild viral infection or an immunization.

gumma a soft, gummy, necrotic mass with surrounding inflammatory and fibrotic zones that develops in patients who have tertiary syphilis.

gyromagnetic ratio a constant for a given nucleus expressed in megahertz/tesla; the ratio of the magnetic moment to the angular momentum of the nucleus.

habitus bodily appearance; form and structure of the body.

hamartoma a malformation that resembles a tumor but is composed of a tissue or mixture of tissues normally found in its region.

Haygarth's nodes periarticular nodules found at the dorsal aspect of the metacarpophalangeal joints.

hemoptysis expectoration of blood in sputum.

hernia a rupture or protrusion of part of an organ through the tissue in which it is normally contained.

heterogeneous differing in kind or nature; composed of unlike elements.

high signal intensity indicated by bright pixels on an magnetic resonance image. Fat demonstrates a high signal intensity on T1-weighted images, and water demonstrates a high intensity on T2-weighted images.

hilum, hilus a depression on a gland or organ marking the entrance and exit of vessels and nerves to and from the structure; root of an organ or gland.

hitchhiker's thumb a characteristic of diastrophic dwarfism in which the thumb is malpositioned and tilted laterally because of a short first metacarpal.

homogeneous same in kind or nature; composed of like elements.

honeycomb lung the radiologic and gross appearance of the lung during end-stage diffuse interstitial fibrosus.

hot spots a term used in scintigraphy to designate areas of increased gamma emission caused by increased radioisotope absorption.

Hounsfield number (CT number) the normalized value of a pixel's (picture element's) x-ray attenuation during computed tomography. The attenuation is expressed in Hounsfield units.

Hounsfield unit a normalized scale of x-ray attenuation used in computed tomography where 11000 (air) to +1000 or more (bone) and water is 0.

hydrocephalus a condition marked by an excessive amount of cerebrospinal fluid in cerebral ventricles; accompanied by ventricle dilation and brain atrophy.

hydromyelia a pathologic accumulation of fluid in the central canal of the spinal cord.

hydronephrosis an accumulation of urine in the kidney pelvis caused by obstructed urine flow.

hydrosyringomyelia a condition in which the patient has coexisting syringomyelia and hydromyelia; the term applied when the location of a fluid accumulation cannot be pinpointed to the central canal or the cord.

hyper- a prefix meaning over, beyond, or excessive; opposite of hypo-.

hyperplasia a nonneoplastic increased number of cells in a tissue or organ.

hypertrichosis excessive hair growth. The localized form often accompanies spinal dysraphism and is known as *faun's tail*.

hypertrophy a nonneoplastic increased body part size caused by increased cell size.

hypo- a prefix meaning under, below, or deficient; opposite of hyper-.

-iasis a suffix meaning diseased state.

iatrogenic caused or induced by treatment; a term typically used to describe unsuccessful results of treatment.

incontinence involuntary discharge of any excretion, particularly urine or feces.

indium-111 (^{111}In) a radionuclide bone marrow and tumor-localizing tracer.

infarct an area of tissue necrosis caused by an obstructed local blood supply.

inferior situated lower or nearer the bottom.

infiltration a term commonly used to describe any shadow on a chest radiograph, especially an ill-defined opacity.

inflammation the vessel and tissue response to injury. The cardinal signs of redness (rubor), heat (calor), swelling (tumor), pain (dolor), and loss of function (functio laesa) are usually noted.

insufflation the act of blowing air or gas into a body cavity.

intervertebral chondrosis degeneration of the intervertebral disc; usually manifests primarily at the inner regions of the disc and is seen as reduced disc height on the radiograph.

invert to turn inward.

involucrum a sheath of new bone that surrounds a sequestrum.

involuntary independent of will.

ipsilateral on the same side.

-itis a suffix denoting inflammation.

ivory vertebra a densely radiopaque vertebra.

jaundice a morbid condition caused by obstruction of the biliary tract and characterized by a yellow discoloration, particularly of the skin and eyes.

jelling phenomenon articular stiffness caused by periods of inactivity.

joint mouse a small moveable calcific body in or near a joint.

kilovolts peak (kVp) a measurement of peak potential difference between the cathode (filament) and anode voltage. The kilovolts peak determines the penetrability or quality of the x-ray beam.

Kirner's deformity congenital medial curvature of the distal fifth finger.

knife-clasp defect an elongated L5 spinous process with a concurrent cleft defect of the S1 sacral arch.

KUB the abbreviation for kidney, ureter, and bladder; the recumbent frontal radiograph of the abdomen.

Kveim reaction a reaction in which noncaseating granuloma develops after an intradermal injection of an antigen derived from a known sarcoidosis-containing lymph node. The reaction indicates the presence of sarcoidosis.

Kveim test an intradermal test used to confirm the diagnosis of sarcoidosis by a positive Kveim reaction.

kyphoscoliosis lateral and posterior curvature of the spine.

kyphosis sagittal curvature of the spine with posterior convexity.

labrum any lip-shaped structure, especially the cartilaginous structure that outlines the perimeter of the acetabular and glenoid cavities.

lamina a thin, flat plate or layer; lamina of vertebrae is a flat section extending between the pedicles and the midline at the base of the spinous process.

laminectomy the excision of the vertebral lamina or posterior region of the vertebral arch.

Larmor equation the basis of magnetic resonance imaging physics, which states that the frequency of spin/precession of the hydrogen nuclei is proportional to the strength of the magnetic field and depends on the gyromagnetic ratio of the atom imaged.

Lannois deformity fibular deviation of the digits with dorsal subluxation at the metatarsal phalangeal joints, sometimes seen in advanced rheumatoid arthritis.

latent not apparent or manifest.

lateral pertaining to the side, opposite of midline; in radiography, a projection taken with the patient facing perpendicular to the central ray.

leptomeningeal cyst a cyst formed by cerebrospinal fluid accumulations in a dural sac extending into a skull fracture.

Lhermitte's sign sudden, transient, shocklike or lightninglike sensations extending into the extremities and occurring when the head is flexed forward; often seen in patients who have multiple sclerosis, cervical cord neoplasms, radiation myelopathy, trauma, and advanced spondylosis.

licked-candy-stick bone tapered distal bone ends caused by atrophic bone resorption.

limbus bone a small ossicle located at the edge or corner of a vertebra that results from an intravertebral herniation of nuclear material separating the secondary growth center of the vertebral endplate from the primary growth centers of the vertebral body.

lipo- a prefix meaning fat.

lipohemarthrosis the leakage of fat and blood into joint spaces as a result of intraarticular fractures; creates a fat–blood interface (FBI sign) on radiographs taken of limbs in a gravity-dependent position.

Lisfranc's joint a tarsometatarsal joint.

-lith a suffix meaning concretion or calculus.

Lofgren syndrome an acute onset of sarcoidosis with high fever, arthralgia, lymphadenopathy, and erythema nodosum.

long (tall) vertebra a vertebral body that appears taller than normal vertebrae as a result of altered mechanical stresses; usually found caudal to a gibbus formation.

lordosis sagittal curvature of the spine with anterior convexity.

low signal intensity indicated by dark pixels on a magnetic resonance image. Fat demonstrates low signal intensity on T2-weighted images, water demonstrates low signal intensity on T1-weighted images, and cortical bone demonstrates low signal intensity on all images.

lumbarization a congenital anomaly of the lumbosacral junction in which the first sacral segment develops as a lumbar vertebra, producing a total of six lumbar vertebrae.

Magnevist trade name for gadopentetate dimeglumine, an intravenous magnetic resonance imaging contrast agent that lowers T1 and T2, resulting in decreased signal intensity on T2-weighted images and increased signal intensity on T1-weighted images.

magnetic resonance imaging (MRI) a diagnostic imaging modality based on magnetic nuclei (especially protons), which become aligned in a strong magnetic field, absorb energy from pulsed radiofrequency, and emit radiofrequency signals as the excitation decays. These signals vary according to proton density and the relaxation times of the tissue. A tomographic image that can be three-dimensional is constructed from the signal information.

mal- a prefix meaning ill or bad.

malignant resistant to treatment; tending to cause death; virulent.

mallet deformity a flexion abnormality of the distal interphalangeal joint of a finger or toe.

mallet finger chronic flexion deformity of the distal interphalangeal joint caused by rupture or avulsion of the extensor digitorum common tendon at the base of the distal phalanx.

Marjolin's ulcer a squamous cell carcinoma in or around the sinus draining an osteomyelitis.

McCune-Albright's syndrome a syndrome characterized by a triad comprising polyostotic fibrous dysplasia, precocious puberty, and skin pigmentations.

medial situated in or pertaining to the midline.

median central position; midline.

median sagittal plane a vertical plane that passes through the center of the body and divides the subject into right and left halves.

mediastinum the space between the pleural sacs of the lungs, sternum, and thoracic spine.

medulla the soft material in the center of a part; marrow of bones.

metaphysis the section of long bone between the epiphysis and diaphysis.

metastasis a transfer or seeding of disease from one part of the body to another.

milliampere-seconds (mAs) measurement of filament current over time; determines the number or quantity of x-rays produced in the beam.

Mitchell markers lead markers used in radiography to orient interpreters to the patient's anatomy. By convention the side of the patient closest to the film is usually marked. Either side may be marked for frontal projections.

monoarticular involving one joint.

Morton disease a disease in which the metatarsal arch is flattened, causing pressure neuropathy of the lateral plantar nerve's digital branches.

Morton's foot (metatarsalgia) pain in the forefoot caused by shortening of the first metatarsal.

myelitis inflammation of the spinal cord or bone marrow.

myoma a benign tumor in the muscle tissue.

myxoid (mucoid) degeneration degeneration of connective tissue into a gelatinous or mucoid substance.

myxoma a benign neoplasm of connective tissue found in the subcutaneous tissues, bones, genitourinary tract, and retroperitoneal area.

nasion the midpoint of the frontonasal suture.

negative ulnar variance an offset at the articular surfaces of the ulna and radius because of a short ulna.

nephrolithiasis accumulation of calculi in the kidney.

nephroptosis abnormal dropping or downward movement of the kidney.

nidus the central point, origination, or focus of a disease process, especially an infection.

nonspondylolytic spondylolisthesis forward displacement of one vertebra over the one immediately below resulting from an etiology other than unilateral or bilateral disruption of the pars interarticularis at the same level; usually caused by degeneration of the posterior vertebral joints.

nuclear magnetic resonance (NMR) the phenomenon of absorption or emission of radiofrequency by atomic nuclei precessing about an axis of a strong external magnetic field at a certain frequency (the Larmor frequency). The frequency can be predicted from a specific atomic constant (the gyromagnetic frequency) and the strength of the external magnetic field.

occult fracture a fracture not detected immediately; may become detected in the future.

Omnipaque trade name for a water-soluble nonionic myelographic contrast agent that is commonly used; less toxic than fat-soluble agents (e.g., Pantopaque).

opera-glass hand (main en lorgnette) a hand deformity associated with destructive arthritis in which the fingers and wrist are shortened and the overlying skin undulates into transverse folds. The fingers appear telescoped like an opera glass.

opisthion the midpoint of the posterior margin of the occipital bone's foramen magnum.

Oppenheimer's erosions pressure erosions from an enlarged abdominal aortic mass seen as erosive gouge defects occurring along the anterior margin of the middle lumbar vertebrae.

Oppenheimer's ossicle a nonunion of the secondary growth center of the inferior articular process of a vertebra.

Ortolani's test an orthopedic maneuver used to evaluate the hip stability in infants. With the infant in a supine position, the knees and hips are flexed 90 degrees and abducted. While abducted, the femur is rotated internally and externally. Asymmetry of movement or a palpatory clicking (Ortolani's sign) constitutes a positive test, suggesting lateral dislocation of the femoral head from the acetabulum.

-osis suffix denoting a state or condition (usually an abnormal one).

osteolysis degeneration and destruction of bone caused by disease.

osteomyelitis inflammation of bone marrow and the medullary portion of bone.

osteopenia a condition in which the bone is subnormally mineralized. The term does not imply causality.

osteophyte a bony outgrowth or bone protuberance at a joint margin caused by degeneration.

osteoporosis circumscripta cranii; a localized, geographic resorption of the skull that develops in patients in the osteolytic phase of Paget's disease; most predominately develops in the frontal and occipital areas.

otosclerosis a hereditary condition in which the bony labyrinth of the inner ear is ossified, especially the stapes.

overhanging margin sign an extensive osseous erosion with an overhanging bone margin that develops in patients who have tophaceous gout.

pachy- a prefix meaning thick or dense.

pannus the granulation tissue affecting the joint during chronic inflammation, especially rheumatoid.

paramedian sagittal plane a plane situated near but not at the midline, dividing the subject into right and left sections.

parathyroid hormone (parathormone, PTH) a hormone produced by the parathyroid glands that increases serum calcium by promoting bone, kidney, and intestinal calcium resorption.

parenchyma the essential, specific, or functional cells of a gland or organ.

pars interarticularis the part of the vertebral arch located between the ipsilateral superior and inferior articular processes, especially in the lumbar spine.

patent open; not occluded; exposed.

pauciarticular involvement of a few joints.

pectus carinatum an outward deformity of the middle of the anterior chest wall.

pectus excavatum an inward deformity of the middle of the anterior chest wall.

Pelken's spurs perpendicular bony outgrowths from metaphyseal margins of patients who have scurvy.

Pellegrini-Stieda disease ossification of the upper portion of the medial collateral ligament.

permanent magnets a magnet system in which the magnetic field is created using ferromagnetic material that is permanently magnetized.

pes cavus foot deformity characterized by an excessively high arch with concurrent toe hyperextension.

pes equinus (talipes equinus) foot deformity characterized by extreme foot hyperextension.

pes planus foot deformity characterized by a flattened longitudinal plantar arch.

phakomatosis (phacomatosis) a group of hereditary neuroectodermal disorders characterized by benign, tumorlike nodules (hamartomas) of the skin, bones, eyes, and brain. Four diseases are recognized: tuberous sclerosis, neurofibromatosis, Sturge-Weber syndrome, and von Hippel-Lindau disease.

Phemister's triad the radiographic findings of tuberculous arthritis: progressive loss of joint space, juxtaarticular osteoporosis, and peripheral erosive defects of the joint surfaces.

phlebolith a stone formation in a vein; often seen in the lower pelvis on frontal radiographs.

picture frame vertebra a vertebral body with a squared, enlarged appearance because of thickening of its cortical perimeter as a result of Paget's disease.

pilonidal cyst a cyst most often found in the skin of the sacrococcygeal region. Although this type of cyst is not usually clinically significant, a chance of infection arises if the cyst connects to the surface of the skin by a pilonidal fistula.

Pitt's pit a radiolucent bone defect of the femoral neck resulting from mechanical erosion of femoral capsule irregularities.

pixel an abbreviation for picture element, which is a two-dimensional representation of a volume element (voxel) in the digital display of a computed tomographic (512×512 pixels) or magnetic resonance (256×256 pixels) image; the tiny squares that make up the image.

pleurisy inflammation of the pleura.

plica a fold.

pneumocephalus air in the cranium, especially air in the subarachnoid space secondary as a result of a fracture with dissection of air from the paranasal sinuses.

pneumoconiosis a condition in which particulate matter is permanently deposited in pulmonary tissues; lung fibrosis caused by dust inhalation.

pneumothorax an accumulation of air or other gas in a pleural cavity.

podagra gout of the great toe.

polyarticular (multiarticular) involving many joints.

polydactyly congenital anomaly characterized by more than five fingers or toes.

polydipsia a prolonged period of excessive thirst; characteristic of diabetes mellitus.

polyp any bump or projection of tissue that projects above or outward from the surface.

popliteal pertaining to the posterior area of the knee.

posterior back surface (e.g., the back surface of the body); opposite of anterior.

precession the wobbling and gyroscopic-like motion of hydrogen protons' magnetic fields in the presence of a static magnetic field.

prespondylolisthesis unilateral or bilateral disruption of the pars interarticularis without forward displacement of the vertebrae.

primary center of ossification the site at which ossification begins, either the shaft of a long bone or the body of an irregularly shaped bone.

primary magnets the assembly constituting the bulk of the magnetic resonance imaging unit and producing the strong main magnetic field, as opposed to the secondary and weaker gradient magnets.

pro- a prefix meaning forward or before.

pronation of hand medial rotation of hand so that it faces downward.

prostate-specific antigen (PSA) a glucoprotein normally found in the prostate that can be detected in all males. Its levels are increased in patients who have prostatic hypertrophy and adenocarcinoma, which often aids in the early diagnosis of these diseases.

proximal toward the beginning; the source or origin of a part.

pseudo- a prefix meaning false or illusory.

pseudofracture (Looser's lines, Milkman syndrome, increment fracture, umbau zonen) an osseous defect that is not a true fracture; often seen in patients who have Paget's disease, rickets, osteomalacia, and fibrous dysplasia.

pseudogout acute or subacute arthralgia associated with calcium pyrophosphate dihydrate (CPPD) deposition disease.

pseudohemangioma appearance of diffuse osteopenia mimicking multiple levels of vertebral hemangioma.

pseudospondylolisthesis forward displacement of one vertebra over the one immediately below as a result of posterior spinal joint degeneration and not a disruption of the pars interarticularis.

ptosis prolapse, or dropping, of an organ or part from its normal position.

purulent consisting of pus.

pyelogram a radiographic projection or series of projections taken of the kidneys and ureters after intravenous injection of radiopaque dye that collects in the urinary system and allows visualization of the urinary tract anatomy.

rachi- a prefix denoting a relationship to the spine.

radiofrequency (RF) coils RF waves excite the nuclear spins. The RF coils serve as both the transmitters and the receivers of the magnetic resonance imaging signal. Manipulation of the radiofrequencies allows for changes in the repetition times and the echo times. Radiofrequency surface coils are placed directly on the anatomic being imaged.

radiolucent offers little resistance to the passage of x-rays used in diagnostic imaging. Radiolucent substances appear black on radiographs.

radiopaque offers resistance to the passage of x-rays used in diagnostic imaging. Radiopaque substances appear white on radiographs.

radiopharmaceutical a radioisotopic particle with an unstable nucleus that undergoes radioactive decay. The consequent emission of gamma radiation is used in radionuclide imaging (e.g., gallium-67); any radioactive pharmaceutical.

Raynaud's phenomenon intermittent attacks of ischemia that are most pronounced in the fingers, toes, nose, and ears; brought on by cold or emotional stimuli and mediated by a dysfunctional sympathetic nervous system. Attacks begin with vasoconstriction and blanching and are followed by cyanosis, vasodilation, and redness.

repetition time (TR) the time interval between successive 90-degree pulses in a spin-echo sequence; represents the primary determinant of T1 relaxation. Longer repetition times reduce T1-dependent image contrast.

resistive electromagnets a system in which the magnetic field originates from a current flowing through an electrical conductor. It is not supercooled.

Reynold's phenomenon the development of central vertebral endplate defects secondary to hypoperfusion of vertebral body centrum seen in sickle-cell anemia; also known as "H-shaped," "Lincoln log," or "step-down" vertebrae.

rhizomelic pertaining to the root of a limb; the proximal region of the humerus and femur.

rhizotomy surgical resection of the spinal nerve root.

Risser's sign used to determine skeletal maturity. The iliac crest apophysis is observed; the apophysis ossifies from lateral to medial along the superior margin of the ilium. The extent of fusion is graded by fourths, from Grade I to Grade IV. Grade V indicates complete fusion of the iliac apophysis.

Romanus lesion an erosion found at the insertion of the outer anulus fibrosus into the anterior corners of the vertebral bodies; seen in patients who have ankylosing spondylitis.

rotator cuff a structure comprising four muscles that arise from the scapula and insert into the humeral head. From anterior to posterior the muscles are the subscapularis, supraspinatus, infraspinatus, and teres minor. The rotator cuff provides dynamic stability for the glenohumeral joint.

rugger jersey spine a spine in which uniform condensation occurs subjacent to the vertebral endplates; seen in patients who have hyperparathyroidism.

saber shin deformity anterior bowing of the tibia seen in patients who have Paget's disease and syphilis.

saccular aneurysm a large (usually more than 5 cm in diameter) spherical outpouching of one side of a vessel; usually caused by trauma.

sacralization the transition of the last lumbar vertebra into the first sacral segment, producing a total of four lumbar segments.

salt-and-pepper skull a skull that has undergone granular deossification and has a resulting finely mottled appearance; seen in patients who have hyperparathyroidism.

Salter-Harris classification a system for classifying growth plate fractures into five classes based on the appearance of the fracture.

sarcomatous transformation the malignant degeneration of benign lesion to a fibrous, osseous, or cartilaginous sarcoma.

sausage digit a single digit experiencing soft-tissue swelling, which occurs during the early stages of psoriatic disease.

sausage finger fingers that appear swollen as a result of acromegaly.

Schmorl's node an intravertebral herniation of the nucleus pulposus through the vertebral body endplate into the spongiosa of the vertebra; often seen on radiographs as a focal defect of the vertebral endplate.

scoliosis abnormal lateral curvature of the spine.

Scotty dog the name given to the appearance of the vertebral arch's anatomy on an oblique lumbar radiographic projection. The shape is similar to that of a Scottish terrier (Scotty) dog. The parts of the dog are as follows: pars interarticularis, dog's neck; ipsilateral pedicle, dog's eye; superior articular process, dog's ears; inferior articular process, dog's forelimbs; lamina, dog's body.

sequestrum a necrotic fragment of tissue, especially bone, that is separated from the surrounding normal tissue.

seronegative arthritis arthritis in patients who do not contain the rheumatoid antigen in their serum (e.g., ankylosing spondylitis).

seropositive arthritis arthritis in patients who have the rheumatoid antigen in their serum (e.g., rheumatoid arthritis).

serum calcium level the amount of calcium in the blood; used to monitor parathyroid function and calcium metabolism. Normally, total serum calcium levels are 9 to 10.5 mg/dl. Although uncommon, increased serum calcium levels may be seen in malignancy resulting from massive osteolysis or a tumor that is producing a substance similar to parathyroid hormone. Decreased levels are associated with conditions such as hypoparathyroidism, renal failure, rickets, and osteomalacia.

serum phosphorus level the amount of phosphorus in the blood; used to indicate parathyroid function and calcium metabolism. Serum phosphorus and calcium levels are inversely related. Normally serum phosphorus levels are 3 to 4.5 mg/dl. Increased levels may be a result of renal dysfunction, increased dietary intake, acromegaly, or hypoparathyroidism; decreased levels may be caused by conditions such as hyperparathyroidism, dietary deficiencies, and hypercalcemia.

shepherd's crook deformity a varus deformity of the hip caused by a decreased femoral angle.

shiny corner sign bone sclerosis at the anterior vertebral margins associated with Romanus lesions in patients who have ankylosing spondylitis.

soft-tissue window the window level and width in a computed tomographic study that emphasizes soft-tissue anatomy. Soft tissues appear light gray, and distinguishing between cortical and medullary bone is difficult.

SPECT single photon emission computed tomography; creates cross-sectional radionuclide images.

spicule a small, needlelike fragment.

spin density (proton-weighted, hydrogen-weighted, balanced) image a magnetic resonance image primarily based on the number of hydrogen nuclei within the sampled volume; T1 and T2 contrast is minimized. A spin density image is obtained by using long repetition time (TR) and short echo time (TE) pulse sequences.

spin-echo (SE) sequence the most common magnetic resonance imaging pulse sequence. Lengthening and shortening of pulses (spin) and "listening" (echo) times create either T1-weighted (short), T2-weighted (long), or proton-density–weighted images. Spin-echo sequences use pulse angles of 90 degrees.

spina bifida a congenital malformation of the vertebral arch of one or more levels resulting in a cleft with or without herniation of the spinal cord and meninges.

spina bifida occulta a cleft in the vertebral arch with no associated herniation of the spinal cord or meninges.

spondylitis inflammation of the vertebral joints.

spondylolisthesis forward displacement of one vertebra over the one immediately below. The term does not specify etiology or amount of displacement.

spondylolysis a condition in which the pars interarticularis is interrupted. Defects may be bilateral or unilateral, and most are caused by stress fractures.

spondylolytic spondylolisthesis forward displacement of one vertebra over the one immediately below as a result of unilateral or bilateral disruption of the pars interarticularis at the same level.

spondylophyte the osteophyte of a spinal joint.

spondylosis degeneration of a vertebral joint, particularly the intervertebral disc.

spondylosis deformans degeneration of the intervertebral disc; primarily manifests at the outer regions of the disc and presents as osteophytes.

spot projection a tightly collimated projection of a specific portion of the anatomy. It is smaller than a routine projection of the same area.

square vertebra a vertebra that has lost its concavity; most characteristic of ankylosing spondylitis.

Srb's anomaly dysplasia of the first rib(s) with synostosis to the second rib.

stroma supportive, connective, nonfunctional tissue of an organ.

structural scoliosis a fixed lateral curvature that is not compensatory or positional.

subarachnoid hematoma an intracranial collection of blood internal to the arachnoid and external to the pia mater of the brain and spinal cord in the space normally occupied by cerebrospinal fluid.

subdural hematoma an intracranial collection of blood between the dura mater and arachnoid mater of the brain and spinal cord.

Sudeck's atrophy (reflex sympathetic dystrophy) an exaggerated neurovascular-mediated response to trauma or other stimulus resulting in pain, vasomotor instability, and trophic disturbances.

summation effect of rheumatoid arthritis a term referring to the vertical subluxation, atlantoaxial impaction, or cranial settling of the upper cervical spine that develops in patients who have advanced rheumatoid arthritis. When extensive, the effects can be fatal.

super scan a bone scan that reveals skeletal uptake that is so diffuse it may be interpreted as normal because of its lack of obvious radionuclide uptake regions. It is most often seen in patients who have a generalized skeletal metastasis. Less uptake is noted in the bladder because of the marked skeletal uptake.

superconductive magnets a magnet system that has been supercooled by cryogens such as liquid helium or liquid nitrogen.

supination of the hand lateral rotation of the hand so that it faces upward.

swan-neck deformity flexion of the distal interphalangeal joint with concurrent extension of the proximal interphalangeal joint.

synchondrosis a joint between two bones that has been formed by hyaline cartilage or fibrocartilage.

syndactyly congenital webbing or fusion of adjacent fingers or toes.

syndesmophyte a radiodense ossification of the outer annulus fibrosis as a result of inflammatory joint disease (e.g., ankylosing spondylitis).

synostosis osseous union of adjacent bones.

syringomyelia a pathologic longitudinal accumulation of fluid within the spinal cord.

T1 a term used in magnetic resonance imaging to denote the time for 63% of the excited hydrogen nuclei to undergo longitudinal relaxation. The time depends on the strength of the external magnet and chemical environment of the hydrogen. Fat demonstrates a bright signal on T1-weighted images. Generally, T1-weighted images provide good anatomic detail.

T2 a term used in magnetic resonance imaging to denote the time for 63% of the excited hydrogen nuclei to undergo transverse relaxation. The time depends on the strength of the external magnet and chemical environment of the hydrogen. Water demonstrates a bright signal on T2-weighted images. Generally, T2-weighted images are more "grainy"-appearing than T1-weighted images. Because most pathologic conditions have associated edema (fluid accumulations), T2-weighted images are sensitive for disease processes.

Tarlov's cyst a perineural cyst in the proximal portion of the spinal nerve roots of the lower spinal cord.

technetium-99m (^{99m}Tc) an artificial radioactive element with an atomic number of 43 and an atomic weight of 99; widely used as a tracer in nuclear imaging. Technetium-99m diphosphonate is one of the more common complexes used for bone scans.

tennis elbow (lateral humeral epicondylitis) pain radiating from the elbow at the origin of the wrist extensors resulting from repetitive muscular strains.

theca a protective case or sheath.

thecal sac a term usually used in a radiologic context referring to the dura and arachnoid mater of the spinal cord.

three-phase bone scan the common bone scan that is interpreted in three phases. The first, or flow, phase uses a radionuclide angiogram taken the first minute after injection. The second phase is the blood pool scan, which takes place 1 to 3 minutes after injection. The third phase is the static bone scan, which takes place 2 to 4 hours after injection. With increased blood flow, the first and second phases demonstrate prominent collection. Collection of radionuclide in the third phase corresponds to osteogenic activity and blood flow and is the most useful portion of the radionuclide bone scan study.

thrombus a plug or clot formed in the heart or a blood vessel that remains at its formation site.

tophus the chalky, white calculi of sodium urate deposits in and around joints of patients who have gout.

tortuous winding or curving.

trident hand a hand that has a widening space between the third and fourth digits; slight flexion of digits of nearly equal length.

trolley track sign ossification of the zygapophyseal joints bilaterally and the supraspinatus and interspinous ligaments along the median, forming three, nearly parallel, vertical lines on frontal lumbar radiographs of some patients who have ankylosing spondylitis.

tube-film distance (TFD) the distance between the x-ray tube and the film; also referred to as focal-film distance (FFD).

tubercle a small nodule or prominence, especially one that is nonpathologic.

tuberosity a large tubercle or process on a bone extending from the surface.

turret exostosis a subperiosteal hemorrhage resulting in a bony protuberance from the ulnar and dorsal aspects of the base of the proximal or middle phalanx.

ureteric colic spasmodic pain in the abdomen causing obstruction or disease of the ureter.

urography radiographic examination of the urinary tract with contrast medium.

vacuum phenomenon (Knuttson's sign) a radiolucent defect caused by nitrogen gas accumulations in anular and nuclear degenerative fissures of the intervertebral disc. The nitrogen gas is thought to arise from the extracellular spaces. Because the gas accumulates in areas of lower pressure, they often are seen in fissures of the anterior portion of the disc on extension radiographs. The presence of a vacuum phenomenon virtually excludes the possibility of an infection being the cause of a narrowed intervertebral disc space. The presence of gas-forming infections is a rare exception to this general rule. Vacuum phenomena are normal in synovial joints under slight distraction.

valgus describes the abnormal position or deviation of a part lateral to the midline.

Valsalva's maneuver the act of forcing a deep breath when the glottis is closed, a hand is over the mouth and nose, or the airway is blocked in some other way.

varix a permanently dilated and tortuous vessel, especially a vein.

varus describes the abnormal position or deviation of a part medial to the midline.

ventral pertaining to the front or anterior side (e.g., the front side of the body).

vertebra plana a flattening compression deformity of the vertebral body height.

vertex the top or highest part of the head.

voxel an abbreviation for volume element; a three-dimensional version of a pixel; the basic unit of computed tomography or magnetic resonance imaging reconstruction.

wedged vertebra compression deformity of the vertebra in which the vertebra has a decreased anterior body height but maintains its posterior body height.

Wilkinson syndrome unilateral disruption of the pars interarticularis with contralateral sclerosis of the pedicle.

Wimberger's sign (ring epiphysis) the radiodense appearance of the epiphyseal circumference that is seen in patients who have scurvy.

window level the midpoint of the window width; expressed in Hounsfield units. The window level determines which tissues are displayed. For example, a window level of 1500 Hounsfield units excludes bone and soft tissues and emphasizes pulmonary anatomy.

window width the range of computed tomography numbers, expressed in Hounsfield units, that are included in the gray-scale image.

xanthoma a benign plaque, nodule, or tumor of fatty and fibrous origin found in the subcutaneous layer of skin, often around tendons.

xeroradiography a diagnostic imaging technique in which an image is produced electrically rather than chemically using a specially coated charged plate instead of x-ray film. It requires less exposure time and lower radiation doses than radiography and provides inherent edge enhancement. It is used primarily for mammography.

zone of provisional calcification a thin line of increased radiodensity at the junction of the physis and metaphysis representing the region of physis cartilage calcification.

Index

A

F

L

P

W

Radiology Mnemonics

A cronyms and mnemonics are useful aids for learning and remembering differential diagnoses for particular radiographic presentations. Most of the following mnemonics are from Wolfgang Dähnert's Radiology Review Manual.* Many of these differential lists vary from those provided in the pattern chapters of this book—certain items have been added, and others have been omitted. Although differences exist among sources, the most important entries remain constant.

Bone

Basilar invagination: "COOP"

Congenital, Osteogenesis imperfecta, Osteomalacia, Paget's disease

Solitary lytic defect in the skull: "TORMENT"

Tuberculosis, Osteomyelitis, Radiation, Metastasis/Multiple myeloma, Epidermoid/dermoid, Neurofibromatosis/Necrosis (radiation), Trauma

Multiple lytic defects in the skull: "BAMMAH"

Brown tumor, Arteriovenous malformation, Multiple myeloma, Metastases, Amyloidosis, Histiocytosis

Button sequestrum of the skull: "TORE ME"

Tuberculosis, Osteomyelitis, Radiation, Eosinophilic granuloma, Metastasis, Epidermoid

Hair-on-end appearance of the skull: "SHITE"

Sickle-cell disease, Hereditary spherocytosis, Iron deficiency anemia, Thalassemia major, Enzyme deficiency (glucose-6-phosphate dehydrogenase)

Absent greater wing of the sphenoid: "M FOR MARINE"

Meningioma, Fibrous dysplasia, Optic glioma, Relapsing hematoma, Metastasis, Aneurysm, Retinoblastoma, Idiopathic, Neurofibromatosis, Eosinophilic granuloma

Wormian (sutural) bones: "PORK CHOPS"

Pyknodysostosis, Osteogenesis imperfecta, Rickets (healing phase), Kinky hair syndrome, Cleidocranial dysplasia, Hypothyroidism/Hypophosphatasia, Otopalatodigital syndrome, Pachydermoperiostosis/Primary acro-osteolysis, Syndrome of Down

Increased skull thickness: "HIPFAM"

Hyperostosis frontalis interna, Idiopathic, Paget's disease, Fibrous dysplasia, Anemia, Metastasis

Atlantoaxial subluxation: "JAP LARD"

Juvenile rheumatoid arthritis, Ankylosing spondylitis, Psoriatic arthritis, Lupus erythematosus, Accident (trauma), Retropharyngeal abscess/Rheumatoid arthritis, Down syndrome

Ivory vertebra: "My Only Sister Left Home On Friday Past"

Myelosclerosis, Osteoblastic metastasis, Sickle-cell anemia, Lymphoma, Hemangioma, Osteopetrosis, Fluorosis, Paget's disease

Vertebra plana: "FETISH"

Fracture, Eosinophilic granuloma, Tumor (metastasis, multiple myeloma), Infection, Steroids, Hemangioma

Bullet-shaped vertebra: "HAM"

Hypothyroidism, Achondroplasia, Morquio's disease

Posterior vertebral body scalloping: "HAMENTS"

Hurler's syndrome/Hydrocephalus, Achondroplasia/Acromegaly, Marfan's syndrome, Ehlers-Danlos syndrome, Neurofibromatosis, Tumor (meningioma, ependymoma), Syringomyelia

---

*Dähnert W: Radiology review manual, ed 3, Baltimore, 1996, Williams & Wilkins.

Anterior vertebral body scalloping: "MALT"

Multiple myeloma (paravertebral soft-tissue mass), Aortic aneurysm, Lymphadenopathy (lymphoma), Tuberculosis

Expansile lesions in the vertebral arch: "GO APE"

Giant cell tumor, Osteoblastoma, Aneurysmal bone cyst, Plasmacytoma, Eosinophilic granuloma

Tumor predisposed to the vertebral body: "CALL HOME"

Chordoma, Aneurysmal bone cyst, Leukemia, Lymphoma, Hemangioma/Hydatid cyst, Osteoblastoma, Multiple myeloma/Metastasis, Eosinophilic granuloma

Neoplasms of the sacrum: "CAGE"

Chordoma/Chondrosarcoma, Aneurysmal bone cyst, Giant cell tumor, Ewing's tumor

Protrusio acetabuli: "PORT"

Paget's disease, Osteomalacia/Otto pelvis, Rheumatoid arthritis, Trauma

Aberrant development of the pubic bone: "CHIEF"

Cleidocranial dysostosis, Hypospadias/epispadias, Idiopathic, Exstrophy of bladder, F for syringomyelia

Widened symphysis pubis: "EPOCH"

Exstrophy of bladder, Prune belly syndrome, Osteogenesis imperfecta, Cleidocranial dysostosis, Hypothyroidism

Widened sacroiliac joint: "CRAP TRAP"

Colitis, Rheumatoid arthritis, Abscess (infection), Parathyroid disease, Trauma, Reiter's syndrome, Ankylosing spondylitis, Psoriasis

Calcification of the intervertebral disc: "DO IT"

Degeneration, Ochronosis, Idiopathic, Trauma

Chondrocalcinosis: "WHIP A DOG"

Wilson's disease, Hemochromatosis/Hemophilia/Hypothyroidism/Hyperparathyroidism/Hypophosphatasia, Idiopathic, Pseudogout, Amyloidosis, Diabetes mellitus, Ochronosis, Gout

Premature osteoarthritis: "COME CHAT"

Calcium pyrophosphate dihydrate crystal deposition, Ochronosis, Marfan's syndrome, Epiphyseal dysplasia, Charcot's (neurotrophic) arthropathy, Hemophilic arthropathy, Acromegaly, Trauma

Arthritis with demineralization: "HORSE"

Hemophilia, Osteomyelitis, Rheumatoid arthritis/Reiter's syndrome, Scleroderma, Erythematosus (systemic lupus)

Arthritis without demineralization: "PONGS"

Psoriatic arthritis, Osteoarthritis, Neuropathic joint, Gout, Sarcoidosis

Arthritis involving distal interphalangeal joints: "POEM"

Psoriatic arthritis, Osteoarthritis, Erosive osteoarthritis, Multicentric reticulohistiocytosis

Premature closure of the epiphyseal plate: "JB HIT"

Juvenile rheumatoid arthritis, Battered child syndrome, Hemophilia, Infection, Trauma

Radiology Mnemonics—cont'd

Epiphyseal lesions: "CAGGIE"
Chondroblastoma, Aneurysmal bone cyst, Giant cell tumor, Geode, Infection, Eosinophilic granuloma/Enchondroma

Epiphyseal lesions: "GELCO"
Giant cell tumor, Eosinophilic granuloma/Enchondroma, Lipoma, Chondroblastoma/Cyst (degenerative), Osteomyelitis

Diaphyseal tumors: "FEMALE"
Fibrous dysplasia, Ewing's sarcoma, Metastasis, Adamantinoma, Lymphoma/Leukemia, Eosinophilic granuloma

Frayed metaphyses: "CHARMS"
Congenital infections (rubella, syphilis), Hypophosphatasia, Achondroplasia, Rickets, Metaphyseal dysostosis, Scurvy

Rhizomelic dwarfism: "MA CAT"
Metatrophic dwarfism, Achondrogenesis, Chondrodysplasia punctata, Achondroplasia (heterozygous), Thanatophoric dysplasia

Short fourth metacarpal: "TOP"
Turner's syndrome/Trauma, Osteomyelitis, Pseudohypoparathyroidism

Radiolucent metaphyseal bands: "SLING"
Systemic illness (rickets, scurvy), Leukemia, Infection (congenital syphilis), Neuroblastoma metastasis/Normal variant, Growth lines

Dense metaphyseal bands: "Heavy Cretins Sift Scurrilously through Rickety Systems"
Heavy metal poisoning (lead, bismuth), Cretinism, Syphilis (congenital), Scurvy, Rickets (healed), Systemic illness

Periosteal reaction in child: "PERIOSTEAL SOCKS"
Physiological/Prostaglandin, Eosinophilic granuloma, Rickets, Infantile cortical hyperostosis, Osteomyelitis, Scurvy, Trauma, Ewing's sarcoma, A-hypervitaminosis, Leukemia, Syphilis, Osteosarcoma, Child abuse, Kinky hair syndrome, Sickle-cell disease

Expansile rib lesion: "THELMA"
Tuberculosis, Hematopoiesis, Eosinophilic granuloma/Ewing's sarcoma/Enchondroma, Leukemia/Lymphoma, Multiple myeloma/Metastasis, Aneurysmal bone cyst

Destruction of the medial end of the clavicle: "FEMALE"
Fibrous dysplasia, Ewing's sarcoma, Metastasis, Adamantinoma, Lymphoma/Leukemia, Eosinophilic granuloma

Thick heel pad: "MAD COP"
Myxedema, Acromegaly, Dilantin therapy, Callus, Obesity, Peripheral edema

Acroosteolysis: "RADISH"
Raynaud's phenomena, Arteriosclerosis, Diabetes, Injury (thermal), Scleroderma/Sarcoidosis, Hyperparathyroidism

Cystic bone lesions: "FEGNOMASHIC"
Fibrous dysplasia, Enchondroma, Giant cell tumor, Nonossifying fibroma, Osteoblastoma, Multiple myeloma/Metastasis, Aneurysmal bone cyst, Simple bone cyst, Hyperparathyroidism/Hemophilic pseudotumor, Infection, Chondroblastoma

Multiple lytic lesions: "FEEMHI"
Fibrous dysplasia, Enchondroma, Eosinophilic granuloma, Metastasis/Multiple myeloma, Hyperparathyroidism (brown tumors)/Hemangioma, Infection

Lytic lesion surrounded by sclerosis: "BOOST"
Brodie's abscess, Osteoblastoma, Osteoid osteoma, Stress fracture, Tuberculosis

Generalized bone sclerosis: "3 M's PROF"
Metastasis (blastic), Mastocytosis, Myelofibrosis, Paget's disease, Rickets, Osteopetrosis, Fluorosis

Moth-eaten bone destruction: "LEMON"
Lymphoma, Ewing's sarcoma/Eosinophilic granuloma, Metastasis/Multiple myeloma, Osteomyelitis, Neuroblastoma

Avascular necrosis: "PLASTIC RAGS"
Pancreatitis/Pregnancy, Lupus erythematosus, Alcoholism, Sickle cell anemia, Trauma, Idiopathic, Caisson disease, Rheumatoid arthritis/Radiation, Atherosclerosis, Gaucher's disease, Steroids

Failed back surgery: "ABCDEF"
Arachnoiditis, Bleeding, Contamination (infection), Disc (residual, recurrent, new level), Error (wrong level or side), Fibrosis (scar formation)

Chest

Diffuse air-space disease: "AIRSPACED"
Aspiration, Inhalation, Renal disease, Swimming (near drowning), Pneumonia, Alveolar proteinosis, Cardiovascular disease, Edema, Drug reaction

Diffuse air-space disease: "BEPT"
Blood, Edema, Pus, Tumor

Opacification of hemithorax: "FAT CHANCE"
Fibrothorax, Adenomatoid malformation, Trauma (hematoma), Collapse/Cardiomegaly, Hernia, Agenesis of lung, Neoplasm (mesothelioma), Consolidation, Effusion

Perihilar (bat-wing) infiltrates: "Please, Please, Please, Study Light, Don't Get All Uptight"
Pulmonary edema, Proteinosis, Periarteritis, Sarcoidosis, Lymphoma, Drugs, Goodpasture's syndrome, Alveolar cell carcinoma, Uremia

Interstitial lung disease: "LIFE lines"
Lymphangitic spread, Inflammation/Infection, Fibrosis, Edema

Interstitial lung disease: "SHIPS & BOATS"
Sarcoidosis, Histiocytosis, Idiopathic, Pneumoconiosis, Scleroderma, Bleomycin/Busulfan, Oxygen toxicity, Arthritis (rheumatoid)/Amyloidosis/Allergic alveolitis, Tuberous sclerosis/Tuberculosis, Storage disease (Gaucher's disease)

Acute interstitial lung disease: "HELP"
Hypersensitivity, Edema, Lymphoproliferative, Pneumonitis (viral)

Chronic infiltrates in child: "ABC'S"
Asthma/Agammaglobulinemia/Aspiration, Bronchiectasis, Cystic fibrosis, Sequestration (intralobular)

Advanced interstitial lung disease (honeycomb lung): "B CHIPS"
Bronchiectasis, Collagen vascular disease, Histiocytosis X, Interstitial pneumonia (viral), Pneumoconiosis, Sarcoidosis

Multiple pulmonary cavities: "CAVITY"
Carcinoma (especially squamous cell), Autoimmune (Wegener's granulomatosis, rheumatoid arthritis), Vascular (septic emboli), Infection (abscess, fungal disease), Trauma, Young (congenital sequestration or bronchogenic cyst)

Reticulonodular pattern in the upper lung: "TAPE"
Tuberculosis, Ankylosing spondylitis, Pneumoconiosis, Eosinophilic granuloma

Reticulonodular pattern in the lower lung: "STAR"
Sarcoidosis/Scleroderma, Talcosis, Asbestosis, Rheumatoid disease